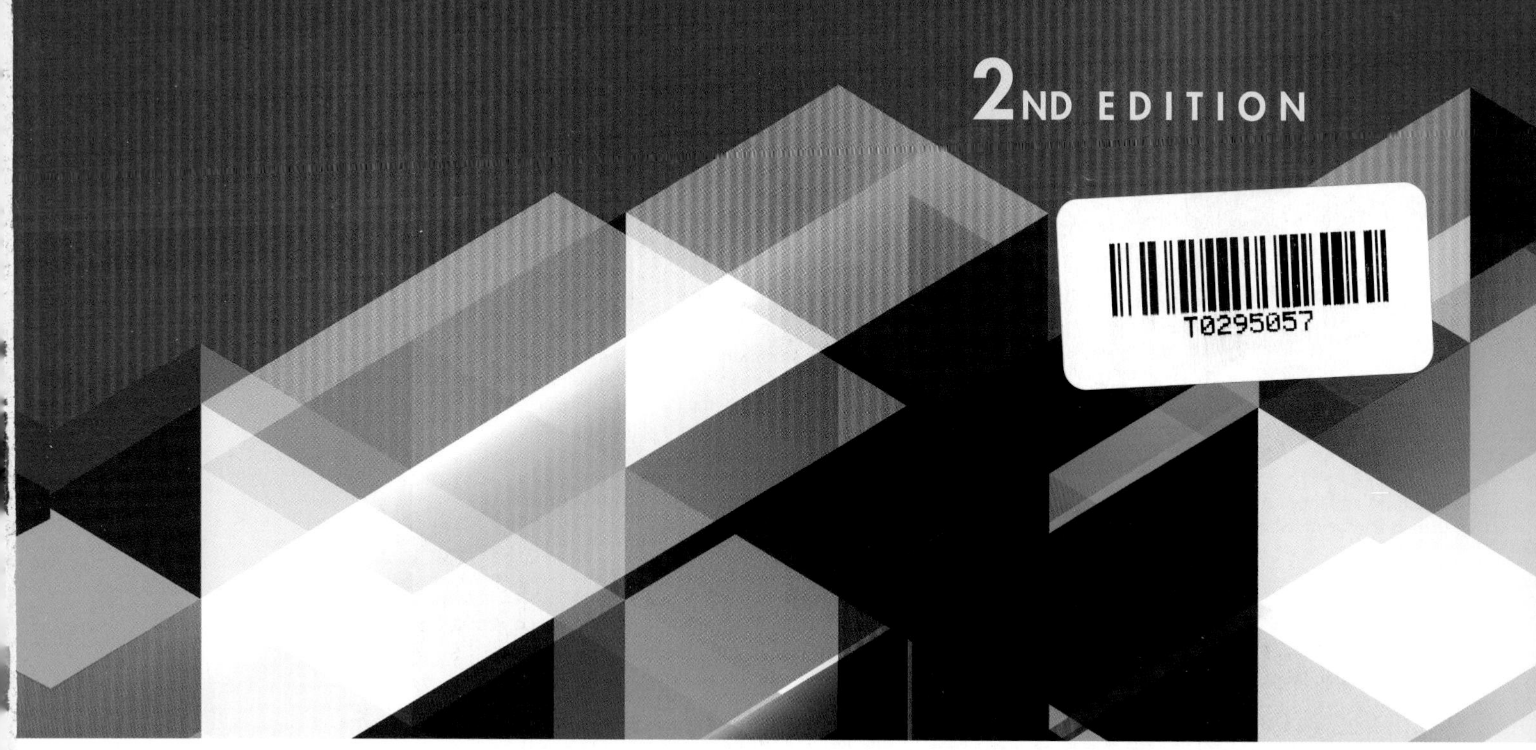

ADVANCED CRITICAL CARE NURSING

EDITORS

VICKI S. GOOD, DNP, RN, CENP, CPPS
System Director Clinical Quality/Safety
CoxHealth
Springfield, Missouri

PEGGY L. KIRKWOOD, MSN, RN, ACNPC, CHFN, AACC
Cardiovascular and Palliative Care Nurse Practitioner
Mission Hospital
Mission Viejo, California

ELSEVIER

ELSEVIER

3251 Riverport Lane
St. Louis, Missouri 63043

ADVANCED CRITICAL CARE NURSING, SECOND EDITION ISBN: 978-1-4557-5875-3

Notices

Knowledge and best practice in this field are constantly changing. As new research and experience broaden our understanding, changes in research methods, professional practices, or medical treatment may become necessary.

Practitioners and researchers must always rely on their own experience and knowledge in evaluating and using any information, methods, compounds, or experiments described herein. In using such information or methods they should be mindful of their own safety and the safety of others, including parties for whom they have a professional responsibility.

With respect to any drug or pharmaceutical products identified, readers are advised to check the most current information provided (i) on procedures featured or (ii) by the manufacturer of each product to be administered, to verify the recommended dose or formula, the method and duration of administration, and contraindications. It is the responsibility of practitioners, relying on their own experience and knowledge of their patients, to make diagnoses, to determine dosages and the best treatment for each individual patient, and to take all appropriate safety precautions.

To the fullest extent of the law, neither the Publisher nor the authors, contributors, or editors, assume any liability for any injury and/or damage to persons or property as a matter of products liability, negligence or otherwise, or from any use or operation of any methods, products, instructions, or ideas contained in the material herein.

Previous edition copyrighted 2009.

Library of Congress Cataloging-in-Publication Data
Names: Good, Vicki, 1965- editor. | Kirkwood, Peggy L., 1951- editor.
Title: Advanced critical care nursing / editors, Vicki Good, Peggy L. Kirkwood.
Other titles: AACN advanced critical care nursing.
Description: Second edition. | St. Louis, Missouri : Elsevier, [2018] | Preceded by AACN advanced critical care nursing / [edited by] Karen K. Carlson. 2009. | Includes bibliographical references and index.
Identifiers: LCCN 2016056255 | ISBN 9781455758753 (pbk. : alk. paper)
Subjects: | MESH: Critical Care Nursing--methods
Classification: LCC RT120.I5 | NLM WY 154 | DDC 616.02/8--dc23 LC record available at https://lccn.loc.gov/2016056255

Executive Content Strategist: Lee Henderson
Senior Content Developmental Manager: Laurie Gower
Content Developmental Specialist: Laura Goodrich
Publishing Services Manager: Jeff Patterson
Senior Project Manager: Mary Pohlman
Designer: Brian Salisbury

Printed in Canada.

Last digit is the print number: 9 8 7 6 5 4 3 2 1

CONTRIBUTORS

Roy Ball, MS, RN, ACNP-BC
Trauma Program Manager
Legacy Emanuel Medical Center
Portland, Oregon

Patricia A. Blissitt, PhD, ARNP-CNS, CCRN, CNRN, SCRN, CCNS, CCM, ACNS-BC
Neuroscience Clinical Nurse Specialist
Clinical Education
Harborview Medical Center
Associate Professor, Clinical Faculty
Biobehavioral Nursing and Health Systems
University of Washington School of Nursing
Seattle, Washington

Diane Byrum, MSN, RN, CCRN, CCNS, FCCM
Quality Improvement Consultant
Innovative Solutions for Healthcare Education
Oak Island, North Carolina

Lisa Carriger, MSN, RN, CCRN
Cardiac Intensive Care Unit
Mission Hospital
Mission Viejo, California

Debra J. Carter, MS, CRNP
Heart Transplant Nurse Practitioner, Surgery
The Johns Hopkins Hospital
Baltimore, Maryland

Jooyoung Cheon, BSN, RN, PhD(c)
Doctoral Student
School of Nursing
University of Maryland
Baltimore, Maryland

Julie Culmone, DNP, RN, ANP-C, APRN, CCCN
Nursing
University of Connecticut
Storrs, Connecticut;
Director of Surgical Care Transitions and Quality Improvement, Lead Nurse Practitioner
Surgery
Saint Francis Hospital and Medical Center
Hartford, Connecticut

Theresa Marie Davis, PhD, RN, NE-BC
Clinical Operations Director
enVision, eICU
Inova Health System
Falls Church, Virginia

Erica Deboer, BSN, MA, RN
Clinical Nurse Leader
Sanford USD Medical Center
Sioux Falls, South Dakota

Anna Dermenchyan, BSN, RN, CCRN-K
Senior Clinical Quality Specialist
Department of Medicine
UCLA Health
UCLA School of Nursing
Los Angeles, California

Sharon Dickinson, MSN, CNS
Nursing
University of Michigan
Ann Arbor, Michigan

Joni L. Dirks, MSN, RN-BC, CCRN-K
Manager Clinical Educators & ICU Educator
Department of Educational Services
Providence Health Care
Spokane, Washington

Diane K. Dressler, MSN, RN, CCRN
Clinical Assistant Professor
Nursing
Marquette University
Milwaukee, Wisconsin

Andrea Efre, DNP, ARNP, FNP
Owner, Nurse Practitioner, and Educator
Healthcare Education Consultants
Tampa, Florida

Eleanor Fitzpatrick, MSN, RN, ACNP-BC, AGCNS-BS, CCRN
Clinical Nurse Specialist
Surgical Critical Care
Thomas Jefferson University Hospital
Philadelphia, Pennsylvania

Vicki S. Good, DNP, RN, CENP, CPPS
System Director Clinical Quality/Safety
CoxHealth
Springfield, Missouri

Rosemarie Hirsch, MSN, CCRN, CNE
Professor; Department Chairperson, Health Sciences
Nursing
Santa Ana College
Santa Ana, California

Roberta Kaplow, PhD, AOCNS, APRN-CCNS, CCRN
Clinical Nurse Specialist
Oncology
Emory University Hospital
Atlanta, Georgia

Mary Jo Kelly, BSN, MSN, RN
Clinical Nurse Specialist/Sepsis Coordinator
Clinical Education
Harborview Medical Center/UW Medicine
Seattle, Washington

Serena Phromsivarak Kelly, MSN, CPNP-AC, FNP-BC, CCRN, CPEN
Pediatric Nurse Practitioner Acute Care
Pediatric Critical Care
OHSU Doernbecher Children's Hospital
Portland, Oregon

Mary King, MSN/CNS, MSN/Ed, RN, ACNS-BC, CNRN, CCRN
Clinical Nurse Specialist
Neuro Critical Care
Barrow Neurological Institute
Phoenix, Arizona

Peggy L. Kirkwood, MSN, RN, ACNPC, CHFN, AACC
Cardiovascular and Palliative Care Nurse Practitioner
Mission Hospital
Mission Viejo, California

Julene (Julie) B. Kruithof, MSN, RN, CCRN
Adult Critical Care Nurse Educator
Spectrum Health
Grand Rapids, Michigan

Nicole Kupchik, MSN, RN, CCNS, CCRN, PCCN, CMC
Independent Clinical Nurse Specialist
Nicole Kupchik Consulting, Inc.
Staff Nurse
Critical Care
Harborview Medical Center
Seattle, Washington

Dana M. Kyles, MSN, RN
Hospital Administrator
Patient Care Services
Harborview Medical Center
Seattle, Washington

Barbara Leeper, MSN, RN-BC, CNS M-S, CCRN, FAHA
Clinical Nurse Specialist
Cardiovascular Services
Baylor University Medical Center at Dallas
Dallas, Texas

Megan Liego, DNP, APRN, ACNP-BC, CNS
Manager of Clinical Operations for Nurse Practitioner Services
Nursing Administration
Long Beach Memorial
Long Beach, California

Karen March, MSN, RN
Adjunct Faculty
Biobehavioral Nursing
University of Washington
KSM Global
Seattle, Washington

Rhonda K. Martin, MSN, RN, CCRN, MLT(ASCP), CNS/ANP-C
Nurse Practitioner/CNS
Interventional Radiology
UCSD Medical Center Instructor
School of Medicine
University of California, San Diego
San Diego, California

Paula McCauley, DNP, APRN, ACNP-BC, CNE
Associate Clinical Professor
School of Nursing
University of Connecticut
Storrs, Connecticut

Michelle A. McKay, MSN, RN, CCRN
SICU Charge RN
Nursing
Thomas Jefferson University Hospital
Philadelphia, Pennsylvania;
Adjunct Clinical Instructor
School of Nursing
Villanova University
Villanova, Pennsylvania

Denise O'Brien, DNP, RN, ACNS-BC, CPAN, CAPA, FAAN
Perianesthesia Clinical Nurse Specialist
Department of Operating Rooms/PACU
University of Michigan Hospitals and Health Centers
Adjunct Clinical Instructor
School of Nursing
University of Michigan
Ann Arbor, Michigan

Carol Olff, MSN, RN, CCRN-K, NEA-BC
Director
Critical Care Services
John Muir Health
Concord, California

Mary Frances D. Pate, BSN, MSN, PhD
Assistant Professor
College of Nursing
East Carolina University
Greenville, North Carolina

Sara Paul, DNP, FNP, CHFN, FAHA
Director
Heart Function Program
Catawba Valley Cardiology/Catawba Valley Medical Center
Conover, North Carolina

Kristine Peterson, MSN, RN, CCRN-K, CCNS-CMC
Cardiac Clinical Nurse Specialist
Patient Care Services
Aspirus Wau Hospital
Wau, Wisconsin

Carmela M. Pontillo, MSN, RN, CBN
Bariatric Program Manager
Bariatric Services
Overlake Hospital Medical Center
Bellevue, Washington

Patricia Radovich, PhD, CNS, FCCM
Director
Nursing Research
Loma Linda University Medical Center,
Loma Linda, California;
Adjunct Professor
School of Nursing
Azusa Pacific University
Azusa, California

Daria C. Ruffolo, MSN, RN, DNP
Acute Care Nurse Practitioner
Anesthesia
Loyola University Medical Center
Maywood, Illinois

Maureen A. Seckel, RN, APRN, MSN, ACNS-BC, CCNS, CCRN, FCCM
Clinical Nurse Specialist Medical Pulmonary Critical Care
Christiana Care Health System
Affiliated Instructor
College of Health Sciences, School of Nursing
University of Delaware
Newark, Delaware

Sandra L. Siedlecki, PhD, RN
Senior Nurse Scientist
Nursing Research & Innovation
Cleveland Clinic
Cleveland, Ohio;
Contributing Faculty
School of Health Sciences
Walden University
Minneapolis, Minnesota

Diane Vail Skojec, DNP, MS, ANP-BC
Lead Nurse Practitioner
Department of Surgery
Johns Hopkins Hospital
Clinical Instructor
Johns Hopkins University School of Nursing
Baltimore, Maryland

Julie A. Stanik-Hutt, BSN, MA, MSN, PhD, RN
Professor
University of Iowa, College of Nursing
Iowa City, Iowa

Mary Fran Tracy, PhD, RN, APRN, CNS, FAAN
Nurse Scientist
University of Minnesota Medical Center
Associate Professor
University of Minnesota School of Nursing
Minneapolis, Minnesota

Charles Walker, PhD, MSN, BSN
Professor
Harris College of Nursing & Health Sciences
Texas Christian University
Fort Worth, Texas

Teresa A. Wavra, MSN, RN, CNS, CCRN
Cardiovascular Clinical Nurse Specialist
Nursing Center of Excellence
Mission Hospital
Mission Viejo, California

Maria Fe White, MSN, FNP-BC, ACNP-BC
Nurse Practitioner
Cedars-Sinai
Los Angeles, California

Debra L. Wiegand, RN, MSN, MBE, PhD
Associate Professor
School of Nursing
University of Maryland
Baltimore, Maryland

Mary Zellinger, APRN-CCNS, MN, ANP-BC, CCRN-CSC
Clinical Nurse Specialist
Cardiovascular Critical Care
Emory University Hospital
Atlanta, Georgia

The editors would also like to thank the writers who contributed to the previous edition of this title.

Nancy Albert, RN, PhD, CCNS, CCRN, CAN, FCCM, FAHA
Cleveland, Ohio

Kathleen M. Baldwin, PhD, RN, ANP, GNP, CNS
Fort Worth, Texas

Laurie Baumgartner, RN, MSN, CNS, ACNP, CCRN
Newport Beach, California

Patricia A. Blissitt, PhD, ARNP-CNS, CCRN, CNRN, SCRN, CCNS, CCM, ACNS-BC
Durham, North Carolina

Jo Ann Brooks, RN, DNS, FAAN, FCCP
Indianapolis, Indiana

Denise Buonocore, RN, MSN, APRN-BC, CCRN
New Haven, Connecticut

Suzanne M. Burns, RN, MSN, RRT, ACNP, CCRN, FAAN, FCCM
Charlottesville, Virginia

Diane Byrum, MSN, RN, CCRN, CCNS, FCCM
Charlotte, North Carolina

Debra J. Carter, MS, CRNP
Baltimore, Maryland

Dennis J. Cheek, RN, BSN, MSN, PhD, FAHA
Fort Worth, Texas

Molly Clark, MS, RD, CD
Seattle, Washington

Laura M. Criddle, RN, MS, CCRN, CCNS
Portland, Oregon

Lori A. Dambaugh, RN-BC, BSN, PCCN
Rochester, New York

Michael W. Day, RN, MSN, CCRN
Spokane, Washington

Sharon Dickinson, MSN, CNS
Ann Arbor, Michigan

Joni L. Dirks, RN-BC, CCRN-K
Spokane, Washington

Diane K. Dressler, MSN, RN, CCRN
Milwaukee, Wisconsin

Margaret M. Ecklund, RN, MS, CCRN, APRN-BC
Rochester, New York

Eleanor Fitzpatrick, MSN, RN, ACNP-BC, AGCNS-BS, CCRN
Philadelphia, Pennsylvania

Mary Beth Flynn Makic, RN, PhD, CNS, CCRN
Denver, Colorado

John J. Gallagher, RN, MSN, CCNS, CCRN
Philadelphia, Pennsylvania

Vicki S. Good, DNP, RN, CEMP, CPPS
Springfield, Missouri

Tarek Hassanein, MD
San Diego, California

Richard Henker, RN, PhD, CRNA
Pittsburgh, Pennsylvania

June Howland-Gradman, RN, MS, MBA
Orland Park, Illinois

Carol E. Jacoby, RN, MSN, ANCP
Portland, Oregon

Roberta Kaplow, PhD, AOCNS, APRN-CCNS, CCRN
Decatur, Georgia

Peggy L. Kirkwood, MSN, RN, ACNPC, CHFN, AACC
Mission Viejo, California

Julene (Julie) B. Kruithof, MSN, RN, CCRN
Grand Rapids, Michigan

Dana M. Kyles, MSN, RN
Seattle, Washington

Denise M. Lawrence, RN, BSN, MS, ACNP
Hartford, Connecticut

Barbara Leeper, MSN, RN-BC, CNS M-S, CCRN, FAHA
Dallas, Texas

Terry A. Lennie, RN, PhD, FAHA
Lexington, Kentucky

Carol S. Manchester, RN, MSN, APRN, BC-ADM, CDE
Minneapolis, Minnesota

Andrea P. Marshall, MN (Research), BN, RN, IC Cert
Sydney, Australia

Rhonda K. Martin, MSN, RN, CCRN, MLT(ASCP), CNS/ANP-C
San Diego, California

Rhonda S. Milam, MS, RD, CD, CNSD
Spokane, Washington

Nancy C. Molter, RN, MN, PhD, CCRC
Fort Sam Houston, Texas

Debra K. Moser, DNSc, RN, FAAN
Lexington, Kentucky

Nancy Munro, RN, MN, CCRN, ACNP
Baltimore, Maryland

Denise O'Brien, DNP, RN, ACNS-BC, CPAN, CAPA, FAAN
Ann Arbor, Michigan

Mary Frances D. Pate, RN, DSN
Greenville, North Carolina

Sara Paul, DNP, FNP, CHFN, FAHA
Conover, North Carolina

Kristine Peterson, MSN, RN, CCRN-K, CCNS-CMC
Wau, Wisconsin

Jan Powers, RN, MSN, FCCM, CCRN, CCNS, CNRN, CWCN
Indianapolis, Indiana

Patricia Radovich, PhD, CNS, FCCM
Azusa, California

Jeannette Richardson, RN, MS
Portland, Oregon

Barbara Riegel, RN, DNSc, FAAN, FAHA
Philadelphia, Pennsylvania

Sophia Chu Rodgers, RN, MSN, ACNP, NP-C
Albuquerque, New Mexico

Robert Rothwell, RN, MN, CCRN
Seattle, Washington

Polly Sather, RN, MSN
New Haven, Connecticut

Michael L. Schlicher, RN, MSN, PHN
Miami, Florida

Christine Smith Schulman, RN, MS, CNS, CCRN
Portland, Oregon

Sandra L. Schutz, RN, MSN
Seattle, Washington

Brenda K. Shelton, RN, MS, CCRN, AOCN
Baltimore, Maryland

Sandra L. Siedlecki, PhD, RN
Minneapolis, Minnesota

Diane Vail Skojec, DNP, MS, ANP-BC
Baltimore, Maryland

Julie A. Stanik-Hutt, BSN, MA, MSN, PhD, RN
Iowa City, Iowa

Louis R. Stout, RN, MS, CEN
Fort Sam Houston, Texas

Kathleen H. Toto, RN, MSN, ACNP
Dallas, Texas

Mary Fran Tracy, PhD, RN, APRN, CNS, FAAN
Minneapolis, Minnesota

Deborah Tuggle, MN, RN, CCNS
Louisville, Kentucky

Charles A. Walker, PhD, MSN, BSN
Fort Worth, Texas

Debra J. Lynn-McHale Wiegand, RN, MSN, MBE, PhD
Baltimore, Maryland

Laura D. Williams, RN, MBA, CHPN
Atlanta, Georgia

REVIEWERS

Patrice C. Al-Saden, RN, BS, CCRC
Senior Clinical Research Associate
Northwestern University
Comprehensive Transplant Center
Chicago, Illinois

Marie K. Arnone, MSN, RN, CCRN
Professional Development Specialist Cardiovascular Services
Swedish Medical Center
Seattle, Washington

Mary-Liz Bilodeau, RN, MS, CCRN, ACNP-BC
Acute Care Nurse Practitioner
Massachusetts General Hospital Burn Associates
Boston, Massachusetts

Cheryl Bittel, MSN, APRN, CCNS, NP-C, CCRN
Clinical Nurse Specialist
Emory Saint Joseph's Hospital
Atlanta, Georgia

Marylee Bressie, DNP, RN, CCNS, CCRN-K, CEN
Graduate Faculty
Capella University
Minneapolis, Minnesota

Damon B. Cottrell, DNP, RN, NP-C, CCNS, ACNS-BC, CEN
Clinical Professor
Texas Woman's University
Dallas, Texas

Micheal W. Day, MSN, RN, CCRN, TCRN
Trauma Clinical Practice Specialist
Northeast Georgia Medical Center
Gainesville, Georgia

Linda DeStefano, CNS, NP, FCCM
Associate Clinical Professor
University of California, Los Angeles
Los Angeles, California

Margaret M. Ecklund, MS, RN, CCRN, ACNP-BC
Clinical Nurse Specialist
Legacy Health
Portland, Oregon

Cheryl Edwards, RN, MSN, CCRN, CPTC
Senior Donation Coordinator
Regional Team Lead, Connecticut
New England Organ Bank
Waltham, Massachussets

Jennifer L. Embree, DNP, RN, NE-BC, CCNS
Clinical Assistant Professor
Coordinator MSN Leadership in Health Systems Program
Interim Coordinator DNP Leadership in Health Systems Program
Indiana University School of Nursing
Magnet Coordinator
Eskenazi Health
Indianapolis, Indiana

Maurice Espinosa, RN, MSN, CNS, CCRN
Critical Care Clinical Nurse Specialist
University of California Irvine Health
Orange, California

David Goede, DNP, MEd, ACNP-BC
Assistant Professor of Clinical Nursing, University of Rochester School of Nursing
Nurse Practitioner, Cardiac Surgery, Strong Memorial Hospital
Rochester, New York

Kiersten Henry, DNP, ACNP-BC, CCNS, CCRN-CMC
Chief Advanced Practice Provider
MedStar Montgomery Health Center
Olney, Maryland

Melissa L. Hutchinson, MN, RN, CCNS, CCRN
Clinical Nurse Specialist MICU/CCU
VA Puget Sound Health Care System
Seattle, Washington

Jennifer Joiner, MSN, RN, CCRN-CSC
Clinical Nurse Educator, CTICU and CCU
Robert Wood Johnson University Hospital
New Brunswick, New Jersey

Alice S. Kerber, MN, APRN, ACNS-BC, AOCN, AGN-BC
Oncology and Genetics Nurse Specialist
Georgia Center for Oncology Research and Education
Atlanta, Georgia

Andrea M. Kline-Tilford, MS, CPNP-AC/PC, FCCM
Pediatric Nurse Practitioner
Children's Hospital of Michigan
Detroit, Michigan

Barbara Konopka, RN, MSN, CCRN, CEN, CNE
Staff Nurse
Endless Mountains Health Systems
Montrose, Pennsylvania

Julene (Julie) B. Kruithof, MSN, RN, CCRN
Adult Critical Care Nurse Educator
Spectrum Health
Grand Rapids, Michigan

Dana Kyles, MS, RN
Assistant Administrator
Harborview Medical Center
Seattle, Washington

Rosemary K. Lee, DNP, ARNP, CNS, ACNP-BC, CCNS, CCRN
Clinical Nurse Specialist
Intensive Care & Progressive Care Unit
Homestead Hospital
Homestead, Florida

James P. McMurtry, MSN, APRN, CNS-BC, CCRN
Clinical Nurse Specialist, Medical Intensive Care Unit
Emory University Hospital Midtown
Atlanta, Georgia

Jennifer Milligan, MS, RN, CCRN
Assistant Clinical Professor
Texas Woman's University
Dallas, Texas

Michaelynn Paul, RN, MS, CCRN
Associate Professor of Nursing
Walla Walla University School of Nursing, Portland
Portland, Oregon

Janice Powers, PhD, RN, CCRN, CCNS, CNRN, FCCM
Director of Clinical Nurse Specialists and Nursing Research
Trauma ICU Clinical Nurse Specialist
St. Vincent Hospital, Indianapolis
Indianapolis, Indiana

Patricia Radovich, PhD, CNS, FCCM
Director
Nursing Research
Loma Linda University Medical Center
Loma Linda, California;
Adjunct Professor
School of Nursing
Azusa Pacific University
Azusa, California

Cynthia Rebik Christensen, MSN, CVN, ARNP-BC
Nurse Practitioner
TeamMD
Des Moines, Iowa

Kathryn B. Reid, RN, PhD, FNP-C
Associate Professor
University of Virginia School of Nursing
Charlottesville, Virginia

Julia Reteleski, MSN, RN, CCRN, SCRN, CCNS
Clinical Nurse Specialist Critical Care Network
Carolinas Healthcare System
Charlotte, North Carolina

Hildy Schell-Chaple, PhD, RN, CCRN, CCNS, FAAN
Clinical Nurse Specialist, Adult Critical Care
University of California, San Francisco Medical Center
Associate Clinical Professor
Department of Physiological Nursing
UCSF School of Nursing
San Francisco, California

Margaret (Peggy) Surratt, MSN/MBA, RN, CCRN, CTRN, CPEN, TCRN
Registered Nurse
Emergency Medicine and Trauma Center Children's National Medical Center
Washington, DC

Lenise Taylor, RN, MN, AOCNS, BMTCN
Hematologic Malignancies/BMT CNS
Seattle Cancer Care Alliance/University of Washington Medical Center
Seattle, Washington

Andrea Kline Tilford, MS, CPNP-AC/PC, FCCM
Faculty, AC PNP Program
Rush University College of Nursing
Chicago, Illinois

Kathleen S. Whalen, PhD, RN, CNE
Associate Professor
Loretto Heights School of Nursing
Regis University
Denver, Colorado

Judith Young, DNP, RN, CNE
Clinical Assistant Professor
Indiana University School of Nursing
Indianapolis, Indiana

ACKNOWLEDGMENTS

As we began discussing taking on the editing of this second edition, our thoughts and hearts went out to Karen Carlson. Although she is no longer with us, Karen had the vision and commitment to create the first *Advanced Critical Care Nursing* textbook. We therefore wish to acknowledge and thank her for her guidance, coaching, and mentoring of the three section editors she chose to help her with that task. None of us were editors at the time, but Karen had faith in us and taught us how to edit and produce an extremely successful resource for experienced nurses. When we were approached to work on the second edition, we felt a strong commitment to preserve Karen's vision and her memory, knowing that what she taught us would serve us well in this edition.

Of course, we were not alone in this journey. It has been our privilege to work with a number of talented editorial staff at Elsevier. Lee Henderson, Executive Content Strategist; Laura Goodrich, Content Development Specialist; and Mary Pohlman, Senior Project Manager, have been our main contacts and support through this project. Their guidance and expertise have been instrumental in producing a quality textbook. We are forever grateful for their support and encouragement throughout this process.

We also want to thank the staff at AACN, especially Michael Muscat, Publishing Manager, and Ramon Lavandero, Senior Director. They were extremely helpful in sorting out some confusing and convoluted issues. We are very appreciative for their "clear as mud" answers that helped us to be accurate in our content.

And, of course, we extend an extremely heartfelt thanks to all the contributors and reviewers for the various chapters. Their commitment and attention to detail made our job much easier. Whether the contributors were staff nurses, advanced practice nurses, or educators, they were also experts in their field. Their hard work and dedicated effort toward making the second edition a resource that will be valuable to our colleagues is deeply appreciated. To those who wrote, thank you for accepting the challenge to aim for a higher level. To those who reviewed, thanks for helping us ensure we were meeting our goal of creating an excellent resource for experienced critical care nurses.

Our personal support systems were also instrumental in our success. Peggy would like to thank her work colleagues, especially her director, Linda Standiford, who was very supportive and flexible in allowing her the time and energy to stay on target with time lines. Other colleagues at work assisted with brainstorming issues, taking on troublesome chapters, and generally providing sounding boards and encouragement during crunch times. Vicki would like to thank her managers, team members, and colleagues near and far who were supportive, allowing me to focus on the book and providing encouragement during difficult times.

Lastly, we want to thank our family and friends who provided personal support and encouragement throughout this endeavor. Peggy would especially like to thank her sister, Patricia, for her support and assistance with the detail work, and her husband, Art, for allowing her to take on this "third job." His encouragement, patience, and love were keys to being able to spend the long weekend hours working on the book. Vicki would like to thank her husband, Daniel, and kids, Meagan and Nathan. They were incredibly supportive throughout the process, especially when mom needed to "lock herself in the office." This dream would have never come to a reality without their support!

We are very proud of the outcome of this project and are extremely thankful for the team of people with whom we had the privilege to work throughout this journey. We are forever thankful to all of you!

Vicki S. Good
Peggy L. Kirkwood

PREFACE

Written by critical care experts, *Advanced Critical Care Nursing,* Second Edition, is a comprehensive, nursing-focused resource that helps experienced nurses in bedside and advanced practice roles care effectively for critical care patients in any clinical setting. The second edition provides key updates from the first edition based on newly developed research and changes in the practice environment. The book's foundation is the clinical reasoning process: the comprehension, analysis, synthesis, and application of knowledge. In addressing patient conditions, each body system is considered separately, emphasizing complex scientific, anatomic, pharmacologic, and pathophysiologic concepts. An interprofessional, evidence-based approach is taken in determining an appropriate course of action for each condition and potential complication.

Anatomy, physiology, and pathophysiology are presented in an application format, rather than as a dry recitation of facts. Assessment focuses on recognizing unusual or life-threatening signs and symptoms and on interpreting out-of-range laboratory values and other abnormal test results. Then the emphasis shifts to linking those findings to diagnoses and interventions. While the chapter text provides a wealth of background information on each condition and its treatment, the book's approach is hands-on and relentlessly practical—it highlights both expected and unexpected clinical events and invites nurses to draw on their own experience and knowledge of the topic in addressing evolving multisystem complications.

Advanced Critical Care Nursing, Second Edition, begins with a look at the current critical care environment and the varied settings in which critical care is practiced. The text then turns focus to a systems approach in addressing disorders affecting key body systems such as cardiovascular, respiratory, gastrointestinal, renal, and metabolic. Additionally, the book underscores its interprofessional approach by addressing topics that affect all critical care patients, whether they are being treated for trauma, having an organ transplant, or recovering from surgical complications. The book concludes with examining special patient populations, including critically ill pregnant patients, pediatric patients who are being cared for in adult critical care units, patients with severe neuropsychiatric disorders, bariatric surgery patients, oncology patients, patients with chemical dependencies, and patients at the end of life.

Wherever possible, the chapters follow a consistent format. *Case Studies* in many chapters challenge nurses to think critically in applying the information presented on each topic. Hundreds of full-color illustrations complement the core chapter content.

Many features found in the first edition have been continued in this second edition. Nutrition information, current research utilization, as well as evidence-based practice and treatment plans are now incorporated into the chapter content (rather than called out in boxes) to provide comprehensive coverage of each topic. Medication tables continue to provide detailed pharmacologic information accessible to readers at a glance. The full-color artwork, which demonstrates complex concepts in an easy-to-understand way, is again a highlight of this edition.

CONTENTS

UNIT VI Renal

1

The Critical Care Environment

Vicki S. Good

Critical care has roots dating back to the early 20th century. One of the earliest critical care units was developed in 1923 at the Johns Hopkins Hospital in Baltimore, Maryland.[11] In the 1940s there was an explosive growth in technology advancements used for the care of the critically ill. These early advancements included increased knowledge of anesthesia, the development of the first successful dialysis machine, new resuscitative measures with intravenous (IV) fluids and blood products, and the introduction of the first external defibrillator. External cardiopulmonary resuscitation (CPR) was first introduced in the 1960s, leading to decreased mortality.[11] All of these factors supported the development of critical care as a specialty within the acute care setting.

As a result of the ever-growing number of critical care units and the new specialty of critical care nursing, the American Association of Critical-Care Nurses (AACN) was established in 1971. AACN and its members helped develop guidelines and define best practice for the care of acute and critical care patients. Recognizing the need to address the empowerment of bedside nurses and demonstrate the skills and competency of critical care nurses, AACN became the industry leader in certification. Certified nurses demonstrate greater empowerment in their position and higher retention.[19] In recent years, AACN has expanded its critical care certification programs to include areas such as progressive care, tele–intensive care unit (ICU), educators, cardiac care, and, in partnership with the American Organization of Nurse Executives (AONE), the nurse manager. Additionally, AACN continues to seek ways to serve nurses and patients beyond the walls of a traditional intensive care unit, recognizing that critical care is now provided in multiple environments.

In addition to the increasing complexity of both the critical care environment and the acuity of critically ill patients, the US healthcare system is experiencing transformational changes. Patients and families along with payers, accreditation organizations, and the government are demanding a safe healthcare environment, positive patient outcomes, and high-quality care. The experienced acute and critical care nurse plays a primary role in meeting these demands. A fundamental key to the success of positive outcomes for critically ill patients is the critical care environment.[1,28,31,55] This chapter will discuss the evolving physical and cultural environment of the acute and critical care patient.

PHYSICAL ENVIRONMENT OF CARE

Since the first critical care units were conceived, the physical environment where this level of care is delivered has evolved. Boundaries have dissolved and critical care patients are now located throughout the acute care, chronic care, and home care settings, challenging nurses to maintain a wide range of skills to care for these patients. Acute and critical care nurses spend the majority of their time engaged in four categories of activities: documentation, medication administration, locating equipment and supplies, and communicating with team and family members. Therefore the environment of care must improve the care-giving experience, create a secure environment that promotes patient safety, contribute to the health and wellness of the patient and nurse, and preserve the human and capital resources for the acute and critically ill patient.[56] Acuity adaptable units, progressive care units, telemedicine, long-term acute care hospitals, ambulatory settings, and home care are a few of the physical environments where critical care is delivered.

Acuity Adaptable Units

Acuity adaptable units serve patients who need both critical care and long-term care in the same facility. In an acuity adaptable unit, the room begins with all equipment needed to care for a critically ill patient. As the patient improves, the room evolves to meet the lower acuity needs of the patient. Acuity adaptable rooms offer advantages of continuity, coordination of care, and flexibility as the patient remains in the same environment with the same nursing staff. The challenge is that the patient requires diverse nursing skill competency within the same nursing staff. The design of an acuity adaptable unit must meet the changing needs of the patient with regard to mobility, sensory needs, sleep quality, and a variety of clinical conditions.[37] The success of the acuity adaptable room has been variable across the United States.

Progressive Care Units

As defined by AACN, *progressive care* is the care delivered to patients whose needs fall along the acute end of the continuum of care and is used to describe areas that may be referred to as intermediate care units, direct observation units, step-down units, telemetry units, or transitional care units.[5] Progressive care units may specialize in certain patient populations (e.g., cardiac, surgical, neurologic, or pulmonary) or may encompass a broader spectrum of general diagnoses. The progressive care patient is moderately stable with less complexity and requires moderate resources and intermittent nursing vigilance. These units provide care with the same interprofessional patient care team as seen in the ICU. The team often includes the staff nurse, advanced practice nurse, nurse manager, clinical educator, pharmacist, respiratory therapist, social worker, occupational therapist, physical therapist, speech therapist, dietitian, and chaplain or pastor. This interprofessional approach is a benefit to the complex nature of these patients.

Characteristics defining the differences in progressive care patients versus traditional critical care patients include decreased risk of a life-threatening event, decreased need for invasive monitoring, increased stability, and increased ability to participate in care. Progressive care patient venues are not limited by geography, but by the needs and required interventions for the patient.

Telemedicine

According to the American Telemedicine Association, telemedicine is "the use of medical information exchanged from one site to another via electronic communications to improve patients' health status."[20] Telemedicine is referred to by several different terms such as *tele-ICU, virtual ICU, remote ICU,* or *e-ICU*. The model was introduced to address supply issues of critical care: too few ICU beds and too few specialty trained nurses and providers. The tele-ICU requires robust collaboration between the virtual and on-site critical care staff. The patient's room and medical record are virtually connected to the telemedicine staff via cameras, audio communication, central monitor and real-time waveforms, clinical information software, and alert systems. The telemedicine nurse and provider make virtual rounds on patients every 1 to 4 hours based on patient acuity.[20]

Telemedicine has been successful in increasing compliance with best practice recommendations, such as deep venous thrombosis prevention, stress ulcer prevention, cardiovascular protection, and hospital-acquired infection prevention. Several positive clinical outcomes for critically ill patients have been demonstrated with this model of care, including decreased mortality, decreased length of stay in the ICU, and decreased hospital-acquired infections. Additionally hospitals have had financial gains by keeping patients in their facilities versus transferring them to other facilities and improving case mix index and case margin.[20,22,30,35] While success has been demonstrated, the challenge is the utilization and acceptance of the additional telemedicine clinicians. Initially the traditional critical care staff showed an ambivalence towards telemedicine, but over recent years greater acceptance has been demonstrated as clinical outcomes improved.[30,61,63]

Long-Term Acute Care Hospitals

Long-term acute care hospitals (LTACHs) provide care to patients with medically complex conditions, such as prolonged mechanical ventilation, multiple organ failure, and complex wound and medication regimens needing long-term acute hospital care, with respiratory system compromise being the most frequent diagnosis. Patients benefit from daily provider visits, 24-hour respiratory therapy, nursing care, pharmacy, physical, speech, and occupational therapy, as well as other services. LTACHs may be free standing or located within a hospital setting. However, LTACH facilities are not evenly distributed across the United States, with higher concentrations in the Midwest and with some states not having any facilities.[42,54]

Ambulatory Settings

Critical or progressive care may also be delivered in ambulatory venues. Therapies supporting ongoing or chronic illnesses, such as respiratory care, medication therapy, and physical and occupational therapy, can be delivered episodically in an outpatient ambulatory setting. Medications that have been limited to critical care or hospital settings in the past may now be provided in an outpatient setting. With prescribed criteria for the levels of resilience and stability, a patient can be seen as an outpatient for assessment and treatment by a critical care team with competence to manage acute and critical illnesses. This affords disease management with a potential for increased quality of life and decreased hospital admissions.[17]

Home Care

Home care is a desired choice of many patients and families; however, this option creates the most challenges for those delivering care. For example, individuals requiring mechanical ventilation need 24-hour supervision, 7 days a week (unless they are independent enough to manage airway and ventilation needs). Additional therapies that may be managed at home include, but are not limited to, peritoneal dialysis, total parenteral nutrition, and complex wound management. Peritoneal dialysis may be initiated in the hospital and taught to patients and caregivers by the dialysis team. If total parenteral nutrition is managed at home, caregivers are instructed how to access and maintain central lines and administer IV therapy. Training related to dressing changes and site assessment may be managed with the assistance of the home care nurse. Outpatient wound ostomy nurses and home care agencies provide patients the option to return home with complex surgical wounds or existing pressure ulcers. Coordination is essential to determine appropriate supplies and insurance coverage for equipment.[17]

The hospital, skilled nursing care facility, or long-term care institution team assesses the feasibility of discharging the patient to home, using input from patients and their support systems. When the patient and family choose home care as the appropriate venue for care, extensive education and training must be completed with the patient and all caregivers. A teaching plan is established and educational sessions coordinated with patients and their chosen caregivers. A complex discharge plan follows to meet the specialized needs of the patient.[17]

HEALTHY WORK ENVIRONMENT STANDARDS

In response to the overwhelming concern expressed about providing quality care to critical care patients, AACN originally published standards for establishment of a healthy work environment in 2005 with an update in 2015. In the *AACN Standards for Establishing and Sustaining Healthy Work Environments: A Journey to Excellence*,[6] AACN defined six fundamental standards for establishing and sustaining healthy work environments (Table 1.1). The standards are a foundation for creating a healthy work environment and are not considered all-inclusive (i.e., clinical practice, patient outcomes, and regulatory requirements for the environment are not discussed in these standards); however, they must be met to provide safe, quality patient care.[6]

The six standards are interdependent of one another. For example, to make effective patient care decisions, the nurse must possess skilled communication and true collaboration. If a healthcare team embraces all six healthy work environment standards, the likelihood of enhancing clinical excellence, increasing clinician engagement, and achieving optimal patient outcomes increases (Fig. 1.1).[6]

By implementing healthy work environment standards, individual units have demonstrated positive clinician engagement outcomes, such as increased retention and decreased absenteeism, as well as increased patient satisfaction and clinical outcomes, such as decreased falls, decreased healthcare-associated infections, decreased safety events, and increased pain management.[29,44] Nurses working in healthy work environments report fewer healthcare-associated infections than nurses who report working in unhealthy environments.[29] Since the introduction of the *AACN Healthy Work Environment Standards*, work has been done to improve the healthcare environment. Despite this focused work, the 2013 AACN study on the work environment of the critical care nurse indicated that the environment has declined since the original study in 2008.[58,59] To be most effective in implementing and sustaining a healthy work environment, there must be a strong commitment from all levels of leadership and staff in the organization. The implementation of the healthy work environment standards requires changes in cultural norms, clinical practices, and philosophies of leadership.[6,60]

TABLE 1.1 AACN Standards for Establishing and Sustaining Healthy Work Environments

Skilled communication	Nurses must be as proficient in communication skills as they are in clinical skills.
True collaboration	Nurses must be relentless in pursuing and fostering true collaboration.
Effective decision-making	Nurses must be valued and committed partners in making policy, directing and evaluating clinical care, and leading organizational operations.
Appropriate staffing	Staffing must ensure an effective match between patient needs and nurse competencies.
Meaningful recognition	Nurses must be recognized and must recognize others for the value each brings to the work of the organization.
Authentic leadership	Nurse leaders must fully embrace the imperative of a healthy work environment, authentically live it, and engage others in its achievement.

Data from References 6 and 44.

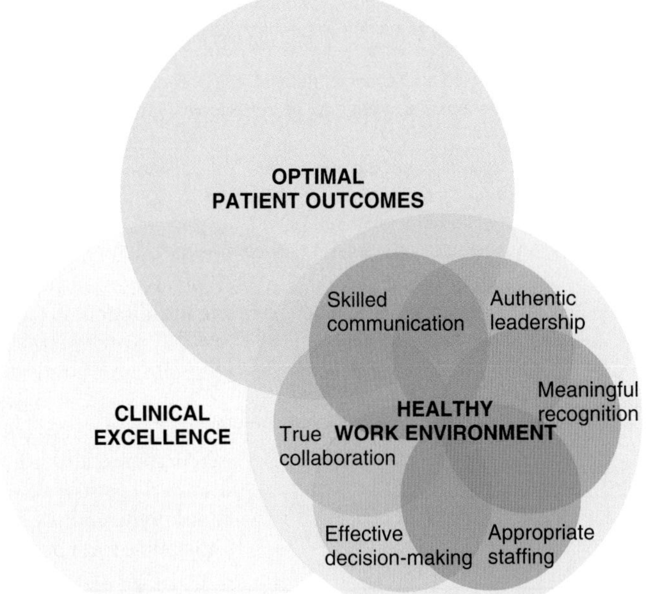

FIG. 1.1 Interdependence of healthy work environments, clinical excellence, and optimal patient outcomes.

Skilled Communication

Nurses must be as proficient in communication skills as they are in clinical skills (Box 1.1). One of the major challenges facing the healthcare team is the lack of respectful, effective communication.[60] Communication is as critical to the provision of safe patient care as clinically competent staff. Silence, a detrimental form of communication, results when nurses do not feel safe or fear that others will not listen.[21,39] Communication (written, spoken, and nonverbal) is the foundation of a healthy work environment and will reduce patient care errors and improve job satisfaction.[6]

Crucial Conversations

According to Merriam Webster,[43] communication is defined as "the act or process of using words, sounds, signs, or behaviors to express or exchange information or to express your ideas, thoughts, feelings, etc. to someone else." The healthcare environment is full of special symbols and language unique only to the healthcare profession. Within the healthcare environment, numerous pieces of information are exchanged continuously.

Communication seems clear and simple; why, therefore, do healthcare professionals struggle with communication? According to research completed by VitalSmarts and Kerry Patterson, most communication in healthcare surrounds "crucial conversations"—conversations that can be difficult to handle. According to VitalSmarts, a crucial conversation is a discussion between two or more people where stakes are high, opinions vary, and emotions run strong.[39,46] Each of these elements is present every day in the critical care setting and complicates the communication between healthcare professionals. Table 1.2 provides coaching strategies for having crucial conversations.

BOX 1.1 Critical Elements of Skilled Communication

- The healthcare organization provides team members with support for and access to education programs that develop critical communication skills, including self-awareness, inquiry/dialogue, conflict management, negotiation, advocacy, and listening.
- Skilled communicators focus on finding solutions and achieving desirable outcomes.
- Skilled communicators seek to protect and advance collaborative relationships among colleagues.
- Skilled communicators invite and hear all relevant perspectives.
- Skilled communicators call upon goodwill and mutual respect to build consensus and arrive at common understanding.
- Skilled communicators demonstrate congruence between words and actions, holding others accountable for doing the same.
- Skilled communicators have access to appropriate communication technologies and are proficient in their use.
- The healthcare organization establishes zero-tolerance policies and enforces them to address and eliminate abuse and disrespectful behavior in the workplace.
- The healthcare organization establishes formal structures and processes that ensure effective information sharing among patients, families, and the healthcare team.
- The healthcare organization establishes systems that require individuals and teams to formally evaluate the impact of communication on clinical and financial outcomes, and the work environment.
- The healthcare organization includes communication as a criterion in its formal performance appraisal system, and team members demonstrate skilled communication to qualify for professional advancement.

From Reference 6. Used with permission.

To make the greatest impact on the critical care environment, institutions should focus on seven areas that impact conversations the most. These include broken rules, mistakes, lack of support, incompetence, poor teamwork, disrespect, and micromanagement.[39,46] Many of these areas involve the need to hold crucial conversations with colleagues who may be at a different hierarchical level. Crucial conversations in a hierarchical structure are very difficult to conduct because of trust and power concerns. Failure to address these concerns may lead to patient harm; therefore, it is important for the healthcare environment to be conducive to open communication *before* concerns occur.[39,46,47] Despite having tools to address communication gaps in the clinical environment, bedside clinicians struggle to communicate concerns as identified by the Silent Treatment Study conducted by VitalSmarts and AACN. Organizations must address the problem of organizational silence in order to improve the work environment and the safety of care to patients.[40]

Interprofessional Communication

Many institutions have increased the efficiency of interprofessional communication by using the *s*ituation, *b*ackground, *a*ssessment, and *r*ecommendation (SBAR) model that flattens the hierarchy among caregivers. The SBAR model has demonstrated improvement in communication and reduction in

TABLE 1.2 Coaching for Crucial Conversations

Principle	Skill	Crucial Question
Start with heart.	Focus on what you really want. Refuse the sucker's choice.	Am I acting like I really want? What do I really want? For me? For others? For the relationship? How would I behave if I really did want this? What do I not want? How should I go about getting what I really want and avoiding what I don't want?
Learn to look.	Look for when the conversation becomes crucial. Look for safety problems. Look for your own style under stress.	Am I going to silence or violence? Are others?
Make it safe.	Apologize when appropriate. Contrast to fix misunderstandings. CRIB to get to mutual purpose: Commit to seek mutual purpose. Recognize the purpose behind the strategy. Invent a mutual purpose. Brainstorm new strategies.	Why is safety at risk? Have I established a mutual purpose? Am I maintaining mutual respect? What will I do to rebuild safety?
Master my stories.	Retrace my path to action. Separate fact from stories. Watch for three clever stories. Tell the rest of the story.	What is my story? What am I pretending not to know about my role in the problem? Why would a reasonable, rational, and decent person do this? What should I do right now to move toward what I really want?
State my path.	Share your facts. Tell your story. Ask about others' paths. Talk tentatively. Encourage testing.	Am I talking about the real issue? Am I really open to others' views? Am I confidently expressing my own views?
Explore others' paths.	Ask. Mirror. Paraphrase. Prime. Agree. Build. Compare.	Am I actively exploring others' views? Am I avoiding unnecessary disagreement?
Move to action.	Decide how you'll decide. Document decisions and follow up.	How will we make decisions? Who will do what by when? How will we follow up?

From Reference 46. Reprinted with permission.

patient care errors.[40] There are four key elements to the SBAR model:[34]

- **Situation:** This includes patient identification data, code status, vital signs, and the chief complaint or the nurse's concern(s).
- **Background:** Data in this section include the patient's mental status, skin condition, and respiratory status.
- **Assessment:** In this section, the clinician defines what she believes to be the problem.
- **Recommendation:** This includes provider orders and recommended actions.

The key to the success of the SBAR model is the gathering of consistent assessment and diagnostic data by clinical staff before initiating communication with any other discipline. The SBAR model uses a standardized approach for all communication, thus decreasing the likelihood of omitting key information.

Written Communication—Electronic Medical Record

Patient care is guided by numerous pieces of data coming together and being communicated to all healthcare team members. Patient care decisions are made on the basis of the data, but if caution is not exhibited, unintended consequences of electronic health records may occur. The exchange of the data becomes the key function of the communication processes between team members. A critical objective in the critical care environment is to determine the most effective and efficient way to communicate the patient care data.[18]

A major challenge to patient safety is the hybrid medical record (electronic platform with some items remaining on paper) that exists in many acute care settings. Healthcare organizations must continue to partner with and challenge information technology industry experts to ensure a seamless process to exchange patient care information in order to eliminate the hybrid model.[36] The degree of use of information systems varies drastically from organization to organization. Some healthcare systems are using voice recognition for charting and order entry, teleradiology, and telemedicine.

The electronic medical record (EMR) has been shown to positively influence the flow of information.[18] When key data are effectively and efficiently communicated, improvements in quality, safety, and efficiency of patient care will result. The EMR improves the interprofessional flow of information across the healthcare team by allowing access to the information in a variety of locations in real time as care is delivered. Many organizations have patients' medical records and key monitoring information available to the providers at his/her home and/or office, increasing efficiency and safety of care.

The primary components of a clinical information system must include providers order entry, diagnostic testing retrieval, clinical documentation, pharmacy monitoring, and medication documentation. Many of these components are operated from multiple different platforms; therefore there must be one overall information system managing all clinical information in order to provide consistency. Clinical information systems continue to grow in efficiency and effectiveness.[9]

Computerized providers order entry (CPOE) is considered the standard for communicating provider orders of care. CPOE offers key standardization to the medication delivery process, specifically the communication of medication orders. CPOE is a valuable tool to decrease adverse drug events (ADEs) within the healthcare environment compared to a manual order approach with the providers, nurse, and pharmacist.[3,9] The impact of CPOE on ADEs is primarily on the medication delivery component of writing and transmitting orders. After implementation of CPOE, Potts et al.[48] demonstrated a decrease in ADEs by 40.9%. These two aspects of medication delivery (writing orders and transmitting orders) are the most error prone for nurses, providers, and pharmacists. Both writing orders and transmitting orders involve a huge potential for human error surrounding illegible handwriting.[9,48] CPOE computerizes these aspects of medication delivery, thereby demonstrating a decrease in ADEs.

Despite all the advances in technology, verbal communication remains the most common way to communicate information in the critical care environment.[13] Verbal communication is the most problematic form of communication because of the potential for interpretations, biases, and misperceptions. Therefore, high priority must be maintained on the development and maintenance of effective communication skills. Through effective communication, organizations will experience greater patient safety and increased employee satisfaction.

True Collaboration

Nurses must be relentless in pursuing and fostering true collaboration (Box 1.2). Collaboration among the healthcare team is an essential element in a healthy work environment. The presence of true collaboration in the critical care environment has been directly linked to increased job satisfaction of nursing staff, decreased patient care errors, and increased quality of care delivered to patients.[23,31,51] During a market research study performed by AACN, 90% of members and constituents reported that collaboration is among the most important elements in creating a healthy work environment. There are three primary

BOX 1.2 Critical Elements of True Collaboration

- The healthcare organization provides team members with support for and access to education programs that develop collaboration skills.
- The healthcare organization creates, uses, and evaluates processes that define each team member's accountability for collaboration and how unwillingness to collaborate will be addressed.
- The healthcare organization creates, uses, and evaluates operational structures that ensure the decision-making authority of nurses is acknowledged and incorporated as the norm.
- The healthcare organization ensures unrestricted access to structured forums, such as ethics committees, and makes available the time needed to resolve disputes among all critical participants, including patients, families, and the healthcare team.
- Every team member embraces true collaboration as an ongoing process and invests in its development to ensure a sustained culture of collaboration.
- Every team member contributes to the achievement of common goals by giving power and respect to each person's voice, integrating individual differences, resolving competing interests, and safeguarding the essential contribution each makes in order to achieve optimal outcomes.
- Every team member acts with a high level of personal integrity.
- Team members master skilled communication, an essential element of true collaboration.
- Each team member demonstrates competence appropriate to his or her role and responsibilities.
- Nurse managers and medical directors are equal partners in modeling and fostering true collaboration.

From Reference 6. Used with permission.

opportunities for collaboration within the critical care environment: nurse to provider, nurse to nurse/other clinicians, and nurse to patient/family.

Collaboration is an ongoing process and is developed over time versus a one-time interaction. For a nurse to effectively engage in collaboration, effective communication, trust, knowledge, respect, and integration must be demonstrated.[6,50] This challenge sounds simple, but when examining the educational preparation of nursing and provider staff, most practitioners have not received formal training in these collaboration and communication skills. It is essential for nursing and provider leaders to mentor others so that true collaboration can occur.

Nurse-Provider Relationship

It is vitally important that the critical care environment have a healthy nurse-provider relationship for true collaboration to grow. An unhealthy relationship between the key professionals caring for the critical care patient leads to increased errors, decreased quality, and decreased staff retention and satisfaction.[23,31,51] To establish true collaboration, the nurse-provider relationship must be addressed, yet this is a difficult relationship to understand.

Mutual respect between all disciplines is one of the fundamental elements that must be present in order to nurture a collaborative work environment. The nurse and provider must demonstrate this mutual respect for each other's unique knowledge and competence. Lack of respect for one's colleagues leads to disharmony in the workplace, ultimately leading to decreased quality of care provided to patients.[14,23,31,38,51]

Mutual respect and establishment of positive nurse-provider collaboration has been cited as one of the top reasons for nurse retention and empowerment within an organization.[32,39,53] However, it is important to recognize that true collaboration will not occur overnight, nor will it be sustained if it is not given constant attention and resources.

Nurse-to-Nurse Collaboration

The ability to collaborate with other nurses before making both clinical and nonclinical decisions has been shown to prevent errors, increase nurse confidence, and increase nurse retention.[10] As the complexity of the critical care patient increases, the need for the critical care nurses to collaborate on decisions increases as well.[10,16]

Bucknall determined that critical care nurses had an increased confidence level and looked more confident when making decisions when they had the opportunity to collaborate with other nurses.[10] Synergy is built as nurses collaborate together on complex patient issues. That same synergy can be experienced when nurses work together on other issues.

Nurses need to work collaboratively among themselves as well as with the nursing leadership to resolve issues on the unit. Nurses' ability to collaborate with the nurse administrator on more than just clinical decisions positively impacts employee satisfaction. To increase nurse satisfaction and retention, the bedside critical care nurse must be actively involved in operational issues, which include scheduling, quality improvement processes, policy development, and participation in organizational decisions that impact professional nursing practice.[10,31]

Nurse-to-Family Collaboration

Not only is collaboration between the healthcare team important, but the collaborative relationship between the nurse and the patient and family must also be considered. Research indicates that when there is a harmonious relationship among staff, patient, and family, the patient will experience a decreased length of stay, increased patient satisfaction, and increased sense of overall collaboration.[23,26,50]

Effective Decision-Making

Nurses must be valued and committed partners in making policy, directing and evaluating clinical care, and leading organizational operations (Box 1.3). The line between collaboration and effective decision-making is exceedingly blurred. To make effective decisions, nurses cannot stand alone. The complexity of the critical care environment continues to expand, which necessitates that all practitioners collaboratively engage in clinical decision-making.[25] All decisions made regarding patient care must be sound in reasoning and grounded in the institution's mission, vision, and values as well as available evidence and industry standards of care. Therefore the bedside clinician, ancillary personnel, provider, and administration personnel must all work together in effective decision-making.

Collaborative Interprofessional Decision-Making

In addition to seeking the opinions of nursing colleagues, the complexity of the critical care patient demands that all disciplines collaborate to make the most effective and efficient decisions. The interprofessional critical care team includes, but is not limited to, the bedside nurse, the advanced practice nurse, and the provider, as well as personnel specializing in the following areas: social work, physical therapy, occupational therapy, speech therapy, nutrition, pharmacy, pastoral care, and anesthesia. Interprofessional decision-making takes many forms, including clinical protocols, order sets, team meetings, and face-to-face communications.[14,16,50]

Nurses who have the ability to participate in decision-making on their unit are more likely to demonstrate higher job satisfaction.[12,31] When nurses are involved in the decision-making process, both of unit operations and of patient care, their job satisfaction and retention increases. Research demonstrates a clear relationship between nurse retention and the level in which the clinical nurse has a voice in organizational and clinical

BOX 1.3 Critical Elements of Effective Decision-Making

- The healthcare organization clearly articulates organizational values, and team members incorporate these values when making decisions.
- The healthcare organization provides team members with support for and access to ongoing education and development programs focusing on strategies that ensure collaborative decision-making. Program content includes mutual goal setting, negotiation, facilitation, conflict management, systems thinking, and performance improvement.
- The healthcare organization has operational structures in place that ensure the perspectives of patients and their families are incorporated into every decision affecting patient care.
- Individual team members share accountability for effective decision-making by acquiring necessary skills, mastering relevant content, assessing situations accurately, sharing fact-based information, communicating professional opinions clearly, and inquiring actively.
- The healthcare organization establishes systems, such as structured forums involving appropriate departments and healthcare disciplines, to facilitate data-driven decisions.
- The healthcare organization establishes deliberate decision-making processes that ensure respect for the rights of every individual, incorporate all key perspectives, and designate clear accountability.
- The healthcare organization has fair and effective processes in place at all levels to objectively evaluate the results of decisions, including delayed decisions and indecision.

From Reference 6. Used with permission.

decision-making.[12,31] Opportunities for the staff nurse to participate in decision-making must be continuously cultivated.

Appropriate Staffing

Staffing must ensure an effective match between patient needs and nurse competencies (Box 1.4). Attempting to match the skills of caregivers with the needs of patients in any environment is challenging without a model of care on which to base decisions. Evidence supports the negative impact to the patient and the nurse when effective staffing is not maintained.[2,45,62] The AACN Synergy Model is a framework for patient care that matches the competency and skills of the nurse (Table 1.3) to the needs and characteristics of the patient (Table 1.4). Eight patient characteristics are identified in the model. These include the following: resiliency, vulnerability, stability, complexity, resource availability, participation in care, participation in decision-making, and predictability. Levels of need range from 1 to 5, with 5 representing the highest level.

Nursing characteristics include clinical judgment, clinical inquiry, facilitation of learning, collaboration, systems thinking, advocacy and moral agency, caring practices, and response to diversity. Levels again range from 1 to 5, with 1 defining a competent nurse and 5 defining an expert nurse. The underlying principle of the AACN Synergy Model is that positive outcomes will occur when nurses' characteristics and competencies are matched with the needs of the patients for whom they are caring.[15,24,27]

The AACN Synergy Model provides a framework for outcome analysis. The outcomes of patient-nurse synergy are threefold: patient-derived, nurse-derived, and system-derived outcomes, as illustrated in Fig. 1.2.[15] As a nurse develops within these areas, the natural outcome is an increased ability to create a compassionate and therapeutic environment in which skilled, knowledgeable professionals care for patients. As patients and

BOX 1.4 Critical Elements of Appropriate Staffing

- The healthcare organization has staffing policies in place that are solidly grounded in ethical principles and support the professional obligation of nurses to provide high-quality care.
- Nurses participate in all organizational phases of the staffing process from education and planning—including matching nurses' competencies with patients' assessed needs—through evaluation.
- The healthcare organization has formal processes in place to evaluate the effect of staffing decisions on patient outcomes. The evaluation includes analysis of both patient and system outcomes. This evaluation includes analysis of when patient needs and nurse competencies are mismatched and how often contingency plans are implemented.
- The healthcare organization has a system in place that facilitates team members' use of staffing and outcome data to develop more effective staffing models.
- The healthcare organization provides support services at every level of activity to ensure nurses can optimally focus on the priorities and requirements of patient and family care.
- The healthcare organization adopts technologies that increase the effectiveness of nursing care delivery. Nurses are engaged in the selection, adaptation, and evaluation of these technologies.

From Reference 6. Used with permission.

TABLE 1.3 Nurse Characteristics of the AACN Synergy Model for Patient Care

Characteristic	NURSES' COMPETENCIES FALL ALONG CONTINUUM REPRESENTED BY THESE THREE CATEGORIES		
	Level 1 (Competent)	Level 3	Level 5 (Expert)
Clinical judgment: Clinical reasoning, which includes clinical decision-making, critical thinking, and global grasp of situation, coupled with nursing skills acquired through a process of integrating formal and experiential knowledge.			
Advocacy/moral agency: Working on another's behalf and representing concerns of patient, family, and community; serving as a moral agent in identifying and helping to resolve ethical and clinical concerns within clinical setting.			
Caring practices: Constellation of nursing activities that are responsive to uniqueness of patient and family and that create a compassionate and therapeutic environment, with aim of promoting comfort and preventing suffering. These caring behaviors include, but are not limited to, vigilance, engagement, and responsiveness.			
Collaboration: Working with others (e.g., patients, families, and healthcare providers) in a way that promotes and encourages each person's contributions toward achieving optimal and realistic patient goals. Collaboration involves intradisciplinary and interdisciplinary work with colleagues.			
Systems thinking: Body of knowledge and tools that allow nurse to appreciate care environment from a perspective that recognizes holistic interrelationship that exists within and across healthcare systems.			
Response to diversity: Sensitivity to recognize, appreciate, and incorporate differences into provision of care. Differences may include, but are not limited to, individuality, cultural differences, spiritual beliefs, gender, race, ethnicity, disability, family configuration, lifestyle, socioeconomic status, age, values, and beliefs surrounding alternative/complementary medicine involving patients, families, and members of the healthcare team.			
Clinical inquiry to innovator/evaluator: Ongoing process of questioning and evaluating practice, providing informed practice, and innovating through research and experiential learning. Nurse engages in clinical knowledge development to promote best patient outcomes.			
Facilitator of learning or patient/family educator: Ability to facilitate patient and family learning.			

From Reference 24. Used with permission.

TABLE 1.4 Patient Characteristics of the AACN Synergy Model for Patient Care

Characteristic	Level 1	Level 3	Level 5
Resiliency: Capacity to return to a restorative level of functioning using compensatory coping mechanisms; ability to bounce back quickly after an insult	Minimally resilient	Moderately resilient	Highly resilient
Vulnerability: Susceptibility to actual or potential stressors that may adversely affect patient outcomes	Highly vulnerable	Moderately vulnerable	Minimally vulnerable
Stability: Ability to maintain steady-state equilibrium	Minimally stable	Moderately stable	Highly stable
Complexity: Intricate entanglement of two or more systems (e.g., body, family, therapies)	Highly complex	Moderately complex	Minimally complex
Resource availability: Extent of resources (e.g., psychologic, social) that patient, family, and community bring to situation	Few resources	Moderate resources	Many resources
Participation in care: Extent to which patient and family engage in aspects of care	No participation	Moderate participation	Full participation
Participation in decision-making: Extent to which patient and family engage in decision-making	No participation	Moderate participation	Full Participation
Predictability: Summative characteristic that allows one to expect a certain trajectory of illness	Not predictable	Moderately predictable	Highly predictable

From Reference 24. Used with permission.

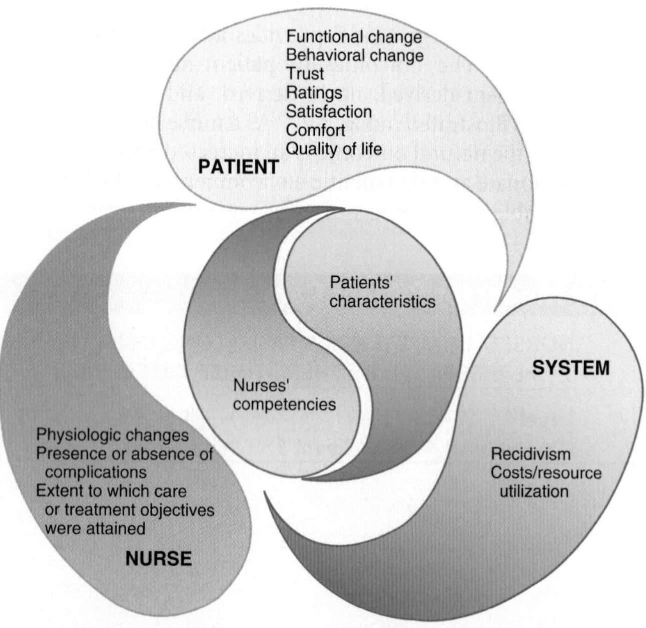

FIG. 1.2 Three levels of outcomes delineated by the AACN Synergy Model for Patient Care: those derived from the patient, those derived from the nurse, and those derived from the healthcare system.

nurses develop these caring relationships, trust develops and information is then easily exchanged, allowing for mutual participation in care. As nurses work to coordinate care for complex patients, using a high degree of collaboration, mortality is lower, patient satisfaction is higher, and nosocomial complication rates are lower.[15] Continuity of care and strong clinical judgment stabilize care within the chaotic critical care environment, leading to higher clinical effectiveness and optimal patient outcomes.

There is little debate on the impact of appropriate staffing levels in building and sustaining a healthy work environment. The bedside nurse has been referred to as the *front line* in providing patient surveillance, assessing the patient, and intervening when problems develop, as well as the one key practitioner prepared to rescue patients when they are in trouble. The nurse plays a vital role in patient care, with studies citing decrease in mortality, length of stay, and infections when a higher nurse ratio is maintained.[52] It is important to also recognize that nurse staffing is the highest expense in the acute care hospital budget. Therefore, it is essential for organizations to ensure safe staffing levels with competent practitioners while monitoring expenses.[2] Because of the complexity of this issue, nurses and organizations must work together to ensure appropriate staffing.

Meaningful Recognition

Nurses must be recognized and must recognize each other for the value each nurse brings to the work of the organization (Box 1.5). One of the fundamental keys to developing a healthy work environment is to ensure satisfied employees.[53] A key human desire is the need to be recognized for our contributions, both in our personal and in our professional lives. Recognition should continuously acknowledge, honor, and celebrate the contribution of individuals or groups; it should never be a singular event.[31,33,41,49,57]

The type of recognition desired by individuals varies from person to person. Recognition can be tangible or intangible. Examples of tangible recognition include gift cards, bonus payments, and gifts, whereas intangible examples are verbal expressions of thanks, recognition in unit/hospital newsletters, and recognition at department meetings.[57] One of the most successful recognition programs is the Disease Attacking the Immune System (DAISY) award. After the death of their 33-year-old son, Patrick, from idiopathic thrombocytopenic purpura (ITP), the Barnes family wanted to recognize the extraordinary acts of compassion that nurses give every single day to their patients. The award is tailored by individual institutions and consists of a statue, a DAISY pin, and Cinnabon rolls (one of Patrick's favorite treats).[8,31]

A second key form of recognition is group recognition for achievements. Examples include the Magnet Recognition Program from the American Nurses Association (ANA) for organizations and the Beacon Award from AACN for individual units. Both of these recognize hospitals and units for excellence in nurse retention, health work environments, and optimal clinical outcomes.[4,7]

Key Aspects of Individual Recognition

Why is recognition so important? The simplest reason is the fact that all individuals appreciate a simple "thank you" for

BOX 1.5 Critical Elements of Meaningful Recognition

- The healthcare organization has a comprehensive system in place that includes formal processes and structured forums that ensure a sustainable focus on recognizing all team members for their contributions and the value they bring to the work of the organization.
- The healthcare organization establishes a systematic process for all team members to learn about the institution's recognition system and how to participate by recognizing the contributions of colleagues and the value they bring to the organization.
- The healthcare organization's recognition system reaches from the bedside to the boardroom, ensuring individuals receive recognition consistent with their personal definition of meaning, fulfillment, development, and advancement at every stage of their professional career.
- The healthcare organization's recognition system includes processes validating that recognition is meaningful to those being acknowledged.
- Team members understand that everyone is responsible for playing an active role in the organization's recognition program and meaningfully recognizing contributions.
- The healthcare organization regularly and comprehensively evaluates its recognition system, ensuring effective programs that help to move the organization toward a sustainable culture of excellence that values meaningful recognition.

Data from references 6. Used with permission.

their hard work and dedication. When an employee feels valued, that individual is more likely to think favorably of the organization, stay at the organization longer, and have increased productivity.

The type of recognition provided is not as important as the fact that recognition is being provided. The key to meaningful recognition is that it must be sincere, timely, and visible. Simple forms of recognition are the best, such as thank you notes, announcements of achievements in staff meetings, bulletin boards, or emails of key achievements. Many institutions have adopted simple ways to provide staff immediate recognition by patients, families, and co-workers. These include documents for individuals to complete noting the special activities that the staff member has performed and small tokens of appreciation such as movie tickets or gift certificates to the cafeteria. All of these items provide instant recognition to the staff member and make a lasting impression on employees of their contribution.[57]

Team Recognition

It is equally important to recognize the critical care team as a whole as it is to recognize the individuals within the critical care unit. As mentioned, the two key recognition programs that recognize hospitals and units for providing and sustaining a healthy work environment are the ANA's Magnet Recognition Program[7] and AACN's Beacon Award.[4]

The Magnet Recognition Program was developed by the American Nurses Credentialing Center (a division of the ANA) to recognize healthcare organizations that provide the best in nursing care. This program was started after the ANA studied hospitals that appeared to be a "magnet" in recruiting and retaining registered nurses. Hospitals are evaluated based on nursing quality indicators and their ability to provide nursing care based on the standards of nursing practice defined by the ANA. Key indicators evaluated include nurse vacancy rates, patient outcome data such as skin breakdown and patient falls, clinical ladder programs, patient satisfaction, nurse engagement, and the percentage of staff with certification and advanced degrees.[7] The recognition is prestigious and exemplifies the provision of a healthy work environment.

AACN launched the Beacon Award for Critical Care Excellence to recognize individual critical care units that have led and sustained the journey toward excellence in the work environment. The Beacon Award is granted to critical care units exhibiting high-quality standards, exceptional care of patients and families, and healthy work environments. The award requires that the unit submit an application demonstrating how they have met and sustained the defined criteria for a Beacon Unit. An expert review panel evaluates the application and the unit is awarded a Bronze, Silver, or Gold level recognition.[4]

Authentic Leadership

Nurse leaders must fully embrace the imperative of a healthy work environment, authentically live it, and engage others in its achievement (Box 1.6). The role of the frontline nurse leader is the foundation for a successful healthcare organization. The frontline nurse leader is continually balancing the demands of the organizational executive leaders with the needs of the critical care patients and the critical care nursing personnel. The goal before the nurse leader is to provide high-quality care while decreasing the length of patient stay and improving the financial performance of the unit. Additionally, the nurse leader faces the challenging role as the primary influence on staff satisfaction and, ultimately, staff retention. Therefore the value of an authentic nurse leader is priceless.

Key Characteristics of a Nurse Leader

The first topic that must be addressed is the educational preparation of a nurse entering a leadership position. Many nurse managers were at one time great bedside nurses who were promoted to the position of nurse leader. Some of these individuals have had formal training regarding management and leadership skills, but many of these individuals have had little or no training. Therefore it is essential that organizations make a commitment to ensure adequate development of individuals in this role. This development must include both formal training and mentoring by senior nurse leaders. Skills that must be addressed include financial issues, quality, clinical safety, regulatory requirements, customer service initiatives, and employee satisfaction.[6]

It can take several years for a nurse leader to develop these skills. To prevent interruption in unit leadership, succession management is important. Succession management encourages hospitals to recognize future leaders and begin their development so they will be ready to take over when a vacancy occurs.

An authentic leader must be committed to empower staff in order to increase effectiveness. Empowered staff has access to resources, information, and support to help them perform their jobs. The nurse leader plays a pivotal role in assisting critical care staff nurses to access each of these key items. Not having the resources to care for acute and critically ill patients is a major source of frustration for a bedside nurse. The most necessary resources can be minor, such as having a copier on the unit, or major, such as having enough bedside nurses on a given shift, yet both have equally important roles in staff satisfaction and the provision of safe patient care.[31,57] An authentic leader encourages staff to work together to define their needs and to develop solutions to meet those needs. By having increased involvement, the staff nurse will have increased satisfaction and retention.

BOX 1.6 Critical Elements of Authentic Leadership

- The healthcare organization provides support for and access to educational programs to ensure that nurse leaders develop and enhance knowledge and abilities in skilled communication, effective decision-making, true collaboration, meaningful recognition, and ensuring resources to achieve appropriate staffing.
- Nurse leaders demonstrate an understanding of the requirements and dynamics at the point of care, and within this context successfully translate the vision of a healthy work environment.
- Nurse leaders excel at generating visible enthusiasm for achieving the standards that create and sustain healthy work environments.
- Nurse leaders lead the design of systems necessary to effectively implement and sustain standards for healthy work environments.
- The healthcare organization ensures that nurse leaders are appropriately positioned in their pivotal role in creating and sustaining healthy work environments. This includes participation in key decision-making forums, access to essential information, and the authority to make necessary decisions.
- The healthcare organization facilitates the efforts of nurse leaders to create and sustain a healthy work environment by providing the necessary time and financial and human resources.
- The healthcare organization provides a formal mentoring program for all nurse leaders. Nurse leaders actively engage in the mentoring program.
- Nurse leaders are role models for skilled communication, true collaboration, effective decision-making, meaningful recognition, and authentic leadership.
- The healthcare organization includes the leadership contribution of creating and sustaining a healthy work environment as a criterion in each nurse leader's performance appraisal. Nurse leaders must demonstrate leadership in creating and sustaining a healthy work environment in order to achieve professional advancement.
- The healthcare organization ensures that measurement of the organization's progress toward creating and sustaining a healthy work environment is evaluated at regular intervals using tools designed for that purpose. The AACN Healthy Work Environment Assessment tool is available at http://www.aacn.org/hwe.
- Nurse leaders and team members mutually and objectively evaluate the impact of leadership processes and decisions on the organization's progress toward creating and sustaining a healthy work environment.

Data from Reference 6. Used with permission.

Role of Accountability

Critical care nurses desire to work with staff who are competent to perform their jobs, are active patient advocates, and have a desire to serve their patients. When nurses encounter other staff members not performing their duties adequately, resulting in compromised patient quality and safety, nurses want leaders who hold colleagues accountable for their actions.

The authentic nurse leader must ensure that the practice expectations of the critical care unit are consistently followed. The practice expectations have been developed by evidence-based research and nursing standards of care from key nursing organizations such as AACN and ANA. Consequences for not following unit expectations must be defined and implemented. When a nurse leader does not consistently hold staff accountable for practice, the unit's success falters. The foundation for success is consistent accountability within a unit by the designated leader.

Power of an Authentic Nurse Leader

The nurse leader must have a support system and the necessary resources to influence the critical care unit, and ultimately the healthcare organization. The authentic nurse leader must possess skills such as communication, decision-making, collaboration, finance, and leadership. The nurse leader becomes the glue holding the critical care unit together and the branch reaching out to other departments in the organization to effectively care for the acute and critically ill patients.

CONCLUSION

Healthy work environments are vital for the provision of optimal patient outcomes regardless of the location in which the care is provided. Building and sustaining a healthy work environment is a process that is never ending. The healthcare environment is a dynamic setting in which technology, research, and patient disease states are in constant change. As more is learned regarding the nursing care of our acute and critically ill patients, more is also learned on how to create a healthy work environment and thus create optimal outcomes for the patient.

The six healthy work environment standards discussed in this chapter merely provide a framework for creating and sustaining a healthy work environment. Each standard is interdependent on the other. A team cannot demonstrate true collaboration when the team is lacking skilled communication. Effective decisions cannot be made without having a collaborative team caring for the patient. Therefore when developing a healthy work environment, do not view each standard exclusively, but view them inclusively.

Each individual acute and critical care nurse must accept responsibility for the physical and cultural environment. Change must occur one person, one unit, and one system at a time in order to be most effective. Each individual nurse must authentically contribute to the physical and cultural environment in order to sustain and create a healthy work environment that results in optimal patient outcomes.

REFERENCES

1. Adomat, R., & Hicks, C. (2003). Measuring nursing workload in intensive care: an observation study using closed circuit video cameras. *J Adv Nurs, 42*(4), 402–412.
2. Aiken, L. H., et al. (2011). Effects of nurse staffing and nurse education on patient deaths in hospitals with different nurse work environments. *Med Care, 449*(12), 1047–1053.
3. Alsweed, F., et al. (2014). Impact of computerized provider order entry system on nursing workflow, patient safety, and medication errors: perspectives from the front line. *Int J Electron Healthc, 7*(4), 287–300. http://dx.doi.org/10.1504/IJEH.2014.064328.
4. American Association of Critical-Care Nurses. (2005). *Beacon award for clinical excellence.* http://www.aacn.org/AACN/ICURecog.nsf/vwdoc/MainPage.
5. American Association of Critical-Care Nurses. (2009). *Progressive care fact sheet.* http://www.aacn.org.
6. American Association of Critical-Care Nurses. (2015). *AACN standards for establishing and sustaining healthy work environments: a journey to excellence.* Aliso Viejo, CA: AACN.
7. American Nurses Credentialing Center. (2005). *ANCC magnet recognition program: recognizing excellence in nursing services.* http://www.ana.org/ancc/magnet/index.html.
8. Barnes, B., & Lefton, C. (2013). The power of meaningful recognition in a healthy work environment. *AACN Adv Crit Care, 24*(2), 114–116.
9. Bria, W. F., & Shabot, M. M. (2005). The electronic medical record, safety, and critical care. *Crit Care Clin, 21*(1), 55–79.
10. Bucknall, T. (2003). The clinical landscape of critical care: nurses' decision-making. *J Adv Nurs, 43*(3), 310–319.

11. Calvin, J., Habet, K., & Parrillo, J. (1997). Critical care in the United States: who are we and how did we get here? *Crit Care Clin North Am, 13*, 363–376.
12. Choi, J., et al. (2004). Perceived nursing work environment of critical care nurses. *Nurs Res, 53*(6), 370–378.
13. Collins, S. A. (2011). Clinician preferences for verbal communication compared to EHR documentation in the ICU. *Appl Clin Inform, 2*(2), 190–201. http://dx.doi.org/10.4338/ACI-2011-02-RA-0011.
14. Cook, A. F., et al. (2004). An error by any other name. *Am J Nurs, 104*(6), 32–43.
15. Curley, M. A. Q. (1998). Patient nurse synergy: optimizing patients' outcomes. *Am J Crit Care, 7*, 64–72.
16. Dougherty, M. B., & Larson, E. L. (2010). The nurse-nurse collaboration scale. *J Nurs Adm, 40*(1), 17–25. http://dx.doi.org/10.1097/NNA.ob3e3181c47cd6.
17. Ecklund, M. M. (2006). Homecare management of ventilator-assisted patients. In S. M. Burns (Ed.), *AACN's practice protocols: Care of the mechanically ventilated patient*. Sudbury, MA: Jones and Bartlett.
18. Erdley, W. S. (2005). Concept development of nursing information: a study of nurses working in critical care. *Comput Inform Nurs, 23*(2), 93–99.
19. Fitzpatrick, J. J., et al. (2010). Certification, empowerment, and intent to leave current position and the profession among critical care nurses. *Am J Crit Care, 19*(3), 218–229. http://dx.doi.org/10.4037/ajcc2010442.
20. Goran, S. F. (2010). A second set of eyes: an introduction to tele-ICU. *Crit Care Nurse, 30*(4), 46–55. http://dx.doi.org/10.4037/ccn2010283.
21. Gordon, S., Mendenhall, P., & O'Connor, B. B. (2013). *Beyond the checklist: What else health care can earn from aviation teamwork and safety*. Ithaca, NY: Cornell University Press.
22. Gorman, M. J. (2011). Tele-ICU comes of age: studies, hospital five-year results validate effectiveness of the technology. *Health Manag Technol, 32*(12), 8–11.
23. Greene, J. (2002). The medical workplace: no abuse zone. *Hosp Health Netw, 76*(3), 26–28.
24. Hardin, S. R., & Kaplow, R. (2005). *Synergy for clinical excellence: The AACN synergy model for patient care*. Sudbury, MA: Jones and Bartlett.
25. Houser, J., et al. (2012). Involving nurses in decisions: improving both nurse and patient outcomes. *J Nurs Adm, 42*(7–8), 375–382.
26. Kaplow, R. (2002). Applying the synergy model to nursing education. *Crit Care Nurse, 22*(3), 77–81.
27. Kaplow, R. (2003). AACN synergy model for patient care: a framework to optimize outcomes. *Crit Care Nurse, Feb*(Suppl), 27–30.
28. Kelley, M. A., et al. (2004). The critical care crisis in the United States: a report from the profession. *Chest, 125*(4), 1514–1517.
29. Kelly, D., et al. (2013). The critical care work environment and nurse-reported health care-associated infections. *Am J Crit Care, 22*(6), 482–489. http://dx.doi.org/10.4037/ajcc2013298.
30. Khunlertkit, A., & Carayon, P. (2013). Contributions of tele-intensive care unit (Tele-ICU) technology to quality of care and patient safety. *J Crit Care, 28*, 315.e1–e12.
31. Larrabee, J. H., et al. (2003). Predicting registered nurse job satisfaction and intent to leave. *J Nurs Admin, 33*(5), 271–283.
32. Leape, L. L., et al. (2012). A culture of respect, part 1 and part 2: the nature and cause of disrespectful behavior by physicians. *Acad Med, 87*(7), 845–858.
33. Lefton, C. (2014). Nursing perspectives: transforming NICU culture: the power of meaningful recognition. *Neoreviews, 15*, e221–e224.
34. LeRoy, W., Bauman, E., & Parvati, D. E. V. (2012). SBAR 'flattens the hierarchy' among caregivers. *Medicine Meets Virtual Reality, 19*, 175–182. http://dx.doi.org/10.3233/978-1-61499-022-2-175.
35. Lilly, C. M., et al. (2011). Hospital mortality, length of stay, and preventable complications among critically ill patients before and after tele-ICU reengineering of critical care process. *J Am Med Assoc, 305*(21), 2175–2183. http://dx.doi.org/10.1001/jama.2011.697.
36. Lugtu, T. (2014). When hybrid records cause harm: how to avoid putting yourself at risk when making the switch to an EHR. *Minn Med, 97*(11–12), 44–45.
37. Mammen, J., & Costello, B. (2014). Relational sustainability: environments for long-term critical care patients. *Crit Care Nurs Q, 37*(1), 53–66.
38. Manojlovich, M., & DeCicco, B. (2007). Healthy work environments, nurse-physician communication, and patient outcomes. *Am J Crit Care, 16*(6), 536–545.
39. Maxfield, D., et al. (2005). *Silence kills: The seven crucial conversations for healthcare* (pp. 1–16). Provo, UT: VitalSmarts.
40. Maxfield, D., et al. (2010). *The silent treatment: Why safety tools and checklists aren't enough to save lives* (pp. 1–12). Provo, UT: VitalSmarts.
41. McCauley, K. (2005). President's address: live your contribution: Our quest for excellence. In *National teaching institute and critical care exposition*. New Orleans, LA: American Association of Critical Care Nurses.
42. Medicare Payment Advisory Commission. (2012). *Report to Congress: Medicare Payment Policy 2012 Report*. http://www.medpac.gov/documents/reports/march-2012-report-to-the-congress-medicare-payment-policy.pdf?sfvrsn=0.
43. Merriam Webster. (2015). *Merriam Webster on-line dictionary*. http://www.merriam-webster.com/dictionary/communication.
44. Nayback-Beebe, A. M., et al. (2013). Using evidence-based leadership initiatives to create a healthy nursing work environment. *Dimens Crit Care Nurs, 32*(4), 166–173. http://dx.doi.org/10.1097/DCC.0b013e3182998121.
45. Needleman, J., et al. (2011). Nurse staffing and inpatient mortality. *N Engl J Med, 364*(11), 1037–1045.
46. Patterson, K., et al. (2002). *Crucial conversations: Tools for talking when stakes are high* (pp. 240). New York: McGraw-Hill.
47. Patterson, K., et al. (2005). *Crucial confrontations: Tools for resolving broken promises, violated expectations, and bad behavior* (pp. 284). New York: McGraw-Hill.
48. Potts, A. L., et al. (2004). Computerized physician order entry and medication errors in a pediatric critical care unit. *Pediatrics, 113*, 59–63.
49. Psychological Associates and DAISY Foundation. (2009). *Literature review on meaningful recognition in nursing*. http://daisyfoundation.org/daisy-award/meaningful-recognition-literature-review/Literature ReviewonMeaningfulRecongnitionNursing.pdf.
50. Revta, B. (2004). NICU—The "I" stands for integrated. *J Neurosci Nurs, 36*(3), 174–176.
51. Rosenstein, A. H. (2002). Nurse-physician relationships: impact on nurse satisfaction and retention. *Am J Nurs, 102*(6), 26–34.
52. Sakr, Y., et al. (2014). The impact of hospital and ICU organizational factors on outcome in critically ill patients: results from the extended prevalence of infection in intensive care study. *Crit Care Med, 43*(3), 519–526 2015.
53. Schmalenberg, C., & Kramer, M. (2009). Nurse-physician relationships in hospitals: 20,000 nurses tell their story. *Crit Care Nurse, 29*(1), 74–83.
54. Seneff, M. G., et al. (2000). The impact of long-term acute-care facilities on the outcome and cost of care for patients undergoing prolonged mechanical ventilation. *Crit Care Med, 28*(2), 342–350.
55. Smith, A. P. (2004). Partners at the bedside: the importance of nurse-physician relationships. *Nurs Econ, 22*(3), 161–164.
56. Stroupe, J. M. (2014). Design for safety in the critical care environment: an evidence-based approach: considering the caregiver-patient-family experiences. *Crit Care Nurse Q, 37*(1), 103–114.
57. Studer, Q. (2003). *Hardwiring excellence: Purpose, worthwhile work, making a difference*. Gulf Breeze, FL: Fire Starter Publishing.
58. Ulrich, B. T., et al. (2006). Critical care nurses' work environments: a baseline status report. *Crit Care Nurse, 26*(5), 46–50, 52–57.
59. Ulrich, B. T., et al. (2009). Critical care nurses' work environments 2008: a follow-up report. *Crit Care Nurse, 29*(2), 93–102. http://dx.doi.org/10.4037/ccn2009619.
60. Ulrich, B. T., et al. (2014). Critical care nurse work environment 2013: a status report. *Crit Care Nurse, 34*(4), 64–79.
61. Ward, M., et al. (2015). Factors affecting staff perceptions of tele-ICU service in rural hospitals. *Telemed J E Health, 21*(6), 459–466. http://dx.doi.org/10.1089/tmj.2014.0137.
62. Wiltse Nicely, K. L., Sloane, D. M., & Aiken, L. H. (2013). Lower mortality for abdominal aortic aneurysm repair in high-volume hospitals is contingent upon staffing. *Health Serv Res, 48*(3), 972–991.
63. Young, L. B. (2011). Staff acceptance of tele-ICU coverage: a systematic review. *Chest, 139*(2), 279–288.

2

Advanced Dysrhythmias

Kristine Peterson

Observation of a patient's cardiac rhythm is one of the most important aspects of critical care nursing. Early detection and accurate diagnosis of dysrhythmias or ST-T wave changes may prevent adverse consequences for the patient. The goal of this chapter is to provide information on select cardiac dysrhythmias that have important implications for patient care. An understanding of basic electrocardiography is required.

THE CARDIAC ACTION POTENTIAL

Normal Cardiac Cell Function

The cardiac *action potential* is the electrical activity occurring in individual cardiac cells during one cardiac cycle. It is the result of movement of charged ions across the cell membrane *(sarcolemma).* All cardiac muscle cells are electrically active; however, the morphology of their action potential depends on their unique characteristics. The arrangement and balance of positively and negatively charged ions on both sides of the sarcolemma create a net charge on each side of the membrane. When ready to conduct an impulse, the net charge inside the cell is called the *resting membrane potential* (–90 mV). This is a period of electrical stability also known as *electrical diastole.* The electrical potential at which the cell discharges and conducts an electrical impulse is called the *threshold potential* (–70 mV). Most atrial and ventricular muscle cells (as well as other muscle cells) cannot conduct an impulse without an outside stimulus. That is, when they are at their resting membrane potential, they require an electrical impulse to allow ionic movement to drive the charge inside the cell to threshold. Cardiac pacemaker cells, on the other hand, have a unique characteristic called *automaticity.* Automaticity is the capability of a cell to depolarize spontaneously and propagate an impulse. Although primarily found in the cells of the sinoatrial (sinus or SA) node, atrioventricular (AV) node cells and His-Purkinje cells also possess this characteristic. The SA node and conduction system and the phases of the action potentials of ventricular muscle cells are illustrated in Fig. 2.1.

Action Potential of Ventricular Muscle Cells

Phase 0: Rapid Depolarization

In the normal heart, an electrical impulse is initiated at the SA node and is propagated through the entire muscle via the conduction system. Once it reaches a muscle cell, it causes an influx of sodium (Na^+) that drives the net charge to threshold. Because Na^+ is a positively charged ion, when Na^+ ions move into the cell the net charge inside the cell increases (changes from –90 mV to –70 mV). At threshold, there is a brief (1–2 ms) opening of the Na^+ channels, allowing a further rapid influx of Na^+. The charge inside the cell rapidly increases to between approximately +30 mV and +40 mV. The speed of conduction is directly related to the amount of negativity at activation and the number of Na^+ channels that open. In addition, calcium (Ca^{2+}) channels begin opening in clustered bursts, which allows the influx of Ca^{2+} and also causes the sarcoplasmic reticulum to release Ca^{2+} for muscle contraction.

Phase 1: Early Repolarization

Phase 1 is the beginning of repolarization and is caused chiefly by the closing of inward Na^+ and Ca^{2+} channels. The outward potassium (K^+) channel opens, allowing K^+ to exit the cell. This results in a slight decrease in charge (repolarization) of the cell to approximately +10 mV.

Phase 2: Plateau

During phase 2, inward and outward ion flows are in balance so the charge stays relatively stable. Ca^{2+} and Na^+ continue to flow into the cell while K^+ flows out of the cell. The flow of K^+ builds until the outward flow of K^+ exceeds the inward flow of Na^+ and Ca^{2+}. At this point, contraction ends and repolarization begins. During phase 2, the cell is refractory or unable to respond to another stimulus. The property of cardiac *refractoriness* prevents tetany. The plateau phase does not occur in skeletal muscle action potentials.

Phase 3: Rapid Repolarization

Slow Ca^{2+} channels close while outward movement of K^+ continues, making the inside charge increasingly negative. Na^+ channels are readied to respond to another impulse.

Phase 4: Electrical Diastole

During phase 4, muscle cells are permeable to K^+. The K^+ rectifier current returns K^+ and Na^+ to normal proportions and the charge reaches its resting potential, ready to receive another impulse. Outward K^+ movement and inward Na^+ movement continue during phase 4. If not depolarized by an impulse from a higher pacemaker, a muscle cell could conceivably reach threshold potential through this influx of Na^+ ions.

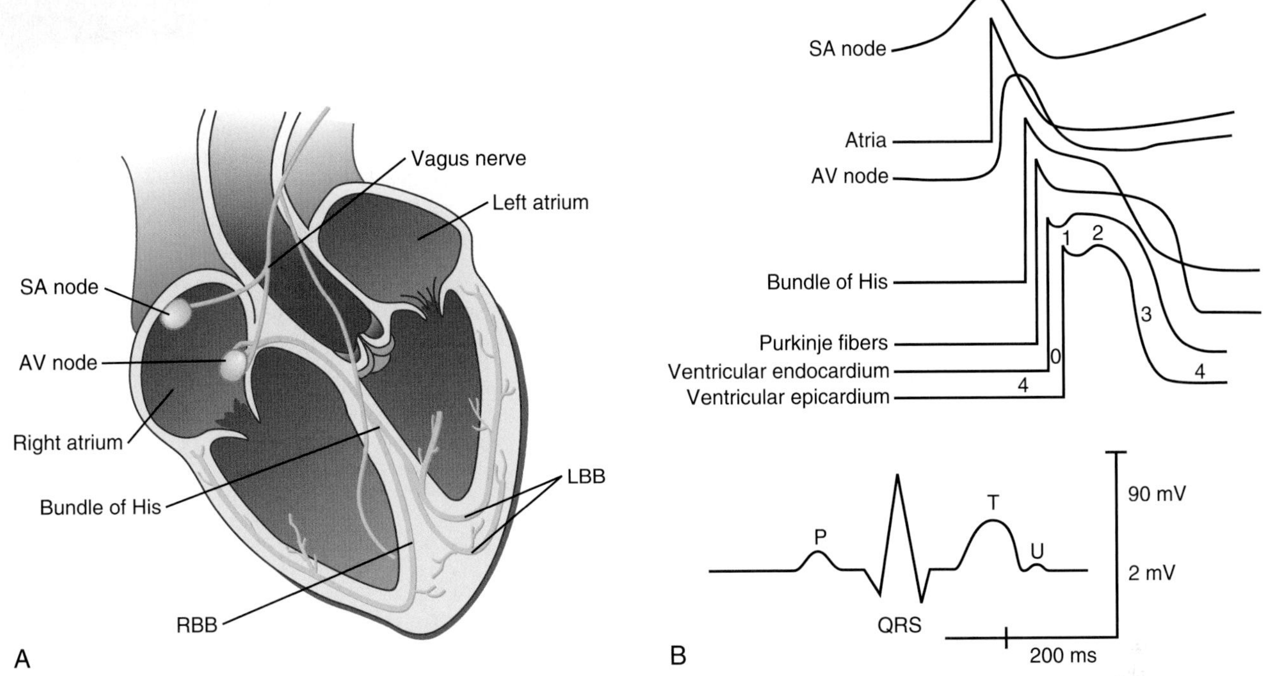

FIG. 2.1 **A,** Sinus node and conduction system. **B,** Action potentials. *AV,* Atrioventricular; *LBB,* left bundle branch; *RBB,* right bundle branch; *SA,* sinoatrial (sinus).

Action Potential of Pacemaker Cells

The action potential in the SA node, AV node, and His-Purkinje cells differs in many respects from the action potential of a working myocardial cell. The action potential here begins in phase 4.

Phase 4: Slow Diastolic Depolarization

As noted earlier, pacemaker cells have the property of automaticity, meaning that they do not require an outside stimulus to bring them to threshold potential. At the end of phase 3, the charge inside the pacemaker cell reaches its most negative *(maximum diastolic potential).* At this point, outward K^+ flow slows and there is a slow inward flux of Na^+ and then Ca^{2+}. This inward flow slowly raises the charge inside the cell to threshold potential, which initiates phase 0. The slope of phase 4 is steeper in pacemaker cells, meaning that threshold potential is reached sooner here than in other cells. Under normal conditions, the SA node controls the heart rate because the SA node cells generate threshold potential faster than other conductive tissue.

Phases 0–4

In pacemaker cells, phase 0 is the result of Ca^{2+} influx rather than Na^+, and the change in potential between phase 4 and phase 0 is not as abrupt. The upstroke is shorter and not as steep. phase 1 is absent in pacemaker cells. After maximum positive voltage is reached, a slow outward K^+ current begins repolarization. Phases 2 and 3 are present but brief. The rate of phase 3 repolarization is slower and results in a maximum diastolic potential that is less negative than in muscle cells. At the maximum diastolic potential, phase 4 begins.

Ionic Channels and Pumps

Ions move across the cell membrane according to the permeability to that ion, as well as the electrical and diffusion forces on that ion. Equilibrium is a state of no net movement of ions, although transmembrane movement can still occur. The electrical difference between areas, such as the inside and outside of a cell membrane, is called the *potential difference.* This difference creates an electromotive force that is measured in volts (1 mV = 0.001 V).

The movement of ions is closely regulated via permeability of the cell membrane and molecular pumps. Ion movement is either passive or active. Cell membranes are able to control which ions move across the membrane. This is called *selective permeability* and is the result of protein pores in the membrane, or channels. The channels are composed of several proteins encoded by specific genes. One membrane protein traverses the membrane while others act as gates. These channels open and close like gates via electrical or chemical signals. When a channel is open, specific ions are permitted to cross according to the electrical and concentration gradients. When the channel closes, movement of those ions stops. Effective cardiac conduction depends on the correct timing, sequence, and voltage activation of the membrane channels. A more detailed description of ion movement and channels may be found in other sources.[48,68,101]

Ionic Channels

I_{Na} is the fast inward Na^+ channel responsible for phase 0. It opens at threshold potential (–70 mV) for 1–2 ms. There are many Na^+ channels that open sequentially, producing a large, rapid influx of Na^+. The more Na^+ channels open, the faster the speed of conduction. The Na^+ channel is inactivated by the positive voltage caused by the Na^+ influx. It cannot be reactivated again until the cell repolarizes. I_{Na} channels are not present in pacemaker cells of the SA and AV nodes.

I_{Ca} produces a slow influx of Ca^{2+} during slow diastolic depolarization and during Phase 2 plateau. The inward Ca^{2+} channel also activates Ca^{2+} release from the sarcoplasmic reticulum. I_{Ca} opens at positive potentials and inactivates at negative potentials.

K^+ currents generally produce the opposite effects of Na^+ channels. The timing of activation and inactivation directly influences the length of the refractory period. Opening early predisposes the cell to premature excitation while late activation shortens repolarization. The outward K^+ current increases with time during phase 2 until it is inactivated. This terminates the plateau phase. Furthermore, outward K^+ channels can be activated by acetylcholine. This outward K^+ current creates a more negative maximum diastolic potential than would be present without the influence of acetylcholine. From this voltage it takes longer to reach threshold potential, which accounts for the parasympathetic effect of slowing the heart rate. Some K^+ channels are sensitive to adenosine triphosphate (ATP) and are activated by ischemia, anoxia, or contractile failure.

hERG1 is a gene encoding a protein that forms *hERG1* channels that conduct the potassium channel (I_{Kr}). As such the *hERG1* gene is a major determinant of repolarization. Mutations of this gene delay repolarization and are a major cause of inherited long QT syndromes. Medications that alter the *hERG1* channel may cause dysrhythmias.[85,86] The pacemaker current (I_f) is actually a combination of several effects. This current is present in SA and AV node cells and in Purkinje fibers. I_f activates at the end of phase 3 at maximum negative diastolic potential and produces a net inward positive current via movement of Na^+ and K^+. Inward Na^+ and Ca^{2+} currents activating at specific voltages are also involved.

Ionic Pumps

While ion movement through channels is passive, not requiring energy, pumps move ions against electrochemical gradients and are dependent upon the presence of ATP. Two pumps have direct effects on the action potential.

Na^+-K^+-ATPase pump. The Na^+-K^+-ATPase pump moves Na^+ ions outside of the cell in exchange for K^+ ions moved into the cell at a ratio of 3:2. This pump maintains the negative resting potential by returning the concentrations of Na^+ and K^+ to the resting state. The pump continually moves K^+ to the inside of the cell, creating a large K^+ gradient, and removes the Na^+ that enters during depolarization, thus ensuring that the cell is excitable.[46]

Sodium-calcium exchange pump. The purpose of the Na^+-Ca^{2+} exchange pump is to remove the free Ca^{2+} transported into the cell to activate contraction. Na^+ is pumped down the concentration gradient, which produces energy to move Ca^{2+} out of the cell against the concentration gradient.

Implications for Patient Care

Classifications and Actions of Antidysrhythmic Agents

The Vaughan Williams classification lists antidysrhythmic agents according to the types of effects (Table 2.1). Table 2.2 lists common antidysrhythmic agents and their points of action.

TABLE 2.1 The Vaughan Williams Classification of Antidysrhythmic Agents

Class	Actions	Examples*
Ia	Moderate fast Na^+ channel blockade Effects significant only at rapid heart rates Decreased conduction velocity Prolonged action potential duration	Disopyramide Procainamide Quinidine
Ib	Mild fast Na^+ channel blockade Decreased action potential duration Effects minimal on normal tissue but significant in depolarized tissue	Lidocaine Mexiletine Phenytoin
Ic	Potent fast Na^+ channel blockade Decreased conduction velocity Prolonged vulnerable period	Flecainide Propafenone
II	Beta receptor blockade Decreased conduction velocity Decreased heart rate Negative inotrope	Atenolol Carvedilol Esmolol Metoprolol Propranolol
III	K^+ channel blockade (I_{Kr}) Prolonged action potential duration	Amiodarone Dofetilide Dronedarone Ibutilide Sotalol
IV	Calcium slow channel blockade Decreased AV conduction	Diltiazem Nifedipine Verapamil

*Adenosine and digitalis are not classified.
Data from References 25, 26, 40, 79, 80, and 83.

Prodysrhythmia

Antidysrhythmic medications affect specific points in the action potential. In addition, antidysrhythmics may be negative inotropes and prodysrhythmic. *Prodysrhythmia* is defined as "the generation of new or worsened arrhythmias with drug therapy."[26] The paradox of most antidysrhythmic agents is that instead of suppressing dysrhythmias, these agents may actually worsen the dysrhythmia or precipitate a new one. Prodysrhythmic effects have been noted for many years; however, it was not until after the publication of the Cardiac Arrhythmia Suppression Trial (CAST), 1989, and CAST-II, 1992, that the lethal consequences of these effects were fully realized and demonstrated. These trials demonstrated that suppression of ventricular premature ectopic beats did not reduce risk of sudden cardiac death and, in fact, increased mortality.[35,50,83] Three common prodysrhythmia syndromes are digitalis toxicity, drug-induced torsade de pointes (TdP), and sodium channel block toxicity.[26] Prodysrhythmic effects are produced through several electrical and chemical mechanisms. The result of these mechanisms is that tissue that can conduct normally is changed into areas of depressed conduction. Such areas are then subject to dysrhythmogenic mechanisms such as triggered activity or reentry. Medications that slow conduction and suppress lethal dysrhythmias are not selective to only ischemic or depressed tissue. Therefore, while eliminating abnormal conduction in abnormal tissue, the same effects can turn normal tissue into areas of slowed conduction capable of sustaining dysrhythmias. Medications that prolong refractory periods and vulnerable periods make the same tissue susceptible to afterdepolarizations or reentry circuits. In addition, acid pH states can change the binding of agents to channels and alter their effects. In particular, binding and dissociation of medications to the Na^+ channel may be involved.[26]

To date, research has not identified reliable clinical predictors of prodysrhythmia. Recently, recognition of the importance of genetic predisposition to this reaction has prompted more research into the pharmacogenomics of dysrhythmias.[26,82,83]

DYSRHYTHMOGENIC MECHANISMS

Dysrhythmias fall into two categories: abnormalities of impulse formation and abnormalities of impulse conduction. Abnormal impulse formation can result from alterations in automaticity or from triggered activity, while abnormal impulse conduction can result from reentry or ischemia.

TABLE 2.2 Effects of Antidysrhythmic Medications

Drug	Class	Effect on Action Potential	Clinical Effects	Usual Dose Range	Indications	Adverse Effects
Adenosine (Adenocard)		Opens ATP-dependent K^+ channel I_{KAdo} Inhibits I_f pacemaker current in SA and AV nodal cells	Slows SA node Shortens atrial action potential Slows heart rate Slows AV conduction	6 mg rapid IV push, followed by 12 mg and 12 mg at 2-min intervals PRN Maximum total dose is 30 mg	PSVT, including accessory pathways and WPW Not effective for atrial fibrillation, flutter, or VT Effective in macro reentry circuits using AV node	Flushing, chest pain, hypotension, headache, dyspnea Long sinus pauses or increased conduction block possible Bronchoconstriction if asthma Effects may be antagonized by methylxanthines such as caffeine and theophylline Not to be used in patients with bronchospastic disease
Amiodarone (Cordarone)	III	Blocks K^+ channels I_{Kr} and I_{Ks} Blocks I_{Na} and I_{Ca} Potent alpha and beta blockade	Prolongs action potential and repolarization Decreases AV conduction velocity	Pulseless VT or VF: 300 mg IV push, 150 mg IV push if needed, follow with infusion Breakthrough VF or VT: 150 mg IV over 10 min Infusion: 1 mg/min for 6 h, then 0.5 mg/min	Useful for reentrant dysrhythmias Treatment and prophylaxis for unstable VT and VF Symptomatic supraventricular tachycardias, including AF	Hypotension, bradycardia, dysrhythmias Photosensitivity Many drug interactions Can increase AV block Liver toxicity Lengthening QT interval
Budiodarone		Multichannel blocker	Prolongs repolarization	Investigational	Conversion of AF to sinus rhythm	Investigational
Diltiazem (Cardizem)	IV	Inhibits slow inward L-type Ca^{2+} channels	Slows AV conduction and prolongs AV node refractory period	0.25 IV mg/kg/actual body weight, given over 2 min Infusion at 5–15 mg/h for 24 h	Atrial fibrillation or flutter, PSVT NOT for tachycardias of WPW	Dizziness, hypotension, edema, AV block Do not use in presence of sick sinus syndrome or high-degree AV block
Disopyramide (Norpace)	Ia	Blocks fast Na^+ channels Blocks K^+ channels Anticholinergic	Decreases excitability Decreases conduction velocity Prolongs QT	150 mg PO every 6 h (immediate release form) or 300 mg PO every 12 h (controlled release form)	Ventricular ectopy, atrial fibrillation and flutter, PAT	Prolonged QT, torsades de pointes, anticholinergic effects, hypotension, HF
Dofetilide (Tikosyn)	III	Blocks K^+ channel I_{Kr}	Prolongs refractory period (QT) atrium > ventricle	Inpatient initiation of therapy 125–500 mcg PO daily with QTc monitoring during first 3 days	Symptomatic atrial fibrillation or flutter	Prolonged QT, AV blocks, torsades de pointes Dose must be adjusted for renal impairment
Dronedarone (Multaq)	III	Blocks K^+ channels Relative of amiodarone without iodine	Prolongs action potential, refractory period and QTc Prolongs AV conduction	Reduce rate of hospitalization in patients with history of paroxysmal or persistent AF who are in sinus rhythm	Atrial fibrillation, ICD patients	Prolonged QT Black box warning: doubles mortality risk in patients with symptomatic HF
Esmolol (Brevibloc)	II	Blocks beta receptors ($beta_1$ > than $beta_2$ activity)	Slows SA rate Slows AV conduction Negative inotrope	Loading: 500 mcg/kg/min IV for 1 min, then 50 mcg/kg/min IV for 4 min Increase infusion by 50 mcg/kg/min up to 200 mcg/kg/min until desired effect May repeat loading dose with each increase PRN	SVT Atrial fibrillation or flutter	Hypotension, dizziness, HF, bradycardia, bronchospasm, nausea

Continued

TABLE 2.2 **Effects of Antidysrhythmic Medications—cont'd**

Drug	Class	Effect on Action Potential	Clinical Effects	Usual Dose Range	Indications	Adverse Effects
Flecainide (Tambocor)	Ic	Blocks fast Na^+ channels	Slows AV conduction Prolongs ventricular action potential and QT Negative inotrope	100 mg PO every 12 h, maximum dose 400–600 mg/day	Life-threatening ventricular dysrhythmias SVT including AVNRT, AVRT, and accessory pathway tachycardias, atrial flutter, and AF Catecholaminergic polymorphic VT	Exacerbation of HF, prolonged QT, visual disturbances, dyspnea
Ibutilide (Corvert)	III	Blocks K^+ channel I_{Kr} Increases inward Na^+ channel	Prolongs action potential Prolongs refractory period and QT Slows conduction velocity in bypass tracts	For patients ≥ 60 kg, 1 mg IV given over 10 min, may repeat dose in 10 min PRN For patients < 60 kg, 0.01 mg/kg given over 10 min	Conversion of new or recent onset AF or atrial flutter to sinus rhythm. AF due to preexcitation	AV blocks, bradycardia, torsades de pointes-must be given in hospital; prolonged QT, ventricular dysrhythmias
Ivabradine (Corlanor)		Blocks I_f channel (pacemaker channel)	Decreases sinus node firing rate	2.5–7.5 mg BID	Inappropriate sinus tachycardia	Bradycardia Sinus arrest AF AV blocks
Lidocaine	Ib	Blocks fast Na^+ channels Increases electrical threshold	Decreases automaticity Local anesthetic	1.0–1.5 mg/kg IV over 2 min, repeat 0.5–0.75 mg/kg every 5–10 min up to total dose of 3 mg/kg Continuous infusion of 1–4 mg/min	Ventricular dysrhythmias Not recommended as first-line agent	Heart blocks, confusion (especially in elderly patients), agitation, anxiety
Metoprolol (Lopressor)	II	Blocks beta receptors ($beta_1$ > $beta_2$ activity)	Slows SA rate Slows AV conduction Negative inotrope	100–450 mg/day IV divided into 2–3 doses	Atrial fibrillation and flutter	Bradycardia, HF, insomnia, impotence, bronchospasm
Mexiletine (Mexitil)	Ib	Blocks fast inward Na^+ channel Slows rate of rise of Phase 0	Decreases refractory period	200–300 mg PO every 8 h, maximum dose 1.2 g/day	Ventricular dysrhythmias, suppression of PVCs May be useful in sodium-channel type long QT syndrome	AV blocks, dizziness, GI distress, nausea/vomiting, tremor Prodysrhythmic agent Give with food Black box warning: restrict to life-threatening ventricular dysrhythmias.
Procainamide (Pronestyl)	Ia	Blocks fast Na^+ channels Blocks K_{Kr} channel	Prolongs refractory period Decreases conduction velocity Negative inotrope Decreases automaticity	15–18 mg/kg IV over 30 min or 100–200 mg IV, repeated every 5 min to total dose of 1 g Follow by infusion of 1–4 mg/min	VT, PVCs, PSVT, AF	Hypotension, prolonged QT, prodysrhythmic agent, lupus-like syndrome, blood dyscrasias, nausea, vomiting, diarrhea, taste disturbances

TABLE 2.2 Effects of Antidysrhythmic Medications—cont'd

Drug	Class	Effect on Action Potential	Clinical Effects	Usual Dose Range	Indications	Adverse Effects
Propafenone (Rythmol)	Ic	Blocks fast inward Na^+ current Mild beta blockade	Slows conduction velocity Prolongs action potential Decreases automaticity	150–300 mg PO every 8 h	Life-threatening ventricular dysrhythmias	Prodysrhythmic agent, HF, AV blocks, syncope, prolonged QT, dizziness, headache, GI complaints Black box warning for patients with AMI within 6 days to 2 years and if structural heart disease
Quinidine (Quinaglute)	Ia	Blocks I_{Na} Blocks I_{Kr} and I_{Ks} channels Has alpha blocking effects	Depresses Phase 0 Decreases excitability Decreases conduction velocity Decreases contractility Prolongs vulnerable period Vagolytic	Depends on formulation Quinidine sulfate 200–400 mg PO every 4–6 h Quinidine gluconate 324–648 mg PO every 8–12 h Quinidine polygalacturonate 275 mg PO every 6–8 h Must adjust doses when switching from one form to another	Prophylaxis after conversion of atrial fibrillation or flutter, PSVT, VT, idiopathic VF, and Brugada syndrome	Prolonged QT, hypotension, syncope, prodysrhythmic agent, Decreases digoxin clearance, dizziness, diarrhea, taste disturbance, nausea, vomiting, anorexia, heartburn, cramping
Ranolazine (Ranexa)		Multichannel blocker, primarily inward sodium current	Increases atrial refractoriness		Antianginal Investigational for prevention of torsades de pointes in long QT syndromes, prevention of atrial fibrillation, and ICD shocks	Dose-related prolonged QTC Dizziness, bradycardia, GI symptoms, headache
Sotalol (Betapace)	II, III	Beta blocker Blocks K^+-I_{Kr} channels	Slows heart rate Decreases AV conduction velocity Increases AV refractory period Prolongs refractory period	80 mg PO 2 times per day, maximum of 240–320 mg/day	AF and atrial flutter, preventing recurrence of atrial tachycardias First-line antidysrhythmic agent for patients with ICDs	Prolonged QT, bradycardia, palpitations, fatigue, dizziness, weakness, respiratory distress Dose must be adjusted for renal impairment
Vanoxerine		Potent hERG blocker Blocks calcium and sodium channels	Prolongs QT	Investigational	Investigational Conversion of recent-onset AF to sinus rhythm	Sinus pause, GI effects
Verapamil (Calan)	IV	Blocks slow Ca^{2+} channels Decreases automaticity	Slows heart rate Slows AV conduction Relaxation of coronary vascular smooth muscle	2.5–5 mg IV over 2 min, followed by 5–10 mg in 15–30 min, maximum total dose of 20 mg	PSVT, atrial fibrillation, flutter, angina Not for use in rhythms with accessory pathway	AV blocks, bradycardia, hypotension, gingival hyperplasia, constipation
Vernakalant		Multichannel blocker Prolongs action potential duration, atrial > ventricle	Suppresses atrial fibrillation	3 mcg/kg IV over 10 min	Atrial fibrillation > 3 days and ≤ 7 days duration	Altered taste, atrial flutter This drug is in use in Europe but is not in development in the United States

AF, Atrial fibrillation; *AMI*, acute myocardial infarction; *ATP*, adenosine triphosphate; *AV*, atrioventricular; *AVNRT*, atrioventricular nodal reentrant tachycardia; *AVRT*, atrioventricular reentrant tachycardia; *BID*, twice per day; *GI*, gastrointestinal; *HF*, heart failure; *ICD*, implantable cardioverter-defibrillator; *IV*, intravenous; K^+, potassium; *Na+*, sodium; *PAT*, paroxysmal atrial tachycardia; *PO*, per os, *PRN*, as needed; *PSVT*, paroxysmal supraventricular tachycardia; *PVC*, premature ventricular contraction; *QTc*, QT interval corrected; *SA*, sinoatrial; *SVT*, supraventricular tachycardia; *VF*, ventricular fibrillation; *VT*, ventricular tachycardia; *WPW*, Wolff-Parkinson-White.

Data from References 26, 55, 65, and 80.

Alterations in Impulse Formation

Altered Automaticity

Enhanced normal automaticity. As discussed, automaticity is the ability of a cardiac cell to depolarize spontaneously and propagate an impulse. Automaticity is due to slow diastolic depolarization during phase 4. In cells other than the SA and AV nodes, it is the result of an inward positive current through the fast Na^+ channel during phase 4. This inward movement of Na^+ stimulates the Na^+-K^+-ATPase pump. Na^+ is rapidly moved out of the cell, which causes a brief hyperpolarization (very negative charge) of the cell. In pacemaker cells, automaticity is the result of an inward Na^+ movement, I_f, and a slow influx of Ca^{2+}. Normal automaticity responds to physiologic need, increasing with increased oxygen demand and decreasing with lower oxygen demand.

All pacemaker cells, such as those in the SA node, AV node, and His-Purkinje system, have automaticity. The SA node has the fastest rate of automaticity and therefore normally controls the heart rate. Pacemaker cells located farther down the conduction system are depolarized by the sinus impulse before they can reach threshold. This is known as *overdrive suppression.* Sites usually suppressed by the SA impulse are known as *subsidiary* or *latent pacemakers.* Fig. 2.2 illustrates the action potential of altered automaticity.

Enhanced normal automaticity is the result of accelerated generation of action potentials by normal pacemaker tissue.[75] The slope of phase 4 becomes steeper, meaning that it takes less time for the cell to reach threshold potential. The action potential produced is otherwise normal. Enhanced normal automaticity can occur when the sinus node rate increases or decreases, by an increase in another pacemaker cell's automatic rate, if the sinus node is unable to generate impulses, or if the sinus impulse is unable to activate the myocardium.[75] A major cause of enhanced normal automaticity is increased sympathetic activity that increases the sinus rate, such as fever, exercise, or anxiety. Other conditions that increase subsidiary pacemaker cell automaticity include sympathomimetic agents, chronic pulmonary disease, coronary artery disease, and hormones such as aldosterone, angiotensin, thyroid hormone, and insulin.[75,94]

Conditions that may depress normal sinus automaticity include increased vagal (parasympathetic) stimulation, drug levels, abnormal electrolyte levels, and disease of the sinus node.[75] In these situations, overdrive suppression of latent pacemakers does not occur, so a subsidiary pacemaker cell reaches threshold potential and usurps control of the heart rate. This can be protective, as happens in escape rhythms.

Rates produced from altered normal automaticity are seldom much higher than 160 beats per minute (bpm) in adults who are not exercising and include inappropriate sinus tachycardia, atrial tachycardias, multifocal atrial tachycardia, junctional tachycardia, and accelerated idioventricular rhythms.[44,45,94]

Abnormal Automaticity

Abnormal automaticity is the accelerated generation of action potentials in abnormal myocardial tissue.[94] In depressed tissue, such as ischemic areas, the resting membrane potential is reduced (it is less negative than normal). The less negative the membrane potential becomes, the fewer fast Na^+ channels are available because they are voltage-dependent. Depressed cells will not have enough Na^+ channels available to create the conditions described to hyperpolarize.[68] In such situations, any atrial or ventricular cell may reach threshold and fire spontaneously via the normally occurring slow calcium influx during phase 4. The action potential produced is abnormal (see Fig. 2.2).

Abnormal automaticity may be caused by anything that makes the inside of the cell more positive or that impairs the Na^+-K^+-ATPase pump, such as decreased permeability to K^+ or increased permeability to Na^+ or Ca^{2+}. Factors that lead to abnormal automaticity include hypoxia, ischemia, infarction, hyperkalemia, hypocalcemia, abnormal myocardial stretch, increased catecholamines, decreased parasympathetic tone, and digitalis. Atrial tachycardias, accelerated idioventricular rhythms, ventricular tachycardia associated with acute myocardial infarction (MI), and junctional tachycardias may all be the result of abnormal automaticity.[68,95] Tachycardias produced by abnormal automaticity typically are faster than those produced by normal automaticity. The less negative the resting potential, the faster the resulting rate. Abnormal automaticity produces rates between 100 and 200 bpm.

Triggered Activity

Triggered activity is a result of *afterdepolarizations.* Afterdepolarizations are fluctuations in the membrane potential that occur in late repolarization or just after repolarization. If these fluctuations reach threshold, a new action potential is "triggered."

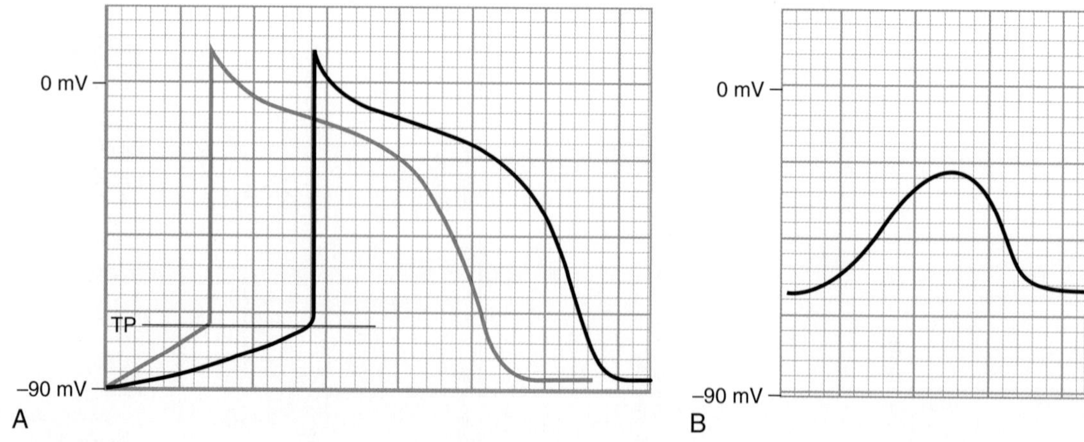

FIG. 2.2 Two types of altered automaticity. **A,** Enhanced normal automaticity (caused by catecholamines) occurs in pacemaker cells such as His-Purkinje cells. Note that the phase 4 slope is steeper in enhanced automaticity. **B,** Abnormal automaticity resulting from ischemia or injury may occur anywhere in the heart. The membrane potential is only –60 mV. *TP,* Threshold potential.

Early afterdepolarizations. Early afterdepolarizations (EAD) occur during phase 3 repolarization and result from a change in the inward positive current, probably because of activation of one type of slow Ca^{2+} channel. If an EAD reaches threshold, it causes a new upstroke depolarization and an early beat. EAD differs from abnormal automaticity in that it is dependent on (triggered by) the previous action potential (Fig. 2.3). EAD activity is associated with long QT intervals, bradycardia, sinus pauses, or anything that prolongs repolarization. Such conditions include hypoxia, acidosis, hypokalemia, hypomagnesemia, hypothermia, hypercapnia, and increased catecholamines. TdP and reperfusion dysrhythmias are the result of EAD activity.

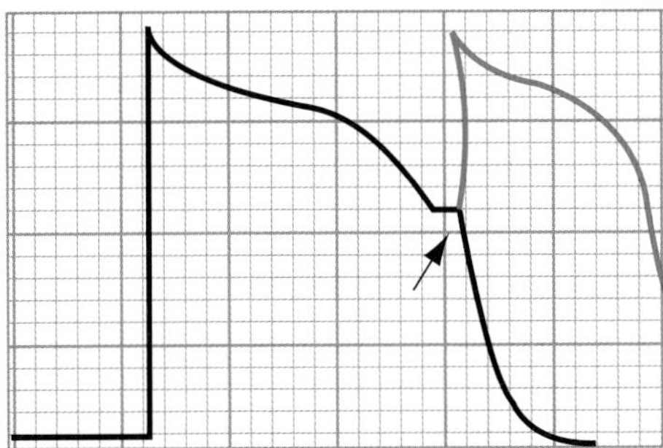

FIG. 2.3 Early afterdepolarization distorts the action potential during phase 3, reaches the threshold potential, and produces a triggered beat.

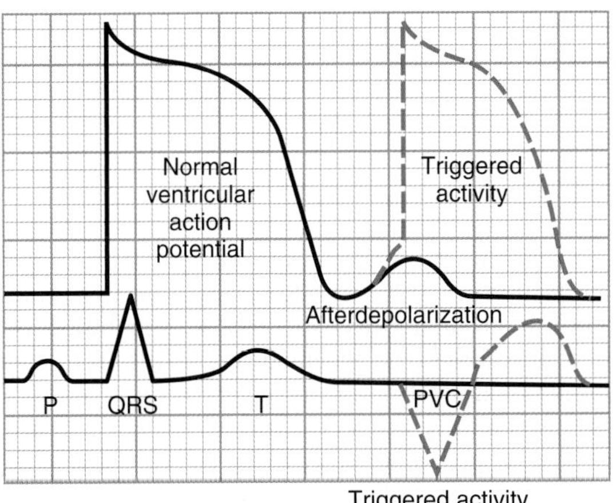

FIG. 2.4 Delayed afterdepolarization shown following the action potential. When the threshold potential is reached, a triggered beat is produced. *PVC,* Premature ventricular contraction.

Delayed afterdepolarizations. Delayed afterdepolarizations (DADs) are fluctuations in the membrane potential that occur after complete repolarization. Again, should this activity reach threshold, another action potential will be triggered (Fig. 2.4). Increased intracellular calcium levels predispose to DADs. Fast heart rates, hypercalcemia, digitalis toxicity, and increased catecholamines can result in DADs.

Alterations in Impulse Conduction

Reentry

Reentry means that an impulse repeatedly depolarizes the same area of tissue (Fig. 2.5). Several conditions are required for reentry to occur: an area with unidirectional conduction block, an area of delayed conduction, and an area of unexcitable tissue. Essentially, the impulse travels down one branch of tissue while being blocked in another branch. Tissue beyond the area of unidirectional block is not depolarized, which allows the impulse to activate that tissue from the opposite direction and conduct slowly through it. By the time the impulse reaches the previously depolarized area, the tissue has repolarized, which allows the original impulse to reenter and stimulate it again. As long as the refractory period is short enough and the conduction is slow enough to allow the depolarized area to recover, the impulse can continue to traverse the circuit. If the refractory period lengthens or the conduction velocity increases, the impulse will reach refractory tissue and die out. *Microreentry* refers to a reentry circuit that is too small for its activation to be seen on a surface electrocardiogram (ECG). *Macroreentry* is reentry that can be seen on a surface ECG or that encompasses depolarization of an entire chamber.[47,96] Recent research demonstrates that reentry is a three-dimensional phenomenon and can have many patterns of "spread."[37,49,100]

Reentry has been variously termed *circus movement, reciprocal tachycardia, echo beats,* and *reentrant tachycardia.* Many common dysrhythmias may be the result of reentry, including the tachycardia of Wolff-Parkinson-White syndrome, paroxysmal supraventricular tachycardia, scar-related ventricular tachycardia, intraatrial reentrant tachycardia, AV nodal reentrant tachycardia, various types of atrial flutter, atrial fibrillation, and ventricular tachycardia.[47,96]

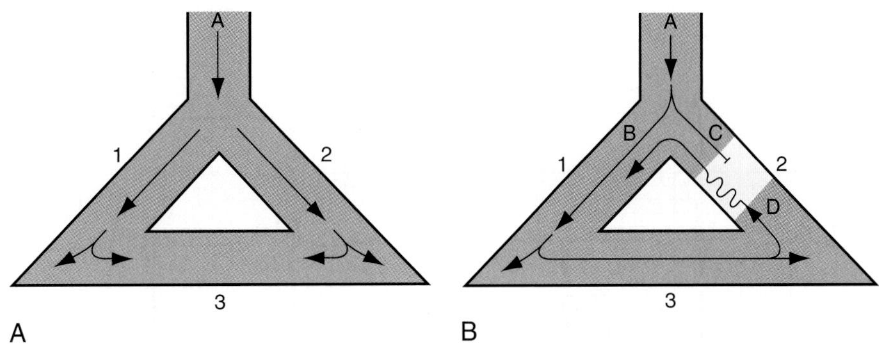

FIG. 2.5 **A,** Normal conduction of an impulse through cardiac muscle with limbs *1* and *2* being depolarized simultaneously. **B,** Shaded area demonstrates unidirectional block. Impulse begins at point *A* and depolarizes limb *1* but is blocked in limb *2* at point *C*. The impulse continues from limb *1* to depolarize limb *3* and enters limb *2* at *D*. At point *D*, the impulse is able to conduct backward through the depressed segment and reenter limb *1* at point *B*.

Ischemia

Cardiac ischemia alters the action potential in several ways. The resting membrane potential becomes less negative; then the upstroke and amplitude of phase 0 decreases, phases 2 and 3 are shortened, and fast Na^+ channels are inactivated. Because of these changes, the cell never reaches the normal resting membrane potential. The result is a slow-response action potential and an area of depressed conduction. Within minutes, cells become unexcitable. Ischemia inactivates the Na^+-K^+ pumps, cell membranes are damaged, and K^+ leaves the cell.

Because sympathetic activity is increased during ischemia, norepinephrine accumulates. During ischemia the effect of norepinephrine is to prolong both the action potential and the vulnerable period. Normally the cardiac muscle contracts in an all-or-nothing manner because the junctions between cells are low resistance and enhance conduction between fibers. During ischemia, "electrical uncoupling" occurs because the junctions between cells become more resistant and do not conduct. The calcium pump is impaired, resulting in an intracellular accumulation of calcium, which further impairs both conduction and contraction. Ischemic tissue may support reentry circuits or become a focus for automaticity, even if it would not normally possess this capability. Conditions that result in hypokalemia, hypomagnesemia, hypocalcemia, hypercalcemia, or ischemia predispose patients to dysrhythmias.

Differentiation among the various mechanisms of dysrhythmias via the surface ECG is difficult. Management depends to a large extent on how well the patient tolerates the tachycardia. Most of the tachycardias resulting from these mechanisms respond to vagal maneuvers, overdrive pacing, medications that block AV conduction, or cardioversion.

SUPRAVENTRICULAR TACHYCARDIAS

Supraventricular tachycardia (SVT) is defined as any tachycardia that originates above the bifurcation of the bundle of His. Atrial tachycardias, atrial flutter, atrial fibrillation, junctional tachycardia, sinus tachycardia, atrioventricular nodal reentry tachycardia (AVNRT), and atrioventricular reciprocating tachycardia (AVRT) can all be termed *SVT*. Most often, SVT has a narrow QRS complex; however, aberrant conduction of a supraventricular rhythm may cause a wide QRS. The term *paroxysmal supraventricular tachycardia* (PSVT) is used when the rhythm begins and ends abruptly.

Inappropriate Sinus Tachycardia

Inappropriate sinus tachycardia is an unusual condition that occurs in persons without underlying heart disease. It is defined as a sinus heart rate greater than 100 bpm with an average of greater than 90 bpm over 24 hours, accompanied by severe palpitations.[51,88] The etiology is not well understood but possible mechanisms include enhanced sinus node automaticity, beta-adrenergic hypersensitivity, decreased parasympathetic activity, or impaired neurohormonal modulation. Treatment involves eliminating other causes of tachycardia and attempting to control the sinus rate with ivabradine (Corlanor) or beta antagonists. Sinus node modulation, ablation, or sympathetic denervation may be used. To date, there is no prospective, randomized, placebo-controlled trial of any intervention that has resulted in improvement in outcomes.[88]

Wolff-Parkinson-White Syndrome

Wolff-Parkinson-White (WPW) syndrome is a specific ECG pattern found in persons with repeated episodes of symptomatic PSVT. These findings indicate ventricular preexcitation and consist of a short PR interval, delta wave, and a regular tachycardia of greater than 200 bpm.[93] Preexcitation is defined as early activation of the ventricles via conduction down an accessory pathway (AP). Many such APs may exist; however, the most common AP location in WPW is an AV bypass tract located in the left ventricular free wall or posteroseptal region. During sinus rhythm the ventricle is activated prematurely via the AP while the impulse is simultaneously conducted down the AV-His-Purkinje system. The AP conduction time is faster than the AV node and because there is no AV delay, like that which occurs in the AV node, the AP impulse reaches the ventricle first. The AP impulse produces a characteristic slurring of the upstroke of the QRS, known as a *delta wave*. The ventricle is then activated by two simultaneous impulses, resulting in a fusion beat. Fig. 2.6 illustrates the characteristic features of WPW. Delta waves are only visible when conduction is occurring over the accessory pathway. WPW is thought to be caused by a genetic defect that leads to abnormal fetal development of the fibrous ring (annulus fibrosus) that keeps the atria and ventricles electrically separate. An accessory pathway is a congenital abnormal connection between the atria and ventricle. A variety of accessory pathways are present during intrauterine life but usually disappear at birth. Any existing AP represents potential for myocardial preexcitation.[93] There is a genetic predisposition to such connections.

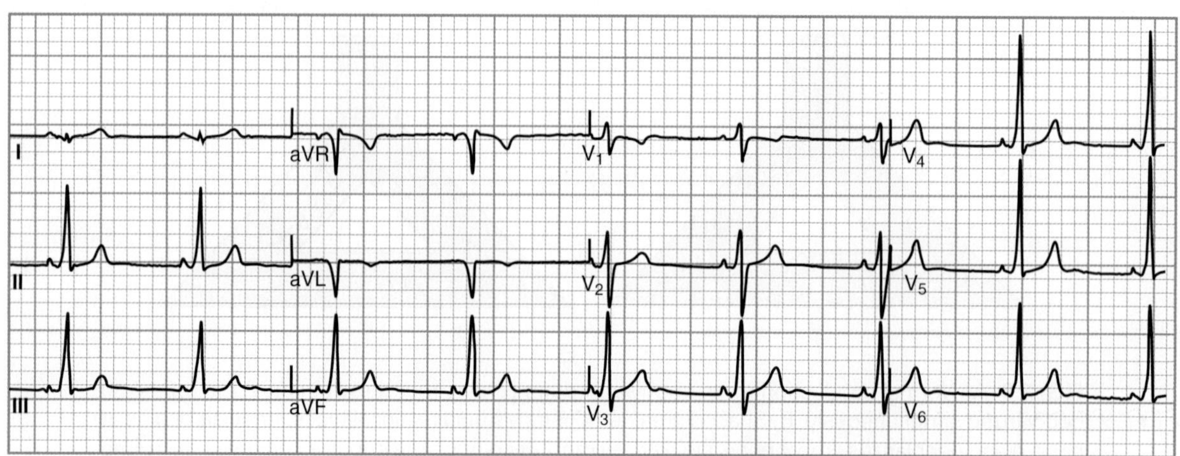

FIG. 2.6 Wolff-Parkinson-White pattern. Note the short PR interval and delta wave in leads II, III, aVF, and V3-V6.

ECG Characteristics

In sinus rhythm of a patient with WPW the PR interval is usually less than 120 ms, and a delta wave is present at the beginning of the QRS, resulting in a QRS slightly broader than normal. The size of the delta wave varies depending on the speed of conduction down the AP and the location of the AP. Because of the abnormality in conduction, abnormal repolarization, represented by inverted T waves, is often present as well. Sinus rhythm and the tachycardias can be present without the characteristic ECG findings when the AP is not used for anterograde conduction. This is called *latent* or *concealed accessory pathway*. Most WPW patients seen clinically have a history of PSVT. WPW tachydysrhythmias are usually rapid and regular.[93]

There are different degrees of preexcitation, depending on the conduction time of the atria, AV node, and the AP. This manifests in differing widths and degrees of visibility of the delta waves. Similarly, depending on the location of the AP, sinus rhythm in WPW may resemble hypertrophy, bundle branch block (BBB), or an acute MI. WPW may be asymptomatic or, rarely, the first symptom may be sudden cardiac death. The most frequent dysrhythmia associated with WPW is orthodromic AV reentrant tachycardia, although atrial fibrillation may be seen as well.[28] Episodes may be so frequent as to be disabling. Severity depends on the duration and rate of the tachycardia.

Atrial flutter and fibrillation that occur in the presence of an AP can result in a ventricular rate as fast as 250–300 bpm and can potentially degenerate into ventricular fibrillation. The precise mechanism for the development of atrial fibrillation in WPW is unknown. Atrial fibrillation with antegrade conduction over an AP manifests as an irregular, rapid, wide-complex tachycardia with varying degrees of preexcitation. These episodes of atrial fibrillation may require intervention to terminate.

Atrioventricular Nodal Reentry Tachycardia

Atrioventricular nodal reentry tachycardia (AVNRT) is a tachycardia resulting from a reentry circuit using two separate pathways into the AV node. Multiple pathways into the AV node are possible, although abnormal. These include the fast and slow pathways, accessory pathways, and others. Any combination of pathways with differing conduction velocities and refractory periods can maintain a reentry circuit. AVNRT tachycardia involves the "fast pathway," which conducts rapidly but has a long refractory period and the "slow pathway," which conducts more slowly but has a shorter refractory period. AVNRT is most commonly initiated by a premature atrial complex that is blocked at the fast pathway and conducted through the AV node via the slow pathway. The delay in conduction through the slow pathway allows the impulse to traverse the AV node through to the ventricle and simultaneously back to the atria retrograde through the fast pathway. The impulse can then reactivate the slow pathway and initiate a tachycardia.[19,56,58] There are two distinguishing ECG features for AVNRT. First, because conduction is delayed in the slow pathway, the interval from the premature P wave to the corresponding R wave is usually greatly prolonged to longer than 300 ms.[58] Additionally, because the atria and ventricles are activated simultaneously, the *retrograde P (P′)* occurs at the end of the QRS complex, which often distorts the final portion and creates a pseudo–right bundle branch block (RBBB) pattern in lead V_1. Best seen as a small, late, positive deflection in V_1 and a small terminal negative component in the inferior leads, this distortion can often be mistaken for part of the QRS (Fig 2.7).[19,58] Fig. 2.8 illustrates the development of AVNRT. Sometimes detection of a P′ wave is recognized only upon careful comparison of the sinus rhythm ECG with the SVT ECG.

ECG Characteristics

Heart rate is 120–220 bpm. Rhythm is most often regular. P′ waves are, if seen, within the terminal portion of the QRS and are negative in inferior leads (leads II, III, and aVF) because of retrograde conduction into the atria. The initiating PR interval is prolonged and the QRS is of normal duration unless aberrant conduction is also present. Often the P′ distorts the terminal portion of the QRS. This resembles a terminal S wave in the inferior leads and a terminal R wave in V_1. AVNRT is benign and paroxysmal and represents approximately two-thirds of cases of PSVT in adults.[19,47,58] It is more common in adult women than in men. AVNRT can be terminated by inducing a temporary block in the AV node through a vagal maneuver or adenosine (Adenocard). Verapamil (Calan) or diltiazem (Cardizem) may be useful if the QRS is narrow. Unstable AVNRT should be treated with adenosine or DC cardioversion.[58,79] Once normal rhythm is restored, a definitive diagnosis can sometimes be made by comparing the 12-lead ECG of the tachycardia to the 12-lead ECG of the patient's normal rhythm. An electrophysiology study is often needed to determine the exact mechanism of the tachycardia. AVNRT may also be termed *AV junctional reciprocating tachycardia* or *reciprocating AV nodal reentrant tachycardia.*

AV Reentrant Tachycardia

AV reentrant tachycardia (AVRT) (or AV reciprocating tachycardia) is a reentry circuit that uses both the normal AV node

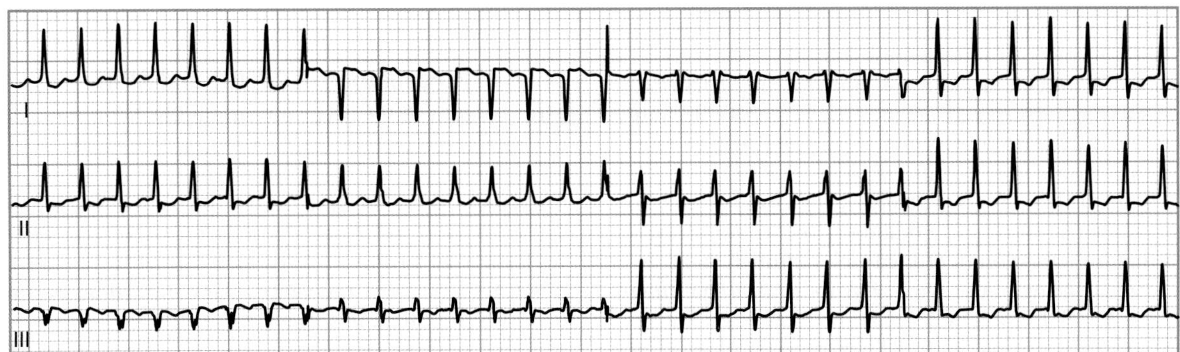

FIG. 2.7 AV nodal reentry tachycardia. Note the pseudo right bundle branch block pattern in V_1 that was not present during normal sinus rhythm, representing the P wave at the end of the QRS complex.

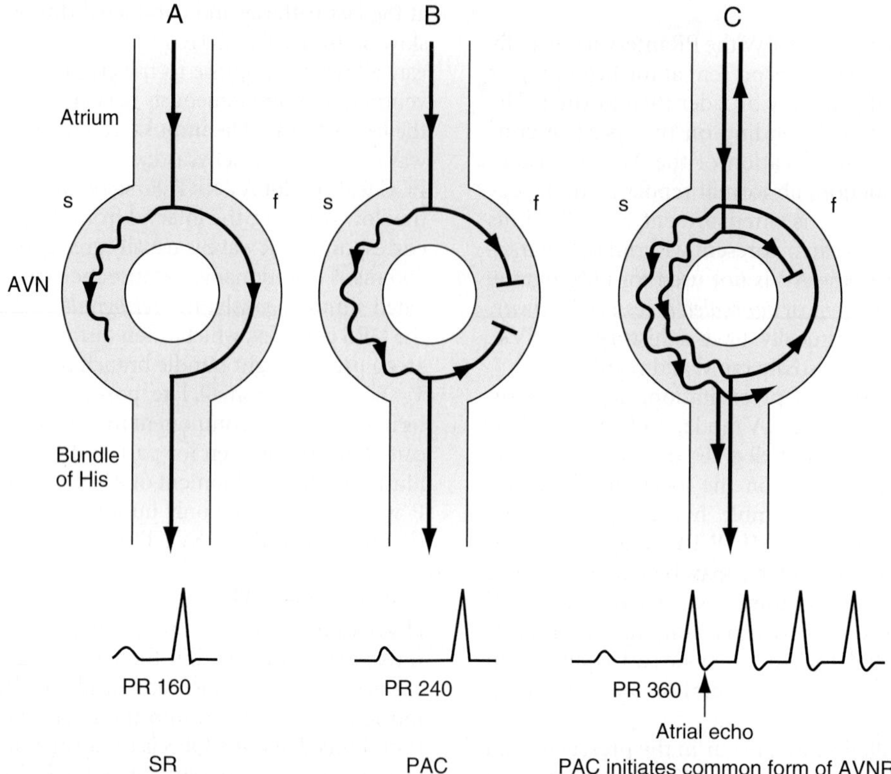

FIG. 2.8 Premature atrial contraction *(PAC)* initiation of AV nodal reentry tachycardia *(AVNRT)*. **A,** Sinus rhythm *(SR)*: atrial impulse reaches the bundle of His via the fast *(f)* pathway, resulting in a normal PR interval. **B,** *PAC* is conducted over a slow *(s)* pathway because of the block in the fast pathway, resulting in the sudden prolongation of the PR interval. **C,** A *PAC* with slower conduction reenters the fast pathway and initiates AV nodal reentry tachycardia. Atrial echo represents the retrograde atrial conduction; also called a *retrograde P wave. AVN,* Atrioventricular node.

pathways and an AP. In orthodromic reciprocating tachycardia (ORT), the impulse is conducted down the AV node with retrograde conduction up the AP resulting in a regular narrow-complex tachycardia. Much less commonly, antegrade conduction occurs down the AP with retrograde conduction through the AV node, resulting in a wide-complex tachycardia (antidromic reciprocating tachycardia).[45,58] ORT AVRT is the most common mechanism for the tachycardias of WPW.[28,47]

In ORT the reentry circuit is usually initiated by a premature atrial contraction (PAC) or premature ventricular contraction (PVC). The premature impulse is blocked by the accessory pathway, but is conducted through the AV node to the ventricles. The accessory pathway is now nonrefractory and the impulse uses it to travel retrograde back to the atria. Thus an orthodromic reentry circuit is formed with the impulse activating the ventricles through normal conduction pathways and traveling backward up the accessory pathway to activate the atria (Fig. 2.9). Because the atria and ventricles are activated in sequence, P′ will be after the QRS, rather than connected to it as in AVNRT. The faster the conduction up the accessory pathway, the closer P′ will be to the QRS. A characteristic ECG finding is *ventricular preexcitation*—premature activation of the ventricles through an accessory pathway seen during sinus rhythm.[28] Another distinguishing factor between AVNRT and AVRT is that the PR interval initiating the tachycardia is normal in AVRT while it is prolonged in AVNRT.[19,28] Fig. 2.9 illustrates an orthodromic AVRT, and Fig. 2.10 shows an antidromic AVRT.

ECG Characteristics

The rate of AVRT is typically 130–250 bpm with a narrow QRS complex and a regular rhythm. The rate can be faster than 200 bpm, and as the rate becomes faster, AV node conduction may vary, producing an irregular rhythm and possible aberrant conduction. The initiating PR interval is normal and P′ is always separate from the QRS. The polarity of P′ waves varies depending on the location of the accessory pathway. The RP′ interval is usually less than half the RR rate of the tachycardia, and there is most often a constant RP′ interval.[28,47] Antidromic AVRT most commonly has a rate of 150–200 bpm, a wide QRS complex with inverted P waves, an RP′ interval that is greater than half the RR interval of the tachycardia, and a constant RP′ interval.[28,44]

Clinical Presentation of AVNRT and AVRT

Most types of PSVT occur intermittently. Symptoms depend on the rate and duration of the rhythm. Patients may experience palpitations, anxiety, angina, syncope, heart failure, or shock. Changes in atrial pressure during the tachycardia are thought to cause release of atrial natriuretic factor (ANF), causing polyuria. A classic sign of PSVT is "cannon" atrial waves in the jugular pulse. Because atrial and ventricular contractions occur simultaneously rather than in sequence, the atria contract against closed tricuspid and mitral valves. This causes a rise in atrial pressure that is reflected back into the central venous circulation and is seen as regular, visible pulsations in the jugular veins.

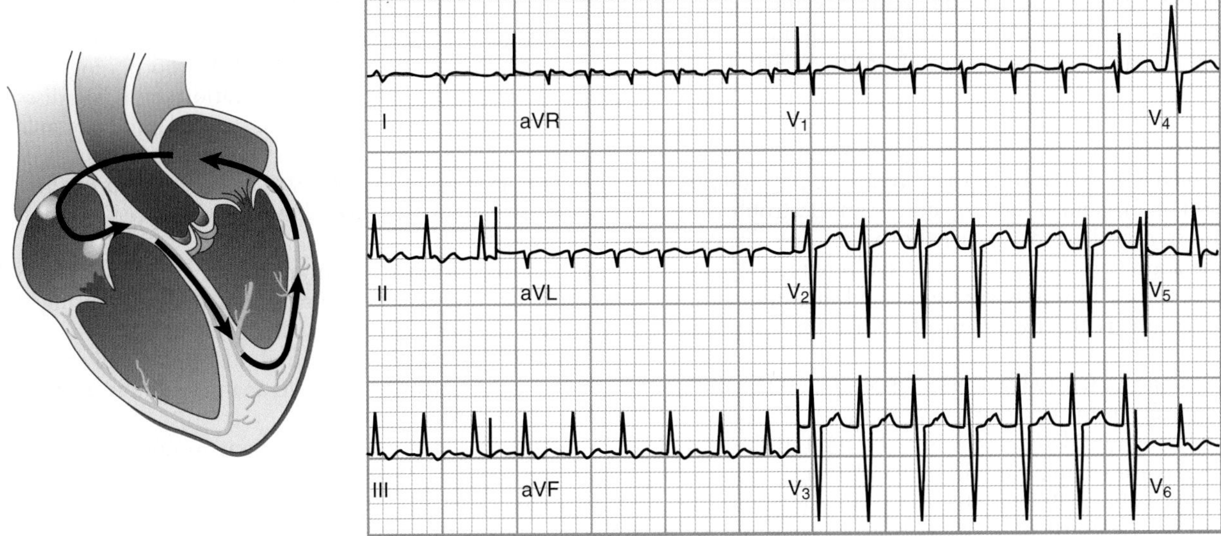

FIG. 2.9 Conduction and ECG in orthodromic AV reentry tachycardia. P waves are visible in the ST segment, especially in V_2 and V_3, and are inverted in leads I, III, and aVF.

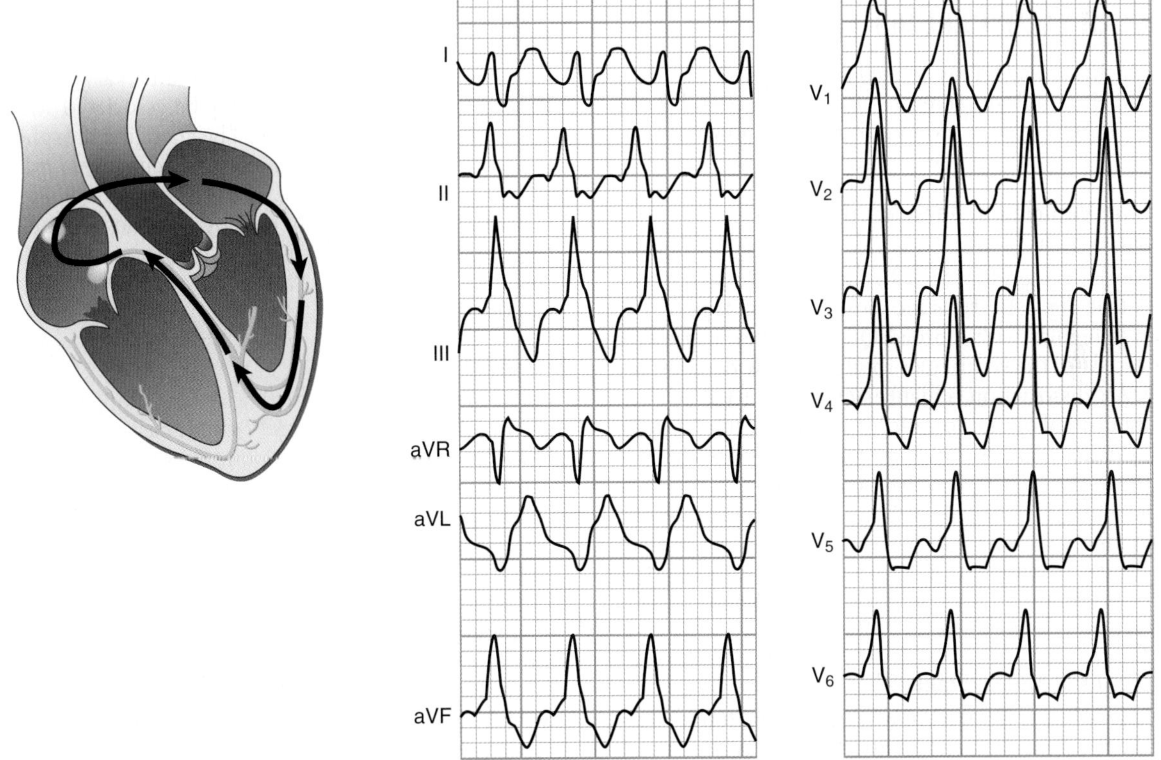

FIG. 2.10 Conduction and ECG in antidromic circus movement tachycardia with AV conduction over a left posterior accessory pathway.

Management of AVNRT and AVRT

Unstable AVNRT or AVRT should be managed with intravenous adenosine and/or DC cardioversion.[28,58,79] Dysrhythmias that use an AP for antegrade conduction (such as atrial fibrillation with rapid ventricular response) should be terminated as soon as possible because they may deteriorate into ventricular fibrillation.

Because the AV node is actively involved in the reentry circuit of AVNRT, blocking the AV node will usually terminate the tachycardia. Acute use of vagal maneuvers is particularly effective for these rhythms. Vagal stimulation causes a release of acetylcholine, which prolongs the refractory period of the AV node, terminating the rhythm. The vagus nerve also affects the sinus node, so a possible adverse effect of vagal stimulation is sinus bradycardia or sinus pauses. Examples of vagal maneuvers that patients can use include coughing, blowing out against a closed glottis, gagging, or squatting. Most patients should be taught several vagal maneuvers so that they are likely to find an effective one when the tachycardia occurs. Carotid sinus massage should be reserved for patients with no symptoms of transient ischemic attacks and no carotid bruits. Eyeball pressure should never be used.[42,58]

If the patient has stable hemodynamics, the recommended sequence of treatment for a narrow QRS complex rhythm is vagal maneuvers, adenosine, then verapamil, or diltiazem. Long-term management often requires an electrophysiology study to identify the exact dysrhythmia and then locate and ablate the source of the tachycardia. Radiofrequency ablation of the accessory pathway is very successful in eliminating the tachycardia and is the treatment of choice for symptomatic WPW.[19]

Antidromic AVRT (wide QRS complex) is often difficult to distinguish from ventricular tachycardia. Procainamide (Pronestyl) or ibutilide (Corvert) may be used in this case. If the rhythm is known to be antidromic AVRT, treatment would be the same as above. Because diltiazem and verapamil may be used to treat atrial fibrillation, WPW must be ruled out before using them. When a patient presents with a very fast, very broad, and irregular tachycardia, the 12-lead ECGs should be carefully checked for the presence of preexcitation.[19,79]

VENTRICULAR TACHYCARDIAS

Ventricular tachycardia (VT) is defined as at least three consecutive ventricular complexes at a rate of faster than 100 bpm.[45] There are two types of VT: monomorphic and polymorphic. TdP is a specific variant of polymorphic VT.

Monomorphic Ventricular Tachycardia

Monomorphic VT arises from one reentrant circuit or pathway in the ventricle; therefore all QRS complexes have the same morphology (see Fig. 2.10). It is the most common type of VT. The rhythm is regular with a broad QRS. P waves, if present, are dissociated from the ventricular rhythm. In a wide-complex tachycardia, AV dissociation is highly suggestive of VT.

The mechanism of monomorphic VT is reentry, altered automaticity of a ventricular fiber, or it may be triggered by delayed afterdepolarizations. Acute MI is the most common precipitant for monomorphic VT. Dilated cardiomyopathy, hypokalemia, hypomagnesemia, hypoxia, and ischemia may all predispose to this dysrhythmia. Sustained monomorphic VT usually requires treatment to prevent hemodynamic compromise and deterioration into ventricular fibrillation (VF).

Alternative Forms of Monomorphic VT

Monomorphic VT may arise from a variety of anatomic locations in either the right or the left ventricle and may occur with or without structural heart disease. Many of these dysrhythmias occur in overtly structurally normal hearts. One form originates in either ventricular outflow tract, most commonly in the right ventricular outflow tract (RVOT VT). The morphology is that of left bundle branch block (LBBB) with an inferior axis. It is thought that this type of VT is the result of a triggered or automatic focus and is characterized by repetitive short bursts of VT. There is an association with caffeine, emotional stress, or exercise. Treatment depends on the severity of symptoms. Most outflow tract VT responds to beta blockers or calcium channel blockers.[91]

Bundle branch reentry tachycardia arises from a reentry circuit in the bundle branches. It is typically fast (200–300 bpm), monomorphic, occurs in the presence of heart disease, and results in sudden cardiac death.[69] Common electrocardiographic characteristics include LBBB morphology, prolonged PR interval, prolonged QRS duration, and AV dissociation. Catheter ablation has successfully treated bundle branch reentry tachycardia or other fascicular tachycardia, although long-term data is lacking. Even after successful ablation of this rhythm, patients with cardiomyopathy are at high risk for sudden cardiac death.[69]

Another form of monomorphic VT is fascicular VT. The most common mechanism is macro reentry using the right or left bundle. This VT usually presents in young adulthood, is more common in males, and does not usually cause sudden cardiac death. Intravenous verapamil will terminate most fascicular VTs.[41]

The significance of these variants is not well understood. It is important to distinguish VT that occurs in the absence of a definable cause (idiopathic) from VT that occurs in patients with dysrhythmogenic right ventricular dysplasia or Brugada syndrome, because these syndromes carry a higher risk of sudden cardiac death. Catheter ablation is rapidly becoming the treatment of choice for alternative forms of monomorphic VT and boasts excellent results.[41]

Polymorphic Ventricular Tachycardia

This type of VT has an irregular and varying morphology. Polymorphic VT (Fig. 2.11) may be associated with a normal QT or prolonged QT interval. The changing morphology is due to differing foci and reentry circuits. Acute myocardial ischemia is the most common cause of polymorphic VT. Fig. 2.12 illustrates polymorphic VT. In patients with no structural heart disease, polymorphic VT strongly suggests an inherited disorder such as long or short QT, Brugada syndrome, or early repolarization syndrome.[73]

Torsades de Pointes

Polymorphic VT associated with a prolonged QT interval is known as *torsades de pointes (TdP)*. It has a continuously varying QRS that appears to rotate around a central line. TdP is pause-dependent (slowing of HR before initiation) and paroxysmal, is associated with a prolonged QT interval, and is commonly drug-induced. There is a genetic component to drug-induced TdP.[36] It may also occur in the setting of electrolyte abnormalities, ischemia, subarachnoid hemorrhage, bradydysrhythmias, or insecticide poisoning.[45] ECG manifestations include a prolonged QT interval, merging of the T and U waves, initiation by an R-on-T PVC with a long coupling interval, and irregular, wide, bizarre QRS complexes with continuously changing morphology that are often notched. It may resemble coarse VF. The short-long-short cycle initiating sequence is classic for TdP. The initiating PVC comes on the T wave of a beat after a long cycle. The varying cycle lengths set up differing refractory periods and predispose to TdP. The rate is usually 200–250 bpm and occurs in paroxysmal, repeating episodes (Fig. 2.13).[36]

TdP is very closely associated with drugs or electrolyte disturbances and it is critical to identify and correct any underlying cause. Diagnosing via the ECG clues is important because it does not respond to the usual VT therapies. Treatment of TdP includes stopping any offending agents and correcting any underlying electrolyte disturbances. Unsynchronized defibrillation is the first intervention for unstable TdP. First-line antidysrhythmic therapy is intravenous magnesium

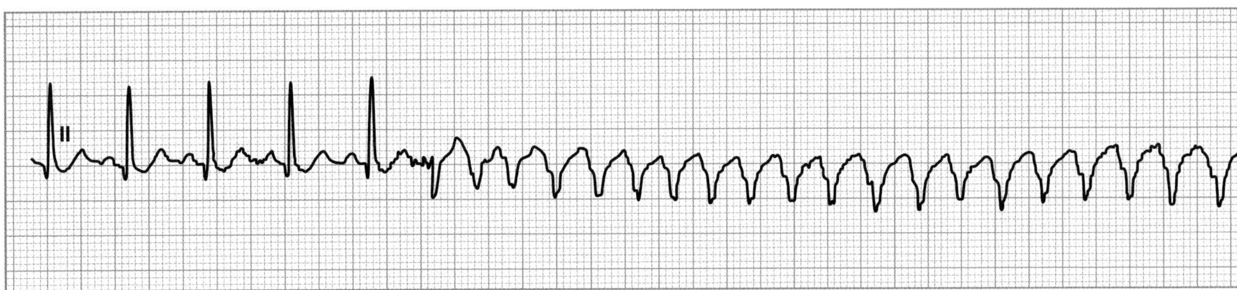

FIG. 2.11 Monomorphic ventricular tachycardia.

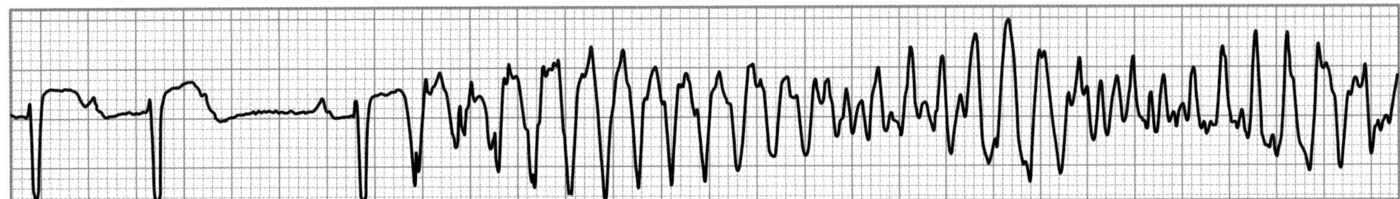

FIG. 2.12 Polymorphic ventricular tachycardia. The QT interval is normal (400 ms).

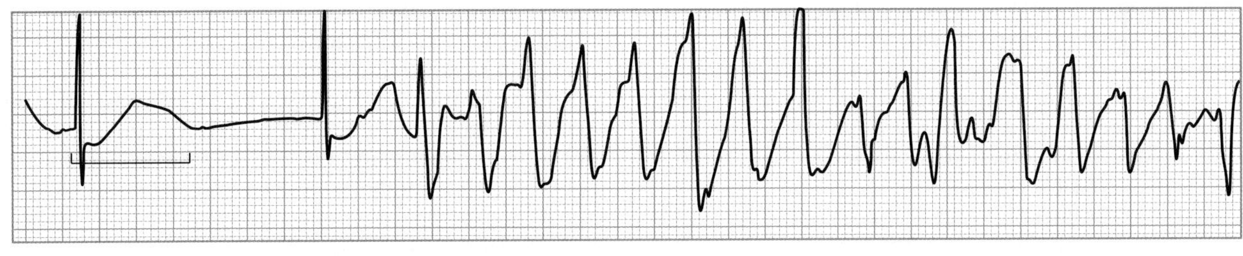

A

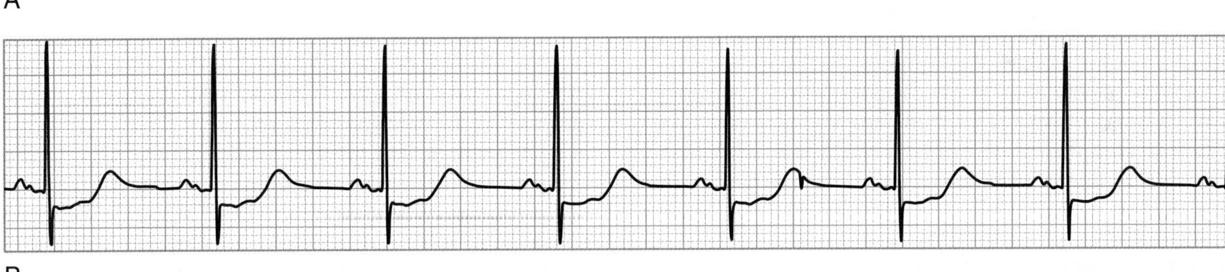

B

FIG. 2.13 A, Torsades de pointes. Note the longer QT interval of 800 ms at the beginning of the strip. B, Same patient in normal sinus rhythm. QT interval is approximately 560 ms.

sulfate. Other therapies include overdrive pacing and intravenous isoproterenol.[9,47]

MANAGEMENT OF VENTRICULAR TACHYCARDIAS

Regardless of the mechanism and origin of the VT, expert consensus documents and best-practice guidelines are available for the management of sustained VT.[4,38,73,78]

For stable sustained monomorphic VT, 2014 guidelines recommend obtaining a 12-lead ECG during the dysrhythmia whenever possible.[72] If there is no evidence of structural heart disease (SHD), further evaluation may be required, including electrophysiology study. Patients with SHD and sustained monomorphic VT (SMVT) should receive an implantable cardioverter-defibrillator (ICD). In addition, management with amiodarone (Cordarone), mexiletine (Mexitil) or sotalol (Betapace), catheter ablation, and/or antitachycardia pacing are recommended for consideration.[73]

Heart Rhythm Society consensus recommends a thorough cardiac evaluation for patients with sustained polymorphic VT or VF.[73] Antidysrhythmics are most commonly used in addition to device therapy rather than as a standalone therapy. Specific agents include quinidine or sodium channel blockers. Specific recommendations for management can be found in the consensus document on management of inherited dysrhythmia syndromes.[78]

VT storm is considered to be three or more separate episodes of sustained VT within 24 hours, with all requiring intervention.[4] Recommendations for VT storm include correcting reversible causes, beta blockers and amiodarone, and catheter ablation.[73,76]

In general, device therapy is becoming the mainstay of treatment for ventricular dysrhythmias. Device therapy is considered after the patient has had a thorough evaluation to determine the cause of the dysrhythmia and correction of reversible causes.

The guidelines for device-based therapy for rhythm abnormalities recommend ICD implantation (usually with antitachycardia pacing capability as well) for survivors of a VF cardiac arrest or unstable VT; patients with SHD and spontaneous sustained VT; and patients with nonsustained VT due to MI, a left ventricular ejection fraction (LVEF) less than 40%, and inducible VF or sustained VT during electrophysiology study.[38,76]

Catheter ablation is an additional viable option for recurrent episodes of VT. Knowledge of this therapy is evolving rapidly. A 2009 consensus document recommends that ablation be used in patients with SHD and symptomatic sustained monomorphic VT that recurs despite device placement and antidysrhythmic medications; control of VT storm that is not due to a reversible cause; patients with ventricular dysrhythmias, which are presumed to cause impaired ventricular function; for bundle branch reentrant or fascicular VT; and for recurrent sustained polymorphic VT for which a trigger point amenable to ablation is suspected.[4] In addition, it is recommended that ablation be considered for patients who have SHD and recurrent episodes of SMVT despite pharmacologic therapy or SMVT due to myocardial infarction with LVEF greater than 30% and expected survival of at least 1 year.[4]

For patients without SHD, ablation should be considered for monomorphic VT that is severely symptomatic or when pharmacologic agents are not a good option, or for VT storm for which an ablatable trigger is suspected. These authors suggest that ablation should not be considered for patients with a ventricular thrombus, asymptomatic nonsustained VT, or for VT due to transient, reversible causes.[4]

The wearable cardioverter-defibrillator (WCD) approved in 2002 is used as temporary prophylaxis for sudden cardiac death in patients who meet criteria for an ICD but must wait due to delays mandated for reimbursement or conditions such as infection when implantation is temporarily not appropriate. A 2010 study by Chung et al. tracked use of the WCD through the manufacturer's registry. This study confirmed a very high rate of patient compliance with the device, a very high first-shock success rate, and low sudden cardiac death (SCD) rates in patients using this device.[20]

DISORDERS OF REPOLARIZATION

The QT Interval

The QT interval represents the time of ventricular depolarization and repolarization, including the refractory period. The QT interval is measured from the time the QRS complex leaves the isoelectric line to the time the T wave returns to the isoelectric line. The most precise method to determine the end of the QT is to draw a tangent line at "the end of the T wave's steepest portion of its terminal point crossing the isoelectric line."[95] Its duration varies with gender, age, autonomic activity, and time of day; and it varies inversely with heart rate. The QRS has a different morphology in each lead; therefore, the QT interval should be measured in multiple limb leads to determine the exact duration.[95]

Because of the variation in QT, it is customary to correct for the heart rate (QTc) to give a more precise measure of refractoriness. Bazett's formula, first introduced in 1920,[95] is the most commonly used formula for this purpose:

$$\text{QTc} = \text{QT (ms)} \div \sqrt{\text{preceding RR interval (ms)}}$$

There is considerable variation in the length of the QT interval in individuals with and without SHD. An interval of 460 ms or greater is generally considered abnormal, although the exact limits of normal remain unknown. Intervals of greater than 500 to 550 ms predispose a patient to malignant dysrhythmias.[95] A long-standing undocumented rule-of-thumb has been commonly used to evaluate the QT interval. This rule states that the QT interval should be no longer than half the preceding RR interval and applies to heart rates of 60 to 100 bpm. The rule was first described by Marriott.[53,68]

Long QT Syndrome

Long QT syndrome (LQTS) is divided into two types: acquired and congenital. Acquired or iatrogenic LQTS is more common and may be caused by any factor that prolongs the QT interval, such as bradycardia, hypomagnesemia, hypokalemia, heart failure, cardiac hypertrophy, hypocalcemia, thyroid disorders, liver disease, renal disease, and subarachnoid hemorrhage. It may be induced by drugs such as Class Ia and III antidysrhythmics, antibiotics, psychotropic drugs, antihistamines, and many others. Box 2.1 lists selected drugs that can prolong the QT interval.

Congenital LQT syndromes are the result of a variety of genetic disorders of ion channels, specifically the I_K and I_{Ks} channels that are responsible for repolarization in phase 3.[8,87] These types of disorders cause bradycardia, prolonged refractory periods, and abnormal T-U waves, which predispose the patient to reentry and triggered activity. Because of variation in penetration of the genetic mutations, the characteristic ECG manifestations may appear intermittently on the same patient's ECGs.[8,87]

Prolonged repolarization equals prolonged refractoriness. Repolarization rate is related to heart rate, and sets up the refractory period for the next beat. A long beat-to-beat interval results in the next beat having a longer refractory time. The repolarization rate normally varies somewhat from cell to cell. Prolonged repolarization increases the disparity of refractoriness within the ventricular muscle cells. This is called *dispersion of repolarization.* The greater the disparity of refractoriness, the more dysrhythmogenic the situation.[68] Thus increased disparity in refractory times among ventricular cells is one adverse consequence of prolonged refractory periods, represented on the ECG by a prolonged QT interval. The second consequence of prolonged refractory periods is the potential for early afterdepolarizations. EADs occurring during the vulnerable period can result in triggered activity and reentrant tachycardias. It is the combination of EADs and dispersion of refractoriness that is dysrhythmogenic.

Clinical Significance

Individuals with LQTS are susceptible to TdP, VF, and sudden cardiac death (SCD), which in some patients is the first symptom.[24,87] Known risk factors include postcardiopulmonary resuscitation, spontaneous TdP, QTc greater than 500 ms, and syncope. A family history of sudden, unexplained death should raise the index of suspicion. Any patient presenting with LQTS, and their family members, should be referred for genetic testing.[8,87] It is important to teach patients with known LQTS about risk factors, potential drug interactions, and symptoms of tachycardia.

Intravenous haloperidol (Haldol) is increasingly used to manage acute confusion in acutely and critically ill patients. Intravenous haloperidol has been associated with prolongation of the QT interval and TdP. Haloperidol blocks the K^+ channel, I_K, and therefore prolongs repolarization and QT. This

BOX 2.1 Selected Drugs That Prolong the QT Interval

Acrivastine	Diphenhydramine	Moricizine
Almokalant	Disopyramide	*N*-Acetylprocainamide
Amantadine	Dofetilide	Nortriptyline
Amiodarone	Doxepin	Papaverine, intracoronary
Amitriptyline	Droperidol	Pentamidine
Amoxapine	Erythromycin	Phenothiazines
Ampicillin	Flecainide	Procainamide
Aprindine	Fludrocortisone	Prochlorperazine
Astemizole	Fluoroquinolones	Propafenone
Azimilide	Fluphenazine	Protriptyline
Bepridil	Haloperidol	Quetiapine
Chloral hydrate	Hydroxyzine	Quinidine
Chloroquine	Ibutilide	Quinine
Chlorpromazine	Imidazole	Risperidone
Cisapride	Imipramine	Sotalol
Citalopram	Ipecac	Tamoxifen
Clemastine	Itraconazole	Terfenadine
Clomipramine	Ketoconazole	Thioridazine
Cocaine	Lithium	Thiothixene
Co-trimoxazole	Loratadine	Trifluoperazine
Desipramine	Milrinone	Trimethoprim sulfamethoxazole

From Reference 23.

effect is dose-related.[24,97] The incidence of TdP in patients who receive intravenous haloperidol is greater in those who have a prolonged QT interval than in those patients who do not. QT dispersion is increased in patients who develop TdP as well. The new generation antipsychotic drugs, such as ziprasidone (Geodon), risperidone (Risperdal), olanzapine (Zyprexa), and quetiapine (Seroquel), may also cause QT prolongation. Several studies of first- and second-generation antipsychotic medications have reported an increased risk of SCD and ventricular dysrhythmias (VD) with the use of these drugs, although not necessarily associated with a prolonged QT. Atypical antipsychotics may have a more favorable safety profile than traditional agents. These drugs should be used with caution in patients with LQTS and the QT monitored carefully.[59,62,97,98] Patients who receive IV haloperidol should have baseline and daily ECGs for measurement of the QTc. K^+ and magnesium levels should be closely monitored.[98,99] Zareba and Lin[99] recommend categorizing patients on antipsychotics into three groups: those with QTc of 410 ms or less, who are unlikely to develop prodysrhythmia; those with borderline risk at QTc of 420–440 ms; and those with a QTc of 450 ms or greater. Those patients at low risk should have a baseline ECG with further ECGs required only if other QT-prolonging drugs are added. Borderline patients are at low risk, and a regular ECG for monitoring QTc is sufficient. Those with prolonged QTc intervals need regular 12-lead ECGs for monitoring the QTc and close monitoring of serum K^+ and magnesium levels. Because a QTc of greater than 500 ms is associated with the greatest risk of TdP, haloperidol should be discontinued if the QTc reaches 500 ms or if multiple QTc-prolonging drugs are needed.[24,90,97,98,99]

Because so many drugs and medical conditions can affect the QT interval, clinicians must be very alert to possible drug interactions. Of special interest are interactions involving drugs that inhibit the cytochrome P450 system (i.e., diltiazem, erythromycin, fluconazole [Diflucan] and methylprednisolone given concurrently with cisapride [Propulsid] or pimozide [Orap]).[27,30,43,60,63,92] The cytochrome P450 system is an enzymatic drug metabolism system expressed in the liver and in the intestinal endothelium. In this system, drugs are metabolized by binding to receptors for the system enzymes. Drugs may be either inducers or inhibitors of the system. Inducing drugs essentially speed up the metabolism of the drug, which can lead to either a decrease in the drug's effect or an accumulation of metabolites. In contrast, inhibitors slow down the metabolism of the drug, which can lead to toxicity if the drug accumulates.[60] Using drugs that affect the cytochrome P450 system concomitantly can lead to unanticipated effects of the drugs and adverse patient reactions. Many drugs can affect this system and there are many genetic polymorphisms that affect reactions to these agents. Because of this, drugs should be examined carefully for drug interactions and particular care taken with those patients who have known propensity for genetic alterations in drug metabolism or for long QT syndrome.[24,60]

Fruit juices have also been found to interact with drugs through the cytochrome P450 system and through the organic anion-transporting peptides (OATs).[27] Drug interactions with the cytochrome P450 system, OATs, and fruit juices can affect any patient and are highly variable among individuals. Avoiding concomitant administration of drugs that prolong QT intervals, monitoring electrolyte levels, and decreasing dosage in individuals with multiple risk factors are all important for prevention of adverse effects related to the QT interval. More information on these interactions and grapefruit juice interactions, in particular, can be found at http://www.fda.gov/Drugs/DrugSafety.[40]

Treatment

Events that cause a sudden increase in sympathetic activity are likely triggers of dysrhythmias in patients with congenial LQTS. Such events might include exercise, emotion, alarm clocks, or telephones. Beta adrenergic blockade is the first-line therapy for all congenital LQTS, with propranolol (Inderal) and nadolol (Corgard) the most widely used. Cardiac sympathetic denervation has demonstrated significant increases in survival in high-risk patients. An ICD is recommended for patients who have had a documented cardiac arrest. It remains controversial for those without cardiac arrest.[87,89]

Lifestyle counseling should include avoidance of competitive sports, especially swimming, and avoidance of sudden events that increase sympathetic tone, such as exercise, alarm clocks, doorbells, or telephones. Patients should be advised to use potassium supplements when they experience vomiting, diarrhea, or excessive sweating. In addition, an updated list of drugs that prolong the QT interval is maintained at www.crediblemeds.org.[23] Patients should be given this website and the list and advised to discuss it with the provider for any new medications. Gene therapy is still evolving.[87]

Short QT syndrome (SQTS) is a genetic disorder involving potassium and calcium channels. QT intervals tend to be between 330 and 370 ms. Clinical presentation is variable, ranging from no symptoms to atrial fibrillation, and there is a high risk of SCD. Implantation of an ICD is the therapy of choice for symptomatic SQTS. There is limited data on pharmacologic therapies.[87]

Brugada Syndrome

Brugada syndrome is an inherited genetic disorder of the Na^+ channels that leads to shortened repolarization in the right ventricle and VF. First described in 1992, it is diagnosed by a characteristic cluster of ECG signs in otherwise healthy young adults with no SHD.[13] Brugada syndrome leads to a propensity for SCD, which is often the first symptom.[14,89]

In Brugada syndrome, the inward Na^+ current in the right ventricle is reduced, shortening repolarization. This increases the dispersion of refractoriness over the myocardium, which is dysrhythmogenic. The characteristic ECG signs (Fig. 2.14) occur most prominently in V_1 to V_3 and include a coved ST elevation greater than 2 mm, followed by a descending negative T wave in at least one right precordial lead and a normal QT. An RBBB pattern is also common. The ECG signs may be transient and there is an association with increased vagal tone (the "full stomach" test).[14] Certain antidysrhythmic drugs are used to elicit the ECG signs of Brugada syndrome and include flecainide and procainamide.[14,77]

Individuals with Brugada syndrome are typically young patients and are prone to syncope and life-threatening dysrhythmias that appear to be mediated via the vagus nerve. Quinidine (Quinidex) and isoproterenol (Isuprel) may be useful in specific circumstances; however, the only therapy with documented success in prevention of SCD in patients with Brugada syndrome is the ICD.[14,78]

A 2013 consensus statement recommends ICD for Brugada syndrome in patients who are survivors of SCD or have documented spontaneous sustained VT. Other recommendations include avoidance of drugs that induce or aggravate ST elevation, avoidance of excessive alcohol intake, and vigorous treatment of fevers with antipyretics. ICD can be considered in patients with a history of syncope or induced VF, but is not recommended for drug-induced symptoms or only on the basis of a family history of SCD.[78]

Patients with Brugada syndrome should be advised to avoid certain drugs that can precipitate characteristic ECG signs. An updated list of medications is maintained at http://www.brugadadrugs.org.[77]

ATRIAL FIBRILLATION

Electrophysiologic Features

The most common dysrhythmia in the United States is atrial fibrillation (AF) with an estimated 2.7–6.1 million people affected. A primary diagnosis of AF accounts for over 467,000 hospitalizations annually and it is associated with over 99,000 deaths per year. Incidence increases with age. Approximately 8% of Medicare fee-for-service beneficiaries have AF and the incidence is expected to more than double in the next 25 years. It is associated with a fivefold increase in incidence of stroke, a threefold increase in risk of heart failure, and a twofold increase in risk of both dementia and death.[54] It adds approximately

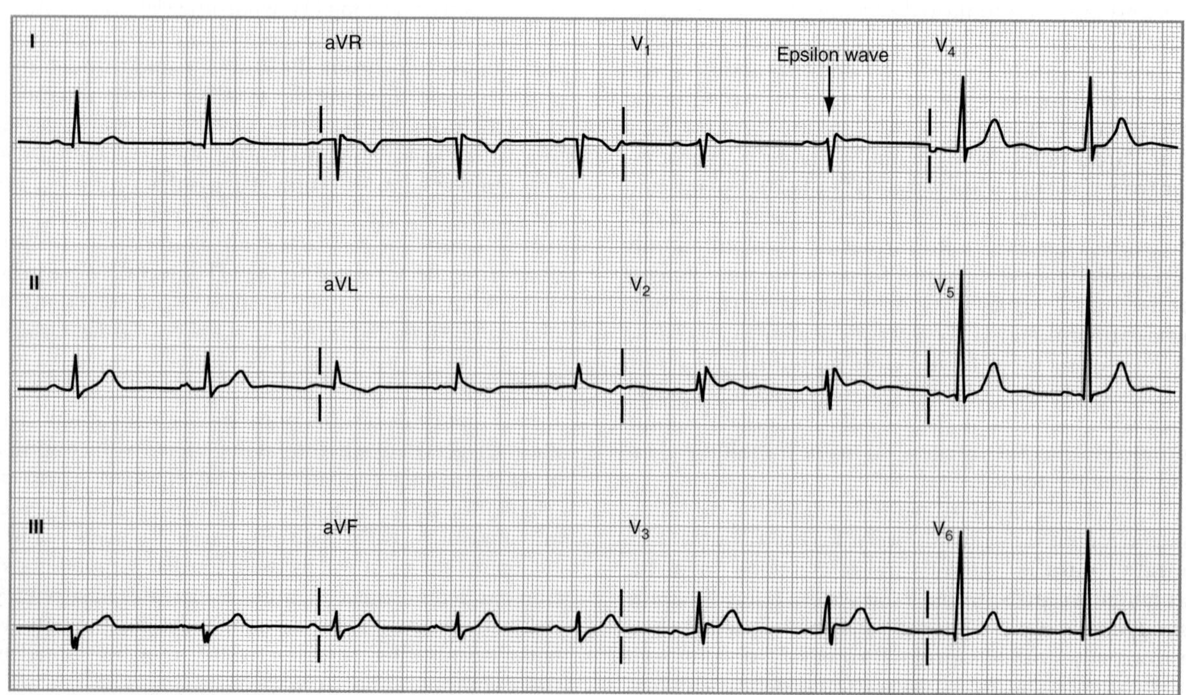

FIG. 2.14 Brugada syndrome. Note the epsilon waves in V_1-V_3 and the absence of S waves in leads I, aVL, and V_6.

$26 billion in healthcare costs each year.[54] AF is a rhythm characterized by rapid and disorganized depolarization in the atria with an irregularly irregular ventricular response. The result is an absence of effective atrial contractions, abnormal heart rates, variable ventricular filling and stroke volumes, sympathetic activation, and stasis of blood in the atria.[54]

The generation of AF is not yet well understood, although knowledge is advancing rapidly. The rhythm requires both a trigger (such as an ectopic foci or reentry wave) and substrate (abnormal atrial tissue capable of sustaining the rhythm).[84] One theory regarding the origin of AF maintains that the driver is often an ectopic focus in specific areas of atrial tissue that trigger the rhythm, such as the tissue around the pulmonary veins, the coronary sinus, or the superior vena cava. The local drivers could be automatic, triggered, or reentry. The focal triggers result in high-frequency three-dimensional rotors that sustain the rhythm.[17] The multiple-wavelet hypothesis states the AF is generated by multiple wandering wavelets that do not reenter their own pathway but can randomly reexcite other pathways that have been previously excited by another wavelet.[84] In either case, multiple, random, three-dimensional reentry circuits (known as *rotors*) seem to be involved.[7,72,84] There is evidence that the presence of AF can alter the atrial electrophysiology and structure in ways that perpetuate AF. This is termed *atrial remodeling*. Atrial remodeling decreases the effective refractory period, shortens the action potential duration, increases the heterogeneity of refractoriness, and alters ion channel expression. In addition, fibrosis develops. Multiple episodes of AF increase both the generation of atrial ectopic foci and create atrial tissue capable of sustaining the rhythm.[7,17] Interventions to prevent remodeling is an area of vigorous research.

The intrinsic cardiac autonomic nervous system (ICANS) is part of the autonomic nervous system and consists of clusters of autonomic cell bodies (ganglia) and axons, which are located on the heart and great vessels. Stimulation of these ganglionic plexi can induce AF, leading to the development of multiple techniques that attempt to ablate these nerve cell bodies.[70]

The American Heart Association (AHA) recommends classifying new AF that is unassociated with a reversible cause (not secondary to cardiac surgery or pericarditis, for example) into one of four types: (1) paroxysmal, in which episodes last 7 days or less with or without intervention; (2) persistent, or continuous AF for at least 7 days; (3) long-standing persistent, in which there is continuous AF for at least 12 months; and (4) permanent. This term is used when the patient and provider jointly decide to make no further attempts to restore or maintain sinus rhythm.[54,70]

Management of Atrial Fibrillation

Goals of management of AF are symptom alleviation and prevention of stroke. A great deal of study has been devoted to the question of whether to restore sinus rhythm (rhythm control) or to control the ventricular response but allow the AF to continue (rate control). Multiple studies have indicated that either therapy is acceptable. Rate control will alleviate many of the hemodynamic symptoms associated with AF and is considered a rate of less than 100 bpm at rest and 90–115 bpm with moderate exercise. Rhythm control has been associated with improvements in ejection fraction, atrial size, and quality of life. It involves cardioversion and antiarrhythmic drugs, and often a nonpharmacologic therapy. It has the advantage of avoiding atrial remodeling. The decision regarding which strategy is appropriate will depend on patient factors, such as age, type of AF, duration, severity of symptoms, and comorbidities.[54,70,84]

Pharmacologic Therapy is the First-line Treatment for Either Management Strategy

Guidelines for the management of AF recommend intravenous beta blockers, nondihydropyridine calcium channel blockers, or amiodarone as a first strategy for rate control for paroxysmal, persistent, or permanent AF in patients without preexcitation in the acute setting. A rate of less than 80 bpm is a reasonable target or less than 110 bpm for asymptomatic patients. Calcium channel blockers should not be used in decompensated heart failure. The 2014 AHA/ACC/HRS guidelines recommend against use of dronedarone (Multaq) for rate control in permanent AF, against the use of AV nodal ablation without a trial of pharmacologic therapy, and against use of digoxin (Lanoxin), calcium channel blockers, and amiodarone for AF with preexcitation.[54]

For rhythm control, guidelines suggest cardioversion to restore sinus rhythm, with attention to the need for anticoagulation. A common practice is to perform a transesophageal echocardiogram to rule out atrial thrombus before performing cardioversion. Cardioversion is also recommended for hemodynamic instability. Flecainide (Tambocor), dofetilide (Tikosyn), propafenone (Rythmol), intravenous ibutilide (Corvert), and amiodarone are useful for pharmacologic conversion to sinus rhythm in the acute setting. Dofetilide should not be initiated outside of the hospital setting.[54,70]

Once in sinus rhythm, amiodarone, dofetilide, dronedarone, flecainide, propafenone, or sotalol are reasonable agents for maintenance of sinus rhythm. The decision for which drug to use depends on analysis of the risk/benefit ratio and on patient characteristics, such as age, presence of SHD, ischemia, ventricular hypertrophy, left ventricular function, and presence of hypertension and/or coronary disease.[54,70] A study published in 2014 indicated that ranolazine (Ranexa) can be effective in suppressing AF in patients with heart failure.[16]

Vanoxerine is a *hERG1* blocker with sodium- and calcium-channel blocking effects. It is investigational in the United States but has shown efficacy in converting recent-onset AF to sinus rhythm with minimal adverse effects and has been used in patients with SHD.[29] Vernakalant is used to convert recent-onset AF and has been used in patients with heart failure. It is reported to be well-tolerated. This drug is in use in Europe but is not in development in the United States.[18,55] Budiodarone is an analog of amiodarone but with a shorter half-life and reported more favorable side-effect profile. It has been used to convert paroxysmal AF to sinus rhythm but is still investigational.[39,100]

Management of Anticoagulation in Atrial Fibrillation

A primary goal of AF therapy is to prevent atrial thrombus and reduce the risk of embolization and stroke. Most AF patients will need long-term anticoagulation. Warfarin is the most common anticoagulant prescribed for this purpose. There are a number of newer anticoagulants in use as well. A more thorough discussion of anticoagulation in AF may be found in other sources.[6,54,64,67]

An estimated 15% of AF patients have left atrial thrombus and 86–90% of these are located in the left atrial appendage (LAA).[6] Eliminating the LAA is a common strategy to prevent thrombus. This may be accomplished via surgery to remove the appendage or various exclusion devices. Long-term safety of the devices is still under study. The 2014 AHA/ACC/HRS guidelines recommend that surgical excision of the LAA be considered in patients undergoing cardiac surgery.[54]

Nonpharmacologic Approaches to Management of Atrial Fibrillation

There are significant disadvantages to pharmacologic options for conversion of AF to sinus rhythm, notably recurrence of AF and side-effect profiles. Because of this, there is growing interest in nonpharmacologic approaches to restoring sinus rhythm. Sinus rhythm offers several advantages, such as symptom alleviation, avoidance of atrial remodeling, and decreased risk of thromboembolism. Nonpharmacologic techniques offer the additional advantage of avoiding drug side-effects.

Surgery for atrial fibrillation. Cox[22] developed the Maze procedure in the 1980s. In this procedure, incisions in the atria isolate parts of the atria and interrupt the reentry circuits. The procedure has evolved dramatically since that time. The surgeon uses various media to create carefully placed lines of block on the epicardial surface of the atria to eradicate the sources of AF, prevent sustained AF, and maintain atrial contraction. In addition the LAA, which is thought to be a major source of emboli, can be closed off or excised using a variety of techniques.[100] Ganglionated plexi can be mapped and ablated. These procedures can now be done through a completely endoscopic procedure or via a median sternotomy.

The first prospective randomized trial to compare catheter and surgical ablation was the FAST trial, reported in 2012. This trial demonstrated significantly higher freedom from AF with surgical ablation than with catheter ablation.[11,100]

Ablative procedures. Catheter ablation for AV evolved from surgical techniques. In this procedure, lines of block are created on the endocardial surface of the atria. A variety of media can be used, including radiofrequency and cryoablation. Catheter ablation is regarded to be more effective for paroxysmal AF than for persistent AF.[17]

Usually catheter and surgical ablation are attempted after a patient has failed at least one trial of an antidysrhythmic mediation. An expert consensus statement from the HRS/EHRA/ECAS released in 2012 recommends catheter ablation for symptomatic refractory paroxysmal AF and persistent AF, with consideration for ablation for long-standing persistent AF. In addition catheter ablation is regarded as reasonable for symptomatic AF prior to initiation of drug therapy.[17]

The same statement recommends surgical ablation for all symptomatic patients who are undergoing cardiac surgery for other indications. Surgical ablation may also be considered for symptomatic patients with paroxysmal, persistent, or long-standing persistent AF who prefer a surgical approach or who have failed one or more catheter ablations.[17,81]

In general, new surgical techniques for treatment of AF have been more successful than catheter ablation. However, there are difficulties in creating transmural lines of ablation via the epicardial technique. Recently, a hybrid approach has been more successful than either approach alone for long-standing persistent AF. This is a staged procedure wherein patients first undergo a thoracoscopic epicardial ablation procedure including pulmonary vein isolation, creation of specific lines of block, ablation of ganglionated plexi, and LAA exclusion when indicated. After recovery from this procedure, the patient undergoes catheter ablation from 4 to 8 weeks later. This approach shows great promise in achieving freedom from AF.[10,15]

Pacing therapies. Pacing in AF has largely been used to maintain acceptable ventricular rates in patients with slow ventricular response. There is substantial evidence that, especially in patients with sinus node dysfunction, physiologic pacing using atrial or dual-chamber pacing modes also decreases the occurrence of AF.[17,57]

The AHA published a *Science Advisory* in 2005 making the following recommendations:[12,21,57]

1. Patents who have a history of AF and who need a pacemaker for bradycardia should receive a physiologic pacemaker (dual-chamber or atrial) rather than a single-chamber ventricular pacemaker.
2. For patients who need a pacemaker for bradycardia and also have AF, there are no consistent data to support alternative single-site atrial pacing, multisite RA pacing, bi-atrial pacing, overdrive pacing, or antitachycardia atrial pacing.
3. Currently, pacing to prevent AF in patients without a bradycardia indication for pacing is not indicated.

HEART RATE VARIABILITY

Measurement

Heart rate variability (HRV) is a measure of the beat-to-beat variability between cardiac cycles in normal sinus rhythm. The sinus node firing rate is based chiefly on the balance of sympathetic or parasympathetic influence on the SA intrinsic rate. Normally, the parasympathetic system has the most influence. Periods of sympathetic predominance occur intermittently over 24 hours; however, sustained sympathetic dominance is abnormal. Normal heart rates vary even at rest, and this variability has been referred to as *respiratory variation.* Conditions that affect the amount of parasympathetic and sympathetic stimulation, such as sleep-wake state, age, gender, body position, activity level, pain, and sleep apnea, influence the normal variability in heart rates.[66]

Clinical Significance

Depressed HRV (less variability than expected) is associated with increased sympathetic activity. To date, research indicates that depressed HRV over 24 hours is an independent predictor of mortality and risk of sustained ventricular tachycardia after MI. Combined with other risk factors, HRV is a powerful predictor of mortality. Chronic activation of the sympathetic system is seen in patients with heart failure, and depressed HRV is associated with worse left ventricular function and peak oxygen consumption, and is an independent predictor of survival in heart failure. It has also been recommended as a method to clearly identify patients who would benefit from ICD implantation by identifying those with left ventricular ejection fraction less than 30% who are at most risk for dsyrhythmias.[61,66]

MONITORING IN CRITICAL CARE

Accurate Lead Placement

Precise placement of the ECG electrodes is critical for accurate rhythm monitoring. Studies indicate that misplacement by as little as one intercostal space can alter the morphology of the QRS enough to change a diagnosis.[31,33]

Skin preparation is important both for accuracy and for prevention of erroneous alarms. Proper skin preparation includes clipping excess hair, washing the site with soap and water, drying vigorously with a dry cloth or gauze, and using a skin-prep paper or sandpaper. Isopropyl alcohol should not be used. Electrodes should be carefully examined for a "use by" date and changed daily.[1,2,3,71,74]

Choosing a Monitoring Lead

Ischemia

Because of the localized nature of ischemia, multiple leads are necessary to monitor for ischemia across a variety of areas. Thus studies have focused on associating coronary arteries with specific leads that are best at detecting ischemia in that area. The monitoring lead should be chosen to correlate with the area at risk. If the patient's particular pattern of ST elevation (ST fingerprint) is known, choose the lead with the highest ST segment elevation. If the footprint is not known, leads III and V_3 are recommended. V_5 can be used to monitor for silent ischemia for non-ACS patients.[1,2,53] Locate the J point and set the monitor to measure the ST segment 60–80 ms after the J point and set the alarm parameter 1–2 mm above and below the patient's baseline.[1] The J point is defined as the point where the QRS and ST segment join.

Reduced-lead configuration methods have been developed that may be used for ischemia monitoring. Technology such as this enables the clinician to obtain 12 ECG leads from a smaller number of electrodes. This creates a practical means of continuously monitoring 12 leads. These systems are considered diagnostically comparable to a standard 12-lead ECG for several purposes. These include analysis of wide-complex tachycardias, acute MI, angioplasty-induced ischemia, transient ischemia, and dysrhythmias.[31,32,34,52]

Dysrhythmia Detection

Lead II is a good diagnostic lead for a variety of atrial dysrhythmias since P waves are easily visible. Leads I, III, and V_1 or V_6 are also very good general monitoring leads. To detect Wellens' syndrome, a marker of critical proximal left anterior descending coronary artery stenosis, V_2 or V_3 should be used. Therefore these leads are also useful for monitoring unstable angina. For wide-complex tachycardia or detecting bundle branch blocks, V_1 should be used, with findings confirmed using V_2 and V_6.[2,31]

QT monitoring

The QT interval is an indication of ventricular repolarization. Lengthening of the QT is considered a marker of increased risk for TdP. There is clinical utility in monitoring the interval since many drugs and patient situations can change the measurement. There is little consensus in the literature about details of QT monitoring. Drew et al. recommend manual measurement of the QT. Because of the limitations with Bazett's formula and the effects of drugs on heart rate, QT measurement should be done before administering an antidysrhythmic agent and every 8 hours thereafter, as well as before and after changes in dosage. The QT should be measured in the same lead over time and the interval documented on a rhythm strip in the patient's record.[31]

Given the variety of patients and conditions that require monitoring, using a standard monitoring lead is illogical. It may be dangerous if incorrect monitoring results in a delay in detection or diagnosis of changes. Choice of a monitoring lead should be based on the patient's clinical condition and the goals of monitoring. More information on clinical monitoring can be found in other sources.[1,2,3,31,53]

CONCLUSION

Diagnosis and management of dysrhythmias require understanding of normal cardiac electrophysiology and dysrhythmogenic mechanisms, and knowledge of pharmacologic effects on cardiac electrophysiology. Given the adverse effects possible if a dysrhythmia is misdiagnosed or missed, and given that the nurse is the constant presence at the bedside, the critical care nurse must have extensive knowledge of all these areas in order to ensure safe passage of dysrhythmia patients through their stay.

REFERENCES

1. AACN. (2009). *Practice alert: ST segment monitoring.* http://www.aacn.org.
2. AACN. (2008). *Practice alert: Dysrhythmia monitoring.* http://www.aacn.org.
3. AACN. (2013). *Practice alert: Alarm management.* http://www.aacn.org.
4. Aliot, E. M., et al. (2009). EHRA/HRS expert consensus on catheter ablation of ventricular arrhythmias. *Heart Rhythm, 6*(6), 886–933.
5. Reference removed in page proof.
6. Armaganijan, L., Chin, A., & Connolly, S. J. (2014). Prevention of stroke in patients with atrial fibrillation. In D. P. Zipes, & J. Jalife (Eds.), *Cardiac electrophysiology: From cell to bedside* (6th ed.). Philadelphia: Saunders.
7. Atienza, F., & Berenfeld, O. (2014). Dominant frequency and the mechanisms of initiation and maintenance of atrial fibrillation. In D. P. Zipes, & J. Jalife (Eds.), *Cardiac electrophysiology: From cell to bedside* (6th ed.). Philadelphia: Saunders.
8. Behare, S. P., Shubkin, C. D., & Weindling, S. N. (2014). Recent advances in the understanding and management of long QT syndrome. *Cur Opin Pediatr, 26*, 727–733.
9. Berul, C. I., et al. (2015). *Acquired long QT syndrome.* http://www.-uptodate.com.
10. Bisleri, G., et al. (2013). Hybrid approach for the treatment of long-standing persistent atrial fibrillation: electrophysiological findings and clinical results. *Eur J Cardiothorac Surg, 44*, 919–923.
11. Boersma, L. V., et al. (2012). Atrial fibrillation catheter ablation versus surgical ablation treatment (FAST): a 2-center randomized clinical trial. *Circulation, 125*, 23–30.
12. Boriani, G., & Padeletti, L. (2015). Management of atrial fibrillation in bradyarrhythmias. *Nature Reviews. Cardiology, 12*(6), 337–349.
13. Brugada, P., & Brugada, J. (1992). Right bundle branch block, persistent ST segment elevation and sudden cardiac death: a distinct clinical and electrocardiographic syndrome. A multicenter report. *J Am Coll Cardiol, 20*, 1391–1396.
14. Brugada, P., Brugada, J., & Roy, D. (2014). Brugada syndrome 1992–2012: twenty years of scientific progress. In D. P. Zipes, & J. Jalife (Eds.), *Cardiac electrophysiology: From cell to bedside* (6th ed.). Philadelphia: Saunders.
15. Bulava, A., et al. (2015). Sequential hybrid procedure for persistent atrial fibrillation. *J Am Heart Assoc, 4*(3), e001754. http://dx.doi.org/10.1161/JAHA.114001754.
16. Burashnikov, A., et al. (2014). Ranolazine effectively suppresses atrial fibrillation in the setting of heart failure. *Circ Heart Fail, 7*, 627–633.
17. Calkins, H., et al. (2012). 2012 HRS/EHRA/ECAS expert consensus statement on catheter and surgical ablation of atrial fibrillation: recommendations for patient selection, procedural techniques, patient management and follow-up, definitions, endpoints, and research trial design. *Heart Rhythm, 9*(4), 632–696.e21.
18. Camm, A. J., et al. (2011). A randomized active-controlled study comparing the efficacy and safety of vernakalant to amiodarone in recent-onset atrial fibrillation. *J Am Coll Cardiol, 57*(3), 313–321.
19. Chugh, A., & Morady, F. (2014). Preexcitation, atrioventricular reentry, and variants. In D. P. Zipes, & J. Jalife (Eds.), *Cardiac electrophysiology: From cell to bedside* (6th ed.). Philadelphia: Saunders.

20. Chung, M. K. (2010). Aggregate national experience with the wearable cardioverter-defibrillator: event rates, compliance, and survival. *J Am Coll Cardiol, 56*, 194–203.
21. Connolly, S. J., et al. (2000). Effects of physiologic pacing versus ventricular pacing on the risk of stroke and death due to cardiovascular causes. *N Engl J Med, 342*, 1385–1391.
22. Cox, D. L. (1991). The surgical treatment of atrial fibrillation. IV. Surgical technique. *J Thorac Cardiovasc Surg, 101*(4), 584–592.
23. *CredibleMeds*. (2015). http://www.crediblemeds.org.
24. Crouch, M. A., et al. (2003). Clinical relevance and management of drug-related QT interval prolongation. *Pharmacotherapy, 23*(7), 881–908.
25. Darbar, D. (2009). Arrhythmia pharmacogenomics: methodological considerations. *Curr Pharm Des, 15*(32), 3734–3741.
26. Darbar, D. (2014). Standard antiarrhythmic drugs. In D. P. Zipes, & J. Jalife (Eds.), *Cardiac electrophysiology: From cell to bedside* (6th ed.). Philadelphia: Saunders.
27. Dolton, M. J., Roufogalils, B. D., & McLachlan, A. J. (2012). Fruit juices as perpetrators of drug interactions: the role of organic anion-transporting polypeptides. *Clin Pharm Ther, 92*(5), 622–630.
28. DiBiase, L. (2014). *Atrioventricular reentrant tachycardia (AVRT) associated with an accessory pathway*. http://www.uptodate.com.
29. Dittrich, H. C., et al. (2015). COR-ART: a multicenter, randomized, double-blind, placebo-controlled dose-ranging study to evaluate single oral doses of vanoxerine for conversion of recent-onset atrial fibrillation for flutter to normal sinus rhythm. *Heart Rhythm, 12*(6), 1105–1112.
30. Dresser, G. K., et al. (2000). Pharmacokinetic-pharmacodynamic consequences and clinical relevance of cytochrome P450 3A4 inhibition. *Clin Pharmacokinet, 38*, 41–57.
31. Drew, B. J., et al. (2005). Practice standards for electrocardiographic monitoring in hospital settings. An American Heart Association scientific statement from the councils on cardiovascular nursing, clinical cardiology, and cardiovascular disease in the young: endorsed by the International Society of Computerized Electrocardiology and the American Association of Critical-Care Nurses. *J Cardiovascul Nurs, 20*(2), 76–106.
32. Drew, B. J., et al. (2002). Comparison of a new reduced lead set ECG with the standard ECG for diagnosing cardiac arrhythmias and myocardial ischemia. *Journal of Electrocardiology, 35*(Suppl.), 13–21.
33. Drew, B. J. (2002). Celebrating the 100th birthday of the electrocardiogram: lessons learned from research in cardiac monitoring. *American J Crit Care, 11*(4), 378–388.
34. Drew, B. J., et al. (1999). Accuracy of the EASI 12-lead electrocardiogram compared to the standard 12-lead electrocardiogram for diagnosing multiple cardiac abnormalities. *J Electrocardiol, 32*(Suppl.), 38–47.
35. Echt, D. S., et al. (1991). Mortality and morbidity in patients receiving encainide, flecainide or placebo: the cardiac arrhythmia suppression trial. *N Engl J Med, 324*, 781.
36. Eckardt, L., & Breithardt, G. (2014). Drug-induced ventricular tachycardia. In D. P. Zipes, & J. Jalife (Eds.), *Cardiac electrophysiology: From cell to bedside* (6th ed.). Philadelphia: Saunders.
37. Ellenbogen, K. A., & Stambler, B. S. (2014). Atrial tachycardia. In D. P. Zipes, & J. Jalife (Eds.), *Cardiac electrophysiology: From cell to bedside* (6th ed.). Philadelphia: Saunders.
38. Epstein, A. E., et al. (2008). ACC/AHA/HRS 2008 guidelines for device-based therapy of cardiac rhythm abnormalities. *Heart Rhythm, 5*(6), 934–955.
39. Ezekowitz, M. D. (2012). A randomized trial of budiodarone in paroxysmal atrial fibrillation. *J Interv Card Electrophysio, 34*(1), 1–9.
40. *FDA*. (2015). http://www.fda.gov/Drugs/DrugSafety.
41. Frankel, D. S., & Marchlinski, F. E. (2014). Fascicular ventricular arrhythmias. In D. P. Zipes, & J. Jalife (Eds.), *Cardiac electrophysiology: From cell to bedside* (6th ed.). Philadelphia: Saunders.
42. Frisch, D. R., & Zimetbaum, P. J. (2013). *Vagal maneuvers*. http://www.uptodate.com.
43. Garvan, C. K., & Lipsky, J. J. (2000). Drug-grapefruit juice interactions. *Mayo Clin Proc, 75*, 933–942.
44. Gilbert, M., Wagner, G. S., & Strauss, D. G. (2014). Reentrant junctional tachyarrhythmias. In G. S. Wagner, & D. G. Strauss (Eds.), *Marriott's practical electrocardiography* (12th ed.). Philadelphia: Wolters Kluwer.
45. Gilbert, M., Wagner, G. S., & Strauss, D. G. (2014). Reentrant ventricular tachyarrhythmias. In G. S. Wagner, & D. G. Strauss (Eds.), *Marriott's practical electrocardiography* (12th ed.). Philadelphia: Wolters Kluwer.
46. Glitsch, H. G. (2001). Electrophysiology of the sodium-potassium-ATPase in cardiac cells. *Physiol Rev, 81*, 1791–1826.
47. Goldberger, A. L., Goldberger, Z. D., & Shvilkin, A. (Eds.). (2013). *Goldberger's clinical electrocardiography* (8th ed.) Philadelphia: Elsevier.
48. Grant, A. O. (2009). Cardiac ion channels. *Circ Arrhythm Electrophysiol, 2*(2), 185–194.
49. Gray, R. A. (2014). Theory of rotors and arrhythmias. In D. P. Zipes, & J. Jalife (Eds.), *Cardiac electrophysiology: From cell to bedside* (6th ed.). Philadelphia: Saunders.
50. Greene, H. L., et al. (1992). The cardiac arrhythmia suppression trial: first CAST… then CAST II. *J Am Coll Cardiol, 19*(5), 894–898.
51. Homoud, M. K. (2015). *Sinus tachycardia: Evaluation and management*. http://www.uptodate.com.
52. Horacek, B. M., et al. (2000). Diagnostic accuracy of derived versus standard 12-lead electrocardiograms. *J Electrocardiol, 33*(Suppl.), 155–160.
53. Jacobson, C., Marzlin, K., & Webner, C. (2014). *Cardiovascular nursing practice*. Burien, WA: Cardiovascular Nursing Education Associates.
54. January, C. T. (2014). AHA/ACC/HRS guideline for the management of patients with atrial fibrillation. A report of the American College of Cardiology/American Heart Association Task Force on practice guidelines and the Heart Rhythm Society. Developed in collaboration with the Society of Thoracic Surgeons. *Circulation, 3*, e199–e267.
55. Kirchhof, P. (2014). New antiarrhythmic drugs and new concepts for old drugs. In D. P. Zipes, & J. Jalife (Eds.), *Cardiac electrophysiology: From cell to bedside* (6th ed.). Philadelphia: Saunders.
56. Kistler, P. (2014). *Focal atrial tachycardias*. http://www.uptodate.com.
57. Knight, B. P., et al. (2005). Role of permanent pacing to prevent atrial fibrillation: Science advisory from the American Heart Association Council on Clinical Cardiology (Subcommittee on Electrocardiography and Arrhythmias) and the Quality of Care and Outcomes Research Interdisciplinary Working Group, in collaboration with the Heart Rhythm Society. *Circulation, 111*(2), 240–243.
58. Knight, B. P. (2015). *Atrioventricular nodal reentrant tachycardia*. http://www.uptodate.com.
59. Kowey, P. R., & Malik, M. (2007). The QT interval as it relates to the safety of non-cardiac drugs. *Eur Heart J*, (Suppl. 9), G3–G8.
60. Krau, S. D. (2013). Cytochrome p450 part 3: drug interactions, essential concepts and considerations. *Nurs Clin North Am, 48*(4), 697–706.
61. LaRovere, M. T. (2012). Autonomic markers and cardiovascular and arrhythmic events in heart failure patients: still a place in prognostication? Data from the GISSI-HF trial. *Europ J Heart Fail, 14*(12), 1410–1419.
62. Leonard, C. E., et al. (2013). Antipsychotics and the risks of sudden cardiac death and all-cause death: Cohort studies in Medicaid and dually-eligible Medicaid-Medicare beneficiaries of five states. *J Clin Exp Cardiolog, 10* (Suppl. 6), 1–9.
63. Lilja, J. J., et al. (2000). Duration of effect of grapefruit juice on the pharmacokinetics of the CYP3A4 substrate simvastatin. *Clin Pharm Ther, 68*, 384–390.
64. Lip, G. Y. H., & Lane, D. A. (2015). Stroke prevention in atrial fibrillation: a systematic review. *J Am Med Assoc, 313*(19), 1950–1962.
65. Makielski, J. C. (2013). *Myocardial action potential and action of antiarrhythmic drugs*. http://www.uptodate.com.
66. Malik, M., & Schmidt, G. (2014). Autonomic testing and cardiac risk. In D. P. Zipes, & J. Jalife (Eds.), *Cardiac electrophysiology: From cell to bedside* (6th ed.). Philadelphia: Saunders.
67. Manning, W. J., Singer, D. E., & Lip, G. Y. H. (2015). *Atrial fibrillation: Anticoagulant therapy to prevent embolization*.http://www.uptodate.com.
68. Marriott, H. J. L., & Conover, M. B. (1998). Membrane channels; and Arrhythmogenic mechanisms and their modulation. In *Advanced concepts in arrhythmias* (3rd ed.). (Ch. 2 & 5). St. Louis, MO: Mosby.

69. Nogami, A., & Olshansky, B. (2014). Bundle branch reentry tachycardia. In D. P. Zipes, & J. Jalife (Eds.), *Cardiac electrophysiology: From cell to bedside* (6th ed.). Philadelphia: Saunders.
70. Oral, H., & Latchamsetty, R. (2014). Atrial fibrillation: paroxysmal, persistent, and permanent. In D. P. Zipes, & J. Jalife (Eds.), *Cardiac electrophysiology: From cell to bedside* (6th ed.). Philadelphia: Saunders.
71. Oster, C. D. (2005). Proper skin preparation helps ensure ECG trace quality. *3M Medical.* http://multimedia.3m.com/mws/media/358372O/proper-skin-prep-ecg-trace-quality-white-paper.pdf .
72. Pandit, S. V. (2013). Rotors and the dynamics of cardiac fibrillation. *Circ Res, 112*, 849–862.
73. Pedersen, C. T., et al. (2014). EHRA/HRS/APHRS Expert consensus on ventricular arrhythmias. *Heart Rhythm, 11*(10), e166–e196.
74. Philips. (2008). *Improving ECG quality: Application note.* http://www.mysupplies.philips.com/Documents/lit/453564119681.pdf.
75. Podrid, P. J. (2013). *Enhanced cardiac automaticity.* http://www.uptodate.com.
76. Podrid, P. J. (2014). *Approach to diagnosis and treatment of wide QRS complex tachycardia.* http://www.uptodate.com.
77. Postema, P. G., et al. (2009). Drugs and Brugada syndrome patients: review of the literature, recommendations, and an up-to-date website. *Heart Rhythm, 6*(9), 1335–1341.
78. Priori, S. G., et al. (2013). HRS/EHRA/APHRS expert consensus statement on the diagnosis and management of patients with inherited primary arrhythmia syndromes: document endorsed by HRS, EHRA, and APHRS in May 2013 and by ACCF, AHA, PACES, and AEPC in June 2013. *Heart Rhythm, 10*(12), 1932–1963.
79. Prutkin, J. M. (2014). *Overview of the acute management of tachyarrhythmias.* http://www.uptodate.com.
80. *Physicians' Desk Reference.* (2015). http://www.pdr.net.
81. Robertson, J. O., Saint, L. L., & Damiano, R. J. (2014). Surgery for atrial fibrillation and other SVTs. In D. P. Zipes, & J. Jalife (Eds.), *Cardiac electrophysiology: From cell to bedside* (6th ed.). Philadelphia: Saunders.
82. Roden, D. M. (2009). Arrhythmia pharmacogenomics: methodological considerations. *Curr Pharm Des, 15*(32), 3734–3741.
83. Roden, D. M. (2014). Pharmacology and toxicology of Na_V1.5-Class 1 antiarrhythmic drugs. *Card Electrophyisol Clin, 6*, 695–704.
84. Romero, I., et al. (2014). Diagnosis and management of atrial fibrillation: an overview. *Cardiovasc Ther, 32*, 242–252.
85. Sanguinetti, M. C., Tristain-Firouzi, M., & Sachse, F. B. (2014). Structural determinants and biophysical properties of hERG1 channel gating. In D. P. Zipes, & J. Jalife (Eds.), *Cardiac electrophysiology: From cell to bedside* (6th ed.). Philadelphia: Saunders.
86. Sanguinetti, M. (2014). HERG1 channel agonists and cardiac arrhythmia. *Curr Opin Pharmacol, April, 15*, 22–27.
87. Schwartz, P. J., & Crotti, L. (2014). Long and short QT syndromes. In D. P. Zipes, & J. Jalife (Eds.), *Cardiac electrophysiology: From cell to bedside* (6th ed.). Philadelphia: Saunders.
88. Sheldon, R., et al. (2015). Heart rhythm society expert consensus statement on the diagnosis and treatment of postural tachycardia syndrome, inappropriate sinus tachycardia, and vasovagal syncope. *Heart Rhythm, 12*(6), e41–63.
89. Tadros, R., et al. (2015). Pharmacotherapy for inherited arrhythmia syndromes: mechanistic basis, clinical trial evidence and practical application. *Expert Rev Cardiovasc Ther, 13*(7), 769–782.
90. Tisdale, J. E., et al. (2001). The effect of intravenous haloperidol on QT interval dispersion in critically ill patients: comparison with QT interval prolongation for assessment of risk of torsades de pointes. *J Clin Pharmacol, 41*, 1310–1318.
91. Tseng, Z. H., & Gerstenfeld, E. P. (2014). Outflow tract ventricular tachyarrhythmias: mechanisms, clinical features and management. In D. P. Zipes, & J. Jalife (Eds.), *Cardiac electrophysiology: From cell to bedside* (6th ed.). Philadelphia: Saunders.
92. Vieweg, W. V. R. (2003). New generation antipsychotic drugs and QTc interval prolongation. *Prim Care Companion J Clin Psychiatry, 5*(5), 205–215.
93. Wagner, G. S. (2014). Ventricular preexcitation. In G. S. Wagner, & D. G. Strauss (Eds.), *Marriott's practical electrocardiography* (12th ed.). Philadelphia: Wolters Kluwer.
94. Wagner, G. S. (2014). Accelerated automaticity. In G. S. Wagner, & D. G. Strauss (Eds.), *Marriott's practical electrocardiography* (12th ed.). Philadelphia: Wolters Kluwer.
95. Wagner, G. S., et al. (2014). Interpretation of the normal electrocardiogram. In G. S. Wagner, & D. G. Strauss (Eds.), *Marriott's practical electrocardiography* (12th ed.). Philadelphia: Wolters Kluwer.
96. Wagner, G. S., & Strauss, D. G. (Eds.), (2014). Introduction to arrhythmias. In *Marriott's practical electrocardiography* (12th ed.). Philadelphia: Wolters Kluwer.
97. Wu, C. S., Tsai, Y. T., & Tsai, J. J. (2015). Antipsychotic drugs and the risk of ventricular arrhythmia and/or sudden cardiac death: a nation-wide crossover study. *J Am Heart Assoc, 4*(2) e001568. http://dx.doi.org/10.1161/JAHA.114.001568.
98. Yap, Y. G., & Camm, J. (2000). Risk of torsades de pointes with non-cardiac drugs. Doctors need to be aware that many drugs can cause QT prolongation. *Br Med, 320*, 1158–1159.
99. Zareba, W., & Lin, D. A. (2003). Antipsychotic drugs and QT interval prolongation. *Psychiatr Q, 74*(3), 291–306.
100. Zembala, M. O., & Suwalski, P. (2013). Minimally invasive surgery for atrial fibrillation. *J Thorac Dis, 5*, S704–S712.
101. Zimetbaum, P. (2012). Antiarrhythmic drug therapy for atrial fibrillation. *Circulation, 125*(2), 381–389.

3

Acute Coronary Syndromes

Megan Liego

ACUTE CORONARY SYNDROME

Acute coronary syndrome (ACS) is an evolving term, found in the literature as early as 1972.[85] However, terminology is changing as scientific information about ruptured and eroded athermanous plaque from cardiovascular disease (CVD) increases. The extent of CVD in the United States is staggering. Over 85 million, or one in three, Americans have one or more types of CVD leading to ACS. With advances in care for CVD, the death rate from CVD and ACS has declined from 2001 to 2011, but it still remains the leading cause of death in men and women. One in seven Americans die each year from some form of CVD.[65] In 2010, the direct and indirect costs were estimated to be over $320 billion and are expected to triple by 2030.[65] ACS conditions include unstable angina (UA), non-ST segment myocardial infarction (NSTEMI), and ST segment elevation myocardial infarction (STEMI). In the 2014 American College of Cardiology/American Heart Association (ACC/AHA) Clinical Practice Guidelines, UA and NSTEMI are combined into a new category called "non-ST elevation acute coronary syndrome" (NSTE-ACS) to show that both should be treated similarly in diagnosis and treatment. This chapter follows these guidelines and refers to ACS as either NSTE-ACS or STEMI when discussing diagnosis and treatment.[4]

ACS results from a spectrum of events at the cellular level that ultimately leads to ischemia or infarction from a reduction in coronary blood flow to the myocardium both at the microvascular and endovascular levels.[4] ACS is a condition resulting from an imbalance between myocardial oxygen demand and consumption. This imbalance can be the consequence of (1) coronary artery obstruction, (2) increased myocardial demand from a nonobstructive lesion and microvascular disease, (3) acute coronary insufficiency from coronary spasms (Prinzmetal angina), (4) arterial inflammation (arteritis), or (5) noncoronary and multifactorial causes (hypotension, severe anemia, aortic stenosis, Takotsubo cardiomyopathy, severe heart failure, cardiotoxic drugs, pulmonary embolism, etc. If the imbalance of supply and demand persists, cell death or myocardial infarction (MI) occurs.[4]

Women with Heart Disease

Historically, CVD has been viewed as a man's disease. However, it is now recognized as the number one cause of death of women in the United States.[62,65] One in three women has some form of CVD.[65] Coronary artery disease (CAD) typically becomes evident in men in their mid-50s, the prime of their life. However, in women it is generally not recognized until 10 to 20 years later. This delay has been attributed to the protection women receive from endogenous estrogen. By the age of 75, the rates of cardiovascular (CV) morbidity and mortality in men and women are almost equal.[64]

Women who develop ACS experience more morbidity and disability than men. The clinical outcomes of women with ACS are sobering. For example, in 2015 the AHA reported the following:[65]

- Within 1 year of a recognized MI, 30% of women (vs. 25% of men) over age 65 years of age will die.
- Fifty-three percent of women MI survivors over the age of 65 will die within 5 years, versus 46% of men.
- Within 5 years, 23% of women MI survivors become disabled with heart failure, versus 19% of men over the age of 65 years of age.

Until the last several decades, subjects in research studies on heart disease were primarily men. Our knowledge of the manifestations of heart disease in women has been extrapolated from these studies. Based on this research, improvements have been made in the treatment of heart disease, mostly in decreased mortality rates in men. However, similar gains have not been seen in decreasing mortality rates in women with heart disease. With the aging population, increased rate of obesity, and other risk factors, such as diabetes, women now have a higher mortality rate after an MI than men and they are more likely to die of sudden cardiac arrest before arriving to the hospital (42% vs. 25%).[65,77,92] Studies find that women more often have recurrent symptoms requiring hospitalizations, contributing to decreased quality of life and inability to perform daily activities. Research shows this leads to different symptom presentation, different risk assessment, diagnostic, and treatment of ACS in women compared to men.[6,77,92]

PATHOPHYSIOLOGY

As the science of vascular biology and cellular functions advances, the understanding of the pathophysiology of ACS has evolved. The concept of "hardened arteries" of atherosclerosis is now known to be more complicated and encompasses the hematologic, immunologic, and inflammatory responses of the body. The theory of atherosclerosis proposes that the initiation of this process may start asymptomatically as early as the teenage years.[65,96] Diets high in saturated fats and cholesterol contribute to the collection of lipids in the arterial wall.[65] With high levels of lipoproteins circulating, accumulation occurs in the intricate collagen fibers of the intima of the arterial wall, developing into an atheroma. This insidious process reflects the "chronic" component of ACS, as it may take years to develop and even longer before symptoms occur.[17]

Inflammatory responses play a key role in the pathogenesis of ACS and in the past were accepted as the main culprit in the instability of plaque in patients. Recent studies show that C-reactive protein (CRP) levels are low in 40% of patients with ACS.[17] In addition, angiography studies fail to demonstrate obstructive atherosclerosis in over one-third of all ACS patients. Obstructive atherosclerosis is more prevalent in men than in women. This suggests the involvement of the coronary microcirculation and epicardial arteries. To better understand the causes of ACS, researchers have divided the pathophysiology of ACS into three separate subclasses: (1) obstructive atherosclerosis (ATS) with systemic inflammation, (2) obstructive ATS without systemic inflammation, and (3) nonobstructive ATS.[4,17,54]

Obstructive Atherosclerosis with Systemic Inflammation

The inflammatory response in obstructive ATS is a nonspecific, protective response to tissue damage elicited by various triggers, such as pathogens, chemical irritations, or disturbance in cellular homeostasis (Fig. 3.1). The acute phase of ATS involves the formation of a thrombus actually occluding arterial blood flow. The fibrous cap protects the inner endothelial cell content but is not impervious to damage itself. During the inflammatory phase, the T cells and macrophages accumulated in the collagen fibers release cytokines and matrix metalloproteinases, decreasing synthesis and degrading the collagen fibers, thereby thinning the cap. This interaction links the inflammatory response with the development of the atheroma at the cellular level. As the fibrous cap becomes thinner, it eventually ruptures and exposes the foam cells. These cells display tissue factor, a potent procoagulant initiating the activation of the extrinsic pathway of the coagulation cascade. Plaque formation, erosion, and fissure, in which there is a break in the plaque, continue as the inflammatory process continues and is enhanced by other mediators. CRP is a marker of inflammation and has high sensitivity. In patients with obstructive and systemic inflammation, higher levels of CRP are detected. This correlates to the disruption of plaque and widespread acute coronary inflammation attributing to the thrombi and stenosis scene with angiography.[17,53,54]

Obstructive Atherosclerosis without Systemic Inflammation

In individuals who have ACS with obstructive ATS, but without systemic inflammation or elevation of CRP, other mechanisms are likely to influence the formation of plaque. The precise cause is poorly understood but is believed to be related to extreme physical, emotional, or environmental stressors.[17,53,54] The ability to form thrombi or have unstable plaque and fissures is related to the activation of the sympathetic nervous system and surge of catecholamines. This leads to vasoconstriction and an increased workload of the heart, which leads to plaque rupture. The sympathetic nervous system also increases platelet activation and a hypercoagulable state leading to the further formation of thrombi and plaque.[17,71] In these patients, it has been found that there are actual chemical alterations in the cholesterol and plaque that make them more susceptible to fissure during exposure to stressors.[17,95]

Nonobstructive ATS

ACS without obstructive ATS is due to the alterations of the epicardial coronary arteries and microcirculation of the heart. This phenomenon occurs in approximately 30% of patients who present with ACS and is more prevalent in women. In these patients, instability may be due to coronary spasms that can cause ACS symptoms. Microvascular constrictions cause decrease in blood flow, cardiac necrosis, electrocardiogram (ECG) ST changes, and release of cardiac biomarkers. Coronary flow is regulated by several endothelium-dependent and independent factors influenced by the microvascular tone. The decreased flow causes ischemia without obstructive disease.[17,76] Microvascular tone and spasm may also promote the acute formation of a coronary thrombosis at the site of suspected plaque, and may be the primary cause of instability in patients found to have obstructive disease via angiography.[17]

With all three pathways, coronary thrombus is the final outcome leading to instability. Ideally blood flow should be quickly restored by various interventions so that cellular activity can be returned to normal. Many outside factors influence and enhance these abnormal cellular disruptions and are considered risk factors in ACS. Thus it is extremely important to identify these risk factors and implement the appropriate preventive measures and treatments in order to reduce the likelihood of thrombus formation.[17]

Pathophysiology of ACS in Women

Several areas of pathogenesis may differ in women: smaller vessel size, plaque characteristics, endothelial integrity, lipid profile, and effects of hormones. Furthermore, ACS without obstructive ATS appears to be a predictor of increased mortality in women, but not among men.[17,91] In several angiographic studies, 20% to 30% of women presenting with elevated biomarkers and ACS symptoms did not have obstructive disease. The Woman's Ischemia Syndrome Evaluation (WISE) study documented that women who have angina and do not have obstructive ATS have a relatively poor prognosis compared with women who have obstructive coronary disease and no myocardial ischemia.[41] Therefore, it would seem that this condition should be recognized early and addressed aggressively.[106]

Several theories surround this phenomenon including perhaps other mechanisms, such as spasm, enhanced coagulation, impaired fibrinolysis, and microvascular disease.[78,86,106] Angina in women is often due to microvascular dysfunction rather than significant epicardial coronary stenosis.[76] These differences in the pathophysiology of ACS in women versus men have led to the development of gender related treatments and guidelines in care for CAD.[62]

PATIENTS AT RISK

Timely treatment of patients presenting with possible symptoms of ACS relies on an accurate risk assessment of the patients for CVD in order to expedite treatment and reduce adverse outcomes. In 2010, the AHA recognized that although treatment of CVD has improved, the aging population and continued unhealthy behaviors and obesity epidemic in America continues to make CVD the number one killer of both men and women in the United States. This led to the focus on prevention and improvement of modifiable factors for overall CV health in the treatment of CVD with a focus on seven health metrics, including three health factors (hypertension, diabetes mellitus (DM), cholesterol) and four health behaviors.[57,65] These same behaviors have been identified in recent studies as significant risk factors for mortality and morbidity from ACS (smoking, weight, physical activity, diet).[48,56,86]

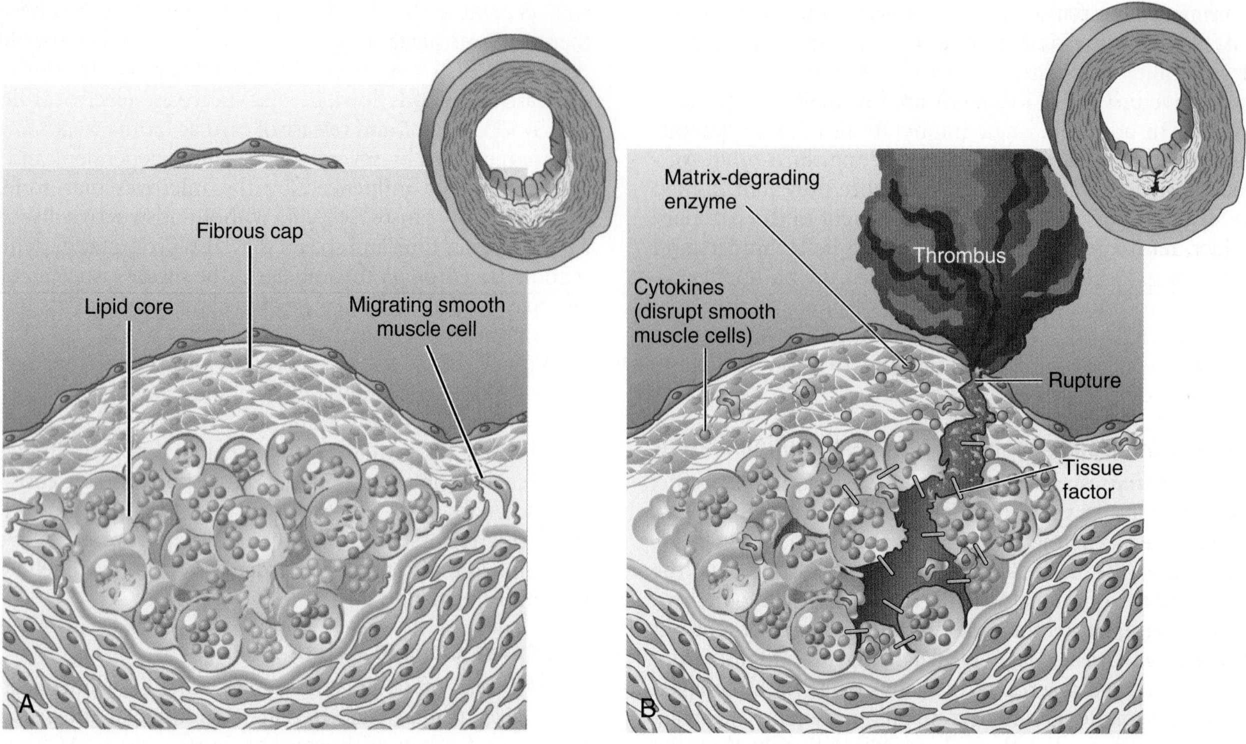

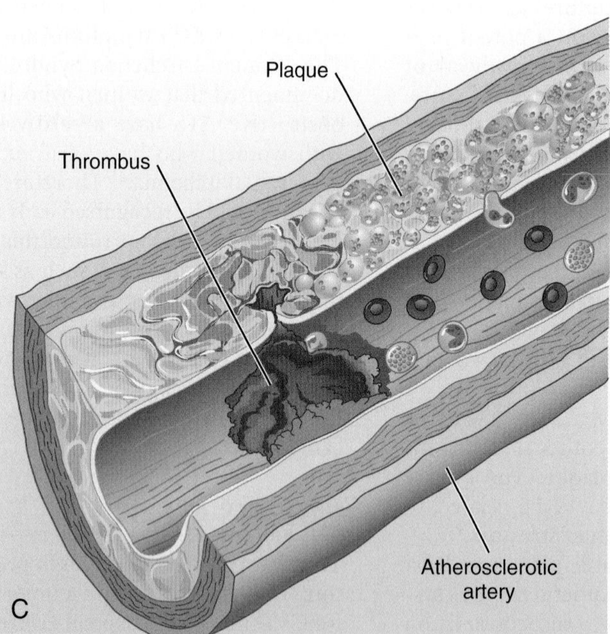

FIG. 3.1 Role of inflammation in coronary artery disease (CAD). A, Inflammation encourages growth of plaque, which becomes covered by a fibrous cap when smooth muscle cells move into the intima. The cap enlarges the size of the plaque deposit. **B,** Over time, inflammatory substances weaken the cap and damage smooth muscle. If the weakened plaque ruptures, a thrombus may form and block blood flow to the heart. **C,** Narrowing of an artery by plaque and thrombus.

Conventional risk factors, such as tobacco use, DM, high triglycerides, and low high-density lipoprotein portend a greater risk in women than in men.[77]

Hypertension (HTN) is the leading CVD risk factor when it comes to ACS and contributes to over 40% of all CVD deaths.[65] HTN is defined as a systolic blood pressure (SBP) greater than 140 mm Hg and a diastolic blood pressure (DBP) greater than 90 mm Hg.[38,65] Hypertensive patients with ACS are more likely to be older, female, of non-white ethnicity, and have a higher rate of comorbidities, such as DM, dyslipidemia, and chronic kidney disease (CKD).[19,31,51] The connection between HTN and ACS can be explained by two factors: (1) common risk factors and comorbidities shared by the two diseases, and (2) accelerated atherogenesis from increased stress and endothelial dysfunction leading to the development of vulnerable plaque whose instability can lead to rupture and ACS.[80,81]

Diabetes mellitus (DM) is another health factor associated with increased incidence of ACS. Individuals with DM have a two to four times higher rate of mortality from ACS compared to those without DM.[65] DM results in an elevation of blood glucose levels, enhancing the glycation of low-density lipoproteins (LDLs) and triggering the initial stages of the inflammatory response. In addition to this increased inflammatory response, increased hyperglycemia, insulin deficiency, metabolic conditions, and other cellular abnormalities cause platelets to be hyperreactive leading to increased activation and aggregation leading to ACS.[28]

Hyperlipidemia is commonly recognized as a major contributor to ACS.[57,65] The insidious process of accumulating lipoproteins in the intima of the arterial wall is postulated to occur over many years. If hyperlipidemia is recognized and controlled in the early stages, ACS could be decreased. With the increased use of cholesterol-lowering medications, cholesterol levels have declined over the years.[29] Unfortunately, hyperlipidemia still remains a large contributor to ACS due to lack of change in dietary patterns. Over 31 million Americans aged 20 or older have total cholesterol levels greater than or equal to 240 mg/dL.[14,65]

Smoking cessation or abstinence from smoking is the ideal health state in order to prevent ACS. Cigarette smoking is thought to elicit the early inflammatory process by the formation of oxidants causing the platelets to become stickier and damage the inner lining of the vessels, which decreases blood flow and potentiates ischemia.[103] Smoking cessation significantly reduces the risk of mortality and morbidity in persons with and without coronary heart disease (CHD). There is no evidence that smoking fewer cigarettes will reduce risk of CHD, but completely quitting significantly lowers one's risk at any age. The longer a person abstains from smoking, the larger the decline in mortality.[65,101,103] Secondhand smoke can also increase risk of developing ACS. Just a few exposures to secondhand smoke have been shown to increase the risk of ACS, especially if the individual has multiple other risk factors for ACS.[65,103] Electronic cigarettes have recently come onto the market as a healthier alternative to smoking and a possible smoking cessation tool. There are few studies on these products and some individuals see them as a possible gateway drug to potential smokers. Until further studies are done on these products, public health advocates advise the public to avoid them.[7,27,103]

Weight, physical activity, and diet are important healthy elements to consider in determining the risk of CVD and ACS. These factors all work together to predispose individuals to other CV risks such as HTN, DM, and dyslipidemia.[57,65] In 2012, over 69% of US adults were overweight or obese. Physical inactivity, as well as dietary patterns, play a large part in this epidemic.[68] Obesity and lack of physical exercise contribute to intravascular inflammation. Studies show that physical activity decreases inflammatory markers in individuals with CHD and decreases overall CV risk.[65,83] Over the years, the changing dietary patterns of Americans have contributed to the increasing obesity problem, as well as to the development of other CV risk factors. Increasing caloric intake and energy imbalance from increased portion sizes has a large impact on CV health and other risk factors, such as obesity and hyperlipidemia.[57,65,66]

TABLE 3.1 Diagnosis of Metabolic Syndrome

TO DIAGNOSE METABOLIC SYNDROME PATIENTS NEED THREE OUT OF THE FIVE RISK FACTORS BELOW	
Blood pressure	• BP ≥130 mm Hg systolic or ≥85 mm Hg diastolic or • Undergoing drug treatment for hypertension or antihypertensive drug treatment in a patient with a history of hypertension
Blood glucose	• Fasting plasma glucose ≥100 mg/dL or • Undergoing drug treatment for elevated glucose
Lipids	• HDL cholesterol <40 mg/dL in men or <50 mg/dL in women or • Undergoing drug treatment for reduced HDL cholesterol
Triglycerides	• Triglycerides ≥150 mg/dL or • Undergoing drug treatment for elevated triglycerides
Waist circumference	• Waist circumference >102 cm in men or >88 cm in women for people of most ancestries living in the United States • Ethnicity and country-specific thresholds can be used for diagnosis in other groups, particularly Asians and individuals of non-European ancestry who have predominantly resided outside the United States

Data from References 2, 35, and 65

Metabolic syndrome is defined as a cluster of individual risk factors for ACS combined into one syndrome[2] and is diagnosed when at least three out of the five risk factors are present (Table 3.1). Besides ACS, metabolic syndrome can lead to a number of other adverse health conditions. Women have been shown to have higher rates of ACS related to metabolic syndrome when compared to men. Unless lifestyle changes occur, metabolic syndrome has been shown to significantly increase an individual's risk of mortality and death from ACS.[64,65]

Other modifiable risk factors include CKD and peripheral vascular disease (PVD). CKD is defined as a reduced glomerular filtration rate (GFR), or increased urine protein, or both. As the incidences of obesity, HTN, and DM rise, so does the incidence of CKD. ACS is the leading cause of mortality in patients with CKD and end-stage renal disease (ESRD). The exact reasons why CKD and ESRD increase the risk of CVD and ACS is not completely understood, but are multifactorial and may be related to the similar risk factors (HTN and DM), as well as other inflammatory causes that may be seen in ACS.[30,65]

PVD affects over 8.5 million people in the United States. Risk factors for PVD and ACS are similar, including smoking, HTN, DM, and hyperlipidemia. This makes patients with PVD at increased risk of mortality and complications from ACS.[65]

TABLE 3.2 **Differential Diagnosis of Episodic Chest Pain**

Diagnosis	Duration	Quality	Provocation	Relief	Location	Comment
Exertional angina	5–15 min	Visceral (pressure)	During effort or motion	Rest, nitroglycerin (NTG)	Substernal, radiates	First episode vivid
Rest angina	5–15 min	Visceral (pressure)	Spontaneous	NTG	Substernal, radiates	Usually nocturnal
Mitral prolapse	Minutes to hours	Superficial	Spontaneous	Time	Left anterior	No pattern, variable character
Esophageal reflux	10–60 min	Visceral	Recumbency, lack of food	Food, antacids	Substernal, epigastric	Rarely radiates
Esophageal spasm	50–60 min	Visceral	Spontaneous, cold liquids, exercise	NTG	Substernal, radiates	Mimics angina
Peptic ulcer	Hours	Visceral (burning)	Lack of food, "acid food"	Food, antacids	Epigastric, substernal	
Biliary disease	Hours	Visceral (wax and wane)	Spontaneous, food	Time, analgesia	Epigastric, radiates	Colic
Cervical disk	Variable (gradually subsides)	Superficial	Head and neck movement, palpation	Time, analgesia	Arm, neck	Not relieved by rest
Hyperventilation	2–30 min	Visceral	Emotion, tachypnea	Stimulus removed	Substernal	Facial paresthesia
Musculoskeletal	Variable	Superficial	Movement, palpation	Time, analgesia	Multiple	Tenderness
Pulmonary	>30 min	Visceral (pressure)	Often spontaneous	Rest, time, bronchodilator	Substernal	Dyspneic

Data from References 1 and 16.

Non modifiable risk factors, such as familial history of CHD, age, race, and gender need to be considered when looking at an individual's risk for ACS. Premature family history of CHD is a strong predictor of ACS. CHD and ACS events increase with age for both men and women.[4,65]

ASSESSMENT OF PATIENTS WITH ACS

History of Patient's Chest Pain

A complete and detailed history of a patient presenting with ACS is the cornerstone to diagnosis and proper treatment. Diagnosis begins with the clinical evaluation of symptoms and potential ischemic chest pain, also known as angina pectoris.[10,16] Ischemic chest pain usually lasts longer than 10 minutes and presents as a pressure-like, retrosternal pain that occurs at rest or with minimal exertion. The pain may radiate to other areas of the body and may include many other variables, including nausea, vomiting, diaphoresis, jaw pain, back pain, and dyspnea.[4,10,16]

Classic chest pain is not as prevalent in women, diabetic patients, and older individuals (over 75 years of age). They typically present with nonspecific chest pain syndromes. Unexplained new onset or increased dyspnea is the most common symptom. Other symptoms may include nausea, epigastric pain, indigestion, pleuritic pain, and syncope. Diabetic patients may not experience pain because of neuropathy associated with the disease. It becomes important to recognize these variances and understand the differential diagnosis.[4] Table 3.2 summarizes chest pain syndromes.

Physical Exam

In addition to the symptoms, the physical exam of the patient can vary and may be nonspecific. Vital signs should be taken and assessed for hemodynamic compromise. The physical exam in many patients may be completely normal. Other patients who have had ischemic events may show signs of heart failure with jugular vein distension (JVD) or edema. A triad of hypotension, JVD, and clear lungs on auscultation are characteristic of right ventricular infarction. Auscultation of the heart may reveal a splitting S2, S3, or S4 sound. A new murmur from mitral regurgitation from ischemic dysfunction of papillary muscle may also be heard.[4,10]

The physical exam can also help determine alternative diagnosis. Pain that occurs with palpitation of chest or movement of upper extremities could indicate musculoskeletal origin. Auscultation of a friction rub could indicate pericarditis. Decreased breath sounds could indicate a pneumothorax or pneumonia. Absent or decreased pulses or pulsus paradoxus could indicate more life-threatening events such as aortic dissection or tamponade.[1,4,74]

It is very important to remember that there is no absolute symptomatology or physical exam for ACS. The clinician should maintain a high index of suspicion with any type of chest pain. The initial evaluation should focus on two initial questions:[4]

1. What is the likelihood that the symptoms and signs represent ACS?
2. What is the likelihood of adverse outcomes?

To help further guide evaluation and treatment, the clinician must determine the likelihood of ACS through utilization of clinical risk scores. The stratification of the patient to either a low, intermediate, or high risk for ACS will help to determine treatment options (Table 3.3). Several risk calculators have been developed, but the most widely used risk calculator is the Thrombolysis in Myocardial Infarction (TIMI) risk score (Box 3.1). When assessing the patient, their risk factors, physical exam, evaluation of cardiac troponins, and ECG help to determine the risk of ACS, as well as risk of adverse outcomes.[4,5,90]

Laboratory Tests

Measurement of cardiac troponins is the mainstay in the diagnosis and risk stratification of ACS.[4] Troponin is a protein found in the cardiac muscle that covers the binding site for the actin and myosin filaments. Troponins are released into the blood as a result of muscle destruction and ischemia. There are two troponin components specific for cardiac muscle: troponin I and troponin T. Cardiac troponin I (cTnI) inhibits muscle

TABLE 3.3 Risk Stratification for Acute Coronary Syndrome

Feature	High Likelihood	Intermediate Likelihood	Low Likelihood
History	Chest or left arm pain or discomfort as chief symptom with known history of CAD including MI	Chest or left arm pain or discomfort as chief symptom; age >70 years; male sex and diabetes mellitus	Probable ischemic symptoms in absence of any of intermediate likelihood characteristics; recent cocaine use
Exam	Transient mitral regurgitation, hypotension, diaphoresis, pulmonary edema, or rales	Extracardiac vascular disease	Chest discomfort reproduced by palpation
ECG	New or presumed new transient ST segment elevation ≥1 mm or T wave inversion in multiple precordial leads	Fixed Q waves; abnormal ST depression of 0.5–1.0 mm or T-wave inversion >1.0 mm	No changes in ECG
Cardiac markers	Elevated cardiac troponins	Normal	Normal

CAD, Coronary artery disease; *ECG*, electrocardiogram; *MI*, myocardial infarction.
Data from References 1, 4, and 49.

BOX 3.1 Thrombolysis in Myocardial Infarction (TIMI) Risk Score

The TIMI risk score is determined by the sum of the presence of seven variables at admission.
One point is given for each of the following variables:

- ≥65 yrs of age
- ≥3 risk factors for CAD
- Prior coronary stenosis ≥50%
- ST deviation on ECG
- ≥2 anginal events in prior 24 hours
- Use of aspirin in prior 7 days
- Elevated cardiac biomarkers

TIMI Risk Score	All-cause mortality, new or recurrent MI, or severe recurrent ischemia requiring urgent revascularization through 14 days after randomization (%)
0–1	4.7
2	8.3
3	13.2
4	19.9
5	26.2
6–7	40.9

CAD, Coronary artery disease; ECG, electrocardiogram; *MI*, myocardial infarction. Modified with permission from References 4 and 5.

contraction, and cardiac troponin T (cTnT) connects the troponin complex to tropomyosin. After injury to the muscle, both of these biomarkers rise in 3 to 4 hours, peak in 10 to 24 hours, and can remain elevated from a couple days to weeks depending on the severity of the ischemia.[4,90] According to the ACC/AHA 2014 guidelines, specific cardiac troponins levels should be checked upon presentation and again 3 to 6 hours after initial presentation. Usually an MI can be excluded in patients within 6 hours after initial presentation. Traditional serial cardiac troponins levels are only recommended if the patient has continued symptomatology and a high suspicion of MI.[4,44,84,99]

Even though troponins are specific to the cardiac muscle, other factors can cause their elevation and they should not be utilized alone in the diagnosis of an MI. Other conditions, such as tachyarrhythmias, hypotension, HTN, pericarditis, recent cardiothoracic surgery, acute heart failure, sepsis, burns, structural cardiac abnormalities from left ventricular (LV) hypertrophy, or dilation common in renal insufficiency and ESRD may also cause elevations. The clinician must look at the risk stratification of the patient, as well as the overall clinical presentation, in order to determine if the patient is having an ACS event.[4,10]

Other biomarkers such as creatine kinase (CK), CK-MB, and myoglobin have had a role in the detection of ACS. Their use is now limited due to their lack of specificity to the cardiac muscle. With the availability of a cardiac sensitive troponins, these biomarkers are no longer recommended for use by clinicians in the detection of ACS.[4]

CRP has developed a role in the prediction of ACS. CRP is a peptide produced by the liver in response to inflammation, infection, or tissue damage. Highly elevated levels may be more predictive of the inflammatory pathway with ACS and ischemic heart disease, especially in individuals with known ACS. CRP levels should be used in conjunction with other data, such as risk factors and family history, because specificity with this marker can be an issue. Levels could be high with an infection or other tissue damage.[8,45,47,90] Standard laboratory testing including electrolytes, blood urea nitrogen (BUN), creatinine, hematocrit, lipid profile, and glucose should also be obtained to establish a baseline for the patient to monitor any changes when treatments are initiated.[1,4]

Electrocardiogram

The 12-lead electrocardiogram (ECG) is the other classic diagnostic tool used in ACS. The ECG should be performed and interpreted by an experienced healthcare provider within 10 minutes of the patient presenting with chest discomfort.[4] The ECG is most helpful for diagnosis of ischemia or infarction and to guide the specific pathway the clinician should take in the treatment of the patient. Immediate reperfusion is indicated when a patient presents with an ECG that has ST elevation at the J point in at least 2 contiguous leads of greater than or equal to 2 mm (0.2 mV) in men or greater than or equal to 1.5 mm (0.15 mV) in women in leads V_2–V_3, and/or of greater than or equal to 1 mm in more than two other contiguous chest or limb leads.[73] This is considered a STEMI. However, there may be marked ST depression or marked T wave inversion (≥2 mm), which can indicate a NSTE-ACS. A patient may also have ACS and show nonspecific ST-T wave findings, or no ECG changes. In these cases the clinical assessment, risk stratification, and serial ECGs become important in the treatment and diagnosis of the patient.[1,4,9,73]

Imaging

Depending on the severity of the symptoms and clinical assessment of the patient, other imaging studies may be appropriate to help in the diagnosis of ACS. A chest radiograph (CXR) should be obtained to look at potential pulmonary causes of chest pain, such as pneumonia or a pneumothorax. CXR also shows the heart and aorta size. If the heart size is enlarged and the CXR shows pulmonary congestion, the patient may have heart failure. If the chest pain is the result of an aortic dissection, the aortic size could be notably increased.[1,4]

An echocardiogram is frequently used as a noninvasive imaging study of the heart. Two-dimensional echocardiography can evaluate for abnormal cardiac wall motion, ejection fraction (EF), and valvular motion and can also be performed with stress testing technology discussed hereafter. Three-dimensional technology has also become available, but is not readily used in most institutions at this time. An echocardiogram is the preferred method of evaluation for LV function. It is recommended that all patients have an assessment of their LV function and EF to help guide treatment.[4,82]

Further evaluation of low- to intermediate-risk patients can be done using stress testing. Under controlled conditions, the workload of the heart is increased, while heart rate (HR), BP, and the ECG are monitored for any changes in the ST segment, T waves, or the development of dysrhythmias or angina. The workload of the heart can be increased by exercise, or if the patient is unable to exercise, pharmacologic agents, such as dobutamine (Dobutrex), dipyridamole (Persantine), adenosine (Adenocard), or regadenoson (Lexiscan), can be administered while the patient remains stationary. Stress testing combined with cardiac imaging, such as an echocardiogram, assists in the diagnosis of ischemic heart disease. Radionuclides (e.g., thallium-201 or technetium-99m sestamibi) can also be injected during maximal stress and traced to determine how myocardial blood flow is distributed for that patient. These tests are very sensitive and accurate.

Computed tomography (CT) and magnetic resonance imaging (MRI) are also being adapted as diagnostic tools for ACS. Noninvasive testing for low to intermediate risk can also be done by CT.[4,11,82] ACT of the chest can be done to rule out any suspicion of pulmonary embolism or aortic dissection.[4] With advances in technology, visualization of coronary arteries has become easier and CT technology can now be used to help identify individuals at risk of ACS. Electron beam CT (EBCT) and multidetector CT (MDCT) are utilized to visualize increased calcium. A calcium score is calculated from the area and density of calcium deposition in the coronary arteries. A score of 11–399 indicates an intermediate risk and a score greater than 400 indicates there is a high risk of ACS.[11,82] Coronary CT angiography (CTA) is another alternative that can identify possible stenosis in the coronary arteries. Even though it is still considered inferior to cardiac catheterization, coronary CTA can provide a noninvasive visualization of the arteries in individuals who are considered low to intermediate risk for ACS.[82,105] Cardiac MRI has become more readily available over the years and has the advantage of less radiation, isotopes, and contrast than CT. Visualization of anatomy, as well as myocardial viability, can be valuable, especially in individuals with a previous history of ACS. The downside to an MRI is that anyone with a pacemaker, intra-aortic balloon pump (IABP), or metal implants cannot undergo the test.[37,60,82] However, the gold standard for evaluation of coronary artery anatomy and obstructive atherosclerosis is coronary angiography, discussed later in this chapter.

Presentation of Women with ACS

Women with ACS may present with different and more diverse symptoms than men. Women's initial manifestation of heart disease may be chest discomfort, rather than an MI. However, that chest discomfort often does not predict prognosis in women. Although women may describe classic chest pain, some do not experience any type of chest discomfort with ACS. When women with classic chest pain were studied angiographically, they did not have significant occlusions as frequently as men. They may describe the pain as more transient, sharp, or stabbing. The most frequent acute symptoms reported are shortness of breath, weakness, and fatigue. Women are also more likely to have neck pain, back pain, jaw pain, paroxysmal nocturnal dyspnea, epigastric pain, nausea, vomiting, indigestion, and loss of appetite than are men. In addition, women are less likely to report diaphoresis, but equally likely to report dizziness, fainting, or syncope.[6,77,92]

Confounding the issue is that women tend to deny their symptoms might be heart-related by thinking their symptoms are not serious, waiting for symptoms to go away, and worrying about troubling others. Also, women tend to place a different meaning on chest pain than do men. Some older women perceive angina as natural, and they may interpret the onset of exertional angina as a normal symptom of fatigue. Failure to recognize nonspecific symptoms may be reasons that women, compared with men, experience a greater proportion of sudden cardiac deaths, have more unrecognized ACS events, or are mistakenly diagnosed and discharged from emergency departments.[62,65]

Diagnostics in Women with ACS

The accuracy and limitations of stress testing in women are confusing. This may be attributable to the higher prevalence of nonobstructive CAD and single-vessel disease in women, as well as the limitation of various forms of stress testing.[77] Standard exercise ECG is the most commonly used and least costly of the noninvasive tests. However, exercise ECG is not as predictive in women as men because of lower sensitivity and specificity and higher false-positive rates than in men.[77] When women have symptoms suggestive of CAD, stress echocardiography, either physiologically on a treadmill or pharmacologically, can be effective to detect CAD and assess prognosis. Stress myocardial perfusion imaging using nuclear scanning provides direct imaging of the myocardium and is not dependent on the ECG to diagnose ischemia. Technical limitations in women have been reported, including false-positive results because of breast attenuation and small left ventricular chamber size; however, current innovations have improved the accuracy in high-risk women.[76] For women with intermediate to high likelihood of CAD, noninvasive diagnostic studies, such as exercise ECG or cardiac imaging studies are recommended.[60,77]

Cardiac positron emission tomography (PET) uses radiolabeled glucose to differentiate between ischemic and infarcted myocardium.[60,82] PET imaging is now performed in an increasing number of centers worldwide and has an excellent diagnostic performance for the detection of CAD in women. With improved imaging quality, reduced artifact, and low radiation, the PET exam may provide a better visualization of microvascular disease in women. Kay et al.[42] recently looked at the influence of risk stratification in women with stress myocardial perfusion testing with new technology utilizing Rb-82 PET imaging. The study showed that improved risk stratification of women was seen with Rb-82 PET imaging compared to traditional studies.

TREATMENT OF ACS

Management and treatment of ACS is based on the initial assessment and risk stratification. The clinician then assigns the patient to one of four categories to help guide treatment. The categories include a noncardiac diagnosis with low or intermediate risk of cardiac event, stable ischemic heart disease, NSTE-ACS (unstable angina and NSTEMI), and STEMI. In this chapter the focus will be on the management and treatment of NSTE-ACS and STEMI patients.

NSTE-ACS (Unstable Angina and NSTEMI)

NSTE-ACS affects over 625,000 people annually, which is approximately three-fourths of all people with ACS.[4,65] NSTE-ACS refers to a pattern of ischemic changes with possible ST depression, T wave inversion (≥2 mm), or no changes depending on the timing of ischemia. It is further subdivided into either unstable angina (UA) or NSTEMI based on the elevation of cardiac biomarkers. UA can have ST-T wave changes, but they are usually transient and biomarkers are not usually elevated. If biomarkers are elevated and meet clinical criteria, the patient is considered to have a NSTEMI. With NSTEMI, the ischemia is severe enough to cause sufficient myocardial damage for detectable levels of biomarkers to be released. This condition was previously referred to as a "non Q wave MI" because there were ST-T wave abnormalities with elevated biomarker levels but no Q wave development. When a patient has any type of chest discomfort, it is important to consider these diagnoses immediately and to initiate an evidence-based plan of care. Fast and appropriate interventions can save myocardial muscle and improve outcomes.[4]

Care of Patients with NSTE-ACS

Once NSTE-ACS is recognized, the immediate goals are relief of ischemic symptoms and prevention of infarction and death.[4] Patient placement is generally on an intermediate cardiac or telemetry floor. If the patient is experiencing hemodynamic compromise or continued ischemia, they may be placed in the critical care unit for further observation. Routine nursing care includes frequently taking vital signs per unit policy and cardiac monitoring. Supplemental oxygen should be administered in the presence of arterial oxygen saturation less than 90% or pulmonary distress.[4] Recent data suggest routine supplemental oxygen in patients with MI with normal oxygen saturation may have negative effects, including increased coronary vascular resistance, reduced coronary blood flow, and increased risk of death.[12,61] The clinical goal should be to keep the oxygen saturation greater than 90% and wean oxygen as symptoms improve.[4]

The nurse should have the basic knowledge required for placing and interpreting a 12-lead ECG. The preferred cardiac monitoring using five electrodes allows the clinician to obtain a true V_1 lead, whereas a three-electrode system produces a modified chest lead (MCL_1). Lead V_1 is the optimal lead for diagnosing bundle branch blocks and confirming proper right ventricular pacemaker location when using temporary pacing, and can be used to distinguish supraventricular tachycardia versus ventricular tachycardia. However, monitoring can only provide valid data if used appropriately. Skin preparation and lead placement are vital steps and, when properly performed, optimize the monitoring data and lessen the likelihood of false alarms. Skin preparation includes shaving electrode sites and removing skin oils and debris with alcohol or a rough washcloth. Once the skin is prepared, proper lead placement has been shown to assist in the differentiation of rhythms. Fig. 3.2 shows the correct five-electrode lead placement. It is important to emphasize that the right and left leg leads should be placed *below* the rib cage. Consistency of lead placement improves the information gained from bedside monitoring, as well as when obtaining a 12-lead ECG. Education and standard methods should be employed to ensure consistent placement of the precordial leads. These evidence-based practices facilitate accurate, efficient nursing practice.[24,46]

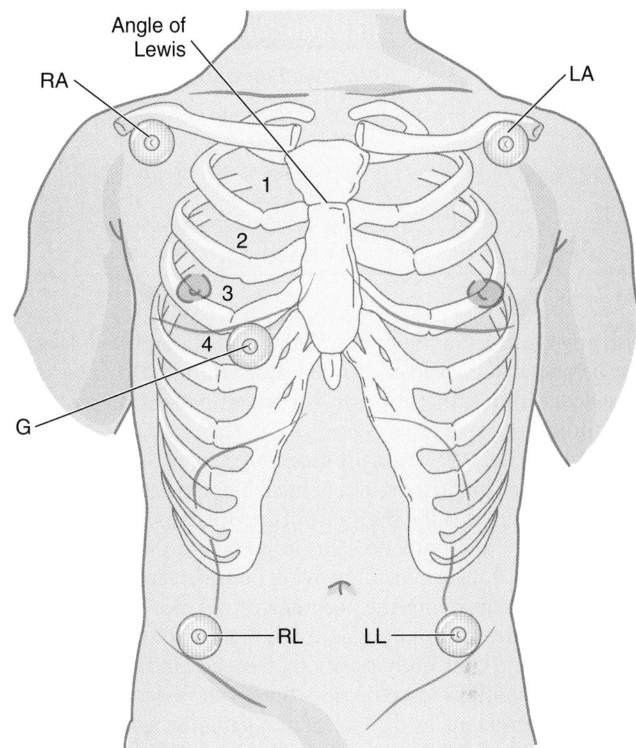

FIG. 3.2 Correct five-electrode lead placement. Commonly used five-electrode lead system that allows for recording any of the six limb leads plus one precordial (V) lead. Shown here is lead placement for recording V_1. A limitation of this system is that only one precordial lead can be recorded. *G,* Ground; *LA,* left arm; *LL,* left leg; *RA,* right arm; *RL,* right leg.

Initial interpretation of a 12-lead ECG helps the nurse anticipate possible interventions. Knowledge of the anatomy of the coronary arteries is needed to understand the relationship between the leads and the anatomic area of the heart represented. Table 3.4 describes the coronary artery system, regions of blood supply, and their corresponding leads. Lesions involving the left anterior descending artery (LAD) usually include the anterior wall of the left ventricle and can lead to pump failure and if extensive damage occurs, cardiogenic shock. The right coronary artery (RCA) supplies the inferior and posterior wall of the left ventricle and the conduction system in the majority of the population. Lesions in this artery can lead to conduction disorders and possible right ventricular dysfunction. Right ventricular dysfunction can be detected by evaluating right-sided chest leads via a 15-lead ECG.[4,73] ST segment elevation may be seen in these leads during an acute right ventricular MI. The lateral wall is usually supplied by the left circumflex artery (LCA). Depending on the individual's coronary anatomy, lateral wall damage rarely occurs alone; it is typically found in conjunction

TABLE 3.4 **Chest Leads**

Lead	Positive Electrode Position	Heart Surface Viewed
V_1	Right side of sternum, fourth intercostal space	Septum
V_2	Left side of sternum, fourth intercostal space	Septum
V_3	Midway between V_2 and V_4	Anterior
V_4	Left midclavicular line, fifth intercostal space	Anterior
V_5	Left anterior axillary line; same level as V_4	Lateral
V_6	Left midaxillary line; same level as V_4	Lateral

From reference 1a.

with any of the other types of wall damage. Lateral wall damage can be associated with sinus node dysrhythmias. This baseline knowledge allows the nurse to anticipate patient presentation and clinical needs.[25]

Unfortunately, ST segment monitoring is widely underused in hospitals, even if the system is available. One reason this tool is not widely used is the high rate of false alarms, as well as lack of understanding about how to properly use this technology. Many of the strategies for improving bedside cardiac monitoring apply to improving the accuracy of ST monitoring. Some of the strategies recommended by the AHA are the following: (1) understand that body position changes can cause ST fluctuations, (2) follow careful skin preparation techniques, (3) maintain consistent lead placement, (4) tailor alarm parameters to the patient's baseline ST level, (5) understand the goals of monitoring, and (6) analyze ECG printout rather than just graphic trends.[4,24,25,73] Using this technology effectively may help improve patient care.

Antiplatelet and Anticoagulation Therapy

Medications administered during the initial treatment of NSTE-ACS include antiplatelet and anticoagulant, along with anti-ischemic agents. Antiplatelet intervention includes dual antiplatelet therapy (DAPT) with administration of aspirin and a $P2Y_{12}$ inhibitor. This important intervention disables the coagulation cascade at two levels in an effort to increase blood flow to the compromised cardiac muscle. Disabling platelet activity has been shown to be an effective treatment and should be initiated immediately. Once the plaque is disrupted, platelets are one of the major participants in thrombus formation. Aspirin (ASA) irreversibly inhibits the cyclooxygenase-1 within platelets, thereby preventing the formation of thromboxane A_2, disabling platelet aggregation. ASA should be administered as soon as possible after patient presentation and should be continued on a daily basis indefinitely.[4] However, some patients may not tolerate ASA because of hypersensitivity, gastric intolerance, or bleeding.

$P2Y_{12}$ inhibitors are another type of medication that effectively inhibit ADP-induced platelet aggregation by selectively and irreversibly blocking the $P2Y_{12}$ receptor. Clopidogrel (Plavix) is one of the first $P2Y_{12}$ inhibitors used as an adjunctive therapy with ASA or when the patient has an ASA intolerance. $P2Y_{12}$ inhibitors and aspirin inhibit platelet aggregation through different pathways; therefore, combined antiplatelet therapy provides complementary and additive benefits compared to either agent.[4] Clopidogrel should be given when there is serious suspicion of myocardial injury. The findings of the Clopidogrel in Unstable Angina to Prevent Recurrent Events (CURE) trial demonstrated a 20% decrease in the combined end point of CV death, nonfatal MI, and stroke when administering a loading dose of 300 mg followed by 75 mg daily to the patients.[4,32] Of note, these results were achieved with an increased risk of bleeding; therefore, this consequence must be considered in centers using aggressive interventional strategies.

Ticagrelor (Brilinta) is a newer $P2Y_{12}$ inhibitor and several studies, including the Platelet Inhibition and Patient Outcomes (PLATO) trial, have shown it to have some superiority over clopidogrel in the treatment of ACS.[39,58] Patients with NSTE-ACS in the trial who received ticagrelor had a lower mortality rate and a reduction in outcomes of death from MI, stroke, and vascular causes. Compared to clopidogrel, ticagrelor has a shorter half-life (12 hours) with a faster recovery of platelet function. Because of the short half-life, twice-a-day dosing is required, which could impact compliance. When combined with ASA, an increase in bleeding was observed, therefore it is recommended that the dose of ASA be decreased to 81 mg daily. Some side effects unique to ticagrelor include dyspnea and bradycardia; however, they are usually not severe enough to treat but still should be monitored.[4]

Prasugrel (Effient) is another newer $P2Y_{12}$ inhibitor. It is usually reserved for use in patients after the anatomy is known and possible interventional revascularization is performed.[4] Despite the major benefits of clopidogrel, there is substantial variability in response by patients due to its metabolism. The enzymes involved in the breakdown of clopidogrel can be genetically altered in many individuals. Prasugrel is not affected by these alterations and can be directly broken down. Therefore, more rapid and consistent drug levels can be found in the body compared to clopidogrel. Due to the rapid metabolism of the drug, caution needs to be used in the elderly and the dosage should be decreased in anyone over age 75 or anyone who weighs less than 65 kg.[107] The drug is also contraindicated in anyone with a history of transient ischemic attack (TIA) or stroke due to the risk of bleeding.[4,107] Similar to the other $P2Y_{12}$ inhibitors, education on potential side effects, especially bleeding, should be provided to the patient and family.[4,52,107]

If more immediate action against platelet aggregation is needed, intravenous glycoprotein IIb/IIIa (GP IIb/IIIa) receptor antagonists are administered. They are indicated when troponins are elevated and the patient is high risk for infarction and a catheterization or percutaneous coronary intervention (PCI) is planned.[4] Since the PCI will cause further endothelial disruption, a GP IIb/IIIa inhibitor should be administered just before the procedure to achieve optimal platelet aggregation antagonism. There are three GP IIb/IIIa inhibitors that may be used in clinical practice: abciximab (ReoPro), eptifibatide (Integrilin), and tirofiban (Aggrastat). Eptifibatide and tirofiban affect different peptide sequences of fibrinogen and are highly specific for the GP IIb/IIIa receptors. Therefore, they are recommended over other GP IIb/IIIa inhibitors in the 2014 ACC/AHA guidelines for the management of NSTE-ACS patients with DAPT and early invasive strategy.[4]

Pharmacologic interventions are aimed at decreasing thrombus formation at various levels in the clotting cascade. Anticoagulation interventions are recommended in addition to antiplatelet therapy. Unfractionated heparin (UFH) and low molecular weight heparins

(LMWHs) are the most commonly used anticoagulation agents. Heparin accelerates the action of antithrombin, which inactivates factor IIa (thrombin), whereas LMWH inactivates both thrombin and factor Xa. Heparin activity requires partial prothrombin time (PTT) monitoring while LMWHs do not require laboratory monitoring. It is important to remember that heparins prevent thrombi formation, but do not lyse existing thrombi.[4,10]

With the increased use of heparins, heparin-induced thrombocytopenia (HIT) has become a more common clinical syndrome. HIT, a platelet disorder associated with development of a drug-induced thrombocytopenia, can be frequently complicated by life-threatening thrombotic events. HIT may be seen in patients who receive heparin, and should be an early consideration in the cardiac patient with new thrombocytopenia that develops 5 to 8 days after the initiation of heparin therapy. If HIT is suspected, argatroban, a direct thrombin inhibitor, can be substituted for heparin.[4,55] Other direct thrombin inhibitors, including bivalirudin (Angiomax) and fondaparinux (Arixtra), have been used in recent studies during PCI. Patients randomly received either bivalirudin with provisional (if necessary during the procedure) GP IIb/IIIa blockade or heparin with planned GP IIb/IIIa blockade. The long-term outcomes are comparable to those of heparin and have been added to the ACC/AHA guidelines.[4,97] Fondaparinux can be given subcutaneously, similar to LMWH. In the Organization to Assess Strategies in Acute Ischemic Syndromes (OASIS) trial,[94] patients who had an NSTE-ACS had similar outcomes to patients who were given LMWH. Caution is advised in patients with creatinine clearance (CrCl) of less than 30 mL/min.[4,94]

The antiplatelet and anticoagulation medications discussed are summarized in Table 3.5. Once the patient's condition stabilizes, long-term therapy can be implemented. It is important to note that even though the cause of myocardial injury in NSTE-ACS may be a nonocclusive thrombus, thrombolysis has not been shown to improve outcomes and is not recommended.[4]

Anti-Ischemic Medication Therapy

Nitrates are one of the first medications given to reduce myocardial oxygen demand. Nitroglycerin (NTG) is a potent vasodilator, reducing preload, ventricular wall tension, and myocardial oxygen consumption. It also dilates large coronary arteries and increases collateral flow to ischemic areas. NTG can be administered sublingually, but when the patient has marginal hemodynamic parameters, intravenous administration may be preferred to better control patient response. Hypotension can occur as a result of hypovolemia, poor myocardial function, or the combination of pharmacologic agents given quickly. The patient's home medications should be reviewed carefully for other drugs that may exacerbate hypotension.[4] Alpha agonists, such as sildenafil (Viagra), are commonly prescribed for erectile dysfunction or pulmonary HTN and can have vasodilatory effects up to 24 hours after a dose.

The 2014 AHA guidelines include morphine sulfate in this category as an adjunct therapy if there is continued ischemia. Morphine sulfate is a potent analgesic and anxiolytic that may be given concurrently with NTG to control chest pain or acute pulmonary congestion. Morphine causes vasodilation, decreased preload, and decreased workload of the compromised myocardium, indirectly assisting with anti-ischemic effects of other drugs. Administer with caution as hypotension and respiratory distress are serious side effects that could further compromise a patient who may already be hemodynamically compromised.[4]

Beta blockers also decrease myocardial ischemia by blocking the effects of catecholamines at beta-receptor sites on cell membranes. In the myocardium, this action decreases HR and contractility, thereby decreasing myocardial oxygen consumption. Adequate beta blockade is achieved by decreasing the HR, which increases diastolic time, resulting in an increased coronary artery filling time. Beta blockers with selective $beta_1$ receptor activity are preferred because they interact primarily with cardiac cells and have minimal activity on beta receptors in the bronchial airways and pancreatic cells. The use of beta blockers was originally shown to decrease morbidity or mortality in patients with MIs and heart failure in the 1980s,[109] and remains an important intervention in the 2014 AHA guidelines. Beta-blockers should be initiated within the first 24 hours of presentation with NSTE-ACS unless the patient has: (1) signs of heart failure, (2) evidence of low output state, (3) increased risk of cardiogenic shock, or (4) other contraindications such as prolonged PR interval, heart block, or reactive airway disease. If beta blocker use is contraindicated at initial presentation, the clinician should reassess later in the patient's treatment course for eligibility.[4]

Calcium channel blockers (CCB) can decrease myocardial ischemia by inhibiting myocardial contractility and slowing atrioventricular (AV) node conduction, reducing the inward calcium flux across the cell membrane. This action decreases myocardial oxygen consumption. If patients have already received nitrates and beta blockers in adequate doses and are still experiencing symptoms or cannot tolerate those drugs, a nondihydropyridine calcium antagonist can be added, such as verapamil or diltiazem. If there is evidence of LV dysfunction, cardiogenic shock, or prolonged PR intervals with possible heart block, these CCBs should be avoided.[4]

Another medication classification associated with decreased mortality in patients with LV systolic dysfunction and EF less than 40% is the angiotensin-converting enzyme (ACE) inhibitor. ACE inhibitors have also been found to be beneficial in patients with NSTE-ACS who have DM, HTN, and stable CKD. In these patients, the addition of an ACE inhibitor has been associated with a decrease in mortality and increase in survival at 30 days. If the patient does not tolerate ACE inhibitors, angiotensin receptor blockers (ARBs) can be used. Combinations of these medications can be used to control symptoms and limit ischemia.[4,73]

Statin therapy should be initiated or continued in all patients presenting with ACS. In the initial studies in PROVE IT-TIMI 22 (Pravastatin or Atorvastatin Evaluation and Infection Therapy-Thrombolysis In Myocardial Infarction) and MIRACL (Myocardial Ischemia Reduction With Acute Cholesterol Lowering) trials, high-dose atorvastatin provided the most benefit in reducing MI, stroke, and death.[4,13,14,73,88] A lipid panel should be obtained within 24 hours of presentation to provide a baseline for care. Once statins are initiated, careful monitoring for myopathy and hepatic toxicity should be done periodically. The FDA recommends that liver enzyme tests should be performed before starting statin therapy and as clinically indicated thereafter.[4,73,104] If the patient complains of muscle pain and weakness, myopathy should be considered and a creatine kinase (CK) level should be obtained to determine whether treatment should be discontinued or changed.[4,73] Table 3.6 summarizes information on the anti-ischemic drugs.

Treatment Pathways of NSTE-ACS

Pending patients' risk stratification, symptomatology, and hemodynamic state, the clinician may decide upon two

TABLE 3.5 **Medications Used for Antiplatelet and Anticoagulation Therapy**

Medication	Actions	Dosage	Special Considerations
Oral Antiplatelet Therapy			
Aspirin (ASA)	Blocks production of thromboxane A_2, which induces platelet aggregation	Initial dose 162–325 mg PO nonenteric followed by 81–325 mg PO daily	Important for first dose to be nonenteric for better absorption
Clopidogrel (Plavix)	$P2Y_{12}$ inhibitor	Loading dose 300 mg; followed by 75 mg PO daily	Loading for more rapid onset • Discontinue at least 5 days prior to surgery
Ticagrelor (Brilinta)	$P2Y_{12}$ inhibitor	180 mg loading dose, then 90 mg BID	Shorter half-life • Need to decrease ASA to 81 mg daily • Discontinue at least 5 days prior to surgery
Prasugrel (Effient)	$P2Y_{12}$ inhibitor	60 mg loading dose, then 10 mg daily (5 mg if >75 years or <65 kg)	Once-a-day therapy • Do not start until anatomy is known via angiography • Need to decrease ASA to 81 mg daily • Do not use in TIA or stroke patients • Discontinue at least 5 days prior to surgery
Intravenous Antiplatelet Therapy			
Tirofiban (Aggrastat)	Prevents platelet aggregation by preventing fibrinogen binding	0.4 mcg/kg/min IV for 30 min followed by 0.1 mcg/kg/min for 48–96 hr	Monitor for occult bleeding (retroperitoneal or groin) Monitor platelet count
Eptifibatide (Integrilin)	Prevents platelet aggregation by preventing fibrinogen binding	180 mcg/kg IV bolus followed by 2 mcg/kg/min infusion for 72–96 hr Can give second bolus 10 min after first bolus if needed	Monitor for occult bleeding (retroperitoneal or groin) Monitor platelet count
Anticoagulant Therapy			
Enoxaparin (Lovenox)	Increases action of antithrombin, inactivating thrombin, but more potent on inhibition of factor Xa Increases action of antithrombin, inactivating thrombin, but more potent on inhibition of factor Xa	1 mg/kg SC q 12 hr (reduce dose to 1 mg/kg SC once daily in patients with creatinine clearance <30 mL/min) May use loading dose 30 mg IV in selected patients	No lab parameter to measure effects (can check anti-Xa levels if using long term) Dose should be adjusted for renal impairment Monitor platelet count
Heparin (UFH)	Increases action of antithrombin, inactivating thrombin	Bolus 60 units/kg IV (max is 4000 units) followed by 12 units/kg/h (max is 1000 units/h)	Adjust per PTT Monitor platelet count Should be continued for 48 hours or until PCI
Bivalirudin (Angiomax)	Direct thrombin inhibitor	0.10 mg/kg loading dose followed by 0.25 mg/kg/h	
Fondaparinux (Arixtra)	Selected inhibitor of factor Xa	2.5 mg SC daily	Do not use if CrCl <30 mL/min
Argatroban (Argatroban)	Direct thrombin inhibitor used if patient has HIT	Usual dose is 2 mcg/kg/min adjust to keep PTT 1.5–3 times the baseline but not over 100	

ASA, Aspirin; *BID*, twice daily; *CrCl*, creatinine clearance; *IV*, intravenous; *PCI*, percutaneous coronary intervention; *PO*, per os; *PTT*, partial prothrombin time; *SC*, subcutaneous; *TIA*, transient ischemic attack.
Data from Reference 4.

different strategies: ischemia-guided strategy versus early invasive strategy. The ischemia-guided strategy is chosen when the patient is hemodynamically stable and does not have objective evidence of ischemia, such as acute ECG changes or ongoing angina at rest. The patient undergoes a noninvasive evaluation and is medically optimized with medication therapy. The advantage of this therapy is that the patient may be stabilized with medical therapy and avoid invasive coronary angiography. If the patient has a high-risk score, DM, and/or renal insufficiency, the clinician may decide to take the patient for a delayed coronary angiogram with possible PCI within 72 hours of medical optimization.[4]

If the patient is hemodynamically unstable or has refractory angina, they may be taken for early invasive therapy via primary PCI. This may be done within 2 hours of presentation or may be delayed for 24–72 hours to medically optimize the patient and allow the plaque to stabilize with the aid of antiplatelet, anticoagulation, and anti-ischemic therapy. The advantage of the invasive treatment pathway is that early revascularization could prevent further complications or infarction, and the patient could potentially discharge earlier from the hospital. Risk assessment, and continued symptomatology, as well as the clinician's clinical assessment are all important pieces to the ultimate pathway chosen and overall outcomes of the patient.[4]

ST-ELEVATION MYOCARDIAL INFARCTION

Of all patients presenting with ACS, approximately 29–38% will present with ST-elevation myocardial infarction (STEMI).[64]

TABLE 3.6 **Medications Used for Anti-Ischemic Therapy**

Medication	Actions	Dosage	Special Considerations
Nitrates			
Nitroglycerin (NTG)	Potent vasodilator of capacitance vessels; reduces preload, thereby reducing ventricular wall tension and myocardial oxygen consumption	Administer sublingual or spray as needed every 5 min × 3 as needed; if IV needed, start at 10 mcg/min and increase 10 mcg every 3–5 min	Monitor for hypotension Contraindicated with recent phosphodiesterase inhibitor intake
Beta Blockers			
Metoprolol (Lopressor)	Blocks effects of catecholamines on cell membrane beta receptors; $beta_1$ selective	50–200 mg PO twice daily; IV with chest pain, 5 mg IV every 5 min × 3	Monitor for bradycardia; hypotension; bronchospasm less likely
Carvediol (Coreg)	Blocks effects of catecholamines on cell membrane beta receptors; alpha-1–, beta-1– selective, and beta-2–receptor	3.125–50 mg twice a day or extended release Coreg (Coreg CR) dose 10–80 mg daily	Monitor for bradycardia and hypotension
Atenolol (Tenormin)	Blocks effects of catecholamines on cell membrane beta receptors; $beta_1$ selective	50–200 mg PO daily	Monitor for bradycardia; hypotension; bronchospasm less likely
Angiotensin-Converting Enzyme (ACE) Inhibitors			
Captopril (Capoten)	Inhibits formation of converting enzyme, thus formation of aldosterone	6.25–50 mg PO 1-3 times a day Max dose is 450 mg/day	Cough is side effect, not allergy; monitor for hyperkalemia and decreased renal function
Enalapril (Vasotec)	Inhibits formation of converting enzyme, thus formation of aldosterone	2.5–40 mg PO once or twice daily	Cough is side effect, not allergy; monitor for hyperkalemia and decreased renal function
Lisinopril (Prinivil, Zestril)	Inhibits formation of converting enzyme, thus formation of aldosterone	2.5–40 mg PO once daily	Cough is side effect, not allergy; monitor for hyperkalemia and decreased renal function
Angiotensin Receptor Blockers (ARB)			
Losartan (Cozaar)	Inhibits formation of angiotensin II and formation of aldosterone	25–50 mg once daily	Monitor for hyperkalemia and renal function
Valsartan (Diovan)	Inhibits formation of angiotensin II and formation of aldosterone	20–40 mg once daily	Monitor for hyperkalemia and renal function
Calcium Channel Blockers			
Diltiazem (Cardizem)	Reduces influx of transmembrane calcium influx, thus decreasing vascular wall contraction	180–360 mg/day; timing of dosages based on whether immediate or sustained release	Caution in patients with LV dysfunction and patients with heart block
Verapamil (Calan)	Reduces influx of transmembrane calcium influx, thus decreasing vascular wall contraction	120–240 mg/day; timing of dosages based on whether immediate or sustained release	Caution in patients with LV dysfunction and patients with heart block
High-Intensity Statin			
Atorvastatin (Lipitor)	HMG CoA reductase inhibitors	10–80 mg/day High dose 80 mg/day recommended in high-risk ACS patients who can tolerate	Caution with drugs metabolized via CYP3A4, fibrates Monitor for myopathy, hepatotoxicity

ACS, Acute coronary syndrome; *LV*, left ventricular; *NTG*, nitroglycerin; *PO*, per os.
Data from References 4 and 73.

As treatment and identification of patients with STEMI has improved, the number of mortalities and adverse outcomes has decreased.[65,73] A patient presenting with a STEMI is characterized by persistent ST elevation or a new left bundle branch block (LBBB) on the ECG, and an elevation of troponins. A STEMI is indicative of an acute MI and cell death is immediate. Therefore, urgency in implementing interventions becomes crucial. Education of the public focuses on entering the healthcare system as soon as possible by calling the emergency medical services (EMS).[73] All EMS and paramedics responding to a patient with chest pain should assess the patient's symptoms and obtain a 12-lead ECG as quickly as possible. A STEMI is defined as ST elevation at the J point in at least two contiguous leads of greater than or equal to 2 mm (0.2 mV) in men or greater than or equal to 1.5 mm (0.15 mV) in women in leads V_2–V_3 and/or of greater than or equal to 1 mm in more than two contiguous limb leads.[73] Fig. 3.3 summarizes ECG changes for ischemia and infarction. If the patient is suspected of having

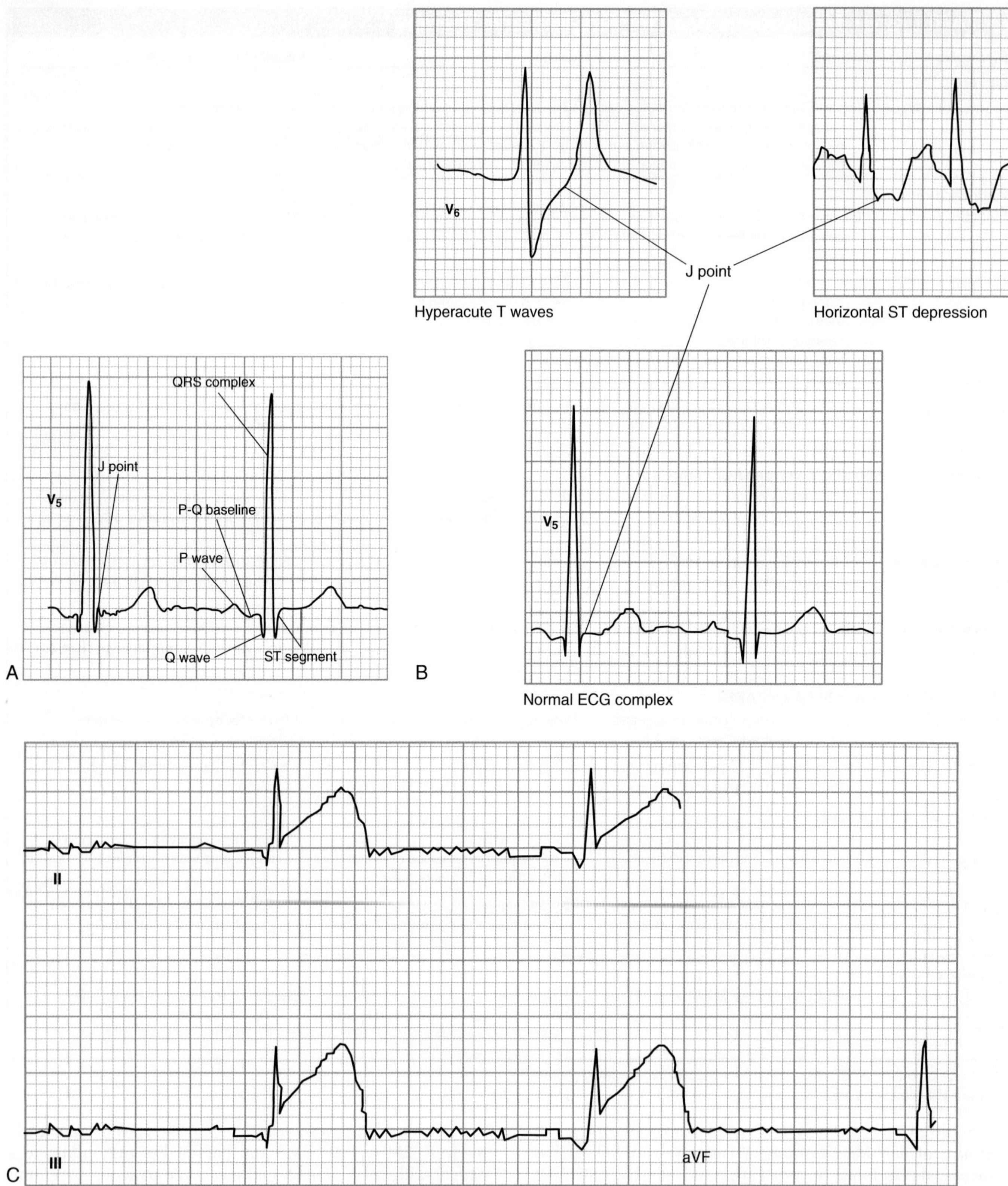

FIG. 3.3 Summary of electrocardiogram (ECG) changes for ischemia and infarction. **A,** Normal ECG. **B,** ST depression and hyperacute T waves. **C,** ST elevation.

BOX 3.2 Contraindications and Cautions for Fibrinolysis

Absolute contraindications

- Any prior intracranial hemorrhage
- Known structural cerebral vascular lesion
- Known malignant intracranial neoplasm (primary or metastatic)
- Ischemic stroke within 3 months EXCEPT acute ischemic stroke within 3 hours
- Suspected aortic dissection
- Active bleeding or bleeding diathesis (excluding menses)
- Significant closed head or facial trauma within 3 months
- Severe uncontrolled hypertension refractory to medications
- Prior treatment with streptokinase in past 6 months

Relative contraindications

- History of chronic, severe, poorly tolerated hypertension
- Severe uncontrolled hypertension on presentation (SBP >180 mm Hg or DBP >110 mm Hg)
- History of prior ischemic stroke greater than 3 months, dementia, or known intracranial pathology not covered in contraindications
- Traumatic or prolonged (>10 min) CPR or major surgery (<3 weeks)
- Recent (within 2–4 weeks) internal bleeding
- Noncompressible vascular punctures
- For streptokinase: prior exposure (>5 days ago) or prior allergic reaction to these agents
- Pregnancy
- Active peptic ulcer
- Current use of anticoagulants

CPR, Cardiopulmonary resuscitation; *DBP,* diastolic blood pressure; *SBP,* systolic blood pressure. Modified from Reference 72.

a STEMI, the EMS should take the patient to a PCI-capable hospital. All communities should have a regional system that includes a plan for the care of STEMI patients and maintain quality performance measures, especially on transport time and timing to treatment.[73]

Treatment of STEMI

The plan of care is similar to that discussed for NSTE-ACS. However, the one major difference is that urgent reperfusion therapy becomes the priority. It is presumed that the atheromatic plaque has ruptured and initiated the coagulation cascade, forming a thrombus large enough to completely obstruct blood flow in one or several coronary arteries. The ECG should be done within 10 minutes of first medical contact. Anti-ischemic therapy should be initiated similar to NSTE-ACS as indicated. Oxygen should be administered if the oxygen saturation of arterial blood is less than 90%. NTG should be administered in the presence of chest pain if the patient is hemodynamically stable. However, nitrates should not be given if: (1) the SBP is less than 90 mm Hg, (2) the SBP is greater than or equal to 30 mm Hg below baseline, (3) there is severe bradycardia (<50 beats/min) or tachycardia (>100 beats/min), (4) a right ventricular infarction is suspected, or (5) the patient has taken a phosphodiesterase inhibitor for erectile dysfunction (e.g., sildenafil [Viagra]) within the last 24 hours.[73] Since STEMI patients may have experienced significant myocardial muscle damage, they may be prone to cardiogenic shock and preload reduction with nitrates could exacerbate that situation. If STEMI or new LBBB is captured on the ECG and duration of symptoms has been less than 12 hours, reperfusion therapy either via primary PCI or fibrinolytic therapy is indicated.[73]

With the advances in technology and increased access to PCI centers, primary PCI is preferred over fibrinolytic therapy and should be performed as soon as possible. The optimum timeline goal is 90 minutes from "door to balloon," especially if congestive heart failure, pulmonary edema, or cardiogenic shock is present. Timing is essential for patients to achieve the greatest improvement in outcomes. Similar to NSTE-ACS, antiplatelet and anticoagulant therapy should be administered after completion of the procedure. PCI is best supported in hospitals that have on-site cardiac surgery programs. If cardiac surgery is not immediately available, a plan should be in place to expedite rapid transport to an appropriately equipped institution.[20,21,73]

Fibrinolytic therapy may be considered if PCI is not immediately available; however, the risk of bleeding is a major concern and evaluation needs to be thorough to avoid major complications. If the patient is initially seen in an emergency department, the goal for initiation of fibrinolytic therapy is 30 minutes "door to needle." Ideally, fibrinolytic therapy should be administered within the first 2 hours of onset of chest pain. The longer the time between onset of symptoms and presentation, the less likely fibrinolytic therapy will be successful.[73]

The goal of fibrinolytic therapy is early clot lysis by attacking the fibrin component of the clot, hence the term *fibrinolysis.* According to the classic work by Topol,[100] this pharmacologic intervention is achieved using thrombolytic agents that can be divided into two categories: (1) fibrin selective, which activates the fibrin-bound plasminogen and lyses clots quickly, and (2) nonselective agents, which provide more systemic plasminogenolysis and fibrinogenolysis at a slower rate and a more prolonged systemic lytic state. Before choosing a thrombolytic agent, it is imperative that a risk assessment for bleeding be completed. Absolute and relative contraindications are summarized in Box 3.2. A complete focused assessment, including neurologic history, becomes essential to establish a baseline and provide clues to possible contraindications for fibrinolysis. A summary of the more commonly used thrombolytics can be found in Table 3.7.[10,73]

Combinations of pharmacologic therapies with thrombolytic agents have been tested to help maintain arterial flow. Continuous IV heparin, enoxaparin (Lovenox), or fondaparinux (Arixtra) is recommended for up to 48 hours to maintain arterial patency. The patient should receive ASA and a $P2Y_{12}$ inhibitor, such as clopidogrel (Plavix), for at least 14 days.[73]

Obvious complications can be avoided by close monitoring of all disruptions in skin integrity, including mucous membranes, wounds, and vascular access sites. Monitoring for adequate tissue perfusion should include specific attention to certain body systems. One of the most devastating consequences can be intracranial hemorrhage (ICH). Neurologic assessment skills should be refined to detect more subtle changes in level of consciousness. Change in cognitive processes, subtle changes in speech, or minor motor deficits may be early signs of cerebral bleeding. If there is any suspicion of ICH, the institution's stroke protocol should be initiated, including neurology or neurosurgery consults, and any type of anticoagulation or fibrinolytic therapy should be discontinued until there is radiologic evidence of the

TABLE 3.7 **Medications Used as Thrombolytic Agents**

Medication	Action	Dosage	Special Considerations
Fibrin Selective			
Alteplase (rt-PA)	Increased affinity to fibrin, which activates fibrin-bound plasminogen	Up to 100 mg in 90 min based on weight	Monitor for occult bleeding (retroperitoneal or groin)
Reteplase (r-PA)	Increased affinity to fibrin, which activates fibrin-bound plasminogen	Two 10-megaunit IV bolus given 30 min apart	Monitor for occult bleeding (retroperitoneal or groin)
Tenecteplase (TNKase)	Increased affinity to fibrin, which activates fibrin-bound plasminogen; very fibrin specific	30–50 mg based on weight	Monitor for occult bleeding (retroperitoneal or groin)
Nonselective			
Streptokinase (SK)	Combines with circulating plasminogen, forming complexes that catalyze plasmin formation	1.5 million units infused over 30–60 min	Monitor for occult bleeding (retroperitoneal or groin); monitor for allergic reaction

Data from References 10 and 73.

absence of ICH.[72] Hypovolemia and hypotension can exacerbate myocardial perfusion issues and can lead to increased frequency or intensity of chest pain, ECG changes, or associated respiratory distress. Renal perfusion may also be compromised because of hypoperfusion or myocardial dysfunction. Careful monitoring of urine output and renal function, including trending BUN, creatinine, and calculated creatinine clearance values, should be integrated into nursing care. Testing all body secretions for blood, measuring and accurately recording blood loss, and participating in interventions to prevent injury, such as use of soft mouth care utensils, minimal blood sampling, and avoidance of invasive procedures (e.g., nasogastric tubes, rectal tubes), are all standard nursing interventions.[10]

Interventional Reperfusion Therapy

Coronary angiography is the gold standard in studying coronary artery anatomy and flow. Early invasive therapy is recommended via coronary angiography if the patient has a STEMI, is high risk with NSTE-ACS, or continues to have angina despite medical therapy. The timing depends on a number of factors. If immediately available, coronary angiography with possible PCI should be performed on STEMI patients with the goal of 90 minutes from door to balloon. “Rescue PCI” may also be performed within 12 hours after failed fibrinolysis and is used in patients who continue to have myocardial ischemia. If the patient has a NSTE-ACS, the timing of angiography may be delayed depending on the patient’s risk and symptoms.[4,52,73]

A coronary angiography study usually includes a left-sided heart catheterization consisting of a ventriculogram that can determine ventricular anatomy and function (ejection fraction), as well as visualize valve structure and function. The usual access site for any angiographic intervention is the right common femoral artery, but the left femoral artery, radial artery, or brachial artery may also be used. A right-sided heart catheterization can be performed by accessing the femoral, internal jugular, or subclavian veins. This study is obtained to evaluate the right heart performance, pressures, and valve function, as well as to detect the presence of a pathologic left to right shunt by measuring progressive oxygen saturation in the vessels, right atrium, and right ventricle.[20,52] The same technique is used for men and women. However, the technical difficulty is somewhat increased in women because of the smaller vessel size. Because of the potential for increased complications, the benefit of invasive strategies in women with ACS is limited to high-risk women.[4,52]

If the information obtained in the catheterization indicates a need for further intervention, a PCI may be performed at that time. The expertise of the operator plays an important role. The ACC/AHA guidelines for PCI, revised in 2011,[52] recommend that the operator maintain an acceptable volume of interventions (more than 75 procedures per year) with cardiac surgery capabilities. The most common procedures available are (1) percutaneous transluminal coronary angioplasty (PTCA), (2) coronary stent placement with bare metal stent (BMS), and (3) coronary stent placement with drug eluting stent (DES).[20,52]

PTCA is an intervention often transitioned to during the catheterization. A guide catheter is placed with a wire across the lesion. A prepared balloon is inserted over the wire, placed across the lesion, and inflated multiple times at various pressures depending on the physician’s preference (Fig. 3.4). Because early outcomes of PTCA initially included acute or delayed restenosis, the coronary stent was introduced to counteract the elastic recoil that occurred in the coronary artery after PTCA (Fig. 3.5). The BMS was designed to be mounted on a balloon that, when expanded, would deploy the device and implant it into the lesion of the coronary artery. Various designs are available (e.g., mesh, coil, slotted tube, ring) and are composed of several materials (e.g., stainless steel, cobalt alloy, tantalum). Initial stenting procedures also had variable outcomes. The stent may produce injury to the endothelium of the artery and may initiate or worsen the inflammatory process, leading to hyperplasia, restenosis, or thrombosis.[20]

To counteract the complications of the BMS, the DES was developed and is now used over 80% of the time. These stents are coated with a drug or material with antiproliferative properties to prevent or lessen the insult to the arterial endothelium and maintain blood flow through the lumen. The first DES was approved in 2003 for use in PCI and was the CYPHER, BX VELOCITY stent. It is a stainless steel stent that has a polymer coating and is impregnated with the drug sirolimus, which is an immunosuppressant that allows normal growth of the endothelium. The polymer coating of the stent decreases the cytokine response and inflammation of the smooth muscle cell.[20,63] These two actions decrease the restenosis rate associated with this intervention. The second DES was approved in 2004 and was the TAXUS paclitaxel-eluting stent. The TAXUS is a polymer-coated stent in which the paclitaxel is a biphasic treatment that has its initial bolus in the first 2 days followed by a sustained-release dose for 10 days.[20,34]

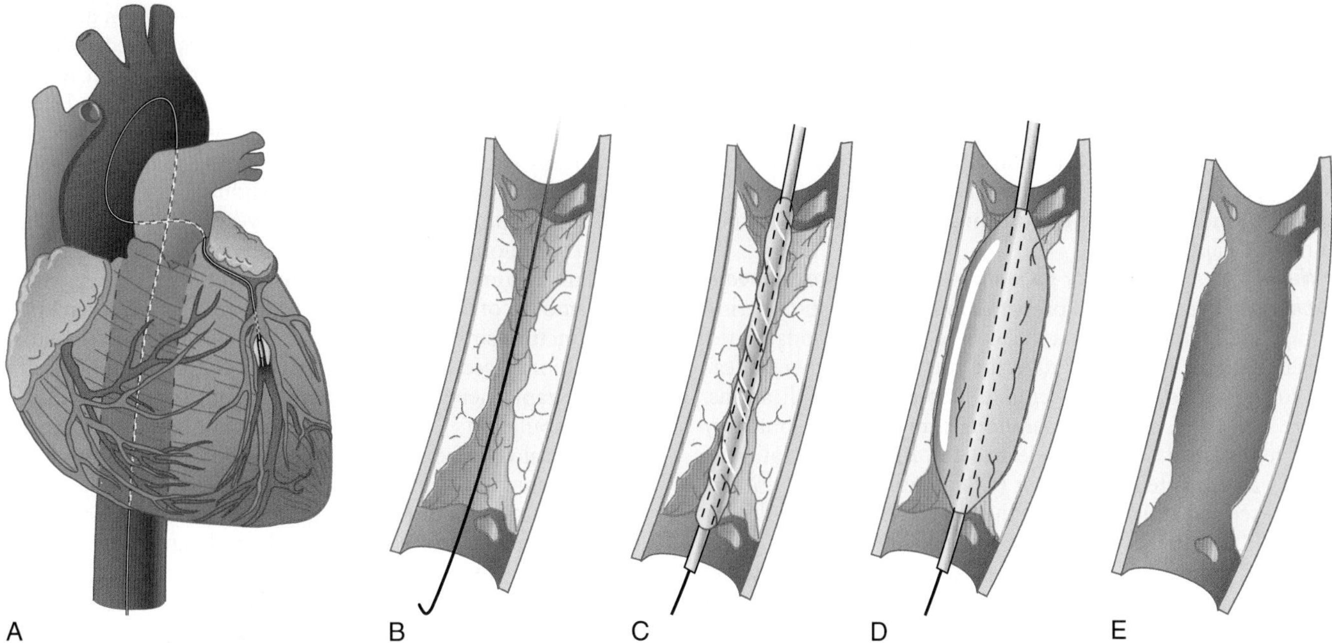

FIG. 3.4 Percutaneous transluminal coronary angioplasty (PTCA). Mechanism of intracoronary balloon angioplasty. **A,** The balloon catheter is introduced into the coronary artery via the catheter in the aorta. **B,** A guidewire is advanced across the area of narrowing. **C,** The balloon catheter is advanced over the wire across the lesion. **D,** The balloon is inflated. **E,** The opened coronary artery as it appears after the PTCA.

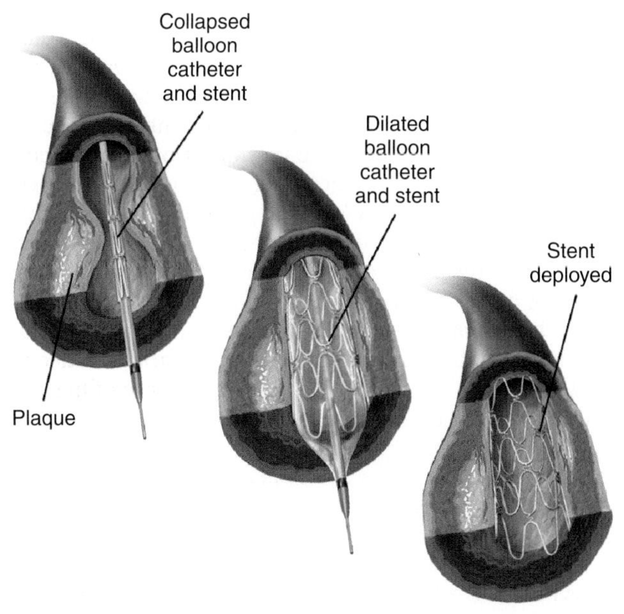

FIG. 3.5 Cardiac stent.

The CYPHER and TAXUS stents are considered first-generation DES and in 2008 new technology brought a second generation of stents called the zotarolimus-eluting stent (ZES) and the everolimus-eluting stent (EES). The platform of these two stents is made of a cobalt-chromium or platinum-chromium alloy and is thinner and more deliverable than the first-generation DES. The second-generation DES are also more biocompatible than first-generation DES and therefore generate less inflammatory response and have more rapid vessel endothelialization or healing.[43,91,93,94] In a meta-analysis of 33 randomized control trials, second-generation stents offer similar efficacy to reduce risk of revascularization, and showed a significant decrease in risk of having a myocardial infarction after placement.[69]

Several other interventional techniques have been developed to help create arterial patency and restenosis. Coronary atherectomy is a technique in which the atheromatous plaque is removed by either a cutter or a burr rotating at a high speed. Because the technique also causes damage to the endothelial wall, cell hyperplasia and restenosis may occur. This intervention may be accompanied by a stent placement to enhance the likelihood that the lumen remains patent.[20]

The presence of intracoronary thrombus may be the main reason for the total obstruction of blood flow in the artery. Thrombectomy devices have been developed to help remove thrombotic material. The angiojet and aspiration catheters have been developed to extract thrombus. Since the thrombus and fragments can move down the coronary system and further obstruct the artery, distal protective devices have been created to help protect the artery from becoming further occluded.[20]

Restenosis is a major complication of any PCI and interventions have been developed to treat the complication. Laser angioplasty was originally used to remove atherosclerotic lesions, but had poor outcomes. However, it is being evaluated again. Tissue ablation is thought to be achieved using a combination of photochemical, localized thermal, and mechanical effects.[20] Brachytherapy provides local radiation treatment to the coronary artery wall to decrease the formation of hyperplastic cells. Any of these techniques can have complications, including perforation or late thrombosis. Other complications associated with these interventions are recurrent chest pain, abrupt closure, vascular spasm, stroke, TIA, NSTEMI, STEMI, dysrhythmias or conduction disorders, and contrast-related complications.[20]

Revascularization of the coronary arteries can also be achieved surgically. Coronary artery bypass graft (CABG) surgery has been used for revascularization for many years and continues to be a viable option even with the development of PCIs.[4,73] A more complete discussion of cardiac surgery can be found in Chapter 5.

Nursing interventions for patients treated with percutaneous coronary interventions. The preparation for, observation period during, and follow-up after a PCI can be pivotal periods for the cardiac patient. It is imperative the nurse has proper education in the care of these patients to help avoid complications. Before the study, the nurse should ensure baseline laboratory tests are obtained, including electrolytes, BUN and creatinine, glucose, a complete blood count (CBC), and, if the patient has been prescribed anticoagulation therapy, coagulation studies. A baseline 12-lead ECG should also be available. If there is a suspicion of ongoing ischemic events, cardiac biomarkers may also be measured. Evaluation of the intravascular volume status of these patients is critical to maintaining adequate renal function. Because the patient will be NPO, intravenous fluids should be ordered. Diuretics may be withheld, depending on the patient's volume status. Oral hypoglycemic agents, especially metformin (Glucophage), are withheld because their use is associated with an increased risk of renal dysfunction. Metformin should also be withheld 48 hours after the intervention.[3] Blood glucose levels should be monitored and insulin ordered to maintain good blood glucose control. Refer to Chapter 24 for more information on glucose control.[3,20]

Renal function is an important parameter that may be compromised, especially with the contrast administered during a PCI. Adequate intravascular volume must be maintained to protect renal function. Assessment of intravascular volume includes HR, BP, and other hemodynamic parameters as available. HR may not be a reliable parameter if a beta blocker is used. There are different types of contrast available for these procedures. The low osmolar nonionic agents are most commonly used to lessen intravascular depletion from the contrast. N-acetylcysteine (Mucomyst) and/or sodium bicarbonate infusion may be used before and after the infusion of contrast to help avoid acute kidney injury related to contrast infusion in patients with CKD. More recent literature suggests that the most effective intervention is adequate hydration before and after the procedure. If the patient has a contrast or iodine allergy, premedication with an antihistamine and steroids can be used.[52]

After the PCI, the same laboratory values (electrolytes, CBC, BUN, and creatinine) that were measured as baselines are obtained concomitant with a 12-lead ECG. Close observation for chest pain, any type of dysrhythmia, and hemodynamic instability should be maintained. If not removed in the catheterization laboratory, the femoral sheath should be removed within 4 to 6 hours after the procedure. An activated clotting time (ACT) is used to monitor anticoagulation status; it should be less than 180 seconds before pulling the sheath. The sheath can be discontinued using either manual compression or a compression device. Pressure should be maintained for 20 minutes, observing for distal circulation, hemodynamic stability, and bleeding at the site.[20] Visualization of the insertion site is very important. Equipment obscuring the site (such as sandbags) can limit the ability to detect bleeding. To help avoid a vagal reaction during sheath removal, adequate hydration and femoral site pain control should be addressed. Pain medication can decrease painful stimuli and tendency of the patient to "bear down," which increases vagal tone. The head of the bed should be less than 30 degrees to ensure hemostasis and comfort. Once the sheath is removed, frequent neurovascular checks of the affected extremity and puncture site should be performed as per institutional protocol. Initial checks every 15 minutes for 1 hour would commonly be included in observation guidelines.[10,87]

Manual compression is still considered the "gold standard" for removal of arterial sheaths.[87,108] Proper management of the puncture site can allow faster mobilization of this patient population. Vascular closure devices (VCDs) are now used to achieve rapid hemostasis, improve patient comfort, and allow early ambulation.[108] Passive VCDs enhance hemostasis through mechanical compression (e.g., Femostop compression device) or prothrombotic material applied via pads or other material over the puncture site (e.g., D-stat Dry). However, they do not actually prompt hemostasis and have not shown to decrease time to ambulation. Active VCDs facilitate hemostasis through either a suture (e.g., Perclose) or a collagen plug (e.g., Angioseal). They have shown to decrease time to ambulation, thus decreasing hospitalization time. VCDs do not reduce the risk of infection or vascular complications and still need to be monitored for complications and bleeding.[88,108]

Complications related to angiography and arterial puncture include hematoma, retroperitoneal bleeding, arterial thrombosis, pseudoaneurysm, and arteriovenous fistula. A high index of suspicion should be maintained when observing these patients. Gentle palpation of the groin puncture site may assist with hematoma detection. Auscultation over the site for a vascular bruit can help with early detection of an arteriovenous fistula. Monitoring hemoglobin and hematocrit provides trends indicating increased bleeding. Monitoring of flank areas near the sheath site should be done to evaluate for retroperitoneal bleeding. Subtle changes, such as increased numbness and tingling of the effected extremity, may indicate pressure from an expanding hematoma on nerves in the groin.[52,87,108] Astute observations may help detect issues earlier, leading to interventions that may lessen devastating complications.

Post procedure pharmacotherapy. Antiplatelet and antithrombotic agents are administered before, during, and after the PCI. ASA should be administered indefinitely after the PCI. In addition to ASA, a $P2Y_{12}$ inhibitor, such as clopidogrel (Plavix), ticagrelor (Brilinta), or prasugrel (Effient), should be administered for up to 1 year after a DES placement, or for at least 30 days after a BMS. Unfractionated heparin or glycoprotein Iib/IIIa inhibitors may be used intravenously during an angioplasty and for a short period after the procedure to prevent platelet aggregation and platelet formation. Bivalirudin (Angiomax) is an alternative anticoagulant that can be used alone or with unfractionated heparin and has been shown to reduce bleeding rates compared to glycoprotein Iib/IIIa inhibitors.[52,73,108]

Other pharmacologic interventions for the STEMI patient are similar to those discussed concerning the NSTE-ACS patients. Medications to decrease myocardial workload, including beta blockers and ACE inhibitors, should be considered as soon as BP and cardiac function are within normal parameters. Statin therapy should be initiated or continued in all patients presenting with ACS. Treatment with statins lowers the risk of death, recurrent MI, stroke, and future need for coronary revascularization.[73]

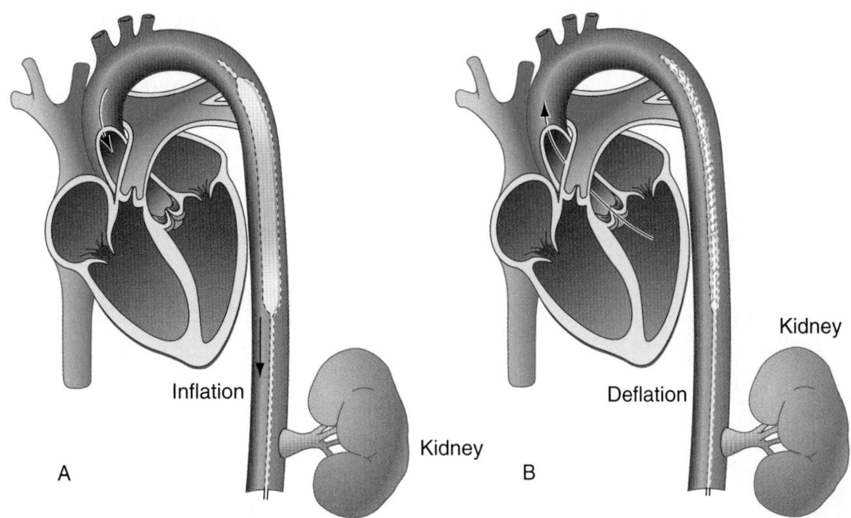

FIG. 3.6 Intra-aortic balloon pump movement. **A,** Inflation during diastole moves blood toward the heart. **B,** Deflation during systole moves blood away from the heart.

Complications of STEMI

If myocardial muscle is deprived of blood flow, cardiac function will deteriorate and cardiogenic shock occurs (Chapter 28). The degree of dysfunction is somewhat dependent on the amount of muscle lost and the anatomic region of the damage. Anterior wall damage can result in major pump failure and cardiogenic shock. Recommended interventions for shock are (1) volume management using a pulmonary artery catheter (PAC) and (2) inotropic support, if needed with sympathomimetic drugs, such as dobutamine (Dobutrex) or milrinone (Primacor). These agents have $beta_1$ and $beta_2$ activity that improve myocardial contractility, as well as decrease afterload. If shock is severe, alpha agonists such as norepinephrine (Levophed) are used to maintain adequate perfusion. Patients with inferior wall STEMI should be assessed for right ventricular infarction using right precordial chest leads, as well as echocardiography. STEMI patients with right ventricular infarctions are dependent on adequate preload and atrial-ventricular synchrony for optimal function.[73]

Mechanical interventions can also support myocardial muscle as it recovers from a significant insult. Current AHA/ACC guidelines recommend a hemodynamic support device for patients with cardiogenic shock and heart failure after an ACS event who do not quickly stabilize with pharmacologic or interventional therapy.[52] The IABP is one device that employs the concept of counterpulsation to improve myocardial performance. Counterpulsation is inflation during ventricular diastole and deflation during isometric ventricular contraction—"counter" balloon movement in relation to ventricular activity. The balloon is placed in the aorta just below the left subclavian artery and above the renal artery via percutaneous insertion in the femoral artery. The device actually displaces volume while moving in the aorta. With balloon inflation, volume is displaced proximally, which increases aortic root pressure while the aortic valve is closed. This action improves the perfusion of the coronary arteries, increasing oxygen delivery to the myocardial muscle. Blood volume is also displaced distally during balloon inflation, which can improve renal perfusion. Deflation of the balloon causes a decrease in intra-aortic blood volume, thereby decreasing impedance of blood flow out of the ventricle or reducing afterload of the left ventricle (Fig. 3.6). Increasing oxygen delivery to compromised myocardial muscle improves contractility and cardiac output (CO). With increased CO, intraventricular pressures decrease, thereby decreasing preload. Afterload reduction also improves CO and function. It is the mechanical equivalent of pharmacologic inotropic support and arterial vasodilation, and is used alone or in conjunction with pharmacologic agents if the myocardium is severely compromised.[15,73]

If the patient has severe ventricular dysfunction from the ischemic event, an IABP may not be sufficient to maintain the patient's hemodynamic status. In this case, a short-term mechanical circulatory support (MCS) device may be needed for support. In recent years, a newer and smaller ventricular assist device (VAD) called the *Impella* has been developed to help support the pumping mechanisms of the heart. Similar to the IABP, the device can be placed through the femoral artery. A single cannula is threaded up the aorta across the aortic valve into the left ventricle with the assistance of fluoroscopy. Through the blood inlet and outlet, the device aspirates blood in the left ventricle and expels it to generate a flow of 2.5 L/min or 5.0 L/min depending on the device placed (Fig. 3.7). The device improves CO by providing continuous flow from the left ventricle. In severe cardiogenic shock cases related to pump failure, this device may provide significantly more flow compared to the IABP, which only generates 500 to 800 mL/min.[15]

Recent studies have evaluated the outcomes of patients undergoing PCI needing either an IABP or Impella device. The PROTECT II trial compared the 30-day and 90-day major adverse event (MAE) for patients who were supported with IABP or Impella. The study showed there was no difference in mortality between the two devices or MAE at 30 days. At 90 days, though, the Impella showed significantly fewer MAEs than the IABP. The procedural hemodynamics were also analyzed and showed maintenance of CO and arterial pressure were superior with the Impella.[18,75] Further studies need to be performed, but the Impella now has a place in the care of cardiogenic shock and treatment of ACS.

Dysrhythmias are another complication of the STEMI patient. Serious ventricular dysrhythmias, such as ventricular tachycardia (VT) and ventricular fibrillation (VF), can be

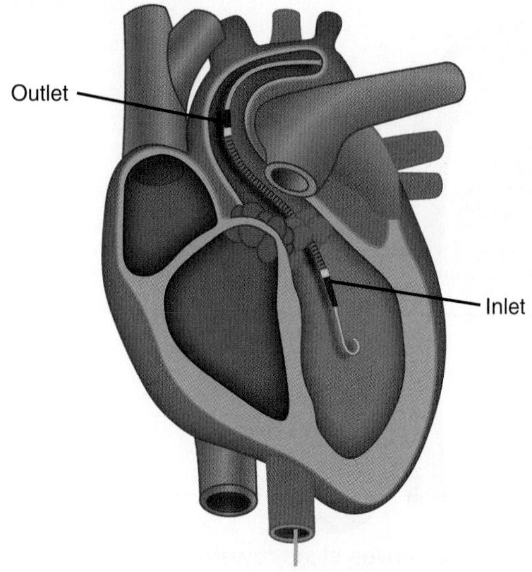

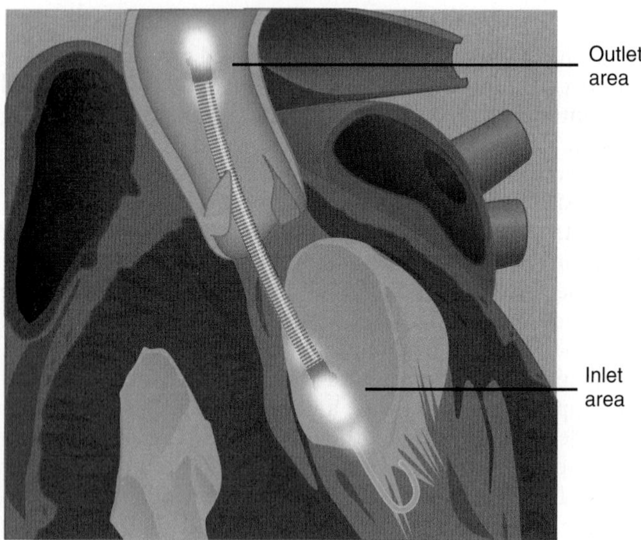

FIG. 3.7 Impella device. (From Urden, L., Stacy, K.M., Lough, M.E. (2014). *Critical care nursing* (7th ed.). St. Louis: Mosby.)

treated using various methods. Emergent deterioration resulting in VF or pulseless VT requires immediate, unsynchronized electric shock following advanced cardiac life support (ACLS) algorithms.[70,73] Amiodarone (Cordarone) is a drug recommended to control these life-threatening rhythms. If the patient continues to experience VF or sustained pulseless VT for more than 2 days after the STEMI, placement of an implantable cardioverter-defibrillator (ICD) is recommended.[73]

Atrial fibrillation is another rhythm that can complicate the post-STEMI course. Treatment priorities are to control the heart rate and convert to sinus rhythm. Lifelong anticoagulation to decrease the risk of stroke may be indicated if the patient remains in atrial fibrillation. Bradycardia and conduction defects are complications of inferior and anterior MIs. Depending on the severity of the disorder, a permanent pacemaker may be inserted to maintain adequate atrial-ventricular synchrony. A complete discussion of dysrhythmias and associated interventions can be found in Chapter 2.[73]

Another complication seen in patients after the STEMI patient is pericarditis (inflammation of the pericardium), which can be treated with ASA. If ASA is not sufficient, the administration of acetaminophen, colchicine, or narcotic analgesic can be used to improve symptomatology and outcomes. Nonsteroidal anti-inflammatory drugs (NSAIDs) should be avoided due to potential for bleeding. If a pericardial effusion develops, anticoagulation should be discontinued immediately to avoid cardiac tamponade.[73] The critical care nurse should always be alert for signs of these complications and initiate institutional protocols early.

INTERVENTIONS IN WOMEN WITH ACS

Women have a higher rate of in-hospital and long-term outcomes after having an ACS event than men. Despite worse outcomes, women with ACS events are under-prescribed guideline-directed therapy, both during the acute event and at discharge.[4,106] This under treatment is possibly related to diagnostic uncertainty and delays in symptom recognition. In general, following an ACS event, women should receive the same pharmacologic and lifestyle interventions as men.[4,22,102]

After an ACS event, women are less likely to receive thrombolytics, antidysrhythmics, antiplatelet agents, beta blockers, and ACE inhibitors. Women derive the same treatment benefit as men from ASA, $P2Y_{12}$ inhibitors, anticoagulants, beta blockers, ACE inhibitors, and statins.[4,22,102] Women metabolize drugs differently than men, which may produce clinically relevant adverse drug reactions. Women have a 50% higher risk of adverse drug reactions, which could be related to the response differences attributable to dosing not being corrected for a lower body weight, the higher percent of body fat in women than in men, and a 10% lower glomerular filtration rate in women. This accounts for the higher risk of potential bleeding in women when utilizing antiplatelet and anticoagulant agents.[4,50] In the 2014 ACC/AHA guidelines on management of patients with NSTE-ACS, it is a Class I recommendation that clinicians pay close attention to weight and/or renally calculated doses of antiplatelet and anticoagulant agents to reduce bleeding risk.[4]

Evidence indicates that high-risk women who present with symptoms of ACS and have elevated troponins benefit the most from early intervention versus ischemia-guided therapy. Amsterdam et al.[4] in the 2014 ACC/AHA guidelines based their decisions on meta-analysis and *post hoc* gender analyses clinical trials. At 1 year, women with early invasive versus ischemia-guided therapy had better outcomes and decreased mortality.[4,23] However, women have a higher risk of procedure and vascular complications after PCI attributed to the smaller body surface area (BSA), smaller coronary arteries, sheaths that are too large for the vessel, and nonweight-adjusted anticoagulant dosing.[4,20,72] As discussed earlier, less aggressive anticoagulation regimens and increased use of weight-adjusted heparin dosing have helped to decrease the incidence of these complications.[20,23]

The benefit of primary PCI over fibrinolytic therapy in women presenting with STEMI has been clearly demonstrated. In observational registries, women are reported to have similar or lower target-lesion revascularization (TLR) rates after balloon angioplasty and stenting.[23,52] It has been shown that DESs are effective in reducing restenosis and enhancing event-free survival in women as well as men.[4,52] Restenosis rates may be slightly higher in women because of the presence of other risk factors as previously described.[4] Given the evidence at this point, it seems that early invasive management of ACS with a PCI in women is beneficial, especially in those with elevated troponin values, which puts them in a higher risk category.[4]

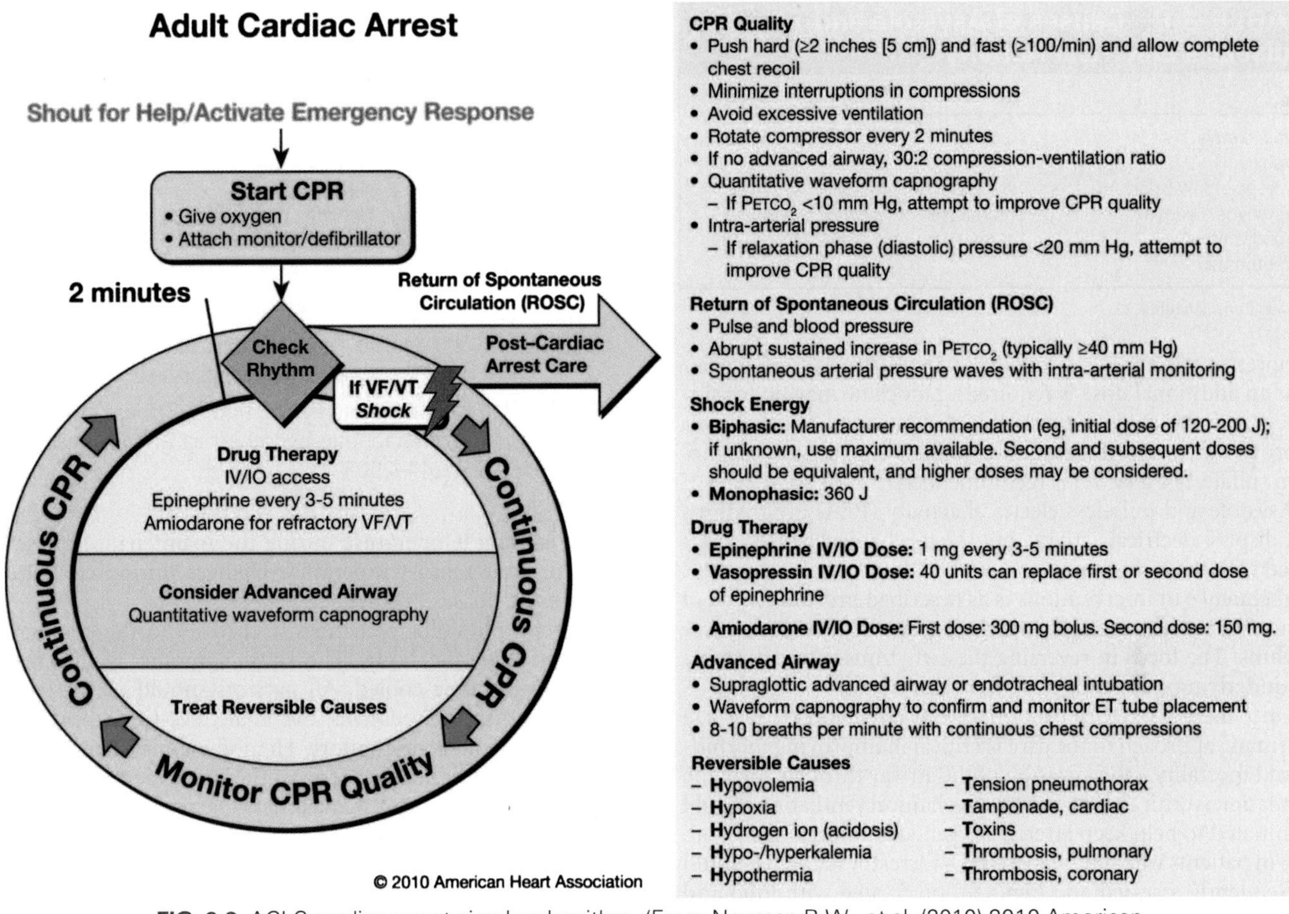

Adult Cardiac Arrest
Shout for Help/Activate Emergency Response
Start CPR
• Give oxygen
• Attach monitor/defibrillator
2 minutes
Return of Spontaneous Circulation (ROSC)
Check Rhythm
Post-Cardiac Arrest Care
If VF/VT Shock
Drug Therapy
IV/IO access
Epinephrine every 3-5 minutes
Amiodarone for refractory VF/VT
Consider Advanced Airway
Quantitative waveform capnography
Treat Reversible Causes
Continuous CPR
Continuous CPR
Monitor CPR Quality
© 2010 American Heart Association
CPR Quality
• Push hard (≥2 inches [5 cm]) and fast (≥100/min) and allow complete chest recoil
• Minimize interruptions in compressions
• Avoid excessive ventilation
• Rotate compressor every 2 minutes
• If no advanced airway, 30:2 compression-ventilation ratio
• Quantitative waveform capnography
– If P_{ETCO_2} <10 mm Hg, attempt to improve CPR quality
• Intra-arterial pressure
– If relaxation phase (diastolic) pressure <20 mm Hg, attempt to improve CPR quality
Return of Spontaneous Circulation (ROSC)
• Pulse and blood pressure
• Abrupt sustained increase in P_{ETCO_2} (typically ≥40 mm Hg)
• Spontaneous arterial pressure waves with intra-arterial monitoring
Shock Energy
• Biphasic: Manufacturer recommendation (eg, initial dose of 120-200 J); if unknown, use maximum available. Second and subsequent doses should be equivalent, and higher doses may be considered.
• Monophasic: 360 J
Drug Therapy
• Epinephrine IV/IO Dose: 1 mg every 3-5 minutes
• Vasopressin IV/IO Dose: 40 units can replace first or second dose of epinephrine
• Amiodarone IV/IO Dose: First dose: 300 mg bolus. Second dose: 150 mg.
Advanced Airway
• Supraglottic advanced airway or endotracheal intubation
• Waveform capnography to confirm and monitor ET tube placement
• 8-10 breaths per minute with continuous chest compressions
Reversible Causes
– Hypovolemia
– Hypoxia
– Hydrogen ion (acidosis)
– Hypo-/hyperkalemia
– Hypothermia
– Tension pneumothorax
– Tamponade, cardiac
– Toxins
– Thrombosis, pulmonary
– Thrombosis, coronary

FIG. 3.8 ACLS cardiac arrest circular algorithm. (From Neumar, R.W., et al. (2010) 2010 American Heart Association guidelines for cardiopulmonary resuscitation and emergency cardiovascular care science. Part 8: Adult advanced cardiovascular life support. *Circulation, 122,* S729–S767.)

As discussed previously, women often present with nonobstructive disease, most likely related to endothelial dysfunction, coronary spasm, and/or plaque rupture. Other studies, such as intracoronary ultrasound and/or optical coherence tomography, may be used to further study the arteries. If coronary spasm has not been ruled out, provocation testing during angiography with agents such as acetylcholine or methacholine may assess for atherosclerosis versus vasospasms. If vasospastic angina is suspected, treatment with calcium channel blocker and/or nitrates may be considered.[4]

EMERGENCY INTERVENTIONS

If the myocardium sustains significant damage, function is severely compromised and the patient may become hemodynamically unstable and experience a cardiac arrest. In 2010 the AHA published updated guidelines for cardiopulmonary resuscitation (CPR) and emergency CV care (ECC). The guidelines have been updated in an attempt to reflect the most recent scientific evidence and expert consensus opinion when evidence is limited. A major theme in the update emphasizes minimal interruption of CPR, especially after defibrillation, in order to enhance coronary perfusion pressure. The most critical intervention when a pulseless arrest is recognized is to initiate CPR and prepare for defibrillation. The three successive ("stacked") shocks have been replaced with one shock because first-shock success rate has improved, especially with biphasic defibrillators. When stacked shocks were used, researchers found that seconds were lost (up to 37 seconds) in charging the defibrillator, releasing the shock, and checking a pulse. Evidence suggests that one shock immediately followed by effective CPR may improve patient outcomes (Fig. 3.8).[70]

The amount of energy used depends on the type of defibrillator. Biphasic devices have individual effective joule levels ranging from 120 J to 200 J, but if the provider is unsure of the appropriate machine level, 200 J is an acceptable dose. If a monophasic machine is used, 360 J is the appropriate dose. If VF reoccurs, the previously successful energy level is delivered. Automated electrical defibrillators (AEDs) are now being used more frequently and are preset to deliver a set electrical dose. Once the shock is delivered, CPR is resumed for five cycles, although that time period may be altered in a hospital-monitored situation at the discretion of a physician.[70]

When VF/pulseless VT persists after at least one shock and a 2-minute CPR period, a vasopressor can be given. Epinephrine is the drug of choice at the dose of 1 mg IV/intraosseous (IO) every 3 to 5 minutes. Vasopressin 40 units IV/IO can be given once to replace the first or second dose of epinephrine. It is important not to interrupt CPR when administering any drug. Antidysrhythmics may be needed if electrical therapy is not successful in converting VF. Amiodarone should be administered when VF/VT is unresponsive to CPR, defibrillation, and

TABLE 3.8 Causes of Asystole and Pulseless Electrical Activity

Hs	Ts
Hypovolemia	Toxins
Hypoxia	Tamponade (cardiac)
Hydrogen ion (acidosis)	Tension pneumothorax
Hypo/hyperkalemia	Thrombosis (coronary or pulmonary)
Hypoglycemia	Trauma
Hypothermia	

Modified from Reference 70.

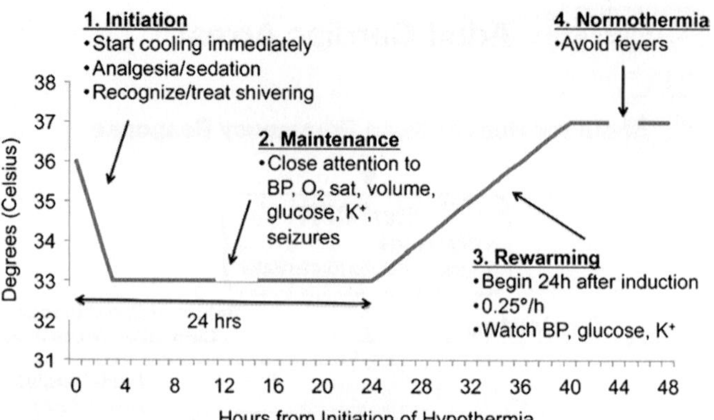

FIG. 3.9 Phases of hypothermia. (From Scirica, B.M. (2013) Clinician update: therapeutic hypothermia after cardiac arrest. *Circulation, 127,* 244–250.)

vasopressor therapy (first dose of 300 mg IV/IO and 150 mg IV/IO if an additional dose is required). Lidocaine may be considered if amiodarone is not available, but has not been shown to improve outcomes. If torsades de pointes is observed, magnesium sulfate 1–2 g IV/IO is recommended.[70]

Asystole and pulseless electrical activity (PEA) are rhythms that display electrical activity, but the mechanical activity associated with these rhythms is too weak to detect a palpable pulse. The sequence of interventions is as described previously except without electrical therapy, which is not effective with these rhythms. The focus in reversing these rhythms is to determine the underlying cause of the rhythm (Table 3.8).[70]

Once there is a return of spontaneous circulation (ROSC), a systematic approach to the care is critical in improving morbidity and mortality. Optimization of the airway through adequate ventilation is critical. If necessary, mechanical ventilation should be initiated to help keep arterial oxygen saturation greater than 94% in patients who have had a cardiac arrest. Vital signs should be frequently assessed and hypotension treated with fluid and inotropic therapy. Continuous ECG monitoring should be continued. Arrhythmias should be treated and an ECG reviewed for possible ACS events. Reperfusion therapy should be initiated immediately if an ACS event is suspected.[73,79]

Neurologic status should be assessed and if the patient does not follow commands, hypothermia therapy should be initiated.[79] Damage from cerebral anoxia starts within seconds of cardiac arrest and important cerebral activities are compromised. When ROSC is achieved, reperfusion of oxygen occurs to the brain, but injury continues to the cells due to the inflammatory processes that lead to endothelial dysfunction, vasomotor dysregulation, edema, and cellular-level hypoxia. Hypothermia helps decrease the inflammatory process as well as the cerebral metabolic rate of oxygen, cerebral blood volume, and intracranial pressure, thereby improving the oxygen supply-and-demand mismatch. Current studies and guidelines recommend therapeutic hypothermia (TH) for individuals who fail to meaningfully respond to verbal commands post cardiac arrest.[89]

TH should be initiated as soon as possible after ROSC. Studies show there is a 20% increase in mortality for every hour of delay in TH. There are four stages to TH: initiation, maintenance, rewarming, and return to normothermia (Fig. 3.9). Target temperature is 32° to 34°C. There are few contraindications to TH, but they include pregnancy, severe sepsis, hypotension refractory to vasopressors, excessive bleeding, major surgery within past 14 days, and ICH.[79,89] There are multiple ways to initiate cooling. Usually the initial cooling begins with cool saline infused over a period of time and ice packs. Temperature-regulating devices, such as the Artic Sun, are utilized by many institutions. These devices help better control and maintain temperature during the maintenance phase and help prevent rapid temperature changes during cooling and rewarming phases.[36,89]

Several physiologic changes occur due to the cooling and rewarming of the body. The most common is shivering as the body is being cooled. All patients should receive continuous infusions of sedatives and analgesics to prevent shivering and potential discomfort. Hemodynamic changes during cooling initially include tachycardia and hypertension due to the vasoconstriction of the arteries. Once cooled, bradycardia is the most common arrhythmia together with PR prolongation. It should only be treated if refractory hypotension occurs. Hypotension should be aggressively treated as it will further the decrease of cerebral circulation. All patients with TH require mechanical ventilation, and fraction of inspired oxygen (Fio_2) should be titrated to maintain an oxygen saturation between 94% and 96%.[89]

Electrolyte imbalance is a common problem with TH, specifically lower serum potassium and magnesium levels due to the inward cellular potassium flow. This is further complicated by hypothermia-induced diuresis. Electrolytes should be measured every 4 to 6 hours and replaced as needed. During the rewarming process, shifting will again occur and will need to be monitored closely.[89]

Hyperglycemia is also common during TH. As the temperature of the body decreases, so does insulin secretion, and insulin resistance increases. Patients should be on a continuous insulin drip during this period and monitored hourly to avoid extreme shifts in blood glucose levels. During the rewarming process, the insulin drip needs to be titrated slowly to keep blood sugars less than 200 mg/dL and hypoglycemia should be avoided.[89]

Hypothermia decreases cellular immunity. Infection is common and patients should be monitored for potential pulmonary and/or bloodstream infections. If infection is suspected, cultures should be sent and broad-spectrum antibiotics should be started.

Rewarming begins 12 to 24 hours after the initiation of cooling measures. Rewarming should be done slowly at a rate of 0.25°C/h until a temperature of 37°C is reached. Close attention should be paid to hypotension, electrolyte imbalances, and hypoglycemia during the rewarming phase. Family members should be educated on the possible prognosis, as well as the potential delay of 72 hours before neurologic prognosis

TABLE 3.9 Risk Factors and Lifestyle Modifications

Risk Factor	Goal	Patient Education and Care
Blood pressure[38]	≤60 years of age and CKD SBP <140 and DBP <90 >60 years of age and CKD SBP <150 and DBP <90	• Reinforce medication and lifestyle adherence. • Provide education on individual patient BP goal • Encourage self-monitoring at home and keep a log of BP readings
Cholesterol[98]	Start therapy in individuals with LDL >80–190 with goal of 50% reduction	• Reinforce medication and lifestyle adherence • Access secondary causes of elevated LDL levels: diet, medications, diseases that alter the states of metabolism (i.e., pregnancy, nephrotic syndrome, biliary obstruction, hypothyroidism) • Check baseline lipid panel, hepatic panel, and CK; only need to recheck liver or CK panel again if hepatoxicity or myopathy is suspected • Evaluate therapy with lipid panel initially 4–12 weeks after initial treatment then 3–12 months as clinically indicated
Diabetes mellitus[3]	HgA1c <7% Premeal blood sugar 80–130 mg/dL 2 h-postmeal <180 mg/dL	• Reinforce medication and lifestyle adherence • Education on self-monitoring of blood glucose and targeted blood sugar goals • HgA1c should be done 2–4 times a year
Diet[26]	Dietary guidelines emphasize • Intake of vegetables, fruits, and whole grains; includes low-fat dairy products, poultry, fish, legumes, nontropical vegetable oils, and nuts • Limits intake of sweets, sugar-sweetened beverages, and red meats (DASH, USDA Food Pattern, AHA) • Sodium intake <2400 mg/day • 5% to 6% of calories from saturated fat	• Reinforce dietary adherence
Weight management[40]	Overweight BMI 25–29.9 kg/m^2 Obese BMI >30 kg/m^2 (Class I) BMI >35 kg/m^2 (Class II) BMI >40 kg/m^2 (Class III)	• Reinforce adherence to lifestyle and diet modifications • Assess and treat CV risk factors
Physical activity[26]	40 min 3–4 times/week of moderate-to-vigorous intensity activity	• Reinforce lifestyle adherence
Smoking[65,103]	• Complete smoking cessation is recommended • Avoid secondhand smoke	• Reinforce lifestyle adherence • Avoid e-cigarettes • Avoid smokeless tobacco products

AHA, American Heart Association; *BMI*, body mass index; *BP*, blood pressure; *CKD*, chronic kidney disease; *CV*, cardiovascular; *DASH*, Dietary Approaches to Stop Hypertension diet; *DBP*, diastolic blood pressure; *HbA1c*, hemoglobin A1c; *LDL*, low-density lipoproteins; *SBP*, systolic blood pressure; *USDA*, United States Department of Agriculture.

can be fully assessed. Neurologic testing relies on physical examination, electroencephalography, neuroimaging, and sensory stimulatory evoked potentials. Further research is needed on specific tools and neurologic assessments during and after TH to help predict outcomes in the ROSC period.[89]

DISCHARGE AND LONG-TERM CARE

In preparation for discharge it is important to remember education and care should surround medications, risk factor modification, and return to activities of daily living.[4,10,73] Discharge instructions should be in written and verbal formats as patients and caregivers may be under extreme stress. Absorption of verbal education will need to be reinforced at home with written instructions. Education on medications should include the reason the individual is taking each medication, possible side effects, dosage, timing, and adherence especially with ASA and $P2Y_{12}$ inhibitors. Education should also focus on risk factors, lifestyle modifications, BP, cholesterol, DM, diet, weight management, physical activity, and smoking cessation (Table 3.9).

A referral to cardiac rehab should be initiated prior to discharge for all eligible candidates.[4,73] Studies show that individuals who undergo cardiac rehabilitation after having a PCI have a 20% to 26% reduction in mortality compared to individuals who do not attend a cardiac rehab program.[33,73] Comprehensive cardiac rehab programs provide patient education, enhance regular exercise, monitor risk factors, and address lifestyle modifications. Aerobic exercise training begins 1 to 2 weeks after discharge. During the program, supervised training may target a heart rate 70% to 85% of the age-predicted maximum heart rate. Adjustments may be made if there is a significant change in BP or if angina is present. Even though there is a significant decrease in mortality in ACS patients with cardiac rehab programs, they are still publically underutilized.[4,73]

Return to physical activity depends on the patient's previous functional status as well as whether the course of treatment has been complicated or uncomplicated. For an uncomplicated STEMI, the patient should start walking immediately and driving within 1 week. Return to sexual activity is usually when the patient can walk up a flight of stairs or when they resume their normal activities. Return to work will vary from patient to patient depending on the physical demand, stress of the job, financial state, and company policies. Exercise treadmill testing may be used to determine when the patient can return to work by measuring the metabolic equivalent of task (MET) level achieved and comparing that to the needed energy level required to perform different activities. Patients with an uncomplicated course may return to work within approximately 2 weeks as long as the aforementioned factors do not interfere.[52]

There is an increased focus on the prevention of readmissions after an ACS event. Focus is on outpatient care coordination with the transition of care from the hospital setting. Scheduling of outpatient appointments should be done prior to discharge from the hospital. This helps facilitate the timely follow-up needed with a healthcare provider. This also helps ensure compliance with prescribed medications and treatments, as well as the early identification of potential complications that could cause an unnecessary readmission.[10] Several insurance carriers and organizations, such as the Centers for Medicare and Medical Services (CMS), are now financially penalizing healthcare providers and hospitals for hospital readmissions within 30 days of discharge.[4,73]

Hormone Replacement Therapy

Hormone replacement therapy (HRT) is used to treat menopausal symptoms (e.g., hot flashes and vaginal dryness). Although epidemiologic evidence was originally thought to be strong for postmenopausal use of estrogen in the prevention of heart disease, current clinical trial evidence does not support these findings. The 2014 AHA/ACC NSTE-ACS guidelines now indicate that HRT should not be utilized as secondary prevention in individuals with ACS and should be discontinued if previously utilized for that purpose.[4]

Several hypotheses have been developed on why HRT does not help in postmenopausal patients. The first is the timing and the fact that HRT was started several years after menopause thus leading to lack of improvement. The other is related to age and the changes that occur with aging. The body can no longer metabolize it, so it does not improve vascular health or reduce cardiomyocyte death. The age-related changes also lead to increase in atherosclerosis and cholesterol metabolites leading to acute inflammation and endothelium damage. Both of these effects may aggravate plaque instability and increase thrombotic risk and the potential for reinfarction.[67]

Studies continue to suggest that postmenopausal women who initiate HRT have an increased risk of cardiac events.[4,59] It is important to remember that the primary indication approved by the FDA for the use of HRT is for the treatment of menopausal symptoms. If HRT is needed for treatment of menopausal symptoms and the benefits outweigh the risks, women should take the lowest dose for the shortest period of time.[4]

CONCLUSION

The concepts of the pathophysiology and treatment of ACS are rapidly evolving. Discovery of new cellular processes of atherosclerosis continues to affect the treatment and prevention of the condition. The focus of treatment is centered on disabling the coagulation system at all levels, reestablishing blood flow, and maintaining adequate blood flow long term. PCIs are coupled with anticoagulation and implemented as early as possible. With earlier interventions, less myocardial muscle damage is incurred and better outcomes are achieved. These efforts, along with preventive interventions and aggressive patient education, will hopefully contribute to the eventual demise of ACS.

CASE STUDY 3.1 Acute Coronary Syndrome

Mrs. H. is a 65-year-old female presenting to the emergency department with complaints of increasing epigastric pain. Past medical history includes hypertension, obesity, and type 2 diabetes. Family history includes father and brother with a history of MI. She is a lifetime nonsmoker and does not drink. She also complains of nausea and increasing fatigue over the last month. Vital signs are BP 160/90 and HR 120. Due to her family history and increased risk for possible ACS, an ECG is done and shows nonspecific ST changes. Labs are drawn and troponin indicates possible NSTE-ACS.

Mrs. H. is taken to the cardiac catheterization laboratory the next day for possible interventional therapy. A coronary angiogram reveals 80% occlusion of the mid LAD, which was stented at the time. She also has some diffuse distal lesions (<50%) in the remaining left coronary system that are not amenable to interventions. A vascular closure device is placed after the sheath is removed. One hour later, she becomes hypotensive (BP = 80/50 mm Hg) and her ECG does not show any new ST changes. She is given a fluid bolus with minimal improvement. The nurse discovers a large hematoma in the right femoral groin area. Manual pressure is placed over the femoral artery and the cardiologist is notified. A fluid bolus is given and stat labs show a hemoglobin level of less than 7g/dL and hematocrit of 21%. A CT scan of the pelvis and abdomen shows a retroperitoneal bleed. Blood is transfused and a vascular surgeon is consulted.

Following postsurgical repair by the vascular surgeon and several days in the hospital, Mrs. H is ready to be discharged home. Her medications include ASA, clopidogrel (Plavix), metoprolol (Toprol), and atorvastatin (Lipitor). She is given an appointment to see her cardiologist and her PCP. She has also received a referral to cardiac rehab. Medication education, including reason for taking, side effects, and compliance, is provided by the nurse. Additional education is provided on the benefits of exercise, weight reduction, cholesterol monitoring, and improving the control of her DM.

Decision Point:

What medication interventions should be instituted immediately on admission and prior to discharge?

Decision Point:

Should Mrs. H. be taken for early interventional therapy versus ischemia-guided therapy?

Decision Point:

Why do women more often than men have increased vascular complications with interventional revascularization?

Decision Point:

Mrs. H has been taking HRT for her menopausal symptoms. What education should be provided to the patient on the continuation of the HRT treatment?

REFERENCES

1. Abid, S., et al. (2015). Chest pain assessment and imaging practices for nurse practitioners in the emergency department. *Adv Emerg Nurs J*, *37*(1), 12–22.
1a. Aehlert B. (2012). *ACLS Study Guide* (4th ed.). St Louis: Mosby.
2. Alberti, K. G., et al. (2009). Harmonizing the metabolic syndrome: a joint interim statement of the International Diabetes Federation Task Force on Epidemiology and Prevention; National Heart, Lung, and Blood Institute; American Heart Association; World Heart Federation; International Atherosclerosis Society; and International Association for the Study of Obesity. *Circulation*, *120*, 1640–1645.

3. American Diabetes Association. (2015). Standards of medical care in diabetes – 2015. *J Clin Appl Res Educ, 38*, s1–s94.
4. Amsterdam, E. A., et al. (2014). 2014 AHA/ACC guideline for the management of patients with Non–ST-Elevation acute coronary syndromes: a report of the American College of Cardiology/American Heart Association task force on practice guidelines. *Circulation, 130*, e344–e426.
5. Antman, E., et al. (2000). The TIMI risk score for unstable angina/non-ST elevation MI, a method for prognostication and therapeutic decision making. *J Am Med Assoc, 284*(7), 835–842.
6. Bairey Merz, C. N., Shaw, L. J., & Reis, S. E. (2006). Ischemic heart disease in women: insights from the NHLBI-sponsored Women's Ischemia Syndrome Evaluation (WISE) Study. Part II: Gender differences in presentation, diagnosis, and outcome with regard to sex-based pathophysiology of atherosclerosis, macro- and micro-vascular CAD. *J Am Coll Cardiol, 47*, 21s–29s.
7. Benowitz, N. L., & Goniewicz, M. L. (2013). The regulatory challenge of electronic cigarettes. *J Am Med Assoc, 310*, 685–686.
8. Biasucci, L. M., Liuzzo, G., & Crea, F. (2008). Acute coronary syndromes: to CRP or not to CRP? *J Am Coll Cardiol, 52*(18), 1500.
9. Birnbaum, Y., et al. (2014). ECG diagnosis and classification of acute coronary syndromes. *Ann Noninvas Electro, 19*(1), 4–14.
10. Blue Verrier, J. M., & Deelstra, M. H. (2010). Acute coronary syndromes. In S. L. Woods, E. S. Sivarajan Froelicher, S. U. Motzer, & E. J. Bridges (Eds.), *Cardiac nursing* (6th ed.) (pp. 511–536). Philadelphia, PA: Wolters Kluwar Health/Lippincott Williams & Wilkins.
11. Bunch, A. M. (2012). A systematic review of the predictive value of a coronary computed tomography angiography as compared with coronary calcium scoring in alternative noninvasive technique in detecting coronary artery disease and evaluating acute coronary syndrome in an acute care setting. *Dimens Crit Care Nurs, 31*(2), 73–83.
12. Cabello, J. B., et al. (2013). Oxygen therapy for acute myocardial infarction. *Cochrane Database Syst Rev, 8*, CD007160.
13. Cannon, C. P., et al. (2002). Design of the pravastatin or atorvastatin evaluation and infection therapy (PROVE IT)-TIMI 22 trial. *Am J Cardiol, 89*(7), 860–861.
14. Carroll, M. D., et al. (2013). Total and high-density lipo-protein cholesterol in adults: National Health and Nutrition Examination Survey, 2011–2012. *NCHS Data Brief, 132*, 1–8.
15. Chen, M. A. (2010). Mechanical circulatory assist device. In S. L. Woods, E. S. Sivarajan Froelicher, S. U. Motzer, & E. J. Bridges (Eds.), *Cardiac nursing* (6th ed.) (pp. 623–637). Philadelphia, PA: Wolters Kluwar Health/Lippincott Williams & Wilkins.
16. Christie, L. G., & Conti, C. R. (1981). Systematic approach to the evaluation of angina-like chest pain. *Am Heart J, 102*, 899.
17. Crea, F., & Liuzzo, G. (2013). Pathogenesis of acute coronary syndromes. *J Am Coll Cardiol, 61*(1), 1–11.
18. Dangas, G. D., et al. (2014). Impact of hemodynamic support with Impella 2.5 versus intra-aortic balloon pump on prognostically important clinical outcomes in patients undergoing high-risk percutaneous coronary intervention (from the PROTECT II randomized trial). *American J Cardiol, 113*(2), 222–228.
19. D'Ascenzo, F., et al. (2011). Comparison of mortality rates in women versus men presenting with ST-segment elevation myocardial infarction. *Am J Cardiol, 107*(5), 651–654.
20. Deelstra, M. H. (2010). Interventional cardiology techniques: percutaneous coronary intervention. In S. L. Woods, E. S. Sivarajan Froelicher, S. U. Motzer, & E. J. Bridges (Eds.), *Cardiac nursing* (6th ed.) (pp. 537–555). Philadelphia, PA: Wolters Kluwar Health/Lippincott Williams & Wilkins.
21. Dehmer, G. J., et al. (2014). SCAI/ACC/AHA Expert Consensus Document: 2014 update on percutaneous coronary intervention without on-site surgical backup. *Circulation, 129*, 2610–2626.
22. Diercks, D. B., et al. (2010). Gender differences in time to presentation for myocardial infarction before and after a national women's CV awareness campaign: a temporal analysis from the Can Rapid Risk Stratification of Unstable Angina Patients Suppress Adverse Outcomes with Early Implementation (CRUSADE) and the National Cardiovascular Data Registry Acute Coronary Treatment and Intervention Outcomes Network-Get with the Guidelines (NCDR ACTION Registry-GWTG). *Am Heart J, 160*, 80–87.
23. Dolor, R. J., et al. (2012). *Treatment strategies for women with coronary artery disease. Comparative effectiveness review no. 66*. Rockville, MD: Agency for Healthcare Research and Quality. AHRQ publication no. 12-EHC070-EF. http://www.effectivehealthcare.ahrq.gov/ reports/final.cfm.
24. Drew, B. J., & Funk, M. (2006). Practice standards for electrocardiographic monitoring in hospital settings: executive summary and guide for implementation. *Crit Care Nurs Clin North Am, 18*(2), 157–168.
25. Dubin, D. (2000). *Rapid interpretation of EKGs: An interactive course* (6th ed.). Tampa, FL: Cover Publishing.
26. Eckel, R. H., et al. (2013). AHA/ACC guidelines on lifestyle management to reduce cardiovascular risk. *Circulation, 129*(25), S76–S99.
27. Fairchild, A. L., Bayer, R., & Colgrove, J. (2014). The renormalization of smoking? E-cigarettes and the tobacco endgame. *N Eng J Med, 370* 293–84.
28. Ferreiro, J. L., & Angiolillo, D. J. (2011). Diabetes and antiplatelet therapy in acute coronary syndrome. *Circulation, 123*, 798–813.
29. Ford, E. S., & Capewell, S. (2013). Trends in total and low-density lipoprotein cholesterol among U.S. adults: contributions of changes in dietary fat intake and use of cholesterol-lowering medications. *PloS One, 8*, e65228.
30. Fox, C. S., et al. (2010). Use of evidence-based therapies in short-term outcomes of ST-segment elevation myocardial infarction and non-ST-segment elevation myocardial infarction in patients with chronic kidney disease: a report from the National Cardiovascular Data Acute Coronary Treatment and Intervention Outcomes Network registry. *Circulation, 121*, 357–365.
31. Frazier, C. G., et al. (2005). Prevalence and management of hypertension in acute coronary syndrome patients varies by sex: observations from the sibrafiban versus aspirin to yield maximum protection from ischemic heart events postacute coronary syndromes (SYMPHONY) randomized clinical trials. *Am Heart J, 150*(6), 1260–1267.
32. Gerschutz, G. P., & Bhatt, D. L. (2002). The CURE trial: using clopidogrel in acute coronary syndromes without ST-segment elevation. *Cleveland Clin J Med, 69*, 1326–1331.
33. Goel, K., et al. (2011). Impact of cardiac rehabilitation on mortality and cardiovascular events after percutaneous coronary intervention in the community. *Circulation, 123*, 2344–2352.
34. Grube, E., et al. (2003). TAXUS I: six and twelve month results from a randomized, double-blind trial on a slow-release paclitaxel-eluting stent for de novo coronary lesions. *Circulation, 107*(1), 38–42.
35. Hari, P., et al. (2012). A gender-stratified comparative analysis of various definitions of metabolic syndrome and cardiovascular risk in a multiethnic U.S. population. *Metab Syndr Relat Disord, 10*, 47–55.
36. Heard, K. J., et al. (2010). A randomized controlled trial comparing the Arctic Sun to standard cooling for induction of hypothermia after cardiac arrest. *Resuscitation, 81*, 9–14.
37. Hundley, W. G., et al. (2010). ACCF/ACR/AHA/NASCI/SCMR 2010 expert consensus document on cardiovascular magnetic resonance: a report of the American College of Cardiology Foundation Task Force on Expert Consensus Documents. *J Am Coll Cardiol, 55*(23), 2416–2662.
38. James, P. A., et al. (2014). 2014 evidence-based guideline for the management of high blood pressure in adults: report from the panel members appointed to the Eighth Joint National Committee (JNC 8). *J Am Med Assoc, 311*(5), 507–520.
39. James, S. K., et al. (2011). Ticagrelor versus clopidogrel in patients with acute coronary syndromes intended for non-invasive management substudy from prospective randomised PLATelet inhibition and patient Outcomes (PLATO) trial. *Brit Med J, 342*, d3527.
40. Jensen, M. D., et al. (2013). 2013 AHA/ACC/TOS/ guidelines for the management of overweight and obesity in adults. *Circulation, 129*, S102–S138.
41. Johnson, B. D., et al. (2004). Prognosis in women with myocardial ischemia in the absence of obstructive coronary disease: results from the National Institutes of Health-National Heart, Lung, and Blood Institute-sponsored women's ischemia syndrome evaluation (WISE). *Circulation, 109*(24), 2993–2999.
42. Kay, J., et al. (2013). Influence of sex on risk stratification with stress myocardial perfusion Rb-82 positron emission tomography: results

from the PET (Positron Emission Tomography) Prognosis Multicenter Registry. *J Am Coll Cardiol, 62*(20), 1866–1876.
43. Kedhi, E., et al. (2010). Second-generation everolimus-eluting and paclitaxel-eluting stents in real-life practice (COMPARE): a randomized trial. *Lancet, 375*(9710), 201–209.
44. Keller, T., et al. (2011). Serial changes in highly sensitive troponin I assay and early diagnosis of myocardial infarction. *J Am Med Assoc, 306*(24), 2684–2693.
45. Kelly, C. R., et al. (2014). Relation of c-reactive protein levels to instability of vulnerable acute coronary plaques (from the PROSPECT study). *J Am Cardiol, 114*(3), 376–383.
46. Khunti, K. (2014). Accurate interpretation of the 12-lead ECG electrode placement: a systematic review. *Health Ed J, 73*(5), 610–623.
47. Krintus, M., et al. (2012). Value of C-reactive protein as a risk factor for acute coronary syndrome: a comparison with apolipoprotein concentrations and lipid profile. *Mediators of Inflamm*. http://dx.doi.org/10.1155/2012/419804.
48. Kul, S., et al. (2014). Metabolic syndrome and long-term cardiovascular outcome in NSTEMI with unstable angina. *Nutr Metab Cardiovasc Dis, 24*(2), 176–182.
49. Kumar, A., & Cannon, C. P. (2009). Acute coronary syndromes: diagnosis and management, part 1. *Mayo Clin Proc, 84*(10), 917–938.
50. Lansky, A. J., et al. (2009). Impact of gender and antithrombin strategy on early and late clinical outcomes in patients with non-ST-elevation acute coronary syndromes (from the ACUITY trial). *Am J Cardiol, 103*, 1196–1203.
51. Lazzeri, C., et al. (2012). Uric acid in the early risk stratification of ST-elevation myocardial infarction. *Intern Emerg Med, 7*(1), 33–39.
52. Levine, G. N., et al. (2011). 2011 ACCF/AHA/SCAI guideline for percutaneous coronary intervention. *J Am Coll Cardiol, 58*(24), e44–e122.
53. Libby, P., Ridker, P. M., & Hansson, G. K. (2011). Progress and challenges in translating the biology of atherosclerosis. *Nature, 473*, 317–325.
54. Libby, P., Ridker, P. M., & Hansson, G. K. (2009). Inflammation in the atherosclerosis: from pathophysiology to practice. *J Am Coll Cardiol, 54*, 2129–2138.
55. Linkins, L. A., et al. (2012). Treatment and prevention of heparin-induced thrombocytopenia: antithrombotic therapy and prevention of thrombosis, (9th ed.) American College of Chest Physicians evidence-based clinical practice guidelines. *Chest, 41*(suppl. 2), e495S–e530S.
56. Li, X., et al. (2013). The prevalence and awareness of cardiometabolic risk factors in Southern Chinese population with coronary artery disease. *ScientificWorldJournal*, Article ID 416192, 1-9. http://dx.doi.org/10.1155/2013/416192.
57. Lloyd-Jones, D. M., et al. (2010). Defining and setting national goals for cardiovascular health promotion and disease reduction: the American Heart Association's strategic impact goal through 2020 and beyond. *Circulation, 121*, 586–613.
58. Mahaffey, K. W., et al. (2011). Ticagrelor compared with clopidogrel by geographic region in the Platelet Inhibition and Patient Outcomes (PLATO) trial. *Circulation, 124*, 544–554.
59. Manson, J. E., et al. (2013). Menopausal hormone therapy and health outcomes during the intervention and extended poststopping phases of the women's health initiative randomized trials. *J Am Med Assoc, 310*(13), 1353–1368.
60. Mieres, J. H., et al. (2014). Role of noninvasive testing in the clinical evaluation of women with suspected ischemic heart disease: a consensus statement from the American Heart Association. *Circulation, 130*, 350–379.
61. Moradkhan, R., & Sinoway, L. I. (2010). Revisiting the role of oxygen therapy in cardiac patients. *J Am Coll Cardiol, 56*, 1013–1016.
62. Mosca, L., et al. (2011). Effectiveness-based guidelines for the prevention of cardiovascular disease in women—2011 update. *Circulation, 123*, 1243–1262.
63. Moses, J. W., et al. (2003). Sirolimus-eluting stents versus standard stents in patients with stenosis in a native coronary artery. *New Eng J Med, 349*(14), 1315–1323.
64. Mottillo, S., et al. (2010). The metabolic syndrome and cardiovascular risk: a systematic review and meta-analysis. *J Am Coll Cardiol, 56*, 1113–1132.
65. Mozaffarian, D., et al. (2015). Heart disease and stroke statistics – 2015 update: a report from the American Heart Association. *Circulation, 131*, e1–e292.
66. Mozaffarian, D., Appel, L. J., & Van Horn, L. (2011). Components of a cardioprotective diet: new insights. *Circulation, 123*, 2870–2891.
67. Murphy, E. (2011). Estrogen signaling and cardiovascular disease. *Circulation Res, 109*, 687–696.
68. National Center for Health Statistics. (2013). *National Health Interview Survey, 2013. Public-use data file and documentation*. http://www.cdc.gov/nchs/.
69. Navarese, E. P., et al. (2014). First-generation versus second-generation drug-eluting stents in current clinical practice: updated evidence from a comprehensive meta-analysis of randomized clinical trials comprising 31,379 patients. *Open Heart, 1*, e000064. http://dx.doi.org/10.1136/openhrt-2014-000064.
70. Neumar, R. W., et al. (2010). Part 8: Adult advanced cardiovascular life support. 2010 American Heart Association guidelines for cardiopulmonary resuscitation and emergency cardiovascular care. *Circulation, 122*(Suppl. 3), S729–S767.
71. Newby, D. E. (2010). Acute coronary syndromes: triggering of acute myocardial infarction: beyond a vulnerable plaque. *Heart, 96*, 1247–1251.
72. Ng, V. G., et al. (2011). Three-year results of safety and efficacy of the everolimus-eluting coronary stent in women (from the SPIRIT III randomized clinical trial). *Am J Cardiol, 107*, 841–848.
73. O'Gara, P., et al. (2013). ACCF/AHA guidelines for the management of ST-elevation myocardial infarction. *J Am Coll Cardiol, 61*(4), e78–e140.
74. Ondrus, T., et al. (2013). Right ventricular myocardial infarction: from pathophysiology to prognosis. *Exp Clin Cardiol, 18*(1), 27–30.
75. O'Neill, W. W., et al. (2012). A prospective, randomized clinical trial of hemodynamic support with impella 2.5 versus intra-aortic balloon pump in patients undergoing high-risk percutaneous coronary intervention: the PROTECT II study. *Circulation, 126*, 1717–1727.
76. Park, K. E., & Pepine, C. J. (2011). Microvascular dysfunction: what have we learned from WISE? *Expert Rev Cardiovasc Ther, 9*, 1491–1494.
77. Patel, A. R., & Kramer, C. M. (2013). Accessing cardiovascular risk in women: a growing body of evidence. *J Am Coll Cardiol, 62*(20), 1877–1879.
78. Pauly, D. F., et al. (2011). In women with symptoms of cardiac ischemia, non-obstructive coronary arteries, and microvascular dysfunction, ACE inhibition is associated with improved microvascular function: A double-blind randomized study from the NHLBI Women's Ischemia Syndrome Evaluation (WISE). *Am Heart J, 162*(4), 678–684.
79. Perberdy, M. A., et al. (2010). Part 9: Post-cardiac arrest care 2010 American Heart Association Guidelines for Cardiopulmonary Resuscitation and Emergency Cardiovascular Care. *Circulation, 122*(suppl), S768–S786.
80. Picariello, C., et al. (2011). The impact of hypertension on patients with acute coronary syndromes. *Int J Hypertens*, 1–7.
81. Rakugi, H., et al. (1996). Links between hypertension and myocardial infarction. *Am Heart J, 132*(1), 213–221.
82. Ramos, L. M. (2014). Cardiac diagnostic testing: what bedside nurses need to know. *Crit Care Nurs, 34*(3), 16–28.
83. Ranković, G., et al. (2009). Effects of physical exercise on inflammatory parameters and risk for repeated acute coronary syndrome in patients with ischemic heart disease. *Vojnosanit Pregl, 66*, 44–48.
84. Reichlin, T., et al. (2011). Utility of absolute and relative changes in cardiac troponin concentrations in the early diagnosis of acute myocardial infarction. *Circulation, 124*(2), 136–145.
85. Rogers, W. R. (1972). Maximal QS 2-interval shortening in acute coronary syndromes: experience with a simple method in fifty patients. *Northwest Med, 71*, 605–608.
86. Salehi, R., Motemavele, M., & Goldust, M. (2013). Risk factors of coronary artery disease in women. *Pakistan J Biologic Sci, 16*(4), 195–197.
87. Schwartz, B. G., et al. (2010). Review of vascular closure devices. *J Invas Cardiol, 22*, 599–607.
88. Schwartz, G. G., et al. (2001). Effects of atorvastatin on early recurrent ischemic events in acute coronary syndromes: the MIRACL study: a randomized controlled trial. *J Am Med Assoc, 285*(13), 1711–1718.
89. Scirica, B. M. (2013). Clinician update: therapeutic hypothermia after cardiac arrest. *Circulation, 127*, 244–250.

90. Scirica, B. M. (2010). Acute coronary syndrome: emerging tools for diagnosis and risk assessment. *J Am Coll Cardiol*, *55*(14), 1403–1415.
91. Shaw, L. J., et al. (2010). Sex differences in mortality associated with computed tomographic angiographic measurements of obstructive and nonobstructive coronary artery disease: an exploratory analysis. *Circulation Cardiovasc Imag*, *3*, 473–481.
92. Shaw, L. J., Bugiardini, R., & Merz, N. B. (2009). Women and ischemic heart disease. *J Am Coll Cardiol*, *54*(17), 1561–1575.
93. Smits, P. C., et al. (2011). 2-year follow-up of a randomized controlled trial of everolimus and paclitaxel-eluting stents for coronary revascularization in daily practice. COMPARE (Comparison of everolimus eluting XIENCE-V stent with paclitaxel eluting TAXUS stent in all-comers: a randomized open label trial). *J Am Coll Cardiol*, *58*(1), 11–18.
94. Steg, P. G., et al. (2010). Low-dose vs. standard-dose unfractionated heparin for percutaneous coronary intervention in acute coronary syndromes treated with fondaparinux: the FUTURA/OASIS-8 randomized trial. *J Am Med Assoc*, *304*(12), 1339–1349.
95. Stone, G. W., et al. (2011). Randomized comparison of everolimus and paclitaxel-eluting stents. 2-year follow-up from the SPIRIT (Clinical Evaluation of the XIENCE V Everolimus Eluting Coronary Stent System) IV trial. *J Am Coll Cardiol*, *58*(1), 19–25.
96. Stone, G. W., et al. (2011). A prospective natural-history study of coronary atherosclerosis. *New Eng J Med*, *364*(3), 226–235.
97. Stone, G. W., et al. (2007). Bivalirudin in patients with acute coronary syndromes undergoing percutaneous coronary intervention: a subgroup analysis from the Acute Catheterization and Urgent Intervention Triage strategy (ACUITY) trial. *Lancet*, *369*(9565), 907–919.
98. Stone, N. J., et al. (2014). 2013 ACC/AHA guidelines on the treatment of blood cholesterol to reduce atherosclerotic cardiovascular risk in adults. *Circulation*, *129*(25), S1–S45.
99. Than, M., et al. (2012). 2-hour accelerated diagnostic protocol to assess patients with chest pain symptoms using contemporary troponins as the only biomarker: the ADAPT trial. *J Am Coll Cardiol*, *59*(23), 2091–2098.
100. Topol, E. J. (1990). *Thrombolytic intervention. Textbook of interventional cardiology*. Philadelphia: Saunders.
101. Thun, M. J., et al. (2013). 50-year trends in smoking-related mortality in the United States. *New Eng J Med*, *368*, 351–364.
102. Truong, Q. A., et al. (2011). Benefit of intensive statin therapy in women: results from PROVE IT-TIMI 22. *Circulation Cardiovasc Qual Outcomes*, *4*, 328–336.
103. US Department of Health and Human Services. (2010). *How tobacco smoke causes disease: The biology and behavioral basis for smoking attributable disease: A report of the surgeon general*. Atlanta, GA: US Department of Health and Human Services. Centers for Disease Control and Prevention, National Center for Chronic Disease Prevention and Health Promotion, Office on Smoking and Health.
104. US Food and Drug Administration. (2012). *FDA Drug Safety Communication: Important safety label changes to cholesterol-lowering statin drugs*. http://www.fda.gov/Drugs/DrugSafety/ucm293101.htm.
105. Weissman, G., & Weigold, G. (2009). Cardiac computed tomography. *J Radiol Nurs*, *28*(3), 96–103.
106. Wenger, N. K. (2012). Women and coronary heart disease: a century after Herrick understudied, underdiagnosed, and undertreated. *Circulation*, *126*, 604–611.
107. Wiviott, S. D., Antman, E. M., & Braunwald, E. (2010). New drugs and technologies: prasugrel. *Circulation*, *122*, 394–403.
108. Young, S. (2014). Coronary angioplasty: patient management and nursing care. *Brit J Card Nurs*, *9*(9), 430–435.
109. Yusuf, S., Wittes, J., & Friedman, L. (1988). Overview of results of randomized clinical trials in heart disease, II: unstable angina, heart failure, primary prevention with aspirin and risk factor modification. *J Am Med Assoc*, *260*, 2259–2263.

4

Heart Failure

Peggy L. Kirkwood and Sara Paul

INTRODUCTION

Heart failure (HF) is a clinical syndrome that occurs as a final manifestation of other cardiac diseases or risk factors, such as ischemic heart disease or hypertension. The prevalence of HF is high, with an estimated 5.7 million Americans currently affected, and greater than 8 million projected to be affected by 2030.[155] There are 870,000 new HF cases diagnosed annually in the United States, with 75% of cases having antecedent hypertension.[155] HF is mentioned on the death certificate of one in every nine deaths. While survival after HF diagnosis has improved over time,[16,127] the death rate remains high, with approximately 50% of people diagnosed dying within 5 years.[185,203] HF is a costly disease, estimated at $30.7 billion in 2012, with most of that attributable to direct medical costs.[98] By the year 2030, the total cost of HF is projected to increase almost 127% to $69.7 billion.

The high cost of caring for patients with HF is largely attributable to hospitalizations for exacerbations of chronic heart failure. HF is the primary diagnosis for over 1 million hospitalizations per year, and approximately 25% of those patients are readmitted within 1 month of discharge.[155] Three-month readmission rates are as high as 20% to 30%, while 6-month readmission rates among symptomatic patients are approximately 50%. Hospitalization for heart failure is the number one admitting diagnosis in patients over age 65 years.[91] As age increases, so does the incidence of HF.[51]

HEART FAILURE DEFINED

Heart failure is a chronic condition that becomes worse over time, progressing in a downward trajectory, culminating in the patient's premature death, regardless of the original cause. It is not a specific disease, but rather, a clinical syndrome that is the end result of other disease states, such as coronary artery disease (CAD), hypertension, valve dysfunction, or other cardiovascular disorders. It may arise from disorders of the pericardium, myocardium, endocardium, heart valves, great vessels, or from certain metabolic abnormalities, but it most commonly arises from impaired left ventricular (LV) myocardial function.[227] Noncardiac causes of HF may include excessive alcohol use, cocaine use, thyroid disorders, certain chemotherapeutic agents, or peripartum cardiomyopathy.[227]

Overall, a confluence of pathophysiologic processes are initiated that result in reshaping or remodeling of the ventricle (dilation or hypertrophy), and alter myocardial function (systolic or diastolic), resulting in decreased circulatory capability to perfuse body organs and tissues. CAD and hypertension are the chief contributors to the development of HF, both of which are found in 40% of HF patients.[203] Hypertensive individuals are at substantially greater risk of developing HF than the normotensive population,[128] and long-term treatment of hypertension can reduce the risk of developing HF by 50%.[102] Diabetes mellitus is also an independent risk factor for heart failure, and the incidence of diabetes has increased dramatically over the last several decades.[223]

Heart failure can be divided according to a variety of functional abnormalities of the LV, ranging from normal LV size and preserved contractility to severely dilated LV and reduced contractility.[227] The strength of cardiac contractility is measured as the ejection fraction (EF), which is the percentage of blood ejected from the LV with each contraction, based on a ventricle that is 100% full at the end of diastolic filling. The left ventricle usually ejects 60% or more of the blood volume in the LV with each contraction, but anything below 40% is considered HF with reduced EF (HFrEF). Ejection fraction of 50% or greater in the presence of HF symptoms is considered HF with preserved EF (HFpEF). Patients with an EF between 40% and 50% are an intermediate group, and are often treated with the same therapies as patients with HFrEF, while managing risk factors and comorbidities.[227] It is estimated that among all individuals with symptomatic HF, 55% have preserved EF.[31]

Whether HF is due to reduced EF or preserved EF, it is a chronic condition that is marked by exacerbations of clinical decompensation. These exacerbations consist of worsening HF symptoms such as dyspnea, swelling, fatigue, orthopnea, and cough. Hospitalization is often required to manage the symptoms and correct physiologic derangements. Decompensated HF can be defined as "new or worsening signs and symptoms of the HF syndrome, frequently leading to emergency room visits or hospitalization."[173] In recent years, considerable effort has been expended by hospitals to prevent patients from requiring readmission to the hospital following a discharge with a diagnosis of HF.[29]

PATHOPHYSIOLOGY OF HEART FAILURE

In order to understand the progression of HF and the treatments that have been shown to improve outcomes, it is imperative to consider the physiologic processes that conspire to change the shape and function of the heart. These processes may be initiated by an event such as myocardial infarction (MI) or hypertension, but they are perpetuated by a complicated combination of neurohormonal and inflammatory activation, as well as adrenergic stimulation. Additionally, there is an overgrowth of myocardial muscle and an overproduction of the interstitial matrix that holds myocytes in proper alignment. These processes ultimately result in alterations of the hemodynamics involved in ventricular contraction (systole) and/or relaxation (diastole), and impact long-term prognosis.

Regardless of the initiating cause or index event, the development and progression of HF is the result of a process known as "ventricular remodeling," which is a change in the size and shape of the cardiac muscle. This occurs as a result of changes at the cellular level and within the extracellular matrix that supports the alignment of cardiac myocytes. Fibroblasts proliferate and cause interstitial fibrosis of myocardial tissue, leading to stiffening of the ventricle and eventual alterations in cardiac performance. These are all compensatory mechanisms to maintain cardiac output and support perfusion of organs in the presence of an index event, such as MI or long-standing hypertension. These systems initially compensate for decreased myocardial function and preserve cardiovascular homeostasis. However, over time cardiac performance suffers from the deleterious effects on myocardial structure.[132] Factors that contribute to ventricular remodeling include neurohormonal activation, dysregulation of the immune system, and alterations in the extracellular matrix (or "scaffolding" that holds myocardial cells in alignment). Vasoconstriction, sodium and water retention, and added sympathetic activity place the failing myocardium in further jeopardy by further increasing preload and afterload and by promoting ventricular dysrhythmias, subendocardial ischemia, hyponatremia, and hypokalemia.

Neurohormonal Activation

Neurohormonal mechanisms are activated in response to an injury or insult that causes a decline in cardiac function. These compensatory mechanisms are intended to maintain cardiac output in the presence of decreased cardiac function and to maintain systemic pressure through vasoconstriction, distributing blood flow to vital organs. Cardiac output is restored by increasing myocardial contractility and heart rate, and by expanding extracellular fluid.

The renin-angiotensin-aldosterone system (RAAS) is activated early in HF by a variety of factors (Fig. 4.1). Renin is released from the juxtaglomerular apparatus of the kidneys and breaks down circulating angiotensinogen (secreted from the liver) to produce angiotensin I. Angiotensin I is converted to angiotensin II when it comes in contact with angiotensin-converting enzyme (ACE), which is secreted by endothelial cells of the blood vessels in the lungs and kidneys. ACE also breaks down bradykinin that would otherwise be a potent vasodilator. Actions of angiotensin II include arteriolar vasoconstriction, aldosterone release from the adrenal cortex, vasopressin arginine release, increased reabsorption of sodium, stimulation of thirst, and increased release of norepinephrine from postganglionic nerve terminals. Norepinephrine stimulates further secretion of renin.[42] Angiotensin II also promotes myocyte hypertrophy, apoptosis (programmed cell death), and fibroblast proliferation. Angiotensin II is also produced locally within tissue via non-ACE dependent mechanisms at sites such as the kidney, blood vessels, adrenal gland, brain, and myocardium.[199] Myocardial stretch from increased ventricular wall stress increases the release of angiotensin II. Inhibiting the effects of ACE results in decreased formation of angiotensin II and decreased metabolism of bradykinin, leading to dilation of arteries and veins.

Aldosterone is produced in the adrenal glands as a response to stimulation from angiotensin II, although there is also production of aldosterone in the failing heart.[152] Aldosterone

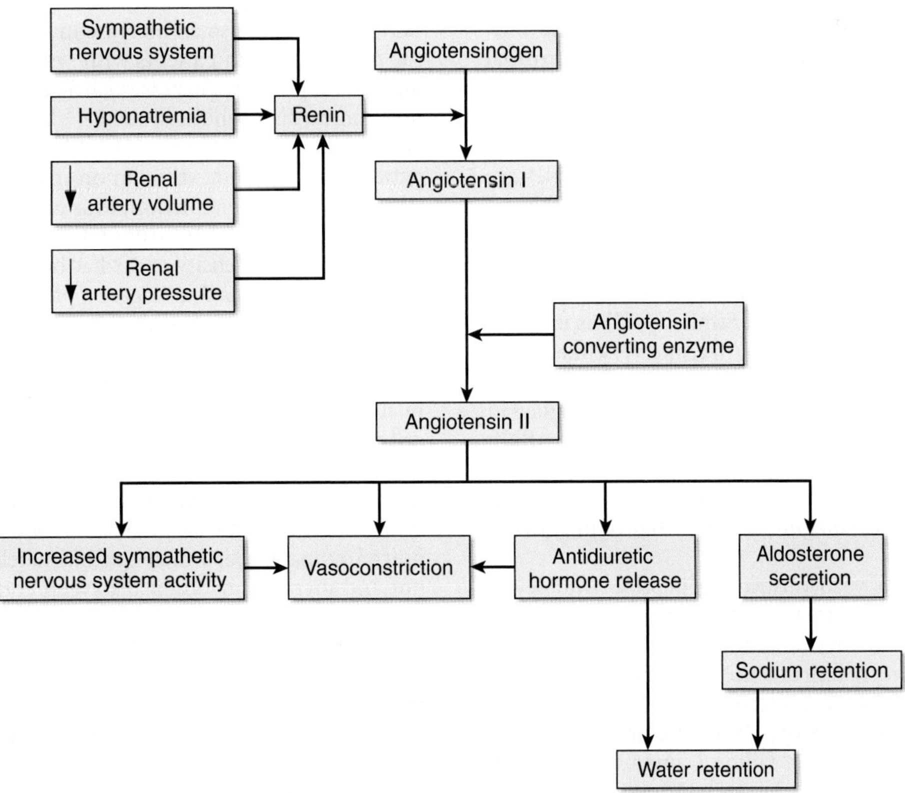

FIG. 4.1 Activation of the renin-angiotensin-aldosterone system leading to vasoconstriction and volume retention.

promotes potassium excretion and additional sodium and water reabsorption in the distal renal tubule. This leads to clinical fluid retention and hypokalemia in HF patients. Aldosterone contributes to myocardial fibrosis by stimulating fibroblast proliferation and collagen accumulation, which promotes stiffness of the myocardium. In patients with HF, plasma aldosterone levels are much higher than in age-matched control subjects without heart failure.[206]

Arginine vasopressin, also known as antidiuretic hormone (ADH), is released in response to activation of carotid sinus and aortic arch baroreceptors in the presence of low cardiac output. Elevated levels of ADH contribute to increased systemic vascular resistance in HF patients by stimulating receptors on vascular smooth muscle cells and causing vasoconstriction. ADH also contributes to decreased water excretion and increased thirst drive, leading to fluid retention and reduced plasma sodium concentration. Hyponatremia is a predictor of survival in HF patients; serum sodium levels parallel the severity of HF. Lower serum sodium levels confer a worsened prognosis.

Natriuretic peptides include atrial natriuretic peptide (ANP), C-type natriuretic peptide, B-type natriuretic peptide (BNP), and urodilatin. ANP and BNP are released by atrial and ventricular cells in response to wall stress from myocardial stretch, as occurs with circulatory volume overload. These peptides promote natriuresis, diuresis, and arterial and venous vasodilation. They also reduce norepinephrine release and sympathetic activation in HF, and inhibit the RAAS.[221] While ANP and BNP should serve as compensatory mechanisms in HF, the effects of these peptides are attenuated either through natriuretic peptide receptor downregulation or through increased ANP and BNP degradation.[63]

BNP is synthesized as a prehormone (proBNP), but once it is released into the circulation, it is cleaved into the biologically active BNP and the biologically inactive N-terminal fragment (NT-proBNP). The half-life of BNP is 20 minutes, whereas NT-proBNP has a half-life of 120 minutes. This causes the NT-proBNP serum values to be approximately 6 times higher than BNP values.[21] BNP and NT-proBNP are elevated in patients with HF, and are related to disease severity, left ventricular ejection fraction (LVEF), and LV diastolic function.[59] As a marker of HF, BNP values less than 100 pg/mL indicate that HF is unlikely, whereas values over 500 pg/mL are very likely to represent HF.[134] Similarly, HF is unlikely with NT-proBNP values under 300 pg/mL, and very likely with values greater than 450 pg/mL (>900 pg/mL in patients over 50 years of age).[104] BNP and NP-proBNP values are higher in females and in the older age group.[180] BNP and NT-proBNP values are increased in patients with reduced renal function, but NT-proBNP is affected more than BNP. Both markers have been found to have similar diagnostic performance in patients with renal disease.[131]

Endothelin (ET) is a vasoconstricting peptide with levels that are increased in patients with HF, and may contribute to the progression of LV dysfunction.[183] ET is expressed in the myocardium, where it has potent inotropic activity, but, in the failing heart, may have a negative inotropic effect.[133] It may also be pro-arrhythmic in the presence of HF.[14] Chronic stimulation of ET-A receptors in failing human myocardium can result in myocyte hypertrophy and fibroblast proliferation. Myocardial ET synthesis is stimulated by hypoxia, ischemia, neurohormones such as norepinephrine, angiotensin II, arginine vasopressin,[38,146] and inflammatory cytokines[160]; all of which are increased in the failing human myocardium and contribute to ventricular remodeling.

In patients with chronic HF, arterial flow-mediated vasodilation is attenuated due to arterial endothelial dysfunction, probably due to reduced nitric oxide (NO) synthesis as well as decreased endothelial release of and response to NO.[111,112,122] In contrast, venous endothelial function, tone, and NO release are preserved. Decreased NO effect to stimulate flow-mediated vasodilation during exercise results in muscle fatigue in patients with HF, and is one factor that limits functional capacity and physical activity in this population.

Sympathetic Nervous System Activation

The sympathetic nervous system (SNS) is activated early in HF in response to a decrease in cardiac output. There is increased norepinephrine release and decreased reuptake at adrenergic nerve endings, which results in catecholamine-driven increase in ventricular contractility and heart rate. This is a compensatory mechanism to maintain cardiac output, but as ventricular function deteriorates with worsening HF, this mechanism loses effectiveness (Fig. 4.2). Sympathetic activation also causes systemic and pulmonary vasoconstriction, as well as increased venous tone, to promote preload and blood pressure and enhance tissue perfusion. Norepinephrine and angiotensin II cause constriction of the renal efferent arterioles, which increases filtration in the glomerulus and preserves renal function, at least temporarily, despite a decrease in renal blood flow in HF. Plasma norepinephrine levels correlate directly with the degree of LV dysfunction (higher levels are associated with worse function) and correspond inversely with survival.[44]

Sympathetic activation is not limited to the systemic circulation, but there is also an increase in sympathetic activity within the myocardium in patients with systolic HF. Elevated ventricular filling pressure increases cardiac norepinephrine spillover into the cardiac venous system.[113] Information about chronic sympathetic stimulation in HFpEF is limited. In hypertensive patients, sympathetic stimulation may be contributory to ventricular diastolic dysfunction, thus increasing the risk for HF.[101]

Chronic sympathetic stimulation leads to down regulation and reduction in density of cardiac beta receptors and desensitization of the signals that trigger a physiologic cardiac response. This results in impaired inotropic (strength of contractility) and chronotropic (heart rate) responses to physiologic stimuli.[161] Additionally, chronic stimulation of beta receptors may result in the loss of cardiomyocytes due to apoptosis (programmed cell death) and necrosis.[46]

Sympathetic adrenergic stimulation begins as a compensatory mechanism, but leads to decompensation. Because sympathetic activation causes vasoconstriction, afterload is significantly increased, which can ultimately reduce cardiac output and increase myocardial oxygen consumption, leading to worsening ischemia. Venoconstriction increases venous return to the heart, thereby increasing preload and ventricular filling pressures, contributing to pulmonary congestion and increased myocardial wall stress. Beta adrenergic stimulation increases heart rate, which decreases ventricular diastolic filling time and diastolic coronary perfusion, while increasing myocardial oxygen consumption. Chronic catecholamine stimulation promotes interstitial fibrosis and induces contractile dysfunction via LV dilatation.[28,165]

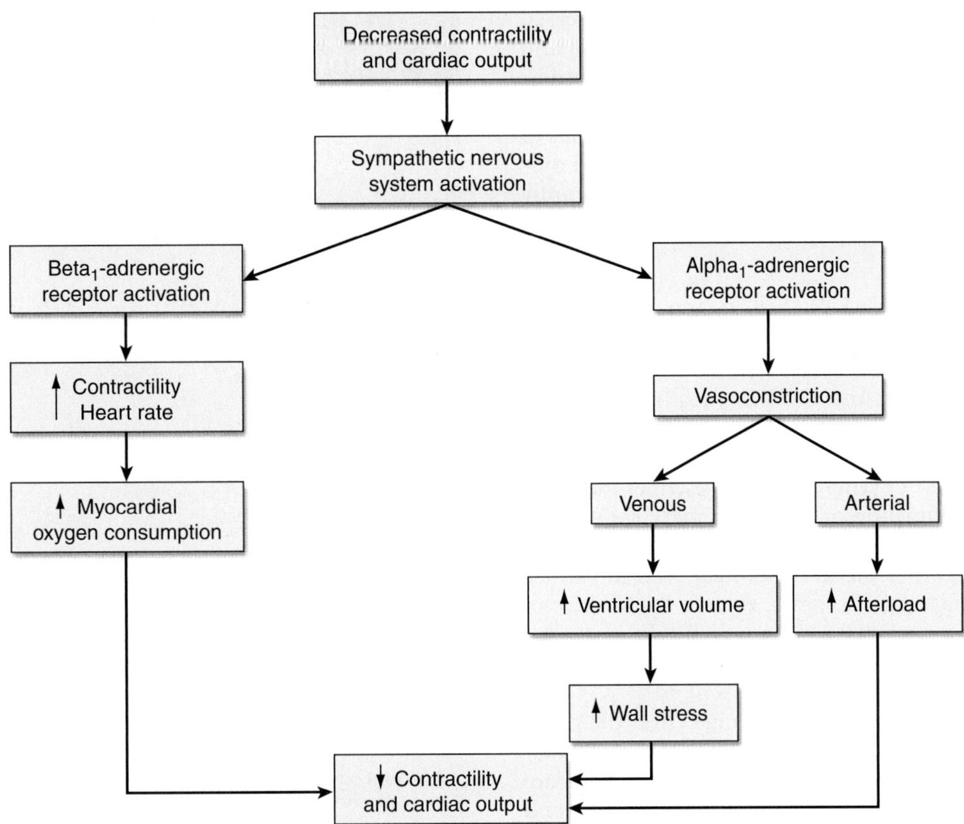

FIG. 4.2 Continued activation of the sympathetic nervous system leads to progression of ventricular dysfunction through several mechanisms.

Disregulation of the Immune System: Cytokines

Proinflammatory cytokines such as tissue necrosis factor alpha (TNFα) and interleukin-6 (IL-6) are elevated in patients with heart failure, and become more pronounced as myocardial function declines, even in the absence of an inflammatory or infectious process in the body.[212] The clinical significance of increased cytokine levels is not clearly understood, but it is known that these cytokines have deleterious effects on myocardial function. At high levels, cytokines can promote LV dysfunction, ventricular remodeling, and apoptosis. TNFα and IL-6 levels correlate with the New York Heart Association (NYHA) functional class, and patients with the highest levels have increased mortality compared to those with lower levels.[212]

Cytokines may be expressed directly from the myocardium in the failing heart, but not in a nonfailing heart. In the failing heart, TNFα is possibly produced in response to myocyte stretch or pressure and volume overload in the LV, although the mechanism is not clearly understood.[109,110] One mechanism suggests that endotoxin release in patients with altered gut permeability due to edema may be a source of chronic inflammation that stimulates activation of cytokines.[157] Deleterious effects of cytokines include toxic effects on the myocardium, and elevated levels of TNFα and IL-6 are associated with an adverse prognosis.[26,30,60,214] Effects such as ventricular fibrosis, chamber dilatation, and LV dysfunction have been seen with elevated levels of TNFα.[26,30] A prominent consequence of inflammatory activation associated with HF is the development of cardiac cachexia. Researchers have established a positive relationship between proinflammatory cytokine levels and severity of cardiac cachexia.[9,10]

Alterations in Extracellular Matrix

Cardiac cells (myocytes) are surrounded by an extensive and highly organized network weave of collagen that binds the cells together to hold them in proper alignment for an organized contraction during systole. Known as the extracellular matrix (ECM), this weave also holds capillaries adjacent to myocardial cells for oxygen and nutrient transfer. Bound together by this matrix, the myocardium has elastic properties that allow equal and appropriate stretch of myocytes during diastolic filling, and prevents slippage of adjacent cardiac cells during the cardiac cycle.[25]

The ECM is made of cardiac fibroblasts, which is the largest cell population in the myocardium. One of the main functions of cardiac fibroblasts is to maintain the integrity of the ECM. In HF or cardiac injury, cardiac fibroblasts can differentiate into myofibroblasts, which can produce more proteins to increase the ECM.[171] Myofibroblasts are not found in healthy myocardium but are only found after cardiac injury,[19] when their proliferation is increased and there is excess production of the ECM.[71] Myofibroblasts produce and secrete cytokines, including TNFα and IL-6, which maintain an inflammatory response to injury[19] and play a key role in reparative fibrosis with myocardial infarction and formation of hypertrophic scar in other cardiac injuries.[34]

In heart disease, the ECM becomes remodeled. If the matrix is disrupted, the connection among myocardial cells and between myocardial cells and blood vessels can compromise cardiac function. Without the ECM to hold them together, slippage of myocytes alters the organized fashion in which cells contract and leads to ventricular dysfunction.[21] Conversely, increased collagen production or fibrosis of the ECM results in increased myocardial stiffness and impaired ventricular contraction and relaxation.[21] Pressure overload in the ventricle triggers cardiac hypertrophy and fibrosis that leads to adverse ECM remodeling with areas of disrupted ECM network adjacent to regions of fibrotic lesions.[108] This further promotes LV dilation and dysfunction. In patients with HF, increased fibrosis is significantly associated with poor outcome.[20]

CARDIOMYOPATHY

The term "cardiomyopathy" was first used in 1957 and is often used interchangeably with "heart failure," but the definition of these two terms is not the same. Cardiomyopathy is a disease of the myocardium, often associated with failure of myocardial performance, either mechanical or electrical. Heart failure is a syndrome or confluence of symptoms that describes the experience of cardiac malfunction and/or pulmonary congestion, which may be a result of cardiomyopathy. Cardiomyopathy may have other effects on the heart as well, such as cardiac dysrhythmias or sudden cardiac death, even in the absence of clinical HF.

Definitions and Classifications

The definition of cardiomyopathy has changed over the years, and the criteria to differentiate it from other cardiovascular conditions continues to evolve. Contemporary definitions are based on the molecular genetics of cardiovascular disease and have clinical applications and implications for diagnosis. As cardiomyopathies are defined by genomics, the dilated-hypertrophic-restrictive classification has become less relevant.

Cardiomyopathy is defined as "a heterogeneous group of diseases of the myocardium associated with mechanical and/or electrical dysfunction that usually (but not invariably) exhibit inappropriate ventricular hypertrophy or dilatation and are due to a variety of causes that frequently are genetic."[140] In 2008, the European Society of Cardiology (ESC) defined cardiomyopathy as "a myocardial disorder in which the heart muscle is structurally and functionally abnormal in the absence of coronary artery disease, hypertension, valvular disease, and congenital heart disease sufficient to explain the observed myocardial abnormality."[66] The World Heart Federation published a phenotype-genotype nomenclature of cardiomyopathy in 2013.[11]

Cardiomyopathies are either confined to the heart or are part of generalized systemic disorders, often leading to cardiovascular death or progressive heart failure–related disability.[140] Originally, cardiomyopathies were defined as disorders that were idiopathic. However in current clinical practice, the term "cardiomyopathy" is often combined with the terms "ischemic," "valvular," and "hypertensive" to describe various heart diseases. Unfortunately, this expands the term cardiomyopathy, which was created to reflect genetically determined diseases with recognized phenotypes.[49]

Cardiomyopathies can be categorized as primary and secondary (Table 4.1). Primary cardiomyopathies include those that are solely or predominantly confined to heart muscle, and can be divided into genetic, mixed, or acquired. Secondary cardiomyopathies were previously known as specific cardiomyopathies or specific heart muscle diseases, and have pathologic myocardial involvement as a component of a variety of other generalized multi-organ disorders.

TABLE 4.1 AHA Classification of Cardiomyopathies

Primary Cardiomyopathies

Genetic
- Hypertrophic Cardiomyopathy
- Arrhythmogenic Right Ventricular Cardiomyopathy/Dysplasia
- Noncompaction
- Conduction System Disease
- Ion Channelopathies
  - Long QT Syndrome
  - Brugada Syndrome
  - Short-QT Syndrome
  - Catecholamine Polymorphic Ventricular Tachycardia

Mixed
- Dilated Cardiomyopathy
- Restrictive Nonhypertrophied

Acquired
- Myocarditis
- Stress Cardiomyopathy (Tako-Tsubo)

Secondary Cardiomyopathies

Infiltrative
- Amyloidosis
- Gaucher disease
- Hurler disease
- Hunter disease

Storage
- Hemochromatosis
- Fabry disease
- Glycogen storage disease
- Niemann-Pick disease

Toxicity
- Drugs, heavy metals, chemical agents

Endomyocardial
- Endomyocardial fibrosis
- Hypereosinophilic syndrome

Inflammatory
- Sarcoidosis

Endocrine
- Diabetes mellitus
- Hyperthyroidism
- Hypothyroidism
- Hyperparathyroidism
- Pheochromocytoma
- Acromegaly

Cardiofacial
- Noonan syndrome
- Lentiginosis

Neuromuscular/neurologic
- Friedreich ataxia
- Duchenne-Becker muscular dystrophy
- Emery-Dreifuss muscular dystrophy
- Myotonic dystrophy
- Neurofibromatosis
- Tuberous sclerosis

Nutritional deficiencies
- Beriberi, pellagra, scurvy, selenium, carnitine, kwashiorkor

Autoimmune/collagen
- Systemic lupus erythematosus
- Dermatomyositis
- Rheumatoid arthritis
- Scleroderma
- Polyarteritis nodosa

Electrolyte imbalance

Secondary to cancer therapy
- Anthracyclines: doxorubicin (Adriamycin), daunorubicin
- Cyclophosphamide
- Radiation

From Reference 66.

Primary Cardiomyopathies – Genetic

Hypertrophic Cardiomyopathy

Hypertrophic cardiomyopathy (HCM) is the most frequently occurring cardiomyopathy and the most common cause of sudden cardiac death in the young.[138,140] HCM can be described as a hypertrophied, nondilated LV in the absence of another systemic or cardiac cause that could produce such a magnitude of wall thickening, such as hypertension or aortic stenosis. Diagnosis is made by 2D echocardiography; however, cardiovascular magnetic resonance is being used with increasing frequency.[141] HCM is associated with a very low mortality rate and normal life expectancy with little or no disability. Some HCM patients may have higher morbidity and mortality related to complications of sudden death, progressive HF, and embolic stroke due to atrial fibrillation.[138] Most patients with HCM may develop dynamic obstruction to the LV outflow tract that occurs with systolic anterior motion of the mitral valve (known as SAM) with septal contact.[140]

Treatment of HCM depends on the degree of patient symptoms. Treatment for exertional dyspnea may include beta blockers, verapamil, or disopyramide. Treatment for severe refractory symptoms with marked outflow obstruction includes the septal myotomy-myectomy operation, but alcohol septal ablation and pacing are alternatives to surgery. High-risk patients may require an implantable defibrillator for sudden death prevention.[138]

Arrhythmogenic Right Ventricular Cardiomyopathy/Dysplasia

Arrhythmogenic right ventricular cardiomyopathy/dysplasia (ARVC/D) is a relatively newly described form of nonischemic cardiomyopathy involving mainly the right ventricle (RV). There is a progressive loss of myocytes, which are replaced with fibrofatty tissue, causing regional areas of hypokinesis and arrhythmias.[140] The LV is involved in approximately 75% of cases with fibrofatty deposits, chamber enlargement, and myocarditis. The prevalence of ARVC/D is 1 in 10,000 in the general US population, and accounts for up to 17% of sudden cardiac deaths in young people.[103] Noninvasive testing to diagnose ARVC/D includes family history, 12-lead ECG, echocardiogram, RV angiography, cardiac magnetic resonance imaging (MRI), and computerized tomography (CT). Biopsy from the RV free wall can be diagnostic if fibrofatty infiltration is seen.[140]

Ventricular arrhythmias that occur with ARVC/D include premature ventricular complexes (PVCs), ventricular tachycardia, and ventricular fibrillation, all of which most commonly arise from the RV.[35,53] Symptomatic ventricular arrhythmias are initially treated with beta blocker therapy, but antiarrhythmic agents such as sotalol or amiodarone may be considered if further treatment is needed.[35] Other HF medications such as ACEIs, as well as devices such as implantable defibrillators, are also used in the management of these patients.[35]

LV Noncompaction

Noncompaction of the LV is a congenital condition described as a spongy appearance of the myocardium. The distal apical section of the LV is marked by deep intertrabecular recesses that occur due to abnormalities of embryogenesis.[140] Diagnosis is made through echocardiography, cardiac MRI, CT, and LV angiography.[215] Conditions that may arise in patients with LV noncompaction include ventricular arrhythmias, thromboembolism, heart failure, and sudden cardiac death.[215]

Conduction System Disease

Primary progressive cardiac conduction defect is marked by development of conduction defects in the His-Purkinje system that lead to widening of the QRS complex, pauses, and bradycardia that may cause syncope.[140] Structural heart abnormalities may or may not be present, but there is a familial occurrence with an autosomal dominant pattern of inheritance.

Ion Channel Disorders

There are many diseases related to ion channels. Many uncommon inherited and congenital arrhythmias are caused by mutations in genes encoding defective ionic channel proteins that control cell membrane transfer of sodium and potassium ions.[140] Although these are discussed as cardiomyopathies in the AHA/ACC Scientific Statement, structural myocardial abnormalities may be absent. These disorders include long QT syndrome, short QT syndrome, and catecholaminergic polymorphic ventricular tachycardia. Brugada syndrome represents a distinct electrocardiographic pattern of right bundle branch block (BBB) and ST-segment elevation in the anterior leads that is associated with sudden cardiac death in young people.[140]

Mixed (Genetic and Nongenetic)

Dilated Cardiomyopathy

Dilated cardiomyopathy is marked by ventricular chamber size enlargement and systolic dysfunction without an increase in LV wall thickness. The dilatation is often severe and is accompanied by an increase in total cardiac mass.[48] The LV cavity becomes less ovoid and more spherical in shape. This leads to progressive HF and decreased LV contractility, arrhythmias, conduction system abnormalities, thromboembolism, and sudden death or HF-related death.[140] Causes include viruses and genetic mutations that are fairly common in idiopathic dilated cardiomyopathy.

Primary Restrictive Nonhypertrophied Cardiomyopathy

Primary restrictive nonhypertrophied cardiomyopathy is a rare form of heart muscle disorder that is characterized by normal or decreased volume of both ventricles, bi-atrial enlargement, normal LV wall thickness, impaired ventricular filling with restrictive pattern, and nearly normal systolic function.[140]

Acquired

Myocarditis (Inflammatory Cardiomyopathy)

Myocarditis is an inflammatory process that affects the myocardium. It may be acute or chronic and is caused by a variety of toxins such as cocaine, IL-2, viral or bacterial infections, fungal or parasitic infections, or a hypersensitivity reaction to certain drugs.[140] The clinical presentation of myocarditis spans a broad range from minimal symptoms, fatigue, chest pain, heart failure, cardiogenic shock, and arrhythmias to sudden death.[162,164] Clinical presentation depends on the histologic disease severity, the cause, and the stage of disease when it is first diagnosed. Inflammation of the myocardium may involve all four cardiac chambers or it may be localized to one area. Rapid onset of severe diffuse myocarditis may cause acute dilated cardiomyopathy. Approximately 10% of unexplained cardiomyopathies are thought to be due to myocarditis.[48] Typically, myocarditis evolves through active, healing, and healed stages, starting with inflammatory cell infiltrates that lead to interstitial edema and focal myocyte necrosis, ultimately ending with fibrosis.[140] This process creates electrical instability in the ventricles and can predispose to ventricular arrhythmias.

Echocardiography is the main method to detect myocarditis, revealing LV dilation, remodeling, and usually global wall motion abnormalities.[158,174] Endomyocardial biopsy may show diagnostic inflammatory infiltrates and necrosis, but it is limited by insensitivity and false-negative results.[140] The Dallas criteria are a standard for the United States Myocarditis Treatment Trial, and are used to define the disease. The criteria define active myocarditis as "an inflammatory infiltrate of the myocardium with necrosis and/or degeneration of adjacent myocytes not typical of the ischemic damage associated with coronary artery disease."[12] However, this criteria is controversial among expert pathologists due to low sensitivity and disagreement on the interpretation of myocardial biopsy material.[18]

Stress ("Tako-Tsubo") Cardiomyopathy

Tako-Tsubo (or sometimes called takotsubo) cardiomyopathy is characterized by acute LV systolic dysfunction triggered by profound psychological distress. It typically affects older women and specifically involves the distal portion of the LV chamber, known as apical ballooning, with hypercontractility of the basal LV.[196] Patients often present with what appears to be an ST-segment elevation myocardial infarction, but generally do not have atherosclerotic coronary artery disease.[196] The pathogenesis of this disorder is not well understood. Also is not understood, why it disproportionately affects postmenopausal women and why it affects the mid-cavity and apical LV. One theory suggests that stress-related catecholamine release may cause diffuse catecholamine-induced microvascular spasm or dysfunction that results in myocardial stunning.[87] Another hypothesis describes direct catecholamine-associated myocardial toxicity.[156] The diagnosis of Tako-Tsubo cardiomyopathy generally requires coronary angiography to rule out atherosclerotic etiology, serial assessment of LV systolic function, with subsequent assessment usually by echocardiography, an electrocardiogram, and cardiac troponin levels. Fortunately, Tako-Tsubo cardiomyopathy is generally a transient disorder that resolves with supportive therapy such as standard medications for HFrEF, including ACEI or angiotensin receptor blockers (ARB), beta blockers, aldosterone antagonists, and diuretics.

Others

Peripartum or postpartum cardiomyopathy can occur during the third trimester of pregnancy or the first 5 months after delivery. It is a rare dilated form of cardiomyopathy associated with LV systolic dysfunction and HF symptoms. Approximately 50% of cases will have full recovery within 6 months, but the remaining cases may have clinical deterioration requiring advanced therapies such as transplantation.[140]

Other, less common, cardiomyopathies that lead to LV dysfunction may include prolonged tachycardias or excessive alcohol consumption. Both of these conditions are potentially reversible when the cause of the cardiomyopathy is removed.

Secondary Cardiomyopathies

A long list of systemic conditions that involve the myocardium may lead to cardiomyopathy. These arise from multiple sources, ranging from infiltrative conditions, toxicities, inflammatory conditions, endocrine or nutritional deficiencies, autoimmune or neuromuscular disorders, and secondary to cancer treatments (see Table 4.1).

ASSESSMENT OF THE PATIENT PRESENTING WITH HEART FAILURE

Physical Findings

Initial evaluation of the HF patient should include a thorough history to determine any cardiac and noncardiac disorders or behaviors that might have caused or accelerated the development or progression of the condition.[114,227] History should include the patient's current health status, focusing on current signs and symptoms, as well as past medical history and related conditions. Focus should be paid to cardiac-related conditions, such as CAD, cardiac surgeries, hypertension, dysrhythmias,

BOX 4.1 Signs and Symptoms of Heart Failure

Signs

- Edema (peripheral, sacral)
- Jugular venous distention or elevated venous pressure (>16 mm Hg)
- Rales (although can be absent in most patients with heart failure because of compensation by pulmonary lymphatic system)
- Cardiomegaly
- Hepatojugular reflex
- Displaced apical pulse
- Ascites
- Third heart sound

Symptoms

- Dyspnea or orthopnea
- Paroxysmal nocturnal dyspnea
- Nocturnal cough
- Activity intolerance, fatigue
- Anorexia or other gastrointestinal symptoms

BOX 4.2 New York Heart Association Functional Classification

Based on patient's report of dyspnea or fatigue during physical activity
Class I: No limitation during physical activity
Class II: Slight limitations during ordinary physical activity, comfortable at rest
Class III: Marked limitations during any physical activity; only comfortable at rest
Class IV: Inability to carry out physical activities without discomfort and symptoms; symptoms at rest

and hereditary diseases. In addition, noncardiac conditions that should be noted include hyper- or hypothyroidism, diabetes mellitus, peripheral vascular disease, connective tissue diseases, hepatitis C, human immunodeficiency virus, chronic pulmonary diseases, renal insufficiency, and chronic kidney disease.

Many symptoms of HF are nonspecific and do not discriminate between HF and other problems, especially in the obese individual.[147] Other comorbidities may mimic HF, such as anemia, pulmonary disease, or renal failure. Presenting symptoms may include breathing problems such as shortness of breath (SOB), dyspnea on exertion (DOE), or paroxysmal nocturnal dyspnea (PND). Patients may also report coughing, wheezing, exercise intolerance, generalized fatigue, chest pain, gastrointestinal problems, peripheral edema, palpitations, dizziness, lightheadedness, mental status changes, and sleep disturbances. Symptoms are generally related to sodium and fluid retention in lungs, gut, and peripheral extremities, or hypoperfusion of various organs (brain, gut, kidneys, peripheral muscles)[147] (Box 4.1). Because of the nonspecific nature of these symptoms, it is important to maintain a high level of suspicion and to confirm findings with objective evidence of structural or functional cardiac abnormality. Functional status of the patient can be evaluated using the New York Heart Association (NYHA) Functional Classification based on the patient's report of dyspnea and fatigue at various levels of activity as outlined in Box 4.2.

Stages of Heart Failure

The American College of Cardiology Foundation/American Heart Association (ACCF/AHA) guideline for the management of heart failure emphasizes prevention at several levels

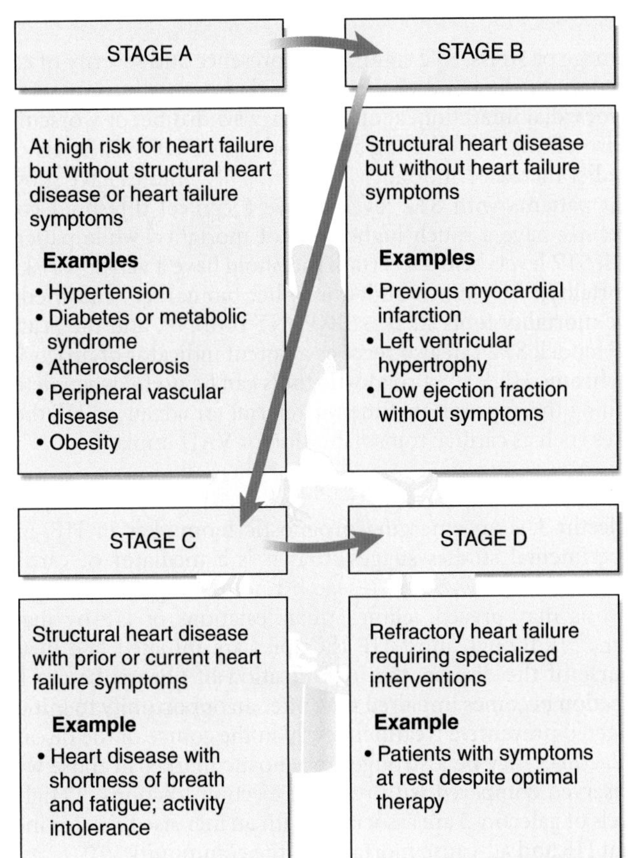

FIG. 4.3 The four stages in the development of heart failure as described by the American College of Cardiology Foundation/ American Heart Association.

in the development and progression of heart failure by conceptualizing heart failure in four progressive stages (Fig. 4.3 and Box 4.3). Those patients in stage A are considered to be in "pre-heart failure," meaning they do not yet have structural heart disease or symptoms, but are at risk for the development of such. The goal of therapy for patients in this stage is the prevention of heart failure. Individuals with stage B heart failure have developed structural heart disease, but do not have symptoms of heart failure. The goal for stage B is to prevent both HF symptoms and further cardiac remodeling. As their HF progresses, patients in stage C develop overt symptoms of HF. The goal at this stage is to control symptoms, improve quality of life, and prevent hospitalizations and mortality. Stage D HF is refractory HF in which specialized interventions are needed. The goal for stage D patients is similar to those for stage C patients with the addition of establishing the patient's end-of-life goals. Therapy for each stage is outlined in Box 4.3.[227]

It is important to remember that the stages move in only one direction reflecting the progressive nature of HF, and can be linked with treatment strategies. Communicating the current stage with patients might help them to recognize the progressive nature of their condition, even when asymptomatic, especially if the communication is coupled with management strategies, including self-care.

BOX 4.3 Management of Stages of Heart Failure from the American College of Cardiology/American Heart Association Heart Failure Guidelines

Stage A Therapy: Treat Risk Factors for Heart Failure and Its Precursors

- Treat hypertension aggressively
- Treat dyslipidemias
- Control diabetes and metabolic syndrome
- Smoking cessation
- Promote regular exercise
- Obesity control
- Other measures to prevent atherosclerosis and coronary artery disease
- Discourage excess alcohol intake, illicit drug use
- Angiotensin-converting enzyme inhibitors or angiotensin receptor blockers in at-risk patients

Stage B Therapy: Treat Structural Heart Disease

- All measures in stage A
- Beta blockers in appropriate patients

Stage C Therapy: Treat Heart Failure

- All stage A and stage B lifestyle measures
- Dietary sodium restriction
- Angiotensin-converting enzyme inhibitors or angiotensin receptor blockers in at-risk patients
- Beta-adrenergic receptor blockers
- Diuretics
- Digoxin
- Aldosterone antagonists
- Hydralazine/nitrates
- Biventricular pacing or implantable defibrillators in select patients

Stage D Therapy: Treat Refractory Heart Failure Requiring Specialized Interventions

- All measures under stages A, B, C
- Mechanical assist devices
- Heart transplantation
- Palliative/hospice care

Diagnostic Testing

Differentiation of ischemic versus nonischemic cardiomyopathy is important since prognosis in CAD–induced cardiomyopathy is improved when the treatment plan includes revascularization in addition to medical management. Segmental (and global) wall motion abnormalities visible by echocardiography are present in both dilated and ischemic cardiomyopathy; thus a definitive etiology cannot be determined by echocardiogram alone. Coronary artery evaluation is needed and cardiac catheterization may be helpful to assess for the presence of ischemic disease, the cardiac output, degree of LV dysfunction, and LV end-diastolic pressure.

Making a diagnosis of HFpEF is much more difficult than HFrEF because there is not a clear diagnostic marker to identify patients, but rather it is diagnosed through exclusion of other potential causes for HF symptoms. Several criteria that have been proposed to define HFpEF include: clinical signs or symptoms of HF, normal or preserved LVEF, and abnormalities of LV diastolic function evidenced by echocardiogram or cardiac catheterization.[218]

There is no single test that definitely diagnoses acute decompensated HF (ADHF); rather the diagnosis is made based on clinical judgment after consideration of a number of factors. The following diagnostic tests may be employed to assist in the decision-making process.

B-Type Natriuretic Peptide or NT-proBNP

As previously mentioned, the natriuretic peptides have diverse cardiovascular, renal, and endocrine system effects. BNP or its amino-terminal equivalent, NT-proBNP, is released from the cardiomyocytes as a result of increased myocardial pressure and stretch. Endogenous BNP causes natriuresis (i.e., urinary loss of sodium and water) and vasodilation. These effects are not adequate to overcome the adverse effects of the counter-regulatory hormones of the neurohormonal system activated in HF. Thus, BNP is released in HF as a protective response to fluid overload and, therefore, is a useful diagnostic and prognostic tool.

The Breathing Not Properly study was the first large multinational prospective study using BNP levels to evaluate the causes of dyspnea.[134] In this study, BNP levels were found to be better at accurately predicting presence of heart failure than history, physical findings, or laboratory values. A BNP level greater than 100 pg/mL had a 90% sensitivity and 76% specificity for differentiating heart failure from other causes of dyspnea.

The level of BNP can be determined from serum assays of BNP or of NT-proBNP, the biologically inactive N-terminal fragment of proBNP cleavage that produces the biologically active BNP. Both BNP and NT-proBNP assays perform equally well in clinical situations. The cut-point for BNP for the best negative predictive value is 100 pg/mL, while the similar cut-point for NT-proBNP is 300 pg/mL. NT-proBNP and BNP values are not comparable and there is no conversion factor for one to the other.[221] There is marked inter-individual variation in repeat BNP and NT-proBNP levels, and BNP and NT-proBNP are affected by age (higher at older ages), gender (women have higher levels), renal failure (higher levels seen with worse renal function), body weight, and the presence of other comorbidities (e.g., diabetes and hypertension). BNP levels may not be elevated in cases of "flash pulmonary edema" from ADHF, and BNP levels are most predictive in ADHF patients with new symptoms. More research is needed to clarify level norms in various subgroups.

BNP levels are now commonly used in the emergency department (ED) to determine whether heart failure is the cause of dyspnea. A BNP level is usually measured when the patient first presents to the hospital with symptoms of ADHF and again before discharge. If BNP levels do not fall after 24 hours of therapy, this may indicate that the patient needs more aggressive treatment or that there may be another cause such as elevated RV end-diastolic volume in the presence of pulmonary embolus. This may mimic the symptoms of LV HF. Failure of BNP to improve with treatment is a poor prognostic sign.[221] The frequency of BNP evaluation throughout the hospitalization depends on the provider's clinical judgment. Although BNP levels are associated with disease severity and prognosis in patients with heart failure, there are as yet no definitive data demonstrating that BNP levels can be used for determining optimization of therapy. Therefore, the 2013 ACCF/AHA Guideline for the Management of HF recommends BNP and NT-proBNP levels to support clinical decision-making during diagnosis, disease severity, and prognosis in acute and chronic HF. However, the usefulness of serial measurements for guided therapy is not well established.[227]

ST2

The ST2 cardiac biomarker is a recently described soluble protein biomarker released from the heart in the presence of damage or stress. ST2 signifies the presence and severity of cardiac remodeling and tissue fibrosis that occurs in response to myocardial infarction, acute coronary syndrome, or worsening heart failure.[181,195] During an episode of ADHF, ST2 levels can predict increased mortality at 1 year.[105,181] Studies have shown that patients with ST2 levels above a clinical threshold consistently have a much higher risk of mortality, while patients with ST2 levels below a certain threshold have a very low risk of mortality.[118,124] When added to other biomarkers and predictive mortality tools such as BNP, NT proBNP, and the Seattle HF model, ST2 can also serve as a potent indicator of prognosis in chronic HF.[124,202] Prognostic tools can be useful when determining the appropriate time for referral for advanced HF therapies such as cardiac transplantation or VAD implant.

Galectin-3

Galectin-3 is an emerging prognostic biomarker in HF, and experimental studies suggest that it is a mediator of cardiac fibrosis.[58,130,194,216] Some research findings suggest that active fibrosis may precede clinical manifestations of HF by many years.[99] Although most HF therapies are initiated late in the course of the disease, the identification of fibrosis before LV function becomes impaired may offer an opportunity to initiate targeted preventive treatment early in the course of the disease. Galactin-3 may be a stronger prognostic marker in those with preserved compared with reduced ejection fractions.[56] Higher levels of galectin-3 are associated with an increased risk for incident HF and all-cause mortality in the community.[57,99]

Other Laboratory Testing

Laboratory testing in patients who present with HF includes a complete blood count, electrolyte panel, blood urea nitrogen (BUN), serum creatinine, and urinalysis. Patients should be tested for diabetes mellitus, or if already diagnosed with diabetes, a hemoglobin A1c level should be obtained. A fasting lipid panel, liver function tests, and thyroid panel should also be evaluated. Based on the patient's history and presenting symptoms, specific tests to screen for hemochromatosis, HIV, rheumatologic diseases, amyloidosis, or pheochromocytoma are reasonable.[227] These laboratory tests are helpful to evaluate comorbidities that contribute to etiology or worsening HF (i.e., anemia, diabetes, renal insufficiency, hyperlipidemia, and thyroid abnormalities).

Chest Radiograph

In the context of the clinical presentation, the chest radiograph (x-ray) can be an important part of the assessment of ADHF. Despite the absence of rales on physical exam, findings of pulmonary congestion may be seen on x-ray.[79,114] An early sign of fluid accumulation in the interstitium is the presence of Kerley B lines, which represent fluid accumulation in the interlobular septa. The findings of cardiomegaly, pulmonary edema, or pleural effusion on the chest x-ray are indicative of heart failure, but these findings alone do not confirm the diagnosis and must be correlated with clinical findings.[177,227]

Electrocardiogram

The electrocardiogram (ECG) is of limited use in establishing a diagnosis of heart failure. However, a normal ECG may rule out HF based on the high negative predictive value for systolic dysfunction.[114] In addition, it may be helpful in determining the onset of new dysrhythmias that may precipitate or exacerbate ADHF, and may provide evidence of myocardial ischemia or infarction, and conduction abnormalities such as BBB.[107]

Echocardiogram

The most useful diagnostic test in the patient with or at risk for HF is the 2-D echocardiogram with Doppler flow studies. Echocardiography can identify the LVEF, abnormalities of myocardium, heart valves, and pericardium, as well as subclinical HF.[227] However, repeated assessment of LV function in patients with HF does not affect or alter the treatment plan unless significant changes in the patient's cardiac function or clinical status have occurred. Thus echocardiography is indicated in ADHF only when there is evidence that changes in patients' myocardial performance or valvular integrity may have precipitated ADHF. It may also provide information about the presence of an acute ischemic syndrome and the status of the pericardium.[6]

Coronary Angiography

Coronary angiography may be appropriate in the evaluation of ADHF if it appears that acute MI or unstable acute coronary syndrome amenable to intervention precipitated the patient's ADHF. In patients with known CAD and angina, angiography is appropriate. If the patient has no prior diagnosis of CAD, but LV dysfunction is present, CAD should be considered as a possible etiology. Evaluation of coronary ischemia, which may include cardiac catheterization, is indicated. It is important to speak with the patient and outline possible interventions before proceeding to the catheterization lab, to determine the patient's wishes for future therapy.

MEDICATIONS USED IN THE MANAGEMENT OF HEART FAILURE

The cornerstone of HF medical treatment is neurohormonal blockade. Guideline-directed medical treatment (GDMT)[227] centers around three neurohormone pathways, as well as other various medications, each with its unique properties. Recommended therapies are based on the evidence provided from many clinical trials.[40] Table 4.2 summarizes the medications, doses, and special considerations for many of the classes of medications.

While the recommendations for HF therapy may seem straightforward, it is imperative to remember that all patients respond to therapy and medication combinations differently. Therefore, HF therapy should be individually tailored to provide optimal symptom management and benefit while minimizing adverse effects and response to therapy.

Angiotensin-Converting Enzyme Inhibitors

Angiotensin-converting enzyme inhibitors (ACEIs) affect the RAAS by inhibiting the conversion of angiotensin I to angiotensin II, thus decreasing vasoconstriction and enhancing afterload reduction and subsequently decreasing the workload on the heart. ACEIs are indicated for the symptomatic and asymptomatic patients with LVEF of less than or equal to 40%. Doses should be titrated to those used in clinical trials and as tolerated by the patient based on laboratory data and symptoms (see Table 4.2).[227] Clinical trials have shown that ACEIs significantly decrease the morbidity, mortality, hospitalizations, and symptoms, as well as increase the quality of life for HF patients.[144,172]

Angiotensin Receptor Blockers

ARBs affect the RAAS by blocking angiotensin II type 1 receptors to mediate most of the detrimental effects of angiotensin II. Similar to ACEIs, they also promote afterload reduction and vasodilation, thus decreasing the workload on the heart. ARBs are indicated to treat symptomatic and asymptomatic patients with LVEF less than or equal to 40% who are intolerant of ACEIs due to a cough. Clinical trials have shown no difference in effectiveness between ACEIs and ARBs.[144,172] GDMT recommends ACEIs as the first choice for inhibition of the RAAS in systolic HF, but ARBs can be considered a reasonable alternative.[227]

Neprilysin Endopeptidase Inhibitor/ARB (Sacubitril/Valsartan)

A medication that is a combination of sacubitril and valsartan (Entresto) was approved in 2015 for use in patients with systolic HF and NYHA Class II to IV. It is given in combination with other HF therapies in place of an ACEI or ARB alone, and combines a neprilysin inhibitor (sacubitril) with an ARB (valsartan). While ARBs have been widely used in treating HF, sacubitril is a new agent in the HF armamentarium. This type of drug inhibits the effects of neprilysin, which is an endopeptidase that degrades endogenous peptides, such as BNP, bradykinin, and adrenomedullin.[52,178,224] By inhibiting neprilysin, the levels of these peptides increase, counteracting the harmful neurohormones that cause vasoconstriction, sodium and water retention, and remodeling of the myocardium.[123,136] Sacubitril/valsartan was evaluated directly against ACEI therapy (enalapril) in patients with HFrEF and NYHA Class II-IV. The trial was stopped early due to an overwhelming benefit with sacubitril/valsartan in reducing the risk of death and hospitalization for HF patients.[148]

Dosing for sacubitril/valsartan is 49/51 mg twice daily, with the goal of titrating to the maximum dose of 97/103 mg after 2 to 3 weeks. The unusual dosage of medications in this combination pill varies from the usual ARB dose due to differences in bioavailability of an ARB alone. It is extremely important to avoid concomitant use of this drug with an ACEI, and there needs to be at least a 36-hour washout period between the time a patient takes an ACEI or ARB and sacubitril/valsartan. Angioedema is a potential problem with this medication due to the neprilysin inhibition, which prevents the degradation of bradykinin.[80] If the patient has ever experienced angioedema, they may be at higher risk of experiencing it with this drug, and it should not be initiated in that patient, particularly if angioedema was related to previous ACEI or ARB use.

Beta Adrenergic Receptor Blockers

Beta-blocking agents work by blocking the effects of the catecholamines epinephrine and norepinephrine, which are activated in HF. They are indicated for patients with LVEF less than or equal to 40% in addition to ACEI or ARB to lessen the symptoms of HF, improve the patient's clinical status, and reduce the risk of death and hospitalizations.[92,167] Beta blockers significantly reduce all-cause mortality rates by 23% to 32%, as well as result in reverse cardiac remodeling and increased LVEF.[54,70,217] They should not be initiated in the setting of acute decompensated HF. However, it is recommended that if the patient is currently on beta blocker therapy, it should be continued during an episode of decompensation whenever possible, even if lower dosages are used. Abrupt withdrawal of treatment with a beta blocker can lead to clinical deterioration.[82]

TABLE 4.2 Medications for Chronic Drug Therapy

Medication	Initial Dose	Maximum Dose	Side Effects	Special Considerations
Angiotensin-Converting Enzyme Inhibitor Therapy				
Captopril (Capoten) Enalapril (Vasotec) Lisinopril (Zestril) Quinapril (Accupril) Ramipril (Altace)	6.25 mg TID 2.5 mg BID 2.5–5 mg daily 5 mg BID 1.25–2.5 mg qd	50 mg TID 10–20 mg BID 20–40 mg daily 20 mg BID 10 mg daily	Hypotension, hyperkalemia, renal insufficiency, cough, angioedema	Efforts to avoid sodium retention or depletion should be made, because volume imbalance affects effectiveness of ACEI therapy; fluid retention decreases benefits and fluid depletion increases potential for hypotension or renal insufficiency. NSAIDs adversely affect ACEI effectiveness and should be avoided
Angiotensin Receptor Blocking Agents				
Candesartan (Atacand) Losartan (Cozaar) Valsartan (Diovan)	4–8 mg daily 25–50 mg daily 20–40 mg BID	32 mg daily 50–100 mg daily 160 mg BID	Hypotension, hyperkalemia, worsening renal function, angioedema (less often than ACEIs, but still occurs)	ACEIs are first choice renin-angiotensin system antagonism. ARBs are an alternative in patients intolerant to ACEIs because of refractory cough. ARBs appear to cause hypotension, worsening renal function, and hyperkalemia as often as ACEIs
Sacubitril/valsartan (Entresto)	49/51 mg BID	97/103 mg BID	Hypotension, angioedema	Washout period of 36 hours required between stopping ACEI/ARB and starting sacubitril/valsartan
Aldosterone Antagonists				
Spironolactone (Aldactone) Eplerenone (Inspra)	12.5-25 mg daily 25 mg daily	25 mg daily or BID 50 mg daily	Hyperkalemia, gynecomastia (spironolactone)	Monitor electrolytes and renal function closely, per protocol (monthly for first 3 months, then every 3 months)
Beta-adrenergic Blocking Agents				
Bisoprolol (Zebeta) Carvedilol (Coreg) Carvedilol CR (Coreg CR) Metoprolol CR/XL (Toprol XL)	1.25 mg daily 3.125 mg BID 10 mg daily 12.5–25 mg daily	10 mg 25 mg BID; 50 mg BID for patients >85 kg; 50 mg BID for patients ≥85 kg 80 mg daily 200 mg	Hypotension, bradycardia and heart block, fatigue, fluid retention, and worsening heart failure	Use with ACEIs, but if hypotension a problem, consider giving ACEIs and beta blocker at different times of day. In patients with fluid overload, diuretics improve action of beta blockers by maintaining fluid and sodium balance. May increase fluid retention during initiation of therapy; close monitoring of fluid status by patient with daily weights is necessary. May take weeks to months for symptoms to improve, and beta blockers should be continued even if symptom status is unchanged because they protect against future adverse cardiac events
Ivabradine (Corlanor)	5 mg BID	7.5 mg BID	Bradycardia	Add only after guideline directed medical therapy has been optimized. Initial starting dose may be lowered to 2.5 mg BID if bradycardia is issue
Diuretic Therapy				
Loop Diuretics				
Bumetanide (Bumex) Furosemide (Lasix) Torsemide (Demadex)	0.5–1 mg daily or BID 20–40 mg daily or BID 10–20 mg daily	10 mg 600 mg 200 mg	Electrolyte depletion, hypotension, azotemia	Diuretics cannot be used alone for management of heart failure. By promoting fluid and sodium balance, diuretics enhance effectiveness of other heart failure medications. Care should be taken to avoid over- and under diuresis. Diuretic equivalencies: bumetanide 1 mg = furosemide 40 mg = torsemide 10–20 mg
Thiazides				
Chlorothiazide (Diuril) Chlorthalidone (Hygroton) Hydrochlorothiazide (Microzide) Indapamide (Lozol) Metolazone (Zaroxolyn)	250–500 mg daily or BID 25–50 mg daily 25 mg daily or BID 2.5 mg daily 5 mg daily	1000 mg 200 mg 100 mg 5 mg 20 mg	Electrolyte depletion, hypotension, azotemia, photosensitivity	
Sequential Nephron Blockade				
Metolazone (Zaroxolyn)	2.5–10 mg once plus loop diuretic			

ACE, Angiotensin-converting enzyme; *ACEI*, angiotensin-converting enzyme inhibitor; *ARB*, angiotensin receptor blocker; *BID*, twice per day, *NSAIDs*, nonsteroidal antiinflammatory drugs; *TID*, three times per day.
Modified from Reference 227.

Aldosterone Receptor Antagonists

Aldosterone antagonists inhibit aldosterone which is activated in HF causing sodium and water retention, as well as an inflammatory response causing myocardial fibrosis and ventricular remodeling. The landmark Randomized Aldactone Evaluation Study (RALES) trial[176] showed a 30% reduction in all-cause mortality, sudden cardiac deaths, and HF hospitalizations when spironolactone was added to the patient's treatment regimen.[219] Close monitoring of renal function, potassium, and diuretic dosing is required to minimize risk of hyperkalemia and renal insufficiency.[176,230,231]

Isosorbide Dinitrate and Hydralazine

The combination of hydralazine and isosorbide dinitrate act as direct vasodilators to reduce afterload and decrease cardiac workload. They can be useful to reduce morbidity and mortality for patients with current or prior symptomatic HFrEF who cannot be given an ACEI or ARB because of medication intolerance, hypotension, hyperkalemia, or renal insufficiency.[227] In addition, the combination is recommended for African Americans with NYHA Class III-IV HFrEF who are already on ACEI and beta blocker therapy.[210]

Digoxin

Digoxin is a neurohormonal modulator that reduces the effects of the sympathetic nervous system and suppresses renin secretion from the kidneys. Several trials have shown that treatment with digoxin for 1 to 3 months can improve symptoms, quality of life, and exercise tolerance in patients with mild to moderate HF.[3,179] Treatment for 2 to 5 years had no effect on mortality but modestly reduced the combined risk of death and hospitalization.[94]

Ivabradine

Elevated resting heart rate is a risk factor for adverse outcomes in HF patients. Ivabradine was approved in 2015 for use in HF patients with an elevated heart rate to reduce the likelihood of hospital readmissions. Unlike beta blockers or calcium channel blockers, ivabradine slows heart rate by inhibiting certain pacemaker currents in the sinoatrial node. Diastolic duration is prolonged, which also acts to decrease chronic stable angina in patients with ischemic heart disease. In patients with HFrEF and heart rate above 70 beats/min, ivabradine was shown to significantly reduce the primary composite endpoint of cardiovascular death and hospitalization for worsening HF in the Systolic Heart Failure Treatment with I_f inhibitor ivabradine Trial (SHIFT) study.[207] Ivabradine is only added after GDMT has been optimized. The starting dose is 5 mg twice a day, and, after 2 weeks, the dose may be adjusted upward to the maximum dose of 7.5 mg twice daily if the heart rate is not below 70 bpm. If there is any concern about the potential for bradycardia, the initiating dose may be lowered to 2.5 mg twice daily.

ACUTE DECOMPENSATED HEART FAILURE

Acute decompensated heart failure (ADHF) is defined as evidence of fluid volume overload or increased left ventricular filling pressures with an abrupt worsening of NYHA functional status by at least one class.[228] Patients may present with new onset HF or an exacerbation of existing chronic HF. ADHF is characterized by acute onset of dyspnea and rapid accumulation of fluid within the interstitial and alveolar spaces of the lungs, resulting in elevated cardiac filling pressures, known as pulmonary edema.[220] Patients are often readmitted to the hospital for repeated episodes of ADHF, contributing to soaring direct and indirect healthcare costs. Twenty-five percent of discharged HF patients are at high risk for all-cause hospital readmission within 1 month.[121] Eighty percent of hospital admissions for ADHF occur in patients with previously diagnosed heart failure.[93] Heart failure with preserved systolic function accounts for approximately one-third to one-half of ADHF admissions.[226] In the Acute Decompensated Heart Failure National Registry (ADHERE registry), nearly half of patients admitted with HF had blood pressure greater than 140/70 mm Hg and more than 30% had atrial fibrillation.[2,5,86]

Precipitating factors of ADHF may arise from many directions, but can most commonly be categorized as adherence, care issues, cardiac, or noncardiac causes (Table 4.3). Additionally, there are a number of medications that can precipitate acute HF exacerbation (Box 4.4). It is important to identify precipitating factors of ADHF in order to prevent recurrence. Patients often do not recognize their own escalating symptoms, and postpone seeking help until symptoms are at their peak. Many patients

TABLE 4.3 Precipitating Factors of ADHF

Type of Issue	Examples
Adherence	Dietary indiscretion Nonadherence with medications Financial constraints to afford medications or other care items Excessive fluid intake
Care	Drug interactions/side effects Discharged from hospital too soon Excessive fluid infusion during medical procedures
Social	Lack of transportation Access to care Depression Health illiteracy
Cardiac	Myocardial infarction/ischemia/acute coronary syndrome Valvular disease Atrial fibrillation, particularly if rapid ventricular response Worsening LV dysfunction - excessive right ventricular pacing in HFrEF Stress-induced (i.e., Tako-Tsubo cardiomyopathy)
Noncardiac	Severe hypertension Renal failure Comorbidities - anemia, thyroid disorders, pneumonia, COPD Pulmonary emboli

BOX 4.4 Medications That May Precipitate Acute Heart Failure

- Calcium channel blockers
- Antiarrhythmic agents
- Glucocorticoids
- Nonsteroidal antiinflammatory drugs (NSAIDs)
- Cyclooxygense-2 inhibitors (Cox-2 inhibitors)
- Thiazolidinediones
- Pseudoephedrine

delay days before seeking treatment, when earlier recognition of symptoms might have prevented hospitalization.[69]

Symptoms

Patients with ADHF often come to the hospital with symptoms of fluid volume overload. They describe rapid onset of their symptoms, from minutes to days before admission. The most common presenting signs and symptoms in patients with ADHF include dyspnea, rales, and peripheral edema.[5] It is important to note that the absence of rales or peripheral edema in patients with chronic HF does not indicate an absence of elevated filling pressures in ADHF.[205] Other presenting symptoms may include cough, orthopnea, edema, chest pain, abdominal fullness, and early satiety.

Physical Findings

Physical assessment findings of patients presenting with ADHF are listed in Box 4.5. Patients may present with any combination of signs and symptoms. The patient's clinical profile should be assessed to determine appropriate treatment strategies. Hemodynamic parameters can be assessed in the context of being wet, dry, warm, or cold (Fig. 4.4). Elevated filling pressures (elevated pulmonary artery occlusion pressure [PAOP] also called pulmonary artery wedge pressure [PAWP]) and decreased cardiac output make up the most common hemodynamic profile in decompensated heart failure. "Wet" or "dry" pertains to the patient's volume status, whereas "warm" or "cold" refers to the patient's cardiac output and peripheral perfusion. Wet patients have signs of congestion, such as dyspnea, edema, and elevated jugular venous pressure. Dry patients are those who are euvolemic, or are volume depleted. Warm patients have adequate peripheral perfusion and adequate cardiac output, whereas cold patients have hypoperfusion of body organs or extremities. The patient's profile is predictive of outcomes and postdischarge mortality.[159]

Of the four hemodynamic profiles, warm and wet is the most commonly seen in hospitalized patients. This means that the patient's perfusion is adequate (warm), but that congestion is present (wet). Patients who are admitted to the hospital with a diagnosis of ADHF but are warm and dry without volume overload or poor perfusion should be evaluated for some other cause besides HF, such as pulmonary disease. Patients who are wet and cold have more advanced HF than those who are wet and warm who, in turn, have more severe HF than those who are warm and dry.[159] Mortality is higher in patients who are warm and wet or cold and wet, as opposed to those who are warm and dry. Patients do not commonly present in the cold and dry category, but those may be the patients who would most benefit from advanced therapies such as biventricular pacing or mitral valve repair.[159]

BOX 4.5 Possible Assessment Findings of Patients with ADHF

- Edema in feet, legs, hands, or periorbital space
- Ascites
- Jugular venous distention
- Positive hepatojugular reflux/abdominojugular test
- Third heart sound (S3)
- Crackles and/or wheezing on auscultation of lungs
- Hypoxia
- Excessive work of breathing/tachypnea
- Peripheral cyanosis
- Liver palpated or percussed below costal margin
- Pulsatile liver
- Right upper quadrant tenderness with palpation
- Tachycardia

Criteria for Admission to the Hospital

Hospitals are initiating programs to decrease HF readmissions in order to avoid financial penalties incurred when an excessive number of patients return to the hospital within 30 days following a HF discharge. The decision to admit a patient, as opposed to treating as an outpatient, carries more weight than ever before. Many factors affect the decision for admission. Some patient characteristics, such as the patient's degree of available services or the level of social support, resources, and self-care ability, may impact whether a patient can be managed on an outpatient basis. Hospitalization is recommended when there is evidence of severely decompensated HF such as signs of shock, dyspnea at rest, hemodynamically significant arrhythmias, or

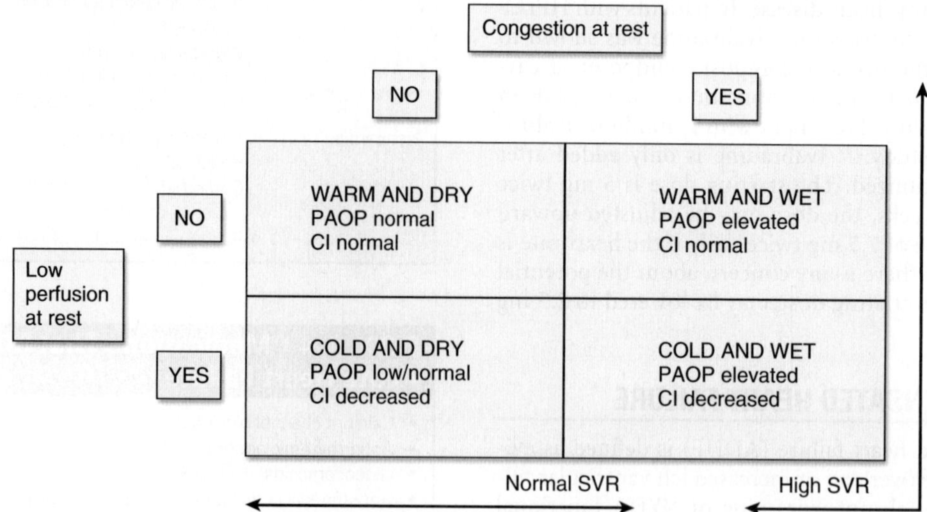

FIG. 4.4 Clinical assessment of patient hemodynamic profiles that occur in acute decompensated heart failure. *CI*, Cardiac index; *PAOP*, pulmonary artery occlusion pressure; *SVR*, systemic vascular resistance.

acute coronary syndrome.[81] Hospitalization should be considered when there is new onset of HF with signs of pulmonary or systemic congestion, significant electrolyte disturbance, or comorbid conditions that put the patient at increased risk for further harm. These would include: pneumonia, pulmonary embolus, diabetic ketoacidosis, cerebrovascular ischemia, or repetitive defibrillations of an implantable defibrillator.[81]

The goals of treatment during a hospitalization are aimed at improving clinical symptoms and physical derangements, preferably within the 4-day period of time that is allowed within the Diagnostic Related Group. The etiology of the onset or exacerbation should be defined in order to avoid future decompensated HF, and the patient should be stabilized and treatments should be optimized (Box 4.6).

Diagnostic Testing

Diagnostic testing is critical to identify the cause and any reversible conditions that may contribute to worsening HF. Most of the diagnostic tests are the same as those conducted in the outpatient setting, such as the electrocardiogram, echocardiogram, chest radiograph, and lab studies. In addition to routine chemistries that are often obtained in outpatient HF management, renal function should be evaluated daily, particularly in patients who are diuresing. Elevated serum creatinine and/or BUN may be a marker for intravascular volume depletion due to overdiuresis. Decreased renal function may also be secondary to low cardiac output state, underlying renal disease, renal artery stenosis, or renal venous congestion.[175] Chest radiograph, electrocardiogram, and echocardiogram have been previously addressed.

Pulmonary Artery Catheterization

Pulmonary artery catheters (PACs), also known as Swan-Ganz catheters, are occasionally used for the management of critically ill patients, although use of these catheters has dramatically decreased. The indications for use of a PAC are limited, and most patient care guidelines do not recommend routine use.[227] Numerous studies have confirmed that the use of PACs in patient management does not improve survival or days in the hospital,[96,193] and may even increase mortality.[47] There are a few situations in which a PAC may be an appropriate approach to guide therapeutic decisions, such as unexplained or unknown volume status in patients with shock, severe cardiogenic shock, suspected pulmonary hypertension, and severe cardiopulmonary disease in patients undergoing surgery to correct congenital heart defects.[222] Additionally, patients being considered for cardiac transplantation or placement of a mechanical circulatory support (MCS) device may be candidates for right heart catheterization.[227] Hemodynamic information that can be obtained with a PAC is listed in Box 4.7.

Laboratory Testing

As previously mentioned, laboratory testing is done to gather a baseline assessment of the patient's status on admission, guide management decisions, evaluate comorbidities, and determine time for discharge. Changes in lab results may alter the plan of care, for example, a reduction in BNP would indicate successful diuresis, or an elevation of creatinine may indicate overdiuresis. It is important to note that troponin levels may be elevated in ADHF, and do not necessarily indicate acute coronary syndrome. Elevated cardiac troponins are associated with worse outcomes and mortality in ADHF.[169] According to the ADHERE registry data, 20% of patients admitted for ADHF have a serum creatinine greater than 2 mg/dL, indicating some level of renal insufficiency.[77] BUN greater than 43 mg/dL was the strongest predictor of in-hospital mortality, followed closely by serum creatinine greater than 2.75 mg/dL and initial systolic blood pressure under 115 mm Hg.[75]

Implanted Device Interrogation

If the patient already has an implantable pacemaker or defibrillator, it should be interrogated in an attempt to identify factors that could contribute to their decompensated clinical condition. Precipitating arrhythmias such as atrial fibrillation with rapid ventricular response or nonsustained ventricular tachycardia may have occurred prior to the patient's presentation with ADHF, but the rhythm may or may not be active once the patient arrives at the hospital. Additionally, excessive pacing in the right ventricle in patients with HFrEF can worsen HF,[209] leading to a decompensated state. Inappropriate timing between left and right ventricular pacing impulses as well as between atrial and ventricular pacing impulses can worsen HF.[125] If the device offers impedance monitoring, reviewing recent trends can be helpful in diagnosing fluid volume overload.[229] Interrogating the patient's device can reveal details that might not be obvious at the time of presentation to the hospital. Optimizing the performance of the device may help to prevent hospitalizations.

Other Imaging Modalities

Other modalities that measure cardiac function include cardiac MRI, multigated acquisition (MUGA) scan, nuclear stress test, and catheterization ventriculogram. If acute myocardial infarction or unstable coronary syndrome is suspected as a precipitant for the patient's ADHF, coronary angiography with percutaneous intervention and/or initiation of reperfusion therapy is indicated. If there is suspicion of new coronary lesions or worsening of existing lesions, interventions should be initiated as appropriate. If the patient is unwilling to undergo any intervention to reduce or bypass the lesions, then it is questionable as to the benefit of doing a diagnostic catheterization that has its own inherent risks. It is important to speak with the patient and to outline possible interventions before proceeding to the catheterization laboratory and to determine the patient's wishes for future therapy, particularly in elderly or frail patients.

BOX 4.6 Goals of Treatment for Patients with ADHF

- Support hemodynamics
- Optimize volume status
- Support oxygenation and ventilation
- Promote symptom relief
- Identify etiology and treat if possible
- Identify and address precipitating factors
- Optimize chronic oral therapy
- Minimize side effects
- Identify patients appropriate for surgical intervention
- Identify patients who could benefit from device therapy
- Identify risk of thromboembolism and initiate anticoagulant therapy if needed
- Educate patients about medications, diet, and self-management of HF
- Refer to a HF disease management program
- Address comorbidities if possible

From Reference 81.

TREATMENT OF ACUTE DECOMPENSATED HEART FAILURE

Basic Therapies

If the patient has been previously diagnosed with HF and is on GDMT, the medication should be continued in the hospital if possible. Continuation of ACEIs, ARBs, and beta blockers in the hospital is associated with better outcomes.[78,150] ACEIs, ARBs, or aldosterone antagonists may be decreased in dosage or temporarily discontinued in patients admitted with significant worsening of renal function or hyperkalemia.[227] Decreasing dosage or withholding beta blocker therapy should only be considered in the presence of marked volume overload or low cardiac output.[227] If possible, GDMT should be resumed or titrated upward prior to discharge from the hospital.

Patients admitted with ADHF should receive anticoagulant prophylaxis for venous thromboembolism, unless contraindicated. The American College of Chest Physicians recommends that acutely ill HF patients who have one or more additional risk factor should receive thromboprophylaxis with low molecular weight heparin, low-dose unfractionated heparin, or fondaparinux.[83] As long as renal function is reasonably preserved (serum creatinine < 2.0 mg/dL), current ACCF/AHA guidelines recommend the use of enoxaparin 40 mg administered subcutaneously daily.[227] Alternatively, unfractionated heparin 5000 units subcutaneously every 8 hours may be used. If anticoagulant thromboprophylaxis is contraindicated, mechanical thromboprophylaxis with graduated compression stockings or intermittent pneumatic compression may be used,[83] although some authors have not demonstrated prophylactic efficacy with compression stockings.[126]

Patients hospitalized with ADHF should be monitored with telemetry to assess for new onset or intermittent arrhythmias and rapid heart rate with activity. Daily weights are mandatory as an assessment tool to evaluate diuresis. Careful intake and output of all liquids should be accounted for each day. If the patient is wet, fluid restriction of 1500 to 2000 mL per 24 hours may assist in promoting diuresis. Diet should be limited to 2000 to 3000 mg sodium per day.[182] If the patient has other comorbidities such as CAD or diabetes, additional alterations to the diet should be prescribed. Supplemental oxygen therapy may be used to maintain saturation above 90%, but it is not recommended as routine therapy in patients unless hypoxemia is present. When the patient is ambulatory, cardiac rehabilitation may improve muscle strength and tone.

BOX 4.7 Hemodynamic Information Obtained with a Pulmonary Artery Catheter

- Central venous pressure (CVP)
- Right-sided intracardiac pressures (right atrium, right ventricle)
- Pulmonary artery pressure (PAP)
- Pulmonary capillary wedge pressure (PCWP)
- Cardiac output (CO)
- Mixed venous oxyhemoglobin saturation (Svo_2)
- Systemic vascular resistance (SVR = 80 × [mean artery pressure – CVP]/CO)
- Pulmonary vascular resistance (PVR = [mean PAP – PCWP]/CO)
- Cardiac index (CI = CO/body surface area)
- Stroke volume index (SVI = CI/heart rate)
- Left ventricular stroke work index (LVSWI = [mean systemic artery pressure – PCWP] × SVI × 0.136)
- Right ventricular stroke work index (RVSWI = [mean Pap – CVP] × SVI × 0.136)
- Oxygen delivery (Do_2 = CI × 13.4 × hemoglobin concentration x arterial oxygen saturation)
- Oxygen uptake (Vo_2 = CI × 13.4 × hemoglobin concentration x [arterial oxygen saturation – venous oxygen saturation])

From Reference 222.

Pharmacologic Treatment

Diuretics

Loop diuretics are the mainstay of symptom management for patients with fluid volume overload. These agents do not treat the pathologic derangements that occur in the remodeling process, but rather manage the symptoms that occur with pulmonary vascular congestion. There is limited clinical trial data to demonstrate mortality benefit from diuretic use in patients with chronic HF.[45] Diuretics that have an effect in the loop of Henle are the most commonly used in treating HF patients, including furosemide (Lasix), torsemide (Demedex), and bumetanide (Bumex). In the hospital or ED, diuretics should be given intravenously without delay to reduce LV filling pressures and intravascular pressure. Additionally, diuretics cause venodilation that decreases pulmonary congestion, even before the patient begins to diurese.[62] Once fluid is mobilized from the interstitium into the vascular space, it can be filtered by the kidney and excreted in the urine.

Loop diuretics are short acting and provide approximately 6 hours of diuresis. After that, the RAAS becomes activated due to the decrease in sodium excretion when diuretic effectiveness wears off. Because of this, subsequent daily doses of diuretic may become less effective, but concomitant use of neurohormonal blocking agents such as ACEIs or ARBs will decrease this effect. In patients who are resistant to initial doses of diuretics, steps to intensify the regimen may include giving higher doses of intravenous loop diuretics or adding a second type of diuretic such as a thiazide diuretic.[227] Extreme caution must be used when administering thiazide diuretics, as electrolyte depletion may be accelerated, particularly sodium and potassium.

The dosage of diuretic is individualized to the patient, and should be titrated upward to elicit an acceptable diuretic response. For patients who have not previously been on loop diuretics, lower doses may be effective. If there is little or no response to the diuretic, the dose should be doubled and administered 2 to 3 hours later. It is important to consider that patients with reduced renal function or severe HF may require higher maximum doses of diuretic in order to have an adequate response.[227] Patients who are already on diuretic therapy may need a higher dose in the acute phase of HF. Their initial diuretic dose in the hospital should be equal to or greater than their maintenance dose prior to admission.[72] Oral diuretics often lose effectiveness due to poor absorption, particularly if the patient has become volume overloaded. Bolus doses of loop diuretic should be administered two or more times per day as needed initially. A continuous infusion of diuretic may be used, but data is limited as to whether this method is superior to bolus doses.[189] Once the patient's symptoms are stabilized, they may be converted to oral dosing.

Patients receiving diuretic therapy need frequent assessment of volume status via daily weights, serum electrolytes (potassium, magnesium, sodium), oxygenation, fluid intake and output, renal function assessment, and lung auscultation. Assessment of dyspnea level should be done regularly; the frequency depends upon the patient's level of acuity. The patient should be monitored for signs of overdiuresis, such as hypotension, orthostatic blood pressure changes, worsening renal function, and metabolic or contraction alkalosis. Patients on diuretic therapy may develop gout, so they should be assessed for red, inflamed, and painful joints. Patients with HFpEF may be more sensitive to overdiuresis and reduction in preload, so caution should be used when removing fluid in these patients.[45]

Vasodilators

Vasodilating agents do not directly improve cardiac function, but reduce preload and afterload, thus improving forward blood flow and relieving pulmonary congestion. Patients receiving vasodilators, particularly when administered intravenously, should undergo frequent or continuous blood pressure and cardiac telemetry monitoring.

Nitroglycerin. Nitroglycerin is the most commonly used vasodilator in ADHF. It lowers preload and congestion primarily through venodilation, but at higher doses can lower systemic vascular resistance and reduce LV afterload, allowing for increased stroke volume and improved cardiac output. Patients who would benefit from the use of nitroglycerin include those with hypertension, coronary ischemia, or significant mitral regurgitation.[65] It is generally given intravenously, has a rapid onset of action within 3 to 5 minutes, and is readily titrated to achieve predetermined hemodynamic goals. The dose is usually initiated at 5 mcg/min and increased every 3 to 5 minutes as needed to alleviate symptoms or lower blood pressure, to a maximum dose of 160 mcg/min. It is possible for patients to develop nitrate "tolerance," which can be managed by titrating to a higher dose. Side effects include headache, tachyphylaxis, and hypotension. Nitrates should not be initiated in patients who have recently used PDE-5 inhibitors such as sildenafil (Viagra or Revatio).[45]

Nitroprusside. Nitroprusside has both arterial and venous vasodilating effects. It has a short half-life of approximately 2 minutes, so the dosage is easily titrated up or down by increasing or decreasing the rate of infusion. Patients receiving nitroprusside are usually placed in a critical care setting with hemodynamic monitoring and an intra-arterial catheter inserted for frequent blood pressure monitoring due to the potential for hypotension. The starting dose of 0.3 to 0.5 mcg/kg/minute is titrated upward by 0.5 mcg/kg/minute every 5 minutes as tolerated until the desired blood pressure is achieved or symptoms are improved, to a maximum dose of 10 mcg/kg/minute. Nitroprusside is generally used for less than 24 to 48 hours due to the possibility of the accumulation of metabolites that can lead to cyanide toxicity, which can be fatal.[45] Side effects of nitroprusside include nausea, vomiting, and disorientation, especially if the infusion continues for more than 48 hours. Cardiac monitoring is recommended due to the fact that nitroprusside can cause reflex tachycardia, similar to nitroglycerin. Rebound vasoconstriction is a potential complication when the infusion is discontinued.[168]

Nesiritide. Nesiritide (Natrecor) is an arterial and venous dilator, but it is less potent than nitroprusside and has a slower onset and offset of action when titrated. With a longer half-life, complications such as hypotension may persist. Nesiritide is usually given as an initial bolus of 2 mcg/kg followed by a continuous infusion of 0.01 mcg/kg/minute, titrated in a similar fashion to nitroglycerin. Because of the longer half-life and higher cost of the medication, nesiritide is not widely used as a first-line vasodilator in ADHF. Because nesiritide is a form of BNP, serum BNP levels will be elevated due to the infusion, so serum BNP levels should not be used to make clinical management decisions.

Morphine. Morphine can occasionally relieve dyspnea by reducing anxiety and promoting venodilation, thus decreasing cardiac filling pressures. Data are limited on the effects of morphine in patients with ADHF, and this medication is not mentioned in the current ACCF/AHA heart failure guidelines. The ESC HF guidelines include the consideration of opiates in some patients with pulmonary edema in order to reduce anxiety and distress associated with dyspnea; however, nausea and depression of respiratory drive are frequent adverse effects.[145]

Inotropic Infusions

Intravenous inotropic agents have not been demonstrated to improve outcomes in patients with ADHF, but are an option in patients with systolic dysfunction who have low cardiac index and depressed end-organ perfusion.[227] Inotropes are not indicated in patients with preserved EF. Intravenous inotrope therapy should be used as a temporary measure until the patient's acute episode has resolved or until definitive therapy can be applied, such as coronary revascularization, MCS, or cardiac transplantation.[45] Patients receiving intravenous inotropes should have continuous blood pressure and cardiac rhythm monitoring.

Dobutamine. Dobutamine is a direct-acting agent with the primary effect of stimulating $beta_1$ receptors in the heart. This exerts a potent inotropic effect to increase contractility, stroke volume, and cardiac output. It also provides a modest decrease in systemic vascular resistance and PCWP. Situations that may require inotropic support include significant hypotension, inadequate renal perfusion, or multiorgan dysfunction until cardiac transplantation or MCS device insertion can be performed. Dobutamine also may be used in the short term following cardiac surgical procedures. The infusion starts at 2.5 mcg/kg/minute and can be gradually increased to 20 mcg/kg/minute.

Inotropic therapy should be used only in situations in which improved contractility is the desired endpoint and should be used for as short duration as possible and with the lowest effective dose. While dobutamine does not usually markedly increase heart rate, it can increase oxygen demand of the myocardium, leading to ischemia. Occasionally, patients may become dependent on inotropic infusion for palliative support in end-stage heart failure and may be discharged from the hospital with a permanent intravenous catheter for home infusion.

Milrinone. Milrinone is a phosphodiesterase inhibitor that increases contractility by inhibiting degradation of cyclic adenosine monophosphate. It produces positive inotropic effects in the myocardium, reduces systemic and pulmonary vascular resistance, and improves LV diastolic relaxation.[200] These effects can increase cardiac index and decrease LV afterload and filling pressures. In contrast to dobutamine, milrinone is not a beta agonist, so its effects are not as diminished in patients taking beta blockers. Milrinone may be given as a loading dose of 50 mcg/kg administered slowly over 10 minutes, followed with an infusion initiated at 0.2 to 0.3 mcg/kg/minute with a maximum dose of 0.75 mcg/kg/minute. Dosage may be titrated to the maximum desired hemodynamic effect.

Hypotension may occur with milrinone, so the patient's blood pressure should be monitored frequently. If hypotension is the reason for inotropic support in a patient with ADHF, milrinone would not be an appropriate choice. As with other inotropes, milrinone may increase the frequency of tachydysrhythmias and ischemic events. It may slightly shorten AV node conduction time, potentially increasing the ventricular rate in atrial flutter or fibrillation if patients are not adequately rate controlled. The primary route of excretion of milrinone is in the urine, so in the presence of decreased renal function, elimination half-life may be prolonged and the dosage may need to be reduced. After weaning off milrinone, patients should continue to be observed for 48 hours.

Vasopressors

Dopamine. At low doses, dopamine stimulates alpha and beta receptors in the heart and dopaminergic receptors that cause vasodilation in the renal and mesenteric artery beds. At slightly higher doses, it increases stroke volume and cardiac output. At higher doses, dopamine also stimulates alpha adrenergic receptors. It has long been thought that at low doses, dopamine may enhance decongestion and preserve renal function in patients with ADHF, but data from the Renal Optimization Strategies Evaluation (ROSE) trial showed that low-dose dopamine did not enhance decongestion or improve renal function when combined with diuretic therapy.[37]

The starting dosage of dopamine is 0.5 to 1 mcg/kg/minute and is increased until the desired effect is achieved, such as increased urine output or improved blood pressure. The maximum dose is 10 mcg/kg/minute. At low doses of 1 to 3 mcg/kg/minute, dopamine is predominantly vasodilatory. However, when a dosage of 5 mcg/kg/minute is reached, alpha receptors are stimulated and it becomes a vasoconstrictor. When dopamine is used as a vasoconstricting agent, weaning may have to be discontinued at 5 mcg/kg/minute, because lower doses may promote vasodilation and lower blood pressure. It may be necessary to expand blood volume while weaning to prevent hypotension. Like other inotropic agents, dopamine may promote tachydysrhythmias and ischemia. Extravasation of the drug into subcutaneous tissue may cause tissue necrosis and sloughing, so a large vein is recommended for infusion.

Other vasoactive agents. Occasionally, patients with ADHF require additional vasoconstricting agents in order to support blood pressure and organ perfusion. In patients with life-threatening hypoperfusion, dopamine is the initial agent for blood pressure support. If dopamine fails to improve the patient's clinical status, intravenous epinephrine or vasopressin infusion may be necessary for short-term therapy. These agents provide profound vasoconstriction for stabilization of blood pressure until the acute episode is resolved or more definitive action may be taken, such as percutaneous coronary intervention, surgery, insertion of a ventricular assist device, or cardiac transplantation. Epinephrine is given at a starting dose of 1 mcg/minute and titrated until the patient's hemodynamics are stabilized. Vasopressin may be used in hypotensive patients who maintain a systolic blood pressure below 70 mm Hg despite maximum vasopressor therapy. It may be used for short periods at doses of 0.05 to 0.1 unit/min. Powerful vasoconstricting agents may contribute to dysrhythmias and worsening ischemia, as well as necrosis of organs and extremities, so they should be used with careful deliberation and caution. Dosages may need to be adjusted during aggressive diuresis in order to prevent hypotension.

Other Medications

Beta blockers must be used with caution in patients with ADHF and HFrEF. If the HF is severely decompensated, beta blocker therapy should be withheld in the initial period of treatment. If the patient is hemodynamically stable with mild decompensation, beta blocker therapy may be continued.[33,150] Withdrawal of beta blocker therapy in patients hospitalized with ADHF has been associated with worse risk and propensity adjusted mortality.[76] Patients who have not previously been on beta blocker therapy should not be started during the acute phase of their hospitalization for ADHF. Once the patient is stabilized and euvolemic, beta blockers may be started at low doses before discharge. This may improve the likelihood of compliance with taking these drugs after discharge.

Aldosterone antagonists such as spironolactone (Aldactone) have been found to decrease mortality when added to beta blockers and ACEI or ARB therapy in patients with HFrEF. Patients who have previously been on these agents should be continued on them in the hospital setting if possible, as long as renal function and electrolytes are stable. If the patient has not been on these agents, initiation prior to or soon after discharge is recommended.[45] If the patient is initiated on ACEI or ARB therapy just prior to discharge, the aldosterone antagonist should not be started until after discharge, after evaluation of serum potassium.

Digoxin may be added to other oral HF medications if symptoms persist despite maximal HF therapy in HFrEF or in the presence of atrial fibrillation with rapid ventricular response despite maximal beta blocker therapy. Serum digoxin levels should be maintained at or below 1.0 mg/dL, and blood sampling should not be done within 6 hours of the last dose. Potassium and magnesium levels should be maintained in order to avoid arrhythmias.[81]

Anticoagulants are not inherently used in the treatment of ADHF unless the patient has a comorbid condition that requires anticoagulation, such as atrial fibrillation or an artificial heart valve. Anticoagulation is not recommended in patients with HFrEF without atrial fibrillation, a prior thrombotic event, or a cardioembolic source.[142] Antiarrhythmic agents may be used in patients whose HF is made worse by the presence of an arrhythmia, such as atrial fibrillation or flutter, or ventricular tachycardia. Amiodarone and dofetilide (Tikosyn) are the only antiarrhythmic agents that have a neutral effect on mortality in patients with HF, so these are the preferred agents for treating arrhythmias in HF patients.[64,211]

Patients with HF who are hypervolemic with a low serum sodium level may have some improvement with fluid restriction and maximized GDMT, but may also benefit from a vasopressin antagonist if cognitive symptoms due to hyponatremia are present.[192] The long-term safety and benefit of vasopressin antagonists for hyponatremia in patients with HF are not known.

Other Treatments

Ultrafiltration

In patients who are refractory to diuretic therapy, hemofiltration/ultrafiltration provides a treatment option to reduce fluid volume and pulmonary congestion. This procedure is similar to hemodialysis; however, during ultrafiltration, water is the only substance extracted from the circulation. Blood is pumped from the patient and passed through a porous filter where fluid is removed. The blood is then returned to the patient without fluctuations in electrolytes (such as potassium or sodium) or acid-base balance. Patients with ADHF and volume overload that is refractory to diuretics tolerate this therapy well because it does not produce wide swings in blood pressure when a venous-venous pump is used. During the ultrafiltration process, the patient is given a "diuretic holiday," meaning that oral and intravenous diuretics are withheld until ultrafiltration is discontinued. During ultrafiltration, 100 mL to 200 mL of water per hour is removed, though 500 mL/hour has been shown to be well tolerated.[188] Fluid removal volume and rate are adjustable and neurohormonal activity is not enhanced. As short-term therapy for diuretic-refractory ADHF, hemofiltration relieves symptoms of pulmonary edema, reduces ascites and peripheral edema, and enhances the subsequent response to diuretics.[50] While this procedure is effective in removing fluid, no benefit has been established over diuretic therapy[17] (see Chapter 23).

Mechanical Circulatory Support

Circulatory support used for HF patients with cardiogenic shock or circulatory collapse include counterpulsation (intra-aortic balloon pump [IABP]) and ventricular assist devices (VAD).

Intra-aortic balloon pump. The IABP is the most common method for cardiac support in acutely ill patients, and has been widely used for many years. It is easily inserted for temporary use, can be removed at the bedside, and is the least expensive of the three choices for circulatory support. Indications for inserting an IABP include cardiogenic shock, intractable angina/ischemia, complicated angioplasty, poor LV function after cardiopulmonary bypass, refractory HF, and intractable ventricular arrhythmias.[73,190] It benefits the myocardium by increasing blood flow to the coronary arteries, decreasing the workload of the heart, and reducing myocardial oxygen demand (see also Chapter 3).

A balloon inserted through a common femoral artery into the proximal descending aorta (distal to the left subclavian artery) rapidly inflates with helium gas immediately after aortic valve closure in diastole, thus displacing blood forward to perfuse the periphery and backward into the coronary arteries. The balloon deflates abruptly just before the aortic valve opens and LV contraction begins, thus creating a suction to "pull" the blood out of the ventricle and augment forward blood flow out of the LV. This greatly reduces the workload of the myocardium by reducing afterload and improves cardiac output by 20% to 40%. Left ventricular filling pressures are also lowered with IABP therapy.[106,191] The timing of balloon inflation and deflation is controlled via the electrocardiogram and arterial pressure monitoring. This therapy can be used in patients as a bridge to transplant and as temporary support until hemodynamic parameters stabilize.

Patients with IABPs must be monitored closely in a critical care unit. A chest x-ray is obtained after insertion for catheter position, and daily chest x-ray films are recommended while the IABP is in place to make sure the catheter remains in the correct position. Intravenously administered heparin must be started after placement to prevent clot formation. The pressure waveform for balloon inflation/deflation timing should be evaluated twice daily, and a complete blood count and renal function labs should be drawn daily. Urine output should be measured continuously. Patients must be kept supine in bed, and pedal pulses must be checked prior to insertion, after removal, and three times daily while in place. Removal of the balloon pump depends on several factors, including hemodynamic status of the patient, LV function, and duration of therapy. Usually, patients are weaned by decreasing the frequency of inflations to 1:2 (one inflation per every two cardiac cycles) for several hours and then 1:3, 1:4, and 1:8. If weaning is tolerated hemodynamically, the balloon pump can be removed. Contraindications to IABP therapy include aortic dissection, abdominal or thoracic aortic aneurysm, severe peripheral vascular disease, coagulopathy or contraindication to heparin, and moderate to severe aortic insufficiency. Disadvantages of prolonged IABP therapy include risk of infection and complications related to extended bed rest.

Ventricular assist device (VAD). VADs are used for both short-term management of ADHF with reduced EF and long-term management of stage D chronic HFrEF (Fig. 4.5). When used as a temporary measure, VADs offer hemodynamic support and allow time to make decisions about definitive treatments such as cardiac reparative surgery or transplantation. VAD completely unloads the LV while supporting the pulmonary or systemic circulation. Candidates for assist devices typically have an EF less than 25%, systolic blood pressure less than 90 mm Hg, PAOP greater than 18 mm Hg, and oliguria despite maximal medical therapy. Contraindications to VAD therapy include aortic regurgitation or prosthetic aortic valve, aortic aneurysm or dissection, severe aortic or peripheral vascular disease, LV or left atrial thrombus, bleeding, or uncontrolled sepsis[13] (see also Chapters 5 and 8).

The use of VADs falls into one of several general categories: bridge to transplantation (until a donor heart is available),

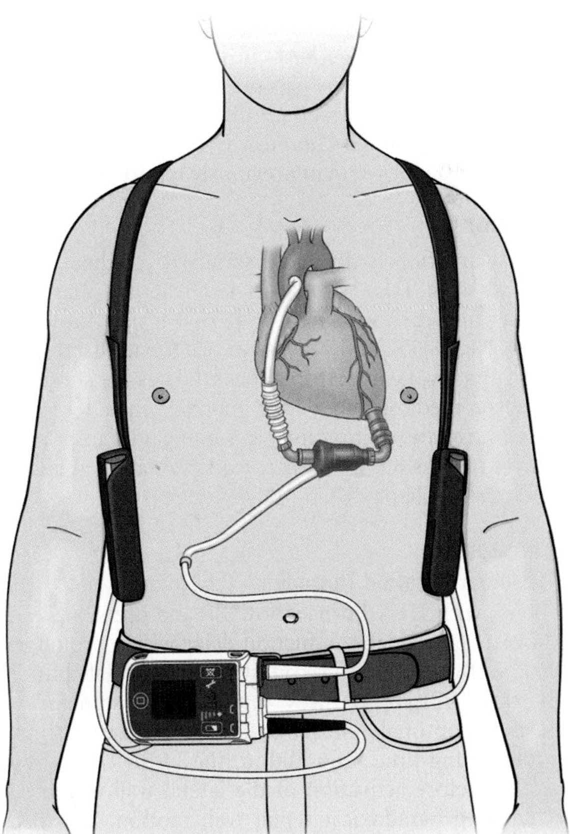

FIG. 4.5 Thoratec Heartmate II ventricular assist device (Courtesy St. Jude Medical.)

bridge to decision (deciding on transplant eligibility or other definitive treatment), destination therapy (permanent), and as a bridge to recovery of myocardial function. Most VADs are implanted in the LV but a small percent of VADs are implanted in both ventricles, termed biventricular. [41] Bridge to transplantation VADs are implanted in patients with deteriorating clinical condition, despite inotrope therapy and often IABP insertion. These patients cannot wait without circulatory support for an available donor heart. In this situation, a VAD may improve body organ function prior to transplantation, lower pulmonary pressures, and allow for improvement in the patient's nutritional status; all of which will improve survival after transplantation.

Bridge to decision is an opportunity to support hemodynamics while determining if a patient is a candidate for transplantation. Support from a VAD may improve or resolve reversible conditions that make transplantation contraindicated. Some third party payers do not recognize this category of VAD use.

Destination therapy refers to long-term use of a VAD in patients with end-stage HF who are not transplant candidates. These patients may have contraindications such as older age, renal dysfunction, obesity, permanent pulmonary hypertension, or other end-organ comorbidities.[115] Nearly 10% of patients with destination VAD therapy will end up undergoing cardiac transplantation within one year after VAD implant.[115] Unloading the LV with VAD therapy can promote recovery of cardiac function, such that the VAD may be removed and the patient may survive without undergoing transplantation. This is termed "bridge to recovery," and may be most successful in patients with acute onset myocarditis.[22] The premise involves maximizing HF medications such as neurohormonal blockade agents while the patient has a VAD in place. Higher doses of the medications may be given than prior to VAD implant, so remodeling may be reduced and cardiac function improved. When the VAD is explanted, durability of myocardial recovery has been found to be higher than previously reported.[23,24]

Transplantation

Cardiac transplantation is the "gold standard" of therapy for refractory end-stage HF. Long-term survival has markedly improved over the years, with 1-, 3-, and 5-year posttransplant survival at 87.8%, 78.5%, and 71.7% survival for adults, respectively.[204] Fortunately, heart transplant candidates are surviving with the use of medical and device therapy, such that survival on the transplant waiting list has significantly improved. Indications and exclusions for cardiac transplantation are listed in Box 4.8 (see also Chapter 8).

Device Therapy

Cardiac Resynchronization Therapy

Many patients with HF who have low EF and are symptomatic also have a ventricular conduction delay with a prolonged QRS (>0.12 sec) on ECG. This conduction delay (left bundle branch block [LBBB]) produces ventricular dyssynchrony, which causes suboptimal ventricular filling because of shortened diastolic filling time. In addition, the LBBB causes septal contraction before activation of the lateral wall of the left ventricle, creating paradoxical septal wall motion. The prolonged QRS causes a more severe mitral regurgitation, resulting in greater impairment of LV contractility. The hemodynamic consequences of the left atrioventricular mechanical delay are a decreased stroke volume and increased left atrial pressure as a result of the mitral regurgitation. Ventricular dyssynchrony has also been associated with an increased mortality and sudden death in heart failure patients.[89,154]

Cardiac resynchronization therapy (CRT), or biventricular (BiV) pacing, coordinates the right and LV contractions to resynchronize the ventricles, thus enhancing ventricular contraction and reducing the degree of mitral regurgitation. The pulse generator device used is approximately the same size as a standard pacemaker, but it allows for three lead connections to the right atrial lead, RV lead, and left ventricular lead. The leads are placed transvenously, similar to a traditional pacemaker, with the addition of the LV lead inserted through the coronary sinus into the coronary vein (Fig. 4.6). Other than standard pacemaker insertion risks, specific risks of this implant procedure are that the left ventricular lead implant is unsuccessful approximately 8% of the time and that dissection or perforation of the coronary sinus occurs approximately 6% of the time. Patients with BiV pacemakers should be afforded the same cautions as those with standard pacemakers: avoid MRI, diathermy, high sources of radiation, electrosurgical cautery, lithotripsy, and radiofrequency ablation. External defibrillation pads should not be placed directly over the device. The patient's ECG after CRT will depend on the conduction delay before implantation and device settings (Fig. 4.7). The device should capture both the right and left ventricles, which will produce a smaller and narrower QRS, ST segment, and T wave.

BOX 4.8 Heart Transplantation Inclusion/Exclusion Criteria

Inclusion Criteria

- Cardiogenic shock requiring either continuous intravenous inotropic support or circulatory support with an intra-aortic balloon pump counterpulsation device or mechanical circulatory support.
- Persistent New York Heart Association functional Class IV heart failure (HF) symptoms refractory to maximal medical therapy (left ventricular ejection fraction <20%; peak Vo_2 <12 mL/kg/min).
- Intractable or severe anginal symptoms in patients with coronary artery disease not amenable to percutaneous or surgical revascularization or severe transplant coronary artery disease.
- Intractable life-threatening arrhythmias unresponsive to medical therapy, catheter ablation, surgery, and/or implantable cardioverter-defibrillator.
- Congenital heart disease with New York Heart Association functional Class III to IV HF not amenable to palliative or corrective surgery. Patients with complex intracardiac abnormalities and significant pulmonary vascular obstructive disease may require heart/lung transplantation.

Exclusion Criteria

- Nonreversible pulmonary vascular resistance >6 Wood units
- Malignancy diagnosed within 5 years
- Active infection
- Diabetes with end-organ damage
- Age > 70 years (relative contraindication)
- Advanced hepatic disease
- Impaired renal function (creatinine > 2.0mg/dL)
- Morbid obesity (body mass index > 35 kg/m²)
- Advanced peripheral vascular disease
- Active peptic ulcer disease
- Psychiatric illness
- Active drug, alcohol, or tobacco abuse
- Renal dysfunction unlikely to recover
- Extra-cardiac life-limiting disease
- Documented history of nonadherence to medical therapy

From Reference 135.

It has been shown that when added to optimal medical therapy in persistently symptomatic patients, CRT results in significant improvements in quality of life, functional class, exercise capacity, CO, EF, and decreased hospitalizations.[89,129] Therefore the current recommendation is that symptomatic patients who have an EF less than or equal to 35%, are in sinus rhythm, have a QRS greater than 0.15 sec, and are NYHA functional Class II, III, or IV despite optimal medical therapy should receive CRT.[227]

Implantable Cardioverter-Defibrillators

Patients with HFrEF frequently manifest ventricular tachydysrhythmias, both nonsustained and sustained. Although mortality is high in these patients, sudden cardiac death (SCD) has been substantially decreased in patients receiving GDMT of neurohormone antagonists.[67,227] Implantable cardioverter-defibrillators (ICDs) have been found to reduce the risk of sudden death in patients with marked left ventricular dysfunction, regardless of etiology.[67] ICDs are recommended treatment for primary prevention of SCD in selected patients with left ventricular dysfunction; who have symptomatic sustained ventricular tachycardia; and have asymptomatic nonsustained but inducible ventricular tachycardia; or have an ischemic cardiomyopathy with an LVEF less than 30% and are on GDMT.[227] ICDs are also effective for prevention of SCD in patients with hypertrophic cardiomyopathy.[139]

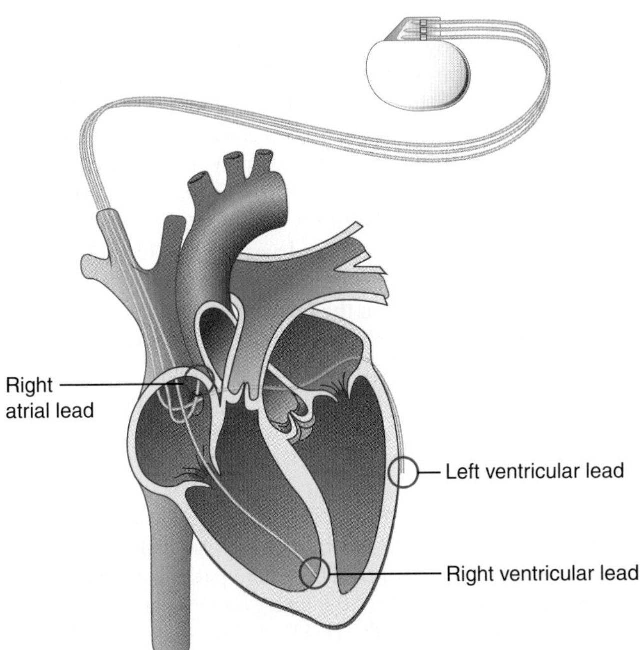

FIG. 4.6 Biventricular pacemaker with lead placement.

Wearable Cardioverter-Defibrillator

Current guidelines recommend ICD implantation 3 to 6 months after the patient with HFrEF has been on appropriate GDMT or waiting at least 40 to 90 days after myocardial infarction (MI).[232] This gap of vulnerability puts patients at risk for SCD. The wearable cardioverter-defibrillator (WCD) is an option to protect these patients who are waiting implantation.[68] The WCD has two defibrillation electrode pads, four sensing electrodes, a monitoring and defibrillation unit incorporated into a lightweight patient-worn vest. The Zoll Life Vest provides a safe and effective approach for patients known to be at high risk of SCD before they receive an ICD.[117]

Wireless Pulmonary Artery Monitoring

More than 90% of hospitalizations for acutely decompensated HF are due to signs and symptoms of congestion. Monitoring daily weights, assessing edema, and asking simple symptom questions are not sensitive to early changes in volume that increase the risks of decompensation.[36] Recent technologic advancements now allow the possibility of frequently monitoring cardiopulmonary filling pressures with implantable devices.[4] Recent studies of the CardioMEMS (St. Jude's Medical) pressure sensor device that is permanently implanted in the pulmonary artery during right heart catheterization demonstrated reduction in hospitalizations for patient with NYHA Class III HF, as well as those with HFpEF.[1,4]

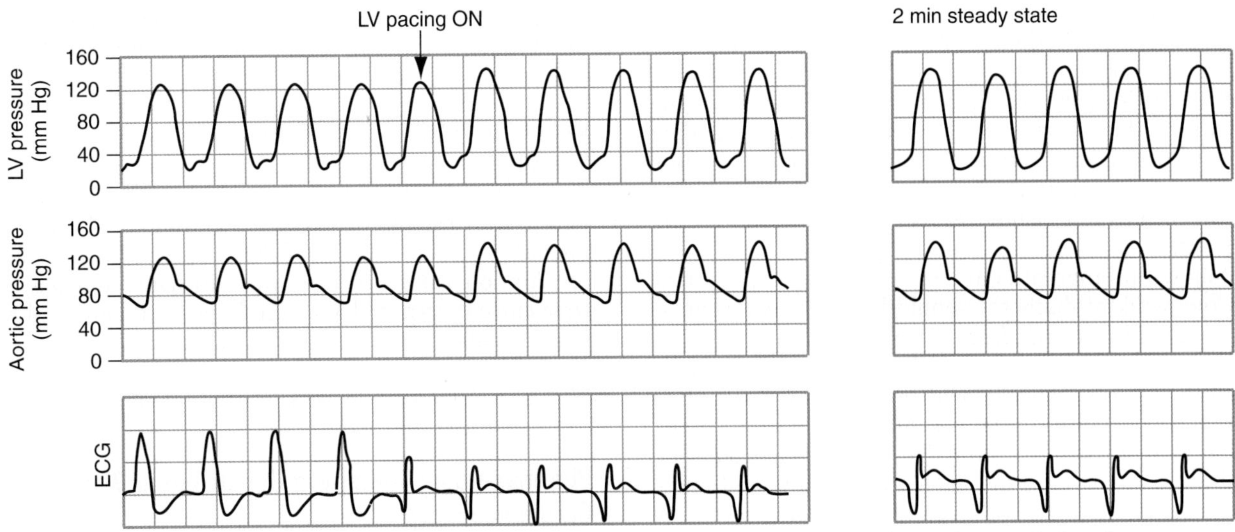

FIG. 4.7 Raw data tracings before, immediately on initiation of biventricular pacing, and after 2 minutes of steady-state left ventricular stimulation in a patient with LBBB. *ECG,* Electrocardiogram; *LV,* left ventricle.

TRANSITION FROM HOSPITAL TO HOME

Assessing Readiness for Discharge

Nearly one out of every four patients admitted to the hospital with a diagnosis of HF will be readmitted within 1 month of discharge.[61] Failure to prepare the patient to meet adequate discharge criteria contributes to this readmission rate.[143] Before considering the patient for discharge, the patient should be stable on an oral regimen for 24 hours, have resolution of symptoms from fluid volume overload, and have adequate blood pressure and renal function. Discharging patients before their ADHF is resolved generally results in another hospitalization in the near future. Renal function and electrolytes should be assessed and comorbidities should be under control, or at least scheduled for management in the outpatient setting soon after discharge. GDMT should be initiated before the patient leaves the hospital, even if it is at small doses.

Transitional Care

The transition from the inpatient to the outpatient setting can be a particularly vulnerable period for patients due to the progressive nature of HF, complex medical regimens, multiple comorbidities, and the many clinicians who participate in the patient's care. Transitional care is a set of actions designed to ensure coordination and continuity of healthcare as patients transfer between different locations, different levels of care, and different providers.[88] HF patients are at risk for fragmented care due to the complexity of their disease. Incorporating comprehensive discharge planning, collaboration and communication between patients and care providers, and planned follow-up may reduce readmissions. Transitional care and preparation for discharge should start at admission by correctly reconciling medications, identifying other family members or caretakers to include in care planning, collaborating among multiple disciplines, and projecting potential post-discharge needs.

Precipitating causes of ADHF that led to the admission, barriers to transitions, and limitations to post-discharge support need to be identified. The patient and their family or caregivers should be educated regarding medications, dietary restrictions, symptoms of worsening HF, and self-care strategies to manage symptoms. Assurance should be made that prescriptions can be filled, or medications should be sent home with the patient until they are able to obtain medications. If the patient is too frail or unable to manage their own care at home, a skilled rehabilitation facility or palliative care referral should be considered.

A follow-up appointment to reevaluate the patient within one week of discharge should be scheduled prior to the patient's hospital discharge. The patient may return to their primary care provider or cardiologist, or they may be referred to a disease management program for close monitoring, further education, and medication titration. If the patient is at high risk for readmission, a follow-up telephone call within 72 hours after discharge may identify and manage early symptoms that could lead to rehospitalization. A report outlining the details of the patient's admission should be sent to all pertinent providers who participate in the patient's care.

CHRONIC HEART FAILURE

Pharmacologic Therapy: Chronic Management

Once patients with ADHF are stabilized, it is important to assess their current chronic medication therapy, begin to take steps to optimize therapy using current guidelines, and ensure that inappropriate medications are discontinued to avoid further episodes of decompensation. Starting appropriate medications during hospitalization or making sure that they are continued after discharge is one method of ensuring optimal outpatient medication therapy.[78]

It is essential that critical care nurses advocate for use of evidence-based pharmacologic therapy in their patients. The appropriate therapy improves symptoms, enhances functional status, reduces the risk of hospitalization, and increases survival,[227] yet too many patients still do not receive appropriate therapy.[170] Routine pharmacologic therapy for patients with heart failure with HFrEF consists of an ACEI (or ARB if ACEI is contraindicated), a beta-adrenergic blocking agent, and diuretics. Aldosterone antagonists, digoxin, and hydralazine/nitrates are added in appropriate patients. Details of outpatient medication therapy are outlined in Table 4.2. The importance of neurohumoral activation to the pathophysiology of heart failure is demonstrated by the finding that only neurohumoral blocking drugs (i.e., ACEIs, beta-adrenergic blockers, and aldosterone antagonists) increase survival. Thus, their use is essential in the management of HF.[227]

Nondihydropyridine calcium channel blockers, such as verapamil (Calan) or diltiazem (Cardizem), should be avoided in patients with reduced EF because they stimulate neurohumoral activation and cause myocardial depression.[227] Several clinical trials have demonstrated either no clinical benefit or worse outcomes in HF patients when receiving these medications.[163] Second-generation dihydropyridine derivatives, amlodipine (Norvasc), and felodipine (Plendil) have also failed to demonstrate any functional or survival benefit in patients with HF; however, they may be considered to manage hypertension or ischemic heart disease in patients with HFrEF and patients with HFpEF.[227]

Antidysrhythmic agents (with the exception of amiodarone [Cordarone]) are also to be avoided in heart failure because they have cardiodepressant and prodysrhythmic effects that negatively affect survival. Nonsteroidal antiinflammatory medications (NSAIDs) should also be avoided because they can cause sodium retention leading to fluid volume overload, and decrease the efficacy of ACEIs.[90]

Underuse of Optimal Therapy

Several investigative teams have demonstrated a consistent failure of providers to use clinical guidelines.[78,163] In one study, only 55% of a cohort of 960 patients hospitalized with HF were discharged on an ACEI.[32] Of these, only 77.1% had filled the prescription within 30 days after discharge and only 63.3% were current users at 1 year. An important additional finding was that patients who were not started on an ACEI during hospitalization were unlikely to have started the medication after discharge. Adherence to guidelines is a predictor of better outcomes in patients with HF.[119]

Pharmacologic Therapy in Hypertrophic Obstructive Cardiomyopathy

Pharmacologic treatment for symptomatic hypertrophic obstructive cardiomyopathy (HOC) centers around beta blockers as the first choice, and the nondihydropyridine calcium channel blocker, verapamil, as the second choice to block the effects of catecholamines that exacerbate the outflow tract obstruction[84,198] These medications enhance diastolic filling by slowing the heart rate. If symptoms are not controlled with a beta blocker, disopyramide (Norpace) should be considered to decrease inotropy and further decrease the outflow gradient, thereby improving or relieving symptoms.[84]

Managing Comorbidities

Most patients with HF have at least one comorbid condition complicating their treatment plan and negatively impacting outcomes. In patients older than age 65, approximately 66% have two noncardiac comorbidities and over 25% have more than six.[15,225] Older adults hospitalized for HF have a high incidence of hypertension (73-84%), anemia (50%), diabetes (25-46%), arthritis (43-62%), chronic pulmonary disease (30%), atrial fibrillation (28%), and dementia (27%).[227] Those with multiple comorbid conditions have more frequent hospitalizations and a relatively higher mortality rate.

Chronic Pulmonary Disease

Chronic pulmonary diseases, including chronic obstructive pulmonary disease (COPD), asthma, and other lower respiratory tract diseases, are some of the most common comorbid conditions found in patients with HF.[27] Refining the medication regimen in patients with these conditions can be challenging. Most problematic are bronchodilators, corticosteroids, loop diuretics, and digoxin (Lanoxin). Beta blockers, important in HF therapy, are traditionally contraindicated in those with COPD. However, newer evidence demonstrates that these medications can be used in persons with mild to moderate COPD.[149] Bronchodilators are important in treating COPD. Once thought to be detrimental in HF patients, recent studies have shown that inhaled bronchodilators may have the potential to improve pulmonary function in patients with obstructive airway and HF because of their potential to improve pulmonary function.[151] Corticosteroids used in COPD may cause fluid retention, which makes fluid management more difficult. Digoxin may cause pulmonary vasoconstriction, dysrhythmias secondary to hypoxia, and acidosis in persons with COPD. Loop diuretics can cause acidosis in those with COPD because patients have increased minute ventilation, which can decrease respiratory drive and accentuate the risk of metabolic acidosis. Patients with both heart failure and chronic lung disease should be taught to seek care immediately with escalating dyspnea not relieved by their usual measures.

Renal Dysfunction

Renal dysfunction is a common comorbidity and is one of the strongest predictors of mortality in patients with HF.[186] When the glomerular filtration rate (GFR) decreases, sodium and water accumulate, causing increased intravascular filling pressures. Elevated blood pressure causes increased afterload and left ventricular hypertrophy. Chronic kidney disease (CKD) patients have more coronary artery disease and two-thirds of dialysis patients develop HF within three years.[201] Chronic renal insufficiency, anemia, and HF commonly occur together as part of the cardio-renal syndrome. The goals of treatment are to relieve congestion by increasing diuresis, decreasing neurohormone activity, and restore hemodynamic stability.[213]

Anemia

Anemia is present in 15% to 55% of patients with HF and is associated with worse functional status, malnutrition, and increased morbidity and mortality.[225] Although early studies suggested improvement in NYHA class, decreased hospitalizations, and slight improvement in EF when patients were treated with darbepoetin alfa, subsequent studies ([Study of Anemia in Heart Failure Trial [STAMINA-HeFT] and Reduction of Events by Darbepoetin Alfa in Heart Failure [RED-HF]) showed no improvement in exercise tolerance, NYHA class, mortality, or hospitalizations.[85,208] Treatment with intravenous iron suggests improvement in symptoms, functional capacity, and quality of life.[74]

Diabetes Mellitus

Various sources report that 25% to 46% of patients with HF also have diabetes.[227] The metabolic consequences of diabetes (i.e., elevated proinsulin level, hyperinsulinemia, and hyperglycemia) adversely affect the vascular endothelium to cause accelerated atherosclerosis and diabetic cardiomyopathy.[233] Insulin resistance has been linked with cardiovascular remodeling.[233] When diabetes and HF coexist, morbidity and mortality are significantly increased, especially in heart failure patients with an ischemic etiology.

ACEIs, the first line of medication therapy for HF, have additional benefits for patients with diabetes because they improve glucose handling. Another important component of medication therapy in HF, beta-adrenergic blockade, was formerly contraindicated in diabetic patients. However, with careful monitoring, studies have demonstrated reduced death, HF hospitalizations, and incidence of acute myocardial infarction in HF patients with diabetes who are taking a beta blocker.[95,116] Although thiazolidinediones (TZDs) control glucose by increasing insulin sensitivity and improving endothelium-dependent vasodilation, there is concern that they may cause edema or weight gain as a result of fluid retention, which may increase hospitalizations. Overall, insulin and metformin are generally considered well-tolerated options to control glucose in the HF patient.

Sleep Disordered Breathing

Sleep disordered breathing (SDB) includes obstructive sleep apnea (OSA) and central sleep apnea (CSA). It is characterized by repetitive periods of apnea and hypopnea greater than 10 seconds. SDB is found in up to 50% of HF patients.[213] Treatment for OSA is continuous positive airway pressure (CPAP). CSA is treated with an adaptive servo-ventilator, which improves exercise capacity, quality of life, and cardiac function in HF patients.[197]

Depression

Anxiety and depression are the most common expression of emotional distress, and are common in HF. Approximately 11% to 35% of HF outpatients, and 35% to 70% of those hospitalized, are depressed.[187] HF patients with depression have a substantially greater risk of functional decline, rehospitalization, and death than those who are not depressed.[7] To date, no research trial has demonstrated a difference in morbidity and mortality outcomes between patients treated for depression and those not treated.[213]

Nonpharmacologic Therapy

Nonpharmacologic therapy assumes its greatest importance after the initial acute phase has passed. Nonpharmacologic therapies are essential to slowing HF progression, improving quality of life, and preventing rehospitalization. There is also evidence that comprehensive education and counseling, the cornerstone of nonpharmacologic therapy, improve survival.[120] Improving these outcomes depends in large part on adoption of good self-care practices by patients and their families. Although critical care nurses may feel that they have only cursory responsibility for promoting self-care, as it is largely an outpatient activity, all nurses must understand the complexity of self-care before they can adequately teach patients to adopt it. Education and counseling, along with reinforcement of what has already been learned, needs to begin as soon as possible after the patient is admitted. This process consists of maintenance behaviors to maintain physiologic stability, including adherence to their treatment plan, as well as management activities, such as recognizing and managing escalating symptoms.

Self-Care and Patient Education

Healthy behaviors keep the patient with HF physiologically stable and must be taught to each patient or his or her caregivers. Adherence is a fundamental element of self-care, but one that is very difficult for patients. Many patients struggle with following recommendations to weigh daily, monitor symptoms, and follow low-sodium diets.[153] Recognizing a patient's willingness and ability to accept and understand the information provided and then helping them to embrace the changes necessary for optimal self-care practices is a challenge. Factors that influence the patient's readiness to learn include their health literacy level, cognitive function, emotional/psychological state, fatigue level, and support system/caregiver availability. Helping the patient and caregivers understand the purpose of the recommendations, as well as incorporating activities to evaluate learning, such as utilizing teach-back (having the patient explain concepts in their own words), recording weight and symptoms, or role playing, may help the patient integrate important activities into their daily routine.

Disease State and Symptoms

Patients with HF have difficulty recognizing their own worsening symptoms usually because of lack of education and understanding and their failure to follow recommendations.[184] Increasing success is seen in patients who are more highly educated, have experience with the diagnosis, have received patient education, and have a strong support system. Patients should be provided with information regarding normal and abnormal heart function, causes of HF, progressive process of HF, treatment options, and symptoms of decompensated HF. They should be able to demonstrate understanding of the signs and symptoms that should be reported to their healthcare provider. Symptoms to monitor and report include increased shortness of breath with activity or when supine, increased lower extremity or abdominal edema, weight increase, worsening fatigue, increased cough, new heart beat irregularities, or increased confusion.

Daily Weighing

Daily weighing is useful for monitoring fluid status, yet fewer than half of all patients weigh themselves daily, even when newly discharged from a hospitalization for ADHF.[153] Patients should be taught the fundamentals of daily weighing at each hospitalization: weigh every day under similar conditions, log weight, and call provider with increases in weight.

Dietary Sodium and Fluid Restriction

Fluid overload secondary to excess dietary sodium intake is one of the most common proximate causes of ADHF. Patients have difficulty adhering to dietary changes for a number of reasons including the following: (1) inadequate knowledge about how to follow a low-sodium diet; (2) lack of helpful instructions; (3) lack of skill in applying knowledge gained; (4) difficulties eating with family and friends, or eating out; (5) age-related changes in smell and taste that add to the unpalatability of salt restriction; and (6) lack of motivation.[20]

When discussing sodium intake, important aspects to include are:

- Include both the patient and the family/caregiver in the discussion
- Begin with an assessment of the current sodium intake and eating habits
- Assess the patient's knowledge of the sodium content of foods
- Recommend daily sodium of between 2 and 3 g/day
- Remember that eating is a social endeavor and address eating out in restaurants and at social gatherings
- Refer for dietary counseling, if needed

Patients with advanced HF, persistent recurrent fluid retention despite sodium restriction and high-dose diuretic, or who are hyponatremic may also need to limit their fluid intake to around two liters per day.[227] This fluid restriction enhances volume management with diuretics and may improve serum sodium concentration. However, it is difficult to maintain and achieve, especially in hot or low-humidity climates. Suggestions to help patients include monitoring fluid intake, including foods that are liquid at room temperature, and using sugar-free hard candies or chewing gum or frozen fruits to address their thirst.

Medication Adherence

Medication nonadherence is common and has been demonstrated in more than half of HF patients.[100] Poor medication adherence is associated with increased rates of hospitalization, longer lengths of hospital stay, and higher mortality.[100] Patients who should be screened carefully for medication nonadherence are those who:

- Lack access to healthcare systems that provide continuity of care
- Have an asymptomatic chronic disease or mental health disorder
- Have physical or cognitive impairment
- Are younger or of a nonwhite race
- Have a complex regimen of medications
- Have low health literacy, high medication costs, live alone, or have poor social support

Techniques to improve medication adherence include:

- Assess potential barriers to medication adherence (lack of knowledge, memory/cognition, literacy, depression, financial)
- Educate patient as to the specific purpose of each HF medication, (i.e., the effect of ACEIs and beta blockers in treating HF, not simply for lowering blood pressure)
- Engage patient to take role in managing heart failure
- Use one-a-day dosing whenever possible
- Use pill dispensers when possible and assist with preparing
- Do not assume patients are taking all of their medicines

Preventive Behaviors

All patients with HF should receive an annual influenza vaccination, and a pneumonia vaccination every 5 years. They should avoid exposure to people with infectious diseases, especially upper respiratory infections. Smoking cessation and avoidance of second-hand smoke should be recommended and reinforced. Patients should avoid extremes in temperature, both heat and cold. Patients with HCM should be encouraged to initiate familial genetic counseling to evaluate relatives at risk.

Alcohol Restriction

There are no prospective studies of the impact of alcohol consumption on HF, and providers differ in their advice. Therefore, controversy exists on how to educate patients. Patients with HF are commonly asked to abstain totally from drinking alcohol because of its presumed myocardial depressant effects, although these effects have not been demonstrated in heart failure and are thought to be minor and transient. Recommendations for alcohol intake include:

- If cause of HF is ischemic, one ounce occasionally is acceptable. Women should drink less than men.
- If cause of HF is alcoholic related or if patient has major depression, anxiety disorder, or behavioral disorder, patient should abstain.
- If patient has recurrent dysrhythmias, history of hypertension, or diabetes, alcohol should be avoided.

Exercise

An important goal for patients with HF is maintenance of functional capacity and quality of life. A Cochrane review concluded that exercise training improved short-term aerobic capacity and quality of life, and reduced hospitalizations in persons with mild to moderate HF.[55] Exercise is beneficial for those with mild to moderate heart failure, and ongoing studies are defining its role in patients with severe heart failure. Although questions may remain about the specifics of prescribing activity for patients with heart failure, it is clear that inactivity is damaging and activity should be encouraged. It is recommended that exercise training or regular physical activity be recommended for patients with HF who are able to participate in order to improve functional status.[227] Patients with stable, chronic systolic HF and NYHA Class II to IV symptoms should be referred to cardiac rehabilitation for 6 weeks of therapy.

Hypertrophic cardiomyopathy is the most common cause of sudden death in young people.[139] Triggers of life-threatening ventricular tachydysrhythmias and sudden cardiac death during sports include emotional stress, environmental factors, myocardial ischemia, sympathetic-vagal imbalance, and hemodynamic changes. Additionally, intense exercise and athletic training could promote disease progression or worsening of the dysrhythmia substrate.[137] Cardiovascular screening initiatives to identify at-risk student athletes include history, physical, and occasionally 12-lead ECGs; however, there is no clear evidence of the value of such screening. Wider dissemination of automatic external defibrillators for secondary prevention is encouraged.[139]

Activity and exercise instructions for patients with HCM and ARVCM include but are not limited to:

- *Not advised, especially if high intensity:* basketball, body building, weightlifting, ice hockey, rock climbing, racquetball, soccer, tennis, touch football, windsurfing, scuba diving, skiing (downhill and cross-country)
- *Assess on an individual basis, especially if moderate intensity:* baseball/softball, skiing, surfing, hiking, sailing, jogging, motorcycling, horseback riding
- *Probably permitted when low intensity:* bowling, golf, skating, lifting weights, brisk walking, jogging, snorkeling, treadmill/stationary bicycling, doubles tennis, swimming
- *Avoid:* burst exertion or sprinting, adverse environmental conditions, exercise programs that escalate in exertion, amusement park rides if intensely stressful or frightening[22]

Nonprescription Medications

Over-the-counter (OTC), complementary, and alternative medicines are used by HF patients to treat a variety of conditions, including colds, musculoskeletal conditions, and stomach illnesses.[8] Patients should be encouraged to report all medications, including herbal therapies and vitamins, to their healthcare provider. Medications known to pose risks to patients with HF include:

- NSAIDs which may cause fluid retention and renal dysfunction
- Ephedrine, pseudoephedrine, diet pills, ma huang, especially in patients with HCM or ARVCM
- Herbal preparations: garlic can inhibit platelet aggregation, ginseng can cause hypertension, hellebore can cause hypotension and bradycardia

Surgical Options

Surgical and percutaneous interventions commonly integrated or considered in HF management include coronary revascularization (CABG or percutaneous coronary interventions); aortic valve replacement; mitral valve replacement or repair; septal myectomy or alcohol septal ablation for HCM; surgical ablation of ventricular arrhythmia; mechanical circulatory support; and cardiac transplantation.[227] CAD is the most common reason for intervention with either revascularization surgery or procedure. Studies on HF patients with an ischemic cause who are treated surgically or medically with GDMT have similar outcomes.[39] Therefore, guidelines recommend revascularization for HF patients on GDMT with angina and suitable coronary anatomy, especially with left main disease.[227] In addition, aortic valve replacement is reasonable for patients with critical aortic stenosis and a predicted surgical mortality of no greater than 10%.[227]

Candidates for surgical septal myectomy include HOC patients with a resting outflow gradient greater than 50 mm Hg and symptoms that limit daily activities. If successful, the gradient and mitral regurgitation will be immediately and completely abolished, leading to near-normal exercise capacity and freedom from symptoms of dyspnea, angina, and exertional syncope.[139] The effects are long-lasting, without recurrence of outflow tract obstruction. Percutaneous alcohol septal ablation has become an alternative to surgical myectomy in selected patients (advanced age, significant comorbidity, and patient preference). Alcohol-induced septal ablation is performed in the cardiac catheterization laboratory. The rate of complete abolition of obstruction and relief of symptoms is less than with myectomy and has inherent risks, including complete heart block requiring permanent pacemaker therapy, large myocardial infarction, ventricular septal defect, intractable ventricular fibrillation, and myocardial perforation.[139]

Disease Management Programs

Disease management has been defined as a comprehensive, integrated system for managing patients across the healthcare continuum by using best practices, clinical practice improvement, information technology, and other tools to improve measurable outcomes.[97] Although most critical care nurses are not involved directly in heart failure disease management, they should understand its usefulness and advocate for its use in patients at risk for rehospitalization. Disease management has been shown to: (1) improve patients' HF knowledge, (2) facilitate health behavior change that improves self-care, including treatment adherence and symptom management, (3) improve symptoms and functional status, and (4) improve clinical outcomes such as rehospitalization rates, costs, and mortality. The principles of successful HF disease management can be adopted and used by critical care nurses. The components of a comprehensive disease management program include:[97]

- Comprehensive education and counseling to patient and caregivers
- Promote patient self-care, including diuretic titration
- Quality of life and functional assessments
- Optimization of medical therapy and evaluation of adherence
- Mechanism to ensure appropriate follow-up
- Coordination with other providers and agencies
- Quality assessment

PALLIATION OF STAGE D HEART FAILURE PATIENTS

Patients with advanced HF are those with persistent symptoms that limit daily activity despite maximum GDMT. These patients are ACCF/AHA Stage D patients with refractory HF who might be eligible for specialized, advanced treatment strategies, such as MCS, procedures to facilitate fluid removal, continuous inotropic infusions, cardiac transplantation, experimental surgical procedures, or end-of-life care, such as hospice.[20] Advanced therapies such as fluid removal procedures, MCS, and cardiac transplantation for select patients have been addressed earlier in this chapter. Patients who are not candidates for those advanced therapies generally receive care to relieve symptoms, known as palliation.

Chronic Inotropic Support

Positive inotropic agents have not demonstrated improved outcomes in patients with advanced HF either in the hospital or when used for chronic support.[43,166] Although there is risk for increased mortality due to arrhythmic events, parenteral inotropes may be useful for a subset of patients with Stage D HFrEF who are refractory to other therapies and are suffering from end-organ failure. Inotropic infusions may be given while the patient lives at home. While often used for palliation of symptoms, patients awaiting more advanced therapies such as heart transplantation may have continuous inotrope infusions as an outpatient.

Palliative Care/Hospice

Comprehensive, ongoing care of advanced HF patients includes assessment and management of symptoms, psychosocial distress, quality of life, caregiver support, access to evidence-based interventions, and end-of-life preferences. Data suggest that advanced directives specifying limitations in end-of-life care are associated with positive impact on survival and quality of life. Chapter 43 describes the concepts of palliative care, hospice, and end-of-life issues. Issues specific to HF include:

- Prognostication is difficult due to erratic and/or prolonged HF disease trajectory.
- Preferences for resuscitation are often difficult since the patient may have survived multiple advanced medical interventions, including ICD placement. Discussion regarding deactivation of ICD timing should be initiated at implantation of the device.
- Concurrent cardio-renal disease may complicate hospice referral if the patient is on hemodialysis since hospices often do not accept patients on dialysis.

CONCLUSION

The care of patients with HF is complex, and ensuring optimal patient outcomes demands that nurses who care for these patients have a full grasp of appropriate care. Optimal short- and long-term outcomes can be achieved only when attention is given to optimizing both pharmacologic and nonpharmacologic therapies. Ultimately an integrated interprofessional approach is needed to deliver such care to these patients and prevent further exacerbations from occurring. Educating patients and their family members about lifestyle changes, medications, and dietary restrictions can assist them in improving self-care. Some patients will be candidates for advanced therapies to prolong life, while others may require palliation of symptoms without aggressive therapies. Either way, these are complicated patients whose welfare is dependent upon the knowledge of their nursing care providers.

CASE STUDY 4.1

R.S. is a 56-year-old African-American woman with a history of prior poorly controlled hypertension, type 2 diabetes, and heart failure. She was brought to the ED because of shortness of breath at rest. She does not follow a low-sodium and low-carbohydrate diet because she does not want to impose her diet on anyone else. Her body mass index is 32 kg/m^2. Medications before admission were: furosemide 20 mg twice per day, digoxin 0.125 mg once per day, and metformin (Glucophage) 500 mg once per day.

In the ED, she is observed to be anxious and in moderate respiratory distress. Heart rate is 126 beats/minute, respiratory rate is 32 breaths/minute, and blood pressure is 160/96 mm Hg. Pulse oximetry reveals an oxygen saturation of 82%. She has distended neck veins with elevated venous jugular pressure, an S3 gallop with a systolic ejection murmur, and 4+ pedal edema. Lung sounds include crackles at both bases. She was placed on oxygen and given furosemide 80 mg IV. Diagnostic studies revealed: Hgb 8.3, creatinine 1.8 mg/dL, BUN 42 mg/dL, glucose 350 mg/dL, BNP 1325 pg/mL. Chest x-ray showed pulmonary congestion; there was no evidence of pulmonary infection or other abnormality to account for dyspnea; ECG showed old infarction, moderate ventricular hypertrophy, and no signs of acute ischemia. Given a diagnosis of ADHF, R.S. was transferred to the critical care unit and placed on nitroglycerin infusion at a rate of 30 mg/h with orders to titrate to blood pressure less than 130/80 mm Hg. Intravenous furosemide was ordered at 40 mg every 12 hours. She was started on lisinopril (Zestril) 10 mg daily. Sliding-scale insulin was used to control blood glucose level.

R.S. met criteria for the warm and wet profile of ADHF. After 24 hours she had diuresed 3 liters of urine; her blood pressure was 126/66 mm Hg, her respiratory rate was 20 breaths/minute with no complaints of dyspnea, and heart rate was 80 beats/minute. She no longer had jugular venous distention, and her lungs were clear. Oxygen was discontinued. Echocardiography revealed left ventricular dysfunction with an ejection fraction of 30% and left ventricular hypertrophy.

Patient and family education and counseling were begun to assist the patient to assume greater self-care responsibility. The fundamentals and rationale of daily weighing as well as instruction on monitoring for symptoms of worsening heart failure were given. A dietitian was consulted to begin teaching R.S. to make low-sodium diet choices. Strategies for medication adherence were also taught. Lisinopril was increased to 20 mg daily, and carvedilol (Coreg) 3.125 mg twice a day was begun.

Decision Point:
What signs and symptoms of heart failure was R.S. exhibiting?

Decision Point:
What causes, risk factors, and lifestyle choices does R.S. have for heart failure?

Decision Point:
What pathophysiologic mechanism contributed to the left ventricular hypertrophy and left ventricular dysfunction?

Decision Point:
What pathophysiologic mechanism contributed to the fluid retention?

REFERENCES

1. Abraham, W., et al. (2011). Wireless pulmonary artery haemodynamic monitoring in chronic heart failure: a randomised controlled trial. *Lancet, 355*(9766), 658–666.
2. Adams, K. F., et al. (2005). Characteristics and outcomes of patients hospitalized for heart failure in the United States: rationale, design, and preliminary observations from the first 100,000 cases in the Acute Decompensated Heart Failure National Registry (ADHERE). *Am Heart J, 149,* 209–216.
3. Adams, K., et al. (2005). Relationship of serum digoxin concentration to mortality and morbidity in women in the digitalis investigation group trial: a retrospective analysis. *J Am Coll Cardiol, 46,* 497–50.
4. Adamson, P., et al. (2014). CHAMPION Trial rationale and design: the long-term safety and clinical efficacy of a wireless pulmonary artery pressure monitoring system. *J Cardiac Fail, 17,* 3–10.
5. ADHERE. (2003). *First quarter 2003 national benchmark report.* Fremont, CA: Scios.
6. Agha, S., et al. (2009). Echocardiography and risk prediction in advanced heart failure: incremental value over clinical markers. *J Card Fail, 15,* 586–592.
7. Albert, N., et al. (2009). Depression and clinical outcomes in heart failure: OPTIMIZE-HF analysis. *Am J Med, 122,* 366–373.
8. Albert, N. M., et al. (2009). Predictors of over-the-counter drug and herbal therapies use in elderly patients with heart failure. *Journal of Cardiac Failure, 15*(7), 600–606.
9. Anker, S. D., et al. (1997). Hormonal changes and catabolic/anabolic imbalance in chronic heart failure and their importance for cardiac cachexia. *Circulation, 96*(2), 526–534.
10. Anker, S. D., & Sharma, R. (2002). The syndrome of cardiac cachexia. *Int J Cardiol, 85*(1), 51–66.
11. Arbustini, E., et al. (2013). The MOGE(S) classification for a phenotype-genotype nomenclature of cardiomyopathy: endorsed by the World Heart Federation. *J Am Coll Cardiol, 62,* 2046.
12. Aretz., et al. (1987). Myocarditis: a histopathologic definition and classification. *Am J Cardiovasc Pathol, 1*(1), 3–14.
13. Aroesty, J. M., Jeevanandam, V., & Eisen, H. J. (2015). *Circulatory assist devices: cardiopulmonary assist device and short-term left ventricular assist devices.* Up To Date, Wolters Kluwer Health.
14. Aronson, D., & Burger, A. J. (2003). Neurohumoral activation and ventricular arrhythmias in patients with decompensated congestive heart failure: role of endothelin. *Pacing Clin Electrophysiol, 26*(3), 703.
15. Azad, N., & Lemay, G. (2014). Management of chronic heart failure in the older population. *J Geriatr Cardiol, 11,* 329–337.
16. Barker, W. H., Mullooly, J. P., & Getchell, W. (2006). Changing incidence and survival for heart failure in a well-defined older population, 1970-1974 and 1990-1994. *Circulation, 113,* 799–805.
17. Bart, B. A., et al. (2012). Ultrafiltration in decompensated heart failure with cardiorenal syndrome. *N Engl J Med, 367*(24), 2296–2304.
18. Baughman, K. L. (2006). Diagnosis of myocarditis: death of Dallas criteria. *Circulation, 113*(4), 593–595.
19. Baum, J., & Duffy, H. S. (2011). Fibroblasts and myofibroblasts: what are we talking about? *J Cardiovasc Pharmacol, 57,* 376–379.
20. Bentley, B., et al. (2005). Factors related to nonadherence to a low sodium diet in heart failure patients. *Eur J Cardiovasc Nur, 4,* 331–336.
21. Bergman, M. R., et al. (2007). Cardiac matrix metalloproteinase-2 expression independently induces marked ventricular remodeling and systolic dysfunction. *Am J Physiol Heart Circ Physiol, 292,* H1847–H1860.
22. Birks, E. (2015). *Intermediate- and long-term mechanical circulatory support.* Up To Date, Wolters Kluwer Health.
23. Birks, E. F., et al. (2011). Reversal of severe heart failure with a continuous-flow left ventricular assist device and pharmacological therapy: a prospective study. *Circulation, 123*(4), 381–390.
24. Birks, E., et al. (2006). Left ventricular assist device and drug therapy for the reversal of heart failure. *N Engl J Med, 355*(18), 1873–1884.
25. Borg, T. K., & Caulfield, J. B. (1981). The collagen matrix of the heart. *Fed Proc, 40*(7), 2037–2041.
26. Bozkurt, B., et al. (1998). Pathophysiologically relevant concentrations of tumor necrosis factor-alpha promote progressive left ventricular dysfunction and remodeling in rats. *Circulation, 97*(14), 1382.
27. Braunstein, J., et al. (2003). Non-cardiac comorbidity increases preventable hospitalizations and mortality among Medicare beneficiaries with chronic heart failure. *J Am Coll Cardiol, 42,* 1226–1233.
28. Brouri, F., et al. (2004). Blockade of beta 1 and desensitization of beta 2 adrenoceptors reduce isoprenaline-induced cardiac fibrosis. *Eur J Pharmacol, 485,* 227–234.
29. Brown, J. R., & Gottlieb, S. S. (2012). Acute decompensated heart failure. *Cardiol Clin, 30*(4), 665–671.
30. Bryant, D., et al. (1998). Cardiac failure in transgenic mice with myocardial expression of tumor necrosis factor-alpha. *Circulation, 97*(14), 1375–1381.
31. Bursi, B. F., et al. (2006). Systolic and diastolic heart failure in the community. *JAMA, 296,* 2209–2216.
32. Butler, J., et al. (2004). Outpatient utilization of angiotensin-converting enzyme inhibitors among heart failure patients after hospital discharge. *J Am Coll Cardiol, 43,* 2036–2043.
33. Butler, J., et al. (2006). Beta-blocker use and outcomes among hospitalized heart failure patients. *J Am Coll Cardiol, 47*(12), 2462–2469.
34. Calderone, A., et al. (2006). Scar myofibroblasts of the infarcted rat heart express natriuretic peptides. *J Cell Physiol, 207,* 165–173.
35. Calkins, H. (2006). Arrhythmogenic right ventricular dysphasia/cardiomyopathy. *Curr Opin Cardiol, 21,* 55–63.
36. Chaudhry, S., et al. (2007). Patterns of weight change preceding hospitalizations for heart failure. *Circulation, 116,* 1549–1554.
37. Chen, H. H., et al. (2013). Low-dose dopamine or low-dose nesiritide in acute heart failure with renal dysfunction: the ROSE acute heart failure randomized trial. *JAMA, 310*(23), 2533–2543.
38. Clavell, A. L., et al. (1996). Angiotensin converting enzyme inhibition modulates endogenous endothelin in chronic canine thoracic inferior vena caval constriction. *J Clin Invest, 97*(5), 1286–1292.
39. Cleland, J. C., et al. (2011). Survival after biventricular assist device implantation: an analysis of the interagency registry for mechanically assisted circulatory support. *J Heart Lung Transplant, 30*(8), 862–869.
40. Cleland, J., et al. (2011). Clinical trials update from the American Heart Association meeting 2010: EMPHASIS-HF, RAFT, TIM-HF, Tele-HF, ASCEND-HF, ROCKET-HF, and PROTECT. *Eur J Heart Fail, 13,* 460–465.
41. Cleland, J., et al. (2011). The Heart Failure Revascularisation Trial (HEART). *Eur J Heart Fail, 13*(2), 227–233.
42. Cody, R. (1997). The integrated effects of angiotensin II. *Am J Cardiol, 79*(5A), 9–11.
43. Cohn, J., et al. (1998). A dose-dependent increase in mortality with vesnarinone among patients with severe heart failure. vesnarinone trial investigators. *N Engl J Med, 339,* 1810–1816.
44. Cohn, J. N., et al. (1984). Plasma norepinephrine as a guide to prognosis in patients with chronic congestive heart failure. *N Engl J Med, 311*(13), 819–823.
45. Colucci, W. S. (2015). *Treatment of acute decompensated heart failure: Components of therapy.* Up To Date, Wolters Kluwer Health.

46. Communal, C., et al. (1998). Norepinephrine stimulates apoptosis in adult rat ventricular myocytes by activation of the beta-adrenergic pathway. *Circulation, 98*(13), 1329–1334.
47. Connors, A. F., et al. (1996). The effectiveness of right heart catheterization in the initial care of critically ill patients. SUPPORT Investigators. *JAMA, 276*(11), 889–897.
48. Cooper, L. T. (2015). Clinical manifestations and diagnosis of myocarditis in adults. http://www.uptodate.com/contents/clinical-manifestations-and-diagnosis-of-myocarditis-in-adults?source=search_result&search=myocarditis&selectedTitle=1%7E150.
49. Cooper, L. T. (2015). Definition and classification of the cardiomyopathies. http://www.uptodate.com/contents/definition-and-classification-of-the-cardiomyopathies?source=search_result&search=cardiomyopathy&selectedTitle=1%7E150.
50. Costanzo., et al. (2007). Ultrafiltration versus intravenous diuretics for patients hospitalized for acute decompensated heart failure. *J Am Coll Cardiol, 49*(6), 675–683.
51. Curtis, L. H., et al. (2008). Incidence and prevalence of heart failure in elderly persons, 1994–2003. *Arch Intern Med, 168*, 418–424.
52. Cruden, N. L., et al. (2004). Neutral endo-peptidase inhibition augments vascular actions of bradykinin in patients treated with angiotensin-converting enzyme inhibition. *Hypertension, 44*, 913–918.
53. Dalal, D., et al. (2005). Arrhythmogenic right ventricular dysphasia: a United States experience. *Circulation, 112*, 3823–3832.
54. Dargie, H. J. (2001). Effect of carvedilol on outcome after myocardial infarction in patients with left-ventricular dysfunction: the CAPRICORN randomised trial. *Lancet, 357*, 1385–1390.
55. Davies, E. J., et al. (2010). Exercise training for systolic heart failure: cochrane systematic review and meta-analysis. *Eur J Heart Fail, 12*(7), 706–715.
56. de Boer, R. A., et al. (2011). Predictive value of plasma galectin-3 levels in heart failure with reduced and preserved ejection fraction. *Ann Med, 43*, 60–68.
57. de Boer, R. A., et al. (2012). The fibrosis marker galectin-3 and outcome in the general population. *J Intern Med, 272*, 55–64.
58. de Filippi, C., et al. (2009). Clinical validation of a novel assay for galectin-3 for risk assessment in acutely destabilized heart failure. *J Card Fail, 15*, S9.
59. de Lemos, J. A., McGuire, D. K., & Drazner, M. H. (2003). B-type natriuretic peptide in cardiovascular disease. *Lancet, 362*, 316–322.
60. Deswal, A., Petersen, N. J., Feldman, A. M., et al. (2001). Cytokines and cytokine receptors in advanced heart failure: an analysis of the cytokine database from the Vesnarinone trial (VEST). *Circulation, 103*(16), 2055.
61. Dharmarajan, K., et al. (2013). Diagnoses and timing of 30-day readmissions after hospitalization for heart failure, acute myocardial infarction, or pneumonia. *JAMA, 309*, 355–363.
62. Dikshit, K., et al. (1973). Renal and extrarenal hemodynamic effects of furosemide in congestive heart failure after acute myocardial infarction. *N Engl J Med, 288*(21), 1087–1090.
63. Dillingham, M., & Anderson, R. (1986). Inhibition of vasopressin action by atrial natriuretic factor. *Science, 231*, 1572–1573.
64. Doval, H. C., et al. (1994). Randomised trial of low-dose amiodarone in severe congestive heart failure. Grupo de Estudio de la Sobrevida en la Insuficiencia Cardiaca en Argentina (GESICA). *Lancet, 344*, 493–498.
65. Elkayam, U., et al. (2004). Comparison of effects on left ventricular filling pressure of intravenous nesiritide and high-dose nitroglycerin in patients with decompensated heart failure. *Am J Cardiol, 93*, 237–240.
66. Elliott, P., et al. (2008). Classification of the cardiomyopathies: a position statement from the European Society of Cardiology Working Group on Myocardial and Pericardial Diseases. *Eur Heart J, 29*(2), 270–276.
67. Epstein, A., et al. (2013). 2012 ACCF/AHA/HRS focused update incorporated in the ACCF/AHA/HRS 2008 guidelines for device-based therapy of cardiac rhythm abnormalities. *J Am Coll Cardiol, 61*(3), 6–75.
68. Epstein, A. E., et al. (2013). Wearable cardioverter-defibrillator use in patients perceived to be at high risk early post-myocardial infarction. *J Am Coll Cardiol, 62*(21), 2000–2007.
69. Evangelista, L. S., Dracup, K., & Doering, L. V. (2000). Treatment-seeking delays in heart failure patients. *J Heart Lung Transplant, 19*, 932–938.
70. Exner, D., et al. (1999). Beta-adrenergic blocking agent use and mortality in patients with asymptomatic and symptomatic left ventricular systolic dysfunction: a post hoc analysis of the studies of left ventricular dysfunction. *J Am Coll Cardiol, 33*, 916–920.
71. Fan, D., et al. (2012). Cardiac fibroblasts, fibrosis and extracellular matrix remodeling in heart disease. *Fibrogenesis Tissue Repair, 5*(15). http://www.fibrogenesis.com/content/5/1/15.
72. Felker, M., et al. (2011). Diuretic strategies in patients with acute decompensated heart failure. *N Engl J Med, 364*(9), 797–805.
73. Ferguson, J. J., et al. (2001). The current practice of intra-aortic balloon counterpulsation: results from the benchmark registry. *J Am Coll Cardiol, 38*(5), 14561462.
74. Filippatos, G., et al. (2013). Intravenous ferric carboxymaltose in iron-deficient chronic heart failure patients with and without anaemia: a subanalysis of the FAIR-HF trial. *Eur J Heart Fail, 15*, 1267–1276.
75. Fonarow, G., et al. (2005). Risk stratification for in-hospital mortality in acutely decompensated heart failure: classification and regression tree analysis. *JAMA, 293*, 572–580.
76. Fonarow, G. C., et al. (2008). Influence of beta-blocker continuation or withdrawal on outcomes in patients hospitalized with heart failure: findings from the OPTIMIZE-HF program. *J Am Coll Cardiol, 52*, 190–199.
77. Fonarow, G., & Committee, for the ASA (2003). The Acute Decompensated Heart Failure National Registry (ADHERE): opportunities to improve care of patients hospitalized with acute decompensated heart failure. *Rev Cardiovasc Med, 4*(Suppl. 7), S21–S30.
78. Fonarow, G., et al. (2008). Heart failure care in the outpatient cardiology practice setting: findings from IMPROVE HF. *Circ Heart Failure, 2*, 98–106.
79. Francis, G., & Tang, W. (2004). Clinical evaluation of heart failure. In D. Mann (Ed.), *Heart failure: A companion to Braunwald's heart disease*. Philadelphia: Saunders.
80. Fryer, R. M., et al. (2008). Effect of bradykinin metabolism inhibitors on evoked hypotension in rats: rank efficacy of enzymes associated with bradykinin-mediated angioedema. *Br J Pharmacol, 153*, 947–955.
81. Galvao, M., & Rasmusson, K. (2015). Acute decompensated heart failure. In (2nd ed.). S. Paul, & P. Kirkwood (Eds.), *Heart failure nursing certification: Core curriculum review*. Mt. Laurel, NJ: American Association of Heart Failure Nurses.
82. Gattis, W., et al. (2004). Predischarge initiation of carvedilol in patients hospitalized for decompensated heart failure: results of the Initiation Management Predischarge: Process for Assessment of Carvedilol Therapy in Heart Failure (IMPACT-HF) trial. *J Am Coll Cardiol, 43*, 1534–1540.
83. Geerts, W., et al. (2008). Prevention of venous thromboembolism: American College of Chest Physicians Evidence-based Clinical Practice Guidelines. *Chest, 133*, 381S.
84. Gersh, B., et al. (2011). 2011 ACCF/AHA guideline for the diagnosis and treatment of hypertrophic cardiomyopathy: executive summary: a report of the American College of Cardiology Foundation/American Heart Association Task Force on Practice Guidelines. *Circulation, 124*, 2761–2796.
85. Ghali, J., et al. (2008). Randomized double-blind trial of darbepoetin alfa in patients with symptomatic heart failure and anemia. *Circulation, 117*, 526–535.
86. Gheorghiade, M., et al. (2006). Systolic blood pressure at admission, clinical characteristics, and outcomes in patients hospitalized with acute heart failure. *JAMA, 296*, 2217–2226.
87. Gibbs, A. (2015). Transitional care for heart failure patients. In S. Paul, & P. Kirkwood (Eds.), *Heart failure nursing certification: Core curriculum review*. Mt. Laurel, NJ: American Association of Heart Failure Nurses.
88. Reference removed in page proof.
89. Gillis, A., et al. (2014). Impact of cardiac resynchronization therapy on hospitalizations in the resynchronization-defibrillation for ambulatory heart failure trial. *Circulation, 129*, 2021–2030.
90. Gislason, G., Rasmussen, J., & Abildstrom, S. (2009). Increased mortality and cardiovascular morbidity associated with use of nonsteroidal antiinflammatory drugs in chronic heart failure. *Arch Intern Med, 169*, 141–149.

91. Go, A. S., et al. (2013). Heart disease and stroke statistics: 2013 update: a report form the American Heart Association. *Circulation, 127* e6–245.
92. Goldstein, S., et al. (2001). Metoprolol controlled release/extended release in patients with severe heart failure: analysis of the experience in the MERIT-HF study. *J Am Coll Cardiol, 38*(4), 932–938.
93. Greenberg, B., & Hermann, D. (2002). *Contemporary diagnosis and management of heart failure.* Newton, PA: Handbooks in Health Care.
94. Group, T. D. I. (1997). The effect of digoxin on mortality and morbidity in patients with heart failure. *N Engl J Med, 336*, 525–533.
95. Haas, S., et al. (2003). Are beta-blockers as efficacious in patients with diabetes mellitus as in patients without diabetes mellitus who have chronic heart failure? A meta-analysis of large-scale clinical trials. *Am Heart J, 146*, 848–853.
96. Harvey, S., et al. (2005). Assessment of the clinical effectiveness of pulmonary artery catheters in management of patients in intensive care (PAC-Man): a randomised controlled trial. *Lancet, 366*, 472–477.
97. Hauptman, P. J., et al. (2008). The heart failure clinic: a consensus statement of the Heart Failure Society of America. *J Card Fail, 14*(10), 801–815.
98. Heidenreich, P. A., et al. (2013). Forecasting the impact of heart failure in the United States: a policy statement from the American heart Association. *Circ Heart Fail, 6*, 606–619.
99. Ho, J. E., et al. (2012). Galectin-3, a marker of cardiac fibrosis, predicts incident heart failure in the community. *J Am Coll Cardiol, 60*(14), 1249–1256.
100. Ho, P. M., Bryson, C. L., & Rumsfeld, J. S. (2009). Medication adherence: its importance in cardiovascular outcomes. *Circulation, 119*(23), 3028–3035.
101. Hogg, K., & McMurray, J. (2005). Neurohumoral pathways in heart failure with preserved systolic function. *Prog Cardiovasc Dis, 47*, 357–366.
102. Isso, J. L., & Gradman, A. H. (2004). Mechanisms and management of hypertensive heart disease: from left ventricular hypertrophy to heart failure. *Med Clin North Am, 88*, 1257–1271.
103. Jain, R. (2010). Athletic status and arrhythmogenic right ventricular dysphasia/cardiomyopathy: from physiological observations to pathological explanation. *Hypothesis, 8*(1), e2–e9.
104. Januzzi, J. L., et al. (2005). The N-terminal pro-BNP investigation of dyspnea in the emergency department (PRIDE) study. *Am J Cardiol, 95*, 948–954.
105. Januzzi, J. L., et al. (2008). Measurement of the interleukin family member ST2 in patients with acute dyspnea: results from the PRIDE (Pro-Brain Natriuretic Peptide Investigation of Dyspnea in the Emergency Department) study. *J Am Coll Cardiol, 50*, 607–613.
106. Jeevanandum, V., et al. (2002). Circulatory assistance with a permanent implantable IABP: initial human experience. *Circulation, 106*, 183–188.
107. Jones, R. C., Francis, G. S., & Lauer, M. S. (2004). Predictors of mortality in patients with heart failure and preserved systolic function in the digitalis investigation group trial. *J Am Coll Cardiol, 44*(5), 1025–1029.
108. Kandalam, V., et al. (2011). Lack of tissue inhibitor of metalloproteinases 2 leads to exacerbated left ventricular dysfunction and adverse extracellular matrix remodeling in response to biomechanical stress. *Circulation, 124*, 2094–2105.
109. Kapadia, S. R., et al. (1997). Hemodynamic regulation of tumor necrosis factor-alpha gene and protein expression in adult feline myocardium. *Circ Res, 81*(2), 187–195.
110. Kapadia, S. R., et al. (2000). Elevated circulating levels of serum tumor necrosis factor-alpha in patients with hemodynamically significant pressure and volume overload. *J Am Coll Cardiol, 36*(1), 208–212.
111. Katz, S. D., et al. (1996). Exercise-induced vasodilation in forearm circulation of normal subjects and patients with congestive heart failure: role of endothelium-derived nitric oxide. *J Am Coll Cardiol, 28*(3), 585–590.
112. Katz, S. D., et al. (1999). Decreased activity of the L-arginine-nitric oxide metabolic pathway in patients with congestive heart failure. *Circulation, 99*(16), 2113–2117.
113. Kaye, D. M., et al. (1994). Neurochemical evidence of cardiac sympathetic activation and increased central nervous system norepinephrine turnover in severe congestive heart failure. *J Am Coll Cardiol, 23*(3), 570–578.
114. Kelder, J. C., et al. (2011). The diagnostic value of physical examination and additional testing in primary care patients with suspected heart failure. *Circulation, 124*(25), 2865–2873.
115. Kirklin, J. K., et al. (2014). Sixth INTERMACS annual report: a 10,000 patient database. *J Heart Lung Transplant, 33*(6), 555–564.
116. Kirpichnikov, D., McFarlane, S., & Sowers, J. (2003). Heart failure in diabetic patients: utility of beta-blockade. *J Card Fail, 9*, 333–344.
117. Klein, H., Goldenberg, I., & Moss, A. (2013). Risk stratification for implantable cardioverter defibrillator therapy: the role of the wearable cardioverter-defibrillator. *Eur Heart J, 34*(29), 2230–2242.
118. Kohli, P., et al. (2011). Role of ST2 in non-ST-elevation acute coronary syndrome in the MERLIN-TIMI 36 trial. *Clin Chem, 58*(1), 257–266.
119. Komajda, M., et al. (2005). Adherence to guidelines is a predictor of outcome in chronic heart failure: the MAHLER survey. *Eur Heart J, 26*, 1653–1659.
120. Krumholz, H., et al. (2002). Randomized trial of an education and support intervention to prevent readmission of patients with heart failure. *J Am Coll Cardiol, 39*, 83–89.
121. Krumholz, H. M., et al. (2009). Patterns of hospital performance in acute myocardial infarction and heart failure 30-day mortality and readmission. *Circ Cardiovasc Qual Outcomes, 2*, 407–413.
122. Kubo, S. H., et al. (1991). Endothelium-dependent vasodilation is attenuated in patients with heart failure. *Circulation, 84*(4), 1589–1596.
123. Kuhn, M. (2004). Molecular physiology of natriuretic peptide signaling. *Basic Res Cardiol, 99*, 76–82.
124. Ky, B., et al. (2011). High-sensitivity ST2 for prediction of adverse outcomes in chronic heart failure. *Circ Heart Fail, 4*(2), 180–187.
125. Leclercq, C., et al. (2002). Comparative effects of permanent biventricular and right-univentricular pacing in heart failure patients with chronic atrial fibrillation. *Eur Heart, 23*, 1780–1787.
126. Lederle, F. A., et al. (2011). Venous thromboembolism prophylaxis in hospitalized medical patients and those with stroke: a background review for an American College of Physicians Clinical Practice Guideline. *Ann Intern Med, 155*, 602–615.
127. Levy, D., et al. (2002). Long-term trends in the incidence of and survival with heart failure. *N Engl J Med, 347*, 1397–1402.
128. Levy, D., et al. (1996). The progression from hypertension to congestive heart failure. *JAMA, 275*, 1557–1562.
129. Linde, C., et al. (2010). REVERSE study group. Cardiac resynchronization therapy in asymptomatic or mildly symptomatic heart failure patients in relation to etiology: results from the REVERSE (Resynchronization reVErses Remodeling in Systolic Left Ventricular Dysfunction) study. *J Am Coll Cardiol, 56*, 1826–1831.
130. Lok, D. J., et al. (2010). Prognostic value of galectin-3, a novel marker of fibrosis, in patients with chronic heart failure. *Clin Res Cardiol, 99*, 323–328.
131. Luchner, A., et al. (2005). Effect of compensated renal dysfunction on approved heart failure markers: direct comparison of brain natriuretic peptide (BNP) and N-terminal pro-BNP. *Hypertension, 46*, 118–123.
132. Lymperopoulos, A., Rengo, R. G., & Koch, W. J. (2013). Adrenergic nervous system in heart failure. *Circ Res, 113*, 739–753.
133. MacCarthy, P. A., et al. (2000). Contrasting inotropic effects of endogenous endothelin in the normal and failing human heart: studies with an intracoronary ET(A) receptor antagonist. *Circulation, 101*(2), 142–147.
134. Maisel, A. S., et al. (2002). Rapid measurement of B-type natriuretic peptide in the emergency diagnosis of heart failure. *N Engl J Med, 347*, 161–167.
135. Mancini, D. (2015). *Indications and contraindications for cardiac transplantation.* Up To Date, Wolters Kluwer Health.
136. Maric, C., Zheng, W., & Walther, T. (2006). Interactions between angiotensin ll and atrial natriuretic peptide in renomedullary interstitial cells: the role of neutral endopeptidase. *Nephron Physiol, 103*, 149–156.
137. Maron, B., et al. (2004). Recommendations for physical activity and recreational sports participation for young patients with genetic cardiovascular disease. *Circulation, 109*, 2807–2816.
138. Maron, B. J. (2002). Hypertrophic cardiomyopathy: a systematic review. *JAMA, 287*(10), 1308–1310.

139. Maron, B. J., et al. (2014). Hypertrophic cardiomyopathy: present and future, with translation into contemporary cardiovascular medicine. *J Am Coll Cardiol, 64*(1), 89–99.
140. Maron, B. J., et al. (2006). Contemporary definitions and classification of the cardiomyopathies: an American Heart Association scientific statement from the Council on Clinical Cardiology, Heart Failure and Transplantation Committee; Quality of Care and Outcomes Research and Function. *Circulation, 113*(14), 1807–1816.
141. Maron, M. S., et al. (2009). Hypertrophic cardiomyopathy phenotype revisited after 50 years with cardiovascular magnetic resonance. *J Am Coll Cardiol, 54*, 220–228.
142. Massie, B. M., et al. (2009). Randomized trial of warfarin, aspirin, and clopidogrel in patients with chronic heart failure: the Warfarin and Antiplatelet Therapy in Chronic Heart Failure (WATCH) trial. *Circulation, 119*, 1616–1624.
143. McDonald, K., et al. (2001). Elimination of early rehospitalization in a randomized, controlled trial of multidisciplinary care in a high-risk, elderly heart failure population: the potential contributions of specialist care, clinical stability and optimal angiotensin-converting enzyme. *Eur J Heart Fail, 3*, 209–215.
144. McKelvie, R., et al. (1999). Comparison of candesartan, enalapril, and their combination in congestive heart failure: randomized evaluation of strategies for left ventricular dysfunction (RESOLVD) pilot study: the RESOLVD Pilot Study Investigators. *Circulation, 100*, 1056–1064.
145. McMurray, J. J., et al. (2012). ESC guidelines for the diagnosis and treatment of acute and chronic heart failure 2012: the Task Force for the Diagnosis and Treatment of Acute and Chronic Heart Failure 2012 of the European Society of Cardiology. *Eur Heart J, 33*(14), 1787.
146. McMurray, J. J., et al. (1992). Plasma endothelin in chronic heart failure. *Circulation, 85*(4), 1374–1379.
147. McMurray, J. J., et al. (2013). ESC guidelines for the diagnosis and treatment of acute and chronic heart failure 2012: the Task Force for the Diagnosis and Treatment of Acute and Chronic Heart Failure 2012 of the European Society of Cardiology. *Revista Portuguesa de Cardiologia, 32*(7-8) e1–641–e61.
148. McMurray, J., et al. (2014). Angiotensin-neprilysin inhibition versus enalapril in heart failure. *N Eng J Med, 371*(11), 993–1004.
149. Mentz, R., et al. (2013). Association of beta-blocker use and selectivity with outcomes in patients with heart failure and chronic obstructive pulmonary disease (from OPTIMIZE-HF). *Am J Cardiol, 111*, 582–587.
150. Metra, M., et al. (2007). Should beta-blocker therapy be reduced or withdrawn after an episode of decompensated heart failure? Results from COMET. *Eur Heart J, 9*(9), 901–909.
151. Minasian, A., et al. (2013). Bronchodilator responsiveness in patients with chronic heart failure. *Heart Lung, 42*, 208–214.
152. Mizuno, Y., et al. (2001). Aldosterone production is activated in failing ventricle in humans. *Circulation, 103*(1), 72–77.
153. Moser, D., Doering, L., & Chung, M. (2005). Vulnerabilities of patients recovering from an exacerbation of chronic heart failure. *Am Heart J, 150*, 984.
154. Moss, A., et al. (2009). Cardiac-resynchronization therapy for the prevention of heart failure events. *N Engl J Med, 361*(14), 1329–1338.
155. Mozaffarian, D., et al. (2015). Heart disease and stroke statistics - 2015 update: a report from the American Heart Association. *Circulation, 131*, e29–e322.
156. Nef, H. M., et al. (2007). Tako-Tsubo cardiomyopathy: intraindividual structural analysis in the acute phase and after functional recovery. *Eur Heart J, 28*(20), 2456–2464.
157. Niebauer, J., et al. (1999). Endotoxin and immune activation in chronic heart failure: a prospective cohort study. *Lancet, 353*, 1838–1842.
158. Nieminen, M. S., Heikkila, J., & Karjalainen, J. (1984). Echocardiography in acute infectious myocarditis: relation to clinical and electrocardiographic findings. *Am J Cardiol, 53*(9), 1331–1337.
159. Nohria, A., et al. (2003). Clinical assessment identifies hemodynamic profiles that predict outcomes in patients admitted with heart failure. *J Am Coll Cardiol, 41*(10), 1797–1804.
160. Noll, G., Wenzel, R. R., & Luscher, T. F. (1996). Endothelin and endothelin antagonists: potential role in cardiovascular and renal disease. *Mol Cell Biochem, 157*(1-2), 259–267.
161. Nozawa, T., et al. (1998). Dual-tracer assessment of coupling between cardiac sympathetic neuronal function and downregulation of beta-receptors during development of hypertensive heart failure of rats. *Circulation, 97*(23), 2359–2367.
162. O'Connell, J. B. (1998). Diagnosis and medical treatment of inflammatory cardiomyopathy. In E. Topol, & J. Nissen (Eds.), *Cardiovascular medicine*. Philadelphia: Lippincott-Raven.
163. O'Connor, C., et al. (2008). Predictors of mortality after discharge in patients hospitalized with heart failure: an analysis from the Organized Program to Initiate Lifesaving Treatment in Hospitalized Patients with Heart Failure (OPTIMIZE-HF). *Am Heart J, 156*, 662–673.
164. Olinde, K. D., & O'Connell, J. B. (1994). Inflammatory heart disease: pathogenesis, clinical manifestations and treatment of myocarditis. *Annu Rev Med, 45*, 481–490.
165. Osadchii, O. E., et al. (2007). Cardiac dilatation and pump dysfunction without intrinsic myocardial systolic failure following chronic beta adrenoreceptor activation. *Am J Physiol Heart Circ Physiol, 292*, H1898–H1905.
166. Packer, M., et al. (1991). Effect of oral milrinone on mortality in severe chronic heart failure. The PROMISE Study Research Group. *N Engl J Med, 325*, 1468–1475.
167. Packer, M., et al. (2001). Effect of carvedilol on survival in severe chronic heart failure. *N Engl J Med, 344*, 1651–1658.
168. Packer, M., et al. (1979). Rebound hemodynamic events after the abrupt withdrawal of nitroprusside in patients with severe chronic heart failure. *N Engl J Med, 301*(22), 1193–1197.
169. Peacock, F., DeMarco, T., & Fonarow, G. C. (2008). Cardiac troponin and outcome in acute heart failure. *N Engl J Med, 358*, 2117–2126.
170. Peterson, P., et al. (2013). Practice-level variation in use of recommended medications among outpatients with heart failure: insights from the NCDR PINNACLE program. *Circ Heart Fail, 6*, 1132–1138.
171. Petrov, W., Fagard, R. H., & Lijnen, P. J. (2002). Stimulation of collagen production by transforming growth factor-beta$_1$ during differentiation of cardiac fibroblasts to myofibroblasts. *Hypertension, 39*, 258–263.
172. Pfeffer, M., et al. (2003). Valsartan, captopril, or both in myocardial infarction complicated by heart failure, left ventricular dysfunction, or both. *N Engl J Med*, 1883–1890.
173. Piano, M. R. (2008). Pathophysiology of heart failure. In D. K. Moser, & B. Riegel (Eds.), *Cardiac nursing* (pp. 897–915). St. Louis: Elsevier.
174. Pinamonti, B., et al. (1988). Echocardiographic findings in myocarditis. *Am J Cardiol, 62*(4), 258–291.
175. Pinto, D. S., & Kocial, R. D. (2015). Evaluation of acute decompensated heart failure. http://www.uptodate.com/contents/evaluation-of-acute-decompensated-heart-failure?source=search_result&search=evaluation+of+decompensated+heart+failure&selectedTitle=1%7E150.
176. Pitt, B., et al. (1999). Randomized Aldactone evaluation study investigators. the effect of spironolactone on morbidity and mortality in patients with severe heart failure. *N Engl J Med, 341*, 709–717.
177. Porcel, J. M. (2010). Pleural effusions from congestive heart failure. *Semin Respir Crit Care Med, 31*(6), 689–697.
178. Rademaker, M. T., et al. (1996). Neutral endopeptidase inhibition: augmented atrial and brain natriuretic peptide, haemodynamic and natriuretic responses in ovine heart failure. *Clin Sci, 91*, 283–291.
179. Rathore, S., et al. (2003). Association of serum digoxin concentration and outcomes in patients with heart failure. *JAMA, 289*, 871–879.
180. Redfield, M. M., et al. (2002). Plasma brain natriuretic peptide concentration: impact of age and gender. *J Am Coll Cardiol, 40*, 976–982.
181. Rehman, S. U., Mueller, T., & Januzzi, J. L. (2008). Characteristics of the novel interleukin family biomarker ST2 in patients with acute heart failure. *J Am Coll Cardiol, 52*(18), 1458–1465.
182. Reilly, C., et al. (2015). American Association of Heart Failure Nurses best practices paper: literature synthesis and guideline review for dietary sodium restriction. *Heart Lung, 44*(4), 289–298.

183. Rich, S., & McLaughlin, V. V. (2003). Endothelin receptor blockers in cardiovascular disease. *Circulation, 108*(18), 2181–2190.
184. Riegel, B., & Carlson, B. (2002). Facilitators and barriers to heart failure self-care. *Patient Educ Couns, 46*, 287–295.
185. Roger, V. L., et al. (2004). Trends in heart failure incidence and survival in a community-based population. *JAMA, 292*, 344–350.
186. Ronco, C., & Di Lullo, L. (2014). Cardiorenal syndrome. *Heart Fail Clin, 10*(2), 251–280.
187. Rutledge, T., et al. (2006). Depression in heart failure: a meta-analytic review of prevalence, intervention effects, and associations with clinical outcomes. *J Am Coll Cardiol, 48*, 527–537.
188. Sackner-Bernstein, J., & Obeleniene, R. (2003). How should diuretic-refractory, volume overloaded heart failure patients be managed? *J Invasive Cardiol, 15*, 585–590.
189. Salvador, D. R., et al. (2005). Continuous infusion versus bolus injection of loop diuretics in congestive heart failure. *Cochrane Database Systematic Review, 209*(3) CD003178.
190. Santa-Cruz, R. A., Cohen, M. G., & Ohman, E. M. (2006). Aortic counterpulsation: a review of the hemodynamic effects and indications for use. *Catheter Cardiovasc Interv, 67*(1), 68–77.
191. Scheidt, S., et al. (1973). Intra-aortic balloon counterpulsation in cardiogenic shock. Report of a co-operative clinical trial. *N Engl J Med, 288*(19), 979–984.
192. Schrier, R. W., et al. (2006). Tolvaptan, a selective oral vasopressin V2-receptor antagonist, for hyponatremia. *N Engl J Med, 355*, 2099–2112.
193. Shah, M. R., et al. (2005). Impact of the pulmonary artery catheter in critically ill patients: meta-analysis of randomized clinical trials. *JAMA, 294*(13), 1664–1670.
194. Shah, R. V., et al. (2010). Galectin-3, cardiac structure and function, and long-term mortality in patients with acutely decompensated heart failure. *Eur J Heart Fail, 12*, 826–832.
195. Shah, R. V., & Januzzi, J. L. (March 2010). ST2: a novel remodeling biomarker in acute and chronic heart failure. *Curr Heart Fail Rep, 7*(1), 9–14.
196. Sharkey, S. W., et al. (2005). Acute and reversible cardiomyopathy provoked by stress in women from the United States. *Circulation, 111*, 472–479.
197. Sharma, B., McSharry, D., & Malhotra, A. (2011). Sleep disordered breathing in patients with heart failure: pathophysiology and management. *Curr Treat Options Cardiovasc Med, 13*(6), 506–516.
198. Sherrid, M., et al. (2013). Treatment of obstructive hypertrophic cardiomyopathy symptoms and gradient resistant to first-line therapy with beta blockade or verapamil. *Circ Heart Fail, 6*, 694–702.
199. Simko, F., & Simko, J. (1999). Heart failure and angiotensin converting enzyme inhibition: problems and perspectives. *Physiol Res, 48*, 1–8.
200. Simonton, C. A., et al. (1985). Milrinone in congestive heart failure: acute and chronic hemodynamic and clinical evaluation. *J Am Coll Cardiol, 6*(2), 453–459.
201. Smith, G., et al. (2006). Renal impairment and outcomes in heart failure: systematic review and meta-analysis. *J Am Coll Cardiol, 47*, 1987–1996.
202. Socrates, T., et al. (2010). Interleukin family member ST2 and mortality in acute dyspnoea. *J Intern Med, 268*(5), 493–500.
203. Centers for Disease Control and Prevention. (2011). Mortality multiple cause micro-data files. http://www.cdc.gov/nchs/data_access/Vitalstatsonline.htm#Mortality_multiple.
204. Stehlik, J., et al. (2011). The Registry of the International Society for Heart and Lung Transplantation: twenty-eighth Adult Heart Transplant Report-2011. *J Heart Lung Transplant, 30*, 1078–1094.
205. Stevenson, L., & Perloff, J. (1989). The limited reliability of physical signs for estimating hemodynamics in chronic heart failure. *JAMA, 261*, 884–888.
206. Swedberg, K., et al. (1990). Hormones regulating cardiovascular function in patients with severe congestive heart failure and their relation to mortality (follow-up of the CONSENSUS trial). *Am J Cardiol, 66*, 40D–45D.
207. Swedberg, K., et al. (2010). Ivabradine and outcomes in chronic heart failure (SHIFT): a randomized placebo-controlled study. *The Lancet, 376*(9744), 875–885.
208. Swedberg, K., et al. (2013). Treatment of anemia with darbepoetin alfa in systolic heart failure. *N Engl J Med, 368*, 1210–1219.
209. Sweeney, M., et al. (2003). Adverse effect of ventricular pacing on heart failure and atrial fibrillation among patients with normal baseline QRS duration in a clinical trial of pacemaker therapy for sinus node dysfunction. *Circulation, 107*, 2932–2937.
210. Taylor, A., Ziesche, S., & Yancy, C. (2004). A combination of isosorbide dinitrate and hydralazine in blacks with heart failure. *N Engl J Med, 351*(20), 2049–2057.
211. Torp-Pedersen, C., et al. (1999). Dofetilide in patients with congestive heart failure and left ventricular dysfunction. Danish Investigations of Arrhythmia and Mortality on Dofetilide Study Group. *N Engl J Med, 341*, 857–865.
212. Torre-Amione, G., et al. (1996). Proinflammatory cytokine levels in patients with depressed left ventricular ejection fraction: a report from the Studies of Left Ventricular Dysfunction (SOLVD). *J Am Coll Cardiol, 27*(5), 1201–1206.
213. Triposkiadis, F. K., & Skoularigis, J. (2012). Prevalence and importance of comorbidities in patients with heart failure. *Curr Heart Fail Rep, 9*(4), 354–362.
214. Tsutamoto, T., et al. (1998). Interleukin-6 spillover in the peripheral circulation increases with the severity of heart failure, and the high plasma level of interleukin-6 is an important prognostic predictor in patients with congestive heart failure. *J Am Coll Cardiol, 31*(2), 391–398.
215. Udeoji, D. U., et al. (2013). Left ventricular noncompaction cardiomyopathy: updated review. *Ther Adv Cardiovasc Dis, 7*(5), 260–273.
216. Ueland, T., Aukrust, P., & Broch, K. (2011). Galectin-3 in heart failure: high levels are associated with all-cause mortality. *Int J Cardiol, 150*, 361–364.
217. Vantrimpont, P., et al. (1997). Additive beneficial effects of beta blockers to angiotensin-converting enzyme inhibitors in the Survival and Ventricular Enlargement (SAVE) study: SAVE Investigators. *J Am Coll Cardiol, 29*, 229–236.
218. Vasan, R. S., & Levy, D. (2000). Defining diastolic heart failure: a call for standardized diagnostic criteria. *Circulation, 101*, 2118–2121.
219. Vizzardi, E., et al. (2010). Effect of spironolactne on left ventricular ejection fraction and volumes in patients with class I or II heart failure. *Am J Cardiol, 106*, 1292–1296.
220. Ware, L. B., & Matthay, M. A. (2005). Clinical practice. Acute pulmonary edema. *N Engl J Med, 353*(26), 2788–2796.
221. Weber, M., & Hamm, C. (2006). Role of B-type natriuretic peptide (BNP) and NT-proBNP in clinical routine. *Heart (British Cardiac Society), 92*(6), 843–849.
222. Weinhouse, G. L. (2015). Pulmonary artery catheterization: indications, contraindications and complications in adults. http://www.uptodate.com/contents/pulmonary-artery-catheterization-indications-contraindications-and-complications-in-adults?source=see_link.
223. Wilhelmsen, L., et al. (2001). Heart failure in the general population of men-morbidity, risk factors and prognosis. *J Intern Med, 249*(3), 253–261.
224. Wilkinson, I. B., et al. (2001). Adrenomedullin (ADM) in the human forearm vascular bed: effect of neutral endopeptidase inhibition and comparison with proadrenomedullin NH2-terminal 20 peptide (PAMP). *Br J Clin Pharmacol, 52*, 159–164.
225. Wong, C., et al. (2011). Trends in comorbidity, disability, and polypharmacy in heart failure. *Am J Med, 124*, 136–143.
226. Yancy, C., & Chang, S. (2003). Clinical characteristics and outcomes in patients admitted with heart failure with preserved systolic function: a report from the Acute Decompensated Heart Failure National Registry (ADHERE). *J Am Coll Cardiol, 3*(47), 76–84.
227. Yancy, C. W., et al. (2013). 2013 ACCF/AHA guideline for the management of heart failure: a report of the American College of Cardiology Foundation/American Heart Association Task Force on Practice Guidelines. *J Am Coll Cardiol, 62*(16), e147–e239.

228. Young, J., & Mills, R. (2004). *Clinical management of heart failure.* West Islip, NY: Professional Communications.
229. Ypenburg, C., et al. (2007). Intrathoracic impedance monitoring to predict decompensated heart failure. *Am J Cardiol, 99*(4), 554–557.
230. Zannad, F., et al. (2000). Limitaion of excessive extracellular matrix turnover may contribute to survival benefit of spironolactone therapy in patients with congestive heart failure: insights from the randomized Aldactone evaluation study (RALES). *Circulation, 102,* 2700–2706.
231. Zannad, F., et al. (2011). Eplerenone in patients with systolic heart failure and mild symptoms. *N Engl J Med, 364,* 11–21.
232. Zei, P. (2013). Is the wearable cardioverter-defibrillator the answer for early post-myocardial infarction patients at risk for sudden death? *J Am Coll Cardiol, 62*(21), 2008–2009.
233. Zhang, P. (2014). Cardiovascular disease in diabetes. *Eur Rev Med Pharmac, 18,* 2205–2214.

5

Cardiac Surgery

Mary Zellinger

More than 300,000 coronary artery bypass graft surgeries are performed in the United States each year.[18] As cardiac surgery has evolved over the last 5 decades, there have been improvements in traditional techniques, including myocardial protection, graft selection, and fast-track recovery, as well as increasing opportunities for less invasive surgical procedures (e.g., port access and smaller incisions for sternotomy). These advances, along with improvements in medical management and increased options for percutaneous intervention, have changed the characteristics of patients undergoing cardiac surgery. Today's patients are older, with more comorbid conditions and higher risk profiles than previous surgical candidates. As a result, the care of patients following cardiac surgery presents special challenges for the critical care team. This chapter will review surgical revascularization procedures as well as procedures performed for structural problems following myocardial infarction. Valvular surgery is addressed in Chapter 6.

CORONARY ARTERY BYPASS GRAFTING

Coronary artery bypass grafting (CABG) provides a new conduit for blood flow to a coronary artery distal to the site of an occlusion or stenosis. This procedure results in improved myocardial oxygen supply and is performed to improve both quality of life (by ameliorating symptoms) and length of life (by reducing mortality associated with coronary events). CABG may be performed alone or in conjunction with other surgical procedures (e.g., valve repair).

Indications

CABG is indicated for patients with refractory angina when a percutaneous coronary intervention (i.e., stenting or angioplasty) either is not feasible—because of lesion morphology or location—or is not successful. In addition, certain subsets of patients with coronary artery disease (CAD) have been found to have improved outcomes following surgical revascularization.[47] CABG is the treatment of choice for patients with significant stenosis of the left main coronary artery or the equivalent of left main stenosis, created by greater than 70% stenosis of both the proximal left anterior descending (LAD) and the circumflex arteries. CABG is also recommended for patients with multivessel (three or more vessels) disease, especially if there is evidence of ventricular dysfunction or inducible ischemia, or if the patient has diabetes. Surgery is also recommended for patients with two-vessel disease when there is involvement of the proximal LAD. Evidence-based indications for CABG have been well-delineated and are described in joint guidelines published by the American College of Cardiology Foundation and the American Heart Association (Table 5.1).[47]

The decision to perform CABG is generally based on data obtained during cardiac catheterization (see Chapter 3). Atherosclerotic lesions narrowing the lumen of an artery by at least 50% are considered significant. Lesions of greater than 70% prevent increases in blood flow distal to the stenosis despite maximal coronary vasodilation, and thus are a priority for bypass. Target vessels for revascularization are also assessed during the cardiac catheterization to ensure that they are of adequate size (1.5–2.0 mm) to support flow through the graft. Other preoperative assessments may include stress testing to verify areas of ischemia, nuclear studies to determine myocardial viability and ventricular function, and echocardiography to detect valvular problems and ventricular wall motion abnormalities.

Selection of Conduits

Conduits for bypass include either native arteries or veins. Sections of a vessel (free grafts) can be attached between an arterial blood source (e.g., the aorta) and the target vessel on the surface of the myocardium. Certain arteries can be left attached at their site of origin (*in situ* or pedicle grafts), dissected from the surrounding tissue, and reattached to the distal end of the coronary vessel. The selection of a particular conduit for CABG is influenced by several factors, including patient age, location of the vessel requiring bypass, conduit availability, degree of stenosis, and surgeon preference. Because improved patency rates and event-free survival have been shown with the use of arterial conduits, they are preferred over venous grafts whenever feasible.[47] Also, arteries are more vasoresponsive to changes in pressure and volume than are veins. Frequently, a combination of grafts is required to achieve the goal of total revascularization (Fig. 5.1).

The saphenous vein is the most commonly used venous conduit. It may be harvested directly, through an open leg incision, or endoscopically, through small (3–4 cm) incisions (Fig. 5.2). Although more time consuming, endoscopic vein harvesting (EVH) has been shown to decrease the incidence of postoperative leg wound complications (e.g., cellulitis and hematoma).[6] Patients also report less pain and improved appearance with EVH.[36] Lesser-used veins include the cephalic vein and the lesser saphenous vein. Major limitations of the saphenous vein include the presence of valves, which hinder blood flow through the vein, and the progressive atherosclerosis seen in all venous grafts. Patency rates have improved slightly with the aggressive use of statins and antiplatelet agents, but still remain at approximately 60% at 10 years after surgery.[47]

The left internal mammary artery (also known as the internal thoracic artery) is the conduit of choice and is used in the majority of elective cases. It has long been shown to provide not

TABLE 5.1 ACC/AHA Guidelines: Class I Recommendations for Coronary Artery Bypass Graft Surgery

Clinical Indication	Coronary Anatomy or Symptoms
Asymptomatic or mild angina	Left main stenosis ≥50% Left main equivalent* Three-vessel disease, especially if EF < 50%
Stable angina	Left main stenosis ≥50% Left main equivalent* Three-vessel disease, especially if EF < 50% Two-vessel disease with >70% stenosis of proximal LAD and EF < 50% or inducible ischemia One- to two-vessel disease without proximal LAD, but with a large area of ischemic myocardium Disabling angina on maximal medical therapy
Unstable angina or non-ST elevation MI	Left main stenosis ≥50% Left main equivalent* Refractory ischemia on maximal medical therapy
Emergent or urgent CABG following STEMI	Refractory ischemia and hemodynamic instability after failed PCI or in patients who are not candidates for PCI or fibrinolysis Performed in conjunction with repair of postinfarction mechanical defects Cardiogenic shock within 36 h of STEMI, as long as surgery can be performed within 18 h of developing shock and patient is <75 years
Poor left ventricular function	Left main stenosis ≥50% Left main equivalent* Two- to three-vessel disease with >70% stenosis of proximal LAD
Ventricular dysrhythmias	Life-threatening ventricular dysrhythmias in presence of left main stenosis ≥50% or three-vessel disease
Failed PCI	Ongoing ischemia, hemodynamic instability, or threatened occlusion
Reoperation after prior CABG	Disabling angina despite optimal nonsurgical therapy No patent grafts with Class I indications in native vessels (left main stenosis, left main equivalent, or three-vessel disease) (Class I: evidence shows CABG to be useful and effective)

*Left main equivalent describes greater than 70% stenosis of both the LAD and the circumflex arteries.
CABG, Coronary artery bypass grafting; *EF,* ejection fraction; *LAD,* left anterior descending; *MI,* myocardial infarction; *PCI,* percutaneous coronary intervention; *STEMI,* ST elevation myocardial infarction.
Data from Reference 25.

only superior patency (>90% at 10 years) but also improved survival with less risk of reoperation or myocardial infarction (MI).[27] Recent data suggest that left internal mammary artery (LIMA) grafting may have a protective effect on perioperative mortality as well.[27] The LIMA is anatomically well positioned to bypass lesions in the LAD artery. The right internal mammary artery (RIMA) can be used as an *in situ* graft to bypass the right coronary artery (RCA) or as a free graft to bypass other vessels. Because of superior patency rates, some surgeons advocate for bilateral use of the internal thoracic artery (BITA). Recent studies have demonstrated improved survival rates and no greater independent risk of deep sternal wound infection with BITA.[7]

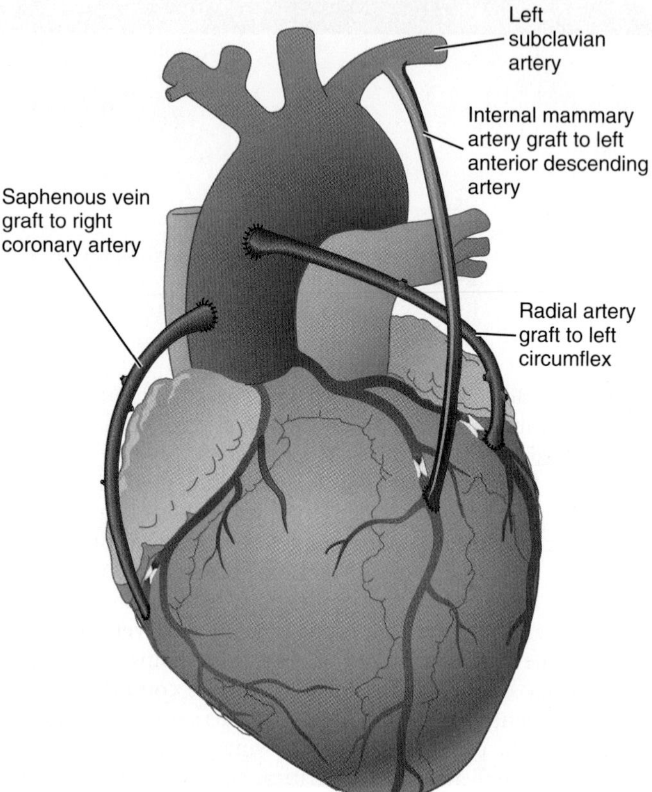

FIG. 5.1 Coronary artery bypass grafting. Conduits for coronary artery bypass grafts may include segments of saphenous vein or radial artery that are anastomosed to the aorta and then to the coronary artery at a point distal to the lesion. The internal mammary artery may also be dissected from the chest tissue and attached directly to the coronary artery.

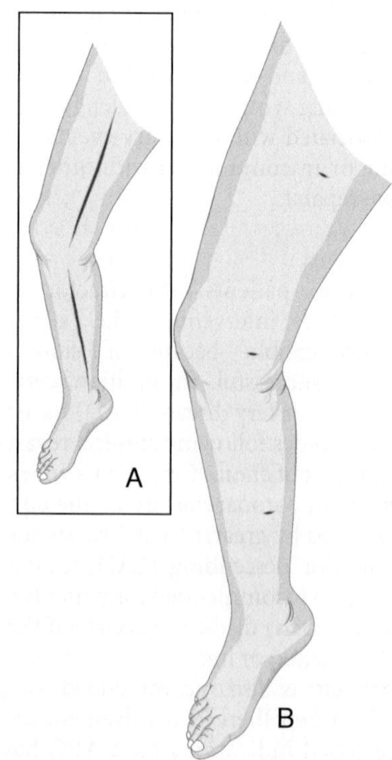

FIG. 5.2 Techniques for harvesting the saphenous vein. Techniques for procuring saphenous veins include an open incision **(A)** and endovascular harvesting **(B)**. There may be one, two, or three incisions. There is usually one on the thigh and one near the knee.

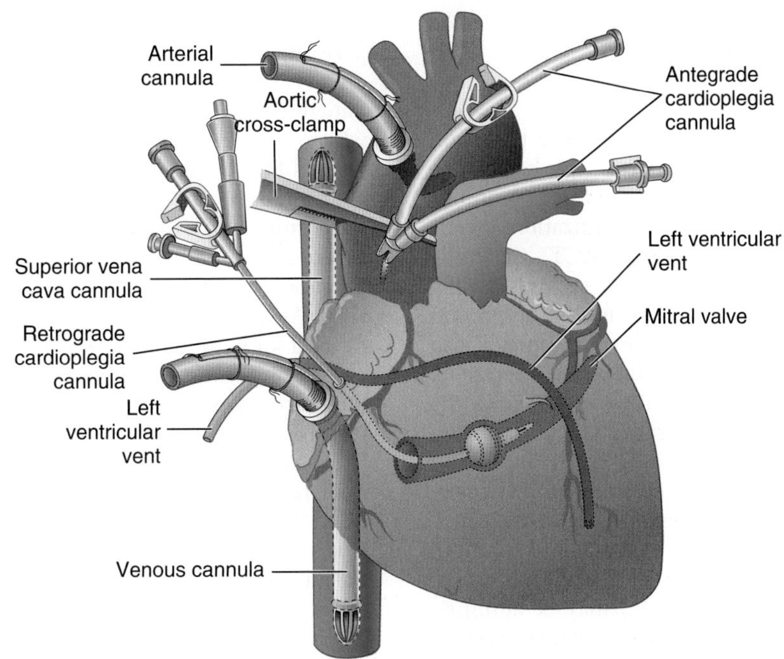

FIG. 5.3 Cannulation for cardiac surgery with cardiopulmonary bypass includes arterial and venous cannulae, as well as cardioplegia cannulae (antegrade and possibly retrograde). A vent may be placed in either the left ventricle or the aortic root. The cross-clamp is applied to the aorta, proximal to the arterial cannula but distal to the cannula that is used to deliver the cardioplegic solution.

The use of the radial artery as a conduit for CABG has increased in the last decade, partially as a result of improved harvesting techniques and medications to prevent vasospasm. This artery is usually harvested from the nondominant hand, either through an open incision or endoscopically, and used as a free graft from the aorta or the LIMA.[8] Patency rates of greater than 90% at 10 years have been reported for radial artery grafts.[54] Multiple studies have shown that the use of a second arterial graft, either of the radial artery or the RIMA, improves long-term outcomes.[21,57]

Other options for arterial conduits include the gastroepiploic artery and the inferior epigastric artery. These may be used in younger patients when the goal of bypass is total arterial revascularization, or in patients in whom other conduits are not available (e.g., patients undergoing reoperation).[50]

Surgical Procedure

Conventional CABG surgery is performed through a median sternotomy on an arrested heart. Cardiopulmonary bypass (CPB) is used to preserve end-organ function during the temporary absence of cardiac and pulmonary function, as well as to provide hemodynamic stability during the surgery. CPB involves diverting venous blood from the right atrium or vena cava to an extracorporeal oxygenator, which removes carbon dioxide from the blood and returns the oxygenated blood to the arterial system of the patient—bypassing the heart and lungs in the oxygenation process. The advantage of this approach is that it allows the surgeon to operate on a relatively bloodless, motionless heart. Currently the majority of CABG procedures are performed "on pump" using CPB.[47]

Cardiopulmonary Bypass

The extracorporeal circuit used for CPB consists of a cannula for blood removal and return, a centrifugal or roller pump providing nonpulsatile flow, and an oxygenator allowing for the exchange of oxygen and carbon dioxide (CO_2). In addition, a heat exchanger controls body temperature by heating or cooling blood passing through the perfusion circuit; filters are located throughout the circuit to remove air and particulate matter.

Cannulation

Venous drainage is usually accomplished by cannulation of the right atrial appendage, with the distal end of the cannula positioned in the inferior vena cava. Arterial return from the bypass pump is accomplished by inserting a cannula through purse-string sutures in the ascending aorta, proximal to the innominate artery. A cross-clamp is applied to the aorta to isolate the heart from blood being returned through the arterial cannula. A vent may be placed in the left atrium or the ventricular apex to decompress the heart, preventing distention of the left ventricle while the aorta is cross-clamped (Fig. 5.3).

Cardioplegia

During cannulation for bypass, one or more catheters are also placed for infusion of a cardioplegic solution into the coronary circulation. This solution is high in potassium and induces rapid diastolic arrest. Additional components vary, but typically include buffering agents and substrates that optimize cellular metabolism and minimize cell damage. Blood is frequently added to the cardioplegic solution to increase oxygen delivery to the myocardial cells.[30] The solution can be either 4°C ("cold" cardioplegia) or 37°C ("warm" cardioplegia), and may be administered continuously or intermittently.

Antegrade cardioplegia is delivered under pressure through a catheter in the ascending aorta that is positioned proximal to the aortic cross-clamp. The distribution of antegrade cardioplegia may be limited by severe coronary artery stenosis, leaving portions of the myocardium at risk for ischemic injury. As an alternative, retrograde cardioplegia allows for perfusion through the venous system of the heart, and is accomplished through a catheter placed in the coronary sinus.

Cardiopulmonary Bypass Adjuncts

A number of adjuncts are used to enhance tissue perfusion while on bypass. Patients are anticoagulated with heparin to minimize clotting as the blood encounters the foreign components of the bypass machine. Adequate heparinization is verified by monitoring the activated clotting time (ACT). Generally the ACT is maintained between 400 and 480 seconds during bypass. After weaning from CPB, protamine is administered to reverse the effect of the heparin. Systemic hypothermia is also used during bypass to protect the body's tissues by decreasing metabolic demands. The decreased metabolic rate allows the tissues to tolerate lower perfusion flow rates. The temperature is usually decreased to between 32°C and 34°C. Hemodilution during bypass helps to counteract the increased blood viscosity that is normally produced by hypothermia. The extracorporeal circuit is primed with 1 L to 1.5 L of crystalloid solution, resulting in a hematocrit (Hct) of 20% to 25% while on bypass. Mannitol (Osmitrol) or furosemide (Lasix) may be administered to promote postoperative diuresis, which helps reverse the hemodilution.

Complications of Cardiopulmonary Bypass

Although bypass supports the body's tissues during the surgical procedure, it is associated with a number of undesired physiologic responses. During CPB, the blood is exposed to a number of foreign surfaces, which damages blood elements (i.e., white cells, red cells, and platelets). In addition, extracorporeal circulation produces a generalized inflammatory response. This initiates a cascade of physiologic changes, including increased capillary permeability, increased circulating catecholamines, and impaired coagulation. The body's response to CPB contributes to the clinical problems encountered in the early postoperative period. Potential complications associated with CPB are summarized in Box 5.1.

"Off-Pump" Surgery

In an effort to avoid the adverse effects of CPB, there was previously significant interest in developing technology to allow for surgical revascularization on a beating heart. The use of off-pump coronary artery bypass (OPCAB), which peaked at 23% in 2002 in the United States, declined to 17% in 2012.[3,4]

Unlike cardiac surgery performed with CPB, off-pump procedures require that the patient's own heart provide adequate perfusion to the body's tissues.[23] The heart's hemodynamic performance may be compromised during the procedure, secondary to positioning of the heart, dysrhythmias, or ischemia. Patients require vigilant monitoring during the operation, which is generally facilitated by transesophageal echocardiography (TEE). Pulmonary artery catheters (PAC) that provide continuous cardiac output (CO) and mixed venous oxygen saturation (Svo_2) data are also frequently employed. Fluids, vasopressors, or inotropic agents may be needed during the operation to maintain an adequate CO and blood pressure (BP). At times, an intra-aortic balloon pump (IABP) may also be used for hemodynamic support.

At this point, there is variance in reported outcomes in the literature regarding OPCAB versus CABG. Some recent studies have concluded that OPCAB patients had worse long-term (>5 years) survival, received fewer grafts, and had inferior graft patency than patients who received on-pump CABG.[49] In addition, the number of grafts and the index of completeness of revascularization were greater for patients who received on-pump procedures, while the need for repeat surgery, rate of recurrent angina, and rate of rehospitalization were significantly greater after the OPCAB procedure.[24] However, other meta-analyses and large observational studies have reported equivalent and, in some cases, improved surgical outcomes for the performance of OPCAB over conventional CABG.[3] Similar revascularization rates, shorter lengths of hospital stay, reduced transfusion requirements, and less myocardial injury were reported. Currently OPCAB is offered to only one in five patients who undergo surgical coronary revascularization.[3]

BOX 5.1 Complications Related to Cardiopulmonary Bypass

- Bleeding
- Dysrhythmias
- Electrolyte imbalances
- Emboli (air, plaque, or denatured proteins)
- Fluid shifts
- Hemodilution
- Hemodynamic instability
- Hypothermia
- Myocardial depression
- Neurocognitive dysfunction
- Pulmonary dysfunction
- Systemic inflammatory response

HYBRID CORONARY REVASCULARIZATION

The data clearly show that freedom from atherosclerosis and long-term graft patency are greatly attributable to using the LIMA to bypass the LAD. Hybrid coronary revascularization is an option for patients needing bypass surgery that does not require an invasive sternotomy. Hybrid surgery involves surgically bypassing the LAD and performing percutaneous coronary intervention (PCI) to the non-LAD vessels. In this procedure, the LIMA is harvested with a robotic surgical system. The pericardium is then opened, and the optimal target site on the LAD is identified. Once the target site for the LAD has been identified, a small thoracotomy incision is made without rib spreading to allow exposure for an off-pump LIMA-LAD anastomosis. A minimally invasive stabilizer is used to secure the target vessel.[22] The LAD is bypassed without CPB or the need for aortic manipulation, with its potential complications. The PCI can be completed either the same day or the next day, after the patient has recovered in the critical care unit. Optimal antiplatelet therapy plus imaging of the LIMA-LAD graft is possible if the PCI is performed as a separate procedure after the surgical bypass. If patent LIMA-LAD is demonstrated, PCI of high-risk targets is possible.

VENTRICULAR ANEURYSM REPAIR

Ventricular aneurysms develop as a result of a large transmural MI, most commonly in the anterolateral wall of the left ventricle.[19] The damaged tissue becomes thin and less contractile, moving paradoxically during contraction. This results in a decrease in stroke volume. Over time, this may lead to dilation of the ventricle and symptoms of heart failure. In addition, thrombi may accumulate in this area. Finally, scar tissue at the border of the aneurysm may serve as a focus for dysrhythmias. When an aneurysm is associated with one or more of these problems, an aneurysmectomy may be performed.

Procedure

The goal of an aneurysmectomy is to correct the size and geometry of the left ventricle, reduce wall tension and paradoxical movement, and improve systolic function. Aneurysmectomy is performed through a median sternotomy with CPB. The standard approach to aneurysm repair is to open and excise the thin aneurysmal tissue, removing any visible thrombus at that time. The healthy ventricular tissue is sutured together, using felt strips to reinforce the suture line. This linear approach may have suboptimal results for large aneurysms, because the normal shape of the ventricle is not maintained.[19] To create a more physiologic ventricular shape, a patch (composed of either Dacron or bovine pericardium) can be attached to the viable tissue at the edge of the aneurysm, with the ventricle closed over the patch. The Dor and Jantene procedures are slightly modified versions of this approach, in which a purse-string suture is placed around the entire circumference of the base of the aneurysm and then tightened to restore a normal ventricular cavity shape.

VENTRICULAR SEPTAL DEFECT

Necrosis and subsequent rupture of the ventricular septum is a rare and frequently fatal complication of acute MI. The frequency of postinfarction rupture of the septum has declined in the era of reperfusion, and is now estimated to occur in less than 1% of patients with ST elevation.[9] Ventricular septal defects (VSDs) allow shunting of blood from left to right, producing acute pulmonary edema and cardiogenic shock. Clinical signs of acute VSD include the presence of a holosystolic murmur and an increase in oxygen saturation in the right ventricle.[9] A cardiac echo can be performed to confirm the diagnosis of VSD.

Surgical repair of an acute VSD is challenging, especially in patients who are hemodynamically unstable. However, because mortality for medically managed patients is greater than 90%, surgery is currently recommended for virtually all patients with postinfarction VSD.[9] Preoperatively patients require inotropic support as well as afterload reduction to improve forward flow from the left ventricle. Generally an IABP is used to support the patient, both before and after the operation.

Procedure

Repair of a VSD is performed through a median sternotomy on an arrested heart. The ventricle is opened, and a prosthetic patch is applied to the intraventricular septum. The ventriculotomy is then closed, using felt strips for reinforcement. Surgical repair is usually performed in conjunction with coronary artery grafting to improve myocardial perfusion. Surgical mortality with this procedure remains high, with reported levels as high as 47%.[9]

INTERPROFFESIONAL PLAN OF CARE

Initial postoperative management of patients following cardiac surgery is similar, regardless of the specific procedure performed. Proper hand-off of care is essential to ensure that information transferred between the operating room (OR) staff and the critical care staff is accurate. If the patient is stable and alarms are on with parameters set, the report can take place at the bedside. Ideally, this five-way report will include the primary registered nurse, the OR anesthesiologist, the critical care provider, the respiratory therapist, and the surgeon or surgical representative. The report will be initiated by the surgical representative, followed by the anesthesiologist, with questions from the team to follow. All team members should verbally confirm that the report is complete and that transfer of care has occurred.

The primary goals of treatment during this time are to prevent complications associated with the surgery (e.g., hypothermia, bleeding, and dysrhythmias) and to optimize the patient's cardiac and pulmonary function. The patient requires frequent assessment, with interventions based on trends rather than absolute numbers. Routine assessment criteria for patients immediately following cardiac surgery are described in Table 5.2.

Patient- and family-centered care is important for the comfort and recovery of the patient. Family members should be incorporated into daily bedside shift reports so that they and

TABLE 5.2 Routine Postoperative Assessment Criteria

Parameter	Criteria Assessed
ECG	Select appropriate leads for dysrhythmia detection and ST analysis
Hemodynamic measurements	Level and zero transducers Obtain baseline measurements for BP, CVP, PAP, and CO/CI Calculate SVR and PVR
Intravenous lines	Have medications infusing and properly labeled; dressings should be dry and occlusive
Lab work	Obtain stat CBC, ABG, electrolytes, and blood glucose measurements Obtain stat coagulation studies if bleeding (PT/aPTT, platelets)
Pacemaker	Verify correct lead attachment or ensure lead wires are electrically dressed and covered If attached, confirm proper functioning of generator and settings as ordered
Physical assessment	Auscultate heart sounds, noting murmurs or abnormal heart sounds Auscultate breath sounds, noting absent or adventitious sounds Assess capillary refill and peripheral pulses Assess LOC, pupil reactivity, and ability to move extremities
Portable chest x-ray	Review position of ETT, central lines, or pulmonary artery catheter Note width of mediastinum and presence of pneumothorax or pleural effusion
Pulse oximeter	Validate adequate signal and correlate with current ABG
Tubes	Ensure ETT tube secured Confirm patency of chest tubes and placement to suction, noting character and quantity of output Verify correct position of NG tube and placement to suction Place Foley to gravity drainage, noting quantity of output

ABG, Arterial blood gas; *aPTT*, activated partial thromboplastin time; *BP*, blood pressure; *CBC*, complete blood cell count; *CVP*, central venous pressure; *CO*, cardiac output; *ECG*, electrocardiogram; *ETT*, endotracheal tube; *LOC*, level of consciousness; *NG*, nasogastric; *PAP*, pulmonary artery pressure; *PT*, prothrombin time; *PVR*, pulmonary vascular resistance; *SVR*, systemic vascular resistance.

the patient have a clear understanding of the status, plan of care, and goals for the patient. Patients are comforted by the presence of and communication with family members, and family members can participate in patient care activities. Interprofessional rounds should be conducted daily with the family member present, where short- and long-term goals are developed and agreed upon by all present.

Hypothermia

Although patients are generally rewarmed to 37°C before coming off of bypass, they frequently have mild hypothermia upon arrival to the critical care unit. This results from continued heat loss while the chest is open, cooler ambient temperatures in the OR, and peripheral vasoconstriction, which limits heat distribution. Negative physiologic effects of hypothermia include impaired coagulation, an increased propensity for dysrhythmias, and increased systemic vascular resistance (SVR). In addition, hypothermia may precipitate shivering, resulting in increased oxygen demand and CO_2 production, and impaired coagulation.[10] Hypothermia has also been associated with prolonging time to extubation.

Measures that can be taken to correct hypothermia include rewarming, with conventional or forced-air blankets or heat lamps. To avoid overwarming, blankets should be removed when the patient reaches 36°C to 36.5°C. Fluid warmers may also be helpful, especially if large quantities of blood products are being administered. Shivering in the postoperative period is a normal compensatory response to body cooling, and may result from anesthesia, drugs, cold cardioplegic solution, and the cool OR environment. Shivering increases oxygen consumption, heart rate, mean arterial pressure (MAP), and CO_2 production. If it continues, shivering may be effectively treated with meperidine (Demerol) administered intravenously in doses of 12.5 mg to 25 mg.[10]

Bleeding

A number of factors place patients at risk for bleeding after cardiac surgery. Sequelae from bypass (i.e., dilution of clotting factors, damage to platelets, and hypothermia) may impair coagulation. Inadequate reversal of the effects of heparin may also contribute to a coagulopathy, or heparin rebound may occur with rewarming as heparin sequestered in the tissues is released into circulation. Postoperative hypertension can increase the risk of bleeding by placing additional stress on surgical suture lines and cannulation sites.

Chest tubes placed at the end of the operation allow for monitoring of mediastinal bleeding. These may be either conventional chest tubes (32 to 36 French [Fr]) or smaller silastic (Blake) drains. The smaller drains provide comparable drainage efficiency and less discomfort for the patient.[17] Chest tubes are usually placed to suction (–20 cm H_2O), and patency is maintained by gently manipulating the tubes when clots are present. Vigorous stripping of conventional chest tubes is avoided, because the high pressures produced by stripping may exacerbate bleeding problems. Hourly milking of the silastic tubes may be necessary to prevent tubes from clotting off, due to their small size. Patients will typically have 50 mL to 150 mL of chest tube output for the first several hours following surgery, and this will gradually taper over time. Persistent, excessive bleeding (>500 mL in 1 hour or >300 mL/h for 2–3 hours) requires surgical reexploration in the OR, but this occurs in less than 3% of cases.

General measures used to promote hemostasis include rewarming and aggressive treatment of postoperative hypertension with vasodilators. Coagulation studies are obtained in patients who are actively bleeding so that appropriate therapy can be instituted. This may include administration of blood products (packed red blood cells [PRBCs] or platelets), replacement of coagulation factors (fresh frozen plasma [FFP] or cryoprecipitate), or medications as needed.

Treatment of postoperative bleeding may be initiated before laboratory results are available, based on the most likely hemostatic disorder. For example, platelets may be administered empirically in patients who have received aspirin (ASA), clopidogrel (Plavix), or glycoprotein IIb/IIIa inhibitors preoperatively. FFP may be used to replenish clotting factors in patients with known hepatic dysfunction or those who have received multiple transfusions of PRBCs intraoperatively. Once coagulation studies become available, more definitive treatment of the bleeding disorder can be selected.

A number of pharmacologic agents are used to manage postoperative bleeding (Table 5.3). Protamine sulfate is administered at the end of the operation to neutralize circulating heparin. Additional protamine may be prescribed in critical care if the activated partial thromboplastin time (aPTT) remains elevated or if the patient receives additional cell-saver blood.[13] Antifibrinolytic agents, including aminocaproic acid (Amicar) and tranexamic acid (Cyklokapron), are administered intraoperatively to decrease blood loss by preventing normal clot breakdown. These agents may also be administered postoperatively when fibrinolysis is suggested by continued bleeding and abnormal coagulation studies—typically a prolonged prothrombin time (PT) or international normalized ratio (INR), increased aPTT, and decreased fibrinogen level. Desmopressin acetate (DDAVP) promotes platelet adhesion and may be beneficial in patients with disorders that affect platelet function (e.g., uremia or von Willebrand disease).

Red blood cell transfusion in cardiac surgical patients has been strongly associated with increased infection, increased ischemic postoperative events, prolonged hospital stay, increased mortality, and increased hospital costs.[34] Cardiac surgery programs should have a uniform evidenced-based protocol for red cell transfusion for cardiac surgical patients.

Although the threshold for administering blood transfusions varies among practitioners, red blood cells are not typically replaced until the patient's hemoglobin (Hgb) level is 7% or lower. The postoperative Hgb is often decreased, secondary to hemodilution in patients receiving nonblood infusions (e.g., colloids, crystalloids, or FFP). The decision to transfuse should be based on the patient's clinical condition and signs of impaired tissue oxygenation, rather than on a specific Hgb level.[14,56] In patients who are actively bleeding, red blood cell transfusion may be warranted to maintain a hemoglobin level that is adequate to maintain tissue oxygenation.

Autotransfusion of shed mediastinal blood can be used to provide the patient with volume and return of red cells. Autotransfusion can produce a coagulopathy, because the shed blood has lower levels of clotting factors and platelets, as well as elevated levels of fibrin split products. When performed, it is usually limited to the first 6 hours postoperatively to minimize the risk of infection. Longer duration of autotransfusion places patients at risk for developing mediastinitis.[42]

Patients are monitored for signs of cardiac tamponade, which may occur if blood is not evacuated effectively from the

TABLE 5.3 Medications Used to Promote Hemostasis After Cardiac Surgery

Drug	Actions	Dose	Special Considerations
Desmopressin acetate (DDAVP)	Synthetic form of vasopressin that promotes platelet adhesion by increasing release of von Willebrand factor from platelets and factor VIII from tissue stores	0.3–0.4 mcg/kg IV over 20 min	Beneficial in patients with disorders that affect platelet function (uremia, von Willebrand disease) and in reoperations Repeat doses not effective
Aminocaproic acid (Amicar)	Antifibrinolytic agent that stabilizes clots by inhibiting conversion of plasminogen to plasmin	Bolus of 5–9 g IV while on CPB, followed by infusion of 1 g/h for 5 h	May be used if fibrinolysis is present (detected by low fibrinogen levels and high fibrin degradation products, or decreased clot lysis time) May require dose adjustment for renal impairment
Tranexamic acid (Cyklokapron)	Antifibrinolytic agent with actions similar to aminocaproic acid	100 mg/kg IV preop; if needed, can give 50 mg/kg postop 9–15 mg/kg IV, or 0.5–1 g IV every 4–6 h	Less expensive than aprotinin, so may be used in lower-risk patients Adjust dose for renal impairment
Protamine	Neutralizes heparin in a dose-related fashion (1 mg of protamine for every 90 units of heparin)	25–50 mg IV slowly,* at a rate of 5 mg/min Remainder of calculated dose can be administered by IV infusion over 8–16 h	May be given postoperatively with reinfusion of cell-saver blood or if aPTT remains elevated Half-life of protamine is only 5 min, so "heparin rebound" may occur if sequestered heparin is released from body tissues; for this reason, doses >25 mg are given IVPB over 20–30 min Risk for anaphylaxis is greatest in patients with IDDM or fish allergies
Activated factor VII (Novoseven)	Promotes formation of thrombin via extrinsic coagulation pathway	2–5 mg via IV push	Obtained from blood bank to be mixed at bedside Risk of systemic thrombosis
Prothrombin complex concentrates (Kcentra)	Contains vitamin K-dependent clotting factors (II, VII, IX, and X)	25 units/kg (rounded to nearest vial size) IVPB	Delivered from pharmacy Reserved for refractory bleeding

*May cause hypotension if administered too rapidly.
ACT, Activated clotting time; *aPTT,* activated partial thromboplastin time; *CPB,* cardiopulmonary bypass; *IDDM,* insulin-dependent diabetes mellitus; *IV,* intravenous; *IVPB,* intravenous piggyback (IV short-term infusion).

mediastinal space. Signs of tamponade include decreased CO that is refractory to inotropes and hypotension, along with elevated and equalized filling pressures. As blood accumulates in the pericardial space, pressure increases around the heart, so that the right atrial pressure, pulmonary artery diastolic (PAD) pressure, and left atrial pressure equilibrate. Pulmonary artery occlusion pressure (PAOP) also called pulmonary artery wedge pressure (PAWP) readings should not be performed routinely, due to the high risk for complications such as pulmonary rupture. If PAD and PAOP correlate, PAD pressures should be used. Physical assessment may reveal jugular venous distention, diminished pulses, *pulsus paradoxus,* and muffled heart sounds. Tamponade usually occurs in patients with significant mediastinal bleeding and is often preceded by a sudden cessation of chest tube drainage. If time permits, a widened cardiac silhouette on chest x-ray or evidence of pericardial fluid on an echocardiogram can provide additional confirmation of cardiac tamponade. Interventions for tamponade include returning to the OR for surgical evacuation of the clot or, if the patient exhibits extreme hemodynamic instability, emergency sternotomy in critical care.

New guidelines specific to cardiopulmonary resuscitation after cardiac surgery have been endorsed by the European Resuscitation Council (ERC), and are under consideration in the United States. There are key differences between the ERC recommendations and American Heart Association Advanced Cardiac Life Support (ACLS) guidelines. The ERC recommends defibrillation or pacing prior to chest compressions to avoid damage to the sternum. Judicious use of epinephrine is advocated because of the potential for rebound hypertension, the pressure on the suture sites, and the exacerbation of bleeding that can occur. If these measures are unsuccessful, rapid resternotomy with internal massage should be initiated.[28] All staff caring for the postcardiac surgery patient should be well versed in protocols for open chest resuscitation, and semi-annual competency checks are recommended.

Dysrhythmias

Dysrhythmias occur frequently following cardiac surgery and include both supraventricular and ventricular rhythms. Rhythm disturbances may occur as a result of the patient's underlying cardiac disease or from surgical sequelae (i.e., edema of the conduction system, electrolyte imbalances, hypoxemia, or hypothermia). In addition, patients who take beta blockers preoperatively may have an inadequate heart rate postoperatively.

Strategies for managing postoperative dysrhythmias include interventions that target prevention as well as treatment. Serum potassium and magnesium levels should be monitored frequently, especially during periods of diuresis, and replaced to adequate levels. Continuous ST analysis should be performed to detect and treat episodes of ischemia. Arterial blood gases (ABGs) are monitored, and ventilator settings adjusted as needed to correct hypoxemia and acidosis. Hemodynamically compromising dysrhythmias are treated immediately with temporary pacing, antidysrhythmic agents, cardioversion, or defibrillation, as described in ACLS protocols.[2]

Atrial fibrillation (AF) is the most common dysrhythmia following cardiac surgery, with a reported incidence ranging from 15% to 40% of patients in the early postoperative period.[38] Although initially it was theorized that AF would occur less frequently with off-pump procedures, studies have not shown a

BOX 5.2 Strategies for Managing Postoperative Atrial Fibrillation

Prophylaxis
Amiodarone
Atrial pacing (AAI or biatrial)
Beta blockers (metoprolol or carvedilol)
Magnesium sulfate
Corticosteroids
Vitamin C
Statins

Treatment
Synchronized cardioversion
Rapid atrial pacing
Beta blockers
Calcium channel blockers
Amiodarone
Ibutilide
Magnesium

significant difference between the two approaches.[3] A number of protocols have been developed for prophylaxis against AF. Preoperative or early postoperative (12–24 hours) administration of beta blockers has proven effective at decreasing the incidence of AF, and is currently recommended as standard therapy in the American College of Cardiology/American Heart Association (ACC/AHA) guidelines.[47] Preoperative statin use has also been associated with reduced rates of postoperative AF, neurologic dysfunction, renal dysfunction, and infection.[47] Other strategies for managing postoperative AF are described in Box 5.2.

Pacing

Temporary epicardial pacing wires are frequently placed on the right atrium and ventricle at the conclusion of the surgical procedure, and can be used for both therapeutic and diagnostic purposes in the postoperative period. Pacing can be used to optimize CO by providing a heart rate of 90 to 100 beats/minute. If possible, patients are paced in synchronous modes that allow for maintenance of atrioventricular synchrony (e.g., AAI or DDD). If the patient has AF or atrial flutter, ventricular pacing (VVI) is used. Atrial pacing is most beneficial, as it allows for an increased heart rate and the maintenance of the atrial kick, which accounts for 25% to 30% of CO.

A temporary pacemaker may also be used to terminate rapid reentrant supraventricular tachycardias (SVTs) that occur postoperatively (e.g., atrial flutter). This is accomplished with special pacemakers that can deliver impulses at rates of up to 800 pulses per minute. Atrial pacing is performed at a rate faster than the patient's intrinsic SVT to capture the atrial tissue, and then abruptly discontinued to allow the sinus node to resume control.

Atrial epicardial wires can be used for diagnostic purposes as well, by providing an amplified view of atrial electrical activity. Either one or both of the atrial wires can be attached to an electrocardiogram (ECG) monitor to obtain an atrial electrogram (AEG), which can be helpful in differentiating between some of the more common postoperative dysrhythmias.[13] An example of an AEG is shown in Fig. 5.4.

Myocardial Depression

Myocardial depression is common in the first 6 to 8 hours following surgery, as the heart recovers from a period of ischemia.

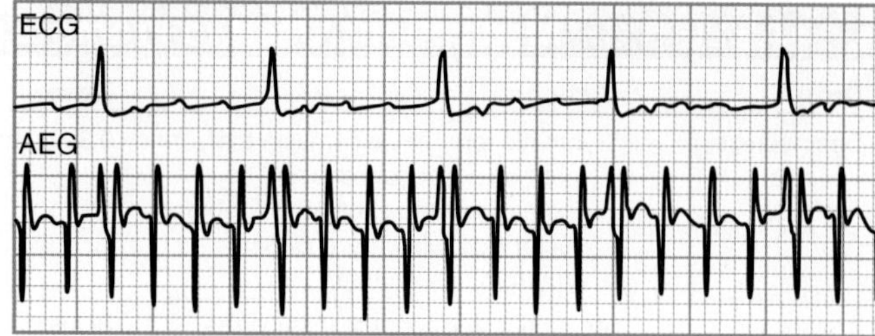

FIG. 5.4 Atrial electrogram. Atrial flutter with 4:1 AV block. The unipolar AEG demonstrates an atrial rate of approximately 300, with a ventricular response of approximately 75/min. *AEG,* Atrial electrogram; *ECG,* electrocardiogram.

Cardiac cellular function may be impaired by hypothermia, cellular edema, or inadequate myocardial protection during the operative procedure. Initial interventions are aimed at optimizing preload and afterload to enhance cardiac contractility, with the goal of maintaining a cardiac index (CI) greater than or equal to 2.2 L/min/m^2 and Svo_2 greater than 65%. Additional measures for CABG patients are directed at maintaining graft patency to ensure adequate myocardial perfusion. If optimizing these parameters fails to produce an adequate CI, inotropes may be used to enhance contractility. Finally, if pharmacologic interventions prove inadequate, patients may be supported with mechanical circulatory assist devices (e.g., IABP). See Chapter 3 for more on IABP.

Preload

Preload is the amount of stretch or volume in the ventricle at the end of diastole, and determines how much blood is available to be ejected during the next ventricular ejection. Preload is altered by a change in the amount of blood delivered to the heart from the venous system. Although patients are usually total body fluid overloaded following CPB, they frequently require fluids to maintain adequate intravascular volume. This occurs in part because of the capillary leak induced by the systemic inflammatory response to bypass. In addition, a relative hypovolemia may occur as the patient vasodilates during rewarming or as a result of various medications. Patients with normal preoperative ventricular function can have their preload assessed with only a central venous catheter. For patients with more complex problems, a PAC is helpful to evaluate postoperative problems. Rarely, a left atrial line may be placed during surgery to monitor left-sided filling pressure in patients with severe pulmonary hypertension (HTN) or patients with a ventricular assist device (VAD). These lines require meticulous handling to minimize the risk of air emboli, including frequent assessment and aspiration of any bubbles and use of an in-line air filter.

Fluids used to treat hypovolemia may vary based on institutional protocol and provider preference. Generally, crystalloids (e.g., normal saline or lactated Ringer's) are used first, and followed by colloids if the crystalloids are insufficient at raising the filling pressures to the required level. Colloid choices include albumin and hetastarch, although both are associated with potential challenges. Albumin administration may cause a greater drop in Hgb than crystalloids, and the effects may last as long as 6 days postoperatively.[45] Hetastarch may increase the risk of renal injury, as well as increased bleeding, following CPB.[15] The end point for fluid resuscitation should be based on achieving an adequate CO, rather than just reaching a target value for central venous pressure (CVP) or PAD. Excessive fluid

TABLE 5.4 Implications of Ventricular Function on Filling Pressures

Ventricular Function	Associated Conditions	Postoperative Implications
Normal LV function		Usually require PAD or LAP of 12–15 mm Hg May need vasodilators short-term to decrease SVR
Hyperdynamic LV	Aortic stenosis Hypertension Hypertrophic cardiomyopathy	Often require higher filling pressures (PAD or LAP of 18–25 mm Hg) Pacing may be helpful to maintain AV synchrony, which optimizes stroke volume Beta blockers may be used if patients are "hyperdynamic" (HTN and tachycardic) postoperatively
Dilated LV	Congestive heart failure Aortic regurgitation Chronic mitral regurgitation	Usually require higher filling pressures (PAD or LAP of 18–25 mm Hg) Afterload reduction is important to maintain CO
RV failure	Pulmonary hypertension Acute RV infarct	Require high CVP (15–20 mm Hg) to increase RV output Vasodilators may be needed to decrease PVR

AV, Atrioventricular; *CO*, cardiac output; *CVP*, central venous pressure; *HTN*, hypertension; *LAP*, left atrial pressure; *LV*, left ventricle; *PAD*, pulmonary artery diastolic; *PVR*, pulmonary vascular resistance; *RV*, right ventricle; *SVR*, systemic vascular resistance.

administration may increase lung water and delay extubation, as well as dilute clotting factors and Hct.

Preload requirements are usually influenced by the patient's preoperative ventricular function. The cardiac catheterization report can provide important information regarding the patient's preoperative function, including the ejection fraction and the right and left ventricular filling pressures. Patients with normal ventricular function will typically require lower filling pressures than those with dilated or hypertrophied ventricles. A comparison of postoperative care for patients with differing ventricular function is provided in Table 5.4.

Afterload

Afterload is the pressure or resistance against which the ventricle pumps blood. Afterload is frequently increased after cardiac surgery, secondary to vasoconstriction induced by hypothermia and the catecholamines released as part of the sympathetic nervous system response to surgery. Patients with well-preserved ventricular function and preoperative HTN are likely to manifest an elevated BP postoperatively. Other patients may have increased SVR accompanied by low or normal BP, secondary to impaired myocardial function. Treatment is usually required to prevent adverse effects of increased afterload, including increased myocardial work and risk of bleeding at surgical sites. Usually, the goal is to keep the patient's systolic BP between 100 and 130 mm Hg and the MAP between 65 and 85 mm Hg. The target MAP must be individualized for patients with a history of HTN or cerebral or renal vascular disease. Lower MAPs are preferred if the patient is bleeding, to minimize pressure on the cannulation sites.

A number of interventions are used to manage postoperative vasoconstriction and HTN. Hypothermic patients are rewarmed in an effort to decrease peripheral vasoconstriction. Analgesics and sedatives are administered as needed to minimize catecholamine outpouring associated with discomfort and emotional stress. A variety of vasodilators may be prescribed to maintain the desired BP and SVR. These agents may be used alone or in conjunction with inotropic agents in patients with marginal CO. Frequently used vasodilators are described in Table 29.3 in Chapter 29. Agents that have an effect primarily on the arterial system may be more advantageous than mixed arterial and venous dilators, especially when hypovolemia is present.

Approximately 10% of patients may present with profound vasodilation following cardiac surgery. This is presumed to be the result of the systemic inflammatory response to CPB.[1] These patients present with hypotension and low SVR, accompanied by signs of decreased perfusion (e.g., lactic acidosis and low urine output). Treatment usually includes volume resuscitation in conjunction with alpha-adrenergic agents (e.g., phenylephrine or norepinephrine). Vasopressin, which induces vasoconstriction through stimulation of V_1 receptors in vascular smooth muscle, has also been shown to be effective when administered as a continuous infusion at 0.01 to 1 unit/minute.[1]

Contractility

Because ventricular function is depressed following cardiac surgery, optimizing preload and afterload may not be sufficient to ensure adequate oxygen delivery to the tissues. Ventricular contractility, the ability of the muscle fibers to shorten and contract when stimulated often needs augmentation with inotropic agents. Inotropes are drugs that alter the force of contractility, and can either increase or decrease the force of contractility depending on the type selected. Positive inotropes increase the strength of contractility, while negative inotropes decrease the strength of contractility. Positive inotropes can be initiated in the OR to wean the patient off CPB or in the critical care unit to maintain a CI of greater than 2.2 L/minute and an Svo_2 greater than 65%. First-line inotropic agents include catecholamines (e.g., epinephrine, dopamine, and dobutamine). If these fail to improve CO, phosphodiesterase inhibitors (e.g., milrinone [Primacor]) may be employed. Inotropic agents are described in Table 29.3 in Chapter 29.

Graft Patency

Ischemia may be a cause of impaired myocardial function in the immediate postoperative period. Patients are monitored for ST segment elevation, which may indicate acute vasospasm or graft closure. Intravenous nitroglycerin has been shown to dilate coronary arteries, increase coronary collateral blood flow, and relax areas of coronary artery spasm. Unfortunately, nitroglycerin may also worsen hypotension and decrease CO, especially when hypovolemia is present. For this reason, it should be administered cautiously in patients who are experiencing active ischemia. Prophylactic use of nitroglycerin has not been shown to be effective at preventing myocardial ischemia in postoperative patients.[47] If a radial artery graft is used or spasm in other arterial conduits is suspected, calcium channel blockers, such as nicardipine (Cardene) or diltiazem (Cardizem), may also be prescribed.

Aspirin (acetylsalicylic acid [ASA]) inhibits platelet aggregation and has been shown to improve graft patency. The latest

BOX 5.3 Indications for Intra-Aortic Balloon Pump in Cardiac Surgery Patients

Preoperative

Mechanical complications post–myocardial infarction (ventricular septal defect or papillary muscle rupture)
Ongoing ischemia (despite medical management)
Hemodynamic instability (cardiogenic shock)
Prophylactic placement for high-risk patients
Left main disease
Severe left ventricular failure (ejection fraction <25%)

Intraoperative

High-risk patients undergoing off-pump coronary artery bypass
Failure to wean from cardiopulmonary bypass

Postoperative

Low cardiac output unresponsive to moderate doses of inotropes
Myocardial ischemia

guidelines on antithrombotic therapy recommend that 75 mg to 325 mg of ASA should be administered within 6 hours after surgery, or as soon as mediastinal bleeding has decreased, and continued indefinitely. If initiated within 48 hours, the administration of ASA reduces cardiovascular events, improves saphenous vein graft patency, decreases mortality, and reduces ischemic complications in other organs, such as brain, kidneys, and gastrointestinal tract.[31,38]

Cardiac Assist Devices

If the aforementioned measures fail to improve CO, an IABP or VAD may be inserted. These devices provide mechanical support to improve tissue perfusion without placing additional demands on the injured myocardium. The selection of a cardiac assist device is influenced by the patient's condition, the capabilities of a particular device, and the availability of the equipment within the healthcare institution.

The IABP is the most commonly used assist device in cardiac surgery.[26] This device consists of a 40-mL to 50-mL polyurethane balloon positioned in the descending aorta and a console that controls inflation and deflation of the balloon in synchrony, but out of phase, with the cardiac cycle. Inflation of the balloon during diastole provides increased coronary perfusion, while deflation just before systolic ejection decreases the afterload. Indications for IABP insertion in cardiac surgery patients are described in Box 5.3.

The intra-aortic balloon is usually inserted percutaneously in the femoral artery, but for patients with severe vascular disease, surgical insertion may be required. Nursing care involves assessment of proper IABP functioning to achieve the desired hemodynamic effects, as well as monitoring the patient for potential complications. Details of nursing care are provided in the *AACN Procedure Manual for Critical Care.*[58]

VADs can provide short- or long-term support, and many types of devices are available. They have three main clinical applications: bridge to transplant, bridge to recovery, and destination therapy for patients with end-stage heart failure. VADs implanted after cardiac surgery are typically placed in patients who are unable to be successfully weaned from CPB despite maximal pharmacologic and IABP support. The different types of devices available include pneumatic or electrically driven pumps that generate pulsatile flow, and rotary pump designs that generate continuous flow. A VAD can be placed in either the left ventricle (LVAD) or the right ventricle (RVAD), or both (BiVAD), depending on where the ventricular failure is occurring.

Tremendous advances have been made in the development of mechanical circulatory support for patients with advanced heart failure. Now, smaller and more durable continuous-flow rotary blood pumps are available, resulting in fewer device-related complications and improved outcomes. These devices are also silent, and create less motion and vibration when operating. The smaller pumps are also better suited for smaller patients, have greater durability, provide greater patient comfort, and reduce the risk of infection. These continuous-flow devices continuously unload the left ventricle throughout the cardiac cycle.[46,52]

Postoperative management of patients with an LVAD is similar to that provided to patients after other types of cardiac surgery, with a few additions. These patients typically require intensive nursing care, including maintaining adequate preload to allow for VAD filling and heparinization to prevent clotting in the device. Complications associated with VADs include bleeding, infection, and device failure. Right ventricular function must be closely monitored, as high pump speeds can cause a significant leftward septal shift and abnormal RV geometry, affecting RV function. Because of the reduced pulse pressure during continuous-flow LVAD support, the arterial pulse is diminished or absent, so BP assessment is more challenging and frequently assessed via Doppler.[52]

Patient and family education is essential for ongoing LVAD success, and includes understanding the system operation, especially care of the percutaneous lead and exit site. Careful immobilization of the lead at the exit site will prevent disruption of the subcutaneous tissue ingrowth in the velour lining of the lead, which can result in infection. Volume status must be monitored post implant, and should include daily weights and other symptoms of dehydration, as oral intake restriction and sodium restriction are often required. Avoidance of power interruption is also necessary, as this could lead to loss of support. Patients and families must be able to recognize and respond to emergencies, and essential contact numbers should be with the patient at all times.

ECMO (extracorporeal membrane oxygenation) is another alternative for decreasing the workload of the heart to allow recovery of cardiac function from injury. ECMO is used as a temporary support until organ recovery occurs, and may also be used as a bridge to a VAD or to cardiac transplantation.[55]

Pulmonary Support

All patients will have some degree of pulmonary dysfunction postoperatively, as a result of the effects of anesthesia, CPB, and surgical methods (i.e., dissection of the internal mammary artery and median sternotomy).[48] Postoperatively, patients experience varying degrees of ventilation/perfusion (V/Q) mismatch and intrapulmonary shunting. Despite these changes, early extubation (either in the OR or within the first 4–6 hours) is feasible in the majority of patients. Studies have shown that early extubation shortens the length of stay and can be achieved without an increase in pulmonary complications.[32,48] Protocols for anesthesia and immediate postoperative sedation have been developed to facilitate fast-tracking patients to extubation.

Initial ventilator settings in critical care usually include a tidal volume of 6 to 8 mL/kg, a respiratory rate of 8 to 10 breaths/

BOX 5.4 Signs of Failure to Tolerate Ventilator Weaning

Changes in neurologic status (agitation or somnolence)
Diaphoresis
Significant changes in heart rate or blood pressure
Increase in respiratory rate >35 breaths/min
Decrease in Pao_2 < 60 mm Hg or Sao_2 < 90% (on an Fio_2 of 0.5)
Increased $Paco_2$ (>50 mm Hg) in conjunction with respiratory acidosis
Sudden increase in pulmonary pressure, which may indicate CO_2 retention

Fio_2, Fraction of inspired oxygen; *$Paco_2$,* partial pressure of carbon dioxide in arterial blood; *Pao_2,* partial pressure of oxygen in arterial blood; *Sao_2,* oxygen saturation of arterial blood.

minute, a fraction of inspired oxygen (Fio_2) of 0.7, low levels (5 cm H_2O) of positive end-expiratory pressure (PEEP), and pressure support (PS). The first ABG is obtained approximately 20 minutes after arrival in the critical care unit, to allow for equilibration after placement on the ventilator. The Fio_2 is usually weaned to maintain an Sao_2 level of greater than 92%, and the respiratory rate is adjusted based on the partial pressure of carbon dioxide ($Paco_2$) and pH results. When adjusting the ventilator settings, the patient's degree of hypothermia should be considered, because the $Paco_2$ will generally rise as the patient rewarms, which can lead to acidosis. Ongoing assessment of the patient's ventilatory status can be accomplished with noninvasive measures of Sao_2 and end-tidal CO_2, with ABGs obtained only if the noninvasive data suggest a problem.

Criteria for weaning from the ventilator (see Chapter 10) include awakening with minimal stimulation, reversal of neuromuscular blockade, satisfactory ABGs or end tidal CO_2 ($ETco_2$) and Sao_2, hemodynamic stability, control of severe bleeding, and rewarming to normothermia. Patients need to be carefully assessed during the weaning process for signs of failure (Box 5.4). If the patient exhibits signs of failure, weaning should be stopped and ventilator settings resumed for a period of time. Prolonged ventilation may be required in patients with hemodynamic instability, advanced pulmonary disease, or severe neurologic damage.

After extubation, patients continue to require vigilant respiratory assessment. Oxygenation may be compromised by fluid overload or atelectasis. Most patients are provided supplemental oxygen via nasal cannula for the first 24 to 48 hours. Patients with a median sternotomy may tend to splint or take shallow breaths, thus retaining CO_2. Patients should be encouraged to cough, use the incentive spirometer every 1 to 2 hours, and get out of bed to a chair as soon as possible. Whether the patient is extubated or remains intubated, increasing activity is important to prevent complications. Getting the patient out of bed and advancing to early mobilization will help prevent deep venous thrombosis and pulmonary complications. Adequate pain medication and a "cough pillow" are important to facilitate these goals.[48]

A nasogastric (NG) tube may be used for gastric decompression, inserted either after the patient's transfer to critical care or upon arrival in the OR. Insertion after admission may cause HTN and dysrhythmias if the patient is not well sedated, or bleeding if the patient has a coagulopathy. The NG tube is removed with extubation, and patients may gradually begin oral intake, usually with ice chips or clear liquids. Patients should be observed during initial oral intake to evaluate for the potential risk of aspiration. Although swallowing difficulties are rare in patients with short-term intubation, aspiration can have devastating consequences.

Antiembolic stockings or sequential compression devices are used routinely in cardiac surgery patients to decrease the risk of deep vein thrombosis and pulmonary embolism. Early mobilization is important to further reduce this risk. If the patient's condition requires prolonged periods of immobility (i.e., hemodynamic instability or prolonged intubation), low molecular weight heparin may also be used.

Sedation/Analgesia

Adequate analgesia and sedation are important to minimize the physiologic and psychological problems associated with pain and anxiety. Myocardial function is impacted by the sympathetic nervous system's response to pain, which includes an increase in myocardial oxygen demand and automaticity. Pulmonary function may also be adversely affected as a result of decreased lung expansion and retention of secretions.[5,33]

Patients generally arrive in critical care sedated from agents they have received in the OR. Some institutions maintain patients on either a propofol (Diprivan) or a dexmedetomidine (Precedex) infusion for a period of time postoperatively. Current evidence supports the avoidance of deep sedation, as maintaining lighter levels of sedation is associated with improved clinical outcomes (e.g., shorter duration of mechanical ventilation and a shorter critical care length of stay).[5] Although maintaining light levels of sedation increases the physiologic stress response, it is not associated with increased incidence of myocardial ischemia. Avoiding benzodiazepines and using sedation scales and sedation protocols designed to minimize sedative use are all associated with improved critical care patient outcomes.

When patients meet criteria for weaning, the propofol (or other sedative infusion) is discontinued, and the patient is allowed to awaken. Propofol causes respiratory depression and must be weaned off prior to ventilator weaning. Dexmedetomidine sedates without respiratory depression, and patients may be more easily aroused while the infusion continues. Dexmedetomidine may be discontinued prior to extubation, or maintained until the infusion is completed. A bispectral index (BIS) monitor has been used in some institutions to evaluate the patient's level of sedation both during and immediately following the surgical procedure. The BIS provides a value derived from the patient's electroencephalograph (EEG), measured via a probe attached to the patient's forehead, that correlates with the patient's level of sedation.

Table 5.5 describes some of the sedative and analgesic agents commonly prescribed for cardiac surgical patients. Most of these medications may be given in small doses or by continuous infusion. Continuous infusions have the advantage of producing less respiratory depression and providing more consistent pain control. As patients progress, other pain options (e.g., patient-controlled analgesia or oral agents) can be used. Adequate analgesia is essential to facilitate increasing activity levels and pulmonary exercises (e.g., coughing and deep breathing). An assessment of pain should be performed during activity as well as at rest, as researchers have found that pain levels are highest with coughing, turning, and getting out of bed.[33] In addition to promoting recovery activities, analgesics are also warranted during procedures (e.g., chest tube removal). Both opioids and nonsteroidal antiinflammatory agents have been

TABLE 5.5 **Medications (Sedatives and Analgesics) Used in Cardiac Surgery Patients**

Drug	Actions	Dose	Special Considerations
Fentanyl (Sublimaze)	Stimulates opiate receptors in central nervous system to produce analgesia and sedation	25–90 mcg IV bolus, or 1–5 mcg/kg/h infusion	More rapid-acting than morphine, with a shorter duration of action; may accumulate with prolonged infusions May cause chest wall rigidity
Dexmedetomidine (Precedex)	Produces anxiolysis and sedation through its effects on alpha 2 receptors	0.2–1.5 mcg/kg/h	Reduces anxiety without sedation; works synergistically with opioids to decrease dosage required
Ketorolac (Toradol)	Nonsteroidal antiinflammatory with analgesic effects	15–60 mg IV every 6 h (not to exceed 72 h)	Avoid in patients with renal dysfunction or active bleeding Inhibits platelet function Does not produce respiratory depression or alter hemodynamics
Midazolam (Versed)	Benzodiazepine that produces sedation, anxiolysis, and amnesia Does not produce analgesia, but may reduce analgesic requirements	2.5–5 mg IV every 1–2 h, or 0.5–4 mg/h infusion	Rapid onset and short duration of action, but may accumulate with prolonged infusion (48 h) or in older adults May cause respiratory depression in some patients
Morphine sulfate	Stimulates opiate receptors in central nervous system to produce analgesia and sedation	2–10 mg IV every 2–4 h, or 1–5 mg/h infusion	Active metabolite of morphine, can accumulate in renal failure Promotes histamine release, which causes vasodilation (may cause hypotension)
Propofol (Diprivan)	Sedative-hypnotic that can be used for induction of anesthesia or sedation	5–50 mcg/kg/min	This agent has no analgesic effects Short duration of action (5–9 min) allows for rapid reversal of effects May cause hypotension, especially in hypovolemic patients Lipid medium may increase triglyceride levels and presents a risk for bacterial growth Prolonged sedation may occur in obese patients
Ketamine	NMDA receptor antagonist	1–20 mg/h via continuous infusion	Both sedative and analgesic effects My cause hypertension and tachycardia Can be used in nonintubated patients

IV, Intravenous; *NMDA*, N-methyl-D-aspartate.

found to be effective in reducing the pain associated with this procedure.[40] Pain that goes untreated can result in both physiologic and psychological stress. These consequences can lead to a decreased immune response, poor wound healing, anxiety, and depression, which may increase length of stay and decrease patient satisfaction. One week after discharge from the intensive care unit (ICU), 82% (*n* = 120) of cardiac surgery patients reported pain as the most common traumatic memory of their ICU stay.[33] Multimodal pain management, combining either two medications or a medication and nonpharmacologic intervention, can minimize the side effects of drugs and contribute to synergistic analgesic effects. An article released by the American Society of Health-System Pharmacists, as a result of their 2003 symposium, supports the use of nonpharmacologic interventions, including massage, guided imagery, music therapy, and relaxation.[53]

NUTRITION AND SPECIAL CONSIDERATIONS

Generally, a diet low in cholesterol and fat is prescribed. The diet may need to be less restrictive in the immediate postoperative period to ensure adequate nutritional intake to support healing, ideally around 25 Kcal/kg/day and protein intake of 1.2 to 1.5 g/kg/day. Ensuring adequate electrolyte replacement is important, as potassium and magnesium level fluctuations may have a significant impact on cardiac rhythms. If the patient has heart failure or is fluid-overloaded, fluid restriction and sodium restriction may be necessary. Diabetic patients will usually resume their preoperative diabetic diet. Increases in morbidity and mortality have been associated with hyperglycemia, and in the past, protocols have driven tight glycemic levels to between 90 and 112 mg/dL. Recent studies, however, recommend a more liberal approach, with targets of 121 to 180 mg/dL, to achieve the same outcome.[39]

A number of standardized protocols have been developed to improve glycemic control, using both continuous insulin infusions and sliding-scale coverage. These protocols allow for titration of insulin based on frequent assessments of blood glucose level, as well as specifying interventions for hypoglycemia, should it occur. Nursing care also includes increased frequency of blood glucose monitoring when alterations in metabolism are anticipated (such as an interruption of feeding or titration of catecholamine infusions).[29, 41]

Complications

The overall mortality associated with coronary artery bypass surgery is reported to be 1.7% at 30 days and 4.3% at 1 year.[25] Operative mortality is influenced by patient demographics, the extent of cardiac disease, the urgency of the operation, and the presence of comorbid conditions. Factors found to be predictive of operative mortality and morbidity are listed in Box 5.5. These criteria are considered by surgeons during their preoperative assessment to determine the patient's surgical risk. The Society of Thoracic Surgeons (STS) uses risk models to adjust cardiac surgery outcomes for preoperative patient characteristics and disease severity. These risk-adjusted outcomes have been widely used for research and patient counseling. In addition, they are used to provide benchmark comparisons among providers and to serve as the basis for public reporting and pay-for-performance reimbursement.[43]

BOX 5.5 Predictors of Cardiac Surgery Mortality and Morbidity

Emergent procedure
Older age (>75)
Poor ventricular function (ejection fraction <30% or elevated beta-type natriuretic peptide levels)
Reoperation
Female gender
Left main disease
Presence of comorbidities: renal dysfunction (especially if dialysis-dependent)
COPD
Diabetes mellitus
Cerebrovascular disease

Perioperative Myocardial Infarction

Perioperative MI is reported to occur in 1% to 7% of patients following surgical revascularization.[25,47] Potential causes include inadequate myocardial protection, arterial spasm in grafts or native arteries, or prolonged hypotension in the perioperative period. Diagnosis may be difficult, because cardiac surgery is usually associated with nonspecific T wave and ST changes postoperatively, as well as elevations in myocardial-specific enzymes such as creatine kinase MB (CKMB) and troponin. The diagnosis is frequently made based on new and persistent ECG changes and new regional wall abnormalities on the echocardiogram.[12] Following CABG, elevations in CKMB and/or troponin levels are common; however, values greater than 1 show a strong, graded association of elevated mortality. Furthermore, the mortality rate more than doubles if the CKMB ratio is greater than 4.4. The data show that CKMB values less than 1 have an associated mortality of 3.4%, whereas for ratios higher than 20%, mortality climbed to 20.2%.[12] Patients in this high-risk group should receive aggressive medical management postoperatively, including administration of antiplatelet agents, beta blockers, angiotensin-converting enzyme (ACE) inhibitors, and statins.[47]

Renal Dysfunction

Renal dysfunction, defined by one large multicenter study as a postoperative serum creatinine level greater than 2 mg/dL or an increase from preoperative level of greater than 0.7 mg/dL, occurs in approximately 8% of patients.[31] Renal failure requiring dialysis occurs less frequently (i.e., in 1% to 2% of patients), but is associated with mortality levels approaching 60%.[47] Risk factors for renal complications include preexisting renal disease, prolonged periods of hypotension or low CO perioperatively, and exposure to nephrotoxic agents.

Pulmonary Complications

Long-term pulmonary complications following cardiac surgery are rare and occur primarily in patients with severe underlying pulmonary disease. Patients with chronic lung disease may also require prolonged ventilation (i.e., >48 hours) in the postoperative period. Acute lung injury progressing to acute respiratory distress syndrome occurs in less than 1% of patients, but carries a high risk of mortality. Diaphragmatic failure may occur in a small number of patients, secondary to intraoperative injury to the phrenic nerve. Signs include failure to wean from the ventilator, vital capacity of less than 500 mL, and paradoxical movement of the diaphragm. Pleural effusions are common, but are generally small and left-sided and resolve spontaneously over time without treatment. Leaving a small Silastic (Blake) drain for several days following surgery has been shown to decrease the incidence of pleural effusions.[17,37]

Neurologic Complications

Neurologic complications after cardiac surgery have a reported incidence of between 0.4% and 80%, depending on how they are defined.[35] Older adult patients (older than 70) and those with HTN, diabetes, or preoperative neurologic dysfunction have an increased risk for adverse outcomes. The risk for altered cerebral tissue perfusion, with resultant neurologic dysfunction, is also increased with prolonged bypass times, perioperative hypotension, calcification of the aorta, and AF. More serious Type 1 complications, which include fatal and nonfatal stroke and transient ischemic attacks, occur in approximately 3% of patients. Type 2 complications, which describe a more subtle impairment of cognitive function (i.e., concentration, short-term memory, and speed of mental or motor responses), occur more frequently, with some studies reporting an incidence of up to 80%.[18]

Gastrointestinal Complications

Gastrointestinal complications occur infrequently following cardiac surgery (i.e., in <1% of patients), but are associated with a high mortality when they do occur.[20] The most common problem encountered is gastroduodenal bleeding. The prophylactic use of histamine H_2-receptor antagonists (H_2 blockers) or proton pump inhibitors may be prescribed by some physicians. Intestinal ischemia or infarction may occur, secondary to compromised blood flow to the mesenteric arteries. Patients typically exhibit persistent acidosis despite correction of CO. Other signs include a persistently elevated white blood cell count, abdominal tenderness, and signs of sepsis.

Wound Infection

Superficial leg incision infections occur in 2% to 20% of patients who undergo open harvesting of saphenous vein grafts, with the highest risk occurring in patients who are obese, who have diabetes, or who have compromised peripheral circulation.[51] The risk for infection with endovascular vein harvest is much lower. Patients typically present with cellulitis at the incisional site, possibly with wound breakdown and purulent drainage. Treatment usually consists of antibiotics, drainage of the wound, and potential debridement.

Sternal wound infections may be superficial or deep; most cases present within the first 2 to 4 weeks after surgery.[42] Deep sternal wound infection (i.e., mediastinitis and sternal osteomyelitis) occurs in 1% to 4% of patients and is associated with high mortality.[47] Risk factors include obesity, diabetes mellitus, chronic obstructive lung disease, longer CPB times, and use of both internal mammary arteries. Antibiotic use within 2 weeks before surgery, reexploration, and longer duration of autotransfusion may also place patients at increased risk for developing mediastinitis.[11]

Superficial infections are associated with symptoms of tenderness, erythema, and serous drainage, while the sternum remains stable. In deep infections, purulent discharge is generally present, along with increased pain and sternal instability. Symptoms of systemic infection (e.g., fever, leukocytosis, and bacteremia) are also common. Positive blood cultures, especially if the organism is *Staphylococcus aureus,* further support the diagnosis of mediastinitis.[16]

BOX 5.6 Prevention of Infections

Preoperative Interventions

Antiseptic skin preparation and hair clipping (no shaving) at surgical site
Prophylactic antibiotics × 24 hours, first dose within 1 hour prior to incision

Postoperative Interventions

No prolonged use of antibiotics
Prompt removal of all lines and catheters
Early extubation
Daily assessment of incision sites
Blood glucose control*

*Recent studies indicate that a more liberal range for a blood glucose target of 121 to 180 mg/dL is safer and more advantageous than a tight target range (90–120 mg/dL) in both diabetic and nondiabetic patients.
From Reference 44.

Treatment of mediastinitis includes opening the incision to allow for drainage and irrigation of the wound, and possible sternal debridement, if warranted. The wound is usually kept open for a period of time to allow for irrigation and packing. Negative-pressure wound therapy with a vacuum-assisted closure (VAC) system has also been used to help expedite wound healing.[44] After the infection clears, the wound may be closed by either primary closure or using a reconstructive flap composed of muscle or omentum. See Box 5.6 for infection prevention strategies.

Sternal nonunion, when the two halves of the sternum or breastplate fail to heal together properly, may also occur. If this occurs in the early postoperative period, surgery may be required to resecure the sternum, depending on the presence or extent of infection. If the nonunion is present after the chest is healed, it may be treated with sternal plating, or even left alone, depending on symptoms. A computerized tomography (CT) scan of the chest will confirm the diagnosis. A rigid plate and screw fixation may be used instead of wires when closing the sternum, to promote more rapid healing and decrease rates of nonunion or infection.

CONCLUSION

Mortality associated with cardiac surgery has not increased over the past several years, despite the fact that patients undergoing surgical procedures are increasingly older and sicker. This is partly attributable to the comprehensive care provided in the immediate postoperative period by the critical care team. The ability of skilled practitioners to anticipate problems and initiate prompt intervention remains an essential component of ensuring successful patient outcomes following cardiac surgery.

CASE STUDY 5.1

Ms. Smith is an 82-year-old woman with an active lifestyle who has complained of dyspnea and fatigue for the past 2 months. She was determined to have had an MI in the past. Coronary angiogram revealed 90% occlusion to the LAD artery, 95% occlusion to the RCA, and 85% occlusion to the posterior descending artery (PDA). She subsequently had CABG surgery with three bypasses using the LIMA to the LAD, RIMA to the RCA, and saphenous vein graft to the PDA. She was admitted to the cardiovascular ICU with a BP of 146/82 mm Hg, MAP of 103 mm Hg, heart rate of 90 bpm, temperature of 35.2°C, pulmonary artery systolic/pulmonary artery diastolic (PAS/PAD) of 28/12 mm Hg, pulmonary artery mean (PAM) of 18 mm Hg, CVP of 7 mm Hg, SVR of 2200 dynes, CO/CI of 4.2/2.2 L, and BSA = 1.9. Dexmedetomidine (Precedex) was infused for sedation.

Two hours later Ms. Smith's temperature rose to 36.9 C, SVR was 700, CI was 1.9 L/min, MAP 60 mm HG, PAD 8 mm Hg, CVP 5 mm Hg. Her chest tube drainage for the past 2 hours has been 300 mL and 125 mL, and her hemoglobin (HgB) was 8.4. Mrs. Smith was weaned and extubated without difficulty, and the dexmedetomidine was weaned off. One hour after extubation she was dangled on the side of the bed, and 4 hours later she was assisted to sit in the chair. She was transferred from the CVICU early the next morning without difficulty.

Decision Point:

Upon admission, what problems required interventions for Ms. Smith?

Two hours later Ms. Smith's temperature rose to 36.9°C, SVR was 700, CI was 1.9 L/min, MAP was 60 mm Hg, PAD was 8 mm Hg, and CVP was 5 mm Hg. Her chest tube drainage for the past two hours was 300 mL and 125 mL, and her hemoglobin (Hgb) was 8.4.

Decision Point:

What do the updated parameters reveal, and what actions are necessary?

Mrs. Smith was weaned and extubated without difficulty, and the dexmedetomidine was weaned off. One hour after extubation, she was dangled on the side of the bed, and 4 hours later she was assisted to sit in the chair. She was transferred from the CVICU early the next morning without difficulty.

REFERENCES

1. Albright, T. N., et al. (2002). Vasopressin in the cardiac surgery intensive care unit. *Am J Crit Care, 11*(4), 326–332.
2. American Heart Association. (2010). Guidelines for cardiopulmonary resuscitation and emergency cardiovascular care. *Circulation, 122*(suppl. 3), 18.
3. Angelini, G. D., et al. (2009). Effects of on-and off-pump coronary artery surgery on graft patency, survival, and health-related quality of life: long-term follow-up of 2 randomized controlled trials. *J Thorac Cardiovasc Surg, 137*(2), 295–303.
4. Bakaeen, F. G., et al. (2014). Trends and use of off-pump coronary artery bypass grafting: results from the Society of Thoracic Surgeons Adult Cardiac Surgery Database. *J Thorac Cardiovasc Surg, 148*(2014), 856–864.
5. Barr, J., & Fraser, G. (2013). Clinical practice guidelines for the management of pain, agitation, and delirium in adult patients in the intensive care unit. *Crit Care Med, 41*(1), 263–306.
6. Bitondo, J. M., et al. (2002). Endoscopic versus open saphenous vein harvest: a comparison of postoperative wound infections. *Ann Thoracic Surg, 73*, 523–528.
7. Choo, S. (2015). The bottom line is completeness of revascularization. *J Thorac Cardiovasc Nurs, 149*, 1034–1035.
8. Connelly, M. W., et al. (2002). Endoscopic radial harvesting: results of the first 300 patients. *Ann Thoracic Surg, 74*, 502–505.
9. Crenshaw, B. S., et al. (2000). Risk factors, angiographic patterns, and outcomes in patients with ventricular septal defect complicating acute myocardial infarction for the GUSTO (Global Utilization of Streptokinase and TPA for Occluded Coronary Arteries) trial investigators. *Circulation, 91*, 27–32.
10. DeWitte, J. & Sessler, D. I. (2002). Perioperative shivering: physiology and pharmacology. *Anesthesiology, 96*, 467–484.
11. Dial, S., Nguyen, D., & Menzies, D. (2003). Autotransfusion of shed mediastinal blood. A risk factor for mediastinitis after cardiac surgery? Results of a cluster investigation. *Chest, 124*, 1847–1851.
12. Domanski, M., et al. (2011). Association of myocardial enzyme elevation and survival following coronary artery bypass graft surgery. *JAMA, 305*(6), 585–591.
13. Drew, B. J., et al. (2004). Practice standards for electrocardiographic monitoring in hospital settings: an American Heart Association scientific statement from the Councils on Cardiovascular Nursing, Clinical Cardiology, and Cardiovascular Disease in the Young. *Circulation, 19*, 2721–2746.

14. Erhman, B. L. & Moore, H. A. (2004). Blood conservation strategies in cardiovascular surgery. *Dimensions Crit Care Nurs, 23*(6), 244–252.
15. FDA Safety Communication. (2013). Boxed warning on increased mortality and severe renal injury, and additional warning on risk of bleeding, for use of hydroxyethyl starch solutions in some settings. US Food & Drug Administration. http://www.fda.gov/BiologicsBloodVaccines/SafetyAvailability/ucm358271.htm.
16. Fowler, V. G., et al. (2003). *Staphylococcus aureus* bacteremia after median sternotomy: clinical utility of blood culture results in the identification of postoperative mediastinitis. *Circulation, 98*, 73–78.
17. Frankel, T. L., et al. (2003). Silastic drains vs. conventional chest tubes after coronary artery bypass. *Chest, 124*, 98–113.
18. Go, A. S., et al. (2014). Executive summary: heart disease and stroke statistics—2014 update: a report from the American Heart Association. *Circulation, 129*, 399–410.
19. Gregoric, I. D. & Cooley, D. A. (2004). Ventricular aneurysms. In S. C. Yang (Ed.), *Current therapy in thoracic and cardiovascular surgery* (pp. 675–677). Philadelphia: Mosby.
20. Guler, M., et al. (2011). Risk factors for gastrointestinal complications in patients undergoing coronary artery bypass graft surgery. *J Cardiothorac Vasc Anesth, 25*(4), 637–641.
21. Halkos, M. & Guyton, R. (2014). Coronary bypass: is it time to take the next step—the routine use of the second arterial graft? *J Thorac Cardiovasc Surg, 148*, 1149.
22. Halkos, M. & Walker, P. (2014). Clinical and angiographic results after hybrid coronary revascularization. *Ann Thorac Surg, 97*(2), 484–490.
23. Houlind, K. & Fenger-Gron, M. (2014). Graft patency after off-pump coronary artery bypass surgery is inferior even with identical heparinization protocols: Results from the Danish On-pump Versus Off-pump Randomization Study (DOORS). *J Thorac Cardiovasc Surg, 148*(5), 1812–1819.
24. Hravnak, M., et al. (2004). Short-term complications and resource utilization in matched subjects after on-pump or off-pump primary isolated coronary artery bypass. *Am J Crit Care, 13*, 499–508.
25. Jakobsen, C., et al. (2015). 30 day mortality after coronary artery bypass grafting and valve surgery has greatly improved over the last decade, but the 1 year mortality remains constant. *Ann Card Anaesth, 18*(2), 138–142.
26. Landoni, G., et al. (2012). A survey on the use of intra-aortic balloon pump in cardiac surgery. *Ann Card Anaesth*, 274–274.
27. Leavitt, B. J., et al. (2001). Use of internal mammary artery graft and in-hospital mortality and other adverse outcomes associated with coronary artery bypass surgery. *Circulation, 93*, 507–512.
28. Ley S. J. (2015). Standards for resuscitation after cardiac surgery. *Crit Care Nurse, 35*(2), 30–38.
29. Lorenz, R. A., Lorenz, R. M., & Codd, J. E. (2005). Perioperative control of blood glucose during adult coronary artery bypass surgery. *AORN J, 81*, 125–150.
30. Louagie, Y. A., et al. (2004). Continuous cold blood cardioplegia improves myocardial protection: a prospective randomized study. *Ann Thoracic Surg, 77*(2), 664.
31. Mangano, C. M., et al. (1998). Renal dysfunction after myocardial revascularization: risk factors, adverse outcomes, and hospital resource utilization. For the Multicenter Study of Perioperative Ischemia Research Group. *Ann Intern Med, 128*, 194–203.
32. Meade, M. O., et al. (2001). Trials comparing early vs. late extubation following cardiovascular surgery. *Chest, 120*, 445S–453S.
33. Milgrom, L. B., et al. (2004). Pain levels experienced with activities after cardiac surgery. *Am J Crit Care, 13*(2), 116–125.
34. Napolitano, L. M., et al. (2009). Clinical practice guideline: red blood cell transfusion in adult trauma and critical care. *Crit Care Med, 37*, 12.
35. Newman, M. F., et al. (2001). Longitudinal assessment of neurocognitive function after coronary artery bypass surgery. *N Engl J Med, 344*(6), 395–402.
36. O'Hanlon, J. V. (2000). Minimally invasive saphenous vein harvesting. *Crit Care Nurs Q, 23*(1), 42.
37. Payne, M., et al. (2000). Left pleural effusions after coronary artery bypass decrease with a supplemental pleural drain. *Ann Thoracic Surg, 73*, 149–152.
38. Peretto, G. & Durante, A. (2014). Postoperative arrhythmias after cardiac surgery: incidence, risk factors, and therapeutic management. *Cardiol Res Pract*, Article ID 615987.
39. Pezella, T. & Holmes, S. (2014). Impact of perioperative glycemic control strategy on patient survival after coronary bypass surgery. *Ann Thorac Surg, 1283*(98), 1281–1285.
40. Puntillo, K. & Ley, J. (2004). Appropriately timed analgesics control pain due to chest tube removal. *Am J Crit Care, 13*, 292–302.
41. Robinson, L. E. & van Soren, M. H. (2004). Insulin resistance and hyperglycemia in critical illness: role of insulin in glycemic control. *AACN Clin Issues, 15*, 45–62.
42. Schlossberg, D. (2015). Mediastinitis. In *Clinical Infectious Disease*. (2nd ed.). (pp. 268–272). Cambridge: Cambridge University Press.
43. Shahian, D. M., et al. (2009). The Society of Thoracic Surgeons 2008 cardiac surgery risk models: part 1—coronary artery bypass grafting surgery. *Ann Thorac Surg, 88*(1), S2–S22.
44. Sjogren, J., et al. (2005). The impact of vacuum-assisted closure on long-term survival after post-sternotomy mediastinitis. *Ann Thoracic Surg, 80*, 1270–1275.
45. Skhirtladze, K., et al. (2013). Comparison of the effects of albumin 5%, hydroxyethyl starch 130/0.4 6%, and Ringer's lactate on blood loss and coagulation after cardiac surgery. *B J Anaesth 112*(2), 255–264.
46. Slaughter, M., et al. (2010). Clinical management of continuous-flow left ventricular assist devices in advanced heart failure. *J Heart Lung Transplant, 29*(Suppl), S1–39.
47. Smith, P. K., et al. (2011). ACCF/AHA Guideline for Coronary Artery Bypass Graft Surgery. *Circulation, 124*, e652–735.
48. Soltis, L., et al. (2013). Early extubation after cardiac surgery leads to decreased returns to ICU and pulmonary complications. *Crit Care Med, 41*(12), A75.
49. Takagi, H., Umemoto, T., All-Literature Investigation of Cardiovascular Evidence (ALICE) Group (2014). Worse long-term survival after off-pump than on-pump coronary artery bypass grafting. *J Thorac Cardiovasc Surg, 148*, 1820–1829.
50. Tavilla, G., et al. (2004). Long-term follow-up of coronary artery bypass grafting in three-vessel disease using exclusively pedicled bilateral internal thoracic and right gastroepiploic arteries. *Ann Thoracic Surg, 77*(3), 794.
51. Thimour-Bergstron, L., et al. (2013). Triclosan-coated sutures reduce surgical site infection after open vein harvesting in coronary artery bypass grafting patients: a randomized controlled trial. *Eur J Cardiothorac Surg, 44*(5), 931–938.
52. Thunberg, C., et al. (2010). Ventricular assist devices today and tomorrow. *J Cardiovasc Vasc Anes, 24*(4), 656–680.
53. Trail-Mahan, T. & Mao, C. (2013). Complementary and alternative medicine: nurses' attitudes and knowledge. *Pain Manag Nurs, 14*(4), 277–286.
54. Tranbaugh, R. F., et al. (2010). Radial artery conduits improve long-term survival after coronary artery bypass grafting. *Ann Thorac Surg, 90*, 1165–1172.
55. Turner, D. (2013). Extracorporeal membrane oxygenation for adult respiratory failure. *Respir Care, 58*(6), 1038–1052.
56. Van der Linden, P., et al. (2001). A standardized multidisciplinary approach reduces the use of allogenic blood products in patients undergoing cardiac surgery. *Can J Anesth, 48*, 894–901.
57. Weiss, A. J., et al. (2013). A meta-analysis comparing bilateral internal mammary artery with left internal mammary artery for coronary artery bypass grafting. *Ann Cardiothorac Surg, 2*, 390–400.
58. Wiegand, D. (2011). *AACN Procedure Manual for Critical Care* (6th ed.). (pp. 443-463). St Louis: Saunders.

6

Valvular Disease and Surgery

Barbara Leeper

The picture of valvular heart disease has changed significantly in the last 50 years. The impact of rheumatic heart disease as the most common cause of valve dysfunction was lessened by the widespread use of prophylactic penicillin.[37,40] In recent years, two factors have contributed to changing the epidemiology of valvular heart disease: the aging of the population and improvement in echocardiography technology, which has increased the ability to diagnose valvular heart disease.[1] Breakthroughs in the medical management and surgical interventions for this potentially life-threatening situation have significantly changed patients' long-term outcomes. However, in spite of the improvements in medical management, the incidence of heart valve surgical procedures has continued to increase.

The purpose of this chapter is to review the etiology and emerging trends in the management of valvular heart disease. The pathophysiology, assessment, medical management, and surgical interventions for each of the valve conditions will also be discussed.

PREVALENCE

The exact incidence of valvular heart disease is unknown. However, a recent population-based epidemiologic study using echocardiography on 16,501 subjects found an age-adjusted prevalence of clinical valvular heart disease (moderate or greater) of 1.8%. The largest prevalence is in individuals 75 years and older (11.7%; 95% [confidence interval] CI, 11.0–12.5%). The investigators suggested the prevalence of any valve disease in the United States is 2.5%, with no significant difference between males and females.[1] Valvular heart disease makes up 10% to 20% of all cardiac surgical procedures in the United States and the numbers are growing. Aortic valvular replacement makes up two thirds of the surgical procedures, primarily for aortic stenosis.[5] Newer transcatheter techniques have emerged and these procedures are increasing in frequency.

ETIOLOGY

Disease processes affecting heart valves will cause either a "stenosis" or an "insufficiency" of the valve. Valvular insufficiency may also be called "regurgitation." A valve is said to be stenotic when it is narrowed and does not open properly. Pure stenosis will block the flow of blood from one heart chamber (atrium to ventricle) or may prevent adequate ejection of the blood from the ventricle into the circulation (pulmonary or peripheral). Insufficiency indicates the valve is leaking, allowing blood to leak back (or regurgitate) into the previous heart chamber. Frequently patients with valvular heart disease will have a combination of stenosis and regurgitation involving one or more valves. The most common diseases that cause valve problems are rheumatic fever and bacterial endocarditis.[5]

Rheumatic Fever

Rheumatic heart disease is one of the most common causes of valvular heart disease, especially mitral stenosis and aortic regurgitation.[5] The disease was thought to have been eradicated in the 1970s; however, there was a resurgence in the 1980s.[31] The American Heart Association (AHA) reported the prevalence of rheumatic heart disease is increasing in all areas of the world with the exception of Europe. Acute rheumatic fever is increasing slightly in North and South America.[1] African Americans, Puerto Ricans, Mexican Americans, and Native Americans have a higher incidence than other populations.[1]

Endocarditis

Endocarditis is a microbial infection of the lining of the heart, most commonly affecting the cardiac valves, but also affecting the endocardium adjacent to an infected valve.[24] Congenital defects (such as patent ductus arteriosus, ventricular septal defect, and bicuspid aortic valves) or acquired defects from rheumatic heart disease are predisposing factors.[17,23] The lesion, or vegetation, is a mass of platelets and fibrin containing abundant microorganisms. The most common causative microorganisms are streptococci, staphylococci, enterococci, and gram-negative coccobacilli.[24] Patients with mitral valve prolapse and those with a history of intravenous drug abuse seem to be at the greatest risk.[24] Fig. 6.1 shows an example of endocarditis affecting the aortic valve. Note the thickened valve leaflets from the vegetations.

Other Etiologies

Table 6.1 lists a variety of other etiologies for valvular heart disease. Of note are congenital defects, such as mitral valve clefts and unicuspid or bicuspid aortic valves, which may produce stenosis or insufficiency. In adults, aortic stenosis and regurgitation are often caused by the build-up of calcium on the valve leaflets, referred to as "senile degenerative" disease. In the setting of acute myocardial infarction, abrupt rupture of the chordae tendineae or papillary muscle will cause acute mitral regurgitation. A similar, but less frequent, event can occur with a right ventricular infarction causing acute tricuspid regurgitation.[5]

Appetite suppressants, including fenfluramine, dexfenfluramine, and phentermine, have also been linked to the development of valvular heart disease.[42] Some researchers have demonstrated a 31% incidence of valvular disease associated with one or more of these drugs.[42] As a result, the US Federal Drug Administration (FDA) asked the pharmaceutical companies making fenfluramine and dexfenfluramine to voluntarily take these drugs off the market. Phentermine continues to be available. Individuals who have previously taken these medications are still affected by them. The most common valvulopathies reported include (in order of frequency) aortic regurgitation, tricuspid regurgitation, and mitral regurgitation.[42] However, a systematic review of the literature demonstrated a wider variation, leading the investigators to conclude that the actual risk is undetermined and may be lower than once thought.[42]

EMERGING TRENDS IN SURGICAL MANAGEMENT OF VALVULAR HEART DISEASE

Valve Repair Versus Valve Replacement

With recent improvements in surgical techniques and devices, valve repair has become an important option for many patients. Valve repair offers patients the advantage of retaining the native valve, having a normal valve orifice, and avoiding the challenges that might be associated with long-term anticoagulation therapy normally required with mechanical valves. Valve repair may include the insertion of a valve ring to repair the annulus, removal of abnormal tissue from the valve leaflets, restoration of the commissures, shortening of the chordae tendineae, or repair of the papillary muscle.[46] Fig. 6.2 illustrates valve repair using a valve ring. Valve repair has been found to be an especially effective treatment for the mitral and aortic valves.[30,45–48]

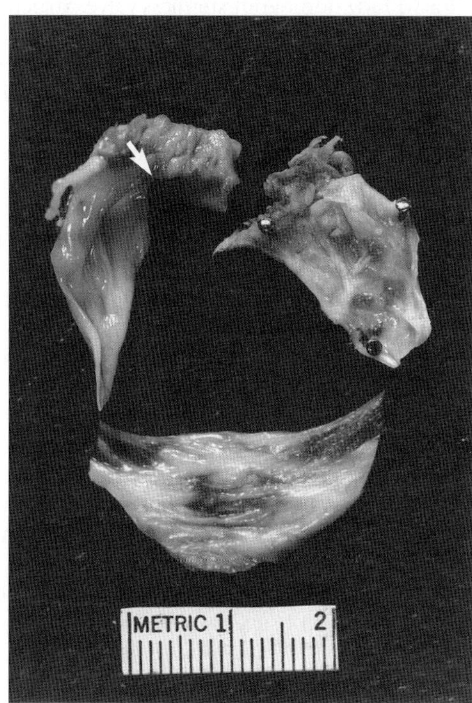

FIG. 6.1 Aortic valve with endocarditis. Note the vegetations on the thickened valve leaflets. The valve leaflet has been partially destroyed by the infectious process *(arrow)*. (Reprinted with permission from Baylor Medical Center.)

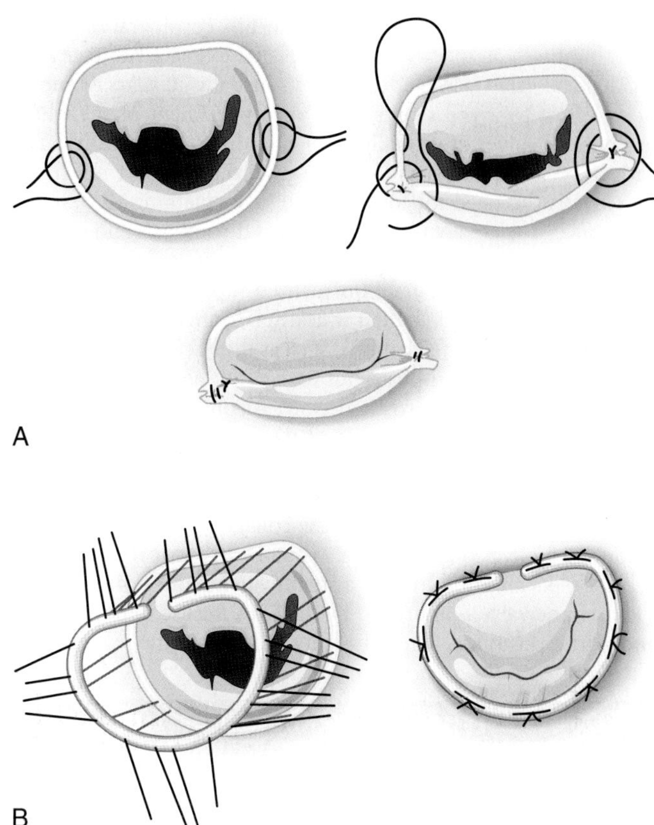

FIG. 6.2 Valve repair replacing the valve ring. **A,** Using valve annulus sutures, the mitral valve is repaired. **B,** This dilated mitral valve annulus is shown being reshaped by use of an annuloplasty ring.

TABLE 6.1 Etiologies of Valvular Heart Disease

MITRAL VALVE		TRICUSPID VALVE	
Stenosis:	**Insufficiency:**	**Stenosis:**	**Insufficiency:**
Rheumatic fever	Infective endocarditis	Rheumatic fever	Right ventricular dilation
Congenital	Myocardial infarction	Atrial myxoma	Pulmonary hypertension
	Systemic lupus erythematosus		Right ventricular infarction
	Rheumatoid arthritis		Bacterial endocarditis
PULMONIC VALVE		**AORTIC VALVE**	
Stenosis:	**Insufficiency:**	**Stenosis:**	**Insufficiency:**
Congenital	Pulmonary hypertension	Congenital bicuspid valve	Rheumatic fever
	Bacterial endocarditis	Rheumatic fever	Endocarditis
		Senile degenerative stenosis	Enlargement of aortic root, stretching valve cusps
		Atherosclerosis	

Data from Reference 5.

Types of Prosthetic Valve

There are two types of prosthetic valve: mechanical and tissue (Box 6.1). Mechanical valves can be caged ball valves, monoleaflet valves, or bileaflet valves. Caged-ball valves are no longer implanted today. The most common mechanical valves now used are low-profile bileaflet disk valves, which offer less impedance to blood flow through the orifice. Fig. 6.3 shows the St. Jude bileaflet mechanical valve, one of the more commonly implanted valves in the United States.[3] Low-profile disk valves have leaflets that open anywhere from 55 to 80 degrees, depending on the type and maker of the valve.[3] The wider the opening, the less the obstruction of blood flow, which is an important consideration when selecting the type of valve to be implanted. The advantage of a mechanical valve is longer durability—usually 20 years or more. In an effort to avoid reoperation for replacement of the valve, mechanical valves are usually implanted in younger individuals with a longer life expectation. The disadvantage of a mechanical valve is the need for long-term anticoagulation. Mechanical valves are associated with a higher risk of thrombosis and peripheral embolization, including stroke. These patients require close monitoring of international normalized ratio (INR)/prothrombin time (PT) to regulate their warfarin (Coumadin) dose. There are newer classes of medications, such as the Factor Xa inhibitors, that will prevent thrombosis, but have yet to be approved by the FDA for prevention of prosthetic valve thrombosis.

There are also several types of tissue valves. These include the heterograft (porcine and bovine), homograft, and autograft valves. The porcine and bovine heterograft valves are sterilized by glutaraldehyde, which stabilizes the collagen for durability. The glutaraldehyde also changes the tissue to be bioacceptable. The valve leaflets are mounted on a stent, which has a sewing ring.[20] The porcine valve is approved by the FDA for use in both mitral and aortic positions. The durability of the porcine valve is less than that of the mechanical valve. There are reports of porcine valves deteriorating 10 years after implant, requiring reoperation in 20% to 40% of patients who had a mitral bioprosthesis and in 15% to 20% who had an aortic bioprosthesis.[20,22]

Bovine valves are made from bovine pericardium and are approved for placement in the aortic position. Durability is somewhat longer than porcine valves, approximately 12 to 15 years, with reoperation occurring in 4% to 9% of patients at the 10-year mark.[22]

A homograft valve is a tissue valve that has been harvested from a donor, cleaned, mounted on a support device (with or without stent), and made available for implantation. The stentless valve that is implanted in the aortic position has a larger orifice, allowing for less impedance of blood flow. All prosthetic valves produce some stenosis, ranging from mild to moderate.[20] Therefore, the stentless valve offers a little more opening for blood flow. Fig. 6.4 shows the St. Jude homograft stentless valve. Structural valve deterioration is lower in this type of valve when compared with other tissue valves.[20] Pulmonary homografts have not been found to do well in the aortic position.[10] Studies show that this type of valve may not be as durable as the porcine valve.[15,20]

An autograft valve is one that is taken from the patient's pulmonic position and reimplanted in the aortic position as part of the Ross procedure. This procedure will be discussed in more detail later in this chapter. The pulmonic valve has been found to function extremely well in the aortic position, with 85% of patients being free from reoperation 20 years following placement.[20]

Older adult patients usually receive tissue valves because of the durability of the valve and the lack of anticoagulation needed. However, a study examining valve-related complications 15 years after mitral valve replacement found no difference in valve-related reoperation and mortality and thus favored mechanical prostheses in patients up to age 70.[20,22] There are some recent studies suggesting that some types of tissue valves may be better for younger age groups, such as using a pulmonary autograft valve in younger and pediatric patients with the Ross procedure. More data with longer-term studies are needed to fully support this type of surgery.[12,15,36]

BOX 6.1 Types of Prosthetic Heart Valve

Mechanical Valves
- Caged-ball (no longer implanted)
- Bileaflet disk

Tissue Valves
- Heterograft valves porcine
- Bovine pericardial
- Homograft valves
- Autograft valves

Complications of Prosthetic Valves

Complications associated with prosthetic heart valves include structural valve deterioration and peripheral embolization related

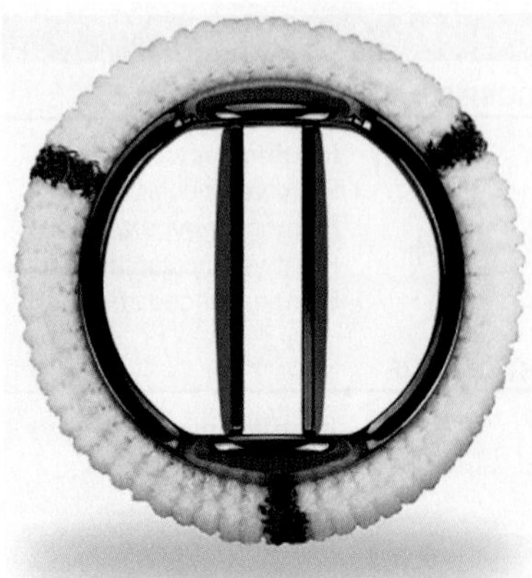

FIG. 6.3 The St. Jude bileaflet mechanical valve. (Reprinted with permission from St Jude Medical, www.sjm.com.)

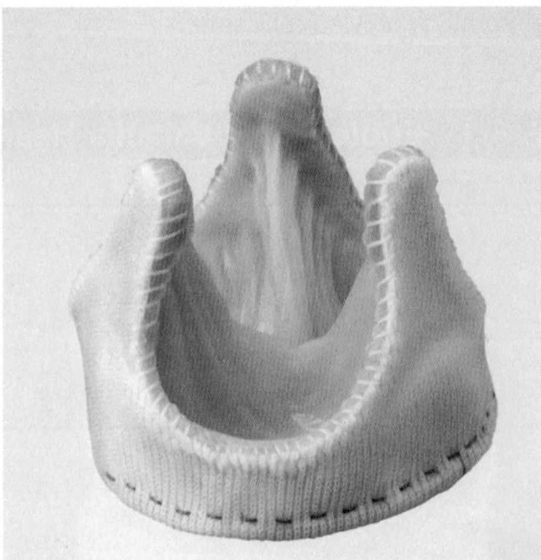

FIG. 6.4 The St. Jude Toronto stentless porcine valve (SPV) homograft stentless valve. (Reprinted with permission from St Jude Medical, www.sjm.com.)

to thrombus generation on the valve structure. Additional complications include prosthetic endocarditis, prosthetic dehiscence, bleeding, perivalvular regurgitation, and primary valve failure. Hemolysis also occurs with all mechanical prosthetic valves, but not with tissue valves. An increase in the concentration of lactic acid dehydrogenase (LDH) has been found to be reliable as an indicator of hemolysis. Patients should be monitored closely for prosthesis dysfunction, perivalvular leak, or cloth tear, which may produce a sudden increase in the LDH concentration.[20]

Surgical Approach

With the development of new instruments and technologies, the surgical approach to repairing or implanting a heart valve has changed. The traditional median sternotomy, considered to be the gold standard, is still routinely performed in many centers. However, this approach is being challenged because of the longer bone-healing time, requiring more time away from work and increased risk for deep sternal wound infections. Younger patients often prefer a less invasive surgical approach to avoid the more visible sternotomy scar. The advantage of the traditional approach is better visualization for the surgeon. Nevertheless, there is a trend to move toward less invasive approaches.

There are a variety of minimally invasive approaches that are being used. Some include a partial sternotomy with a lower transverse division (transsternal) for aortic and mitral valve procedures (Fig. 6.5). Another approach is a parasternal incision for a mitral procedure. Mini-thoracotomies, either from the left or from the right side, are also being used. Many of these approaches require video assistance.[8] Proposed advantages of the minimally invasive approaches are reduction in patient morbidity and mortality. Generally, the literature suggests that the biggest benefit from the minimally invasive approach is the shorter length of hospital stay.[8]

The use of robotics to perform minimally invasive valve surgery continues to increase. The da Vinci system (Intuitive Surgical, Inc.) is one example of this evolving technology (Fig. 6.6). In addition, new instruments and clips have been developed to replace some suture material. The technology continues to undergo evaluation to determine its usefulness and impact on patient outcomes.[25]

Transcatheter Valve Replacement

Over the last 20 years, percutaneous approaches have been used to perform commissurotomies of the mitral valve and valvuloplasties of the aortic valve.[45] In the mid-1990s investigational work began on percutaneous catheter-based valve replacements of the aortic valve, in which a tissue valve is sutured into a stent and implanted in the desired valve position just below the coronary orifices, and the native valve is pushed to the side.[45] This approach offers hope for some patients who are not surgical candidates but may benefit from replacement of their aortic valve.[7,43,44] Transcatheter aortic valve replacement (TAVR) has emerged as an innovative approach for patients with aortic

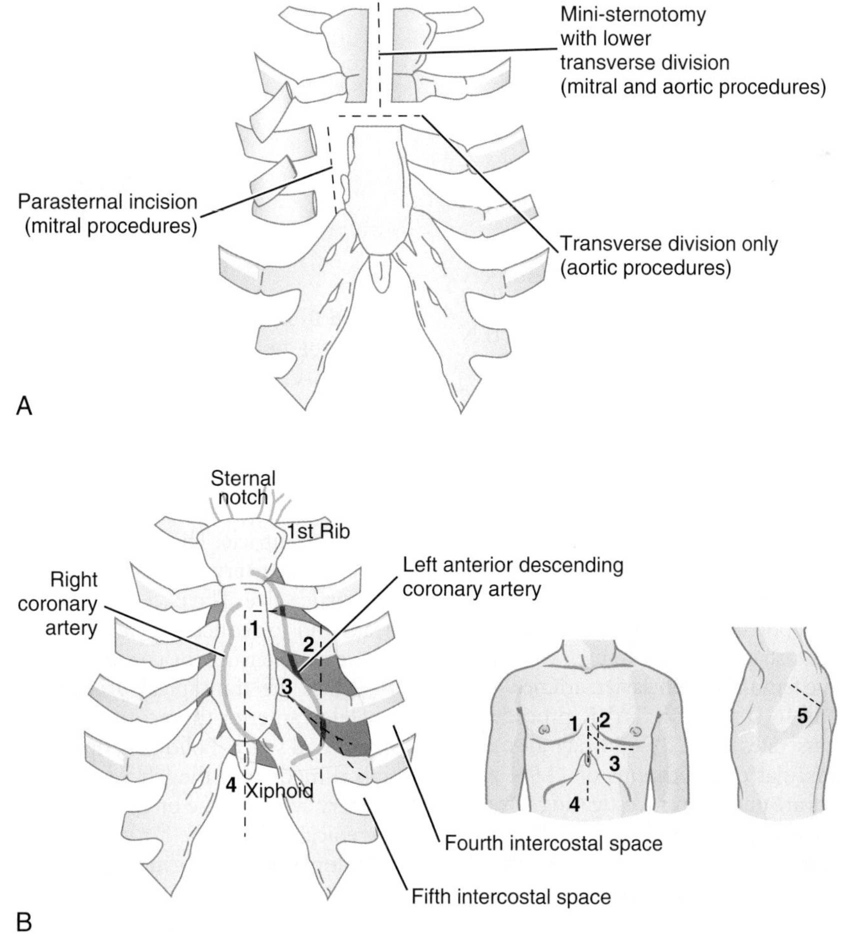

FIG. 6.5 Minimally invasive surgical approaches. **A,** Incision lines. **B,** *1,* Mini-sternotomy approach; *2,* parasternal approach; *3,* anterior mini-thoracotomy approach; *4,* subxiphoid approach; *5,* posterolateral approach.

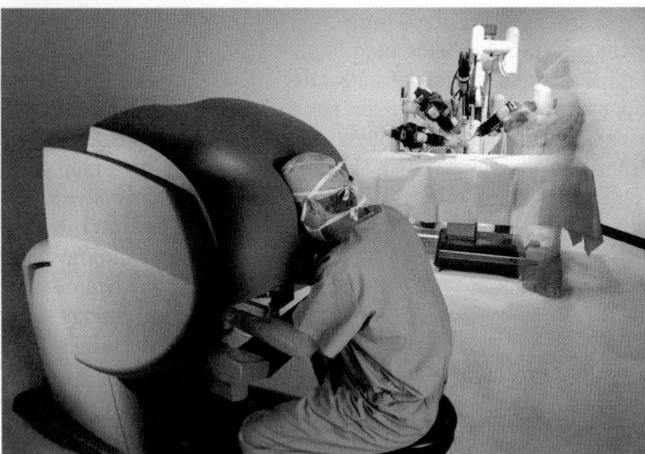

FIG. 6.6 The Intuitive da Vinci robotic system. (Reprinted with permission from Intuitive Surgical Inc., www.davincisurgery.com.)

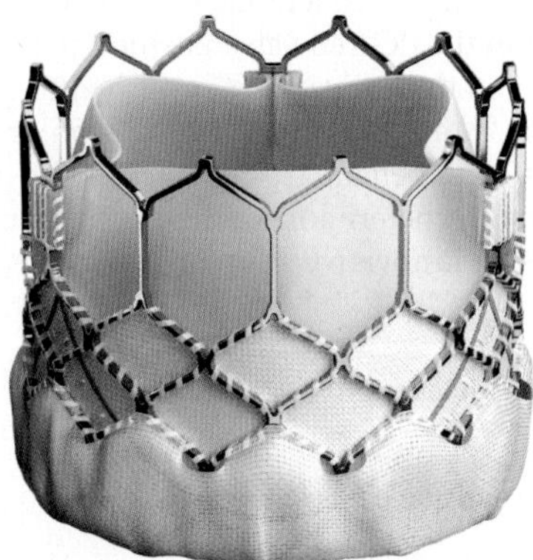

FIG. 6.7 The Edwards SAPIEN XT transcatheter heart valve system. (Courtesy Edwards Lifesciences LLC, Irvine, CA.)

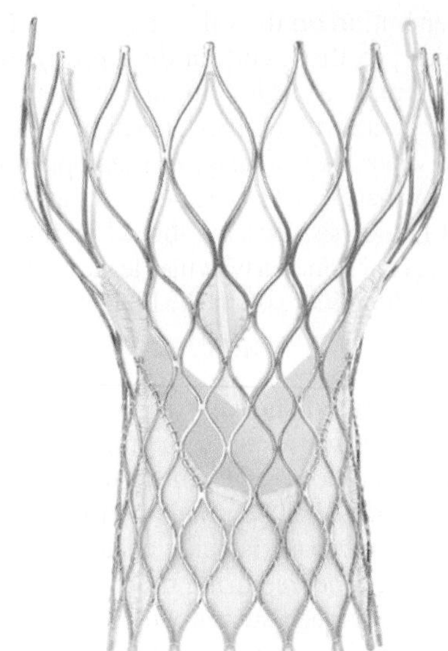

FIG. 6.8 The Medtronic CoreValve system. (Courtesy Medtronic.)

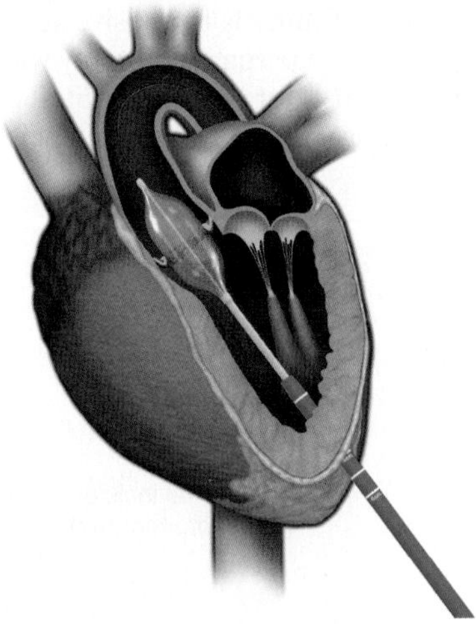

FIG. 6.9 Transapical deployment of Edwards SAPIENT transcatheter heart valve. (Courtesy Edwards Lifesciences LLC, Irvine, CA.)

stenosis and for patients who are at high risk for cardiac surgery and cardiopulmonary bypass. There are two types of valves presently in use in the United States: the Edwards SAPIEN transcatheter heart valve system (Edwards Lifesciences, Irvine, CA) approved by the FDA in 2011 and the Medtronic CoreValve (Medtronic, Inc.) approved by the FDA in 2014.[16] The Edwards SAPIEN valve (Fig. 6.7) is a bovine pericardial valve mounted within an expandable stainless steel stent. This device can be inserted via a femoral approach or a transapical approach. The transapical approach is used when the femoral artery does not meet the size requirement. It is wider and shorter than the CoreValve requiring a femoral arterial vessel lumen of 7 mm.[35]

The CoreValve (Fig. 6.8) is a porcine pericardial valve mounted on a self-expanding hour glass-shaped nitinol frame. This valve may be implanted through the femoral or subclavian arteries.

A systematic review from 16 studies on TAVR procedures demonstrated surgical success rates of 91.2%; 30-day all-cause mortality of 7.8%; major vascular complications of 11.9% and major stroke of 3.2%.[1] Studies are underway investigating a "valve in valve" procedure. This involves performing the TAVR procedure in someone who previously had an aortic valve replacement. Research is just beginning on percutaneous approaches for mitral valve repair and pulmonic valve replacement.

The TAVR procedure is performed in a hybrid operating suite, which is a combination operating room and cardiac catheterization laboratory. In addition to the operating room equipment, there is fluoroscopy. Patients have a central line inserted through which a transvenous pacemaker is inserted into the right ventricle. The balloon valvuloplasty is advanced through the femoral artery up through the aorta until it is positioned in the aortic valve. The pacemaker is turned on at a rate of 150–220 beats/min to reduce the cardiac output. The valve is positioned with care to ensure the coronary artery orifices are not blocked.[28]

When the transapical procedure is performed (Fig. 6.9), a small left anterior thoracotomy is performed, usually in the sixth intercostal space. Following opening of the pericardium, a small stab is made into the left ventricular apex to accommodate the delivery system. One or two bipolar pacing wires are attached to the epicardial surface for pacing during the procedure. Balloon valvuloplasty is performed, pacing initiated as previously mentioned, and the new valve is inserted into the orifice.[28] Following the procedure, the patient will have a chest tube left in overnight. This procedure produces significant relief of symptoms and has resulted in a marked reduction in mortality and hospitalization.[5]

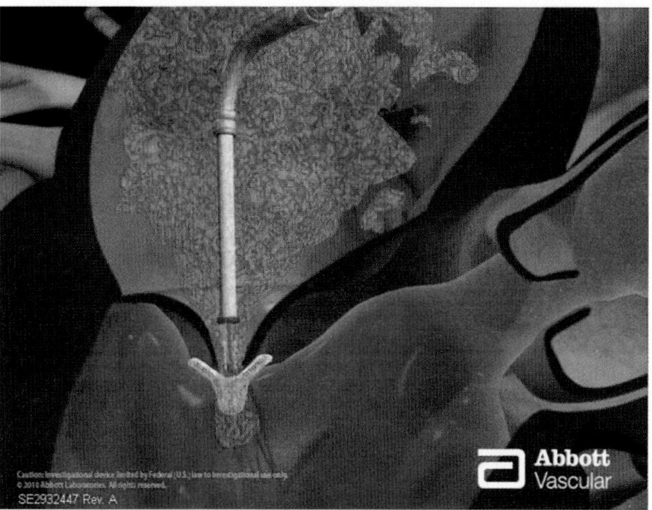

FIG. 6.10 Abbott Vascular MitraClip transcatheter device.

A transcatheter delivery system was recently approved for mitral valve repair in patients with degenerative mitral insufficiency who are considered to be at extremely high risk for surgery. The MitraClip (Abbott Vascular, Menlo Park, CA) device permanently attaches to the mitral valve leaflets, causing a double opening of the mitral valve, and reduces mitral regurgitation by promoting greater closure of the valve (Fig. 6.10).

AORTIC REGURGITATION

Aortic regurgitation is a backflow of blood into the left ventricle after the ventricular contraction is complete because of an incompetent aortic valve. The incidence of aortic regurgitation is approximately 5% of the general population, increases with age, and is more common in men than in women.[14] Patients with aortic regurgitation tend to have higher mortality and morbidity rates than the general population. Heart failure usually occurs within 10 years after the onset.[5] The valvular disease process may be associated with primary disease of the valve or the aortic wall above the valve. Dilation of the aortic root (usually from age-related degeneration, Marfan syndrome, or aortic dissection[5]) occurs more commonly than a primary disease process of the valve leaflets.

Pathophysiology

Aortic root dilation causes the aortic annulus to enlarge, subsequently separating the valve leaflets and causing aortic regurgitation. The dilation causes tension and bowing of the individual valve cusps, further intensifying the regurgitation.[5]

The insufficient aortic valve allows a backflow of blood into the left ventricle during ventricular diastole contributing to a larger left ventricular end-diastolic volume and end-diastolic pressure. This results in a larger stroke volume with the next ventricular ejection causing an increased systolic pressure and wider pulse pressure. The large stroke volume can produce dilation of the ascending aorta. Left atrial pressure and pulmonary vascular pressures increase later in the disease process resulting in a delay of the onset of symptoms of dyspnea and angina.[14]

Regardless of the cause, over time the left ventricle hypertrophies, increasing the patient's risk for sudden death. Patients with an ejection fraction (EF) less than 55% are also at greater risk for sudden cardiac death.[14]

Testing

Aortic regurgitation is identified by the presence of a diastolic murmur. Doppler echocardiography has proven to be indispensable, providing quantification of the regurgitant volume and determining the cause of the regurgitation and the degree of pulmonary hypertension.[4]

The ECG may reflect left ventricular hypertrophy, left axis deviation, and patterns consistent with diastolic overload (i.e., down-sloping, depressed ST segments). The chest x-ray may show left ventricular enlargement; however, the actual changes are related to the severity of the regurgitation. Dilation of the aortic root may or may not be apparent. The presence of an aneurysm in the ascending aorta is suggestive of Marfan syndrome.[5]

Signs and Symptoms

A patient may have aortic regurgitation for many years before symptoms appear. Common symptoms the patient may experience include shortness of breath or chest tightness.[31] The patient will clinically present with bounding arterial pulses, sometimes described as a "water hammer" pulse, indicating an abrupt distention of the pulse followed by a quick collapse. Another classic sign is de Musset sign, described as head bobbing with each heartbeat.[5,31] The peripheral arterial pulse is usually bounding and can be appreciated by palpating the radial artery with the arm elevated above the head.[5]

A widened pulse pressure is also characteristic of aortic regurgitation. The large stroke volume increases the systolic pressure, and the insufficient valve allows backflow of blood into the left ventricle, causing the diastolic pressure to be very low. The Korotkoff sounds may be heard down to zero; however, one should note the point at which muffling of the Korotkoff sounds occurs. This point has been found to correlate with the diastolic pressure.[5]

A third heart sound may be present, along with the diastolic murmur. The murmur is best heard with the patient leaning forward in an upright position. Generally the murmur tends to be harsh sounding. The Austin Flint murmur occurs late in diastole, often described as a rumble, and is heard best at the apex.[5]

Management

Medical management consists of prophylactic antibiotic therapy for prevention of bacterial endocarditis. If the patient has signs and symptoms of volume overload, vasodilators, such as hydralazine (Apresoline), nifedipine (Procardia), felodipine (Plendil), and angiotensin-converting enzyme (ACE) inhibitors, seem to have beneficial effects.[5] If the regurgitation is severe, the patient should be managed similar to severe heart failure. However, beta blockers should be avoided to prevent bradycardia. The patient should be followed with echocardiograms at least annually and more frequently if symptomatic.[4,5] Serial radionuclide ventriculograms to assess left ventricular volume and function at rest have been found to be an accurate, cost-effective alternative to the echocardiogram.[4]

Surgery will relieve symptoms and correct the mechanical problem. Although there are no studies comparing nonsurgical therapy with surgical intervention, most experts agree that surgery is indicated for patients who have no contraindications.[12] The American Heart Association/American College of Cardiology (AHA/ACC) Class I recommendations state that indications for surgery are severe symptoms or a left ventricular end-diastolic volume (LVEDV) or dimension greater than or equal to 75 mm, an end-systolic diameter greater than or equal to 50 mm, and an EF less than 50%.[4]

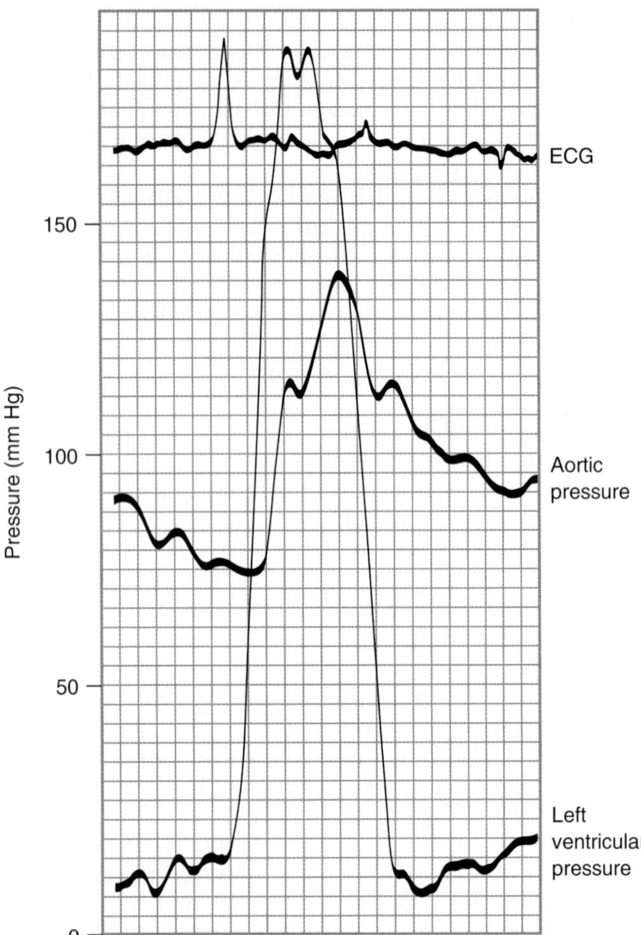

FIG. 6.11 Left ventricular (LV) aortic pressure gradient associated with aortic stenosis. The LV systolic pressure is approximately 45 mm Hg higher than the aortic systolic pressure, which is a significant gradient.

AORTIC STENOSIS

Aortic stenosis is an acquired or congenital narrowing of the aorta or its orifice attributable to lesions of the wall with scar formation. Congenital aortic stenosis is a condition in which there are two valve cusps versus the normal three. Acquired aortic stenosis can be caused by rheumatic heart disease or by calcification and degeneration of the valve cusps associated with the aging process. Degenerative aortic stenosis often coexists with calcification of the mitral valve. Statin medications have been shown to lower the rate of progression of senile aortic calcification, confirming that the process may have elements in common with the development of atherosclerosis.[5] Risk factors for the development of degenerative aortic stenosis include atherosclerosis, diabetes, and hypertension.[5]

Pathophysiology

In the setting of aortic stenosis, the left ventricle hypertrophies over time, maintaining an adequate cardiac output. Eventually, the valve becomes critically stenotic and cardiac output will fall. Severe aortic stenosis is defined as a peak systolic pressure gradient greater than 40 mm Hg and a valve area less than 1 cm^2, or less than one fourth of the normal aortic valve area (3 to 4 cm^2).[4,5] Fig. 6.11 illustrates the pressure gradient that occurs with aortic stenosis. The left ventricle may develop a concentric hypertrophy as an adaptive response to the higher intracavitary pressures. Coronary blood flow may be reduced in relationship to the increased muscle mass. Additionally, as the heart rate increases with exercise, maldistribution of blood flow may occur, resulting in ischemia and the onset of chest pain.[4]

The left atrial waveform will have large "a" waves reflecting the higher end-diastolic pressure in the left ventricle. Atrial contraction is very important in the setting of aortic stenosis, as it serves to increase the left ventricular end diastolic pressure (LVEDP) and support the pressure needed to eject the stroke volume. The cardiac output is generally normal at rest and will usually be diminished during exercise.[5]

Testing

The ECG may show signs of left ventricular and left atrial hypertrophy. The chest x-ray may reveal a heart that is slightly enlarged, with rounding of the left ventricular border and apex.[5] Left heart angiography is associated with some risk in these patients, in that it may be difficult to introduce a catheter across the valve if significant stenosis is present. Also, the injection of a large bolus of dye into a high-pressure left ventricle can be hazardous because of the negative inotropic effect of the dye. Therefore left ventriculography is recommended only when noninvasive tests are inconclusive.[4] Right heart catheterization may be performed to assess the presence of pulmonary and right-sided hypertension.[5]

Echocardiography is considered to be the best assessment tool for aortic stenosis.[5] It provides reliable information about dimensions of the left ventricle and atrium, the size of the valve orifice, pressure gradients across the valve, and the dilation of the aortic root.

Signs and Symptoms

A murmur is often the first and only sign of aortic stenosis.[31] As the valve becomes more stenotic, the patient will begin to complain of dyspnea, angina, and dizziness or near-syncopal episodes. When the valve becomes critically narrowed, these patients are at risk for sudden death. The onset of atrial fibrillation with the loss of the atrial contribution to ventricular filling can cause syncope or sudden death.[31]

With senile aortic stenosis, the onset of symptoms usually occurs in the fifth or sixth decade. Patients will begin to experience shortness of breath with exertion, angina, syncope, and heart failure.[5] The arterial pulse waveform is characterized by *pulsus parvus et tardus,* in which the pressure rises slowly and is sustained (Fig. 6.12). Aortic stenosis produces a systolic murmur heard best at the base of the heart, and may also be transmitted to the carotids.[5]

Management

Patients with aortic stenosis should be instructed to immediately report any onset of symptoms (angina, exertional dyspnea, dizziness, syncope), as well as to avoid vigorous physical activity.[5] Patients need to receive instruction about bacterial endocarditis prophylaxis. They should be followed closely with echocardiographic evaluations every 6 to 12 months, depending on the severity.[5] Generally, medical therapy offers very little for these patients. Therefore surgery becomes the treatment of choice for symptomatic patients (Class I recommendation).[4]

Surgical intervention usually involves replacement of the valve, although in some instances the valve may be repaired. The average perioperative mortality rate associated with isolated aortic valve replacement is 3% to 4%.[4] Since many of these patients are older, research has been done to determine outcomes and quality of life of these patients following surgery.[31] Investigators have demonstrated that outcomes of individuals beyond 80 years of age undergoing aortic valve replacement were associated with a 30-day mortality rate of 11%.[43] Survival at 1 year and 5 years was 80% and 55%, respectively, and quality of life assessments were comparable to those predicted for the general population older than 75 years.[31] It was concluded that surgery should not be withheld from older adults if age is the only determining factor.[43]

The Ross procedure is a surgical option for some adult patients who have isolated aortic valve stenosis. This procedure was first described by Donald Ross in 1967 and is done primarily in children. Recently, there has been growing acceptance of performing this procedure in adults up to 60 years and older. Additionally, it has proven to be beneficial for women of child-bearing age.[31,33] The procedure involves the removal of the native aortic root, aortic valve, pulmonic valve, and pulmonary artery root. The native pulmonary valve is implanted in the aortic position (autograft), and the coronary arteries are reimplanted into the trunk of the newly implanted root. A prosthetic tissue (homograft) is implanted in the pulmonic position (Fig. 6.13).[39] Preoperative evaluation includes right and left cardiac catheterization, as well as transesophageal echocardiography for the purpose of assessing the structure and size of the aortic and pulmonic valves. During the surgery, care must be taken to avoid injury to the coronary arteries, specifically the left main and left anterior descending coronary arteries. The left main coronary artery is near the posterior surface of the pulmonary artery, and the first septal branch of the left anterior descending coronary artery is adjacent to the pulmonary artery outflow tract.[39] Postoperatively patient management is similar to that of any patient undergoing cardiac surgery.

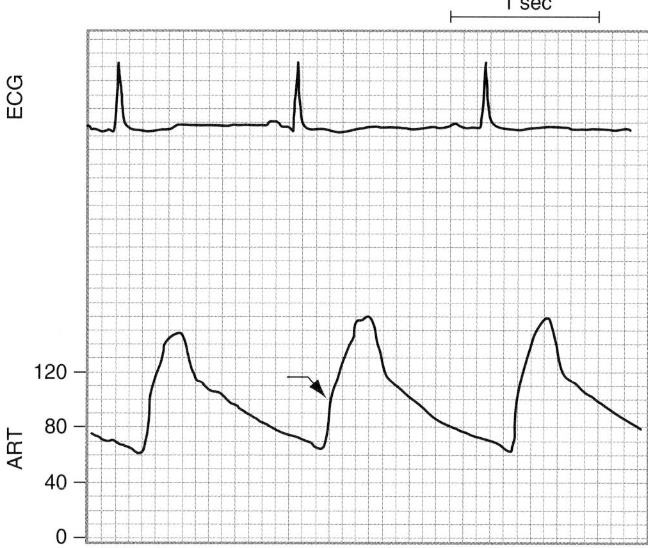

FIG. 6.12 Arterial pressure waveform demonstrating aortic stenosis. The slurred upstroke of the systolic pressure and the delayed peak are characteristic of aortic stenosis. *ART*, Arterial; *ECG*, electrocardiogram.

MITRAL REGURGITATION

Mitral regurgitation is a backflow of blood from the left ventricle into the left atrium, resulting from imperfect closure of the mitral or bicuspid valve. Common causes of mitral regurgitation include rheumatic heart disease, bacterial endocarditis, mitral valve prolapse, dilated cardiomyopathy, and acute myocardial infarction.[5]

Pathophysiology

In dilated cardiomyopathy, the mitral valve annulus may dilate, or degenerate and become calcified. Calcification commonly occurs in patients with hypertension, diabetes, or atherosclerosis.[5]

In the presence of left ventricular dilation, the chordae tendineae may stretch, causing mitral regurgitation. In the setting of acute myocardial infarction, the chordae and the papillary muscle may rupture. The posterior papillary muscle is perfused by the posterior descending coronary artery and the anterior lateral papillary muscle is supplied by the left anterior descending and left circumflex coronary arteries. Rupture of the posterior papillary muscle occurs more frequently than rupture of the anterior lateral papillary muscle.[5]

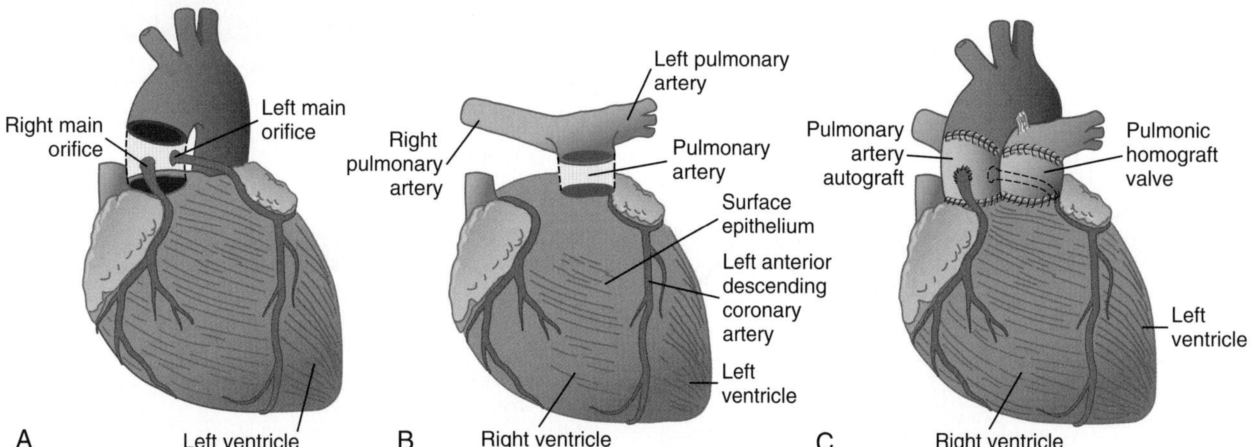

FIG. 6.13 Ross procedure. **A**, The aortic valve and aortic root are removed. **B**, The pulmonic valve and pulmonary artery root are removed. **C**, The pulmonic autograft valve is implanted into the aortic position and the coronary arteries are reimplanted. A homograft valve is implanted in the pulmonic position.

The regurgitant flow of blood back into the left atrium during systole enhances left ventricular emptying. As the ventricle dilates and hypertrophies over time, the LVEDV will increase. This process can cause the mitral regurgitation to worsen by increasing the size of the valve annulus. Eventually, as compliance is reduced, the ventricle begins to decompensate, left ventricular filling pressures start to increase, and cardiac output falls.[5]

Testing

The ECG may indicate left atrial hypertrophy and, in some patients, signs of right ventricular hypertrophy are present. Lateral views of a chest x-ray will reveal left atrial hypertrophy.[5]

Echocardiography, including Doppler, two-dimensional, and transesophageal, is useful for assessing the presence and severity of mitral regurgitation (Class I recommendation).[4] The size of both the left atrium and the left ventricle can be determined, and the regurgitant volume and regurgitant orifice area can be measured. Echocardiography has proven to be more reliable than performing left heart angiography.[5] Magnetic resonance imaging (MRI) is useful in providing accurate measurements of the regurgitant flow as well.[5] Left ventriculography and hemodynamic assessments are recommended when noninvasive tests are inconclusive (Class I recommendation).[4]

Signs and Symptoms

Mitral regurgitation produces a holosystolic murmur and may resemble that of ventricular septal defect (VSD). The distinguishing factor is that the murmur of mitral regurgitation is heard loudest at the base of the heart, whereas the murmur of a VSD will be loudest at the sternal border. Mitral regurgitation produces a large "v" wave in the pulmonary artery occlusion pressure (PAOP) also called pulmonary artery wedge pressure (PAWP) waveform (Fig. 6.14); therefore one must be careful to take the PAOP reading at the "a" wave to avoid overestimation of the pressure.

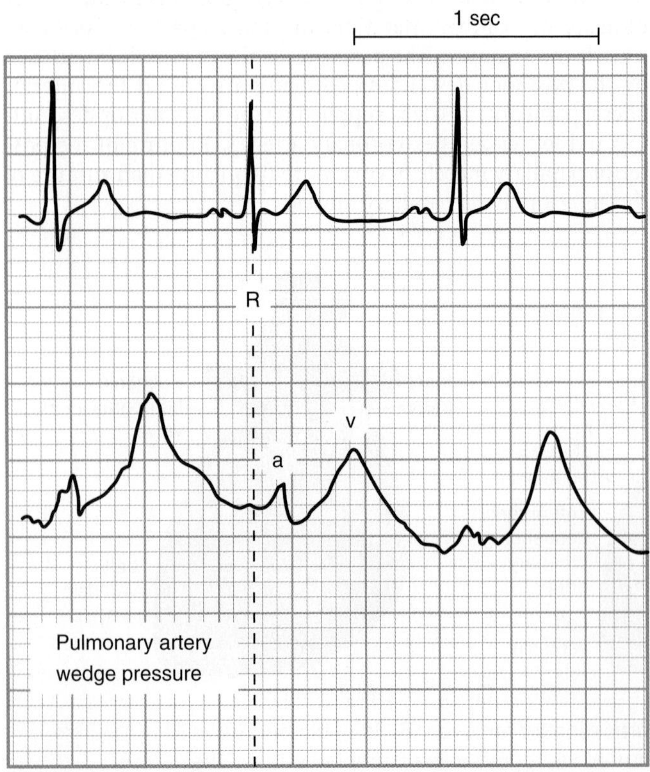

FIG. 6.14 Pulmonary artery wedge pressure tracing with increased amplitude of "v" wave associated with mitral regurgitation.

Management

Acute versus chronic onset of mitral insufficiency will determine the best medical management of mitral regurgitation. With acute onset following myocardial infarction, afterload reduction is important. This can be accomplished pharmacologically with the use of sodium nitroprusside (Nipride), nitroglycerin, or ACE inhibitors.[4,5] Use of intra-aortic balloon pumping provides mechanical unloading of the left ventricle.

Medical management of chronic mitral regurgitation is not as clear. Small studies indicate some benefit from the use of ACE inhibitors, but there has not been a large randomized trial supporting this as definitive therapy.[5] Some suggest that the use of beta blockers may be more beneficial than the use of ACE inhibitors.[5] Anticoagulation therapy should be considered if the patient has a history of rheumatic heart disease and atrial fibrillation or a history of embolism.[38] If the patient has mitral valve prolapse, anticoagulation therapy is not recommended unless there is a history of unexplained transient ischemic attacks. Table 6.2 outlines specific anticoagulation recommendations.

Surgical interventions should be considered for patients who have impaired activities of daily living (ADLs) from severe symptoms and for those who have progressive deterioration of the left ventricle.[4,5] Left ventricular EF is one of the best predictors for timing of surgery. Recommendations are to consider surgery if the EF falls below 55%.[6] The surgeon must consider whether to repair or replace the valve, weighing the costs and benefits of each procedure. Valve repair may consist of repairing the valve ring (annuloplasty) or using a prosthetic ring (see Fig. 6.2). The chordae may be repaired and the surgeon can excise abnormal tissue material off of the valve leaflets, restoring them to near-normal functioning. Data suggest mitral valve repair is applicable for all forms of mitral regurgitation and preferable over mitral valve replacement in patients with chronic severe mitral regurgitation (Class I recommendation).[4] Studies are currently underway in the United States for using a transapical

TABLE 6.2 Recommendations for Anticoagulation Therapy in Mitral Valve Disease

	Antithrombotic Therapy	Target INR
Rheumatic heart disease plus atrial fibrillation or history of embolism	Long-term oral anticoagulation (warfarin [Coumadin])	2.5 (range 2–3)
If systemic embolization develops	Add ASA 75–100 mg daily, or if unable to take ASA, dipyridamole (Persantine) 400 mg/day or clopidogrel (Plavix) 75 mg/day	
Mitral valve prolapse	No therapy is recommended	
Mitral valve prolapse with unexplained TIAs	Long-term therapy is recommended: ASA 50–162 mg/day	

ASA, Aspirin; *INR*, international normalized ratio; *TIA*, transient ischemic attack.
Data from Reference 27.

approach for surgical implantation of chordae tendineae for mitral valve prolapse.

Replacement of the valve with a mechanical or tissue valve has been performed for many decades. The actual operative time for replacement may be shorter than when the valve is repaired, but the major disadvantage is the need for anticoagulation therapy.[4] Studies indicate, however, that repair of the valve is associated with better valve performance because of the intact chordae and papillary muscles.[5]

MITRAL STENOSIS

Mitral stenosis is a narrowing of the mitral orifice, obstructing free flow from the atrium to the ventricle. Rheumatic heart disease is the predominant cause of 99% of stenotic mitral valves excised at time of replacement.[5]

Pathophysiology

Following the initial rheumatic fever disease process, the mitral valve may become deformed by thickening and calcification of the valve leaflets. The pressure in the left atrium increases as higher pressures are needed to drive flow through the stenotic valve. Eventually the left atrium hypertrophies and becomes calcified, and the left main stem bronchus rises. Over time, the higher left atrial pressure causes increased pressure in the pulmonary vascular bed, resulting in moderate, and often severe, pulmonary hypertension. Clinically the patient will complain of exertional dyspnea.[5]

The normal mitral valve orifice is 4 to 6 cm^2. When the orifice is narrowed to 2.5 cm^2, a small pressure gradient will occur, in which the left atrial pressure will be higher than the left ventricular filling pressure.[5] A valve orifice of 1 cm^2 is considered critical mitral stenosis. In this situation, the left atrial to left ventricular pressure gradient is often as high as 20 mm Hg. The clinical implication is that a mean left atrial pressure of 25 mm Hg may be required to maintain a normal cardiac output at rest.[5]

It is interesting to note that the left ventricle (LV) may remain "protected" in the setting of isolated mitral stenosis. In 25% of patients with mitral stenosis, the LV EF and end-diastolic volumes are below normal.[5] This has been attributed to the chronic reduction in preload.

Hemodynamic changes associated with elevation of the left atrial pressure cause an increased amplitude of the "a" wave in the left atrial and PAOP tracings (Fig. 6.15). Therefore the use of PAOP as an indicator of left ventricular filling pressure is misleading in this situation.

The left atrial hypertrophy will contribute to disorganized conduction velocities during depolarization and repolarization, contributing to the development of atrial fibrillation. The atrial fibrillation aggravates the atrial hypertrophy. The outcome is irreversible atrial fibrillation.[5]

Testing

Left atrial enlargement will be present in the lateral views of the chest x-ray. There may also be interstitial edema if PAOP is greater than 20 mm Hg.[5]

Right and left heart catheterization is often performed for the purpose of assessing the appearance of the mitral valve structures, the left ventricular performance, and the presence of coronary artery disease. Right heart catheterization will assess for high pulmonary vascular bed pressures.

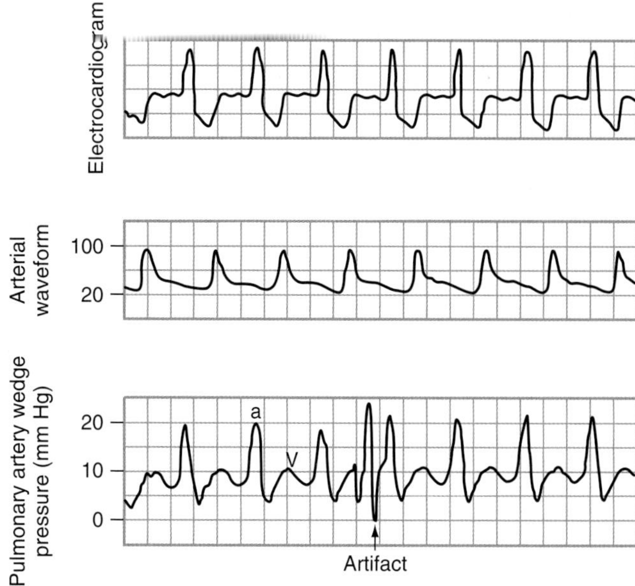

FIG. 6.15 Pulmonary artery wedge waveform with large "a" wave associated with mitral stenosis.

The gold standard for assessment of mitral stenosis is 2D and Doppler echocardiography, which provides information about the thickened valve leaflets and hypertrophied left atrial chamber (Class I recommendation).[4] This exam also provides information about the presence of a left atrial thrombus and left ventricular contractile performance.[5]

Signs and Symptoms

The main symptom of mitral stenosis is dyspnea, which may be accompanied by a cough and wheezing. Orthopnea may develop as the disease progresses, and the patient is at risk for developing episodes of frank pulmonary edema with any increase in exertion. All of these can be attributed to the reduction in pulmonary compliance associated with the higher pressures. A few patients (15%) will complain of chest discomfort, which has been attributed to a marked increase in right ventricular pressure.[5]

Additional symptoms include the onset of hoarseness caused by the greatly enlarged left atrium and lymph nodes as well as a dilated pulmonary artery compressing the left recurrent laryngeal nerve. This is called *Ortner syndrome*.[5]

Physical examination will reveal a prominent "a" wave in the jugular venous pulse. With auscultation, an accentuated first heart sound (S_1) and a low-pitched, rumbling diastolic murmur, heard best at the apex using the bell of the stethoscope, may be heard.[5]

Management

Medical management focuses on prophylaxis for endocarditis, especially if the patient has a history of rheumatic fever. Sodium restriction and use of diuretics have been shown to improve the symptoms.[5] Monitoring for the onset of atrial fibrillation is important, and, if present, beta blockers and calcium channel blockers may be used to slow the sinus rate or control the ventricular rate.[5] Also, anticoagulant therapy is indicated to prevent systemic embolization.[5]

Surgical interventions include a valvotomy, valve repair, and valve replacement. A balloon mitral valvotomy can be performed using a percutaneous approach. This has been found to be effective in younger patients who do not have marked thickening or calcification of the valve leaflets.[5] A surgical valvotomy can be performed with or without the use of cardiopulmonary bypass. This low-risk procedure is a palliative procedure, but will provide the patient with 10 to 15 years of clinical improvement.[5]

Mitral valve replacement is indicated for patients who have a mitral valve area less than 1.5 cm^2 and New York Heart Association (NYHA) Class III or IV symptoms of heart failure; it is also recommended for patients who have critical mitral stenosis (valve area >1 cm^2), NYHA Class II symptoms, and pulmonary artery pressure (PAP) greater than 70 mm Hg.[4]

TRICUSPID VALVE

Isolated tricuspid stenosis is rare. These patients usually have coexisting mitral or aortic valvular disease. Rheumatic heart disease is the most common cause (approximately 90%) of tricuspid stenosis. Other causes are right atrial myxomas and vegetations on the valve leaflets. Tricuspid regurgitation is most commonly caused by right ventricular dilation associated with right ventricular failure. When the right ventricular pressure exceeds 55 mm Hg, tricuspid regurgitation occurs. Other common causes include bacterial endocarditis, right ventricular infarction, and pulmonary hypertension.[5]

Pathophysiology

Tricuspid stenosis causes an elevated right atrial pressure (RAP), which causes a pressure gradient across the valve. If the disease becomes severe, there will also be a marked increase of peripheral venous pressures.

Tricuspid regurgitation worsens right ventricular failure. The insufficient valve contributes to an increased blood volume in the right atrium. Subsequently, the atrium delivers a higher volume of blood into the right ventricle and can contribute to further distention of the chamber.[5]

Testing

ECG changes seen in tricuspid stenosis are tall, peaked P waves when the patient is in a sinus rhythm. Tricuspid regurgitation produces an incomplete right bundle branch block. A chest x-ray will show marked cardiomegaly. Echocardiography is used to identify the presence and severity of tricuspid stenosis or regurgitation.[5]

Signs and Symptoms

The signs and symptoms of tricuspid stenosis may be masked because it is often associated with mitral valve disease. Auscultation will disclose a diastolic murmur at the lower left sternal border, which becomes louder on inspiration. Hemodynamically, the RAP is elevated, causing increased neck vein distention and an increased "a" wave on the right atrial waveform. Additional signs of peripheral venous congestion may be present, including hepatomegaly, ascites, and peripheral edema.

Generally, tricuspid regurgitation is well tolerated. However, when pulmonary hypertension is present, cardiac output falls and there are signs and symptoms of right heart failure. Hemodynamically, the right atrial waveform will have increased amplitude of the "v" wave (Fig. 6.16). The patient will have a systolic murmur that is loudest in the fourth intercostal space, along the left sternal border, and may also be heard in the neck veins.[5] It is common for the patient to have a right ventricular S_3.

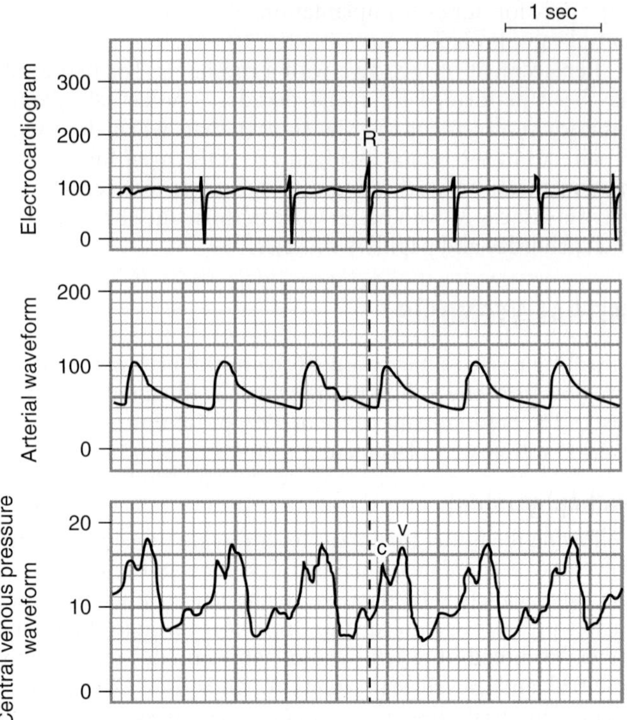

FIG. 6.16 Central venous pressure (CVP) waveform and tricuspid regurgitation. Note the increased "v" wave amplitude in the CVP tracing.

Management

Medical management of tricuspid stenosis includes restriction of sodium and administration of diuretics to relieve the venous congestion. The primary treatment, however, should be surgical intervention.

If pulmonary hypertension is present with tricuspid regurgitation, the intensity of symptoms of right heart failure is increased, and therefore more aggressive treatments should be considered. Surgical interventions may include an annuloplasty or valve replacement. Generally, an annuloplasty is performed using a prosthetic valve ring. However, it can also be done without a valve ring and is then called the *De Vega procedure.*[5] A recent study contradicts this practice of performing tricuspid valve annuloplasty, finding that the procedure does not consistently eliminate the regurgitation and, over time, the regurgitation increases.[27] The investigators suggest that these patients eventually require a high-risk reoperation and should be referred for surgery only when their symptoms are disabling.[27]

PULMONIC VALVE

Pulmonic stenosis is usually a congenital defect, and not the result of rheumatic fever. Pulmonic regurgitation is commonly caused by dilation of the valve ring in the setting of pulmonary hypertension. Pulmonic regurgitation can also be caused by endocarditis.[5]

Testing

The ECG may show signs of diastole overload, such as right ventricular hypertrophy or incomplete right bundle branch block (rSR').[5] If pulmonary hypertension is present, a chest x-ray may show a prominent pulmonary artery. An echocardiogram is useful for assessing a dilated or hypertrophied right ventricle in the setting of pulmonary hypertension. A right heart catheterization may be performed to establish the diagnosis.[5]

Signs and Symptoms

Pulmonic regurgitation causes volume overload of the right ventricle and, as a result, can worsen right ventricular failure. If pulmonary hypertension is not present, most patients will tolerate pulmonic regurgitation for many years.[5]

Auscultation will disclose a diastolic murmur heard best at the third or fourth intercostal spaces along the left sternal border. As PAP increases, a characteristic Graham Steell murmur may be heard. This is a high-pitched murmur that is loudest along the left sternal border between the second and fourth intercostal spaces.[5]

Management

Pure pulmonic regurgitation seldom requires medical intervention. Treatment should be directed toward the primary cause, (e.g., antibiotic therapy) if endocarditis is present. Inotropic agents have been shown to be beneficial if right ventricular failure is present.[5] Surgical replacement of the valve may be considered when right ventricular failure becomes severe.

MULTIVALVULAR DISEASE

Rheumatic fever and endocarditis are the most common causes of multivalvular disease. The patient's clinical presentation as well as the specific valves that are involved will determine the medical or surgical approach to be undertaken.

POSTOPERATIVE MANAGEMENT

Postoperative management of the patient following open chest valve surgery as well as those who undergo a TAVR procedure is similar to the postoperative management of any patient after cardiac surgery. Patients are cared for in the critical care unit and hemodynamic monitoring in conjunction with continuous ECG monitoring is done. Patients who have a femoral approach for a TAVR procedure may bypass the ICU and go directly to the acute care area. However, this is dependent on the facility where the procedure is performed.

Care specific to the TAVR patient includes a temporary pacemaker to be connected and on standby due to an increased risk for heart block related to the position of the stent against the intraventricular septum. Patients who receive TAVR procedures are also at high risk for stroke due to embolization of vegetation or plaque from the native valve. Consistent neurologic assessments are important for these patients. In addition to routine care, these patients also require close monitoring for limb ischemia. An echocardiogram will be performed to ensure the valve is in good position. These patients usually only require a 24- to 48-hour stay in the critical care unit.[26,35]

Immediate postoperative issues specific to open chest valve surgery patients may include the management of pulmonary hypertension and increased frequency of atrial dysrhythmias, such as atrial flutter and fibrillation. Pulmonary hypertension may be present as a complication of aortic or mitral valve disease and may contribute to right ventricular failure. If pulmonary hypertension is severe, postoperative pulmonary artery systolic pressures may range from 70 to 100 mm Hg. The use of pulmonary artery vasodilator agents may be required to lower the pressures and reduce right ventricular afterload. The short-term use of nitric oxide or aerosolized epoprostenol in the immediate postoperative period has been shown to effectively lower PAPs and improve the hemodynamic performance of the heart.

The postoperative incidence of atrial flutter and fibrillation tends to be higher in this group of patients (60%) when compared with coronary artery bypass surgery patients (25% to 40%).[11] Atrial fibrillation has been found to increase hospital costs by as much as $10,000 and length of stay by 4.9 days.[11] Valvular heart disease is associated with atrial hypertrophy, affecting the pulmonary veins coming off the left atrium. This causes electrophysiologic changes to the area and increases the incidence of atrial fibrillation. There have been many studies investigating pharmacologic prophylaxis of atrial fibrillation.[11] The use of beta blockers before, during, and after surgery has been shown to have some effect. There has also been an increase in the use of amiodarone. Atrial pacing in one or both atria has been used as a nonpharmacologic prevention. The rationale is that atrial fibrillation may be prevented by overdrive suppression of atrial ectopy. Investigators have shown that atrial pacing, regardless of the site, is safe and effective for preventing postoperative atrial fibrillation.[11]

Another difference is the initiation of anticoagulant therapy within 1 to 2 days following surgery, particularly if a mechanical valve has been implanted. The warfarin dosing will be regulated to achieve a target INR (Box 6.2). Caution must be used when initiating warfarin therapy in the older adult patient because of the increased risks for bleeding. There are published recommendations for warfarin dosing in this group of patients.[19,21,38]

Before discharge, patients should be encouraged to consider attending cardiac rehabilitation at a facility near where they reside. Cardiac rehabilitation in patients following heart valve surgery has been proven to have beneficial effects.[41] Researchers have demonstrated that women with mitral valve replacement improve their peak metabolic equivalent capacity by 19% and physical working capacity by 25%.[41] The increase in aerobic capacity in the exercise group was 38% higher when compared with a control group at 6 months and 37% higher after 12 months.[41] For most patients, participation in an outpatient cardiac rehabilitation program will improve their functional capacity and their ability to perform activities of daily living. The Centers for Medicare and Medicaid Services will reimburse cardiac rehabilitation costs for Medicare patients who have only had valve replacement.

Following discharge from the hospital, the first outpatient visit is usually within 3 to 4 weeks after the date of surgery. During this visit a chest x-ray, ECG, Doppler echocardiogram, and various laboratory tests are performed. The main focus is to evaluate the function of the repaired or prosthetic valve and assess for infection or valvular disorder. The Doppler echocardiogram will serve to provide baseline measurements for comparison of subsequent measurements.[4] Further follow-up outpatient visits are determined by the patient's needs. It is important to remember that replacement or repair of the valve is not curative. The patient must be followed carefully as with a patient before surgery. Annual visits are appropriate for those patients who are asymptomatic and uncomplicated.[4]

BOX 6.2 Warfarin Sodium (Coumadin) and Valvular Heart Disease

Indications

Prevention of thromboembolic complications associated with:
1. Cardiac valve replacement
2. Atrial fibrillation

Pharmacokinetics

1. Onset of action: 1 to 3 days
2. Duration of action: 4 to 5 days
3. Peak effect: 3 to 6 days
4. Half-life: 20 to 60 hours

Metabolism

Metabolized by cytochrome P-450 enzymes in the liver. NOTE: This implies that the risk for drug-drug interaction is high. Patients should be educated regarding informing their healthcare provider when taking new medications, including those that are prescribed, over-the-counter, and herbal supplements. Impaired renal function will not significantly affect the excretion of warfarin.

Dosing

Recommended initial dosing is 2 to 10 mg daily to achieve a therapeutic international normalized ratio (INR), usually within 2 to 4 days. Adjust the dose thereafter to maintain the therapeutic INR.

Laboratory Monitoring

Complete blood counts, INR, and prothrombin time (PT) should be monitored. Daily INR levels are obtained until the desired level of anticoagulation is achieved, usually while an inpatient following surgery. Following stabilization of the INR, the duration between tests is gradually lengthened from weekly to every 3 to 4 weeks.

Adverse Effects

Bleeding, microembolization, purple toe syndrome, gastrointestinal disturbances, and elevated liver function tests can occur. Abnormal skin reactions, including dermatitis, alopecia, skin necrosis, vasculitis, and local thrombosis, may occur.

Special Groups

1. Asians appear to be more sensitive than Caucasians to the effects.
2. Older adults are more sensitive to warfarin and may require smaller doses.
3. Hepatic insufficiency may intensify the effects of warfarin by inhibiting the metabolism of the drug. Warfarin should be used with caution in this group of patients and INR levels monitored closely.

Overdose

1. Vitamin K may be used to reverse the effects of warfarin.
2. Blood transfusions, clotting factors, and fresh frozen plasma may be administered if significant bleeding is present.

Data from References 18 and 29.

PATIENT EDUCATION ISSUES

Subacute Bacterial Endocarditis Prophylaxis

The risk for development of prosthetic valve endocarditis is greatest during the first 6 weeks to 6 months after surgery. *Staphylococcus epidermidis* is a common cause. Should valvular endocarditis occur, the infection often spreads beyond the valve into the surrounding tissue. Abscesses are formed and eventually the valve itself can dehisce.[24] There are recommendations for therapy (prevention and treatment) based on the patient's risk for endocarditis, type of organism, and resistance issues.[24,32]

Prosthetic valve endocarditis is associated with higher mortality regardless of whether it is managed medically or surgically.

BOX 6.3 Conditions Associated with Increased Risk of Bacterial Endocarditis

- Tonsillectomy or adenoidectomy
- Professional teeth cleaning
- Bronchoscopy
- Surgery of gastrointestinal tract, urinary tract, or upper respiratory system
- Gallbladder or prostate surgery
- Surgery on infected tissue

Data from Reference 17.

TABLE 6.3 Recommendations for Anticoagulation Therapy for Patients with Prosthetic Heart Valves

	Antithrombotic Therapy	Target INR (Range)
All patients with mechanical heart valves St. Jude bileaflet valve in aortic position Tilting-disk valves and bileaflet mechanical valves in mitral position	Warfarin (Coumadin)	2.5 (2–3) 3 (2.5–3.5) 3 (2.5–3.5)
Caged-ball or tilting-disk valves	Add ASA 75–100 mg/day	
Bioprosthetic valves	Warfarin for first 3 months after insertion in aortic and mitral position	2.5 (2–3)
For patients in sinus rhythm and no atrial fibrillation	Long-term ASA 75–100 mg/day	

ASA, Aspirin; *INR*, international normalized ratio.
Data from Reference 38.

Some recommend surgical management if the infection occurs within 3 months after valve replacement.[15] If the infection occurs later, medical management is appropriate. If the infection does not respond to antibiotic therapy, surgery may be required.

Box 6.3 provides a list of conditions associated with an increased risk of bacterial endocarditis. General recommendations for conditions that are associated with a higher risk for development of bacterial endocarditis are presented in Table 6.3. Patients should be instructed to contact their primary care provider or cardiologist for specific antibiotic prophylaxis (Table 6.4) that may be required. It is helpful to give patients written information about endocarditis and what their responsibility should be. The AHA has printed materials that are available for patient and family education.

Anticoagulation Issues

Patients receiving a mechanical valve will require chronic anticoagulation with warfarin for prevention of embolic events, such as ischemic stroke. General recommendations for a bileaflet aortic valve are an INR of 2 to 3, and for a bileaflet mitral valve, a slightly higher INR of 2.5 to 3.5.[38] Higher INR levels may be desirable if the patient has more than one prosthetic valve or if atrial fibrillation is present. Few randomized clinical trials have examined the relationship between the risk/benefit and INR levels associated with anticoagulant therapy. One such study that reviewed the medical records of more than 1600 patients with a follow-up of more than 6000 patient-years demonstrated the optimal INR range to be 2.5 to 4.9.[9] Adverse events associated with this target range were 2 per 100 patient-years. If the INR level was higher than 4.9 or less than

TABLE 6.4 Medications for Treatment of Native Valve Bacterial Endocarditis (Adults)

Drug	Dosage/route	Duration	Comments
Penicillin Susceptable:			
Aqueous crystalline penicillin G sodium	12–18 million units/24 hr IV continuously OR in 6 equally divided doses	4 weeks	Preferred in patients older than 65 years
OR			
Ceftriaxone sodium	2 gm/24 hr IV/IM in 1 dose	4 weeks	
Patients without Cardiac Disease or Extracardiac Abscesses:			
Aqueous crystalline penicillin G sodium	12–18 million units/24 hr IV continuously OR in 6 equally divided doses	2 weeks	Not for those with creatinine clearance < 20 ml/min or impaired eighth cranial nerve function
OR			
Ceftriaxone sodium	2 mg/kg per 24 hr IV/IM in 1 dose	2 weeks	
PLUS			
Gentamicin sulfate	3 mg/kg per 24 hr IV/IM in 1 dose	2 weeks	
OR			
Vancomycin hydrochloride	30 mg/kg per 24 hr IV in 2 equally divided doses not to exceed 2 gm/24 hr (unless vancomycin serum concentrations are not at target)	4 weeks	Recommended for patients unable to tolerate penicillin or ceftriaxone Recommended peak concentration 1 hour after administration 30–45 mcg/mL Recommended trough concentration 10–15 mcg/mL
Penicillin Resistant*			
Aqueous crystalline penicillin G sodium	24 million units / 24 hr IV continuously or in 4–6 equally divided doses	4 weeks	
OR			
Ceftriaxone sodium	2 g/24 hr IV/IM in 1 dose	4 weeks	
PLUS			
Gentamicin sulfate	3 mg/kg per 24 hr IV/IM in 1 dose	2 weeks	
OR			
Vancomycin hydrochloride	30 mg/kg per 24 hr IV in 2 equally divided doses not to exceed 2 gm/24 hr (unless vancomycin serum concentrations are not at target)	4 weeks	Recommended for patients unable to tolerate penicillin or ceftriaxone Recommended peak concentration 1 hour after administration 30–45 mcg/mL Recommended trough concentration 10–15 mcg/mL

*Therapy for penicillin-resistant streptococci including *S. bovis* and viridans group.
IM, Intramuscular; *IV,* intravenous.
Data from References 2 and 4.

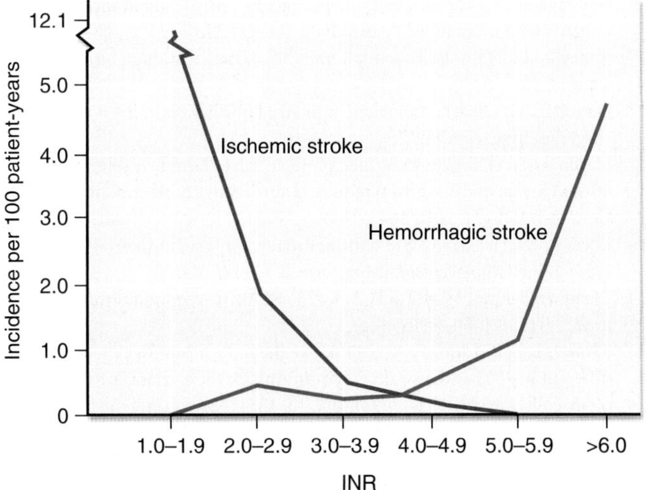

FIG. 6.17 Incidence of ischemic and hemorrhagic stroke related to international normalized ratio (INR) levels.

2.5, the adverse event incidents rose sharply.[9] Fig. 6.17 demonstrates the incidence of ischemic and hemorrhagic stroke according to the INR level. Some suggest that close monitoring by an anticoagulation clinic will help ensure that the target INR range is maintained. Others report the use of home testing of the INR and patient self-monitoring using standardized protocols may be successful.[13] Regardless of the method, a systematic approach to patient management is essential to prevent bleeding complications. Table 6.5 provides a summary of anticoagulation recommendations for patients with prosthetic heart valves.

Patient and family education about the anticoagulation regimen is crucial. They should verbalize understanding of the purpose, dosing, side effects, and need for close follow-up of lab testing for INR values. They should be taught which over-the-counter medications to avoid, and they should be encouraged to be aware of their dietary intake of foods high in vitamin K, such as green, leafy vegetables (spinach, kale, broccoli, etc.). General recommendations indicate avoiding excessive intake of these foods as they may decrease the effect of the drug.

Echocardiography Following Valve Surgery

An echocardiogram is obtained 3 to 4 weeks after the surgical procedure to provide baseline information about the valve, heart chamber dimensions, and systolic function. It is suggested that repeat echocardiograms be obtained every 1 to 3 years initially. Patients with tissue valves that have been implanted for 10 years or longer should have repeat studies performed more frequently

TABLE 6.5 General Recommendations for Conditions Associated with a Higher Risk for Development of Bacterial Endocarditis

Procedure	Recommendation
Dental, oral, and upper respiratory tract procedures	Amoxicillin 2 g 1 h before procedure, clindamycin 600 mg 1 h before procedure, or azithromycin 500 mg 1 h before procedure
Genitourinary and gastrointestinal procedures	Ampicillin 2 g IV/IM plus gentamicin 1.5 mg/kg within 30 min of procedure; repeat ampicillin 1 g IV/IM or give amoxicillin 1 g 6 h later If allergic to penicillin: vancomycin 1 g IV over 1–2 h plus gentamicin IM/IV 30 min before procedure; second dose not recommended

IM, Intramuscular; *IV*, intravenous.
Data from References 4 and 24.

because of the limited durability of the valves.[34] Other routine follow-up visits should be dependent on the patient's needs.[4]

CONCLUSION

Valvular heart disease remains a significant cardiovascular problem with serious implications if the patient is not managed appropriately. Bacterial endocarditis prophylaxis is very important for both medically and surgically managed patients. Advances in surgical techniques and the development of newer types of heart valves offer promising treatment options for patients.

Case Study 6.1

Mrs. J. is a 76-year-old female who arrived at the emergency department with acute respiratory distress and pulmonary edema. She has known aortic stenosis and reported episodes of shortness of breath during the last 3 to 4 months while walking. She denied any episodes of chest pain or feeling faint. Her physical examination revealed a loud systolic murmur, grade V/VI, at the second intercostal space, right sternal border. Her blood pressure was 156/86 mm Hg, heart rate 110 beats/min and regular sinus rhythm, and respiratory rate 32 breaths/min. Her pulse oximetry was 88%. Oxygen was started at 5 L per nasal cannula and furosemide (Lasix) 40 mg was given intravenously. She was admitted to the cardiac telemetry unit. Her echocardiogram 6 months previously reported her aortic valve orifice was 1 cm^2. She was asymptomatic at that time, and her cardiologist recommended continued observation. The etiology of her aortic stenosis was thought to be senile degeneration with calcification of the valve.

On admission, the echocardiogram indicated her aortic valve orifice to be 0.5 cm^2 with significant thickening and hypertrophy of the left ventricular wall. The cardiac catheterization revealed normal coronary arteries. She was referred for an aortic valve replacement.

The following day she received a bovine pericardial tissue valve. On arrival to the critical care unit, she was intubated and sedated. Her BP was somewhat labile during the first few hours after surgery, and albumin was given to increase her intravascular volume and RAP. She was fully awake and extubated within 4 hours after arrival to critical care

The next morning, her arterial line and PAC were removed. She was transferred to the telemetry unit. She was encouraged to cough and deep breathe, and she began to ambulate but complained of shortness of breath and the inability to cough. Her breath sounds were diminished in the lower bases, more so on the left than on the right. She remained in a sinus rhythm with a rate of 90 beats/min. During her second postoperative night, she became increasingly short of breath and anxious. Her BP increased to 164/85 mm Hg and her respiratory rate was 32 breaths/min. Pulse oximetry was 91%. The provider was notified and a portable chest x-ray was obtained. It was noted that she had a significant left pleural effusion, and a thoracentesis was performed, with 750 mL of dark red fluid removed. The patient immediately stated she could breathe much better.

Following this event, she continued to increase her ambulation and improve clinically. She was started on aspirin 325 mg daily, irbesartan (Avapro) 150 mg daily, and furosemide 40 mg PRN. The decision was made not to start warfarin (Coumadin) because of her age.

She was discharged on her sixth postoperative day on the same medications as listed previously. Outpatient cardiac rehabilitation was encouraged with the suggestion that she begin after her follow-up visit to her surgeon 2 weeks post-discharge. She continued to improve clinically and functionally with no adverse events.

Decision Points:

1. When is the narrowed aortic valve considered to be critical?
2. What are key symptoms a patient with aortic stenosis should be taught to report to their healthcare provider?
3. How frequently should a patient with aortic stenosis be seen by their healthcare provider once the aortic valve orifice is 1.0 cm^2?
4. Is sinus tachycardia common following cardiac surgery? Why?
5. What discharge instructions should be provided for this patient?

REFERENCES

1. American Heart Association. (2015). *Heart disease and stroke statistics—2015 update.* Dallas, TX: American Heart Association.
2. Baddour, L. M., et al. (2005). Infective endocarditis: diagnosis, antimicrobial therapy, and management of complications. A statement for healthcare professionals from the Committee on Rheumatic Fever, Endocarditis, and Kawasaki Disease, Council on Cardiovascular Disease in the Young, and the Councils on Clinical Cardiology, Stroke, and Cardiovascular Surgery and Anesthesia, American Heart Association—executive summary. *Circulation, 111*, 3167–3184.
3. Bloomfield, P. (2002). Choice of heart valve prosthesis. *Heart, 87*, 583–589.
4. Bonow, R. O., et al. (2014). 2014 ACC/AHA guideline for the management of patients with valvular heart disease. *Circulation, 129*, e521–643.
5. Bonow, R. O. & Otto, C. (2015). Valvular heart disease. In D. C. Mann, et al. (Ed.), *Braunwald's heart disease* (10th ed.) (pp. 1446–1523). Philadelphia: Elsevier Saunders.
6. Borer, J. S. & Bonow, R. O. (2003). Contemporary approach to aortic and mitral regurgitation. *Circulation, 108*, 2432–2438.
7. Boudjemline, Y. & Bonhoeffer, P. (2001). Percutaneous aortic valve replacement: will we get there? *Br Heart J, 86*(6), 705–706.
8. Caffarelli, A. D. & Robbins, R. C. (2004). Will minimally invasive valve replacement ever really be important? *Curr Opin Cardiol, 19*, 123–127.
9. Cannegieter, S. C., et al. (1995). Optimal oral anticoagulant therapy in patients with mechanical heart valves. *N Engl J Med, 333*(1), 11–17.
10. Dacey, L. J. (2000). Pulmonary homografts: current status. *Curr Opin Cardiol, 15, 8*, 6–90.
11. Daoud, E. G. (2004). Management of atrial fibrillation in the post-cardiac surgery setting. *Cardiol Clin, 22*, 159–166.
12. Degenais, F., et al. (2004). Which biologic valve should we select for the 45- to 65-year-old age group requiring aortic valve replacement? *J Thorac Cardiovasc Surg, 129*(5), 1041–1049.
13. Ebell, M. H. (2005). A systematic approach to managing warfarin doses. *Family Pract Management*. http://www.aafp.org/fpm.
14. Enriquez-Sarano, M. & Tajik, A. J. (2004). Aortic regurgitation. *N Engl J Med, 351*(15), 1539–1546.
15. Fann, J. I., & Burdon, T. A. (2001). Are the indications for tissue valves different in 2001 and how do we communicate these changes to our cardiology colleagues? *Curr Opin Cardiol, 16*, 126–135.
16. US Food and Drug Administration. MitraClip Clip Delivery System – P100009. http://www.fda.gov/MedicalDevices/ProductsandMedicalProcedures/DeviceApprovalsandClearances/Recently-ApprovedDevices/ucm375149.htm.
17. Ferguson, E., Reardon, M. J. & Letsou, G. V. (2000). The surgical management of bacterial valvular endocarditis. *Curr Opin Cardiol, 15*, 82–85.
18. Frishman, W. H., Cheng-Lai, A. & Nawarskas, J. (2005). *Current cardiovascular drugs* (4th ed.). Philadelphia: Current Medicine LLC, 114–116.

19. Gage, B. F., Fihn, S. D., & White, R. (2001). Warfarin therapy for an octogenarian who has atrial fibrillation. *Ann Intern Med, 134*(6), 465–474.
20. Grunkemeier, G. L., Starr, A. & Rahimtoola, S. H. (2004). Clinical performance of bioprosthetic heart valves. In V. Fuster, R. W. Alexander, & R. A. O'Rourke (Eds.), *Hurst's the heart* (11th ed.) (pp. 1723–1736). New York: McGraw-Hill.
21. Hamilton, R. J. & Sanchez, M. (2006). Oral anticoagulation management. *US Pharmacist, 27.* http://www.uspharmacist.com.
22. Hardin, S. R. & Kaplow, R. (2010). *Cardiac surgery essentials for critical care nursing.* Sudbury, MA: Jones and Bartlett Publishers.
23. Jamieson, W. R. E., et al. (2005). Performance of bioprostheses and mechanical prostheses assessed by composites of valve-related complications to 15 years after mitral valve replacement. *J Thorac Cardiovasc Surg, 129*(6), 1301–1308.
24. Karchmer, A. W. (2005). Infective endocarditis. In D. P. Zipes, et al. (Eds.), *Braunwald's heart disease* (7th ed.). Philadelphia: Elsevier Saunders.
25. Kypson, A. P., et al. (2004). Robotics in valvular surgery: 2003 and beyond. *Curr Opin Cardiol, 19,* 128–133.
26. Mark, J. B. (1998). *Atlas of cardiovascular monitoring.* New York: Churchill Livingstone.
27. McCarthy, P. M., et al. (2004). Tricuspid valve repair: durability and risk factors for failure. *J Thorac Cardiovasc Surg, 127,* 674–685.
28. McRae, M. E., et al. (2009). Transcatheter and transapical aortic valve replacement. *Critical Care Nurse, 29*(1), 22–36.
29. Messerli, F. H. (1996). *Cardiovascular drug therapy.* Philadelphia: Saunders, 1517–1521.
30. Minakata, K., et al. (2004). Is repair of the aortic valve regurgitation a safe alternative to valve replacement? *J Thorac Cardiovasc Surg, 127*(3), 645–653.
31. Nishimura, R. A. (2002). Aortic valve disease. *Circulation, 106,* 770–772.
32. Nishimura, R. A. (2008). ACC/AHA 2008 guideline update on valvular heart disease: focused update on infective endocarditis. *Circulation, 118,* 887–896.
33. Oswalt, J. D. (1990). Acceptance and versatility of the Ross procedure. *Curr Opin Cardiol, 14*(2), 90.
34. Otto, C. M. (2004). *Valvular heart disease* (2nd ed.). Philadelphia: Saunders.
35. Pannos, A. M. & George, E. L. (2014). Transcatheter aortic valve implantation options for treating severe aortic stenosis in the elderly. *Dimensions in Critical Care, 33,* 49–56.
36. Potter, D. D., et al. (2005). Operative risk of reoperative aortic valve replacement. *J Thorac Cardiovasc Surg, 129,* 94–103.
37. Rahimtoola, S. H. & Frye, R. L. (2000). Valvular heart disease. *Circulation, 102* IV-24IV-33.
38. Salem, D. N., et al. (2004). Antithrombotic therapy in valvular heart disease—native and prosthetic. The Seventh ACCP Conference on Antithrombotic and Thrombolytic Therapy. *Chest, 126,* 457S–482S.
39. Scott, C., Schactman, M. & Graver, L. M. (1997). Aortic valve replacement with a pulmonary autograft: case studies of the Ross procedure. *Am J Crit Care, 6*(6), 418–422.
40. Soler-Soler, J. & Gaive, E. (2000). Worldwide perspective of valve disease. *Heart, 83,* 721–725.
41. Stewart, K. J., et al. (2003). Cardiac rehabilitation following percutaneous revascularization, heart transplant, heart valve surgery, and for chronic heart failure. *Chest, 123*(2), 2104–2111.
42. Teremae, C. Y., et al. (2000). Diet drug-related cardiac valve disease. The Mayo Clinic echocardiographic laboratory experience. *Mayo Clin Proc, 75*(5), 456–461.
43. Unic, D., et al. (2005). Early and late results of isolated and combined heart valve surgery in patients > 80 years of age. *Am J Cardiol, 95,* 1500–1503.
44. Vahanian, A. & Palacios, I. F. (2004). Percutaneous approaches to valvular disease. *Circulation, 109,* 1572–1579.
45. Vassiliades, T. A., et al. (2005). The clinical development of percutaneous heart valve technology. A position statement of the Society of Thoracic Surgeons (STS), the American Association for Thoracic Surgery (AATS), and the Society for Cardiovascular Angiography and Interventions (SCAI). *J Thorac Cardiovasc Surg, 129,* 970–976.
46. Walkes, J. M. & Reardon, M. J. (2004). Status of mitral valve surgery. *Curr Opin Cardiol, 19,* 117–122.
47. Wiegand, D. L. (2003). Advances in cardiac surgery: valve repair. *Crit Care Nurse, 23*(2), 72–90.
48. Yacoub, M. H. & Cohn, L. H. (2004). Novel approaches to cardiac valve repair, from structure to function: Part I. *Circulation, 109,* 942–950.

7

Vascular Emergencies and Surgery

Joni L. Dirks

Patients with aortic and peripheral vascular disease are at high risk for cardiovascular-related morbidity and mortality. Fortunately, advances in medical, interventional, and surgical procedures have increased treatment options for these complex patients. Patients who undergo major vascular surgery or urgent/emergent procedures generally require critical care monitoring. Vascular emergencies occur as a result of an acute occlusion or disruption of blood flow to organs or tissues, and can have catastrophic results. Disruption of flow in the aorta may be caused by dissection or rupture of an aneurysm, whereas occlusion of peripheral veins or arteries typically occurs secondary to acute thrombosis. Regardless of the cause, prompt intervention is required to restore blood flow to the affected area and preserve end-organ function. The majority of patients who present with a vascular crisis have peripheral artery disease (PAD), a broad term that encompasses the pathophysiologic processes that alter the structure and function of the aorta and its branch arteries. The prevalence of this disease increases with age and exposure to atherosclerotic risk factors such as smoking, diabetes, hyperlipidemia, and hypertension.[3] This chapter will review the pathophysiology, diagnosis, and treatment of patients with vascular pathologies that involve the aorta and the peripheral vessels.

DISEASES OF THE AORTA

Vascular emergencies of the aorta can occur as a result of aortic dissection or rupture of an aneurysm. Although these two conditions are often described as a single entity—a dissecting aneurysm—they actually represent two different pathologies. Blunt trauma to the chest can also create a tear in the aorta. Although uncommon, these conditions are highly lethal. Aortic dissection and aneurysms result in approximately 10,000 deaths each year.[70] A significant number of patients with an acute aortic condition die before reaching the hospital.[18] For those who do present for treatment, accurate diagnosis may be hindered by the fact that the symptoms mimic other more common conditions such as acute coronary syndrome or stroke.[33,47] Treatment strategies for these other conditions differ significantly, because anticoagulants and thrombolytics are contraindicated in the setting of acute dissection. Patient survival thus depends on accurate diagnosis and rapid intervention.

Aortic Dissection

Aortic dissection is the most common vascular emergency involving the aorta, with an incidence of approximately 3000 cases each year in the United States.[61] In most cases the aortic dissection results from a tear in the intimal layer of the aorta that allows blood to flow into the medial layer, creating a false channel. The rate of pressure change in the aorta (dP/dT) created by ejection of blood from the left ventricle plays a significant role in the propagation of the dissection.[75] With the force of pressure generated by ventricular contraction and systemic blood pressure (BP), the dissection can extend either proximally or distally. As blood flows into the false lumen, perfusion to major arteries arising from that section of the aorta may be reduced or eliminated. Specific complications depend on the location and extent of the dissection, but many can be lethal, especially when the dissection impairs perfusion of the coronary arteries or the extracranial cerebral vessels (Fig. 7.1). The dissection is described as "acute" for the first 2 weeks—the period associated with the greatest morbidity and mortality. For patients who survive this initial period, the dissection is referred to as sub-acute (2 weeks to 2 months) or chronic (>2 months).[45]

Etiology

Aortic dissection occurs secondary to iatrogenic injuries, trauma, or disease processes that weaken the vessel wall. Arteries consist of three layers: the intima, the media, and the adventitia. Weakening of the middle layer, or medial degeneration, is believed to contribute to the formation of aortic dissections and aneurysms.[39] The media consists of smooth muscle cells, collagen, and elastic fibers. Changes such as plaque formation and decreased elasticity may increase the risk for dissection. Hereditary connective tissue disorders, such as Marfan syndrome and Ehlers-Danlos syndrome, affect the medial layer and are a primary cause of aortic dissection in younger people.[75] Atherosclerosis and long-standing hypertension increase stress on the aorta and are most likely responsible for weakening of the medial layer in older patients. Cocaine use has also been implicated as a cause in otherwise healthy people, presumably because of the acute rise in BP.[32] Other risk factors for aortic dissection are listed in Box 7.1.

Classification

Two types of classification systems are used to describe aortic dissections, based on anatomic location (Fig. 7.2).[18] In the DeBakey system, aneurysms are classified as type I if they involve the entire aorta; type II, the ascending aorta only; and type III, the descending aorta distal to the left subclavian artery. The Stanford system simplifies this somewhat, with type A involving the ascending or proximal aorta (DeBakey types I and II) and type B including the descending or distal aorta (DeBakey type III). The Stanford classification is widely used in determining both prognosis and a strategy for treatment.[96]

The most common site of dissection is the ascending aorta (Stanford type A), with the majority occurring just centimeters from the aortic valve.[61] Because the ascending aorta contains

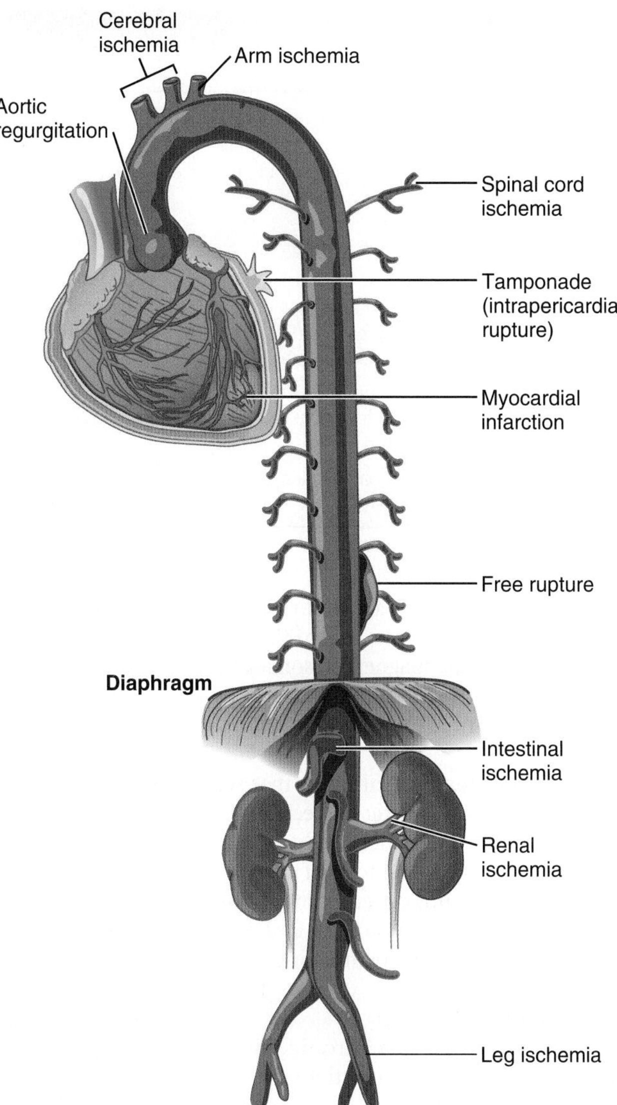

FIG. 7.1 Potential complications of aortic dissection.

important structures such as the aortic valve and the coronary arteries, patients with type A dissections are at significant risk for death from complications such as acute aortic regurgitation and pericardial tamponade. As a result, urgent surgical intervention is recommended to reduce mortality, which is estimated to be as high as 1% to 2% per hour from the time of symptom onset.[75] Generally, type B dissections (distal aorta) are considered less lethal, and are initially managed medically, unless they are associated with ischemic complications or refractory hypertension. For patients with complicated type B dissections, endovascular repair is associated with improved survival.[74]

Clinical Presentation

The clinical presentation of an aortic dissection varies with the location of the dissection, and its associated complications stem from the resultant loss of perfusion to involved arteries or compression of adjacent tissues. The most common symptom of an aortic dissection is the sudden onset of severe pain, which occurs in up to 90% of patients.[39,42,45] Pain is usually described as tearing or ripping, and is typically substernal in an ascending dissection and intrascapular if the descending aorta is affected. As the dissection progresses, pain can propagate into the neck,

BOX 7.1 Conditions Associated with Aortic Dissection

Atherosclerosis
Chronic hypertension
Congenital heart defects
- Bicuspid aortic valve
- Coarctation of the aorta

Connective tissue disorders
- Marfan syndrome
- Ehlers-Danlos syndrome
- Loeys-Dietz syndrome

Vascular inflammation
- Giant cell arteritis
- Takayasu's arteritis

Trauma
- Motor vehicle crashes
- Falls
- High-intensity weight lifting

Iatrogenic events
- Cardiac catheterization
- Cannulation for cardiopulmonary bypass
- Aortic cross-clamping

Crack-cocaine use
Pregnancy (rare)

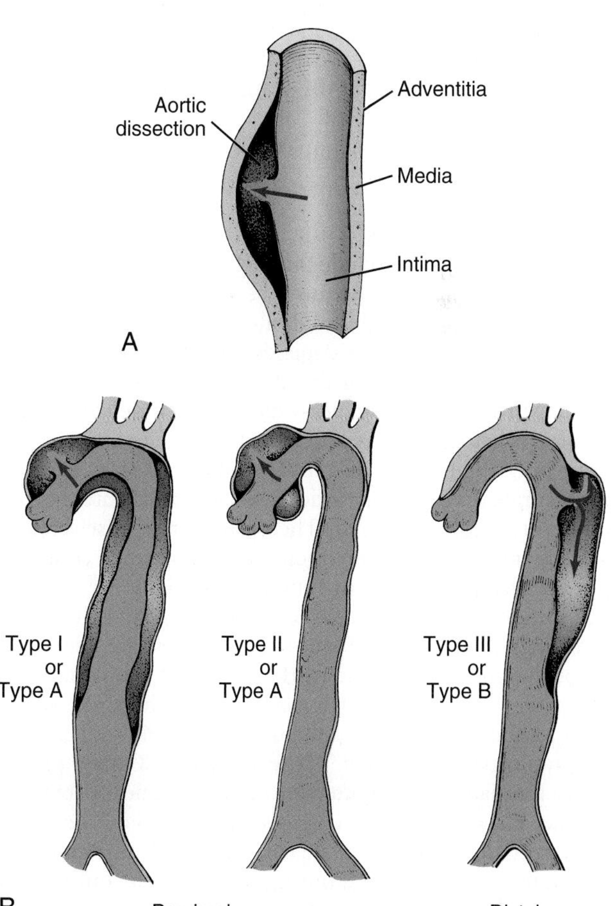

FIG. 7.2 **A,** Separation of vascular layers. **B,** Stanford (types A and B) and DeBakey (types I, II, III) classifications of aortic dissections. Types I and II are in the proximal aorta and type III is in the distal aorta. Arrows indicate path of blood flow. (From Urden, L.D., Stacy, K.M., & Lough, M.E. (2014). *Critical care nursing* (7th ed.). St Louis: Mosby.)

TABLE 7.1 Potential Signs and Symptoms of Aortic Dissection

Location of Dissection	Impairment/Problem	Symptoms
Ascending aorta	Damage to aortic valve Impaired coronary blood flow Cardiac tamponade Laryngeal nerve compression Bleeding into pleural space	Diastolic murmur Chest pain indicative of MI Muffled heart sounds, *pulsus paradoxus,* JVD, hypotension Hoarseness Dyspnea, hemothorax
Aortic arch	Reduced blood flow to brain Interruption of cervical sympathetic ganglia Impaired brachiocephalic flow	Syncope, altered mental status Ptosis, miosis, anhidrosis (Horner syndrome) Blood pressure differential, asymmetric pulses in upper extremities
Descending aorta	Spinal cord ischemia Mesenteric artery ischemia	Limb paresthesia or paralysis Acute abdominal pain, melena, hyperactive bowel sounds
Thoracoabdominal aorta	Renal artery ischemia Lower limb ischemia	Flank pain, oliguria Diminished or absent pulses in lower extremities

JVD, Jugular venous distention; *MI,* myocardial infarction.

lower back, abdomen, or flanks. Hypertension is present in up to 70% of patients with descending aneurysms, but hypotension may occur in up to 25% of ascending aneurysms, secondary to aortic insufficiency, cardiac tamponade, or myocardial infarction.[33] A diastolic murmur secondary to aortic regurgitation may be present in up to 50% of patients with dissection of the ascending aorta.[18] If the dissection involves the brachiocephalic vessels, significant BP variation between the arms (> 20 mm Hg) may be present. Table 7.1 outlines other possible symptoms based on the location of the dissection.

Diagnostic Tests

In a patient with suspected aortic dissection, one of the first priorities is to confirm or exclude the diagnosis so that appropriate therapy can be initiated. Because the presenting symptoms of aortic dissection are variable and often shared by other pathologies, an accurate diagnosis depends on clinicians maintaining a high level of suspicion for this disorder.[47] Physical examination may provide helpful clues—such as pulse deficits or focal neurologic deficits—but is generally not sufficient to prove the diagnosis.[95] A number of diagnostic studies can be used to facilitate accurate diagnosis of aortic dissection, and more than one study is frequently required. The particular tests selected are generally influenced by the urgency of the patient's condition, provider preference, and institutional availability.[47,96]

Common diagnostic tests, such as chest x-ray, 12-lead electrocardiogram (ECG), and laboratory studies, are generally a part of the initial diagnostic workup. A chest x-ray may show signs of acute dissection, such as changes in the aortic silhouette or a widened mediastinum, but in 10% to 40% of cases the radiograph may be normal.[45] The 12-lead ECG may provide clues to the diagnosis, but often the findings are nonspecific. For example, a lack of ischemic changes on the ECG can be helpful in differentiating between acute coronary syndrome and aortic dissection in some patients, but if the dissection compromises flow through the coronary arteries, ischemic changes will be present. Similarly, troponin and creatine phosphokinase (CPK) levels can be elevated if the dissection has extended into the coronary arteries and caused myocardial injury.

Because of the need for a definitive diagnosis, the presence of aortic dissection is usually established by either enhanced computed tomography (CT) or transesophageal electrocardiography (TEE). These imaging studies can confirm the diagnosis of dissection by visualization of an intimal flap that separates the two lumens. Other tests, such as magnetic resonance imaging (MRI), may be used in some settings. Advantages and disadvantages of imaging tests commonly used to diagnose aortic dissection are summarized in Table 7.2.

Research is ongoing for a test that will allow for more rapid diagnosis of acute aortic dissection. A recent meta-analysis found that serum D-dimer levels of less than 500 ng/mL could be used to rule out a diagnosis of aortic dissection.[86] An elevated D-dimer level cannot differentiate aortic dissection from other pathologies, such as pulmonary embolism, but can confirm the need for urgent diagnostic imaging.

Aortic Aneurysm

An aortic aneurysm is a chronic dilatation of the vessel wall, and is typically 50% greater than the normal aortic diameter.[29] The progressive dilatation involves all three layers of the vasculature, and may occur in one or more segments of the aorta. As the aneurysm increases in size, the vessel wall weakens, and the chance of rupture increases. The size of the aneurysm has proved to be the major risk factor for dissection, rupture, and, ultimately, survival.[25] As a result, patients with known aneurysms are followed with serial exams to determine the need for elective repair. Mortality levels from ruptured aneurysms are estimated to be as high as 90%, and emergent repair is the only chance for survival.[51,92]

Aneurysms are generally described based on their position in the aorta. Thoracic aneurysms occur in sections of the aorta above the diaphragm. Those that begin in the thorax but extend distally below the level of the diaphragm are referred to as *thoracoabdominal.* Abdominal aneurysms occur below the diaphragm and may be located either above (suprarenal) or below (infrarenal) the renal arteries. Aneurysms may be further described based on their morphology, which includes either fusiform or saccular. Fusiform aneurysms are symmetrical and involve the entire circumference of the aorta, whereas saccular aneurysms involve a local ballooning of a portion of the vessel wall.

Thoracic aneurysms may occur in one or more segments of the thoracic aorta—the ascending aorta, the aortic arch, and the descending thoracic aorta—and are classified by location.

TABLE 7.2 Diagnostic Tests for Aortic Dissection

Test	Advantages	Disadvantages
Chest x-ray	May provide diagnostic evidence of AD, such as mediastinal widening or pleural effusions Performed at bedside	May be normal in 10% to 40% of patients with AD[45]
Computed tomography (CT)	High sensitivity and specificity (> 90%) for detection of AD, and accuracy is increased with helical CT[45] Widely available Demonstrates proximal and distal extent of dissection	Does not provide information regarding aortic valve and coronary artery involvement Requires use of IV contrast for improved accuracy
Magnetic resonance imaging (MRI)	Multiple views facilitate determination of extent of aortic dissection and assessment of branch vessels Allows for evaluation of complications of AD, such as AR MRI contrasts are less nephrotoxic	Not available on an emergent basis in some institutions Requires more time than CT May interfere with monitoring and medication infusions in unstable patients Contraindicated in patients with metallic implants, such as pacemakers
Transesophageal echocardiogram (TEE)	Complete visualization of ascending and descending aorta Allows for assessment of complications of AD, such as AR and status of LV function Performed at bedside No radiation or contrast exposure	Does not allow for visualization of abdominal aorta Requires use of procedural sedation that may induce hypotension Operator-dependent Contraindicated in patients with esophageal varices or strictures
Transthoracic echocardiogram (TTE)	Noninvasive Performed at bedside No sedation required	Limited visualization of descending thoracic aorta Suboptimal studies in obese patients and those with pulmonary emphysema

AD, Aortic dissection; *AR*, aortic regurgitation; *IV*, intravenous; *LV*, left ventricle.

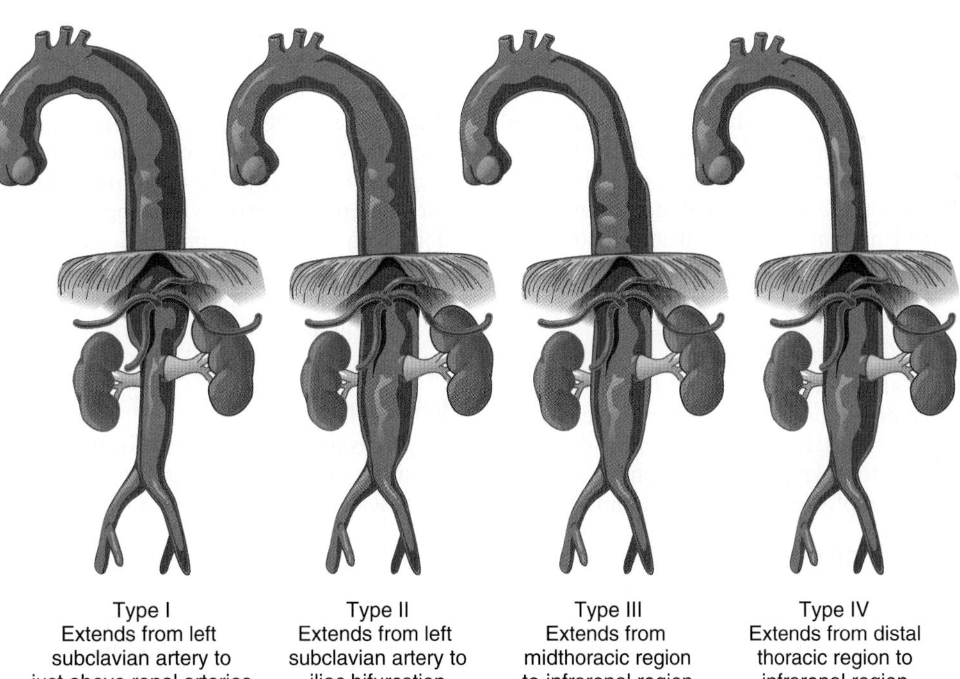
Type I
Extends from left subclavian artery to just above renal arteries
Type II
Extends from left subclavian artery to iliac bifurcation
Type III
Extends from midthoracic region to infrarenal region
Type IV
Extends from distal thoracic region to infrarenal region

FIG. 7.3 Crawford classification of thoracoabdominal aneurysms.

When the aneurysm involves the aortic root, the term *annuloaortic ectasia* is used. Crawford and colleagues developed a system for classifying thoracoabdominal aneurysms based on the extent of the aneurysm (Fig. 7.3).[26] This classification has proved useful in defining treatment modalities, potential complications, and mortality associated with operative repair for various types of thoracoabdominal aneurysms.

Abdominal aortic aneurysms (AAAs) are much more common than thoracic aneurysms, with the infrarenal location being the most common site.[51] Age is considered an important risk factor, with one study revealing an incidence of 5% in men over the age of 65 screened by ultrasound.[71] While AAAs are less common in women, the risk of rupture is four times greater in women than in men.[68] For this reason, current guidelines suggest that elective repair of aneurysms in women should be performed earlier than in men, when the aneurysm diameter is less than 5.5 cm.[25,103]

Etiology

The causes of aortic aneurysm are similar to the causes for aortic dissection, and an aortic aneurysm may occur at more than one location within the aorta in some patients.[12] Although atherosclerosis and its related risk factors (smoking, hypertension, and hyperlipidemia) have long been considered the cause of abdominal aneurysms, genetics and inflammation play a significant role as well.[54,92] Smoking has been implicated as a significant risk factor for aortic aneurysm formation, and has also been linked to accelerated rates of aneurysm expansion.[59] The incidence of chronic obstructive pulmonary disease (COPD) is also more prevalent in patients with aortic aneurysms, and may be related to a common pathogenic mechanism for both diseases, specifically, elastin degradation caused by tobacco smoking.[92] Aneurysm formation secondary to chronic dissection can occur at any location along the aorta.

Clinical Presentation

Many patients with aortic aneurysms are asymptomatic; the aneurysm is detected during a routine chest x-ray or imaging study performed for some other reason. Patients may present with pain in the chest, back, or flank, depending on the location of the aneurysm. Other symptoms may result from compression of adjacent structures because of the size of the aneurysm, or ischemia secondary to altered perfusion. Rupture of the aneurysm is generally associated with an abrupt onset of pain, unrelieved by changes in position. A ruptured thoracic aneurysm produces symptoms similar to those of an aortic dissection. The classic symptoms of a ruptured abdominal aneurysm include sudden onset of severe abdominal pain, hypotension, and the presence of a palpable pulsatile mass. It is recommended that patients who present with these symptoms undergo immediate surgical evaluation.[6] Unfortunately, this diagnostic triad of symptoms is only present in approximately half of patients.[8]

Diagnostic Tests

A number of imaging tests can be performed to define the size and extent of an aortic aneurysm. Ultrasound of the aorta is preferred for initial diagnosis because it is noninvasive and is readily available in most settings. If time permits, more detailed studies such as computed tomography angiography (CTA) or magnetic resonance angiography (MRA) can be obtained.

Traumatic Injury to the Aorta

Tears in the aorta may result from blunt trauma to the chest, such as a motor vehicle accident or a fall from a significant height. The tear usually occurs at the aortic isthmus—the junction between the aortic arch and the descending aorta—or the aortic root.[66] This type of injury carries a high mortality, as 80% to 85% of patients die at the scene of the accident or in transport, usually secondary to pericardial tamponade or massive exsanguination.[23] If the rupture is contained by the adventitial layer of the aorta, the chance for initial survival is much improved.[66]

Clinical Symptoms

Patients who survive to reach the emergency department may have signs of hypovolemic shock, as well as evidence of injury to the ascending aorta (aortic valve insufficiency, coronary artery ischemia, and tamponade) and impaired perfusion through the main branches of the thoracic aorta (upper extremity or cerebral ischemia). In addition, there may be signs of trauma to the chest wall such as bruising and fractures of the ribs or sternum. A chest x-ray may indicate a widened mediastinum and hemothorax. If the patient's condition allows, the diagnosis can be confirmed by CT angiography. Urgent intervention with open surgery was once thought to be the only option for survival, but since 2006 there has been a shift to endovascular repair, with resultant decreases in mortality and procedure-related paraplegia.[66] If definitive therapy is delayed, strict control of BP is needed to reduce further stress on the injured aorta.

TREATMENT STRATEGIES FOR AORTIC DISEASE

Treatment options for aortic disease include open surgical or endovascular repair or medical management. Because disease of the aorta is progressive, lifestyle modification and ongoing surveillance are also essential components of care in this patient population.

Surgical Treatment

Surgery on the aorta may be performed for dissection, aneurysm, or traumatic tears. For dissections, surgery involves resecting the area of the intimal tear to "exclude" the false lumen from high-pressure blood flow, and positioning a graft to reinforce the damaged aorta.[16] In some cases tissue adhesives or glue may be used to repair the dissected layers of the aortic vasculature.[90] For aneurysm repair, surgery involves interposition of a Dacron graft and attaching it both proximally and distally to nondiseased segments of the aorta. If the aortic valve is damaged by either dissection or an aneurysm, it is repaired or replaced at the time of surgery. If the aneurysm is extensive and includes both the ascending and the descending segments of the aorta, the repair may take place in stages. Surgery for an aortic tear involves isolating the tear and anastomosing the aorta with or without a prosthetic graft. The procedure is usually performed through a left posterolateral incision with a "clamp and sew" technique to allow for rapid repair.[2] A description of some of the surgical procedures performed on the aorta is provided in Table 7.3.

Indications

Surgery is performed urgently for type A dissections, aortic tears, or any type of ruptured aneurysm. Generally type B dissections are more stable and can either be managed medically or treated with an endovascular stent graft. The exception to this is type B dissections that present with a rapidly expanding aortic diameter, or evidence of decreased perfusion to a major branch vessel, or chronic dissections in patients with connective tissue disorders.[47,108] To prevent the high mortality and morbidity associated with rupture, surgical repair of an aortic aneurysm is performed electively when an aneurysm reaches a critical size. The decision to perform surgery is based on a number of factors, including the size and shape of the aneurysm, the rate of expansion, the type of aortic disease present (i.e., Marfan syndrome, bicuspid aortic valve, or familial disease), and the general health and age of the patient.[25,47] Indications for aortic surgery are given in Box 7.2.

The risks of surgery increase with the urgency of the procedure. For example, operative risk for mortality with a ruptured AAA ranges from 30% to 65%, compared with 4% to 5% in elective repairs.[67,83] Mortality for elective repair of a thoracic

TABLE 7.3 Surgical Procedures Performed on the Aorta

Surgical Procedure	Description	Indications
Simple tube graft	Dacron tube graft is used to replace damaged portion of aorta	May be used for aneurysms in ascending aorta in patients with a normal aortic root
Bifurcated graft	Dacron tube graft bifurcates into two branches at the distal end; used to replace the damaged aorta where it intersects with the iliac arteries	Used in repairs of aortic aneurysms that extend into the iliac arteries, or when there is severe calcification of the aortic bifurcation
Composite graft (Bentall procedure[36])	Damaged section of ascending aorta is replaced with a Dacron graft, which has a valve incorporated into one end; coronary arteries are removed from diseased aorta and reimplanted in graft	Generally required in severe connective tissue disorders such as Marfan syndrome; also indicated whenever there is a combined dilation of aortic root, valve annulus, and ascending aorta, or dissection of these structures
Valve-sparing: reimplantation (David procedure[31])	Native aortic valve leaflets are reimplanted inside a Dacron tube graft, followed by reattachment of coronary arteries to graft	Primarily suitable for patients with bicuspid or trileaflet aortic valves with minimal aortic insufficiency
Valve-sparing: remodeling (Yacoub procedure[4])	Involves resecting aneurysmal sinus tissue while maintaining tissue along valve leaflets and scalloping Dacron graft to form new sinuses to reconstruct root; this procedure also requires reimplantation of coronary arteries	Indicated for use in same group of patients as valve-sparing reimplantation procedure
Pulmonary autograft (Ross procedure)	Native pulmonary valve is placed in aortic valve position, and a homograft (human donor) valve replaces pulmonary valve	Ideal operation for a young or middle-aged patient who requires aortic valve replacement; extensiveness of surgery may be beyond tolerance of unstable patients.
Staged repair of ascending and descending aorta ("elephant trunk" procedure[63])	First operation involves placement of a Dacron graft in ascending aorta, with an additional segment of graft left extending into distal lumen, like an elephant trunk; in second operation, distal end of graft is used to repair defect in descending thoracic aorta	Used for extensive aneurysms involving ascending aorta, aortic arch, and descending thoracic or thoracoabdominal aorta; first procedure is done via median sternotomy and second via thoracotomy

BOX 7.2 Indications for Aortic Surgery

Ascending aorta/aortic arch
- Symptomatic or rapidly expanding (> 0.5 cm/y) aneurysm[47]
- Aneurysm > 5.5 cm (or 4.0-5.0 cm in Marfan syndrome patient)[47]
- Aneurysm > 4.5 cm if surgery needed for AI or AS[47]
- All acute type A dissections

Descending thoracic
- Chronic dissection > 5.5 cm in patients with connective tissue disorders[47]

Thoracoabdominal
- Symptomatic or rapidly expanding aneurysm
- Aneurysm > 6 cm in patients with limited endovascular options[47]

Abdominal
- Symptomatic or rapidly expanding aneurysm[25]
- Aneurysm > 5.5 cm in low-risk patients[25]
- Aneurysm > 5 cm in women[25]

AI, Aortic insufficiency; *AS*, aortic stenosis.

aneurysm is somewhat higher, ranging from 8% to 12%.[46] For urgent repair of a dissection, the mortality can be as high as 30%. This is still considered an acceptable risk, however, as the mortality for patients managed medically is more than twice that of patients managed surgically.[96]

Surgical Procedures

Surgery on the aorta presents special challenges because of the risks associated with compromising circulation to major organs and tissues. Unlike traditional cardiac surgery, the use of cardiopulmonary bypass (CPB) may be limited in some cases where clamping of the aorta is hindered by the location of the injury. A number of techniques have been developed to minimize risks and improve outcomes associated with these high-risk procedures, including hypothermic circulatory arrest (HCA), left heart bypass, and separate cerebral perfusion catheters. The incisional approach, the use of CPB, and specialized techniques used to provide neurologic protection vary depending on the type of aortic surgery being performed.

When surgery is performed on the ascending aorta for repair of either a type A dissection or an aneurysm, the goals are similar. These include maintaining myocardial blood flow via the coronary ostia, restoring function of the aortic valve, and preventing rupture into the pericardium, which could lead to tamponade and death.[16] The ascending aorta is accessed via a median sternotomy. The patient is placed on CPB, usually via cannulation of the right atrium and either the aorta distal to the surgical site or one femoral artery. The degree of damage to the aorta and the aortic valve is then assessed. If the dissection or aneurysm involves the aortic valve, or the aortic tissue has deteriorated (common in Marfan syndrome), a composite graft is used for repair (Bentall procedure). This consists of a Dacron tube with an aortic valve sewn into one end. The graft is attached to the aortic annulus, and the coronary arteries are then reimplanted in the graft. If the aortic tissue is structurally viable and the valve leaflets are intact, a valve-sparing procedure may be performed.[4,31] Although technically more demanding, this approach is preferred by some because it avoids the long-term anticoagulation therapy required with prosthetic valves.

Surgical repair of dissections or aneurysms involving the aortic arch is more complicated, because the vessels branching from this area—the innominate, carotid, and subclavian arteries—supply blood flow to the upper body, including the brain. During repairs to the arch, the brachiocephalic vessels must first be removed from the diseased section of the aorta, and then reimplanted in the graft. This is typically performed with a period of circulatory arrest to allow for operation on a bloodless field.

Circulatory arrest is performed under deep hypothermia, with the patient cooled systemically to 15°C to 18°C—the point at which electroencephalographic (EEG) silence is thought to occur. Systemic cooling is performed through the bypass circuit until the desired temperature is reached and EEG silence is confirmed. CPB is then halted, and the surgical repair completed as quickly as possible. The goal is to perform the procedure in 40 minutes or less, because periods of HCA beyond this time are associated with increased neurologic dysfunction.[109]

During HCA, a variety of cerebral protection techniques are employed to minimize the neurologic damage that can occur secondary to emboli or from global ischemia. These include packing the head in ice, providing antegrade or retrograde cerebral circulation with strategically positioned catheters, and administering cerebral protective medications.[84] These techniques are listed in Box 7.3. Of these methods, the use of antegrade cerebral perfusion is currently believed to convey the most neurologic benefit. Studies suggest that the use of this adjunct may allow for circulatory arrest to be safely performed using more moderate temperatures (24°C), thus avoiding some of the complications associated with deep hypothermia.[62]

BOX 7.3 Techniques for Cerebral Protection

Hypothermia
- Systemic cooling
- Packing the head in ice

Cerebral perfusion
- Antegrade via the innominate or carotid artery
- Retrograde via the superior vena cava

Pharmacologic
- Barbiturates
- Steroids
- Magnesium
- Mannitol

Repairs to the descending aorta are typically done via a left thoracotomy and may be performed with full, partial, or no CPB in an attempt to minimize ischemia to the spinal cord and the kidneys. When full CPB is used, femoral cannulation is generally performed. Distal perfusion may be augmented with left heart bypass, in which a centrifugal pump is used to circulate oxygenated blood between the left atrium and a point in the aorta distal to the surgical repair. For traumatic injuries or aneurysm rupture, a clamp-and-go technique may be used, in which clamps are applied on both sides of the damaged area and the graft is quickly interpositioned. This method may also be used for uncomplicated aneurysm repairs in which the anticipated period for clamping the aorta is 30 minutes or less.[2]

The most devastating complication of surgery on the distal aorta is paraplegia, which occurs secondary to interruption of blood flow to the spinal cord. Patients with extensive thoracoabdominal aneurysms (Crawford I and II) and those with active dissection are at greatest risk, with a reported incidence as high as 20% in some studies.[106] The process for injury to the spinal cord is complex, and involves several factors—perfusion, metabolic demand, and reperfusion injury. Several interventions have been used in an attempt to mitigate the risk of spinal cord injury, including regional hypothermic cooling of the spinal cord, perioperative drainage of cerebral spinal fluid, maintenance of distal aortic perfusion with left heart bypass, and reimplantation of critical intercostal arteries into the graft. These techniques are briefly described in Table 7.4.

Pulmonary complications are the most common sequelae following surgery on the descending or thoracoabdominal aorta. These include postoperative ventilation longer than 48 hours, pleural effusion, pneumonia, and tracheostomy.[28] This is partially attributable to the high prevalence of smoking and COPD in this patient population. In addition, the surgery typically requires a period of one-lung ventilation, as well as a thoracotomy incision and the need to cut through the diaphragm to access the aorta. The use of lung-protective ventilator strategies and surgical approaches that protect the phrenic nerve and

TABLE 7.4 Perioperative Strategies to Reduce Paraplegia

Intervention	Description	Rationale
Hypothermia	Local cooling of spinal cord is accomplished by a continuous infusion of cold (20°C) isotonic saline into an epidural catheter inserted at the T11 to T12 level	Hypothermia decreases metabolic demands of tissues and increases tolerance to decreased perfusion
Steroids	Intravenous boluses of steroids may be administered intraoperatively as well as postoperatively if patient exhibits signs of neurologic deficit	Stabilizes cell membranes and inhibits inflammatory cell mediators
Naloxone (Narcan)	Naloxone infusions are administered intravenously throughout surgery	Antagonizes effects of endogenous opiates, which are believed to play a role in development of spinal cord ischemia
Reattachment of spinal arteries	Anterior radicular artery is believed to be primary artery supplying spinal cord, but there is significant variability in perfusion among patients	All patent lower intercostal arteries from T8 to T12 are reattached at time of surgery to supplement perfusion to spinal cord[107]
Left heart bypass	Centrifugal pump is used to circulate blood from a cannula placed in left atrium to one positioned in femoral artery or descending aorta	Oxygenated blood from left heart can improve perfusion to spinal vessels from distal aorta during surgery
Cerebrospinal fluid (CSF) drainage	Lumbar catheter is inserted into subarachnoid space to allow drainage of CSF to maintain a prescribed pressure (usually < 10 mm Hg)[15]	CSF pressure rises with aortic cross-clamping and may impair perfusion to spinal cord; drainage of CSF during and after surgery may improve blood flow into spinal cord, by relieving opposing pressure created by pressure in subarachnoid space

preserve as much diaphragm as possible have helped to improve outcomes somewhat.

The risk of compromised blood flow to the kidneys occurs as a consequence of the dissection/aneurysm itself, from the absence of perfusion during cross-clamping, and because of hypotension during the perioperative period. In addition, preoperative renal insufficiency and ruptured aneurysms are known predictors of acute postoperative renal failure.[89] Outcomes can be improved with adequate hydration, judicious use of contrast dye, distal perfusion techniques, and renal artery reconstruction when needed.[28]

During repair of an AAA, access is obtained via a midline incision or through a retroperitoneal approach. The latter approach is associated with a decrease in pulmonary complications.[89] In elective cases, heparinization is used to minimize the risk of embolic complications, but this is not feasible for repair of a ruptured aneurysm. Open repair consists of clamping the aorta, first proximally, to stop the flow of blood into the aneurysm, and then distally, to prevent flow of intra-arterial debris into distal arteries. The aneurysm is then incised, and a Dacron tube graft is anastomosed to the proximal and distal aorta. If the iliac arteries are involved, a bifurcated graft may be used. Cross-clamping the proximal aorta is associated with an increase in cardiac workload, and prevents blood flow to the lower body and mesenteric vessels. If the aneurysm is below the renal arteries, an effort is made to clamp below these vessels to allow continued perfusion to the kidneys during surgery. Complications for this procedure include myocardial infarction, spinal cord and colon ischemia, renal failure, and lower extremity emboli/thrombosis.[89]

Endovascular Options

Since the mid-1990s a number of endovascular options have emerged as less invasive and potentially safer alternatives to open surgical repair for many aortic pathologies. Options to restore flow through the aorta now include endovascular stents and catheter-guided fenestration, as well as hybrid procedures that combine open repair with endovascular techniques.[108] Initially reserved for patients who were deemed too high risk for surgery, studies have shown that endovascular procedures may offer improved outcomes even in high-risk patients.[37,67,74]

Percutaneous balloon fenestration is an endovascular technique used in aortic dissection to restore flow into the aorta by creating a tear in the dissection flap between the true and false lumen. A needle attached to a guidewire is positioned within the false lumen at the desired location, and a balloon catheter is used to create a tear. Although this may restore flow to compromised arterial branches, it carries the risk of embolism from thrombosis within the false lumen, as well as an increased risk for future arterial rupture.[104] An alternative is to use a fenestrated stent graft designed with openings that can be positioned to allow flow into branch arteries while maintaining patency of the aortic lumen.

Endovascular stent grafts were first used in the abdominal aorta in 1990. Initially used only in the elective repair of abdominal aneurysms, stent use has now evolved to include treatment of thoracic aneurysms, complicated type B dissections, traumatic injuries, and even ruptured aneurysms.[92] Aortic stent grafts are available in a variety of configurations—straight tube, bifurcated, and branch graft—depending on the area of the aorta that requires repair. All of the grafts are deployed via the femoral artery and positioned with the use of fluoroscopy. Fig. 7.4 shows an endovascular graft positioned in the thoracic aorta.

Generally this procedure can be performed under epidural anesthesia, with minimal blood loss. As a result, these procedures may be performed in patients who would otherwise be deemed inoperable because of comorbid conditions. Advantages of endovascular repair include lower rates of pulmonary and cardiovascular complications and shortened length of stay. Whereas the initial operative mortality and morbidity are lower with endovascular stents, randomized studies have shown no significant difference in long-term survival between open and endovascular interventions in patients with AAA.[10,13,41,60] Despite these findings, the use of endovascular aneurysm repair (EVAR) has increased, and now accounts for the majority of procedures performed on the abdominal aorta.

There has also been continued expansion in the use of thoracic endovascular aneurysm repair (TEVAR) since the mid-2000s. Guidelines now recommend TEVAR for complicated Type B aortic dissection, as well as degenerative or traumatic thoracic aneurysms, when feasible.[47] The endovascular approach in patients with suitable anatomy has reduced the complication rate by 50% for both operative mortality and spinal cord injury, when compared to open repair.[12] In addition to decreased morbidity in the initial postoperative period, there is some evidence that thoracic stents may offer improved outcomes on a long-term basis. For example, a recent study showed improved 5-year survival when thoracic endovascular aortic repair was added to medical management in patients with stable Type B dissection.[73]

There are some complications that are unique to endovascular graft repair. These include endoleaks (defined as remaining blood flow within the aneurysmal sac) and graft migration.[20] Postprocedural imaging studies are done on a scheduled basis to evaluate flow through the graft and monitor for potential complications. As a result, costs associated with life-long surveillance and reintervention are greater for endovascular repair than for open surgery.[34]

Medical Management

Patients with uncomplicated Type B dissections, along with those patients with Type A dissections or aortic tears who are

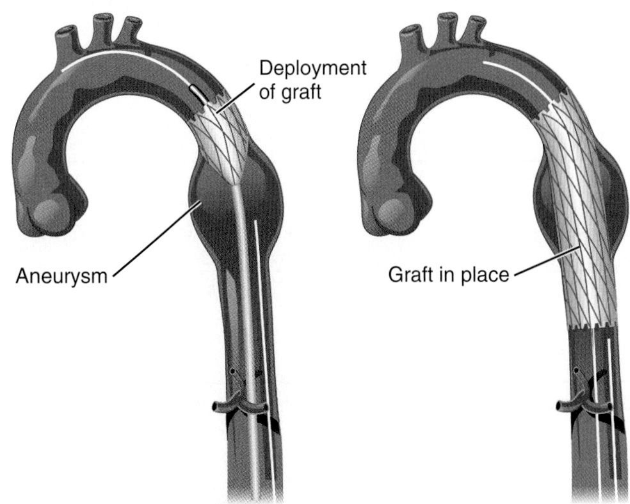

FIG. 7.4 Endovascular graft of the thoracic aorta.

deemed too high a risk to undergo surgery, are usually managed medically (Table 7.5). The goals of therapy include stabilizing the dissection or tear to prevent rupture and allow for healing, as well as reducing the risk of complications. Treatment consists of BP control and reduction in the force of cardiac contraction, accomplished initially with intravenous agents such as beta blockers and vasodilators, and later with oral medications. These pharmacologic options are listed in (Table 7.5). Long-term therapy with beta blockers to reduce the rate of aneurysm expansion is controversial. The beneficial effect of beta blockade on slowing aneurysmal growth has only been validated in one study of patients with Marfan syndrome.[87] However, beta blockers are believed to be beneficial for the majority of patients with aortic disease, especially since they generally have concomitant hypertension and coronary artery disease—both well-established indications for beta-blocker therapy.[51,91] BP control is essential, and may include beta blockers, angiotensin-converting enzyme (ACE) inhibitors, or calcium channel blockers to maintain the systolic pressure within a range of 100 to 110 mm Hg. Aggressive treatment of hypercholesterolemia and smoking cessation are also important management strategies for patients with either a dissection or an aneurysm.

Routine follow-up is performed both for medically managed patients and for those who have undergone either surgical or endovascular repair. This is to monitor for disease progression, as well as complications such as late dissection, development of additional aneurysms, and leaks from the endovascular stent.

INTERPROFESSIONAL CARE FOR AORTIC DISEASE

Patients with suspected aortic dissection or acute rupture of an aortic aneurysm are admitted to critical care for aggressive control of BP and vigilant monitoring. Frequent assessment, titration of vasoactive medications to targeted parameters, and pain management are essential nursing functions while the patient undergoes diagnostic tests and preparation for surgery, as warranted. Support of the patient and family are important in light of the life-threatening nature of acute aortic syndromes.

Aortic aneurysms and dissection frequently occur in older adult patients with multiple comorbid conditions. At

TABLE 7.5 Medications Used in the Treatment of Aortic Emergencies

Drug	Dose	Actions	Special Considerations
Enalapril (Vasotec)	0.625 mg IV over 5 min, then every 6 h	Decreases blood pressure by inhibiting conversion of angiotensin I to angiotensin II (potent vasoconstrictor)	Especially useful in treatment of refractory HTN caused when AD impairs flow to kidneys, resulting in activation of RAAS
Esmolol (Brevibloc) Metoprolol (Lopressor)	500 mcg/kg bolus, followed by infusion of 50–200 mcg/kg/min 2.5–5 mg IV over 2 min; repeat up to total dose of 15 mg	Cardioselective agents block beta$_1$ receptors to decrease contractility and heart rate, thus decreasing BP	Used alone or in combination with arterial vasodilators to decrease blood pressure and force of contraction
Labetalol (Trandate)	Intermittent boluses of 20–40 mg administered over 2 min, or as infusion at 1–4 mg/min	Combined alpha and beta blocker; blocks alpha receptors to decrease SVR and BP; blocks beta$_1$ receptors to prevent reflex tachycardia	Helpful in setting of aortic dissection to decrease BP without reflexive increases in CO and HR; may be used intravenously in acute setting or as oral agent for long-term management; maximum recommended cumulative dose per 24 h is 300 mg
Diltiazem (Cardizem)	Bolus dose of 0.25 mg/kg IV over 2 min, followed by infusion of 5–15 mg/h	Blocks calcium channels in myocardial tissue, decreasing both heart rate and contractility	May be used to decrease heart rate and myocardial contractility in patients with contraindications to beta blockers
Nicardipine (Cardene)	2.5 mg over 5 min (may repeat × 4), followed by infusion at 2–4 mg/h	Blocks transport of calcium into smooth muscle cells lining vasculature, causing vasodilation and decrease in SVR	A titratable intravenous calcium channel blocker with onset of action between 5 and 15 min and duration of 4–6 h;[104] may induce reflex tachycardia; use cautiously in patients with renal/hepatic impairment
Fentanyl (Sublimaze) Morphine sulfate	25–100 mcg IV bolus OR 50–200 mcg/h infusion 2–10 mg IV every 2 to 4 h OR 1–5 mg/h infusion	Stimulate opiate receptors in central nervous system to produce analgesia and sedation	Pain control helps prevent exacerbations of tachycardia and hypertension
Sodium nitroprusside (Nipride)	0.1–8 mcg/kg/min infusion	Relaxes arterial and venous smooth muscle to decrease both preload and afterload	Commonly used because of rapid onset and short duration of action; may induce reflex tachycardia, may cause cyanide toxicity
Phenylephrine (Neo-Synephrine)	10–100 mcg/min	Stimulates alpha receptors in vasculature to cause vasoconstriction	May be used in setting of hypotension if fluid resuscitation fails to restore adequate blood pressure; maximum rate is 300 mcg/min

AD, Aortic dissection; *BP*, blood pressure; *CO*, cardiac output; *HR*, heart rate; *HTN*, hypertension; *IV*, intravenous; *SVR*, systemic vascular resistance; *RAAS*, renin-angiotensin-aldosterone system.

a minimum, most of these patients will have hypertension (HTN) and diffuse atherosclerosis. Others may have diabetes mellitus, renal insufficiency, or chronic lung disease. The plan of care must also address preventing problems related to these conditions in order to optimize patient outcomes.

Assessment

In the initial evaluation, the patient's hemodynamic status should be assessed with the establishment of ECG monitoring and evaluation of BP in both arms. This allows for the detection of "pseudohypotension," which may occur in one arm if the dissection involves the brachiocephalic vessels. An arterial line should be placed to allow for continuous monitoring of BP. Generally pressures are followed in the arm with the higher pressure, to allow for more accurate control of systemic BP. Careful physical assessment is performed to obtain clues to the possible location of the dissection and to establish a baseline for comparison with ongoing assessments. Bilateral pulses are assessed, and a rapid neurologic assessment is performed to detect gross motor or sensory deficits, as well as signs of impaired cerebral circulation, such as confusion or decreased level of consciousness. Cardiac assessment focuses on the presence of a diastolic murmur (indicative of an incompetent aortic valve) and the symptoms of cardiac tamponade, such as increased jugular venous pressure, muffled heart sounds, or *pulsus paradoxus*. Stable patients who are able to maintain adequate gas exchange are provided supplemental oxygen to optimize delivery to the tissues. Patients with respiratory compromise may require urgent intubation. A urinary catheter may be inserted to measure hourly changes in urine output, which can provide clues to decreased renal perfusion.

Lab work typically includes hemoglobin and hematocrit to evaluate blood loss secondary to potential rupture and hemorrhage. Blood urea nitrogen (BUN) and creatinine levels are used to evaluate renal function. Cardiac enzymes can be used to detect myocardial damage secondary to involvement of the coronary arteries.

Blood Pressure Control

The initial therapeutic goal for a patient who presents with hypertension is reduction of systolic BP to the lowest level commensurate with adequate vital organ (e.g., cardiac, cerebral, renal) perfusion. Intravenous pharmacologic agents are used to reduce the systolic BP to approximately 100 to 120 mm Hg and the heart rate to 60 beats or less per minute.[47,105] Typically, beta blockers such as esmolol (Brevibloc) or metoprolol (Lopressor) are used first, with the addition of vasodilators as needed to achieve the desired BP.[47] The sequence is important, because the initiation of a vasodilator before beta blockade can result in a reflexive increase in heart rate and contractility. This response, mediated by the sympathetic nervous system, could increase the dP/dT in the aorta and lead to extension of the dissection or aortic rupture. If beta blockers are contraindicated, calcium channel blockers that decrease heart rate and contractility, such as diltiazem (Cardizem), may also be used.[63]

Hypotensive patients require assessment for pseudohypotension, which may occur if the dissection involves the brachiocephalic vessels. In this case there may be a significant difference in BP between the two arms; therefore, bilateral BP should be evaluated in a patient with suspected aortic dissection. If hypotension is confirmed, then the patient is assessed for myocardial causes (acute ischemia, aortic regurgitation, or tamponade) as well as acute rupture (hypovolemia and decreased hematocrit). These patients typically require fluid resuscitation and may need vasopressor support until they can be taken to the operating room.

Pain Control

Pain control is often difficult in the setting of acute aortic emergencies, because it occurs secondary to ischemia or pressure on adjacent organs. Morphine or fentanyl (Sublimaze) may be prescribed to help blunt the pain response, and may be administered either intermittently or by continuous infusion. These may be combined with sedative agents such as midazolam (Versed) or propofol (Diprivan), especially if deeper sedation is required to achieve hemodynamic stability.

Postoperative Management

If the patient undergoes surgery for aortic repair, postoperative care will include monitoring for complications related to the procedure. This care is similar to that required for patients following cardiac surgery (see Chapter 5), although the mortality and morbidity associated with surgery on the thoracic aorta, especially if performed urgently, are much greater.[28] This chapter will address primarily those postoperative issues that are unique to surgery performed on the aorta, including sequelae of HCA and ischemic risks related to interrupting blood supply to the distal aorta.

HCA Complications

Although patients are rewarmed at the end of surgery, they may experience a significant drop in temperature after initial rewarming and present to critical care with hypothermia. To counteract the problems associated with hypothermia (hypertension, dysrhythmias, and coagulopathy), aggressive interventions are used to rewarm the patient. The patient's core temperature is monitored continuously through the pulmonary artery catheter, and warming blankets and fluid warmers are used as needed. If the patient exhibits shivering, meperidine (Demerol) may be administered intravenously in doses of 12.5 mg to 25 mg every 20 minutes until shivering is controlled.

The extensive operative time required for cooling and warming the patient increases the risk for significant coagulopathy. Bleeding is monitored via chest tube drainage, and interventions include rewarming the patient, administering antifibrinolytic medications, and transfusing blood products as necessary. Hematocrit, platelet count, and coagulation studies are obtained in bleeding patients to guide appropriate therapy. The threshold for blood transfusion in this patient population is controversial, but many surgeons prefer to keep the hematocrit at 28% or the hemoglobin level between 9 and 10 g/dL to optimize tissue perfusion.[89] Studies suggest that avoiding blood transfusions may reduce postoperative morbidity and mortality, leading some to advocate for a more restrictive transfusion strategy (see also Chapter 26).[77]

Because HCA also increases the risk for neurologic deficits, patients are allowed to awaken as soon as feasible postoperatively to evaluate their neurologic status. After a gross assessment of central and peripheral neurologic function is performed, patients may be resedated to promote hemodynamic stability and facilitate hemostasis.

Neurologic Complications

Following surgical repair of the descending and thoracoabdominal aorta, patients are assessed for potential injury to the spinal cord.

A number of interventions are used to mitigate the risk of paraplegia. For example, the patient's mean arterial pressure (MAP) may be maintained somewhat higher than preoperative levels (80–90 mm Hg) to optimize organ perfusion, especially to the spinal cord.[11] Blood products are administered as needed to maintain a hemoglobin level that is adequate to supply oxygen to vital tissues. Supplemental oxygen is provided to prevent hypoxemia.

If a lumbar drain is placed to improve spinal cord perfusion, nursing care includes maintaining the drain at the proper level (generally the level of the insertion site) and draining the cerebrospinal fluid (CSF) via gravity, either continuously or intermittently, to maintain the pressure within the subarachnoid space at the prescribed level. Studies have shown improved neurologic outcomes when the pressure within the spinal column is maintained at 10 mm Hg.[11] Patients are also assessed for complications related to the lumbar drain (such as infection, elevated temperature, nuchal rigidity, headache, or cloudy CSF). Typically, the drain is maintained for 48 to 72 hours, but may be used for a longer period of time if the patient presents with neurologic impairment. Delayed neurologic deficits may also occur, typically preceded by hypotension, hypoxemia, or a low hemoglobin level. If recognized immediately, these deficits may sometimes be reversed by increasing MAP and draining CSF.[84]

Myocardial Infarction

Because atherosclerosis is a risk factor for aneurysm and dissection, patients with aortic disease generally have coronary artery disease as well. Patients are monitored for myocardial infarction (MI) during the perioperative period, with continuous ECG monitoring that includes ST segment analysis (see Chapter 2). Patients taking beta blockers preoperatively should continue this therapy postoperatively, as beta blockers have been shown to decrease the risk of MI in the high-risk vascular patient population.[38] Postoperative patients are also at risk for atrial dysrhythmias and may receive additional benefits from the antidysrhythmic effects of beta blockers.

Pulmonary Dysfunction

Patients generally arrive in the critical care unit intubated, with the goal of weaning to extubation as soon as feasible. Unstable patients may be sedated for a period of time, until hemodynamic stability and hemostasis are achieved. As patients are allowed to awaken, adequate pain management is important to facilitate respiratory efforts, especially in patients who have undergone a thoracotomy.

Patients with poor preoperative pulmonary function may require prolonged mechanical ventilation and tracheostomy placement to facilitate weaning. In addition, patients who have received large quantities of blood products as a result of hemorrhage from the aortic injury or a perioperative coagulopathy are at increased risk for acute lung injury. These patients may develop signs of acute respiratory distress syndrome (ARDS) in the postoperative period, and require complex ventilatory management.

Gastrointestinal Dysfunction

A nasogastric tube is usually placed intraoperatively, especially if the abdominal cavity is entered during surgery. Once patients are extubated, they can generally resume oral intake, as long as bowel sounds are present. If the patient requires mechanical ventilation for a prolonged period, a feeding tube is placed to allow for enteral feeding when bowel activity returns.

Although rare, patients may develop a paralytic ileus postoperatively, especially when an abdominal aneurysm is repaired. Approximately 10% of patients who survive a ruptured abdominal aneurysm will develop some degree of ischemic colitis, which may be limited to the mucosa or may involve the full thickness of the colon.[79] Symptoms include abdominal distention, bloody diarrhea, leukocytosis, fever, and persistent acidosis. If the colitis is superficial, it usually resolves on its own. If necrosis occurs, rapid surgical repair is required to limit contamination of the peritoneal cavity.

Renal Dysfunction

Urine output is monitored hourly, along with cardiac filling pressures such as central venous pressure (CVP) or pulmonary artery pressure (PAP), as available. Adequate hydration and maintenance of an adequate MAP are essential to preserving renal function. Daily BUN and creatinine values are helpful in identifying renal dysfunction. If acute renal failure occurs, continuous renal replacement therapy is often employed to assist with fluid and waste removal while minimizing hemodynamic instability.

Lower-Extremity Thrombosis

Following surgery on the aorta, patients are also monitored for signs of embolization to the lower extremities. Thrombosis may occur in arterial vessels—leading to diminished or absent pulses—or in the microcirculation, where it causes cutaneous necrosis. Toes and feet are often affected, and the condition may be referred to as "trash foot" or "blue toe syndrome." Patients present with painful, mottled areas on the plantar surface of the feet or with cyanotic toes. Treatment generally includes antiplatelet agents, as well as supportive wound care and pain control.

DISEASES INVOLVING ARTERIES AND VEINS

Vascular disease also occurs in peripheral vessels, most often affecting the lower extremities. The most common cause is progressive atherosclerosis in medium to large arteries. As the vessel lumen narrows, blood flow is limited and can result in tissue ischemia. In addition to chronic changes, an acute compromise in peripheral perfusion can occur secondary to plaque rupture, emboli, or trauma.

Peripheral Arterial Disease

PAD affects approximately 8.5 million Americans, and results from progressive atherosclerosis that leads to narrowing of all arteries.[70] The symptoms for this chronic disease range from mild decreases in blood flow to critical limb ischemia manifested by pain at rest and nonhealing ulcerations. Because atherosclerosis is a systemic disease, patients with PAD have a significant risk for other cardiovascular events such as MI and stroke.

Etiology

Recognized risk factors for atherosclerosis impact the onset, progression, and severity of PAD. These include smoking, diabetes mellitus, hypertension, and hyperlipidemia, with smoking posing the greatest risk.[3] The incidence of PAD increases with age, and is estimated to affect up to 10% of patients over 40 years of age and 20% of patients over the age of 70.[21]

Clinical Presentation

Many patients with PAD are asymptomatic due to the slow progression of the disease. The most common presenting symptom is intermittent claudication, leg pain brought on by exertion as a result of decreased blood flow to the muscles that is relieved with rest. Approximately 50% of patients will have atypical leg pain that must be distinguished from other possible causes such as a peripheral neuropathy or musculoskeletal disorders.[43] Patients with more advanced disease may present with ischemia at rest or tissue loss characterized by nonhealing ulcerations or gangrene.

General assessment of patients with suspected PAD should include a history of symptoms, with targeted questions addressing the presence of leg pain (quality, duration, and precipitating events) or numbness in the extremities, along with assessment of pulses by palpation and Doppler. Physical examination findings may include cool skin, abnormal capillary refill time, bruits over the major arteries, and distal extremity pallor on elevation. Other indications of chronically impaired perfusion include hair loss, *stasis dermatitis*, and thickened toenails. Since many patients present without symptoms of intermittent claudication, some groups recommend screening high-risk patients with a resting ankle brachial index (ABI), as described hereafter.[7,82]

Critical limb ischemia (CLI) is the most advanced form of peripheral arterial disease, and is defined by limb pain that occurs at rest or impending tissue loss from ulceration or gangrene.[35] Although CLI occurs in only a small percentage of patients with PAD, it is associated with significant morbidity and mortality. Within 1 year of diagnosis, it is estimated that 40% to 50% of patients with CLI will require amputation, and up to 25% will die.[35] Further diagnostic evaluation is essential to confirm the diagnosis, localize the responsible lesion, gauge the relative severity, and assess the hemodynamic requirements for successful revascularization and endovascular or operative risk.

Traditionally two classification systems—Fontaine and Rutherford—have been used to categorize the risk of amputation in patients with CLI, based on the presence of ischemic rest pain and degree of tissue loss. These systems have limitations in modern practice, since they were not originally intended for use in patients with diabetes, and treatment options for revascularization have expanded rapidly since the mid-1990s. The Society for Vascular Surgery recently developed a new, more detailed classification system to determine the possibility of limb salvage that incorporates three factors: wound, ischemia, and foot infection.[65] It is hoped that this system will provide more precise stratification of patients at greatest risk for amputation and identify those most likely to benefit from revascularization.[35]

Diagnostic Tests

Noninvasive tests can provide useful information regarding extremity anatomy, as well as the severity and progression of the disease. Doppler ultrasound can be used to detect sound waves as blood moves through a vessel. Diminished sound waves are caused by arterial obstruction. Arterial and venous Doppler signals provide important information that can be used to identify the clinical category of acute limb ischemia (Table 7.6).[80]

ABI, the ratio of the BP in the leg to the BP in the arm, has been found to be quite accurate for detecting arterial stenosis of greater than or equal to 50%. The ankle BP is obtained by inflating the cuff above the ankle and detecting the return of the *dorsalis pedis,* or posterior tibial pulse, by Doppler as the cuff is slowly deflated. Normally, the BP in the ankle is the same as or higher than the BP in the arm. The ABI is calculated by dividing the higher systolic pressure of the tibial measurement by the highest of the brachial pressures to determine the ratio. ABIs as high as 1.4 can be normal; abnormal values of less than 0.9 indicate PAD (Table 7.7). Diabetes and heavily calcified vessels can produce an artificially elevated ankle pressure, which can underestimate disease severity. In these patients, toe pressure determinations more accurately reflect perfusion.[6] Continuous wave Doppler ultrasound performed in combination with pressure measurements may also provide more accurate information about flow in noncompressible arteries.[94]

Imaging of the arteries in the lower extremities may be accomplished using duplex ultrasound, digital subtraction angiography (DSA), MRA, or CTA. Typically these tests are reserved for patients who are being considered for revascularization procedures, to identify the location and severity of the lesion(s).[43] Arteriography delineates the proximal site of arterial occlusion and provides precise information about arterial inflow and outflow. This more invasive evaluation is associated with a risk of bleeding, infection, vascular access complications, atheroembolization, contrast allergy, and contrast nephropathy. It can be useful to differentiate thrombotic from embolic disease.

TABLE 7.6 Rutherford Classification of Acute Limb Ischemia

Rutherford Class	Prognosis	Sensory Examination	Motor Examination	Arterial Doppler Signal	Venous Doppler Signal	Skin Examination
Class I: Viable/Not threatened	Not threatened	Normal	Normal	Audible	Audible	Normal capillary return
Class IIa: Marginally threatened	Salvageable with prompt therapy	Minimal (toes are involved)	Normal	Often audible	Audible	Decreased capillary return
Class IIb: Immediately threatened	Salvageable if treated immediately	Mild sensory loss (more than toes) and rest pain	Normal	Usually inaudible	Audible	Pallor
Class III: Irreversible	Irreversible tissue and nerve damage	Profound sensory loss	Paralysis and rigor	Inaudible	Inaudible	No capillary return, skin marbling

From Reference 80.

TABLE 7.7 Interpreting Ankle/Brachial Index for Diagnosing Peripheral Arterial Disease (PAD)

Ankle-Brachial Index	Diagnosis of PAD
≤ 0.90	Peripheral arterial disease
0.91–0.99	Borderline
1.0–1.4	Normal
> 1.4	Concern for noncompressible arteries

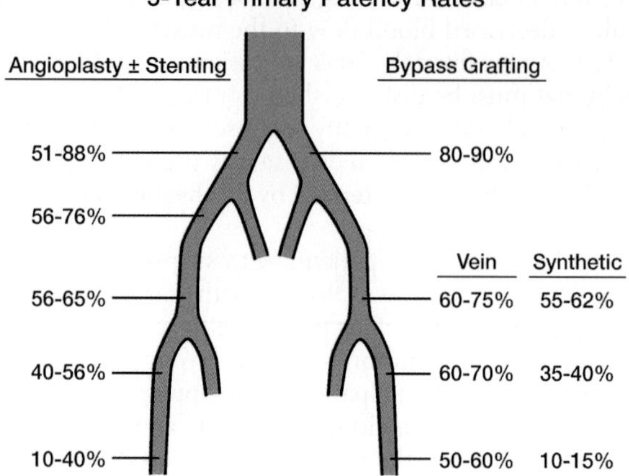

FIG. 7.5 Patency rate for peripheral revascularization. (From Shamoun, F.E., Fankhauser, G.T., & Mookadam, M. (2013). Vascular medicine: aortic and peripheral arterial disease. *Prim Care Clin Office Pract* 40:169-177.)

Treatment

General treatment goals for patients with PAD include aggressive risk factor reduction, relief from the symptoms of intermittent claudication, and prevention of amputation. Lifestyle modification and medications are vital to reduce the increased risk of MI and stroke associated with this disease. This includes smoking cessation, control of hypertension and diabetes, and administration of statins. Guidelines also recommend antiplatelet therapy (either aspirin or clopidogrel) for all patients with PAD.[5]

The most effective treatment for intermittent claudication is exercise, which is theorized to improve perfusion through a combination of angiogenesis, enhanced endothelial function, and increased muscle strength.[3] Supervised exercise therapy has better outcomes than an unstructured program, when that option is available.[56] The phosphodiesterase inhibitor cilostazol (Pletal) may be prescribed if risk factor modification and an exercise program have not improved symptoms. Cilostazol does not improve overall mortality in patients with PAD, and is contraindicated in patients with heart failure. Pentoxifylline (Trental), which improves flow by decreasing blood viscosity, may be considered as a second-line therapy to improve walking distances, although there is limited research supporting its effectiveness.[5,6] Medications used in the treatment of PAD are described in Table 7.10.

Patients with significant claudication that does not respond to treatment and patients who present with critical limb ischemia should be considered for endovascular or surgical revascularization. Outcomes of revascularization are influenced by anatomic aspects of the vascular lesions (location, size, and length of the diseased segment), patient comorbidities, and the type of procedure performed. Long-term patency rates for endovascular versus surgical procedures vary by location and type of conduit (Fig. 7.5). A working group with representatives from several societies developed the TransAtlantic Inter-Society Consensus Classification (TASC II) system to offer treatment recommendations based on specific types of lesions (A, B, C, or D).[76] This group recommends endovascular treatment for short, focal type A lesions and open surgical treatment for more diffuse type D lesions. Types B and C intermediate lesions may be treated with either modality, based on patient preference, comorbidities, and life expectancy. The question of whether endovascular treatment should be attempted prior to surgery was addressed in a multicenter trial. Results suggest that angioplasty should be performed in patients with a life expectancy of less than 2 years, since it is associated with decreased cost and morbidity, while surgical intervention is preferable for patients with longer longevity because of better patency rates.[17]

Endovascular procedures include transluminal angioplasty, atherectomy, and stenting (Fig. 7.6). Stenotic lesions from the iliac to the tibial arteries may be treated with endovascular techniques, and the choice of strategy is based on access to the site and the characteristics of the lesion.[21] Possible contraindications to endovascular treatment include lesions that are likely to cause atheroemboli, lesions that are not amenable to dilation, and patients with severe renal insufficiency who are at high risk for contrast-induced nephropathy.

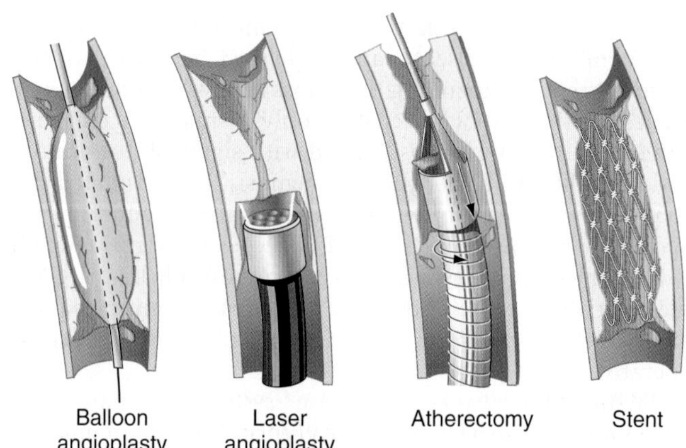

FIG. 7.6 Endovascular procedures.

Percutaneous transluminal angioplasty (PTA) is performed most often, with provisional stenting used in lesions that fail balloon dilation. Stenting may also be used in vessels that show evidence of dissection following PTA. Balloon-expandable stents are at risk for external compression, which generally limits their use to the iliac arteries. Self-expanding stents are more flexible and may offer more options for smaller vessels. Adjunctive devices such as laser and atherectomy catheters are used infrequently in peripheral arteries.[14]

Surgical intervention entails bypassing the occluded or ulcerated arterial segment by using autogenous vein or synthetic graft material such as Dacron or polytetrafluoroethylene (Teflon). Generally, vein grafts have improved patency and less risk of infection that synthetic grafts.[85,93] The procedure involves the anastomosis of the graft from an area proximal to the lesion to an area distal to the disease. Regardless of the type of procedure selected, inflow is always established first through

BOX 7.4 Causes of Acute Limb Ischemia

Embolism
- Atrial fibrillation
- Severe LV dysfunction
- Valvular heart disease
- Aneurysmal disease
- Venous embolism via PFO
- Catheter-related (air, dislodged thrombus)
- Tumor

Thrombosis
- Atherosclerotic plaque rupture
- Hypercoagulable states
- Hypoperfusion (hypovolemia, cardiogenic shock)
- Arterial dissection

LV, Left ventricular; *PFO,* patent foramen ovale.

repair of vascular defects that compromise flow into the femoral vessels. If symptoms persist, this is followed by repair of outflow lesions in vessels in the lower leg.[99]

Acute Peripheral Arterial Occlusions

Acute limb ischemia (ALI) is a sudden decrease in perfusion (<14 days) that threatens the tissue viability of the effected extremity.[76] Since there is no time to develop collateral circulation, the tissue beyond the point of occlusion suffers severe hypoperfusion. Irreversible muscle damage can occur in as little as 6 hours, so early diagnosis and rapid intervention are essential to restore perfusion and preserve the limb. Despite advances in treatment, ALI is associated with greater morbidity than other syndromes associated with PAD, with mortality rates as high as 18%.[48]

Etiology

Acute occlusion of the artery can occur as a result of thrombosis, emboli, dissection, or trauma. Thrombosis frequently occurs at the site of a ruptured atherosclerotic plaque in native vessels, but may also occur in bypass grafts. The majority of emboli (>80%) originate in the heart and travel downstream, where they lodge in a narrow portion of a distal vessel. Common causes of acute peripheral arterial occlusion are described in Box 7.4.

Clinical Presentation

Acute occlusion can cause severe ischemia with sensory and motor loss in the affected limb. Patients with acute arterial occlusion often present with a hallmark set of symptoms known as the 6 Ps: *pain, pulselessness, paresthesias, pallor, poikilothermia* (impaired temperature regulation resulting in a cool limb), and *paralysis.*

Diagnosis

The diagnosis of ALI is made based on history, presenting symptoms, and the physical examination, which should include bilateral measurement of the ankle-brachial index and pulses via Doppler, as well as assessment of motor and sensory status. These criteria are used to categorize the severity of the ischemia (see Table 7.6) and determine appropriate interventions. Patients who present with a cool distal extremity, an ABI less than 0.4, a flat pulse volume recording waveform, and absent pulses require emergent referral to a vascular specialist to prevent limb loss.

Imaging studies are performed to establish the extent of the occlusion and the status of inflow and outflow arteries, and are selected based on the clinical status of the patient. Options include CTA, MRA, duplex ultrasonography, and contrast arteriography. Laboratory and diagnostic tests should be considered to assess for possible etiology of the occlusion, including assessment of renal function, coagulation studies, and an ECG.

TABLE 7.8 Percutaneous Mechanical Thrombectomy Devices

Mechanism/Description	Devices
Suction: Uses suction to aspirate and remove the thrombus	Export Advance Pronto LP
Rheolytic: Saline instilled at high velocity through jets enclosed in catheter lyse the thrombus and use the Venturi-Bernoulli principle to create a vacuum for fragment removal	Angiojet
Rotational Fragmentation: Mechanically fragments the thrombus into microscopic fragments and disperses it within the vessel	Helix
Ultrasound: Delivers thrombolytic with low-energy ultrasound to enhance delivery into the thrombus	EKOS
Isolated: Delivers thrombolytic infusion between two occluding balloons with an oscillating wire to promote lysis, followed by aspiration of lytic agent and the clot fragments	Trellis-8 and -6

Treatment

The goal of treatment in ALI is to restore blood flow to a viable or threatened limb as soon as possible, using medications, mechanical devices, or surgery, either alone or in combination. While the patient is being evaluated, intravenous anticoagulation with unfractionated heparin should be initiated to prevent thrombotic propagation and further embolization, if no contraindications exist.[78]

Catheter-directed thrombolysis (CDT) is an effective therapy that is recommended for eligible patients with ALI (see Rutherford's classes I and IIa: Table 7.6) of less than 14 days' duration.[6,78] CDT therapy offers a low-risk alternative to open surgery in complex patients with severe comorbidities. Intra-arterial administration of thrombolytics results in better clinical outcomes and decreased bleeding complications when compared to intravenous infusion.[81]

After obtaining arterial access, angiography is performed to confirm the diagnosis, assess the nature and length of the thrombus, and assess both inflow and outflow vessels. The occlusion is then crossed with a guidewire, and a catheter with side holes is inserted to deliver the thrombolytic agent directly into the clot. Commonly used medications include tissue plasminogen activator (t-PA) and reteplase (Retavase).[27] While local administration helps minimize systemic fibrinolysis, there is still a 5% risk of major bleeding with CDT.[80]

Percutaneous mechanical thrombectomy (PMT) devices can be used as adjunctive therapy for ALI to hasten reperfusion. These devices use a variety of mechanisms to avoid the need for thrombolysis or to permit the use of decreased doses of thrombolytic drugs (Table 7.8). Of all of the PMT devices

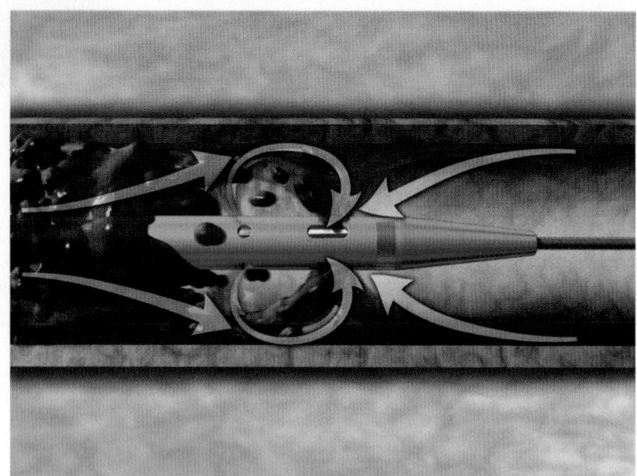

FIG. 7.7 AngioJet thrombectomy device. Saline jets enclosed in the catheter create strong vacuum at inflow windows indicated by the arrows.

currently available, the largest clinical experience has been with the AngioJet (Fig. 7.7). Technical success rates for this device range from 56% to 95%.[55]

Patients who have contraindications to thrombolytics or anatomy that is not amenable to endovascular access can be treated with open surgical embolectomy or bypass grafting. Unfortunately, surgical treatment in this group is associated with high rates of adverse perioperative events, as well as increased mortality and rates of amputation during the first year following the procedure.[9,53]

Acute Peripheral Venous Occlusions

Venous thromboembolism (VTE) refers to the formation of thrombi in the veins and includes both deep vein thrombosis (DVT) and pulmonary embolism (PE). VTE is the cause of death in over 100,000 US patients each year and is estimated to account for 5% to 10% of all deaths among hospitalized patients.[57] The majority of patients with DVT are treated in the outpatient setting with low molecular weight heparin (LMWH) or oral anticoagulants. Patients with extensive proximal DVTs may be treated with more aggressive therapy in an effort to reduce the incidence of post-thrombotic syndrome, which is associated with pain, edema, and venous stasis ulceration.[52] Up to 30% of untreated DVT may embolize and lead to a PE, a partial or complete occlusion of a pulmonary arterial vessel that can be life threatening.[95]

Etiology

Venous thrombus formation depends upon the interaction of three factors, which are described as Virchow's triad: vessel wall trauma with endothelial injury, hypercoagulability, and stasis. Clinical risk factors include dehydration, prolonged immobility (bed rest or paralysis), cancer, sepsis, cardiac or respiratory failure, and orthopedic surgery (hip or knee replacement). Additional risk factors are described in Box 7.5.[95] Most venous thrombi begin in the valve cusps of deep calf veins, but emboli may also come from sources outside the vasculature, such as air, amniotic fluid, fat, or an infectious source. Twenty percent of PEs have no identified risk factors and are considered idiopathic.[69]

Clinical Presentation

Classic symptoms of DVT include unilateral pain and limb edema, but symptoms vary in severity based on the size and location of the thrombus. For example, thrombus that does not cause a net venous outflow obstruction is often asymptomatic, while thrombus that involves the iliac bifurcation, the pelvic veins, or the vena cava produces leg edema that is usually bilateral rather than unilateral. Patients may also have red or purple discoloration of the lower extremity, secondary to venous engorgement. The most severe forms of DVT, *phlegmasia cerulea dolens* ("painful blue leg") and *phlegmasia alba dolens* ("milk leg"), result from massive iliofemoral obstruction of venous drainage and present with extreme pain, edema, and discoloration of the leg.[30]

The clinical presentation of PE also varies widely, based on the size of the embolism and the patient's underlying physical status. Pulmonary emboli should be suspected if the patient presents with sudden onset of dyspnea, lightheadedness, pleuritic chest pain, and cyanosis. Some patients may also report cough or hemoptysis. Physical exam may identify tachycardia, as well as signs of acute right ventricular failure, such as distended neck veins. Massive PE can present with severe hemodynamic instability or even cardiac arrest.

Patient history can be helpful in identifying risk factors for VTE. A well-validated clinical prediction rule known as the Wells model provides a reliable estimate of the pretest probability of DVT and PE.[100,102] These tools can be used to help guide further evaluation and treatment (Boxes 7.6 and 7.7).

BOX 7.5 Risk Factors for Venous Thromboembolism (VTE)

Patient-related	Situational
• Advanced age	• Immobility during travel
• Previous VTE	• Bone fracture
• Hypercoagulable diseases	• Pregnancy
• Smoking	• Spinal cord injury
• Hormone replacement therapy	• Chemotherapy
• Oral contraceptives	• Central venous catheterization
• Obesity	

BOX 7.6 Wells Model for Predicting Probability of Deep Vein Thrombosis

Active cancer (treatment ongoing or within previous 6 months or palliative)	1
Paralysis, paresis, or recent plaster immobilization of lower extremity	1
Recently bedridden for more than 3 days or major surgery within 4 weeks	1
Localized tenderness along the distribution of the deep venous system	1
Entire leg swollen	1
Calf swollen by more than 3 cm when compared to asymptomatic leg (measured 10 cm below tibial tuberosity)	1
Pitting edema (greater in symptomatic leg)	1
Collateral superficial veins (nonvaricose)	1
Alternative diagnosis as likely or greater than that of deep vein thrombosis (DVT)	1

Scoring

If both legs are symptomatic, score the more severe side
High risk = 3 or more
Moderate risk = 1 or 2
Low risk = 0 or less

From Reference 100.

BOX 7.7 Wells Model for Predicting Probability of Pulmonary Embolism

Clinical signs and symptoms of deep vein thrombosis (DVT) (minimum of leg swelling and pain with palpation of deep veins)	3
An alternative diagnosis is less likely than pulmonary embolism (PE)	3
Heart rate > 100 beats/min	1.5
Immobilization or surgery in previous 4 weeks	1.5
Previous DVT/PE	1.5
Hemoptysis	1
Malignancy (on treatment, treated in last 6 months, or palliative)	1

Score < 2 = low clinical pretest probability
Score 2–6 = moderate clinical pretest probability
Score > 6 = high clinical pretest probability

From Reference 101.

Diagnostic Tests

In patients with low risk for VTE, a D-dimer assay can be used to determine the need for subsequent tests. A negative D-dimer has been proven to have a strong negative predictive value for patients with a low probability of DVT or PE. In patients with a low probability of DVT (Wells score of 0) or PE (Wells score < 2), a negative D-dimer can rule out the possibility of DVT/PE, and no further testing is needed. If warranted, further testing for DVT may include duplex ultrasound with compression, or a venogram. Venography with contrast is limited by the risk of pain, phlebitis, and hypersensitivity or toxic reactions to contrast agents. DVTs may also develop in a small number of patients who undergo this procedure.

In patients with a moderate probability and clinical symptoms indicative of PE, additional diagnostic tests should be performed. This can include arterial blood gases, a chest x-ray, and an ECG to differentiate PE from alternative diagnoses such as acute coronary syndrome, pneumonia, or pericarditis. An echocardiogram is useful to evaluate for right ventricular (RV) dysfunction and may be used to visualize clots in patients too unstable for transport. Multidetector (spiral) CT angiography is the preferred imaging study in patients who are clinically stable, since it has greater diagnostic accuracy in identifying the location of emboli and can also assess RV enlargement.[24]

Classification

Once the diagnosis of PE is made, patients can be classified according to their level of risk. PE was historically classified based on the amount of thrombus in the pulmonary vasculature.[69] More recently, PE has been reclassified based on the degree of hemodynamic compromise and RV dysfunction induced by the PE (Fig. 7.8). The new guidelines define three categories of PE—massive, submassive, and nonmassive—based on symptoms of hemodynamic instability and RV dysfunction.[49] These classifications are helpful in determining treatment options and predicting the prognosis of acute PE (Table 7.9). Massive PE has a very high mortality rate within the first 6 hours of symptom onset; therefore, rapid diagnosis and intervention are essential to improve patient survival.[69]

Treatment

Prevention is the best treatment strategy for VTE, but despite strong evidence supporting the use of prophylaxis, studies show that compliance is only approximately 40% to 60%.[57] Identifying those patients at risk and starting anticoagulants can prevent thrombi from forming or extending. VTE can be prevented by counteracting increased blood coagulation with medications or by reducing venous stasis with external pneumatic compression, a venous foot pump, or graduated compression stockings.[19] In patients at moderate or high risk, anticoagulant prophylaxis is preferred. Despite intensive study, antiplatelet drugs have not proved to be effective for prevention.

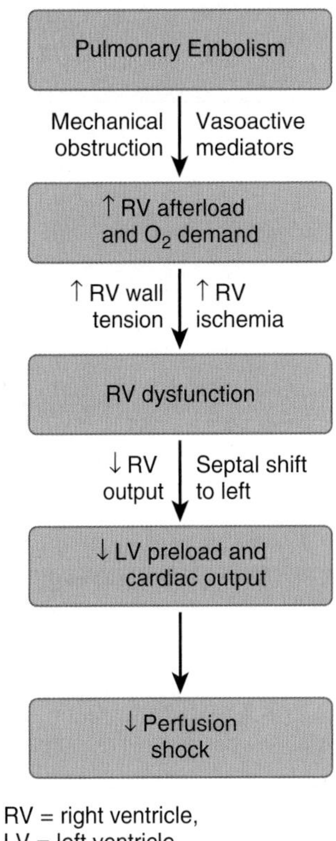

FIG. 7.8 Hemodynamic effects of acute pulmonary embolism.

In patients diagnosed with acute, symptomatic VTE, anticoagulation is the first line of therapy.[24] Unless there is a strong contraindication, parenteral anticoagulation is started with one of the agents described later. Intravenous unfractionated heparin (UFH) is indicated in patients with increased risk of bleeding or when thrombolytics are being considered, because it is short acting and can be reversed with protamine if needed. UFH is also preferred in patients with severe renal impairment or extreme obesity. LMWH is associated with less risk of major bleeding than UFH, as well as greater efficacy in preventing recurrent VTE.[102] Two new oral agents, both factor Xa inhibitors, have been approved for initial treatment of acute VTE. These newer agents have the advantages of increased ease of administration and a predictable dose-dependent response that eliminates the need for routine monitoring. Medications used in the treatment of VTE are described in Table 7.10.

Other strategies may be used in conjunction with anticoagulants to hasten clot breakdown, such as systemic thrombolysis, catheter-directed thrombolytics, PMT, or surgical embolectomy. These therapies are usually reserved for patients with clinically significant VTE, such as iliofemoral DVT, and submassive or massive PE. Rapid breakdown of the thrombus is warranted in these cases to preserve limbs or restore end-organ perfusion. In addition, employing these techniques helps to reduce the amount of residual thrombus, which correlates strongly with the risk of recurrent VTE.[49]

Thrombolytic therapy is most effective when initiated within 48 hours of symptoms, but may have some efficacy for up to 14

TABLE 7.9 Classification and Treatment Recommendations for Pulmonary Embolism

Classification	Presentation	Recommended Treatment
Small to moderate PE	Normal hemodynamics Normal RV size and function	Anticoagulation with parenteral therapy as a bridge to warfarin or other oral agents
Submassive PE	Stable blood pressure (SBP > 90 mm Hg) Evidence of moderate to severe RV dysfunction or enlargement	Anticoagulation with intravenous UFH In patients with worsening RV failure, consider systemic thrombolysis, PMT or surgical embolectomy
Massive PE	Sustained hypotension (SBP < 90 mm Hg or requiring inotropes) Evidence of poor tissue perfusion or organ failure Extensive right and/or left main pulmonary artery thrombus	Anticoagulation with intravenous UFH Systemic thrombolysis PMT or surgical embolectomy in patients with bleeding risk

PE, Pulmonary embolism; *PMT*, percutaneous mechanical thrombectomy; *RV*, right ventricle; *SBP*, systolic blood pressure; *UFH*, unfractionated heparin.

TABLE 7.10 Medications Used in the Treatment of PAD and VTE

Drug	Dose	Actions	Special Considerations
Aspirin	81–325 mg/day	Inhibits synthesis of thromboxane A2, resulting in irreversible inhibition of platelet activation	Given to reduce the risk of cardiovascular events (stroke, MI) in patients with PAD Lower doses are recommended when given with other antithrombotics
Clopidogrel (Plavix)	75 mg/day	Irreversibly inhibits the ADP P2Y12 platelet receptor to block platelet activation	Given to reduce the risk of cardiovascular events (stroke, MI) in patients with PAD Should be withheld 5 to 7 days before elective surgery to decrease risk of bleeding Some patients may have a genetic resistance to clopidogrel, resulting in inadequate platelet inhibition
Cilostazol (Pletal)	100 mg twice a day	Inhibits cellular phosphodiesterase to inhibit platelet aggregation and promote vasodilation	Contraindicated in patients with congestive heart failure of any severity
Pentoxifylline (Trental)	400 mg 3 times per day	Precise mode of action not known, but thought to improve blood flow by lowering blood viscosity and improving erythrocyte flexibility	Second-line alternative to cilostazol in patients with claudication Should not be used in patients with recent cerebral and/or retinal hemorrhage Administration with theophylline may lead to theophylline toxicity
Unfractionated heparin (UFH)	Initial bolus 80 units/kg (max dose 5000 U) followed by 18 units/kg/h infusion	Enhances activity of antithrombin III, a natural anticoagulant, to prevent clot formation	Effectiveness of treatment may be monitored by aPTT or ACT Response is variable because of binding with plasma proteins Effects may be reversed with protamine sulfate Risk of developing HIT Protamine can be used to reverse the effects
Low molecular weight heparin (LMWH) Enoxaparin (Lovenox)	30 mg IV bolus, followed by 1 mg/kg SC every 12 h	Enhances activity of antithrombin III	More predictable dose response than heparin, so monitoring not usually required Anti-Xa levels may be measured if monitoring is needed Lower risk of HIT than with UFH Not recommended in severe renal dysfunction (CrCl < 30 mL/min)
Dabigatran (Pradaxa)	150 mg twice a day after using a parenteral agent for at least 5 days	Directly inhibits both circulating and clot-bound thrombin	Not recommended for patients with CrCl <30 mL/min) Does not require routine anticoagulant monitoring
Fondaparinux (Arixtra)	Prophylaxis: 2.5 mg subcutaneously daily Treatment: 5 mg daily if weight < 50 kg; 7.5 mg daily if weight 50–100 kg; 10 mg daily if weight >100 kg	Selective inhibitor of factor Xa	May be used in conjunction with fibrinolytics or warfarin for treatment of acute DVT or PE[1] Long half-life (> 17 h) Contraindicated in patients with renal failure

TABLE 7.10 **Medications Used in the Treatment of PAD and VTE—cont'd**

Drug	Dose	Actions	Special Considerations
Warfarin sodium (Coumadin)	Initial: 2–5 mg/day Maintenance: 2–10 mg/day, titrated to maintain target INR of 2 to 3	Antagonizes vitamin K to reduce the production of factors II, VII, IX, and X	Drugs, dietary changes, and other factors affect INR Contraindicated in pregnancy and in patients with HIT
Rivaroxaban (Xarelto)	15 mg twice a day × 21 days, then 20 mg/day	Inhibits factor Xa to decrease generation of thrombin; indirectly inhibits thrombin-induced platelet aggregation	Not recommended for initial treatment of PE in hemodynamically unstable patients who may receive thrombolytics Contraindicated in patients with severe liver disease or renal insufficiency (CrCl < 30 mL/min) Avoid in patients who are pregnant or nursing Does not require routine anticoagulant monitoring
Apixaban (Eliquis)	10 mg twice a day × 7 days, then 5 mg twice a day	Inhibits factor Xa to decrease generation of thrombin; indirectly inhibits thrombin-induced platelet aggregation	Not recommended for initial treatment of PE in hemodynamically unstable patients who may receive thrombolytics No adjustment needed for patients with renal insufficiency Does not require routine anticoagulant monitoring
tPA (alteplase)	IV: 100 mg infusion over 2 h Intra-arterial or catheter-directed dosage varies	Binds to fibrin at the clot and promotes activation of plasminogen to plasmin	Anticoagulants are given concurrently
rPA (reteplase)	IV: 10 units given as a bolus over 2 min, repeated in 30 min Intra-arterial or catheter-directed dosage varies	Binds to fibrin at the clot and promotes activation of plasminogen to plasmin	Anticoagulants are given concurrently

ACT, Activated clotting time; *ADP*, adenosine diphosphate; *aPTT*, activated partial thromboplastin time; *CrCl*, creatinine clearance; *DVT*, deep vein thrombosis; *HIT*, heparin-induced thrombocytopenia; *INR*, international normalized ratio; *IV*, intravenous; *MI*, myocardial infarction; *PAD*, peripheral arterial disease; *PE*, pulmonary embolism; *VTE*, venous thromboembolism.

days.[69] The benefits from this therapy must be balanced with the risk of bleeding complications. Current guidelines recommend that thrombolytic therapy be used for patients with massive PE, or unstable patients with submassive PE with an acceptable risk of bleeding, but not in low-risk patients.[49]

Catheter-based techniques similar to those described in the treatment of ALI (see Table 7.8) can also be used to recanalize the pulmonary arteries during PE. These interventions can be used in patients with contraindications to thrombolysis, or to increase the rate of lysis in patients with continued hemodynamic instability. The three types of PMT used in the treatment of PE include aspiration embolectomy, thrombus fragmentation, and rheolysis.[49] Some researchers have also achieved success with ultrasound-accelerated thrombolysis.[40,58]

For patients with peripheral DVT, the use of thrombolytics and PMT is more controversial. Systemic thrombolysis is associated with a significant risk of major bleeding (up to 14%), and is therefore not recommended by current guidelines. Catheter-directed thrombolysis is currently only recommended in patients with limb-threatening DVT or rapidly expanding thrombus despite anticoagulation.[49] However, many clinicians advocate for a broader application of CDT, since more rapid clot lysis is associated with lower rates of post-thrombotic syndrome—the development of chronic venous insufficiency following DVT that results in pain, edema, and possibly venous stasis ulcers. A multicenter study is currently being conducted to determine if the use of CDT in acute proximal DVT prevents post-thrombotic syndrome and improves quality of life.[98]

Inferior vena cava (IVC) filters were introduced decades ago, and have seen increased usage more recently as a result of improved technology. Temporary devices can now be placed percutaneously in patients at high risk for DVT who present with contraindications to anticoagulation, or those with recurrent emboli despite anticoagulation. The filters are usually placed in the infrarenal IVC in an effort to capture embolization of DVT before it enters the pulmonary and renal vasculature.[69] Potential candidates include trauma patients with significant head or organ injury, and patients with spinal cord injury. Anticoagulation should be resumed as soon as feasible, and the filters can be removed once the period of highest risk for PE is over.[97]

TRAUMATIC INJURY OF THE PERIPHERAL VASCULATURE

Injuries to the peripheral arteries are the most common type of vascular injury seen in trauma patients. Although seldom lethal, there is a high risk for amputation, especially when there is a delay in diagnosis.[23] The majority of these injuries occur in the lower limbs.[72] Although vascular injuries can occur in isolation, they often occur in patients with severely compromised extremities.

Blunt trauma can result from motor vehicle accidents, falls, assaults, and crush injuries. Fractures of the long bones or dislocated joints can increase the chance for vascular injuries. Penetrating trauma can be caused by gunshot and stab wounds, as well as industrial accidents and intravenous (IV) drug use. Vascular injuries can also be a result of iatrogenic complications

TABLE 7.11 Assessment of Vascular Injury

Hard Signs	Soft Signs
Signs of acute limb ischemia (6 Ps)	Delayed capillary refill, pulse deficit without ischemia
Rapidly expanding, contained hematoma	Small, nonexpanding hematoma
Active external bleeding	History of arterial bleeding at scene or during transport
Palpable thrill or audible bruit over suspected injury	Neurologic deficit or wound immediately proximal to vascular distribution

of vascular access medical procedures, such as cardiac catheterization, arteriography, and balloon angioplasty.[64] Traumatic injury to the extremities accounts for up to 75% of all combat injuries, secondary to increased exposure to improvised explosive devices.[23]

Clinical Presentation

Signs of hemorrhagic shock are clues to vascular trauma. Vessel injuries may be nonsevered, partially severed, or completely severed. Patients may present with large lacerations or open wounds and hemorrhage. Signs include differences in BP between extremities, diminished or absent distal pulses, pallor, and paresthesia of the extremity. "Hard" and "soft" signs are used to identify appropriate treatment (Table 7.11). Hard signs identify patients requiring surgical intervention. A finding of a cold or pulseless extremity in a hemodynamically stable patient generally indicates underlying proximal vascular injury that requires definitive repair. Patients with one or more soft signs require close observation, since the severity of the vascular injury may not be overtly obvious. If the patient has an associated orthopedic injury or a history of vascular disease, further imaging is warranted.[23]

When patients present with extensive soft tissue injury or fractures, the decision to perform vascular repair becomes more complicated and must be weighed against the probability of long-term success. Poor prognostic signs for limb salvage are a major soft tissue injury, an ischemic time in excess of 6 hours, the presence of significant neurologic deficit, especially of the tibial nerve, and other major organ injuries.[23]

Several scoring systems have been developed and are utilized to evaluate the degree of injury and predict amputation and functional outcome. One example is the Mangled Extremity Severity Score (MESS), which examines degrees of skeletal/soft tissue injury, limb ischemia, symptoms of shock, and patient age (Table 7.12).[44] Traditionally, a MESS score of 8 or higher was predictive of the need for amputation.[50] This cut-off may not be definitive, since some clinicians have reported acceptable salvage rates of greater than 50% for patients with early revascularization (<5 hours after injury) and the use of fasciotomy in patients with a MESS score greater than or equal to 8.[22]

Diagnosis

Lab studies include baseline blood work consisting of complete blood count (CBC), platelet count, electrolytes, BUN, and creatinine. Typing and cross-matching of four to eight units of packed red blood cells (PRBCs) should be considered in a patient with obvious vascular trauma. In acute hemorrhage,

TABLE 7.12 Mangled Extremity Severity Score

Skeletal/Soft Tissue Injury	
Low energy (e.g., stab, simple fracture, gunshot wound)	1
Medium energy (e.g., open or multiple fractures, dislocation)	2
High energy (e.g., shotgun, crush injury)	3
Very high energy (as above plus gross contamination, soft tissue avulsion)	4
Limb Ischemia	
Pulse reduced or absent, but normal perfusion	1
Pulseless, paresthesias, reduced capillary filling	2
Cool, paralyzed, insensate limb (score doubled if longer than 6 hours)	3
Shock	
Systolic blood pressure maintained >90 mm Hg	0
Transient hypotension	1
Persistent hypotension	2
Age	
< 30	0
30–50	1
> 50	2

See text for scoring instructions.
From Reference 44.

the hematocrit and hemoglobin levels may appear within the normal range, even though there may be signs of cellular volume loss.

Additional diagnostic tests are performed to evaluate the presence and extent of vascular injury. These are done to prevent unnecessary operations, document the presence of a surgical lesion, and localize the surgical lesion to plan an operative approach. The ABI can be used to evaluate vascular insufficiency, and a result of less than 0.9 warrants further evaluation. Transcutaneous oxygen monitoring of the extremity can also provide clues to decreased perfusion. Duplex ultrasonography is a rapid, noninvasive method of assessing vascular injury. Plain x-ray of the injured extremity can determine the presence of fractured bones and foreign bodies. Arteriogram can be performed in hemodynamically stable patients without renal compromise, if there is a need to evaluate the extent of the injury prior to repair.

Treatment

The first priority of care is to control bleeding and maintain an adequate BP. Frequent monitoring of circulation—including the presence and quality of pulse, capillary refill, color and temperature of the extremity, and sensation and motor ability—should be continued until further decisions are made regarding definitive treatment of the vascular injury. Antibiotics, tetanus toxoid, and analgesics are provided to help with infection and pain.

Unstable patients generally require immediate surgical exploration. Temporary vascular shunts may be placed to provide limb salvage in patients with complex multisystem injuries, until a more definitive procedure can be performed.[23] There has also been an increased interest in the use of endovascular techniques in the setting of vascular trauma.[72] Although potentially promising, further research is needed to establish the use of catheter-based interventions in this population.

INTERPROFESSIONAL CARE FOR PERIPHERAL VASCULAR DISEASE

Patients with acute vascular occlusion or critical limb ischemia require frequent monitoring during and immediately after therapy to evaluate the effectiveness of treatment and identify potential complications. Lower extremity revascularization is associated with increased risk for MI, with mortality ranging from 2% to 8% following peripheral bypass procedures.[28] As in patients with aortic disease, it is important to continue preoperative beta blockers, antiplatelet agents, and statins throughout the perioperative course to optimize patient outcomes.[88]

Assessment

Monitoring of patients following lower limb revascularization is similar to that described for aortic procedures. Continuous ECG monitoring is needed to detect myocardial ischemia. Potential alterations in circulation to the involved extremity are assessed with frequent pulse checks and inspection of skin color and temperature. Adequate BP and hydration are important to promote flow through a reopened vessel or new bypass graft, as well as to prevent renal complications, especially when patients have received contrast dye. The patient's level of pain is also evaluated and treated with analgesics as needed.

Patients who are receiving anticoagulants or thrombolytic therapy require frequent monitoring of the appropriate coagulation studies to ensure that they remain within the prescribed therapeutic range. For patients receiving UFH, this might include aPTT or ACT, as well as monitoring platelet levels to evaluate for potential HIT. Patients are also assessed for evidence of bleeding, both systemically and at vascular access sites. Serial hemoglobin and hematocrit levels provide important clues to blood loss, especially with less obvious bleeding that may occur into the peritoneal cavity.

Compartment Syndrome

Patients who have undergone revascularization procedures for ALI are at increased risk for compartment syndrome. This occurs when reperfusion edema causes increased tissue pressure within a closed muscle compartment. The increased pressure exceeds the perfusion pressure, resulting in muscle and nerve ischemia. The risk is greatest in patients with limited collateral circulation (acute occlusion or trauma) or prolonged ischemia before revascularization. The most common symptom is pain disproportional to injury or pain with passive extension of muscles in the involved compartment. Patients with these symptoms should have compartment pressure measurements performed to confirm the diagnosis and undergo immediate fasciotomy to prevent permanent neurologic injury.[14]

Rhabdomyolysis

Patients with ALI for more than 6 hours are at risk for rhabdomyolysis, due to necrotic breakdown of muscle and the associated release of myoglobin. Recirculation of myoglobin can overwhelm the kidneys, resulting in acute tubular necrosis. Symptoms include oliguria and pink urine, and the diagnosis can be confirmed with a urine myoglobin level. Treatment includes intravenous hydration and forced diuresis with either mannitol or furosemide (Lasix). Alkalinization of the urine with bicarbonate may also prove helpful.

Right Ventricular Support

Acute RV dysfunction is the main cause of death in patients with massive PE. Interventions to support RV function are needed while efforts are undertaken to remove the embolism. Management of RV failure in this setting generally consists of administering volume to ensure optimal preload, as well as administering inotropic agents to increase contractility. In intubated patients, positive end expiratory pressure should be minimized if possible to avoid further increases in afterload. Inhaled nitric oxide may also prove beneficial in vasodilating the pulmonary vasculature without worsening systemic hypotension.[69]

CASE STUDY 7.1 Thoracic Aortic Dissection

R.B. is a 62-year-old man who presented in the emergency department after sudden onset of tearing pain in his chest and upper back. The pain was unrelieved by changes in position and was not associated with shortness of breath, nausea, or vomiting. He had a history of hyperlipidemia and long-standing hypertension. On admission, R.B.'s BP was 168/92 mm Hg, his respiratory rate (RR) was 28 breaths/min, and he was afebrile. The ECG monitor showed sinus tachycardia without ectopy at a heart rate (HR) of 122 beats/min, and the pulse oximeter reading was 98% on room air. Lungs were clear to auscultation bilaterally, and there were no abnormal heart sounds or murmurs. Neurologically, the patient was alert and oriented, but he presented with numbness and significant weakness in his left lower leg.

R.B. had two large-bore peripheral intravenous catheters inserted and was placed on oxygen via nasal cannula at 2 L/min. A 12-lead ECG was obtained, which showed nonspecific ST/T wave changes. Lab work was initiated immediately, and the troponin test was negative. Electrolytes, hematocrit, and hemoglobin were all within normal limits. A chest x-ray was also normal, except for an abnormal aortic contour. A transesophageal echocardiogram performed at the bedside revealed a thoracic aortic dissection with true and false lumens extending from the left subclavian artery into the distal aorta. A CT scan of the aorta confirmed the presence of an aortic dissection that extended from the subclavian artery into the distal abdominal aorta. Vital signs at this time were as follows: HR 124 beats/min, BP 176/92 mm Hg in the left arm and 184/88 mm Hg in the right arm, RR 30 breaths/min, Spo_2 97%.

Decision Point:

What interventions should be implemented at this time?

CONCLUSION

The management of patients undergoing major vascular surgery and urgent procedures to restore blood flow is challenging. The combination of advanced age, multiple comorbidities, and the systemic impact of atherosclerosis significantly increases the risk of adverse events during hospitalization. Implementation of a comprehensive plan of care to restore perfusion, maintain hemodynamic stability, and prevent complications is essential to optimize outcomes.

REFERENCES

1. Abraham, P., et al. (2013). A review of current agents for anticoagulation for the critical care practitioner. *J Crit Care, 28*(5), 763–777.
2. Acher, C. & Wynn, M. (2012). Paraplegia after thoracoabdominal aortic surgery: not just assisted circulation, hypothermic arrest, clamp and sew, or TEVAR. *Ann Cardiothorac Surg, 1*(3), 365–372.
3. Agrawal, K. & Eberhardt, R. T. (2015). Contemporary medical management of peripheral arterial disease: a focus on risk reduction and symptom relief for intermittent claudication. *Cardiol Clin, 33*, 111–137.
4. Aicher, D., et al. (2007). Aortic root remodeling: ten-year experience with 274 patients. *J Thorac Cardiovasc Surg, 134*, 909–915.
5. Alonso-Coello, P., et al. (2012). Antithrombotic therapy in peripheral artery disease: antithrombotic therapy and prevention of thrombosis

(9th ed). American College of Chest Physicians evidence-based clinical practice guidelines. *Chest, 141*(2)(suppl.), e669S–e690S.
6. Anderson, J. L., et al. (2013). Management of patients with peripheral artery disease (compilation of 2005 and 2011 ACCF/AHA guideline recommendations). *J Am Coll Cardiol, 61*, 1555–1570.
7. Ankle Brachial Index Collaboration, Fowkes, F. G., et al. (2008). Ankle brachial index combined with Framington risk score to predict cardiovascular events and mortality: a meta-analysis. *JAMA, 300*, 197–208.
8. Azhar, B., Patel, S. R., Holt, J. E., et al. (2014). Misdiagnosis of ruptured abdominal aortic aneurysm: systematic review and meta-analysis. *J Endovasc Ther, 21*, 568–575.
9. Baril, D. T., Patel, V. I., Dejah, R., et al. (2013). Outcomes of lower extremity bypass performed for acute limb ischemia. *J Vasc Surg, 57*(1), 296–297.
10. Becquemin, J. O. (2009). The ACE trial: a randomized comparison of open versus endovascular repair in good risk patients with abdominal aortic aneurysm. *J Vasc Surg, 50*(1), 222–224.
11. Berg, K. B. & Janelle, G. M. (2012). Descending thoracic aortic surgery: update on mortality, morbidity, risk assessment and management. *Curr Opin Crit Care, 18*, 393–398.
12. Bicknell, C. D. & Powell, C. T. (2013). Thoracic aortic aneurysms. *British J of Surg, 100*, 850–852.
13. Blankensteijn, J. D., de Jong, S. E., Prinssen, M., et al. (2005). Two-year outcomes after conventional or endovascular repair of abdominal aortic aneurysms. *N Engl J Med, 352*(23), 2398–2405.
14. Blecha, M. J. (2013). Critical limb ischemia. *Surg Clin N Am, 93*(4), 789–812.
15. Bobadilla, J. L., Wynn, M., Tefera, G., et al. (2013). Low incidence of paraplegia after thoracic endovascular aneurysm repair with proactive spinal cord protective protocols. *J Vasc Surg, 57*, 1537–1542.
16. Bonser, R. S., Ranasinghe, A. M., Loubani, M., et al. (2011). Evidence, lack of evidence, controversy and debate in the provision and performance of surgery of acute type A aortic dissection. *J Am Coll Cardiol, 58*, 2455–2474.
17. Bradbury, A., Adam, D., Bell, J., et al. (2010). Bypass versus angioplasty in severe ischemia of the leg (BASIL) trial: an intervention to treat analysis of amputation-free and overall survival in patients randomized to bypass surgery-first or a balloon angioplasty-first revascularization strategy. *J Vasc Surg, 51*, 5S17S.
18. Braverman, A. C. (2010). Acute aortic dissection: clinician update. *Circulation, 122*, 184–188.
19. Brunelli, A. (2012). Deep vein thrombosis, pulmonary embolism: prophylaxis, diagnosis and management. *Thorac Surg Clin, 22*, 25–28.
20. Buckley, S. D. & Buckley, C. J. (2014). Endovascular aortoiliac aneurysm repair: surgical progress through new treatment paradigms and innovative endograft design. *AORN, 100*(3), 271–279.
21. Bujak, M., Gamberdella, J. & Mena, C. (2014). Management of atherosclerotic aortoiliac occlusive disease. *Intervent Cardiol Clin, 3*, 531–543.
22. Callcut, R. A., Acher, C. W., Hoch, J., et al. (2009). Impact of intraoperative arteriography on limb salvage for traumatic popliteal artery injury. *J Trauma, 67*(2), 252–257.
23. Callcut, R. A. & Mell, M. W. (2013). Modern advances in vascular trauma. *Surg Clin N Am, 93*, 941–961.
24. Castillo, C. & Tapson, V. F. (2012). Right ventricular responses to massive and submassive pulmonary embolism. *Cardiol Clin, 30*(2), 233–241.
25. Chaikof, E. L., Brewster, D. C., Dalman, R. L., et al. (2009). The care of patients with an abdominal aortic aneurysm: the Society for Vascular Surgery practice guidelines. *J Vasc Surg, 50*(85), 2S–49S.
26. Crawford, E. S., et al. (1986). Thoracoabdominal aortic aneurysms: preoperative and intraoperative factors determining immediate and long-term results of operations in 605 patients. *J Vasc Surg, 3*, 389–404.
27. Creager, M. A., Kaufman, J. A. & Conte, M. S. (2012). Acute limb ischemia. *N Engl J Med, 366*(23), 2198–2206.
28. Crimi, E. & Hill, C. C. (2014). Postoperative ICU management of vascular surgery patients. *Anesthesiology Clin, 32*, 735–757.
29. Danyi, P., Elefteriades, J. A. & Jovin, I. S. (2011). Medical therapy of thoracic aortic aneurysms: are we there yet? *Circulation, 124*, 1469–1476.
30. Dardik, A. (2014). Phlegmasia alba and cerulean dolens. http://www.emedicine.medscape.com/article/461809, updated Feb 25, 2014.
31. David, T. E., Armstrong, S., Manlhiot, C., et al. (2013). Long-term results of aortic root repair using the reimplantation technique. *J Thorac Cardiovasc Surg, 145*, S22–S25.
32. Dean, J. H., Woznicki, E. M., O'Gara, P., et al. (2014). Cocaine-related aortic dissection: lessons from the International Registry of Acute Aortic Dissection. *Am J Med, 127*(9), 878–885.
33. Dixon, M. (2011). Misdiagnosing aortic dissection: a fatal mistake. *J Vasc Nurs, 29*(4), 139–146.
34. Dolinger, C. & Strider, D. V. (2010). Endovascular interventions for descending thoracic aortic aneurysms: the pivotal role of the clinical nurse in postoperative care. *J Vasc Nurs, 28*(4), 147–153.
35. Elsayed, S. & Clavijo, L. C. (2015). Critical limb ischemia. *Cardiol Clin, 33*, 37–47.
36. Etz, C. D., Bischoff, M. S., Bodian, C., et al. (2010). The Bentall procedure: is it the gold standard? A series of 597 consecutive cases. *J Thorac Cardiovasc Surg, 140*, 564–570.
37. Faure, E. M., Canaud, L., Marty-Ane, C., et al. (2015). Endovascular management of rupture in acute type B aortic dissection. *Eur J Vasc Endovasc Surg, 49*, 655–660.
38. Flu, W. J., van Kuijk, J. P., Chonchol, M., et al. (2010). Timing of preoperative beta-blocker treatment in vascular surgery patients: influence on post-operative outcome. *J Am Coll Cardiol, 56*, 1922–1929.
39. Goldfinger, J. Z., et al. (2014). Thoracic aortic aneurysm and dissection. *J Am Coll Cardiol, 64*, 1725–1739.
40. Graif, A., Niesen, T. J., Gakhal, M., Kimbiris, G., et al. (2015). Comparison of percutaneous ultrasound-accelerated endovascular thrombolysis (EKOS) with pigtail catheter directed thrombolysis for the treatment of acute pulmonary embolism. *J Vasc Interven Radiol, 26*(2), S75.
41. Greenhalgh, R. M. (2005). Endovascular aneurysm repair versus open repair in patients with abdominal aortic aneurysm (EVAR trial 1): randomized controlled trial. *Lancet, 365*, 2179–2186.
42. Hagan, P. G., et al. (2000). International Registry of Acute Aortic Dissection (IRAD): new insights into an old disease. *JAMA, 283*, 897–903.
43. Hennion, D. R. & Siano, K. A. (2013). Diagnosis and treatment of peripheral arterial disease. *Am Fam Physician, 88*(5), 3060310.
44. Helfet, D. L., Howey, T., Sanders, R., et al. (1990). Limb salvage versus amputation: preliminary results of the mangled extremity severity score. *Clin Orthop Relat Res, 256*, 80–86.
45. Hines, G., Dracea, C. & Katz, D. S. (2011). Diagnosis and management of acute type A aortic dissection. *Cardiol Review, 19*, 226–232.
46. Hoel, A. W. (2013). Aneurysmal disease: thoracic aorta. *Surg Clin N Am, 93*, 893–910.
47. Hiratzka, L. F., Bakris, G. L., Beckman, J. A., et al. (2010). 2010 ACCF/AHA/AATS/ACR/ASA/ SCA/SCAI/SIR/STS/SVM guidelines for the diagnosis and management of patients with thoracic aortic disease: executive summary: a report of the American College of Cardiology Foundation/American Heart Association Task Force on Practice Guidelines, American Association for Thoracic Surgery, American College of Radiology, American Stroke Association, Society of Cardiovascular Anesthesiologists, Society for Cardiovascular Angiography and Interventions, Society of Interventional Radiology, Society of Thoracic Surgeons, and Society for Vascular Medicine (developed in collaboration with the American College of Emergency Physicians). *J Am Coll Cardiol, 55*(14), 1509–1544.
48. Hynes, B. G., Margey, R. J., Ruggiero, N., et al. (2012). Endovascular management of acute limb ischemia. *Ann Vasc Surg, 26*, 110–124.
49. Jaff, M. R., McMurtry, M. S., Archer, S. L., et al. (2011). American Heart Association Council on Cardiopulmonary, Critical Care, Perioperative and Resuscitation, American Heart Association Council Peripheral Vascular Disease, American Heart Association Council on Arteriosclerosis, Thrombosis and Vascular Biology: management of massive and submassive pulmonary embolism, iliofemoral deep vein thrombosis, and chronic thromboembolic pulmonary hypertension: a scientific statement from the American Heart Association. *Circulation, 123*(16), 1789–1793.
50. Johansen, K., et al. (1990). Objective criteria accurately predict amputation following lower extremity trauma. *J Trauma, 30*, 568–573.
51. Kapur, V. & Gray, W. A. (2014). Management of aneurysmal disease of the aorta. *Intervent Cardiol Clin, 3*, 545–555.

52. Karthikesalingam, A., Young, E. L., Hinchliffe, R. J., et al. (2011). SA systematic review of percutaneous mechanical thrombectomy in the treatment of deep venous thrombosis. *Eur J Vasc Endovasc Surg, 41*, 554–565.
53. Kempe, K., Starr, B., Stafford, J. M., et al. (2014). Results of surgical management of acute thromboembolic lower extremity ischemia. *J Vasc Surg, 60*, 702–707.
54. Kuzmik, G. A., Sang, A. X. & Elefteriades, J. A. (2012). Natural history of thoracic aortic aneurysms. *J Vasc Surg, 56*, 565–571.
55. Landry, G. J. (2014). Acute peripheral arterial and bypass graft occlusion: thrombolytic therapy. In J. L. Cameron, & A. M. Cameron (Eds.), *Current Surgical Therapy* (11th ed.). (pp. 909–914). Philadelphia: Saunders.
56. Lane, R., Ellis, B., Watson, L., et al. (2014). Exercise for intermittent claudication. *Cochrane Database Syst Rev* (7), CD000990.
57. Lau, B. D. & Haunt, E. R. (2014). Practices to prevent venous thromboembolism: a brief review. *BMJ Qual Saf, 23*, 187–195.
58. Laurich, C., Kelly, P., Santos, A., et al. (2014). Safety and efficacy of ultrasound accelerated catheter–directed lytic therapy in acute pulmonary embolism. *J Vasc Surg, 60*(4), 1109.
59. Lederle, F. A., et al. (2000). The aneurysm detection and management study screening program: validation cohort and final results. Aneurysm Detection and Management Veterans Affairs Cooperative Study Investigators. *Arch Intern Med, 160*, 1425–1430.
60. Lederle, F. A., et al. (2012). Long-term comparison of endovascular and open repair of abdominal aortic aneurysm. *N Engl J Med, 367*(21), 1988–1997.
61. Lederle, F. A., Powell, J. T. & Nienaber, C. A. (2014). Does intensive medical treatment improve outcomes in aortic dissection? *BMJ, 349*, 33–34.
62. Leshnower, B. G., Myung, R. J., Kilgo, P. D., et al. (2010). Moderate hypothermia and unilateral selective antegrade cerebral perfusion: a contemporary cerebral protection strategy for aortic arch surgery. *Ann Thorac Surg, 90*(2), 547–554.
63. Li, J. Z., Eagle, K. A. & Vaishnava, P. (2013). Hypertensive and acute aortic syndromes. *Cardiol Clin, 31*, 493–501.
64. Merriweather, N. & Sulzbach-Hoke, L. M. (2012). Managing risks of complications at femoral vascular access sites in percutaneous coronary intervention. *Crit Care Nurse, 32*(5), 16–29.
65. Mills, J., Conte, M., Armstrong, D., et al. (2014). The Society for Vascular Surgery Lower Extremity Threatened Limb Classification System: risk stratification based on wound, ischemia and foot infection. *J Vasc Surg, 59*, 220234.
66. Mitchell, J., Bogar, L. & Burton, N. (2014). Cardiothoracic surgical emergencies in the intensive care unit. *Crit Care Clin, 30*(3), 499–525.
67. Mohan, P. P. & Hamblin, M. H. (2014). Comparison of endovascular and open repair of ruptured abdominal aortic aneurysm in the United States in the last decade. *Cardiovasc Intervent Radiol, 37*, 337–342.
68. Moll, F. L., Powell, J. T., Fraedrich, G., et al. (2011). Management of abdominal aortic aneurysms clinical practice guidelines of the European Society of Vascular Surgery. *Eur J Vasc Endovasc Surg, 41*, S1–S58.
69. Moorjani, N. & Price, S. (2013). Massive pulmonary embolism. *Cardiol Clin, 31*(4), 503–518.
70. Mozaffarian, D., Benjamin, E. J., Go, A. S., et al. (2015). On behalf of the American Heart Association Statistics Committee and Stroke Statistics Subcommittee: heart disease and stroke statistics—2015 update: a report from the American Heart Association. *Circulation, 131*, e29–e322.
71. Multicentre Aneurysm Screening Study Group. (2002). Multicentre aneurysm screening study (MASS): cost-effectiveness analysis of screening for abdominal aortic aneurysms based on four year results from a randomized controlled trial. *BMJ, 325*, 1135–1138.
72. Nagarsheth, K. H. & Dubose, J. J. (2015). Endovascular management of vascular trauma. *Trauma, 17*(2), 93–101.
73. Nienaber, C. A., Kische, S., Rousseau, H., et al. (2013). For the INSTEAD-XL trial: endovascular repair of type B aortic dissection: long-term results of the randomized investigation of stent grafts in aortic dissection trial. *Circ Cardiovasc Interv, 6*, 407–416.
74. Nienaber, C. A., Divchev, D., Palisch, H., et al. (2014). Early and late management of type B aortic dissection. *Heart, 100*, 1491–1497.
75. Nienaber, C. A. & Clough, R. E. (2015). Management of acute aortic dissection. *Lancet, 385*, 800–811.
76. Norgren, L., Hiatt, W. R., Dormandy, J. A., et al. (2007). On behalf of the TASC Working Group: inter-society consensus for the management of peripheral arterial disease (TASC II). *Eur J Vasc Endovasc Surg, 33*, S1–S70.
77. Obi, A. T., Park, Y. J., Bove, P. C., et al. (2015). Clinical research study: the association of perioperative transfusion with 30-day morbidity and mortality in patients undergoing major vascular surgery. *J of Vasc Surg, 61*(4), 1000–1009.
78. Patel, N. H., Krishnamurthy, V. N., Kim, S., et al. (2013). Quality improvement guidelines for percutaneous management of acute lower-extremity ischemia. *J Vasc Interv Radiol, 24*, 3–15.
79. Perry, R. J., Martin, M. J., Eckert, M. J., et al. (2008). Colonic ischemia complicating open vs endovascular aortic aneurysm repair. *J Vasc Surg, 48*, 272–277.
80. Purushottam, P., Karthik, G., Zalewski, A. & Krishnan, P. (2014). Acute limb ischemia. *Intervent Cardiol Clin, 3*, 557–572.
81. Robertson, I., Kessel, D. O. & Robertson, I. (2013). Infusion techniques for peripheral arterial occlusion. *Cochrane Database Syst Rev, 12*, CD001099.
82. Rooke, T. W., Hirsch, A. T., Misra, S., et al. (2011). 2011 ACCF/AHA Focused update of the guideline for the management of patients with peripheral artery disease (updating the 2005 guidelines): a report of the American College of Cardiology Foundation/American Heart Association Task Force on Practice Guidelines. *J Am Coll Cardiol, 58*, 2020–2045.
83. Schermerhorn, M. L., Giles, K. A., Sachs, T., et al. (2011). Defining perioperative mortality after open and endovascular aortic aneurysm repair in the US Medicare population. *J Am Coll Surg, 212*, 349–355.
84. Seco, M., Edelman, J. B., Van Boxtel, B., et al. (2015). Neurologic injury and protection in adult cardiac and aortic surgery. *J Cardiothorac Vasc Anesth, 29*(1), 185–195.
85. Shamoun, F. E., Fankhauser, G. T. & Mookadam, M. (2013). Vascular medicine: aortic and peripheral arterial disease. *Prim Care Clin Office Pract, 40*, 169–177.
86. Shimony, A., Filion, K. B., Mottillo, S., et al. (2011). Meta-analysis of usefulness of D-dimer to diagnose acute aortic dissection. *Am J Cardiol, 107*(8), 1227–1234.
87. Shores, J., Berger, K. R., Murphy, E., et al. (1994). Progression of aortic dilatation and the benefit of long-term beta-adrenergic blockade in Marfan's syndrome. *N Engl J Med, 330*, 1335–1341.
88. Singh, S., Maldonado, M. D. & Taylor, M. A. (2014). Optimal perioperative management of the vascular surgery patient. *Anesthesiology Clin, 32*(3), 615–637.
89. Stone, D. H. & Cronenwett, J. L. (2013). Surgical treatment of abdominal aortic aneurysms. In M. A. Creager, J. A. Beckman, & J. Loscalzo (Eds.), *Vascular Medicine: A Companion to Braunwald's Heart Disease* (2nd ed.). (pp. 479–492). Philadelphia: Saunders.
90. Suzuki, S., Munetaka, M. & Imoto, K. (2014). The use of surgical glue in acute type A aortic dissection. *Gen Thorac Cardiovasc Surg, 62*, 207–213.
91. Suzuki, T. (2012). Type-selective benefits of medications in treatment of acute aortic dissection (from the International Registry of Acute Aortic dissection [IRAD]). *Am J Cardiol, 109*(1), 122–127.
92. Takayama, T. & Yamanouchi, D. (2013). Aneurysmal disease: the abdominal aorta. *Surg Clin N Am, 93*, 877–891.
93. Tatterton, M. R. & Homer-Vanniasinkam, S. (2011). Infections in vascular surgery. *Injury Int J Care Injured, 42*, S35–S41.
94. Tehan, P. E., Bray, A. & Chuter, V. H. (2016). Non-invasive vascular assessment in the foot with diabetes: sensitivity and specificity of the ankle brachial index, toe brachial index and continuous wave Doppler for detecting peripheral arterial disease. *J Diabetes Complications, 30*(1), 155–160. http://dx.doi.org/10.1016/j.jdiacomp.
95. Truong, T. T., Jones, D. S. & Dunn, A. S. (2014). Pulmonary embolism. *Hosp Med Clin, 3*, 479–493.
96. Upadhye, S. & Schiff, K. (2012). Acute aortic dissection in the emergency department: diagnostic challenges and evidence-based management. *Emerg Med Clin N Am, 30*, 307–327.
97. Velopulos, C. G. & Haut, E. R. (2014). Venous thromboembolism: prevention diagnosis and treatment. In J. L. Cameron, & A. M. Cameron (Eds.), *Current Surgical Therapy* (11th ed.). (pp. 958–963). Philadelphia: Saunders.

98. Vendantham, S., Goldhaber, S. Z., Kahn, S. R., et al. (2013). Rationale and design of the ATTRACT study: a multicenter randomized trial to evaluate pharmacomechanical catheter-directed thrombolysis for the prevention of postthrombotic syndrome in patients with proximal deep vein thrombosis. *Am Heart J*, *165*, 523–530.
99. Weinberg, M. D., Lau, J. F., Rosenfield, K., et al. (2011). Peripheral artery disease. Part 2: medical and endovascular treatment. *Nat Rev Cardiol*, *8*, 429–441.
100. Wells, P. S., et al. (1997). Value of assessment of pretest probability of deep vein thrombosis in clinical management. *Lancet*, *350*, 1795–1798.
101. Wells, P. S., Anderson, D. R., Rodger, M., et al. (2000). Derivation of a simple clinical model to categorize patients' probability of pulmonary embolism: increasing the model's utility with the SimpliRED D-dimer. *Thromb Haemostasis*, *83*(3), 416–420.
102. Wells, P. S., et al. (2014). Treatment of venous thromboembolism. *JAMA*, *311*, 717–728.
103. White, A. & Broder, J. (2012). Aortic emergencies—Part 1. *Adv Emergency Nurs J*, *34*(3), 216–229.
104. White, A., Broder, J., Mando-Vandrick, J., et al. (2013). Aortic emergencies—Part 2. *Adv Emergency Nurs J*, *35*(1), 28–52.
105. Wittels, K. (2011). Aortic emergencies. *Emerg Med Clin N Am*, *29*, 789–800.
106. Wong, C. S., Healy, D., Canning, C., et al. (2012). A systematic review of spinal cord injury and cerebrospinal fluid drainage after thoracic endografting. *J Vasc Surg*, *56*, 1438–1447.
107. Wynn, M. M. & Archer, C. A. (2014). A modern theory of spinal cord ischemia/injury in thoracoabdominal aortic surgery and its implication for prevention of paralysis. *J Cardiothorac Vasc Anesth*, *28*(4), 1088–1099.
108. Ziganshin, B. A. & Elefteriades, J. A. (2014). Surgical management of thoracoabdominal aneurysms. *Heart*, *100*, 1577–1582.
109. Ziganshin, B. A., Rajbanshi, B. G., Tranquilli, M., et al. (2014). Straight deep hypothermic circulatory arrest for cerebral protection during aortic arch surgery: safe and effective. *J Thorac Cardiovasc Surg*, *148*, 888–900.

8

Heart and Lung Transplantation

Julie A. Stanik-Hutt, Debra J. Carter, and Diane Vail Skojec

For nearly 50 years, transplantation has been the last therapeutic option for patients suffering end-stage heart or lung disease despite maximal medical therapy. Thoracic organ (i.e., heart, lung, or combined heart-lung) transplantation can prolong life, as well as enhance its quality. Over the years, improvements in donor and recipient selection, organ preservation, operative techniques, postoperative care, and immunosuppression have increased both patient and graft survival. Outcomes after heart transplant are good, and both short- and long-term outcomes after lung transplant continue to improve.

Optimal outcomes with thoracic transplantation require the collaborative efforts of a interprofessional team of healthcare professionals, including, but not limited to: critical care and transplant nurses; physicians; clinical pharmacists; respiratory, physical, occupational, and speech therapists; dietitians; social workers; psychologists; home care specialists; and financial coordinators. Medical specialties involved include cardiology, pulmonology, thoracic surgery, anesthesiology, pathology, immunology, and infectious disease specialists. The patient and the patient's family are also vital members of the team. They have a significant impact on the patient's preparation for, and recovery from, this major surgery. The interprofessional team approach is used to evaluate and select candidates for transplant, prepare them for the procedure, and provide care to the recipient after the transplant procedure.

This chapter will provide the critical care nurse with an understanding of the physiology and pathophysiology related to heart and lung transplantation, as well as implications for patient care during recovery from these procedures. Care of patients with end-stage heart or lung disease before transplantation, complex rules for posting candidates to national transplant lists, care of solid organ donors, care of donor organs between harvest and implantation, and heart-lung transplant procedures are not included. Combined heart-lung transplant is done in only a very limited number of individuals who have both heart and lung failure (e.g. Eisenmenger syndrome). Most of these patients can be successfully treated with simultaneous repair of their heart defect at the time of lung transplant. Information regarding long-term post-transplant monitoring, care, complications, and prognosis is also beyond the scope of this chapter.

More than 29,450 lung and 69,363 heart transplants have been performed since 1988.[113,114] At any given time, approximately 6000 Americans are waiting for a thoracic organ transplant: approximately 4200 for a heart and approximately 1500 for a lung.[113,114] Whereas the use of allocation systems takes into account severity of illness, there is still a shortage of usable donor organs, which contributes to between 6% and 11% of lung and 12% and 15% of heart transplant candidates dying before a donor organ is found.[32,114,126] Out of 100 patients evaluated as a potential organ donor, only 15 can ultimately be used as a lung donor.[104] Therefore, a little more than 2600 heart and 1900 lung transplants are performed in the United States annually. One-year survival after lung transplant is 83%, and by year 5, only 46% of lung transplant recipients are still alive. Conversely, 1- and 5-year survival rates after heart transplant are 87% and 72%, respectively.[114]

EVALUATION AND CANDIDACY FOR THORACIC TRANSPLANTATION

Because of the lack of an adequate number of thoracic organ donors, it is imperative that pretransplant conditions are optimized so that every transplanted thoracic organ and recipient has the highest chance for success and long-term survival. This process begins with careful evaluation of all potential thoracic transplant candidates before listing (Box 8.1).

The first goal of the evaluation is to confirm that the patient's disease is irreversible and would be likely to cause the individual's death within 2 years (Table 8.1 and Box 8.2).[111,120,125] It is also essential to determine that no conditions exist that would significantly increase the morbidity or mortality of the transplant procedure or the subsequent required immunosuppression (Box 8.3).[56,120,125]

The perfect thoracic transplant candidate is an individual who has life-threatening, irreversible heart or lung disease and no comorbidities. Debilitated patients with multiple comorbid conditions, those who are significantly overweight or underweight, and those colonized with pan-resistant microorganisms would be unlikely to survive the transplant procedure. They would probably be among the 13% of heart or 17% of lung recipients who do not survive the first year after transplantation.[113,114] Individuals with psychosocial characteristics (history of noncompliance, major uncontrolled psychiatric problems, active substance abuse, poor social support, and inadequate financial/insurance coverage) that would interfere with adherence to complex posttransplant regimens are also not good candidates. Age criteria may also be used to determine eligibility for thoracic transplantation. Although physiologic age may be taken into account, heart transplantation is generally not offered to individuals more than 70 years of age.[71] Traditionally, the age limits for combined heart and lung, bilateral lung, and single lung transplants were 55, 60, and 65, respectively,[63] but today nearly 30% of lung recipients are older than 65.[39,48,114]

In the past, patients who were ventilator dependent or receiving extracorporeal membrane oxygenation (ECMO) were rarely offered transplantation. Recently, some sites have offered transplants to a growing number of these critically ill individuals and

BOX 8.1 Heart and Lung Transplant Candidate Evaluation Procedures

Diagnostic Tests	Consultations
Electrocardiogram	Transplant cardiology/pulmonology
Echocardiogram	Transplant surgeon
MUGA scan*	Physical and occupational therapy
Cardiac catheterization*	Dietitian
Cardiopulmonary stress testing†	Social worker
PA and lateral chest x-ray	Transplant psychologist
Chest CT*	Transplant nurse coordinator
Complete pulmonary function tests (spirometry, volumes, and diffusion testing)	Financial/insurance adviser
Differential quantitative ventilation/perfusion scan	Dental examination and clearance
Arterial blood gases‡	
6-minute walk test‡	
Peripheral Doppler†	
Carotid ultrasound†	
QuantiFERON-TB Gold test	

Laboratory Testing	Disease Prevention Screening
CBC, PT/PTT	Pelvic exam with Pap smear
Mammogram	Prostate-specific antigen§
Basic metabolic panel with liver function tests	Digital rectal exam§
Lipid profile	Bone density scan
24-hour urine for creatinine clearance	Colonoscopy/sigmoidoscopy§
Blood typing and antibody testing	
Human leukocyte antigen tissue typing	
Panel of reactive antibody testing	
Antibody serologies: CMV, EBV, HSV, VZV, MMR	
Screening for hepatitis B, hepatitis C, HIV, toxoplasmosis	
Sputum for culture and sensitivity‡	

*All heart candidates; lung candidates older than 40 years of age or multiple risk factors.
†Heart candidates only.
‡Lung candidates only.
§If older than 50 years of age.
CBC, Complete blood cell count; *CMV,* cytomegalovirus; *CT,* computerized tomography; *EBV,* Epstein-Barr virus; *HIV,* human immunodeficiency virus; *HSV,* herpes simplex virus; *MMR,* measles, mumps, rubella, *MUGA,* multiple gated acquisition; *PA,* posteroanterior; *Pap,* Papanicolaou; *PT,* prothrombin time; *PTT,* partial thromboplastin time; *TB,* tuberculosis; *VZV,* varicella zoster virus.
From Reference 63.

TABLE 8.1 Indications of End-Stage Heart and Lung Disease

Heart	
Maximum V_{O_2} < 10 mL/kg/min with achievement of anaerobic metabolism	
Dependence on IV inotropic agents to support adequate organ perfusion	
Refractory cardiogenic shock	
Severe ischemia consistently limiting routine activity and not amenable to revascularization	
Recurrent symptomatic ventricular dysrhythmias refractory to all accepted therapeutic modalities	
Lung	
Life expectancy of less than 2 years	
Patients with COPD	BODE index ≥ 7 FEV_1< 15–20% predicted ≥ 3 severe exacerbations in preceding year One severe exacerbation with acute hypercapnic respiratory failure Moderate pulmonary hypertension
Patients with cystic fibrosis	FEV_1< 30% predicted Pa_{CO_2} < 60 mm Hg or Pa_{CO_2} > 50 mm Hg Pulmonary hypertension Frequent hospitalization Rapid decline in lung function
Patients with restrictive disease	6 month decline FVC ≥ 10% over 6 months or FEV_1 < 30% predicted 6 month decline DLCO ≥ 15% Pa_{O_2} < 50 mm Hg or Pa_{CO_2} > 55 mm Hg Desaturation or decline in 6-minute-walk distance Pulmonary hypertension Increased hospitalizations Massive hemoptysis
Patients with pulmonary vascular disease	6-minute-walk test of < 350 m. Mean RA pressure >15 mm Hg Cardiac index < 2 L/min/m² NYHA Class III or IV despite 3 months combination therapy including prostanoids Significant hemoptysis, pericardial effusion, or progressive right heart failure

COPD, Chronic obstructive lung disease; *BODE index,* body-mass index, airflow obstruction, dyspnea, and exercise; *FEV_1,* forced expiratory volume in 1 second; *FVC,* forced vital capacity; *DLCO,* carbon monoxide diffusion capacity; *PAP,* pulmonary artery pressure; *mm Hg,* millimeters of mercury; *RA,* right atrial; *NYHA,* New York Heart Association.
From References 44, 67 and 120.

reported satisfactory outcomes.[6,54,117,126] Living donor lobar transplantation remains controversial, but is another option for selected patients in urgent need of transplantation. Donors and recipients are typically the parents or family members of children with cystic fibrosis. Currently available data indicate that 1-year recipient survival is 70% and donor outcomes are also satisfactory.[24]

Once accepted and listed, candidates are seen at the transplant center every few months to monitor their status and to be sure no new condition has developed that would preclude transplantation. At these visits, progression of the patient's disease may prompt a change in their listing status and move them higher on the priority list. Candidates may wait up to a year between listing and transplantation.[114,126] During this time, it is not uncommon for a candidate to be requested to come to the hospital for transplant, only to be sent home when some problem with the donor organ is discovered.

SURGICAL APPROACHES TO THORACIC TRANSPLANTATION

When an appropriate organ is identified, the patient is taken to the operating room (OR) to begin preparation for transplantation. Family members generally accompany the patient as far as possible and are reminded about the length of the surgery. At intervals, usually after specific landmarks in the procedure (for example, after the surgical incision is made, after organs arrive in the room, after implantation is complete, and after weaning from cardiopulmonary bypass [CPB]), someone from the surgical team will inform the family of the patient's condition and progress of surgery. After the completion of the surgery, the surgeon will meet the family to provide specific information about the procedure.

BOX 8.2 Diagnoses Amenable to Thoracic Transplantation

Heart Diseases

- Ischemic cardiomyopathy
- Nonischemic cardiomyopathy (peripartum, inflammatory, familial, toxic, idiopathic)
- Miscellaneous (congenital, refractory ventricular dysrhythmias, valvular disease, retransplantation)

Lung Diseases

- Obstructive (COPD, emphysema, α_1-antitrypsin deficiency)
- Restrictive (sarcoidosis, scleroderma, idiopathic pulmonary fibrosis)
- Suppurative (cystic fibrosis, bronchiectasis)
- Pulmonary vascular (primary pulmonary hypertension, Eisenmenger's syndrome)

COPD, Chronic obstructive lung disease.
From References 44, 67, 72, and 126.

BOX 8.3 Contraindications to Thoracic Transplantation

Absolute

- Age greater than 70 years
- Active malignancy in last 2–5 years
- Other significant irreversible organ system dysfunction
  - Renal: creatinine clearance < 40 mg/mL/min
  - Hepatic
  - Bone marrow
  - Diffuse advanced cerebrovascular disease
  - Severe pulmonary hypertension (unless combined heart-lung transplant planned)
- Chronic colonization with pan-resistant microorganisms
- Active hepatitis or tuberculosis
- Massive pulmonary mycetoma
- Active substance abuse/dependence including smoking or alcohol
- Major psychiatric problems
- Weight greater than 140% (or BMI > 30–35 kg/m^2) or less than 70% of ideal body weight
- Severely limited functional status with poor rehabilitation potential
- Social/behavioral problems (e.g., noncompliance)
- Inadequate social support

Relative

- Human immunodeficiency virus
- Significant chest wall or spinal deformity, or previous thoracic surgery or pleurodesis
- Chronic dependence on mechanical ventilation or extracorporeal life support
- Chronic high-dose steroids
- Symptomatic osteoporosis
- Severe malnutrition/cachexia
- Advanced dementia
- Financial problems

BMI, body mass index.
From References 63 and 120.

Heart Transplantation

The two surgical procedures used during heart transplantation are *orthotopic* and *heterotopic* implantation. The most common, orthotopic, requires explantation of all but parts of the atria of the recipient's native heart (Fig. 8.1). This is followed by biatrial or bicaval implantation of the donor heart along with end-to-end anastomosis between the recipient and donor aorta and pulmonary artery (Figs. 8.2 and 8.3). Heterotopic implantation occurs when the recipient's heart is not explanted. Rather, the donor heart is implanted alongside the recipient's native heart (Fig. 8.4).

Once the donor organs have been inspected and accepted for transplantation, explantation of the native heart proceeds. The recipient's chest is opened via sternotomy, which may be extended into the abdomen. The pericardium is opened, and preparations are made for CPB. At this point, adhesions formed after previous cardiac surgeries may present considerable challenges to dissection and cause significant hemorrhage. Dissection and preparation are necessary so that rapid explantation can proceed once the donor organs are in the room and ready for implantation. Precise timing is important in order to limit the ischemic time to less than 6 hours for the donor organs. When both donor and native hearts are ready, the native heart is removed and the donor heart is placed into the thoracic cavity. CPB is used to support the patient while implantation of the donor heart is completed. Cooled lap pads and continuous cold pericardial irrigation are also used to insulate and preserve the unperfused organ.

The biatrial and bicaval approaches are the two most commonly used techniques for orthotopic heart transplant. The biatrial technique was the standard method of implantation for more than 35 years.[53,70] This method required the recipient's heart to be dissected, leaving cuffs of the right and left atria at the base of the heart. The donor and native atrial cuffs were joined and end-to-end anastomoses performed on the aorta and pulmonary artery.[5] Postoperative atrial dysfunction and dysrhythmias were common after this procedure.

The second method of implantation, the bicaval technique, has become more common since 2004.[110] It requires explantation of the entire native right atrium with subsequent bicaval anastomosis on the right. With this technique, the donor right atrium is preserved intact. The left atrial anastomosis is performed in the traditional manner. This method reduces the incidence of postoperative dysrhythmias and atrioventricular valvular regurgitation,[5] as well as increases postoperative survival and decreases hospital length of stay.[70]

A third orthotopic technique, the total heart transplant procedure, is the newest procedure being used at approximately 8% of transplant centers at this time.[70] This procedure requires total explantation of the recipient's native heart, preserving only a small amount of common atrial tissue surrounding the two left and right pulmonary veins (Fig. 8.5). The bicaval technique is used to anastomose the right atrium, and the donor heart left atrium is anastomosed to the preserved patch of the recipient's left atrial tissue adjacent to the pulmonary veins. Because there are six anastomoses, operative time is significantly increased. The posterior pulmonary vein anastomosis sites are difficult to reach and may result in pulmonary vein stenoses.[70] Heterotopic implantation may be used for recipients who have fixed pulmonary hypertension, or if the donor heart is too small to fully support the recipient. The donor heart is implanted without explanting the native heart. Anastomoses are performed with the superior vena cava, pulmonary artery, and aorta. This technique requires lifelong anticoagulation and, because the native heart is not removed, the patient may still experience debilitating anginal pain. This technique is rarely used, and accounts for less than 1% of heart transplants.[10]

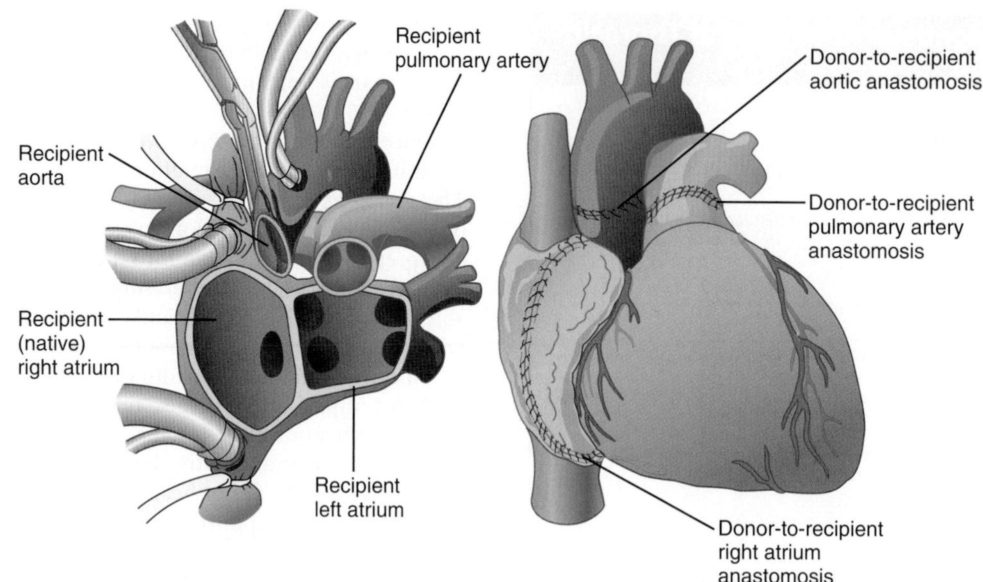

FIG. 8.1 Before and after view of biatrial technique for donor heart implantation.

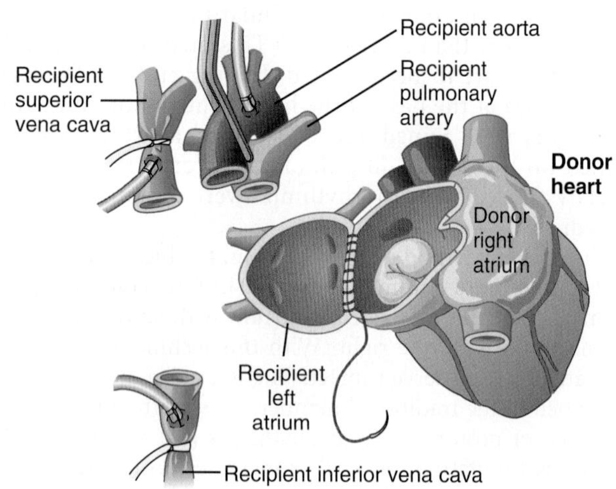

FIG. 8.2 Bicaval anastomotic technique. Bicaval implantation proceeds with left atrial anastomosis followed by superior and inferior vena cava anastomoses. After the pulmonary arteries are joined, caval snares are released, air is vented from the heart, and blood is allowed to circulate through the heart and lungs. Finally, aortic anastomoses are performed.

After implantation is complete, the patient is weaned from CPB. Once the patient is stabilized, transported, and settled in critical care, the family is invited to visit.

Lung Transplantation

Lung implantation procedures differ based on the number of lungs being transplanted. Single lung transplant is accomplished via a standard posterolateral thoracotomy incision. Double lung transplant requires a much larger anterior thoracosternotomy, also called a clamshell incision (Fig. 8.6). Patients may or may not require support from CPB during lung implantation. During the surgery, the recipient's native pulmonary artery, left atrium, and bronchi are dissected away from supporting structures. Great care is taken to avoid injury to the heart, aorta, thoracic duct, and thoracic nerves (phrenic, vagus, and recurrent laryngeal nerves) (Figs. 8.7 and 8.8). This dissection is necessary in order to mobilize the native structures and facilitate their rapid explantation once the donor organs are in the room so that ischemic time can be limited to less than 6 hours.[108] As the tissues are dissected, adhesions from previous thoracic or cardiac surgery may cause significant hemorrhage. Once the donor organs are prepared for implantation, the native lung is removed and the donor organ placed into the thoracic cavity. Ice slush or cold surgical lap pads are used to cool the organs in the chest while the donor bronchus and pulmonary artery are anastomosed to corresponding recipient structures (Figs. 8.9 and 8.10).[16] Finally, the donor pulmonary veins and the area adjacent to the recipient's left atrial-pulmonary vein junction are incised to create one large donor pulmonary vein and one large atrial-pulmonary cuff. These two reshaped structures are then joined, completing the transplantation (Fig. 8.11).

After implantation is complete, the surgeon inspects the bronchial anastomosis and clears any blood or debris from the airway via bronchoscopy. Unless independent lung ventilation is planned, the double-lumen endotracheal tube used during the surgery is exchanged for a single-lumen tube. The patient is then transported intubated, with mechanical ventilator support, to critical care. The family is informed of the outcome of surgery. Once the patient has been stabilized, the patient's family is encouraged to visit.

ALTERED PHYSIOLOGY IN THE TRANSPLANTED HEART AND LUNG

In addition to consequences that may accompany thoracotomy (such as pain, pneumothorax, hemothorax, atelectasis, pneumonia, or wound infection) and CPB (such as hemodynamic instability, bleeding, change in mental status, stroke, or renal insufficiency), thoracic transplant recipients can experience untoward effects related to physiologic derangements as a result of the transplant procedure.

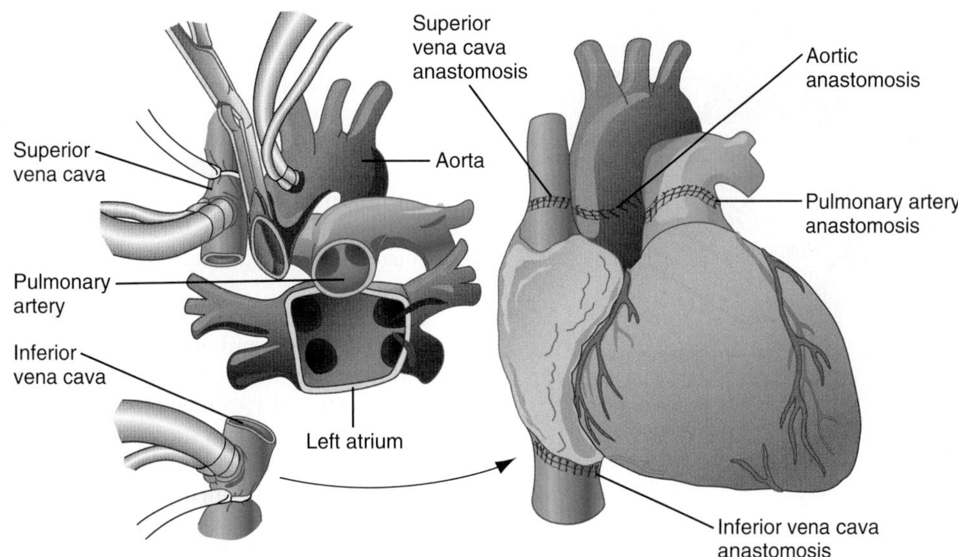

FIG. 8.3 Before and after view of bicaval technique for donor heart implantation. Bicaval technique proceeds with left atrial anastomoses followed by superior and inferior vena caval anastomoses.

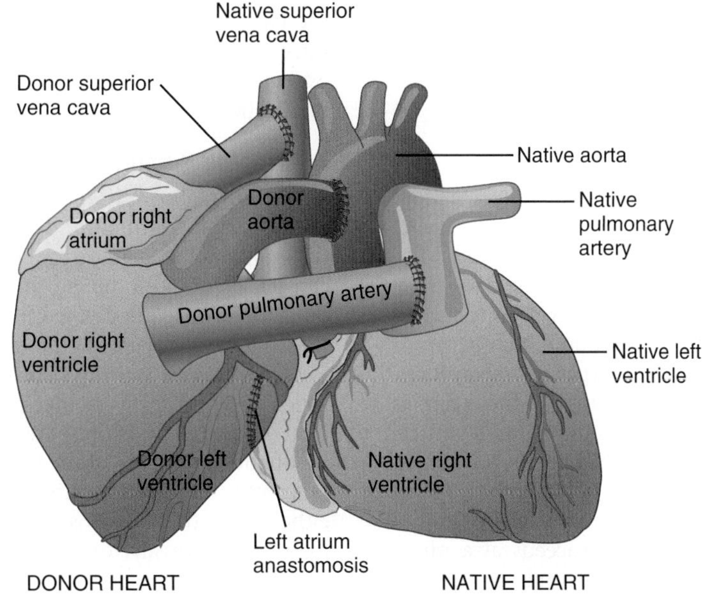

FIG. 8.4 Heterotopic heart transplantation. The donor heart is placed in the recipient chest and positioned next to the native heart. The superior vena cava, aorta, pulmonary arteries, and left atrial anastomoses join the donor heart to that of the recipient.

Heart transplant recipients are vulnerable to postoperative problems related to denervation of the heart. Postoperative problems specifically related to lung transplantation include pulmonary denervation, disruption of lymphatic drainage, and ciliary paralysis.[73]

The Denervated Transplanted Heart

During harvesting, connections between the donor heart and nerves are severed. As a result, the donor heart is denervated and abnormalities of heart rhythm and contractility occur. Normally, heart rate (HR) is regulated via neural and hormonal systems. The parasympathetic and sympathetic nervous systems maintain HR within certain limits and produce an increase in the rate when metabolic demand is increased. These systems control the rate of firing of the sinoatrial (SA) node as well as depolarization and repolarization of the myocardium. They also modulate the contractility of the heart to meet metabolic demands.

The denervated heart is not subject to direct efferent neural stimulation. Vagal tone is lost, causing a resting HR of between 90 and 110 beats per minute (beats/min). However, circulating hormones, such as the catecholamines, epinephrine, and norepinephrine, can still stimulate the heart. This stimulation proceeds at a much slower pace than typically seen with direct autonomic stimulation of a native heart. Consequently, the chronotropic response that typically increases the HR during stress and exercise is blunted.[123] Because these chronotropic responses are slow, reliance on tachycardia as an indication of

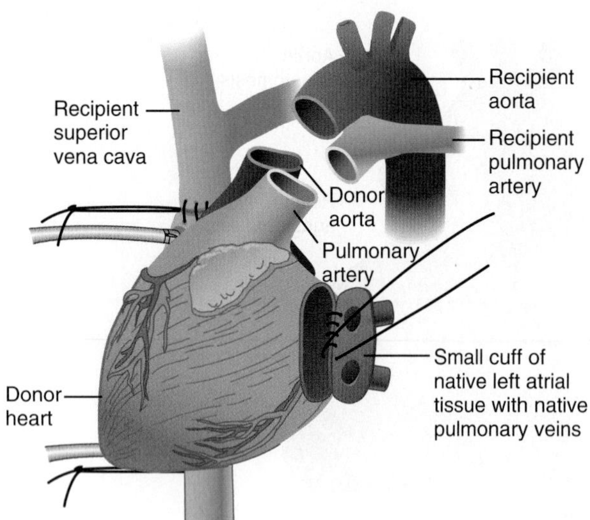

FIG. 8.5 Total orthotopic heart transplantation proceeds after total excision of the recipient heart, leaving only a very small amount of native atrial tissue surrounding the pulmonary vein insertion sites of left atrial "cuffs" on the native pulmonary veins. Consequently, the native pulmonary veins must be anastomosed directly to the donor heart, requiring four pulmonary vein anastomoses. (From Mora, B. N., Patterson, G. A. (2002). Lung preservation. In W. Baumgartner, B. Reitz, E. Kasper, J. Theodore (Eds.), *Heart and lung transplantation* (2nd ed.). Philadelphia: Elsevier.)

hypovolemia, hemorrhage, hypoxia, and fever can delay recognition of these problems and, subsequently, delay life-saving interventions.

Cardiac output (CO) is the product of heart rate and stroke volume (SV). SV is determined by preload, afterload, and contractility. If one of the contributors to CO is reduced, another must increase or CO will fall and the patient will experience symptoms.

Preload is reduced when venous return to the heart is reduced. When a patient rises from the recumbent to a vertical position, preload falls. To maintain CO with position changes, exercise, or other physical stresses, the transplanted heart must rely on circulating catecholamines to increase inotropic and chronotropic function. This stimulation proceeds at a much slower pace than that provided by direct neural stimulation. Consequently, a heart transplant recipient must allow the transplanted heart time to "warm up" before activities, such as position changes or exercise. Conversely, after stress or activity, the HR will return to resting levels more slowly because of the time required for circulating catecholamines to decline. As a result, "cool down" periods must be extended.

Afferent and efferent sensory fibers are also severed. This prevents the transmission of nociceptive impulses associated with cardiac ischemia. Without these afferent impulses, the experience of ischemic angina is absent. Patients may not be aware of episodic myocardial ischemia and therefore may fail to seek medical attention when needed. The loss of these afferent impulses also explains the lack of reflex autonomic responses to position changes (i.e., peripheral vasoconstriction), which normally maintain blood pressure (BP).[66]

Standard medications used to manipulate cardiac function may not have the desired effect on a denervated transplanted heart. The treatment of atrial tachydysrhythmias and bradycardias requires careful drug choices. For example, the use of digoxin (Lanoxin) to control atrial fibrillation or paroxysmal atrial tachycardia has little or no effect on the SA or atrioventricular (AV) nodes after heart transplant. Adenosine (Adenocard) may still be used to treat a paroxysmal supraventricular tachycardia, but an exaggerated response and profound bradycardia may occur. If atrial fibrillation occurs, Class III antiarrhythmic medications such as sotalol (Betapace), amiodarone (Cordarone), or nondihydropyridine calcium channel blockers such as diltiazem (Cardizem) may be used for rhythm and/or rate control.[17]

More importantly, after heart transplant, atropine's vagolytic effects are lost and may actually cause asystole or AV block if used to treat bradycardia.[7] In the past, isoproterenol (Isuprel) was the preferred treatment for symptomatic bradycardia. It may still be used in addition to oral or intravenous theophylline (Aminophylline) for persistent bradycardia. However, these beta stimulant medications have been associated with increased myocardial oxygen demand and can precipitate myocardial ischemia. Therefore the current treatment of choice for posttransplant bradydysrhythmias is temporary atrial or AV sequential pacing.[52,100] Compensatory reflex tachycardia, which maintains CO when antihypertensive medications such as hydralazine (Apresoline) are used, may not occur. As a result, the use of these medications after heart transplant may produce more profound decreases in CO and BP than are typically expected. If hypotension should occur with the use of these medications, epinephrine would be the drug of choice.[52,100]

Interrupted Pulmonary Lymphatics After Lung Transplant

Under normal conditions, the lymphatic system drains 10% of pulmonary interstitial fluid, including an average of 100 mL/h through the thoracic duct. These lymphatic drainage systems can be interrupted during the lung transplant surgical procedure.[38,69] Consequently, excess interstitial fluid can only leave the lung parenchyma via the capillary networks.

According to Starling's law of fluid dynamics, movement of fluids between intravascular to extravascular spaces is dependent on the relationships between intravascular and extravascular oncotic and hydrostatic pressures.[38] In order for interstitial (extravascular) fluid to enter the capillary (intravascular space), either interstitial hydrostatic pressure must exceed capillary hydrostatic pressure or capillary oncotic pressure must exceed interstitial oncotic pressure. These circumstances rarely occur. The loss of lymphatic drainage, therefore, leaves the transplanted lung vulnerable to interstitial fluid retention.

Interstitial fluid retention causes altered gas diffusion, loss of compliance, and increased work of breathing. The loss of lymphatic drainage also interferes with elimination of infectious organisms from the interstitial space, predisposing the lung to infection.

Pulmonary Ciliary Dysfunction After Lung Transplant

Pulmonary cilia in transplanted lungs do not function properly.[40,109,115] The cause of this dysfunction is not clearly understood; however, epithelial abnormalities, specifically ciliary depletion and cellular death, have been described.[40,109,115] As a result, mucus does not move up out of the small terminal airways and can accumulate, causing mucous plugs. Small airways become obstructed, resulting in postobstructive atelectasis and ultimately loss of gas-exchanging units. The result may be hypoxemia and hypercarbia. Accumulated mucus also creates media for bacterial growth and predisposes the patient to infection.[35]

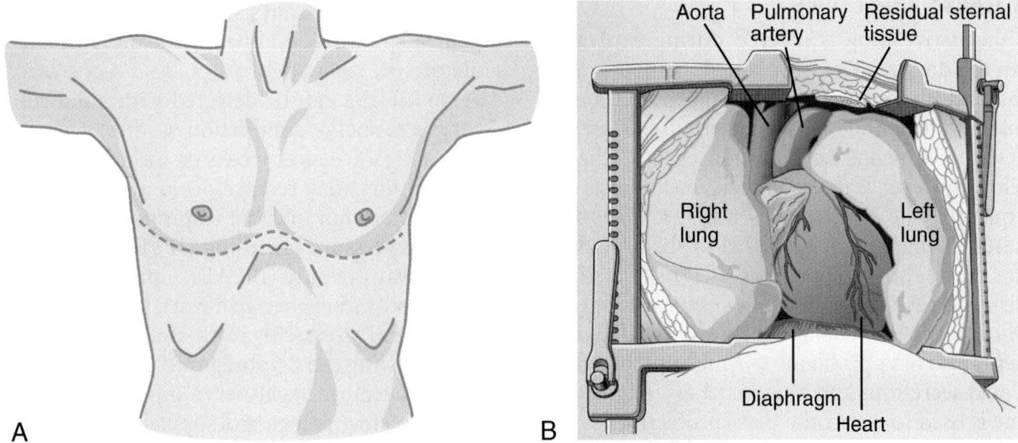

FIG. 8.6 Clamshell incision for lung transplantation. **A,** Bilateral thoracosternotomy or clamshell incision used for bilateral lung transplantation, **B,** Exposed right and left lungs, heart, and great vessels with retraction of ribs and soft tissue via clamshell incision. Sternum has been transected and temporarily removed during the procedure.

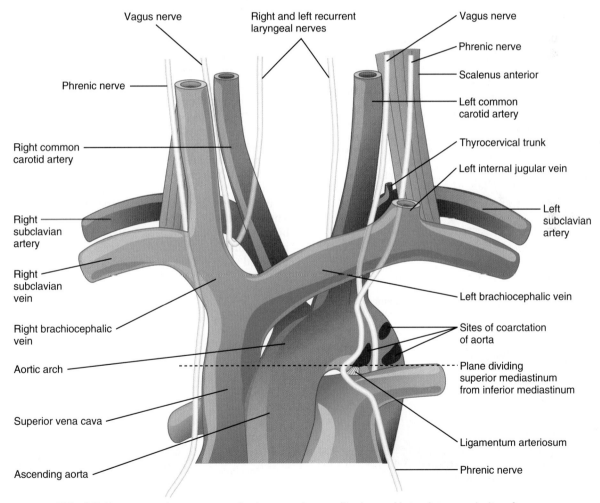

FIG. 8.7 Neurovascular structures in the superior mediastinum. Note close proximity of vagus and phrenic nerves to the heart, great vessels, and lungs. These nerves can easily be injured during heart or lung transplantation.

The Denervated Transplanted Lung

Nerve supply to the native lung is severed during explantation.[40,109,115] When the donor lung is implanted, these thoracic nerves cannot be anastomosed. As a result, the transplanted lung does not transmit or respond to nervous impulses from the central nervous system. Bronchial reflex responses to mechanical stimulation below the level of the bronchial anastomosis are absent.[4,41] Consequently, the patient does not spontaneously cough to expel materials that are aspirated below the bronchial anastomosis.[27] This places the patient at increased risk for silent aspiration. This risk is greatest in patients with preexisting gastroesophageal reflux disease or esophageal disorders related to scleroderma. Patients also have problems sensing, and therefore clearing, accumulated secretions and mucous plugs. Aggressive pulmonary hygiene is used to overcome these problems.

Peripheral Nerve Injuries

During transplant surgery, peripheral nerve injuries may also occur. The phrenic, vagus, and recurrent laryngeal nerves are all vulnerable to injury during dissection and reimplantation (see Figs. 8.7 and 8.8). Injury to the phrenic nerve can produce diaphragmatic paralysis.[29] This complication may present as poor inspiratory volumes or weaning parameters on the ventilator, or, after extubation, as a very weak cough. Phrenic nerve injuries can be detected with a fluoroscopic sniff test or peripheral nerve conduction studies. They may be permanent or may resolve after weeks or months. Patients with a phrenic nerve injury may require prolonged mechanical ventilation or intermittent noninvasive respiratory assistance via intermittent positive pressure breathing (IPPB) or bilevel continuous positive airway pressure (BiPAP). Upright positioning, for example, chair rest (rather than bed rest), helps to decrease the impact of this injury by reducing intra-abdominal pressure on the thorax, thus allowing the diaphragm to move more freely.

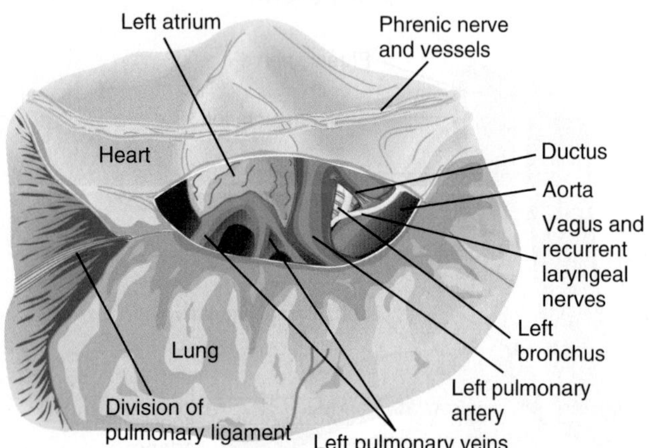

FIG. 8.8 Proximity of peripheral nerves to cardiopulmonary and vascular structures.

Laryngeal or vagal nerve injuries may also occur, producing problems with gastroesophageal reflux, gastroparesis, vocal cord function, and dysphagia.[3,105,124] Injuries to these nerves are more difficult to detect, and although they usually resolve after a few days to weeks, they can produce significant problems.

Injury to the recurrent laryngeal nerve can produce vocal cord paralysis, leaving the patient's airway unprotected. Vocal cord paralysis causes hypophonia or a hoarse voice. It can also interfere with airway protection reflexes, especially during swallowing. After extubation, and before oral hydration or nutrition is started, patients undergo bedside swallow evaluation by a speech therapist. If evidence of vocal cord dysfunction, aspiration, or inability to clear laryngeal penetrations is found, the patient continues without oral intake. A video swallow can be performed to further evaluate functional swallowing. Postpyloric or parenteral nutrition and appropriate speech therapy (swallowing instructions and maneuvers, and recommendations regarding dietary consistency) are provided until the patient can safely swallow. Ear, nose, and throat consult for direct laryngoscopy and vocal cord injection may also be required.

Injuries to the vagus nerve can be more difficult to identify. The patient may complain of heartburn, nausea, early satiety, bloating, or abdominal pain. Patients may present with hoarseness, vomiting, or ileus. Direct laryngoscopy sometimes reveals inflamed vocal cords as a result of acid reflux. Barium swallow

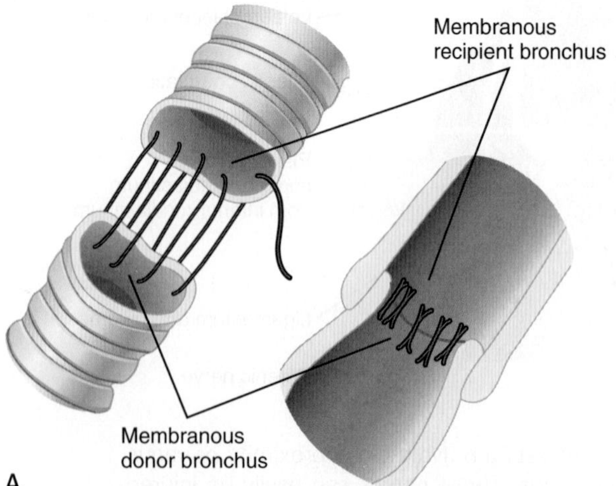

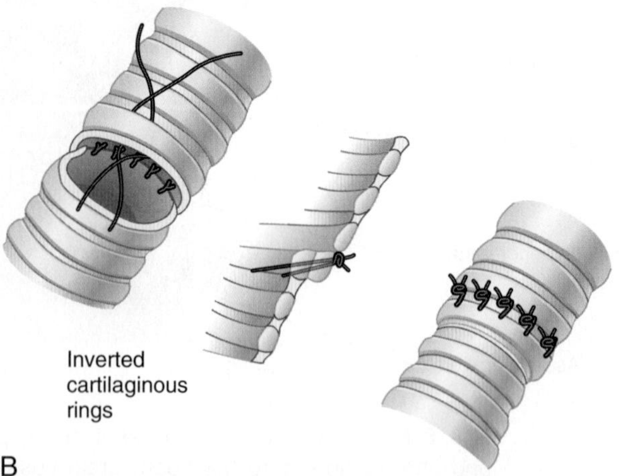

FIG. 8.9 Techniques for membranous and cartilaginous bronchial anastomoses. **A,** Bronchial anastomosis is shown here using an inverted technique that uses continuous sutures on the membranous bronchus and interrupted sutures on the cartilaginous bronchus. **B,** The interrupted sutures used on the cartilaginous bronchus are sewn in a figure-eight pattern. The donor and recipient bronchi are drawn together when the sutures are tightened. Sutures are tied on the external surface.

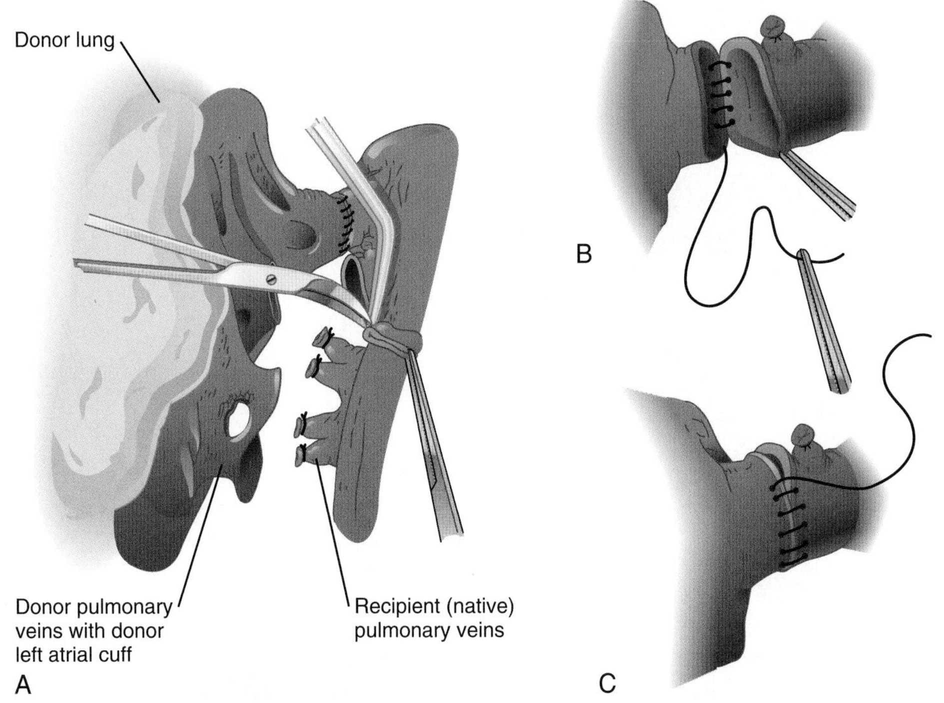

FIG. 8.10 Techniques for pulmonary artery anastomosis in lung transplantation. **A**, Donor and recipient arteries are trimmed to appropriate lengths. **B** and **C**, End-to-end anastomoses of donor to recipient pulmonary arteries.

or endoscopy may be required to rule out esophageal emptying problem or reflux. Gastric emptying studies can determine if emptying times are prolonged. If new to the patient, any of these findings could be evidence of vagal nerve injury. However, the symptoms, signs, and test findings could also have a variety of other causes. Levels of serum electrolytes, especially potassium, magnesium, and calcium, are monitored and maintained within normal limits. Patient mobility should be encouraged. Time in bed is minimized to periods of sleeping, and the patient is assisted out of bed to a chair for all meals. Gastric acid can be controlled with proton pump inhibitors or histamine 2 blockers, and promotility agents can be used to provide symptomatic relief. Small, frequent feedings may be needed to ensure adequate nutrition.

THE IMMUNE SYSTEM AND TRANSPLANTATION

A basic understanding of the immune system is essential when caring for patients who have undergone heart or lung transplantation. Increased survival in this population may be attributed in part to the improved understanding of transplant immunology and the development of more specific immunosuppressive agents to prevent and treat rejection.

The immune system functions to allow the recognition of *self* vs. *nonself*. In this context, a transplanted organ is viewed as a foreign pathogen or antigen, which initiates the immune response directed at the allograft.[38] The location of the major histocompatibility complex (MHC) that codes for the antigens on all cell surfaces is chromosome 6. In humans, these antigens are called human leukocyte antigens (HLAs).[106] HLAs are divided into Class I and Class II antigens. Class I antigens (HLA A, B, and C) are located on all nucleated cells. Class II antigens (HLA DP, DQ, and DR) are found only on antigen-presenting cells (i.e., B lymphocytes, macrophages), activated T lymphocytes, and endothelial cells.[38]

Before being listed for transplantation, patients are HLA typed to identify their preexisting Class I and II antigens. A panel-reactive antibody (PRA) assessment is also obtained to identify preformed antibodies that may have developed after a previous blood transfusion, pregnancy, use of left ventricular assist devices, or a previous transplant.

The immune response to foreign antigens consists of a cellular response and a humoral response. The cellular response is mediated by the T lymphocytes, and the humoral response is mediated by the B lymphocytes. In order for the immune response to be initiated, the foreign antigen must be recognized as nonself by presenting it in the context of the MHC by antigen-presenting cells (APCs). A transplanted organ is different from a foreign pathogen in that it has two sets of APCs capable of stimulating the activation of a recipient's T lymphocytes.[80,105] The direct pathway is thought to be dominant in transplantation and is a result of the donor's cells directly stimulating the recipient's T cells. The intensity of the rejection response is believed to be related to this direct pathway. The indirect pathway involves the recipient's APCs activating T lymphocytes to recognize the donor cell as nonself MHC.[116] Fig. 8.12 illustrates the rejection response that occurs when an allograft cell is identified by the immune system.[80]

IMMUNOSUPPRESSION

Management of immunosuppression is critical to long-term outcomes after transplantation. Intense immunosuppression prevents rejection, but increases the risk of infection and malignancy, and may contribute to dysfunction of other organ systems.[28] Weak immunosuppression decreases the risk of

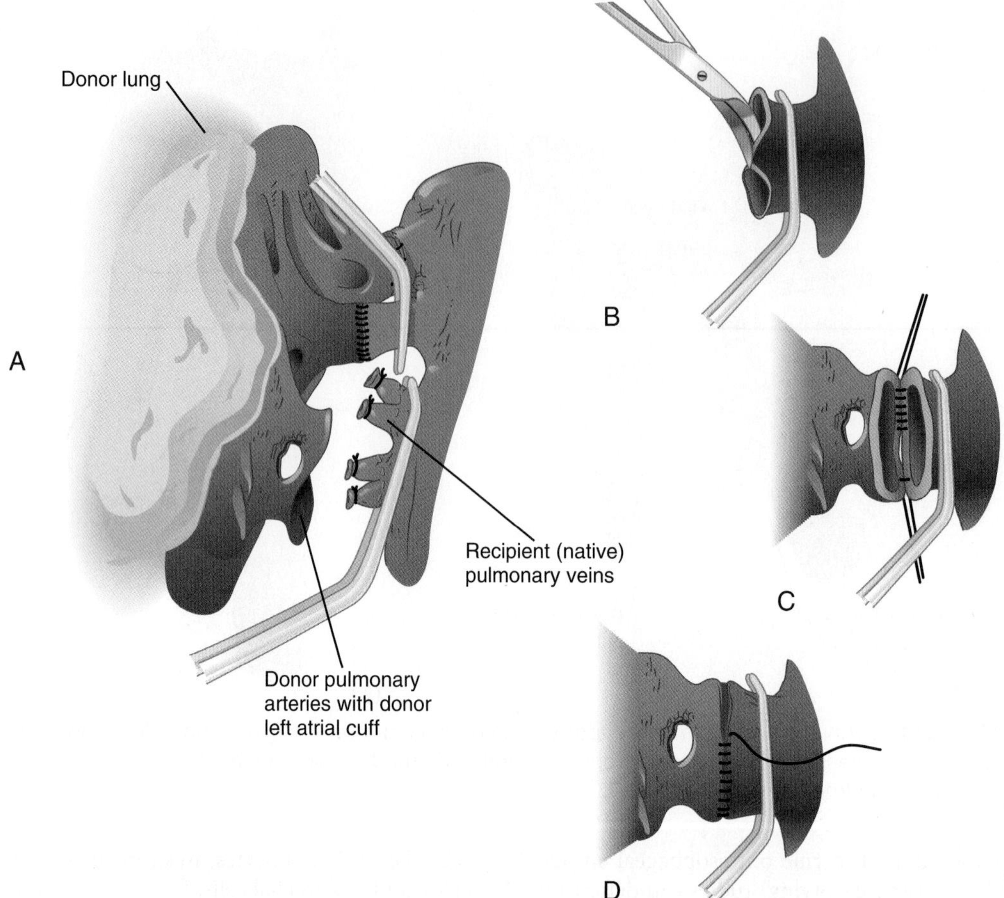

FIG. 8.11 Technique for anastomosis of donor pulmonary vein cuff and recipient left atrial cuff in lung transplantation. **A,** Large recipient left atrial cuff is created by trimming remaining pulmonary vein tissue and incising left atrial tissue between the superior and inferior pulmonary vein insertions into left atria, creating a larger insertion cuff for the donor pulmonary vein cuff. **B-D,** The donor and newly created recipient pulmonary vein cuffs are joined.

infection and malignancy, but increases the risk of rejection and subsequent transplanted organ dysfunction. Consequently, appropriate immunosuppression requires careful attention and close monitoring and is always individualized.

It was not until the introduction of cyclosporine in the 1980s that thoracic transplantation became a viable option for individuals with end-stage heart and lung disease. During the ensuing 35 years, the development of stronger and more specific immunosuppressive agents has allowed clinicians to individualize medication regimens.[78] This has resulted in decreased side effects from the various agents. Immunosuppression regimens are divided into three forms: induction, maintenance, and rescue therapy (Fig. 8.13). Agents in each category are listed in Table 8.2.

During an induction regimen, potent intravenous medications are used to initiate immunosuppression.[68] Induction immunosuppression is provided at the time of surgery, and its goal is to delay the onset of the first episode of acute rejection. Induction protocols are controversial, but are used in 50% of heart and up to 63% of lung transplant centers.[58,125,126] When used, induction protocols begin either in the OR or on the day after surgery.

Intravenous steroids such as methylprednisolone sodium (Solu-Medrol) are used to begin induction and are commonly administered intraoperatively just before removal of arterial cross-clamps. Other agents commonly used for induction include cytolytic agents, such as the polyclonal antibodies antithymocyte immune globulin (equine, ATGAM; rabbit, Thymoglobulin) and the newer interleukin-2 (IL-2) receptor blocker basiliximab (Simulect). Induction agents are also used early after transplant as "renal sparing" therapies to allow for the delay in initiating the use of a calcineurin inhibitor. Calcineurin inhibitors frequently contribute to renal dysfunction. By delaying the use of calcineurin inhibitors until the kidneys have recovered from intraoperative insults, renal function may be preserved or "spared." They are also used for high-risk individuals when donor or recipient characteristics place the recipient at greater than usual risk for rejection.

Antithymocyte cytolytic agents can be associated with several adverse effects, including pancytopenia and bronchospasm. During therapy, patients are monitored closely with daily complete blood counts (CBCs) and CD3 counts to guide dosing. These agents may produce a serum sickness–like syndrome, which presents as fever, chills, and hypotension. It is difficult to differentiate this syndrome from the onset of infection. Premedication with a steroid, acetaminophen (Tylenol), and diphenhydramine (Benadryl) can minimize the severity of this

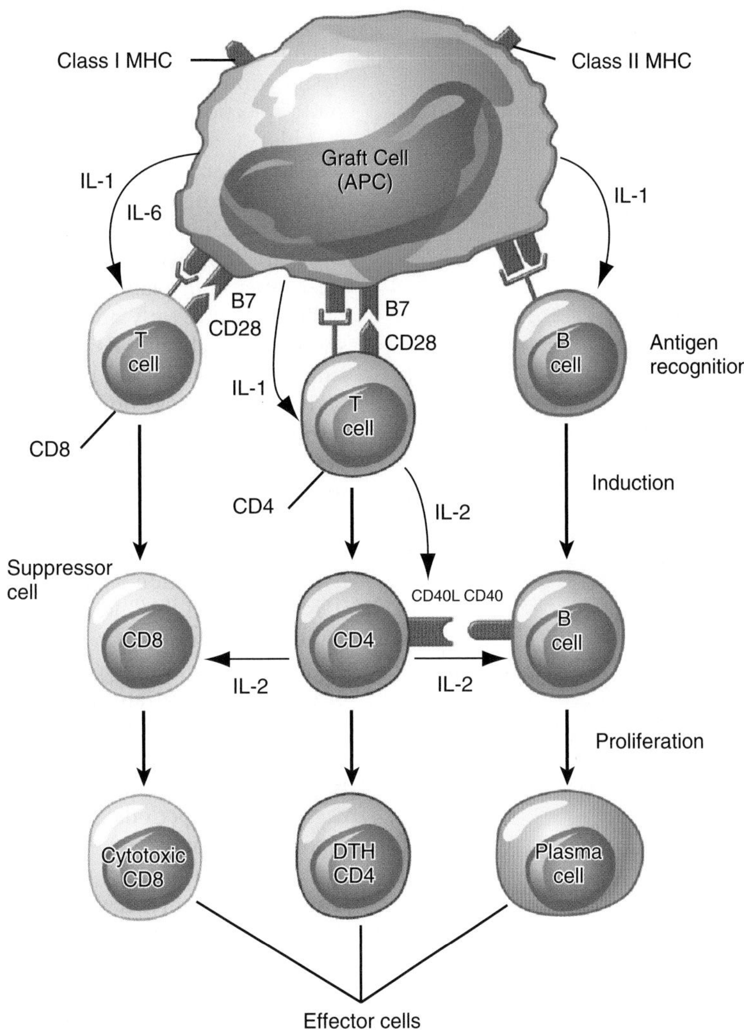

FIG. 8.12 Generation of primary allograft rejection responses. *APC,* Antigen-presenting cell; *MHC,* major histocompatibility; *DTH,* delayed-type hypersensitivity; *IL,* interleukin; *T cell,* T lymphocyte; *B cell,* B lymphocyte.

syndrome. In addition, the use of cytolytic agents increases the risk of infection and malignancy.[81,106]

The IL-2 receptor blockers primarily affect the activated T lymphocytes and are generally well tolerated. They have been found to reduce cellular rejection without increasing infections or malignancy.[26,60,81,97]

The second regimen, maintenance immunosuppression, is a daily medication cocktail designed to allow long-term graft survival and prevent acute rejection episodes. Maintenance immunosuppression is usually lifelong and begins immediately after surgery or after initial induction therapy. Most institutions use what is called "triple therapy" for maintenance immunosuppression.[56,86] Triple therapy consists of simultaneous use of medications from three drug categories: a corticosteroid, a calcineurin inhibitor, and an antimetabolite. Abnormal renal and hepatic function during the immediate postoperative period, as well as low blood cell counts from the use of cytolytic induction agents, requires careful attention when using maintenance immunosuppressants. Dosages are reduced over time, and consideration of rejection history, time since transplant, and other rejection risk factors are used to determine the tapering of each agent.

The most common steroid used for long-term maintenance therapy is prednisone. Cyclosporine (Sandimmune, Neoral, Gengraf) and tacrolimus (Prograf, FK-506) are calcineurin inhibitors. Azathioprine (Imuran) and mycophenolate mofetil (CellCept) are antimetabolites. Many institutions begin maintenance immunosuppression by administering an oral loading dose of a calcineurin inhibitor and an antimetabolite preoperatively. A newer class of immunosuppression agents, inhibitors of the mammalian target of rapamycin (mTOR), specifically Sirolimus (Rapamune) or Everolimus (Zortress) may be used in combination with a drug from another immunosuppressive class. However, use of mTOR agents is avoided early (within the first 3 months) after heart and lung transplant because of the risk of delayed sternal wound healing, or tracheobronchial anastomosis dehiscence.[37,50,86]

The use of immunosuppressive agents to reverse an established rejection is called rescue therapy. Rescue immunosuppression includes the use of potent immunosuppression medications to augment existing immunosuppression, followed by changes to the patient's maintenance regimen to optimize immunosuppression. It typically employs the use of short-course intravenous or increased dose of oral steroids.[56]

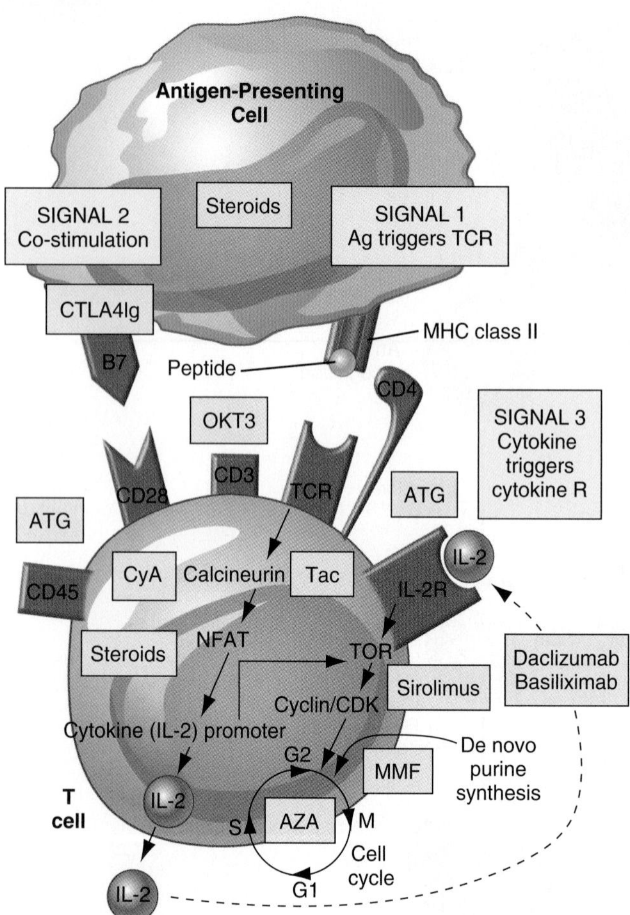

FIG. 8.13 US Food and Drug Administration–approved immunosuppressive agents and sites of action. *APC,* Antigen-presenting cell; *MHC,* major histocompatibility; *IL,* interleukin; *TOR,* target of rapamycin; *TCR,* T-cell receptor; *ATG,* polyclonal antithymocyte globulin; *AZA,* azathioprine; *CyA,* cyclosporine; *MMF,* mycophenolate mofetil; *Tac,* tacrolimus.

Depending on the patient's history, severity of the rejection, and clinical findings, cytolytic agents may be employed. Rescue immunosuppression is not used during the initial posttransplant period unless acute rejection is suspected or diagnosed.

REJECTION

Rejection occurs when the recipient's immune system recognizes the transplanted tissue as foreign and activates complex processes to attack the grafted organ. Rejection can damage and ultimately destroy the transplanted organ. Despite the advances in management of individuals undergoing transplant and the improved survival statistics, rejection continues to be a major cause of morbidity and mortality. Rejection occurring early after transplant can be divided into three categories: hyperacute, acute cellular, and acute antibody-mediated rejection (AMR) (previously known as humoral or vascular rejection).[5,118] Chronic rejection, manifested as accelerated vasculopathy in heart transplants and as bronchiolitis obliterans in lung transplants, develops over several months to years and is not a problem in the acute and critical care recovery period after thoracic transplant surgery.

Signs and symptoms of rejection may be subtle, such as fatigue or fever, or may present as more specific signs of organ dysfunction (Box 8.4). The most reliable method of detecting acute rejection in heart transplant recipients is endomyocardial biopsy, and in lung transplant recipients is transbronchial biopsy. Because many patients do not experience symptoms until rejection is advanced, many transplant centers perform surveillance biopsies on a specific schedule.[34,56,62,103]

Heart transplant recipients undergo biopsy as early as 1 week after transplant. However, pulmonary biopsy is rarely performed this early after transplant, as tissue will invariably show diffuse alveolar damage related to ischemia and reperfusion, and therefore is of little help in guiding further treatment.

Hyperacute rejection is an antibody-mediated or humoral response that may occur within minutes to hours following graft revascularization.[106] This type of rejection is a result of preformed antibodies to donor HLA. These antibodies react to the endothelia of the graft, resulting in the development of microemboli that leads to graft thrombosis and necrosis. Because hyperacute rejection leads to rapid graft dysfunction and loss, it is often fatal.[18,121] Retransplantation is the only treatment option, and death from heart or pulmonary failure typically occurs before another organ can be found. Fortunately, because of the intense pretransplant screening for preformed antibodies, this type of rejection is rare.

Acute cellular rejection is a T lymphocyte mediated response to an allograft. It is uncommon during the acute and critical care recovery periods after thoracic transplant surgery and accounts for only 1.3% and 4.9% of early deaths after heart and lung transplant, respectively.[9,57,105] It is the most prevalent within the first few months posttransplant, and the incidence decreases dramatically after the first year.[106] Despite a decrease in the incidence of acute cellular rejection after the first year, recipients will always be susceptible to the development of this form of rejection and, therefore, will require lifelong immunosuppression.

Initial treatment of acute cellular rejection with rescue immunosuppression includes corticosteroids, either intravenous (IV) methylprednisolone or an increased dose of oral prednisone.[59] If treatment with IV methylprednisolone is used, it is followed by increased doses of oral prednisone that are then rapidly tapered back to the baseline dose over several days (e.g., methylprednisolone 500–1000 mg IV daily for 3 doses, then prednisone 40 mg orally daily for 7 days, followed by a 5 mg/day taper back to the previous daily prednisone dose). If the rejection is steroid resistant or there is severe cardiopulmonary or hemodynamic compromise, cytolytic agents (antithymocyte immune globulin, alemtuzumab) may be used (see Fig. 8.13). In addition, the maintenance immunosuppression is maximized.

Acute antibody-mediated rejection (AMR) is less frequently diagnosed, but this may be because many transplant centers fail to screen for it.[92] For many years, the clinical significance of AMR (previously known as humoral rejection) was disputed. Recently, however, the International Society for Heart Lung Transplantation has recognized AMR as a distinct clinical entity.[81] It is usually seen in the early posttransplant phase. This type of rejection may be correlated with the development of HLA antibodies to the donor but has also been seen without identified HLA antibody formation.[33,107] It is manifested by vascular inflammation and damage.[65] Biopsy immunofluorescence stains disclose immunoglobulin G (IgG), IgA, or IgM depositions with C3d, C4d or C1q.[18,95] This type of rejection

TABLE 8.2 **Immunosuppressant Medications Used after Heart or Lung Transplant**

Medication	Actions	Dosage	Special Considerations
Cyclosporine (Neoral, Gengraf, Sandimmune)	Inhibition of T lymphocytes through suppression of interleukin-2 production and release	PO dose based on baseline creatinine (creatinine < 1.4 = 10 mg/kg to max of 800 mg; creatinine 1.4–2 = 5 mg/kg; creatinine >2 = none) Note: Many centers choose to delay initiating calcineurin inhibitors until after transplantation. Postop: IV infusion 0.25–1 mg/kg/min or 1 mg/h and then adjust dose daily to reach goal blood level before transition to PO. Rising creatinine may preclude aggressive titration to goal. PO dosing adjusted to reach goal level based on morning 12-hour trough levels.	Monitor serum concentrations Monitor for nephrotoxicity (25%–37% incidence); hepatotoxicity (4%–7% incidence); usually responsive to dose reduction. May cause hypertension, tremors, confusion, seizures, hyperkalemia, hypomagnesemia hemolytic-uremic syndrome, and hyperlipidemia. Multiple drug, food, and herbal interactions. Use of NSAIDs can increase nephrotoxicity. Brands are not bioequivalent and should not be used interchangeably. Oral dose will depend on formulation.
Tacrolimus (Prograf)	Inhibition of T lymphocytes through suppression of interleukin-2 (IL-2) production	Note: Many centers choose to delay initiating calcineurin inhibitors until after transplantation. Postop: IV tacrolimus: 0.01 mg/kg/day as continuous infusion: dose based on trough levels. Note: Many centers start postop immunosuppression with IV infusion of tacrolimus to establish goal blood level before transition to PO dosing. Rising creatinine may preclude aggressive titration to goal. PO: 0.015–0.03 mg/kg/day given BID: PO dosing adjusted to reach goal level based on morning 12-hour trough levels	Monitor serum concentrations. Monitor for nephrotoxicity, glucose intolerance. May cause hypertension, tremors, confusion, seizures, hyperkalemia, hemolytic-uremic syndrome, and hyperlipidemia. Multiple drug, food, and herbal interactions. Use of NSAIDs can increase nephrotoxicity.
Sirolimus (Rapamune)	Inhibition of IL-2, IL-4, and IL-5 activation and proliferation of T lymphocytes	PO: 6 mg loading dose. Maintenance: 2–5 mg/day. Doses adjusted based on 24-hour trough levels. Not recommended within 3 months after lung transplant due to impact on healing.	Monitor serum concentrations. Monitor CBC, renal function tests, and lipids. May cause hypertension and hyperlipidemia, bone marrow suppression, hemolytic-uremic syndrome, bronchiolitis obliterans organizing pneumonia.
Everolimus (Zortress)	Inhibits IL-2 and -15 activation and proliferation of both T and B lymphocytes.	PO: 0.75–1 mg given BID. Maintenance: BID dosing based on trough levels. Doses adjusted based on trough levels. Not recommended within 3 months after heart or lung transplant due to impact on healing.	Monitor serum concentrations. Monitor CBC, lipids, glucose tolerance, renal and liver function. May cause hypertension, hyperlipidemia, bone marrow suppression, proteinuria, hemolytic-uremic syndrome, interstitial lung disease.
Mycophenolate mofetil (CellCept)	Inhibits inosine monophosphate dehydrogenase in purine synthesis pathway, thereby inhibiting T and B lymphocytes	Cardiac: 1–1.5 g BID IV/PO. Lung: 1 g BID IV/PO.	Compatible only with D_5W infusions. May cause bone marrow suppression, diarrhea, and vomiting. Monitor CBC, LFTs. Blood levels may be monitored.
Azathioprine (Imuran)	Interferes with DNA and RNA synthesis, inhibition differentiation and proliferation of both T and B lymphocytes	Lung: 2 mg/kg/day to max of 200 mg daily IV/PO.	May cause bone marrow suppression, hepatotoxicity, nausea, and vomiting. Monitor CBC and LFTs.
Methyl-prednisolone (Solu-Medrol)	Suppression of migration of leukocytes; inhibits lymphokine-mediated amplification of macrophages and lymphocytes	Induction protocols are frequently a set dose, e.g., 250–1000 mg IV intraoperatively, followed by POD 1–125 mg IV q 8 h, POD 2–125 mg IV q 12 h, POD 3–switch to prednisone PO dosing 0.1–0.5 mg/kg daily or in divided doses, etc.	Monitor for hyperglycemia, hypokalemia, fluid retention, hypertension, impaired wound healing, myopathy, osteoporosis, gastric ulcers, sleep disturbances, and psychosis.
Prednisone	Suppression of migration of leukocytes; inhibits lymphokine-mediated amplification of macrophages and lymphocytes	PO: 0.1 to 0.5 mg/kg daily or in divided doses. Dose will depend on time since transplant, rejection history, infection history.	Monitor for same adverse effects as for methylprednisolone.

BID, Twice a day; *CBC*, complete blood cell count; *IV*, intravenous; *LFTs*, liver function tests; *PO*, by mouth; *POD*, postoperative day; *OR*, operating room.

BOX 8.4 Signs and Symptoms of Acute Rejection in Thoracic Transplant Recipients

Heart Transplant	Lung Transplant
Fatigue	Fatigue
Shortness of breath	Increased shortness of breath
Low-grade fever	More than 10% decrease in FEV_1
Atrial dysrhythmias	Low-grade fever
Decreased ejection fraction	Increased cough or sputum production
Peripheral edema	Decreased exercise tolerance
Third heart sound	Hypoxemia
Increased jugular venous pressure	Pulmonary infiltrates on CXR
	New pleural effusion

CXR, Chest x-ray; *FEV_1*, forced expiratory volume at 1 second.
From Reference 45.

may occur in the presence or absence of acute cellular rejection. It is often manifested in heart recipients by significant hemodynamic compromise and in lung recipients by pulmonary dysfunction. Treatment may include the use of corticosteroids, the employment of plasmapheresis, and the administration of intravenous immunoglobulin. Rituximab may also be added to the above options to decrease the chance of recurrent AMR episodes.[17]

SURGICAL COMPLICATIONS AFTER THORACIC TRANSPLANT

Common complications and causes of perioperative mortality after thoracic transplant include hemorrhage, infection, early graft failure, cardiac rhythm disturbances, right ventricular failure, acute renal failure, and gastrointestinal disturbances. In addition, lung transplant recipients may also suffer complications related to bronchial, arterial, or venous anastomoses[105,111] (Table 8.3; Fig. 8.14).

Hemorrhage and infection can occur after any surgical procedure. Patients who have had previous thoracic surgeries (e.g., open heart surgery, lobectomy) are at higher risk for bleeding because of the presence of vascular-rich scar tissue from previous surgeries. This may increase bleeding during the dissection required to remove the diseased native organ. CPB, with associated anticoagulation use, also contributes to hemorrhage.

Infections

Infection is a leading cause of early death (within 1 year of transplant) for both heart and lung transplant recipients.[85,93,99,112] Infection control procedures are incorporated into processes for patient evaluation before patients are listed for transplantation.[31,99] These include surveillance activities that occur while the patient is waiting for transplant as well as protocols followed during the perioperative period to minimize infectious exposures and risks. At the time of surgery, infectious risks include incisions, the transplanted organ, systems breached with invasive devices (bloodstream, bladder), and unrelated preoperative infections.

Before being listed for transplantation, transplant candidates are carefully evaluated for the presence of infections or conditions that would increase their risk of infection. Some preexisting infections, such as tuberculosis and hepatitis C, may require treatment before listing. Patients with these potentially life-threatening organisms may be deferred from listing. Candidates are also tested for antibodies to common viral infections (such as herpes simplex virus [HSV]; varicella-zoster virus [VZV]; mumps, rubella, rubeola [MMR]; cytomegalovirus [CMV]; Epstein-Barr virus [EBV]; hepatitis B virus [HBV]; and toxoplasma gondii). Patients who lack immunity to viruses that can be prevented with immunization (VZV, MMR, and HBV) are immunized during the waiting period. Identification of CMV status is used to select appropriate posttransplant prophylaxis. Some centers avoid transplanting EBV-positive organs into an EBV-negative recipient because of the increased risk for posttransplant lymphoproliferative disorder.

Patients found to be chronically colonized with pan-resistant organisms may be deferred from listing.[77,99] Patients with preexisting septic lung processes, such as cystic fibrosis and bronchiectasis, provide sputum specimens for culture at intervals during routine preoperative clinic visits. This culture and sensitivity information is available at the time of transplant and is incorporated into decision making regarding antibiotic therapies.

The use of a mechanical circulatory support (MCS) to bridge a failing heart to transplantation can also present infectious risks.[30] Implanted devices increase the incidence of subacute, device-related (ventricular assist device [VAD] hardware, pocket, and percutaneous driveline) infections, and the risk of colonization with nosocomial microorganisms that may be resistant to standard antibiotics.[119] Multidrug resistance can also be a problem if the patient has required hospitalization or has been exposed to long-term antibiotic therapy before transplantation.

At the time of transplant, the presence of any active infection can significantly increase surgical morbidity and mortality. Most transplant centers will defer the offer of transplantation until an infection is cleared. During the postoperative period, nosocomial infections, caused by the same organisms that plague all critically ill patients, are frequent in solid organ recipients.[112] To minimize the risk of these infections, scrupulous attention is paid to infection control procedures during this period of profound immunosuppression. To minimize exposure to pathogens in critical care after the procedure, the patient is admitted to a private room; careful hand washing is essential; protective equipment, such as gowns, gloves, and masks, is worn during patient contact per institutional policy; and staff and visitors who are ill are asked to avoid patient contact. Strict sterile technique must be observed during line and drain placement and during dressing changes.

Institutional protocols specify initial empiric surgical antibiotic prescriptions. Cephalosporins or vancomycin (Vancocin) are typically used for surgical prophylaxis with heart transplantation to prevent *Staphylococcus aureus* wound infections. Sternal wound infections are very serious and carry a 25% to 31% mortality rate in this population.[1,30] Lung transplant recipients can develop nosocomial pulmonary infections related to donor microorganisms.[99] During the period of ventilatory support before the determination of donor brain death and organ harvest, donor lungs frequently become colonized with gram-negative bacteria. During donor evaluation, sputum is collected for culture to determine if colonization has occurred. At the time of implant, donor and recipient

TABLE 8.3 **Causes of and Complications After Thoracic Transplantation**

Complication	Heart Transplant Causes	Lung Transplant Causes
Hemorrhage	Adhesions from previous cardiac surgery Anticoagulation from CPB	Adhesions from previous thoracic surgery Adhesions from previous pneumothoraxes Adhesions from previous pleurodeses High pulmonary artery or venous pressures Extracorporeal membrane oxygenation
Infections	Sternal wound Invasive lines or drains	Thoracic wound Pneumonia from donor organisms
Early graft failure	Pericardial tamponade Poor myocardial preservation Myocardial stunning, ischemia, or infarction Donor-recipient size mismatch (can prolong surgical procedure or preclude closing the chest)	Ischemia reperfusion injury Pneumonia from preoperative recipient colonization with organisms or septic lung disease Bronchial anastomosis site dehiscence or wound infection Silent aspiration Inability to clear secretions because of poor cough reflex and ciliary paralysis Invasive lines or drains Poor preservation Volume overload Flooding grafted lung with entire cardiac output because of high pulmonary artery pressures in native lung Compression of grafted lung from overexpanded native lung Pulmonary arterial or venous anastomosis stenosis or kinking (may prompt invasive interventions to correct) Dehiscence of bronchial anastomosis Phrenic nerve injury-related diaphragmatic paralysis
Disturbances of cardiac rhythm	Poor preservation Surgical trauma during implantation Interruption of sinoatrial node blood supply Loss of direct neural control Electrolyte imbalance Preoperative use of amiodarone	Postthoracotomy atrial irritability Irritability of pulmonary veins Volume overload and dilation of atria Hypoxemia, hypercarbia, or acidosis Circulating catecholamines Electrolyte imbalance
Right ventricular failure	Preexisting pulmonary hypertension Poor preservation Hypoxemia Acute hypercapnia Left ventricular dysfunction Pericardial tamponade Pulmonary embolism	Ischemia reperfusion injury Persistent pulmonary hypertension Pulmonary arterial or venous anastomosis stenosis or kinking Pulmonary embolism
Renal failure	Preexisting renal insufficiency Ischemia during CPB Nephrotoxic medications Hypertension	Ischemia during CPB Hypoxia because of early graft failure Nephrotoxic medications
Gastrointestinal problems	Pancreatitis "Shock liver" or bowel ischemia/infarction because of CPB	Paralytic ileus, gastroparesis, and gastroesophageal reflux disease related to vagal nerve injury Cystic fibrosis patients: malabsorption resulting from failure to provide pancreatic enzymes, distal intestinal obstruction syndrome

CPB, Cardiopulmonary bypass.

bronchi are swabbed for culture specimens.[16] In the absence of preexisting recipient septic lung disease, broad-spectrum antibiotics are administered during the perioperative period to minimize the risk of infection caused by donor organisms. If gram-negative organisms, such as *Pseudomonas,* are found in the sputum cultures, inhaled tobramycin (Tobi) or colistin (Polymyxin E) is often added to intravenous antibiotics. Once available, the results of both donor and recipient cultures are used to guide specific antibiotic therapy. If all cultures remain negative, and the recipient remains free of signs or symptoms of infection, these empiric antibiotics may be discontinued after 1 week.

Use of multiple invasive devices also increases the risk of infection (such as central vascular catheters or urine catheters) and should be removed as soon as possible. Patients are monitored for any sign or symptom of infection (i.e., temperature elevation, leukocytosis, purulent sputum, inflammation of any wounds). Any evidence of possible infection should prompt an immediate search for a cause with blood, urine, sputum, and drainage specimens for culture, and chest x-ray for infiltrates. Potentially contaminated devices should be removed or replaced using sterile technique. Early consultation with the transplant infectious disease team should also occur to further evaluate the patient and obtain recommendations regarding appropriate antimicrobial therapies.

Opportunistic infection is a well-known complication of immunosuppression in heart and lung transplant recipients. Risk of opportunistic infection is greatest during the period starting approximately 4 weeks after transplant and continuing until approximately 6 months after transplant.[51]

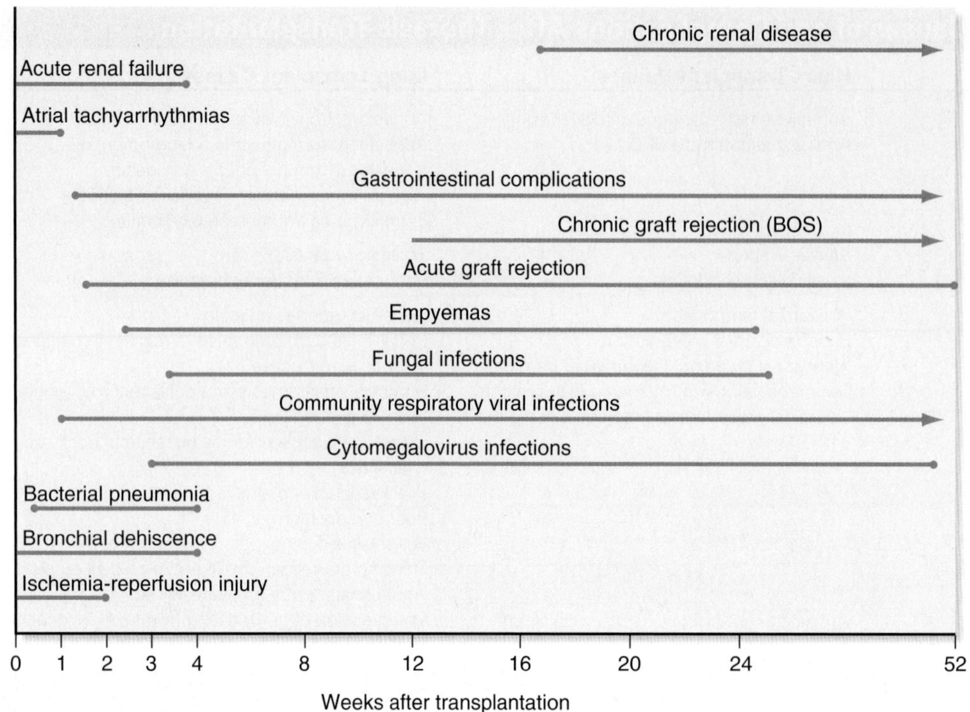

FIG. 8.14 Complications timeline after lung transplantation. *BOS*, Bronchiolitis obliterans syndrome.

Therefore antibiotic prophylaxis for opportunistic infections is instituted during critical care hospitalization (Box 8.5).[68] Prophylactic antimicrobial protocols include medications to prevent *Pneumocystis jiroveci* pneumonia and oral *Candida albicans*. Lung recipients are also vulnerable to aspergillus, particularly at the bronchial anastomosis site,[75] therefore nebulized amphotericin B (Fungizone) is used as prophylaxis.[56,69]

CMV infection can be particularly devastating to heart and lung recipients and contributes to long-term graft loss. Universal prophylaxis with an antiviral has been found to reduce CMV and non-CMV viral disease[46], time from transplant to onset of CMV disease[42], acute rejection, and mortality.[46] Most transplant centers have specific antiviral prophylaxis protocols based on the donor and recipient antibody status for this disease (Table 8.4). CMV immune globulin (CytoGam) is used in the highest-risk patients, in addition to oral or intravenous ganciclovir (Cytovene) or oral valganciclovir (Valcyte). Valacyclovir (Valtrex) may be used for lower-risk patients who need anti–herpes simplex virus prophylaxis.[17]

BOX 8.5 Alternatives for Opportunistic Infection Prophylaxis After Thoracic Transplant*

- *Candida albicans* esophagitis (until daily prednisone dose < 5 mg)
  Nystatin (Mycostatin) solution 500,000 units PO swish and swallow 4 times a day
  Clotrimazole (Mycelex) troches 10 mg PO after meals and before bed
- *Pneumocystis jiroveci* pneumonia (lifelong)
  SS (trimethoprim/sulfamethoxazole [Bactrim]) PO daily or DS (trimethoprim/sulfamethoxazole) every other day
  Dapsone 100 mg PO daily
  Atovaquone (Mepron) 750 mg PO BID
  Pentamidine (NebuPent) nebulization monthly
- *CMV* infection or reactivation (drug protocol and duration varies by risk stratification)
  CytoGam cytomegalovirus immune globulin 150–100 mg/kg for 7 doses
  Ganciclovir 5–10 mg/kg IV daily for 14 days induction followed by 5 mg/kg daily for maintenance period
- Ganciclovir 3 gm PO daily for maintenance period
- Valganciclovir 900 mg PO BID for 14 days induction followed by 900 mg PO daily for maintenance period; acyclovir 2 gm PO in divided doses daily or valacyclovir 500–1000 mg PO daily (after GCV/valganciclovir completed)

*Doses adjusted as needed based on creatinine clearance.
BID, Twice a day; *CMV*, cytomegalovirus; *GCV*, ganciclovir; *IV*, cytomegalovirus; *PO*, by mouth.
From References 42 and 89.

Primary Graft Failure

Primary graft failure (PGF) (previously called early or primary graft dysfunction) is a problem for both heart and lung transplant recipients and accounts for up to 30% of deaths within the first 30 days of heart transplantation.[1] It may occur during weaning from CPB in the OR and can produce right or left ventricular failure. Pharmacologic support may be necessary to successfully wean from bypass. In cases of severe graft dysfunction, atrial pacing, intra-aortic balloon counterpulsation, or single or bilateral VAD may be required. Cardiac graft dysfunction can also present in the initial postoperative phase,[8] and may be caused by poor myocardial protection at the time of procurement, hyperacute cardiac rejection, or pericardial tamponade.

PGF in lung transplant recipients (previously referred to as ischemia reperfusion injury, or IRI) is a common type of acute lung injury that occurs within hours after lung transplant. It is similar to adult respiratory distress syndrome (ARDS) and is associated with high mortality (Fig. 8.15).[13,49]

TABLE 8.4 **Sample Cytomegalovirus Universal Prophylaxis Protocol Based on Donor/Recipient CMV Status**

	Recipient CMV Negative	Recipient CMV Positive
Donor CMV negative	Low risk: Oral valganciclovir or ganciclovir or IV ganciclovir × 6 weeks	Moderate risk: Reactivate recipient's strain of CMV oral valganciclovir IV ganciclovir × 8–12 weeks
Donor CMV positive	Highest risk: Development of new active CMV infection during immunosuppression IV ganciclovir or PO valganciclovir × 12 weeks plus full course CMV immune globulin: CytoGam 150 mg/kg IV on days 0, 14, 28, 42, 56 CytoGam 100 mg/kg IV on days 84 and 112	Moderate risk: Reactivate recipient's strain of CMV or develop new infection from donors strain IV ganciclovir or oral valganciclovir × 8–12 weeks plus full course CMV immune globulin

CMV, cytomegalovirus.
From References 42, 46, and 89.

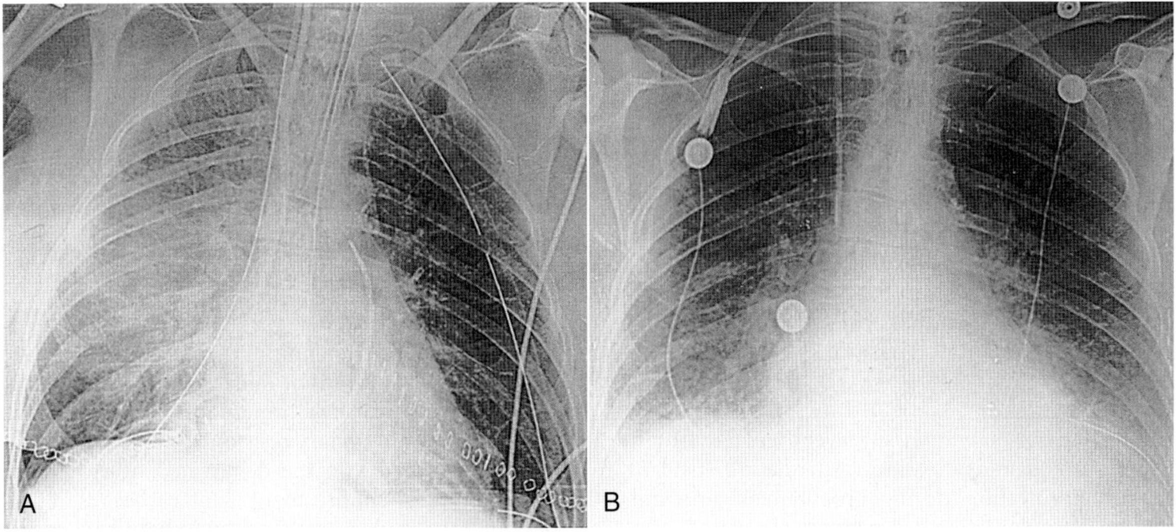

FIG. 8.15 Unilateral ischemia-reperfusion lung injury. **A**, Significant unilateral lung edema and diffuse interstitial infiltrates characteristics of ischemia reperfusion injury. **B**, Same patient several days later with complete resolution of ischemia reperfusion injury after supportive care. From Mora, B.N. & Patterson, G.A. (2002). Lung preservation. In W. Baumgartner, et al. (Eds.). *Heart and lung transplantation* (2nd ed.). Philadelphia: Elsevier.

The causes of pulmonary PGF are not fully understood; however, it is associated with procedural risks, such as prolonged (more than 6 hours) ischemic time, inadequate lung preservation, hyperinflation between harvest and implant, and use of CPB.[12,22] Donor-related risks include increased age, smoking history, aspiration pneumonia, and lung contusions before harvest.[55,69,82,108] Recipient risks of PGF include history of pulmonary arterial hypertension.[122] Loss of lymphatic pulmonary drainage in the transplanted lung and volume overload may also contribute.

Pulmonary PGF presents as a progressive, sometimes rapid decline in lung function. On biopsy, pathologic changes indicative of increased pulmonary capillary permeability, increased interstitial lung water, and occasionally diffuse alveolar damage can be seen.[105] The chest radiograph usually resembles the diffuse pulmonary infiltrates seen in pulmonary edema or ARDS. Clinical signs and symptoms include decreased lung compliance, hypercapnia, hypoxemia, increased pulmonary artery pressures, right ventricular failure, and even systemic shock.[14,69] The appearance of PGF demands immediate attention, including ensuring a negative fluid balance, maximal ventilator support, and occasionally use of inhaled nitric oxide (iNO) and extracorporeal membrane oxygenation (ECMO).[23,55,64,79,91,98]

Airway Problems

After lung transplantation, the area of bronchial anastomosis is particularly vulnerable to injury and infection because it has a poor blood supply and is dependent on retrograde flow from the pulmonary circulation.[96,111] Consequently, the bronchial anastomosis is a relatively ischemic wound, with necrotic tissue subject to infection and dehiscence. The use of complex bronchial revascularization procedures have not been shown to significantly alter outcomes.[83,84] Early use of sirolimus has also been associated with bronchial wound healing problems.[37] Pulmonary PGF and early episodes of acute rejection have also been found to be associated with problems at the bronchial anastomosis.[96]

To decrease the interstitial edema related to the interruption to pulmonary lymphatics, patients are actively diuresed, fluid intake is restricted, and pulmonary hypertension is avoided, which will reduce the capillary hydrostatic pressure and allow interstitial fluid to return to the intravascular compartment.[87] Nursing and respiratory therapy interventions focus on facilitating coughing to assist with mucus clearance, which is necessary because of the ciliary dysfunction. Specific therapies include: chest physiotherapy with postural drainage; cupping and clapping; endotracheal suctioning; and therapeutic bronchoscopy. Patients are encouraged to cough and use the incentive spirometer 10 times hourly while awake. They are also taught other mucus mobilization techniques, such as use of a flutter device and huffing. A flutter device is a handheld, pipe-shaped device through which the patient exhales. As the patient exhales, a ball inside the device moves up and down, creating airway resistance and a slight vibration. This vibration helps to mobilize respiratory secretions.[43,90] Huffing is a coughing technique used to move airway secretions to large airways where they can be cleared by coughing. To huff, the patient inspires deeply and then breathes out forcefully through an open mouth and without closing the glottis, causing a blowing "huh" sound.[61] Once mobilized to the upper airway, secretions can be cleared by expectoration.

Dehiscence presents as abrupt respiratory distress, new air leak, subcutaneous emphysema or expanding pneumothorax, and hemoptysis. Sepsis frequently follows these symptoms. Dehiscence is diagnosed with direct bronchoscopy and, if very small, may be repaired with topical fibrin glue. However, if the area of dehiscence is large, surgical repair may be required.[88]

Dysrhythmias

After heart and lung transplantation, supraventricular dysrhythmias are the most frequent dysrhythmia. After heart transplant, inadequate atrial protection during procurement or surgical trauma during implantation can produce sinus node dysfunction (SND), resulting in a bradydysrhythmia. Additional causes of SND include intraoperative disturbance in blood supply to the SA node or the preoperative use of amiodarone (Cordarone).[36] Because of its long half-life, the antidysrhythmogenic and negative chronotropic effects of amiodarone can persist for some time after the last dose. AV sequential pacing, and less often intravenous isoproterenol or theophylline, may be required to support the HR until the bradycardia resolves. If the bradycardia does not resolve on its own, the insertion of a permanent pacemaker may be required.

AV disturbances can also occur, but the AV node's response to exogenous agents is altered from denervation. In addition, any new onset of dysrhythmia, especially atrial flutter, may signify an acute rejection episode in heart recipients.[20] A right bundle branch block caused by surgical trauma is associated with right ventricular dysfunction.[102] Mobitz I rhythm has also been seen with acute graft failure or rejection.[47] Second-degree AV block and complete heart block are also consequences of surgical injury.[19]

For lung transplant patients, uncontrolled tachycardia can degenerate into atrial fibrillation. Vasopressors, such as dopamine (Intropin), and continued endogenous catecholamine discharge resulting from unrelieved pain can increase the risk of supraventricular tachycardias.[74] Electrolyte imbalances can also increase the risk for dysrhythmias. If present, supraventricular tachycardia in lung recipients should be rate controlled with beta blockers or calcium channel blockers, and treated with amiodarone.

Right Ventricular Failure

Right ventricular (RV) failure in the newly transplanted heart can have devastating effects on the postoperative recovery. Because preexisting pulmonary hypertension contributes to this complication, routine right heart catheterizations are done to assess the pulmonary pressures during pretransplant evaluation. Ideally, the pulmonary vascular resistance (PVR) should be well below 5 Wood units and the transpulmonary gradient less than 12 to 15 mm Hg. Progression of congestive heart failure can lead to an increased PVR as the pressures on the left side of the heart rise. The patient may require continuous intravenous milrinone (Primacor) or dobutamine (Dobutrex) therapy, or MCS, such as implantation of a left or bilateral (right and left) VAD to optimize pulmonary pressures before transplantation.

RV failure can also be the result of hypoxemia, acute hypercapnia, pericardial tamponade, pulmonary embolus, or inadequate preservation of the RV during procurement. Treatment involves optimizing RV output and decreasing pulmonary resistance to RV outflow, with a goal of maintaining a transpulmonary gradient of 5 to 10 mm Hg.[15] A systolic murmur in the tricuspid area and prominent V waves when assessing the jugular venous pressure are indicative of tricuspid regurgitation, which is a complication of RV failure. Lower extremity edema with or without hepatomegaly and abdominal bloating may also be present.

Correcting hypoxemia, acidosis, and electrolyte imbalances can improve RV function. Pharmacologic agents of choice include IV preparations of milrinone, nitroprusside (Nipride), nitroglycerin (Tridil), isoproterenol, and dobutamine. Inhaled NO decreases pulmonary resistance and exerts a positive chronotropic influence on the denervated heart.[15] It is preferred over the use of epoprostenol (Flolan) because of its selective pulmonary vasodilator effects and should be made available both perioperatively and postoperatively. Sildenafil (Revatio) used orally twice daily has also been shown in clinical trials to reduce pulmonary hypertension and has now been approved by the Food and Drug Administration (FDA) for this purpose.[127] If the failure is severe, MCS such as an RV assist device should be initiated to support the failing ventricle until the cause can be corrected or minimized.[17]

Renal Failure

Acute renal insufficiency or renal failure can occur during the initial postoperative phase after heart transplant due to effects of preexisting renal insufficiency, CPB, or a compromised postoperative CO.[76] In lung transplant recipients, aggressive diuresis to decrease interstitial lung water also is a contributing factor. Calcineurin inhibitor immunosuppression is frequently implicated as a major contributor to this complication, but no association has been found between the use of calcineurin inhibitor medications and chronic renal failure (CRF).[76] Among patients undergoing nonrenal transplant, the incidence of CRF has been reported to be as high as 16.5%, with nearly one-third of those patients (28.9%) requiring chronic dialysis or transplantation. Five-year risk of CRF is 6.9% among heart-lung recipients, 10.9% in heart recipients, and 15.8% in lung recipients.[76] Careful attention detects decreases in urine output, indicating inadequate renal perfusion, or decreased effectiveness of diuretics, signifying worsening renal function.

If renal dysfunction is present, diuretics may be used to keep the urine output greater than 50 mL/h. Calcineurin inhibitors (cyclosporine, tacrolimus) may be temporarily avoided because of their nephrotoxic effects. Ojo et al studied the role of calcineurin inhibitors in CRF.[76] In this case, induction therapy with cytolytic antibodies is essential in order to prevent early cellular rejection. When calcineurin inhibitors are used, serum creatinine and 12-hour trough drug levels are monitored daily. Based on these data, the dose is adjusted to achieve therapeutic levels and avoid toxic levels.[76]

Other nephrotoxic agents must also be avoided if at all possible. All nonsteroidal antiinflammatory drugs, with the possible exception of low-dose aspirin, are contraindicated. Aminoglycoside antibiotics, intravenous contrast, and systemic amphotericin are avoided unless absolutely necessary. Doses of renally eliminated drugs, such as trimethoprim/sulfamethoxazole (Bactrim) and ganciclovir (Cytovene), are adjusted daily based on fluctuations in creatinine clearance.

Consultation with a transplant nephrologist is warranted for more than minor changes in renal function. Ultrafiltration, continuous veno-veno hemodialysis, or hemodialysis (see Chapter 23) may be required in order to control fluid balance and provide adequate nutrition and necessary IV medications until renal function improves.

Gastrointestinal Complications

Gastrointestinal complications occur frequently after thoracic transplantation. Symptoms include nausea, vomiting, diarrhea, and abdominal pain or discomfort. The cause may be difficult to determine and may stem from residual effects of anesthesia, the surgery itself, infection, or immunosuppressant or other medication side effects. Mycophenolate mofetil and azathioprine can cause anorexia, nausea, vomiting, dyspepsia, abdominal pain, diarrhea, and elevated levels of liver transaminases. Cyclosporine can also contribute to nausea and vomiting. Hypoperfusion to the gut and bowel ischemia or infarction during bypass can also lead to diarrhea. Pancreatitis can be caused by preexisting pancreatic disease, perioperative hypoperfusion, direct trauma, or drugs such as trimethoprim/sulfamethoxazole or azathioprine. Corticosteroids can mask an acute abdominal process, making diagnosis difficult. Prompt evaluation with blood work and radiographic studies is necessary to rule out an acute process. If one is found, immediate gastrointestinal surgical consultation should be obtained and surgical intervention considered.

Diabetes Mellitus

Both heart and lung transplant recipients are vulnerable to short- or long-term diabetes from the immunosuppressant drugs. Posttransplant hyperglycemia and insulin resistance are significant risk factors for cardiovascular disease and postoperative infections. New postoperative hyperglycemia may be steroid-induced and sometimes disappears once steroids are weaned to minimal doses. The incidence of new diabetes during immunosuppression with tacrolimus is five times greater than that with cyclosporine.[25]

Blood glucose levels are monitored several times a day throughout the postoperative period. If results are significantly elevated, treatment with a continuous insulin drip is indicated. Once glycemic control is attained, the insulin drip can be replaced with long-acting insulin. Short-acting insulin is added as needed before meals on the basis of monitoring results. If only mild hyperglycemia is present, patient is taking oral nutrition, and no renal insufficiency exists, oral agents (sulfonylureas, insulin sensitizers) may be used. Chapter 24 provides comprehensive information about glycemic control.

Nutrition

End-stage lung disease and transplant surgery significantly increase metabolic needs. In general, both heart and lung transplant recipients should be on a heart healthy diet due to immunosuppressant-related hyperlipidemia and hypertension. Dietary intake of carbohydrates may also need to be controlled in patients who are diabetic or develop immunosuppressant-related glucose intolerance. Lung transplant recipients may need increased dietary protein and fat and decreased carbohydrate in order to provide adequate nutritional substrate without increasing carbon dioxide production. Dietary consultation and guidance are necessary to tailor exact diet prescriptions to each patient's unique circumstances. Calorie counts and levels of albumin, prealbumin, and transferrin are monitored to determine adequate nutritional intake. Cystic fibrosis (CF) patients must be given their pancreatic enzymes before meals. Special attention is required to avoid severe constipation in patients with CF, who are prone to distal intestinal obstruction syndrome.

Nutrition should be provided via the enteral or parenteral route within 48 hours of transplant. If the enteral route is used, a postpyloric tube is preferred to minimize the risk of aspiration of gastric contents. Patients should be cleared for oral intake with a swallow evaluation. Because of the risks of delayed esophageal and gastric emptying, patients should be out of bed for all meals and should not resume recumbent position for at least 1 hour after eating.[11] If a patient encounters nausea or vomiting, promotility agents and nonsedating anti-emetics should be used.

Hypertension

Controlling postoperative hypertension after heart transplant is important but must be addressed with caution in the presence of renal insufficiency and cardiac denervation.[101] Judicious use of IV hydralazine in patients who remain intubated may be necessary. If the creatinine level permits, an angiotensin-converting enzyme (ACE) inhibitor is the drug of choice. A short-acting version, such as captopril (Capoten), may initially be used until patient tolerance is established. The renal protection properties of this family of drugs are most beneficial to the transplant recipient because of preexisting or steroid-induced diabetes and the nephrotoxic effects of immunosuppression. If the patient is unable to use ACE inhibitors because of allergy or cough, an angiotensin II receptor blocker (ARB) is an appropriate alternative. These drugs should not be used in the presence of hyperkalemia or without nephrology consult if the creatinine level is greater than or equal to 2.5 mg/dL.

Calcium channel blockers are also effective in controlling hypertension after thoracic transplant. However, diltiazem significantly interacts with and increases cyclosporine blood levels. To avoid cyclosporine toxicity, doses should be cautiously reduced and levels monitored frequently. Beta blockers are used with much less frequency during the initial postoperative phase because of the negative inotropic and chronotropic effects. However, they may be used in lung transplant patients who develop atrial fibrillation with rapid ventricular response. Diuretics can be used in all heart and lung transplant recipients if filling pressures and kidney function allow. Central-acting alpha antagonists may also be used in patients who require triple or quadruple therapy.

GENERAL POSTOPERATIVE CARE

In many ways, initial postoperative care delivered to thoracic transplant recipients is similar to that of any patient who has undergone cardiothoracic surgery (see Chapter 5). Goals of postoperative care after thoracic transplant include stabilization of cardiopulmonary function; prevention of postoperative complications including renal failure, infections, malnutrition, and debilitation; attention to alterations in physiologic function related to transplantation; and initiation of immunosuppression. Many transplant centers use critical pathways to guide care and optimize outcomes. Patients require one-to-one and sometimes two-to-one nursing care until cardiopulmonary stability is attained.

Immediate Care

On admission, arterial blood gases, CBC, electrolytes, blood urea nitrogen (BUN), creatinine, coagulation studies, and portable chest x-ray are obtained. If iNO is used, methemoglobinemia can occur, interfering with tissue oxygen delivery. To prevent this, methemoglobin levels are monitored and abnormal values promptly addressed.

Cardiac rhythm is continuously evaluated. Pacing wires implanted during heart transplant are attached to an external pulse generator set in a demand or AV sequential pacing mode. Peripheral arterial and central venous or pulmonary artery pressure (PAP) catheters are used to assess hemodynamic parameters. CO, cardiac index (CI), filling pressures, PAP, and systemic and PVR measurements are obtained. Transcutaneous oxygen saturation monitors are used to track peripheral tissue oxygenation. Core temperature is measured and a warming blanket is applied if the temperature falls below 36°C. Conscientious fluid balance monitoring requires bladder catheterization with hourly urine output measurement. In addition, patients need at least two large-bore peripheral intravenous catheters to administer multiple IV medications.

Vital signs are monitored for evidence of inadequate CO. Decreases in pulse oximetry may herald worsening ventilation/perfusion (V/Q) mismatch resulting from pulmonary PGF. Elevations in PAP can indicate left ventricular failure, PGF, or hypoxemia and may precede RV failure. Chest x-ray is obtained daily until the patient is extubated and all chest tubes are removed. Pulmonary function is assessed clinically and through ventilator-derived parameters, chest x-rays, and arterial blood gases.

Daily laboratory tests will also provide clues to the patient's status. White blood cells (WBCs) are monitored for elevations indicative of infection and for decreases that may occur with administration of T-cell antibodies or other medication effects (trimethoprim/sulfamethoxazole, azathioprine, ganciclovir). Anemia may occur because of surgical blood loss, effects of T-cell antibodies, and calcineurin-related hemolysis or renal insufficiency. Blood chemistries may reveal abnormalities of magnesium, potassium, glucose, blood urea nitrogen, or creatinine. Many electrolyte abnormalities (such as potassium or magnesium) may occur as side effects of calcineurin inhibitors and should be corrected as needed. If the patient is receiving T-cell antibodies, CD3 counts should be checked daily so that the daily dose of the antibody can be adjusted based on effectiveness of the antibodies in reducing the CD3 count. Once calcineurin inhibitors are started, daily 12-hour trough serum levels of these drugs are checked so that therapeutic, rather than subtherapeutic or toxic, levels are attained.

Pulmonary Care

Immediately postoperatively, patients are intubated with positive pressure ventilation and 100% fraction of inspired oxygen (Fio_2). Mechanical ventilation is continued for 24 to 48 hours until the patient is awake, breathing spontaneously, and able to support respiration without assistance. This usually occurs earlier in heart recipients. In lung transplant recipients, it is especially important to avoid high levels of positive pressure, which could compromise the integrity of the bronchial anastomosis site. Use of high ventilation pressures could also interfere with venous return and pulmonary perfusion.

Most patients will have a single-lumen endotracheal tube. However, lung recipients who receive a single lung transplant for end-stage chronic obstructive pulmonary disease are vulnerable to air trapping in the native lung. To avoid this, these patients may have a double-lumen endotracheal tube (ETT) with one lumen providing ventilation to each main bronchus. When a double-lumen ETT is used, two separate ventilators are required to independently ventilate each lung. These patients require closer supervision and collaboration among nurses, respiratory therapists, and physicians in order to achieve optimal synchronization of the ventilators.

Fio_2 and ventilatory support are weaned on the basis of ongoing assessment of lung function. Arterial blood gases, weaning parameters, measures of patient-ventilator interaction, and clinical examination data are analyzed repeatedly to determine patient progress. Once the patient is physiologically stable and awake, attempts are made to first wean supplemental oxygen to 40% followed by reductions in inspiratory support. During weaning, oxygen saturation is kept above 92% and partial pressure of arterial carbon dioxide ($Paco_2$) is kept below 45 mm Hg, unless permissive hypercarbia is acceptable. Once extubated, a humidified oxygen mask or nasal cannula is necessary to keep the oxygen saturation above 92%.

Secretion clearance is an important component of care. Chest physiotherapy and endotracheal suctioning are performed as needed to remove mucous plugs and to maintain a patent airway. During suctioning, soft red rubber catheters, rather than hard plastic catheters, are used to minimize inadvertent perforation of the bronchial anastomosis site in lung transplant recipients. Increasing inspiratory pressures could indicate retained secretions or an obstruction at the bronchial anastomosis site.

Double-lumen ETTs are more prone to displacement, and their smaller internal diameters predispose them to secretion obstruction. Passing a suction catheter through these small lumens is difficult and may cause the tube to be dislodged. To safely perform this procedure, one provider should stabilize the ETT while another applies suction.

Changes in pulmonary compliance, with a progressive fall in static or dynamic compliance, could indicate increasing lung water or the onset of pulmonary PGF. These patients may also develop high PAP and hypoxemia. Inhaled NO is often used to relieve these problems by producing isolated pulmonary vasodilation, relieving a degree of pulmonary hypertension and consequent RV failure, and improving overall CO. At the same time, iNO decreases mismatch and improves oxygenation. Both of these physiologic effects improve systemic perfusion and oxygenation and reduce the likelihood of renal failure and multisystem organ failure.

Pleural and mediastinal chest tubes are inserted at the end of both heart and lung transplantation. Daily chest x-rays are taken until these tubes are removed. Drainage of more than

100 mL/h of serosanguinous fluid may indicate hemorrhage. The water seal chamber of pleural drainage tubes is monitored for evidence of continued air leak. Should air leak abruptly increase, dehiscence of the bronchial anastomosis, a life-threatening complication, is suspected. Pleural and mediastinal chest tubes remain in place until pneumothoraxes are resolved and daily drainage is less than 100 mL. They are usually removed in a stepwise fashion, with mediastinal tubes removed first and pleural tubes removed one at a time as the patient's x-ray improves.

Aggressive pulmonary care is a must throughout hospitalization. Both heart and lung recipients are assisted to use incentive spirometry, cough, breathe deeply, turn every 2 hours while in bed, and ambulate as soon as possible. Lung recipients also learn to use a flutter valve and specific exercises, such as huffing, to facilitate secretion removal.

Hemodynamic Care

Maintenance of adequate right and left ventricular CO and mean arterial pressure is essential to optimal graft function and to overall patient recovery. In the early postoperative phase after heart transplantation, CO may be less than optimum because of pretransplant ischemic injury or intraoperative insult, and may require support from inotropic agents.

Controlling PVR is especially critical in patients with a history of preoperative pulmonary hypertension. The increased resistance that may be present in the pulmonary vasculature stresses the RV, predisposing it to failure. In lung transplant recipients, iNO may be used to reduce pulmonary hypertension, improve oxygenation, and decrease the effects of ischemia-reperfusion injury. It may also be used after heart transplant to minimize pulmonary hypertension and its deleterious effects on the function of the donor RV. Severe, uncontrolled pulmonary hypertension after heart transplant may require the use of a right VAD to prevent further RV insult.

Dysrhythmias and HR abnormalities can also affect hemodynamic homeostasis. Tachycardia in lung transplant recipients can degenerate into atrial fibrillation. Vasopressors, such as dopamine, and continued endogenous catecholamine discharge from unrelieved pain can increase the risk of supraventricular tachycardias. Dysrhythmias in heart transplant recipients may be related to denervation and are treated as described earlier in the chapter.

Systemic hypotension requires immediate attention and investigation for active bleeding, which may require reoperation control. To avoid pulmonary edema from aggressive fluid resuscitation, nonhemorrhagic hypotension is treated with vasopressors such as phenylephrine (Neo-Synephrine), epinephrine, and dopamine. Alternatively, hypertension can contribute to bleeding and exposes arterial and venous anastomoses to additional stress and increased risk for dehiscence.

Recovery

Once the patient is stable with adequate cardiopulmonary function and successfully extubated, therapies to foster overall recovery begin in earnest. Physical therapy to encourage early ambulation and chair rest at least twice a day improve pulmonary function and promote early recovery. Adequate pain control must be provided during therapy. Thoracotomy is known to be associated with severe postoperative pain. If uncontrolled, this pain can interfere with ambulation, recovery of pulmonary function, overall recovery, and rehabilitation. It is specifically associated with hypoventilation, atelectasis, suppressed cough, and pneumonia. Lung transplantation requires thoracotomy in a chronically ill, debilitated patient who will be profoundly immunosuppressed during the postoperative period. Lung transplantation also alters pulmonary function (e.g., ciliary paralysis, cough reflex, diaphragmatic dysfunction), which increases risks for postoperative complications. Therefore, pain control after lung transplant is of greater importance than after even standard thoracotomy. Pain may be greater and last longer after thoracotomy for lung transplant when compared with standard thoracotomy.[94] These patients may need intensified analgesic plans. Effectiveness of analgesic therapies for these patients should be assessed frequently and titrated to effect. Analgesic therapies may also need to be provided for longer periods of time than for patients undergoing standard thoracotomy. Lung transplant patients should also be assessed carefully for the impact of pain on activities important to their recovery (e.g., ability to ambulate, sleep, deep breathe, clear respiratory secretions, and participate in self-care).[94]

Pain should be assessed at rest and during activities and treated appropriately. Analgesic protocols include systemic opioids, epidural opioids, and local anesthetics, as well as peripheral or intercostal nerve blocks to enable patients to tolerate and actively participate in these therapies.[94] Nonsteroidal anti-inflammatory drugs are avoided because they cause vasoconstriction to the afferent renal arterioles and can increase renal insufficiency when coadministered with calcineurin inhibitors.

Nutritional support is an integral part of the recovery phase. The nasogastric tube can be discontinued after extubation if bowel sounds are present and if no vomiting has occurred. Once endotracheal and nasogastric tubes are removed, heart transplant recipients may receive ice chips followed by small amounts of clear liquids. Adequate swallow and airway protection reflexes should be evaluated in lung recipients before initiating oral nutrition or medications. If well tolerated, the diet can then be advanced to a no-added-salt, low-fat diet for cardiac patients. Medications can be transitioned from IV to oral routes. Immunosuppressant-related nausea should be controlled with antinauseants or anti-emetics to prevent vomiting.

Finally, both the thoracic transplant recipient and his or her family members need to begin learning the complexities of living with the new organ.[21] This instruction begins at the time of transplant evaluation and continues after the procedure. Topics for instruction include importance of adherence to medical regimen and medications, signs and symptoms of infection and rejection, how to minimize the risk for infections, when to call the transplant office, wound care, respiratory care, activity expectations, diet modifications, and follow-up routines.[2,21] Information should be provided both orally and in written form. Teaching sessions should be tailored to the individual, and timed to maximize attention and retention of information without overwhelming the learners. Before being discharged home, both the patient and at least one family member should show evidence of mastery of essential educational materials.

CONCLUSION

Thoracic transplantation is a unique and important last option for patients with end-stage heart or lung disease. Careful donor and recipient selection and care at the time of the transplant can make the difference between success and failure. Care after a thoracic transplant starts with standard post-cardiothoracic surgical care, with the addition of specific needs and complications based on the type of transplant and the attendant altered physiology peculiar to that transplanted organ. Common problems include primary graft failure, infections, renal failure, and atrial dysrhythmias. Optimal outcomes require close collaboration among all members of the transplant team, including, but not limited to, the patient, critical care and transplant nurses, advanced practice nurses, all types of therapists, and physicians.

CASE STUDY 8.1

M.J. is a 52-year-old male with diabetes mellitus (DM), hypertension, and a family history of coronary artery disease (CAD) who was diagnosed with ischemic cardiomyopathy. He initially presented with complaints of decreased exercise tolerance and was treated medically. Despite optimal medical therapy, including percutaneous revascularization, M.J. continued to experience angina and his heart function continued to deteriorate. He was experiencing increasing episodes of heart failure and ventricular tachycardia.

He was referred for a transplant evaluation two years later, which revealed an ejection fraction of 15% with severe global hypokinesis. A right heart catheterization showed right atrial (RA) pressure 11 mm Hg, PAP 16/6 mm Hg, pulmonary artery occlusion pressure (PAOP) 7 mm Hg, and CO 4.5 L/min. On exercise testing, his maximum oxygen consumption (Vo_2) was 11 mL/kg/min with achievement of anaerobic metabolism. Medical history was notable for DM for 8 years and hypertension for 6 years; no prior surgeries, no blood transfusions. Social history was notable for remote 10 pack-year smoking history, daily glass of red wine, and no other substance use or abuse. M.J. was disabled from his job in a manufacturing company sales office and is married to a woman who suffers from rheumatoid arthritis. Following completion of the evaluation, he was placed on the heart transplant waiting list as a status 2. After 6 months on the list, an appropriate donor was available and he underwent an orthotopic heart transplant.

Post-Heart Transplant Care

M.J. tolerated the transplant procedure well with a graft ischemic time of 205 minutes. Initially in critical care, he was ventilated, afebrile, HR 66 beats/min, blood pressure 104/68 mm Hg, right atrial pressure 13 mm Hg, PAP 20/10 mm Hg, PAOP 18 mm Hg, CO 3.5 L/min, respiratory rate 18/min with normal ABGs on stable ventilator settings. He was on IV epinephrine 0.3 mcg/kg/min. Creatinine increased from 1.2 mg/dL preoperatively to 2.5 mg/dL the morning after surgery. Other labs included BUN 52 mL/dL, glucose 340 mL/dL, total bilirubin 1.3 μmol/L, AST 43 units/L, ALT 62 units/L, WBCs 15.2, Hgb 10.5 g/mL, Hct 31%. Initial immunosuppression included basiliximab (Simulect) on the day of surgery followed by methylprednisolone (Medrol) 500 mg IV daily × 3 days, tacrolimus infusion, mycophenolate mofetil (CellCept) 1000 mg IV bid thereafter.

On postoperative day (POD) 3, M.J. was transferred to the cardiac surgery step-down unit. The AV pacemaker was gradually weaned off. Chest tubes were discontinued, which decreased his pain significantly. M.J.'s creatinine level decreased to 1.8 mg/dL; he was transitioned to oral medications and ambulated in the hallways. He and his wife completed posttransplant medication and self-care teaching, and for the last 2 days before discharge, M.J. was selecting and self-administering his own medications. Home care follow-up was arranged, and his wife picked up his new immunosuppressant medications from their pharmacy. M.J. continued to do well and was discharged to home on POD 7.

Decision Point:

Is M.J. an appropriate heart transplant candidate?

Decision Point:

What is your assessment of his overall status?

Decision Point:

What interventions might be appropriate?

REFERENCES

1. Alexander, R., & Steenbergen, C. (2003). Cause of death and sudden cardiac death after heart transplantation. An autospy study. *Am J Clin Pathol, 119*(5), 740–748.
2. Augustine, S., & Ohler, L. (2002). Nursing care. In W. Baumgartner, et al. (Ed.), *Heart and lung transplantation* (2nd ed.). Philadelphia: Saunders.
3. Atkins, B., et al. (2007). Assessing oropharyngeal dysphagia after lung transplantation: altered swallowing mechanisms and increased morbidity. *J Heart Lung Transplant, 26*(11), 1144–1148.
4. Baldwin, J., et al. (1985). Bronchoscopy after cardiopulmonary transplantation. *J Thorac Cardiovasc Surg, 89*(1), 1–7.
5. Baumgartner, W. (2002). Operative techniques used in heart transplantation. In W. Baumgartner, et al. (Ed.), *Heart and lung transplantation* (2nd ed.). Philadelphia: Saunders.
6. Bermudez, C., et al. (2011). Extracorporeal membrane oxygenation as a bridge to lung transplant. *Ann Thoracic Surg, 92*(4), 1226–1231.
7. Bernheim, A., et al. (2004). Atropine often results in complete atrioventricular block or sinus arrest after cardiac transplantation: an unpredictable and dose-independent phenomenon. *Transplantation, 77*(8), 1181–1185.
8. Borkon, A., & Stuart, R. (2002). Postoperative care and immunosuppressive monitoring: heart. In W. Baumgartner, et al. (Ed.), *Heart and lung transplantation* (2nd ed.). Philadelphia: Saunders.
9. Burton, C., et al. (2008). Minimal acute cellular rejection remains prevalent up to 2 years after lung transplantation. *Transplantation, 85*(4), 547–553.
10. Campbell, L. (2000). Cardiac transplantation. In S. Marso, B. Griffin, & E. Topol (Eds.), *Cardiovascular medicine*. Philadelphia: Lippincott Williams & Wilkins.
11. Cantu, R., et al. (2004). Early fundoplication prevents chronic allograft dysfunction in patients with gastroesophageal reflux disease. *Ann Thorac Surg, 78*(4), 1142–1151.
12. Cassivi, S., et al. (2002). Thirteen-year experience in lung transplantation for emphysema. *Ann Thorac Surg, 74*, 1663–1669.
13. Christie, J., et al. (2005). Impact of primary graft failure on outcomes following lung transplantation. *Chest, 127*(1), 161–165.
14. Christie, J., et al. (2005). Report of the ISHLT Working Group on Primary Lung Graft Dysfunction: Definition. *J Heart Lung Transplant, 24*(10), 1454–1459.
15. Chowdhary, S., et al. (2002). Chronotropic effects of nitric oxide in the denervated human heart. *J Physiol, 541*(Pt 2), 645–651.
16. Conte, J., & Reitz, B. (2002). Operative technique of single-lung, bilateral lung, and heart-lung transplantation. In W. Baumgartner, et al. (Ed.), *Heart and lung transplantation* (2nd ed.). Philadelphia: Saunders.
17. Costanzo, M., et al. (2010). The International Society of Heart and Lung Transplantation Guidelines for the care of heart transplant recipients. *J Heart Lung Transplant, 29*(8), 914–956.
18. Cotts, W., & Johnson, M. (2001). The challenge of rejection and cardiac allograft vasculopathy. *Heart Failure Rev, 6*(3), 227–240.
19. Cui, G., et al. (2003). Cause of atrioventricular block in patients after heart transplantation. *Transplantation, 76*(1), 137–142.
20. Cui, G., et al. (2001). Increased incidence of atrial flutter associated with the rejection of heart transplantation. *Am J Cardiol, 88*(3), 280–284.
21. Dabbs, A., et al. (2003). Pattern and predictors of early rejection after lung transplantation. *Am J Crit Care, 12*(6), 497–507.
22. Dalibon, N., et al. (2006). Use of cardiopulmonary bypass for lung transplantation: a 10-year experience. *J Cardiothorac Vasc Anesth, 20*(5), 668–672.
23. Date, H., et al. (1996). Inhaled nitric oxide reduces human lung allograft dysfunction. *J Thorac Cardiovasc Surg, 111*(5), 913–919.
24. Date, H., et al. (2015). Living-donor lobar lung transplantation provides similar survival to cadaveric lung transplantation even for very ill patients. *Eur J Cardiothorac Surg, 47*(6), 967–973.
25. Davidson, J., & Wilkinson, A. (2003). New-onset diabetes after transplantation: 2003 International Consensus Guidelines. *Transplantation, 75*(Suppl. 10), SS3–SS24.

26. de la Torre, M., et al. (2005). Basiliximab in lung transplantation: preliminary experience. *Transplant Proceed*, *37*(3), 1534–1536.
27. D'Ovidio, F., et al. (2005). Bile acid aspiration and the development of bronchiolitis obliterans after lung transplantation. *J Thorac Cardiovasc Surg*, *129*(5), 1144–1152.
28. Eisen, H., & Ross, H. (2004). Optimizing the immunosuppressive regimen in heart transplantation. *J Heart Lung Transplant*, *23*(Suppl. 5), S207–S213.
29. Ferdinande, P., et al. (2004). Phrenic nerve dysfunction after heart-lung and lung transplantation. *J Heart Lung Transplant*, *23*(1), 105–109.
30. Filsoufi, F., et al. (2007). Incidence, treatment strategies and outcome of deep sternal wound infection after orthotopic heart transplantation. *J Heart Lung Transplant*, *26*(11), 1084–1090.
31. Fishman, J. (2007). Infection in solid-organ transplant recipients. *N Engl J Med*, *357*(25), 2601–2614.
32. Garrity, E., et al. (2007). Heart and lung transplantation in the United States, 1996-2005. *Am J Transplant*, *7*(5 Pt 2), 1390–1403.
33. Glanville, A. (2010). Antibody-mediated rejection in lung transplantation: Myth or reality. *J Heart Lung Transplant*, *29*(4), 395–400.
34. Glanville, A. (2013). The role of surveillance bronchoscopy post-lung transplantation. *Semin Respir Crit Care Med*, *34*(3), 414–420.
35. Girgis, R., & Theodore, J. (2002). Physiology and function of the transplant lung allograft. In W. Baumgartner, et al. (Ed.), *Heart and lung transplantation* (2nd ed.). Philadelphia: Saunders.
36. Goldstein, D., et al. (2003). Relative perioperative bradycardia does not lead to adverse outcomes after cardiac transplantation. *Am J Transplant*, *3*(4), 484–491.
37. Groetzner, J., et al. (2004). Airway anastomosis complications in de novo lung transplantation with sirolimus-based immunosuppression. *J Heart Lung Transplant*, *23*(5), 632–638.
38. Guyton, A., & Hall, J. (2016). *Textbook of medical physiology* (13th ed.). Philadelphia: Saunders.
39. Hayanga, A., et al. (2015). Contemporary analysis of early outcomes after lung transplantation in the elderly using a national registry. *J Heart Lung Transplant*, *34*(2), 182–188.
40. Herve, P., et al. (1993). Impairment of bronchial mucociliary clearance in long-term survivors of heart/lung and double-lung transplantation. *Chest*, *103*(1), 59–63.
41. Higenbottam, T., et al. (1989). The cough response to ultrasonically nebulized distilled water in heart-lung transplantation patients. *Am Rev Resp Dis*, *140*(1), 58–61.
42. Hodson, E., et al. (2005). Antiviral medications to prevent cytomegalovirus disease and early death in recipients of solid-organ transplants: a systematic review of randomized controlled trials. *Lancet*, *365*, 2105–2115.
43. Hristara-Papadopoulou, A., et al. (2008). Current devices of respiratory physiotherapy. *Hippokratia*, *12*(4), 211–220.
44. Hunt, S. A., et al. (2009). 2009 focused update incorporated into the ACC/AHA 2005 Guidelines for the Diagnosis and Management of Heart Failure in Adults: a report of the American College of Cardiology Foundation/American Heart Association Task Force on Practice Guidelines: developed in collaboration with the International Society for Heart and Lung Transplantation. *Circulation*, *119*(14), e391–e479.
45. Judge, D., & Hare, J. (2002). Management of acute heart rejection. In W. Baumgartner, et al. (Ed.), *Heart and lung transplantation* (2nd ed.). (pp. 325–332). Philadelphia: Saunders.
46. Kalil, A., et al. (2005). Meta-analysis: the efficacy of strategies to prevent organ disease by cytomegalovirus in solid organ transplant recipients. *Ann Int Med*, *143*(12), 870–880.
47. Kertesz, N., et al. (2003). Long-term follow-up of arrhythmias in pediatric orthotopic heart transplant recipients: incidence and correlation with rejection. *J Heart Lung Transplant*, *22*(8), 889–893.
48. Kilic, A., et al. (2012). Lung transplantation in patients 70 years old or older: have outcomes changed after implementation of the lung allocation score? *J Thorac Cardiovasc Surg*, *144*(5), 1133–1138.
49. King, R., et al. (2000). Reperfusion injury significantly impacts clinical outcome after pulmonary transplantation. *Ann Thorac Surg*, *69*(6), 1681–1685.
50. King-Biggs, M., et al. (2003). Airway anastomotic dehiscence associated with use of sirolimus immediately after lung transplantation. *Transplantation*, *75*(9), 1437–1443.
51. Kishman, J. (2007). Infection in solid-organ transplant recipients. *N Engl J Med*, *357*(25), 2601–2614.
52. Kobashigawa, J. (1999). Postoperative management following heart transplantation. *Transplant Proceed*, *31*(5), 2038–2046.
53. Kutarski, A., et al. (2002). Atrial resynchronization in patients after heart transplantation. *Ann Transplant*, *7*(2), 11–17.
54. Lang, G., et al. (2012). Primary lung transplantation after bridge with extracorporeal membrane oxygenation: a plea for a shift in our paradigms for indications. *Transplantation*, *93*(7), 729–736.
55. Lau, C., Patterson, G., & Palmer, S. (2004). Critical care aspects of lung transplantation. *J Intensive Care Med*, *19*(2), 83–104.
56. Levine, S. (2004). A survey of clinical practice of lung transplantation in North America. *Chest*, *125*(4), 1224–1238.
57. Luckraz, H., et al. (2005). Early mortality after cardiac transplantation: should we do better? *J Heart Lung Transplant*, *24*(4), 401–405.
58. Lund, L., et al. (2014). The registry of the International Society for Heart and Lung Transplantation: thirty-first official adult heart transplant report. *J Heart Lung Transplant*, *33*(10), 996–1008.
59. Martinu, T., et al. (2011). Acute allograft rejection: cellular and humoral process. *Clin Chest Med*, *32*(2), 295–310.
60. Mattei, M., et al. (2007). Lower risk of infectious deaths in cardiac transplant patients receiving basilizimab versus anti-thymocyte globulin as induction therapy. *J Heart Lung Transplant*, *26*(7), 693–699.
61. McCool, F., & Rosen, M. (2006). Nonpharmacologic airway clearance therapies: ACCP evidence-based clinical practice guidelines. *Chest*, *129*(Suppl. 1), 250S–259S.
62. McWilliams, T., et al. (2008). Surveillance bronchoscopy in lung transplant recipients: risk versus benefit. *J Heart Lung Transplant*, *27*(11), 1203–1209.
63. Mehra, M. R., et al. (2006). Listing criteria for heart transplantation: International Society for Heart and Lung Transplantation guidelines for the care of cardiac transplant candidates–2006. *J Heart Lung Transplant*, *25*(9), 1024–1042.
64. Meyers, B., et al. (2000). Selective use of extracorporeal membrane oxygenation is warranted after lung transplantation. *J Thorac Cardiovasc Surg*, *120*(1), 20–26.
65. Michaels, P., et al. (2003). Humoral rejection in cardiac transplantation: risk factors, hemodynamic consequences and relationship to transplant coronary artery disease. *J Heart Lung Transplant*, *22*(1), 58–69.
66. Miniati, D., Robbins, R., & Reitz, B. (2001). Heart and heart-lung transplantation. In E. Braunwald, et al. (Ed.), *Heart disease Vol. 1* (6th ed.). Philadelphia: Saunders.
67. Mobindra, V., & Doyle, R. (2002). Clinical evaluation of heart-lung and lung transplantation candidates. In W. Baumgartner, et al. (Ed.), *Heart and lung transplantation* (2nd ed.). (pp. 64–71). Philadelphia: Saunders.
68. Moffatt, S., et al. (2005). Lung transplantation: a decade of experience. *J Heart Lung Transplant*, *24*(2), 145–151.
69. Moon, M., Barlow, C., & Robbins, R. (2002). Early postoperative care of lung and heart-lung transplant recipients. In W. Baumgartner, et al. (Ed.), *Heart and lung transplantation* (2nd ed.). Philadelphia: Saunders.
70. Morgan, J., & Edwards, N. (2005). Orthotopic cardiac transplantation: comparison of outcome using biatrial, bicaval, and total techniques. *J Cardiac Surg*, *20*(1), 102–106.
71. Morgan, J., et al. (2003). Long-term results of cardiac transplantation in patients 65 years of age and older: a comparative analysis. *Ann Thorac Surg*, *76*(6), 1982–1987.
72. Nathan, S. (2005). Lung transplantation: disease-specific considerations for referral. *Chest*, *127*(3), 1006–1016.
73. Nathan, S., & Ohler, L. (2002). Lung and heart-lung transplantation. In S. Cupples, & L. Ohler (Eds.), *Solid organ transplantation: a handbook of primary health care providers*. New York: Springer.
74. Nielsen, T., et al. (2004). Atrial fibrillation after pulmonary transplant. *Chest*, *126*(3), 496–500.
75. Nunley, D., et al. (2002). Saprophytic fungal infections and complications involving the bronchial anastomosis following human lung transplantation. *Chest*, *122*(4), 1185–1191.

76. Ojo, A., et al. (2003). Chronic renal failure after transplantation of a nonrenal organ. *N Engl J Med, 349*(10), 931–940.
77. Olland, A., et al. (2011). Should cystic fibrosis patients infected with Burkholderia cepacia complex be listed of lung transplantation? *Interact Cardiovasc Thorac Surg, 13*(6), 631–634.
78. O'Neill, J., Taylor, D., & Starling, R. (2004). Immunosuppression for cardiac transplantation—the past, present and future. *Transplant Proceed, 36*(Suppl. 2), S309–S313.
79. Oto, T., et al. (2004). Extracorporeal membrane oxygenation after lung transplantation: evolving technique improves outcomes. *Ann Thoracic Surg, 78*(4), 1230–1235.
80. Parslow, T., et al. (2001). *Medical immunology* (10th ed.). New York: Lange Medical Books/McGraw-Hill.
81. Patel, J., & Kobashigawa, J. (2004). Immunosuppression, diagnosis, and treatment of cardiac allograft rejection. *Semin Thorac Cardiovasc Surg, 16*(4), 378–385.
82. Patel, M., et al. (2005). Hyperinflation during lung preservation and increased reperfusion injury. *J Surg Res, 123*(1), 134–138.
83. Pettersson, G., Yun, J., & Norgaard, M. (2010). Bronchial artery revascularization in lung transplantation: techniques, experience and outcomes. *Curr Opin Organ Transplant, 15*(5), 572–577.
84. Pettersson, G., et al. (2013). Comparative study of bronchial artery revascularization in lung transplantation. *J Thorac Cardiovasc Surg, 146*(6), 894–900.
85. Pham, M. (2015). Prognosis after cardiac transplantation. (Topic 3523, Version 13.0). *UpToDate.* Wolters Kluwer. http://www.uptodate.com/contents/prognosis-after-cardiac-transplantation.
86. Pham, M. (2015). Induction and maintenance of immunosuppressive therapy in cardiac transplantation. (Topic 3530, Version 9.0). *UpToDate.* http://www.uptodate.com/contents/induction-and-maintenance-of-immunosuppressive-therapy-in-cardiac-transplantation.
87. Pilcher, D., et al. (2005). High central venous pressure is associated with prolonged mechanical ventilation and increased mortality after lung transplantation. *J Thorac Cardiovasc Surg, 129*(4), 912–918.
88. Pelletier, M., et al. (2005). Successful repair of tracheal dehiscence after heart-lung transplantation. *J Heart Lung Transplant, 24*(1), 99–101.
89. Pirsch, J., Simmons, W., & Sollinger, H. (2003). *Transplantation drug manual* (4th ed.). Austin, TX: Landes Bioscience.
90. Pryor, J. (1999). Physiotherapy for airway clearance in adults. *Eur Resp J, 14*(6), 1416–1424.
91. Rea, R., Ansani, N., & Seybert, A. (2005). Role of inhaled nitric oxide in adult heart or lung transplant recipients. *Ann Pharmacother, 39*(5), 913–917.
92. Reed, E., et al. (2006). Acute antibody-mediated rejection of cardiac transplants. *J Heart Lung Transplant, 25*(2), 153–159.
93. Remund, K., Best, M., & Egan, J. (2009). Infections relevant to lung transplantation. *Proc Am Thorac Soc, 6*(1), 94–100.
94. Richard, C., et al. (2004). Acute postoperative pain in lung transplant recipients. *Ann Thorac Surg, 77*(6), 1951–1955.
95. Rodriguez, E., et al. (2005). Antibody-Mediated Rejection in Human Cardiac Allografts: evaluation of immunoglobulins and complement activation products C4d and C3d as markers. *Am J Transplant, 5*(11), 2778–2785.
96. Ruttmann, E., et al. (2005). Evaluation of factors damaging the bronchial wall in lung transplantation. *J Heart Lung Transplant, 24*(3), 275–281.
97. Segovia, J., et al. (2006). A randomized multicenter comparison of basilizimab and muromonab (OKT3) in heart transplantation. *Transplantation, 81*(11), 1542–1548.
98. Shargall, Y., et al. (2005). Report of the ISHLT working group on primary lung graft dysfunction. Part IV: Treatment. *J Heart Lung Transplant, 24*(10), 1489–1500.
99. Sims, K., & Blumberg, E. (2011). Common infections in the lung transplant recipient. *Clin Chest Med, 32*(2), 327–341.
100. Simsch, O., et al. (2011). The intensive care management of patients following heart transplantation at the Deutsches Herzzentrum Berlin. *Appl Cardiopulm Pathophys, 15*, 230–240.
101. Spinarova, L. (1999). Hypertension after heart transplantation. *Vnitr Lek, 45*(9), 555–558.
102. Spinarova, L. (2003). Changes in the ECG in chronic heart failure and after transplantation. *Vnitr Lek, 49*(9), 730–733.
103. Stehlik, J., et al. (2006). Utility of long-term surveillance endomyocardial biopsy. *J Heart Lung Transplant, 25*(12), 1402–1409.
104. Straznicka, M., et al. (2002). Aggressive management of lung donors classified as unacceptable: excellent recipient survival one year after transplantation. *J Thorac Cardiovasc Surg, 124*(2), 250–258.
105. Studer, S., et al. (2004). Lung transplant outcomes: a review of survival, graft function, physiology, health-related quality of life and cost-effectiveness. *Eur Resp J, 24*(4), 674–685.
106. Szeto, W., & Rosengard, B. (2002). Basic concepts in transplantation immunology and pharmacologic immunosuppression. In W. Baumgartner, et al. (Ed.), *Heart and lung transplantation* (2nd ed.). Philadelphia: Saunders.
107. Taylor, D., et al. (2000). Allograft coronary artery disease: clinical correlations with circulating anti-HLA antibodies and the immunohistopathologic pattern of vascular rejection. *J Heart Lung Transplant, 19*(6), 518–521.
108. Thabut, B., et al. (2005). Graft ischemic time and outcome of lung transplantation. A multicenter analysis. *Am J Resp Crit Care Med, 171*(7), 786–791.
109. Thomas, B., et al. (2012). Persistent disruption of ciliated epithelium following paediatric lung transplantation. *Eur Resp J, 40*(5), 1245–1252.
110. Tonsho, M., et al. (2014). Heart transplantation: challenges facing the field. *Cold Spring Harb Perspect Med, 4*(5), 1–30.
111. Trulock, E., Patterson, G., & Cooper, J. (2005). Lung transplantation. In D. Kasper, et al. (Ed.), *Harrison's principles of internal medicine* (16th ed.). New York: McGraw-Hill.
112. Tucker, P. (2002). Infectious complications. In W. Baumgartner, et al. (Ed.), *Heart and lung transplantation* (2nd ed.). Philadelphia: Saunders.
113. United Network for Organ Sharing. *US transplantation data.* (2015). http://www.unos.org/about/annual-report/
114. US Organ Procurement and Transplantation Network and the Scientific Registry of Transplant Recipients. (2011). *Transplant data 1997-2004.* www.optn.org OPTN/SRTR 2010 annual Data Report. Department of Health and Human Services, Heath Resources and Services Administration. Rockville, Maryland.
115. Veale, D., et al. (1970). Ciliary beat frequency in transplanted lungs. *Thorax, 48*(10), 629–631.
116. Vella, J. (2013). Transplantation immunobiology. (Topic 7346, Version 11.0). *UpToDate.* http://www.uptodate.com/contents/transplantation-immunobiology.
117. Vermeijden, J., et al. (2009). Lung transplantation for ventilator dependent respiratory failure. *J Heart Lung Transplant, 28*(4), 347–351.
118. Wade, C., et al. (2004). Postoperative nursing care of the cardiac transplant recipient. *Crit Care Nurs Q, 27*(1), 17–28.
119. Wang, P., et al. (2004). Heart transplantation in the patient under ventricular assist complicated with device-related infection. *Transplant Proceed, 36*(8), 2377–2379.
120. Weill, D., et al. (2015). A consensus document for the selection of lung transplant candidates: 2014–n update from the Pulmonary Transplantation Council of the International Society for Heart and Lung Transplantation. *J Heart Lung Transplant, 34*(1), 1–15.
121. Whelan, T., & Hertz, M. (2005). Allograft rejection after lung transplantation. *Clin Chest Med, 26*(4), 599–612.
122. Whitson, B., et al. (2006). Risk factors for primary graft dysfunction after lung transplantation. *J Thorac Cardiovasc Surg, 131*(1), 73–80.
123. Wilson, R., et al. (2000). Sympathetic reinnervation of the sinus node and exercise hemodynamics after cardiac transplantation. *Circulation, 101*(23), 2727–2733.
124. Young, L., et al. (2003). Lung transplantation exacerbates gastroesophageal reflux disease. *Chest, 124*(5), 1689–1693.
125. Yusen, R., et al. (2014). The registry of the International Society for Heart and Lung Transplantation: thirty-first adult lung and heart-lung transplant report–2014; focus theme: retransplantation. *J Heart Lung Transplant, 33*(10), 1009–1024.
126. Yusen, R., et al. (2010). Lung transplantation in the United States, 1999 – 2008. *Am J Transplant, 10*(4 pt. 2), 2047–2068.
127. Zhao, L., et al. (2001). Sildenafil inhibits hypoxia-induced pulmonary hypertension. *Circulation, 104*(4), 424–428.

9

Acute Respiratory Failure and Acute Lung Injury

Theresa Marie Davis and Carol Olff

ACUTE RESPIRATORY FAILURE AND ACUTE LUNG INJURY

Acute respiratory failure (ARF) is the most common type of organ failure and a major cause of morbidity and mortality in the adult critical care unit.[23,24] In the United States, the incidence of ARF increased from 1,007,549 in 2001 to 1,917,910 in 2009 with an associated increase in total hospital costs from $30.1 billion to $54.3 billion.[47,48] ARF alone has a good prognostic outcome; however, when a patient has dysfunction in multiple organs, the chance of mortality rises exponentially per dysfunctional organ.

DEFINITION

ARF is the inability of the respiratory system to maintain gas exchange. One of two phenomena may occur. In type 1 failure, the body fails to deliver an adequate supply of oxygen to the arterial blood. Type 1 is also known as *hypoxemic failure* or *oxygenation failure*. In type 2 failure, the body ineffectively eliminates carbon dioxide (CO_2) from the arterial blood. Type 2 is also known as *hypercapnic respiratory failure* or *ventilatory failure*.[23,24]

Defining objective measurements for ARF is a challenge for healthcare professionals. The most common clinical definition of ARF uses set partial pressure of arterial oxygen tension (Pao_2) and partial pressure of arterial carbon dioxide ($Paco_2$) values. The definition of hypoxemic ARF is a Pao_2 value less than 60 mm Hg. Hypercapnic ARF is defined as a $Paco_2$ value greater than 50 mm Hg with a pH less than or equal to 7.30. Others have defined ARF based on the Pao_2/fraction of inspired oxygen (Fio_2) [P/F] ratio. The Acute Lung Injury (ALI)/Acute Respiratory Distress Syndrome (ARDS) section (later in the chapter) provides a comprehensive review of the P/F ratio.

Nursing Assessment

It is crucial that each patient receives a comprehensive assessment that includes respiratory rate, rhythm, depth, symmetry, pattern, and effort of respirations, including accessory muscle use. Auscultation of anterior, lateral, and posterior lung fields is needed to identify the presence of wheezing, crackles, rhonchi, rubs, or diminished or absent lung sounds that may be indicative of disease progression or adverse events. Palpation and percussion assessment techniques are useful to compare to auscultatory findings. Restlessness is a common indication of early hypoxemia, although alteration in level of consciousness is a late finding in acute respiratory failure. Through appropriate assessments, patients requiring noninvasive ventilatory support or intubation and mechanical ventilation will be identified.

MECHANISM OF HYPOXEMIC ACUTE RESPIRATORY FAILURE

The respiratory system consists of the lungs (the gas-exchanging unit), the chest wall (including the respiratory muscles), the respiratory controllers in the central nervous system (CNS), and the spinal and peripheral nerves that connect the CNS to the respiratory muscles. During hypoxemic ARF, the gas-exchange unit becomes dysfunctional, resulting in the inability to diffuse oxygen across the alveoli to the arterial blood supply. Conditions that often result in hypoxemic ARF include chronic obstructive pulmonary disease (COPD), asthma, bronchiolitis, cystic fibrosis, pneumonia, pulmonary emboli, inhalation of toxic gases, and near drowning.[52]

There are five primary mechanisms of hypoxemic ARF. A brief discussion of each will follow.

Ventilation/Perfusion Mismatching

Under normal physiologic conditions, pulmonary blood flows to ventilated areas, resulting in a matching of ventilation ($\dot{V}$) and perfusion($\dot{Q}$). Hypoxemia causes a compensatory localized capillary vasoconstriction, preventing pulmonary blood from flowing past hypoxic alveoli.[43,46] $\dot{V}/\dot{Q}$ mismatch occurs when some perfused alveoli are flooded or collapsed, as occurs with pneumonia and congestive heart failure (pulmonary edema) ($\dot{V} < \dot{Q}$); some alveoli are ventilated, but not perfused because of capillary thrombosis, as occurs in pulmonary embolism ($\dot{V} > \dot{Q}$). Alveoli are relatively unaffected ($\dot{V} = \dot{Q}$) (Fig. 9.1).

Intrapulmonary Shunt

Depending on the amount of blood that does not take part in gas exchange in the lungs, oxygenation may be greatly affected. Shunt refers to the state in which pulmonary capillary perfusion is normal, but alveolar ventilation is lacking. Pulmonary

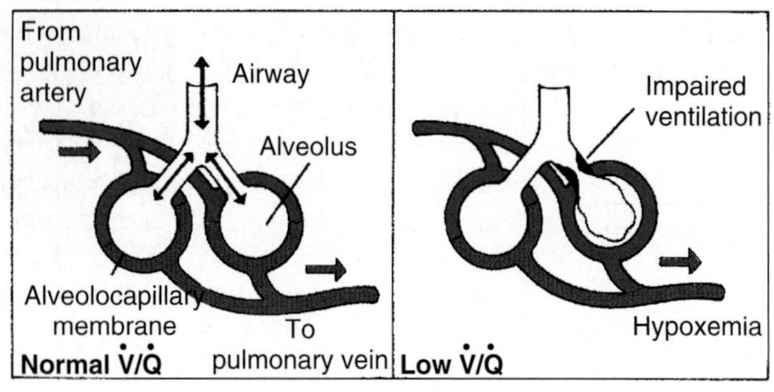

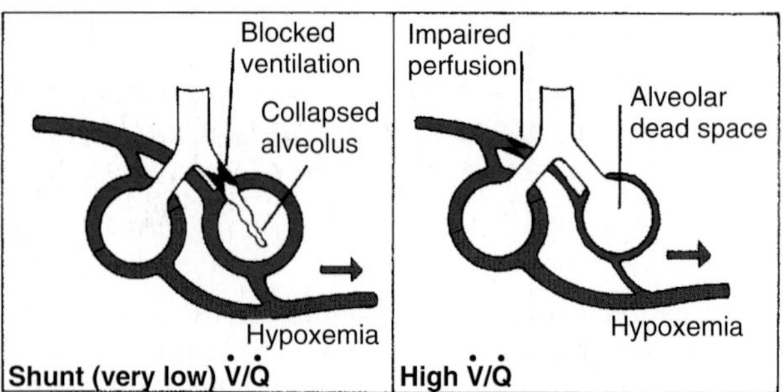

FIG. 9.1 Heterogeneous presentation of alveoli. (From McCance, K. & Huether, S. (2003). *Pathophysiology* (4th ed.). Philadelphia: Mosby.)

capillary blood that passes by a nonfunctioning alveolar unit cannot pick up oxygen from that alveolus. Although some shunting is normal, if too many alveolar units become nonfunctioning, a significant decrease in arterial oxygen saturation (Sao_2) will occur, causing hypoxemia.[42,45]

Indexes of oxygenation are valuable to identify shunting as the primary mechanism of hypoxemia, to assess trends in oxygenation, and to determine effectiveness and titration of therapies. The widening of the partial pressure of the alveolar (*A*) and arterial (*a*) oxygen (*A–a*) gradient, *a*/*A* ratio, and P/F ratio all assist with estimating the degree of intrapulmonary shunt.[52]

The *A–a* gradient is a useful measurement in the evaluation of the hypoxic patient. The *A–a* gradient may be determined by using the following formula:

$$A - a(O_2) = (\%Fio_2/100) * [760 \text{ (atmospheric pressure at sea level)} - 47 \text{ mm Hg (water vapor pressure of humidified air)}] - (Paco_2/0.8) - Pao_2$$

The gradient increases slightly with age and administration of oxygen. An approximation of the normal gradient is (age + 10)/4. The normal *A–a* gradient ranges from 20 to 65 mm Hg. As $Paco_2$ increases, Pao_2 must decrease, but the *A–a* gradient may remain normal. A normal *A–a* gradient implies normal lungs and suggests impaired respiratory control, neuromuscular innervation, or chest wall abnormalities as the etiology of ARF. The three causes of an increased *A–a* gradient are ventilation/perfusion abnormalities (most common), diffusion abnormalities, and arteriovenous shunts.[52]

The *a*/*A* ratio is a commonly used measurement; it is the ratio between the available dissolved oxygen in the arterial bed and the oxygen in the alveolar space. An obtained value greater than 60% is normal and requires no supplemental oxygen. As the *a–A* gradient drops, oxygen supplementation and/or mechanical ventilation may be required. A value less than 60% indicates a worsening intrapulmonary shunt.

The normal P/F value is greater than 350. The minimum clinically acceptable value is 286. As the intrapulmonary shunt worsens, the more this value will drop below normal.

The evaluation of pulmonary vascular resistance (PVR) has been included because of its clinical relevance in the high-acuity patient population. A flow-directed pulmonary artery catheter (PAC) measures PVR. Normal values are 50 to 150 dynes/s cm^{-5}. As respiratory failure is identified, reflex vasoconstriction in the lungs will typically cause an elevation in pulmonary blood pressure, also known as *pulmonary hypertension*.[14] The following factors are associated with increased PVR: decreased Pao_2, decreased pH, increased $Paco_2$, mechanical ventilation, positive end-expiratory pressure (PEEP), pulmonary emboli, scleroderma, emphysema, pneumothorax, and hemothorax; and histamine, prostaglandin, and angiotensin. When respiratory disease produces elevated pulmonary blood pressure, resistance to the ejection of blood from the right ventricle can trigger right-sided failure, resulting in the pathologic condition known as *cor pulmonale* that manifests as venous congestion ranging from distended neck veins to peripheral edema.[52]

Alveolar Hypoventilation

Alveolar hypoventilation may occur with CNS depression that diminishes respiratory drive. "Ondine's curse," or primary alveolar hypoventilation (PAH), is a rare disorder. Both oxygen deprivation and CO_2 accumulation trigger the normal ventilatory drive. PAH patients are thought to have insensitivity to CO_2 accumulation. During periods of sleep apnea, an accumulation of CO_2 does not trigger the respiratory drive. Oxygen therapy may inhibit the ventilatory drive. Obesity, alcohol, and drug overdose may also cause hypoventilation.[39]

Impaired Diffusion

Gas exchange normally occurs rapidly across the narrow alveolar-endothelial interface. However, as fluids accumulate in the interstitium and in the alveolus, respiratory gases are no longer able to diffuse rapidly and gas exchange is impaired. Fick's law of diffusion state that diffusion of gas across a fluid membrane is proportional to the difference in partial pressures of the diffusing gases (oxygen and CO_2), proportional to the area of the membrane, and inversely proportional to the thickness of the membrane. Thus, as the thickness of the air-gas interface increases because of accumulation of fluid and exudates, and the area of the membrane decreases from atelectasis, the ability of the gases to diffuse decreases, leading to shunting throughout the lung. Because CO_2 is more than 22 times more soluble in water compared with oxygen, CO_2 needs less time to diffuse. This is clinically manifested as hypoxemia rather than hypercarbia.

Low Partial Pressure of Inspired Oxygen

Low partial pressure of inspired oxygen (Pio_2) occurs at altitudes above sea level. Low Pio_2 may also occur when gas mixtures are incorrect, which may occur during anesthesia or respiratory therapy.

MECHANISMS OF HYPERCAPNIC ACUTE RESPIRATORY FAILURE

During hypercapnic ARF, the muscles or the respiratory controllers in the CNS have failed and the body is unable to eliminate $Paco_2$ effectively. When ventilation decreases below

4 L/min to 6 L/min, hypercapnia develops. In hypoventilation, the alveolar-arterial oxygen gradient remains relatively normal. Ventilatory pump failure results from primary dysfunction of the CNS respiratory centers, dysfunction of the ventilatory neuromuscular apparatus, or structural abnormalities of the chest wall that prevent effective transmission of respiratory muscle forces. Disorders that can result in hypercapnic ARF include drug overdoses, brain trauma or lesions, Guillain-Barré syndrome, myasthenia gravis, multiple sclerosis, morbid obesity, pneumothorax, COPD, asthma, pneumonia, and acute lung injury (ALI).[52]

Increased dead-space ventilation is the primary pathophysiologic mechanism of hypercapnia (type 2) respiratory failure. Initially, there may be contraction of bronchial smooth muscles as a result either of an immunologically mediated process or of direct stimulation of irritant receptors within the airways, or both. The resistance to airflow occurs primarily during inspiration, which leads to air trapping and hyperventilation. CO_2 retention is a result of diaphragmatic muscle fatigue and wasted ventilation. When hypercapnia occurs in normal lungs, neuromuscular diseases usually cause it. The lungs are normal, but weak respiratory muscles or inadequate neurologic innervation of the muscles decreases the ventilation.

The serum CO_2 level directly relates to the amount of CO_2 the body produces and indirectly relates to the amount of CO_2 the body eliminates. Furthermore, the alveolar ventilation is composed of the expiratory volume minus the dead-space ventilation. If a patient is hypoventilating, the alveolar ventilation decreases and consequently the relative amount of dead space is increased, leading to increased levels of CO_2.

Increased $Paco_2$ will occur if either metabolic CO_2 production increases or alveolar ventilation decreases. Increased CO_2 production may occur during fever, seizure activity, pain, overfeeding, and pregnancy. Decreased alveolar ventilation may occur if there is an increase in dead space or decreased minute ventilation. Some causes of decreased minute ventilation occur with drug overdose, traumatic brain injury, COPD, pneumonia, and atelectasis.

There are three primary mechanisms of hypercapnic ARF. Any condition causing a decrease in lung compliance, an increase in airway resistance, a decrease in chest wall compliance, or a decrease in lung recoil substantially increases the work of breathing, possibly leading to respiratory failure. A brief description of each follows.

Chest Wall/Respiratory Neuromuscular System

The primary muscle of respiration is the diaphragm. It is a dome-shaped muscle that is connected to the sternum anteriorly, the ribs laterally, and the vertebrae posteriorly; the diaphragm separates the thorax from the abdomen. During inhalation, the diaphragm contracts and flattens, pushing down on the abdomen and decreasing the thoracic pressure to below atmospheric pressure, causing a rush of air into the lungs. During exhalation, the diaphragm returns to its dome shape, exerting pressure on the lungs and returning the thorax pressure to a few millimeters of mercury greater than atmospheric pressure. These pressures in combination with the inherent recoil of the lung cause air to exit the lungs passively. Other muscles of inhalation, called *accessory muscles*, include those that elevate and depress the rib cage, back, and shoulder muscles, and those that elevate the sternum and first two ribs. Exhalation is normally passive but may become augmented during exercise or conditions such as asthma or emphysema by using the internal intercostal and abdominal muscles.

Any condition that causes muscular weakness or dysfunction will decrease the ability of these muscles to perform the work of breathing. These conditions include poliomyelitis, amyotrophic lateral sclerosis (ALS), tetanus, muscular dystrophy, myasthenia gravis, stroke, spinal cord injury, scoliosis, and chest wall injury.

Central Nervous System

The CNS controls ventilation. The brainstem in the pons and medulla in the pneumotaxic center, the chemotaxic center, and the dorsal and ventral respiratory groups control ventilation.

Whereas the cerebral cortex controls voluntary ventilation, control of the muscles of respiration occurs in the spinal cord. The phrenic nerve controls the diaphragm. There are central and peripheral chemoreceptors that sense the chemical composition of the blood and extracorporeal fluids and provide information to the CNS about oxygenation, pH, and CO_2 concentrations. Conditions that inhibit these sensors and pneumotaxic and chemotaxic centers include narcotic or sedative overdose, CNS abnormalities, such as tumor or congenital abnormalities, infections of the brain, infections or disruption of the spinal cord, botulism, Guillain-Barré syndrome, myxedema, and obesity (pickwickian syndrome).

Lungs: Airways/Alveoli

Alterations in the airways or alveolar-blood interface (such as from pneumonia, chronic bronchitis and emphysema [COPD], severe asthma, cystic fibrosis, pulmonary edema, pulmonary fibrosis, ALI, and adult respiratory distress syndrome) cause significant alterations of carbon dioxide diffusion. Both high and low $\dot{V}/\dot{Q}$ ratios limit gas exchange. When additional stressors materialize in patients with chronic respiratory conditions (hypoxic or hypercapnic), the patient may succumb to ARF. A Cochrane database meta-analysis of randomized control trials in COPD patients found that noninvasive positive pressure ventilation (NIPPV) reduces the incidence of and morbidities associated with endotracheal intubation and mechanical ventilation.[11]

ACUTE LUNG INJURY/ACUTE RESPIRATORY DISTRESS SYNDROME

ALI and ARDS are life-threatening inflammatory diseases of the lung that manifest in a continuum (Fig. 9.2). Characteristics of

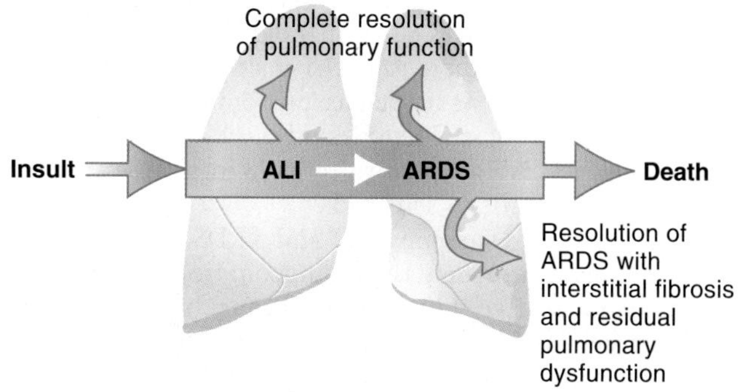

FIG. 9.2 Continuum of lung injury. *ALI*, Acute lung injury; *ARDS*, acute respiratory distress syndrome.

TABLE 9.1 Definition of ALI and ARDS

Onset	Acute and Persistent
Oxygenation criteria	$Pao_2/Fio_2 > 200; \leq 300$ for ALI $Pao_2/Fio_2 \leq 200$ for ARDS
Exclusion criteria	PAOP ≥ 18 mm Hg Clinical evidence of left atrial hypertension
Radiographic criteria	Bilateral opacification representative of pulmonary edema

ALI, Acute lung injury; *ARDS,* acute respiratory distress syndrome; *Fio_2,* fraction of inspired oxygen; *Pao_2,* pressure of arterial oxygen; *PAOP,* pulmonary artery occlusion pressure.
Data from Reference 6.

TABLE 9.2 Results of ALIVE Study

6522 total patients:	463 with ALI (7.1%)
Mechanically ventilated:	16.1% with ALI
Patients presenting with ALI:	55% progressed to ARDS within 3 days
Hospital mortality:	49.4% for ALI, 57.9% for ARDS
Increasing mortality risk with:	Age, immunoincompetence, high severity of illness scores, logistic organ dysfunction, pH less than 7.3, and early air leak (95% confidence interval)

ALI, Acute lung injury; *ALIVE study,* ALI Verification of Epidemiology study; *ARDS,* acute respiratory distress syndrome.
Data from Reference 10.

ALI and ARDS include bilateral pulmonary infiltrates, hypoxemia unresponsive to increasing oxygen supplementation, and decreased pulmonary compliance. In ALI the P/F ratio falls between 200 and 300 mm Hg, and in ARDS the P/F ratio is less than 200 mm Hg.[6]

Vietnam War physicians first described ARDS in the 1960s using names such as shock lung, wet lung, posttraumatic respiratory distress syndrome, and Da Nang lung.[4] These conditions involved common patterns of severe respiratory distress, refractory cyanosis, loss of lung compliance, and diffuse alveolar infiltrates compounded by a variety of clinical contexts including sepsis, pneumonia, aspiration, and major trauma.[50]

Before 1994 a lack of consensus on the defining characteristics of ALI and ARDS impeded epidemiology and outcome research. This problem was partially ameliorated when the North American-European Consensus Conference (NAECC) on ALI and ARDS established the criteria for diagnosis[6] (Table 9.1). The issue is not completely resolved because the definitions provide sensitivity, but still lack specificity, making it difficult to ensure a homogeneous population. The exclusion criterion helps to ensure the absence of heart failure as the cause of pulmonary edema.

EPIDEMIOLOGY AND RISK OF ACUTE LUNG INJURY/ACUTE RESPIRATORY DISTRESS SYNDROME

The incidence and prevalence of ALI and ARDS have historically proven to be elusive numbers, due in part to the lack of definitive definitions. A recent study estimates the annual US ALI incidence to be 64.2 cases per 100,000 persons.[26] The authors of a single hospital study done in Spain using American-European consensus criteria reported the incidence of ARDS (in cases per 100,000 population) as follows: ages 15–29, 4.6; ages 30–44, 13.6; ages 45–59, 21.6; ages 60–74, 51; older than 74, 73.9.[36] In sepsis-induced ARDS, there is a 1.7:1 male preponderance. In nonseptic ARDS, there is no gender predominance.[7] Table 9.2 shows the results of a French study, ALI Verification of Epidemiology (ALIVE),[10] performed in 78 intensive care units (ICUs) with 6522 patients screened.

Risk factors for developing ALI and ARDS are the following: lung transplant patients; immunocompromised patients; patients who receive blood transfusions; severe trauma; increasing age; sepsis; bacterial, viral, and aspiration pneumonia; patients requiring mechanical ventilation; traumatic brain injury; and chronic alcohol abuse.[10,46] The landmark 1993 National Mortality Followback Study for mortality associated with ARDS reported significantly elevated risk for ALI for medical/surgical misadventure, sepsis, nonwhite race, and cirrhosis. Risks were elevated, but not statistically significant, for smokers, former smokers, and those who consume alcohol.[46]

Pathophysiology of Acute Lung Injury/Acute Respiratory Distress Syndrome

It is important to point out that ALI and ARDS are not diseases, but syndromes; they are associated with a number of underlying clinical disease processes, such as pneumonia, trauma, and sepsis. Direct/intrapulmonary injury occurs from damage to the air-alveolus interface. Indirect/extrapulmonary injury happens with damage to the pulmonary vasculature or an event outside the lung. Direct events commonly include pneumonia (bacterial, viral, or fungal) and aspiration. Other, less common direct events include blunt chest trauma, pulmonary contusion, near drowning, oxygen toxicity, gas toxicity, high-altitude edema, drug toxicity, and reperfusion/reexpansion injuries. Indirect contributors to ALI and ARDS include sepsis, systemic inflammatory response syndrome (SIRS), multisystem trauma with fractures, and massive transfusion of blood products resulting in transfusion-related ALI (TRALI). Less common indirect events include disseminated intravascular coagulation (DIC), shock, acute pancreatitis, cardiopulmonary bypass with prolonged bypass time, drug overdose, pulmonary embolism, severe burns, severe malaria, sickle cell crisis, and severe head injury with increased intracranial pressure. Approximately 1 in 20 deaths that occur in patients with ALI are the result of acute arterial hypoxemia respiratory failure.[42,45,50]

The pathophysiology of ALI and ARDS is complex. When the insult is direct, a cascade of inflammation occurs throughout the lung's epithelial, interstitial, and endothelial compartments. When the insult is indirect, the vascular endothelium is the predominant site of inflammation.[42,45] Regardless of the instigating insult, a devastating uncontrolled inflammatory process follows, damaging the alveolar-capillary membrane. This damage causes increased vascular permeability, interstitial edema, plasma protein leakage, and loss of alveolar cellular integrity and function, resulting in diffuse alveolar infiltrates; this is classified as the exudative phase of ALI/ARDS[42,45] (Fig. 9.3).

The normal alveolar-capillary barrier is composed of two layers: the microvascular endothelium and the alveolar epithelium (Fig. 9.4). The normal alveolar epithelial tissue is less permeable than the vascular endothelial tissue. Surfactant decreases the surface tension created by water on the

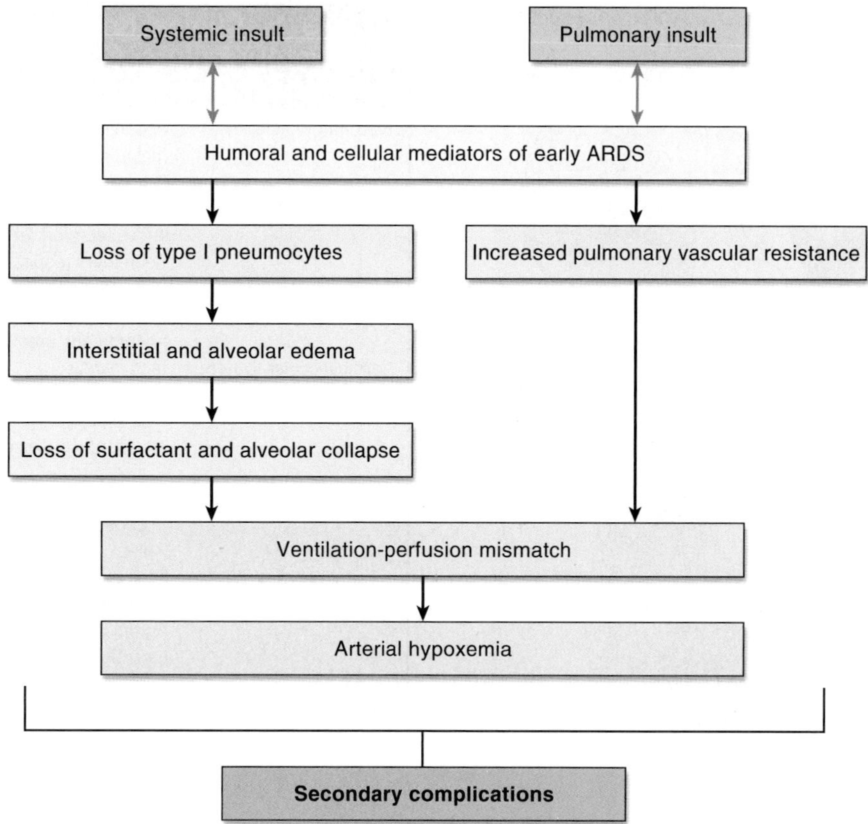

FIG. 9.3 Exudative phase of acute respiratory distress syndrome.

opposing alveolar surfaces. The loss of surfactant as a result of type II pneumocyte dysfunction limits the alveolus from reopening after exhalation. The loss of type II cells inhibits removal of fluids from the alveolus. Hyaline membranes form from the fibrin, blood proteins, alveolar cell debris, and edema on the necrotic and desquamated epithelial basement membranes.[38]

Lung compliance decreases through the loss of surfactant, the accumulation of fluid within the alveoli, and the fibrotic processes that occur as the syndrome progresses to the fibroproliferative stage of ARDS. The loss of functioning epithelium and surfactant prompts the alveoli to collapse, resulting in ventilation/perfusion mismatch and pulmonary shunt. The two major abnormalities in ARDS are the following: pulmonary shunt, blood flowing in unventilated areas (low $\dot{V}/\dot{Q}$ units), and ventilation of areas of limited perfusion (high $\dot{V}/\dot{Q}$ units). ARDS will occur when $\dot{V}/\dot{Q}$ mismatching is severe[39] (see Fig. 9.1).

Host defenses generate an uncontrolled inflammatory response in ALI and ARDS. Both the epithelial and the endothelial cells produce and release proinflammatory and anti-inflammatory mediators, contributing to the inflammatory cascade. Complement activation occurs during bacterial infection; excess production of the proinflammatory mediators C3a and C5a contributes to complement-activated cellular damage and organ failure.[57]

Resident in the normal lung tissue is the alveolar macrophage—a mononuclear phagocyte that engulfs and destroys inhaled particulates, cellular debris, and infectious material. Macrophages promote adaptive immunity as antigen-presenting cells through T-lymphocyte activation.[20] Macrophages express tissue factor, tumor necrosis factor alpha (TNFα), eicosanoids, or macrophage migration inhibitory factor, dependent upon the inciting extracellular milieu.[20,38] Cytokines and chemokines stimulate chemotaxis and cause neutrophil activation. Pathology reports from patients with ARDS show massive pulmonary accumulation of neutrophils.[56] Neutrophils release oxidants, proteases, leukotrienes, and platelet-activating factor (PAF), which damage cellular membranes and cause microthrombosis.[38]

Cytokines IL-1 and TNF activate endothelial cells to upregulate cellular surface protein receptors, increasing extravasation of neutrophils, monocytes, T cells, and B and T memory cells into the tissues. Cytokines and the other inflammatory mediators cause damage to the endothelial layers of the adjacent alveolar capillaries, producing thrombosis, fibrosis, and vascular occlusion. Pulmonary hypertension is a common finding in ARDS resulting from pulmonary vasoconstriction, thromboembolism, and interstitial edema. The pulmonary endothelium controls the vascular smooth muscle tone through the synthesis and release of nitric oxide, thromboxane, prostaglandins, cyclooxygenase (COX) products, leukotrienes, endothelins, and PAF. [14] Prostaglandins and nitric oxide are pulmonary vasodilators. Thromboxane is a potent vasoconstrictor and bronchoconstrictor, and it promotes platelet aggregation.[35] Endothelins are vasoconstrictors; they also increase capillary permeability.[14] Vasoconstrictors predominate in the pulmonary vasculature in ALI/ARDS. Pulmonary hypertension diminishes right heart function and cardiac output, decreasing systemic oxygen delivery and end-organ perfusion. The magnitude of pulmonary hypertension has been positively correlated with severity of lung injury and mortality.[14]

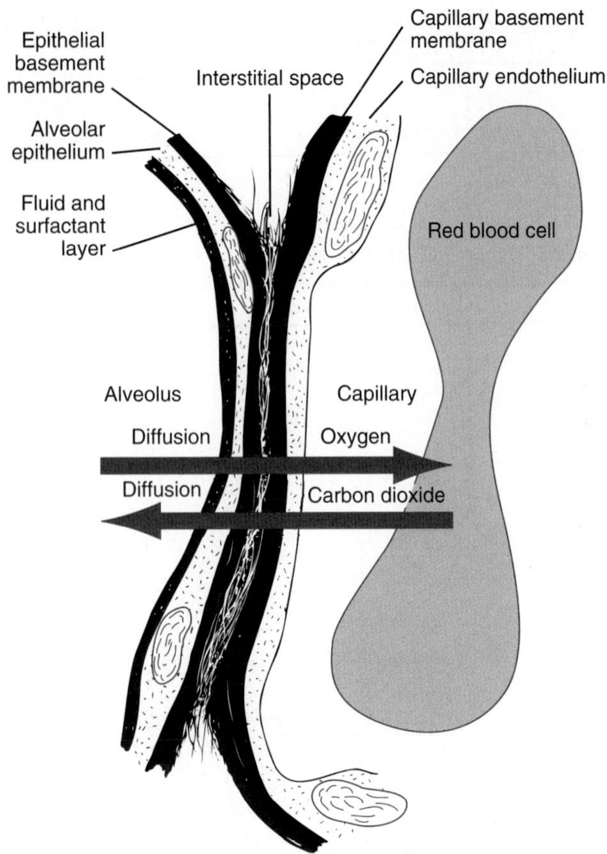

FIG. 9.4 Alveolar endothelial interface. (From Guyton, A. & Hall, J. (2002). *Textbook of medical physiology* (10th ed.). Philadelphia: Saunders.)

Host defenses are mobilized not only by invading organisms (bacterial, viral, fungal), which initiate the inflammatory cascade, but also by iatrogenic complications, such as those injuries caused by mechanical ventilation. Detailed discussion of these concepts appears later in the chapter.

Physical Assessment Findings

The ALI/ARDS patient presents with alterations to many organ systems—respiratory system, cardiovascular system, central nervous system, and integumentary system (Box 9.1).

Respiratory System

The ALI/ARDS patient will exhibit a widening of the *A–a* gradient. The P/F ratio will become elevated as respiratory dysfunction ensues. The P/F is less accurate at FiO_2 values less than or equal to 0.5 than with higher FiO_2 values.[27] Tachypnea results from increased metabolic rate, increased systemic CO_2 production, and decreased alveolar dead space to tidal volume delivered ratio (V_D/V_T), which contributes to high minute ventilation (V_E). Pulmonary hypertension is evidenced by an increase in pulmonary artery pressure, and results from vasoconstriction of the pulmonary capillary bed that is partially caused by hypoxia from the shunt. Right heart strain may be evident on the electrocardiogram. Diffuse bilateral pulmonary infiltrates reflect noncardiogenic pulmonary edema. On exam, the practitioner will detect increased work of breathing, as evidenced by tachypnea, use of accessory muscles, intercostal retractions, and nasal flaring. Decreased respiratory excursion, dullness to percussion, diminished breath sounds in atelectatic areas, and adventitious breath sounds (crackles or rales, rhonchi, wheezes, and rubs) will be evident.[27]

BOX 9.1 Clinical Presentation of the Acute Respiratory Failure/Acute Lung Injury/Acute Respiratory Distress Syndrome Patient

Respiratory system	Widening of the alveolar/arterial gradient
	Tachypnea
	Pulmonary hypertension
	Pulmonary edema
	Increased work of breathing
	Decreased respiratory excursion
	Dullness to percussion
	Diminished breath sounds
	Adventitious breath sounds
Cardiovascular system	Tachycardia
	Decreased pulmonary artery occlusion pressure
	Increased cardiac output and cardiac index in sepsis
Integumentary system	Increased capillary refill time
	Cyanosis
	Pallor
Central nervous system	Early signs: Anxiety
	Forgetfulness, distractibility
	Agitation
	Late signs: Altered level of consciousness
	Coma

Cardiovascular System

The ALI/ARDS patient will exhibit tachycardia because of the increased workload on the heart related to dysfunction in oxygen exchange. Hemodynamics may demonstrate decreased pulmonary artery occlusion pressure (PAOP) also called pulmonary artery wedge pressure (PAWP) in the face of pulmonary edema, pulmonary hypertension, or high-pressure ventilation strategies. The right side of the heart will be working against increased pressures; failure or dysfunction will exacerbate the pulmonary edema and contribute to left-sided dysfunction. With other conditions, such as sepsis, the patient may exhibit increased cardiac output and cardiac index. Septic patients with cardiac dysfunction and those with preexisting cardiac abnormality may obviously not fit within the ALI/ARDS definition limitation of a normal PAOP.

Integumentary System

Capillary refill time is increased with hypoxia. Cyanosis and pallor are late signs.

Central Nervous System

Anxiety, forgetfulness, distraction, and agitation are early signs of hypoxemia. CNS changes ranging from altered level of consciousness to frank coma occur in severe hypoxemia.

DIAGNOSTIC EVALUATIONS

The chest radiograph (CXR) of a patient with ALI/ARDS will change over the course of the disease progression. Early in the course of the disease, the patient will present with hypoxia, while the CXR may be relatively normal. As the disease progresses and fluid accumulates in the interstitial and alveolar spaces, the CXR will begin to have a hazy, white appearance consistent with interstitial fluid accumulation and alveolar flooding. Small lines

(Kerley B) will appear as fissures fill with fluid. Increased vascular markings will appear as the vascular endothelium thickens because of fluid accumulation. Infiltrates and consolidation will become evident as whitened areas appear on the CXR. The silhouette sign is the loss of visibility of a perceived boundary between two elements because of fluid accumulation. Air bronchograms may become evident when an air-filled bronchus traverses a consolidated lung area. ARDS generally progresses to virtual "whiteout" of the CXR as air is absorbed from atelectatic lungs; fluid, foam, and cellular debris fill the alveoli and airways. Atelectasis may become more evident in the resolving phase of ARDS, evidenced by increased density; abnormally placed fissures; and hilar, diaphragmatic, and mediastinal changes in position and size on CXR. The fibroproliferative stage may show an interstitial pattern of irregular branching of the blood vessels and bronchi. The belief that CXRs are nonspecific in volume status interpretation in ALI/ARDS patients has been challenged for several years. One study reported that radiographic changes in vascular pedicle width correlate highly with intravascular volume status.[37]

In 1998 Gattinoni, Pelosi, and Sutter[25] published a landmark paper on ARDS describing the use of computed tomography (CT) scanning of the lungs to differentiate the lung damage associated with direct and indirect insults and explaining how each is impacted by the application of PEEP. The study refutes the commonly held belief that ALI/ARDS lung damage is a homogeneous process within the lung.[25] Morphologic changes evident on CT scan in all ALI/ARDS patients include ground-glass opacification with preservation of bronchial and vascular markings, consolidation, and reticular patterns. The CT scan shows inhomogeneous disease in the craniocaudal and sternovertebral planes, revealing dependent and caudal areas with greater fluid accumulation. CT scanning has enabled the understanding that the tissue mass (tissue and fluid) to gas ratio is doubled in ARDS and that recruitment of collapsed and partially fluid-filled alveoli occurs throughout the entire volume/pressure curve, implying the existence of multiple regions with differing opening pressures. CT scanning allows more definitive diagnosis of effusion, atelectasis, abscesses, and pneumothoraces than CXR.[15]

Laboratory and Microbiology Studies

The arterial blood gas (ABG) is essential in the diagnosis and care of a patient with ALI/ARDS. The ABG is a sensitive test for identifying early ALI/ARDS. Both the P/F ratio and the *A–a* gradient are calculated from the ABG. The *A–a* gradient provides an assessment of alveolar-capillary gas exchange; the larger the gradient, the more serious the respiratory compromise. Alterations in the ABG of an ALI/ARDS patient typically include hypoxemia. Early in the disease process, the patient compensates for hypoxia with tachypnea. Hyperventilation may cause hypocapnia, manifested as respiratory alkalosis. Hypercapnia occurs when shunts have formed, causing $\dot{V}/\dot{Q}$ mismatch and severe impairment of gas exchange. Imbalance in pH is evident when hypercapnia occurs and when end-organ tissue oxygenation is impaired, producing lactic acidosis from anaerobic metabolism (generally producing a mixed metabolic and respiratory acidosis).

When the cause of ALI/ARDS is not evident, the patient should be pan-cultured (wound, blood, urine, and sputum) for all conceivable sources of infection as sepsis is the most common cause of ALI/ARDS.[38] Complete blood cell count, including differential, is useful in identifying infectious causes and a decreased hematocrit contributing to hypoxemia. Chemistry panels monitor for the presence of multiple organ failure, nutritional deficits, fluid status, electrolyte balance, metabolic acidosis, blood glucose control, and effectiveness of treatments and supportive care.

INTERPROFESSIONAL PLAN OF CARE

The desired outcome for patients with ALI or ARDS is the provision of a lung-protective ventilation strategy that prevents further injury while providing oxygenation and ventilation sufficient to sustain the patient until the syndrome resolves. Of significant importance to a positive patient outcome is direct, open communication between all care providers, such that each is aware of the complete plan of care, current difficulties, and potential solutions. Familiarity with guidelines on the care of ALI/ARDS ensures appropriate care by the entire interprofessional team. Deviation from guidelines is appropriate when dictated by comorbidities or unusual circumstances. When this occurs, the team must understand the rationale for the deviation from the guidelines, thus providing the team an opportunity to develop a modified plan. This plan of care should consider the following:

- Ventilator bundle measures, including frequent oral care, head-of-bed (HOB) elevation greater than 30 degrees, daily weaning assessment, deep vein thrombosis (DVT) prophylaxis, stress ulcer prophylaxis, etc. See AACN practice alerts for ventilator-associated pneumonia prevention and oral care at www.aacn.org.
- Monitoring pulmonary function tests (PFTs), vital capacity (VC), maximum inspiratory pressure (MIP), minute volume (V_E), and tidal volume (V_T) to allow for early intervention and early weaning.
- Review of CXR and ABG results for additional diagnostic and monitoring information.
- Positioning, including proning, to alleviate dyspnea and provide optimal ventilation.
- Administration of humidified oxygen, as appropriate, to increase the oxygen pressure gradient for diffusion between alveoli and blood.
- Chest physiotherapy to encourage movement of trapped secretions.
- Bronchodilator administration, as ordered, to increase airway patency and mobilize trapped secretions.
- Analgesia and sedation to minimize anxiety and pain, with daily spontaneous awakening trials.
- Education of patient and family.

Mechanical Ventilation

Intubation and mechanical ventilation are life-saving therapies frequently administered to patients presenting with ALI and ARDS. There have been myriad studies comparing and contrasting ventilator management. There is strong evidence to support the use of lung-protective ventilation, including volume- and pressure-limited strategies and PEEP in adult patients with ALI and ARDS.[46] For a detailed review of mechanical ventilation, see Chapter 10. The following will cover mechanical ventilation techniques pertinent to ALI/ARDS.

As flooding and atelectasis result in alveolar collapse and lung compliance decreases, the patient with ALI experiences greater resistance to lung expansion during inspiration and increased work of breathing. The patient is often unable to meet the metabolic demand associated with the increased work of breathing; in addition, the patient is unable to maintain adequate gas exchange and requires mechanical ventilation. Indications for intubation include airway protection, secretion control, oxygenation, and ventilation. Consideration for intubation should occur when oxygenation fails or when hypercarbia occurs. The nurse monitors the patient for early signs of respiratory compromise, such as restlessness, dyspnea, anxiety, confusion, tachypnea, and tachycardia. Cyanosis, somnolence, and significant alterations in level of consciousness are late signs of respiratory compromise and intubation is emergent.

The ARDSNet ventilator management protocol recommends assist control, volume ventilation with maximum tidal volume of 6 mL/kg of predicted (lean) body weight, maximum plateau pressure less than 30 cm H_2O, maximum respiratory rate of 35 breaths/min, and inspiratory flow rate above patient demand (> 80 L/min). Goals include maintenance of Pao_2 at 55–80 mm Hg or arterial oxygen saturation by pulse oximetry (Spo_2) of 88% to 95%, plateau pressure less than or equal to 30 cm H_2O, pH 7.30 to 7.45, and inspiration/expiration ratio of 1:1 to 1:3.[44]

Authors of the Surviving Sepsis Campaign developed guidelines for the management of septic patients with ALI/ARDS.[44] Synopsis of the recommendations will thread throughout the following paragraphs regarding mechanical ventilation. PEEP should be set on the basis of oxygen deficit, guided by the Fio_2 level required to maintain adequate oxygenation, Pao_2 of greater than 58–60 mm Hg or Sao_2/Spo_2 of greater than or equal to 90%, and adequate pressure to prevent alveolar collapse on exhalation.[44] The ARDSNet protocol provides two Fio_2/PEEP recommendations, both with similar outcomes.[44] High PEEP table is used when patients require high Fio_2 and can tolerate higher PEEP (stable blood pressure, no barotrauma) (Table 9.3). Small tidal volumes (< 6 mL/kg of predicted body weight) and pressure-limiting (30 cm H_2O) ventilation strategies positively affect patient outcome.[44] Body weight formulas are given in Table 9.4. Using these formulas, a 5-foot 5-inch woman has a predicted lean mass of 57 kg and a 6-foot-tall man has a predicted lean mass of 77.6 kg. These weights would dictate tidal volumes of less than or equal to 340 mL and less than or equal to 470 mL, respectively.

The Surviving Sepsis Campaign ALI/ARDS guidelines state that intubation has not positively influenced patient outcomes, but appropriate mechanical ventilation has had a positive influence. Normalization of neither pH (> 7.20) nor $Paco_2$ is necessary in ALI/ARDS. Permissive hypercapnia allows the practitioner to limit tidal volume and airway pressures. It is uncertain whether the prone position improves outcomes. A trial of the prone position should be attempted for patients requiring high levels of pressure or Fio_2. Use of nitric oxide is experimental and should be reserved for controlled clinical trials or as rescue therapy for hypoxemia. There is no recommended fluid management strategy except those currently used in sepsis and shock, although the ARDSNet group is currently testing liberal versus tight fluid control with low tidal volume ventilation in the Fluid and Catheter Treatment Trial (FACTT). Further information is available at http://www.ardsnet.org.[44]

Many ARDS patients require mechanical ventilation and are at risk for ventilator-associated lung injury (VALI), including biotrauma, volutrauma, atelectrauma, barotrauma, and oxygen toxicity. *Biotrauma* is a general term used to describe the upregulation of the inflammatory response within or outside the lung, resulting in pulmonary alveolar and vascular damage from mechanical ventilation.

Volutrauma is a term used to describe the alveolar damage that occurs with large tidal volumes. Early studies of the effect of ARDS on the lungs using CT[15] described the three heterogeneous areas of the lung in ARDS: consolidated, collapsed lung that cannot be ventilated; an area that collapses on expiration, but can be recruited; and normal lung. The delivery of "normal tidal volumes" to the smaller functional area of the lung, commonly referred to as *baby lung*, which can be as small as one-third of the lung size,[33] causes excessive distention of the more compliant lung areas with resultant alveolar stretch and stress failure. Volutrauma causes alveolar fracture, increased alveolar permeability, and increased alveolar fluid accumulation with increased inflammatory response.[45]

Cyclical opening and closing of the recruitable lung area causes *atelectrauma*. PEEP is used to prevent alveolar collapse on exhalation, helping to prevent lung derecruitment and atelectrauma.[1] PEEP is applied and titrated to the lower and upper inflection points in a volume/pressure curve such that a minimum amount of PEEP is applied that opens but does not hyperdistend the lung tissue. Criticism of the use of PEEP involves the phenomenon of auto-PEEP, which may occur during high respiratory rates because of inadequate exhalation time. Auto-PEEP can contribute to lung recruitment, but may also cause barotrauma.[12]

Barotrauma is caused by excess pressure in positive-pressure ventilation as evidenced on radiograph by pneumothorax, pneumomediastinum, pneumatocele, or subcutaneous emphysema. Positive correlation between the application of PEEP and barotrauma and negative association between barotrauma and any other ventilator pressures have been studied.[21] Excessive pressure on the alveolar epithelial cells disrupts the alveolus, and air passes into the interstitial space and accumulates in the mediastinum, pleura, peritoneum, and subcutaneous tissue.[44] Barotrauma can occur after only one high-volume breath.

TABLE 9.3 NIH-NHLBI ARDS Clinical Network Mechanical Ventilation Protocol PEEP

Fio_2	0.3	0.4	0.4	0.5	0.5	0.6	0.7	0.7	0.7	0.8	0.9	0.9	0.9	1.0	1.0	1.0
Low PEEP	5	5	8	8	10	10	10	12	14	14	14	16	18	20	22	24
High PEEP	12–14	14	16	16	18–20	20	20	20	20	20–22	22	22	22	22	22	24

ARDS, Acute respiratory distress syndrome; *NHLBI,* National Heart, Lung, and Blood Institute; *NIH,* National Institutes of Health; *PEEP,* positive end-expiratory pressure.
Data from Reference 44. Used with permission. NIH NHLBI ARDS Clinical Network Mechanical Ventilation Protocol Summary: http://www.ardsnet.org.

TABLE 9.4 Predicted Lean Body Weight

Predicted Body Weight	Formula
Male adult	50 + 2.3 (height [inches] − 60) or 50 + 0.91 (height − 152.4)
Female adult	45.5 + 2.3 (height [inches] − 60) or 45.5 + 0.91 (height − 152.4)

Data from Reference 44. Used with permission. NIH NHLBI ARDS Clinical Network Mechanical Ventilation Protocol Summary: http://www.ardsnet.org.

In 1954 Rebecca Gershman and Daniel L. Gilbert proposed that oxygen, even in atmospheric concentrations, forms oxygen radicals.[29] They also developed the superoxide theory of oxygen toxicity, which states that formation of the superoxide radical in vivo contributes substantially to the toxic oxidant effects of oxygen administration.[28] Delivery of high concentrations of oxygen causes pulmonary toxicity, which results in atelectasis, pulmonary edema, and propagation of the inflammatory response. Therefore, oxygen therapy should be maintained at the minimum effective dose. Safe concentrations of oxygen have been defined as an Fio_2 value less than or equal to 0.5. Reductions of Fio_2 values to less than or equal to 0.5 should be done as expeditiously as the patient is able to tolerate, using techniques such as PEEP, the prone position, and recruitment maneuvers to facilitate improvement in oxygenation.

Positive End-Expiratory Pressure

The goal of PEEP is to recruit previously atelectatic lung alveoli and prevent derecruitment and atelectrauma. The initial study on PEEP by Amato et al.[1] reported that PEEP levels in the range of 14–16 cm H_2O were needed to recruit alveoli. The ARDSNet trial used PEEP, although auto-PEEP could not be ruled out, therefore the actual levels of PEEP were not known. The ARDSNet trial has recommendations for PEEP based on Fio_2 (see Table 9.3). In the ARDSNet ALVEOLI study, all patients received low tidal volume ventilation and were randomly placed in a low or high PEEP group. The separation in PEEP levels was not sufficient to determine a difference in outcomes, making the results of the trial inconclusive.[9]

Permissive Hypercapnia

Normal $Paco_2$ values may be difficult to achieve in ALI/ARDS. Increased respiratory rate or tidal volumes that facilitate gas exchange to normalize $Paco_2$ have detrimental effects on friable, atelectatic, and inflamed lung tissues. Hypercapnia has both beneficial and detrimental physiologic effects. In hypercapnia, myocardial contractility diminishes; the heart rate increases as a compensatory mechanism, improving cardiac output. Hypercapnia causes a right shift in the oxygen dissociation curve, which improves oxygen uptake in the lungs and facilitates release of oxygen at the tissues, increasing tissue oxygenation. Hypercapnia also causes vasodilation, improving the blood volume and hence oxygen supply to the surrounding tissues. Vasodilation may only occur in nonischemic tissues, creating steal, causing further ischemia, especially in the coronary vasculature. Hypercapnia causes cerebral vasodilation, an increase in cerebral blood volume, an increase in intracranial pressure, and redistribution of cerebral blood flow.[45] Permissive hypercapnia with resultant pH change is an acceptable practice to limit VALI.[33,45]

Inverse Ratio Ventilation

The definition of inverse ratio ventilation (IRV) is a ratio of inspiratory to expiratory time greater than one. Prolongation of the inspiratory time creates intrinsic PEEP because of inadequate expiratory time recruiting alveoli early in ALI.[33,45] Historically, patients who require high Fio_2 and exhibit poor oxygenation benefit from IRV. Sedation needs to increase with IRV, as this is a very unnatural ventilatory technique and is very uncomfortable to patients. Neuromuscular blockade may be required, with all its inherent complications. IRV has not been proven to improve gas exchange or mean airway pressure in the few studies performed.[33,45]

Recruitment Maneuvers

Different patterns of atelectasis are seen in ALI/ARDS, depending on whether the cause is direct or indirect. Those patients with direct ARDS have significant consolidation and require high levels of PEEP to recruit, with increased VALI and suboptimal results. Those patients with indirect ARDS, however, have higher percentages of atelectasis, and use of approximately 5 to 12 cm H_2O of PEEP is sufficient to recruit alveoli. The open lung strategy uses various maneuvers to achieve alveolar recruitment, including sustained inflation to high pressures, intermittent sighs and stepwise increases in PEEP, or positive inspiratory pressure (PIP). The use of intermittent sighs, with high plateau pressures (40 cm H_2O for 40 seconds or 60 cm H_2O for 60 seconds) has been shown to increase oxygenation; however, derecruitment occurred at cessation of maneuvers, and the patients were prone to barotraumas. Within the first 24 hours, hyperinflation techniques are beneficial as rescue therapy in ARDS, or routinely for recruitment early in ALI/ARDS. In the fibroproliferative stage of ARDS, little recruitment is achievable and barotrauma is more likely.[12,33,45] It is important to follow recruitment maneuvers with sufficient PEEP above the lower inflection point of the pressure/volume curve of the respiratory system (P_{flex}) to inhibit derecruitment. P_{flex} is technically difficult to measure and is estimated by raising the pressure support and PEEP to 40 cm H_2O and then commencing with alternating reduction of the pressures until the tidal volume drop gives an indication of the lower inflection point that should be used as PEEP to maintain lung recruitment. Several trials have shown improved mortality in ARDS patients treated with low tidal volume and PEEP on the first day at the lower inflection point plus two cm H_2O.[1,53]

High-Frequency Oscillatory Ventilation

High-frequency oscillatory ventilation (HFOV) does not provide standard tidal volume ventilation. Inflation of the lungs occurs with a mean airway pressure high enough to expand the lung field. Gas exchange occurs through dispersion by delivering small tidal volumes with high frequency via vibration through the lung. Patients frequently require heavy sedation and neuromuscular blockade with this technique. Two randomized, controlled trials have shown nonsignificant but positive trends in outcome with this ventilation technique,[19] while Bollen et al.[8] stopped a trial related to mortality with HFOV.

Inhaled Nitric Oxide

Inhaled nitric oxide (iNO) diffuses freely across cell membranes, promotes pulmonary vasodilation, decreases pulmonary artery pressure, and promotes increased right-ventricular ejection fraction. The dose of iNO required to cause pulmonary vasodilation is between 10 and 100 parts per million.[33,45] Dellinger et al. published a randomized, controlled trial in 1998[18] that showed significant oxygenation improvement in the first 24 hours of iNO administration. Not all patients respond to iNO; those with sepsis do not respond as favorably.[33,45] Dellinger et al. recommended that, if available, iNO is a clinically useful intervention to reduce Fio_2 requirements,[18] while the Surviving Sepsis Campaign ALI/ARDS guidelines grade iNO use as experimental (grade A).[33,45] A recent triple-blinded, multicenter, randomized, placebo-controlled trial of low-dose inhaled nitric oxide showed no difference between control and treatment groups in days off mechanical ventilation or mortality, even though they found a statistically significant increase in Pao_2 in the first 48 hours.[51]

Liquid Ventilation

Perfluorocarbon is an inert, colorless, high-density fluid with low vapor pressure, high spreading coefficient, and low surface tension that is minimally absorbed across the alveoli. As such, it is an ideal vehicle to flush out cellular debris from flooded and atelectatic lung fields, promoting oxygenation. It promotes V/Q matching and decreases the inflammatory response. Studies up to 2014 have shown improved oxygenation, without improvement in mortality.[33,45] A 2004 trial reported increased pneumothoraces and hypotensive and hypoxic events; the authors recommended partial liquid ventilation not be used in ARDS patients.[32]

OTHER INTERVENTIONS

Noninvasive Positive Pressure Ventilation

The Surviving Sepsis Campaign guidelines reported uncertainty as to whether NIPPV could safely be used in ALI/ARDS, with the possible exception of patients with respiratory failure and immunosuppression.[46] Additional studies have yielded mixed results since this recommendation. NIPPV limits ventilator-associated pneumonia and other endotracheal tube-associated iatrogenic complications, such as airway trauma and sinusitis. For NIPPV to be successful, patients must be able to cooperate, maintain their own airway, initiate respiration, and clear their secretions. Additionally, patients must show no signs of hemodynamic compromise, dysrhythmias, gastrointestinal bleeding, or facial deformity that would preclude the use of NIPPV. NIPPV is favored over intubation because of the increased tolerance, need for minimal sedation, and greater patient freedom it affords. A French study reported that in 689 patients in 42 ICUs, 108 were initially ventilated with noninvasive ventilation (NIV).[13] In 52 of these patients, discontinuation of NIV occurred because of lack of efficacy; 43 patients required intubation and mechanical ventilation. The other nine patients required NIPPV for an average of 8 hours and needed only supplemental oxygen after discontinuation of NIV. Use of NIV was not shown to be a risk factor associated with death, and failure of the NIV trial was associated with increased acuity. Duration of NIV and critical care length of stay were lower in the NIV patients.[13] A search of the clinical trials database produced many ongoing trials with NIPPV.

Prone Positioning

Many journal articles publicize the oxygenation benefits of the prone position in ALI/ARDS patients.[30,54] Prone positioning affects ventilation by changing the pressures within the chest wall, which enables the recruitment of previously closed alveoli and thus successfully matches ventilation and perfusion in the area. Distribution of fluid and compression of the anterior thorax increase gas distribution to the more dorsal areas of the lung, recruiting areas dependent in the supine patient. The weight of the heart is not borne by the proned lung, and the abdomen exerts less pressure on the diaphragm in the prone patient. Many studies have revealed improved oxygenation while in the prone position, no studies have shown statistical significance in reduction of mortality.[19,31,54] Perhaps this is not surprising because the cause of death for most of the patients is multisystem organ failure, rather than ARDS. The studies would have to be large to show positive mortality benefit under these conditions.

Post-hoc analysis of a study of the prone position showed a trend toward decreased mortality in patients with severe respiratory failure (P/F ratios > 100) and other comorbidities.[33,45] Pressure breakdown can occur in prone-positioned patients if insufficient padding is used in supporting the face and bony prominences. Repositioning of the head and arms every 2 hours is required to counteract joint contractures. If the provisions of planning, appropriate positioning, or use of adequate personnel do not occur during proning maneuvers, iatrogenic complications, such as extubation or loss of intravenous lines or drains may occur. Nonetheless, improvements in oxygenation have been shown, warranting use of prone positioning in those patients who require a high Fio_2 and when conventional means of lung recruitment have failed to correct the hypoxemia.[19,31,54] New equipment advancements have occurred for prone therapy including beds (with rotational therapy) and additional equipment to facilitate prone positioning.

Medication/Fluid Use In ALI/ARDS

It cannot be too strongly stated that treatment of the underlying event must be rapidly instituted to limit catastrophic respiratory compromise; appropriate antibiotic dosing and timing, especially in community-acquired pneumonia and sepsis, are especially important. Preventive treatment strategies to limit DVT, ventilator-associated events, elevated blood glucose levels, and peptic ulcer disease are needed to diminish nosocomial complications frequently seen with critical illness including ALI and ARDS.

There are myriad reports of pharmaceutical agents and various intervention trials in animal models for ALI and in human trials for ALI/ARDS (Table 9.5). Many of the pharmaceutical agents have inadequate clinical data to support their efficacy. This may be due, in part, to the heterogeneity of the disease process in ALI/ARDS patients and the difficulty of achieving representative disease processes in the animal models. As a greater understanding of the pathogenesis of direct and indirect ALI/ARDS is achieved, we may see additional trials of novel immunomodulating agents.

Steroids

Corticosteroids should not be used for prevention or early treatment of ARDS. Trials of steroid administration have improved morbidity in a subgroup of ALI/ARDS patients in the fibroproliferative stage of ARDS. In 1999, Meduri reported a 14-day methylprednisolone protocol trial in patients with unresolving ARDS in which the sustained administration

TABLE 9.5 Pharmaceutical Agents and Interventions Trialed in Acute Lung Injury/Acute Respiratory Distress Syndrome*

Medication/Class	Rationale
Lisofylline/cytokine inhibitor	Trials showed decreased intracellular signaling and neutrophil accumulation; trial stopped for futility.
IL-10/antiinflammatory cytokine	Trials showed reductions in inflammation and trend toward decreased MV.
Sivelestat/elastase inhibitor	No reduction of mortality or duration of MV. Other elastase inhibitors are in trial.
Antioxidants	
Superoxide dismutase	SOD is in trial for neonates; no adult trials.
N-Acetylcysteine and oxothiazolidine	NAC and oxothiazolidine show reduced duration of ALI; less organ failure with oxothiazolidine.
Platelet-activating factor antagonist	No difference in overall survival seen.
Soluble complement receptors TP-10 and TP-20	Trials showed reduction of C3 and C5 with TP-10; development of TP-10 has been suspended. TP-20 is in development.
Corticosteroids	High doses given early in sepsis do not prevent ALI. High doses do not improve established ALI. Small studies report survival benefit in fibroproliferative stage. Studies under way by ARDSNet greater than or equal to 7 days ALI. Preliminary LaSRS results show better oxygenation, increased blood glucose levels, and less pneumonia and septic shock, with no mortality difference.
Prostaglandins/PGE_1	PGE_1 showed shorter time to reverse hypoxemia, had no survival benefit, and caused systemic hypotension requiring dose reduction. PGI_2 causes smooth muscle relaxation, and redistribution of blood flow to well-ventilated areas in extrapulmonary causes of ALI.
Epoprostenol/PGI_2	
Anticoagulants	
Antithrombin, activated protein C, and tissue factor pathway inhibitor	PROWESS trial showed decreased mortality from sepsis with multiorgan failure (generally one of which is the lung) using rhAPC. A phase III trial of TFPI did not show benefit in septic patients; an ALI trial is in progress. There is an ALI/ARDS trial with rhAPC underway.
Surfactant replacement	Plasma surfactant protein levels have shown prognostic value in ALI. Several replacement surfactants are in phase II/III trials with mixed results.
Human growth hormone	HGH worsens survival in ALI.
Granulocyte colony-stimulating factor	G-CSF increases neutrophil accumulation and edema.
Granulocyte macrophage CSF	GM-CSF preserved alveolar epithelium and facilitated fluid clearance.
Keratinocyte growth factor	KGF shows mixed results in animal studies.
Nitric oxide	Inhaled NO is preferentially delivered to well-ventilated areas of lung, causing vasodilation without systemic vasodilation. Multiple trials show increased oxygenation without differences in mortality.
Atrial natriuretic peptide	ANP is elevated in ALI; trials of ANP showed increased oxygenation, urine output, and thoracic compliance without survival improvement.
Liquid ventilation with perfluorocarbons	Trials show improved gas exchange, without survival benefit.
β_2-adrenergic agonists	Demonstrated increased alveolar fluid clearance. β_2-adrenergic agonists are in trial phase.

*NOTE: Study sizes were generally not large enough to make a decision to use these medications in practice or there was no difference in mortality between medication and placebo, so these medications did not receive Food and Drug Administration (FDA) approval for this indication.
ALI, Acute lung injury; *ANP*, atrial natriuretic peptide; *ARDS*, acute respiratory distress syndrome; *AT*, antithrombin; *G-CSF*, granulocyte colony-stimulating factor; *GM-CSF*, granulocyte macrophage colony-stimulating factor; *HGH*, human growth hormone; *KGF*, keratinocyte growth factor; *LaSRS*, late steroid rescue study; *MV*, mechanical ventilation; *NAC*, *N*-acetylcysteine; *NO*, nitric oxide; *rhAPC*, activated protein C; *SOD*, superoxide dismutase.

of prednisone reduced mortality in patients who responded to the steroids versus those who did not.[40] Whereas Meduri reported improved outcomes with sustained methylprednisolone administration, the ARDSNet trial—Late Steroid Rescue Study (LaSRS): The Efficacy of Corticosteroids as Rescue Therapy for the Late Phase of Acute Respiratory Distress Syndrome—did not.[49] The ARDSNet study did not use the same administration protocol as the Meduri study.[41] Trials of steroids in ARDS have had mixed results. Lee et al.[34] studied the efficacy of low-dose steroids in postoperative ARDS patients. Annane et al.[3] studied use of steroids in ARDS patients with sepsis and concluded that a 7-day treatment of low-dose hydrocortisone and fludrocortisone improved survival of patients with hypothalamic-pituitary-adrenal axis deficit. The Surviving Sepsis Campaign guidelines recommend the use of intravenous hydrocortisone for patients in septic shock who do not respond to fluid resuscitation and vasopressor therapy.[17] ALI/ARDS is common in septic patients, but it should not be extrapolated that corticosteroid administration is as effective a treatment for other ALI/ARDS patients. High-dose corticosteroids, aminoglycoside antibiotics, and neuromuscular blockade have been implicated in critical illness polyneuropathy and myopathy in patients with ARDS.[5]

Fluid and Diuretics

Fluid resuscitation in septic patients has been a recent focus, with aggressive resuscitation being recommended.[18,47] Depending upon the causative factors of ALI/ARDS, studies indicate that fluid administration should be aggressive or limited. The Saline versus Albumin Fluid Evaluation (SAFE) study concluded that resuscitation with 4% albumin or 0.9% normal saline was equally efficacious.[22] The FACTT study from the ARDSNet group addressed the use of central venous pressure (CVP) or PAC monitoring. The authors concluded that use of the PAC is not warranted in ALI/ARDS as outcomes between the PAC and CVP groups did not differ and the complications associated with the PAC were greater.[55] The cautious clinician, in light of limited data, will provide adequate fluids to maintain hemodynamic stability and vital organ perfusion, guided by central venous oxygen saturation ($Scvo_2$), lactate clearance, CXR, urine output, and hemodynamic monitoring as available.

RESOLUTION OF ACUTE LUNG INJURY AND ACUTE RESPIRATORY DISTRESS SYNDROME

The initial phase of ARDS is the exudative phase, which lasts approximately 7 days. The disease progresses to the proliferative stage lasting approximately 7 to 14 days. Lastly, the patient experiences a fibrotic stage, which resolves slowly over time.

Resolution of the acute edematous phase of ARDS occurs when type II pneumocytes proliferate and redifferentiate into type I pneumocytes, thus restoring the epithelial surface of the alveoli. Edema resolves when type II cells actively transport sodium to the interstitium. Water follows passively through the type I cell aquaporins. Removal of soluble and insoluble proteins occurs by the alveolus through diffusion, endocytosis, and phagocytosis by macrophages. Resolution of the protein deposition in the alveoli is important to diminish development of fibrosis that the hyaline membranes promote. Neutrophils are cleared from the lung tissue through apoptosis, necrosis, and phagocytosis. During the fibroproliferative stages of ARDS, there is deposition of a fibrin and collagen matrix that promotes angiogenesis and bronchiolization, due, in part, to transforming growth factor β (TGF-β). Overexpression of this growth factor, coagulation disorders, fibrinogen leakage, fibroblast invasion, and abnormalities of the surfactant system result in fibrosis.[38,42,45]

During the fibrotic phase, gradual remodeling and resolution of fibrotic tissues occur. Several studies have shown significantly decreased quality of life in survivors of ALI and ARDS.[2,16] Persistent restrictive and obstructive pulmonary defects, bronchial hyper-reactivity, decreased diffusing capacity, increased exercise *A–a* gradient (Po_2), and post-traumatic stress disorder may persist longer than 1 to 5 years after ARDS survival.[32,45] Deconditioning, resulting from a lengthy ICU and hospital stay, creates functional limitations after discharge. There may be complete resolution of the disease with no residual deficit.

CONCLUSION

ALI and ARDS are high mortality syndromes. Mortality associated with ALI and ARDS occurs more from the underlying disease process or multiorgan failure rather than respiratory failure and inability to ventilate. Lung-protective low-volume ventilation is beneficial because it reduces ventilator-associated lung injury. Research continues on new techniques for ventilating and novel immunomodulating agents for these complex patients. The heterogeneous nature of the instigating insults leading to the thought that perhaps trials of interventions and medication should be performed on subgroups of ALI/ARDS patients, compounds understanding the pathophysiology and efficacy of interventions. It is probable that in the near future subgroups of ALI/ARDS patients will be treated with different therapies, tailored to fit the underlying pathology. New imaging techniques are under development to aid the clinician in earlier diagnosis and definitive ventilatory techniques. At this time, the evidence-based supportive care and management of the ALI/ARDS patient influences survival.

CASE STUDY 9.1

A 35-year-old male presents to the emergency department 6 hours after a motor vehicle crash. His past medical history indicates that he is a 2.5 pack/day smoker of 14 years. He exhibits a chronic cough, worsened in the last week from a viral infection, from which he is producing a moderate amount of thick, off-white secretions.

Nursing assessment. Vital signs: T 38.2°C, HR 108, BP 135/82 mm Hg, RR 26, oxygen saturation 91% on room air. The patient complains of severe left shoulder and chest pain (10/10) with inspiration. He denies shortness of breath, but has shallow respirations.

Clinical findings. X-rays reveal four broken ribs, a fracture of the proximal humerus, pulmonary contusions in the left apex and right base, and consolidation in the right middle lobe.

Interventions. The patient is admitted to the step-down unit for increased monitoring with the following provider orders:

Respiratory secretions for culture and sensitivity; azithromycin (Zithromax) 500 mg IV every 24 hours; 2 mg of morphine IV every 2 hours for pain; nicotine patch and smoking cessation counseling; incentive spirometry; arm immobilization and planned surgical reduction of the fracture in the morning; 5-liter nasal cannula with intermittent oxygen saturation monitoring.

Twelve hours after admission, the patient complains of shortness of breath.

Nursing assessment. T 38.6°C, HR 127, BP 108/64 mm Hg, RR 32, oxygen saturation 92% on 5-liter nasal cannula.

Clinical findings. ABG results on 5 liters: pH 7.49, $Paco_2$ 34 mm Hg, Pao_2 58 mm Hg, HCO_3^- 24 mEq/L.

Interventions. A non-rebreather facemask is prescribed for hypoxemia. Repeat chest radiograph reveals diffuse bilateral infiltrates and cardiac silhouette that is less than half the chest diameter.

Decision Point:
What is the patient's *A–a* gradient, what is normal, and why is this important to know?

Decision Point:
What is the patient's P/F ratio, and does this patient have ALI or ARDS?

Decision Point:
What signs does the patient exhibit that show continued respiratory compromise?

Decision Point:
What changes should occur to the plan of care?

REFERENCES

1. Amato, M. B., et al. (1998). Effect of a protective-ventilation strategy on mortality in the acute respiratory distress syndrome. *N Engl J Med, 338*(6), 347–354.
2. Angus, D. C., et al. (2001). Quality-adjusted survival in the first year after the acute respiratory distress syndrome. *Am J Respir Crit Care Med, 163*(6), 1389–1394.
3. Annane, D., Sebille, V. & Bellissant, E. (2006). Effect of low doses of corticosteroids in septic shock patients with or without early acute respiratory distress syndrome. *Crit Care Med, 34*(1), 22–30.
4. Ashbaugh, D. G., et al. (1967). Acute respiratory distress in adults. *Lancet, 2*(7511), 319–323.
5. Bercker, S., et al. (2005). Critical illness polyneuropathy and myopathy in patients with acute respiratory distress syndrome. *Crit Care Med, 33*(4), 711–,715.
6. Bernard, G. R., et al. (1994). The American-European consensus conference on ARDS: definitions, mechanisms, relevant outcomes and clinical trial coordination. *Am J Respir Crit Care Med, 149*, 818–824.

7. Bindl, L., et al. (2003). Gender-based differences in children with sepsis and ARDS: the ESPNIC ARDS Database Group. *Intensive Care Med, 29*(10), 1770–1773.
8. Bollen, C. W., et al. (2005). High frequency oscillatory ventilation compared with conventional mechanical ventilation in adult respiratory distress syndrome: a randomized controlled trial [ISRCTN24242669]. *Crit Care, 9*(4), R430–R439.
9. Brower, R. G., et al. (2004). Higher versus lower positive end-expiratory pressures in patients with the acute respiratory distress syndrome. *N Engl J Med, 351*(4), 327–336.
10. Brun-Buisson, C., et al. (2004). Epidemiology and outcome of acute lung injury in European intensive care units. Results from the ALIVE study. *Intensive Care Med, 30*(1), 51–61.
11. Burns, K. E., et al. (2013). Noninvasive positive-pressure ventilation as a weaning strategy for intubated adults with respiratory failure. *Cochrane Database Syst Rev, 12*, CD004127.
12. Burns, S. M. (2005). Mechanical ventilation of patients with acute respiratory distress syndrome and patients requiring weaning: the evidence guiding practice. *Crit Care Nurse, 25*(4), 14–23, quiz 24.
13. Carlucci, A., et al. (2001). Noninvasive versus conventional mechanical ventilation. An epidemiologic survey. *Am J Respir Crit Care Med, 163*(4), 874–880.
14. Chemla, D., et al. (2015). Systolic and mean pulmonary artery pressures: are they interchangeable in patients with pulmonary hypertension? *Chest, 147*(4), 943–950.
15. Chiumello, D., et al. (2013). Clinical review: lung imaging in acute respiratory distress syndrome patients—an update. *Crit Care, 17*(6), 243.
16. Cooper, A. B., et al. (1999). Long-term follow-up of survivors of acute lung injury: lack of effect of a ventilation strategy to prevent barotrauma. *Crit Care Med, 27*(12), 2616–2621.
17. Dellinger, R. P., et al. (2013). Surviving sepsis campaign: international guidelines for management of severe sepsis and septic shock: 2012. *Crit Care Med, 41*(2), 580–637.
18. Dellinger, R. P., et al. (1998). Effects of inhaled nitric oxide in patients with acute respiratory distress syndrome: results of a randomized phase II trial. Inhaled Nitric Oxide in ARDS Study Group. *Crit Care Med, 26*(1), 15–23.
19. Derdak, S., et al. (2002). High-frequency oscillatory ventilation for acute respiratory distress syndrome in adults: a randomized, controlled trial. *Am J Respir Crit Care Med, 166*(6), 801–808.
20. Dong, H., et al. (2013). Comparative analysis of the alveolar macrophage proteome in ALI/ARDS patients between the exudative phase and recovery phase. *BMC Immunol, 14*, 25.
21. Eisner, M. D., et al. (2002). Airway pressures and early barotrauma in patients with acute lung injury and acute respiratory distress syndrome. *Am J Respir Crit Care Med, 165*(7), 978–982.
22. Finfer, S., et al. (2004). A comparison of albumin and saline for fluid resuscitation in the intensive care unit. *N Engl J Med, 350*(22), 2247–2256.
23. Flaatten, H., et al. (2003). Outcome after acute respiratory failure is more dependent on dysfunction in other vital organs than on the severity of the respiratory failure. *Crit Care, 7*(4), R72.
24. Garland, A., et al. (2004). Outcomes up to 5 years after severe, acute respiratory failure. *Chest, 126*(6), 1897–1904.
25. Gattinoni, L., et al. (1998). Acute respiratory distress syndrome caused by pulmonary and extrapulmonary disease. Different syndromes? *Am J Respir Crit Care Med, 158*(1), 3–11.
26. Goss, C. H., et al. (2003). Incidence of acute lung injury in the United States. *Crit Care Med, 31*(6), 1607–1611.
27. Gowda, M. S. & Klocke, R. A. (1997). Variability of indices of hypoxemia in adult respiratory distress syndrome. *Crit Care Med, 25*(1), 41–45.
28. Halliwell, B. & Gutteridge, J. M. (1984). Oxygen toxicity, oxygen radicals, transition metals and disease. *Biochem J, 219*(1), 1–14.
29. Heyland, D. K., et al. (2003). Canadian clinical practice guidelines for nutrition support in mechanically ventilated, critically ill adult patients. *JPEN J Parenter Enteral Nutr, 27*(5), 355–373.
30. Hu, S. L., et al. (2014). The effect of prone positioning on mortality in patients with acute respiratory distress syndrome: a meta-analysis of randomized controlled trials. *Crit Care 2014, 18*(3), R109.
31. Kacmarek, R. M., et al. (2005). Partial liquid ventilation in adult patients with the acute respiratory distress syndrome. *Am J Respir Crit Care Med, 173*(8), 882–889.
32. Kapfhammer, H. P., et al. (2004). Posttraumatic stress disorder and health-related quality of life in long-term survivors of acute respiratory distress syndrome. *Am J Psychiatry, 161*(1), 45–52.
33. Keenan, J. C., Formenti, P. & Marini, J. J. (2014). Lung recruitment in acute respiratory distress syndrome: what is the best strategy? *Curr Opin Crit Care, 20*(1), 63–68.
34. Lee, H. S., et al. (2005). Low-dose steroid therapy at an early phase of postoperative acute respiratory distress syndrome. *Ann Thoracic Surg, 79*(2), 405–410.
35. Lone, A. L. & Taskén, K. (2013). Proinflammatory and immunoregulatory roles of eicosanoids in T-cells. *Front Immunol, 4*, 130.
36. Manzano, F., et al. (2005). Incidence of acute respiratory distress syndrome and its relation to age. *J Crit Care, 20*(3), 274–280.
37. Martin, G. S., et al. (2002). Findings on the portable chest radiograph correlate with fluid balance in critically ill patients. *Chest, 122*(6), 2087–2095.
38. Matthay, M. A., Ware, L. B. & Zimmerman, G. A. (2012). The acute respiratory distress syndrome. *J Clin Invest, 122*(8), 2731–2740.
39. McCance, K. L. & Huether, S. E. (2009). *Pathophysiology: the biological basis for disease in adults and children* (6th ed.). St. Louis: Mosby.
40. Meduri, G. U. (1999). Levels of evidence for the pharmacologic effectiveness of prolonged methylprednisolone treatment in unresolving ARDS. *Chest, 116*(Suppl. 1), 116S–118S.
41. Meduri, G. U., et al. (2002). Prolonged methylprednisolone treatment suppresses systemic inflammation in patients with unresolving acute respiratory distress syndrome: evidence for inadequate endogenous glucocorticoid secretion and inflammation-induced immune cell resistance to glucocorticoids. *Am J Respir Crit Care Med, 165*(7), 983–991.
42. Needham, D. M., et al. (2014). Risk factors for physical impairment after acute lung injury in a national, multicenter study. *Am J Respir Crit Care Med, 189*(10), 1214–1224.
43. Neff, T. A., et al. (2003). Long-term assessment of lung function in survivors of severe ARDS. *Chest, 123*(3), 845–853.
44. Pomprapa, A., et al. (2014). Automatic protective ventilation using the ARDSNet protocol with the additional monitoring of electrical impedance tomography. *Crit Care 2014, 18*(3), R128.
45. Ragaller, M. & Richter, T. (2010). Acute lung injury and respiratory distress syndrome. *J Emerg Trauma Shock, 3*(1), 43–51.
46. Rao, M. H., Marulidhar, A. & Reddy, A. K. S. (2014). Acute respiratory distress syndrome. *J Clin Sci Res, 3*, 114–134.
47. Rivers, E., et al. (2001). Early goal-directed therapy in the treatment of severe sepsis and septic shock. *N Engl J Med, 345*(19), 1368–1377.
48. Stefan, M. S., et al. (2013). Epidemiology and outcomes of acute respiratory failure in the United States, 2001 to 2009: a national survey. *J Hosp Med, 8*(2), 76–82.
49. Steinberg, K. P., et al. (2006). Efficacy and safety of corticosteroids for persistent acute respiratory distress syndrome. *N Engl J Med, 354*(16), 1671–1684.
50. Sweatt, A. J. & Levitt, J. E. (2014). Evolving epidemiology and definitions of the acute respiratory distress syndrome and early acute lung injury. *Clin Chest Med, 35*(4), 609–624.
51. Taylor, R. W., et al. (2004). Low-dose inhaled nitric oxide in patients with acute lung injury: a randomized controlled trial. *JAMA, 291*(13), 1603–1609.
52. Urden, L. D., Stacy, K. M. & Lough, M. E. (2013). *Critical care nursing: diagnosis and management* (7th ed.). St. Louis: Mosby.
53. Villar, J., et al. (2006). A high positive end-expiratory pressure, low tidal volume ventilatory strategy improves outcome in persistent acute respiratory distress syndrome: a randomized, controlled trial. *Crit Care Med, 34*(5), 1311–1318.
54. Voggenreiter, G., et al. (2005). Prone positioning improves oxygenation in post-traumatic lung injury—a prospective randomized trial. *J Trauma, 59*(2), 333–341.
55. Wheeler, A. P., et al. (2006). Pulmonary-artery versus central venous catheter to guide treatment of acute lung injury. *N Engl J Med, 354*(21), 2213–2224.

56. Williams, A. E. & Chambers, R. C. (2013). The mercurial nature of neutrophils: still an enigma in ARDS? *Am J Physiol Lung Cell Mol Physiol*, *306*, L217–L230.
57. Xu, Y., et al. (2014). Targeting complement anaphylatoxin C5a receptor in hyperoxic lung injury in mice. *Mol Med Rep*, *10*(4), 1786–1792.

SUGGESTED WEBLINKS

ARDS Clinical Network Website. http://www.ardsnet.org.

Professional Education. http://www.ccmtutorials.com; http://www.emedicine.com.

Patient and Family Support and Education. http://www.ards.org; http://www.ardsusa.com; http://www.nhlbi.nih.gov/health/dci/Diseases/Ards/Ards_WhatIs.html.

Nutrition. http://www.criticalcarenutrition.com.

National Guidelines. http://www.guidelines.gov.

CONSENSUS CONFERENCES

International Consensus Conference in Intensive Care Medicine: Ventilator Associated Lung Injury in ARDS. http://ajrccm.atsjournals.org/cgi/content/full/160/6/2118.

American-European Consensus Conference on ARDS, Part 2: Acute Lung Injury. http://ajrccm.atsjournals.org/cgi/content/abstract/157/4/12.

International Consensus Conferences in Intensive Care Medicine: Non-invasive Positive Pressure Ventilation in Acute Respiratory Failure, Dec 2000. http://ajrccm.atsjournals.org/cgi/content/full/163/1/283.

10

Mechanical Ventilation and Weaning

Maureen A. Seckel

Mechanical ventilation is one of the most commonly used technologies in critical care. Unfortunately, patients who require mechanical ventilation, especially for longer than 3 days, are at risk for many iatrogenic complications, prolonged and costly hospital stays, ventilator dependence, and death.[38,40,50,51,58,68,69,87,90,91,94]

As a result, expedient liberation from the ventilator is the goal. However, in order to ensure timely and effective application of mechanical ventilation and weaning techniques, an in-depth understanding of the science and technology is essential. This chapter covers the evidence related to the ventilation of patients with acute respiratory distress syndrome (ARDS) and patients with acute asthma, invasive and noninvasive positive-pressure mechanical ventilator modes, and monitoring and assessment techniques such as respiratory waveform monitoring. In addition, the chapter discusses the process of ventilator liberation with and without a tracheostomy.

VOLUME VERSUS PRESSURE MODES

Volume ventilation has been the mainstay of mechanical ventilation for more than 50 years, and is still commonly used in critical care.[48,79] However, pressure modes of ventilation are becoming increasingly more popular and prevalent. Knowledge of the characteristics of both volume and pressure ventilation is essential to understanding the specific modes and their application.

Characteristics of Volume Ventilation

Volume ventilators provide a predetermined tidal volume (V_T) to the patient, regardless of changes in compliance or resistance. As a result, the pressure required to deliver the breath varies between breaths. Pressure gradually builds until it reaches a peak (with the end of volume delivery), known as the *peak airway* or *peak inspiratory* pressure. As shown in Fig. 10.1, the associated pressure waveform is commonly referred to as an accelerating pressure waveform (shark fin configuration). The flow pattern (or gas flow) with these breaths is generally stable through the breath and is called *a square flow pattern* (Fig. 10.2).

Because the delivered V_T must overcome both the resistance of the airways and the compliance of the lungs (and chest wall), the peak airway pressure is a reflection of both lung compliance and airway resistance. A plateau pressure is measured to differentiate the two (Fig. 10.3 and Box 10.1). The plateau pressure, also called the *static, alveolar,* or *distending* pressure, reflects the pressure required to hold the lungs open without the contribution of the pressure required to move gases down the airways (thus it is measured in a "static" state). Both peak and plateau pressures are measured when volume ventilation is used to assess the adequacy of therapy, and to ensure that ventilation is adapted to prevent damage to the lungs (i.e., volutrauma, which will be discussed later).

Characteristics of Pressure Ventilation

Pressure ventilation, in contrast to volume ventilation, ensures that the inspiratory pressure level is stable for every breath. The pressure waveform associated with pressure ventilation is called a square pressure waveform (Fig. 10.4). Although the pressure level is maintained throughout inspiration, the volume varies with changes in compliance and resistance. It is this characteristic that manufacturers have responded to in the form of ventilator modes designed to deliver every breath as a pressure breath, while ensuring delivery of a desired volume (specific modes will be described later in this chapter).

In addition to the guaranteed pressure level provided with most pressure modes, an important feature is the associated

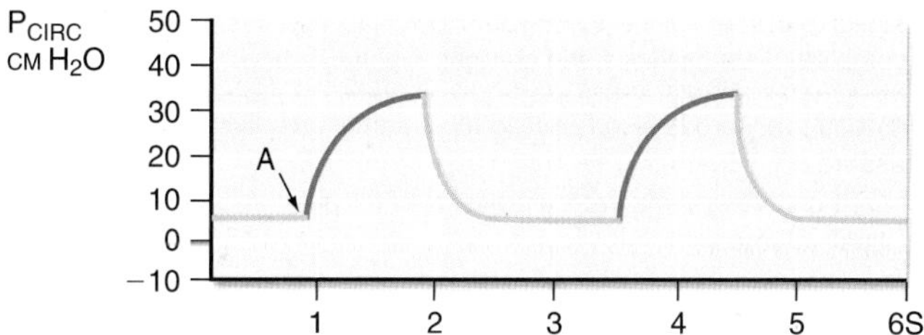

FIG. 10.1 Accelerating pressure waveform associated with volume breath delivery. *A* marks the point at which the mandatory breath is delivered (in contrast, a deflection preceding the positive pressure breath would indicate a spontaneous effort/patient-initiated breath). *P_{CIRC},* Circuit pressure.

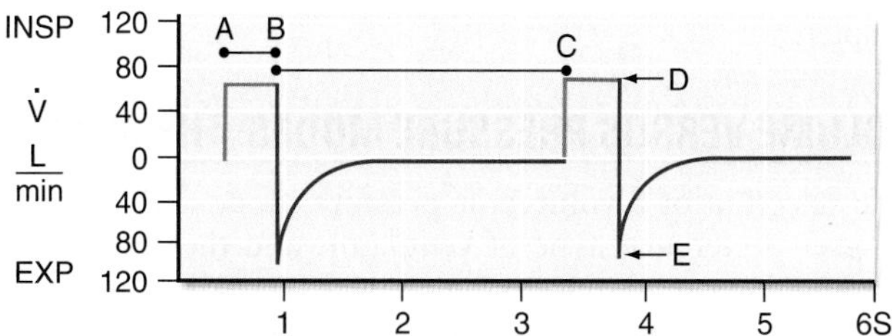

FIG. 10.2 Square flow pattern associated with volume breath delivery. Points *A-B* and *C-D* represent inspiration. The expiratory limb of the waveform is below the baseline. Point *E* indicates the peak expiratory flow. Units are liters per minute. *INSP,* Inspiration; *EXP,* expiration.

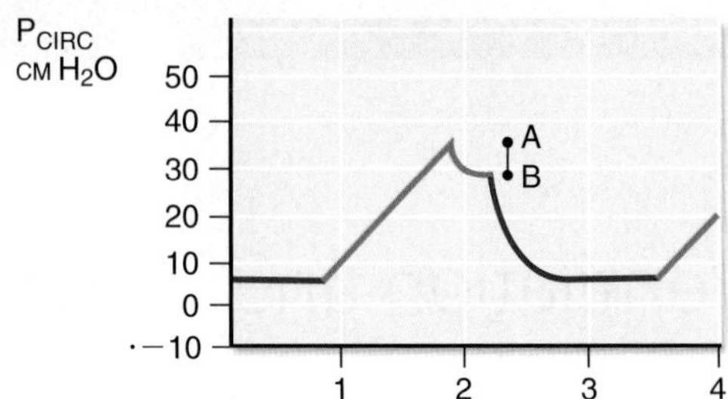

FIG. 10.3 Accelerating pressure waveform (volume breath) with inspiratory hold and demonstration of a plateau pressure. *B* indicates the drop in peak airway pressure *(A)* to plateau pressure *(B)*. P_{CIRC}, Circuit pressure.

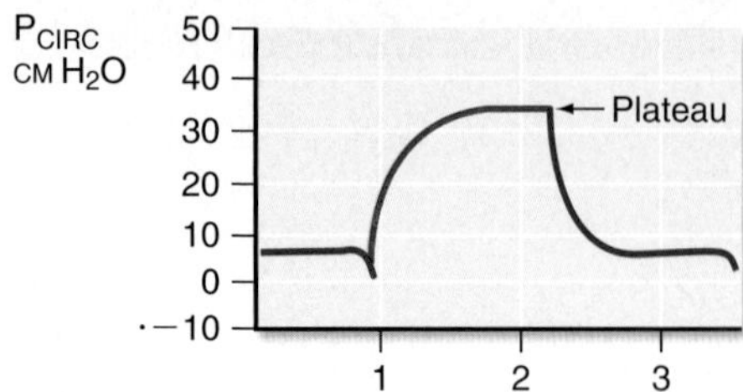

FIG. 10.4 Square pressure waveform associated with a pressure breath. Note the plateau associated with inspiration. P_{CIRC}, Circuit pressure.

BOX 10.1 Measurement of Plateau Pressure* and Calculation of Dynamic Characteristic and Static Compliance

Plateau pressure

A plateau pressure is measured by activating the *end-inspiratory* hold button on the ventilator (at end-inspiration or peak inspiratory pressure). The pressure level will drop to the level that is required to distend the lungs, which is called the *plateau pressure*. Generally the difference between peak and plateau pressures is 10 to 15 cm.

Dynamic characteristic

This measurement is obtained by dividing the V_T by the PIP minus PEEP. This is an overall measure of the compliance and resistance of the system. This measurement is sometimes referred to as *dynamic compliance*. Because the measurement is inclusive of both airway resistance and lung compliance, the term is not exact.

Static compliance

This measurement is obtained by dividing the V_T by the plateau (i.e., static) pressure minus PEEP. Both dynamic characteristic and static compliance are used to trend changes in patient status.

*Plateau pressure is also referred to as static, alveolar, and distending pressure.

PEEP, Positive end-expiratory pressure; *PIP*, peak inspiratory pressure; V_T, tidal volume.

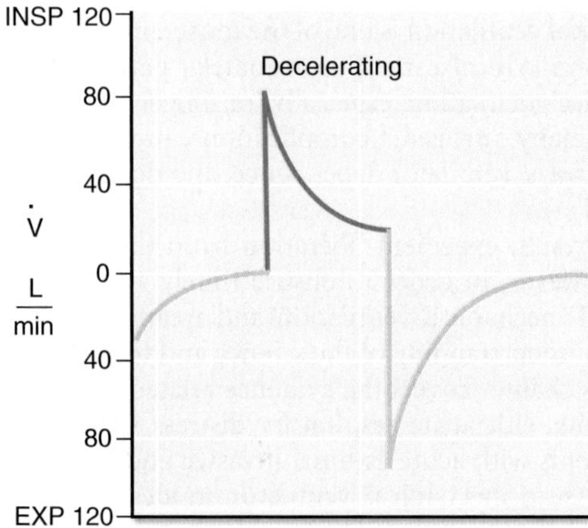

FIG. 10.5 Decelerating flow pattern seen with a pressure breath. *INSP*, Inspiration; *EXP*, expiration.

flow pattern. The flow pattern is called a *decelerating flow* pattern (Fig. 10.5). Flow is initially very high, but gradually slows or tapers as the chest fills. This pattern is thought to be more physiologic (similar to spontaneous breathing) and may provide better gas distribution than is seen with the stable flow (square) pattern of volume ventilation.[77]

These concepts are inherent in the design and function of all ventilator mode options that are discussed throughout this chapter.

VOLUME VERSUS PRESSURE MODES: THE SCIENCE

The selection of a volume or pressure mode is determined by user preference, type of ventilator, and the goals of the therapy. User preference is generally driven by comfort (i.e., exposure and experience), and the type of ventilator limits the availability of some mode options. Regardless, existing research does help guide the selection and application of volume and pressure modes. Specific examples of this include the ventilation of those with ARDS and acute asthma. In both cases, ventilation is adapted to prevent lung injury, with resultant expected and accepted hypercarbia (i.e., *permissive hypercarbia*). These concepts are covered before a description of ventilator parameters and volume and pressure modes because an understanding of the science makes it easier to understand the function of selected modes and how they are applied in practice.

Ventilating the Noncompliant Lung

In ARDS animal models, noncompliant (stiff) lungs, ventilated at large V_T values, experience alveolar injury (fractures) following 72 hours of ventilation.[32,33,41,86] The lungs, which are subjected to repetitive opening and closing during inflation and deflation, are injured by the shear forces of the distending breaths. This type of repetitive opening injury is termed *volutrauma* and is associated with alveolar flooding.[2,32,34,79] The associated plateau pressures in these studies were greater than 35 cm H_2O, and many questioned whether it was volume or pressure that caused the lung injury.[78]

Subsequently, human studies demonstrated that low-volume ventilation, with resultant low plateau pressures, favorably affected mortality.[47,48] In 2000 the National Heart, Lung and Blood Institute of the National Institutes of Health ARDS Network (NIH-NHLBI ARDSnet) reported the preliminary results of a randomized controlled trial designed to compare clinical outcomes of ARDS patients assigned to low-volume (6 mL/kg) versus "traditional" volume (12 mL/kg) ventilation.[85] The study was stopped following a preliminary analysis of 861 patients, which demonstrated significantly lower mortality in the low V_T group compared to the control group (31.0% vs. 39.8%, $p = 0.007$). The plateau pressures associated with the low-volume group were in the range of 26 cm H_2O, considerably less than the 35 cm H_2O that was previously associated with volutrauma in animal models.[64,83]

Lung-protective strategies with the use of lower V_T values (6 mL/kg predicted body weight) and goal plateau pressures (≤ 30 cm H_2O) are the standard of care for ARDS patients.[44,76] However, a recent meta-analysis has suggested that the use of lower V_T values in patients without ARDS may be associated with better outcomes.[67] Additional randomized control trials are needed to determine the optimal V_T for best outcomes in this patient population. Management of patients with ARDS needs to focus on implementing lung-protective strategies that ensure that V_T levels are no greater than 6 mL/kg predicted body weight. This can be done with both volume and pressure ventilation and may be more easily accomplished with selected modes.[26] Regardless of the mode, if V_T and subsequently minute ventilation are decreased, hypercarbia will ensue and is expected (see Permissive Hypercarbia).

Another concept related to ventilation of the ARDS lung is that of recruitment and derecruitment. Computed tomography (CT) scans of the ARDS lung demonstrate that the distribution of air space involvement is not homogeneous; some air spaces are open, whereas others are not.[44,45,46] The aerated areas of the lung (called the *baby lung*) are prone to injury from the distending forces of a breath.[44,45,46] Thus, recruitment of the rest of the lung is important to prevent lung injury and requires that a critical opening pressure be applied.[36,58] Techniques to accomplish this include using a 40/40 or 60/60 maneuver (i.e., applying positive end-expiratory pressure [PEEP] at 40 cm H_2O for 40 seconds [or 60 cm H_2O for 60 seconds]) or using inflection pressures to determine the best level of PEEP. The inflection pressure method requires that PEEP levels be increased while compliance is monitored. As the lung begins to open (*open lung ventilation,* i.e., critical opening pressure), the compliance increases, and a rise in the lower part of the PEEP/compliance graph (the lower inflection point) occurs (Fig. 10.6). Recruitment maneuvers have been associated with short-term improvement in oxygenation, along with risk of adverse events such as hypotension and desaturation, and should be considered on an individualized basis for patients with severe refractory hypoxemia.[38,76] A recent meta-analysis of ten randomized controlled studies demonstrated a small improvement in hospital mortality; however, the authors described the evidence as low and not definitive.[80]

As previously described, recruiting the lung is difficult, and once recruited, derecruitment must be prevented. Monitoring oxygenation is the traditional method for selecting the PEEP. Using oxygenation as the determinant of adequacy of recruitment is somewhat misleading because improved oxygenation may be the effect of either recruitment or redistribution of blood flow to aerated areas of the lung. Prone positioning may help recruit the lung and prevent derecruitment.[43,74]

Research has shown that higher PEEP values in patients with ARDS correlate with decreased intensive care unit (ICU) mortality and hospital mortality.[12] What is not known is the optimal method of titrating PEEP; however, ARDSnet has provided recommendations (Table 10.1).[12,66]

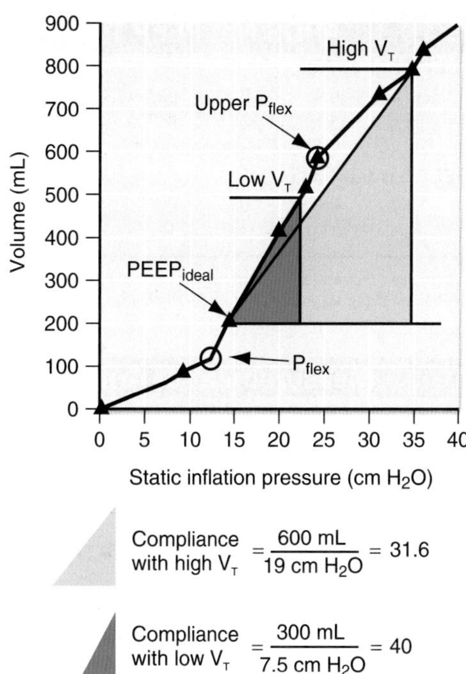

FIG. 10.6 Inspiratory static P/V curve of the respiratory system showing two sharp inflection points (P_{flex}). The lower P_{flex} point represents the critical opening pressure of a large population of alveoli, while the upper P_{flex} point reflects the loss of the elastic properties of the lung due to overdistention of the pulmonary interstitium and elastic fibers. As shown in the figure, the use of a "normal" V_T = 10 mL/kg plus PEEP = 15 cm H_2O ($PEEP_{ideal}$) would certainly cause overdistention of the lung parenchyma in this patient, with inspiratory incursions reaching the upper flat portion of the P/V curve. The choice of a low tidal volume in this patient was accompanied by an increase of the calculated compliance (the tangent curve represented by the triangles), illustrating the basic principle of an open-lung approach to mechanical ventilation—simultaneously avoiding alveolar collapse (keeping PEEP above the lower P_{flex}) and overdistention (keeping inspiratory pressures below the upper P_{flex} by using low tidal volumes and lower inspiratory pressures above PEEP). *PEEP,* Positive end-expiratory pressure; *P_{flex},* inflection pressure; *V_T,* tidal volume.

Ventilating Patients with Severe Airflow Limitation

In patients with acute asthma or chronic obstructive pulmonary disease (COPD), airflow limitation may result in dynamic hyperinflation and auto-PEEP.[62,86] Both phenomena occur when not enough time is allowed for a complete exhalation. The result is a hyperinflated state that can lead to increases in pulmonary vascular resistance and right ventricular afterload, as well as impediments to venous return due to elevations in pleural and right atrial pressures.[62] Additional complications of hyperinflation include barotrauma (e.g., pneumothorax), hemodynamic consequences (e.g., hypotension), and ineffective patient triggering (which will be discussed in the section on ventilator parameters).

Auto-PEEP is common, and results from increased alveolar pressure at end expiration that exceeds the set PEEP and can be measured on the ventilator using an end-expiratory hold maneuver

TABLE 10.1 ARDS Net PEEP Table

Lower PEEP/Higher FiO_2														
FiO_2	0.3	0.4	0.4	0.5	0.5	0.6	0.7	0.7	0.7	0.8	0.9	0.9	0.9	1.0
PEEP	5	5	8	9	10	10	10	12	14	14	14	16	18	18-24
Higher PEEP/Lower FiO_2														
FiO_2	0.3	0.3	0.3	0.3	0.3	0.4	0.4	0.5	0.5	0.5-0.8	0.8	0.9	1.0	1.0
PEEP	5	8	10	12	14	14	16	16	18	20	22	22	22	24

ARDS, Acute respiratory distress syndrome; *FiO_2,* fraction of inspired oxygen.
Excerpt from ARDSnet Protocol. Available at http://www.ardsnet.org/files/ventilator_protocol_2008-07.pdf

BOX 10.2 Measurement of Auto-PEEP

Auto-PEEP is measured by activating the *end-expiratory* hold button (at the end of exhalation just before inspiration) for a few seconds. This closes the system and allows pressures to equilibrate. The baseline pressure (i.e., zero or set PEEP level) will rise, reflecting the level of auto-PEEP above baseline.

PEEP, Positive end-expiratory pressure.

(Box 10.2). Management of auto-PEEP includes decreasing frequency (fx) and V_T (i.e., minute ventilation [V_E], or shortening the inspiratory time to allow for longer exhalation), and relieving bronchospasm. Water in the ventilator circuit, small inner diameter endotracheal tubes, and some expiratory valves also contribute to auto-PEEP, and should be considered as potential causes. An additional way to decrease auto-PEEP (in some cases) is to add set PEEP to allow for better airway opening (Box 10.3).[9,62,88]

Auto-PEEP is difficult to measure in spontaneously breathing patients. Auto-PEEP may not be detected despite long end-expiratory hold maneuvers when hyperinflated alveoli are unable to empty secondary to severe bronchoconstriction or obstruction. In patients with *status asthmaticus,* it is prudent to assume the presence of auto-PEEP, even if auto-PEEP is not detected. Furthermore, with extreme hyperinflation, cardiac output will be decreased. The resultant hypotension may be profound and result in death; brief removal from the ventilator may be life-saving. When the patient is returned to the ventilator, fx and V_T should be decreased to prevent a recurrence of this phenomenon.

Permissive Hypercarbia

As previously noted, hypercarbia may ensue. If hypercarbia occurs, patient management is directed at preventing volutrauma (secondary to high V_T values) and barotrauma (secondary to hyperinflation and auto-PEEP). Generally, the hypercarbia is well tolerated, provided the pH is maintained at approximately 7.25 (lower pH values have been reported). However, some categories of patients are not appropriate for low pH values or high partial pressures of arterial carbon dioxide ($PaCO_2$), such as patients with intracranial pressure concerns and some cardiac states. Sodium bicarbonate infusions or tromethamine may be used to ensure a "safe" pH in hemodynamic instability.[1,76,85] It is important to remember that bicarbonate is converted into carbon dioxide (CO_2) and water, and so the resultant increase in the CO_2 concentration will decrease the pH. The utilization of buffers is considered a temporary solution.

VENTILATOR PARAMETERS

Parameters are options on the ventilator that allow the clinician to configure breath delivery. Not all parameters are required for every mode. The required parameters for each mode will be covered in the section on modes. A description of ventilator parameters is listed in Box 10.3.

INVASIVE MODES OF VENTILATION

Many modes of ventilation are currently available on ventilators (Box 10.4). A discussion of invasive and noninvasive volume and pressure modes follows. Application of the modes is dependent on the condition of the patient and the disease process. Related concepts were discussed earlier.

Volume Modes

Assist Control

Assist control (AC) delivers a set number of breaths at a selected V_T. Between control breaths, the patient may initiate a breath. Upon sensing patient effort, the ventilator delivers a full preset V_T.

- Advantages/disadvantages: AC ventilation is useful as a control mode of ventilation. If flow or sensitivity is inappropriately set, this mode may result in excessive patient work; patient/ventilator dyssynchrony will result. In addition, hypocarbia may ensue if central drive (e.g., head injury) prevents autoregulation of $PaCO_2$ levels. The mode is not used as a weaning mode because a full V_T breath will be delivered with each spontaneous effort.
- Parameters set on the AC mode include V_T, fx, sensitivity, inspiratory time (T_I), fraction of inspired oxygen (FiO_2), and PEEP.

Synchronized Intermittent Mandatory Ventilation

Synchronized intermittent mandatory ventilation (SIMV) delivers a set number of mandatory V_T breaths. Between mandatory breaths, the patient may breathe spontaneously at a patient-determined V_T and fx.

- Advantages/disadvantages: SIMV has traditionally been used as a weaning mode because the mandatory breaths can be gradually decreased, allowing the patient to assume more of the work. However, the workload is substantially increased with low SIMV rates (e.g., 2–4 breaths/min), especially if flow rates are not adequate or if the ventilator response time is slow. It is common for pressure support to be added to assist with spontaneous breathing.
- Parameters set on SIMV include V_T, fx, sensitivity, T_I, FiO_2, and PEEP.

Pressure Modes

Pressure Support Ventilation

Pressure support ventilation (PSV) is a mode of ventilation that augments or supports a spontaneous inspiration with a

BOX 10.3 Ventilator Parameters

- Fraction of inspired oxygen (Fio_2): Variable from 0.21 to 1.0.
- Tidal volume (V_T): Generally set between 8 and 12 mL/kg. However, volumes may need to be set much lower (e.g., 6 mL/kg) to prevent volutrauma when the patient has acute respiratory distress syndrome (ARDS), or in the case of acute asthma when dynamic hyperinflation and auto-PEEP are present.
- Frequency (fx) or respiratory rate (RR): Set between 10 and 20 breaths/min. The combination of fx and V_T results in V_E (the total ventilation in 1 minute). Normal V_E is between 5 and 10 L/min. However, depending on the therapy goals, the V_E may be higher or lower. A high V_E requirement is reflective of inefficient gas exchange.
- Inspiratory (I) and expiratory (E) time and I/E ratio: Inspiratory time is determined by the speed of gas flow. The higher the flow, the faster the speed of the gas and the shorter the inspiratory time (T_I). An average adult T_I is 0.7–1 s; I/E is usually 1:2 or 1:3. I/E ratios are adjusted to ensure clinical goals are met. For example, in a patient with airflow obstruction, the goal is to allow for complete exhalation; thus inspiration will be as short as possible. However, the shorter the T_I, the faster the flow rate and the more turbulent the gas flow. This increases peak inspiratory pressure (PIP) and does not contribute to optimum gas distribution, thus limiting the use of this intervention. In contrast, an inverse I/E ratio may be used in patients with ARDS to lengthen the time the lung is kept open and to prevent derecruitment (alveolar closure). The T_I should always be matched to meet the patient's inspiratory demand or patient-ventilator dyssynchrony will result. When nonphysiologic I/E ratios are used, sedation and paralytic agents are often necessary. Some newer modes of ventilation, discussed later in this chapter, may obviate the need for pharmacologic interventions in these cases.
- Positive end-expiratory pressure (PEEP): The purpose of PEEP is to restore functional residual capacity (FRC), or that volume left in the lungs at the end of a resting exhalation; a pressure of 5 cm H_2O is considered physiologic PEEP. PEEP is increased in increments. In patients with restrictive disease conditions (e.g., ARDS, pulmonary edema, atelectasis, or pneumonia), the loss of FRC results in alveolar closure, shunt, hypoxemia, and an increase in the work of breathing. Thus PEEP is increased to open the lung and improve compliance. Generally, PEEP is increased to attain an acceptable partial pressure of arterial oxygen tension (Pao_2) or saturation of arterial oxygen (Sao_2) with a Fio_2 of less than or equal to 0.5. In patients with ARDS, PEEP levels may need to be very high to ensure that alveolar opening (i.e., recruitment) occurs, and that alveolar closure (i.e., derecruitment) is prevented. Improved mortality rates have been demonstrated using higher levels of PEEP (12–14 cm H_2O).[2,3]
- PEEP may also be used to open airways to allow for complete alveolar emptying (i.e., in asthmatic patients or patients with COPD).[66,83] This is accomplished by measuring auto-PEEP and increasing set PEEP to, or slightly below, the auto-PEEP level. Measurement of plateau pressure is also helpful. If the addition of set PEEP increases plateau pressure, it is contributing to hyperinflation. However, if the addition of PEEP is opening small airways, allowing for alveolar emptying, the plateau pressure may decrease or stay the same. The addition of set PEEP may also result in improved patient triggering (see "sensitivity" hereafter).
- Continuous positive airway pressure (CPAP): CPAP, similar to PEEP, is used to restore FRC. In contrast to PEEP, positive pressure is provided continuously to a spontaneously breathing patient (i.e., no ventilator breaths). CPAP is often used as a last step in the weaning process (more on this in the section on weaning) and also as a noninvasive method of providing a pneumatic splint to the airways of those with obstructive sleep apnea (OSA).
- Sensitivity (trigger sensitivity): Sensitivity allows the ventilator to recognize patient-initiated efforts (i.e., negative pressure), and can be either pressure- or flow-activated. Most ventilators use a pressure-sensing mechanism that is adjusted automatically to the set PEEP level. The most common settings for pressure sensitivity are −1 to −2 cm H_2O (the more negative the number, the harder it is to trigger a breath). When the patient initiates a breath, thus dropping the system pressure, the pressure drop is sensed on the inspiratory side of the ventilator circuit and flow, or a breath, is delivered. In the presence of auto-PEEP, patient triggering may be negatively affected, since the ventilator does not sense the auto-PEEP. In this case, the patient must generate a pressure equal to the auto-PEEP plus the sensitivity level in order to trigger a breath, greatly increasing the work of breathing. The set PEEP may be increased to the level of auto-PEEP (or just slightly below) so that the ventilator senses the patient's efforts. However, the best solution is to try to eliminate auto-PEEP.
- It has been known for quite some time that pressure-triggering mechanisms impose a greater workload for the patient than do systems that provide continuous flow.[4,8,42,48] To that end, "flow triggering" was developed and is available on many newer ventilators. This is a more sensitive option than pressure sensing (if set correctly). With flow triggering, a bias flow is provided for patient-initiated breaths, and a flow drop (in L/min) is set as a "trigger." The flow is sensed on the expiratory side of the circuit. When the patient initiates a spontaneous breath, the drop in flow is sensed downstream, triggering the ventilator to deliver more flow or a breath, depending on the mode.
- Inspiratory pressure level (IPL): Pressure modes of ventilation require a pressure level be selected. The required pressure level is determined by the clinical goal of therapy. In the patient with ARDS, for example, the clinical goal may be to maintain the plateau pressure at 30 cm H_2O. If the goal is to maintain a target V_T, the pressure level is adjusted to attain that V_T (remember, the volume will vary from breath to breath with pressure-targeted ventilation, but an acceptable range is the goal). IPL may be referred to by different names, depending on the mode.

BOX 10.4 Modes of Ventilation: Categories

Invasive modes (require an artificial airway)

Volume Modes

- Assist control (AC)
- Synchronized intermittent mandatory ventilation (SIMV)

Pressure Modes

- Pressure support (PS)
- Pressure control (PC) and pressure-controlled inverse ratio ventilation (PC/IRV)
- Pressure augmentation (PA) (volume-guaranteed pressure option)
- Volume support (VS) and pressure-regulated volume control (PRVC) (volume-guaranteed pressure options)
- Volume ventilation plus (VVP) (volume-guaranteed pressure option)
- Airway pressure release ventilation (APRV) and bi-level ventilation

Nonconventional Mode

- High-frequency oscillation (HFO)

Noninvasive modes (used with a full face mask or nasal mask interface)

- Continuous positive airway pressure (CPAP)
- Bi-level positive airway pressure (BiPAP)

clinician-selected pressure level. With PSV, the preset pressure rises rapidly to a plateau that is maintained throughout inspiration. Termination of inspiration occurs when the flow diminishes to a predetermined level (e.g., one-fourth the original flow). Generally, this mode is thought of as a mode for weaning. The patient must have a reliable ventilatory drive.

- Advantages/disadvantages: The patient controls the T_I, fx, and V_T variables. High levels of PSV (i.e., PSV_{max}) provide nearly total ventilatory support. PSV_{max} is when the PSV level is high enough to result in a respiratory rate (RR) of less than 20 breaths per minute and a V_T between 8 and 12 mL/kg, without accessory muscle use. PSV also allows for gradual respiratory muscle conditioning, or endurance conditioning (discussed under Weaning from Mechanical Ventilation). A disadvantage of PSV is that the RR and V_T are dependent on the patient's condition (i.e., lung compliance/airway resistance).
- Parameters set on PSV include inspiratory pressure level (PS level), PEEP, sensitivity, and Fio_2. Like all pressure modes, V_T and RR are patient-dependent and must be monitored frequently.

Pressure Control and Pressure-Controlled Inverse Ratio Ventilation

Pressure control (PC) is used to control and lower plateau pressures and to optimize gas exchange in patients with ARDS. When used with an inverse ratio, the prolonged T_I allows less opportunity for derecruitment to occur because the expiratory time is abbreviated. This is called *pressure-controlled inverse ratio ventilation* (PC/IRV) (Box 10.5).

Volume-Guaranteed Pressure Modes

Volume-guaranteed pressure modes, or dual modes, combine pressure-supported ventilation with a decelerating flow pattern and a guaranteed volume. These modes were developed because of the widespread interest in using pressure modes in the critically ill unstable patient.[46,85] However, the fact that V_E might be adversely affected because of unanticipated changes in compliance and resistance was of concern. Manufacturers responded with pressure modes that also ensure a set volume. Although the modes have different names depending on the manufacturer, the concept is similar. While it is beyond the scope of this chapter to describe in detail the specific ventilator variations for this mode, descriptions of some of the more common modes that are available follow.

BOX 10.5 Advantages/Disadvantages of Pressure-Controlled Inverse Ratio Ventilation

Pressure control (PC) is often used in patients with ARDS who have oxygenation difficulties. The plateau pressure is controlled, and the decelerating flow associated with the mode may improve gas distribution. However, since the inspiratory time and rate are determined by the clinician, the patient can quickly become dyssynchronous if available flow is not adequate, especially with the use of inverse ratio ventilation (IRV), which is very common with the older ventilator PC mode options. Often heavy sedation and paralytic use are necessary to ensure synchrony. As in any pressure mode, the tidal volume (V_T) must be monitored frequently.

Parameters set on the PC and PC/IRV modes include the following: IPL, fx, T_I, PEEP, and Fio_2. When IRV is used, the I/E ratio is set at 1:1, 2:1, 3:1, or 4:1. Auto-PEEP may be a desired outcome of IRV, and should be routinely monitored.

ARDS, Acute respiratory distress syndrome; *fx,* frequency; *Fio_2,* fraction of inspired oxygen; *IPL,* inspiratory pressure level; *PEEP,* positive end-expiratory pressure; *T_I,* inspiratory time.

Volume Support and Pressure-Regulated Volume Control

Volume support (VS) is designed for spontaneous breathing. This mode adjusts the pressure level in a stepwise fashion (e.g. 3 cm H_2O at a time) to maintain the desired (selected) volume on a breath-to-breath basis. All breaths are pressure breaths. Pressure-regulated volume control (PRVC) is designed as a control mode. As described for VS, this mode adjusts pressure to attain the set volume, but other parameters (e.g., fx and T_I) are set. Thus all breaths are pressure breaths, but the target volume selected by the clinician determines the level of pressure.[28,61]

Volume Ventilation Plus

Volume ventilation plus (VVP) is similar to PRVC in breath delivery, but an active exhalation valve allows unrestricted breathing during the respiratory cycle.[28]

Parameters set for volume-guaranteed pressure modes include V_T (desired for the guaranteed V_T), fx (only for the control options), T_I (only for the control options), inspiratory pressure level (IPL), PEEP, sensitivity, and Fio_2.

Airway Pressure Release Ventilation and Bi-Level Ventilation

Airway pressure release ventilation. Airway pressure release ventilation (APRV) allows for spontaneous breathing on a preset (relatively high) continuous positive airway pressure (CPAP) level interrupted by a short (approximately 1 to 1.5 seconds) release for further expiration.[28,31] The mode was designed for patients with ARDS, because it uses a high level of CPAP to recruit the lung. The brief release allows for emptying of some of the alveolar units that empty slowly (to prevent overdistention), while not allowing complete derecruitment to occur throughout the lung. This mode is different from other modes because spontaneously breathing patients may look quite tachypneic despite adequate oxygenation and ventilation. Discussions of the advantages/disadvantages of this mode and parameter settings follow the discussion of bi-level positive airway pressure (BiPAP) below.[28,31]

Bi-level ventilation. Bi-level ventilation is similar to PCV; however, in this mode the patient's spontaneous breathing is allowed during both the inspiratory and expiratory phases, called *high PEEP* and *low PEEP,* respectively. The ventilator does this by supplying a very high flow of gas to the patient during inspiration and using an active exhalation valve to allow for unrestricted breathing. The mode is considered appropriate for patients with ARDS noncompliant lungs, and in patients in whom it is undesirable to use paralytic agents to ensure acceptable respiratory gas exchange.

- Advantages/disadvantages: There is ambiguity in the terminology between APRV and bi-level ventilation.[30,72] Additionally, no randomized controlled trials have been performed to compare either the APRV or the bi-level modes to more traditional modes using low V_T ventilation in ARDS patients. These modes may allow for optimal recruitment of the lung with high levels of PEEP or open lung ventilation, while still permitting spontaneous breathing, without the risk of derecruitment. Patient workload is unclear and may be a consideration when selecting the mode.
- Parameters set on APRV and bi-level ventilation include fx (frequency release if APRV), T_I (bi-level), select CPAP level (APRV), high PEEP/low PEEP (bi-level), sensitivity (both), and Fio_2 (both).

High-Frequency Oscillation

High-frequency oscillation (HFO) is a very different form of ventilation than both the conventional volume and pressure modes.[25] With HFO, a bias flow of gases is provided, and an oscillator disperses the gases throughout the lung at high frequencies, a process called *augmented dispersion*.[25]

- Advantages/disadvantages: It was thought that this mode might allow for optimal lung recruitment and prevent the potential for the repetitive opening and closing injury associated with most traditional modes. However, this mode is very different from conventional ventilation, and there is a very steep learning curve related to its use in the clinical setting. Recent research has shown that HFO does not improve mortality over conventional ventilation in patients with ARDS, with one randomized control trial demonstrating an increased mortality.[39,56,93] HFO has also been shown to be associated with longer ICU and hospital stays. Additional concerns about the use of HFO are that frequently heavy sedation and paralytics are required to ensure compliance with the mode. HFO should not be used routinely in adult patients with ARDS.[39,56,93]
- Parameters set for HFO include bias flow (approximately 40 to 50 L/min), oscillatory fx (in hertz [Hz], with starting level of 5 Hz), mean airway pressure (slightly above conventional), and ΔP (i.e., change in pressure or pressure amplitude; this is adjusted to achieve chest wall vibration or "wiggle").

Advanced Modes: Patient-Controlled Ventilation

Patient-controlled ventilation modes were developed to improve patient synchrony by delivering ventilator assistance in direct proportion to the patient's efforts. Airway resistance and elastance, or the pressure change that is a measure of the resistance of lung to expand, is measured from breath to breath. The ventilator calculates the pressure needed at any given moment to provide ventilation. The total pressure needed to ventilate (P_{total}) is equal to the tidal volume (V_T) times elastance (E) plus flow (V) times airway resistance (R).[46,49,74,85]

Proportional-Assist Ventilation

Proportional-assist ventilation (PAV) synchronizes the support that is given by the ventilator to the patient's inspiratory effort to adapt to changes in ventilatory demand. Pressure will increase along with flow as patient demand increases. Flow is adjusted at the initiation of inspiratory effort to end expiration, which is thought to improve cycling. There is no set V_T, target flow, ventilation, or airway pressure set; the percentage of assist is selected based on ideal body weight (IBW) along with PEEP.

- Advantages/disadvantages: The settings are complex and require education and familiarity to use safely. In order for PAV to work, the patient's respiratory drive and muscle output must be responsive to changes in pH, $Paco_2$, and Pao_2. PAV is contraindicated in patients who have respiratory depression, need high-dose sedation and are heavily sedated, have a history of central apnea, or have severe neuromuscular weakness. In addition, PAV is not appropriate for patients with bronchocutaneous fistulas and with an exhaled V_T less than 75% of the inhaled volume.[17,85]

Neurally Adjusted Ventilator Assist

Neurally adjusted ventilatory assist (NAVA) uses diaphragmatic electrical activity (Edi) to control ventilation and provide feedback to the lungs. The ventilator assists in synchrony and, similar to PAV, assists in proportion to the patient's respiratory effort.[61] Effort is measured by a catheter inserted into the esophagus nasally or orally with electrodes that measure Edi, the signal is monitored from a display. NAVA can also be used with invasive and noninvasive ventilation. A NAVA level is set along with PEEP, and the NAVA level plus the Edi determines the pressure needed to ventilate the patient's lungs.[44,47,59,83]

- Advantages/disadvantages: The settings are complex and require education and familiarity to use safely. NAVA cannot be used if the patient has a paralyzed diaphragm or a nasogastric or orogastric tube, or if there is no respiratory drive. Unlike PAV, NAVA is unaffected by leaks or by intrinsic PEEP.[49,85]

NONINVASIVE VENTILATOR MODES

Noninvasive ventilation may be performed with a conventional ventilator or with a ventilator designed specifically for noninvasive applications. The use of noninvasive ventilation is encouraged whenever possible because it is correlated with lower ventilator-associated pneumonia rates and lower morbidity and mortality rates.[15,24] However, the selection of patients for the therapy must be conducted carefully. An essential variable is mental status; noninvasive modes do not provide for airway protection as the ventilation is delivered through a nasal mask, full facemask, or nasal pillows. Intact mental status is especially important if a full facemask is used, as vomiting may result in aspiration. Other patients who would be poor choices for the therapy are those requiring very high levels of oxygen (unless noninvasive ventilation is accomplished using a conventional ventilator) and those unable to effectively clear their airway, especially if secretions are copious.

In the past, volume modes (e.g., AC) were preferred because leaks around the mask interface were common, and it was difficult to ensure adequate ventilation with pressure modes. Today, newer ventilators provide leak compensation, making noninvasive ventilation with pressure possible. The most common noninvasive modes used today are CPAP and BiPAP.

CPAP

CPAP is one of the most common forms of noninvasive ventilation, and has been used predominantly to manage patients with obstructive sleep apnea (OSA). The required CPAP level is generally determined in a sleep laboratory. However, other forms of noninvasive mask ventilation may be provided for patients who prefer to avoid more invasive airway management methods (i.e., endotracheal tube or tracheostomy), and are sometimes used to prevent intubation or reintubation following extubation. Additionally, patients with heart failure (HF) may benefit from noninvasive ventilation.[15,24] Advantages of, disadvantages of, and parameters for CPAP are covered following the discussion of BiPAP.

BiPAP

Though a number of equivalent noninvasive methods for BiPAP exist, the term was originally coined by Respironics (Murrysville, PA).[70] This mode provides for two levels of positive pressure—pressure support and PEEP—and is delivered through a nasal mask, nasal pillows, or full facemask.

- Advantages/disadvantages: As described previously, noninvasive mode options may prevent iatrogenic complications and shorten length of stay. However, effective application requires time and patience. Careful selection of the interface size and fit is essential to patient comfort and acceptance. Any mask poses potential skin integrity issues; the fit of the mask around other devices (e.g., nasogastric tubes) may be difficult. A chinstrap may be used to help close the mouth of the patient, thus providing a better seal and decreasing the risk of air leaks. It is important to remember that leaks are expected and acceptable, providing they are not excessive and are compensated for by the ventilator.

- The names of the parameters that are set for CPAP and BiPAP vary by manufacturer. CPAP level and oxygen are the main settings for CPAP. Parameters set for BiPAP are as follows: inspiratory pressure level (IPL, I-PAP), expiratory pressure level (PEEP, E-PAP), and Fio_2 (may be controlled by a dial on the ventilator but most require that oxygen is bled into the system [e.g., 6 L] at the mask interface or between the ventilator and circuit).
- Mode names also vary by manufacturer and include spontaneous (PSV), spontaneous/timed (S/T or AC), and timed (control) modes. With the timed modes, fx and T_I are also set.

RESPIRATORY WAVEFORM MONITORING

A relatively new assessment skill for nurses and respiratory therapists working with mechanically ventilated patients is the interpretation of respiratory waveforms. Years ago, respiratory waveform monitoring was rare; today, it is widely available on ventilators. Unfortunately, the waveforms are poorly understood, and as a result, the technology is not used to full advantage. This section describes the most common waveforms available on ventilators today. The reader is reminded that waveform configurations may vary depending on the manufacturer; however, the concepts are broadly applicable.

Respiratory waveform monitoring is most helpful in monitoring volume or pressure modes of mechanical ventilation. Respiratory waveform monitoring is noninvasive, is undetectable by the patient, and does not interfere with normal ventilator function; no special patient considerations are required for its use. Once the visual display is set up, selected waveforms are available and may be graphed (depending on the equipment). Commonly available waveform graphics include pressure-time, flow-time, volume-time, and "loop" configurations (pressure-volume and flow-volume loops). Respiratory waveform monitoring may be helpful in identifying appropriate modes of ventilation (and patient/ventilator dyssynchrony), detecting auto-PEEP and air leaks, evaluating changes in compliance and resistance, identifying end-expiration during hemodynamic monitoring, and monitoring spontaneous respiratory effort when muscle relaxants are being used. A description of the waveforms and selected applications follows.

Pressure-Time and Flow-Time Waveforms

Volume modes are associated with *accelerating pressure* waveforms (see Fig. 10.1), because pressure gradually builds as the volume of gas is delivered. Examples of pressure waveforms from volume modes of ventilation include AC (Fig. 10.7) and SIMV (Fig. 10.8). Flow waveforms with volume ventilation are generally a *square* configuration (see Fig. 10.2) because flow is stable throughout the breath.

With *pressure modes,* a high flow of gas is delivered until a predetermined pressure is reached. The pressure is maintained throughout inspiration, and the associated waveform is called a *square pressure waveform* (see Fig. 10.4). Examples of pressure waveforms from pressure modes include PSV (Fig. 10.9), PC/IRV (Fig. 10.10), and volume-guaranteed pressure options (Figs. 10.11 and 10.12). Pressure waveforms of mixed volume and pressure modes, such as SIMV plus PSV, demonstrate a combination of the two (Figs. 10.13 and 10.14). In all pressure modes, flow is initially high but tapers as the chest fills; thus the associated flow waveform

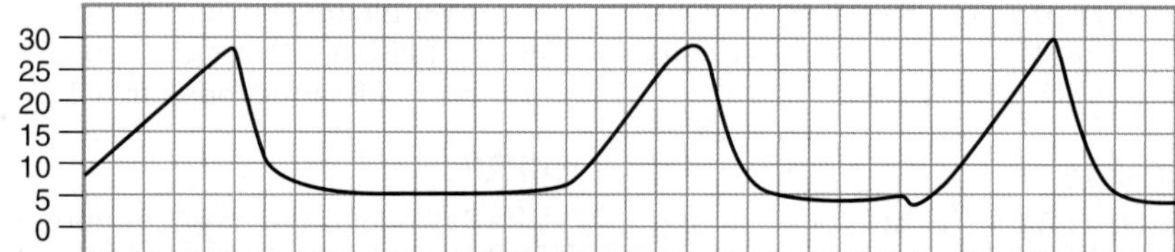

FIG. 10.7 Pressure waveform of the assist-control (AC) mode. Note that the third waveform starts with a negative deflection, which is indicative of patient effort.

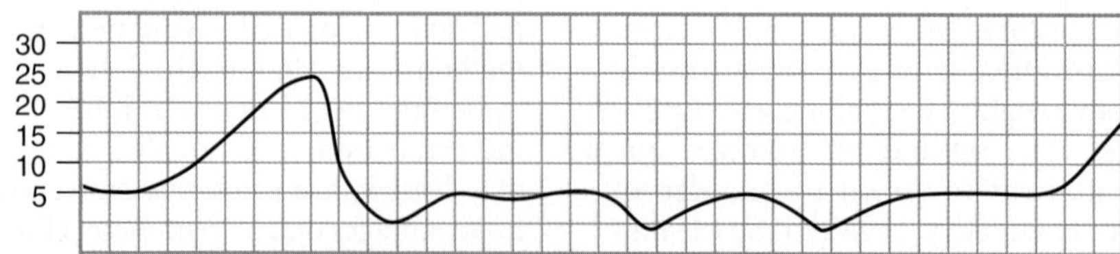

FIG. 10.8 Pressure-time waveform of synchronized intermittent mandatory ventilation (SIMV).

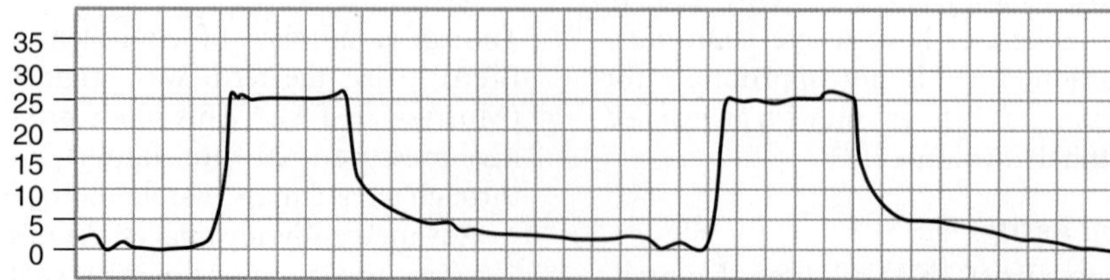

FIG. 10.9 Pressure-time waveform of pressure support ventilation. All breaths have a square pressure configuration.

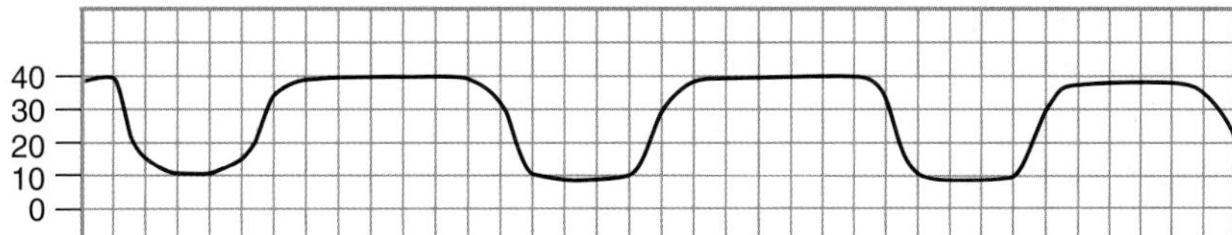

FIG. 10.10 Pressure-time waveform of pressure-controlled inverse ratio ventilation (PC/IRV) (2:1 ratio).

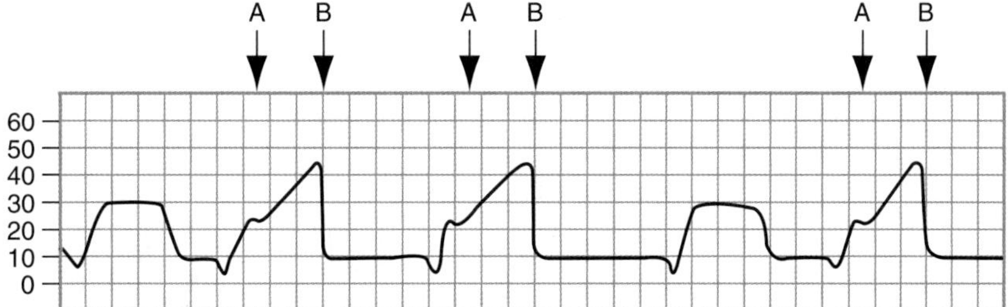

FIG. 10.11 Pressure-time waveform of pressure-controlled inverse ratio ventilation (2:1 ratio). The breath starts as a pressure breath (*A,* square pressure waveform) but ends as a volume breath (*B,* accelerating pressure waveform).

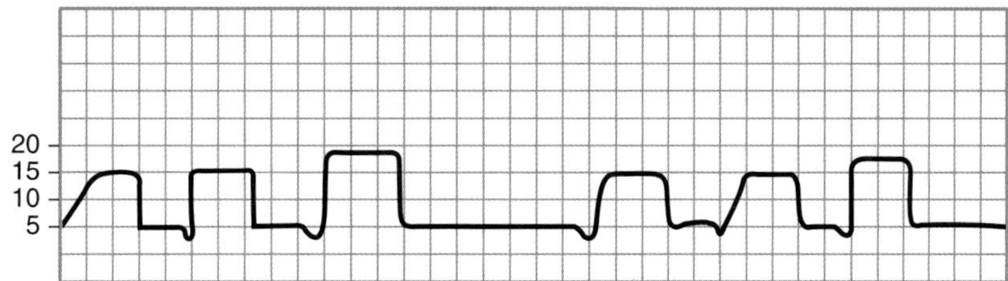

FIG. 10.12 Pressure-time waveform of a volume-guaranteed pressure option: "volume support." The mode adjusts the pressure level to ensure the desired volume.

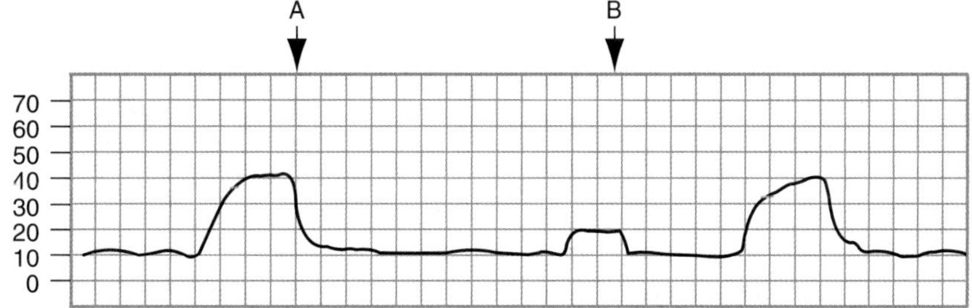

FIG. 10.13 Pressure-time waveform of mixed modes: SIMV *(A)* plus PSV *(B)*. *SIMV,* Synchronized intermittent mandatory ventilation; *PSV,* pressure support ventilation.

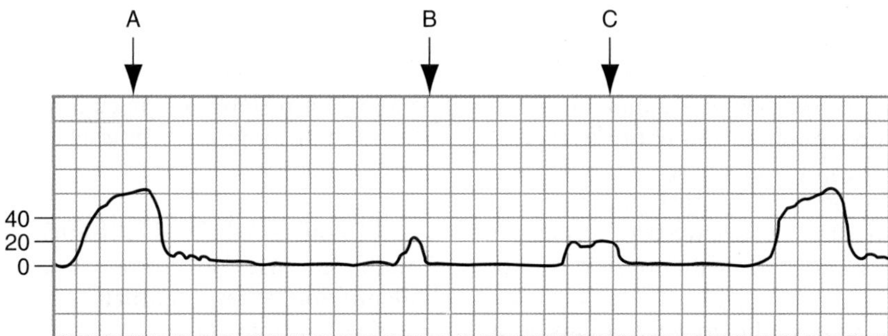

FIG. 10.14 Pressure-time waveform of mixed modes: SIMV (*A*) plus PSV (*B* and *C*). Waveform *B* demonstrates poor inspiratory effort. *SIMV,* Synchronized intermittent mandatory ventilation; *PSV,* pressure support ventilation.

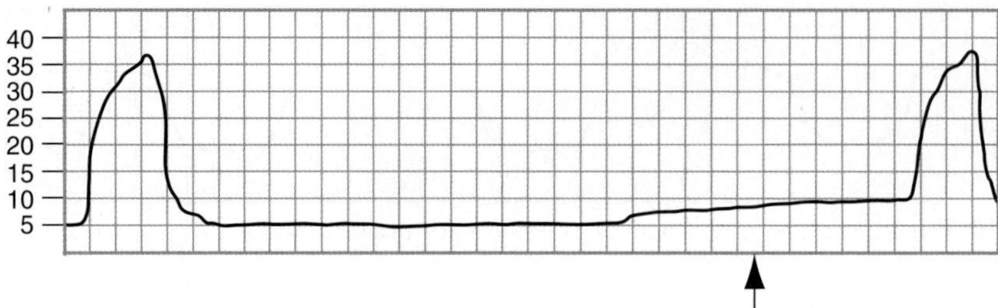

FIG. 10.15 Pressure-time waveform demonstrating end-expiratory hold to measure auto-PEEP. The *arrow* indicates auto-PEEP.

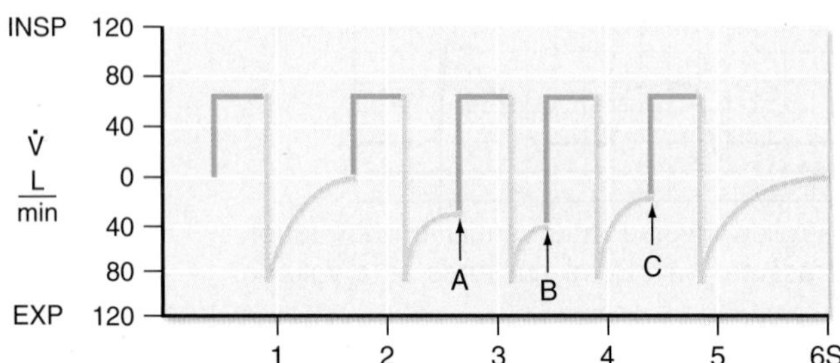

FIG. 10.16 *A, B,* and *C* are all the end-expiratory limbs of the breaths. They do not return to baseline, thus indicating auto-PEEP. *INSP,* Inspiration; *EXP,* expiration.

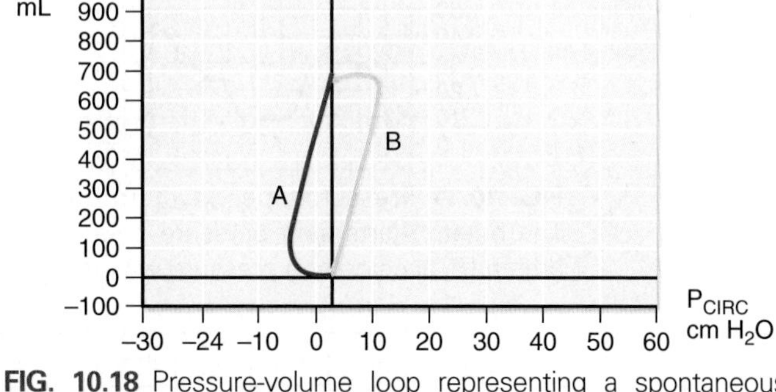

FIG. 10.18 Pressure-volume loop representing a spontaneous breath. The loop is plotted in a clockwise direction. *A,* inspiration (negative portion of the graph); *B,* expiration. P_{CIRC}, Circuit pressure.

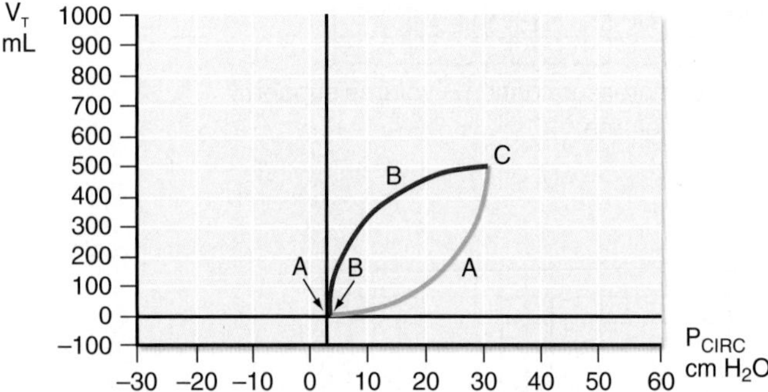

FIG. 10.17 Pressure-volume loop representing a mandatory breath. The loop is plotted in a counterclockwise fashion. *A,* inspiration; *B,* expiration; *C,* peak inspiratory pressure. P_{CIRC}, Circuit pressure.

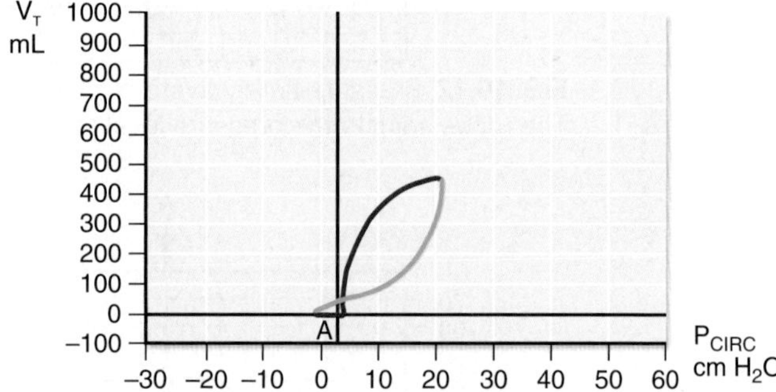

FIG. 10.19 Pressure-volume loop represents a patient-initiated breath. *A,* spontaneous effort (moves to negative portion of the graph). As the ventilator delivers the positive pressure breath, the loop moves to the left. P_{CIRC}, Circuit pressure.

seen with pressure ventilation is called a *decelerating flow waveform* (see Fig. 10.5). Auto-PEEP may be detected with a pressure-time or flow waveform (Figs. 10.15 and 10.16).

Pressure-Volume Loops

Pressure-volume loops vary depending on whether the breath is a spontaneous breath (negative pressure) or a mandatory ventilator breath (positive pressure). Spontaneous effort is reflected on the negative portion of the horizontal axis, and mandatory ventilator breaths are on the right, or positive, portion of the axis (Figs. 10.17, 10.18, and 10.19). Assessment of changes in compliance and resistance is possible with pressure-volume loops.

- *Decreased compliance:* the slope of the pressure-volume loop will shift to the right and down (i.e., a greater pressure is required to obtain a given volume) (Fig. 10.20).
- *Increased resistance:* the beginning portion of the loop will reflect an increase in pressure, which is referred to as increased bowing (Fig. 10.21).

Flow-Volume Loops

Flow-volume loops graph expiration first, followed by inspiration. These loops are helpful in assessing the effect of bronchodilator therapy on peak flow (Fig. 10.22).

Additional Uses of Respiratory Waveforms

Additional uses of respiratory waveform monitoring include identifying patient ventilator dyssynchrony (Figs. 10.23 and 10.24), establishing end-expiration during hemodynamic monitoring (Fig. 10.25), and monitoring spontaneous respiratory effort when muscle relaxants are being used (Fig. 10.26).

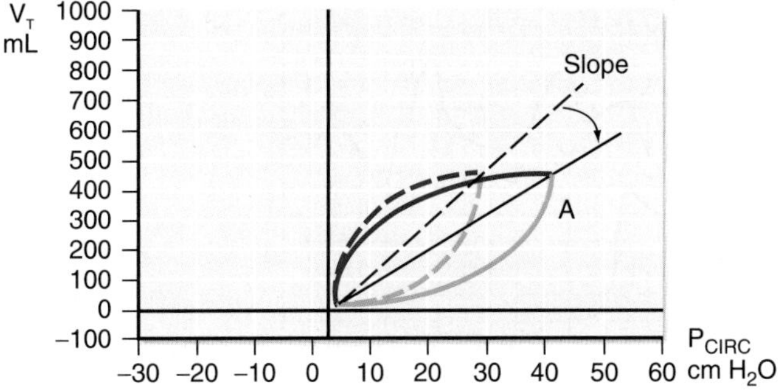

FIG. 10.20 Pressure-volume loop demonstrating the downward movement (slope) of the curve with decreased compliance. Greater pressure is required to deliver the same volume. *A*, same breath as the hatched line. P_{CIRC}, Circuit pressure.

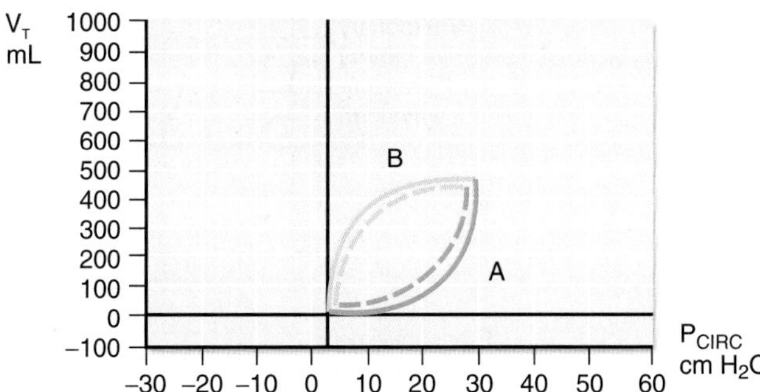

FIG. 10.21 Pressure-volume loop demonstrating increased resistance. In this case, greater pressure is needed to overcome the resistance of the airways. The result is a bowed configuration of the loop (*A* and *B*). P_{CIRC}, Circuit pressure.

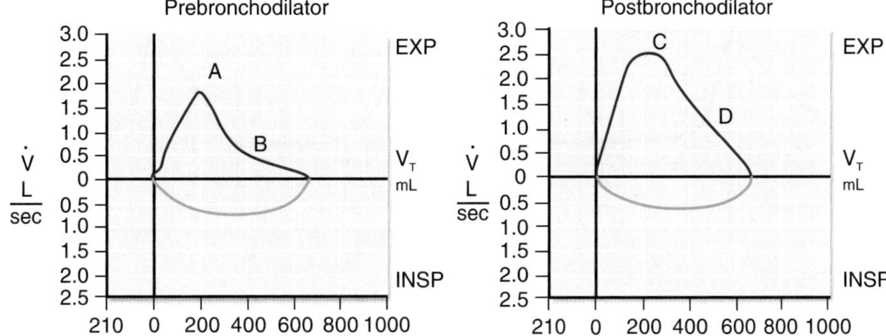

FIG. 10.22 Flow-volume loops demonstrating the difference in peak expiratory flow rate before and after bronchodilator therapy *(A and C)*. In addition, the scalloped shape near the end of the exhalation *(B)* is characteristic of poor airway conductivity before bronchodilator use, which is markedly improved after using the bronchodilator *(D)*. INSP, Inspiration; EXP, expiration.

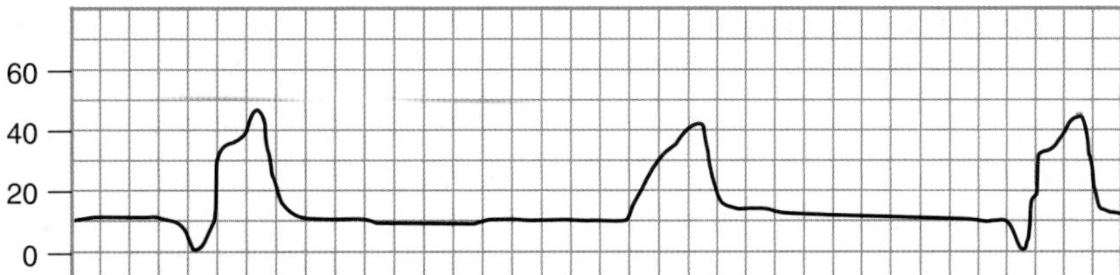

FIG. 10.23 Pressure-time waveform of the AC mode. Note the first and third waveforms, which are initiated by the patient. The deep negative pressure drop preceding the patient-initiated breaths indicates significant breathing effort. The scooped portion of the accelerating waveform suggests that flow is not adequate. The patient is dyssynchronous. *AC,* Assist control.

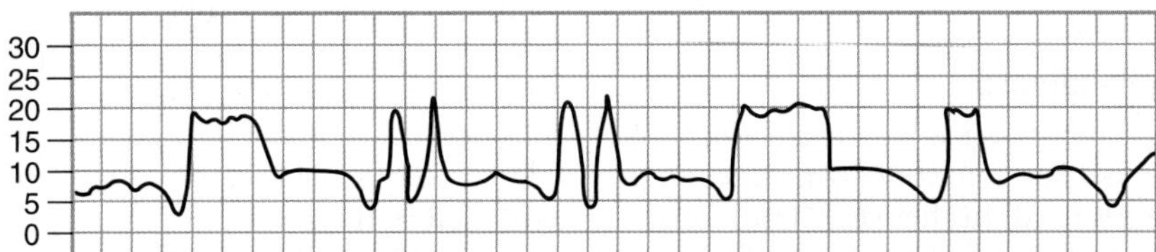

FIG. 10.24 Pressure-time waveform of PSV. The short, choppy waveforms indicate poor inspiration (the patient was hiccoughing). The patient is dyssynchronous. *PSV,* Pressure support ventilation.

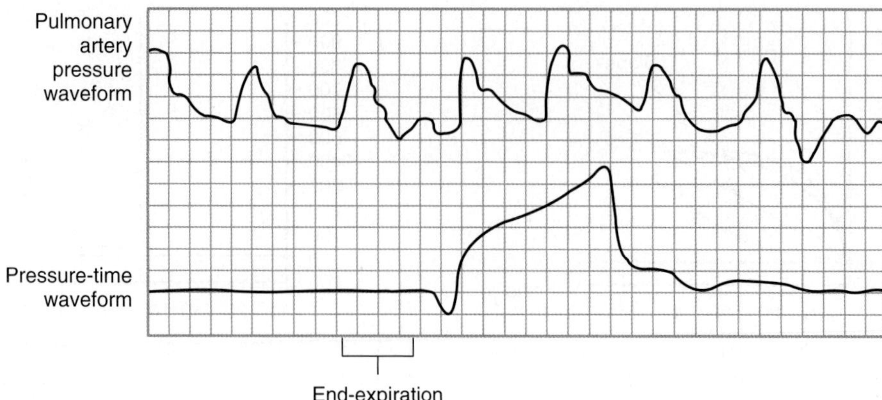

FIG. 10.25 Simultaneous pulmonary artery tracing and pressure-time waveform. Measurement of end-expiration is easy to perform.

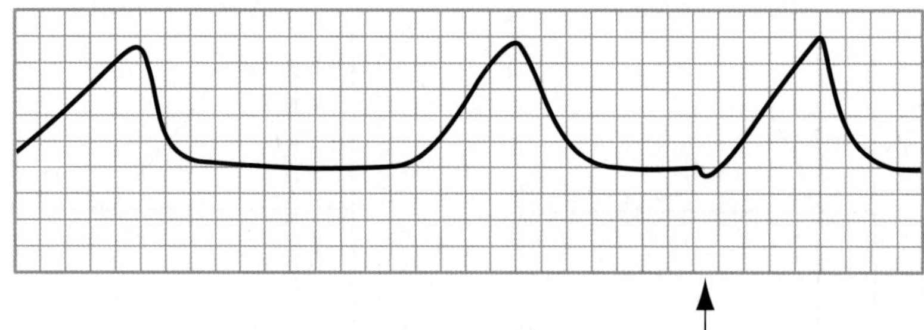

FIG. 10.26 Pressure-time waveform indicating breakthrough breathing *(arrow)* on a patient receiving neuromuscular blockade.

Exposure to the respiratory waveforms increases familiarity and subsequent use as a real-time noninvasive monitoring tool.

WEANING FROM MECHANICAL VENTILATION

The process of ventilator liberation has continued to be of great interest to clinicians charged with the care of the mechanically ventilated patient. Delays in weaning result in increased morbidity and mortality, increased length of stay in hospitals and use of ventilator units, and decreased satisfaction of patients, families, and staff.[19,38,40,50,51,58,69,71,87] Over the last decade, efforts to improve the weaning process have demonstrated that approaches that decrease variability are superior.[4,5,16,21-23,42,58,69] This section of the chapter will cover assessment; respiratory muscle conditioning, rest, and work; modes and methods of weaning; timing of tracheostomy and weaning methods; and interprofessional interventions.

Assessment of Weaning Readiness

Assessment of the weaning patient begins with evaluating stability and determining whether the condition(s) necessitating mechanical ventilation has resolved. In the past, "traditional" or "standard" weaning indexes were relied on to identify weaning readiness (Box 10.6).[58,60] While the indexes are helpful for assessing respiratory muscle strength and endurance, they are not good positive predictors.[18,60] In fact, only the negative inspiratory pressure (NIP) measurement is non–effort-dependent; studies have demonstrated that it is highly variable, dependent on technique.[92] However, the traditional indexes may be useful as negative predictors; a poor value, and especially a poor NIP value, is associated with an inability to wean successfully.

Because of the poor positive predictive value of the traditional weaning indexes, investigators have developed other indexes that integrate additional variables.[23] An example is the index of rapid, shallow breathing (Box 10.7).[82] Unfortunately, this index has not proven to be predictive in many cases. Regardless, the ratio does represent a pattern of breathing that may indicate respiratory muscle fatigue (i.e., rapid, shallow breathing) and subsequently unsuccessful weaning trials.[82] The information may be effectively used as part of a more comprehensive assessment.

While weaning measures may be more effective for their negative prediction value, a good measure of weaning readiness is a "bundle" approach that combines a safety-screening tool with a collaborative weaning protocol. The Awakening and Breathing Controlled trial demonstrated that patients who received a protocol-based spontaneous awakening trial and spontaneous breathing trial had fewer ventilator days and decreased lengths of ICU and hospital stay.[42] An example of a daily safety screening tool is the "Wake Up and Breathe" protocol (Box 10.8).

An additional approach to ensure that the patient is physiologically and psychologically ready to begin weaning trials is to assess both pulmonary and nonpulmonary factors regularly. An example of an assessment tool that has been designed to accomplish this goal is the Burns Weaning Assessment

BOX 10.6 Traditional Weaning Indexes

Negative Inspiratory Pressure (NIP)

Before beginning, the endotracheal or tracheal tube cuff is inflated. Attach a one-way valve and a pressure manometer to the patient's artificial airway, making sure the cuff is inflated. Instruct the patient to try to exhale maximally before attaching the measurement device (to attempt to begin at residual volume). Once the measurement device is attached, instruct the patient to inhale forcefully against the closed system. The best effort (most negative number) is recorded in 20 seconds. Abort the test if the patient becomes unduly agitated or experiences dysrhythmias or desaturation.

$$\text{NIP threshold} \leq 30 \text{ cm } H_2O$$

Positive Expiratory Pressure (PEP)

Inflate the endotracheal or tracheal tube cuff. Measurement is as in NIP, but the measurement device is adapted to allow the patient to inhale but not exhale. The patient is instructed to exhale forcefully against the closed system. The best effort, in this case the most positive number, is recorded in 20 seconds.

$$\text{PEP threshold} \geq 30 \text{ cm } H_2O$$

Spontaneous Tidal Volume (V_T sp)

Attach a respirometer or other volume-measuring device to the expiratory side of a two-way valve and instruct the patient to breathe normally for 1 minute. Average tidal volume (V_T) is calculated by dividing the patient's spontaneous respiratory rate (RR) into the minute ventilation. This measurement may also be performed with the patient on the ventilator at a continuous positive airway pressure (CPAP) level of zero. Observe the digital V_T readout to determine the average V_T.

$$V_T \text{ sp threshold} = 5 \text{ mL/kg}$$

Vital Capacity (VC)

Obtained using the same equipment as with V_T sp (or on the ventilator, as described), but the technique is markedly different and difficult to perform on the intubated patient. The patient must be able to understand and follow the instructions. First, ask the patient to inhale maximally before the measurement device is attached. Once the device is attached, the patient is asked to exhale maximally and forcefully. The maneuver is usually attempted more than once, and the patient is allowed to rest between attempts. Record the best effort.

$$\text{VC threshold} \geq 15 \text{ mL/kg}$$

Minute Ventilation (V_E)

Minute ventilation is obtained by multiplying RR times V_t. It may be measured manually (after 1 minute of spontaneous breathing) using a respirometer (as described for V_T sp). More commonly, the exhaled minute ventilation (also known as *minute volume*) may be observed on the ventilator displays.

$$V_E \text{ threshold} = 5 - 10 \text{L/min}$$

From Reference 18.

BOX 10.7 Rapid Shallow Breathing Ratio*

To calculate the rapid shallow breathing ratio, divide spontaneous respiratory frequency (fx) in 1 minute by tidal volume (V_T) in liters:

Threshold:
- <105 = weaning success
- >105 = weaning failure

*Also known as *frequency to tidal volume (fx/V_T) ratio.*

BOX 10.8 Daily Safety Screen

"Wake Up and Breathe"

1. Daily assessment of safety screen to remove sedation
   - Is sedation for active seizures?
   - Is sedation for alcohol withdrawal?
   - Is a paralytic agent used?
   - Is the patient agitated, as determined by a validated assessment score?
   - Has there been myocardial ischemia in the previous 24 hours?
   - Is intracranial pressure (ICP) elevated?
2. If ready, perform spontaneous awakening trial (SAT)
   - Is there increased agitation, as measured by a validated assessment score?

   Is peripheral capillary oxygen saturation, an estimate of the amount of oxygen in the blood (pulse oximetry [Spo_2]) <88% for 5 minutes or longer?
   - Is respiratory rate >35/min for 5 minutes or longer?
   - Are there new cardiac arrhythmias?
   - Does the patient have two or more of the following?
     - Heart rate increase ≥20 beats per min (bpm)
     - Heart rate <55 bpm
     - Use of accessory muscles
     - Abdominal paradoxical breathing
     - Diaphoresis
     - Dyspnea
3. If ready, coordinate spontaneous breathing trial with respiratory therapist

Adapted from Reference 5.

Program (BWAP) (Box 10.9). The BWAP, which consists of a bedside checklist and a personal digital assistant application, is designed to prompt the clinician to systematically assess factors important to weaning and to encourage interventions to improve them. In addition, the BWAP score may be used to track progress, or lack thereof, and to determine the level of weaning readiness.[21,22]

The effects of sedation (sedation infusions) on weaning along with effects on pain and delirium have recently been clarified, and point to the importance of routinely assessing pain, agitation, and delirium (PAD).[6,7,42,53] As in weaning, there are strong recommendations for ventilator and ICU care to be performed in an integrated, collaborative fashion.

RESPIRATORY MUSCLE FATIGUE, REST, WORK, AND CONDITIONING

Respiratory muscles, like all muscles, fatigue, and once fatigued, require 12 to 24 hours to recuperate.[8] When the muscles are required to work to excess, mitochondrial stores deplete, the muscles do not contract optimally, and hypercarbic respiratory failure ensues.[8,27] Dyspnea, rapid shallow breathing, and chest abdominal asynchrony appear to be compensatory signs heralding fatigue, and should be heeded.[8,27] To that end, decreasing the respiratory muscle workload is essential; mechanical ventilation in these cases is life-saving. However, the method of applying mechanical ventilation to ensure respiratory muscle rest is dependent on the mode and application of ventilation.

Studies by Marini et al. have demonstrated that for muscle work to cease during ventilation, patient effort must cease.[63] For example, consider the case of a patient on a volume mode of ventilation. If the patient on the AC mode of ventilation initiates breaths between the set (i.e., control) breaths, the patient's

BOX 10.9 Burns Weaning Assessment Program (BWAP)*

Patient ______________________

Yes No N/A

General Assessment

___ ___ ___ 1. Hemodynamically stable (pulse rate, cardiac output)?
___ ___ ___ 2. Free from factors that increase or decrease metabolic rate (seizures, fever, sepsis, bacteremia, hypo/hyperthyroid)?
___ ___ ___ 3. Hematocrit >25% (or baseline)?
___ ___ ___ 4. Systemically hydrated (weight at or near baseline, balanced intake and output)?
___ ___ ___ 5. Nourished (albumin >2.5 g/dL, parenteral/enteral feedings maximized)? (If albumin is low and anasarca or third spacing is present, score for hydration should be "no".)
___ ___ ___ 6. Electrolytes within normal limits (including Ca^{2+}, Mg^+, PO_4)? (Correct Ca^{2+} concentration for albumin level.)
___ ___ ___ 7. Pain controlled (subjective determination)?
___ ___ ___ 8. Adequate sleep/rest (subjective determination)?
___ ___ ___ 9. Appropriate level of anxiety and nervousness (subjective determination)?
___ ___ ___ 10. Absence of bowel problems (diarrhea, constipation, ileus)?
___ ___ ___ 11. Improved general body strength/endurance (i.e., out of bed to chair, progressive activity program)?
___ ___ ___ 12. Chest roentgenograph improving?

Respiratory Assessment

Gas Flow and Work of Breathing

___ ___ ___ 13. Eupneic respiratory rate and pattern (spontaneous respiratory rate <25 breaths/min, without dyspnea, absence of accessory muscle use)? *(This is assessed off the ventilator while measuring Items 20–23.)*
___ ___ ___ 14. Absence of adventitious breath sounds (rhonchi, rales, wheezing)?
___ ___ ___ 15. Secretions thin and minimal?
___ ___ ___ 16. Absence of neuromuscular disease/deformity?
___ ___ ___ 17. Absence of abdominal distention/obesity/ascites?
___ ___ ___ 18. Oral endotracheal tube ≥7.5 mm/ID (inner diameter) or trach ≥6.5 mm/ID?

Airway Clearance

___ ___ ___ 19. Cough and swallow reflexes adequate?

Strength

___ ___ ___ 20. Negative inspiratory pressure ≤20 cm H_2O?
___ ___ ___ 21. Positive expiratory pressure >30 cm H_2O?

Endurance

___ ___ ___ 22. Spontaneous tidal volume >5 mL/kg?
___ ___ ___ 23. Vital capacity >10–15 mL/kg?

Arterial Blood Gases

___ ___ ___ 24. pH between 7.30 and 7.45?
___ ___ ___ 25. $Paco_2$ approximately 40 mm Hg (or baseline) with minute ventilation <10 L/min (evaluated while on ventilator)?
___ ___ ___ 26. Pao_2 >60 mm Hg on Fio_2 <0.40?

*To score the BWAP: divide the number of "yes" responses by 26.
N/A, not assessed.
From Reference 20.

respiratory muscles will continue to work throughout the machine-delivered patient-initiated breaths. To ensure respiratory muscle rest with volume ventilation, patient effort must be eliminated. Often, increasing the set rate to eliminate spontaneous effort or the judicious use of sedatives accomplishes this goal.

With a spontaneous mode of pressure ventilation such as PSV, off-loading of muscles may occur with an increase in the PSV level.[13] With this mode, the absence of accessory muscle use, a eupneic breathing pattern, and a spontaneous RR of less than 20 breaths per minute are signs of decreased workload.

Closely related to the concepts of respiratory muscle work and rest are those of conditioning and deconditioning. Respiratory muscles can become deconditioned, and in some cases may atrophy. This is especially true if paralytic agents, steroids, or high levels of sedation are used. Though possible under these conditions, it is indeed rare that a patient does not work at all while on the ventilator. Studies suggest that the type of muscle work (endurance or strengthening) may dictate the application of conditioning regimens.[57,59] In weight lifting, *strength conditioning* works muscles to extreme; indeed, to fatigue. The muscle fibers sustain small muscle tears, and lactic acid production is expected. The fatigued muscles are then rested for more than 24 hours to optimize the training effect. In the ventilated patient, modes and methods that require high-pressure, low-volume work most closely simulate such conditioning. CPAP, t-piece, or "blow-by" are examples of modes and methods that provide this type of work.[57,59]

Endurance conditioning requires that the workload be gradually increased over time. The muscle work is increased slowly and steadily as endurance increases. A form of ventilatory endurance conditioning is PSV, which can be gradually decreased as the patient assumes more and more of the workload. PSV used in this manner provides high-volume, low-pressure work.[57,59]

These concepts, borrowed from the discipline of exercise physiology, are useful. However, the specifics related to how long training intervals should be, how fast to progress them, and what type of conditioning is best are yet to be determined. Studies exploring weaning modes and methods (described later) suggest that short-duration CPAP or t-piece trials (30–120 minutes, once per day) followed by rest may be superior.[57,60] These methods are discussed in the next section on modes and methods of weaning.

MODES AND METHODS OF VENTILATOR WEANING

Studies suggest that protocols for weaning are essential to attain positive outcomes.[29,35,60] In addition, the use of a "safety screen" is an integral component because it ensures early testing of readiness. The use of a spontaneous breathing trial has been shown to be an effective initial weaning strategy for most patients.[42,58,63] While most of the studies used spontaneous breathing modes such as CPAP or t-piece for the trials, others used PSV, and still others used volume modes such as

SIMV.[14,16,36,52] It is as yet unclear whether any one mode is better than the other for weaning; however, how they are used does make a difference. The point is to construct the protocol so that a weaning trial is attempted as soon as the patient is "ready," as identified by the wean screen criteria. Protocol components include the wean screen, the trial mode or method, criteria defining wean trial intolerance, and how to rest the patient between trials (Box 10.10).[45,58,60,85] The components of weaning protocols follow.

BOX 10.10 Example of a Weaning Protocol

Weaning Trial Screen: Assessed Daily

1. Hemodynamic stability (no dysrhythmias, heart rate [HR] ≤ 120 beats per min (bpm), absence of vasopressors—low-dose dopamine and dobutamine are exceptions).
2. Fio_2 ≤50%.
3. PEEP ≤8 cm H_2O.
4. BWAP >45% (in patients ventilated less than 3 days, a BWAP assessment is not necessary).
5. If the patient meets all these criteria, a *weaning trial protocol* is initiated, following discussion with the interprofessional team.

Weaning Trial Protocol: Continuous Positive Airway Pressure (CPAP) (1 trial, 1-hour duration)

1. One trial of CPAP is attempted daily. The trial may last *no more than* 1 hour total, unless previously negotiated with healthcare team.
2. With any signs of intolerance (see definition below), the trial is discontinued, and the patient is returned to a resting mode until the next trial.
3. When the complete trial is sustained without signs of intolerance, the team is approached and extubation is discussed.
4. Full respiratory muscle rest is provided between trials and at night.

Or

Weaning Trial Protocol: Pressure Support Ventilation (PSV) (2 trials, 4-hour duration)

1. Start at PSV_{max} level (level to attain RR ≤ 20 breaths/min with tidal volume [V_T] of 8–10 mL/kg).
2. Decrease PSV by 5 cm H_2O.
3. If no signs of intolerance are evident during the first 4-hour trial, the PSV is decreased by another 5 cm H_2O for the second trial.
4. With any signs of intolerance during trials, the patient is returned to the previous level for the next 4-hour trial.
5. If unable to tolerate, the patient is fully rested until the next day, when the process begins again.
6. Once the patient is able to sustain 5–6 cm PSV without signs of intolerance (for 4 hours), the interprofessional team considers extubation.

Intolerance for Either Protocol Is Defined as Any of the Following (3–5 min sustained)

1. Respiratory rate (RR) ≥35 breaths/min for 5 minutes.
2. O_2 saturation ≤90% or a decrease of 4%.
3. Heart rate (HR) ≥140 bpm or a 20% sustained change of HR in either direction.
4. Systolic blood pressure (BP) ≥180 and ≤90 mm Hg.
5. Excessive anxiety or agitation.
6. Diaphoresis.

Rest for Either Protocol

1. PSV_{max}: PSV_{max} is that pressure level required to attain an RR of 20 breaths/min or less and a V_T of 8–10 mL/kg. Respiratory pattern should be synchronous, and there should be no accessory muscle use.
2. Other modes: With volume modes such as assist control (AC) or synchronized intermittent mandatory ventilation (SIMV), respiratory muscle rest is not ensured unless there is cessation of respiratory muscle activity. Therefore, rest is considered that level of support required to prevent patient-initiated breaths. When SIMV is used, PSV may be added for protection (i.e., as "safety"). Regardless, the goal is cessation of spontaneous effort.

Adapted from the University of Virginia Health System MICU weaning protocol.

COMPONENTS OF WEANING PROTOCOLS

Criteria for Entry ("Wean Screen")

The "wean screen" consists of physiologic criteria that suggest patient stability and readiness to begin a weaning trial. A minimum number of criteria are selected (e.g., Fio_2, PEEP levels, V_E, hemodynamic status, and secretions). Patients who have been ventilated for a long time are generally more debilitated than those who have undergone short-term ventilation. In these patients, the use of a more comprehensive assessment tool (e.g., the BWAP) may be helpful.

Weaning Trial Protocol

Protocol weaning trials that include spontaneous breathing trials (SBTs), reduction of sedation, and providing spontaneous awakening trials have been shown to decrease ventilator days.[11,16,58,60] Patients with tracheostomies generally fall into prolonged mechanical ventilation, use a tracheostomy collar, and have longer trials of spontaneous breathing than those with endotracheal tubes (ETTs). The end point of a trial with an ETT is extubation, whereas the goal with a tracheostomy trial may be extension of the spontaneous breathing interval.

Evidence suggests that long-duration SBTs are not necessary in the majority of patients (except in the tracheostomy patient who requires very prolonged ventilator duration, as noted previously). There is strong evidence that SBTs should be at least 30 minutes but not longer than 120 minutes.[40,60,63,69,85] SBTs may be accomplished by various methods, including t-piece, CPAP on the ventilator, low-level pressure support (5–8 cm H_2O), or the use of automatic tube compensation.[10,58]

Research has also shown that important components of weaning include interprofessional collaboration and communication that includes the patient, family members, and the entire care team.[71,84]

Transitioning from extubation to noninvasive ventilation may be an alternative weaning strategy for patients who may still require ventilatory support. A 2014 meta-analysis identified 16 trials using noninvasive ventilation as a weaning strategy and concluded that, while noninvasive weaning did not affect the length of mechanical ventilation, there was reduction in mortality and pneumonia.[15] The mortality benefits were significantly greater in patients with COPD.[15]

When PSV is used, the PSV level is gradually decreased, and the trials are gradually lengthened. Extubation is attempted once the lowest desired PSV level is reached. PSV is an especially good option for endurance conditioning. Examples of patients who may be good candidates for this mode include those who are profoundly weak and those with poor cardiac reserves. In patients with cardiac problems (e.g., HF), the rapid removal of positive pressure results in an increase in venous return that may overwhelm the heart's ability to compensate.[54,69,75] Attention to preload and afterload reduction in these patients is the key to good outcomes. Gradual PSV reduction may be better tolerated than the more dramatic spontaneous trials with CPAP or t-piece in patients who have difficulty weaning.

Combined modes (e.g., SIMV with PSV) for weaning trials were found to prolong the duration of weaning in at least one study.[37] To date, no studies have been completed testing the validity of this finding; it may be that the use of combined modes simply adds unintended variability to the weaning process. Decisions about how to decrease either the PSV or the SIMV tend to be arbitrary and based on clinician preference. Furthermore, the plan tends to be less aggressive than when a CPAP protocol is used, and clear intolerance thresholds for the combination modes are difficult to identify. If combined modes are used, it is important to carefully construct the protocol so that the patient's weaning is advanced as aggressively as possible.

Signs of Intolerance and How to Rest

For protocols to be interpreted easily and implemented effectively, intolerance must be defined so that a weaning trial is not continued inappropriately. As discussed in the section on respiratory muscle fatigue, signs of impending weaning failure include tachypnea, dyspnea, and chest-abdomen asynchrony. However, other signs of stress may also emerge (e.g., diaphoresis, tachycardia, and blood pressure changes). The protocol not only defines the criteria for stopping a trial, but also describes how to rest the patient. Refer to the content on rest described earlier and to Box 10.8 for an example of a weaning protocol that includes all of these components.

Timing of Tracheostomy and Weaning Trials

The optimal tracheostomy timing for patient outcomes has conventionally been thought to be early (<10 days of mechanical ventilation) if the patient is projected to need more than 14 days of mechanical ventilation.[65,73] In a retrospective review of 124,990 tracheostomy cases, early tracheostomy was associated with decreased length of stay and mortality; decreased VAP and sepsis; increased likelihood of being discharged to home; and decreased charges and hospital costs.[89] In another study by Young et al., 909 patients in the first 4 days of mechanical ventilation who were likely to require at least 7 more days were randomized to early tracheostomy (within 4 days of critical care admission) versus late tracheostomy (day 10 or later).[93] There was no difference in mortality, ICU length of stay, hospital length of stay, or antibiotic use between the two groups. In addition, only 45% of the patients randomized to late tracheostomy received a tracheotomy, due to patient recovery or discharge from the ICU.[93]

There were conflicting results from three recent meta-analysis, possibly due to the lack of heterogeneity among the patient populations studied.[3,55,81] However, the research identified suggested that some benefits are associated with early tracheostomy, including decreased sedation.[55] While the research is conflicted, a process for identification of patients who may benefit from earlier tracheostomy should be considered.

Weaning with a tracheostomy tube in place affords an element of safety that is not possible with an ETT. Because the goal is not extubation, but rather spontaneous breathing for at least 24 hours, the trials can be more aggressive (i.e., longer) with a tracheostomy tube. However, in very difficult cases, trials are best progressed gradually while other rehabilitation plans (e.g., physical mobility) are also activated. A plan incorporating daytime trials with nighttime rest on the ventilator often works well. Progression to spontaneous breathing during the night is accomplished once daytime goals are attained. Concepts of respiratory muscle rest, work, and fatigue apply, as well as the need for systematic assessment (and correction) of impediments.

Interprofessional Plan of Care

System initiatives are programs that incorporate many evidence-based elements of care into a formalized approach. These models vary in scope and design, but the common focus is a systematic, progressive approach to weaning, decreasing variation in the process. In many models, evidence-based clinical pathways are used to clarify when to initiate selected care elements, mobility, prophylaxis (e.g., gastrointestinal bleeding, deep vein thrombosis, and sinusitis), weaning trials, and other aspects of care that affect weaning (e.g., delirium and sedation management).[4-7,11,16,22,38,42,53] Importantly, clinicians (often advanced practice nurses) are identified to manage the process, coordinate the interprofessional approach, and monitor the outcomes.[4,5,21,22,71,84,94] To date, these interprofessional approaches have resulted in positive clinical and financial outcomes and are to be encouraged. However, it is clear that few care processes are successful unless sustained attention to monitoring and managing the care processes are ensured.

Managing the ventilated patient is complex and requires an in-depth understanding of the available modes and methods, as well as the evidence that guides their application. Collaboration among the many disciplines caring for the patient's well being, along with family and significant others, is necessary to produce positive outcomes.

CONCLUSION

Caring for the mechanically ventilated patient requires that the clinician understand the pathophysiology of pulmonary conditions that require the therapy, as well as how to monitor and intervene when appropriate. Knowledge of ventilator parameters and modes, in conjunction with the use of respiratory waveform monitoring, is essential to produce favorable outcomes from the acute stage to the weaning stage of ventilation.

CASE STUDY 10.1

M.C. is a 42-year-old woman who was admitted to the ward following a cholecystectomy. She had been doing well until day 4, when she became increasingly short of breath and hypoxemic. She was placed on a 100% nonrebreather mask and transferred to the surgical intensive care unit (SICU) for diagnosis and management. A rapid evaluation was performed, and a workup for the presence of a deep vein thrombosis and possible pulmonary embolus was initiated. A portable chest x-ray demonstrated diffuse bilateral infiltrates with a normal heart size and no evidence of pneumothorax. During this time she became progressively dyspneic, and an arterial blood gas (ABG) was obtained. The ABG results were as follows: pH = 7.30, $Paco_2$ = 32 mm Hg, and Pao_2 = 46 mm Hg. A heparin infusion was started for presumed pulmonary embolus, and the decision to intubate and ventilate M.C. was made. Initial settings were as follows: mode = A/C, Fio_2 = 1.0, fx = 18 breaths/min, V_T = 500 mL (M.C. weighs 50 kg), T_I = 1.0 s, sensitivity = −1 cm H_2O, and PEEP = 5 cm H_2O. The team scheduled a CT pulmonary angiogram (CTPA) and planned to send M.C. to radiology as soon as she was stable and well oxygenated. M.C.'s oxygen saturation was 89% after 10 minutes on the initial settings.

Decision Point:

What should be done to improve M.C.'s oxygenation status?

Decision Point:

What should be done next?

REFERENCES

1. Adeva-Andany, M. M., Fernández-Fernández, C., Mouriño-Bayolo, D., et al. (2014). Sodium bicarbonate therapy in patients with metabolic acidosis. *Scientific World Journal*. Article ID 627673 http://dx.doi.org/10.1155/2104/627673.
2. Albaiceta, G. M., & Blanch, L. (2011). Beyond volutrauma in ARDS: the critical role of lung tissue deformation. *Crit Care, 15*(2), 304.
3. Andriolo, B. N. G., Andriolo, R. B., Saconato, H., et al. (2015). Early versus late tracheostomy for critically ill patients. *Cochrane Database of Syst Rev*. 1, CD007271. http://dx.doi.org/10.1002/146518.CD007271.pub3.
4. Balas, M. C., Olsen, K. M., Cohen, M. Z., et al. (2014). Effectiveness and safety of the awakening and breathing coordination, delirium monitoring/management, and early exercise/mobility bundle. *Am J Crit Care, 42*, 1024–1036.
5. Balas, M. C., Vasilevskis, E. E., Burke, W. J., et al. (2012). Critical care nurses' role in implementing the "ABCDE Bundle" into practice. *Crit Care Nurs, 32*, 35–47.
6. Barr, J., Fraser, G. L., Puntillo, K., et al. (2013). American College of Critical Care Medicine: clinical practice guidelines for the management of pain, agitation, and delirium in adult patients in the intensive care unit. *Crit Care Med, 32*, 243–248.
7. Barr, J., & Pandharipande, P. P. (2013). The pain, agitation, and delirium care bundle: synergistic benefits of implementing the 2013 pain, agitation, and delirium guidelines in an integrated and interdisciplinary fashion. *Crit Care Med, 41*, S99–S115.
8. Bellemare, F., & Grassiino, A. (1982). Evaluation of human diaphragm fatigue. *J Appl Physiol, 53*, 1196–1206.
9. Berlin, D. (2014). Hemodynamic consequences of Auto-PEEP. *J Intensive Care Med, 29*, 81–86.
10. Bien, M., Liu, Y. S., & Shih, C. (2011). Comparisons of predictive performance of breathing pattern variability measured during T-piece, automatic tube compensation, and pressure support ventilation for weaning intensive care unit patients from mechanical ventilation. *Crit Care Med, 39*, 2253–2262.
11. Blackwood, B., Burns, K. E. A., Cardwell, C. R., & O'Halloran, P. (2014). Protocolized versus non-protocolized weaning for reducing the duration of mechanical ventilation in critically ill adult patients. *Cochrane Database Syst Rev, 5*, CD006904. http://dx.doi.org/10.1002/14651858.CD006904.pub3.
12. Briel, M., Meade, M., Mercat, A., et al. (2010). Higher vs lower positive end-expiratory pressure in adults with acute lung injury and acute respiratory distress syndrome: systematic review and meta-analysis. *JAMA, 303*, 865–873.
13. Brochard, L., Pluskwa, F., & Lemaire, F. (1987). Improved efficacy of spontaneous breathing with inspiratory pressure support. *Am Rev Respir Dis, 136*, 411–415.
14. Brochard, L., Rauss, A., Benito, S., et al. Comparison of three methods of gradual withdrawal from ventilatory support during weaning from mechanical ventilation. *Am J Respir Crit Care Med*, 150, 896–903.
15. Burns, K. E. A., Meade, M. O., Premji, A., & Adhikari, N. K. J. (2014). Noninvasive ventilation as a weaning strategy for mechanical ventilation in adults with respiratory failure: a Cochrane systematic review. *CMAJ, 186*, e112–e122.
16. Burns, K. E. A., Nisenbaum, R., Lessard, M. R., & Friedrich, J. O. (2014). Automated weaning and SBT systems versus non-automated weaning strategies for weaning time in invasively ventilated critically ill adults. *Cochrane Database Syst Rev, 9*, CD008638. http://dx.doi.org/10.1002/14651858.CD008638.pub2.
17. Burns, S. M. (2008). Pressure modes of mechanical ventilation; the good, the bad and the ugly. *AACN Adv Crit Care, 19*, 399–411.
18. Burns, S. M., Burns, J. E., & Truwit, J. D. (1994). Comparison of five clinical weaning indices. *Am J Crit Care, 33*, 42–352.
19. Burns, S. M., Clochesy, J. M., Hanneman, S. K., et al. (1995). Weaning from long-term mechanical ventilation. *Am J Crit Care, 4*, 4–22.
20. Burns, S. M., Fayey, S. A., Barton, D. M., & Slack, D. (1991). Weaning from mechanical ventilation: a method for assessment and planning. *AACN Clin Issues, 2*, 372–387.
21. Burns, S. M., Fisher, C., Tribble, S. S., et al. (2010). Multifactor clinical score and outcome of mechanical ventilation weaning trials: Burns wean assessment program. *Am J Crit Care, 19*, 431–442.
22. Burns, S. M., Fisher, C., Tribble, S. S., et al. (2012). The relationship of 26 clinical factors to weaning outcome. *Am J Crit Care, 21*, 53–58.
23. Burns, S. M. (2012). Weaning from mechanical ventilation; where were we then, and where are we now? *Crit Care Nurs Clin North Am, 24*, 457–468.
24. Cabrini, L., Landoni, G., Oriani, A., et al. (2015). Noninvasive ventilation and survival in acute care settings: a comprehensive systematic review and meta-analysis of randomized controlled trials. *Crit Care Med, 43*, 880–888.
25. Care Fusion. http://www.carefusion.com.
26. Chacko, B., Peter, J. V., Tharyan, P., John, G., & Jeyaseelan, L. (2015). Pressure-controlled versus volume-controlled ventilation for acute respiratory failure due to acute lung injury (ALI) or acute respiratory distress syndrome (ARDS). *Cochrane Database Syst Rev, 1*, CD008807 http://dx.doi.org/10.1002/14651858.pub2.
27. Cohen, C. A., Zagelbaum, G., Gross, D., et al. (1982). Clinical manifestations of inspiratory muscle fatigue. *Am J Med, 73*, 308–316.
28. Covidien. http://www.medtronic.com/covidien/products/acute-care-ventilation/puritan-bennett-pb840-ventilator.
29. Cook, D. (1999). *Evidence report on criteria for weaning from mechanical ventilation*. Rockville, Md: Agency for Health Care Policy and Research. Contract No. 290-97-0017.
30. Daoud, E. G., Farag, H. L., & Chatburn, R. L. (2012). Airway pressure release ventilation: what do we know? *Resp Care, 57*, 282–292.
31. Drager. http://draeger.com/sites/en_me/Pages/Hospital/Advisor.aspx?navID=272.
32. Dreyfuss, D., Basset, G., & Soler, P. (1985). Intermittent positive-end expiratory pressure hyperventilation with high inflation pressures produces pulmonary microvascular injury in rats. *Am Rev Respir Dis, 132*, 880–884.
33. Dreyfuss, D., Soler, P., Basset, G., & Saumon, G. (1988). High inflation pressure pulmonary edema: respective effects of high airway pressure, high tidal volume, and positive end-expiratory pressure. *Am Rev Respir Dis, 137*, 1159–1164.
34. Dreyfuss, D., & Saumon, G. (1993). The role of tidal volume, FRC and end-inspiratory volume in the development of pulmonary edema following mechanical ventilation. *Am Rev Respir Dis, 148*, 1194–1203.
35. Ely, E. W., et al. (1996). Effect on the duration of mechanical ventilation of identifying patients capable of breathing spontaneously. *N Engl J Med, 335*, 1864–1869.
36. Esteban, A. (1995). A comparison of four methods of weaning patients from mechanical ventilation. *N Engl J Med, 332*, 345–350.
37. Esteban, A., Alia, I., Ibanez, J., et al. (1994). Modes of mechanical ventilation and weaning: a national survey of Spanish hospitals. *Chest, 106*, 1188–1193.
38. Fan, E., Cheek, F., Chian, L., et al. (2014). An official American Thoracic Society Clinical Practice Guideline: the diagnosis of intensive care unit-acquired weakness in adults. *Am J Respir Crit Care Med, 190*, 1437–1446.
39. Ferguson, N. D., Cook, D. J., Guyatt, G. H., et al. (2013). High-frequency oscillation in early adult respiratory distress syndrome. *N Engl J Med, 368*, 795–805.
40. Frutos-Vivar, F., & Esteban, A. (2014). Our paper 20 years later: how has withdrawal from mechanical ventilation changed? *Intens Care Med, 40*, 1449–1459.
41. Fu, Z., Costello, M. L., Tsukimoto, K., et al. (1992). High lung volume increases stress failure in pulmonary capillaries. *J Appl Physiol, 73*, 123–133.
42. Girard, T. D., Kress, J. P., Fuchs, B. D., et al. (2008). Efficacy and safety of a paired sedation and ventilator weaning protocol for mechanically ventilated patients in intensive care (Awakening and Breathing Controlled trial): a randomized controlled trial. *Lancet, 371*, 126–134.
43. Guerin, C., Baboi, L., & Richard, J. C. (2014). Mechanisms of the effects of prone positioning in acute respiratory distress syndrome. *Intens Care Med, 40*, 1634–1642.
44. Guo, R., & Fan, E. (2014). Beyond low tidal volumes: ventilating the patient with acute respiratory distress syndrome. *Clin Chest Med, 35*, 729–741.
45. Gupta, P., Giehler, K., Walters, R. W., et al. (2014). The effect of a mechanical ventilation discontinuation protocol in patients with simple and difficult weaning: impact on clinical outcomes. *Resp Care, 59*, 170–177.
46. Haas, C. R., & Bauser, K. A. (2012). Advanced ventilator modes and techniques. *Crit Care Nurs Q, 35*, 27–38.
47. Hu, S. L., He, H. I., Pan, C., et al. (2014). The effects of prone positioning on mortality in patients with acute respiratory distress syndrome: a meta-analysis of randomized controlled trials. *Crit Care, 18*, R109.

48. Kacmarek, R. M. (2011). The mechanical ventilator: past, present, and future. *Resp Care, 56*, 1170–1180.
49. Kacmarek, R. M. (2011). Proportional assist ventilation and neutrally adjusted ventilatory assist. *Resp Care, 56*, 140–152.
50. Klompas, M., Anderson, D., Trick, W., et al. (2015). The preventability of ventilator-associated events: The CDC Prevention Epicenters Wake Up and Breathe Collaborative. *Am J Resp Crit Care Med, 191*, 292–301.
51. Klompas, M., Branson, R., Eichenwald, E. C., et al. (2014). Strategies to prevent ventilator-associated pneumonia in acute care hospitals: 2014 update. *Infect Control Hosp Epidemiol, 35*, 915–936.
52. Kollef, M. H., Shapiro, S. D., Silver, P., et al. (1997). A randomized, controlled trial of protocol-directed versus physician-directed weaning from mechanical ventilation. *Crit Care Med, 25*, 567–574.
53. Kress, J. P., Pohlman, A. S., O'Connor, M. F., Hall, J. B., et al. (2000). Daily interruption of sedative infusions in critically ill patients undergoing mechanical ventilation. *N Engl J Med, 342*, 1471–1477.
54. Lemaire, F., Teboul, J. L., Cinotti, L., et al. (1988). Acute left ventricular dysfunction during unsuccessful weaning from mechanical ventilation. *Anesthesiology, 69*, 171–179.
55. Liu, C. C., Livingstone, D., Dixon, E., & Dort, J. C. (2014). Early versus late tracheostomy: a systematic review and meta-analysis. *Otolaryngology-Head Neck Surg, 152*, 219–227.
56. Maitra, S., Bhattacharjee, S., Khanna, P., & Baidya, D. K. (2014). High frequency ventilation does not provide mortality benefit in comparison with conventional lung-protection ventilation in acute respiratory distress syndrome. *Anesthesiology, 122*, 841–851.
57. MacIntyre, N. R. (1986). Respiratory function during pressure support ventilation. *Chest, 89*, 677–683.
58. MacIntyre, N. R. (2013). The ventilator discontinuation process: an expanding evidence base. *Resp Care, 58*, 1074–1086.
59. MacIntyre, N. R. (1988). Weaning from mechanical ventilatory support: volume-assisting intermittent breaths versus pressure-assisting every breath. *Respir Care, 83*, 1121–1225.
60. MacIntyre, N. R., Cook, D. J., Ely, E. W., et al. (2001). Evidence-based guidelines for weaning and discontinuing ventilatory support: a collective task force facilitated by the American College of Chest Physicians; the American Association for Respiratory Care; and the American College of Critical Care Medicine. *Chest, 120*, 375S–395S.
61. Maquet Critical Care. http://www.maquet.com/int/products/servo-s.
62. Marini, J. J. (2011). Dynamic hyperinflation and auto-positive end-expiratory pressure: lessons learned over 30 years. *Am J Crit Care Med, 184*, 756–762.
63. Marini, J. J., Rodriguez, M., & Lamb, V. (1986). The inspiratory workload of patient-initiated mechanical ventilation. *Am Rev Respir Dis, 134*, 902–909.
64. McMullen, S. M., Meade, M., Rose, L., et al. (2012). Partial ventilatory support modalities in acute lung injury and acute respiratory distress syndrome-a systematic review. *PLoS ONE 7e40190.*
65. McWhorter, A. J. (2003). Tracheotomy: timing and techniques. *Curr Opin Otolaryngol Head Neck Surg, 11*, 473–479.
66. The National Heart, Lung, and Blood Institute ARDS Clinical Trials Network. (2004). Higher versus lower positive end-expiratory pressures in patients with the acute respiratory distress syndrome. *N Engl J Med, 351*, 327–336.
67. Neto, A. S., Cardoso, S. O., Manetta, J. A., et al. (2012). Association between use of lung-protective ventilation with lower tidal volumes and clinical outcomes among patients without acute respiratory distress syndrome: a meta-analysis. *JAMA, 308*, 1651–1659.
68. Penuelas, O., Furtos-Vivar, F., Fernandez, C., et al. (2011). Characteristics and outcomes of ventilatored patients according to time to liberation from mechanical ventilation. *Am J Respir Crit Care Med, 185*, 430–437.
69. Perren, A., & Brouchard, L. (2013). Managing the apparent and hidden difficulties of weaning form mechanical ventilation. *Intens Care Med, 39*, 1885–1895.
70. Respironics. http://www.respironics.com.
71. Rose, L., Dainty, K. N., Jordan, J., & Blackwood, B. (2014). Weaning from mechanical ventilation: a scoping review of qualitative studies. *Am J Crit Care, 23*, e54–371.
72. Rose, L., & Hawkins, M. (2008). Airway pressure release ventilation and biphasic positive airway pressure: a systematic review of definitional criteria. *Intensive Care Med, 34*(10), 1766–1773.
73. Rumbak, M. J., Newton, M., Truncale, T., et al. (2004). A prospective, randomized study comparing early percutaneous dilational tracheotomy to prolonged translaryngeal intubation (delayed tracheotomy) in critically ill medical patients. *Crit Care Med, 32*, 1689–1694.
74. Schmidt, M., Kindler, F., & Cecchini, J. (2015). Neurally adjusted ventilatory assist and proportional assist ventilation both improve patient-ventilator interaction. *Crit Care, 19*, 56. http://dx.doi.org/10.1186/s13054-015-0763-6.
75. Sereika, S. M., & Clochesy, J. M. (1996). Left ventricular dysfunction and duration of mechanical ventilatory support in the chronically critically ill: a survival analysis. *Heart Lung, 25*, 45–51.
76. Silversides, J. A., & Ferguson, N. D. (2013). Clinical review: Acute respiratory distress syndrome-clinical ventilator management. *Crit Care, 17*, 225.
77. Singer, B. D., & Corbridge, T. C. (2011). Pressure modes of invasive mechanical ventilation. *South Med J, 104*, 701–709.
78. Slutsky, A. S. (1994). Consensus conference on mechanical ventilation—January 28–30, 1993, at Northbrook, Ill. Parts 1 and 2. *Intensive Care Med, 20*, 64–79 150–162.
79. Slutsky, A. S. (2015). History of mechanical ventilation; from Vesalius to ventilator-induced lung injury. *Am J Respir Crit Care Med, 191*, 1106–1115.
80. Suzumura, E. A., Figueiro, M., Normilio-Silva, K., et al. (2014). Effects of alveolar recruitment maneuvers on clinical outcomes in patients with acute respiratory distress syndrome: a systematic review and meta-analysis. *Intens Care Med, 40*, 1227–1240.
81. Szakmany, T., Russell, P., Wilkes, A. R., & Hall, J. E. (2014). Effect of early tracheostomy on resource utilization and clinical outcomes in critically ill patients: meta-analysis of randomized controlled trials. *Br J Anaesth*, 114. 396-405. http://dx.doi.org/10.1093/bja/aeu440.
82. Tanios, M. A., Nevins, M. I., Hendra, K. P., et al. (2006). A randomized controlled trial of the role of weaning predictors in clinical decision making. *Crit Care Med, 34*, 2530–2535.
83. The Acute Respiratory Distress Syndrome Network. (2000). Ventilation with lower tidal volumes as compared with traditional tidal volumes for acute lung injury and the acute respiratory distress syndrome. *N Engl J Med, 342*, 1301–1307.
84. Thille, A. W., Boissier, F., Ghezala, H. B., et al. (2015). Risk factors for and prediction by caregivers of extubation failure in ICU patients: a prospective study. *Crit Care Med, 43*, 613–620.
85. Tobin, M. J. (2013). *Principles and Practice of Mechanical Ventilation* (3rd ed.). New York: McGraw-Hill Companies, Inc.
86. Tremblay, L. (1997). Injurious ventilatory strategies increases cytokines and c-fos m-RNA expression in an isolated rat lung model. *J Clin Invest, 99*, 944–952.
87. Vasilevskis, E. E., Ely, E. W., Speroff, T., et al. (2012). Reducing iatrogenic risks: ICU-acquired delirium and weakness-crossing the quality chasm. *Chest, 138*, 1224–1233.
88. Vicente, E. G., Sandoval Almengor, J. C., Diaz Caballero, L. A., & Slagado Campo, J. C. (2011). Invasive mechanical ventilation in COPD and asthma. *Med Intensiva, 35*, 288–298.
89. Villwock, J. A., & Jones, K. (2014). Outcomes of early versus late tracheostomy: 2008-2010. *Laryngoscope, 124*, 1801–1806.
90. Waters, B., & Muscedere, J. (2015). A 2015 update on ventilator-associated pneumonia: new insights on its prevention, diagnosis, and treatment. *Curr Infect Dis Rep, 17*(8), 496.
91. Wunsch, H., Linde-Zwirbie, W. T., Angus, D., et al. (2010). The epidemiology of mechanical ventilator use in the United States. *Crit Care Med, 38*, 1947–1953.
92. Yang, K. L. (1992). Reproducibility of weaning parameters. A need for standardization. *Chest, 102*, 1829–1832.
93. Young, D., Lamb, S. E., Shah, S., et al. (2013). High-frequency oscillation for acute respiratory distress syndrome. *NEJM, 368*, 806–813.
94. Zilberberg, M. D., & Shorr, A. F. (2008). Prolonged acute mechanical ventilation and hospital bed utilization in 2020 in the United States: implications for budgets, plant and personal planning. *BMC Health Serv Res, 8, 242.* http://dx.doi.org/10.1186/1472-6963-8-242.

11

Thoracic Surgery

Julie Culmone

INTRODUCTION

Thoracic surgery, a subspecialty of cardiothoracic surgery, encompasses the operative and perioperative care of conditions within the chest (thorax) including the lungs, chest wall, diaphragm, and esophagus. First developed in the late 19th century, thoracic surgery has become increasingly popular as a result of chronic infections of the lung, upper aerodigestive cancers, and other pulmonary, esophageal, and mediastinal diseases.[49,54,83]

As bronchiectasis and tuberculosis continued to plague the world during the 19th century, surgical techniques for pulmonary resections were explored. In 1901, the first successful lobectomy for bronchiectasis was performed by Themistokles Gluck (1853–1942) in Berlin, Germany; however, it received little attention for many years. In 1933, Evarts A. Graham (1883–1957) performed the first successful single-stage pneumonectomy for carcinoma of the lung at Barnes Hospital in St. Louis, Missouri, paving the way for further advances in thoracic surgery.[8,49,83]

This chapter will discuss thoracic surgery procedures specific to the lung, pleura, chest wall, diaphragm, mediastinum, and esophagus. Since thoracic surgery encompasses a wide range of procedures, only those most commonly performed will be discussed.

THE THORAX

The thorax or chest refers to the upper trunk between the neck and abdomen; it is formed by the 12 thoracic vertebrae, the 12 pairs of ribs, and the sternum. The thorax also includes the thoracic cavity and thoracic wall. The principal organs of the thoracic cavity consist of the heart, along with its major blood vessels and the lungs, and the bronchi and the thymus.[56] The trachea enters the thorax to connect with the lungs and the esophagus travels through the thoracic cavity to connect with the stomach below the diaphragm.[56] Also contained within the thoracic cavity are the aorta, superior vena cava, inferior vena cava, and the pulmonary artery.[56]

PULMONARY RESECTION

Clinical Presentation

Carcinoma of the lung is the most common reason for performing a pulmonary resection; however, respective surgery may be performed for benign masses, acute or chronic infection, or congenital abnormalities.[41,82] According to the World Health Organization, cancer is the leading cause of death worldwide, accounting for 8.2 million deaths in 2012, with carcinoma of the lung being the most common cause of cancer death (1.59 million deaths).[86]

Lung cancer is broadly classified as either non–small cell lung cancer (NSCLC) or small cell lung cancer (SCLC). NSCLC accounts for 85% of all lung cancers, with SCLC accounting for the remaining 15%.[28,70] NSCLC can be further classified according to the following three subtypes: adenocarcinoma, squamous cell or epidermoid carcinoma, and large cell or undifferentiated carcinoma. Adenocarcinoma, the most common type of NSCLC, presents as a peripheral tumor or nodule and frequently metastasizes at an early stage. Squamous cell carcinoma is typically more centrally located, arising more commonly in the segmental and subsegmental bronchi. Large cell, or undifferentiated, carcinoma is a fast-growing tumor that typically arises peripherally. SCLCs occur primarily as proximal lesions, but may arise in any part of the tracheobronchial tree. Most SCLCs develop in the major bronchi and spread by infiltration along the bronchial wall.

In addition to cell type, carcinoma of the lung is staged according to the American Joint Committee on Cancer TNM staging system.[4] *T* indicates the size of the primary *tumor; N* describes the spread of cancer to regional lymph *nodes;* and *M* indicates whether or not the cancer has *metastasized* to other organs of the body.[4] NSCLC is staged as I to IV; stage I is the earliest stage and has the highest cure rate, whereas stage IV designates metastatic disease.[19] SCLCs are classified as small cell undifferentiated carcinoma or oat cell carcinoma.

Stages of NSCLC that may be amenable to surgical intervention include stages I through IIIA. Current literature supports the management of stage I NSCLC with surgery to remove the tumor by lobectomy, sleeve resection, segmentectomy, or wedge resection.[4,49] As further research is needed to determine the effectiveness of segmentectomy or wedge resection, lobectomy remains the management option of choice as it offers the greatest chance for cure. Adjuvant (postsurgical) chemotherapy or radiation therapy has been shown to be effective for tumors 4 cm or larger.[30,33,53] For stages II and IIIA, neoadjuvant (presurgical) chemotherapy or radiation coupled with adjuvant chemotherapy or radiation has proven beneficial.[2] Although surgical intervention is recommended for the management of stages I through IIIA NSCLC, a poor surgical candidate may receive stereotactic body radiation therapy (SBRT), conventional radiation therapy, or radiofrequency ablation as the primary source of treatment.[49,84] Stages IIIB and IV cannot be completely removed by surgical intervention and are therefore treated with chemotherapy and radiation therapy alone.

SCLC the most aggressive type of lung cancer, is staged as either limited or extensive.[55] Regardless of the stage, SCLC is usually managed with chemotherapy rather than surgical intervention; more often than not, when SCLC is found, it has metastasized to the brain, liver, or bone.

Carcinoma of the lung rarely causes symptoms until the disease has progressed. Common symptoms include fatigue, persistent cough, anorexia, dyspnea, hemoptysis, and bone pain. If lung cancer is suspected, initial evaluation begins with a thorough history and physical, laboratory studies (including alkaline phosphatase, alanine aminotransferase [ALT], aspartate aminotransferase [AST], total bilirubin, creatinine, and albumin) and a chest radiograph.[4] If a chest radiograph reveals areas of suspicion, a computed tomography (CT) scan of the chest and pelvis is then performed, marking the beginning of the staging process.

Diagnostic Studies

A variety of other scans may be used to assess for metastasis, including magnetic resonance imaging (MRI), positron emission tomography (PET), CT/PET scan, and bone scan.[24,71] Unlike the CT scan and MRI, which provide images of specific structures of the body, the PET scan provides images of the entire body and distinguishes between benign and malignant lesions. PET is based on the biological activity of the tumor cells in response to an injection of 18-fluorodeoxyglucose.[24,34,71] Cancer cells usually demonstrate a higher glucose uptake and utilization compared to normal lung or lymphatic tissue. However, false-positive results may occur in granulomatous inflammatory diseases and in infection.

Although diagnostic studies may suggest carcinoma of the lung, the actual diagnosis of lung cancer cannot be made without a biopsy (examination of a sample of tissue removed from the body to determine the cause or extent of a disease).[49] A biopsy for the diagnosis and staging of lung cancer may be performed through several different minimally invasive procedures, including bronchoscopy, transthoracic needle biopsy, endobronchial ultrasound (EBUS) guided biopsy, video-assisted thoracic surgery (VATS) biopsy, and thoracotomy[19,49] (Fig. 11.1).

Surgical resection is the preferred method of treating patients with localized NSCLC, no evidence of metastatic spread, and adequate cardiopulmonary function. The cure rate of surgical resection depends on the type and NSCLC stage.[33,87] Surgery is primarily used for NSCLC because small cell cancer of the lung grows rapidly and metastasizes early and extensively.[87] Unfortunately, in many patients with bronchogenic cancer, the lesion is inoperable at the time of diagnosis.

Other malignant tumors of the pulmonary system that may require pulmonary resection include carcinoid and sarcoma.[40] Examples of benign lung tumors include papilloma, fibroma, leiomyoma, hamartoma, teratoma, and inflammatory pseudotumors. Diseases or problems that might require pulmonary resection include empyema, necrotizing pneumonia, bronchiectasis, granulomatous disease, and other infectious processes of the lung.

Preoperative Evaluation

Prior to proceeding with elective surgery, it must be determined whether or not the patient is physiologically capable of undergoing resectional surgery. Preoperative evaluation by an interprofessional team (e.g., a thoracic surgeon, medical oncologist, radiation oncologist, and a pulmonologist) is essential for determining the risk versus benefit of curative intent surgery for the management of lung cancer.[9,69,80] A preoperative cardiovascular risk assessment should be performed on all patients undergoing resectional surgery as the prevalence of underlying coronary artery disease is approximately 17%. This is commonly related to a predisposition to atherosclerotic disease because of cigarette smoking.[80]

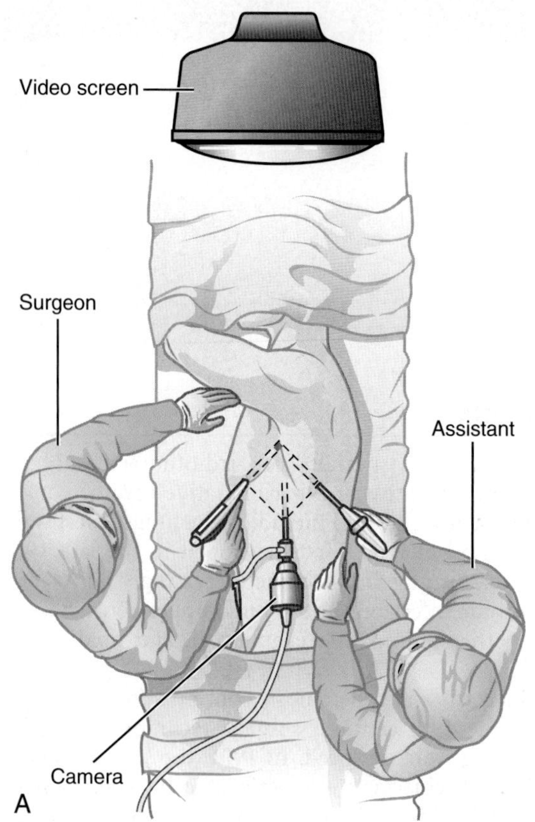

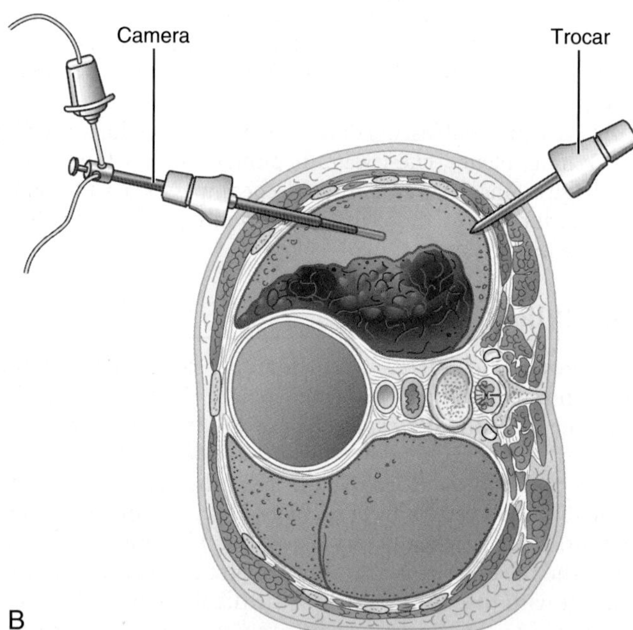

FIG. 11.1 Different views of video-assisted thoracic surgery (VATS). **A,** Patient is positioned in a 30 degree semi-supine position. **B,** Transverse plane view.

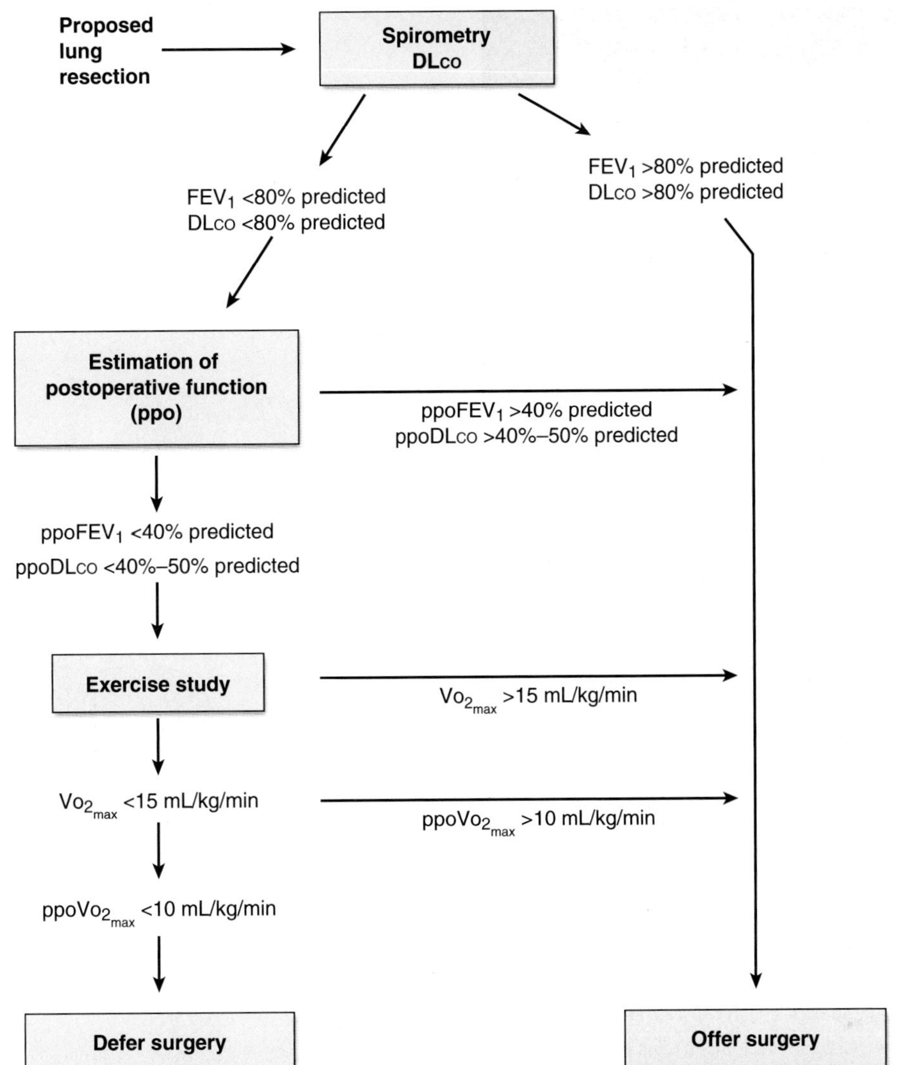

FIG. 11.2 Algorithm for preoperative pulmonary evaluation. *DLco,* Diffusing capacity of the lung for carbon monoxide; *FEV_1,* forced expiratory volume in 1 second; *ppo,* predicted postoperative; *Vo_2,* oxygen consumption.

Spirometry is frequently evaluated and critical values include the predicted postoperative (PPO), forced vital capacity (FVC), and forced expiratory volume in 1 second (FEV_1).[9] In addition, a diffusing capacity (DLCO) may be evaluated to examine the lung's ability to diffuse a test gas across the alveolar-capillary membrane. As part of the evaluation of spirometry, predicted postoperative values for FEV_1 and DLCO may be determined.[9] These values are calculated by determining the amount of lung requiring resection and evaluation of the predicted postoperative values. Specific calculations are available to determine predicted postoperative values. Patients who are considered to be a high risk for pulmonary complications are referred to a pulmonologist for preoperative consultation and optimization of pulmonary function (Fig. 11.2).

APPROACHES AND PROCEDURES

Thoracic surgeries are broadly defined as either open surgery or minimally invasive surgery (Table 11.1). Surgical resections of the lung can be classified as either anatomical or nonanatomical.[53] Anatomical lung resection involves removal of the diseased pulmonary segment, lobe, or lung in conjunction with the draining lymph nodes (segmentectomy, lobectomy, or pneumonectomy). Nonanatomical lung resection involves removal of diseased portions of the lung without complete dissection of the anatomic segment of the lobe of the lung and without removal of the draining lymph nodes (wedge resection).[53] Fig. 11.3 illustrates the most common surgical approaches used for thoracic procedures.

Common surgical procedures used for the treatment of NSCLC include wedge resection, segmentectomy, lobectomy, and pneumonectomy (Table 11.2).

Wedge Resection

A wedge resection is a nonanatomic surgical procedure performed to resect a wedge-shaped section of a lobe to remove a small, well-circumscribed peripheral pulmonary nodule or nodules (benign or metastatic).[43,47] Current studies demonstrate a 5-year survival rate associated with wedge resection, which is significantly lower than that of the lobectomy (58% vs. 70%, respectively). However, it is important to remember that patients who undergo a wedge resection are considered high-risk surgical candidates with numerous comorbidities and

TABLE 11.1 Definitions of Common Thoracic Approaches

Approach	Definition
Thoracoscopy (VATS)	Also known as *VATS*: Minimally invasive approach that uses two or more "ports" or small incisions in chest. Openings used to place instruments into chest, including video camera and other instruments for grasping, cutting, or stapling. Used for diagnostic purposes, pleurodesis, staging procedures, or partial/total lung resection.
Thoracotomy	Incision made between two ribs to gain access to the thoracic cage for exploration or definitive surgical therapy. Location and extent of incision are dependent on specific operation to be performed. Types: lateral, posterolateral, anterior, and muscle-sparing.
Thoracoabdominal	Large incision that provides exposure to both upper abdominal cavity and thorax. Starts in upper abdomen and sweeps up in a crescent shape into thorax and between ribs.
Median sternotomy	Widely used in cardiac surgery, but may be used in thoracic procedures. Sternum is cut in half lengthwise from suprasternal notch to xiphoid process. Sternum reconnected with wires.
Partial sternotomy	Like a sternotomy but only a portion of sternum is cut in a vertical fashion. Example: upper portion of sternum is cut to access thymus for thymectomy.
Hemiclamshell (trapdoor)	Provides wide access to one side of chest. Incision begins mid-axillary in 4th or 5th intercostal space and continues across chest to sternum. Incision then moves vertically upward as a partial sternotomy.
Transverse sternotomy (clamshell)	Provides access to mediastinum and both lungs. Incision begins mid-axillary in 4th or 5th intercostal space and continues across chest (transversely) following line of 4th or 5th rib, through sternum to opposing mid-axillary line.
Cervical	Oblique incision of neck that begins at sternal notch and continues along anterior border of sternocleidomastoid muscle.
Subxiphoid	Vertical incision over lower sternum and xiphoid process with or without removal of xiphoid to gain access to pericardium or lower mediastinum.

VATS, Video-assisted thoracoscopic surgery.

diminished pulmonary reserve.[43] The morbidity after a wedge resection is minimal, with postoperative complications associated with retention of secretions or pleural problems. Persistent pleural airspace occurs in less than 10% of cases and frequently resolves with conservative management.

Segmentectomy

A segmentectomy is an anatomic surgical procedure performed to resect a diseased segment of the lung that has segmental distribution without removing excess normal lung.[53] Complications following a segmentectomy include prolonged air leak (peripheral alveolar pleural fistula or bronchopleural fistula), empyema, and persistent pleural air space.[53,55] Persistent pleural air space may be as high as 33% in specialized populations, such as those with pulmonary tuberculosis. As compared with a lobectomy, persistent pleural air spaces following segmentectomy are small. They may be conservatively treated with prolonged chest tube drainage and, if necessary, talc pleurodesis may be used.[10,20,55]

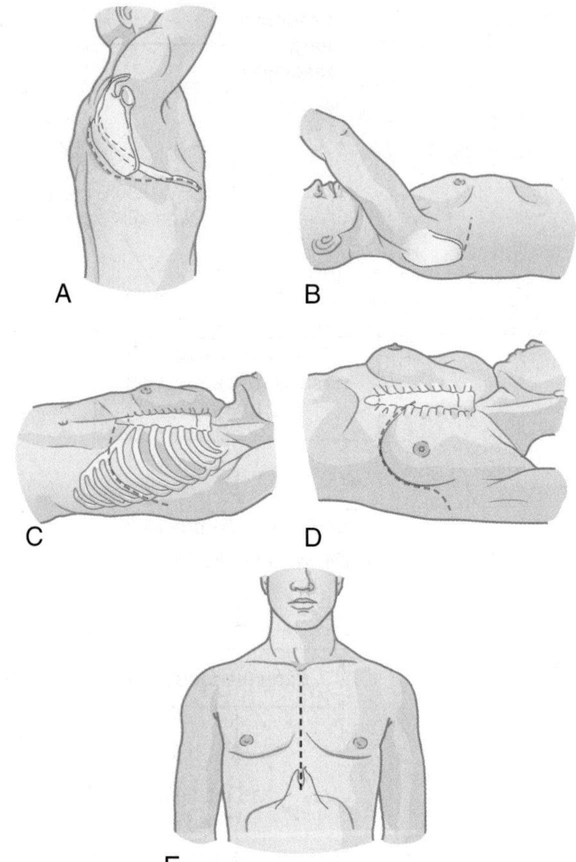

FIG. 11.3 Common surgical approaches for thoracic surgery. **A**, posterolateral approach; **B**, lateral approach; **C**, thoracoabdominal approach; **D**, anterior approach; **E**, median sternotomy approach.

However, when problems in the pleural space arise, they are often septic in nature. Mortality rate following segmentectomy is approximately 1%, but may be as high 4% to 6% in patients with poor pulmonary function or previous pulmonary resection.[47]

Lobectomy

Lobectomy is an anatomic surgical procedure performed to resect a diseased lobe of the lung. Occasionally two lobes of the right lung are removed, either right upper and middle or right lower and middle; this is defined as a bilobectomy.[43,53] Lobectomy remains the treatment of choice for primary NSCLC assuming the patient is not classified as a poor surgical candidate, the primary tumor is confined to one lobe, and there is no distant metastasis.

Physiologic changes following a lobectomy include overinflation of both the contralateral tissue and the remaining lung tissue on the operated side. Functional loss of the lung is dependent upon the preoperative pulmonary function and presence of postoperative complications.[79] Mortality following lobectomy is cited between 2% and 3% and may be greater in those over the age of 75 and those with comorbid conditions.[58]

Avoidance of complete removal of a lung (pneumonectomy) has been shown to reduce both early complications and long-term disability as the result of shortness of breath.[62,76,85] An alternative to a pneumonectomy is the sleeve lobectomy, which may be performed to preserve lung tissue and reduce morbidity

TABLE 11.2 Definitions of Common Thoracic Procedures

Procedure	Definition
Pulmonary	
Wedge resection, single	Removal or resection of a small, wedged-shape area of lung parenchyma. Indicated for well-circumscribed benign tumors, pulmonary metastasis in select patients with small peripheral nodule(s), or a biopsy. Performed by either VATS or thoracotomy.
Segmentectomy	Resection of an anatomic subdivision of a pulmonary lobe (bronchopulmonary segment). Procedure is indicated for a nodule/mass with segmental distribution. Other indications: bronchiectasis, hematoma, or lung abscess. Usually performed using thoracotomy approach.
Lobectomy	Resection of a lung lobe. Frequently performed for treatment of NSCLC, but may also be used for nonmalignant conditions. Performed by either thoracotomy or VATS.
Sleeve lobectomy	Procedure used to save lung parenchyma because of location of a mass that directly involves or protrudes into a major airway. A section of the airway and lobe is removed. Reanastomosis of airway proximal and distal to resected area is performed. Procedure is primarily used for malignancy, but may also be used for more benign conditions such as carcinoid tumors or trauma. Usual approach is thoracotomy.
Bilobectomy	Resection of two lobes of the lung. Is most frequently performed for treatment of NSCLC. Usual approach is thoracotomy.
Pneumonectomy, standard	Removal of entire lung. Primary indication is NSCLC. Other indications: multiple lung abscesses, bronchiectasis, or extensive infection. Occasionally performed for extensive involvement of lung in diseases such as sarcoma, mesothelioma, or metastatic disease to lung. Standard incision is posterolateral thoracotomy. Other approaches are median sternotomy and rarely VATS.
Pneumonectomy, intrapericardial	Similar to standard pneumonectomy, but one or more of the principal lung vessels within pericardial sac must be ligated. May occur when a tumor encroaches on hilum to extent that a standard pneumonectomy is not otherwise possible, the dissection is extremely difficult because of inflammatory tissue, or a vessel is torn close to pericardium. Standard incision is thoracotomy.
Pneumonectomy, sleeve (carinal)	Used when a tumor involves mainstem airway (right, rarely left). Carina and entire lung are resected in one piece. Remaining mainstem bronchus then gets sewn end-to-end to trachea. Right-sided carinal pneumonectomy is usually done either through a right thoracotomy or by a median sternotomy. Left-sided carinal pneumonectomy requires bilateral thoracotomies because left mainstem bronchus cannot be sewn into trachea from left chest (aortic arch prevents access).
Pneumonectomy, extrapleural	Removal of lung within envelope of the parietal pleura. Parietal pleura is separated from chest wall and diaphragm. Indications include malignant disease such as NSCLC, mesothelioma, or extensive infectious processes. Standard incision is thoracotomy and often a rib is resected as well to gain adequate exposure.
Pneumonectomy, completion	Removal of all remaining lung following previous removal of a portion. Standard incision is thoracotomy and often a rib is resected as well to gain adequate exposure.
Lung volume reduction	Removal of lung tissue damaged by emphysema. Provides room for expansion of better functioning lung tissue. Usually upper lobes are targeted. Bilateral approach is generally preferred to provide maximum benefit in one operation. Approaches include sternotomy, VATS, or thoracotomy.
Bullectomy	Removal of bullae from the lung. Bullae are opened and fibrous septa excised. Walls of bulla used to reinforce staple line at base of resected bulla. Usually thoracotomy is used.
Pleura	
Pleurodesis	Procedure to create adhesions between visceral and parietal pleurae. Usually done to prevent recurrent pneumothoraces or reaccumulation of pleural effusion. A sclerosing agent such as talc is instilled to cause inflammation and adhesion between pleurae. VATS or muscle-sparing thoracotomy is used.
Pleurectomy	Removal/excision of lining along inside of chest wall (parietal) and the lung (visceral). Thoracotomy is used.
Decortication	Removal of exudate/scar tissue in pleural space that traps lung. Completed when lung is constricted and cannot be totally expanded. Approach used is VATS or thoracotomy.
Clagett procedure	Resection of rib(s) for drainage of an empyema; skin flap created to maintain an open window for access.
Chest Wall	
Chest wall resection	Performed to remove masses/tumors that invade into/through chest wall. Both ribs and muscular areas adjacent to affected ribs may be removed. Indications include neoplasm, infection, trauma, and radiation burns. Approach is highly dependent upon location and depth of resection required. Following chest wall resection, some type of reconstructive surgery may be necessary.
Chest wall reconstruction	Done to reestablish structural stabilization of chest and protect underlying chest organs. Indications for reconstruction are trauma, reconstruction following chest wall resection for infection, radiation burns, and congenital anomalies. Plates or struts, synthetic materials (Prolene or Vicryl mesh), solid prostheses, or composites may be sutured over defect area to bridge defects in rib cage. Skin or muscle coverage of the mesh may also be used.
Thoracoplasty	Removal of two or more ribs to promote inward collapse of an area of chest wall. Although widely used in past to treat diseases such as tuberculosis, thoracoplasty is used today only to treat patients with chronic pleural space infection where lung cannot be reexpanded.
Sternectomy, complete	Complete removal of sternum. Performed because of a mass or malignancy involving sternum, infection, or severe trauma. Both rigid and soft materials may be used to cover area.
Sternectomy, partial	Partial removal of sternum. Performed because of a mass or malignancy involving sternum, chronic infection, or severe trauma.
Diaphragm	
Diaphragmatic plication	Plicating the diaphragm is tucking the muscle or making folds in the membrane to make it smaller and more functional with respiration.
Diaphragmatic hernia repair	Repair of diaphragm following injury, trauma, or congenital defect. Hole or opening in diaphragm allows abdominal contents to protrude into chest; abdominal contents are repositioned into abdomen and opening in diaphragm is closed by suturing or using a patch.

Continued

TABLE 11.2 Definitions of Common Thoracic Procedures—cont'd

Procedure	Definition
Mediastinum	
Mediastinoscopy	Use of a rigid scope to examine mediastinum and biopsy tissue anterior to trachea; an incision is made at the base of the neck, above sternal notch, and mediastinoscope is passed along trachea.
Anterior mediastinotomy (Chamberlain)	Small horizontal incision between ribs, usually to the left, but sometimes to the right of sternum. This approach is often used to examine lymph nodes in aortopulmonary window or anterior mediastinal masses.
Mediastinal lymph node dissection	Removal of lymph nodes in mediastinum; this procedure indicates removal of most lymph nodes on one side of mediastinum, at all nodal stations. Done for pathologic staging of NSCLC.
Mediastinal lymph node sampling	Same as above, but sampling of lymph nodes on one side of mediastinum. Done for pathologic staging of NSCLC.
Resection, mediastinal mass	Removal of a mass in mediastinum. Type of approach is dependent upon location of mass.
Thymectomy	Excision/removal of thymus gland. Thymus is in anterior mediastinum. Usual approaches are transcervical, VATS, transthoracic (median sternotomy).
Thoracic duct ligation	Tying off of main lymph channel in chest; usually performed at level of diaphragm on right side and commonly done for a chyle leakage (chylothorax); duct is usually visualized near L2 vertebra and is approached using thoracotomy or VATS.

NSCLC, Non–small-cell lung cancer; *VATS*, video-assisted thoracoscopic surgery.

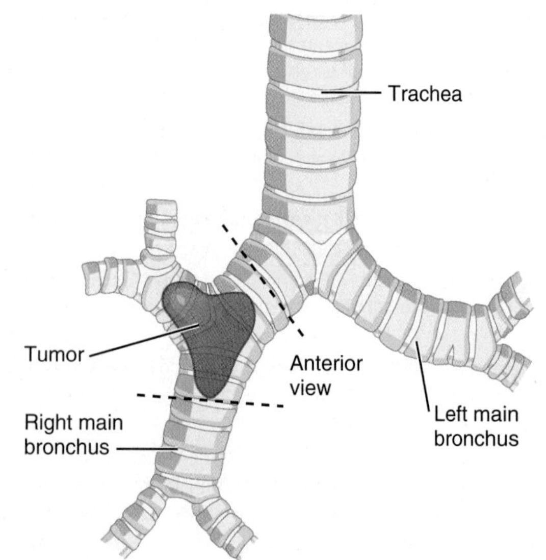

FIG. 11.4 Sleeve lobectomy removing a right main bronchus tumor.

and mortality. Sleeve lobectomy is the complete removal of a lobe of the lung and part of the airway that conducts air to the remaining lobe, then the reconnection of that airway to the remaining lobe.[22] Although studies have shown that this procedure provides the same cure rate as a pneumonectomy, few thoracic surgeons are trained in the sleeve lobectomy[22] (Fig. 11.4).

Pneumonectomy

Pneumonectomy is most commonly performed for malignant disease of the lung. Tumors located in the main stem (proximal bronchus) that are adjacent to the right upper lobe orifice, or that extend across a major fissure may all be indications for a pneumonectomy.[58] Rarely is a pneumonectomy performed for pulmonary metastases or benign inflammatory lung disease (i.e., tuberculosis, mycobacteria, necrotizing pneumonia, lung abscess, bronchiectasis, or extensive fungal infections).

There are two different types of pneumonectomy procedures: standard pneumonectomy, in which only the diseased lung is removed; and extrapleural pneumonectomy, in which portions of the diaphragm, pericardium, and pleura are removed along with the diseased lung.[79] Regardless of which procedure is performed, the anatomical and functional changes following a pneumonectomy can be extensive. During the immediate postoperative period, air fills the space previously occupied by the lung (postpneumonectomy space [PPS]). Eventually, a number of changes result in a decrease in the size of the PPS, including elevation of the hemidiaphragm, hyperinflation of the remaining lung, and shifting of the mediastinum towards the postpneumonectomy space. There is also a progressive reabsorption of air in the PPS and replacement with fluid. The trachea, heart, and mediastinum shift towards the operated side, and the remaining lung expands anteriorly and extends into the pneumonectomy space.

Lung Volume Reduction Surgery

Resective surgeries are performed for reasons other than carcinoma of the lung. Treatment options for patients with end-stage chronic obstructive pulmonary disease (COPD) with a primary emphysematous component may undergo lung volume reduction surgery (LVRS) to reduce hyperinflation and allow for expansion of the functional tissue.

This procedure is an option for those patients with homogenous disease or disease that is focused in one area and not widespread throughout the lungs. LVRS involves the removal of a portion of the diseased lung parenchyma, resulting in improved elastic recoil of the lung and improved elastic recoil of the lung and chest wall.[51] Lung volume reduction surgery does not cure COPD or increase life expectancy, but it may reduce dyspnea and improve the patient's overall quality of life.[51,74] Careful selection of patients for this procedure is essential to minimize morbidity and mortality.[11]

The National Emphysema Treatment Trial (NETT) concluded that the addition of LVRS to optimal medical management and pulmonary rehabilitation led to an overall improvement in exercise tolerance and survival in a subgroup of patients with predominantly upper lobe disease.[57] All eligible persons must be able to complete a preoperative rehabilitation program in preparation for surgery.[16,74] The ideal candidate for LVRS is one with heterogeneous disease with defined targets in the diseased lung. In addition, debate surrounds the type of procedure (unilateral vs. bilateral) and the incisional technique used (median sternotomy vs. VATS). Regardless of technique, the diseased lung is identified and a staple line is used to excise one-half to two-thirds of the upper lobes. Depending upon

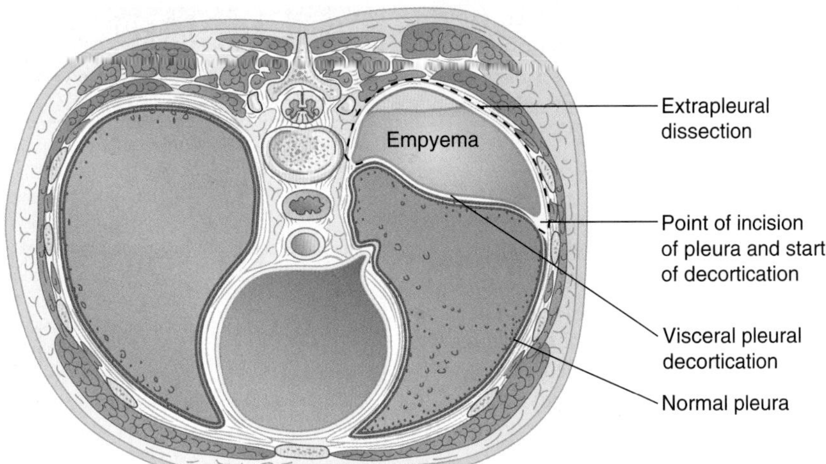

FIG. 11.5 Cross section of thorax with empyema and operative techniques.

the amount of lung excised, there is the potential for a residual postoperative air space that may result in a prolonged air leak. A pleural tent may be used, which involves dissecting the parietal pleura from the chest wall and reducing the size of the pleural space by promoting apposition of the pleural surfaces. Operative mortality following LVRS varies from 5% to 10%, with most deaths related to pulmonary insufficiency, infection, or cardiac complications.[57]

Of the information available regarding LVRS, the following can be concluded at this time: (1) in a select group of patients, this procedure offers an improved quality of life; (2) bilateral resection may provide better results than unilateral resection; (3) VATS results in lower postoperative morbidity; (4) stapling of the tissue may provide more consistent results than laser ablation; (5) pulmonary rehabilitation before and after surgery may be beneficial; and (6) LVRS is a palliative procedure.[39]

PLEURAL SURGERY

The pleura is a membrane that consists of two large, thin layers of tissue. One layer wraps around the outside of the lungs (parietal layer), the other layer lines the inside of the chest cavity (visceral layer).[75,89] Between these two layers of tissue is a very thin space referred to as the pleural space. Normally this space is filled with approximately 5 mL to 10 mL of serous fluid that helps the layers of the pleura glide smoothly past each other during inhalation and exhalation. Pleurisy occurs when the two layers become inflamed or irritated. There are several different surgical procedures that may be performed to treat diseases and conditions of the pleural space, including thoracentesis, VATS, thoracotomy, and wedge resection. Common diseases and conditions of the pleural space include pneumothorax, pleural effusion, empyema, bronchiectasis, lung abscess, pneumatoceles, and mediastinitis.

Conditions of the Pleural Space

Pneumothorax

A pneumothorax is defined as a collection of air in the pleural space as the result of an injury to the lung tissue, a bronchial tear, or chest wall injury. A simple pneumothorax causing respiratory impairment is frequently treated with chest tube insertion and evacuation of air from the pleural space. However, surgery may be indicated for patients who require definitive management of a pneumothorax with a persistent air leak or a pneumothorax that will not resolve. Indications include a massive air leak that prevents lung reexpansion, a persistent air leak, or a recurrent pneumothorax. VATS may be used for examination of the pleural space and the achievement of pleural symphysis.

Pleural Effusion

A pleural effusion is an abnormal accumulation of fluid in the pleural space resulting in excess fluid production or decreased absorption.[37] A pleural effusion is rarely a primary condition, but rather a complication of heart failure, tuberculosis, pneumonia, pulmonary infection, nephrotic syndrome, connective tissue disease, pulmonary embolism, or neoplastic tumors.[77] Carcinoma of the lung is the most common condition associated with a pleural effusion. Once the pleural space is adequately drained, a chemical pleurodesis may be performed to obliterate the pleural space and prevent reaccumulation of fluid. Other treatments for malignant pleural effusions include surgical pleurectomy, Pleur-X catheter, and implantation of a pleuroperitoneal shunt.[37,77,78,90]

Empyema

An empyema is an accumulation of thick, purulent fluid within the pleural space (an infection in the pleural space), often with fibrin development and a loculated (walled-off) area where the infection is located. Most empyemas occur as a complication of bacterial pneumonia or a lung abscess. Other causes include penetrating chest trauma, hematogenous infection of the pleural space, nonbacterial infections, or iatrogenic causes (following thoracic surgery or thoracentesis). Treatment of an empyema includes fluid evacuation, pleural space obliteration, nutritional optimization, and antimicrobial support.[40] An acute empyema may be drained by thoracentesis or placement of a chest tube if fluid reaccumulates. Chronic empyemas may require rib resection, drainage, or decortication. Open chest drainage is usually performed via thoracotomy and includes potential rib resection to remove the thickened pleura, pus, debris, and the underlying diseased pulmonary tissue.[75,81,88]

With long-standing inflammation, a layer of exudate can form over the lung, trapping the lung and interfering with its normal expansion. This exudate, or pleural peel, must be removed surgically in a process called *decortication*[68] (Fig. 11.5). Once the pleural peel is removed, compliance in the chest wall returns, allowing the lung to expand and deflate, which rapidly improves patient symptoms. Although decortication is an effective surgical procedure for the management of a chronic empyema, its success depends upon careful patient selection. Therefore, as with all thoracic surgery procedures, a thorough preoperative evaluation should be performed prior to surgery.

Pleural Tumors

Tumors of the pleural space develop when cancer cells are transferred to the pleural space through the bloodstream, the lymph system, or by direct contact from cancer tissue of the lungs. There are several different types of tumors that can involve the pleura. These include primary pleural tumors (malignant pleural mesothelioma, solitary fibrous tumor, fibrosarcoma, liposarcoma, pleural lymphoma, synovial sarcoma) and secondary lesions (metastases and tumors of the pericardium and chest wall).

The most common primary pleural tumor is malignant pleural mesothelioma, which is attributed to asbestos exposure. Mesothelioma is an aggressive, incurable disease commonly managed with chemotherapy, radiation therapy, or surgical intervention.[59] Surgical procedures included in the management of malignant pleural mesothelioma include wide local excision, pleurectomy and decortication, pleurodesis, and extrapleural pneumonectomy.

Procedures of the Pleural Space

Pleurodesis

Pleurodesis is a procedure performed to artificially obliterate the pleural space to prevent recurrence of a pneumothorax or pleural effusion.[37,78] Pleurodesis may be performed either chemically or surgically; a chemically irritating agent such as bleomycin, tetracycline, povidone-iodine, or talc is introduced into the pleural space via a thoracic catheter; surgical pleurodesis is performed via thoracotomy or thoracoscopy and involves mechanically irritating the parietal pleura with a rough pad.

Pleurectomy

A pleurectomy is a surgical procedure in which the parietal pleura is removed as a palliative approach to relieve symptoms caused by fluid in the thoracic cavity. This procedure creates space in the thoracic cavity and allows for lung expansion, which can relieve chest discomfort and improve breathing.

MEDIASTINAL DISEASE

The mediastinum is the space in the chest (thoracic cavity) between the pleural sacs of the lungs that contains all of the tissues and organs of the chest, except the lungs and pleurae. The mediastinum can be subdivided into two compartments according to boundaries: superior mediastinum (trachea, esophagus, great vessels, veins, thymus, phrenic and vagus nerves, thoracic duct, some lymph glands) and inferior mediastinum, which is further subdivided into three boundaries: anterior mediastinum (residue of thymus, fat, lymph glands), middle mediastinum (heart, pericardium, ascending aorta, lower half of the superior vena cava, trachea, main bronchi, lymph nodes, pulmonary artery and veins, phrenic nerve), and posterior mediastinum (descending aorta, esophagus, azygos vein, hemiazygos veins, lymph glands, thoracic duct). Approximately 25% to 42% of mediastinal masses are malignant, and in the adult the most common masses in order of decreasing frequency are neurogenic tumors, primary cysts, thymomas, lymphomas, and germ cell tumors.[25]

TABLE 11.3 Types of Diaphragmatic Hernias

Type	Description
Morgagni	Retrosternal anterior diaphragmatic defect. Usually on right side (90%). Hernia sac may contain omentum, colon, stomach, and liver. Surgically repaired when symptomatic.
Paraesophageal	Upward dislocation of gastric fundus alongside a normally (type II) positioned gastroesophageal junction. Less common than sliding hernias. Potential for serious complications such as gastric volvulus/obstruction or gastric necrosis. Surgery indicated because of seriousness of potential complications.
Sliding (Type I)	Dome-shaped upward migration of gastroesophageal junction into posterior mediastinum. Treated when symptomatic.

Diagnostic Studies

Diagnostic tests for evaluating mediastinal disease include a CT scan of the chest, MRI, endoscopic ultrasound (EUS), radionuclide agents (e.g., iodine-131 or iodine-123), and biochemical markers (e.g., alpha-fetoprotein, human chorionic gonadotropin beta-subunit, carcinoembryonic antigen).[6] A mediastinoscopy may be used to biopsy nodes or masses anterior to the trachea in the mediastinum, and a mediastinotomy may be used to biopsy masses in the aortopulmonary window area. CT-guided fine-needle aspiration or core biopsies may also be done, if the mass is accessible via this technique.

Surgical Approaches

Surgical approaches to the mediastinum are dependent upon the area of involvement of the mediastinum and the amount of disease present. The anterosuperior mediastinum is accessed by either a median sternotomy or an anterolateral thoracotomy. The superior aspect of the anterosuperior mediastinum is accessed via a transcervical approach, and the middle or posterior mediastinum through a posterolateral thoracotomy.

DIAPHRAGMATIC SURGERY

The diaphragm serves both anatomically as a separation of the thoracic and abdominal cavities and functionally as the major muscle of respiration. The diaphragm has two distinct parts: the costal muscle and the crural aspect. The costal muscle is thin and provides some of the downward displacement of the diaphragm on inspiration. The crural aspect is thicker and supports the heart. In reality, the diaphragm is made of two hemidiaphragms divided by a central tendon and innervated by the phrenic nerve.

Anatomic disorders of the diaphragm are classified as either congenital or acquired. Congenital diaphragmatic hernias occur when the muscles of the diaphragm do not develop normally, which results in displacement of abdominal components into the thorax.[60] Bochdalek hernias represent the majority of congenital diaphragmatic hernias. Acquired diaphragmatic hernias are most commonly caused by blunt and penetrating trauma. Although diaphragmatic hernias have traditionally been managed by laparotomy or thoracotomy, minimally invasive surgery using laparoscopy of VATS have become increasingly more common[42,45] (Table 11.3). Diaphragm eventration refers to an abnormal elevation of the dome of the diaphragm caused by a condition in which all or part of the diaphragm is composed of fibrous tissue with only a few interspersed muscle fibers.[42]

Diaphragm paralysis is the loss of control of one or both hemidiaphragms secondary to traumatic injury or a disease process, which decreases or terminates the respiratory drive. Diaphragmatic plication may be performed when there is paralysis of either the left or the right diaphragm. The goal of plication is to lower the diaphragm into a flat position in order to reduce the paradoxical motion and associated shift in the mediastinum during respiration.[41] Although a thoracotomy or thoracoabdominal approach is most often used for plication, VATS may also be performed.

Primary tumors of the diaphragm are rare. More often, tumors spread from the lung, upper abdominal viscera, or pleura and invade the diaphragm. Benign diaphragmatic tumors include lipoma, cystic masses, and bronchogenic, mesothelial, and teratoid tumors. Examples of malignant tumors include sarcoma, schwannoma, chondroma, pheochromocytoma, and endometriosis.

CHEST WALL DISORDERS

Tumors are the most common disorder of the chest wall observed in adults. Approximately 5% of thoracic neoplasms are primary chest wall tumors, and approximately 85% of these occur in the ribs.[41] Chest wall tumors can be classified as benign or malignant tumors of the bone or soft tissue. Examples of benign tumors are lipomas, osteochondroma, chondroma, and fibrous dysplasia. Malignant tumors of the chest wall include chondrosarcoma, fibrosarcoma, multiple myeloma, and Ewing's sarcoma. Solid tumors may metastasize to the chest wall and include lung, breast, pancreatic, gastric, and colon cancers. Treatment of a chest wall tumor is dependent on the specific tumor and the extent of involvement. Some chest wall tumors are treated in a palliative fashion with radiation therapy. If surgery is indicated, a variety of procedures may be performed, depending on the location and the involvement of surrounding tissues and ribs.

COMPLICATIONS OF THORACIC SURGERY

Intraoperative

There are four primary intraoperative complications associated with thoracic surgery. These include hemorrhage secondary to injury to a major vessel, cardiac dysrhythmia, myocardial ischemia, and development of a contralateral pneumothorax.[58] A contralateral pneumothorax is a rare complication, with an incidence of less than 1%. This intraoperative complication may occur during the positive pressure ventilation of the nonoperative lung as the result of the spontaneous rupture of a bleb. Although the majority of complications related to thoracic surgical procedures are pulmonary in origin, intraoperative cardiac complications can also occur in patients with preexisting cardiac disease (Table 11.4).

TABLE 11.4 Functional Effects and Complications Related to Specific Thoracic Procedures

Procedure	Physiologic Effects	Complications
Wedge resection	Minimal	Retention of secretions Persistent pleural air space
Segmentectomy	Overinflation of contralateral lung and remaining tissue on operated side	Retention of secretions Prolonged air leak Empyema Persistent pleural space
Lobectomy	Similar to segmentectomy	Similar to segmentectomy
Pneumonectomy	Residual pneumonectomy space Mediastinal/tracheal shift toward remaining lung Functional loss of lung tissue Diaphragm elevation on resected side Cardiac output transversions: one pulmonary and one lung	Retention of secretions Bronchopulmonary fistula Empyema Noncardiac pulmonary edema

Pulmonary Complications

Prolonged Air Leak

According to the Society of Thoracic Surgeons, a prolonged air leak is defined as an air leak that lasts beyond postoperative day 5. A prolonged air leak following thoracic surgery is associated with increased length of stay, increased hospital costs, increased rates of empyema, and other postoperative complications. Air leaks are common after lobectomy, especially when incomplete fissures have been divided during the operation and in LVRS.[8,37,57] Most resolve upon reexpansion of the lung and stop within 2 weeks.

There is a lack of evidence-based practice management of chest tubes following pulmonary resection. Recent studies have shown that although the majority of provider favor placing chest tubes to suction when a patient has an air leak following resection, water seal is superior.[10,20,65,81]

The use of tissue glue has been suggested to reduce the incidence and duration of air leak. Fabian et al. conducted a prospective, blinded study and randomized patients to aerosolized spraying of 5 mL of fibrin glue onto raw lung surface.[23] Patients receiving the aerosolized fibrin glue had a reduction in the incidence of air leak, duration of air leak, and duration of chest tube use.[39,48,89] Additional studies are needed to support these results.

For patients with a prolonged air leak who are otherwise ready for discharge from the hospital, options are available. Patients can be discharged with small one-way valves (Heimlich Chest Drain Valve, BD Bard-Parker, Franklin Lakes, NJ; Pneumostat Chest Drain Valve, Atrium Medical Corporation, Hudson, NH). In addition, a small 500-mL chest tube drainage device that also monitors air leak is available (Express Mini 500, Atrium Medical Corp.). If the air leak continues for 2 to 3 weeks, other options should be discussed and may include returning to surgery with a VATS procedure, either to apply a sealant or to perform a pleurodesis.

Bronchopleural Fistula

Tracheal or bronchopleural fistula complications are difficult to prevent and manage in the postoperative patient. Prevention focuses on vigilant management of the tracheobronchial anastomosis. Frequent bronchoscopic evaluation to assess the area for ischemia or necrosis may be used. Some surgeons advocate minimization of deep endobronchial suctioning so that the integrity of the suture line is not compromised.

Unfortunately, the bronchial stump does not always heal following an anatomic lung resection, which may result in a minor complication or progress to a life-threatening event.[15] It is more common after a pneumonectomy (right greater than left) and is a more serious complication following a pneumonectomy compared to that of a lobectomy or segmentectomy. Risk factors for this complication include type of resection, reason for resection (such as resection performed for infection or inflammation), timing of resection (such as following full-dose radiation therapy or prolonged mechanical ventilation), postresection infected space, or technical factors.[62,89]

Management of this complication depends upon the time of development following surgery. Reoperation and repair may be indicated very early in the postoperative period. If the fistula occurs later in the postoperative recovery, the patient will expectorate serosanguineous, frothy fluid from the pleural space. Prompt attention to this complication is needed so that the remaining lung is not flooded with the pleural drainage. The patient should be positioned with the operative side down to protect the remaining lung, and a chest tube should be placed, or a portion of the previous incision site should be opened and a tube placed.

If the bronchopleural fistula persists or occurs in the presence of infection (empyema), more aggressive measures may be indicated. Drainage may be performed by establishing an Eloesser flap or reopening a portion of the original thoracotomy. A flap of skin is sutured to the pleura, creating an epithelium-lined opening into the empyema area to assist in drainage. The bronchial stump is resutured and reinforced. A Clagett maneuver is used to sterilize the pleural space. This involves open drainage and irrigation of the pleural cavity with antibiotics for several months. The chest wall is then closed once the infection has been thoroughly treated and has resolved.

Atelectasis

Atelectasis occurs in all patients in the postoperative period; however, severe atelectasis leading to respiratory insufficiency occurs in 15% to 20% of patients following resection.[72,73] Treatment includes adequate volume while the patient is on mechanical ventilation and intensive volume expansion measures, including secretion management, frequent repositioning, mobilization, and bronchoscopy following extubation.

Pneumonia

Pulmonary infection may occur in association with unresolved atelectasis, aspiration, and in the setting of mechanical ventilation. The incidence with thoracic surgery is cited between 2% and 22%, with larger series ranging from 5% to 8%.[34] Thoracic surgery is listed as a risk factor for nosocomial pneumonia.[72] In the thoracic surgery patient, risk factors for postoperative pneumonia include increased age, preexisting pulmonary disease (chronic lung disease, smoking), poor nutritional status, aspiration, prolonged anesthesia, use of transfusions, presence of a nasogastric tube, prolonged mechanical ventilation, poor volume expansion, poor secretion management, poor pain management, and lack of mobilization.[72]

Pneumonia is often misdiagnosed in the postoperative setting. Treatment includes early identification of patients at risk, early extubation, early identification of pneumonia, appropriate antibiotic treatment, lung volume expansion maneuvers, and aggressive secretion management. Key measures to prevent ventilator-associated pneumonia include initiation of the ventilator bundle of care.

Early identification of this complication is important. Mortality in the postoperative patient can be as high as 30%, and unfortunately, pneumonia may lead to acute respiratory failure or acute respiratory distress syndrome.[71]

Acute Respiratory Failure and Acute Respiratory Distress Syndrome

Respiratory failure and acute respiratory distress syndrome are discussed in detail in Chapter 9.

Postpneumonectomy Pulmonary Edema

Postpneumonectomy pulmonary edema is difficult to predict, prevent, and treat successfully. It is a rapidly occurring, lethal complication that happens in 2% to 5% of cases and, when unrecognized, carries a mortality rate of 60% to 90%.[62] Although the complication is similar to noncardiogenic pulmonary edema, it is refractory to standard therapy and may have devastating consequences for the pneumonectomy patient. The pathophysiologic mechanisms are similar to those for acute respiratory distress syndrome and include the factors of contralateral pulmonary hyperinflation, alveolar rupture, interstitial emphysema, damage to the alveolocapillary membrane, and decreased lymphatic resorption of fluid.[62]

Prevention of postpneumonectomy pulmonary edema involves minimization of fluid infusion in the operative and early postoperative periods, early use of diuretics, and use of vasopressors if fluid volume appears adequate.[62] Prolonged high-pressure ventilation should be minimized if at all possible.

Pleural Effusion

In the acute postoperative period, a small effusion at the base of the lung is common after lobectomy or a lesser resection. Small to moderate effusions are drained via the chest tube or reabsorbed over time. A chronic or recurring effusion that causes symptoms of pulmonary impairment in the postoperative setting may require ultrasound-guided thoracentesis or a return to surgery for drainage and pleurodesis.

Chylothorax

A chylothorax is an accumulation of lymphatic fluid within the pleural space. Chylothorax may occur after pneumonectomy, lobectomy, or extensive hilar and mediastinal dissection. Although injury to the thoracic duct may occur anywhere along its course, injuries to the thoracic duct in the lower chest often result in right-sided chylothorax, and injuries to the upper portion of the duct typically result in left-sided chylothorax. In approximately 50% of cases, the lymphatic fistula will close with nonoperative management.[32,41] Surgical repair should be considered in patients with large volume drainage or drainage that exceeds 2 weeks.

Lobar Torsion

A lobar torsion (lung torsion) occurs when a lobe rotates around hilar structures compromising the airway, arterial blood supply, and venous lymphatic drainage. Although extremely rare (incidence of 0.09% to 0.4%), a lobar torsion is classified as an adverse event following a pneumonectomy or VATS that requires emergent intervention. Early recognition involves hypoxemia and chest radiograph, which demonstrates hilar displacement, bronchial cut-off, and lobar consolidation.[1]

Urgent flexible bronchoscopy is performed to diagnose lobar torsion and to evaluate the airways. Once diagnosed, lobar torsion requires emergent surgical intervention to release the torsion and increase viability of the lobe. If unrecognized and not corrected, infarction of the lobe and gangrene can occur.

Pulmonary Embolism

Pulmonary embolism occurs in approximately 5% of patients following thoracic surgery and is more common following a pneumonectomy (right greater than left) when compared to other thoracic surgery procedures.[62] The Institute for Clinical Systems Improvement published a patient algorithm for risk and prophylaxis of venous thromboembolism.[38] Few studies are available to support specific prophylaxis regimens following thoracic surgery. The American College of Chest Physicians 9th Consensus Conference recommended early initiation of prophylaxis; if elastic stockings or sequential compression devices (SCDs) are used, they should be applied before surgery and continued until the patient is ambulatory, with the same plan for the use of intermittent compression devices.[38] There are several types of SCDs, including foot, calf, and thigh-high compression as well as graduated, asymmetric, and circumferential compression.[31] Studies comparing foot, calf, and thigh-high compression found little difference in effectiveness. Pharmacologic prophylaxis should be used in addition to mechanical means in patients undergoing thoracic surgery.

Cardiac Complications

Cardiac Dysrhythmias

Atrial fibrillation is the most common dysrhythmia following noncardiac thoracic surgery, with a reported incidence of 0.4% to 12%.[14,17] Although the exact causative factors for postoperative atrial fibrillation following noncardiac thoracic surgery remain unknown, proposed causes are nonspecific and multifactorial. They include age, extrapleural or intrapericardial pneumonectomy, right sided procedures, extent of pulmonary resection, and COPD.[14] Although atrial fibrillation is often self-limiting and transient, there can be serious consequences associated with the dysrhythmia. Postoperative atrial fibrillation can lead to disabling symptoms and may have consequences such as stroke, hemodynamic instability, intensive care level of stay, prolonged hospitalization, and increased patient discomfort. Atrial fibrillation occurring after thoracic surgery has been associated with increased mortality.[14,17]

Myocardial Ischemia and Infarction

Although myocardial ischemia and infarction are extremely rare following thoracic surgical procedures, those with preexisting cardiac problems are at an increased risk for both conditions. Appropriate cardiac evaluation prior to surgery is essential to prevent or minimize myocardial infarction.

Cardiac Herniation

If a thoracic resection requires opening the pericardium, cardiac herniation can occur regardless of the location of pulmonary resection (left vs. right). Cardiac herniation usually occurs in the early postoperative period and requires prompt surgical repair. Clinical signs and symptoms include increased venous pressure, sudden hypotension, tachycardia, displaced cardiac impulse, and cardiovascular collapse.[91] Cardiac herniation is confirmed by chest radiograph.[26]

Cardiac Tamponade

Cardiac tamponade risk is increased when the pericardium has been opened and closed during surgery. Undetected bleeding may occur in the pericardium. Signs and symptoms include hypotension, increased central venous pressure, a paradoxical pulse, and slowly developing cardiac failure. Treatment includes drainage of the fluid via a transthoracic, subxiphoid incision, or by a percutaneous catheter.

Neurologic Complications

Although extremely rare, injury to the phrenic nerve during thoracic surgery is a potential complication. The phrenic nerve controls the diaphragm muscle, which regulates breathing. Injury to the phrenic nerve may cause unilateral loss of diaphragmatic function and the loss of ventilation. Even though most patients are at risk for this alteration in breathing, the consequences are significant for patients with limited pulmonary reserve.[62]

This injury occurs more frequently on the left side and results from injury during the surgery or invasion of tumor into the area of the aortopulmonary window. Right-sided injury is rare and seen only in very extensive lymph node dissection. Unilateral damage to the nerve results in hoarseness, and some patients may experience alterations with cough, aspiration, and secretion clearance. Treatment includes a "watch and wait" philosophy to see if the injury is transient because of traction on the nerve during surgery, or a minor procedure for medialization of the vocal cords may be performed.

INTERPROFESSIONAL CARE

Principles of Care

The goal of postoperative management is to prevent or minimize the effects of the most common problems that may lead to poor outcome.[36] Prevention begins during the preoperative phase of care and involves a interprofessional approach. Preoperative patient education is critical for the thoracic surgery population in an effort to improve patient outcomes and reduce preventable hospital readmissions.[53] Preparation for elective surgery includes preoperative teaching, "prehabilitation" with lung volume expansion maneuvers and exercises, smoking cessation, nutritional evaluation with optimization, review of preoperative medications, and psychological preparation of the patient. Setting realistic expectations for the immediate postoperative period is crucial, such as the need for mechanical ventilation, functional compromise, and pain management.[53]

Prehabilitation has been encouraged for those patients deemed high-risk candidates for thoracic surgery. Goals are to optimize quality of life, functional capacity, and overall surgical outcomes.[80] Historically, both presurgery rehabilitation and postoperative rehabilitation have been used with positive results in lung volume reduction surgery and lung transplantation. Lung resection surgery has been added to the list that may benefit from such a program. However, little information is available regarding descriptions of these programs, and minimal data exist to support the use of prehabilitation in patients undergoing lung resection surgery.[80,81] One reason that few data exist is due to the time constraint between diagnosis with NSCLC and the urgency of surgical resection.

Intraoperative Management

Unfortunately, intraoperative management of the thoracic surgery patient cannot be generalized as the type of surgical procedure and the approach used may affect postoperative pain management and hospital length of stay. A muscle-sparing thoracotomy is less invasive than a standard posterolateral thoracotomy because it preserves the latissimus dorsi and serratus anterior muscles.[46] Furthermore, compared to a thoracotomy, a VATS procedure decreases the amount of chest wall involvement, which reduces postoperative pain and improves pulmonary function. VATS has also been associated with improved postoperative immune response by reducing the body's inflammatory response, decreasing length of stay, and producing an earlier return to normal functions when compared to a thoracotomy.[29]

Chest Drainage Management

Chest tubes and drainage systems are used to reexpand the lung and keep the lung expanded, as well as to prevent the development of a space infection. In the past, all chest tubes were placed to suction at −20 cm H_2O; however, in more recent years this practice has been reexamined.[15,68] An important role of the nurse is to assess the drainage tubes regularly for patency, function, air leak, and drainage. A functioning tube is one that shows fluctuation in the fluid within the tubing as the patient breathes, demonstrating pressure changes within the pleural space.[45]

Air leaks are best assessed by observing the water seal chamber during quiet respiration while off suction. The patient is requested to cough and the chamber is assessed. The suction can be applied and then the patient is requested to cough again. Air leaks are assessed by the amount of cough required to expel air. A small leak is one that is intermittent whereas a large leak is continuous. Systems are configured differently among manufacturers; some include a water seal and some are considered dry systems. In addition, the chest tube is evaluated for the extent of air leak and changes that may occur.

Cerfolio et al. have developed a qualitative and quantitative method to measure postoperative air leaks.[12,13] This classification system evaluates an air leak based on when it occurs in the respiratory cycle (qualitative) and how large the air leak appears (quantitative). The air leak is classified as continuous, inspiratory, expiratory, or forced expiratory, and the air leak is scored by evaluating in which chamber on the water seal drainage the bubbles from the air leak appear. Leaks are assigned a numerical value from 1 to 28.[12,13]

The amount, consistency, and character of drainage should be closely monitored. A change from sanguineous to serous is a positive sign, whereas a change from sanguineous to purulent could indicate the development of an empyema or infection. Milky colored fluid may indicate a chylothorax.

Once air leak and drainage have decreased to acceptable levels, the chest tube can be removed. There is little evidence to guide this practice. Different criteria for removal of the chest tube are used by surgeons, ranging anywhere from 100–400 mL of drainage per 24 hours, lack of an air leak, and a volume of 100–150 mL of fluid output per 24 hours. The chest tube is removed as the patient performs a Valsalva maneuver or during the expiratory phase of mechanical ventilation.[32] Routine chest radiographs are not necessary after uncomplicated chest tube removal, and the decision to reinsert a chest tube can be based on the patient's clinical examination.[32] Newer small chest drainage systems are available (500-mL capacity) that facilitate patient ambulation, and patients may be discharged home with such a device if drainage or an air leak persists.

Pain Management

Thoracic surgery can produce intense postoperative pain that can become chronic.[61] Current treatment options for acute postoperative pain include epidural analgesia, intravenous patient-controlled analgesia, intercostal and paravertebral nerve blocks, and oral medications. A multimodality approach with a smooth transition between pain medications should be chosen with the focus of minimizing and preventing pain.

Several considerations must be taken into account when choosing a pain management regimen: route, frequency, and dosage of medications; patient's past medical history and age; and type of surgery. Systemic opioids administered intravenously via patient-controlled mechanisms are a mainstay for acute pain management.[66] Epidural analgesia is also commonly used in the postoperative setting. Studies have demonstrated that patients receiving epidural analgesia following thoracic surgery have less pain, are extubated sooner, have fewer pulmonary complications, and have a decreased length of stay.[27] Questions remain regarding the optimal use of epidural analgesia and include optimal location for placement of the catheter, medications used, timing of the initiation of medications, use of patient-controlled analgesia, and use of adjuvant analgesics.

A newer method of providing continuous infusion of local anesthetic is called the *ON-Q catheter* (ON-Q Pain Buster, I-Flow Corp., Lake Forest, CA). This device delivers anesthetic to the surgical wound site to reduce postoperative pain. The device consists of a small balloon pump that holds a local anesthetic and delivers it through a small catheter directed into the surgical site at the end of surgery. This catheter can be used alone or in conjunction with other pain management strategies.[27] At discharge, patients should be given explicit instructions regarding how and when to use these medications. Pain will exist during the recovery phase of care, but adequate pain management should facilitate recovery by assisting in increased ambulation and improved psychological outlook on recovery.

Nutrition

Fluid management in the thoracic surgery patient is focused on limiting free water that may produce interstitial edema and limit oxygenation. During the first 24 to 48 hours after surgery, urine output will be lower than that for other surgical patients (if < 20 mL/h, notify provider). Fluid intake and renal function are monitored closely in all thoracic surgery patients to prevent fluid overload in the early postoperative phase of care.

Depending upon the surgical procedure and the progress of the patient following extubation, the patient may begin oral fluids and quickly transition to a regular diet. Patients should be monitored closely for sedation, overzealous pain management, and the potential for aspiration. Roberts et al. studied patients undergoing thoracic operations and found that preemptive gastrointestinal tract management (nothing by mouth [NPO] the day of surgery, clear liquids on day 1, and regular diet on day 2) reduced the incidence of aspiration and respiratory failure versus patients who had nutritional orders to "advance as tolerated."[69]

Pneumonectomy patients are generally kept NPO for 24 to 48 hours because of risk of aspiration resulting from mediastinal shift, diaphragmatic elevation, alteration of the esophageal hiatus, and possible damage to the vagus and recurrent laryngeal nerves.[35] For complex patients with hemodynamic instability, ventilatory dependency, preoperative cachexia, and those expected to be NPO for longer than 48 hours, early nutrition should be established via enteral or parenteral routes.[50]

Mechanical Ventilation

Following thoracic surgery, the goal is to extubate the patient in the operating room as soon as possible.[35] However, high-risk patients may require continued intubation and ventilatory support. Potential indications for mechanical ventilation following thoracic surgery include poor preoperative pulmonary function, prolonged intraoperative course, massive fluid administration or blood infusions under anesthesia, cardiac failure, need for postoperative chest wall immobilization/stabilization, inadequate respiratory drive or incomplete recovery of neuromuscular function, fraction of inspired oxygen (Fio_2) requirement greater than 0.50, and visible respiratory distress.[35] In addition, specific types of surgery may require mechanical ventilation in the postoperative period to facilitate healing and recovery (e.g., tracheal resection, sleeve resection, pneumonectomy).

The specific ventilatory needs of the patient will dictate the mode of ventilation; however, the most common mode of ventilation used in the thoracic surgical patient postoperatively is spontaneous intermittent mandatory ventilation (SIMV) with pressure support ventilation (PSV).

Respiratory Care

Early extubation is a priority in the thoracic surgery patient to minimize the risk of ventilator-associated pneumonia and to speed the recovery process. Following extubation, it is critical to promote frequent volume expansion maneuvers (e.g., incentive spirometry, continuous positive airway pressure). Atelectasis is a common complication following thoracic surgery and, if left untreated, can potentially lead to pneumonia.

Secretion management is critical in this population and requires cautious observation and management of secretions, including the amount, color, and consistency of secretions. If standard secretion management techniques do not assist in clearing the airways, then more aggressive measures such as bronchoscopy may be indicated. Positioning may cause an increase in secretions, and the patient must be closely monitored when changing positions.

Mobilization

Early mobilization and ambulation are as important in the thoracic surgery patient as they are in any postoperative patient. Mobilization helps to increase ventilation, improve perfusion, enhance secretion clearance, prevent lower extremity blood stasis, and build stamina in the recovering patient.

Along with mobilization in the postoperative period, it is important for patients to begin both active and passive physical therapy exercises. Prior to discharge from the hospital, the patient should be instructed on simple upper extremity exercises to assist with mobilization on the operative side.[44] Additionally, the patient should be coached on a progressive walking program with daily goals. The treatment combination for optimal postoperative management to prevent pulmonary complications includes pain management, volume expansion, secretion management, and early mobilization.[44]

Critical Care

Although postoperative care of thoracic surgical patients is an essential component of patient recovery, it poses numerous challenges. Thoracic surgery impairs pulmonary function thereby increasing the likelihood of developing postoperative respiratory failure. As of 2016, the literature demonstrates that the incidence of postoperative pulmonary complications following thoracic surgery is 19% to 59% compared to less than 5% following lower abdominal surgery.[40] Unfortunately, these postoperative complications frequently result in critical care admissions, increased lengths of stay, and poor patient outcomes.

Admission to the critical care unit postoperatively is typically decided by the surgeon prior to surgery and is primarily influenced by age and preexisting comorbid conditions. Recovering in the critical care unit utilizes a interprofessional team often comprised of the surgeon, a team of specially trained critical care nurses, physical therapist, occupational therapist, speech therapist, social worker, pharmacist, and nutritionist. Although each member of the team plays an integral part in postoperative care of the thoracic patient, the critical care nurse delivers the vast majority of care and serves as the primary advocate in an effort to optimize recovery and improve outcomes.

ESOPHAGEAL DISEASE

The esophagus is a hollow muscular channel comprised of four layers: mucosa, submucosa, muscularis propria, and adventitia with multiple regional and nonregional lymph nodes surrounding the esophagus. Measuring approximately 25 cm in length, the esophagus extends from the pharynx inferiorly to the stomach and serves as a conduit for saliva, liquids, and food. Anatomically the esophagus originates in the neck at the inferior border of C6, descends anteriorly to the vertebral column, passes through the superior and posterior mediastinum and then through the diaphragm, and enters the abdomen opposite T11. The narrowest part of the esophagus is where it passes into the diaphragm.

Other structures located near the esophagus and sometimes involved in surgery include the recurrent laryngeal nerves, ascending between the esophagus and the trachea (tracheoesophageal groove), and the thoracic duct, located on the left side of the esophagus. The thoracic duct carries the majority of the lymph and chyle into the blood and is the end point for most of the lymphatic vessels of the body except for some of the vessels on the right side. Both of these structures may be involved or injured during the surgical process.

Esophageal disorders may be either benign or malignant (esophageal cancer). Once esophageal cancer is diagnosed, an endoscopic ultrasound is performed to determine the extent of mucosal invasion of the tumor. This begins the staging process for esophageal cancer.

Esophageal Cancer

Esophageal cancer accounts for 1% of all cancers in the United States. According to the American Cancer Society, in 2015, there were an estimated 16,980 newly diagnosed cases of esophageal cancer (13,570 in men and 3410 in women) with 15,590 deaths.[3] There are two main histologic types of esophageal cancer: squamous cell and adenocarcinoma.[21] Squamous cell is usually located in the upper two thirds of the esophagus; adenocarcinoma is found in the distal third of the esophagus and in the gastroesophageal junction. Whereas the incidence of squamous cell carcinoma has remained relatively stable over the past 30 years, the incidence of adenocarcinoma of the esophagus has increased rapidly at an alarming rate.[18,64,92] It now accounts for more than half of all esophageal cancers.[18,64] Barrett's esophagus is thought to be a precursor to esophageal adenocarcinoma. Risk factors have been documented between Caucasian race, increasing age, frequency and duration of gastroesophageal reflux disease, and an incidence of Barrett's esophagus.[18,64]

Esophageal cancer typically occurs in mid to late adulthood, and the incidence increases with age. This cancer is 2.7 times more common in males than in females. Squamous cell cancer is more prevalent in African-American males, whereas Caucasian males have a higher prevalence of adenocarcinoma. Risk factors of squamous cell carcinoma include cigarette smoking, alcohol consumption, limited fruit and vegetable consumption, obesity, gastroesophageal reflux disease, and achalasia. Barrett's esophagus is a risk factor for adenocarcinoma and the risk is further increased with cigarette smoking.[91]

The diagnosis of esophageal cancer is done via an esophagogastroduodenoscopy (EGD). The patient is instrumented with a flexible endoscope, and the lining of the esophagus can be directly visualized for abnormalities and biopsies taken. A CT scan of the chest and abdomen is done to grossly evaluate tumor size, invasion of adjacent structures, potential nodal involvement, and metastatic disease to the chest and abdomen. An endoscopic esophageal ultrasound (EUS) is a staging technique and has provided a significant advancement in the evaluation of esophageal cancer. The EUS provides specific information regarding the depth of tumor invasion through the wall of the esophagus and the lymph nodes involved in proximity to the gastrointestinal wall. With this technique, lymph nodes proximal to the esophagus can be biopsied. A variety of other scans may be used to assess for metastasis of the cancer. These may include bone scans, abdominal scans, PET scans, fusion CT/PET scans, and liver ultrasound. PET scans are now widely used as part of the staging process.

As with lung cancer, esophageal cancer is staged by the TNM system. The *T* evaluates the tumor invasion through the wall of the esophagus, the *N* evaluates lymph node involvement, and the *M* is metastasis. Once esophageal cancer develops, it may spread rapidly. At the time of diagnosis, more than 50% of patients have either unresectable disease or metastases.[67] The overall survival rate at 5 years for localized (contained) esophageal cancer is 40%.[3]

Esophageal Resection Procedures

Patients who present with localized esophageal cancer are treated with surgery alone or with neoadjuvant chemoradiation therapy followed by surgery. Differing surgical procedures can be used to perform an esophagectomy (removal of all or part of the esophagus) or esophagogastrectomy (removal of all or part of the esophagus and removal of a portion of the gastric cardia). Esophagectomy may also be performed following damage to the esophagus from caustic injuries or achalasia that does not respond to more conservative medical or surgical management.

The surgery is most commonly performed through an open approach; however, thoracoscopic and robotic procedures are also completed.[63] No single esophagectomy approach is suited for all patients. There is controversy regarding the optimal surgical approach and the extent and need of regional lymph node dissection. The four common surgical approaches for an esophagectomy are the Ivor-Lewis, 3-field, thoracoabdominal approach, and the transhiatal approach (blunt dissection of the thoracic esophagus) (Table 11.5). Usually, the stomach, or remaining portion of the stomach, is pulled up to take the place of the esophagus (gastric pull-up); however, colon and jejunum may also be used.

Preoperative Evaluation

Since an esophageal resection is considered to be a major thoracic procedure, a patient must be thoroughly evaluated to determine surgical candidacy. Factors to consider regarding surgical risk include age, cardiac and pulmonary function, nutritional status, presence of preoperative chemotherapy or radiation therapy, and understanding of the complexity and long-term recovery following surgery.

Pulmonary complications are the most common problem following esophagectomy and implicated in increased length of stays, poor patient outcomes, and increased morbidity and mortality. Potential increased risk factors include the opening into two body cavities, disruption of the lymphatic system, disruption of pulmonary muscles, placement of a conduit in the chest, and potential recurrent laryngeal nerve injury.[76] Preexisting impaired pulmonary function, cigarette smoking history, alcohol abuse, and poor functional status all contribute to potential preoperative and postoperative complications.

Malnutrition, dysphagia, decreased immune function, and preoperative radiation therapy or chemotherapy may all

TABLE 11.5 Description of Approaches for Esophageal Resection

Approach	Description	Advantages	Disadvantages
Ivor-Lewis	Laparotomy and right thoracotomy Broadly applicable to differing tumor sites Considered the gold standard	Precise esophageal and lymph node dissection under direct vision Anastomosis in chest (low incidence of leaks)	Carries the complications of both a large abdominal and thoracic procedure; increased pain; increased risk for pneumonia due to limited mobility secondary to pain
3-Field	Ivor-Lewis approach plus left cervical incision	Precise esophageal and lymph node dissection under direct vision Anastomosis in neck	Pain from thoracotomy
Thoracoabdominal	Combined laparotomy and left thoracotomy Best suited for tumors of gastric cardia	Excellent exposure to stomach and distal esophagus	Painful incision Anastomosis in chest
Transhiatal	Laparotomy and left cervical incision Best suited for tumor of distal esophagus, but may be used for mid-thoracic tumors	Near-total esophagectomy Anastomosis in neck (less severe leaks)	Imprecision in esophageal and lymph node dissection Reduced pain (no thoracotomy) Risk of recurrent laryngeal nerve injury

contribute to poor outcomes. An extensive nutritional evaluation should be performed; preoperative nutritional supplementation should be considered as optimizing nutritional status is critical for improved outcomes.

Postoperative Care

Pulmonary care. Care following esophagogastrectomy is similar to that for the thoracic surgery patient and focuses on preventing and minimizing pulmonary complications. The clinical care focuses on early extubation, intensive lung expansion maneuvers, secretion management, and frequent repositioning and mobilization. Bronchoscopy may be used to assist in secretion management.

Depending upon the surgical technique used, the patient may have one or two chest tubes in place. If a cervical incision has been made, the patient may also have a drain placed and the amount and type of drainage should be noted every 8 hours. Lastly, early mobilization of the patient is important, just as it is with thoracic surgery patients.

The patient is maintained on intravenous fluids with nothing to eat or drink for 5 to 7 days after surgery. A nasogastric tube remains in place and should be well secured and placed on intermittent suction. On postoperative day 5 to 7, an EGD or Gastrografin swallow is performed to assess the anastomotic integrity. Once the anastomosis is studied and an anastomotic leak is ruled out, the nasogastric tube is removed and a clear liquid diet may be initiated. Oral intake is subsequently started on an incremental basis, beginning with clear liquids and then slowly progressing to solids. Patients may have a jejunostomy tube in place, and feeding will commence once the nasogastric tube is removed (Box 11.1).

Pain management techniques are similar to those used in thoracic surgery. With the differing esophageal approaches, pain may be an important issue in the recovery of the patient. Pain management is also key in assisting the patient in the progression of mobilization and frequent ambulation.[46]

Complications Related to Esophageal Surgery

An anastomotic leak is a breakdown along an anastomosis that causes fluids to leak. Cervical anastomotic leaks may occur and gastric drainage may be noted at the cervical incision or through the drain. Usually, the cervical incision is opened and wound care administered. A cervical anastomotic leak usually heals with conservative approaches and rarely requires surgical closure. Conservative management of an anastomotic leak includes radiologic confirmation of leak, restriction of oral intake, decompression with nasogastric tube, provision of enteral or parenteral nutrition, and administration of antibiotics as indicated. Intrathoracic leaks present a more complex problem and are less likely to heal spontaneously; definitive surgical repair may be necessary.

Approximately 50% of all patients who undergo an esophagectomy will develop an anastomotic stricture within the first 3 months following surgery secondary to scar tissue formation at the site of the anastomosis.[90] Clinical presentation includes complaints of increasing dysphagia or feeling as though food is "sticking." Treatment for an anastomotic stricture includes an endoscopy with dilation of the stricture.

Rarely, there is ischemia with necrosis of the conduit (stomach, colon, or jejunum) because of poor blood flow. Signs include septic toxemia, fever, and foul-smelling secretions. Endoscopy is used to confirm the diagnosis. Once identified, the patient is returned to surgery and the conduit removed.[52] A cervical esophagostomy is performed in which the stomach and the esophageal stump are closed and the remainder of the esophagus is exteriorized at the neck.[52] A pouching system is placed over the opening for containment of saliva and secretions. A feeding tube is placed (often jejunal); placement is dependent upon which area will be used for the subsequent reconstruction of the esophagus. Reconstruction is not attempted for at least 3 to 6 months following this event.

Achalasia

Achalasia is a motor disorder of the esophagus characterized by functional obstruction of the distal esophagus because of incomplete relaxation of the lower esophageal sphincter.[5] This causes a lack of progressive peristalsis in the body of the esophagus. Secondary achalasia (pseudoachalasia) may be caused by a distal obstruction (carcinoma, lymphoma) or be neuropathic in origin. Assessment for achalasia includes a thorough history and physical, barium swallow, and esophageal manometry.[5] Symptoms include dysphagia, regurgitation of undigested food, and retrosternal pain. Surgical treatment is usually attempted following failed medical management. Surgical treatment includes an esophagomyotomy, in which a 5-cm to 7-cm myotomy or cutting of the muscle is performed on the distal esophagus. A variety of approaches may be used to accomplish a myotomy, including a VATS, laparoscopic incision, left thoracotomy, or laparotomy.

Esophageal diverticula are pouches arising from the esophageal lumen. Zenker's diverticulum is the most commonly diagnosed of the esophageal diverticula. Symptoms include dysphagia, halitosis, retrosternal pain, alterations in voice tone or character, and coughing or wheezing following episodes of aspiration.[7] Treatment of Zenker's diverticulum is a cricopharyngeal myotomy.

CONCLUSION

The thoracic surgery patient provides both challenges and opportunities for the experienced critical care nurse to combine advanced knowledge of pathophysiology and specific interventions to prevent or minimize complications following

BOX 11.1 Nutritional Considerations for Esophageal Resection

- Patient should eat in a relaxed state while sitting up and avoid eating 3 hours before bedtime to prevent reflux.
- Patient may expect weight loss following discharge as the body adapts to the new gastrointestinal conduit.
- Weight should be monitored at home and reported to the healthcare provider.
- Foods may not taste or smell appealing as a result of anesthesia and chemotherapy. With time, normal taste and smell will return.
- Appetite may be poor and caloric intake may be a difficult topic at times; patient will require strong support from caregivers.
- Increasing activities will help to stimulate appetite and gastrointestinal motility.
- Patient should be instructed to eat six small meals per day.
- Information regarding dumping syndrome and avoidance of concentrated sweets, which may cause postprandial diarrhea, should be reviewed with patient prior to discharge.
- Intake of high-calorie foods and liquid supplementation may be necessary for nutritional support.

surgery. The critical care nurse plays an essential role as a member of the interprofessional team and serves not only as a caregiver, but also as an educator to ensure improved patient outcomes and decreased preventable readmissions for this surgical population.

CASE STUDY 11.1

M.R. is a 46-year-old male referred to the thoracic surgery clinic with complaints of increasing shortness of breath and intermittent hemoptysis for the past 3 months. M.R. works full-time as a recycling technician and has smoked three packs of cigarettes per day for the past 31 years; he has recently cut down to two packs per day with the onset of his worsening shortness of breath. He reports an unintentional weight loss of 20 lb over the past 6 months as well as increased fatigue and lower back pain, which he associates with his 50-hour work week. Last week, M.R. was evaluated by his primary care provider and underwent a chest radiograph, which demonstrated an abnormality in the apex of the right lung.

Decision Point:
What laboratory studies should be performed?

Decision Point:
What diagnostic study should be performed?

Decision Point:
Should a biopsy be scheduled at this time or should he be referred to an oncologist at this time?

REFERENCES

1. Alassar, A. & Marchbank, A. (2014). Left lower lobe torsion following upper lobectomy-prompt recognition and treatment improve survival. *J Surg Case Rep, 8*, 78.
2. Albain, K., et al. (2009). Radiotherapy plus chemotherapy with or without surgical resection for Stage III non-small cell lung cancer. *Lancet, 374*, 379–386.
3. American Cancer Society. (2015). How is cancer of the esophagus staged? http://www.cancer.org/cancer/esophaguscancer/detailedguide/esophagus-cancer-staging.
4. Asamura, H. (2014). Role of limited sublobar resection for early-stage lung cancer: steady progression. *J Clin Oncol, 32*, 2449–2456.
5. Ates, F. & Vaezi, M. F. (2015). The pathogenesis and management of achalasia: current status and future directions. *Gut Liver, 9*, 449–463.
6. Berania, I., et al. (2015). Endoscopic mediastinal staging in lung cancer is superior to "gold standard" surgical staging. *Ann Thorac Surg, 15*, 431–439.
7. Bizzotto, A., et al. (2013). Zenker's diverticulum: exploring treatment options. *Acta Otorhinolaryngol Ital, 33*, 219–229.
8. Breathnach, C. S. (2016). Evarts Ambrose Graham: doyen of pulmonary surgeons. *Ir J Med Sci, 185*, 265–266.
9. Brunelli, A., et al. (2013). Physiologic evaluation of the patient with lung cancer being considered for resectional surgery. *Chest, 143*, e166S–e190S.
10. Burt, B. M. & Shrager, J. B. (2014). Prevention and management of postoperative air leaks. *Ann Cardiothorac Surg, 3*, 216–218.
11. *Centers for Medicare and Medicaid Services.* (2012). Baltimore, MD: National coverage determination for lung volume reduction surgery.
12. Cerfolio, R. J. (2002). Advances in thoracostomy tube management. *Surg Clin North Am, 82*, 833–848.
13. Cerfolio, R. J. (2002). Chest tube management after pulmonary resection. *Chest Surg Clin North Am, 12*, 507–527.
14. Chelazzi, C., Villa, G. & DeGaudio, A. R. (2011). Postoperative atrial fibrillation. *ISRN Cardiol, 2011*, 1–10.
15. Coughlin, S. M., et al. (2012). Management of chest tubes after pulmonary resection: a systematic review and meta-analysis. *Can J Surg, 55*, 264–270.
16. Criner, G. J. (2012). Lung volume reduction as an alternative to transplantation for COPD. *Clin Chest Med, 32*, 279–397.
17. Danelich, I. M., et al. (2014). Practical management of postoperative atrial fibrillation after noncardiac surgery. *J Am Coll Surg, 219*, 831–841.
18. Dellon, E. S. & Shaheen, J. J. (2005). Does screening for Barrett's esophagus and adenocarcinoma of the esophagus prolong survival? *J Clin Oncol, 23*, 4478–4482.
19. Eberhardt, W. E. & Stuschke, M. (2015). Multimodal treatment of non-small cell lung cancer. *Lancet, 386*, 1018–1019.
20. Elsayed, H., McShane, J. & Shackcloth, M. (2012). Air leaks following pulmonary resection for lung cancer: is it a patient or surgeon related problem? *Ann R Coll Surg Engl, 94*, 422–427.
21. Enzinger, P. C. & Mayer, R. J. (2003). Esophageal cancer. *N Engl J Med, 349*, 2241–2252.
22. Faber, L. P. (2005). Sleeve lobectomy. In T. Shields, et al. (Ed.), *General thoracic surgery* (6th ed.). Philadelphia: Lippincott Williams & Wilkins.
23. Fabian, T., Federico, J. A. & Ponn, R. B. (2003). Fibrin glue in pulmonary resection: a prospective, randomized blinded study. *Ann Thorac Surg, 75*, 1587–1592.
24. Flechsig, P., et al. (2015). PET/MRI and PET/CT in lung lesions and thoracic malignancies. *Semin Nucl Med, 45*, 268–281.
25. Flummerfelt, P. M. (2001). Tumors of the mediastinum. In H. L. Karamanoukian, P. R. Soltoski, & T. A. Salerno (Eds.), *Thoracic surgery secrets.* Philadelphia: Hanley & Belfus.
26. S. Gadhinglajkar, S., et al. (2010). Cardiac herniation following completion pneumonectomy for bronchiectasis. *Ann Card Anaesth, 13*, 249–252.
27. Gebhardt, R., et al. (2013). Epidural versus ON-Q local anesthetic-infiltrating catheter for post-thoracotomy pain control. *J Cardiothorasc Vasc Anesth, 27*, 423–426.
28. Goldstraw, D., et al. (2011). Non-small cell lung cancer. *Lancet, 378*, 1727–1740.
29. Gonzalez-Rivas, D. (2012). VATS lobectomy: surgical evolution from conventional vats to uniportal approach. *Scientific World Journal, 2012*, 1–5.
30. Green, M. R., et al. (2005). Adjuvant therapy choices in patients with resected non-small-cell lung cancer: correlation of doctor's treatment plans and relevant phase III trial data. *J Oncol Pract, 1*, 37–42.
31. Guyatt, G. H., et al. (2012). Antithrombotic therapy and prevention of thrombosis. (9th ed.), College of Chest Physicians evidence-based clinical practice guidelines *Chest, 141*, 7S–47S.
32. Hartigan, P. M., Body, S. C. & Sugarbaker, D. J. (2005). Pulmonary resection. In J. A. Kaplan, & P. D. Slinger (Eds.), *Thoracic anesthesia* (3rd ed.). Philadelphia: Churchill Livingstone.
33. He, J. & Xu, X. (2012). Thoracoscopic anatomic pulmonary resection. *J Thorac Dis, 4*, 520–547.
34. Hetzel, J., Hetzel, M. & Babiak, A. (2005). Staging and early diagnosis of patients with non-small cell lung cancer. *New Directions Treatment Lung Cancer, 1*, 1–10.
35. Higgins, T. L. (2005). Postthoracotomy complications. In J. A. Kaplan, & P. D. Slinger (Eds.), *Thoracic anesthesia* (3rd ed.). Philadelphia: Churchill Livingstone.
36. Hoogeboom, T. J., et al. (2014). Merits of exercise therapy before and after major surgery. *Curr Opin Anaesthesiol, 27*, 161–166.
37. Inoue, T., et al. (2013). Talc pleurodesis for the management of malignant pleural effusions in Japan. *Intern Med, 52*, 1173–1176.
38. Institute for Clinical Systems Improvement (ICSI). (2003). *Venous thromboembolism prophylaxis for surgical/trauma patients.* Bloomington, Minn: ISCI.
39. Ishikawa, K., et al. (2013). Endobronchial closure of a bronchopleural fistula using a fibrin glue-coated collagen patch and fibrin glue. *Ann Thorac Cardiovasc Surg, 19*, 423–427.
40. Iyer, A. & Yadav, S. (2013). Postoperative care and complications after thoracic surgery. In M. S. Firstenberg (Ed.), *Principles and practice of cardiothoracic surgery* (pp. 57–84). Rijeka, Croatia: InTech.

41. Kaiser, L. R. & Singhal, S. (2004). *Surgical foundation: essentials of thoracic surgery*. Philadelphia: Mosby.
42. Kansal, A. P., et al. (2009). Right-sided diaphragmatic eventration: a rare entity. *Lung India, 26*, 48–50.
43. Kent, M., et al. (2013). Segmentectomy versus wedge resection for non-small cell lung cancer in high-risk operable patients. *Ann Thorac Surg, 96*, 1747–1755.
44. Khasanov, A. F., et al. (2015). The program of accelerated rehabilitation after esophagoplasty (fast track surgery) in esophageal cancer surgery. *Khirurgiia (Mosk), 3*, 37–43.
45. Lian, C., et al. (2013). Video-assisted radical thoracoscopic and laparoscopic surgery for esophageal carcinoma. *J Thorac Dis, 5*, 892–894.
46. Lin, J. & Iannettoni, M. D. (2005). Fast-tracking: eliminating roadblocks to successful early discharge. *Thorac Surg Clin, 15*, 221–228.
47. LoCicero, J. (2005). Segmentectomy and lesser pulmonary resections. In T. Shields, et al. (Ed.), *General thoracic surgery* (6th ed.). Philadelphia: Lippincott Williams & Wilkins.
48. Lopex, C., et al. (2013). Efficacy and safety of fibrin sealant patch in the treatment of air leak in thoracic surgery. *Minerva Chir, 68*, 559–567.
49. Loscertales, J., et al. (2010). Video-assisted thoracic surgery: lobectomy results in lung cancer. *J Thoracic Dis, 2*, 29–35.
50. Mashhadi, R., et al. (2015). Early postoperative enteral versus parenteral feeding after esophageal cancer surgery. *Iran J Otorhinolaryngol, 27*, 331–336.
51. Meyers, B. F. & Patterson, G. A. (2003). Chronic obstructive pulmonary disease. 10: Bullectomy, lung volume reduction surgery, and transplantation for patients with chronic obstruction pulmonary disease. *Thorax, 58*, 634–638.
52. Meyerson, S. L. & Mehta, C. K. (2014). Managing complications II: conduit failure and conduit airway fistulas. *J Thorac Dis, 6*, S364–S371.
53. Miyasaka, Y., et al. (2010). Postoperative complications and respiratory function following segmentectomy of the lung-comparison of the methods of making an inter-segmental plane. *Interact Cardio Vasc Thorac Surg, 12*, 426–429.
54. Mountain, C. F. (2000). The evolution of the surgical treatment of lung cancer. *Chest Surg Clin North Am, 10*, 83–104.
55. Mueller, M. R. & Marzluf, B. A. (2014). The anticipation and management of air leaks and residual spaces post lung resection. *J Thorac Dis, 6*, 271–284.
56. Naidu, B. V. & Rajesh, P. B. (2010). Relevant surgical anatomy of the chest wall. *Thorac Surg Clin, 20*, 453–463.
57. National Emphysema Treatment Trial Research Group. (2003). A randomized trial comparing lung-volume reduction surgery with medical therapy for severe emphysema. *N Engl J Med, 348*, 2059–2073.
58. Nwogu, C. E. (2001). Primary malignant neoplasms of the lung. In H. L. Karamanoukian, P. R. Soltoski, & T. A. Salerno (Eds.), *Thoracic surgery secrets*. Philadelphia: Hanley & Belfus.
59. Panadero, R. (2015). Diagnosis and treatment of malignant pleural mesothelioma. *Arch Bronconeumol, 51*, 177–184.
60. Parelkar, S. V., et al. (2012). Traumatic diaphragmatic hernia: management by video-assisted thoracoscopic repair. *J Indian Assoc Pediatr Surg, 17*, 180–183.
61. Peng, Z., et al. (2014). A retrospective study of chronic post-surgical pain following thoracic surgery: prevalence, risk factors, incidence of neuropathic component, and impact on quality of life. *PLoS One, 9*, 1–8.
62. Ponn, R. B. (2005). Complications of pulmonary resection. In T. Shields, et al. (Ed.), *General thoracic surgery* (6th ed.). Philadelphia: Lippincott Williams & Wilkins.
63. Port, J. L., Korst, R. & Altorki, N. K. (2005). Transthoracic resection of the esophagus. In T. Shields, et al. (Ed.), *General thoracic surgery* (6th ed.). Philadelphia: Lippincott Williams & Wilkins.
64. Powers, C. J. & Karamanoukian, H. L. (2001). Esophageal diverticula. In H. L. Karamanoukian, P. R. Soltoski, & T. A. Salerno (Eds.), *Thoracic surgery secrets*. Philadelphia: Hanley & Belfus.
65. Qiu, T. (2013). External suction versus water seal after selective pulmonary resection for lung neoplasm: a systematic review. *PLoS One, 8*, 1–7.
66. Rawal, N. (2012). Epidural technique for postoperative pain: gold standard no more. *Reg Anesth Pain Med, 37*, 310–317.
67. Ricci, M. & Karamanoukian, R. L. (2001). Achalasia. In H. L. Karamanoukian, P. R. Soltoski, & T. A. Salerno (Eds.), *Thoracic surgery secrets*. Philadelphia: Hanley & Belfus.
68. Ris, H. B. & Krueger, T. (2006). Video-assisted thoracoscopic surgery and open decortication for pleural empyema. *Multimed Man Cardiothorac Surg, 2006*, 1–6.
69. Roberts, J. R., et al. (2000). Preemptive gastrointestinal tract management reduces aspiration and respiratory failure after thoracic operations. *J Thorac Cardiovasc Surg, 119*, 449–452.
70. Sack, S. Z. & Glatstein, E. (2005). Non-small cell lung cancer: importance of locoregional tumor control in the era of emerging adjuvant chemotherapy. *Principles Practice Updates Oncol, 19*, 1–15.
71. Schmidt-Hansen, M., Baldwin, D. R. & Zamora, J. (2015). FDG-PET/CT imaging for mediastinal staging in patients with potentially resectable non-small cell lung cancer. *JAMA, 313*, 1465–1466.
72. Segers, P. & DeMol, B. A. (2009). Prevention of ventilator-associated pneumonia after cardiac surgery: prepare and defend. *Intensive Care Med, 35*, 1497–1499.
73. Sengupta, S. (2015). Post-operative pulmonary complications after thoracotomy. *Indian J Anaesth, 59*, 618–626.
74. Shah, A. A. & D'Amico, T. A. (2009). Lung volume reduction surgery for the management of refractory dyspnea in chronic obstructive pulmonary disease. *Curr Opin Support Palliat Care, 3*, 107–111.
75. Sherry, V., Patton, N. & Stricker, C. T. (2010). Diagnosis and management of postpneumonectomy empyema with an Eloesser flap. *Clin J Oncl Nurs, 14*, 553–556.
76. Shields, T. W. (2005). General features of pulmonary resections. In T. Shields, et al. (Ed.), *General thoracic surgery* (6th ed.). Philadelphia: Lippincott Williams & Wilkins.
77. Srour, N., et al. (2013). Management of malignant pleural effusions with indwelling pleural catheters or talc pleurodesis. *Can Respir J, 20*, 106–110.
78. Suárez, P. M. & Gilart, J. L. (2013). Pleurodesis in the treatment of pneumothorax and pleural effusion. *Monaldi Arch Chest Dis, 79*, 81–86.
79. Subotic, D., et al. (2009). Lung function changes and complications after lung cancer in septuagenarians. *Ann Thorac Med, 4*, 54–59.
80. Takaoka, S. T. & Weinacker, A. B. (2005). The value of preoperative pulmonary rehabilitation. *Thorac Surg Clin, 15*, 203–211.
81. Tassi, G. F. (2010). Practical management of pleural empyema. *Monaldi Arch Chest Dis, 73*, 124–129.
82. Tomaszek, S. C. & Wigle, D. A. (2011). Surgical management of lung cancer. *Semin Respir Crit Care Med, 32*, 69–77.
83. Veeramachaneni, N. K., et al. (2012). Management of Stage IIA non-small cell lung cancer by thoracic surgeons in North America. *Ann Thorac Surg, 94*, 922–928.
84. Weksler, B., et al. (2012). Surgical resection should be considered for stage I and II small cell carcinoma of the lung. *Ann Thorac Surg, 94*, 889–894.
85. Win, T., et al. (2007). The effect of lung resection on pulmonary function and exercise capacity in lung cancer patients. *Respir Care, 52*, 720–726.
86. World Health Organization (WHO). (2015). *National Heart, Lung and Blood Institute (NHLBI)*. Lung health and diseases.
87. Wormuth, J. K. & Heitmiller, R. F. (2006). Esophageal conduit necrosis. *Thorac Surg Clin, 16*, 11–22.
88. Xhang, P., et al. (2012). Completion pneumonectomy for lung cancer treatment: early and long term outcomes. *J Cardiothorac Surg, 7*, 1749–8090.
89. Yu, H., & Burke, C. T. (2011). Management of pleural effusion, empyema, and lung abscess. *Semin Intervent Radiol, 28*, 75–86.
90. Zanotti, G. & Mitchell, J. D. (2015). Bronchopleural fistula and empyema after anatomic lung resection. *Thorac Surg Clin, 25*, 421–427.
91. Zarogoulidis, K. (2013). Malignant pleural effusion and algorithm management. *J Thorac Dis, 5*, S413–S419.
92. Zhang, Y. (2013). Epidemiology of esophageal cancer. *World J Gastroenterol, 19*, 5598–5606.

12

Head Injury and Dysfunction

Karen March

Traumatic brain injury (TBI) results from any mechanical disruption of brain tissue from an impact or injury to the head resulting in an activation of a complex series of biochemical responses. Severe head injury can be one of the most complex and challenging conditions with which clinicians must contend, requiring a coordinated, comprehensive, and interprofessional approach.[154]

In the United States, nearly 2.5 million people sustain TBIs each year. Of these, more than 52,000 die, 275,000 are hospitalized, and 2.2 million are treated and released from emergency departments.[62,129] Fifty to eighty percent of the emergency room visits are for mild TBIs.[129,165] Children (0–4 years), older adolescents (15–19 years), and adults aged 75 years and older are more likely than others to sustain a TBI. Adults aged 65 and older sustain 155,000 TBIs each year. Adults aged 75 or older have the highest rates of TBI-related hospitalization and deaths. In every age group, males have a higher incidence of TBI than females.[129] The leading cause of TBI varies among age groups; falls contribute to 40% of TBIs and are most common in those younger than 14 years (55%) or older than 65 years (81%), 29.8% are motor vehicle related (15.5% pedestrian and 14.3% occupant), and 11% are due to assaults (75% of TBIs in 15–44 year age group).[31,129] Unfortunately, even as mortality rates from TBI have decreased in the United States (17.1 per 100,000 population, down from 18.5 per 100,000), there is still significant morbidity and long-term disabilities associated with TBI, leaving some patients in a persistent vegetative state or requiring constant supervision and care. The consequences of TBI are not only physical and cognitive but have significant financial and societal implications. It is estimated that the direct and indirect cost of TBI is 76.2 billion dollars annually.[31] Approximately 5.3 million Americans are living with disabilities resulting from TBI, though these numbers may be underestimated.[31,129,165]

Although there is no universally accepted definition of TBI, severity of injury is commonly classified using the Glasgow Coma Scale (GCS) score (Table 12.1), with a mild TBI being a GCS of 13 to 15, moderate being 9 to 12, and severe being a GCS of 8 or less.[109]

The GCS is a commonly used tool providing a standardized approach for assessment of level of consciousness (LOC) and is used for determination of TBI severity. The GCS has become the most widely used and accepted tool for outcome prediction; however, there are many limitations to the use of this tool and the GCS does not necessarily reflect the extent of injury associated with the TBI. It does not assess pupil response, laterality, or account for subtle changes with strength or movement of extremities. Skewed assessments and inaccurate scoring can result when patients are intubated, have language issues (dominate hemisphere injury or primary language spoken in another language), or have received medications that alter level of consciousness. Trauma patients often have concomitant spinal or other orthopedic injuries that can affect the accuracy of the GCS.[63,121] The GCS, although useful in determining LOC, needs to be used in conjunction with other neurologic assessment methods. A new scoring system called *Full Outline of UnResponsiveness (FOUR) Score* may be more comprehensive and predictive of outcome than GCS.[82,143,181]

The understanding of the underlying mechanisms of injury and the associated intracranial pathophysiology of TBI have been rapidly advancing. Outcomes following TBI can be significantly improved when the activities of all disciplines are integrated into a coordinated systematic approach in caring for the patient.

APPLIED PHYSIOLOGY

Serial neurologic assessment is of utmost importance for any patient with neurologic injuries and is especially true for patients who have sustained a TBI. Because patients with brain injuries can exhibit fluctuating neurologic examination, it is extremely important for the critical care nurse to be aware of how these changes may reflect with brain dysfunction and increased intracranial pressure (ICP).

The purpose of this chapter is not to review the basics of neurologic assessment or anatomy; however, Tables 12.2 through 12.4 and Figs. 12.1 and 12.2 review basic findings associated with traumatic brain dysfunction.

The brain represents 2% of body weight, and utilizes 15% of cardiac output, 20% of total body oxygen, and 25% of total body glucose supplies.[171] Fifty percent of the brain's metabolic function is used for synaptic activity, 25% for maintenance of ionic gradients, and 25% for biosynthesis. Most of the brain's metabolic function (95%) arises from aerobic glucose metabolism and requires a constant cerebral blood flow (CBF). In the acute period following TBI, many patients will have a 50% reduction in their cerebral metabolic rate of oxygen ($CMRO_2$).[18,19] This leads to calcium-mediated impairment of mitochondrial function which may lead to early cell death. A compensatory mechanism is to

TABLE 12.1 Glasgow Coma Scale

Eyes	Open	Spontaneously	4
		To verbal command	3
		To pain	2
		No response	1
Best motor response	To verbal command	Obeys	6
	To painful stimulus	Localizes pain	5
		Flexion—withdrawal	4
		Flexion—abnormal (decorticate rigidity)	3
		Extension (decerebrate rigidity)	2
		No response	1
Best verbal response		Oriented and converses	5
		Disoriented and converses	4
		Inappropriate words	3
		Incomprehensible sounds	2
		No response	1
Total			3–15

From References 63 and 121.

TABLE 12.2 Primary Functions of Brain Lobes

Lobe	Function
Frontal	Prefrontal Short-term memory Emotional responsiveness Abstract thinking Foresight/judgment Behavior/tactfulness Primary motor cortex Broca's speech area (dominant hemisphere)* Expressive speech/vocalization Intellect Personality
Temporal	Primary auditory cortex Visual task learning Dominant hemisphere* Wernicke's speech area Receptive speech/comprehension Interpretive area Intellect Emotion Long-term memory Dominant hemisphere: verbal Nondominant hemisphere: sensory
Parietal	Primary sensory cortex Sensory interpretation Tactile and kinesthetic sense Body awareness Body image Spatial orientation/relations Dominant hemisphere Language Object perception recognition Nondominant hemisphere Neglect syndrome
Occipital	Primary visual cortex Visual association

*Dominance: The majority (80%) of both right- and left-handed people have left hemispheric dominance for speech. A small percentage of left-handed people have both right and left hemispheric speech control. The preponderance of left cerebral dominance is felt to be due to anatomic asymmetry of the human brain. Sixty-five percent of people have a larger speech area (Wernicke's area) surface on the left hemisphere, in 11% the right is larger, and in 24% the right and left sides are equal in size. Hemispheric lateralization or dominance is also found in functions related to mood and affect, as well as verbal, auditory, and visuospatial tasks.
From Reference 116.

TABLE 12.3 Pupil Abnormalities Related to Brain Dysfunction

Pupil Findings	Related Dysfunction	Other Potential Causes
Unilateral fixed and dilated pupil	Ipsilateral oculomotor (CN III) compression or injury	Instillation of mydriatics (e.g., scopolamine, atropine) Orbital injuries
Bilateral fixed and dilated pupils	Severe brain anoxia and ischemia; bilateral CN III compression	Medications (e.g., dopamine, amphetamines, atropine)
Pinpoint, nonreactive pupils	Pons damage	Miotic agents, opiates Overdose
Small, equal, reactive pupils	Bilateral diencephalic damage affecting sympathetic innervation originating from hypothalamus	Metabolic dysfunction
Nonreactive, midpositioned pupils	Midbrain damage	

TABLE 12.4 Respiratory Patterns Associated with Brain Dysfunction

Name	Description	Neuroanatomic Brain Lesions
Cheyne-Stokes respirations	Regular cycles of respirations that gradually increase in depth to hyperpnea and then decrease in depth to periods of apnea	Usually bilateral lesions deep within cerebral hemispheres, diencephalon, and basal ganglia
Central neurogenic hyperventilation	Deep, rapid respiration	Midbrain, upper pons
Apneustic respirations	Prolonged inspirations followed by a 2- to 3-second pause; occasionally may alternate with an expiratory pause	Pons
Cluster respirations	Clusters of irregular breaths followed by an apneic period lasting a variable amount of time	Lower pons and upper medulla
Ataxic or Biot's respirations	Irregular, unpredictable pattern of shallow and deep respirations and pauses	Medulla

From Reference 116.

increase glucose utilization (hyperglycolysis) in order to restore ion gradients. This mechanism, however, is short lived.[178]

Cerebral Hemodynamics

Cerebral blood flow (CBF) is a function of influx pressures (systole), efflux pressures (venous outflow), vascular radius (capacitance), and blood viscosity. Other autoregulatory mechanisms include extravascular pH as influenced by the partial pressure of arterial carbon dioxide ($Paco_2$), the partial pressure of arterial oxygen tension (Pao_2), vasoreactivity, the metabolic need, and neurogenic factors (sympathetic and parasympathetic innervation).[104] CBF averages 50 mL/100 grams of brain tissue per minute (50 mL/100 g/min) with normal CBF being

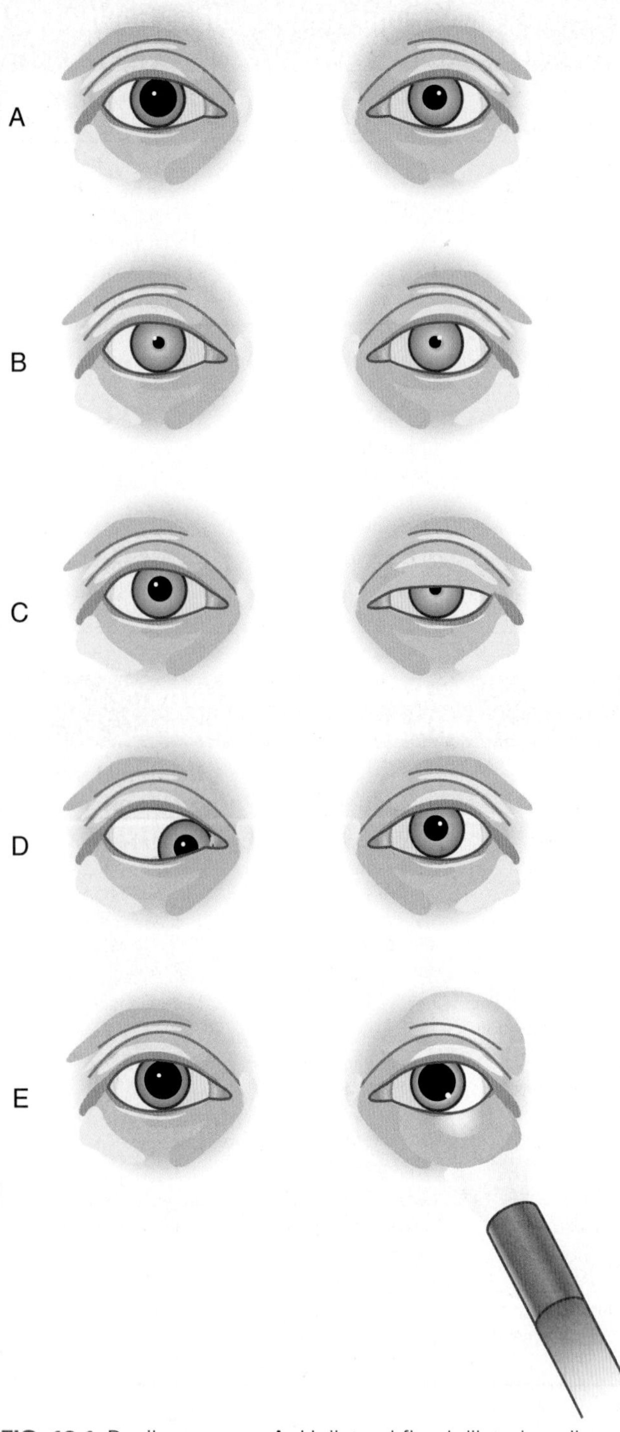

FIG. 12.1 Pupil response. **A,** Unilateral fixed dilated pupil: pressure on cranial nerve (CN) III. **B,** Pinpoint pupils: brain stem hemorrhage. **C,** Unilateral small pupil and ptosis: Horner syndrome with sympathetic/parasympathetic dysfunction. **D,** Failure of eyes to look downward and inward (left eye is normal eye): CN IV palsy. **E,** Bilateral fixed dilated pupils: brain herniation.

higher in the cortex (approximately 80 mL/100 g/min and approximately 20 mL/100 g/min in the white matter).[177] CBF may be markedly reduced within the first few hours after severe brain injury.[18,19] Ischemia levels of CBF (approximately 15 mL/100 g/min) may be seen during the acute phase of TBI (first 24 hours) leading to cell dysfunction. Cell death occurs at 8 to 10 mL/100 g/min.[17,179] CBF greater than 55 to 60 mL/100 g/min is called *hyperemia.* Hyperemia is often associated with impaired autoregulation and vasodilation, leading to increased ICP, and is seen more frequently in children.[176]

The net driving force for the cerebral circulation is cerebral perfusion pressure (CPP), which is defined as the difference between mean arterial pressure (MAP) and ICP. Cerebral autoregulation is the brain's ability to keep cerebral blood flow relatively constant despite changes in CPP. Autoregulation allows the brain to maintain a constant blood flow even in the face of wide variations in systemic mean arterial pressures. A constant CBF is maintained between pressures of 50 to 150 mm Hg by vasoconstriction as CPP increases and vasodilation as CPP decreases (Fig. 12.3). When vasomotor autoregulation is lost, CBF becomes closely correlated with MAP and CPP. CBF will increase with increases in MAP/CPP and decrease with a fall in CPP/MAP.[35] Two other mechanisms that are important in controlling CBF are flow metabolism coupling and metabolic (chemical) need. Flow metabolism coupling is the relationship of CBF with metabolic need. As metabolic need increases, CBF increases. This mechanism is often impaired following injury, either as uncoupling when at-rest flow matches demand but cannot increase when demand increases, or mismatch when flow never meets demand. Both result in cerebral ischemia. Metabolic autoregulation is the result of changes in extravascular pH and may be associated with the changes in $Paco_2$ and Pao_2. Hypoxia and hypercarbia may lead to acidosis (decreased pH) resulting in vasodilation whereas hypercarbia (hyperventilation) leads to alkalosis and vasoconstriction.[86,179]

MECHANISM OF INJURY

All cranial injuries involve the transmission of kinetic energy through the brain. These pressure waves vary in magnitude and duration, resulting in damage to vascular structures from impact, strain, rotation, and compression.

Common mechanisms of injury related to TBI can be divided broadly into two categories: blunt or penetrating injuries. Mechanisms of blunt TBI within these categories include acceleration-deceleration injury, deformation, and rotation (Fig. 12.4). Most blunt injuries are a result of motor vehicle crashes, motorcycle crashes, pedestrian injuries, falls, or assaults. In the pediatric population, shaken baby syndrome and other causes of nonaccidental trauma are a major concern.

Acceleration injury occurs when a moving object hits the stationary skull and brain. Deceleration injury occurs when the moving head hits a stationary object, causing the skull to stop abruptly. As the brain moves within the skull, it collides with the inner cranial surface and its rough bony prominences. The brain then moves backward in the opposite direction colliding with the contralateral skull surface, leading to coup-contrecoup injury (Fig. 12.5).[111] Rotation may also occur with acceleration-deceleration injuries, resulting in a torsion of the brain structures within the skull. Rotational forces produce shearing of brain tissue or vascular structures. Injury severity is dependent upon the speed, direction, force of rotation, and impact.[71,92] Current biomechanical research suggest that most brain injuries result from rotational forces and skull fractures occurring from linear forces.[92]

Penetrating injuries are most commonly related to missile injuries from bullets (gunshot) or stab wounds. However, any object that penetrates the skull into the brain tissue

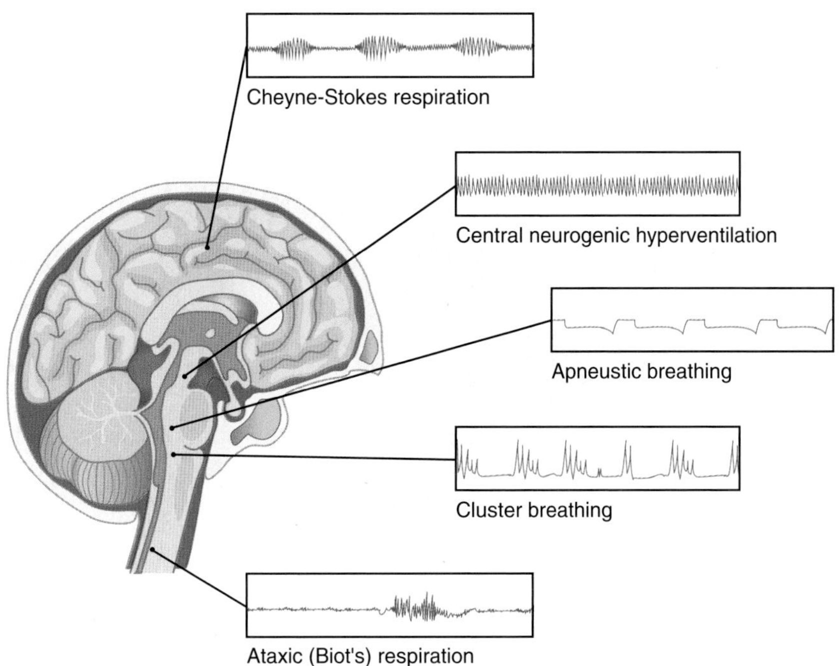

FIG. 12.2 Increased intracranial pressure-associated changes in respiratory patterns.

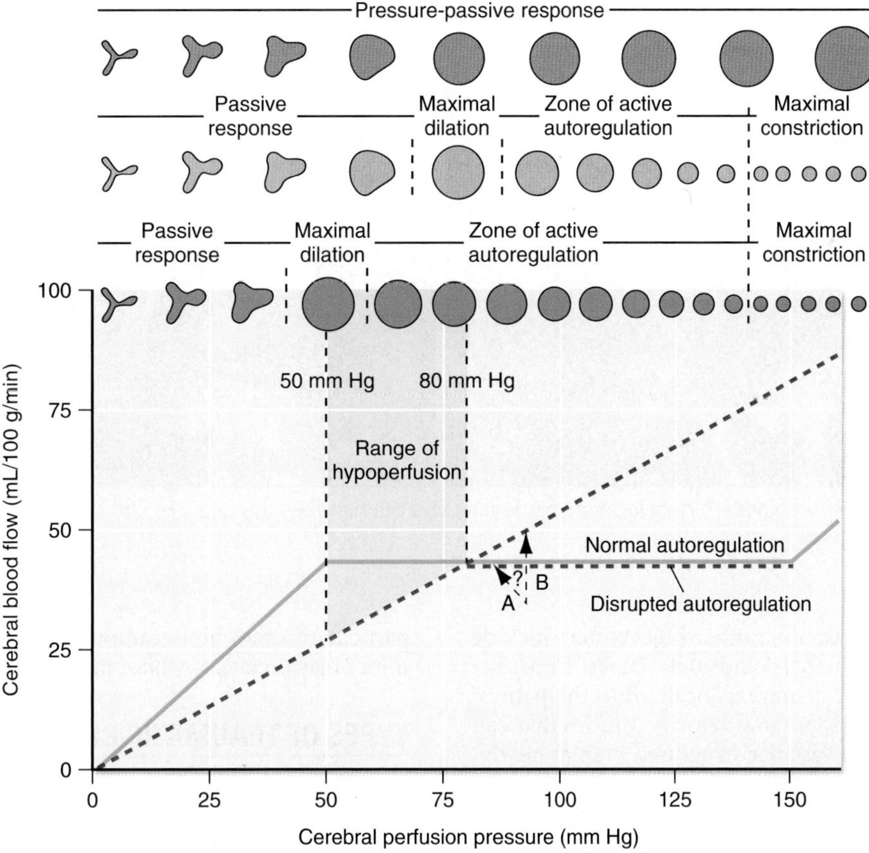

FIG. 12.3 Mechanisms of normal and disrupted autoregulation. The top three rows represent the vascular system. *Bottom row:* Intact autoregulation (AR). *Middle row:* Partially disrupted AR. *Top row:* Complete disruption of AR. On the graph, the *solid line* represents normal pressure AR in the range of 50 to 150 mm Hg *(bottom row above)*. The *broken line* represents disrupted pressure AR and illustrates its pressure-passive nature (line *B*) where cerebral blood flow is directly proportional to cerebral perfusion pressure (CPP). In partial disruption (line *A*), the system is pressure-passive up to 80 mm Hg, followed by pressure AR occurring until pressure exceeds 150 mm Hg. NOTE: The range of hypoperfusion between 50 and 80 mm Hg may represent ischemia even when CPP appears to be normal.

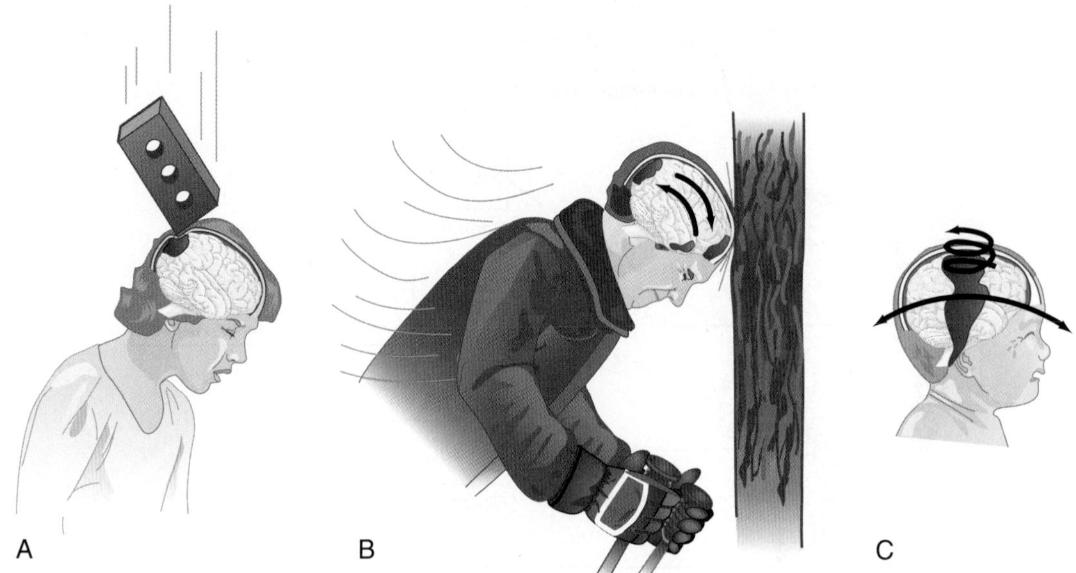

FIG. 12.4 Mechanisms of injury. **A,** Deformation. **B,** Acceleration-deceleration. **C,** Rotation.

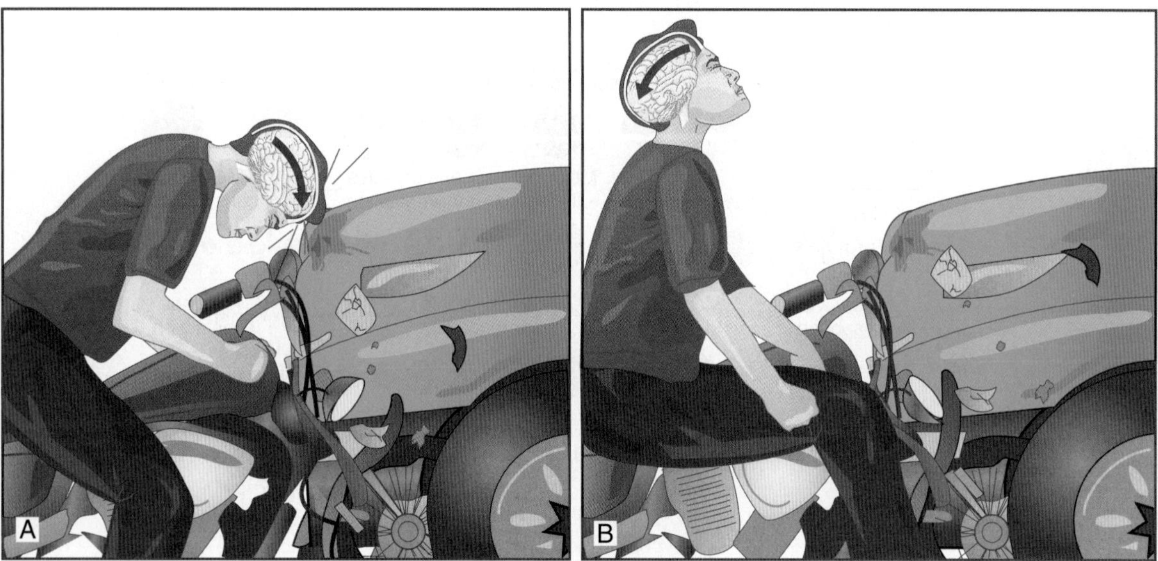

FIG. 12.5 Acceleration-deceleration injuries. **A,** The brain strikes the skull. **B,** The brain rebounds.

can result in penetrating trauma; other objects may include shrapnel, arrows, nails, hatchets, and metal pipes. In a penetrating injury, the area of damage is localized to the path of the object.[57,88] Stab wounds are low-velocity injuries that can cause localized damage to vascular structures, cranial nerves, and white matter fiber tracts along its path. High-velocity injuries such as bullets not only cause damage along its path but also have an expanded injury path from cavitation formed by the conic waves transmitted by the velocity, size, and yaw of the bullet.[58]

Blast injury is another type of injury that may be seen in patients exposed to explosion. Blast waves are changes in atmospheric pressure that are transmitted through soft tissues such as the brain. These pressure changes are the result of pressurization of gases, putting stress and strain on the brain tissues, particularly the hippocampus and brainstem. Penetrating injury may accompany blast injury.[93,105]

TYPES OF TRAUMATIC BRAIN INJURY

Regardless of the underlying mechanism, damage to the brain typically results in focal or diffuse lesions. Diffuse brain injury and focal brain injury can coexist, especially in the severely injured patient.

Focal Injuries

Focal injuries are generally associated with a direct impact to the head. These localized brain injuries are typically easier to identify and some can be treated surgically. Focal injuries generally result in hematomas or contusions. Hematomas are categorized by their location in relation to the brain tissue and meningeal layers.

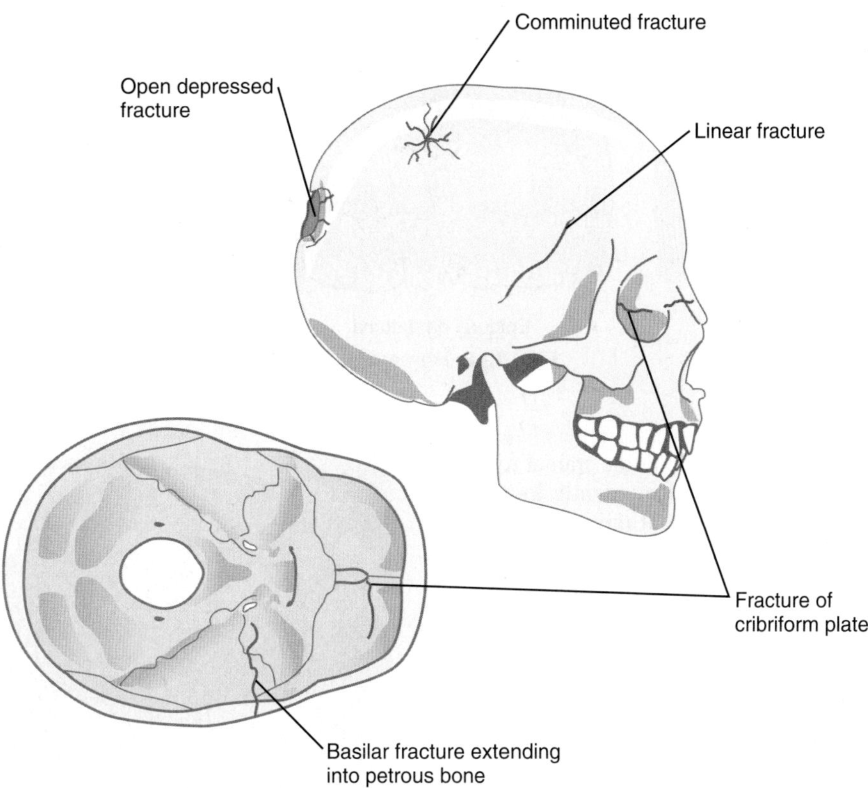

FIG. 12.6 Types of skull fractures.

Symptomatology, morbidity, and mortality from focal injuries are affected by the size, location, and progression of the lesion.

Skull Fractures

Although not technically brain injuries, many skull fractures can cause or accompany underlying brain injury (Fig. 12.6). The more severe the brain injury, the greater likelihood an associated skull fracture may be present.

A simple linear fracture is the most benign type of fracture and typically does not require any specific treatment. However, it is helpful to perform a computed tomography (CT) scan to assess for any associated brain injuries, especially if the fracture is in the temporal region where underlying arteries are present and easily torn.[111]

Depressed skull fractures are more complex, resulting in cranial bone being forced below the normal plane of the skull, and impingement on brain tissue. Depressed skull fractures result in lacerations of the meninges, brain parenchyma, and hematomas. Surgical treatment of this injury is sometimes required for debridement and evacuation of associated clots or bone fragments, repair of dural lacerations, and elevation of the depressed bone fragment. These patients are at high risk of infection and posttraumatic epilepsy.[27]

Basilar skull fractures are located at the base of the cranium, generally in the anterior or middle fossa. These fractures are best diagnosed by using CT bone windows and clinical findings.[67] Fractures of the anterior fossa exhibit periorbital ecchymosis (raccoon eyes), extensive subconjunctival hemorrhage, and cerebrospinal fluid (CSF) otorrhea. Fractures of the middle and posterior fossa will result in ecchymosis over the mastoid process (Battle's sign) and CSF rhinorrhea. Otorrhea and rhinorrhea are concerning because they indicate the presence of a dural tear, which places patients at risk for meningitis. Patients with basal skull fractures should have orogastric (OG) tubes placed rather than nasogastric (NG) tubes to prevent the inadvertent placement of the tube into the brain.[111,139]

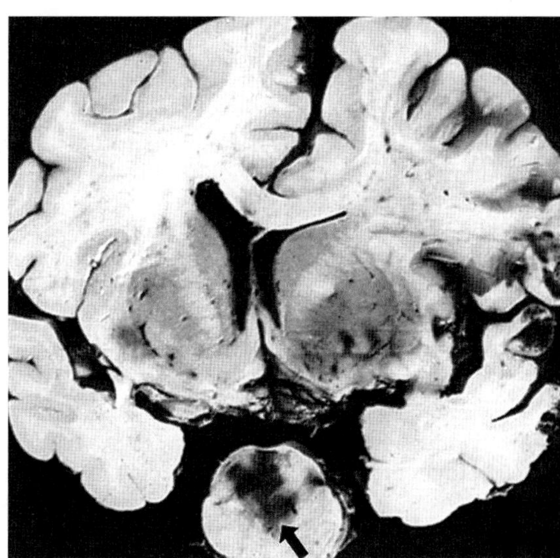

FIG. 12.7 Recent contusions of frontal and temporal lobes, with displacement of cingulate gyrus and lateral ventricles. Secondary hemorrhages are evident.

Contusions

Cerebral contusions are bruising of the subcortical white matter from damage to small blood vessels in the parenchyma (Fig. 12.7). Injury occurs when brain tissue moves across the

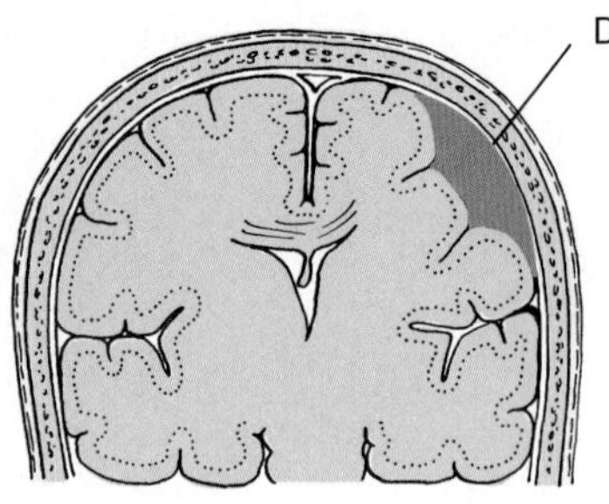
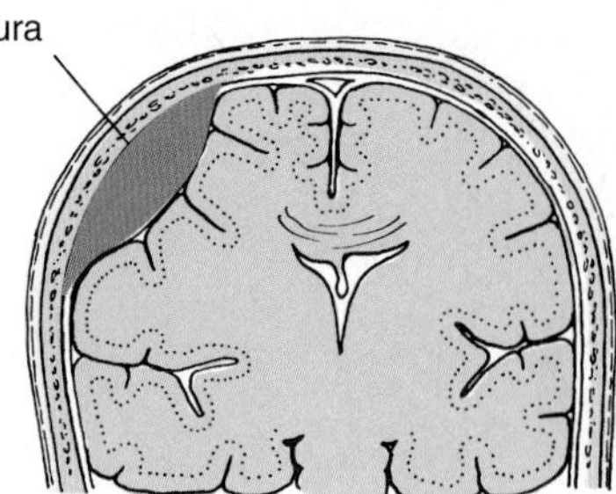

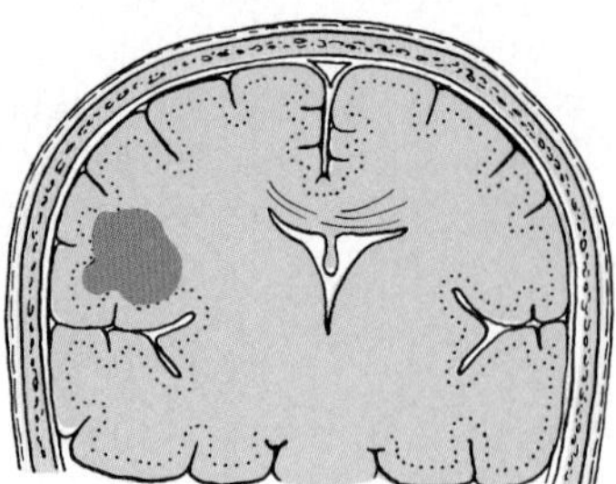
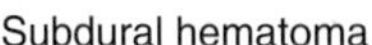

FIG. 12.8 Hematomas.

irregular bony surfaces of the anterior and middle cranial fossa during rapid deceleration. Contusions are frequently located in the inferior frontal lobes and inferolateral temporal lobes. Severity of injury is dependent on the site of injury and the extent of contused brain. Cerebral contusions rarely occur in the occipital lobes and cerebellum. Because contusions often occur in frontal and temporal lobes, patients often present with behavior and personality changes as well as speech and motor deficits. Contusions can resolve with little consequence or may worsen over time, often referred to as *blossoming contusions.* However, expanding lesions may lead to increased mass effect and increased intracranial pressure.[111]

Contusions are classified as gliding or surface. Gliding contusions are seen with rotational forces affecting the parasagittal tissue and are associated with diffuse axonal injuries. Surface contusions are caused by contact related to fractures, coup-contrecoup, and herniation.[111,139]

Hematomas

Epidural, subdural, and intracerebral hematomas are illustrated in Fig. 12.8 and discussed in the sections that follow.

Epidural Hematoma

An epidural hematoma (EDH) is arterial bleeding between the skull and dura mater, giving the EDH its classic lens shape (Fig. 12.9). An EDH occurs in 2.7% to 4% of TBI patients, with approximately 10% being fatal.[24] EDH most commonly occurs in the second decade of life. EDH occurs most frequently in the temporal-parietal region and is associated with laceration of the middle meningeal artery as a result of a temporal skull fracture. Other sources of EDH arise from bleeding from the middle meningeal vein or diploic vein, or bleeding from a venous sinus. Twenty to thirty percent of EDHs are found in the frontal region or posterior fossa. Approximately 50% of patients with an EDH present with a loss of consciousness, followed next by a period of lucidity, and then progress to a loss of consciousness. Patients may present with an ipsilateral dilated and fixed pupil and contralateral motor deficits. In patients with neurologic deterioration (development of coma and/or pupillary abnormality) and clot greater than 30 mL, immediate surgical evacuation will increase chances of a favorable outcome. If surgery is delayed, this injury can be fatal because of rapid arterial bleeding leading to cerebral herniation.[24]

Subdural Hematoma

A subdural hematoma (SDH) involves venous bleeding in the subdural space between the dura and arachnoid meninges (see Fig. 12.8). This produces a classic crescent-shaped collection of blood, with irregular edges visible on CT scan (Fig. 12.10). Acute SDHs occur in approximately 12% to 29% of severe head injuries. SDHs most commonly result from tearing of the tiny, bridging veins located between the cerebral cortex and the venous sinus, and are often the result of acceleration-deceleration injuries. Mortality ranges from 40% to 68%, with the lowest mortality occurring in patients who

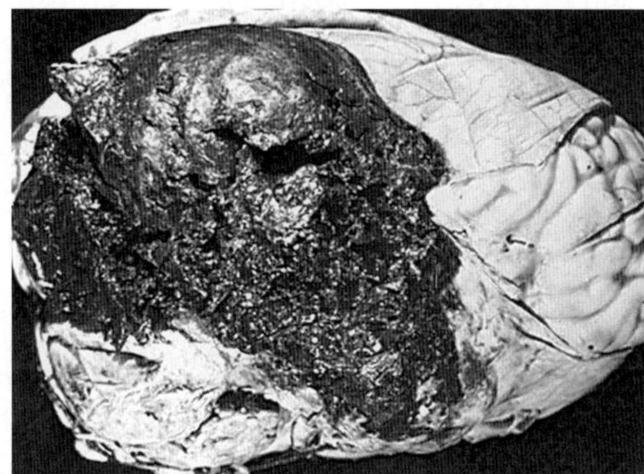

FIG. 12.9 Acute epidural hematoma. Skull fracture with tear of middle meningeal artery and vein.

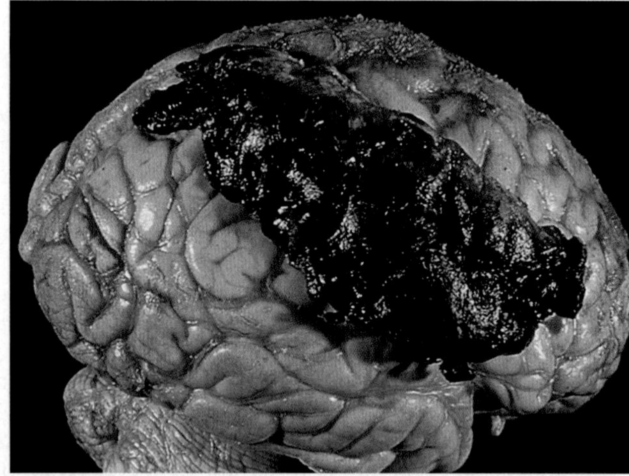

FIG. 12.10 Acute subdural hematoma (dura removed).

undergo surgery within 4 hours of injury. Eighty percent of patients presenting with an SDH have an adjacent parenchymal contusion. This underlying brain injury most strongly influences the patient's course and outcome.[25]

SDHs can be classified based on time from injury to presentation of symptoms. Acute SDH contains clotted blood and occurs either immediately upon impact or up to 48 to 72 hours later. Subacute hematoma contains a mixture of clotted blood and fluid and occurs within several days of the injury up to 3 weeks afterward. Chronic SDH occurs 3 weeks or more after injury and consists mostly of fluid. Older adults, chronic alcohol abusers, and those taking anticoagulants will have a greater incidence of chronic SDH. Presentation of the chronic SDH is most commonly confusion, slowed processing, headache, drowsiness, and seizures.[111]

Intracerebral Hematoma

Intracerebral hematomas (ICHs) are areas of bleeding within the brain parenchyma from contusions or blood vessel injury at the time of the primary injury resulting in a mass lesion (see Fig. 12.8).[26] Some ICHs evolve over time and are called *delayed traumatic ICH* or *DITCH*. When caused by trauma, hematomas are found most commonly in the white matter of the frontal and temporal lobes, whereas hypertensive ICH is deeper in the thalamus, basal ganglia, or parasagittal white matter. Bleeding is caused by rupture of parenchymal blood vessels at the time of injury, and ICHs are noted on CT scan as hyperdense areas representing intraparenchymal hemorrhage. ICH occurs in 13% to 35% of severe head injury patients. One-third to one-half of the patients with an ICH are unconscious on admission, and up to 20% demonstrate a lucid interval between the time of injury and the onset of coma.[26] Frequent (hourly) neurologic assessments are critical to identify signs of mass lesion and intracranial hypertension. Lesions with hematoma volumes greater than 20 mL, with a midline shift of greater than 5 mm, compressed cisterns, or 50 cc with increased ICP, require surgery.[26]

Diffuse Injuries

Diffuse injuries are microscopic neuronal injuries, making them difficult to detect on CT. The most common types of diffuse injuries are concussions and diffuse axonal injuries.

Concussion

A concussion is the onset of transient neurologic dysfunction that results after complex bio-mechanical forces. Patients may or may not have a loss of consciousness (LOC). Other symptoms of a concussion include LOC of less than 30 minutes, amnesia to the event, confusion, headache, disorientation, dizziness, and disturbances with vision.[119,182] Concussions are typically diagnosed clinically and do not present with any identifiable lesions on CT scan. Concussions result from axonal injury and swelling, especially of the hippocampal neurons, disruption of the reticular activating system, alterations in metabolism, neurotransmitter function, and ionic shifts. During this time, the brain is particularly vulnerable to a secondary injury (second impact syndrome). The majority of patients will recover spontaneously.[182]

Diffuse Axonal Injuries

Diffuse axonal injury (DAI) or traumatic axonal injury is the presence of diffuse axonal injury of the frontotemporal white matter; periaqueductal gray, corpus callosum; rostral brainstem; or septum pellucidum. DAI often results in immediate and prolonged unconsciousness. The pathophysiology of DAI is thought to result from stretching and swelling of axons and tearing of microvasculature. Axonal chromolysis (breakdown) and myelin degeneration leads to an influx of extracellular ions, such as calcium, resulting in DAI. Sodium and calcium channels are disrupted leading to cellular edema (cytotoxic) and mitochondrial dysfunction, leading to further cell death. This tissue damage continues to occur for several hours to days after the injury. Accumulation of beta-amyloid precursor protein occurs, which may lead to symptoms later in life.[71]

DAI is not easily seen on CT scans and requires magnetic resonance imaging (MRI) for confirmation. CT scans may reveal small punctate hemorrhages, but often CT scans appear negative and diagnosis is based on clinical exam in which there is a lack of radiographic findings to explain the patient's loss of consciousness. MRI is required to identify and qualify the injury as mild, moderate, or severe. The extent and location of axonal damage will determine the outcome associated with this type of injury. High morbidity and mortality have been associated with DAI, and these patients are often left in a persistent vegetative state.[148]

Traumatic Subarachnoid Hemorrhage

Traumatic subarachnoid hemorrhage (TSAH) is another type of diffuse injury. TSAH is commonly associated with rupture of aneurysms or arteriovenous malformations (AVMs), but also occurs as a result of traumatic injury to the brain. Thirty-three to sixty-eight percent of TBI will have TSAH that increases mortality.[96,166] TSAH involves bleeding into the subarachnoid space and is often associated with an acute SDH and/or contusions. Unlike aneurysmal SAH, which is seen with the blood at the base of the brain, TSAH is seen with the blood over the convexity of the brain. SAH interferes with the normal circulation and reabsorption of CSF, increasing the risk of hydrocephalus and subsequent intracranial hypertension. It is estimated that 2% to 41% of patients with TSAH will develop delayed ischemic events resulting from vasospasm, which is associated with poor outcomes.[96,179]

PATHOPHYSIOLOGY

Damage from TBI occurs via two mechanisms: primary and secondary injury. The initial primary injury to the brain results in cellular damage from mechanical forces discussed previously. These forces produce immediate neuronal dysfunction and death as a result of damage to blood vessels, axons, and neurons. Secondary injury is a more complex set of events activated by a massive neuronal depolarization, which follows the primary injury. These processes include biochemical, metabolic, and inflammatory cascades leading to ischemia, cerebral edema, inflammation, and cell death. Each of these processes will be discussed more in depth later in the chapter.[96,107,155]

Ischemia

Ischemia is a major trigger of the pathophysiologic cascade. In one study, 90% of patients with a fatal TBI showed evidence of regional and global cerebral ischemia on autopsy. Hypotension during the acute phase following TBI has been shown to double the mortality. The effect of hypotension depends on the magnitude, duration (burden), and the ischemia it causes.[36] Areas most affected are those in the distal circulation where vessels are few and smaller referred as *watershed areas*. Patients with multisystem trauma are particularly susceptible because of decreased cerebral perfusion from systemic hemorrhage related to other injuries or shock. CBF is further reduced at the tissue level by such processes as astrocytic swelling, hypotension, and elevated ICP, all of which cause cellular dysfunction and potentiation for secondary brain injury. Hypoxemia tends to have a global effect.[179]

Ischemic areas surrounding hematomas and contusions are called *penumbra*. Brain tissue in this region is particularly vulnerable to inadequate perfusion and is dependent on strategies to optimize treatments to improve perfusion to maintain and salvage viable tissue. Specific neuroprotective strategies are designed to target the cells in the penumbra, preserve cellular function, and limit the area of neuronal death. Neuroprotective strategies will be discussed later in this chapter.[107,155]

Multiple systemic mechanisms may contribute to secondary brain damage after TBI, including hypotension, hypoxemia, hyperthermia, hypercarbia, hypo- and hyperglycemia, and electrolyte imbalances. Intracranial mechanisms contributing to secondary injury are intracranial hypertension, development of delayed hematomas, vascular injury, vasospasm, and seizures.[107,155] At the cellular level, the process leading to secondary brain injury involves a cascade of complex molecular events that, if not recognized and reversed, produce cellular damage and cerebral edema.[74] This can result in increased ICP, inadequate tissue perfusion, neuronal cell death, permanent neurologic impairment, and the initiation of a self-perpetuating cycle of neuronal damage. This secondary damage is potentially preventable and reversible with early recognition and adequate treatment.[107,155]

The downward trajectory often associated with the cellular ischemic cascade and subsequent secondary brain injury begins immediately after the primary impact. Ischemia, excitotoxicity, impaired metabolism, blood-brain barrier (BBB) disruption, loss of autoregulation, and inflammatory factors have all been implicated in secondary brain injury.[79,179]

Neurotoxicity

When there is a decrease in oxygen availability to the cell, tissue hypoxia and lactic acidosis develop. This ischemic damage causes the release of excitatory amino acids (EAAs), glutamate, and aspartate.[60] These amino acids act as excitatory neurotransmitters to influence receptor-operated calcium channels in damaged brain tissue, thereby altering intracellular concentrations of sodium and calcium and leading to neuronal cell death (see Fig. 12.13).[9,179]

Glutamate initiates cell membrane depolarization, allowing movement of calcium and sodium into the cell and an efflux of potassium out of the cell through ion channels such as *N*-methyl-d-aspartate (NMDA) receptors. Activation of glutamate receptors also causes the generation of highly reactive free radical molecules like nitric oxide. Neurotoxicity from activation of glutamate receptors is due to excessive intracellular calcium levels and the subsequent production of toxic levels of nitric oxide.[179]

High levels of intracellular calcium activate phospholipases leading to breakdown of the cell wall and formation of EAA, which lead to the development of reactive oxygen species (ROS) or oxygen free radical. Oxygen free radicals are active in many chemical reactions and are necessary for life, but can also result in cell damage via unwanted side effects. In TBI, oxygen free radicals are associated with the inhibition of cell membrane-mediated ion exchange activity, the release of arachidonic acid, and neuron apoptosis. Associated adenosine triphosphate (ATP) depletion leads to increased calcium levels, triggering further ion permeability at the mitochondrial membrane level.[11,179] The mitochondria swell and trigger oxidative phosphorylation, resulting in more free radicals and cell death. These oxygen free radicals also lead to lipid peroxidation, causing the breakdown of the cell membrane and oxidation of lipoproteins further destroying the cell. This process will spread to adjacent cells, perpetuating the process and killing more cells.[11]

TBI triggers various cellular processes that lead to an excess of intracellular calcium.[120,179] Calcium concentration increases tenfold within seconds of onset of severe ischemia, causing a rapid and massive increase of intracellular free calcium ions within minutes of the initial injury. This overabundance of intracellular calcium activates and sustains additional mechanisms that lead to secondary brain injury via multiple metabolic pathways. The net result is a dangerous increase in intracellular ion concentrations, furthering and perpetuating inflammation, ischemia, and neural damage.[112,120,179] Fig. 12.11 outlines the mechanisms activated by an increase in intracellular calcium concentration. The common final end points of the processes described earlier are neurotoxicity, the release of cellular contents, and neuronal death (Figs. 12.12 and 12.13).

Cerebral ischemic and metabolic changes result in widespread cell membrane depolarization and release of neurotransmitters into the extracellular space. The associated failure of cellular membrane pumps, excess intracellular calcium, and reduction in available ATP provide additional pathways that lead to neuronal swelling (cytotoxic edema) or cell death. The cumulative effects of these pathologic mechanisms affect patients with severe head injury to varying degrees.[11,179]

Impaired Metabolism

The brain depends on the delivery of oxygen and glucose for aerobic metabolism and the production of ATP. Impairment of perfusion and oxygenation frequently follows severe head injury, most likely related to hypermetabolism. This metabolic derangement is a common and important consequence of TBI.[9] Studies have documented an increase in oxygen consumption of up to 89% in sedated patients and 138% in nonsedated patients. Accelerated metabolism further depletes already inadequate oxygen and glucose supplies, potentiating hypoxia, anaerobic metabolism, and secondary brain injury.[11]

Neuronal cell death can also be related to an increase in regional glucose utilization usually noted in the first few days after injury. This early posttraumatic hyperglycolysis may result from cellular efforts to reestablish normal ionic gradients. In the absence of adequate oxygen, the cell shifts to an increase in glucose metabolism, glycolysis. This hyperglycolysis results in an increase in lactic acid formation that is used as temporary fuel for the cells metabolism.[12,179] Lactate generation and anaerobic cerebral metabolism occur even when blood flow is adequate, suggesting that trauma incapacitates mitochondrial activity and causes a shift toward anaerobic metabolism. Evidence suggests a link between increased extracellular fluid (ECF), glutamate, and increased anaerobic glycolysis. Depending on the extent and severity of tissue damage, brain cells may be unable to restore ionic homeostasis despite a maximal increase in glycolytic activity. If tissue blood flow is reduced during an episode of maximal metabolic need, tissue glucose and oxygen levels fall to subthreshold levels. When glucose and oxygen levels fall, tissue swelling is exacerbated and ischemic necrosis will occur.[12,179]

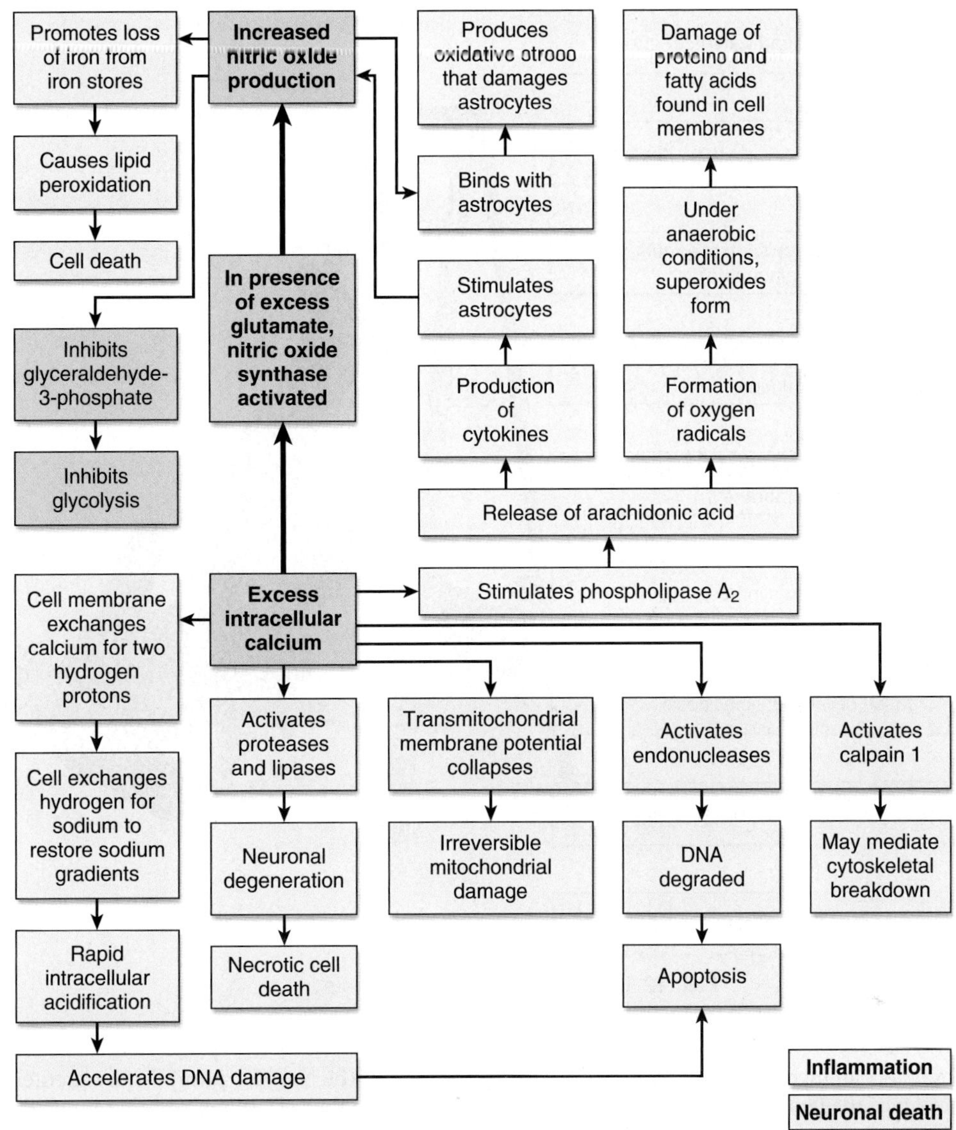

FIG. 12.11 Effects of calcium on brain injury.

Inflammatory Factors

The inflammatory response and the role of cytokines are critical factors in the pathophysiology of TBI. Cytokines are proteins that play a role in the expression of adhesion molecules, cellular filtration, and the release of other inflammatory cells and growth factors that lead to cell regeneration or cell death. Inflammatory mediators are stored intracellularly as precursor proteins and are eventually modified into active molecules. Cytokines are released as a defense response to infection, inflammation, trauma, and ischemia within minutes of TBI. Cytokine production following TBI occurs via intrinsic and extrinsic mechanisms. Intrinsic mechanisms produce cytokines from neurons, astrocytes, and microglia, whereas extrinsic mechanisms generate cytokines by infiltrating leukocytes.[79,164]

Overexpression of cytokines can be harmful to injured tissue and may even cause cell death. Conversely, some research suggests the tumor necrosis factor (TNF), interleukins (IL-1, IL-6, IL-8, IL-10, and IL-12), and nerve growth factor may be neuroprotective.[164] While information regarding cytokines involved in brain injury continues to evolve, the most commonly known cytokines are IL-1 and TNF. Both of these molecules act as mediators in neuronal apoptosis, causing neuronal loss in brain-injured patients.[100,164]

In addition, IL-1 and TNF can disrupt many endothelial cell activities, resulting in vascular endothelial damage and increased permeability. Normally, the vascular endothelium regulates coagulation and inflammatory responses, allowing lymphocytes and monocytes to efficiently adhere and penetrate vessel walls. When the vascular endothelium is damaged, however, the resulting prothrombotic condition causes intravascular coagulation. Furthermore, an overwhelming response by lymphocytes and monocytes causes injury to the vascular endothelium, leading to interstitialization of fluids and additional cytokine release.[79,100,164]

Types of Cerebral Edema

Progressive edema may result from leukotrienes released from white blood cells and platelets. Leukotrienes are chemoattractant agents primarily involved in the activation of inflammatory and immune responses. Brain swelling after head injury results

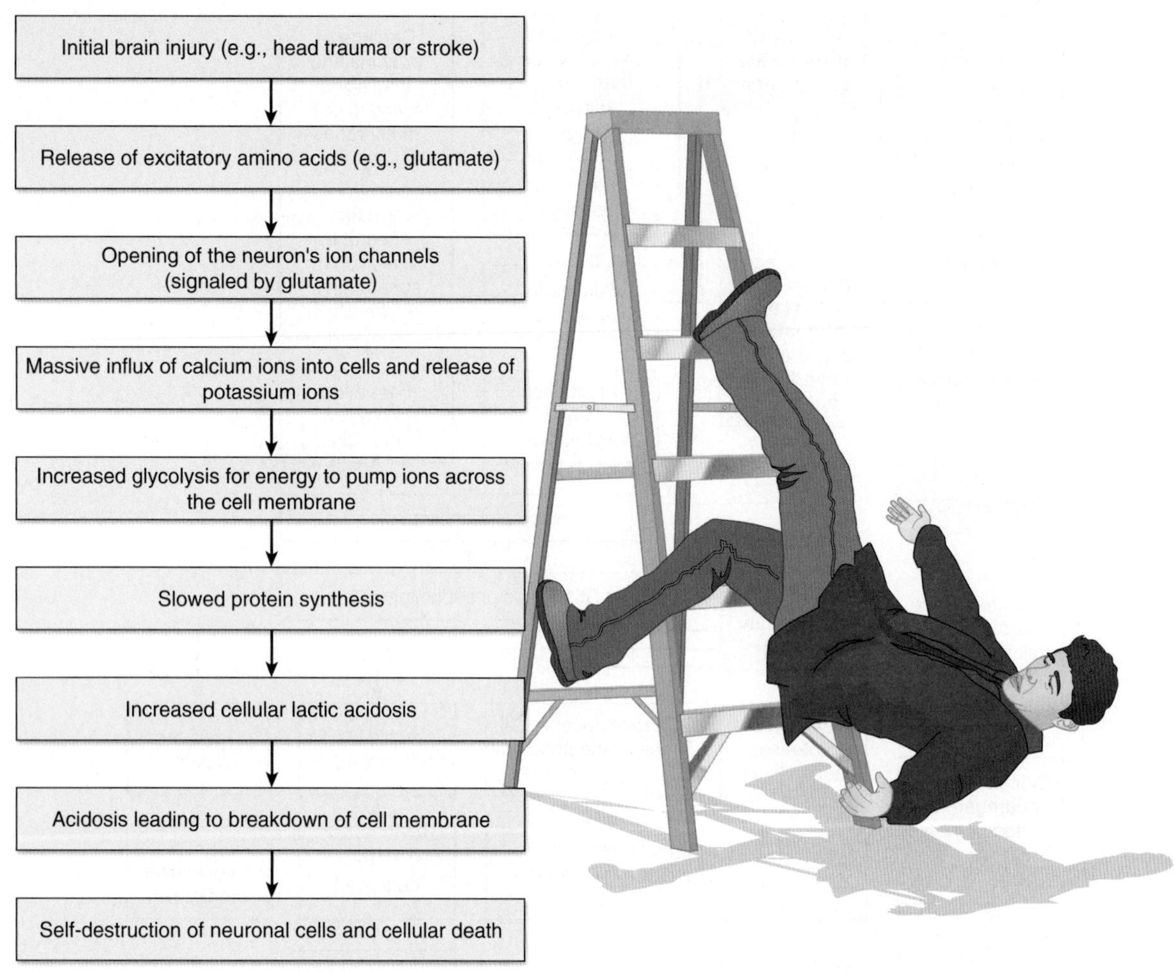
Initial brain injury (e.g., head trauma or stroke)
Release of excitatory amino acids (e.g., glutamate)
Opening of the neuron's ion channels (signaled by glutamate)
Massive influx of calcium ions into cells and release of potassium ions
Increased glycolysis for energy to pump ions across the cell membrane
Slowed protein synthesis
Increased cellular lactic acidosis
Acidosis leading to breakdown of cell membrane
Self-destruction of neuronal cells and cellular death

FIG. 12.12 Metabolic cascade of brain injury.

from cerebral cellular edema, an increase in intravascular blood volume, or a combination of the two.[164]

Though there are five types of cerebral edema, only two play a major role in TBI: cytotoxic and vasogenic. In the first hours after TBI, vasogenic edema occurs. Vasogenic edema occurs with the disruption in the BBB. The BBB is the cellular barrier responsible for the regulation of which substrates can pass from the blood to the brain. Astrocytic feet line the blood vessels forming tight junctions allowing only lipid- soluble compounds to pass into the interstitial space. Disruption in the BBB allows for accumulation of protein-rich fluid in the extracellular space and may occur in response to direct injury, hypoxic injury, significant hypertension, inflammatory mediators, or endotoxins, and is most commonly located around contusions or hematomas.[54,179]

Another contributing factor to interstitial edema are aquaporins (AQP). AQP are water channels that are key regulators of transmembrane water conductance in cell types throughout the body, including the brain. There are 11 subtypes, with Aquaporin4 (AQP4) playing a role in brain edema. Depletion of AQP4 as it acts on the astrocyte foot processes and in ependymal cells plays a major role in regulating the influx of cellular water associated with edema formation.[14,54]

Cytotoxic edema occurs days or weeks after injury as a result of cerebral ischemia and the failure of the sodium (Na^+) potassium (K^+) pump. When there is an energy failure causing a failure in the NA^+/K^+ pump, sodium enters the cell and potassium exits the cell. When sodium enters the cell, water follows, resulting in intracellular edema.[179]

INTRACRANIAL PRESSURE AND CEREBRAL PERFUSION

Elevated ICP has long been associated with a poor outcome. Intracranial hypertension (sustained elevation in ICP) correlates with increased morbidity and mortality. Currently, monitoring ICP is a mainstay of TBI therapy and forms the basis for most interventions and treatments. However, there is considerable controversy over the usefulness of ICP monitoring, monitor types, site of placement, treatment thresholds, and outcome measures.

The Monro-Kellie doctrine or hypothesis (Fig. 12.14) states that the cranial vault is a container with three basic volumes: blood, brain, and CSF. If one of these contents increases, another must decrease in order to allow room for the other to expand. If this does not happen, the brain tissue within the cranial vault will be compressed, displaced, or herniate, leading to irreversible damage.[89,128]

Normal ICP is 0 to 15 mm Hg. Transient, brief elevations in ICP to 30 to 50 mm Hg can occur with activities such as suctioning, turning, and other routine nursing care that cause increases in intrathoracic pressure, but do not necessarily

Trauma
Traumatic disruption of cell membrane
Calcium entry through gaps in cell membrane
Blood-brain barrier disruption
Leukocyte recruitment
Reduction of blood flow
Anaerobic metabolism
Reversal of sodium-calcium exchanger
Calcium enters cell, sodium leaves cell
Inadequate synthesis of ATP
Failure of ATP-dependent calcium extrusion
Cellular acidosis
Failure of ATP-dependent transport of calcium across mitochondrial membrane
Excess intracellular calcium
Failure of NaK-ATPase pumps
Mitochondrial failure
Cell membrane depolarization
Increased calcium sequestration
Magnesium dislodged from NMDA receptors
Glutamate released
Activates metabotropic receptors
Activation of NMDA and AMPA receptors
Second messenger activates inositol triphosphate pathway
Calcium released from endoplasmic reticular stores within cell
Inflammation
Cerebral swelling
Ischemia, excitotoxicity, energy failure

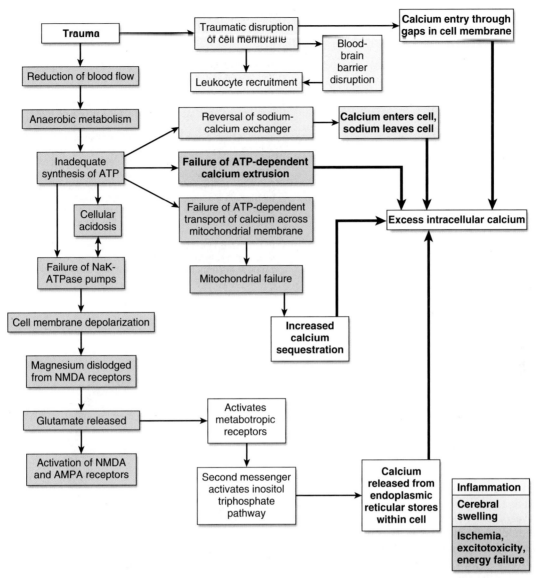

FIG. 12.13 Pathophysiology of secondary brain injury. *AMPA,* Alpha amino-3-hydroxy-5-methylisoxazole-4-propionic acid; *ATP,* adenosine triphosphate; *NMDA, N*-methyl-D-aspartate.

Normal

Brain 80%
Blood 10%
CSF 10%

ICP 10 mm Hg

The intracranial contents are housed in a rigid container: the skull.

Compensated

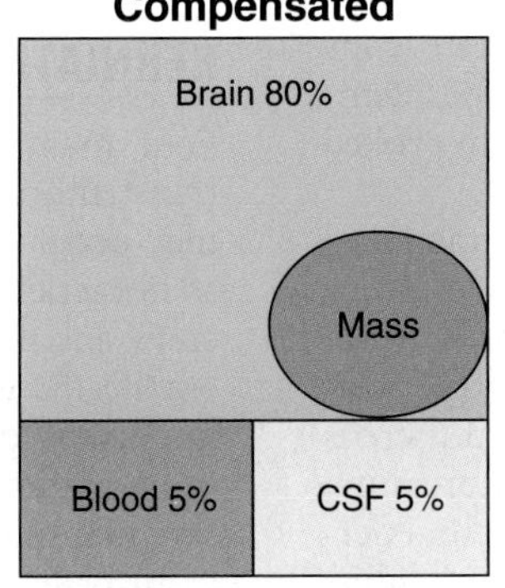

ICP 15 mm Hg

As one of the components increases, there is a reciprocal decrease in the other contents in order to maintain a normal pressure (compensated state). In the compensated state, the pressure remains normal but the brain stiffens (loss of compliance).

Decompensated

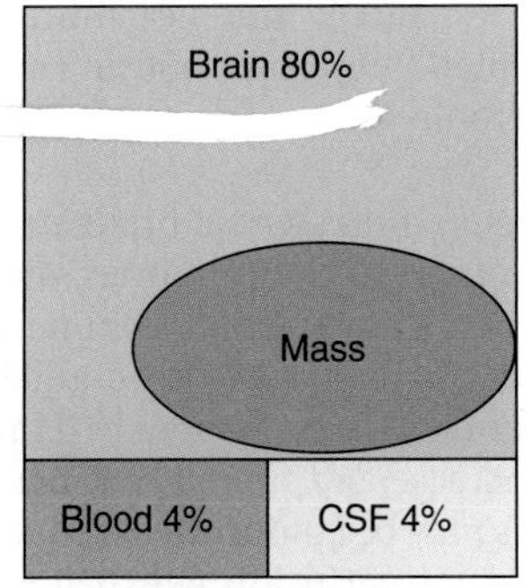

ICP 30 mm Hg

When the contents can no longer adapt to increases in volume, compliance is lost and intracranial pressure increases (decompensated state).

FIG. 12.14 Monro-Kellie doctrine.

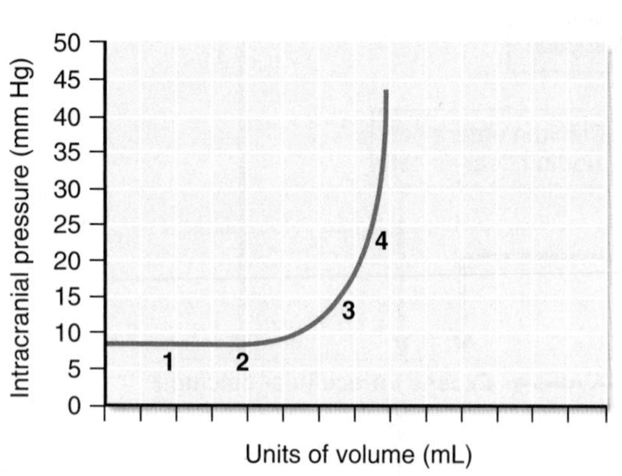

STAGES ON THE PRESSURE-VOLUME CURVE

Stage 1: There is high compliance and low elastance. The brain is in total compensation, with accommodation and autoregulation intact. An increase in volume does not increase ICP.

Stage 2: The compliance is lower and elastance is increasing. An increase in volume places the patient at risk of increased ICP.

Stage 3: There is high elastance and low compliance. Any small addition of volume causes a great increase in pressure. There is a loss of autoregulation, and there may be symptoms indicating increased ICP, such as systolic hypertension with an increasing pulse pressure, bradycardia, and slowing of respiratory rate (Cushing's triad). With the loss of autoregulation and the rise in the systolic blood pressure as a result of the Cushing's response, decompensation occurs. The ICP passively mimics the blood pressure.

Stage 4: Finally, when the patient reaches stage 4, the ICP rises to terminal levels with little increase in volume. Herniation occurs as the brain tissue shifts from the compartment of greater pressure to the compartment of lesser pressure.

FIG. 12.15 Pressure-volume curve.

need treatment unless increased ICP is sustained at greater than 20 to 25 mm Hg for 5 minutes.[23] However, with TBI, ICP increases may occur with these procedures due to brain edema, mass lesions, or vascular congestion (hyperemia) of the brain tissue.

Cerebral perfusion pressure (CPP) is an indirect measure of cerebral perfusion. CPP is calculated by subtracting the ICP from the MAP. The goal for CPP management in TBI is to maintain the CPP greater than 50 mm Hg in children older than 6 years and in adults, and greater than 40 mm Hg in children less than 6 years. CPP of less than 40 mm Hg may result in ischemia and should be avoided.[21,23] It was once thought that attempts should be made to increase CPP to greater than 70 mm Hg with fluids and pharmacologic agents; however, it is now known that this can cause further detriment to the patient by resulting in pulmonary complications.[23] Controversy exists as to what is the best parameter to treat in TBI, ICP or CPP; however, the best outcomes involve multimodality monitoring using oxygen (jugular venous oxygen saturation [Sjvo$_2$], brain tissue oxygen levels [Bto$_2$], and near-infrared spectroscopy [NIRS]), cerebral blood flow, metabolism (microdialysis, temperature), or electrophysiology (electroencephalogram evoked potential).[30,104,137,171]

Increasing pressure on essential brain structures may lead to brain tissue damage. In brain injuries with mass lesion or cerebral edema, small increases in volume are not harmful because blood and CSF flow out of the cranial vault to accommodate increased brain tissue volume.[126] However, if there is further volume increase and there is an increase in pressure, vascular structures may be compressed, reducing cerebral perfusion. When cerebral perfusion falls below a critical value, cerebral ischemia occurs (Fig. 12.15). Ischemia leads to neuronal injury and aggravates cerebral edema, further increasing ICP. As the ICP continues to increase, pressure gradients eventually displace brain tissue from areas of higher pressure to areas of lower pressure. Displacement of brain tissue from one intracranial compartment to another is known as *herniation.*[112]

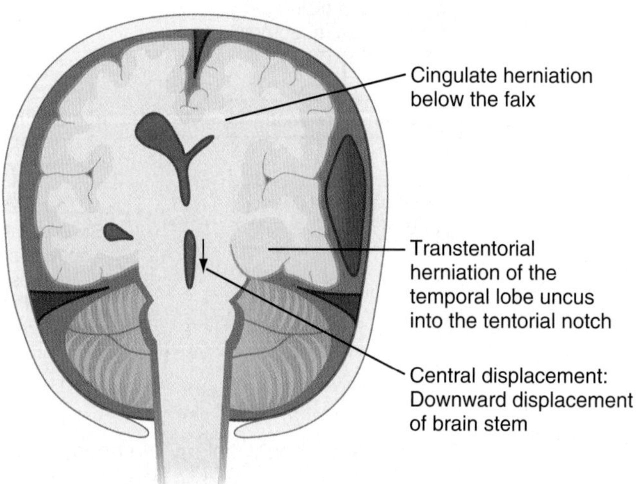

FIG. 12.16 Brain displacement from supratentorial herniation.

HERNIATION

Four main types of herniation can occur: cingulate, uncal, transtentorial or central, and infratentorial (Fig. 12.16). They may occur in isolation from one another or in combination, as intracranial pressure gradients can displace brain tissue laterally and downward at the same time. Herniation syndromes are life-threatening occurrences and can progress rapidly. It is important to remember that rapid identification and treatment of herniation syndromes is critical to reverse these events and save neuronal function. Time is brain.

In order to understand the different types of herniation, it is important to briefly review the basic anatomy within the intracranial compartment. The intracranial compartment is divided into smaller compartments by fibrous dura mater; double folds of the dura are the falx cerebri and the tentorium cerebelli. The falx cerebri divides the supratentorial space into left and right hemispheres along a longitudinal fissure. The tentorium cerebelli separates the supratentorial space (cerebral hemispheres) from the infratentorial space (cerebellum and brain stem).[112]

Cingulate herniation occurs as increasing pressure from an expanding lesion in one cerebral hemisphere pushes brain tissue beneath the falx cerebri. Intracranial volume is displaced across the midline and compresses brain tissue on the opposite side of the brain as well as vascular structures (anterior cerebral artery), potentiating cerebral edema and ischemia. This results in an increase in ICP, but little else is known about the signs and symptoms associated with cingulate herniation (also called *subfalcine herniation*). Uncal herniation occurs when a lesion in a cerebral hemisphere shifts the brain down and toward the midline and the inferior medial temporal lobe pushes over the edge of the tentorium cerebelli.[112,169] Classic signs of uncal herniation include rapid deterioration of consciousness, ipsilateral fixed and dilated pupil, contralateral hemiparesis, and progressive dysfunction of cranial nerves III through XII, though this occurs in less than half the patients. This type of herniation is associated with lesions ipsilateral to the abnormal pupil such as an epidural hematoma and can cause life-threatening brain stem compression.[112,169]

Transtentorial herniation, also called *rostral-caudal* or *central herniation,* is the most common form of herniation. Transtentorial herniation occurs with lesions of the midline structures (i.e., diencephalon), or bilateral hemispheric lesions causing downward displacement of the cerebral hemisphere, basal ganglia, diencephalon, and midbrain through tentorial incisura compressing the posterior cerebral artery. Patients often present with decreasing LOC, bilateral small reactive pupils to fixed and mid-position pupils to fixed and dilated pupils. Motor function progresses from weakness to abnormal motor movements (decorticate to decerebrate posturing) to flaccid. Vital signs change from hypertension with a widening pulse pressure, tachycardia, and irregular respirations at the level of the diencephalon to hypertension with a widening pulse pressure, irregular respirations, and bradycardia, which is known as *Cushing's triad.*[34,51,112]

Infratentorial herniation is the downward displacement of the medulla and cerebellum (cerebellar tonsils) through the foreman magnum. This usually leads to rapid deterioration of the patient with apnea, hypotension, and imminent death.[112]

INTERPROFESSIONAL PLAN OF CARE FOR THE TRAUMATIC BRAIN INJURY PATIENT

In TBI, the goal of treatment is to limit the extent of secondary damage. Current treatment of TBI involves optimization of the ABCs (airway, breathing, and circulation), supportive therapy, neuroprotection, and control of ICP; ongoing research continues to identify new treatment options. Management of the patient with TBI can be divided into various phases of care. These management phases are prehospital, emergency department, critical care, acute care, and rehabilitation.

Prehospital Phase

The prehospital phase starts immediately after injury and continues until arrival in the emergency department (ED). This is an important time interval for determining eventual outcome and preventing irreversible damage. The goals during this phase are to identify, treat, and prevent: hypoxia, hypercarbia, hypocarbia, hypotension, and neurologic decompensation. Basic interventions include airway management and ventilation, spine immobilization, hemodynamic monitoring, fluid resuscitation, and monitoring LOC, followed by rapid transport to a trauma center with neurologic and neurosurgical services.[22,117] Fifty percent of TBI patients are reported to be hypoxic in the field; prehospital intubation has been associated with significant reduction in mortality of TBI patients.[170] It is essential to perform early orotracheal intubation with spine immobilization in any patient with a GCS less than or equal to eight.[15,22,117,180] A recent randomized control trial (RCT) compared rapid sequence intubation (RSI) using sedation and short-acting paralytics to delayed intubation in the ED. Results demonstrated significantly improved outcomes in the prehospital intubated group. Some centers have advocated for intubation being performed without the aid of long-acting paralytics or sedation so as to not interfere with the initial neurologic evaluation, but data suggest low success in intubation and worse outcomes. Patients with O_2 saturation of greater than 90%, a PaO_2 greater than 110 mm Hg, $PaCO_2$ levels of 30 to 49 mm Hg in adults, or $ETCO_2$ maintained at 35 to 44 mm Hg have been shown to have better outcomes.[15]

Permissive hypotension, which has been advocated in the multitrauma patient, should be avoided as delay in treatment of hypotension with volume resuscitation in patients with head injuries has been shown to compromise perfusion and worsen secondary brain injury.[15] Continuous blood pressure (BP) monitoring and volume resuscitation with an isotonic solution (normal saline or Ringer's lactate) is important to maintain a systolic BP of greater than 90 mm Hg in adults. Use of hypertonic solutions, hypertonic saline solution (HTS), or dextran may be considered. The use of hypotonic solutions is not recommended as it may cause or worsen cerebral edema. Research regarding the use of HTS continues.[21]

A brief neurologic assessment using the GCS or AVPU (alert, verbal, pain, unresponsive) to establish a baseline LOC is essential. Continuous monitoring is also necessary, especially before and after interventions such as intubation.

Early Hospital Management

The early hospital management phase consists of the care received in the emergency department, operating room, and initial hours in critical care. Goals during this phase of care are to continue to identify, treat, and prevent: hypoxia, hypercarbia, hypocarbia, hypotension, and neurologic decompensation, while determining the extent and type of brain injury in order to develop the appropriate plan of care. Patients with GCS less than or equal to 8, and those who are otherwise unable to protect their airway, require immediate intubation if this has not been performed. The incidence of concomitant spinal cord injury (SCI) with TBI is 6% to 8%; therefore cervical spine precautions need to be maintained at all times, especially during intubation. Cervical spine precautions include using a rigid cervical collar, backboards, and log-rolling the patient until any damage to the spine is ruled out radiographically.[21] Though sedatives and paralytics will briefly interfere with the neurologic exam, studies show that there is greater success with intubation and improved outcomes with their use. Initially, all TBI patients should be placed on 1.0 fraction of inspired oxygen (FIO_2) and then titrated down to maintain a PaO_2 greater than 60 mm Hg (optimal PaO_2 95–100 mm Hg). The $PaCO_2$ should be maintained between 35 and 40 mm Hg. The use of prophylactic hyperventilation ($PaCO_2 \leq 35$ mm Hg) should be avoided in the first 24 hours following TBI.[21,22] Though hyperventilation may lower ICP by decreasing CBF through severe vasoconstriction, it has been associated with increased tissue ischemia and hypoxia. Clinical studies have demonstrated that patients hyperventilated after head injury experienced worse neurologic outcomes compared to patients kept normocarbic.[134]

After securing an airway and oxygenation, maintaining a BP and restoring normal circulating volume are essential. The current Brain Trauma Foundation (BTF) guidelines[20,21,22] for management of severe head injury state that maintaining a MAP of greater than or equal to 90 mm Hg in adults should be the goal for the TBI patient in order to ensure a cerebral perfusion pressure of 50 to 70 mm Hg.[20,21,22] A single episode of hypotension is associated with a doubling of mortality and an increase in morbidity following TBI. It is extremely important to aggressively restore normal circulating volume to avoid hypotensive episodes.[36] The optimal method for restoring circulating volume is through the use of isotonic fluids. Other fluid options may include the use of packed red blood cells (PRBCs) if the patient has experienced blood loss and hypertonic solutions (HTS).[68] A 2013 RCT found that albumin is detrimental to the TBI patient and should not be given.[44] Should the patient with TBI be unresponsive to fluid resuscitation, norepinephrine may be used to increase MAP without resulting in hyperemia if pressure autoregulation is preserved. Aggressive attempts to maintain CPP greater than 70 mm Hg with fluids or vasopressors should be avoided because of the increased risk of pulmonary complications.[22]

Isotonic fluids, such as normal saline (NS) or lactated Ringer's solution, are used for volume resuscitation of hypotensive, hypovolemic patients because these fluids will remain in the intravascular space and have a limited effect on edema. Hypotonic solutions (e.g., 0.45% NS or D_5W) are dangerous to use because sudden fluid shifts from the intravascular space into brain cells increases cerebral edema and elevates ICP. They should not be administered to head-injured patients. Dextrose solutions should only be given to patients with hypoglycemia.[15]

HTS has been shown to have beneficial effects in head-injured patients. The effects of HTS include expansion of intravascular volume, extraction of water from the intracellular space into the intravascular space, ICP reduction, increased cardiac contractility, stabilization of the cell membrane, and blunting of the immune response.[87,118] Although HTS use appears promising, optimal timing, appropriate concentration, and ideal volume have yet to be determined. Administration of HTS will cause an increase in serum sodium concentrations; levels greater than 160 mEq/L have been associated with side effects such as fluid overload, renal failure, and potentially osmotic demyelination, though it has never been reported.[117] During this phase of care, the prophylactic use of mannitol is not recommended unless the patient is exhibiting signs of transtentorial herniation because of its volume-depleting diuretic effect.[22]

Continued Critical Care Management

Once the patient is stabilized and transferred to critical care, it is important to implement further physiologic monitoring in order to facilitate and direct the ongoing management of these patients. Continued hemodynamic and respiratory resuscitation may be required to manage associated injuries as well as facilitate cerebral perfusion. Early priorities for managing the patient's neurologic injuries are to control intracranial pressure and limit secondary brain injury; ICP monitoring should be instituted as soon as possible in the ED, operating room (OR), or critical care unit. Treatment of TBI patients in critical care is guided by ICP monitoring and focused on reducing elevated pressures according to accepted guidelines. Extended critical care management of these patients will require ongoing fluid resuscitation, ventilator management, and nutritional support. Attention must be focused on preventing and treating complications such as electrolyte derangements, pulmonary problems, deep vein thrombosis, stress ulcers, contractures, and decubitus ulcers. These will be discussed later in this chapter.

Rehabilitation

The last phase of care with the TBI patient is rehabilitation. This is necessary for the majority of moderately and severely injured patients. The goal of rehabilitation is to preserve and promote the patient's functional and cognitive status as much as possible with the goal of returning to preinjury status. This phase of care begins in the ICU by prevention of contractures and decubitus ulcers with proper positioning of extremities, frequent repositioning of the patient, range of motion exercises, and early mobility.[122,135,158]

MONITORING

There are several techniques for monitoring brain tissue for signs of damage related to TBI. Monitoring devices measure ICP, oxygenation of the brain tissue, electroencephalogram (EEG) activity, CBF, electrolytes, and other substrates in the brain tissue. It is the prevalent thought that there is not one method that should be solely relied upon for all treatment decisions, but rather a multimodality approach will best serve the patients with TBI.[104]

Intracranial Pressure Monitoring

The most common monitoring technique is ICP monitoring.[6,37] ICP can be monitored in the intraparenchymal tissue, epidural space, subdural space, and intraventricular sites (Table 12.5 and Fig. 12.17); however, the most reliable sites are intraparenchymal and intraventricular. Intraventricular monitoring has been considered the gold standard for ICP measurement and allows for drainage of CSF.[22,123,145] The catheter used for this method is also the most difficult to place, especially if the ventricles are small or displaced. Insertion of an external ventricular drain (EVD) has a higher rate of infection and hemorrhage compared to other monitors. Placement of an intraparenchymal ICP probe is quick and easy, with very few associated complications (Fig. 12.18).[22,123,145]

Monitoring ICP should encompass more than the mean ICP and should include the interpretation of the ICP waveform and the calculation of the CPP. The ICP waveform has been shown to provide evidence suggestive of changes in cerebral compliance. Compliance is the brain's ability to adapt to physiologic and external challenges to the system, and is sometimes referred to as *stiffness.* Compliance is responsible for maintaining equilibrium and is often expressed as the change in ICP in response to changes in volume. As volume increases and intracranial contents can no longer adapt to changes in volume, compliance decreases, and ICP increases. The ICP waveform represents intracranial and arterial pulsations reflecting the cardiac and respiratory cycles. Waveforms have three peaks: P_1, P_2, and P_3 (Fig. 12.19). P_1 is the percussion wave and originates from arterial pressure transmitted to the intracranial arteries and the choroid plexus.[6,38,171] P_2, the

TABLE 12.5 Comparison of Intracranial Pressure Monitors

Type	Site	Advantages	Disadvantages
Intraventricular catheter	Ventricles	Most accurate, CSF cultures can be collected, CSF can be withdrawn to control ICP, contrast materials can be injected for radiologic studies	Risk of hemorrhage, increased risk of infection, risk of CSF leak at site, artifacts may cause dampening of recordings, more difficult to insert
Subarachnoid bolt	Subarachnoid space	Can be used with small or collapsed ventricles, does not penetrate brain parenchyma, low infection rates, low cost, ease and safety of insertion	Does not allow CSF drainage or withdrawal, becomes occluded, may dampen and give unreliable readings after a few days, brain tissue may herniate into bolt
Epidural sensor	Epidural space	Ease of insertion, least invasive, recommended in cases of meningitis and CNS infections, less risk of infection, does not require recalibration	Slower response time, fragile, can become wedged against skull, affected by heat or febrile patient, diaphragm can rupture, less accurate, unable to drain CSF
Intraparenchymal catheter	Intraparenchymal tissue	Very accurate, yields good waveform patterns, second only to intraventricular based on accuracy and stability, easy and quick to insert even with small ventricles	Fiberoptic catheters can break if kinked or stretched, does not allow CSF drainage or withdrawal, potential complications of infection or hemorrhage

From References 22, 123, and 145.

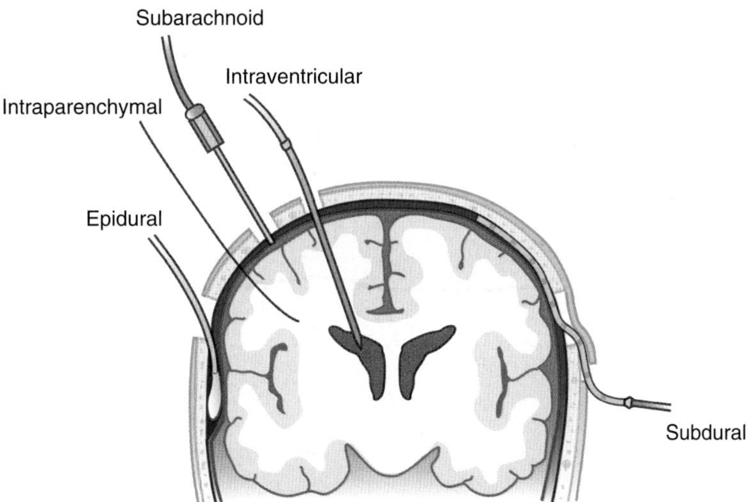

FIG. 12.17 Potential sites for intracranial pressure monitoring devices.

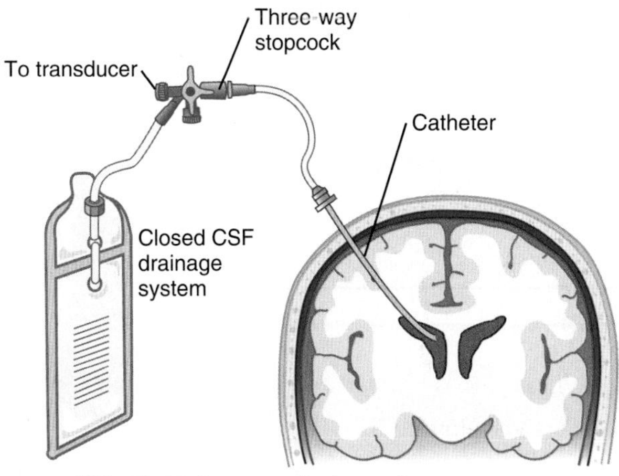

FIG. 12.18 Intraventricular catheter system.

tidal wave, is a venous wave that is influenced by brain tissue and CSF volumes. P_3, the dicrotic wave, also a venous wave, represents aortic valve closure. Pulse amplitude and peak to trough increases with a low compliance and age. Normally P_1 is greater than P_2, with P_2 being 80% of the height of P_1. As P_2 becomes equal to or greater than P_1, compliance is poor.[6,38,171]

Research suggests that those patients with an increase in P_2 will develop an increase in mean ICP. For example, if P_1 and P_2 are of equal amplitude, meaning the compliance is poor, it would be best to limit care activities or space interventions in order to decrease stimulation. Nursing activities such as turning and suctioning may need to be modified based on waveform interpretation. Suctioning may need to be kept brief or require premedication with lidocaine to limit increased ICP response.[6,171] Performing these and other nursing interventions guided by waveform interpretation and assessment of compliance changes may prevent dangerous elevation in ICP that might precipitate herniation syndromes.[6,38]

ICP trends generally fall into one of three different categories: A, B, or C. A waves, referred to as *plateau waves,* are of large amplitude (50 to 100 mm Hg) and variable duration (5 to 20 minutes). Large amplitude waves are clinically significant and indicate dangerously reduced intracranial compliance. A waves indicate increased ICP and demand immediate attention because, if unalleviated, cerebral ischemia and neurologic deterioration will result. B waves are smaller (up to 50 mm Hg), sharper waves, with a dominant frequency of 0.5 to 2 minutes. C waves are small (up to 20 mm Hg), rhythmic oscillations with a frequency of 4 to 8 minutes and are of little clinical significance[6,38,145] (Fig. 12.20).

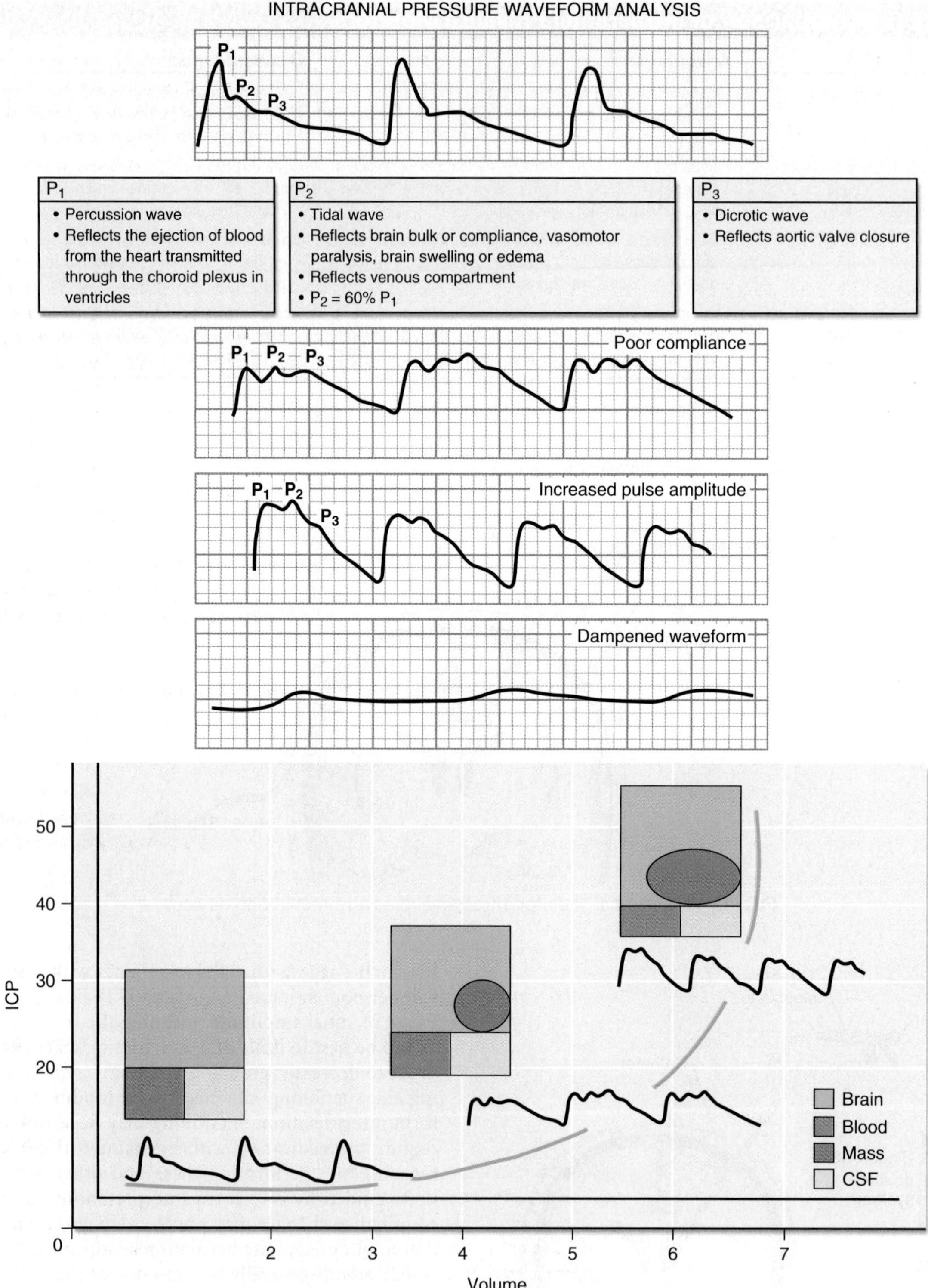

FIG. 12.19 Normal intracranial pressure waveform.

NEUROIMAGING

Early identification of intracranial pathology is essential to determine whether surgery is needed and to guide interventions. The most commonly used method for neuroimaging is the CT scan. The CT scan is helpful for identifying gross abnormalities, bleeding, fractures, hydrocephalus, and edema. MRIs may be used later in the patient's course to identify more subtle lesions such as axonal injury and ischemic changes. If the patient is unavailable for interventions during the MRI, these exams may be deferred until later in the hospital course when the patient is determined to be more stable.[111]

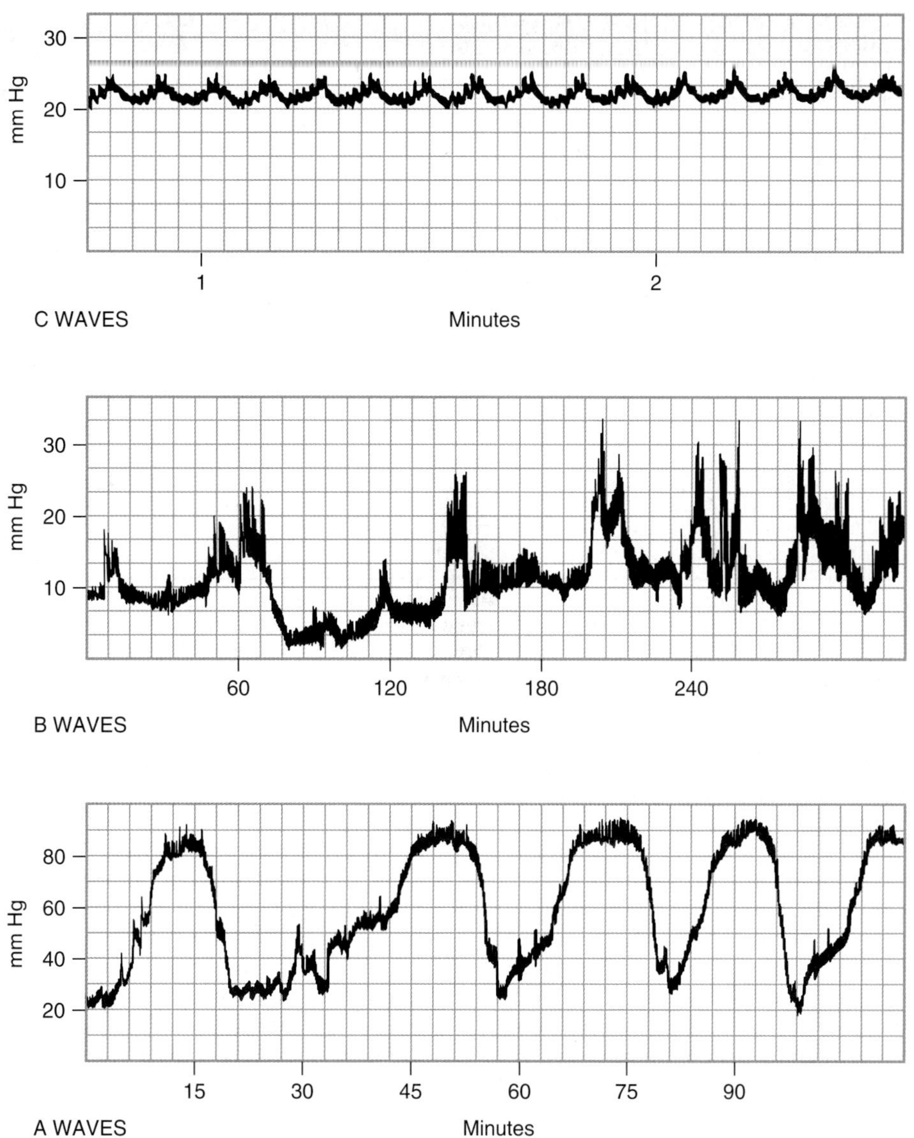

FIG. 12.20 Intracranial pressure (ICP) trend waves or Lund waves.

A CT scan is the diagnostic procedure of choice for the evaluation of acute head trauma. CT scanners are quick and readily available in most institutions. A head CT should be performed on anyone who has a GCS of less than 15 with focal neurologic deficits, clinical signs of a basilar or depressed skull fracture, or any LOC. It is important to remember that a normal initial CT scan does not exclude the presence of significant intracranial hypertension. Therefore, it is important to review the CT scan in context with the clinical examination of the patient. Emergent neurosurgical evaluation is critical for determining whether to proceed with immediate surgical evacuation of hematomas.[55] General guidelines for surgical intervention include the following: all acute subdural hematomas greater than or equal to 1 cm in thickness; epidural hematomas greater than 30 mL with neurologic deterioration, coma, and/or abnormal pupils; intracerebral hematomas greater than 20 mL with mass effect; and depressed, compound skull fractures.[24-27]

Currently there are two techniques to measure global CBF, xenon CT and CT perfusion. Xenon CT measures CBF quantitatively by measuring the brain's uptake and clearance of the diffusible gas xenon. Xenon is a lipid-soluble gas, which diffuses freely across the BBB, allowing it to be used as a tracer to measure CBF. Xenon is administered most commonly by inhalation, but can also be used intravenously. This is a relatively easy method that can be used to determine global and regional CBF. Patient movement, resulting in artifact and inaccurate results, can affect this technique. The xenon concentration can also cause vasodilation and augment CBF, which can also affect the study results.[142] This method can now be done at the bedside with the portable CT scanner. CT perfusion uses an iodine contrast media to quantify CBF, cerebral blood volume (CBV), mean transit time (MTT), and time to peak (time from injection of contrast to maximum enhancement). Both methods only give a snapshot in time.[80,157]

TABLE 12.6 Monitoring Parameters

Parameter	Source	Normal Value	Critical Levels
Parameters Used in TBI			
ICP	Directly measured	0–15 mm Hg	> 20 mm Hg
CPP	Calculated: MAP–ICP	60–100 mm Hg	< 60 mm Hg
CBF	Directly measured	50–55 mL/100 g/min	< 28–20 mL/100 g/min
$CMRo_2$	Calculated	3.2 mL/100 g/min	
$Pbto_2$	Directly measured	25–40 mm Hg	Low: < 20 mm Hg Ischemic values: < 15 mm Hg for 30 min < 10 mm Hg for 10 min
$Sjvo_2$	Directly measured	55–75%	< 50% for 10 min
Cerebral Extraction			
Of oxygen (CEo_2)	Calculated: $Sao_2 - Sjvo_2$	24–40%	< 24% oxygen, supply greater than demand > 40% oxygen, supply less than demand
$AvjDo_2$	Calculated: $Cao_2 - Cjvo_2$ $Cao_2 = (Sao_2 \times 1.34 \times Hb) + (Pao_2 \times 0.0031)$ $Cjvo_2 = (Sjvo_2 \times 1.34 \times Hb) + (Pjvo_2 \times 0.0031)$	4.5–8.5 mL/dL	< 4.5 mL/dL, oxygen supply greater than demand > 8.5 mL/dL, oxygen supply insufficient for demand

$Avjo_2$, Arterio-jugular venous oxygen difference; *Cao_2*, arterial oxygen content; *CBF*, cerebral blood flow; *CEo_2*, cerebral extraction of oxygen; *$Cjvo_2$*, jugular venous oxygen content; *$CMRo_2$*, cerebral metabolic rate of oxygen; *CP*, cerebral perfusion pressure; *Hb*, hemoglobin; *IC*, intracranial pressure; *MAP*, mean arterial pressure; *$Pbto_2$*, partial pressure of brain tissue oxygen; *$Pjvo_2$*, partial pressure of jugular venous oxygen; *Sao_2*, arterial oxygen saturation; *$Sjvo_2$*, jugular venous oxygen saturation *TBI*, traumatic brain injury.
From References 52, 69, 123, and 171.

Other types of imaging techniques for functional neuroimaging include positron emission tomography (PET), single-photon emission computed tomography (SPECT), and MR perfusion. PET and SPECT scanning techniques use radionuclide tracers injected into the patient and then employ different scanning techniques to assess cerebral blood flow and metabolism, allowing for the detection of areas of cerebral dysfunction and brain ischemia that may not be detected on CT scan or MRI.[55,102,111,157] These techniques are helpful in determining changes in CBF and metabolism during recovery. For this reason, they are helpful in determining prognosis after TBI.[55,98,102] MRI perfusion weighted imaging (PW-MRI) is a common imaging scan using gadolinium contrast to enhance T2 weighted images. Perfusion weighted images are often used together with diffusion weighted images and can assess CBF, CBV, and MTT. Studies suggest MR perfusion may be superior to CT perfusion, but the studies take longer to perform.[55,98,157]

Transcranial Doppler ultrasonography (TCD) uses a low-frequency ultrasonic signal to measure velocity of blood flow in the intracranial arteries by insolating the major cerebral blood vessels through thin areas of bone called *windows*.[1] This is most commonly used to detect vasospasm following aneurysms and other vascular disorders, but it may also be helpful in detecting posttraumatic cerebral hemodynamic changes and complications such as hyperemia, vasospasm, emboli, decreased CBF, and intracranial hypertension.[75,124,171] Magnetic resonance angiography (MRA) is another technique that may be beneficial with TBI. MRA, typically used to locate vascular lesions such as aneurysms and AVMs, utilizes flow measurement by oxyhemoglobin spectral shifts and contrast indication transit times to detect flow through the vasculature to identify vascular abnormalities. This is currently being investigated for use in patients with acute severe head injuries. These methods and their value in the critical care management phase require further evaluation.[124]

Cerebral Oxygen Monitoring

There are several methods for monitoring cerebral oxygen in patients with TBI. Methods for monitoring oxygenation include continuous monitoring of jugular venous oxygen, brain tissue oxygen sensors, and near infrared spectroscopy (NIRS). Monitoring of regional saturation of jugular oxygen ($Sjvo_2$) can be done using a jugular bulb catheter. $Sjvo_2$ can be monitored intermittently by placing an intercath into the internal jugular vein or continually with an oximetrics catheter at the level of the jugular bulb. The jugular bulb is a dilated area of the jugular vein as it exits the skull. By placing the catheter in the right jugular, it is believed to measure approximately 80% of the blood exiting the brain. $Sjvo_2$ is a measure of the amount of O_2 remaining in the blood after the brain tissue has extracted the O_2 it needs. Proper placement of the catheter is confirmed by plain radiograph film.[171] Normal $Sjvo_2$ in an adult is approximately 65% (ranging from 55% to 80%).[69,123] In comatose patients, values greater than 50% are considered normal. Whenever $Sjvo_2$ drops below 50% for longer than 15 minutes, the etiology must be sought. A decline in $Sjvo_2$ may be caused by low Pao_2, prolonged hyperventilation, decreased CPP (< 70 mm Hg), vasospasm, or low hemoglobin concentration.[68,123] An increase in $Sjvo_2$ reflects an increased supply of oxygen to the brain (i.e., hyperemia) or decreased oxygen utilization from sedation, barbiturates, hypothermia, or large areas of cerebral infarction.[69,177] Other measures obtained by the retrograde jugular catheter are the cerebral metabolic rate of O_2 (CEo_2), which is calculated by subtracting the $Sjvo_2$ from the mixed venous O_2. The arteriovenous rate of O_2 ($AVDo_2$) is $CMRO_2$ divided by CBF. $AVDo_2$ provides an overall picture of the relationship of cerebral blood flow and oxygen consumption. Normal $AVDo_2$ levels range from 4.5 to 8.5 mL/dL. See Table 12.6 for a summary of all normal and abnormal values for monitoring parameters. Elevations occur as a result of inadequate cerebral blood flow or decreased oxygen consumption. Decreased values reflect an excessive oxygen delivery over the demand for oxygen.[171,177] $Sjvo_2$ reflects global cerebral blood flow and therefore is not used to detect focal ischemic episodes. Because jugular bulb and local oxygen pressure monitoring complement each other by providing distinctly different information, many facilities use these modalities in conjunction with each other.[69]

Monitoring the partial pressure of brain tissue oxygen ($Pbto_2$) is one of the techniques most frequently used as an adjunct to ICP in treating patients with severe TBI. Studies have shown that prolonged episodes of tissue hypoxia (increased burden) are correlated with an unfavorable outcome.[2] $Pbto_2$ is the partial pressure of brain tissue oxygen in a focal area around the sensor. Normal $Pbto_2$ is approximately 30 mm Hg with a $Pbto_2$ of 15 mm Hg being the critical lower limit in patients with severe TBI (Table 12.6).[52,179] Some controversy exists as to whether the most appropriate placement site for the probe is within injured, penumbral, or uninjured tissue. One study showed that placing the probe near injured tissue was more predictive of outcome than placing the probe in uninjured tissue.[147] A recently completed phase 2 clinical trial (BOOST2–brain oxygen or standard therapy) comparing the treatment of TBI using conventional management using ICP/CPP-guided treatment to ICP/ CPP and brain oxygen guided therapy, found patients treated using $Pbto_2$ had less brain hypoxia, lower mortality, and more favorable outcomes (presented September 2015 at Neurocritical Care Society Annual Conference, Seattle, WA). There are two devices currently commercially available to monitor $Pbto_2$.

Microdialysis

Microdialysis has been used as a research tool to identify neurochemical and metabolic changes following TBI. Microdialysis involves the insertion of a tubular dialysis membrane connected to a small pump into the brain tissue to measure lactate, glucose, pyruvate, and glutamate. Correlations have been noted between reduced cerebral oxygenation and elevations in lactate concentration. Microdialysis is currently being used primarily in academic and research settings and is not yet widely used for routine clinical practice.[30,123]

Continuous Electroencephalography

The 2014 International Multidisciplinary Consensus Conference on Multimodality Monitoring advocated that all acute brain injury patients who have unexplained persistent altered LOC should be monitored using continuous EEG monitoring[39] Seizures are common after acute brain injury and most are nonconvulsive. Studies show that up to 48% of patients will have nonconvulsive seizures and 14% will have nonconvulsive status epilepticus.[23,39,123] In order to adequately detect and treat these seizures, it is recommended that patients undergo continuous EEG monitoring for 24 to 72 hours.[23] A growing field of research is using depth EEG electrodes to identify, prognosticate, and potentially treat spreading depolarization (also called *spreading cortical depression*), which are spreading waves of neuronal and astrocytic depolarization that occur spontaneously and are related to structural and ischemic brain injury. These events have been correlated with poor prognosis in TBI.[39,84] Another application of continuous EEG monitoring is in the patient with induced barbiturate/ propofol coma for refractory increased ICP. EEG monitoring facilitates assessment of the extent of burst suppression (4 to 6 bursts/min or 5 to 8 seconds of suppression to 1 second of burst activity).[75] EEG monitoring may also be used to verify of the absence of brain activity in the diagnosis of brain death.[23,39]

Another type of EEG monitoring that may have future applications in TBI is the use of bispectral index (BIS) monitoring. BIS monitoring is a newer technology integrating electromyography (EMG) and EEG waveforms to assess sedation levels.[75,153] This has been used in operative situations to assess sedation levels and absence of recall. A recent exploratory study using bilateral BIS suggests this may be a useful tool to detect pain in nonverbal patients with left hemisphere injury and altered LOC.[7] Another potential use for BIS is monitoring of sedated patients and those in pentobarbital or propofol induced coma.[8,151] The BIS value provides a numerical representation from 0 to 100, with 100 being wide awake. Typically, a BIS value of 40 to 60 represents the absence of recall, and this is the goal in operative situations and in critical care sedation. An additional index on the BIS monitor is the suppression ratio (SR), which is a measurement of the percentage of EEG in the last 63 seconds that is completely suppressed or isoelectric. This number is a measure from 0 to 100, with 0 being no burst suppression of the EEG and a measure of 100 indicating the complete absence of electrical activity.[8,75] When used for therapeutic barbiturate coma, the goal of therapy is to keep BIS less than 20 and SR greater than 70.[8,151] Data suggest that BIS may be a potentially viable assessment tool that is easily applied and interpreted at the bedside and may be particularly valuable to guide titration of barbiturates.[8,151]

TREATMENT OF TRAUMATIC BRAIN INJURY

MANAGEMENT OF HYPOXIA AND HYPOTENSION

The first goal in treating the TBI patient is to reduce initial hypoxic ischemic damage by following standard trauma resuscitation principles. The most important component of early care is prevention of hypoxia and hypotension. Any hypotension and hypoxia must be treated aggressively. Hypoxemia with a Pao_2 of less than 60 mm Hg at the scene of injury has a reported incidence of as high as 55%.[170] Supplemental oxygen and mechanical ventilation may be needed to maintain Pao_2 greater than 60 mm Hg and $Paco_2$ between 35 and 40 mm Hg. Even brief episodes of hypotension are associated with an increased risk of death in trauma patients and may result in a longer critical care recovery phase for those patients who survive. A single episode of hypotension has been shown to double mortality and increase morbidity in patients with severe TBI.[36,66] The goal of BP management should be to keep SBP greater than 90 mm Hg with fluids and vasopressors.

Fluids and vasopressor agents are given to augment CPP and increase blood flow to the brain, preventing ischemia that may result from increased ICP. CPP should be maintained between 50 and 70 mm Hg.[22] Although it was once thought that attempts should be made to increase CPP greater than 70 mm Hg with fluids followed by pharmacologic agents, research has shown that excessive fluid resuscitation increases the incidence of pulmonary complications.[154] Therefore, if TBI patients remain hypotensive despite seemingly adequate fluid resuscitation and filling pressures, vasopressors may be needed to keep BP greater than 90 mm Hg.

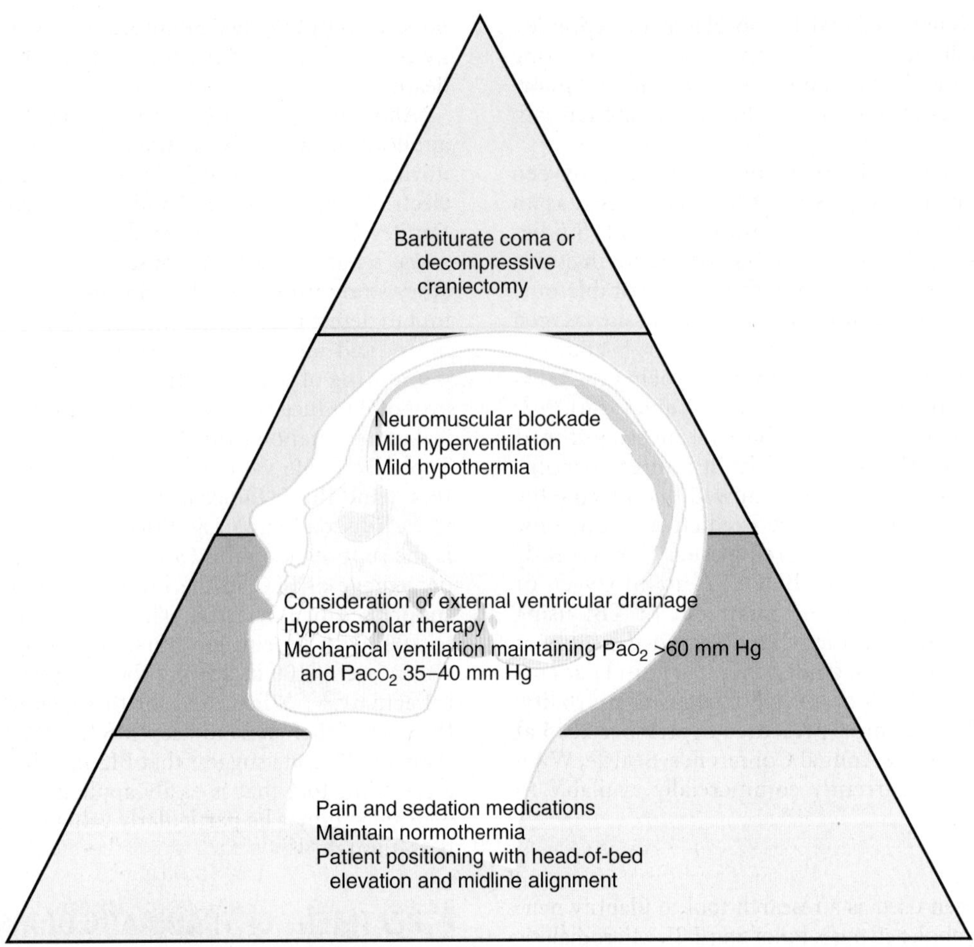

FIG. 12.21 Treatment pyramid for increased intracranial pressure.

MANAGEMENT OF INTRACRANIAL PRESSURE

Management of traumatic brain injuries is primarily aimed at prevention and reduction of elevated ICP to preserve brain function. Fig. 12.21 shows a hierarchy for treating patients with ICP. Treatment of elevated ICP should be initiated when levels are sustained greater than or equal to 20 mm Hg for longer than 5 to 10 minutes.[169] ICP management involves a tiered approach using the TBI guidelines.

First-Level Approaches for Intracranial Pressure Management

The most basic approach to decreasing ICP is to facilitate venous drainage and prevent constriction of venous outflow; this is easily accomplished with appropriate patient positioning. Patients should be positioned with the head of the bed elevated 30 to 45 degrees,[59] avoiding hyperextension, flexion, or rotation of the head and neck; the legs should be straight, and sharp hip flexion avoided. Use of reverse Trendelenburg's (RT) position may be helpful to facilitate venous drainage by preventing femoral constriction. The nurse should also ensure there is no constriction of the jugular veins from endotracheal tube tape, tracheostomy ties, or cervical collars that are too tight.[122]

It is also important to consider other causes of increased ICP unrelated to TBI. Increased levels of positive end-expiratory pressure (PEEP) to treat pulmonary conditions such as acute respiratory distress syndrome (ARDS) can result in increase in the ICP. PEEP may increase intrathoracic pressure, and so impede venous return, resulting in an increased ICP; thus the use of PEEP to improve oxygenation should be used cautiously, and patients closely monitored.[103]

Abdominal compartment syndrome (ACS) may also result in increased ICP due to a compromise in jugular venous outflow, caused by the increased abdominal pressure that constricts the abdominal contents.[28] ACS is characterized clinically by the evolution of a tense, distended abdomen, progressive oliguria, and progressive respiratory compromise.[28] Decreasing environmental stimuli and utilizing sedation and pain medications are additional measures to prevent increased ICP and optimize the oxygen delivery/consumption ratio.

Sedation and Analgesia

Pain control and use of sedation are important interventions in TBI patients. Pain and agitation increase cerebral metabolic demand, resulting in increased CBF and leading to increased ICP. Severe agitation increases intrathoracic pressure and reduces venous outflow. Any noxious stimuli, commonly seen with nursing activities such as turning and suctioning, can increase cerebral metabolic demands and elevate ICP. Pain control and sedation decrease the cerebral metabolic rate of oxygen consumption and reduce CBF and CBV, thereby decreasing ICP. It also facilitates adequate ventilation and maintenance of CPP.[65] These agents can also limit the neurologic exam; therefore, they need to be administered judiciously, especially in patients without intracranial monitoring devices. If possible, a complete neurologic exam should be performed before administration of sedatives or analgesic agents. Current practice recommendation for ICU care encourages the use of pain, agitation, and delirium (PAD) assessment tools to facilitate objective assessment of the clinical status of the patient's PAD; however, these assessments are often difficult in the neurologically impaired patient.[65] A recent exploratory study suggests that the BIS monitor may be a helpful tool for pain and sedation in the TBI patient.[8] Until 2014, the use of daily sedation wake-ups (sedation vacation) to allow for a thorough neurologic exam were controversial. A study by Skoglund in 2014, however, found that although ICP and CPP may be compromised, neurochemistry and brain oxygenation were not, suggesting this practice is safe.[167] Common medications, dosages, and contraindications for the administration of sedation and analgesic agents are presented in the medication table "Selected Sedative Agents" in Chapter 39.

Propofol. Propofol (Diprivan) is an intravenous sedative-hypnotic that is lipid soluble and rapidly crosses the BBB. Propofol can be quickly discontinued in order to assess a patient's neurologic status because of its short effective half-life (< 1 hour), rapid onset, and short recovery time. It can then be restarted, with a rapid onset of action. It is also theorized that there may be a dose-dependent decrease in CBF and cerebral metabolic rate (CMR), thus decreasing ICP. Patients with head injury may be at higher risk of cardiac failure at doses higher than 5 mg/kg/hour; starting the infusion at 0.3 mg/kg/hour, and increasing every 5 to10 minutes to a maximum of 3 mg/kg/hour as needed, may avoid cardiac complications.[69] It is important to monitor liver and pancreatic functions because of the lipid component of propofol when prolonged high doses are used. Prolonged and high-dose (>4 mg/kg/h for longer than 48 hours) use of propofol has been associated with the development of *propofol infusion syndrome,* lactic acidosis, cardiac failure, and "Brugada-like" EKG changes. The syndrome can progress to rhabdomyolysis, renal failure, and cardiovascular collapse.[22,65]

Benzodiazepines. Benzodiazepines have sedative and anticonvulsant properties, making them very useful for the management of TBI patients during anesthesia and critical care treatment. Benzodiazepines commonly used are midazolam (Versed) and lorazepam (Ativan).[22]

Narcotics. Pain has a direct effect on cerebral metabolic rate and subsequent problems of elevated ICP. The healthcare team needs to balance the management of pain versus interference with neurologic assessment and adverse hemodynamic effects. Morphine, fentanyl, alfentanyl, sufentanyl, and remifentanil may be given to patients for their analgesic effects. Morphine, however, may cause vasodilation, which threatens adequate cerebral perfusion. Fentanyl and other shorter-acting synthetic opioids (alfentanyl, sufentanyl, and remifentanil) may cause carbon dioxide–independent ICP increases.[22,65]

Osmotherapy

Osmotic diuretics are frequently used to decrease ICP. The ideal osmotic agent produces a favorable osmotic gradient by remaining largely in the intravascular compartment, being inert and nontoxic, and having minimal systemic side effects. The most common osmotic diuretic used is mannitol.

Mannitol (Osmitrol) is usually given as a 20% solution in bolus doses of 0.25 to 1 g/kg and not as a continuous infusion. ICP will typically decrease within 15 to 20 minutes, with maximum effect occurring in approximately 90 minutes and lasting up to 6 hours. A powerful osmotic diuretic, mannitol draws fluid from the intracellular and interstitial spaces into the vascular compartment. The resulting hemodilution reduces blood viscosity, which improves CBF and cerebral oxygen delivery. Another beneficial effect of mannitol is a reduction in red blood cell (RBC) rigidity, which also facilitates RBC movement into small vessels.[22,159,175]

An intact BBB is relatively impermeable to the effects of mannitol. However, in high serum osmolarity or after prolonged use, the BBB can become damaged, allowing mannitol and other large molecules to enter the extracellular space. Thus it can cause a reverse osmosis and actually draw fluid into brain cells, causing a rebound rise in ICP (Fig. 12.22). A serum osmolality of 300 to 320 mOsm/L has been recommended for patients with poor intracranial compliance. However, in an attempt to obtain maximal benefit from osmotherapy in patients with brain injuries, a serum osmolality greater than 320 mOsm/L can be permitted if used with caution.[22,159,175]

Close monitoring of serum osmolality is essential when using diuretics to prevent inadvertent volume depletion. As osmolality rises, increased blood viscosity causes a decrease in CPP, which subsequently leads to cerebral vasodilation and a rise in ICP. With repeated doses, mannitol may become less effective in reducing ICP. Consequences of prolonged or repeated doses of mannitol include dehydration, hypotension, hypokalemia, and renal failure. It is important to maintain euvolemia with adequate fluid replacement when administering mannitol.[22,175]

Another osmotic agent that is used as an alternative to mannitol is HTS. These two options are compared in Table 12.7. The mechanism of action of HTS is based on the high tonicity of the fluid, which draws water from the cells and interstitial tissues into the vascular spaces. Other benefits include dehydration of erythrocytes and endothelial cells (leads to improved blood flow), vasoregulation (vasoconstriction as a result of decreased viscosity), stabilization of cell membrane (facilitates function of sodium-potassium pump), improved hemodynamic stability, and immune modulation.[159,175] The dose and concentration of HTS that are most effective, most commonly used, and equimolar to mannitol for the treatment of increased ICP is 3%[47]; however, researchers continues to look at concentrations that range from 2% to 24.3%. The current recommended dosage for 3% HTS is between 0.1 and 1.0 mL/kg of body weight per hour given as a bolus for the greatest effect, as the osmotic gradient may be less effective when given as a continuous infusion. Sodium levels should not exceed 165–170 mEq/L. In the patient with refractory increased ICP despite maximal osmotic therapy, other therapies to reduce ICP must be initiated.[90]

Furosemide (Lasix) is a nonosmotic diuretic that can be used alone or in combination with osmotic agents to potentiate the effect. Furosemide acts rapidly and reduces ICP to a lesser extent than mannitol or other osmotic agents, but is not associated with increased cerebral blood flow.[56]

Cerebrospinal Fluid Drainage

EVDs are used for several reasons: to monitor ICP, as a treatment of ICP by facilitating drainage of CSF, and to monitor the color and amount of CSF. By draining CSF, one of the contents of the cranial vault, more space is created within the cranium

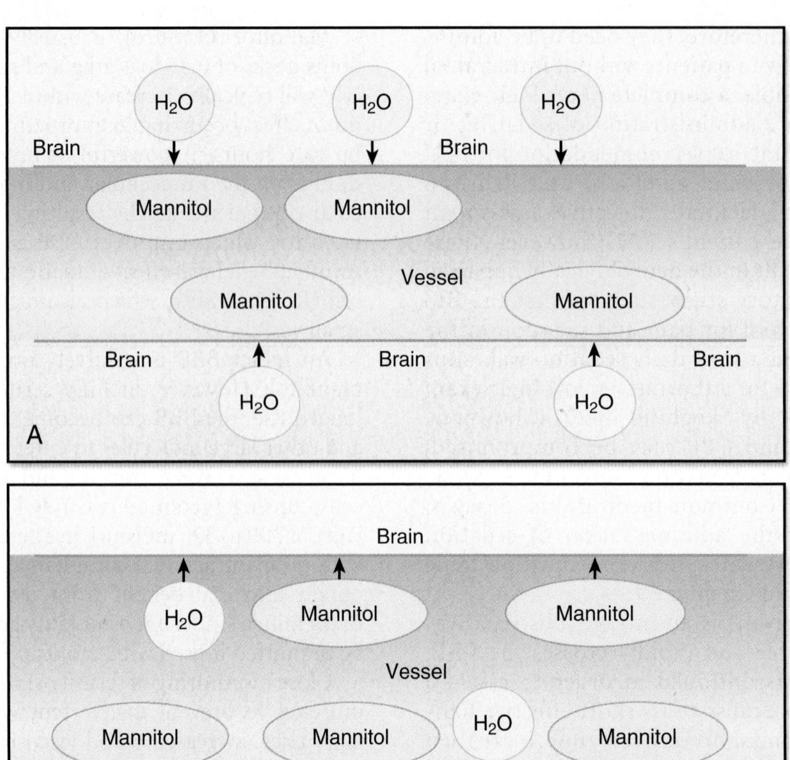

FIG. 12.22 Effect of mannitol on fluid movement in the brain. A, Normal effect of mannitol. B, Reverse effect of mannitol.

TABLE 12.7 Comparison of Mannitol and Hypertonic Saline Solution

	Mannitol	Hypertonic Saline Solution
Bolus dosing	0.25–1 g/kg rapid bolus	None
Infusion dose		0.1–1 mL/kg/h
Maximum serum osmolality	320 mOsm/L	360 mOsm/L
Diuretic effect	Osmotic diuretic; may necessitate volume replacement to avoid hypovolemia	Diuresis through action of atrial natriuretic peptide (ANP)
Proposed beneficial effect	Antioxidant effects	Restoration of resting membrane potential and cell volume, inhibition of inflammation
Adverse effects	Renal failure, hypotension, rebound elevation in ICP	Rebound elevation in ICP, central pontine myelinolysis, bleeding, electrolyte abnormalities

From References 22, 159, and 175.

and ICP will decrease. Removing CSF too quickly can result in ventricular collapse and deterioration in the patient's neurologic status, and lead to upward herniation of the brain stem.[6] Complications of EVDs and CSF drains include dislodgment of the catheter, blockage of the catheter by blood or debris, hemorrhage, and infectious complications. The EVD is leveled and zeroed to an external reference point representing the foramen of Monro. The external auditory canal, or the tragus of the ear, can be used as a visible landmark for this structure. The height of the drainage chamber at a level above zero is determined by the provider to create a pressure gradient that the CSF pressure must exceed, thus controlling the ICP and amount of CSF drainage. The nurse should closely monitor the EVD for appropriate positioning and drainage; CSF drainage decreases if the collection unit is raised and drainage increases if the collection unit is lowered. The provider's orders should state whether the EVD is to remain open to continuous drainage and only monitor the ICP intermittently (hourly) or to monitor ICP continuously and provide intermittent drainage at scheduled intervals or when an ICP measurement is higher than a certain value.[6] One study found that continuous drainage may miss underlying episodes of increased ICP; therefore, pressure should be continuously monitored by a second device or drainage should be intermittent.[141] To avoid infectious complications such as ventriculitis and meningitis, it is imperative that the system remains closed and strict aseptic technique is utilized when any interruption of the system is necessary (e.g., whenever samples are removed or when tubing is changed).[6,64,78] The use of routine antibiotics is not advocated by the BTF Guidelines, but a dose of antibiotic should be administered 30 minutes prior to or up to 2 hours after the procedure.[21,22] There is no strong evidence as to best practice for dressing and care of the EVD site; practices range from no dressing to occlusive dressing with antiseptic cleansing.[6]

Neuromuscular Blocking Agents

The use of neuromuscular blocking agents (NMBAs) is appropriate to facilitate mechanical ventilation and to control intracranial hypertension related to muscle movement such as posturing, or nursing care such as turning and suctioning. The use of NMBAs is only a temporary bridge to more definitive treatments that control problems with agitation and should always be used in conjunction with analgesics and sedation.[160]

NMDAs can only be used in mechanically ventilated patients. They may be especially helpful in the first 24 to 48 hours following injury to prevent asynchronous breathing with the ventilator and other activities that increase intracranial pressure or increase cerebral oxygen demand. Depolarizing and nondepolarizing agents are available as short- and long-acting agents. For routine intubations, depolarizing, short-acting agents, such as succinylcholine (Anectine), are typically the medications of choice. However, succinylcholine can cause increased ICP and should be avoided in patients with TBI.[160] Depolarizing agents should also be avoided for patients who have been immobile or in critical care for a long period of time because these agents cause release of intracellular potassium, which may lead to profound cardiac complications such as ventricular tachycardia and asystole.[115] The best choice for prolonged ICP management is provided by longer-acting, nondepolarizing agents such as cisatracurium or vecuronium.[160] Chapter 39 reviews commonly used NMBAs along with dosing recommendations and duration of action. Although previously believed not to penetrate the brain, it is now known that these agents do cross the BBB and may activate brain acetylcholine receptors. This could lead to central autonomic dysfunction, weakness, and seizures. If used, patients should be carefully monitored using a peripheral nerve stimulator to minimize resistance caused by receptor upregulation.[160]

Second-Level Approaches for Intracranial Pressure Management

For patients with ICP refractory to first-tier therapies, there are various second-tier therapeutic options, including induced barbiturate coma, controlled hyperventilation, mild hypothermia, and surgical decompression (Fig. 12.23).

Barbiturates

Barbiturates, such as thiopental or pentobarbital, may be used to treat patients with refractory ICP. Intravenous barbiturates are administered in anesthetic doses to induce coma and a dose-dependent decrease in CMR and CBF, thus decreasing ICP. With intact autoregulation, the reduction in ICP occurs by decreasing cerebral blood volume by cerebral vasoconstriction. There may also be an effect on decreasing secondary brain injury by stabilizing plasma and lysosomal membranes and reducing the release of excitotoxic amino acids and intracellular calcium concentrations.[114,152]

Despite evidence of cerebral protection in experimental models, there is little evidence that barbiturates improve outcome after severe head injuries. A recent study suggests that younger patients with EDH, contusions, and lower severity of injury treated with barbiturates will have a better outcome.[110] Negative consequences to the use of barbiturates include decreased gastrointestinal motility, decreased protective mechanisms (i.e., suppression of cough and gag reflexes), and immunosuppression, leading to increased susceptibility to pulmonary complications such as pneumonia. High doses of pentobarbital can cause myocardial depression, necessitating the use of vasopressors to maintain BP and CPP. Serum pentobarbital levels may be monitored in order to determine adequacy of dosages and to avoid toxicity, but are often inaccurate.[145] Induction of barbiturate coma should be monitored by continuous EEG or BIS monitoring to attain a burst suppression ratio of 5 to 10 seconds of suppression to 1 second of burst activity.[8]

Targeted Temperature Management – Normothermia Versus Hypothermia

Temperature regulation is an important management strategy in TBI patients in order to prevent and treat ICP. Hyperthermia is detrimental to the brain because it impairs energy metabolism, disrupts the BBB, and increases the release of excitatory neurotransmitters and free radicals, all of which contribute to increased ICP. Increased body temperature has also been associated with increased cytokine release and worse outcomes in TBI. Animal models and small, single site clinical studies of therapeutic hypothermia demonstrated promise, yet multiple RCTs have failed to demonstrate improved outcomes using induced hypothermia.[4,40,41,50,81,109] Side effects of hypothermia include shivering, dysrhythmia, hemodynamic instability, and suppressed immune system. Hypothermia should only be used in patients with primary central nervous system injury because it can cause or exacerbate complications in specific populations. For example, it can lead to coagulopathy and acidosis in the trauma patient because of platelet alterations, enzyme inhibition, and fibrinolysis.[41]

Although the benefit of induced hypothermia in TBI has not been shown in RCTs, there is evidence to demonstrate the detrimental effect of hyperthermia, the relationship to increased ICP, and neurologic deterioration. There is a linear relationship between increased temperature leading to an increase in CBF and a resultant increase in ICP. Early treatment and diagnosis of the underlying cause of fever (>38°C) are critical in TBI patients to minimize its effect on secondary brain injury. Maintenance of normothermia (36.5°C–37.5°C) is essential.[46,109] Several techniques are available for both external and internal cooling.

Controlled Hyperventilation

Hyperventilation, once the cornerstone in the treatment of increased ICP, has been shown to be detrimental to the patient and to brain tissue. Decreased $Paco_2$ is a potent vasoconstrictor; hyperventilation results in vasoconstriction, which subsequently leads to a decrease in intracranial blood volume and ICP. Aggressive hyperventilation ($Paco_2 < 30$ mm Hg) may result in extreme constriction in cerebral blood vessels, severely compromising blood flow to the point of causing ischemia. Current recommendations from the TBI Guidelines suggest maintaining normocarbia in the low-normal level of $Paco_2$ 35 to 40 mm Hg. The use of prophylactic hyperventilation ($Paco_2 \leq 35$ mm Hg) during the first 24 hours after TBI should be avoided because of the potential for compromised cerebral perfusion. Further hyperventilation can severely reduce blood flow and is not recommended without some additional monitoring

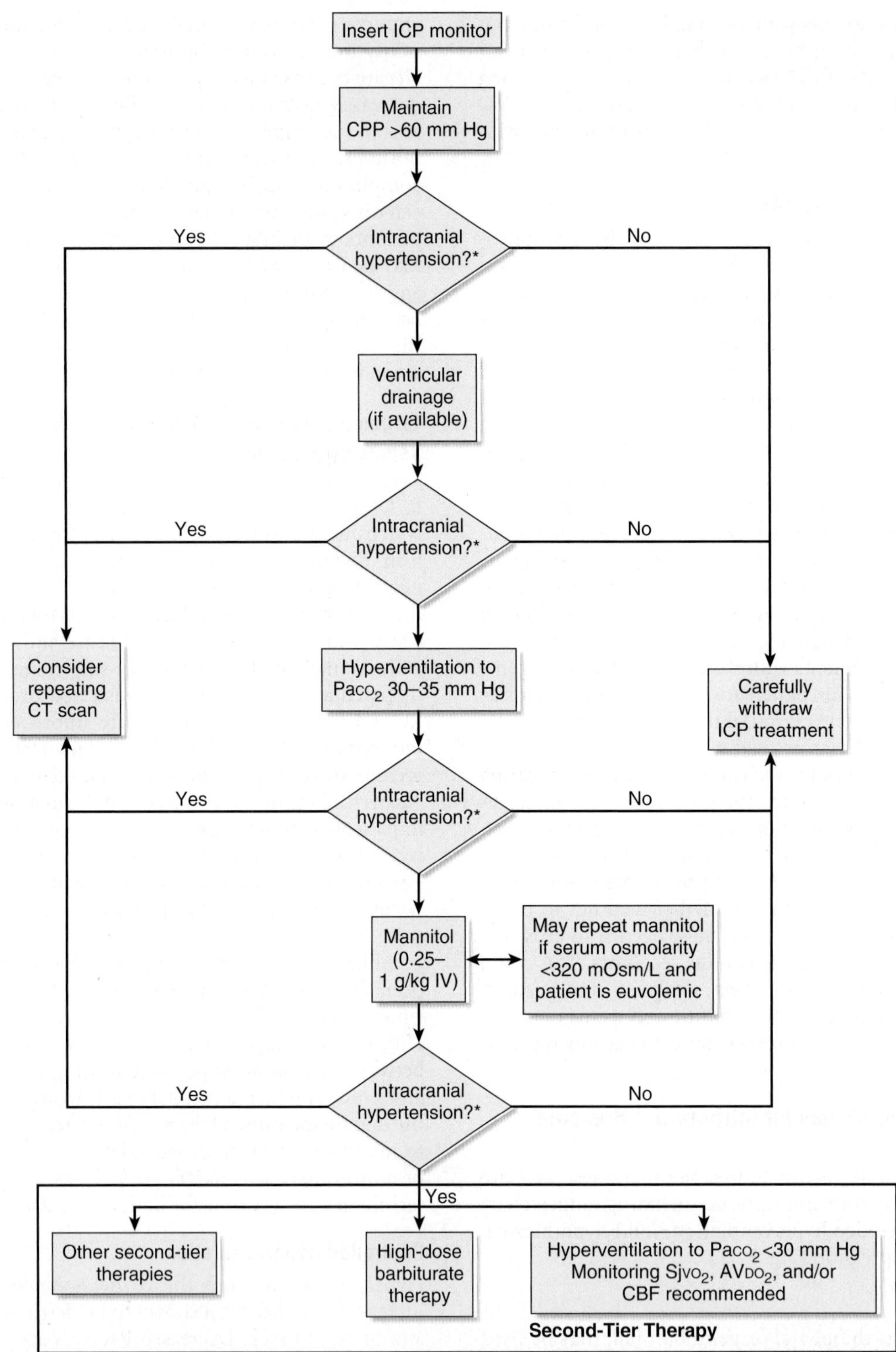

*Threshold of 20–25 mm Hg may be used. Other variables may be substituted in individual conditions.

FIG. 12.23 Algorithm for treatment of increased intracranial pressure. *$AVDO_2$*, Arteriovenous oxygen content difference; *CBF*, cerebral blood flow; *CPP*, cerebral perfusion pressure; *CT*, computed tomography; *ICP*, intracranial pressure; *mOsm/L*, milliosmoles per liter; *$Paco_2$*, partial pressure of arterial carbon dioxide; *$Sjvo_2$*, jugular venous oxygen saturation.

of brain tissue oxygenation via $Sjvo_2$ or Bto_2 or CBF to ensure that any further reduction in $Paco_2$ (values < 30 mm Hg) does not compromise blood flow and cause brain tissue ischemia.[22] $Paco_2$ of 20 to 25 mm Hg may reduce the CBF by 40% to 50%, and, conversely, an increase to greater than 50 mm Hg increases CBF by more than 50%. These changes occur almost immediately in a healthy human, but responses may be altered after head injury.[19]

Decompressive Craniectomy

Decompressive craniectomy (DC) is another treatment for severe, refractory intracranial hypertension that does not respond to first-tier measures. Removal of a large area of the skull allows for an increase in intracranial volume without an increase in pressure.[94] A Cochrane Review published in 2006 concluded that there was no evidence supporting routine use of DC, although it is an option that may improve survival and neurologic outcome in some patients.[161] Several unanswered questions remain regarding which patients are appropriate for this surgery and which surgical technique should be used. There are two approaches to this procedure: a bifrontal craniectomy (removal of both frontal bones) and a hemicraniectomy (removal typically of the frontotemporoparietal bone on one side). In 2011, the controversial results of the Decompressive Craniectomy in Patients with Severe Traumatic Brain Injury (DECRA) RCT were reported, showing no significant improvement of outcome in patients randomized to early bifrontal DC. The surgery was performed for an ICP greater than 20 mm Hg sustained for longer than 15 minutes with patients who failed first-tier therapies compared to those who did not undergo early bifrontal DC, with the DC group having a poor outcome of 70% compared to 51% in the control group.[45] The results are expected on another multicenter RCT, RESCUEicp study (Randomized Evaluation of Surgery with Craniectomy for Uncontrollable Elevation of Intra-Cranial Pressure), which compares the standard medical treatment of refractory ICP greater than 25 for longer than 1 to 12 hours to DCH. This study may provide new evidence on this topic.[150]

STRATEGIES FOR NEUROPROTECTION

All the interventions described previously are aimed at reducing cerebral edema and preventing secondary injury. More definitive treatment strategies for neuroprotection are still in the experimental stages. To date, no studies of neuroprotection have shown beneficial in large human RCTs. Agents studied and being studied include free radical scavengers to prevent lipid peroxidation, *N*-methyl-D-aspartate (NMDA), and alpha amino-3-hydroxy-5-methylisoxazole-4-propionic acid (AMPA) receptor antagonists to limit damage from excitatory amino acids such as glutamate, calcium antagonists to prevent influx of calcium into cells, and hormones such as estrogen and progesterone.[9,100,155]

PREVENTION AND TREATMENT OF COMPLICATIONS AFTER TRAUMATIC BRAIN INJURY

Unfortunately, many problems can occur following a TBI that further complicate the patient's course. It is important for the nurse to be aware of these complications in order to prevent their occurrence or to be able to identify them early so that proper treatment can be instituted. Complications result from the injury itself, immune dysfunction resulting from TBI, and problems related to the patient's immobility.

Coagulopathy

TBI and severe traumatic injuries are associated with activation of the coagulation system from the inflammatory response and damage to the endothelium. Activation of the coagulation system results in increased clotting and consumption of clotting factors that ultimately lead to excessive bleeding. In the TBI patient, clotting issues may develop in the absence of excessive bleeding. This condition occurs from a large release of thromboplastin from the brain parenchyma and from tissue emboli that are produced by circulating factor VII released from vascular endothelium. The severity of coagulopathy has been correlated with the severity of morbidity from TBI.[53,108,168] It is important to monitor coagulation parameters and replace RBCs, clotting factors (fibrinogen and factor XIII), cryoprecipitate, plasma, and platelets as indicated by laboratory tests. The use of factor VIIa to treat coagulopathy remains controversial, as results from RCTs are conflicting regarding benefit, dose, and outcome.[108]

Venous Thrombosis (Deep Vein Thrombosis)

Venous thrombosis occurs at a rate of 1 to 2 per 1000 trauma patients regardless of pharmacologic prophylaxis and increases to 25% in the TBI population.[149,162] Studies suggest that deep vein thrombosis (DVT) develops as early as 24 hours after injury.[83] Studies have found that early prophylaxis using intermittent compression devices and chemoprophylaxis, and unfractionated heparin, or low-molecular-weight heparin, decrease the incidence of DVT. The exact timing of chemoprophylaxis is unclear due to the risk of expansion of hemorrhage. In a meta-analysis by Jamjoom and Jamjoom in 2013, the risk ratio of developing an ICH with early (within 72 hours) prophylaxis compared to late (after 72 hours) prophylaxis was 0.64.[83] Adbel-Aziz found similar risk benefit in providing chemoprophylaxis with a 5.6% risk of hematoma expansion with prophylaxis started within 72 hours and 1.5% risk after 3 days.[3] The risk of developing DVT increased from 2.6% when chemoprophylaxis was started in 1 to 3 days, 2.6% when started within 4 to 5 days, and 14.1% when started in 8 days.[3] Early chemoprophylaxis with consideration for hematoma stability[60,146] and risk of expansion along with use of mechanical devices should be implemented.[42] Use of compression stockings does not appear to have benefit.

Electrolyte Disturbances

An understanding of fluid and electrolyte imbalances associated with head injury is important for optimal patient management. The reader is referred to Chapter 21 for detailed discussions of electrolyte management. This chapter addresses these issues as they relate to TBI, hyper- or hyponatremia resulting from central neurogenic diabetes insipidus (CNDI), syndrome of inappropriate antidiuretic hormone (SIADH), and cerebral salt wasting (CSW). Uncorrected hyper- or hyponatremia may lead to deterioration of neurologic status and a worsening of outcome.

Hyponatremia

A serum sodium (Na) concentration of less than 131 mEq/L, as seen with SIADH or CSW, occurs in approximately 25% to 33% of patients with TBI and is twice as likely to occur in mild and moderate TBI than STBI.[91] Hyponatremia will usually occur in the first week after injury and will most frequently be from SIADH. In SIADH, hyponatremia is often due to excess antidiuretic hormone (ADH) secretion secondary to stimulation of the feedback mechanisms, osmoreceptors and baroreceptors, which are activated by hypovolemia, fluid restriction, or hemorrhage. When serum osmolarity increases and stimulus on the baroreceptors is decreased, ADH is secreted and stimulated by the renal tubules to hold on to free water. Although excess ADH secretion is an appropriate response to hypovolemia, it is in-appropriate when it results in water intoxication and hyponatremia as seen in SIADH.[85]

Syndrome of inappropriate antidiuretic hormone. SIADH occurs as a result of increased ADH secretion leading to water retention, increased ECF volume, decreased urine output, and a dilatational hyponatremia. Diagnosis of SIADH is by clinical signs and laboratory studies. Clinical signs include decreased urine output to less than 500 cc/4 hours, and weight gain due to fluid retention. Laboratory findings include hyponatremia (< 135 mEq/L), decreased serum osmolality (< 275 mOsm/L), elevated urine osmolarity (greater than serum osmolarity), and urine sodium excretion greater than 25 mEq/L. Other clinical signs include headache, nausea, vomiting, fatigue, muscle twitching, confusion, lethargy, decreased LOC, coma, and seizures (latter two signs seen with sodium <120 mEq/L). Conservative treatment involves fluid restriction of less than 1 L/24 hours and sodium replacement for mild hyponatremia. More aggressive therapy includes administration of HTS (3%) and possibly furosemide for diuresis.[85,91,127] Two new vasopressin receptor agonists are available to treat patients with SIADH: Conivaptan, which blocks both V2 receptors and V1A receptors,[113,138] and Tolvaptan, a V2 receptor inhibitor that suppresses AQP expression by the renal collecting ducts.[70]

Cerebral salt wasting. Another form of hyponatremia associated with TBI is CSW which is a true hyponatremia due to a loss of sodium and water. It is hypothesized that this condition occurs when brain injury triggers the stress response and a surge of sympathetic nervous system hormones and catecholamines act on the kidneys to excrete sodium and there is an excessive secretion of atrial natriuretic hormone. As a result, there is an inability to conserve sodium and water, leading to hypovolemia. Other symptoms of this syndrome are tachycardia, dehydration, weight loss, lethargy that may progress to a decreased LOC, coma, and seizures. Laboratory tests will show serum hyponatremia, low serum osmolarity, elevated urine sodium and osmolarity, increased hematocrit, blood urea nitrogen, and urine specific gravity. Unlike SIADH, patients with CSW require fluid volume replacement with a combination of NS and HTS (3%). Caution must be used when administering HTS as rapid correction of the sodium level may lead to central pontine myelinolysis. Restriction of fluids and use of diuretics is contraindicated and could be deadly, as patients are volume depleted. In more severe cases, fludrocortisone (Florinef) may be given to facilitate the absorption of sodium by the renal tubules.[85,91,127] See Table 12.8 for a comparison of CSW with SIADH and diabetes insipidus.

Hypernatremia

Hypernatremia is defined as a plasma sodium level greater than 145 mEq/L. Hypernatremia is associated with hyperosmolality and may be caused by water depletion. In water-depleted states, the thirst mechanism stimulates a conscious individual to drink water, a response frequently impossible for the neurologically impaired or unresponsive patient. Hypernatremia is generally not symptomatic unless plasma sodium concentration is 155 to 160 mEq/L or greater (this equates to water depletion of 6 liters or more in a 70-kg male). Clinical symptoms with hypernatremia include pyrexia, restlessness, weakness, paralysis, irritability, drowsiness, lethargy, confusion, tremor, hyperreflexia, seizures, and coma. These findings are the result of increased osmolality that reduces brain cell volume. Hypernatremia is fairly well tolerated if it develops slowly. However, a sudden drop in the osmolality of the ECF can cause a shift of water into the brain cells, producing cerebral edema.[173]

Diabetes insipidus. Diabetes Insipidus (DI) is characterized by polyuria and polydipsia resulting either from a complete or partial failure of ADH secretion (central or neurogenic DI) or from a decrease in the renal response to ADH (nephrogenic DI); as many as 20% of TBI patients may develop DI. Early-onset DI is typical following major hypothalamic damage and is associated with a high mortality rate. Head-injured patients with fractures involving the base of the skull and sella turcica are at an increased risk for DI. Time of onset of DI in TBI is commonly 5 to 10 days, but can be as early as 12 to 24 hours following injury. DI is characterized by polyuria, hypernatremia, plasma hyperosmolality, and low urine specific gravity.[85]

DI is treated with administration of maintenance fluids along with hourly fluid replacement with 0.45% saline solution equal or greater to the urinary output. Aqueous vasopressin (AVP) 0.5 to 2 units IV administered every 3 hours is given if urine output remains excessive (< 300 mL/h over 2 consecutive hours) in the absence of diuretics or the presence of hyperosmolality. An AVP continuous infusion of 0.2 unit/min may be needed and can be titrated as needed to a maximum dose of 0.9 unit/min. Desmopressin (DDAVP), a synthetic analog of AVP with a longer half-life and fewer vasoconstrictive effects, may also be used. The usual dose of DDAVP is 5 to 40 mcg/day in divided doses. It is important to monitor urine output and to watch for water excess, evidenced by hyponatremia and elevated urinary osmolality.[85]

TABLE 12.8 Differentiation of Diabetes Insipidus from Syndrome of Inappropriate Antidiuretic Hormone and Cerebral Salt Wasting Syndrome

	Serum Sodium	Serum Osmolality	Urine Sodium	Urine Osmolality	Urine Specific Gravity
Diabetes insipidus*	↑	↑	↓	↓	↓
SIADH	↓	↓	↑	↑	↑
Salt wasting syndrome	↓	↑ or normal	↑	↑	↑

*Cerebral salt wasting (CSW) syndrome is associated with dehydration and increased BUN levels, whereas dehydration is absent in SIADH and BUN levels are normal.
From References 9, 91, and 127.

Volume Depletion

Dehydration increases sympathetic stimulation, metabolism, and oxygen demand. The aim of therapy is to maintain euvolemia and normal physiologic indexes, especially CPP. There is no evidence to support fluid restriction as a means of limiting cerebral edema following brain injury, therefore it is no longer considered appropriate to keep TBI patients "dry."[85]

Tonicity defines effective osmolality (i.e., the osmotic force caused by the particles), which cannot permeate between compartments. All body fluids must be in osmotic equilibrium. Changes in tonicity, regardless of their cause, will result in fluid shifts between the ECF and the intracellular fluid (ICF) in order to reestablish osmotic equilibrium. Patients with osmotic hypertonicity will have a contracted intracellular compartment. Because brain expansion is limited by the confines of the skull, severe hyponatremia will result in cerebral edema and increased ICP. Urea increases osmolality but does not affect tonicity, and because it passes freely through biological membranes, it will not alter the intracellular volume.[130]

Fluid used for resuscitation should include isotonic fluids such as NS or lactated Ringer's solution. Both solutions are freely permeable across the vascular membrane and distribute evenly. Hypotonic solutions will decrease serum osmolality, which will promote water to move from the vascular compartment into the interstitial compartment, increasing cerebral edema, and should not be administered to head-injured patients. D_5W is a hypotonic solution and should not be used except to treat hypoglycemia as it encourages fluid movement into the cells, increasing cerebral edema.[68]

Until recently, colloid solutions such as albumin were thought to be beneficial in resuscitation of the TBI patient. Colloid solutions do not cross capillary membranes readily and are confined mainly to the intravascular spaces. The large protein molecules give colloid solutions a very high osmolality, drawing fluid from the interstitial and intracellular compartments into the vascular compartments.[68] Cooper et al. found that patients resuscitated with albumin had negative patient consequences due to increased ICP from albumin. Research concluded that albumin should not be given to TBI patients.[44]

The use of packed RBCs should be considered in TBI, if hemoglobin (Hgb) is less than 7 mg/dL especially in patients with acute blood loss from associated injuries. A recent RCT compared administration of erythropoietin, transfusion threshold with Hgb 7 g/dL, with maintaining Hgb greater than 10 g/dL. The study found no improvement in outcome in patients receiving erythropoietin or having an Hgb greater than 10 g/dL. Patients with an Hgb greater than 10 g/dL were associated with an increased number of adverse events.[153] Global tissue perfusion exacerbates cerebral hypoxia, cerebral ischemia, and increased ICP. RBCs expand circulating volume and may improve oxygen-carrying capacity to the injured brain.

Metabolic Response

As described earlier, the brain is highly dependent on oxygen and glucose for energy. There are adverse consequences when the supply of oxygen and glucose is inadequate to support the increased metabolic requirements of the injured brain.[101] Interestingly, hyperglycemia also adversely affects patient outcomes with TBI and is associated with more pronounced cerebral edema and a deterioration of brain energy metabolism.[156] Studies show that patients with blood glucose levels exceeding 200 mg/dL during the first 10 days postinjury in severe TBI have a 3.6-fold increased risk of death.[72] Current recommendations for TBI patients are to maintain glucose levels between 140 and 180 mg/dL.[10,125] Close monitoring of glucose levels at least every 2 to 4 hours is recommended to maintain normal levels.

Nutrition

Following a TBI, basal metabolic rate may be increased to 120% to 250% above normal, rapidly putting patients into a negative nitrogen balance.[10,43] Härtl et al. report a twofold increase in mortality if patients were not fed in 5 days and a fourfold increase if not fed in 7 days.[76] The Brain Trauma Foundation Guidelines recommend patients be fed as early as possible, ideally on day 1, preferably by enteral feeding, and that they reach their full caloric requirement by 7 days after injury. Protein should compose 15% of the calories.

Infectious Complications

TBI patients, like all ICU patients, are prone to infectious complications such as urinary tract infections (UTIs), bloodstream infections, pneumonia, and other systemic infections.[132] TBI patients are susceptible to developing central nervous system infections such as brain abscesses or meningitis resulting from a breach of the dura mater from penetrating objects or open skull fractures, and ventriculitis from the EVD.[22,27]

Patients with penetrating CNS wounds and open skull fractures may require meticulous cleansing, debridement, closure of their wounds, and appropriate antibiotic coverage to decrease the risk of wound infections, meningitis, and brain abscesses.[24–26,88] The nurse will need to maintain close surveillance of the wound site for evidence of infection.

Patients monitored with an EVD have a 6.6% (range 5.7–15%) risk for infection. Risk factors for developing a ventriculitis are: duration of ICP monitoring, use of prophylactic parenteral antibiotics, other infections, intraventricular hemorrhage or subarachnoid hemorrhage, open skull fracture/basilar skull fracture with CSF leak, leaking CSF around ICP catheter insertion sites, and invasion of EVD for flushing or changing the system. It is recommended that strict aseptic technique be used when inserting and manipulating the EVD and only periprocedural antibiotics be administered.[73] See Box 12.1 for more information on preventing infection with EVDs.

Pulmonary Complications

Pulmonary dysfunction is common in critically ill neurologic patients. Pulmonary complications associated with head injury include prolonged or permanent inadequate airway protection, ventilator-acquired events (VAE), ARDS and acute lung injury (ALI), neurogenic pulmonary edema (NPE), and pulmonary embolism from venous thromboembolism. The most common complication is pneumonia, either caused by aspiration at the time of the initial injury or acquired in the hospital. Ventilator-associated pneumonia (VAP) has the highest incidence in neurotrauma patients, and is related to immobility, loss of protective reflexes, and the immune suppression associated with trauma.[5,74,103] NPE and ALI/ARDS will be discussed here as related to TBI.

Patients with TBI may develop ALI or ARDS that negatively impact outcomes. In one study evaluating the use of CPP to direct goal-oriented management of TBI, the risk of ARDS was reported to be 5 times greater in the CPP-targeted

BOX 12.1 External Ventricular Drain Infection Prevention

Catheter Insertion

- Braid or clip hair with electric or disposable clippers
- Single dose of antibiotic is given before incision
- Hand hygiene
- Sterile gloves
- Sterile gown
- Cap
- Mask
- Large sterile drape
- Skin preparation (Providone iodine. Chlorhexidine gluconate not recommended due to meningeal toxicity per Food and Drug Administration [FDA]). Ensure preparation has completely dried before insertion
- All staff in room wear cap and mask during insertion
- Sterile occlusive dressing with transparent film–no routine dressing change

EVD Manipulation

- Don cap, mask, sterile gown, and sterile gloves
- Access port and surrounding tubing are cleaned with chlorhexidine, alcohol, providone iodine, or any combination of the three
- Port cap is removed and discarded
- Luer fitting inside of port is cleaned and rinsed (multiple times) with sterile, preservative-free normal saline
- CSF fluid draw or flush is performed with strict sterile technique
- New sterile port cap is applied
- Tubing and drainage system should not be routinely changed

From References 6, 29, 31, 64, and 99.

group than in the ICP-targeted group. Therefore, attempts to maintain CPP greater than 70 mm Hg with aggressive administration of fluids or vasopressors should be avoided because of the increased risk of ARDS.[154] Incidence of ALI/ARDS are reported to occur in 20% to 25% of TBI.[103] TBI patients are more susceptible to ARDS because of the central neurogenic mechanism for increased sympathetic activity, resulting in an increased capillary pressure, endothelial damage, and leaking of the capillaries, resulting in NPE. In addition, the inflammatory response to IL-6 inflammatory mediators contributes to NPE. A second theory is that the initial catecholamine surge and systemic inflammatory mediators followed by a second event from infections, transfusion, and mechanical ventilation set the patient up to develop ALI/ARDS. TBI patients who develop ARDS are more likely to develop refractory elevations of ICP and are 3 times more likely to be in a vegetative state or dead at 6 months post-injury.[103]

The treatment of ARDS includes the use of protective lung ventilation with the use of low tidal volume (6–8 mL/kg) and PEEP.[103] Low tidal volume ventilation commonly results in an increase in $Paco_2$, which is problematic for the TBI patient and can result in an elevated ICP. Use of PEEP with ARDS patients is a mainstay of treatment but has been controversial in those with head injuries. Although PEEP improves oxygenation in the head-injured patient, it also alters systemic hemodynamics by increasing intrathoracic pressure, which, in turn, increases CVP and decreases cardiac filling.[103] This results in decreased MAP, reduced CPP, and, subsequently, increased ICP.[133] In patients with intact cerebral autoregulation, the responses to MAP reduction can be tolerated without development of cerebral ischemia. However, when autoregulation is impaired, there is a greater risk of ischemia.[103]

Seizures

Seizures are a known complication in TBI and can occur as early posttraumatic seizures (PTS) within the first 7 days after injury or late PTS after the first week. Early PTS occur at a rate of 2.6% to 16.9%, and late PTS 1.9% to 30%. A recent military series suggest soldiers may have an incidence of 34% to 63% late posttraumatic seizures.[32] Seizures are more likely in patients with penetrating brain injuries with an incidence of 30% to 50%, and in patients with contusions or subdural hematomas.[88,106] Seizure activity increases cerebral metabolism and CBF, exacerbating cerebral ischemia and secondary brain injury in TBI patients.

Benzodiazepines reduce cerebral metabolism and increase the seizure threshold, making them valuable first-line agents for treating seizures. Administration of prophylactic anticonvulsants is controversial, and studies have not shown that they prevent the development of late posttraumatic epilepsy. Anticonvulsant agents such as phenytoin (Dilantin) or fosphenytoin (Cerebyx) are indicated for seizure prophylaxis for the first 7 days postinjury with carbamazepine (Tegretol), or valproate (Depakote) recommend by the TBI Guidelines, but these are less widely studied. Prophylactic treatment beyond the first 7 days after injury is not recommend.[22] Phenytoin is given as a loading dose of 15 mg/kg followed by a maintenance dose of 100 mg every 6 to 8 hours unless a seizure has occurred in the patient. Adverse effects associated with the use of phenytoin are rash, Stevens-Johnson syndrome, leukopenia, and elevated liver enzymes.[33,174] As an alternative, levetiracetam (Keppra) has been found to have comparable efficacy to phenytoin with fewer side effects.[97,140,174]

Gastrointestinal Prophylaxis

TBI is an independent risk factor for the development of gastrointestinal (GI) bleeding resulting from gastric erosion due to high hyperacidity. Development of GI bleeding can be related to elevated cortisol levels, hypothalamic dysfunction, and vagal hyperactivity, which lead to ulcer formation in the stomach, esophagus, and duodenum. Mechanical ventilation as well as coagulopathy and renal dysfunction may potentiate the problem. Proton pump inhibitors (PPI), and histamine receptor antagonists (H2A) (ranitidine) have been found to reduce GI bleeding in the critically ill patient. However, a recent meta-analysis questions these recommendations, citing poor quality of the data.[95] Caution must be used when administering these medications, for they may interact with other medications such as anticonvulsants and antiplatelet agents, and may increase nosocomial pneumonia rates.[163]

Paroxysmal Dysautonomia

Paroxysmal dysautonomia (PD) has been described using many terms, including *diencephalic seizures, storming, sympathetic storming, autonomic dysfunction syndrome,* and others. It is most commonly seen in patients with DAI and may start in the first week to weeks following the injury. Patients with PD have increased days on the ventilator and periods of unconsciousness. Patients exhibit a constellation of symptoms, including tachycardia, hypertension, tachypnea, hyperthermia, motor posturing (decorticate or decerebrate), and diaphoresis.[61,66,77] The syndrome is poorly understood but is thought to be a disconnection between the cortex and the hypothalamus, or an imbalance between excitatory and inhibitory neurotransmitters. Treatment is focused on pharmacologic agents to control symptoms associated with the autonomic instability. There are no RCTs and most publications quote case reports cessation on treatment such as regularly scheduled morphine sulfate administration which appear to show benefit.[16] Other medications found to be useful either alone or in combination include propranolol (Inderal), clonidine (Catapres), chlorpromazine (Thorazine), bromocriptine (Parlodel), dantrolene (Dantrium), atenolol (Tenormin), and labetalol (Normodyne).[144,172]

OTHER MEDICATIONS USED FOR TRAUMATIC BRAIN INJURY

Lidocaine

Lidocaine, a local anesthetic, may be given to prevent ICP spikes during intubation. The dose is 1 to 1.5 mg/kg IV given within 60 to 90 seconds of intubation or as a 4% intra-tracheal aerosol.[114] Bolus doses of 1 mg/kg lidocaine can be given intravenously or via endotracheal tube before suctioning to blunt the increased ICP response to suctioning.[116] In 2009, Bilotta et al. found that the doses could be safely administered down the ETT up 2 mg/kg/hour adjusting the dose up or down by 0.5 mg/kg/hour to blunt the cough.[13]

Steroids

Steroids are contraindicated in the TBI patient. Steroids have been shown in several RCTs to not reduce ICP or improve outcome and to increase death rate when given after severe brain injury. The CRASH (Clinical Randomization of an Antifibrinolytic in Significant Hemorrhage) trial researched the effect of intravenous corticosteroids on death within 14 days. The study was halted early due to clinically significant detrimental effects on traumatic head injury patients. Steroids are effective in the treatment of edema associated with brain tumors and abscesses.[48,49]

OUTCOMES

Outcomes following TBI are often predicted based on initial GCS and functional level. Mortality rates have decreased and there have been improved functional outcomes in the past decades with improved prehospital and in hospital care using the TBI guidelines. However, an accurate prognosis cannot be determined for up to 12 months after injury, and improvement may continue for 3 to 5 years after injury. Because of the heterogeneity of brain injuries, differing age responses, and varying extent of secondary injuries, it is difficult to accurately predict patient outcomes.[36] Two factors shown to negatively impact outcomes following TBI are the presence of hypotension and hypoxia at any point following TBI.[36] Hypotension and hypoxia occurring in the early posttraumatic period are primary determinants of outcome. Even one episode of hypotension increases the morbidity and mortality associated with TBI. The Traumatic Coma Data Bank confirmed this finding when data analysis demonstrated that prehospital hypotension was an independent predictor of poor outcome.[36]

Family decision-making related to prognosis of TBI is extremely difficult because of the differing responses and outcomes. It is extremely difficult for families facing the potential reality of a loved one being left in a persistent vegetative state and making the decision to withdraw life-saving supportive measures. In the cases of TBI resulting in brain death, families are also faced with the decision of organ donation; even if brain death is not determined and the decision to withdraw support is made, the possibility of donation after cardiac death exists. It is important for families to fully understand the implications of all care alternatives in order to make the most informed decisions. Family support regarding all potential options related to outcomes is essential. This is also true when patients are left with long-term disabilities. Family access to community resources is indispensable in assisting with physical, psychological, emotional, and social needs.

CONCLUSION

Patients who recover from severe head injury may have significant cognitive and physical handicaps, producing social disability. The distinction between primary brain damage and damage that develops from secondary events is helpful in explaining the apparent paradox of one patient whose initial injury was relatively mild yet ends up with severe brain damage, whereas another patient whose early condition was life-threatening recovers completely. Patients with the same type of lesion may have markedly different outcomes, depending on the causative lesion and treatment received.

The most commonly used predictors of outcome are based on postresuscitation GCS score, pupil reaction, age, and type of head injury. Computerized tools have been developed and validated by the CRASH trial which include age, GCS, pupils, and presence of major extracranial injury[131] and IMPACT model.[136] TBI is not limited to an isolated event or impact. It is instead an aggregate of many mechanisms involving both primary and secondary damage. It is essential that the critical care nurse be knowledgeable of events contributing to secondary injury in order to aggressively prevent and treat potential causes of further deterioration. Early hemorrhage control, volume resuscitation, tissue oxygenation, optimization of cerebral perfusion, adequate treatment of increased intracranial pressure, temperature management, and prevention of complications are essential components of TBI patient care.

CASE STUDY 12.1

M.P., a 34-year-old male, fell 20 feet from the roof of his house, hitting his head. Emergency medical technicians (EMTs) arrived in 5 minutes to find M.P. walking around his yard disoriented and combative, with a GCS of 14. Within minutes he loses consciousness, develops difficulty breathing, and requires intubation. GCS is now 7; pupils are unequal, right 3 mm and briskly reactive, left 5 mm and sluggishly reactive. On arrival to the emergency department he has a grand mal seizure and is given IV lorazepam and a loading dose of phenytoin. Pupils are still unequal, and both are reacting sluggishly with a GCS of 7. Head CT scan reveals a left SDH, a small left temporal SAH, a left temporal nondepressed skull fracture, and a left basilar skull fracture. He is taken to the OR for evacuation of the SDH. An intraparenchymal ICP monitor is placed in his right cerebral hemisphere, and M.P. is admitted to neuroscience critical care. The next day, M.P. develops sustained increases in ICP to greater than 30 mm Hg on several occasions.

Decision Point:
What should the plan of care look like?

Decision Point:
What are the treatment options?

REFERENCES

1. Aaslid, R., et al. (2003). Dynamic pressure-flow velocity relationships in the human cerebral circulation. *Stroke, 34*, 1645–1649.
2. Adamides, A., Cooper, D. J., Rosenfeldt, F. L., Bailey, M. J., Pratt, N., Tippett, N., et al. (2009). Focal cerebral oxygenation and neurological outcome with or without brain tissue oxygen-guided therapy in patients with traumatic brain injury. *Acta Neurochir, 151*(11), 1399–1409.
3. Adbel-Aziz, H., Dunhuam, C. M., Malik, R. J., & Hileman, B. M. (2015). Timing for deep vein thrombosis chemoprophylaxis in traumatic brain injury: an evidence-based review. *Crit Care, 19*, 96–106.
4. Adelson, P. D., Wisniewski, S. R., Beca, J., Brown, S. D., Bell, M., Muizelaar, J. P., et al. (2013). Paediatric Traumatic Brain Injury Consortium. Comparison of hypothermia and normothermia after severe traumatic brain injury in children (Cool Kids): a phase 3, randomized controlled trial. *Lancet Neurol, 12*(6), 546–553.
5. American Thoracic Society & Infectious Diseases Society of America. (2005). Guidelines for the management of adults with hospital-acquired, ventilator-associated, and healthcare-associated pneumonia. *Am J Respir Crit Care Med, 171*, 388–416.
6. AANN Clinical Practice Guidelines Series, & Thompson, H. J. (Eds.). (2011). *Care of the patients undergoing Intracranial Pressure Monitoring/ External Ventricular Drainage or Lumbar Drainage*. Glenview IL: AANN.
7. Arbour, C., Gelinas, C., Loiella, C., & Bourgault, P. (2015). An exploratory study of bilateral Bispectral Index for pain detection in traumatic-brain-injured patients with altered level of consciousness. *J Neuroscience Nurs, 47*(3), 166–177.
8. Arbour, R. B., & Dissin, J. (2015). Predictive values of Bispectral Index for burst suppression on diagnostic electroencephalogram during drug-induced coma. *J Neurosc Nurs, 47*(3), 113–121.
9. Arundine, M., & Tymianski, M. (2004). Molecular mechanisms of glutamate-dependent neurodegeneration in ischemia and traumatic brain injury. *Cell Mol Life Sci, 61*, 657–668.
10. Badjatia, N., & Vespa, P. (2015). Monitoring nutrition and glucose in acute brain injury. *Neurocrit Care, 21*(Suppl, 2), S159–S167.
11. Bendo, A. A., Kass, I. S., Hartung, J., & Cottrell, J. A. (2005). Anesthesia and neurosurgery. In P. G. Barash, B. F. Cullen & R. K. Stoelting (Eds.). *Clinical Anesthesia* (5th ed.) (pp. 746–789). Philadelphia: Lippincott Williams and Wilkins. http://www.kalbemed.com/Portals/6/KOME-LIB/ANAESTHETICS-LOCAL%20and%20GENERAL/Anestesi/Isoflurane/anesthesia%20in%20neurosurgery.pdf.
12. Bergsneider, M., Hovda, D. A., Shalmon, E., Kelly, D. F., Vespa, P. M., et al. (1997). Cerebral hyperglycolysis following severe traumatic brain injury in humans: a positron emission tomography study. *J Neurosurg, 86*(2), 241–251.
13. Bilotta, F., Giovannini, F., Caramia, R., & Rosa, G. (2009). Glycemia management in neurocritical care patients: a review. *J Neurosurg Anesthesio 21*(1), 2–9.
14. Bloch, O., & Manley, G. T. (2007). The role of aquaporin-4 in cerebral water transport and edema. *Neurosurgical Focus, 22*(5), E3.
15. Boer, C., Franschman, G., & Loer, S. A. (2012). Prehospital management of severe traumatic brain injury: concepts and ongoing controversies. *Curr Opin Anaesthesiol, 25*(5), 556–562.
16. Boeve, B. F., Wijdicks, E. F., Benarroch, E. E., & Schmidt, K. D. (1998). Paroxysmal sympathetic storms ("diencephalic seizures") after severe diffuse axonal head injury. *Mayo Clin Proc, 73*(2), 148–152.
17. Botteri, M., Bandera, E., Minelli, C., & Latronico, N. (2008). Cerebral blood flow thresholds for cerebral ischemia in traumatic brain injury. A systematic review. *Crit Care, 36*(11), 3089–3092.
18. Bouma, G. J., et al. (1991). Cerebral circulation and metabolism after severe traumatic brain injury: the elusive role of ischemia. *J Neurosurg, 75*, 685–693.
19. Bouma, G. J., et al. (1992). Ultra-early evaluation of regional cerebral blood flow in severely head-injured patients using xenon-enhanced computed tomography. *J Neurosurg, 77*, 360–368.
20. Brain Trauma Foundation. (2012). Guidelines for the acute medical management of severe traumatic brain injury in infants, children, and adolescents. *Pediatr Crit Care Med, 13*(Suppl. 1), s1–s82.
21. Brain Trauma Foundation. (2007). Guidelines for prehospital management of traumatic brain injury (2nd ed.). *Prehospital Emergency Care, 12*(1), s1–s52.
22. Brain Trauma Foundation, American Association of Neurological Surgeons & Congress of Neurological Surgeons Joint Section on Neurotrauma and Critical Care (AANS/CNS). (2007). Guidelines for the management of severe traumatic brain injury. *J Neurotrauma*, 24.
23. Brophy, G. M., Bell, R., Claassen, J., Alldredge, B., Bleck, T. P., T, et al. (2012). Guidelines for the evaluation and management of status epilepticus. *Neurocrit Care, 17*(1), 3–23.
24. Bullock, M. R., Chesnut, R., Ghajar, J., Gordon, D., Hartl, R., Newell, D., F, et al. (2006). Surgical management of acute epidural hematomas. *Neurosurgery, 58*(3), S2-7–S2-15.
25. Bullock, M. R., Chesnut, R., Ghajar, J., Gordon, D., Hartl, R., Newell, D., et al. (2006). Surgical Management of Acute Subdural Hematomas. *Neurosurgery, 58*(3), S2-16–S2-25.
26. Bullock, M. R., Chesnut, R., Ghajar, J., Gordon, D., Hartl, R., Newell, D., F, et al. (2006). Surgical management of traumatic parenchymal lesions. *Neurosurgery, 58*(3), S2-25–S2-46.
27. Bullock, M. R., Chesnut, R., Ghajar, J., Gordon, D., Hartl, R., Newell, D., et al. (2006). Surgical management of depressed cranial fractures. *Neurosurgery, 58*(3), S2-56–S2-60.
28. Burch, J. M., et al. (1996). The abdominal compartment syndrome. *Surg Clin North Am, 76*, 833–842.
29. Camacho, E. F., Boszczowski, I., Freire, M. P., et al. (2013). Impact of an educational intervention implanted in a neurological intensive care unit on rates of infection related to external ventricular drains. *PLOS ONE, 8*(2), e50708.
30. Cecil, S., Chen, P. M., E Callaway, S., Rowland, S. M., Adler, D. E., & Chen, J. W. (2011). Traumatic brain injury: advanced multimodal neuromonitoring from theory to clinical practice. *Crit Care Nurse, 31*(2), 25–36.
31. Centers for Disease Control and Prevention (CDC). (2010). Traumatic Brain Injury. From http://www.cdc.gov/TraumaticBrainInjury.
32. Cesnik, E., Casetta, I., & Granieri, E. (2013). Post-traumatic epilepsy: review. *J Neurol Neurophysiol, S2*, 1–5.
33. Chang, B. S., & Lowenstein, D. H. (2003). Practice parameter: antiepileptic drug prophylaxis in severe traumatic brain injury. *Neurology, 60*, 10–16.
34. Chesnut, R. M. (2015). A conceptual approach to managing severe traumatic brain injury in a time of uncertainty. *Ann N Y Acad Sci, 1345*(1), 99–107.
35. Chesnut, R. M. (2015). What is wrong with the tenets underpinning current management of severe traumatic brain injury? *Ann N Y Acad Sci, 1345*(1), 74–82.
36. Chestnut, R. M., Marshall, L. F., & Klauber, M. R. (1993). The role of secondary brain injury in determining outcome from severe head injury. *J Trauma, 34*, 216–222.
37. Chesnut, R., Videtta, W., Vespa, P., & Le Roux, P. (2014). Intracranial pressure monitoring: fundamental considerations and rationale for monitoring. *Neurocritical Care, 21*(Suppl. 2), s1–s26.
38. Chopp, M., & Portnoy, H. D. (1983). Hydraulic model of cerebrovascular bed: an aid to understanding the volume-pressure test. *Neurosurgery, 13*, 5–11.
39. Claassen, J., & Vespa, P. (2014). Electrophysiologic monitoring in acute brain injury. *Neurocrit Care, 21*(Suppl. 2), S129–S147.
40. L Clifton, G., Valadka, A., Zygun, D., Coffey, C. S., Drever, P., Fourwinds, S., et al. (2011). Very early hypothermia induction in patients with severe brain injury (the National Acute Brain Injury Study: Hypothermia II): a randomised trial. *Lancet Neurology, 10*(2), 131–139.
41. Clifton, G. L., Miller, E. R., Choi, S. C., Levin, H. S., McCauley, S., Smith, K. R., et al. (2001). Lack of effect of induction of hypothermia after acute brain injury. *N Engl J Med, 344*, 556–563.
42. CLOTS (Clots in Legs Or sTockings after Stroke) Trials Collaboration. (2013). Effectiveness of intermittent pneumatic compression in reduction of risk of deep vein thrombosis in patients who have had a stroke (CLOTS 3): a multicentre randomized controlled trial. *Lancet, 382*, 516–524.
43. Cook, A. M., Peppard, A., & Magnuson, B. (2008/2009). Nutrition considerations in traumatic brain injury. *Nutr Clin*, 23(6), 608–620.

44. Cooper, D. J., Myburgh, J., Heritier, S., Finfer, S., Bellomo, R., Billot, L., et al. (2013). Albumin resuscitation for traumatic brain injury: Is intracranial hypertension the cause of increased mortality? *J Neurotrauma, 30*(7), 512–518.
45. Cooper, D. J., Rosenfeld, J. V., Murray, L., Arabi, Y. M., Davies, A. R., D'Urso, P., et al. (2011). Decompressive craniectomy in diffuse traumatic brain injury. *N Engl J Med, 364*, 1493–1502.
46. Corry, J. J. (2014). The use of targeted temperature management for elevated intracranial pressure. *Curr Neurol Neurosci Rep, 14*, 453.
47. Cottenceau, V., Masson, F., Mahamid, E., Petit, L., Shik, V., & Sztark, F. (2011). Comparison of effects of equiosmolar doses of mannitol and hypertonic saline on cerebral blood flow and metabolism in traumatic brain injury. *J Neurotrauma, 28*(10), 2003–2012.
48. CRASH trial collaborators. (2004). Effect of intravenous corticosteroids on death within 14 days in 10,008 adults with clinically significant head injury (MRC CRASH trial): randomised placebo-controlled trial. *Lancet, 364*, 1321–1328.
49. CRASH trial collaborators. (2005). Final results of MRC CRASH, a randomised placebo-controlled trial of intravenous corticosteroid in adults with head injury—outcomes at 6 months *Lancet, 365*, 1957–1959.
50. Crossley, S., Reid, J., McLatchie, R., Hayton, J., & Clark, C. (2014). A systematic review of therapeutic hypothermia for adult patients following traumatic brain injury. *Critical Care, 18*, R75 11 pages.
51. Cushing, H. (1901). Concerning a definite regulatory mechanism of the vasomotor centre which controls blood pressure during cerebral compression. *Bulletin of John Hopkins Hospital, 126*, 289–292.
52. DeGeorgia, M. A. (2015). Brain tissue oxygen monitoring in neurocritical care. *J Intensive Care Medicine, 30*(8), 473–483.
53. de Oliveira Manoel, A. L., Neto, A. C., Veigas, P. V., & Rizoli., S. (2015). Traumatic brain injury associated coagulopathy. *Neurocritic Care, 22*(1), 34–44.
54. Donkin, J. J., & Vink, R. (2010). Mechanisms of cerebral edema in traumatic brain injury: therapeutic developments. *Curr Opin Neurol, 23*(30), 293–299.
55. Dubroff, J. G., & Newberg, A. (2008). Neuroimaging of traumatic brain injury. *Semin Neurol Semin Neurol, 28*(4), 548–557.
56. Duhaime, A. C. (1996). Conventional drug therapies for head injury. In R. K. Narayan, J. E. Wilberger, Jr., & J. T. Povlishock (Eds.), *Neurotrauma*. New York: McGraw-Hill.
57. Dutton, R. P., & McCunn, M. (2003). Traumatic brain injury. *Curr Opin Crit Care, 9*, 503–509.
58. Ecklund, J., Ling, G. S. F., & Rengachary, S. S. (2005). Gunshot wounds of the head. In S. E. Rengachary, & R. G. Ellenbogen (Eds.), *Principles of Neurosurgery* (2nd ed.). (pp. 319–327). Philadelphia: Elsevier/Mosby.
59. Fan, J. (2004). Effect of backrest position on intracranial pressure and cerebral perfusion pressure in individuals with brain injury: a systematic review. *J Neurosci Nurs, 36*(5), 278–288.
60. Farooqui, A., Hiser, B., Barnes, S. L., & Litofsky, N. S. (2013). Safety and efficacy of early thromboembolism chemoprophylaxis after intracranial hemorrhage from traumatic brain injury. *J Neurosurg, 119*(6), 1576–1582.
61. Fernandez-Ortega, J. F., A Prieto-Palomino, M., Garcia-Caballero, M., Galeas-Lopez, J. L., Quesada-Garcia, G., & Baguley, I. J. (2012). Paroxysmal sympathetic hyperactivity after traumatic brain injury: clinical and prognostic implications. *J Neurotrauma, 29*(7), 1364–1370.
62. Finkelstein, E., Corso, P., & Miller, T. (2006). *The incidence and economic burden of injuries in the United States*. New York: Oxford University Press.
63. Fischer, J., & Mathieson, C. (2001). The history of the Glasgow coma scale: implications for practice. *Crit Care Nurs Q, 23*(4), 52–58.
64. Flint, A. C., Rao, V. A., Renda, N. C., Faigeles, B. S., Lasman, T. E., & Sheridan, W. (2013). A simple protocol to prevent external ventricular drain infections. *Neurosurgery, 72*(6), 993–999.
65. Flower, O., & Hellings, S. (2012). Sedation in traumatic brain injury. *Emerg Med Int, 2012*, 1–11.
66. Frattalone, A. R., & Ling, G. S. F. (2013). Moderate and severe traumatic brain injury: pathophysiology and management. *Neurosurg Clin N Am, 24*(3), 309–319.
67. Frodel, J. L. (2008). Management of skull fractures. *Op Techniq in Otolaryngol, 19*, 214–223.
68. Gantner, D., Moore, E. M., & Cooper, D. J. (2014). Intravenous fluids in traumatic brain injury. What's the solution? *Curr Opin Crit Care, 20*(4), 385–389.
69. Gopinath, S. P., et al. (1994). Jugular venous desaturation and outcome after head injury. *J Neurol Neurosurg Psychiatry, 57*, 717–723.
70. Graziani, G., Cucchiar, D., Arold, A., Angelini, C., Gaetani, P., & Selmi, C. (2012). Syndrome of inappropriate secretion of antidiuretic hormone in traumatic brain injury when tolvaptan becomes a lifesaving drug. *J Neurol Neurosurg Psychiatry, 83*, 510–512.
71. Greve, M., & Zink, B. (2009). Pathophysiology of Traumatic Brain Injury. *Mt Sinai J Med, 76*, 97–104.
72. Griesdale, D. E., Tremblay, M. H., McEwen, J., & Chittock, D. R. (2009). Glucose control and mortality in patients with severe traumatic brain injury. *Neurocritic Care, 11*(3), 311–316.
73. Hagel, S., Bruns, T., Pletz, M. W., Engel, C., Kalff, R., & Ewald, C. (2014). External ventricular drain infections: risk factors and outcome. *Interdiscip Perspect Infect Dis*. Epub 2014 Nov 17.
74. Hall, S., Kumaria, A., & Belli, A. (2014). The role of vagus nerve overactivity in the increased incidence of pneumonia following traumatic brain injury. *Br J Neurosurg, 28*(2), 181–186.
75. Harris, C. (2014). Neuromonitoring indications and utility in the intensive care unit. *Crit Care Nurse, 34*(3), 30–39.
76. Härtl, R., Gerber, L., Ni, Q., & Ghajar, J. (2008). Effect of early nutrition on deaths due to severe traumatic brain injury. *J Neurosurg, 109*(1), 50–56.
77. Hendricks, H. T., Heerens, A. H., & Vos, P. E. (2010). Dysautonomia after severe traumatic brain injury. *Eur J Neurol, 17*, 1172–1177.
78. Hill, M., Baker, G., Carter, D., et al. (2012). A multidisciplinary approach to end external ventricular drain infections in the neurocritical care unit. *J Neurosci Nurs, 44*(4), 188–193.
79. Hinson, H. E., Rowell, S., & Schreiber, M. (2015). Clinical evidence of inflammation driving secondary brain injury: a systematic review. *J Trauma Acute Care Surg, 78*(1), 184–191.
80. Case, I., Jain, R., Gujar, S. K., Shah, G. V., & Deveikis, J. P. (2004). Cerebral Perfusion CT: technique and clinical applications. *Radiology, 231*, 632–644.
81. Hutchison, J., Ward, R., Lacroix, J., Hebert, P., Barnes, M., Bohn, D., et al. (2008). Hypothermia therapy after traumatic brain injury in children. *N Eng J Med, 358*(23), 2447–2456.
82. Jalali, R., & Rezaei, M. (2014). A Comparison of the Glasgow Coma Scale Score with Full Outline of Unresponsiveness Scale to predict patients' traumatic brain injury outcomes in intensive care units. *Crit Care Res Pract*, 1–4.
83. Jamjoom, A. A., & Jamjoom, A. B. (2013). Safety and efficacy of early pharmacological thromboprophylaxis in traumatic brain injury: systematic review and meta-analysis. *J Neurotrauma, 30*, 503–511.
84. Jeffcote, T., Hinzman, J. M., Jewell, S. L., Learney, R. M., Pahl, C., Tolias, C., et al. (2014). Detection of spreading depolarization with intraparenchymal electrodes in the injured human brain. *Neurocrit Care, 20*(1), 21–31.
85. John, C. A., & Day, M. W. (2012). Inappropriate secretion of antidiuretic hormone and cerebral salt wasting syndrome in Traumatic Brain Injury. *Care Nurse, 32*(2), e1–e8.
86. Joshi, S., & Young, W. E. (2010). Cerebral and spinal blood flow. In J. Cottrell, & W. Young (Eds.), *Anesthesia and Neurosurgery*. Philadelphia: Mosby.
87. G Junger, W., Rhind, S. G., Rizoli, S. B., Cuschieri, J., Baker, A. J., Shek, P. N., et al. (2013). Prehospital hypertonic saline resuscitation attenuates the activation and promotes apoptosis of neutrophils in patients with severe traumatic brain injury. *Shock, 40*(5), 366–374.
88. Kazim, S. F., Shamin, M. S., Tahir, M. Z., Enam, S. A., & Waheed, S. (2011). Management of penetrating brain injury. *J Emerg Trauma Shock, 4*(3), 395–402.
89. Kellie, G. (1824). An account of the appearances observed in the dissection of two of three individuals presumed to have perished in the storm of the third and whose bodies were discovered in the vicinity of Leith on the morning of the 4th, November, 1821, with some reflections on the pathology of the brain. *Transact Medico-Chirugical Soc Edinburgh, 1*, 84–169.

90. Kheirbek, T., & Pascual, J. L. (2014). Hypertonic saline for the treatment of intracranial hypertension. *Curr Neurol Neurosci Rep, 14*, 482.
91. Kirkman, M. A., Albert, A. F., Ibrahim, A., & Doberenz, D. (2013). Hyponatremia and brain injury: historical and contemporary perspectives. *Neurocrit Care, 18*(3), 406–416.
92. Kleiven, S. (2013). Why most traumatic brain injuries are not caused by linear acceleration but skull fractures are. *Front Bioeng Biotechnol, 1*, 15.
93. Kocsis, J. D., & Tessler, A. (2009). Pathophysiology of blast-related brain injury. *J. Rehab Res Dev, 46*(3), 667–672.
94. Kolias, A. J., Kirkpatrick, P. J., & Hutchinson, P. J. (2013). Decompressive craniectomy: past, present and future. *Nat Rev Neurol, 9*(7), 405–415.
95. Krag, M., Perner, A., Wetterslev, J., Wise, M. P., & Hylander, M. (2014). Stress ulcer prophylaxis versus placebo or no prophylaxis in critically ill patients. A systematic review of randomised clinical trials with meta-analysis and trial sequential analysis. *Intensive Care Med, 40*(1), 11–22.
96. Kramer, D. R., Winer, J. L., Matthew Pease, B. A., Amar, A. P., & Mack, W. J. (2013). Cerebral Vasospasm in Traumatic Brain Injury. *Neurol Res Int.* http://dx.doi.org/10.1155/2013/415813 Epub 2013 Jun 19.
97. Kruer, R. M., Harris, L. H., Goodwin, H., Kornbluth, J., Thomas, K. P., & Slater, L. A. (2013). Changing trends in the use of seizure prophylaxis after traumatic brain injury: a shift from phenytoin to levetiracetam. *J Crit Care, 28*(5) 883.e9–13.
98. Kubal, W. S. (2012). Updated imaging of traumatic brain injury. *Radiol Clin N Am, 50*, 15–41.
99. Kubilay, Z., Amini, S., Fauerbach, L. L., Archibald, L., Friedman, W. A., & Layon, A. J. (2013). Decreasing ventricular infections through the use of a ventriculostomy placement bundle: experience at a single institution. *J Neurosurg, 118*(3), 514–520.
100. Kumar, A., & Loane, D. J. (2012). Neuroinflammation after traumatic brain injury: opportunities for therapeutic intervention. *Brain Behav Immun, 26*(8), 1191–1201.
101. Lam, A. M., et al. (1991). Hyperglycemia and neurological outcome in patients with head injury. *J Neurosurg, 75*, 545–551.
102. Lautsch, L., et al. (1999). Incorporation of SPECT imaging in a longitudinal cognitive rehabilitation therapy programme. *Brain Injury, 13*, 555–570.
103. Lee, K., & Rincon, F. (2012). Pulmonary complications in patients with severe brain injury. *Crit Care Res Pract* Article, ID 207247, Epub 2012 Oct 23.
104. Le Roux, P. D., Menon, D. K., Citerio, G., Vespa, P., Bader, M. K., Brophy, G. M., et al. (2014). Consensus Summary Statement of the International Multidisciplinary Consensus Conference on Multimodality Monitoring in Neurocritical Care: A statement for healthcare professionals from the Neurocritical Care Society and the European Society of Intensive Care Medicine. *Neurocritical Care, 21*(Suppl. 2), S1–S25.
105. Ling, G., Bandak, F., Armonda, R., Grant, G., & Ecklund, J. (2009). Explosive blast neurotrauma. *J Neurotrauma, 26*(6), 815–825.
106. Lowenstein, D. H. (2009). Epilepsy after head injury: an overview. *Epilepsia, 50*(Suppl. 2), 4–9.
107. Maas, A. I. R., Stocchetti, N., & Bullock, R. (2008). Moderate and severe traumatic brain injury in adults. *Lancet Neurol, 7*, 728–741.
108. Maegele, M. (2013). Coagulopathy after traumatic brain injury: incidence, pathogenesis, and treatment options. *Transfusion, 53*(Suppl. 1), 28S–37S.
109. Maekawa, T., Yamashita, S., Nagao, S., Hayashi, N., & Ohashi, Y. (2014). Prolonged mild therapeutic hypothermia versus fever control with tight hemodynamic monitoring and slow rewarming in patients with severe traumatic brain injury: a randomized controlled trial. *J Neurotrauma, 32*(7), 422–429.
110. Majdan, M., Mauritz, W., Wilbacher, I., Brazinova, A., Rusnak, M., & Leitgeb, J. (2013). Barbiturates use and its effects in patients with severe traumatic brain injury in five European countries. *J Neurotrauma, 30*(1), 23–29.
111. March, K. S., & Hickey, J. V. (2014). Craniocerebral injuries. In J. V. Hickey (Ed.), *The Clinical Practice of Neurological and Neurosurgical Nursing* (7th ed.). (pp. 343–381). Philadelphia: Lippincott Williams and Wilkins.
112. March, K. S., & Hickey, J. V. (2014). Intracranial hypertension: theory and management of increased intracranial pressure. In J. V. Hickey (Ed.), *The Clinical Practice of Neurological and Neurosurgical Nursing* (7th ed.). (pp. 266–299). Philadelphia: Lippincott Williams and Wilkins.
113. Marik, P. E., & Rivera, R. (2013). Therapeutic effects of Conivaptan bolus dosing in hyponatremic neurosurgical patients. *Pharmacotherapy, 33*(1), 53–55.
114. Marshall, G. T., James, R. F., Landman, M. P., O'Neill, P. J., Cotton, B. A., et al. (2010). Pentobarbital coma for refractory intra-cranial hypertension after severe traumatic brain injury: Mortality predictions and one-year outcomes in 55 patients. *J Trauma, 69*, 275–283.
115. Martyn, J. A., & Richtsfeld, M. (2006). Succinylcholine-induced hyperkalemia in acquired pathologic states: etiologic factors and molecular mechanisms. *Anesthesiology, 104*(1), 158–169.
116. Mathieu, A., Guillon, A., Leyre, S., Martin, F., Fusciardi, J., & Laffon, M. (2013). Aerosolized lidocaine during invasive mechanical ventilation: in vitro characterization and clinical efficiency to prevent systemic and cerebral hemodynamic changes induced by endotracheal suctioning in head-injured patients. *J Neurosurg Anesthesiol, 25*(1), 8–15.
117. Mayglothling, J., M Duane, T., Gibbs, M., McCunn, M., Legome, E., Eastman, A. L., et al. (2012). Emergency tracheal intubation immediately following traumatic injury: an Eastern Association for the Surgery of Trauma practice management guideline. *Trauma Acute Care Surg, 73*(5), Supplement 4, S333–S340.
118. Mazzoni, M. C., et al. (1988). Dynamic fluid redistribution in hyperosmotic resuscitation of hypovolemic hemorrhage. *Am J Physiol, 255*(3 pt 2), H629H637.
119. McCrory, P., Meeuwisse, W., Johnston, K., et al. (2013). Consensus statement on Concussion in Sport 4th International Conference on Concussion in Sport held in Zurich, November 2012. *Br J Sports Med, 47*, 250–258.
120. Mcilvoy, L. H. (2005). The effect of hypothermia and hyperthermia on acute brain injury. *AACN Clin Issues, 16*(4), 488–500.
121. McNett, M. (2007). A review of the predictive ability of Glasgow Coma Scale scores in head-injured patients. *J Neurosci Nurs, 39*(2), 68–75.
122. McNett, M., & Olson, D. M. (2013). Evidence to guide nursing interventions for critically ill neurologically impaired patients with ICP monitoring. *J Neuroscience Nurs, 45*(3), 120–123.
123. Miller, C. (2012). Update on multimodality monitoring. *Curr Neurol Neurosci Rep, 12*, 474–480.
124. Miller, C., & Armonda, R., Participants in the International Multidisciplinary Consensus Conference on Multimodality Monitoring. (2014). Monitoring of Cerebral Blood Flow and Ischemia in the Critically Ill. *Neurocrit Care, 21*(suppl 2), S121–S128.
125. Moghissi, E., Korytkowski, M., Dinardo, M., Einhorn, D., Hellman, R., Hirsch, I., et al. (2009). American Association of Clinical Endocrinologists and American Diabetes Association consensus statement on inpatient glycemic control. *Diabetes Care, 32*(6), 1119–1131.
126. Mokri, B. (2001). The Monro-Kellie hypothesis: Applications in CSF volume depletion. *Neurology, 56*, 1746–1748.
127. Momi, J., Tang, C. M., Abcar, A. C., Kujubu, D. D., & Sim, J. J. (2010). Hyponatremia-Cerebral salt wasting. *Perm J, 14*(2), 62–65.
128. Monro, A. (1783). *Observations on the structure and function of the nervous system.* Edinburgh: Creech & Johnston.
129. Centers for Disease Control and Prevention. Nonfatal traumatic brain injuries related to sports and recreation activities among persons aged ≤19 years - United States, 2001-2009. *MMWR Morb Mortal Wkly Rep* 60(39):1337-1342. http://www.cdc.gov/mmwr/preview/mmwrhtml/mm6039a1.htm?s_cid=mm6039a1_w.
130. Morse, M. L., et al. (1985). Effect of hydration on experimentally induced cerebral edema. *Crit Care Med, 13*(7), 563–565.
131. MRC CRASH Trial Collaborators. (2008). Predicting outcome after traumatic brain injury: practical prognostic models based on large cohort of international patients. *BMJ, 336*, 425–435.
132. Muehlschlegel, S., Carandang, R., Ouillette, C., Hall, W., Anderson, F., & Goldberg, R. (2013). Frequency and Impact of Intensive Care Unit Complications on Moderate-Severe Traumatic Brain Injury: Early Results of the Outcome Prognostication in Traumatic Brain Injury (OPTIMISM) Study. *Neurocrit Care*, Published online: 2 February 2013.

133. Muench, E., et al. (2005). Effects of positive end-expiratory pressure on regional cerebral blood flow, intracranial pressure, and brain tissue oxygenation. *Crit Care Med*, *33*(10), 2367–2372.
134. Muizelaar, J. P., Marmarou, A., & Ward, J. D. (1991). Adverse effects of prolonged hyperventilation in patients with severe head injury: a randomized clinical trial. *J Neurosurg*, *75*, 731–739.
135. Mulkey, M., Bena, J. F., & Albert, N. M. (2014). Clinical outcomes of patient mobility in a neuroscience intensive care unit. *J Neuroscience Nurs*, *46*(3), 156–161.
136. Murray, G. D., Butcher, I., McHugh, G. S., et al. (2007). Multivariable prognostic analysis in traumatic brain injury: results from the IMPACT Study. *J Neurotrauma*, *24*(2), 329–337.
137. Naidech, A. M., Kumar, M. A., & Participants in the International Multidisciplinary Consensus Conference on Multimodality Monitoring. (2014). Monitoring of hematological and hemostatic parameters in neurocritical care patients. *Neurocrit Care*, *21*(Suppl. 2), S168–S176.
138. Naidech, A. M., Paparello, J., Liebling, S. M., Bassin, S. L., Levasseur K, K., & Alberts, M. J. (2010). Use of Conivaptan (Vaprisol) for hyponatremic neuro-ICU patients. *Neurocrit Care*, *13*(1), 57–61.
139. Narayan, R. N., & Kempisty, S. (2005). Closed head injury. In S. E. Rengachary, & R. G. Ellenbogen (Eds.), *Principles of Neurosurgery* (2nd ed.). (pp. 301–318). Philadelphia: Mosby.
140. Nau, K., Divertie, G., Valentino, A., & Freeman, W. (2009). Safety and efficacy of Levetiracetam for critically ill patients with seizures. *Neurocrit Care*, *11*, 34–37.
141. Nwachuku, E. L., Puccio, A. M., Fetzick, A., et al. (2014). Intermittent versus continuous cerebrospinal fluid drainage management in adult severe traumatic brain injury: assessment of intracranial pressure burden. *Neurocrit Care*, *20*(1), 49–53.
142. Obrist, W. D., & Marion, D. W. (1997). Xenon techniques for CBF measurements in clinical head injury. In R. K. Narayan, J. E. Wilberger, & J. T. Povlishock (Eds.), *Neurotrauma*. New York: McGraw-Hill.
143. Patel, F. D., & Lakshmanan, R. (2012). The FOUR Score predicts outcome in patients after traumatic brain injury. *Neurocrit Care*, *16*(1), 95–101.
144. Patel, M. B., McKenna, J. W., Alvarez, J. M., et al. (2012). Decreasing adrenergic or sympathetic hyperactivity after severe traumatic brain injury using propranolol and clonidine (DASH After TBI Study): study protocol for a randomized controlled trial. *Trials*, *26*(13), 177.
145. Perez-Barcena, J., Llompart-Pou, J. A., & O'Phelan, K. H. (2014). Intracranial pressure monitoring and management of intracranial hypertension. *Crit Care Clin*, *30*(4), 735–750.
146. Phelan, H. A., Wolf, S. E., Norwood, S. H., Aldy, K., Brakenridge, S. C., Eastman, A. L., et al. (2012). A randomized, double-blinded, placebo-controlled pilot trial of anticoagulation in low-risk traumatic brain injury: the Delayed Versus Early Enoxaparin Prophylaxis I (DEEP I) study. *J Trauma Acute Care Surg*, *73*(6), 1434–1441.
147. Ponce, L. L., Pillai, S., Cruz, J., et al. (2012). Position of probe determines prognostic information of brain tissue PO2 in severe traumatic brain injury. *Neurosurgery*, *70*(6), 1492–1502.
148. Povlishock, J. T., & Katz, D. I. (2005). Update of neuropathology and neurological recovery after traumatic brain injury. *J Head Trauma Rehabil*, *20*(1), 76–94.
149. Reiff, D. A., Haricharan, R. N., Ramanath, N. M., et al. (2009). Traumatic brain injury is associated with the development of deep vein thrombosis independent of pharmacological prophylaxis. *J Trauma Injury Infection and Crit Care*, *66*(5), 1436–1440.
150. Kolias, A. G., Adams, H., Timofeev, I., Czosnyka, M., Corteen, E. A., Pickard, J. D., et al. (2016). Decompressive craniectomy following traumatic brain injury: developing the evidence base. *Br J Neurosurg*, *30*(2), 246–250. http://dx.doi.org/10.3109/02688697.2016.1159655.
151. Riker, R. R., Fraser, G. L., & Wilkins, M. L. (2003). Comparing the bispectral index and suppression ratio with burst suppression of the electroencephalogram during pentobarbital infusions in adult intensive care patients. *Pharmacotherapy*, *23*, 1087–1093.
152. Roberts, I., & Sydenham, E. (2009). Barbiturates for acute traumatic brain injury. *Cochrane Database Syst Rev*, *3*, CD000033.
153. Robertson, C. S., Hannay, H. J., Yamal, J. M., Gopinath, S., Goodman, J. C., Tilley, B. C., Epo Severe TBI Trial Investigators, et al. (2014). Effect of erythropoietin and transfusion threshold on neurological recovery after traumatic brain injury: a randomized clinical trial. *JAMA*, *312*(1), 36–47.
154. Robertson, C. S., Valadka, A. B., Hannay, H. J., Contant, C. F., Gopinath, S., Cormio, M., et al. (1999). Prevention of secondary ischemic insults after severe head injury. *Crit Care Med*, *27*(10), 2086–2095.
155. Rosenfeld, J. V., Maas, A. I., Bragge, P., Morganti-Kossmann, M. C., Manley, G. T., & Gruen, R. I. (2012). Early management of severe traumatic brain injury. *Lancet*, *380*(9847), 1088–1098.
156. Rostami, E. (2014). Glucose and the injured brain-monitored in the neuro-intensive care unit. *Front Neurol*, *5*(91). http://dx.doi.org/10.3389/fneur.2014.00091.
157. Rostami, E., Engquist, H., & Enblad, P. (2014). Imaging of cerebral blood flow in patients with severe traumatic brain injury in the neurointensive care. *Front Neurol*, *7*(5). http://dx.doi.org/10.3389/fneur.2014.00114.
158. Roth, C., Stitz, H., Kalhout, A., Kleffmann, J., Deinsberger, W., & Ferbert, A. (2013). Effect of early physiotherapy on ICP & CPP. *Neurocrit Care*, *18*, 33–38.
159. Sakellaridis, N., Pavlou, E., Karatzas, S., Chroni, D., Vlachos, K., Chatzopoulos, K., et al. (2011). Comparison of mannitol and hypertonic saline in the treatment of severe brain injuries. *J Neurosurg*, *114*(2), 545–548.
160. SanFlippo, F., Santonocito, C., Veenith, T., Astuto, M., Maybauer, M. O., (2015). The role of neuromuscular blockade in patients with traumatic brain injury: a systematic review. *Neurocrit Care*, *22*(2), 325–334.
161. Sahuquillo, T., (2006). Decompressive craniectomy for the treatment of refractory high intracranial pressure in traumatic brain injury, *Cochrane Database Syst Rev* (Online), Issue 1, pp. CD003983
162 Schaible, E. V., S., & Thal, C. (2013). Anticoagulation in patients with traumatic brain injury. *Current Opinion*, *26*(5), 529–534.
163. Schirmer, C. M., Kornbluth, J., Heilman, C. B., & Bhardwaj, A. (2012). Gastrointestinal prophylaxis in neurocritical care. *Neurocrit Care*, *16*(1), 184–193.
164. Schwarzmaier, S. M., & Plesnila, N. (2014). Contributions of the immune system to the pathophysiology of traumatic brain injury - evidence by intravital microscopy. *Front Cell Neurosci*, *8*, 358.
165. Selassie, A. W., Zaloshnja, E., Langlois, J. A., Miller, T., Jones, P., & Steiner, C. (2008). Incidence of long-term disability following traumatic brain injury hospitalization, United States, 2003. *J Head Trauma Rehabil*, *23*(2), 123–131.
166. Shahlaie, K., Keachie, K., Hutchins, I., Rudisill, N., Madden, L. K., Smith, K., et al. (2011). Risk factors for posttraumatic vasospasm. *J Neurosurg*, *115*(3), 602–611.
167. Skoglund, K., Hillered, L., Purins, K., Tsitsopoulos, P. P., Flygt, J., Engquist, H., et al. (2014). The neurological wake-up test does not alter cerebral energy metabolism and oxygenation in patients with severe traumatic brain injury. *Neurocrit Care*, *20*(3), 413–426.
168. Stein, S. C., & Smith, D. H. (2004). Coagulopathy in traumatic brain injury. *Neurocrit Care*, *1*, 479–488.
169. Stevens, R. D., Huff, J. S., Duckworth, J., Papangelou, A., Weingart, S. D., & Smith, W. S. (2012). Emergency neurological life support: intracranial hypertension and herniation. *Neurocrit Care*, *17*(Suppl. 1), S60–S65.
170. Stochetti, N., Furlan, A., & Volta, F. (1996). Hypoxemia and arterial hypotension at the accident scene in head injury. *J Trauma*, *40*, 764–767.
171. Stocchetti, N., Le Roux, P., Vespa, P., et al. (2013). Clinical review: neuromonitoring - an update. *Crit Care*, *17*(1), 201.
172. Strum, S. (2011). Post head injury autonomic complications. *Medscape*. http://emedicine.medscape.com/article/325994-overview.
173. Thomas, P. D. (1997). Fluid, electrolyte and metabolic management. In P. Reilly, & R. Bullock (Eds.), *Head injury: pathophysiology and management of severe closed injury*. London: Chapman & Hall.
174. Torbic, H., Forni, A. A., Anger, K. E., Degrado, J. R., & Greenwood, B. C. (2013). Use of antiepileptics for seizure prophylaxis after traumatic brain injury. *Am J Health Syst Pharm*, *70*(9), 759–766.
175. Torres-Healy, A., Marko, N. F., & Weil, R. J. (2012). Hyperosmolar therapy for intracranial hypertension. *Neurocrit Care*, *17*, 117–130.

176. Udomphorn, Y., Armstead, W. M., & Vavilala, M. S. (2008). Cerebral blood flow and autoregulation after pediatric traumatic brain injury. *Pediatr Neurol, 38*(4), 225–234.
177. Valadka, A. B., Furuya, Y., Hlatky, R., & Robertson, C. S. (2000). Global and regional techniques for monitoring cerebral oxidative metabolism after severe traumatic brain injury. *Neurosurg Focus, 9*(5), 1–3.
178. Vespa, P., Bergsneider, M., Hattori, N., Wu, H. M., Huang, S. C., Martin, N. A., et al. (2005). Metabolic crisis without brain ischemia is common after traumatic brain injury: a combined microdialysis and positron emission tomography study. *J Cereb Blood Flow Metab, 25*(6), 763–767.
179. Engelhard, W. K. (2007). Pathophysiology of traumatic brain injury. *Brit J Anaesth, 99*(1), 4–9.
180. Wijayatilake, D. S., J, S., & Shepherd (2014). What's new in the management of traumatic brain injury on neuro ICU? *Curr Opin Anesthesiol, 27*, 459–464.
181. Wijdicks, E. F., Kramer, A. A., Rohs, T., et al. (2015). Comparison of the Full Outline of UnResponsiveness Score and the Glasgow Coma Scale in predicting mortality in critically ill patients. *Crit Care Med, 43*(3), 439–444.
182. Young, G. B. (2009). Coma. *Ann N Y Acad Sci, 1157*, 32–47.

13

Cerebrovascular Disorders

Patricia A. Blissitt

INTRODUCTION

Stroke is a neurologic emergency requiring prompt recognition and timely implementation of effective interventions for the best possible outcome.[14,22,80,81,123,124,143] Stroke has long been recognized as a leading cause of death. The Centers for Disease Control and Prevention recently reported a decrease in stroke from fourth to fifth place as a cause of death, but it remains the leading cause of disability in the United States.[205,206,209] Worldwide, statistics are less clear.[246,257] In 2010, stroke was identified as the second most common cause of death and a leading cause of disability globally.[246,257] Failure to respond to the concept that "time is brain" in an efficient and effective manner is all too common, even in the acute care setting.[9,123,124] In the past, both the National Institute of Neurologic Disorders and Stroke (NINDS)[211] and the World Health Organization (WHO) defined stroke as loss of brain function related to inadequate cerebrovascular blood flow for a duration of at least 24 hours.[88,272] Recently, stroke has been defined as inadequate cerebral blood flow resulting in brain infarction, without reference to duration.[212] This is based on work with identification of brain infarction imaging to differentiate stroke from transient ischemic attacks (TIAs). The definition of stroke continues to include both ischemic and hemorrhagic stroke.[77,241] A stroke occurs every 40 seconds in the United States,[205] and up to 17% of all strokes may occur in the inpatient setting.[60] Critical care patients are particularly vulnerable to stroke, frequently having predisposing conditions such as hemodynamic instability, cardiac disease, and coagulopathy. The critically ill also undergo interventions that result in vascular injury, embolism, hypotension or hypertension, and prothrombotic or anticoagulated states.[29] Stroke may be the primary diagnosis, secondary to another illness or injury, or related to a required intervention for another disease or condition.[28,29] Since 1996, awareness in stroke care and research has flourished. New technologies, pharmacologic agents, and procedures have been developed or adapted for stroke intervention. The American Heart Association became the American Heart Association/American Stroke Association (AHA/ASA), demonstrating significant commitment to the care of stroke patients. Additionally, a number of professional organizations developed clinical practice guidelines for stroke care, including AHA/ASA, American Association of Neuroscience Nurses (AANN), and the Neurocritical Care Society (NCS).[7,55,71,135,142,252,259,262,278] In recognition of the need for excellence in stroke care, The Joint Commission (TJC) developed a certification program for both primary and comprehensive stroke centers in collaboration with the Brain Attack Coalition and the ASA.[11,12,211]

Whereas some strokes may be inevitable, the critical care nurse working in a collaborative manner with the interprofessional team is key in minimizing secondary injury and maximizing resources available to lessen disability and mortality.[31,252]

PATIENTS AT RISK

In 2014, the Stroke Council, Council of Cardiovascular and Stroke Nursing, Council on Clinical Cardiology, Council on Functional Genomics and Translational Biology, and Council on Hypertension of the AHA/ASA updated previous evidence-based consensus statements regarding stroke risk factors.[193] The task force categorized stroke risk factors into one of three categories: nonmodifiable; modifiable and well documented; and potentially modifiable or less well documented.[193] Stroke risk is multifactorial. Risk factors identified as nonmodifiable are age, low birth weight, race/ethnicity, and genetics.[193] In regard to age, stroke risk doubles every 10 years after age 55.[10] Low birth weight refers to stroke in adults, not perinatal stroke. Low birth weight as a nonmodifiable risk factor is based on both European and North American studies. The risk of stroke doubles for individuals who weighed less than 2500 g (5.5 lb) at birth compared to those who weighed more than 4000 g (8.8 lb) at birth.[193] The relationship of birth weight to stroke is not clear.[193] Blacks and some Hispanic Americans share a higher incidence of all stroke types and stroke-related mortality than whites, in part related to the prevalence of prehypertension, hypertension, diabetes, and obesity in these ethnicities.[193] Genetics not only contributes to stroke incidence in regard to one's familial predisposition to hypertension, diabetes, and hyperlipidemia, but is also related to inherited coagulopathies and vascular disease.[193] A number of chromosomal variants increase stroke risk. Autosomal dominant traits such as protein C and S deficiencies and the Leiden (factor V) mutations increase the risk of thrombosis.[193] Familial tendencies have been noted in arterial dissections, moyamoya syndrome, and fibromuscular dysplasia.[193] Autosomal dominant polycystic kidney disease, and connective tissue diseases, Ehlers-Danlos type IV, and Marfan syndrome have long been associated with increased risk of intracranial aneurysms.[177,193] The presence of apolipoprotein E (APOE) alleles E2 and E4 has been associated with increased intracerebral hemorrhage risk.[135,177]

The modifiable and well-documented risk factors include hypertension; smoking; diabetes; atrial fibrillation and other cardiac conditions; dyslipidemia; high-grade carotid artery stenosis (defined as $> 70\%$ and $< 100\%$);[193] sickle cell disease; a diet high in fat and lacking in fruits and vegetables; physical inactivity; and obesity with abdominal fat.[193] Hypertension and diabetes increase the risk of stroke related to angiopathy. Atrial fibrillation increases the risk of an acute ischemic stroke (AIS) fivefold.[193] Other cardiac disorders include acute myocardial infarction, ischemic and nonischemic cardiomyopathy, valvular heart disease, prosthetic heart valves, endocarditis, patent foramen ovale, atrial septal aneurysms, cardiac tumors, and aortic atherosclerosis.[193] Dyslipidemia refers to increased levels of total cholesterol, total triglycerides, low-density lipoprotein (LDL) cholesterol, and decreased levels of high-density lipoprotein (HDL) cholesterol. Current recommendations include an LDL cholesterol level of less than 70 mg/dL or a 50% reduction from the baseline.[193,233]

Individuals who have TIAs, previous stroke, and symptomatic carotid or intracranial disease are also at increased risk for stroke.[193,233] TIAs are defined as brief episodes of focal neurologic deficits related to inadequate cerebral blood flow but without evidence of cerebral infarction.[77] The risk of stroke after a TIA may be greater than 10%, with the greatest incidence of stroke occurring during the first week after the TIA.[77]

The less well-documented or potentially modifiable risk factors designated by the AHA/ASA include metabolic syndrome, alcohol consumption, drug abuse, sleep-disordered breathing, migraine headaches, hyperhomocysteinemia, elevated levels of lipoprotein(a) (Lp[a]), hypercoagulability, inflammation, and infection.[193]A diagnosis of metabolic syndrome requires three or more of the following: (1) obesity based on abdominal circumference of greater than 102 cm (40 inches) for men and 88 cm (35 inches) for women; (2) hyperlipidemia defined as levels of triglycerides equal to or greater than 150 mg/dL and of HDL cholesterol less than 40 mg/dL; (3) blood pressure (BP) equal to or greater than 130/85 mm Hg; and (4) a fasting glucose level of equal to or greater than 110 mg/dL.[193] Vascular headaches classified as migraines are associated with stroke in women less than 55 years of age, although the mechanism is not clear.[193] The stroke risk in men with migraine headaches is less substantiated.[193] Hyperhomocysteinemia increases the risk of stroke by two to three times related to associated atherosclerotic vascular disease.[193,233] An elevated Lp(a) also contributes to atherosclerosis. Hypercoagulability may be inherited or acquired.

Many individuals with sleep-disordered breathing, formerly known as *sleep apnea,* have established risk factors for stroke, including age, male gender, smoking, and alcohol consumption. However, sleep-disordered breathing may also increase the probability of stroke independent of these risk factors. Sleep-disordered breathing has been found to reduce cerebral blood flow, alter vascular tone and cerebral autoregulation, and contribute to systemic hypertension and atrial fibrillation.[59,181,193,233]

A number of other systemic diseases/conditions increase stroke risk. Whereas cardiac disease is a well-documented risk factor for stroke,[119,193,233] other diseases also increase risk, including hepatic and renal disease and cancer.[57,138,261] Patients with hepatic disease, particularly end-stage liver disease, are at great risk for hemorrhagic stroke. Associated coagulopathies include impaired synthesis of clotting factors, excessive fibrinolysis, disseminated intravascular coagulation (DIC), thrombocytopenia, and platelet dysfunction.[138,253]

Ischemic stroke in patients with chronic renal failure is primarily the result of atherosclerosis, thromboembolic disease, or hypotension during dialysis.[260,261] Hyperhomocysteinemia, an independent risk factor for atherosclerosis, is estimated to be present in 85% to 100% of the patients with chronic renal failure.[283] High doses of folic acid and vitamin B may reduce homocysteine levels, but endothelial function is not improved in this patient population.[283] Hemorrhagic stroke in patients with chronic renal failure is multifactorial, including the following: impaired platelet dysfunction and platelet-vessel wall interaction associated with uremia; systemic hypertension; the use of anticoagulation during hemodialysis;[260] and a 5% to 10% increased risk of cerebrovascular anomalies in polycystic kidney disease compared to the general population.[131]

Stroke in oncology patients may be the result of a coagulopathy induced by the cancer, cerebral metastasis, or oncology treatment. Coagulopathic mechanisms resulting in ischemic stroke include nonbacterial thrombotic endocarditis, intravascular coagulation, and cerebral venous thrombosis (CVT).[121] Coagulopathic mechanisms resulting in hemorrhagic stroke include DIC, thrombocytopenia, and microangiopathic hemolytic anemia. Radiation may cause carotid atherosclerosis and cerebral vasculopathy, and chemotherapy may result in arterial or venous sinus thrombosis or hemorrhage, increasing the risk of stroke.

Stroke Across the Lifespan

Although increased age is a well-documented risk factor in stroke,[193] stroke also occurs during pregnancy and childhood.[100,263] A number of alterations in maternal physiology contribute to stroke in pregnancy. Pregnancy is, in many respects, a hypercoagulable state as a result of platelet hyperaggregability and decreased fibrinolysis; increased clotting factors V, VII, VIII, IX, X, and XII and fibrinogen; decreased levels of proteins C and S and antithrombin III during the last trimester; and increased resistance to protein C.[100,198] This hypercoagulability continues 2 to 3 weeks after childbirth. However, aneurysmal or arteriovenous malformation-related subarachnoid hemorrhage (SAH) and intracerebral hemorrhage (ICH) can occur, as well as AIS.[198] Hemorrhagic stroke is most likely to occur 2 days prior to and 1 day after delivery.[198] Hypertension associated with eclampsia is present in 25% to 45% of all strokes during pregnancy.[198] Preeclampsia increases the risk of stroke during pregnancy by 3 to 12 times.[198] Other pregnancy-related causes of ischemic stroke include cerebral venous thrombosis, choriocarcinoma, amniotic fluid embolism, and peripartum cardiomyopathy. Most aneurysmal SAH occurs during the third trimester.[100,198]

Fortunately, stroke in the pediatric population is rare. The first 30 days of life and even up to the first year have a disproportionate incidence of both ischemic and hemorrhagic stroke, compared to ages 1 to 14 years.[263] Unlike adults, risk factors for stroke, including diabetes, hyperlipidemia, and cardiovascular disease, are not common in the pediatric population. However, the increasing trend of childhood obesity in the United States may result in these risk factors beginning at a much younger age. Congenital heart disease and sickle cell anemia are the most common etiologies of pediatric stroke.[263] Other etiologies of pediatric stroke include hematologic disorders, such as leukemia and polycythemia; prothrombotic states related to decreased levels of protein C, protein S, or antithrombin III, or the presence of antiphospholipid antibodies; arteriovenous malformations (AVMs), aneurysms, cerebral venous thrombosis (CVT), patent foramen ovale (PFO), moyamoya disease, and other intracranial vascular anomalies; metabolic syndromes such as hyperhomocysteinemia; migraine and substance abuse–related vasospasm; infection; and trauma.[72,216,263] Unlike adults, the ratio of pediatric ischemic strokes to hemorrhagic strokes is approximately equal, and long-term outcome in ischemic and hemorrhagic pediatric stroke survivors is the same.[72,216,263]

PREVENTION

Stroke is not entirely preventable. However, concerted efforts to lessen modifiable risk factors decrease stroke risk. Hypertension has been identified as the most modifiable risk factor.[233] Hypertension has been associated with ischemic and hemorrhagic stroke.[233] Strong evidence exists that smoking doubles the risk of ischemic stroke and doubles to quadruples the risk of aneurysmal subarachnoid hemorrhage.[113,193,233] Diabetes mellitus, defined as an HgA1c more than 6.5%, doubles to triples the risk of stroke.[113,193,233] Glycemic control in diabetes, particularly in conjunction with a reduction in BP, has been well substantiated as an effective measure in reducing stroke risk.[193] Statins, along with lifestyle changes, are recommended for the primary prevention of ischemic stroke in patients with an elevated 10-year risk for cardiovascular events.[193] Though not well substantiated, a diet high in folate and vitamins B_6 and B_{12}, or supplementation with these vitamins, may provide some protection against hyperhomocysteinemia-related stroke.[193,233] Patients with prothrombotic and cardioembolic conditions may require antiplatelet agents or anticoagulation for primary and secondary stroke prevention. However, these agents may also increase the risk of intracranial hemorrhage.[113,119,193]

Some neurologic and cardiovascular conditions, such as valvular disease and high-grade carotid stenosis, are amenable to surgery or endovascular surgery, and correction of these abnormalities may provide greater benefit than risk to the patient in regard to stroke prevention. Indications for carotid endarterectomy (CEA) have been well defined by a number of multicenter prospective randomized controlled trials. In addition to a daily aspirin and a statin, CEA is recommended for high-grade, 70% to 99% asymptomatic carotid stenosis[36,37,193] (Box 13.1). Prophylactic carotid stenting (CAS) may also be considered in asymptomatic carotid stenosis of at least 60% to 99% stenosis by angiography or 70% to 99% stenosis by Doppler ultrasound.[193,204]

CEA is recommended for patients with recent TIAs or ischemic stroke, 50% to 99% carotid artery stenosis by angiography, or 70% to 99% carotid artery stenosis by noninvasive imaging.[36,37,97,246] Carotid artery stenting may be considered for symptomatic patients who are not candidates for CEA. The patient's comorbidities and life expectancy and the surgeon's or interventional radiologist's estimates mortality and morbidity rates must be taken into consideration.[193,204,246]

DEFINITION

Stroke is a heterogeneous disease. The two major subtypes are ischemic and hemorrhagic. Hemorrhagic stroke refers to SAH and ICH. Approximately 87% of all strokes are ischemic and approximately 10% of strokes are the result of ICH, with SAH contributing another 3%.[205] Each subtype has a number of mechanisms (Fig. 13.1).

Ischemic stroke may occur as a result of atherothrombotic events, including large-vessel stenosis; artery-to-artery plaque embolization with occlusion of smaller vessels distal to the original site of plaque formation; and small-vessel disease in deep penetrating arteries supplying the basal ganglia, cerebral white matter, thalamus, and pons.[44,258]

Risk factors for small-vessel ischemic stroke, also referred to as lacunar infarct or stroke, are hypertension, diabetes, and smoking.[44,97,202] The carotid, or vertebral, arteries may dissect and shower emboli distal to the dissection, with or without trauma.[288] In cerebral venous thrombosis (CVT), one or more of the cerebral veins or sinuses occlude, resulting in cerebral edema, impaired cerebrospinal fluid (CSF) absorption, and hemorrhagic or nonhemorrhagic infarcts.[42,90,91]Moyamoya disease is a chronic cerebral angiopathy characterized by progressive narrowing of the terminal end of the internal carotid artery and/or the proximal portion of the anterior cerebral or middle cerebral arteries, along with the development of abnormal collateral vasculature at the base of the brain. It is more prevalent among Asians and may result in both ischemic and hemorrhagic stroke. On angiography, moyamoya appears as a "puff of smoke."[126,140]

Cardiac-related stroke refers to cardioembolic atrial fibrillation, valvular disease or mechanical valve thrombogenesis, recent myocardial infarction, infectious endocarditis, cardiomyopathy, and paradoxical emboli associated with PFO[97,119] (Fig. 13.2). Approximately 23% to 40% of all strokes are ischemic strokes of undetermined etiology, or cryptogenic.[21]

BOX 13.1

American Heart Association/American Stroke Association Levels of Evidence and Recommendations

The AHA/ASA has established levels of evidence and recommendation grades for their clinical practice guidelines regarding management of patients with AIS, SAH, and ICH.

Three levels of evidence exist, with Level A being the highest and Level C being the lowest

- Level A evidence constitutes data obtained from multiple randomized clinical trials or meta-analyses.
- Level B evidence constitutes data obtained from a single randomized controlled trial or nonrandomized studies.
- Level C evidence constitutes data obtained from very limited populations or limited to expert opinion by consensus, case studies, or standards of care.

Three classes of recommendations exist with Class I being the highest and Class III being the lowest

- Class I: Benefit outweighs risk and the procedure or intervention should be performed or administered; the procedure or intervention is indicated or useful, effective, or beneficial.
- Class IIa: Benefit outweighs risk less than Class I but more than Class IIb and the procedure or intervention is reasonable, can be useful, effective, or beneficial, and is probably recommended.
- Class IIb: Benefit outweighs risk less than Class IIa but still of benefit. The procedure or intervention may or might be considered reasonable, or the procedure or intervention's usefulness or effectiveness is unknown, unclear, uncertain, or not well established.
- Class III: The procedure or intervention is of no benefit or may be of harm. The procedure or intervention is not recommended, not indicated, not useful, beneficial, or effective, and should not be performed or administered, or the procedure or intervention causes harm or is potentially harmful or associated with increased mortality and morbidity, and should not be performed or administered.

AHA/ASA, American Heart Association/American Stroke Association; *AIS,* acute ischemic stroke; *ICH,* intracerebral hemorrhage; *SAH,* subarachnoid hemorrhage.
From References 55, 135, and 142.

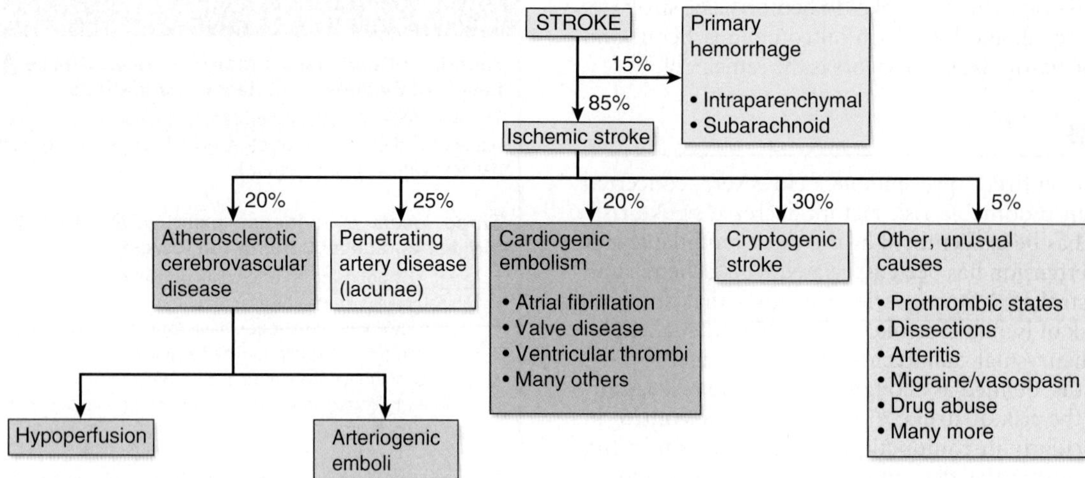

FIG. 13.1 Classification of stroke by mechanism with frequency estimates.

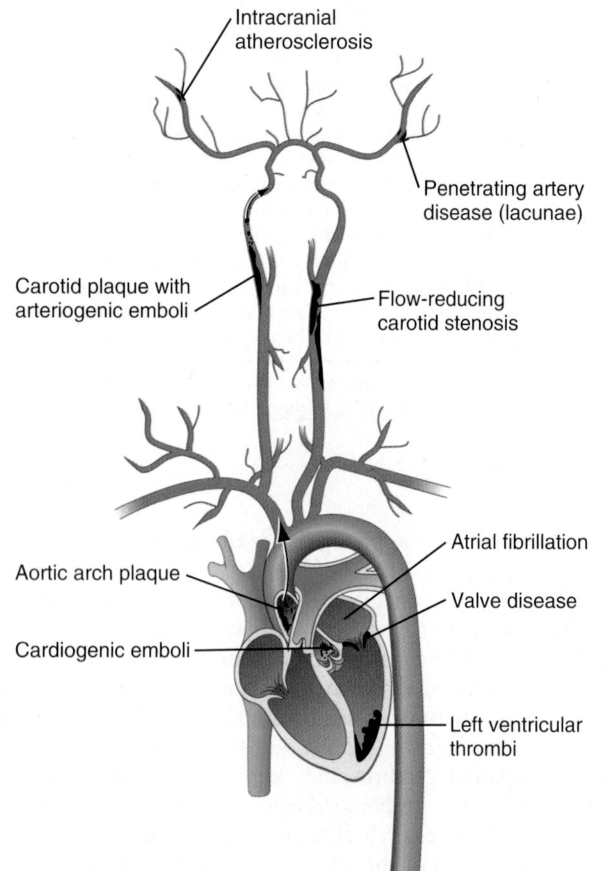

FIG. 13.2 Common sites of arterial and cardiac lesions causing ischemic stroke.

However, every attempt should be made to determine the etiology of a stroke before declaring it cryptogenic. Cardiac or respiratory arrest and generalized hypotensive states may result in a more global ischemia. Patients with systemic hypotension are at risk for watershed infarctions. Watershed, or border-zone infarction, is the term used to describe a subtype of ischemic stroke in nonanastomosing/terminal arterial border zone areas between major vessels of the circle of Willis.[64,185] Normally, blood flow to the most distal branches of the circle of Willis is under a lower amount of arterial pressure than that to the more proximal branches. During hypotensive states, the cerebral perfusion pressure and collateral blood flow to these areas may be inadequate, resulting in infarction.[64,185] The junction of the distal branches of the middle cerebral artery (MCA) and the anterior cerebral artery (ACA) and the junction of the distal branches of the MCA and the posterior cerebral artery (PCA) are two areas prone to watershed infarction[64,185] (Figs. 13.3 and 13.4). Preexisting internal carotid artery disease may contribute to watershed infarction[99] (Table 13.1).

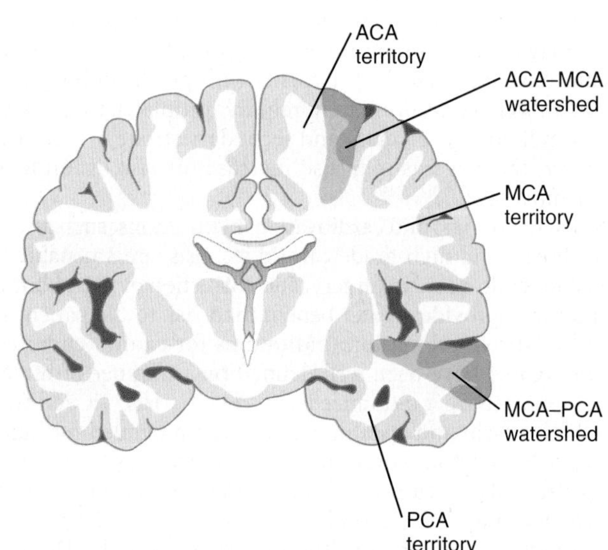

FIG. 13.3 Watershed zone for the major arteries: coronal section. *ACA,* Anterior cerebral artery; *MCA,* middle cerebral artery; *PCA,* posterior cerebral artery.

Spontaneous subarachnoid hemorrhage (SAH) is most often the result of aneurysmal rupture or, less commonly, bleeding from an AVM.[237] An AVM is a vascular anomaly characterized by dilated arteries and veins in the absence of an intervening capillary bed. The AVM typically ruptures

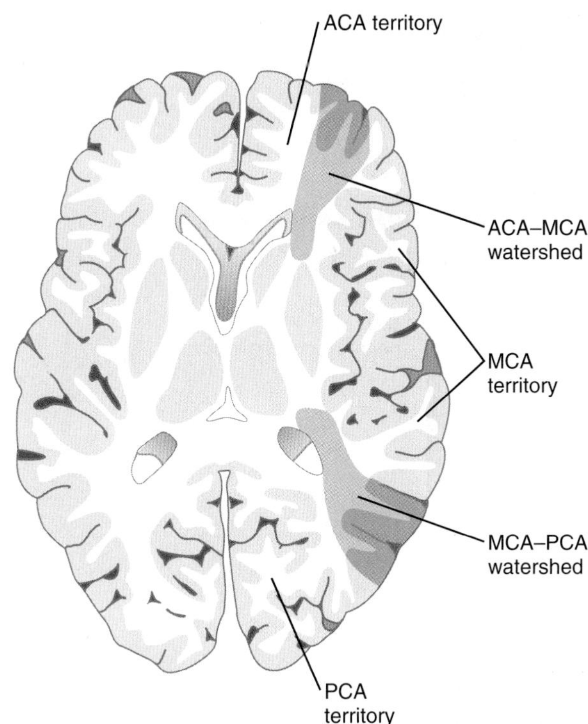

FIG. 13.4 Watershed zone for the major arteries: axial section. *ACA,* Anterior cerebral artery; *MCA,* middle cerebral artery; *PCA,* posterior cerebral artery.

into the subarachnoid space and may extend into the parenchyma from the venous side of the AVM.[168,249] Another form of spontaneous SAH is perimesencephalic (nonaneurysmal) SAH[152] (Fig. 13.5). Perimesencephalic SAH refers to blood in the perimesencephalic and prepontine cisterns, anterior to the midbrain and pons, rather than the more typical location of aneurysmal SAH in the ventricles or lateral sylvian fissures. The cerebral angiogram in perimesencephalic SAH is negative for a vascular anomaly.[152] Up to 90% to 95% of all perimesencephalic SAH patients have a second angiogram that does not reveal a vascular anomaly, and most have a low risk for rebleed or vasospasm.[245] Some small aneurysms may not be seen on angiogram immediately after subarachnoid hemorrhage or in the presence of vasospasm, and a repeat angiogram may be needed later to confirm the absence of a vascular anomaly that must be repaired. Though generally considered benign compared to aneurysmal SAH, perimesencephalic SAH may result in long-term cognitive sequelae.[152]

Spontaneous intracerebral hemorrhage (ICH), or intraparenchymal hemorrhage, is most often associated with systemic hypertension or cerebral amyloid angiopathy (CAA). CAA is associated with lobar, cortical, or subcortical ICH, whereas hypertensive ICH typically occurs in deep structures such as the basal ganglia (putamen and caudate nucleus), thalamus, and pons[168,188] (Fig. 13.6).

PATHOPHYSIOLOGY

All subtypes present according to anatomic and clinical correlation[20,78] (see Tables 13.1 and 13.2; Fig. 13.7). In addition, large artery or posterior fossa infarcts and infarcts with hemorrhagic transformation in AIS, SAH, and ICH may present with additional signs and symptoms related to increased intracranial pressure (ICP) from edema, mass effect, or hydrocephalus.[187,188,255] The clinical presentation of stroke is also impacted by the biochemical events of the ischemic cascade, impaired autoregulation, or uncoupling of the cerebral blood flow (CBF) and cerebral metabolism.[33] Autoregulation, the ability of the cerebral blood vessels to dilate and constrict as needed to maintain adequate cerebral perfusion, is only operational

TABLE 13.1 Arterial Supply to the Brain

Artery	Territory Supplied by Artery
Anterior Circulation (and Branches)	
Internal Carotid Artery (ICA)	
Anterior choroidal	Optic tract, choroid plexus, internal capsule, basal ganglia, hippocampus, cerebral peduncle
Ophthalmic artery	Eye orbits and optic nerves
Middle Cerebral Artery (MCA)	
M1	Sylvian fissure
Lenticulostriate	Basal ganglia, internal capsule
M2	Cerebral cortex in lateral sulcus (insula)
M3	Cerebral cortex above and below the lateral sulcus (opercula)
M4	Lateral cortical surface of brain (except occipital pole), precentral (motor) gyrus supplying arm and face, postcentral (sensory) gyrus supplying arm and face
Anterior Cerebral Artery (ACA)	
A1	Junction of anterior communicating artery (AComA)
A2	
A1 and A2	Corpus callosum
Recurrent artery of Huebner	Medial surfaces of frontal and parietal lobes, cingulate gyrus and precentral (motor) gyrus supplying leg, postcentral (sensory) gyrus supplying leg
Basal ganglia and internal capsule	
Anterior communicating artery (AComA)	Connects two anterior cerebral arteries
Posterior communicating artery (PComA)	Connects carotid (anterior) circulation with vertebrobasilar (posterior) circulation
Posterior Circulation Vertebral Artery (VA)	
Posteroinferior cerebellar artery (PICA)	Undersurface of cerebellum, medulla, and choroid plexus of fourth ventricle
Anterior and posterior spinal arteries	Anterior two-thirds and posterior one-third of spinal cord
Basilar Artery (BA)	
Posterior cerebral artery (PCA)	Thalamus, hypothalamus, medial and inferior surface of temporal lobes, occipital lobes, midbrain, choroid plexuses of third and fourth ventricles
Choroidal artery	Tectum, choroid plexus of third ventricle, medial/superior thalamus
Superior cerebellar artery (SCA)	Undersurface of cerebellum and midbrain
Anterior inferior cerebellar artery (AICA)	Undersurface of cerebellum and lateral pons

From References 20, 96, and 273.

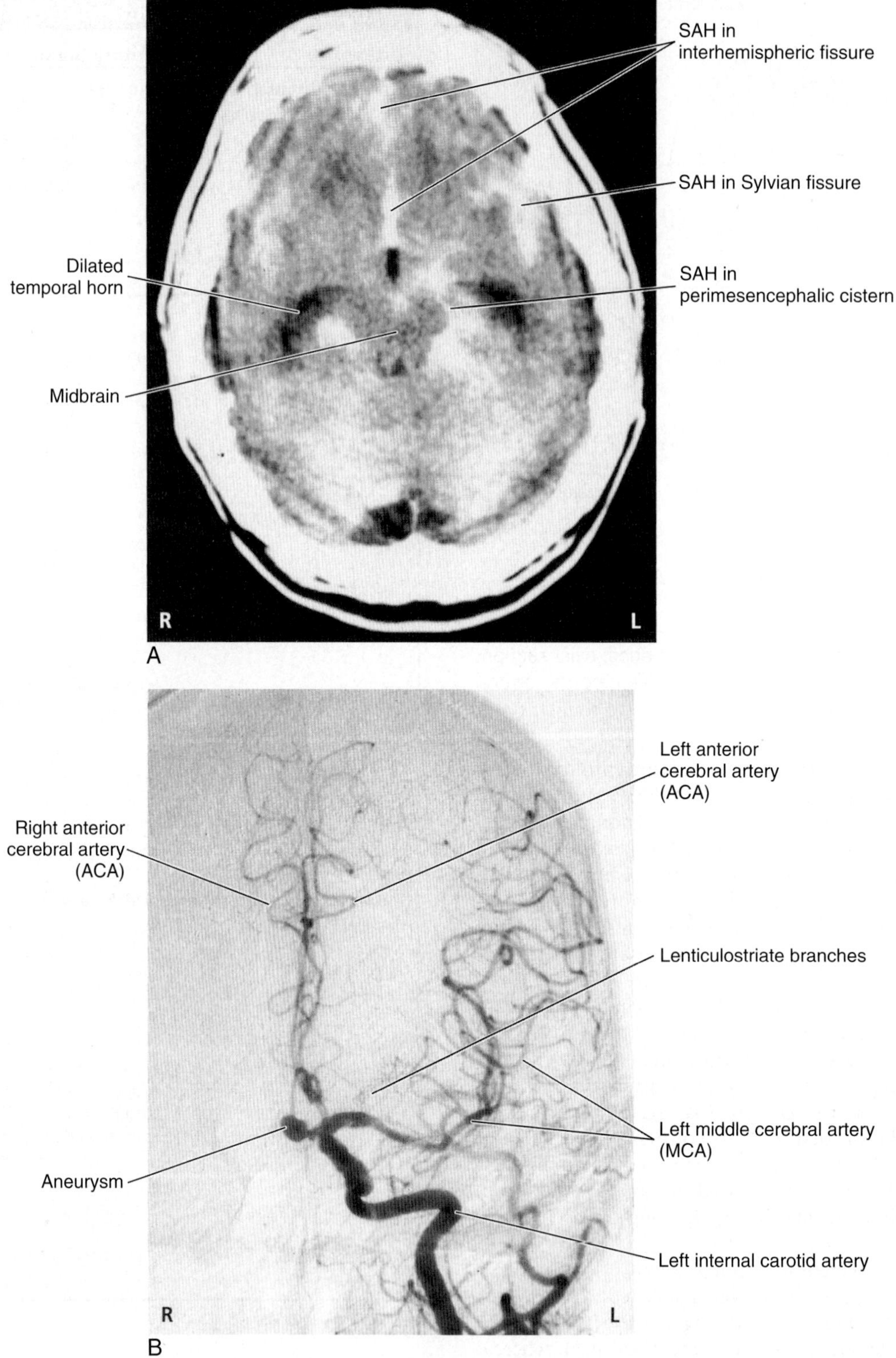

FIG. 13.5 Aneurysmal subarachnoid hemorrhage (SAH). **A,** CT axial image showing subarachnoid blood and hydrocephalus. **B,** Angiogram, anteroposterior view. (From Blumenfeld, H. (2002). *Neuroanatomy through clinical cases.* Sunderland, MA: Sinauer.)

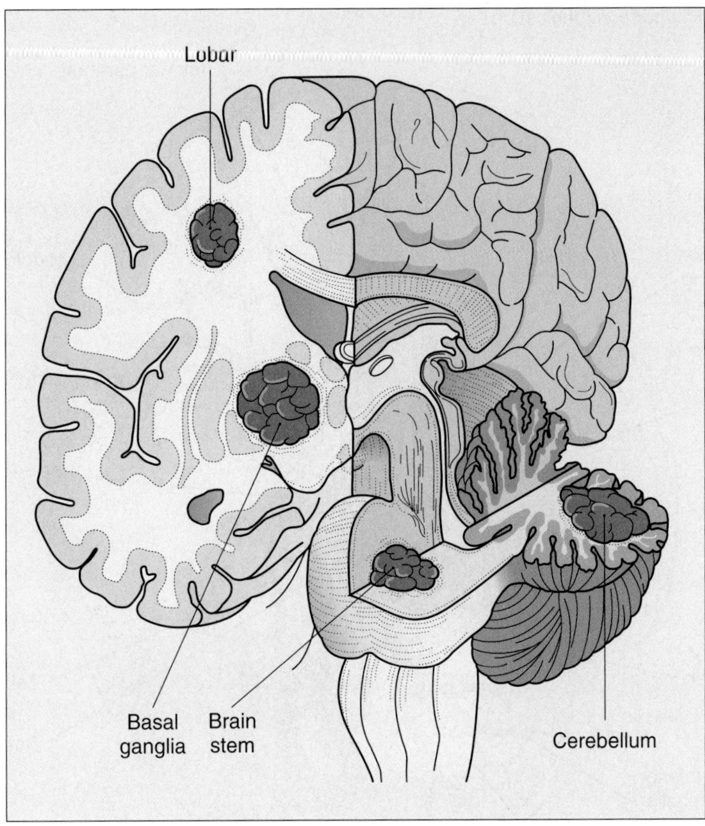

FIG. 13.6 Locations of intracerebral hemorrhage. (From Rengachary, S., & Ellenbogen, R. (2005). *Principles of neurosurgery* (2nd ed.). Philadelphia: Mosby.)

at a mean arterial BP of approximately 60 to 150 mm Hg and may be impaired in chronic hypertension or as a result of the stroke.[33,70,146,223] With impaired autoregulation, the CBF passively follows the systemic BP, resulting in ischemia or hyperemia. Both may cause increased ICP. In chronic hypertension, the BP necessary to adequately perfuse the brain is shifted to the right, requiring a higher baseline BP[33] (Fig. 13.8).

Ischemic Stroke

Glucose is the brain's only energy substrate. As a result, the brain depends on a constant supply of glucose and oxygen for aerobic metabolism. When a blood vessel is occluded, oxygen and glucose delivery to the area of the brain perfused by that vessel is critically decreased or stopped altogether.[108,115,171] The events that follow, referred to as *the ischemic cascade,* begin with the depletion of adenosine triphosphate (ATP), membrane depolarization, and the release of extracellular potassium. These processes are followed by an increase in oxygen extraction and glucose metabolism with the formation of lactic acid. Depolarization of neuronal membranes results in the opening of calcium channels and an influx of intracellular calcium. In addition, the ease of toxic excitatory neurotransmitters, such as glutamate, activates *N*-methyl-D-aspartate (NMDA) receptors to increase the neuron's sodium permeability and cellular swelling. NMDA receptors mediate additional movement of calcium into the cells. Glutamate-activated alpha-amino-3-hydroxy-5-methyl-4-isoxazolepropio acid (AMPA) and metabotropic receptors also participate in the influx of calcium.[108,115,171]

Calcium activates enzymes such as lipases to produce arachidonic acid and free radicals, and stimulates neuronal nitric oxide synthase (nNOS) to increase nitric oxide production. Nitric oxide is a free radical. The production of free radicals and enzymatic perturbations result in lipid peroxidation that result in disruption of the neuronal and endothelial membrane. The release of proinflammatory mediators (cytokines), loss of cytoskeletal integrity, and mitochondrial damage further contribute to cell death[108,115,171](Fig. 13.9).

The core tissue, the area immediately around the blood vessel, infarcts and is no longer salvageable. However, tissue just outside the core area, referred to as the ischemic penumbra, is injured but potentially viable. The ischemic penumbra can be restored to normal function if reperfused within an adequate time.[171,224] Over the next 5 days, cerebral edema increases, peaks, and then typically resolves in the injured and especially the infarcted area[125] (Fig. 13.10). In AIS, this may result in some increased ICP; however, unless the infarct involves the cerebellum or a large portion of a hemisphere (more than 50% of the MCA territory), the increased ICP will likely not result in herniation.[69,154] The mass effect and additional edema associated with hemorrhagic transformation of an AIS may further increase ICP and risk of herniation.[69,154] Infarcts, particularly in the cerebellum or brain stem, may result in respiratory impairment.[65,142,278]

Subarachnoid Hemorrhage

SAH most frequently occurs as a result of an intracranial aneurysm rupture. Intracranial aneurysms most often occur on the circle of Willis or its major arterial branches at the base of the brain in the subarachnoid space[26,56,255] (Table 13.2). The greatest number of intracranial aneurysms are located at the anterior communicating cerebral artery, followed by the posterior communicating and the middle cerebral arteries.[26,56,255] As a result of the aneurysm's rupture, blood is forced into the subarachnoid space and basal

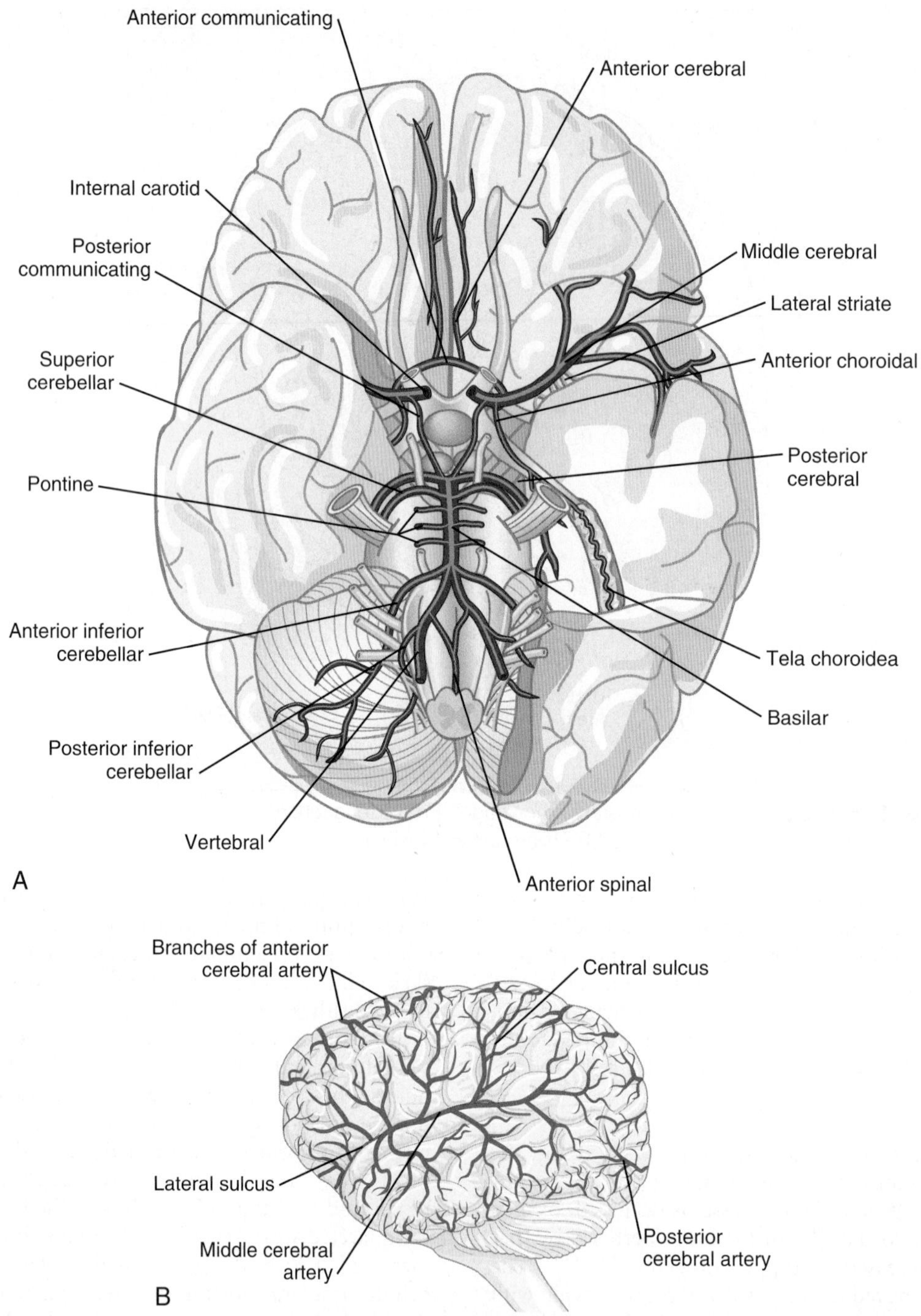

FIG. 13.7 Cerebral circulation **A,** Cerebral arterial circulation at the base of the brain. **B,** Blood vessel distribution on the lateral surface of the cerebral hemisphere.

cisterns, mixing with CSF. The blood may form thick layers or clots intraventricularly but may also extend intraparenchymally and subdurally.[27,250,255]

The pathogenesis of aneurysms is not completely known.[47,196] Although aneurysms are congenital, their growth and rupture may be influenced by conditions such as hypertension and smoking. Hemodynamic stress, genetics, hormones, and the environment are thought to play a role in the development, growth, and rupture of cerebral aneurysms.[26,47] Cerebral aneurysms exhibit features of inflammation and tissue degeneration.[43,196] They are frequently found at the bifurcation of the vessel, and 25% to 50% of individuals with an aneurysm have more than one area of infarcted tissue that may occur at the site of the rupture[26,84,168] (Fig. 13.11). The patient is at risk for rebleeding if the vessel is not repaired, with the greatest risk of rebleeding within the first 24 hours.[43,103,168,255] Mortality associated with rebleeding has been estimated as high as 50% to 70%.[43,168,255] In addition, the extravascular blood and blood clots in the subarachnoid space and ventricles frequently result in hydrocephalus and increased ICP. Hydrocephalus occurs as a result of the blood in the CSF impairing reabsorption of the CSF.[43,103,168,255] The hydrocephalus may resolve over the first couple of weeks after the SAH, or the patient may require a shunt.[43]

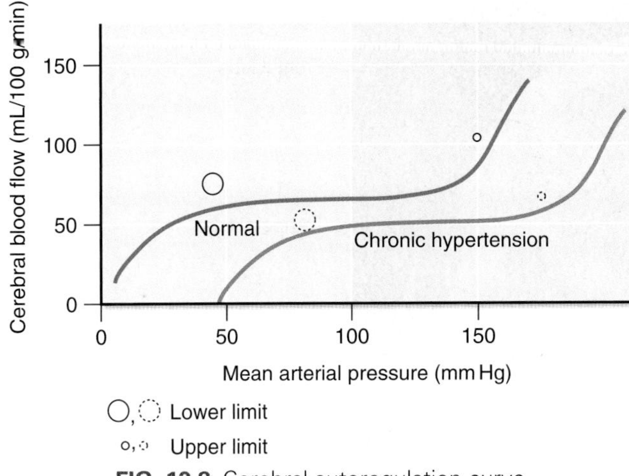

FIG. 13.8 Cerebral autoregulation curve.

At the time of the aneurysmal rupture, a massive transient increased intracranial pressure with a precipitous drop in cerebral perfusion pressure occurs. In addition, a brief period of arterial vasospasm also occurs, which, in combination with the increased ICP, may limit the amount of intracranial hemorrhage but also contribute to the initial infarct.[168] A more sustained cerebral vasospasm may occur from 4 days after the aneurysmal SAH up to 2 or 3 weeks post bleed.[18,62,256]

Up to 80% of all aneurysmal subarachnoid hemorrhage patients will describe a severe headache as "the worst headache of my life."[237] Patients with chronic headaches, such as migraines, may describe a change in the character of the headache.[26,89] If the aneurysm ruptures, the patient may experience syncope, seizures, nausea and vomiting, nuchal rigidity, photophobia, loss of consciousness, or herniation.[26,168,240]

Cerebral vasospasm is sustained constriction of the blood vessel related to the biochemical and histologic changes induced by extravascular blood and may occur at multiple sites simultaneously, at the site of the rupture, and on the contralateral

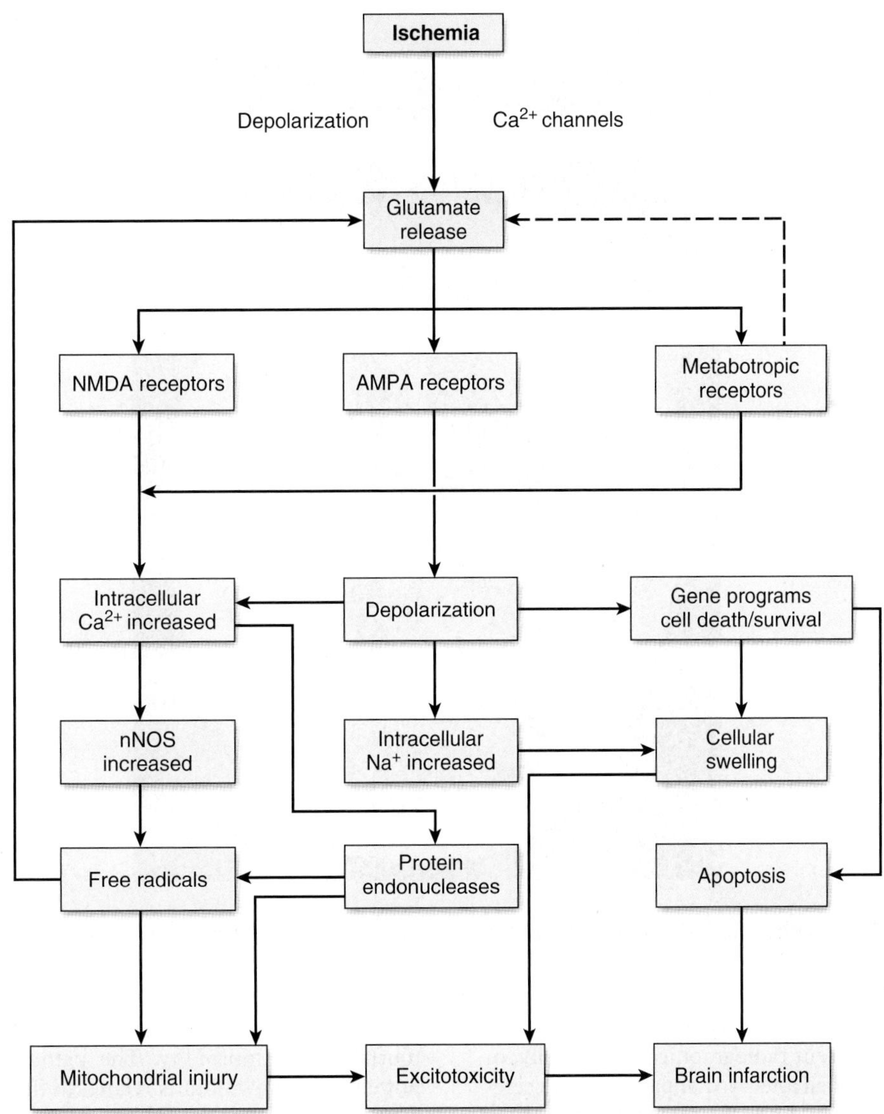

FIG. 13.9 Neurodegenerative cascade. *AMPA,* Alpha-amino-3-hydroxy-5-methyl-4-isoxazolepropionic acid; *Ca^{2+},* calcium; *nNOS,* neuronal nitric oxide synthase.

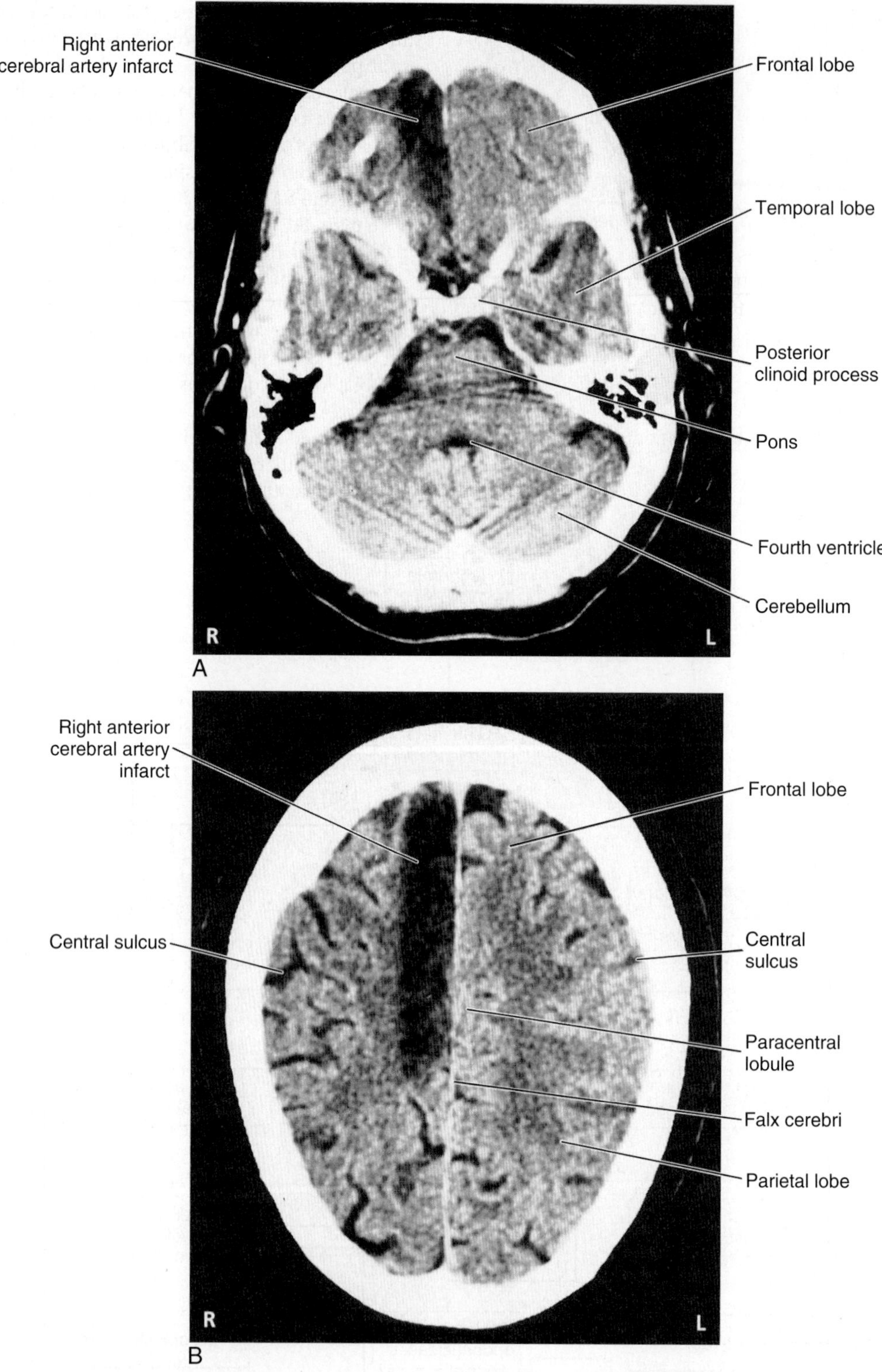

FIG. 13.10 Right anterior cerebral artery infarction: axial CT images progressing from inferior **(A)** to superior **(B)**. (From Blumenfeld, H. (2002). *Neuroanatomy through clinical cases*. Sunderland, MA: Sinauer.)

side. Vasospasm may be present radiographically, clinically, or both. Approximately 70% of all aneurysmal patients have cerebral vasospasm, but only 20% to 30% are symptomatic.[62,103] Clinical cerebral vasospasm is also referred to as delayed cerebral ischemia (DCI). Vasospasm, if allowed to progress, may result in secondary infarct, permanent deficits, and increased mortality and morbidity. The pathogenesis of vasospasm is not entirely known but is related to the sustained extraluminal exposure of subarachnoid blood. The blood and its constituents provoke an inflammatory response, accompanied by a decrease in nitric oxide, and release of endothelin-1, and morphologic changes in the vessels.[38,168] The amount of blood in the

TABLE 13.2 Anatomic and Clinical Correlation: Circle of Willis

Cerebral Vessel/Area	Clinical Presentation
I. Anterior Circulation (frontal lobe, temporal lobes, parietal lobes, occipital lobe)	
Internal carotid artery (ICA)	Contralateral arm and leg weakness/paralysis and sensory loss; contralateral homonymous hemianopsia; expressive and receptive aphasia/dysphasia
Anterior cerebral artery (ACA)	Contralateral leg weakness/paralysis and sensory loss (leg worse than arm); frontal lobe behavioral abnormalities; contralateral hemineglect if lesion on nondominant side
Middle cerebral artery (MCA)	Contralateral arm weakness/paralysis and sensory loss (arm worse than leg); frontal lobe behavioral abnormalities; contralateral homonymous hemianopsia; contralateral lower facial motor and sensory loss; expressive/receptive dysphasia if dominant side
II. Posterior Circulation (occipital lobe, cerebellum, and brain stem)	
Posterior cerebral artery (PCA)	Contralateral hemiplegia and sensory loss; homonymous hemianopsia
Vertebral basilar (VB) arteries	Hemiplegia, ipsilateral facial weakness/numbness; dysarthria, dysphagia, vertigo, nausea, dizziness, ataxic gait, locked-in syndrome
Posterior inferior cerebellar artery (PICA)	Wallenberg syndrome: ataxia, vertigo, nausea and vomiting; contralateral body pain and temperature loss; ipsilateral facial pain and temperature loss; nystagmus, dysarthria, dysphagia, dysphonia, Horner syndrome
Cerebellum	Ataxia, dysarthria, disconjugate gaze, nystagmus
Brain stem	Quadriplegia and sensory loss; ataxia, dysarthria, disconjugate gaze, nystagmus
III. Lacunar Syndromes	Pure motor or pure sensory deficits limited to one side of body only

From References 20, 96, 140, and 273.

subarachnoid space and ventricles is an independent predictor for the amount of postaneurysmal subarachnoid hemorrhage vasospasm.[103,168] Following aneurysmal SAH, cerebral autoregulation is impaired, related to ischemic damage at the time of the hemorrhage, decreased CBF, increased ICP, vasospasm, and preexisting chronic hypertension in some patients.[223]

An AVM is an abnormal cluster of blood vessels that lack the normal capillary connection between arteries and veins necessary for tissue perfusion. The blood is shunted and the area around the shunt, the core of the AVM, is referred to as the nidus.[159] Progressive neurologic deficits may occur as a result of the shunting.[5] In addition, the arterial blood flowing to the venous side under arterial pressure may result in both subarachnoid and intracerebral hemorrhages.[127,168] Most AVMs become symptomatic following hemorrhage. However, they may also cause headaches and seizures before and after hemorrhage.[249] Though thought to be less common than with aneurysmal SAH, vasospasm may occur with ruptured AVMs as well.[122] AVMs vary in size, may be superficial or deep, and may or may not involve functionally important structures of the brain.[249]

Intracerebral Hemorrhage

Spontaneous ICH or intraparenchymal hemorrhage (IPH) occurs with bleeding into the parenchyma of the brain. As the bleeding occurs, additional vessels and planes of tissue in the surrounding area are torn and damaged. Bleeding may be lobar (cortical, subcortical), or it may occur in deeper cerebral structures, such as the basal ganglia or thalamus, or it may be infratentorial, in the cerebellum or brain stem.[48] Lobar bleeds are associated with CAA that increases with age.[48] The intracerebral blood may dissect through brain parenchyma and the walls of the ventricles, causing intraventricular extension (Fig. 13.12). Intraventricular blood carries a poorer prognosis related to obstruction of CSF flow, distention of the ventricles, and compression of adjacent brain tissue, resulting in hydrocephalus and increased ICP.[93] Hydrocephalus and increased ICP are common and herniation is less common at the time of the bleed.[97,107] ICH is frequently the result of hypertension, and secondary enlargement of the hematoma may occur with continued uncontrolled hypertension. The goal of systolic blood pressure is 140 mm Hg if the initial blood pressure is between 150 to 220 mm Hg.[135,143] If the ICH is related to coagulopathy, the hematoma may continue to enlarge until the coagulopathy is reversed.[187,188] A potentially salvageable area of tissue may exist around the hemorrhage. However, the cause of the penumbra is controversial, but may be related to ischemic, altered biochemical change, disruption of the blood-brain barrier, activation of the complement system, and the release of hemoglobin, oxyhemoglobin, or free radicals. Another cause of spontaneous intracerebral hemorrhage includes ingestion of sympathomimetic drugs of abuse such as cocaine and methamphetamines.[48] The drugs may or may not impair autoregulation; attempts at normalization of BP may result in secondary injury.[70,117,219]

ASSESSMENT

Whereas the definitive diagnosis of stroke will be made by a neurodiagnostic study, a bedside assessment with attention to the cardiopulmonary status; airway, breathing, and circulation (ABCs); and neurologic deficits (D) is imperative for the stroke patient. The components of a thorough neurologic exam include level of consciousness, mental status, language and speech, cranial nerves, movement and strength of extremities, sensation, and vital signs.[13,78,142,242,252]

Other key aspects of assessment for the new onset stroke patient include a brief history and assessment of risk factors; the time the patient was last known well and in a normal state of health (if recombinant tissue plasminogen activator [rtPA] is a consideration); and inclusion and exclusion criteria for the administration of rtPA. Stroke mimics conditions such as hypoglycemia, syncope of cardiac origin, seizure, brain tumor, drug or alcohol abuse, complicated migraines, peripheral vertigo, and psychiatric disease and must be considered in the differential diagnosis.[75,78,142,214]

A number of scoring tools are applicable to the acute stroke patient. These include the Glasgow Coma Scale (GCS), the Full Outline of UnResponsiveness (FOUR) Score, the National Institutes of Health Stroke Scale (NIHSS), Hunt and Hess SAH classification, World Federation of Neurological Surgeons (WFNS) SAH scale, Fisher SAH scale, Spetzler and Martin AVM Classification, and the Hemphill ICH score. The ICH scale is

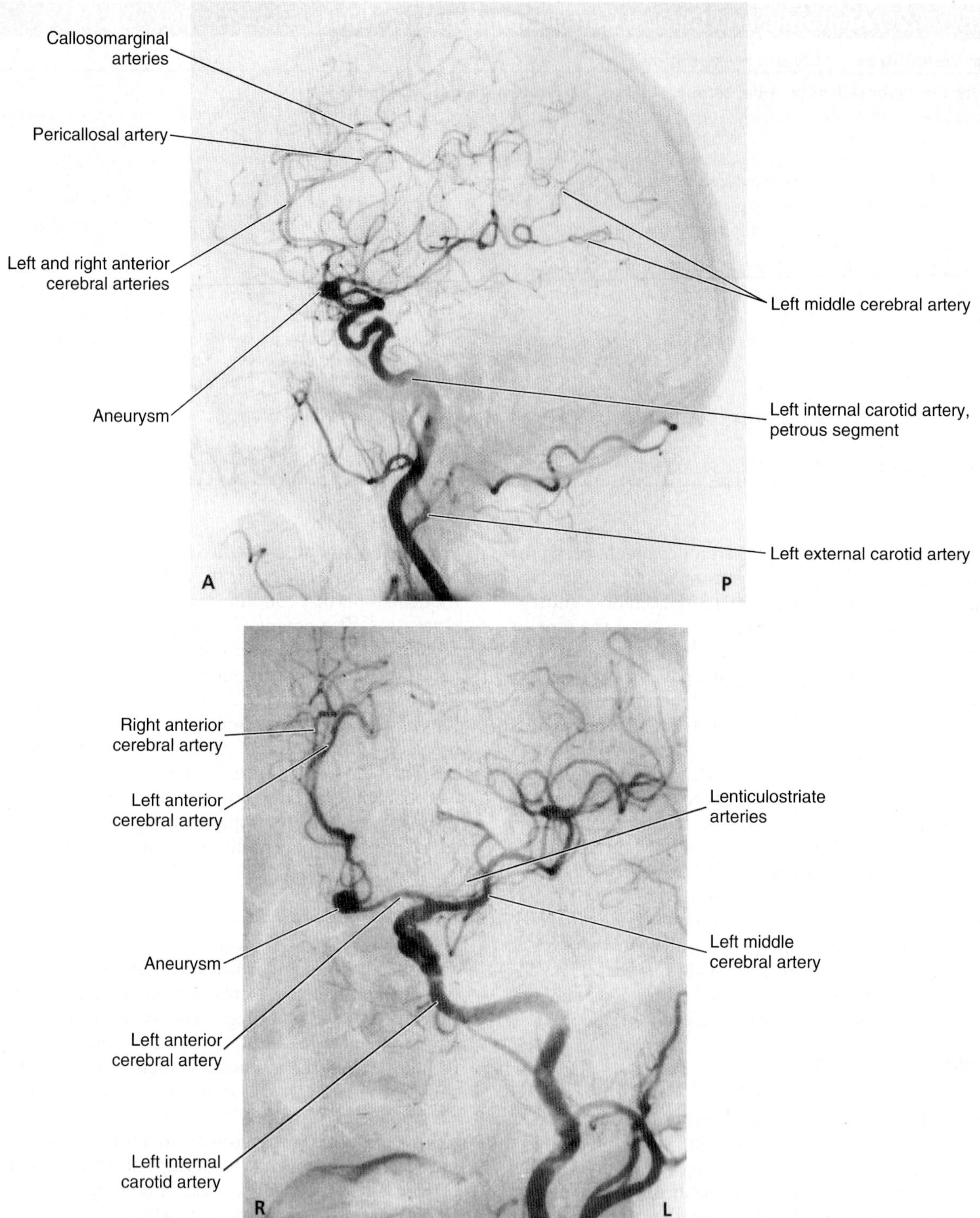

FIG. 13.11 Anterior cerebral artery aneurysm. (From Blumenfeld, H. (2002). *Neuroanatomy through clinical cases*. Sunderland, MA: Sinauer.)

used in combination with the Kothari method of determining intracerebral hemorrhage volume on CT. Other stroke assessment tools include those predictive of stroke, $ABCD^2$, $CHADS_2$, and CHA_2DS_2-VASc and functional recovery scales including the Modified Rankin, Glasgow Outcome Scale, the Barthel Index, and Functional Independence Measure. Functional recovery scales are sometimes used after stabilization of the stroke as a baseline for goal setting for rehabilitation.[1,46,153]

The GCS is a level of consciousness assessment scale, originally developed as a research tool for the assessment of severe traumatic brain injury but later applied to nontraumatic injury as well.[94,166,182] Patients are scored based on eye opening, best

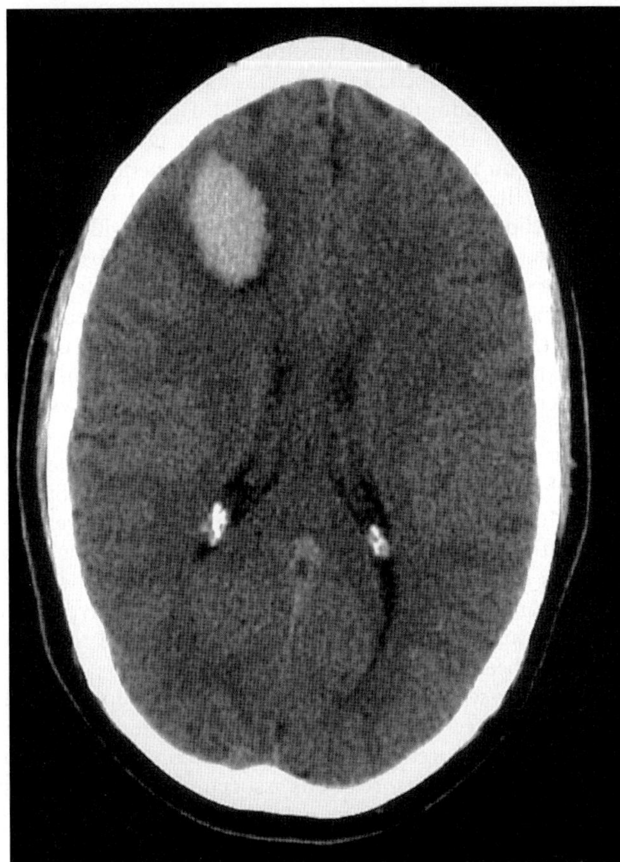

FIG. 13.12 Intracerebral hemorrhage. (From Layon, A., Gabrielli, A., & Friedman, W. (2004). *Textbook of neurointensive care.* Philadelphia: Saunders.)

TABLE 13.3 Glasgow Coma Scale

Response	Score
Eye Opening	
Spontaneous	4
To sound	3
To pain	2
None	1
Motor Response	
Obeys commands	6
Localizes pain	5
Normal flexion (withdrawal)	4
Abnormal flexion	3
Extension	2
None	1
Verbal Response	
Oriented	5
Confused conversation	4
Inappropriate words	3
Incomprehensible sounds	2
None	1

From References 1, 46, and 153.

verbal response, and best motor response to stimuli. GCS values range from 3 to 15; a high GCS score is associated with a better outcome. A GCS score of equal to or less than 8 is associated with severe neuronal injury[1] (Table 13.3). The GCS is

TABLE 13.4 FOUR Score

Eye Response		
4	=	Eyelids open or opened, tracking, or blinking to command
3	=	Eyelids open but not tracking
2	=	Eyelids closed but open to loud voice
1	=	Eyelids closed but open to pain
0	=	Eyelids remain closed with pain
Motor Response		
4	=	Thumbs-up, fist, or peace sign
3	=	Localizing to pain
2	=	Flexion response to pain
1	=	Extension response to pain
0	=	No response to pain or generalized myoclonus status
Brainstem Reflexes		
4	=	Pupil and corneal reflexes present
3	=	One pupil wide and fixed
2	=	Pupil or corneal reflexes absent
1	=	Pupil and corneal reflexes absent
0	=	Absent pupil, corneal, and cough reflex
Respiration		
4	=	Not intubated, regular breathing pattern
3	=	Not intubated, Cheyne-Stokes breathing pattern
2	=	Not intubated, irregular breathing
1	=	Breathes above ventilator rate
0	=	Breathes at ventilator rate or apnea

From References 1, 277, and 278.

more useful in assessing a stroke resulting in an impaired level of consciousness. Limitations of the GCS include moderate interrater reliability, the inability to assess aphasic patients in regard to the verbal component, and difficulty assessing intubated patients.[1,166,275]

The FOUR Score, a more recent level of consciousness assessment tool, specifically addresses brainstem function. Developed in 2005, the FOUR Score addresses eye response, motor response, brainstem reflexes, and respirations. Each component is scored from 0-4 with a best total score of 16 (Table 13.4). Advantages over the GCS include specific consideration for the intubated patient and assessment of the pupil, corneal, and cough reflexes, and respiratory pattern.[166,277] It may be beneficial in detecting locked-in syndrome and persistent vegetative state.[32,166] The FOUR Score has been useful in both acute ischemic and hemorrhagic stroke.[164]

The NIHSS was originally developed to screen and follow patients who receive rtPA for AIS, but is also used for SAH and ICH. The NIHSS is composed of 15 items. The score ranges from 0-42 with 0 being best. An NIHSS score of greater than 20 is predictive of severe disability or death, and a score of less than 5 is associated with good recovery.[1] The NIHSS has established reliability, validity, and prognostic value. However, it does not include a detailed cranial nerve assessment that could lessen attention to the significance of a brainstem or cerebellar stroke.[153] Interrater reliability is variable depending on the clinician's compliance with the scoring instructions.[1,153] Videos and online training and certification to increase the likelihood of correct use of the NIHSS are available through the AHA/ASA (Table 13.5). Yearly retraining to maintain competence is recommended.[112]

The Hunt and Hess classification scale, WFNS scale, and Fisher scale are specific to aneurysmal SAH. The original

TABLE 13.5 National Institutes of Health Stroke Scale

Item	Name	Response
1a	Loss of consciousness	0 = Alert 1 = Not alert, arousable 2 = Not alert, obtunded 3 = Unresponsive
1b	Questions	0 = Answers both correctly 1 = Answers one correctly 2 = Answers neither correctly
1c	Commands	0 = Performs both tasks correctly 1 = Performs one task correctly 2 = Performs neither task correctly
2	Gaze	0 = Normal 1 = Partial gaze palsy 2 = Total gaze palsy
3	Visual fields	0 = No visual loss 1 = Partial hemianopsia 2 = Complete hemianopsia 3 = Bilateral hemianopsia
4	Facial palsy	0 = Normal 1 = Minor paralysis 2 = Partial paralysis 3 = Complete paralysis
5a	Left motor arm	0 = No drift 1 = Drifts before 10 seconds 2 = Falls before 10 seconds 3 = No effort against gravity 4 = No movement
5b	Right motor arm	0 = No drift 1 = Drifts before 10 seconds 2 = Falls before 10 seconds 3 = No effort against gravity 4 = No movement
6a	Left motor leg	0 = No drift 1 = Drifts before 10 seconds 2 = Falls before 10 seconds 3 = No effort against gravity 4 = No movement
6b	Right motor leg	0 = No drift 1 = Drifts before 10 seconds 2 = Falls before 10 seconds 3 = No effort against gravity 4 = No movement
7	Ataxia	0 = Absent 1 = One limb 2 = Two limbs
8	Sensory	0 = Normal 1 = Mild loss 2 = Severe loss
9	Language	0 = Normal 1 = Mild aphasia 2 = Severe aphasia 3 = Mute or global aphasia
10	Dysarthria	0 = Normal 1 = Mild 2 = Severe
11	Extinction/inattention	0 = Normal 1 = Mild 2 = Severe

From References 46, 142, 153, and 210.

intention with the Hunt-Hess grade was to be based on the initial clinical assessment on admission and, despite the patient's course or outcome, the Hunt-Hess classification was to stay the same as an indicator of surgical risk.[137,180] However, in clinical practice today, the Hunt-Hess classification is often changed daily based on the patient's level of improvement or worsening during the first 2 to 3 weeks postaneurysmal SAH.[239] The patient's clinical status is graded from 0 to V, with 0 being unruptured, I to II being good grade, and IV to V being considered poor grade (Table 13.6). The Hunt-Hess Scale is most useful as a predictor of neurologic outcome after aneurysmal SAH.[1] Limitations include its lack of consideration for comorbidities and terminology without clear definition. Some clinicians alter the scale by adding an additional grade for systemic disease.[239]

The WFNS scale combines the GCS, Hunt-Hess classification, and the presence of any neurologic motor deficits. Similar to the Hunt-Hess classification, lower grades (I-II) are associated with better outcomes and grades IV to V have a worse prognosis (Table 13.7). The scale has been said to be more objective and less prone to interobserver variability.[168] The prognostic value of the WFNS scale is in dispute; research on its validity has been conflicting.[46,239]

The Fisher scale is based on the amount of blood visualized by computed tomography (CT) scans. The Fisher score was developed to predict vasospasm based on the amount of SAH blood. A Fisher score of 3 is associated with the greatest risk of vasospasm. However, a Fisher score of 4, denoting intraventricular or intracerebral clot, is also associated with a poor outcome.[46] Fisher scores range from 1 (no blood) to 4 (clot) (Table 13.8). The Fisher score has been criticized for its subjectivity, lack of reproducibility, and inability to differentiate the patients at greatest risk of symptomatic vasospasm.[26,280]

A guide to predicting surgical risk, the Spetzler and Martin score is a 1 to 5 ranking based on angiogram size of the AVM, the pattern of venous drainage (e.g., deep or superficial), and the functional importance of the AVM. The larger the nidus, the deeper the venous drainage; and the greater the functional importance of the area supplied by the AVM, the higher the score and the greater the surgical risk[251] (Table 13.9). Whereas the Spetzler-Martin (SM) grading system has been prospectively and retrospectively validated, it may oversimplify selection of surgical candidates and may not be predictive of radiosurgery outcomes.[174,251]

The ICH score ranges from 0 to 6 and combines the GCS with the ICH volume (Kothari method), the location of blood, and the age of the patient[133,167] (Table 13.10). The lower the score, the better the predicted outcome.[52,132] This scoring system has been externally validated but has demonstrated a lack of predictive ability in regard to poor outcome.[139]

The ABCD^2 score was developed to assist in predicting stroke following a transient ischemic attack (TIA). Each letter represents a predictive variable: Age, Blood pressure, Clinical features of TIA, Duration of TIA, and Diabetes, with scores in each category ranging from 0 through 2[145] (Table 13.11). The tool has been validated and may be predictive of stroke risk at 2, 7, 30, and 90 days after TIA.[78,145] The AHA/ASA has developed guidelines around hospitalization and diagnostic workup within 72 hours following TIA based on the ABCD^2 score.[77] However, at least one large prospective validation study found the tool to be an inaccurate predictor of stroke.[227]

TABLE 13.6 Hunt and Hess Clinical Classification of Subarachnoid Hemorrhage

Grade*	Criteria
Grade I	Asymptomatic or minimal headache and slight nuchal rigidity
Grade II	Moderate to severe headache, nuchal rigidity, no neurologic deficit other than cranial nerve palsy
Grade III	Drowsiness, confusion, or mild focal deficit
Grade IV	Stupor, moderate to severe hemiparesis, possibly early decerebrate rigidity and vegetative disturbances
Grade V	Deep coma, decerebrate rigidity, moribund appearance

*Serious systemic disease such as hypertension, diabetes, severe arteriosclerosis, chronic pulmonary disease, and severe vasospasm seen on arteriography results in placement of the patient in the next less favorable category.
From References 1, 46, 55, and 153.

TABLE 13.7 World Federation of Neurological Surgeons Subarachnoid Hemorrhage Scale

WFNS Grade	GCS Score	Motor Deficit
I	15	Absent
II	14–13	Absent
III	14–13	Present
IV	12–7	Present or absent
V	6–3	Present or absent

GCS, Glasgow Coma Scale; *WFNS*, World Federation of Neurological Surgeons.
From References 1, 55, and 74.

TABLE 13.8 Fisher Grading System of Severity of Subarachnoid Hemorrhage

Fisher Grade	Blood on Computed Tomography
1	No subarachnoid blood detected
2	Diffuse or vertical layers < 1 mm thick
3	Localized clot or vertical layer > 1 mm thick
4	Intracerebral or intraventricular clot with diffuse or no subarachnoid hemorrhage

From References 1 and 95.

TABLE 13.9 Spetzler Martin AVM Grade

Determination of Arteriovenous Malformation (AVM) Grade*

Grade Feature	Points Assigned
Size of AVM	
Small (<3 cm)	1
Medium (3–6 cm)	2
Large (>6 cm)	3
Eloquence of Adjacent Brain	
Noneloquent	0
Eloquent	1
Pattern of Venous Drainage	
Superficial only	0
Deep	1

*Grade = (size) + (eloquence) + (venous drainage)
For example (1, 2, or 3) + (0 or 1) + (0 or 1)
From References 1 and 248.

TABLE 13.10 ICH Score

GCS	Points Assigned
3-4	2 pts
5-12	1 pt
13-5	0 pts
ICH volume	
Yes	1 pt
No	0 pts
Location	
Intratentorial	1 pt
Supratentorial	0 pts
Age	
≥80 yrs	1 pt
<80 yrs	0 pts

From Reference 1.

TABLE 13.11 ABCD² Score

Clinical Feature		Points Assigned
Age	> 60 years	1 point
Blood pressure	≥ 140/90 mm Hg	1 point
Clinical features	Speech disturbance without weakness	1 point
	Unilateral weakness with or without speech impairment	2 points
Duration	< 10 minutes	0 points
	10–59 minutes	1 point
	> 60 minutes	2 points
Diabetes	Present	1 point

From References 22, 106, 111, and 156.

The $CHADS_2$ and CHA_2DS_2-VASc scoring classifications were designed to predict stroke (and thromboembolic) risk in patients with nonvalvular atrial fibrillation. Similar to the $ABCD^2$ score, the letters represent the risk factor: Congestive heart failure, *H*ypertension, *A*ge, *D*iabetes, prior *S*troke (or TIA or thromboembolism). The score for each variable is 1 with the exception of those followed by a "2" (Table 13.12). The CHA_2DS_2-VASc score adds vascular disease; peripheral, arterial, and myocardial infarction and aortic plaque. The composite score for each provides an annual stroke risk for the patient who also has atrial fibrillation[23,226] (Table 13.13). CHA_2DS_2-VASc may provide greater identification of patients at low risk and better discrimination of those at moderate risk of stroke.[50] However both scores may underestimate stroke risk for patients who have experienced a recent TIA or ischemic stroke yet have no other risk factors.[156] The risk stratification provided by these tools may assist in determining management such as antithrombotic versus anticoagulation pharmacologic management.[178]

Once the patient's stroke has stabilized, functional scales provide a baseline in critical care for later comparison as functional recovery progresses. The Glasgow Outcome Score (GOS) is among the earliest functional assessment tools. Similar to the GCS, it is not specific to stroke. The scores range from 1 (death)

TABLE 13.12 $CHADS_2$ Score

Clinical Feature	Points Assigned
Congestive heart failure	1
Hypertension	1
Aged ≥ 75 years	1
Diabetes mellitus	1
Stroke/TIA/TE	2
Maximum Score	6

From References 22, 50, and 156.

TABLE 13.13 CHA_2DS_2-VASc Score

Clinical Feature	Points Assigned
Congestive heart failure/Ld dysfunction	1
Hypertension	1
Aged ≥ 75 years	2
Diabetes mellitus	1
Stroke/TIA/TE	2
Vascular disease (prior MI, PAD, or aortic plaque)	1
Aged (65–74 years)	1
Sex category (i.e., female gender)	1
Maximum Score	10

LV, left ventricle; *MI*, myocardial infarction; *PAD*, peripheral artery disease; *TE*, thromboembolic events; *TIA* transient ischemic attack.
From References 23, 50, and 226.

TABLE 13.14 Glasgow Outcome Scale

Outcome	Score
Good Recovery	5
(A) Full recovery without symptoms or signs	
(B) Capable of resuming normal activities but has minor complaints	
Moderate Disability	4
Independent but disabled	
(A) Signs present but can resume most former activities	
(B) Independent in activities of daily living but cannot resume previous activities	
Severe Disability	3
Conscious but dependent	
(A) Partial independence in activities of daily living but cannot return to previous activities	
(B) Total or almost total dependency for activities of daily living	
Vegetative State	2
Death	1

From References 1 and 23.

TABLE 13.15 Barthel Index

Activity	Points Assigned
Feeding	0 = dependent
	5 = needs help (e.g., cutting, spreading butter)
	10 = independent in all actions
Bowels	0 = incontinent
	5 = occasional accident
	10 = continent
Bladder	0 = incontinent/catheterized and unable to manage
	5 = occasional accident
	10 = continent
Grooming	0 = needs help
	5 = independent for face/hair/teeth/shaving
Toilet use	0 = dependent
	5 = needs some help
	10 = independent
Transfers (bed-chair)	0 = unable with transfers
	5 = major help with transfers, but sits without support
	10 = minor help (verbal or physical)
Walking	0 = unable
	5 = independent in wheelchair
	10 = walks with help of person (verbal or physical)
	15 = independent (may use aide)
Dressing	0 = dependent
	5 = needs help, but does half
	10 = independent (including buttons, zippers, and laces)
Stairs	0 = unable
	5 = needs help (verbal or physical)
	10 = independent
Bathing	0 = dependent
	5 = independent

Instructions: Record information about function for the 24 hours before the assessment. Take the information from the best available source (i.e., nurses, relatives, the patient). Comatose patients are given a score of "0" even if they have not yet been incontinent of feces.
From References 1, 23, and 235.

TABLE 13.16 Modified Rankin Scale

Findings	Score
No symptoms present at all	0
No disability despite some symptoms	1
Slight disability but does not require assistance	2
Moderate disability but can walk	3
Moderately severe disability	4
Severe disability, usually bedridden	5
Dead	6

From references 1 and 23.

to 5 (good recovery).[46] The GOS does not delineate activities of daily living but focuses on general categories of recovery, which likely lessen interrater reliability[153] (Table 13.14). It has been used extensively to report outcomes in both ischemic stroke and subarachnoid hemorrhage research.[1]

In contrast, the Barthel Index (BI) is an ADL, self-care, and mobility-specific score and includes 10 activities for which the assessor rates the stroke patient as dependent, partially dependent, or independent in their ability to perform. The score ranges from 0 to 100 with 100 being fully independent[23,235] (Table 13.15). It does not include assessment of cognition, language, vision, or emotional impairment.[1,153,235]

The modified Rankin scale (mRS) is similar to the GOS in that it defines function status by category from 0 (asymptomatic) to 6 (dead) with variable levels of disability between 0 and 6 (Table 13.16). Similar to the GOS, it lacks detail and is not specific to stroke.[1,153] The mRS is the designated functional scale of choice for The Joint Commission (TJC) Comprehensive Stroke Center Performance Standards at 90 days and is often designated as the outcome measure post-stroke in the conduct of clinical research.[256]

The Functional Independence Measure (FIM) is perhaps the most detailed functional scoring system, with items including ADLs but also language, social interaction, problem solving, and memory. Scores in each category may range from 1 to 4 with 4 being best[1,118] (Table 13.17). Administering the FIM requires

TABLE 13.17 Functional Independence Measure

Each routine daily task is rated on a 7-point scale of dependency.

No helper

7. Complete independence
6. Modified independence

Helper (Modified dependence)

5. Supervision
4. Minimal assistance
3. Moderate assistance

Helper (Complete dependence)

2. Maximal assistance
1. Total assistance

Self-Care							
Eating	7	6	5	4	3	2	1
Grooming	7	6	5	4	3	2	1
Bathing	7	6	5	4	3	2	1
Dressing—upper body	7	6	5	4	3	2	1
Dressing—lower body	7	6	5	4	3	2	1
Toileting	7	6	5	4	3	2	1
Sphincter Control							
Bladder management	7	6	5	4	3	2	1
Bowel management	7	6	5	4	3	2	1
Transfers							
Bed, chair, wheelchair	7	6	5	4	3	2	1
Toilet	7	6	5	4	3	2	1
Tub, shower	7	6	5	4	3	2	1
Locomotion							
Walk, wheelchair	7	6	5	4	3	2	1
Stairs	7	6	5	4	3	2	1
Communication							
Comprehension	7	6	5	4	3	2	1
Expression	7	6	5	4	3	2	1
Social Cognition							
Social interaction	7	6	5	4	3	2	1
Problem solving	7	6	5	4	3	2	1
Memory	7	6	5	4	3	2	1

From Reference 1. Adapted from Granger, C. V., Hamilton, B. B., Linacre, J. M., et al. (1993). Performance profiles of the functional independence measure. *Am J Phys Med Rehabil, 72*, 84–89.

training and is primarily used in the rehabilitation setting. The FIM is considered a valid measure of post-stroke outcome.[53,118]

None of the clinical stroke scales discussed are comprehensive, but each provides a standardized and clinically practical format for assessing and communicating the stroke patient's condition. They may be helpful in predicting the patient's outcome, but the limitations of each tool should be recognized.[46,109]

Laboratory Findings

The most basic laboratory workup of the stroke patient consists of serum chemistry, complete blood count, coagulation, and toxicology studies. Other tests may be indicated, depending on the patient's systemic disease, general condition, and potential etiologies, including arterial blood gas, creatine kinase-myocardial bands (CK-MB), troponin, cholesterol, triglycerides, glycosylated hemoglobin (HbA1c), antiphospholipid antibodies (anticardiolipin), hemoglobin electrophoresis, lipid profile, factor V Leiden (FVL), lupus anticoagulant, homocysteine, disseminated intravascular coagulation panel, partial thromboplastin time (PTT), platelet assays, proteins C and S, prothrombin time, thrombin time, INR, fibrinogen, sickle cell test, and an antithrombin III study[57] (Table 13.18).

Routine testing for hypercoagulable states such as FVL mutation, protein C and S deficiencies, antiphospholipid antibody syndrome (APS), and hyperhomocysteinemia is not recommended if the ischemic stroke or TIA can be explained otherwise.[142,149,156] A point of care testing of blood glucose is sufficient prior to administering IV rtPA.[78,142,157] However, prior to administering IV rtPA, current use of anticoagulation medications must be noted and the result of an INR obtained if the patient is on warfarin (Coumadin), or a PTT and platelet count if the patient is on heparin. There are no specific laboratory assays for the oral

TABLE 13.18 Laboratory Testing in Stroke

Laboratory Test	Normal Values	Abnormal Values and Significance in Stroke
Antiphospholipid antibodies	Negative (not prothrombotic)	Present in hypercoagulability; increases risk of ischemic stroke
Anticardiolipin antibody	Negative (not prothrombotic) 3 subtypes: Immunoglobulin A (IgA) Negative = 0–11 APL (units) Immunoglobulin G (IgG) Negative = 0–14 GPL (units) Immunoglobulin M (IgM) Negative = 0–12 MPL (units)	Most common antiphospholipid antibody; positive in hypercoagulability; increases risk of ischemic stroke
Antithrombin III	Plasma: 21–30 mg/dL; 85–115% of standard; greater than 50% of control value	Decreased in ischemic stroke; increased in hemorrhagic stroke
Disseminated intravascular coagulation panel		Underlying etiology may be malignancy, sepsis, surgical or obstetric complications, or trauma Stroke may be thromboembolic or hemorrhagic
• Fibrin degradation products	2–10 mcg/mL	Increased
• Fibrin split products	Negative	Positive
• Fibrinogen level	150–400 mg/dL	Decreased
• Partial thromboplastin time	20–36 sec	Prolonged
• Platelets	150,000–400,000	Decreased
• Prothrombin time	10–15 sec	Prolonged
Factor assays, especially factor V Leiden		Increased clotting factors associated with hypercoagulability and increased risk of ischemic stroke
• V, VII, VIII, IX, X, XII	50–150% of normal (control sample)	
• XI	65–135% of normal (control sample)	
• XIII	Clot is insoluble for 24 hours	Decreased or absent factor VIII or IX with hemophilia
Glucose (fasting)	Adult: 70–115 mg/dL Child: 60–100 mg/dL	Diabetes is associated with increased risk of ischemic stroke
Glycosylated hemoglobin (HgA_{1c})	Normal: 5.5–8.8% Well-controlled diabetes: 3.5–6.0%	Poorly controlled diabetes associated with atherosclerosis and microangiopathy of cerebral arteries; increases risk of thromboembolic strokes
Hemoglobin electrophoresis	Hemoglobin S: negative	Sickle cell hemoglobin greater than 30%, 80–100%
Homocysteine	3–4.7 μmol/L	Increased homocysteine levels are associated with increased ischemic stroke risk related to atherosclerosis
Lipid profile	Recommended coronary heart disease risk levels	Low HDL is associated with ischemic stroke in men
• Total cholesterol	< 200 mg/dL	
• HDL cholesterol	> 35 mg/dL	
• LDL cholesterol	< 130 mg/dL	
• Total triglyceride	< 190 mg/dL	
Lupus anticoagulant	Negative	Present with hypercoagulability; increases risk of ischemic stroke
Partial thromboplastin time	20–36 sec	Prolonged on heparin therapy and hypercoagulability; increases risk of hemorrhagic stroke
Platelet aggregation	60–100% (depends on assay used and laboratory-specific normal values)	Increased values may indicate greater risk of thrombosis, ischemic stroke May be used to monitor effectiveness of antiplatelet agents for primary or secondary prevention of ischemic stroke
Protein C	58–148%	Deficiency increases risk of thrombosis, ischemic stroke
Protein S	74–112 units/dL	Deficiency increases risk of thrombosis, ischemic stroke
Prothrombin time INR	10–15 sec 1.0	Prolonged with warfarin therapy; increases risk of hemorrhagic stroke
Thrombin Time	Less than 20 sec	Greater than 20 seconds for presence of direct thrombin inhibitors (dabigatran)
Ecarin clotting time	Negative	Positive for presence of direct thrombin inhibitors (e.g., dabigatran); highly sensitive; not routinely available
Anti-factor Xa activity	Negative	Positive for presence of factor Xa inhibitors (apixaban, rivaroxaban)
Sickle cell test	Negative	Positive in sickle cell disease or trait; screening test for sickle cell; definitive test is hemoglobin electrophoresis Sickle cell disease increases risk of ischemic stroke
Toxicology screen	Negative	Positive for amphetamines and cocaine metabolites in intracerebral hemorrhage and subarachnoid hemorrhage

HDL, High-density lipoprotein; *INR*, international normalized ratio; *LDL*, low-density lipoprotein.
From References 63, 66, 225, 264, and 266.

direct thrombin or direct factor Xa inhibitors used for the prevention of stroke related to nonvalvular atrial fibrillation at time of publication. A normal thrombin time (TT) or ecarin clotting time (ECT) may rule out the presence of the direct thrombin or direct factor Xa inhibitors, and the provider must obtain a current medication profile before considering rtPA.[63,66,78,142]

A 12-lead electrocardiogram (ECG) is recommended for all critically ill stroke patients because cardiac disease or myocardial injury may be the cause or the result of a stroke. Signs and symptoms of cardiac-related stroke, myocardial infarction, or hemodynamic instability warrant additional studies, including serial CK-MB and troponin laboratory assessments, transthoracic echocardiogram (TTE), transesophageal echocardiogram (TEE), and cardiac catheterization.[142] TTEs reveal valvular disease, left ventricular dysfunction, low ejection fraction, atrial or ventricular thrombi, or PFO as possible sources of stroke.[16,119,154,179] Commercially available contrast agents or agitated saline may be used as contrast media for enhancing the detection of right to left cardiac shunts in PFO.[191] A TEE is more sensitive in the detection of left atrial thrombi, a PFO, some valvular dysfunction, and aortic arch plaques that may be the cardioembolic source for a stroke.[16,119,160] TEE requires the insertion of an esophageal probe, which may not be well tolerated by the patient, and sedation and continuous monitoring may be needed.[2]

Radiographic Findings

The radiographic workup of the stroke patient consists of a number of well-established and newer neuroimaging modalities, utilizing CT, angiography, magnetic resonance imaging (MRI), and single photon emission computed tomography (SPECT) (Table 13.19). The noncontrast CT scan is universally considered a first-line neurodiagnostic tool for stroke.[17,28,142] Whereas the noncontrast CT will not demonstrate an AIS in its earliest stages, it will show the presence of blood as a hemorrhagic stroke subtype, providing quick information regarding a patient's ineligibility for rtPA administration if blood is present.[28,55] If a CT scan is negative for hemorrhage but SAH is suspected, and no mass effect/signs of increased ICP are seen, a lumbar puncture (LP) should be performed.[55,168] An MRI may be performed to detect subarachnoid hemorrhage if the LP is contraindicated.[55] A noncontrast CT may show subtle intraparenchymal injury with loss of gray/white differentiation and effacement in early ischemic stroke within 3 hours of stroke onset.[142] In addition, a thrombus in the middle cerebral artery (hyperdense MCA sign) may be seen within the first few hours of a large MCA stroke.[28,142] CT is also used to determine the volume of an intracerebral hemorrhage.[183]

Perfusion CT (CTP) utilizing contrast media quickly quantifies ischemia and provides color-code graphic displays indicating cerebral blood flow, cerebral blood volume, and mean transit time.[28] CTP may be used as an alternative when MRI is not available or contraindicated; however, it has not been validated for rtPA decision-making.[17]

Whereas the noncontrast CT scan is more efficient at identifying intracranial blood and less costly than an MRI, T2-weighted MRI images are better than CT at detecting acute brain stem and lacunar ischemic stroke.[44,142] However, some patients cannot undergo MRI because of internal ferromagnetic devices/objects. Intraocular foreign bodies from welding or firearms, heart valves made before 1964, older aneurysm clips, shunts, pacemakers, medication pumps, and middle ear prosthetics are contraindications for MRI.[25,151] Some MRI approved devices, such as newer shunts and vagal nerve stimulators, must be reprogrammed or at least interrogated upon return from MRI to determine that the settings have not be affected by the magnet. The presence of ferromagnetic intraocular foreign bodies may be determined with a plain skull x-ray. Medication patches with foil or metal components may burn the patient and must be removed before the test. Monitoring and care of the critically ill patient in MRI is difficult because of the inability to use the usual ferromagnetic-containing equipment and signal interference on the ECG.[25,151] Gadolinium, the contrast agent used for contrast-enhanced MRI, is associated with nephrogenic systemic fibrosis, particularly in patients with acute or severe chronic kidney disease.[58]

Other MRI modalities, such as diffusion-weighted imaging (DWI) and perfusion-weighted imaging (PWI), are gaining favor in regard to sensitivity and specificity relative to the character of AIS. MRI diffusion can differentiate stroke (infarcted tissue) from stroke mimics. MRI diffusion is the most accurate method of detecting cerebral infarction.[17]

MRI perfusion can identify the ischemic penumbra.[28] However, most institutions cannot efficiently complete most of these new modalities for the critically ill patient within the window of opportunity for rapid intervention such as the standard 3- to 4.5-hour time limit for intravenous rtPA administration. Completion and interpretation of DWI and PWI MRIs require more time than noncontrast CT, and assessment and management of the patient are more difficult while the test is performed.[17,142]

Two of the newer, more clinically valuable MRI modalities, DWI and PWI MRIs, may eventually allow intravenous rtPA to be safely administered beyond the 3- to 4.5-hour window from onset of symptoms in AIS patients with a PWI-DWI mismatch. In AIS, PWI identifies the tissue that is hypoperfused (the penumbra) and DWI examines the area that has already infarcted and cannot be salvaged (the infarcted core).[17,28] The difference between the two, PWI minus DWI, is referred to as the PWI-DWI mismatch. If the area of decreased perfusion, PWI, is significantly larger than the diffusion abnormality, DWI, the patient may be at lower risk for hemorrhage from rtPA administration; more likely to benefit from reperfusion therapy; and possibly eligible for rtPA up to 6 hours after symptom onset without worsening outcome. The intricacies of mapping the best PWI and calculating the volume of the hypoperfused but salvageable tissue have not been determined; research continues in this area.[17,125,142]

T2 gradient spin-echo MRI sequences have been found to be valuable in detecting blood breakdown products from small lobar hemorrhages related to CAA in ICH[17,28,142] and may, in the future, determine treatment in regard to a hemorrhagic stroke that initially appears to be ischemic in origin.[17,28,142] Fluid-attenuated inversion recovery (FLAIR) MRI may provide information beyond T2 gradient spine-echo images in regard to infarction.[176] Additionally, FLAIR MRI may detect an acute subarachnoid hemorrhage.[28]

Both CT angiography (CTA) and MR angiography (MRA) provide useful information regarding the cerebral vasculature. Carotid ultrasound and duplex also identify atherosclerotic lesions at the bifurcation of the carotid arteries. However, the four-vessel angiogram or digital subtraction angiography is still considered the gold standard for large-vessel and intracranial vascular anomalies, stenosis, and vasospasm.[4,19,28,125] Complications of diagnostic angiography include stroke, renal failure, arterial occlusion, arteriovenous fistula, hematoma, hemorrhage, and allergic response to the contrast media.[4] A nuclear medicine study that utilizes

TABLE 13.19 Radiographic Tests for Stroke

Radiographic Study	Indication	Advantages	Disadvantages
Cerebral angiography	Demonstrates structure of cerebral vasculature, vascular anomalies, and vasospasm	Detailed Direct arterial access allows endovascular therapy including stenting, embolization, and intra-arterial injection of rtPA and papaverine Gold standard for outline of cerebral vasculature and vasospasm	Requires arterial puncture, risk of dissection of arteries, plaque rupture with embolization, retroperitoneal hemorrhage Contrast material that is potentially nephrotoxic if injected
CT without contrast	Differentiates ischemic vs. hemorrhagic stroke Demonstrates infarction (less acutely), edema, herniation	Rapid Portable scanners are available Does not require injection of contrast material	Less informative regarding infratentorial structures
CT angiography	Demonstrates structure of cerebral vessels	Does not require arterial puncture	Requires peripheral IV access Contrast material that is potentially nephrotoxic is injected
Perfusion CT	Demonstrates qualitative and quantitative maps of CBF, cerebral blood volume, and mean transit time	Allows rapid evaluation of stroke; distinguishes infarcted tissue from ischemic penumbra	Contrast material that is potentially nephrotoxic is injected
MRI	Identifies infarct and hemorrhage, especially in posterior fossa and deep cerebral structures		Longer duration than CT Ferromagnetic metals are not allowed in room (requires special precautions or equipment for monitoring and care during MRA/MRI) No ionizing radiation used but patient has to be screened for MRI Compatible/incompatible metals or devices in body Patient may experience claustrophobia
MRA	Demonstrates structure of cerebral vessels	Does not use x-ray Greater detail in regard to infratentorial area	Longer duration than CT Ferromagnetic metals are not allowed in room (requires special precautions or equipment for monitoring and care during MRA/MRI) Patient has to be screened for MRI Compatible/incompatible metals or devices in body
Magnetic resonance imaging			
• Perfusion-weighted imaging (PWI)	Identifies area of ischemic tissue (area that is still potentially salvageable)	If area of decreased perfusion (PWI) is significantly larger than area of decreased diffusion (DWI), a PWI-DWI mismatch, patient may be less likely to hemorrhage with rt-PA administration and possibly eligible for rt-PA beyond 3-hour limit	Same as MRI Best method to determine volume of salvageable tissue has not been determined
• Diffusion-weighted imaging (DWI)	Identifies area of infarcted tissue (core of stroke)		
Fluid-attenuated inversion recovery (FLAIR) MRI	May detect even more detail regarding infarction than T2 gradient spin-echo sequences		Same as MRI
T2 gradient spin-echo sequences MRI	Detects small lobar ICH related to cerebral amyloid angiography		Same as MRI
SPECT	Provides qualitative information regarding early ischemia (as in early vasospasm)	Noninvasive; radioisotope is injected through an intravenous catheter Nurse may stay in room during scan	Provides qualitative information; scan must be performed within a few hours of injection

CBF, Cerebral blood flow; *CT,* computed tomography; *FDA,* Food and Drug Administration; *ICH,* intracerebral hemorrhage; *IV,* intravenous; *MRA,* magnetic resonance angiography; *MRI,* magnetic resonance imaging; *rtPA,* recombinant tissue plasminogen activator; *SPECT,* single photon emission computed tomography.
From References 55, 135, 142, 225, and 266.

an intravenously injected radioisotope, the SPECT scan, provides qualitative information regarding ischemia and is sometimes used to demonstrate early ischemia related to vasospasm[162,244] (Fig. 13.13).

The value of transcranial Doppler (TCD) in cerebral ischemia related to sickle cell anemia and aneurysmal SAH vasospasm is substantial.[208,274] TCD is also used in emboli detection in carotid dissection, endarterectomy, stenting, and PFO.[28,165,243] Although angiography remains the gold standard for assessing vasospasm, TCD has the advantage of being performed at the bedside, being noninvasive, and not requiring injection of potentially nephrotoxic contrast materials[148] (Figs. 13.14 and 13.15). TCD does not directly measure cerebral blood flow; rather, it measures cerebral blood flow velocity (in centimeters per second). Mean

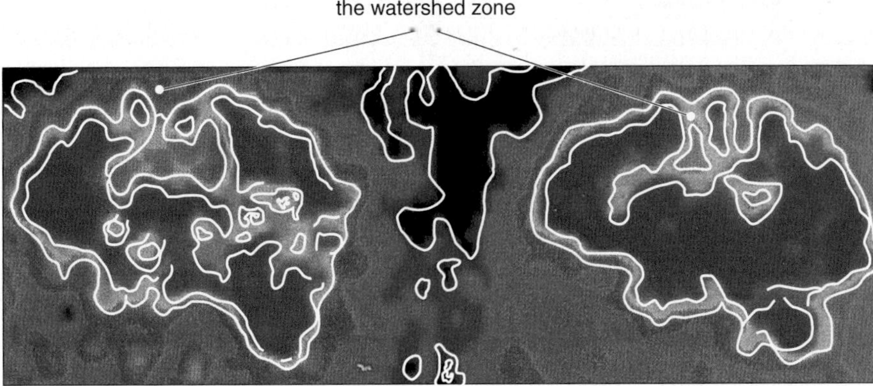

FIG. 13.13 Single photon emission computed tomographic (SPECT) cerebral blood flow scan in a patient with carotid occlusion and frequent spells of hemiparesis but no evidence of infarction on CT or MRI scan.

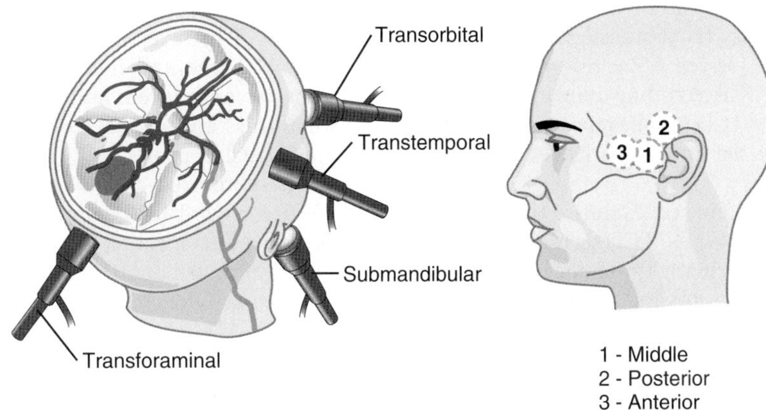

FIG. 13.14 Transcranial Doppler views. The temporal view has three aspects.

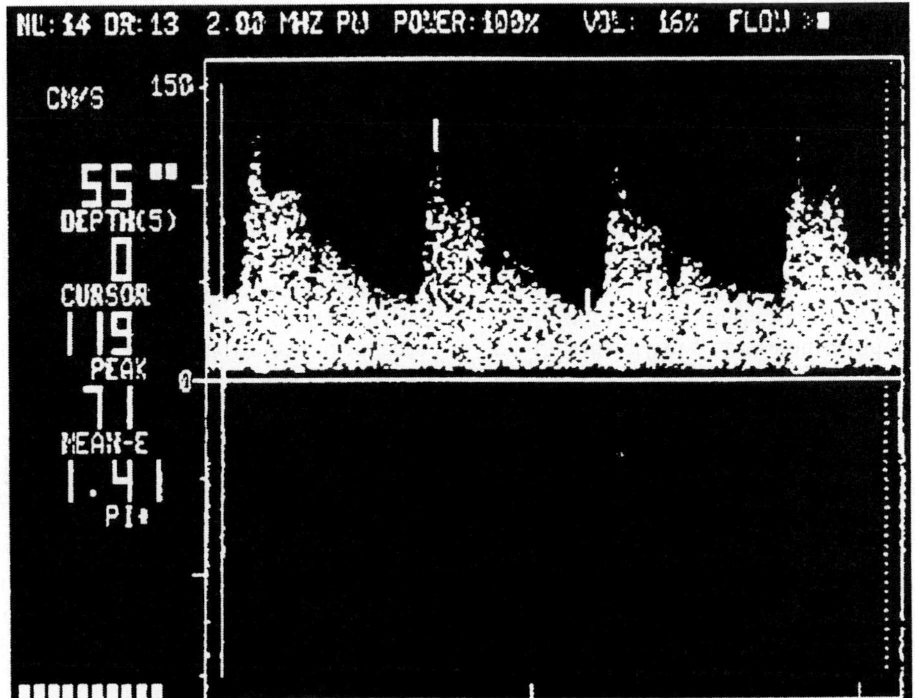

FIG. 13.15 Normal transcranial Doppler waveform. Note the similarity to an arterial pressure waveform. (From Layon, A., Gabrielli, A., & Friedman, W. (2004). *Textbook of neurointensive care.* Philadelphia: Saunders.)

TABLE 13.20 Normal Depth, Direction, and Mean Flow Velocities in the Arteries of the Circle of Willis

Artery	Depth (mm)	Direction	Children	Adults
M1 MCA	45–65	Toward	<170 cm/sec	32–82 cm/sec
A1 ACA	62–75	Away	<150 cm/sec	18–82 cm/sec
ICA siphon	60–64	Bidirectional	<130 cm/sec	20–77 cm/sec
OA	50–62	Toward	Variable	Variable
PCA	60–68	Bidirectional	<100 cm/sec	16–58 cm/sec
BA	80–100+	Away	<100 cm/sec	12–66 cm/sec
VA	45–80	Away	<80 cm/sec	12–66 cm/sec

From Reference 281.

flow velocities (MFVs) are used in the interpretation of TCD (Table 13.20). Upright waveforms indicate the flow of blood toward the probe (e.g., MCA), and inverted waveforms reveal flow away from the probe (e.g., ACA).[148,208] Other cerebrovascular parameters, such as pulsatility index, which is a measure of cerebrovascular resistance, may be obtained. Emboli can be heard and visualized on the TCD screen. Some research has been done in the area of noninvasive ICP recording utilizing TCD, but is inconclusive at this time.[148,208] TCD may be repeated daily, and serial recordings, especially by the same experienced sonographer, are advantageous.

Limitations of TCD include limited expertise and inadequate bone windows to insonate vessels. TCD technology relies on areas of the cranium with sufficiently thin bone or naturally occurring foramina to allow transmission of the ultrasound beam.[82] The following are naturally occurring cranial windows: transtemporal for insonation of the MCA, ACA, PCA, anterior communicating artery, and posterior communicating artery; transforaminal (suboccipital) for insonation of the vertebral artery and basilar artery; transorbital for insonation of the ophthalmic artery and internal carotid artery (ICA) siphon; and retromandibular (submandibular) to insonate the ICA before it enters the skull.[208] Surgical burr holes or craniotomy flaps may serve as additional intracranial windows. Surgical staples, burr hole covers, extracranial and intracranial edema, displacement of vessels from mass effect, patient movement, and naturally occurring hyperostosis of the cranium may complicate transmission of the ultrasound signal.[82]

In the pregnant patient, a brain CT may be safely performed with shielding of the abdomen.[76] A brain MRI, which does not use ionizing radiation, is safe and may be obtained as well.[54] Avoidance of CT and MRI contrast agents is preferable; however, if cerebral angiography is necessary, it may be performed with abdominal shielding.[76] TCD may safely be performed, as it is an application of the same ultrasound technology used in monitoring the fetus.

MANAGEMENT

Initial Management

Before admission to critical care, a number of interventions for patients with stroke may have occurred. These may have happened before arrival at the hospital, in the emergency department, or elsewhere in the hospital if they are already inpatients. Airway, breathing, and circulation are always of higher priority than the neurologic insult because failure to promptly recognize and emergently and aggressively treat respiratory and cardiac instability may worsen the cerebral ischemia or infarct.[13,142] The goal for oxygen saturation is greater than 94%; therefore, some stroke patients will require intubation and mechanical ventilation, particularly if they have a decreased level of consciousness, are unable to maintain their airway, or have aspirated. Others may only need supplemental oxygen with a nasal cannula or face mask.[142] Intravenous access is essential for administration of normal saline and medications as needed. ECG rate and rhythm are monitored, and hemodynamically compromising dysrhythmias are treated according to Advanced Cardiac Life Support (ACLS) protocols.

BP is monitored and is only treated initially if it exceeds 185/110 mm Hg. The BP parameter will need to be lowered if the stroke type is determined to be acute ischemic and (1) rtPA eligible, (2) intra-arterial thrombolysis eligible, or (3) mechanical thrombectomy eligible with a goal of BP less than 180/105 mm Hg during IV rtPA infusion, thrombolysis, or thrombectomy and maintained during at least the first 24 hours.[123,124,142,234] The BP may be liberalized initially if the patient is not IV rtPA or neurointerventional eligible up to 220/120 mm Hg.[123,124,142,147,234]

If the stroke type is determined to be hemorrhagic, the upper BP limits are less clear. However, with aneurysmal subarachnoid hemorrhage and an initially unsecured aneurysm, an upper limit systolic of 160 mm Hg is recommended.[55] After spontaneous (nontraumatic) intracerebral/intraparenchymal hemorrhage, a decrease in the systolic blood pressure to 140 mm Hg is recommended.[135] As soon as the patient's cardiopulmonary status is stabilized and new neurologic deficits are recognized, a systematic approach, including a brief history, physical examination, laboratory tests, and radiographic workup, must be conducted. Each of the following must be determined: (1) when did stroke signs and symptoms begin; (2) has the patient had a stroke in the past; (3) is the patient having a stroke now; (4) if so, is the stroke ischemic or hemorrhagic; and (5) if the stroke is ischemic, does the patient meet inclusion criteria to receive rtPA? The sudden onset of numbness or weakness in an extremity or face; difficulty with speech or dysarthria; visual disturbance in one or both eyes; severe headache; and clumsiness or loss of balance are among the most common assessment findings suggestive of a stroke.[78,142] However, stroke mimics conditions such as hypoglycemia and alcohol/drug ingestion, which must also be ruled out[285] (Table 13.21). An emergency department or inpatient unit should activate a stroke code or a rapid response team when the possibility of a stroke is recognized. The stroke code team members are an interprofessional group of first responders dedicated to assessing and managing stroke during the first few hours after onset and have demonstrated improved outcomes when utilized.[40,254] Although certain signs and symptoms, such as complaints of "the worst headache of my life," seizures, nausea and vomiting,

TABLE 13.21 Stroke Mimics

Condition	Distinguishing Features
Seizure	History of loss of consciousness, seizure activity, postictal state, or history of epilepsy usually present
Somatoform or conversion disorder	Fluctuations in clinical picture, nonanatomic symptoms or signs or history of mental illness Among the most common stroke mimics in patients treated with thrombolysis Reported prevalence of 0.4% to 11.7% Younger age and history of psychiatric disease increases the risk May coexist with stroke One third of patients older than 50 years with features of conversion had a coexisting stroke compared with no patients younger than 50 years with that presentation
Migraine headache	History of similar events, preceding aura and headache Common mimic in persons younger than 50 years
Toxic-metabolic disturbances	Hypoglycemia and drug or alcohol intoxication Nonfocal neurologic examination and laboratory results distinguish from stroke
Systemic infection	Chest is the most common source Acute illness exacerbating a previous deficit
Syncope/presyncope or hypotension	Hypotension is unusual in acute stroke; prevalence of blood pressure < 120/80 mm Hg at initial stroke presentation is 7.1%; symptoms may be transient or respond to hydration
Tumor	Mass noted on neuroimaging
Acute confusional state	May be related to alcohol intoxication, medication adverse effect, or other encephalopathy
Vertigo or dizziness	Prevalence of stroke or transient ischemic attack in adults older than 44 years with isolated dizziness symptoms in emergency setting is 0.7% Stroke prevalence is approximately 25% in patients presenting with acute vestibular syndrome
Dementia	Presence of known cognitive impairment was one of two factors that independently predicted a stroke mimics in an Australian prospective study of patients admitted with suspected stroke
Headache and neurologic deficits with cerebrospinal fluid lymphocytosis (HaNDU) syndrome	Second most common diagnosis in a large case study Requires lumbar puncture for diagnosis and initial presentation may mimic stroke
Encephalitis	Fever, signs of infection
Spinal epidural hematoma	Rare, presenting with quadriparesis, paraparesis or hemiparesis usually in the absence of cranial nerve finding Caused by exercises, trauma, surgery, lumbar puncture, coagulopathy, vascular malformation, or chiropractic spinal manipulation Treatment requires urgent surgical decompression

From References 75, 78, 142, 214, and 285.

and a decreased level of consciousness may strongly suggest hemorrhagic stroke, differentiation of an ischemic stroke from a hemorrhagic stroke can only be confirmed by noncontrast brain CT.[142] An AIS within the first few hours after onset may not be seen on CT scan; however, blood will be evident.[17,285]

Because delays in care may worsen the prognosis and limit treatment options, time targets recommended by the AHA/ASA include a goal of 1 hour after arrival in the emergency department or recognition of an in-hospital stroke to assess, obtain initial labs and CT, determine type of stroke, and initiate treatment. The recommended stroke assessment scale is the NIHSS.[142] The therapeutic window for intravenous rtPA is administration of the medication within 3 to 4.5 hours, since the patient was "last known well."[142] Relative contraindications for administration from 3 to 4.5 hours include age greater than 80 years; NIHSS greater than 25; use of an anticoagulant; and a history of diabetes and previous ischemic stroke.[142] If the patient meets criteria for rtPA administration, administration should begin by the end of the first hour, but only after all invasive devices and lines are inserted and when the BP is within the acceptable range of less than 180/105 mm Hg.[142] Recommended invasive devices and lines include a minimum of two intravenous catheters and a Foley catheter.[105,252] Because of time constraints, rtPA administration typically begins in the emergency department or in the patient's original room if an inpatient and generally concludes in critical care. Invasive devices must be inserted before administration of rtPA. rtPA for acute ischemic stroke is weight-based, 0.09 mg/kg up to 90 mg/kg. The first 10% of medication is given in the first minute and the remainder is given over the next 59 minutes.[142,252] A neurosurgical consult, as appropriate, is to be completed by the second hour. If the stroke is determined to be hemorrhagic, oral or intravenous antihypertensives, as a bolus or as continuous infusions, may be administered before transfer to critical care to prevent additional hemorrhage. In general, the remainder of the neurodiagnostic evaluation and most additional interventions, such as insertion of invasive monitoring devices (for patients not receiving rtPA) will occur after admission to critical care. Transfer to the appropriate level of care, such as critical care, progressive care, or, at minimum, a telemetry floor, is to be completed by the third hour.[9,142]

Many of the interventions for stroke are the same regardless of the stroke subtype. Before a discussion of interventions specific to each subtype, AIS, SAH, and ICH, interventions common to all stroke subtypes are discussed.

Neurologic Interventions

Following stroke, the patient is at risk for secondary neuronal injury related to a number of mechanisms. Cerebral edema occurs with all strokes, and the patient may experience further neurologic deterioration from edema and increased ICP for 96 hours or more after the stroke. Increased ICP may result in further ischemia, infarction, and herniation.[103,147,252] Detailed serial neurologic assessment, including level of consciousness, orientation and mentation, language and speech, cranial nerves, movement, sensation, and vital signs every 1 to 2 hours, is paramount. Deterioration may be subtle or dramatic but must be detected as soon as possible and evaluated with consideration of additional interventions as appropriate.[69,141,252] Signs and symptoms of increased ICP include a decrease in level of consciousness; headache; nausea and vomiting; change in pupil size, shape, and reactivity; and impaired extraocular movements.[69,141]

Nursing interventions to decrease the ICP and maintain an adequate cerebral pressure include elevation of the head of the bed at 30 degrees or as needed to maintain an ICP less than 20 mm Hg and an acceptable cerebral perfusion pressure (CPP).[69,141] Specific recommendations for CPP in stroke have not been established; a goal of 60 to 70 mm Hg is used based on evidence from traumatic brain injury guidelines.[34] If a critical carotid or vertebral stenosis is compromising cerebral perfusion, a head of bed position of 0 degrees may be indicated in rare cases.[142,194] Vasopressors or antihypertensive agents may be needed based on the type of stroke to achieve a target BP that is adequate enough to maintain the goal CPP without increasing the risk of additional ischemia, hemorrhagic transformation, rebleed, or hyperemia.[120,147] More specific BP-related interventions are addressed later in this chapter with regard to each stroke subtype. In general, no attempt should be made to normalize the BP, particularly in a patient with a known history of hypertension. Attempts to scientifically determine the optimal BP for a particular stroke patient or perhaps a subgroup of stroke patients utilizing autoregulatory testing and multimodality monitoring have been conducted.[69,144,232]

Other position-related measures to decrease ICP include maintaining the trunk and neck in alignment to minimize intrathoracic and intra-abdominal pressure and promote jugular venous return. Spacing the timing of nursing activities such as turning, hygiene, and venipunctures may also reduce sustained increases in ICP. Small doses of analgesics such as morphine or fentanyl (Sublimaze) for headache or other discomfort may decrease ICP and assist with BP management in the hypertensive patient. Nausea and vomiting, which may occur as a result of intracranial hemorrhage or increased ICP, also aggravates ICP.[141] Nonphenothiazines such as ondansetron (Zofran) are recommended for nausea and vomiting; agents such as promethazine (Phenergan) and prochlorperazine (Compazine) are not recommended as they lower the seizure threshold and may produce extrapyramidal symptoms with repeated dosing.[163,247] Routine administration of stool softeners assists with comfort and prevents increased ICP and bleeding or rebleeding associated with the Valsalva maneuver and straining with bowel evacuation.[141]

Hyperthermia increases the cerebral metabolic rate (CMR), which consists of the brain's oxygen and energy requirements. Brain temperature is normally 1°C (1.8°F) greater than core temperature and may be even higher when systemic hyperthermia is present. Increased CMR is associated with increased CBF, which increases ICP.[142,186] At the cellular level, fever has been shown to contribute to the ischemic cascade by depleting ATP stores, promoting the release of glutamate, contributing to the synthesis of oxygen free radicals, and facilitating breakdown of the blood-brain barrier. Every attempt should be made to attain and maintain normothermia in the care of the acute stroke patient.[69,161,228] Interventions to achieve normothermia include administering antipyretics, obtaining and monitoring cultures and sensitivities with administration of appropriate antimicrobials, monitoring serum antimicrobial levels, and implementing additional cooling measures. Reduction of ambient temperature, cool baths, and the use of such technologies as intravascular cooling catheters may also facilitate achieving normothermia.[39,71,161,282] Shivering associated with cooling measures will increase the ICP and the CMR, and negate the benefits of fever reduction.[286] A limited number of studies of various research designs have been conducted regarding the use of therapeutic hypothermia in acute stroke.[171] However, methodologies have differed and Level I evidence for controlled hypothermia in stroke is lacking. Many questions remain regarding the optimal cooling process, target temperature, duration, and risks versus benefits.[150,173]

A number of pharmacologic agents, as detailed in the medication table (Table 13.22) may be administered to decrease ICP in acute stroke, including mannitol (Osmitrol), furosemide (Lasix), hypertonic saline (HTS), barbiturates, propofol (Diprivan), opioids, and benzodiazepines. Repeated dosing of mannitol may result in rebound edema and hypovolemia. Renal failure may occur if the serum osmolality exceeds 320 mOsm/L.[92,215] HTS acts rapidly and may be given after maximum serum osmolality has been reached with mannitol. HTS increases the serum sodium concentration, which results in a rapid movement of fluid out of the edematous tissues and into the intravascular compartment. However, pulmonary edema, congestive heart failure, and rebound edema may occur with its use. The target serum sodium level has not been established, although some clinicians have used a goal of 145 to 155 mg/dL. Concentrations of 2%, 3%, 7.5%, and 23.4% HTS have been used;[92] however, the optimal concentration has not been determined, and conclusive evidence regarding its efficacy is lacking.[92]

Sedation of the patient with increased ICP is frequently managed with propofol or barbiturates. Propofol and barbiturates decrease the CMR.[69] Both propofol and barbiturates require intubation and mechanical ventilation and often a vasopressor to maintain adequate cerebral perfusion pressure. The short half-life of propofol makes serial neurologic assessment possible. Barbiturates are generally reserved for refractory increased ICP because they depress the myocardium, induce hypotension, and impede neurologic assessment. Barbiturate coma is associated with an increased risk of pneumonia, sepsis, and hepatic failure.[144] Continuous electroencephalogram monitoring is required to titrate the barbiturate to burst suppression.[98,175] Barbiturates may also lower body temperature.[98,175]

In addition to ICP and CPP monitoring, cerebral oxygenation monitoring may guide therapy. A jugular venous oxygen saturation ($Sjvo_2$) bulb catheter measures global oxygenation. Acceptable values for $Sjvo_2$ are 55 to 75 mg/dL. A brain tissue oxygenation catheter ($Pbto_2$) measures regional brain oxygenation. Acceptable values vary by manufacturer; goal parameters specific to the Licox brain tissue oxygen catheter are 20 to 25 mm Hg.[102,132,218] The $Sjvo_2$ catheter and the $Pbto_2$ catheter may be used together. The $Sjvo_2$ catheter may allow judicious use of hyperventilation in increased ICP refractory to other measures, and placement of the $Pbto_2$ catheter in the ischemic penumbra may facilitate prompt recognition and aggressive treatment of salvageable tissue adjacent to infarction or vasospasm.[132]

In supratentorial ischemic or hemorrhagic stroke with massive edema, surgical decompression with removal of cranial bone and infarcted tissue may be life-saving (Fig. 13.16). The AHA/ASA has endorsed decompressive craniectomy for malignant edema of the cerebral hemisphere.[142,278] However, the procedure is controversial and not without adverse effects;

TABLE 13.22 **Medications Used to Treat Cerebrovascular Disorders**

Medication	Action	Dosage	Special Considerations
Anticonvulsants			
Phenytoin (Dilantin)	Stabilizes neuronal membranes in motor cortex	Loading dose: 15–18 mg/kg IV; maintenance dose: 300–400 mg IV/PO/NG daily Status epilepticus loading dose: 15-20 mg/kg; not to exceed a total dose of 1.5 grams Administer no faster than 50 mg/min IV Use an in-line filter when administering as infusion; avoid using with dextrose-containing diluents/IV solutions (will precipitate)	Prophylactic use of anticonvulsants in stroke is controversial; recommended in hemorrhagic stroke Monitor total and free levels: total therapeutic range, 10–20 mcg/mL; free therapeutic range, 0.1–0.2 mcg/mL Avoid peripheral IV injection (irritating to vein and surrounding tissues with extravasation) or use fosphenytoin (a phenytoin prodrug) Because phenytoin is highly protein bound, it interacts with many other medications. Monitor serum levels closely when initiating other medications.
Fosphenytoin (Cerebyx)	Stabilizes neuronal membranes in motor cortex	Loading dose: 10–20 mg phenytoin equivalents (PE)/kg IV; IV Maintenance dose: 4-6 mg PE/kg/24 h in divided doses Status epilepticus loading dose: 15-20 mg PE/kg IV	Prophylactic use of anticonvulsants in stroke is controversial; recommended in hemorrhagic stroke Monitor total and free levels: total therapeutic range, 10–20 mcg/mL; free therapeutic range, 0.1–0.2 mcg/mL Fosphenytoin is less irritating to tissues than phenytoin when given by peripheral IV injection May cause less hypotension and bradycardia than phenytoin
Levetiracetam (Keppra)	May inhibit neuronal impulses by limiting sodium influx across the motor cortex cell membrane; used in the management of generalized tonic-clonic and partial seizures	PO/IV 500 mg BID; may be titrated up to 3000 mg daily in divided doses	Dizziness, somnolence, psychosis, nonpsychotic behavioral symptoms, headache, ataxia
Anticoagulants			
Enoxaparin (Lovenox)	Low molecular weight heparin for DVT prophylaxis	40 mg subcutaneous daily	Monitor platelets, renal function, and observe for signs and symptoms of bleeding
Heparin	Blocks conversion of prothrombin to thrombin and fibrinogen to fibrin; prevents formation of new clots DVT prophylaxis Prevention of cardioembolic stroke related to prosthetic heart valves, atrial fibrillation Prevention of artery to artery emboli, e.g., carotid or vertebral dissections Management of DVT and pulmonary emboli	5000 units subcutaneously BID to TID for DVT prophylaxis	Monitor aPTT and observe for signs and symptoms of hemorrhage; monitor platelet count for HIT Antidote for prolonged aPTT: protamine sulfate Heparin is of no proven benefit in management of atherothrombotic TIAs
Warfarin (Coumadin)	Interferes with synthesis of vitamin K–dependent clotting factors Prevents formation of new clots Prevention of cardioembolic stroke associated with prosthetic heart valves and atrial fibrillation Prevention of artery-to-artery emboli, e.g., carotid or vertebral dissections Management of DVT/pulmonary emboli	Atrial fibrillation 5–15 mg PO daily initially; then 2–10 mg daily with adjustments according to PT/INR	Monitor PT/INR and observe for signs and symptoms of hemorrhage Repeated and intense patient/family education regarding compliance, PT/INR monitoring, precautions, and food-drug interactions Antidote is vitamin K
Dabigatran (Pradaxa)	Direct thrombin inhibitor (DTI) Used in the management of nonvalvular atrial fibrillation to reduce the risk of stroke and systemic embolism	150 mg PO BID; 75 mg orally BID in renal impairment (creatinine clearance 15–30 mL/min)	Peaks in 1-2 h delayed when taken with food Renal excretion Increases aPTT, thrombin time (TT), and ecarin clotting time (ECT). Recently, a dabigatran-specific reversal agent, idarucizumab (Praxbind), has received FDA approval and is available for use Half life 12–17 h
Rivaroxaban (Xarelto)	Direct factor Xa inhibitor Used in the management of nonvalvular atrial fibrillation to reduce the risk of stroke and systemic embolism	20 mg PO daily; 15 mg PO daily in renal impairment (creatinine clearance 15–30 mL/min)	Peaks in 2–4 h No specific antidote Lack of validated reversal strategy Anticoagulation effect best evaluated with substance-specific-anti-factor Xa activity (PT, aPTT). Follow dose with food or enteral tube feeding (to minimize gastric irritation) Half life 5–9 h

Continued

TABLE 13.22 Medications Used to Treat Cerebrovascular Disorders—cont'd

Medication	Action	Dosage	Special Considerations
Apixaban (Eliquis)	Direct factor Xa inhibitor Used in the management of nonvalvular atrial fibrillation to reduce the risk of stroke and systemic embolism	5 mg PO twice a day; 2.5 mg PO twice a daily with 2 or more of the following: renal impairment (serum creatinine > 1.5 mg/dL; > 80; weight < 60 kg	Peaks in 1–3 h No specific antidote Lack of validated reversal strategy Anticoagulation effect best evaluated with substance-specific-anti-factor Xa activity (PT, aPTT) Half-life approximately 12 h
Antihypertensives			
Hydralazine (Apresoline)	Directly dilates arterioles	10-20 mg IV bolus every 4–6 h as needed. Maximum dose is 300 mg/day	May produce lupuslike syndrome
Labetalol (Trandate)	Blocks alpha$_1$-, beta$_1$-, and beta$_2$-adrenergic receptor sites	20-mg IV bolus given over 2 min Can repeat with boluses of 40–80 mg at 10-min intervals as needed up to 300 mg Alternatively, can give IV infusion of 1 mg/mL labetalol at rate of 2 mg/min; max dose is 300 mg	Contraindicated in asthma, AV heart block, and bradycardia Effects should be observed within 5 min of IV dose
Nicardipine (Cardene)	Calcium channel blocker, depresses cardiac and vascular smooth muscle	Continuous infusion: 25 mg/250 mL or 50 mg/250 mL (central venous catheter concentration); infuse at 5–15 mg/h	Abrupt discontinuation may result in chest pain, particularly in patients with angina
Antiplatelets			
Acetylsalicylic acid (aspirin)	Inhibits platelet aggregation and prostaglandin synthesis For primary and secondary ischemic stroke prevention	80–325 mg PO daily	May cause gastric irritation
Dipyridamole (Persantine)	Inhibits platelet aggregation and prostaglandin synthesis For primary and secondary ischemic stroke prevention	75–400 mg PO daily	May prolong bleeding time; observe for bleeding Monitor platelet count for thrombocytopenia Not typically used as solo therapy
Aspirin/ dipyridamole (Aggrenox)	Aspirin: see above Dipyridamole: inhibits platelet aggregation by inhibiting activity of adenosine deaminase and phosphodiesterase, enzymes that cause adenosine and cyclic AMP accumulation	Each capsule consists of 200 mg dipyridamole and 25 mg aspirin Dose is typically one capsule twice daily	GI distress: heartburn, nausea Alters platelet for life of platelet (approximately 10 days) Patients should avoid aspirin or other products containing aspirin while on Aggrenox therapy
Clopidogrel (Plavix)	Inhibits platelet aggregation by inhibiting binding of ADP to its platelet receptor and ADP-mediated activation of a glycoprotein complex	75 mg PO daily	GI distress: heartburn, nausea Increased risk of gastrointestinal hemorrhage when administered with aspirin
Ticlopidine (Ticlid)	Inhibits platelet aggregation by inhibiting ADP-induced platelet-fibrinogen binding	250 mg PO BID	GI distress: heartburn, nausea Monitor closely during the first 3 months of therapy due to risk of life-threatening neutropenia/agranulocytosis, thrombotic thrombocytopenic purpura, and aplastic anemia
Fludrocortisone (Florinef)	Mineralocorticoid that works at distal renal tubules to increase sodium reabsorption and water retention	0.2 mg PO/NG daily	May aggravate HF Monitor sodium and potassium carefully
Mannitol (Osmitrol)	Osmotic diuretic; pulls cerebral edema into intravascular space Use for increased intracranial pressure	0.25–1 g/kg IV Use inline filter of less than 5 microns if given as infusion (rather than bolus); extract from vial with filtered needle if giving IV bolus	Renal failure; monitor serum osmolality; risk increases with serum osmolality greater than 320 mmol/L Hypotension Hypokalemia Monitor electrolytes
Nimodipine (Nimotop)	Cerebroselective calcium channel blocker; protects neurons during vasospasm	60 mg NG/PO every 4 h; use 18-gauge needle to withdraw solution from the capsule. After adding medication to NG tube, flush with 30 mL NS. Adjust dose to 30 mg NG/PO every 2 h if hypotension occurs	Observe for hypotension; avoid sublingual dosing to minimize large decreases in BP

TABLE 13.22 **Medications Used to Treat Cerebrovascular Disorders—cont'd**

Medication	Action	Dosage	Special Considerations
Recombinant tissue plasminogen activator (Alteplase)	Thrombolytic: enzyme binds to fibrin in clot, converting plasminogen to plasmin, initiating fibrinolysis	Bolus: 10% of 0.9 mg/kg dose over 1 min followed by 90% of 0.9 mg/kg dose over 59 min Recommended within 3–4.5 h from onset of symptoms (time last seen well)	Obtain head CT before administration Obtain baseline labs, CBC, coagulation studies, including fibrinogen, and type and screen before administration Monitor for signs and symptoms of hemorrhage; hemorrhagic transformation of AIS Do not administer heparin, warfarin, or aspirin for at least 24 h after infusion Avoid venipunctures, arterial punctures, and insertion of invasive devices after administration Risk of orolingual angioedema, particularly for patients receiving angiotensin-converting-enzyme inhibitor (ACE inhibitors) prior to Alteplase
Sodium chloride tablets	Use in the management of hyponatremia related to SIADH or CSW	May be crushed for feeding tube administration; use normal saline flush	Oral intake may cause nausea and vomiting Goal serum sodium level is 145–155 mEq/L Monitor serum sodium every 4-6 h
Saline: isotonic (0.9%) and hypertonic (HTS) (2%, 3%, 5%, 7.5%, and 10%) continuous infusions and 23.4% (bolus) for refractory increased intracranial pressure	Pulls cerebral fluid into intravascular space for renal elimination Used for refractory increased intracranial pressure IV bolus amounts vary from 10 to 30 mL 0.9% to 3% used for hyponatremia in CSW or SIADH	Use central venous catheter for 3% or greater concentration	Hypernatremia; transient intravascular fluid overload Calculate sodium deficit to guide dosing Goal serum sodium level is 145–155 mEq/L. Monitor serum sodium every 4-6 h Caution if serum sodium level exceeds 160 mEq/L HTS is irritating to veins and tissues; administer concentrations greater than 2% HTS through central venous catheter Risk of demyelination of the pons with rapid increase of serum sodium, more than 8-12 mEq/L within 24 h

From References 3, 101, 105, 160, 163, 200, 230, 231, and 268.

the optimal time for surgery is unknown, and improvement of outcome in stroke patients has been unsubstantiated. In contrast, emergent surgical decompression in cerebellar stroke may result in good outcomes.[39,65,278]

Pulmonary Interventions

Following stroke, the patient may have a number of pulmonary complications that can contribute to additional neurologic deterioration. These must be managed aggressively because systemic hypoxia worsens cerebral ischemia. Acute stroke patients are at high risk for aspiration, which may result in pneumonia, respiratory distress, or respiratory failure.[161]

Head of bed elevation of 30 to 45 degrees or more is preferred to minimize risk of aspiration.[191,222] Stroke patients who exhibit any signs or symptoms of dysphagia must not receive anything by mouth (NPO) until they are evaluated and deemed safe for oral intake with or without restrictions[142,154] (Box 13.2). Up to 78% of all stroke patients initially present with dysphagia, which will subside over time.[8] An institution-approved, nurse-initiated swallow screen may be performed initially to detect dysphagia. A swallow screen may consist of a brief history and physical assessment, followed by a water test if the patient passes the initial assessment. If the patient fails the nurse-initiated swallow screen, the patient should remain NPO until seen by a speech pathologist for a comprehensive evaluation. Indicators of dysphagia and aspiration risk include choking, absent or weak cough or gag reflex, wet voice, delay in swallow, pocketing of food in buccal mucosa, and inability to retain secretions, oral liquids, or food in the mouth.[141,252] A speech pathologist should be consulted for a formal swallow evaluation or a feeding tube may be indicated. In addition to a bedside evaluation, the speech pathologist may conduct a fiberoptic endoscopic evaluation of swallowing (FEES).[24] Patients should only be given oral intake with the head of the bed upright in a normal sitting position. Drinking straws may increase the risk of aspiration and should be avoided unless approved by the speech pathologist. The speech pathologist may recommend thickened liquids on a case-by-case basis. Momentary decreases in the Spo_2 may indicate micro-aspiration when the patient is swallowing.

Unilateral hemispheric AIS patients rarely require intubation unless they experience a decreased level of consciousness related to cerebral edema. However, brain stem or bilateral hemispheric strokes with cranial nerve dysfunction may require intubation to protect the airway.[154,161] Intubation and mechanical ventilation is indicated with any of the following:[69,154]

1. GCS less than or equal to 8
2. Inability to swallow or clear oral secretions
3. Absent cough and gag reflexes
4. Airway obstruction related to loss of tongue and pharyngeal muscle control
5. Respiratory distress or failure as evidenced by apnea, tachypnea, hypercapnia, oxygen desaturation, and use of accessory muscles
6. Partial pressure of arterial oxygen tension (Pao_2) less than 70 mm Hg despite oxygen therapy by nasal cannula or mask
7. Partial pressure of arterial carbon dioxide ($Paco_2$) greater than 60 mm Hg, or severe respiratory acidosis

In some cases, bronchoscopy may be needed to remove secretions. Other measures to minimize an increase in ICP and

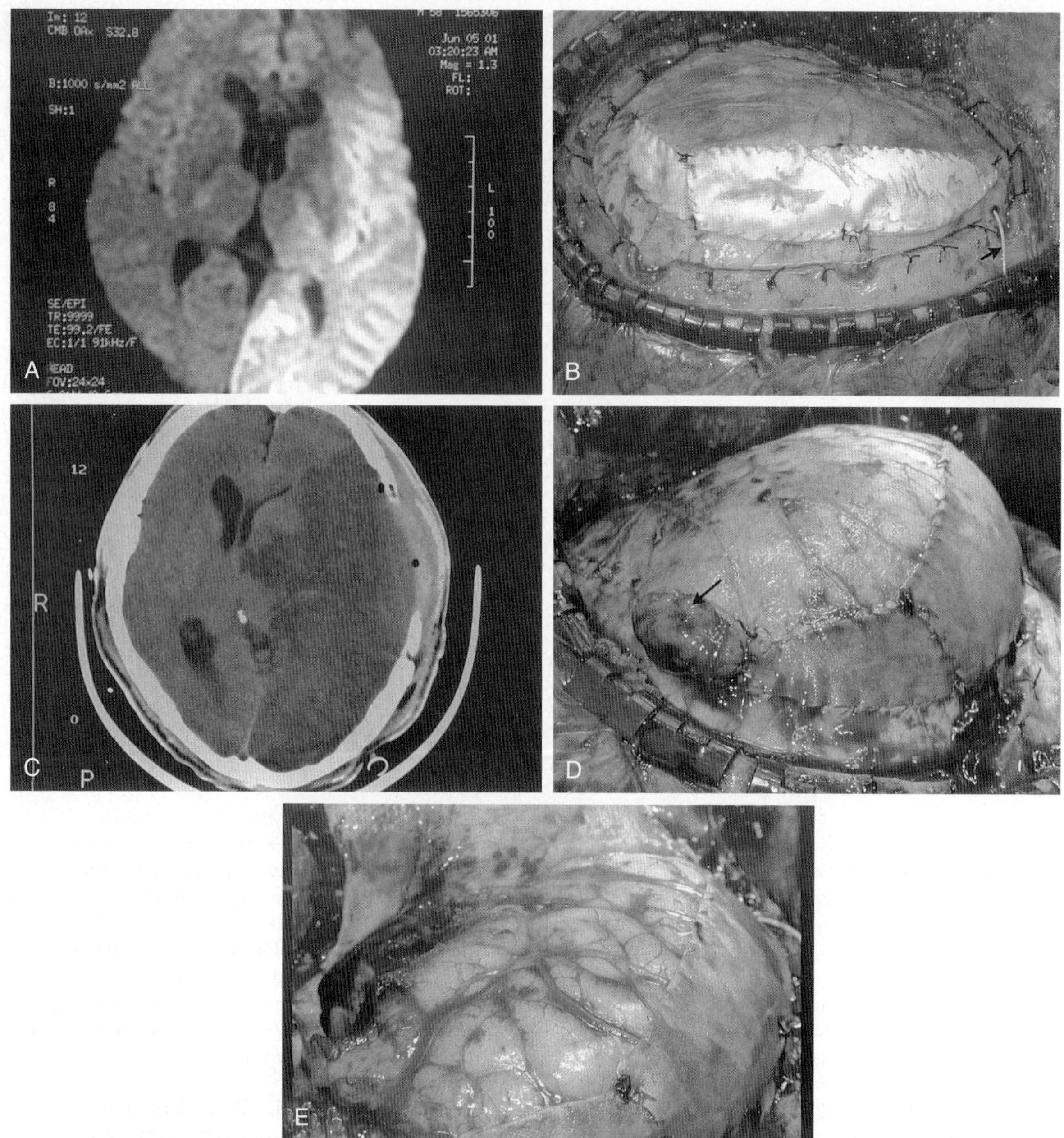

FIG. 13.16 Radiographic changes in a patient with a sudden loss of consciousness and right hemiplegia. **A,** Magnetic resonance imaging (MRI) 4 hours after onset showing large hypersensitivity area at middle and posterior cerebral arteries. **B,** Decompressive craniotomy with duraplasty performed. **C,** Computed tomography (CT) scan shows larger and extended low density with midline shift of the brain at 36 hours. **D,** With return to surgery, brain herniated from the weak point of duraplasty. **E,** Brain edema subsided after enlargement of the craniotomy, opening of the dura, and an anterior temporal lobectomy was performed. (From Cho, D. Y., Chen, T. C., & Lee, H. C. (2003). Ultra-early decompressive craniectomy for malignant middle cerebral artery infarction. *Surg Neurol 60*, 227–233.)

cerebral ischemia include preoxygenation with 100% oxygen before suctioning and limiting suctioning to less than 15 seconds.

For other patients, supplemental oxygen by nasal cannula or facemask may be the only oxygen therapy needed. Patients with sleep-disordered breathing may benefit from continuous positive airway pressure (CPAP) or bi-level positive airway pressure (BiPAP).[154,161] The goal is to maintain arterial oxygen saturation (Sao_2) greater than 94%.[142,161] Serial chest x-rays indicate worsening of the pulmonary status. Aggressive treatment of infection based on the culture and sensitivity is imperative. Pneumonia is the most common infection after stroke, accounting for 15% to 25% of all stroke deaths.[154] For patients who can participate, deep-breathing exercises and use of an incentive spirometer may be effective in minimizing atelectasis. If ICP, CPP, and other intracranial parameters permit, chest physiotherapy may facilitate pulmonary hygiene.[154]

BOX 13.2 Signs and Symptoms of Dysphagia During and Between Meals

- Drooling, excessive secretions
- Excessive tongue movement, tongue thrusting, or spitting food out of the mouth
- Poor tongue control
- Facial weakness
- Pocketing of food in cheek, under tongue, or on hard palate
- Slurred speech
- Coughing or choking while eating*
- Regurgitation through nose, mouth, or tracheostomy tube
- Wet "gurgly" voice after eating or drinking, or frequent throat clearing
- Hoarse or breathy voice
- Complaints of food getting stuck in the throat
- Delay or absence of laryngeal (Adam's apple or thyroid cartilage) elevation
- Recurrent pneumonia (because of aspiration)
- Prolonged chewing or eating time
- Reluctance to consume particular food consistencies or to eat at all

*Caution: Aspiration commonly occurs without coughing. The presence or absence of the gag reflex does not indicate whether the swallowing reflex is intact.
From References 142 and 154.

Cardiac Interventions

Critically ill patients with acute stroke are at risk for cardiac complications for several reasons, including preexisting cardiac disease (a risk factor for stroke), acute myocardial infarction, and dysrhythmias related to autonomic nervous system dysfunction.

The most common dysrhythmia in stroke patients is atrial fibrillation.[116] A 12-lead ECG and at least 24 hours of continuous cardiac monitoring is recommended upon admission for all stroke patients to assess for intermittent atrial fibrillation or lethal arrhythmias.[142,154] Chest pain, unexplained hypotension, and hemodynamically unstable dysrhythmias indicate the need for serial cardiac enzymes, CK-MB, and troponin. An echocardiogram may be beneficial to determine ejection fraction and structural abnormalities, such as PFO, valvular defects, or vegetations.[161] Serial doses of low-dose beta blockers such as metoprolol (Lopressor) may be administered in the absence of bradycardia, atrioventricular blocks, and relative hypotension to blunt the deleterious effects of catecholamines on the heart.[154,161] The patient with acute stroke is also at risk for venous thromboembolism (VTE), deep venous thrombosis (DVT), and pulmonary embolism (PE). Ten percent of deaths in stroke patients occur as a result of PE.[142,161] Factors contributing to VTE include immobility, paralysis, atrial fibrillation, and advanced age. Because administration of subcutaneous prophylactic heparin or low-dose heparinoid may be delayed following hemorrhagic stroke or administration of rtPA (for at least 24 hours), early mobilization and mechanical devices such as sequential compression devices should be initiated as soon as possible.[217] Anti-embolism stockings are of unproven value although they are frequently used, sometimes in addition to sequential compression devices.[142,161,217,222] VTE may occur in the upper extremities as well. Central venous catheters may promote upper extremity thrombosis and emboli formation. Venous Doppler studies are indicated for stroke patients with any unilaterally swollen, inflamed, and painful extremity or signs and symptoms of PE, including tachypnea, chest pain, and oxygen desaturation.[142,154] Low molecular weight heparin may be more effective than unfractionated heparin and aspirin may be used for VTE prophylaxis.[161,217]

Many stroke patients have a known history of hypertension before their stroke, which is a well-documented risk factor. A number of intravenous and oral anti-hypertensive agents are used in the management of acute stroke, as indicated in Table 13.22. Hypertension must be controlled but with consideration for cerebral perfusion. Hypotension and rapid fluctuations in BP may result in additional ischemia and infarction.[69,154,161]

Gastrointestinal Interventions

The impact of stroke on the gastrointestinal system may increase the risk of aspiration related to nausea and vomiting, gastric hypomotility, impaired swallow, and enteral nutrition. Stroke patients with an abnormal gag, impaired or absent cough, inability to swallow saliva, dysphonia, and cranial nerve palsies are at increased risk of aspiration.[69,222] In addition to elevation of the head of the bed, preventive interventions include the following:[69]

1. Maintain NPO status until a dysphagia evaluation is completed
2. Adhere to dietary restrictions based on swallow evaluation
3. Allow oral intake only when the patient is alert and head is elevated
4. Monitor gastric residuals
5. Administer metoclopramide (Reglan) to facilitate gastric emptying

While bedside swallowing assessments are helpful in dysphagia screening, video fluoroscopy and fiberoptic endoscopy during feeding may provide more definitive information.[24,73] Collaboration with speech therapy for dysphagia assessment and management is prudent. Techniques that facilitate swallowing include tucking the chin, turning the head, and checking for pocketing of food. Maintaining head of bed elevation for 30 minutes to 1 hour after eating, particularly for individuals with gastroesophageal reflux, may minimize aspiration.[195]

Nasogastric tubes for gastric emptying and enteral feeding offer only limited protection against aspiration. If tube feedings are required to attain adequate nutrition, small-bowel feedings may lessen the aspiration risk and enable attainment of caloric and protein requirements more quickly.[189] If long-term enteral feeding is required, percutaneous endoscopic placement of a feeding tube is indicated.[73,142] Failure to provide the stroke patient with adequate nutrition may negatively impact outcome; however, the benefit of supplemental nutrition has not been substantiated. While studies have shown traumatic brain injury patients to be hypermetabolic and hypercatabolic, the exact requirements specific to stroke have not been determined beyond basic energy expenditure requirements with the addition of a stress factor.[69,252] However, at a minimum, monitoring intake and output, weight, caloric intake, serum proteins, fluids and electrolytes, and blood count is recommended.[195,252] Collaboration with a registered dietitian is essential to establish dietary requirements and modifications based on other risk factors such as heart disease, renal disease, and diabetes.

Stroke patients are at risk for stress ulcers and gastrointestinal hemorrhage, particularly if they have received anticoagulation, antiplatelet, or thrombolysis agents or experience repetitive vomiting.[222] Whereas oral intake or enteral feeding may provide some protection against stress ulcers, prophylaxis with histamine blockers or proton pump inhibitors is recommended. It should be noted that proton pump inhibitors might reduce the effectiveness of clopidogrel (Plavix).[222] Constipation is to be avoided; straining during bowel movements may result in increased ICP and intracranial hemorrhage. Most patients benefit from stool softeners during the acute phase of stroke.[222]

Genitourinary Interventions

Initially, many critically ill stroke patients will require an indwelling urinary catheter to minimize the risk of retention and incontinence and to maintain accurate intake and output records. Urinary retention may increase the risk of infection, add to the patient's discomfort, and increase the ICP. Incontinence may increase the risk of skin breakdown and decrease the accuracy of output measurements.[154,192] However, the catheter should be removed as soon as possible to decrease the risk of infection and to reestablish voiding.[154,192]

Placing the patient on the bedpan, bedside toilet, or offering urinal routinely may facilitate voiding. Noninvasive monitoring for urinary retention may be facilitated with a bladder scanner. Signs and symptoms of urinary tract infections warrant investigation and appropriate antimicrobial management based on culture and sensitivity.[154,222]

Endocrine Interventions

Hyperglycemia has been associated with poor outcomes after ischemic and hemorrhagic stroke.[142,154,284] Hyperglycemia is thought to increase acidosis, edema, and glutamate release, which result in greater neuronal injury. Hyperglycemia may also contribute to hemorrhagic transformation.[129] However, the acceptable range of blood glucose level varies from publication to publication. Because hypoglycemia is defined as a blood glucose less than 60 mg/dL, and is also detrimental to neurons, attaining and maintaining a blood glucose level of approximately 140 to 180 mg/dL is reasonable.[142] Because intravenous solutions containing dextrose may aggravate hyperglycemia and cerebral edema, some clinicians advocate minimizing their use.[154] If the glucose level cannot be managed with a sliding scale insulin regimen with or without a basal dose, then an infusion of regular insulin with hourly glucose monitoring may be indicated.[142]

Musculoskeletal Interventions

Following stroke, weak or paralyzed extremities are extremely vulnerable to injury.[195,267] At a minimum, care must be taken to maintain the arm and leg in proper alignment when turning and positioning to avoid musculoskeletal complications. Orthotic devices may assist in maintaining alignment of the extremities as well.[73] Although evidence is lacking regarding the best time to start physical and occupational therapy, the nurse has a role in assessing the patient's tolerance to passive range of motion and performing those exercises once the intracranial dynamics and vital signs have stabilized. Progressive early mobility with attention to neurologic status and vital signs, particularly changes in blood pressure, is currently a focus in both acute and critical care for the stroke patient.[154,252] After an initial period of flaccidity, spasticity is likely, which may be uncomfortable and also increase the risk of permanent deformities. Antispasticity medications may be warranted and enhance benefits received from physical and occupation therapy.[73,195] If shoulder subluxation, footdrop, external hip rotation, or contractures occur, they may severely compromise the patient's rehabilitation potential and affect the patient's quality of life.[267] Approaches to hemiplegic shoulder pain include pharmacologic interventions, neural stimulation, biofeedback, blocks, and complementary and alternative medicine therapies.[267]

Integumentary Interventions

Paralysis, impaired sensation, diabetes, peripheral vascular disease, bed rest, incontinence, and poor nutrition may all contribute to skin breakdown. Maintenance of clean and dry skin and frequent turning with attention to alleviating pressure points is essential. Use of pressure-alleviating beds may assist in maintaining skin integrity. A standardized approach to skin assessment, such as the Braden Scale, may predict the risk of skin breakdown for individual patients.[252]

Rest and Comfort Interventions

Following stroke, pain is multifactorial.[222] Initially following stroke, pain presents primarily as headache. If the patient has had an SAH, the headache is frequently accompanied by a painful and stiff neck and backache from the blood in the CSF irritating the meninges. Photophobia may also be present with subarachnoid blood. Hypertension and increased ICP may also contribute to headache.[55] Central pain, which may be perceived as burning, occurs as a result of a lesion in the ventroposterolateral nucleus of the thalamus.[73] Invasive monitoring and therapeutic devices add to the patient's discomfort. If surgical or endovascular therapy is performed, those procedures cause additional discomfort. Analgesics may make neurologic assessment more difficult; however, their judicious use is appropriate as needed for comfort. Multimodal analgesia may include an antiepileptic agent, nonopioid analgesic, and antidepressant.[73] Failure to alleviate pain and discomfort may cause further deterioration in the patient's status. Deteriorations may include depression, anxiety, difficulty sleeping, drug dependence, and social withdrawal.[220]

Once the patient is stable, uninterrupted sleep of at least 1- to 2-hour intervals is essential and may result in an improved neurologic assessment. Fatigue and impaired sleep are common manifestations after stroke, and a prolonged stay in intensive care with repeated neurologic assessments and interventions further deprive the stroke patient of much needed sleep and rest.[73,195] Sleep disordered breathing may occur as a result of the stroke or may have been present as a risk factor prior to the stroke and continues to lessen the quality of a patient's sleep.[222]

Communication Interventions

Following stroke, up to 38% of all stroke patients have impaired communication.[201] The communication disorder may be a language disorder, aphasia, or a problem with the mechanics of speech, such as dysarthria. The term *aphasia* is used interchangeably with the word *dysphasia*. Aphasia may be one of the following: Wernicke's or fluent, formerly known as receptive; Broca's or nonfluent, formerly known as expressive; or more often mixed, a combination of fluent and nonfluent. Global aphasia, a complete inability to communicate, is indicative of poor to no rehabilitation potential. Anomia is difficulty with word finding. Broca's area, responsible for expressive speech (verbalization), is located in the motor strip of the frontal lobe; Wernicke's area, responsible for receptive speech (understanding the spoken word), is located at the junction of the temporal and parietal lobes[201] (Fig. 13.17). A speech therapy consult may

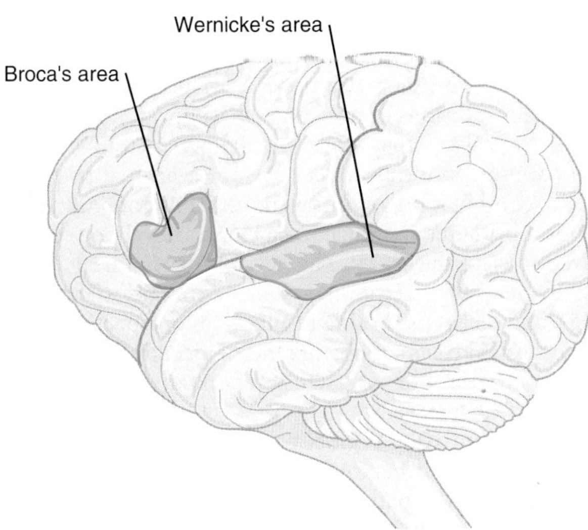

FIG. 13.17 Territories of language areas.

be beneficial before and after extubation to assist with communication in acute stroke patients. Hand-held boards with the alphabet or pictures and visual cueing may facilitate communication and decrease anxiety in the patient with receptive ability.[195]

Perception and Sensory Interventions

Following stroke, patients may have both sensory and perceptual deficits, including visual field cuts and neglect. The field cut most associated with supratentorial strokes is homonymous hemianopsia, in which half of the visual field, contralateral to the side of the brain lesion, is missing. Neglect is also contralateral to the brain lesion. A visual field cut and neglect may exist separately or simultaneously. Immediately after a stroke, communication is most effective if the patient is approached from the side without the deficit or at least from the midline. Later, during recovery, the stroke patient can be taught to compensate for the visual deficit by turning the head from the intact visual field to the missing visual field.[141] Occupation, physical, and speech therapy also work with the patient to teach compensation for visual and perceptual deficits.[61,73,201]

Psychosocial Support

Up to 33% of all stroke survivors have moderate to severe depression.[154,195] The reasons for depression following stroke are psychosocial and physiologic. Most stroke patients have neurologic deficits from which they may never completely recover, and many have difficulty communicating because of cranial nerve deficits, dysphasia/aphasia, intubation, cognition, or sedation. Furthermore, they may not feel well and are sleep-deprived as a result of their stroke and the critical care environment. In addition, some researchers have shown that pathophysiologic changes as a result of left hemispheric infarcts may contribute to poststroke depression.[73] An additional risk factor for depression is a history of depression prior to the stroke.[172]

Tricyclic antidepressants, methylphenidate (Ritalin), or selective serotonin reuptake inhibitors (SSRIs) may be helpful.[73] Depression, in general, has been associated with low serotonin levels, and SSRIs block the reuptake of serotonin. Initiating physical, occupational, and speech therapy as soon as possible may decrease depression as well, particularly if the patient is made aware of his or her progress. Collaboration with the patient's family and a clinical psychologist may provide insight into the patient's thoughts and needs. Poststroke depression is associated with less functional recovery.[172] A number of instruments have been used to screen for poststroke depression, including the 2- and 9-item versions of the Personal Health Questionnaire, PHQ-2 and PHQ-9.[169,190] Both the PHQ-2 and the PHQ-9 have demonstrated validity and reliability as screening tools for poststroke depression in patients who can communicate effectively.[67-69,279] Evidence-based strategies for assessment and management of poststroke depression are needed.[128]

Education

Following stroke, the educational needs are great for both the family and the patient, if the patient is cognitively aware of the diagnosis. Secondary prevention of stroke with focus on the type of stroke and patient's personal risk factors is key. Both family and patient need basic information about stroke pathophysiology, emergency action during stroke, stroke management and rehabilitation, risk factors, and strategies for modification of risk factors.[41] Patient education must be tailored to the patient's readiness and ability to learn, the type of stroke sustained by the patient, and the patient's personal risk factors. Education of the patient and family may empower them to better cope with the illness and focus on the future.[41,221,252]

Palliative Care

Palliative care is a priority for patients and families following a stroke with resulting impairment of function, a decrease in quality of life, or a reduction in life expectancy. A palliative care consult with follow-up promotes patient and family-centered care by the interprofessional team, assists in prognostication, establishes the goals of care, aides in decision-making, and provides expertise regarding symptom detection and management both, physiologic and psychosocial.[136]

ISCHEMIC STROKE

Most AIS patients may not need or benefit from intensive care. However, if they have oxygenation issues, require intubation or mechanical ventilation, experience cardiac instability, require continuous infusions of vasoactive agents, or have neurologic instability, admission to a critical care unit is warranted. A patient who has sustained a large MCA infarct with massive edema needs advanced critical care and consideration of a decompressive craniectomy within 48 hours.[142,259,278] Other more stable AIS patients may benefit from an acute care unit with an aggressive interprofessional approach to stroke care, including early involvement of occupational, physical, and speech therapy. Dedicated stroke units, which are frequently classified as progressive care units, have been shown to have better outcomes than nonneurologic acute care units.[142,154]

Following AIS, BP regulation is a major consideration. BP that is too high may contribute to cerebral edema and hemorrhagic transformation. However, BP that is too low may inadequately perfuse the brain, resulting in an even larger infarct.[70,154] Optimal BP for this subgroup of stroke patients has not been scientifically substantiated. Based on AHA/ASA guidelines for AIS, BP is only to be treated if it exceeds a systolic of greater than 220 mm Hg or a diastolic of greater than 120 mm Hg, unless the patient is a candidate for rtPA.[142] If rtPA is to be administered, the BP must then be lowered cautiously to 185/110 mm Hg prior to administration and down to 180/105 mm Hg during rtPA administration and for the next 24 hours post-rtPA.[123,124,142] Scientific support for the use of intravenous rtPA for thrombolysis in AIS is based on a large multicenter randomized controlled trial conducted by NINDS.[49,104] The use of intravenous rtPA in eligible AIS patients is based on level I evidence. If a patient is being considered for intravenous rtPA, inclusion and exclusion criteria for 3 and 4.5 hours (Boxes 13.3 and 13.4) after the patient is last known well and guidelines for follow-up care must be strictly adhered to in order to minimize the risk of bleeding.[142] Contraindications to rtPA administration include intracranial and systemic hemorrhage.[15,49,104,142] Anticoagulants and antiplatelet agents must not be given for at least 24 hours.[142] Risk factors associated with hemorrhage following rtPA administration include a high NIHSS score, longer time to treatment, hyperglycemia, decreased platelet count, and increased age. Hyperglycemia also decreases recanalization or reopening of the occluded artery.[129] BP is maintained within parameters for post-rtPA administration; invasive monitoring and arterial and venous punctures are minimized. BP is carefully lowered with antihypertensives such as intermittent IV doses of labetalol or continuous nicardipine (Cardene).[142] The use of continuous intravenous infusions of nitroprusside (Nipride), a vasodilator, is controversial as it may contribute to increased ICP.[105,255]

In addition to intravenous rtPA, intra-arterial rtPA (at the clot), a combination of intravenous rtPA and intra-arterial rtPA as a bridging approach, or a clot retrieval device may be utilized to clear the artery. The development of newer devices, such as the stent retrieval systems (Solitaire, Trevo) (Fig. 13.18), and recent promising results from prospective randomized controlled trials supporting mechanical thrombolysis have renewed interest in endovascular treatment of acute ischemic stroke.[158, 203,229,232]

Recombinant rtPA is clot-specific yet may result in intracranial or systemic hemorrhagic tendencies. Following rtPA administration, the patient must be closely watched for signs of intracranial or systemic hemorrhage. Neurologic deterioration related to intracranial hemorrhage after rtPA may be subtle or dramatic, such as a sudden loss of consciousness, seizure, onset of severe headache, or sudden increase in systemic BP. Tachycardia, a decrease in BP, and a downward trend in the hematocrit and hemoglobin levels, as well as visible bleeding may indicate systemic hemorrhage.[15]

Recombinant rtPA has not been approved for use during pregnancy. However, low-dose aspirin, subcutaneous low-dose heparin, low molecular weight heparin, and warfarin have been safely used during pregnancy to prevent thrombosis in hypercoagulable states or to prevent cardiac-related embolization.[15,105]

BOX 13.3 Inclusion/Exclusion Criteria for rtPA Within 3 Hours

Inclusion Criteria:

- Diagnosis of ischemic stroke causing measureable neurologic deficit
- Onset of symptoms less than 3 hours before beginning treatment
- Age greater than or equal to 18 years

Exclusion Criteria:

- Significant head trauma or prior stroke in previous 3 months
- Symptoms suggest subarachnoid hemorrhage
- Intracranial neoplasm, arteriovenous malformation, or aneurysm
- Recent intracranial or intraspinal surgery
- Elevated blood pressure (systolic > 185 mm Hg or diastolic > 110 mm Hg)
- Active internal bleeding
- Acute bleeding risk including but not limited to:
  - Platelet count < 100,000/mm^3
  - Heparin received within 48 hours, resulting in abnormally elevated aPTT greater than the upper limit of normal
  - Current use of anticoagulant with INR > 1.7 or PT > 15 seconds
  - Current use of direct thrombin inhibitor or direct factor IIa inhibitors with elevated sensitive laboratory tests such as aPTT, INR, platelet count, and ECT, TT, or appropriate factor IIa assays
- Blood glucose concentration <50 mg/dL (2.7 mmo/L)
- CT demonstrates multilobal infarction (hypodensity > 1/3 cerebral hemisphere)

Relative Exclusions:

- Recent experience suggests that under some circumstances, with careful consideration and weighting of risk to benefit, patients may receive fibrinolytic therapy despite 1 or more relative contraindications. Consider risk to benefit of IV tPA administration carefully if any of these relative contraindications are present.
- Only minor or rapidly improving stroke symptoms (clearing spontaneously)
- Pregnancy
- Seizure at onset with postictal residual neurologic impairments
- Major surgery or serious trauma within previous 14 days
- Present gastrointestinal or urinary tract hemorrhage (within previous 21 days)
- Recent acute myocardial infarction (within previous 3 months)

From reference 142.

BOX 13.4 Inclusion/Exclusion Criteria for rtPA Within 3–4.5 Hours

Inclusion Criteria:

- Diagnosis of ischemic stroke causing measurable neurologic deficit
- Onset of symptoms within 3 to 4.5 hours before beginning treatment

Relative Exclusion Criteria:

- Age > 80 years
- Severe stroke (NIHSS > 25)
- Taking an oral anticoagulant regardless of INR
- History of both diabetes and prior ischemic stroke

From reference 142.

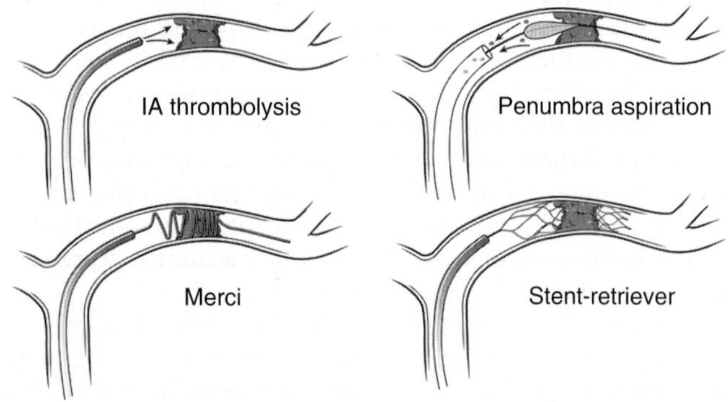

FIG. 13.18 Mechanical thrombolysis: intra-arterial rtPA and clot retrieval devices: Merci, Penumbra, Stent-Retriever Devices (e.g., Solitaire, Trevo). (Copyright University at Buffalo Neurosurgery. Published with permission.)

Surgical CEA or interventional carotid angioplasty with stenting has been shown to be beneficial with asymptomatic carotid stenosis of greater than 70% but less than 100% or symptomatic (recent TIA or AIS) carotid stenosis of greater than 50% but less than 100%.[36,37] CEA is based on Level A evidence, whereas interventional carotid angioplasty with stenting is based on Level B evidence.[36,37] Recanalizing an ICA that is already 100% stenosed may result in ICH because collateral circulation has compensated for the closure of the ICA and reestablishment of ICA flow may result in hyperemia with hemorrhage.[85,86]

Both approaches, surgical and endovascular, have advantages and disadvantages. Surgery is associated with a greater risk of myocardial infarction, DVT, and PE, as well as the complications associated with general anesthesia, including intubation, the systemic effects of muscle relaxants and anesthesia, and pneumonia. Although CEA may be performed under local anesthesia, general anesthesia is more common[85,97] (Fig. 13.19).

In endarterectomy, the artery distal to the stenosis is temporarily clamped to protect the brain from embolic material. Similarly, protective filters and occlusive balloons are used during angioplasty and stenting to prevent embolism. The surgical incision in CEA may injure cutaneous and cranial nerves, result in hematoma formation with life-threatening tracheal compression, or become infected.[85,97]

In contrast, angioplasty with stenting is usually performed under local anesthesia and conscious sedation.[86] Angioplasty with stenting carries the usual risks of angiography. In addition, plaque debris may extrude through the struts of the stent during placement and is potentially thrombogenic until endothelium covers the stent. Restenosis is more common after angioplasty with stenting than with CEA, and the long-term efficacy of endovascular therapy is unknown.[86] Following angioplasty with stenting, the patient may be placed on a heparin or abciximab (ReoPro) infusion and discharged home on aspirin or clopidogrel[86] (Fig. 13.20).

An extracranial-intracranial (EC-IC) bypass of the anterior circulation may be successfully performed for selected patients with such conditions as Moyamoya disease.[197] A branch of the superficial temporal artery (STA) is anastomosed to a branch of the MCA to provide blood flow distal to the ICA occlusion (Fig. 13.21). The saphenous vein or radial artery may also be used.[213,238] Complications include ischemic or hemorrhagic stroke. Immediate postoperative care may include positioning the patient on the side opposite the bypass to avoid compromising flow, avoiding a constricting head dressing, and auscultation of blood flow over the temporal area with a handheld vascular Doppler by the nurse or a TCD by a sonographer to assess patency.[155] If the radial artery is used, circulation to the upper extremity must be assessed and compression with a blood pressure cuff and tourniquet avoided.

Revascularization procedures may also be performed to restore blood flow to the posterior circulation when pharmacologic therapy, including antiplatelet agents, has failed. Treatment options such as vertebrobasilar angioplasty and stenting, endarterectomy, arterial reimplantation, and EC-IC bypass may be performed.[199,213,238] The STA, occipital artery, and external carotid artery can be used to increase blood flow to the superior cerebellar artery, PCA, posterior inferior cerebellar artery, and anterior inferior cerebellar artery.[238] The AHA/ASA has stated that extracranial-intracranial bypass procedures for ischemic stroke are of no proven benefit.

Malignant MCA cerebral or cerebellar infarction may result in refractory increased intracranial pressure and herniation.[65,144,278] If the increased ICP cannot be treated with the usual mannitol, furosemide, HTS, or barbiturate coma, a craniectomy

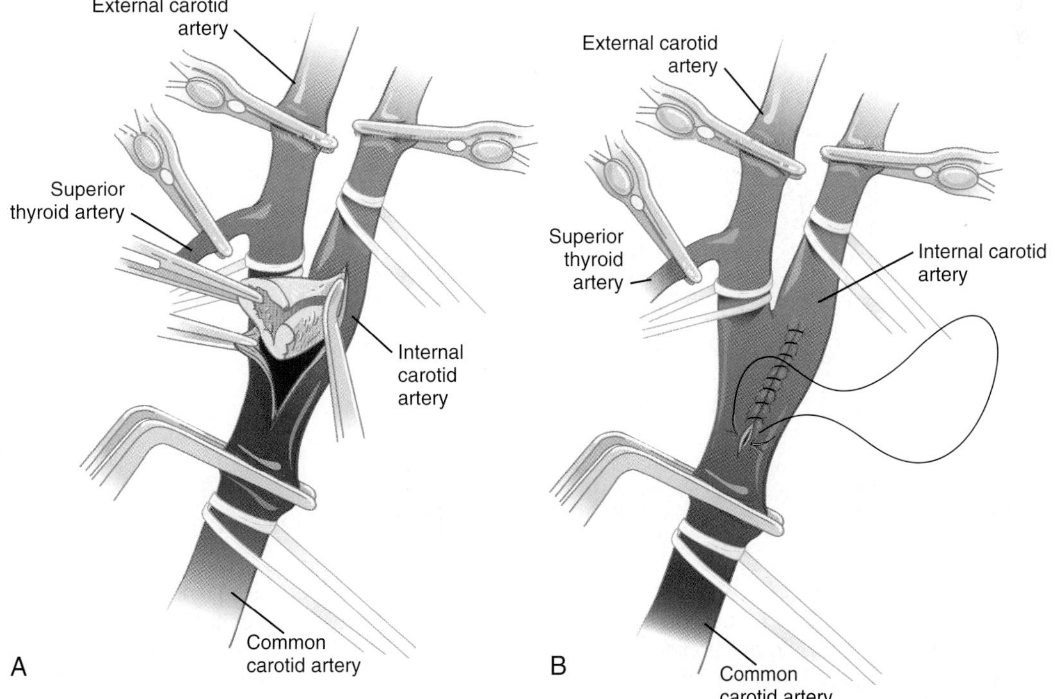

FIG. 13.19 Cross-clamping with carotid endarterectomy **A,** Dissection of plaque within the common carotid artery with extension into the internal carotid artery. **B,** Carotid artery closure following plaque removal.

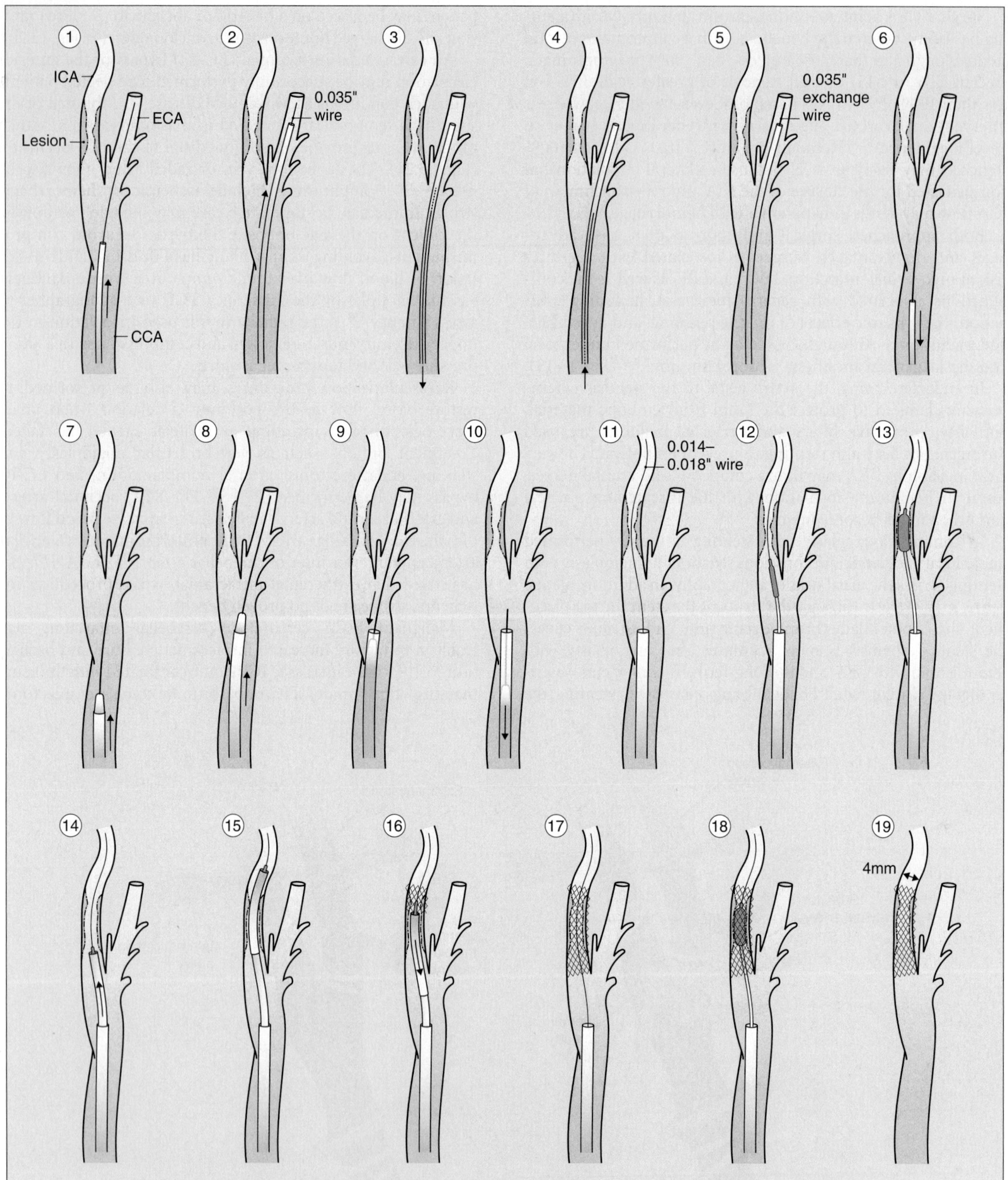

FIG. 13.20 Placement of a carotid stent. *12* and *13,* An angioplasty balloon is advanced across the lesion and inflated. *14,* The balloon is removed. *15,* The stent is advanced over the wire, across the lesion. *16,* Following positioning, the stent is unsheathed. *17,* Completed stent deployment. *18,* Post-stent angioplasty is performed to remove any remaining areas of in-stent stenosis. *19,* Final view showing the carotid following stent-assisted angioplasty. *CCA,* common carotid artery; *ECA,* external carotid artery; *ICA,* internal carotid artery. (From Rengachary, S., & Ellenbogen, R. (2005). *Principles of neurosurgery* (2nd ed.). Philadelphia: Mosby.)

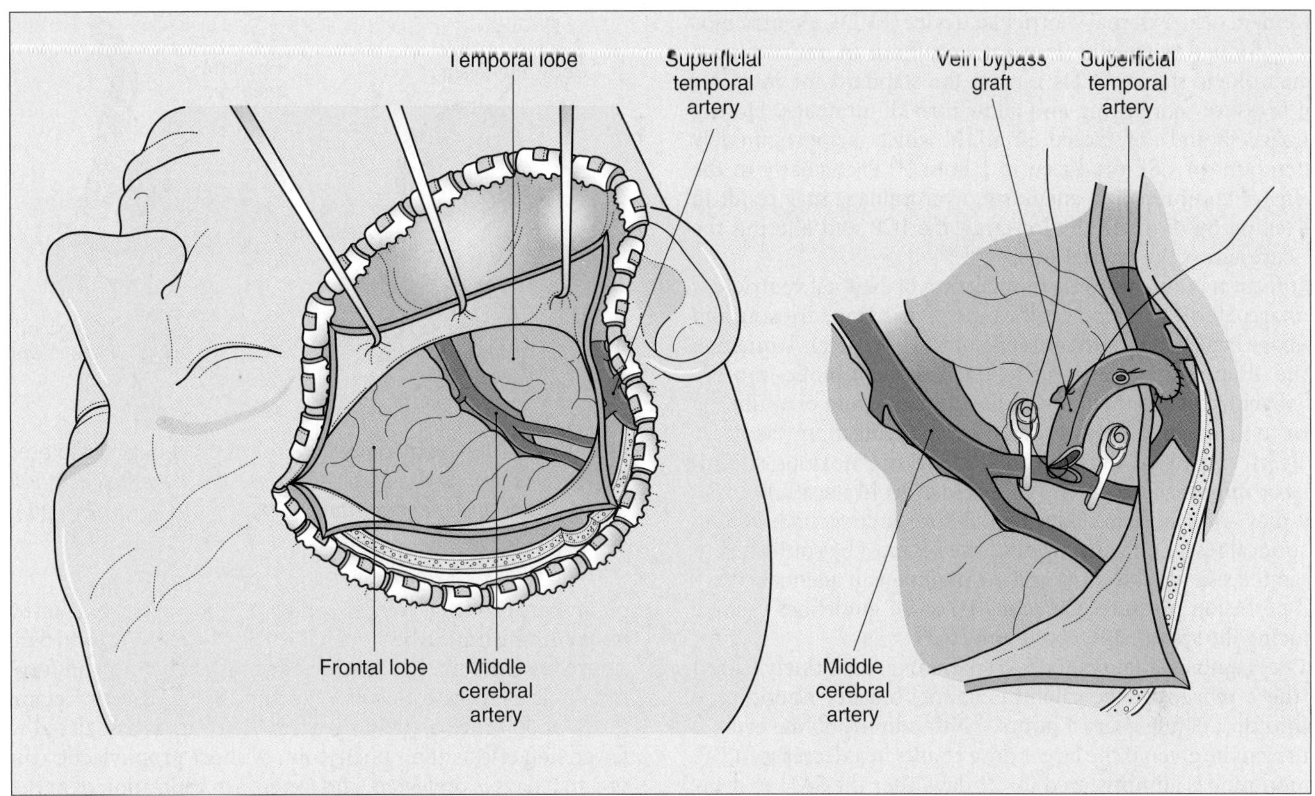

FIG. 13.21 Superficial temporal artery to middle cerebral artery bypass technique. (From Rengachary, S., & Ellenbogen, R. (2005). *Principles of neurosurgery* (2nd ed.). Philadelphia: Mosby.)

or a decompressive craniotomy with removal of infarcted brain within the first 48 hours in patients less than 60 years of age may be life-saving.[144,278] However, if delayed, or if age greater than 60 years, such heroic surgical efforts may not result in an improved quality of life. Prophylactic anticonvulsants are not recommended with acute ischemic stroke. However, if seizures occur, they must be treated emergently with a benzodiazepine and treated long-term with an anticonvulsant.[142]

Anticoagulation with intravenous heparin followed by oral warfarin (Coumadin) has not been shown to be effective after AIS with the exception of cardioembolic sources such as mechanical valves or atrial fibrillation or CVT. In addition to diet and drug interactions, compliance, gender, and ethnicity/race may affect prothrombin time/International Normalized Ratio (PT/INR) levels. The goal INR for prevention of cardioembolic stroke related to atrial fibrillation and bioprosthetic valves is 2.0 to 3.0, or 2.5.[119,142] The target INR for patients with mechanical heart valves is 2.5 to 3.5, or 3.0.[119,142] Attaining and maintaining a therapeutic PT/INR is not straightforward. Patient and family education is critical. An alternative to warfarin for nonvalvular atrial fibrillation only is the newer non-vitamin K-dependent oral anticoagulants, including dabigatran (Pradaxa), apixaban (Eliquis), and rivaroxaban (Xarelto).[79,87,234] These agents require daily (rivaroxaban) to twice daily dosing (dabigatran and apixaban). No routine laboratory testing is advised, as no specific assays exist at this time for any of the direct oral anticoagulants.[79,87,234] Rivaroxaban and dabigatran are primarily excreted through the kidneys. Food may delay absorption of rivaroxaban and dabigatran. Thrombin time has been identified as the trough level test to detect the presence of dabigatran activity, with antifactor XA activity being the trough level test for rivaroxaban and apixaban.[63,66] Fresh frozen plasma and prothrombin complex concentrate (PCC) have been used to manage hemorrhage associated with the use of nonvitamin K anticoagulants.[83,87,234] A dabigatran-specific reversal agent, idarucizumab (Praxbind), has received Food and Drug Administration (FDA) approval and is available for use.[231]

The time to start or resume oral anticoagulants after an ischemic stroke or spontaneous intracerebral hemorrhage is unknown. Administering oral anticoagulants closer to the time of the infarct or in large infarcts increases the likelihood of hemorrhagic transformation. Administration 2 to 3 weeks after the stroke may be prudent; however, the risk of additional ischemic stroke may occur during that time.[87]

Following ischemic stroke, antiplatelet therapy with aspirin, an aspirin and dipyridamole combination (Aggrenox), clopidogrel (Plavix), or aspirin and clopidogrel is generally prescribed.[142] Initial dose of aspirin is 325 mg with a maintenance dose between 30 and 1300 mg daily.[45] If rtPA is administered, antiplatelet agents should not be started until 24 hours after antifibrinolytic therapy.[142] The efficacy of clopidogrel in acute ischemic stroke is not well established and the combined use of clopidogrel and aspirin increases the risk of hemorrhage.[142] Multi-agent or increased dosing of any of the antiplatelet agents may increase the risk of bleeding, systemic or intracranial.[45]

SUBARACHNOID HEMORRHAGE

Following rupture, aneurysmal SAH patients are at risk for rebleed, hydrocephalus, seizures, and vasospasm.[43,80,81,103,237] Blood in the subarachnoid space and ventricles frequently impairs the reabsorption of CSF, resulting in hydrocephalus.

Placement of an external ventricular device (EVD), a ventriculostomy, for hydrocephalus frequently results in an improvement in neurologic status. EVDs remain the standard for intracranial pressure monitoring and allow for CSF drainage. Hourly drainage should not exceed 20 mL/h, which is approximately the amount of CSF produced in 1 hour.[110] Particularly in the setting of an unrepaired aneurysm, overdrainage may result in rebleeding by dramatically lowering the ICP and altering the pressure across the arterial wall.[55,110,168]

Infection is a significant complication of external ventricular drainage. Sterile technique at the time of insertion, dressing and drainage bag change, and sampling of CSF is critical. Tunneling of the drain at the insertion site, the use of antibiotic-impregnated ventricular catheters, and possibly one dose of antibiotic prior to the insertion may lessen the risk of infection.[110]

Before repair of the ruptured aneurysm, noxious stimuli must be minimized as much as possible to avoid elevations in BP that may contribute to rebleeding. Before endovascular coiling or surgical resection with clipping, the BP must be controlled to lessen the risk of rebleeding and yet maintain an adequate cerebral perfusion pressure. Current AHA/ASA guidelines include reducing the systolic BP to 160 mm Hg.[55]

On diagnosis, aneurysmal SAH patients are routinely placed on the cerebroselective calcium channel blocker nimodipine (Nimotop), 60 mg every 4 hours.[55] Nimodipine 30 mg every 2 hours can be given if the larger dose results in a decrease in BP. Nimodipine is administered for 21 days after the SAH to minimize secondary neuronal injury related to vasospasm.[237,244] The exact mechanism of action of nimodipine is not known; it does not decrease angiographic vasospasm as originally thought. Nimodipine may improve collateral circulation or provide a neuroprotective effect. Its use following aneurysmal subarachnoid hemorrhage is associated with improved outcomes.[237]

Optimal head position following aneurysmal subarachnoid hemorrhage is controversial. Some clinicians believe raising the head when the patient is at risk for vasospasm, or is in vasospasm, may worsen cerebral ischemia. As a result, patients may be managed with their head positioned less than or equal to 30 degrees for longer than 2 weeks, which increases their risk for aspiration and the consequences of immobility. Three small interventional studies showed that head-of-bed elevations over a range of 0 to 90 degrees did not increase vasospasm or cause neurologic deterioration. However, additional research is needed.[30,170,286]

The use of prophylactic anticonvulsants after SAH is controversial. The risk of SAH-related seizures has been reported to be as high as 26%, with most occurring at the time of the initial hemorrhage.[55] Anticonvulsants are given to minimize the risk of the deleterious intracranial and systemic effects of a seizure or status epilepticus, including rebleed and increased ICP. However, no research has been published that refutes or substantiates the value of prophylactic anticonvulsants after SAH.[55] If anticonvulsants are prescribed, fosphenytoin (Cerebyx), phenytoin (Dilantin), or levetiracetam (Keppra) are commonly used.[43] A phenytoin or fosphenytoin equivalent dose of 1000 mg or higher is typical. Phenytoin is protein-bound, and both free and total levels may be monitored for therapeutic efficacy. Administration of intravenous phenytoin is associated with hypotension and bradycardia. Purple glove syndrome may occur when phenytoin is given peripherally. Extravasation of Dilantin into a limb may result in tissue necrosis, ischemia, and possibly loss of the extremity.[163,247] Fosphenytoin (Cerebyx), a phenytoin prodrug, may be preferable for peripheral intravenous administration because it is less likely to injure local tissues. A rare but potentially fatal side effect of phenytoin and fosphenytoin is Stevens-Johnson syndrome.[163,247] Levetiracetam in doses of 500 mg to 1000 mg every 12 hours is associated with fewer side effects than phenytoin. A short prophylactic course of 3 to 7 days is preferred, and long-term utilization of anticonvulsants is not recommended.[55,71,237]

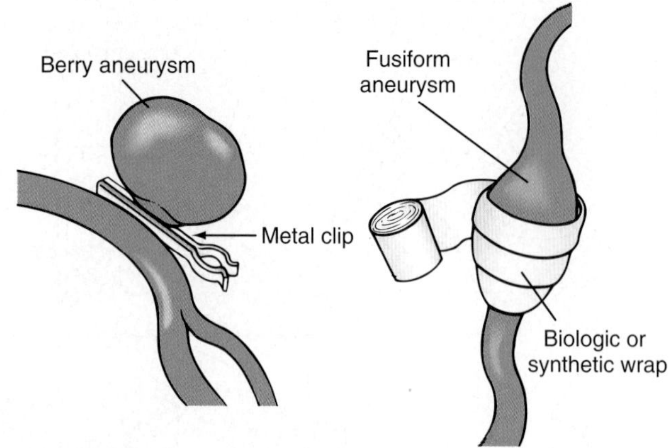

FIG. 13.22 Aneurysm clipping. (From Lewis, S.L., Heitkemper, M.M., Dirksen, S.R., et al. (2007). *Medical-surgical nursing: assessment and management of clinical problems* (6th ed.). St Louis: Mosby.)

Early surgical resection of the aneurysm with placement of a clip, or coil embolization with or without stenting, is standard practice, allowing for the aggressive treatment of vasospasm.[55] The decision to perform endovascular therapy or surgery depends on a number of factors, including the following:[6,270]

1. The efficacy of coiling versus clipping
2. The patient's life expectancy, comorbidities, family history, and clinical presentation (e.g., Hunt and Hess and WFNS scores)
3. Aneurysm size, configuration, and location; neck dimensions; parent vessel anatomy
4. Technical skills of the neurosurgeon and the interventional neuroradiologist

Endovascular occlusion, involving placement of coils in the aneurysmal sac, is less invasive and may be safer, particularly for older patients with comorbidities and poor grade Hunt and Hess and WFNS scores. However, the risk of recanalization after coiling is problematic. When a clip is securely placed across the neck of the aneurysm and completely occludes blood flow to the aneurysmal sac, that aneurysm will never bleed again (Fig. 13.22). In contrast, packing the aneurysmal sac with coils pulls the walls of the aneurysmal sac apart. As a result, endothelialization does not occur, allowing continued exposure of the aneurysmal thrombus or the coils in the sac to the circulating blood. The coils may compress and compartmentalize, allowing blood to flow around their periphery into the aneurysmal sac. This recanalization of the aneurysm makes the patient vulnerable to the possibility of rebleed because blood flow to the aneurysmal sac is no longer blocked by the coils.[6,270]

Placement of coils in the sac of the aneurysm may be performed with general anesthesia or conscious sedation. Coils come in various configurations[287] (Figs. 13.23 and 13.24). Consideration must be given to the size of the aneurysm, the configuration, and

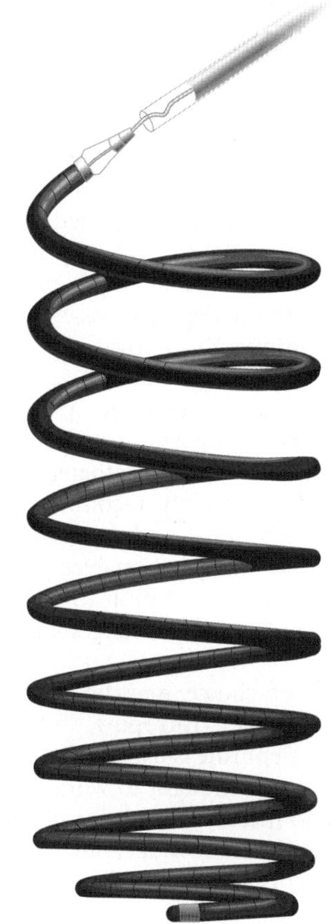

FIG. 13.23 Aneurysm coils: microcoil.

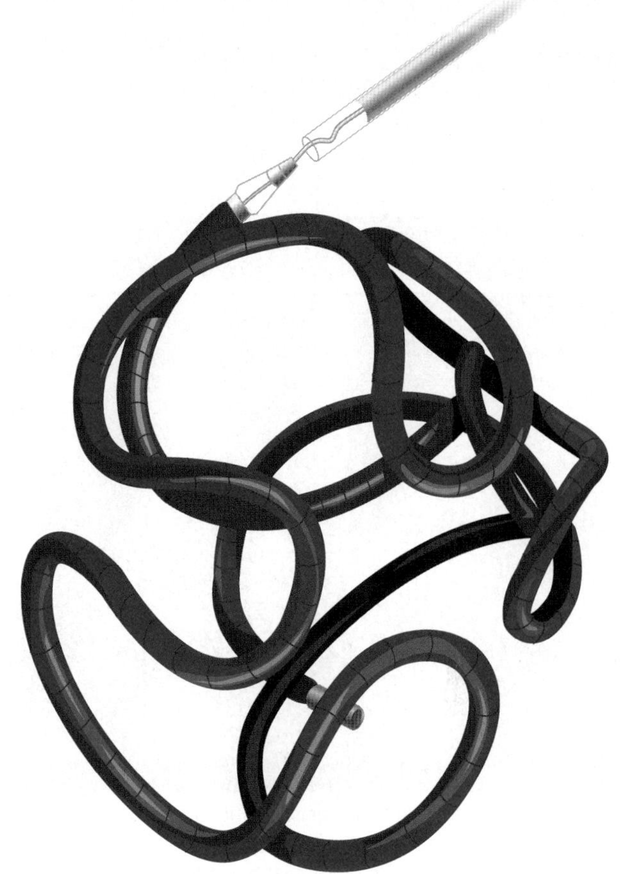

FIG. 13.24 Aneurysm coils: three-dimensional spherical coils.

the dome-to-neck ratio before coiling is performed. A small neck, a small dome size, and a large dome-to-neck ratio are optimal for coiling. Several coils may be placed into the aneurysmal sac to prevent rebleed.[6,270] Placement of a stent at the neck of the aneurysm may prevent migration of coils and lessen the possibility of rebleed[6,270,287] (Fig. 13.25). Endovascular stents and aneurysm coils are thrombogenic, and the patient will require antiplatelet agents following these interventions.[236]

If clipping or coiling of the aneurysm is not possible and collateral circulation is adequate, the parent vessel may be sacrificed by surgical ligation or embolization to prevent rebleed. Before permanently occluding the parent artery surgically or in interventional neuroradiology, blood flow through that vessel may be temporarily stopped utilizing an endovascular balloon during cerebral angiography to determine collateral flow. The patient remains awake and is assessed during the balloon occlusion test so that any neurologic deterioration will be detected.[6,270]

Patients with SAH may benefit from multimodality monitoring, including ICP, CPP measurement, $Pbto_2$, brain temperature, $Sjvo_2$ as a measure of global oxygenation, and, ideally, daily TCD to quantify vasospasm.[175] Sensitivity and specificity for middle cerebral artery vasospasm are high; however, they are less so for the other vessels.[69,175] Diagnosis of MCA vasospasm requires measurement of the MFV not only of the MCA but also of the ICA to determine the MCA/ICA (Lindegaard or hemispheric) ratio. Abnormally high values for grading the severity of the vasospasm in the circle of Willis vessels vary in the literature. Generally, MCA MFV values of 120 cm/sec or greater and MCA/ICA ratios of 3 or greater indicate vasospasm.

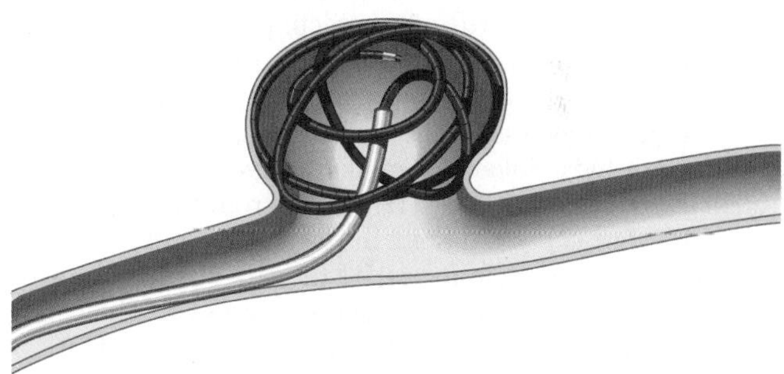

FIG. 13.25 Coils in aneurysm.

Severe vasospasm of the MCA is defined as MCA values of greater than 200 cm/sec and MCA/ICA ratios of greater than 6[69,175] (Fig. 13.26).

A distinction between radiographic or sonographic vasospasm, vessel narrowing visible on angiography or TCD, and clinical vasospasm has recently been made. Cerebral vasospasm may occur without ischemia or infarction just as ischemia and infarction may occur without vasospasm.[43,55,71,237,271] Clinical cerebral vasospasm, vasospasm associated with neurologic deterioration that lasts for more than 1 hour and occurs more than 3 days after aneurysmal rupture and is not attributable to any other cause, is now referred to as delayed cerebral ischemia (DCI).[43,55,71,237,271] Clinical signs and symptoms of vasospasm correlate with the functional area supplied by the constricted vessel(s) and may be subtle or profound. Extremity weakness, for example, may

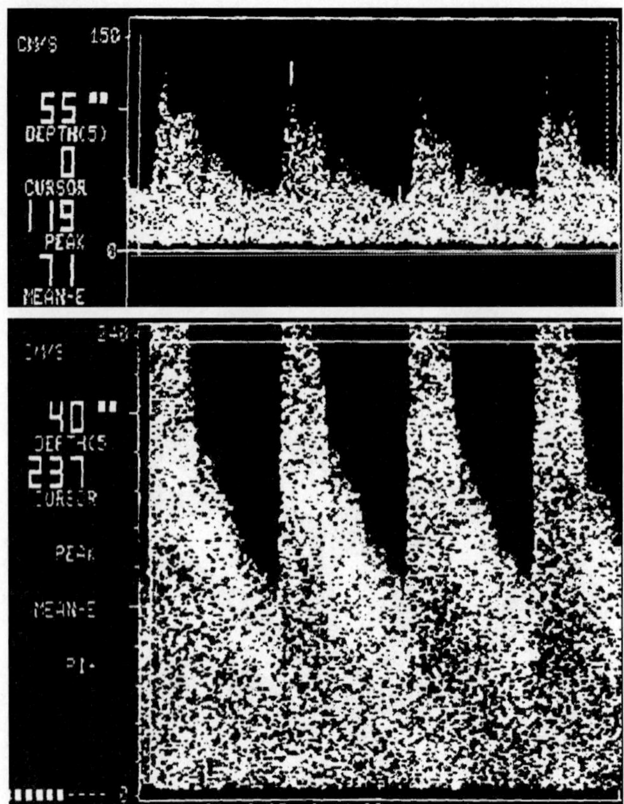

FIG. 13.26 Transcranial Doppler showing severe vasospasm. (From Layon, A., Gabrielli, A., & Friedman, W. (2004). *Textbook of neurointensive care.* Philadelphia: Saunders.)

range from pronator drift to complete paralysis. Vasospasm typically begins after day 3 but may continue for 3 or 4 weeks. The peak incidence of vasospasm is approximately 3 to 5 through 14 days after the hemorrhage.[38,103,237]

Previously hypervolemic hemodilution with or without controlled hypertension therapy (HHH) was routinely used in the treatment of vasospasm despite the lack of evidence regarding its benefit. The rationale for HHH therapy was based on the brain's impaired autoregulatory status after SAH. The CBF is passively dependent on the mean arterial pressure (MAP); by increasing the intravascular volume, diluting the blood, and increasing the systemic BP, an adequate MAP and CBF might be achieved to prevent secondary ischemia and infarct associated with vasospasm.[223] However, a prospective randomized controlled multicenter trial was never published that substantiated the value of HHH therapy in improving outcomes, and the pharmacologic agents and the parameters used varied from publication to publication. HHH therapy, including and especially the extreme hypervolemia and hemodilution aspects of the therapy, was associated with a number of side effects, including heart failure with pulmonary edema, electrolyte abnormalities, coagulopathy, blood transfusion reactions, and cerebral edema.[262]

Consequently, the use of HHH therapy in the management of DCI has been discontinued in favor of euvolemia to slight hypervolemia with emphasis on blood pressure augmentation once the aneurysm has been repaired and the patient is at risk or experiences DCI.[55,262] Hypovolemia, which may be worsened with the cerebral salt wasting (CSW) associated with aneurysmal subarachnoid hemorrhage, has been shown to increase vasospasm-related infarct and should be avoided.[55,71,168]

Systemic hypertension has been associated with increased cerebral blood flow and reversal of neurologic deficits in up to 66% of DCI patients.[262] The exact parameters for BP augmentation are not known. The Neurocritical Care Society recommends a stepwise approach with each assessment of neurologic assessment until the designated MAP level has been achieved.[71,262] However, systolic BP may be used in clinical practice rather than MAP. Goal blood pressure parameters are generally related to the degree of vasospasm. For example, following surgical clipping or endovascular coiling, the target parameters in mild vasospasm might be a systolic BP 140 to 160 mm Hg; in moderate vasospasm, systolic BP 160 to 180 mm Hg; and in severe vasospasm, systolic BP 180 to 200 mm Hg. The use of a pulmonary artery catheter to guide DCI management is no longer routinely recommended.[71,262] Central venous pressure, fluid balance, and the use of minimally invasive hemodynamic monitors that analyze pulse pressure variation (PPV), stroke volume variation (SVV), or continuously measure cardiac output have been suggested to guide the management of DCI.[175]

The vasopressor of choice may be phenylephrine (Neo-Synephrine), dopamine (Intropin), or norepinephrine (Levophed).[168] Phenylephrine is usually the first choice because it is an alpha agonist and thought to work primarily on extracranial vasculature to increase flow to vasospastic cerebral vessels and minimize risk of secondary infarction.[168] Dopamine may result in unacceptable tachycardia. All are ideally administered through a central venous catheter to prevent injury to peripheral tissues.[207,244] Approximately 20% to 30% of patients with intracranial aneurysms have more than one aneurysm; clinicians must be cognizant of this in regard to the risk of increasing BP to treat vasospasm.[262]

SAH patients are at high risk for hyponatremia, primarily related to CSW rather than syndrome of inappropriate antidiuretic hormone (SIADH).[269] The mechanism by which SAH leads to CSW is not completely understood. Central nervous system (CNS)-mediated input to the kidneys is thought to be impaired as a result of the SAH, and atrial and brain natriuretic peptides are released, resulting in hypovolemia, hemoconcentration, and hyponatremia. CSW is a true hyponatremia and managed improperly, specifically with total fluid restriction, may result in hypovolemia with worsening of DCI and infarct.[244]

As serum sodium level drops, patients are also at increased risk for seizures. A serum sodium level below 125 mEq/L may impair the patient's level of consciousness and increase the likelihood of seizures.[168] Supplemental enteral salt (sodium chloride tablets) and fludrocortisone (Florinef) may be given to increase the serum sodium level and maintain a normal to slightly hypervolemic fluid status.[55,168] Free water is restricted and saline is used to flush feeding tubes. HTS of varying percentages may be given to increase the serum sodium level and to decrease intracranial pressure, although large human studies demonstrating efficacy have not been published at time of printing. Rapid correction of hyponatremia may result in central pontine myelinolysis. Therefore, the serum sodium should not be corrected more rapidly than 10 mEq/L in a 24-hour time period.[175] Sustained dosing of hypertonic sodium chloride may result in hypochloremia with metabolic acidosis.[269] A 2% to 3% hypertonic sodium acetate solution may be used as an alternative. Hypervolemia and HTS may increase the risk of

BOX 13.5 Differentiating Cerebral Salt Wasting and Syndrome of Inappropriate Antidiuretic Hormone

Cerebral Salt Wasting (CSW) (true salt wasting)	Syndrome of Inappropriate Antidiuretic Hormone (SIADH) (dilutional hyponatremia)
Serum sodium level < 135 mEq/L	Serum sodium level < 135 mEq/L
Decreased extracellular fluid volume	Increased extracellular fluid volume
Increased hematocrit	Normal hematocrit
Increased plasma albumin concentration	Normal plasma albumin concentration
Normal or increased serum potassium level	Normal serum potassium level
Normal or decreased plasma uric acid level	Decreased plasma uric acid level
Increased blood urea nitrogen/creatinine level	Urine sodium level > 25 mEq/L
Signs of dehydration:	Serum osmolality < 280 mOsm/L
Orthostatic changes	Urine osmolality > serum osmolality
Flat neck veins	Decreased urine output (400–500 mL/24 h)
Dry mucous membranes	Signs of hypervolemia:
Poor skin turgor	Increased body weight
Tachycardia	Elevated central venous pressure and pulmonary artery occlusion pressure readings
Weight loss	
Negative fluid balance	
Central venous pressure < 6 mm Hg or pulmonary artery occlusion pressure < 8 mm Hg	

From Reference 269.

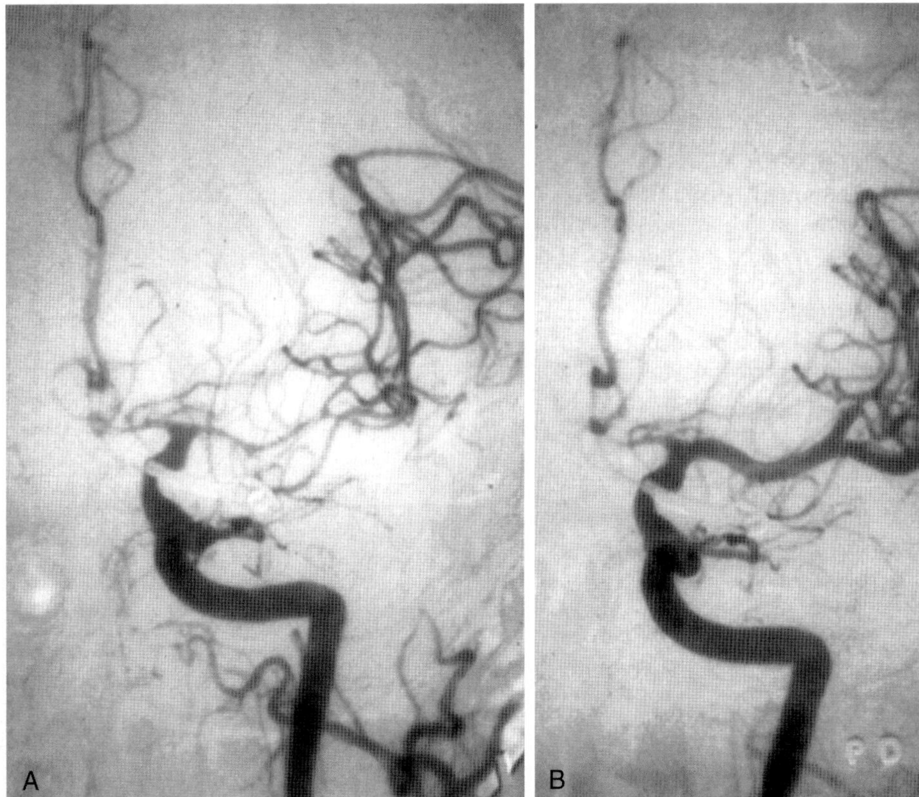

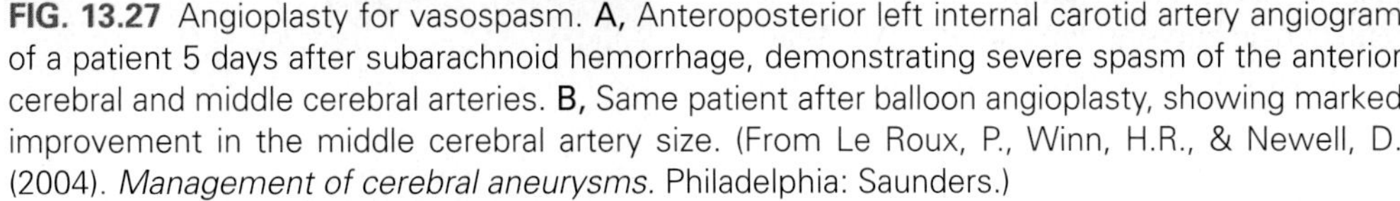

FIG. 13.27 Angioplasty for vasospasm. **A,** Anteroposterior left internal carotid artery angiogram of a patient 5 days after subarachnoid hemorrhage, demonstrating severe spasm of the anterior cerebral and middle cerebral arteries. **B,** Same patient after balloon angioplasty, showing marked improvement in the middle cerebral artery size. (From Le Roux, P., Winn, H.R., & Newell, D. (2004). *Management of cerebral aneurysms.* Philadelphia: Saunders.)

neurogenic pulmonary edema or acute respiratory distress syndrome adding to the patient's pulmonary compromise.[168,269]

In contrast, SIADH is the CNS-mediated release of excess antidiuretic hormone (ADH) or increased renal sensitivity to ADH, resulting in hypervolemia and hyponatremia. Treatment for SIADH is total fluid restriction, which is generally thought to be harmful to patients at risk for cerebral vasospasm[168,175,269] (Box 13.5).

If nimodipine and euvolemia with blood pressure augmentation are insufficient to prevent DCI related to vasospasm, selective cerebral angioplasty may be performed[71] (Fig. 13.27). However, distal vasospasm often cannot be reached without vessel injury, and intra-arterial vasodilators such as nicardipine, papaverine, verapamil, or milrinone are injected into the vasospastic artery to open the vessel.[18,62] Cerebral angioplasty may be repeated, but sometimes once is all that is required. Unfortunately, the results of intra-arterial vasodilators are short-lived, generally lasting less than 24 hours. Attention to the ICP is necessary during the intra-arterial injection of vasodilators because it may result in a massive cerebral vasodilation and a sudden rise in ICP, increasing the risk of hemorrhage or herniation.[103] Risks of angioplasty include dissection, thrombosis, and reperfusion injury.[103]

Ongoing studies regarding vasospasm include the use of nicardipine implants, cisternal irrigation, hypermagnesemia, statins, the role of nitric oxide, and cerebral microdialysis. Nicardipine implants, cisternal irrigation and intraventricular thrombolysis, hypermagnesemia, and nitric oxide are intended to directly decrease vasospasm or protect the neurons from vasospasm-induced ischemia and infarction.[35] Cisternal irrigation, intraventricular thrombolysis, and CSF drainage using a lumbar drain may assist in the removal of blood from the ventricles and around the blood vessels, which in turn may lessen vasospasm.[35,62] A nitric oxide deficiency may contribute to vasospasm.[35] In contrast, microdialysis is a monitoring modality aimed at analyzing biomarkers of cerebral ischemia in vasospasm, including pH, lactate-to-pyruvate ratio, and levels of lactate, pyruvate, and glutamate.[132]

In addition to neurologic interventions, many aneurysmal SAH patients will require intubation and mechanical ventilation associated with decreased level of consciousness, impaired respiratory effort, or neurogenic pulmonary edema.[51,103] They may also present with neurogenic dysrhythmias and 12-lead ECG changes suggestive of a myocardial infarction. ECG changes associated with aneurysmal SAH have been reported to occur from 50% to 100% of the time and include rhythm changes, P wave, repolarization, conduction abnormalities, and pathologic Q waves.[43,51] Disturbances in rhythm are usually benign and are treated only if the patient is hemodynamically compromised.[43,51] A cardiac workup may reveal actual coronary artery occlusion with infarction and abnormal CK-MB and troponin levels, but cardiac damage is more frequently the result of the catecholamine and sympathetic release at the time of the bleed.[43,51] Pathologic changes, though different from true myocardial ischemia, may occur with neurogenic cardiac injury and contribute to pulmonary edema, hypotension, and decreased cardiac output. The myocardium is referred to as "stunned," and the neurogenic-induced cardiac changes may reverse over time. Takotsubo cardiomyopathy with ballooning of the apex and decrease in ejection fraction may occur as well. In severe cases, intra-aortic balloon counterpulsation may be indicated to maintain cerebral and systemic perfusion.[43,51]

Critical care management of AVMs, ruptured or unruptured, is similar to management of aneurysms. Patients with AVMs are also at risk for rebleed, seizures, vasospasm, and hydrocephalus. Definitive treatment of AVMs includes surgical resection, endovascular embolization, and radiosurgery.[130,184] Surgical resection alone was the only definitive treatment for years, and complications, including hemorrhage during and after surgery, cerebral edema, and stroke, were common. Endovascular therapy allows embolic agents (such as polyvinyl alcohol), detachable coils, or liquid polymer to be injected into the feeder arteries at the arteriovenous junction. This halts the flow of blood to the venous side of the AVM, where most AVM bleeding occurs. This procedure may be conducted before surgical resection or radiosurgery to decrease circulation to the AVM and facilitate eradication of the AVM.[130,184] Stereotactic radiation, using gamma knife or linear accelerator with or without endovascular therapy, usually requires several treatments and a time span of up to 2 years before obliteration of the AVM[130,184] (Fig. 13.28).

Aneurysmal or AVM SAH may be treated surgically or endovascularly during pregnancy using an abdominal shield during radiographic procedures. Treatment of the ruptured aneurysm or AVM hemorrhage to minimize the risk of rebleed should take precedence over obstetric concerns if the patient is not in labor and the fetus is not in distress.[100] However, the risk of using prophylactic anticonvulsants, nimodipine, and papaverine in pregnancy may outweigh the benefits.[100]

INTRACEREBRAL HEMORRHAGE

As in aneurysmal SAH, the patient with ICH frequently presents with impaired level of consciousness and inability to protect the airway or inadequate respiratory effort. Also as in SAH, if the patient was found supine, aspiration is a concern.[48,168]

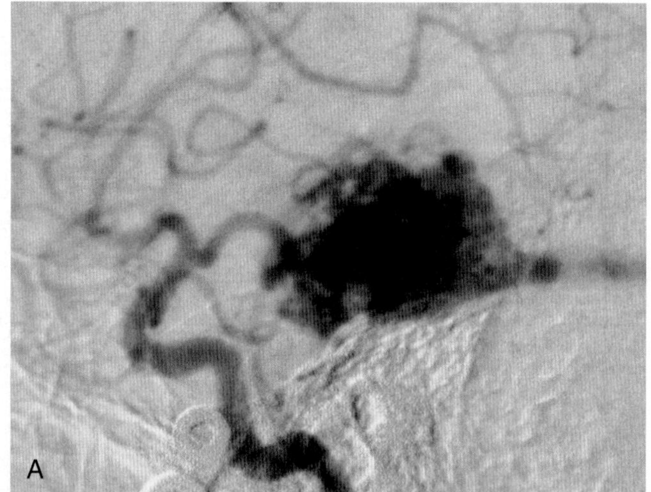

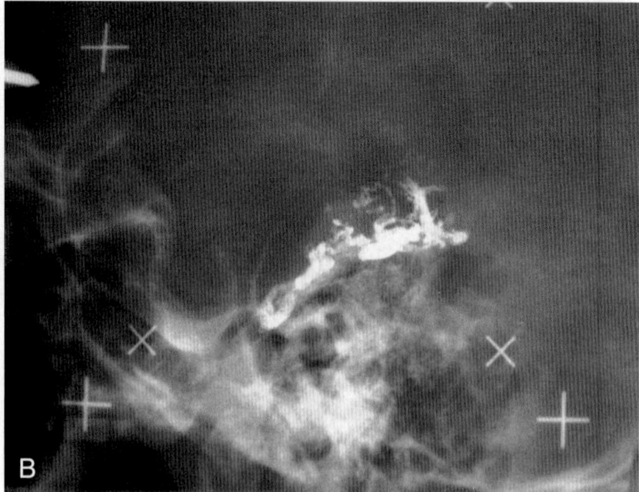

FIG. 13.28 Arteriovenous malformation. **A,** Preoperative angiogram. **B,** After radiation and embolization. (From Mohr, J., Choi, D., Grotta, J., et al. (2004). (From Mohr, J., Choi, D., Grotta, J., et al. (2004). *Stroke: pathophysiology, diagnosis, and management* (4th ed.). London: Churchill Livingstone.)

ICH stroke patients may also present with neurogenic cardiac dysrhythmias and 12-lead ECG changes, as well as neurally mediated pulmonary edema, and the initial cardiopulmonary workup/treatment is similar to that for SAH. ECG changes in patients with ICH have been less documented than those in SAH, but their incidence has been reported as high as 60% to 70%.[48,168,265] The most common ICH-related abnormalities are rhythm disturbances, QT prolongation, T wave inversion, U waves, ST depression, and pathologic Q waves. These cardiac abnormalities are left untreated unless the patient is hemodynamically unstable. ICH of the deeper structures, such as the thalamus and basal ganglia or the posterior fossa, brain stem, or cerebellum, places the patient at increased risk of increased ICP and herniation, or respiratory arrest requiring emergency intubation and mechanical ventilation.[48]

ICH may occur with or without coagulopathy, and the most common reasons are systemic hypertension and CAA.[107,168] If the patient with ICH is being given anticoagulants or antiplatelet agents, they must be discontinued immediately, even if the patient is at risk for cardioembolic events, until the neurologic condition has stabilized.[135] Patients requiring anticoagulation for atrial fibrillation are at less risk for cardioembolic events than those with mechanical cardiac valves.[69] If coagulopathy is present, it must be corrected as soon as possible. Fresh frozen plasma and vitamin K have been most commonly used to correct a coagulopathy. Vitamin K will not be effective in the reversal of the newer nonvitamin K anticoagulants (dabigatran, apixaban, and rivaroxaban). Prothrombin complex concentrate (PCC) has also been used with some success for both vitamin K and nonvitamin K anticoagulants with fewer side effects than FFP.[83,135,284] Recombinant activated factor VII (rfVIIa [Novo-7]) may be more effective in correcting the coagulopathy than fresh frozen plasma and vitamin K with vitamin K anticoagulants. In addition, recombinant activated factor VII does not carry risk of blood transfusion reaction and does not require a large-volume administration. However, repeated administration may be necessary and may increase the risk of thromboembolism.[69,135]

Enlargement of the hematoma may be associated with hypertension; however, the optimal BP has not been determined. AHA/ASA guidelines for intracerebral hemorrhage have been revised. Current guidelines recommend a systolic BP of 140 mm Hg for patients presenting with a systolic BP between 150 to 220 mm Hg. Aggressive reduction of the presenting BP is recommended if the presenting pressure is greater than 220 mm Hg.[135,143] Prescribed antihypertensives include hydralazine, labetalol, and nicardipine.

Mannitol and hypertonic saline are used to reduce intracranial pressure.[168] Monitoring the ICP with a ventriculostomy allows drainage of CSF and blood if ventricular extension of the hemorrhage has resulted in hydrocephalus and increased intracranial pressure. If the patient has a coagulopathy, it must be corrected before insertion of the ventriculostomy. Patients with supratentorial lesions may benefit from ICP/CPP monitoring and perhaps $Pbto_2$ monitoring in ICH. Anticonvulsant therapy is reasonable in lobar and especially cortical lesions.[48,284] Medical versus surgical management is controversial. Surgical management is generally considered appropriate in the young person with a moderate to large lobar hemorrhage and good GCS or early in a cerebellar hemorrhage before long-standing herniation.[135,168] However, a craniotomy or blind aspiration to evacuate a deep hematoma may only worsen the patient's condition.[135] The International Surgical Treatment of ICH (ISTICH) study, a large multicenter prospective randomized controlled trial, was conducted comparing surgical with nonsurgical management of ICH. Surgery was not found to be more beneficial than medical management; however, the study had several design flaws. Surgery was found to be more effective if performed within 21 hours of the bleed in a STICH II subanalyses.[135,168] Less invasive surgical techniques may improve outcomes, such as endoscopic hematoma evacuation using ultrasound and laser coagulation; stereotactic endoscopic ultrasonic aspiration; and stereotactic aspiration with thrombolytics used at the clot.[114]

Resuming anticoagulation administration is controversial. AHA/ASA guidelines include waiting 4 weeks after the ICH before restarting anticoagulation in patients without mechanical heart valves.[135] As with aneurysmal subarachnoid hemorrhage and acute ischemic stroke, fever, nosocomial infections, hyperglycemia, VTE, and seizures are common and increase mortality and morbidity.[168] An aggressive approach to the management of the patient with ICH may result in better outcomes. Care of the critically ill ICH patient in a designated neuroscience critical care unit or stroke unit has been associated with improved outcomes.[142] In contrast, if the ICH patient is managed in an environment where some diagnoses are promptly associated with "do not resuscitate" (DNR) status, attempts to aggressively treat the sequelae of ICH may be viewed as futile and may result in poor outcomes. In one study, the single most important factor in regard to an ICH patient's outcome was the hospital's percentage of all patients with DNR orders. The higher the hospital's percentage of all patients with DNR orders, the higher the mortality rate for patients with ICH.[134,168]

EVIDENCE-BASED CARE

The AHA/ASA has published practice guidelines and advisory statements on the prevention, diagnosis, acute management, and rehabilitation of stroke for more than 25 years. Several of these guidelines have been referenced in this chapter. Since 2010, over 40 new guidelines have been published. These documents are evidence-based consensus statements from task force experts who have reviewed the current evidence. These guidelines include the grade of the recommendation and the level of the evidence.[7,55,135,142,252,259,262,278] The Neurocritical Care Society (NCS) has also published a consensus statement on the management of aneurysmal subarachnoid hemorrhage.[71,262] NCS utilized the GRADES classification system for leveling the evidence and formulating recommendations.[71,262]

ETHICAL CONSIDERATIONS

Many critically ill patients with stroke have a poor prognosis. Regardless of the clinicians' best efforts, the primary injury may be too devastating to restore a quality life. Some patients may present on admission or within the next few hours or days as brain dead. When to consider withdrawal of life support or "do not attempt to resuscitate" status is often not clear and is emotionally laden for both clinicians and family.[240] Neurologic assessment tools have been shown to be of some help in predicting outcome. A poor prognosis is associated with a GCS less than 8, Hunt-Hess grades IV–V, and an NIHSS greater than 20.[1,135,276] However, some stroke patients improve unexpectedly if aggressive care with a proactive cohesive interprofessional approach to the prevention of secondary neuronal injury and the sequelae of stroke is undertaken.[31]

CONCLUSION

Stroke is a heterogeneous disease with many clinical presentations and variable outcomes. A number of pharmacologic agents and technologies are available today that were not available 20 years ago to enhance care. In addition, more is known today about stroke than was known previously. However, none of these advances are of value if knowledgeable, skilled, and caring clinicians do not utilize them, especially and including the critical care or progressive care nurse. The acute and critical care nurse is key in the assessment, planning, intervention, and evaluation of care.

CASE STUDY 13.1

Mrs. S.P. is a 55-year-old Caucasian female who presents with the "worst headache of her life" (10/10), nausea and vomiting, photophobia, and increasing drowsiness. She has a history of migraines but she states that this headache is much worse than her typical migraine. Other pertinent medical history includes smoking 2 packs per day for 30 years, and mild hypertension. Mrs. S.P. is neurologically intact except for a headache 10/10, nuchal rigidity, slight drowsiness, and a slight right lower facial weakness (asymmetric smile). Her vital signs are as follows: temperature 37.5°C (99.5°F); heart rate 78 beats/min (normal sinus rhythm); respirations 16 breaths/min; BP 160/88 mm Hg; Sao_2 95%.

Mrs. S.P.'s GCS is 14 (opens eyes to name, but not spontaneously), NIHSS 1 (not alert, requires minor stimuli), Hunt and Hess Grade II (moderate to severe headache, unequal pupils), WFNS Grade II (GCS 14 and no major focal deficit), and Fisher Grade 3 (localized clot of subarachnoid blood on CT scan > 1 mm). She is sleepy but arouses to name; oriented to name, place, time, and situation; and moves all extremities without difficulty 5/5. She has slightly unequal pupils, with the left being 4 mm and the right being 3 mm, but both are briskly reactive to light and accommodation. Both she and her family claim her pupils are usually equal. No other cranial nerve deficits are detected. Mrs. S.P. has nuchal rigidity and continues to complain of a severe headache with nausea and vomiting. A stat CT reveals diffuse subarachnoid blood, a localized clot of subarachnoid blood greater than 1 mm (Fisher 3), and slightly enlarged ventricles. An angiogram reveals a left middle cerebral artery aneurysm. Her vital signs now are as follows: temperature 37.8°C (100°F); heart rate 74 beats/min (normal sinus rhythm); respirations 16 breaths/min; Sao_2, 92%; BP 170/110 mm Hg. Her laboratory workup is negative for toxicology and coagulopathy.

Decision Point:
What pathophysiology is associated with this stroke?

Decision Point:
What are the initial priorities for her care?

REFERENCES

1. Adams, H. P., Jr. (2011). Clinical scales to assess patient with stroke. In J. P. Mohr, P. A. Wolf, J. C. Grotta, M. A. Moskowitz, M. R. Mayberg, & R. von Kummer (Eds.), *Stroke: pathophysiology, diagnosis, and management* (5th ed.) (pp. 307–333). Philadelphia: Elsevier Saunders.
2. Adams, S., Butas, D., & Spurlock, D. (2015). Capnography ($ETco_2$), respiratory depression and nursing interventions in moderately sedated adults undergoing transesophageal echocardiography (TEE). *J Perianesth Nurs, 30*(1), 14–22.
3. Aguilar, M. I., Kuo, R. S., & Freeman, W. D. (2013). New anticoagulants (dabigatran, apixaban, rivaroxaban) for stroke prevention. *Neurol Clin, 31*(3), 659–675.
4. Ahn, S. H., Prince, E. A., & Dubel, G. J. (2013). Basic neuroangiography: review of technique and perioperative patient care. *Semin Intervent Radiol, 30*(3), 225–233.
5. Ajiboye, N., Chalouhi, N., Starke, R. M., Zanaty, M., & Bell, R. (2014). Cerebral arteriovenous malformations: evaluation and management. *Scientific World Journal, 2014*, 1–6. http://dx.doi.org/10.1155/2014/649036.
6. Alaraj, A., Ti, J., & Dashti, R. (2014). Patient selection for endovascular treatment of intracranial aneurysms. *Neurol Res, 36*(4), 283–307.
7. Alexander, S., Gallek, M., Presciutti, M., & Zrelak, P. (2012). *AANN clinical practice guideline series: care of the patient with aneurysmal subarachnoid hemorrhage.* Chicago: American Association of Neuroscience Nurses.
8. Altman, K. W., Richards, A., Goldberg, L., Frucht, S., & McCabe, D. J. (2013). Dysphagia in stroke, neurodegenerative disease, and advanced dementia. *Otolaryngol Clin North Am, 46*(16), 1137–1149.
9. American Heart Association. (2011). Stroke. In *Advanced cardiovascular life support (ACLS) provider manual.* Dallas: American Heart Association.
10. American Stroke Association. (2012). *Understanding Risk.* http://www.strokeassociation.org/STROKEORG/AboutStroke/UnderstandingRisk/Understanding-Stroke-Risk_UCM_308539_SubHomePage.jsp.
11. American Heart Association and American Stroke Association. (2015). *Primary stroke center certification: overview sheet.* Dallas TX: AHA/ASA. http://www.heart.org/HEARTORG/HealthcareResearch/Hospital AccreditationCertification/PrimaryStrokeCenterCertification/Primary-Stroke-Center Certification_UCM_439155_SubHomePage.jsp.
12. American Heart Association and American Stroke Association. (2015). *Comprehensive stroke center certification: overview sheet.* Dallas TX: AHA/ASA. http://www.heart.org/idc/groups/heart-public/@wcm/@hcm/@gwtg/documents/downloadable/ucm_456297.pdf.
13. Anderson, J. A. (2014). The golden hour: performing an acute ischemic stroke workup. *Nurs Pract, 39*(9), 22–29.
14. Andrews, C. M., Jauch, E. C., Hemphill, J. C., Smith, W. S., & Weingart, S. D. (2012). Emergency neurologic life support: intracerebral hemorrhage. *Neurocrit Care, 17*, S37–S46.
15. Antonios, N., & Silliman, S. (2013). Treatment of acute ischemic stroke. In K. M. Barrett, & J. F. Meschia (Eds.), *Stroke* (pp. 37–54). West Sussex UK: Wiley-Blackwell.
16. Arboix, A., & Alió, J. (2012). Acute cardioembolic cerebral infarction: answers to clinical questions. *Curr Cardiol Rev, 8*(1), 54–67.
17. Arcot, K., Johnson, J. M., Levy, M. H., & Yoo, A. J. (2013). Neurovascular imaging of the acute stroke patient. In K. M. Barrett, & J. F. Meschia (Eds.), *Stroke* (pp. 16–36). West Sussex UK: Wiley-Blackwell.
18. Baggott, C. D., & Aagaard-Kienitz, B. (2014). Cerebral vasospasm. *Neurosurg Clin North Am, 25*(3), 497–528.
19. Bakker, N. A., Groen, R. J. M., Foumani, M., et al. (2014). Repeat digital subtraction angiography after a negative baseline assessment in nonperimesencephalic subarachnoid hemorrhage: a pooled data meta-analysis. *J Neurosurg, 120*(1), 99–103.
20. Balami, J. S., Chen, R. L., & Buchan, A. M. (2013). Stroke syndromes and clinical management. *QJM, 106*(7), 607–615.
21. Bang, O. Y., Ovbiagele, B., & Kim, J. S. (2014). Evaluation of cryptogenic stroke with advanced diagnostic techniques. *Stroke, 45*(4), 1186–1194.
22. Barrett, K. M., & Meschia, J. F. (2013). Preface. In K. M. Barrett, & J. F. Meschia (Eds.), *Stroke* (p. ix). West Sussex UK: Wiley-Blackwell.
23. Barrett, K. M., & Meschia, J. F. (2013). Appendix: practical clinical stroke scales. In K. M. Barrett, & J. F. Meschia (Eds.), *Stroke* (pp. 153–158). West Sussex UK: Wiley-Blackwell.
24. Bax, L., McFarlane, M., Green, E., Miles, A., et al. (2014). Speech-language pathologist led fiberoptic endoscopic evaluation of swallowing: functional outcomes for patients after stroke. *J Stroke Cerebrovasc Dis, 23*(3), e195–e200.
25. Berry, Z. J., & Barr, Z. B. (2015). Addressing magnetic resonance safety using a modified preoperative time-out approach. *Radiol Technol, 86*(5), 574–579.

26. Bershad, E. M., & Suarez, J. I. (2011). Aneurysmal subarachnoid hemorrhage. In J. P. Mohr, et al. (Ed.), *Stroke: pathophysiology, diagnosis, and management* (5th ed.) (pp. 589–615). Philadelphia: Elsevier Saunders.
27. Biesbroek, J. M., van der Sprenkel, J. W. B., Algra, A., & Rinkel, G. J. E. (2013). Prognosis of acute subdural haematoma from intracranial aneurysm rupture. *J Neurol Neurosurg Psychiatry*, *84*(3), 254–257.
28. Birenbaum, D., Bancroft, L. W., & Felsberg, G. J. (2011). Imaging in acute stroke. *West J Emerg Med*, *12*(1), 67–76.
29. Blacker, D. J. (2003). In-hospital stroke. *Lancet Neurol*, *2*(12), 741–746.
30. Blissitt, P. A., Mitchell, P. H., Newell, D. W., Woods, S. L., & Belza, B. (2006). Cerebrovascular dynamics with head of bed elevation in patients with mild or moderate vasospasm after aneurysmal subarachnoid hemorrhage. *Am J Crit Care*, *15*(2), 206–216.
31. Blissitt, P. A. (2016). Interprofessional teams in stroke care. In J. V. Hickey, & S. L. Livesay (Eds.), *The continuum of stroke care: an interprofessional approach to evidence-based care* (pp. 48–66). Philadelphia: Wolters Kluwer.
32. Bordini, A. L., Luiz, T. F., Fernandes, M., Arruda, W. O., & Teive, H. A. G. (2010). Coma scales: a historical review. *Arq Neuropsiquiatr*, *68*(6), 930–937.
33. Bor-Seng-Shu, E., Kita, W. S., Figueiredo, E. G., et al. (2012). Cerebral hemodynamics: concepts of clinical importance. *Arq Neuropsiquiatria*, *70*(5), 352–356.
34. Brain Trauma Foundation, American Association of Neurological Surgeons. (2003). *Guidelines for the management of severe traumatic brain injury update: cerebral perfusion pressure* (3rd ed.). New York: Brain Trauma Foundation. https://www.braintrauma.org/uploads/06/06/Guidelines_Management_2007w_bookmarks_2.pdf.
35. Brathwaite, S., & Macdonald, R. L. (2014). Current management of delayed cerebral ischemia: update from results of recent clinical trials. *Translational stroke research*, 5(2), 207–226.
36. Brott, T. G., Halperin, J. L., Abbara, S., et al. (2011). ASA/ACCF/AHA/AANN/AANS/ACR/ASNR/CNS/SAIP/SCAI/SIR/SNIS/SVM/SVS Guideline on the management of patients with extracranial carotid and vertebral artery disease: executive summary. *Catheter Cardiovasc Interv*, *81*(1), E76–E123.
37. Brott, T. G., Halperin, J. L., Abbara, S., et al. (2011). ASA/ACCF/AHA/AANN/AANS/ACR/ASNR/CNS/SAIP/SCAI/SIR/SNIS/SVM/SVS Guideline on the management of patients with extracranial carotid and vertebral artery disease: executive summary. *Vasc Med*, *16*(1), 35–77.
38. Budohoski, K. P., Guilfoyle, M., Hlemy, A., et al. (2014). The pathophysiology and treatment of delayed cerebral ischaemia following subarachnoid haemorrhage. *J Neurol Neurosurg Psychiatry*, *85*(12), 1343–1353.
39. Burns, J. D., Green, D. M., Metivier, K., & DeFusco, C. (2012). Intensive care management of acute ischemic stroke. *Emerg Med Clin North Am*, *30*(13), 713–744.
40. Busby, L., Owada, K., Dhungana, S., et al. (2015). CODE FAST: a quality improvement initiative to reduce door-to-needle times. *J Neurointerv Surg*, *0*, 1–4. http://dx.doi.org/10.1136/neurintsurg-2015-011806.
41. Cameron, V. (2013). Best practices for stroke patient and family education in the acute care setting: a literature review. *Medsurg Nurs*, *22*(1), 51–55.
42. Canhão, P., & Ferro, J. M. (2012). Presentation and management of acute cerebral venous thrombosis. In E. M. Manno (Ed.), *Emergency management in neurocritical care* (pp. 99–107). West Sussex UK: Wiley-Blackwell.
43. Caplan, J. M., Colby, G. P., Coon, A. L., Huang, J., & Tamargo, R. J. (2013). Managing subarachnoid hemorrhage in the neurocritical care unit. *Neurosurg Clin North Am*, *24*(3), 321–337.
44. Caplan, L. R. (2015). Lacunar infarction and small vessel disease: pathology and pathophysiology. *J Stroke*, *17*(1), 2–6.
45. Castellanos, M., Weksler, B. B., & Benavente, O. R. (2011). Antiplatelet therapy for secondary prevention of stroke. In J. P. Mohr, P. A. Wolf, J. C. Grotta, M. A. Moskowitz, M. R. Mayberg, & R. von Kummer (Eds.), *Stroke: pathophysiology, diagnosis, and management* (5th ed.) (pp. 1147–1172). Philadelphia: Elsevier Saunders.
46. Cavanagh, S. J., & Gordon, V. L. (2002). Grading scales used in the management of aneurysmal subarachnoid hemorrhage: a critical review. *J Neurosci Nurs*, *34*(6), 288–295.
47. Chalouhi, N., Hoh, B. L., & Hasan, D. (2013). Review of cerebral aneurysm formation, growth, and rupture. *Stroke*, *44*, 3613–3622.
48. Chan, S., & Hemphill, J. C. (2014). Critical care management of intracerebral hemorrhage. *Crit Care Clin*, *30*(14), 699–717.
49. Chapman, S. N., Mehndiratta, P., Johansen, M. C., McMurry, T. L., Jonston, K. C., & Southerland, A. M. (2014). Current perspectives on the use of intravenous recombinant tissue plasminogen activator (tPA) for treatment of acute ischemic stroke. *Vasc Health Risk Manag*, *10*, 75–87.
50. Chen, J. Y., Zhang, A. D., Lu, H. Y., Guo, J., Wang, F. F., & Li, Z. C. (2013). $CHADS_2$ versus CHA_2DS_2-VASc score in assessing the stroke and thromboembolism risk stratification in patients with atrial fibrillation: a systematic review and meta-analysis. *J Geriatr Cardiol*, *10*(3), 258–266.
51. Chen, S., Li, Q., Wu, H., Krafft, P., Wang, Z., & Zhang, J. H. (2014). The harmful effects of subarachnoid hemorrhage on extracerebral organs. *Biomed Res Int*, 858496. http://dx.doi.org/10.1155/2014/858496.
52. Cheung, R. T., & Zou, L. Y. (2002). Use of the original, modified, or new intracerebral hemorrhage score to predict mortality and morbidity after intracerebral hemorrhage. *Stroke*, *34*(7), 1717–1722.
53. Chumney, D., Nollinger, K., Shesko, K., Skop, K., Spencer, M., & Newton, R. A. (2010). Ability of Functional Independence Measure to accurately predict functional outcomes of stroke-specific population: systematic review. *J Rehabil Res Dev*, *47*(1), 17–29.
54. Ciet, P., & Litmanovich, D. E. (2014). MR safety issues particular to women. *Magn Reson Imaging Clin N Am*, *23*(1), 59–67.
55. Connolly, E. S., Rabinstein, A. A., Carhuapoma, J. R., et al. (2012). Guidelines for the management of aneurysmal subarachnoid hemorrhage. *Stroke*, *43*(6), 1711–1737.
56. Coppadoro, A., & Citerio, G. (2011). Subarachnoid hemorrhage: an update for the intensivist. *Minerva Anestesiol*, *77*(1), 74–84.
57. Coull, B. M., & Drake, K. (2011). Coagulation abnormalities in stroke. In J. P. Mohr, et al. (Ed.), *Stroke: pathophysiology, diagnosis, and management* (5th ed.) (pp. 772–789). Philadelphia: Elsevier Saunders.
58. Crownover, B. K., & Bepko, J. L. (2013). Appropriate and safe use of diagnostic imaging. *Am Fam Physician*, *87*(7), 494–501.
59. Culebras, A. (2015). Sleep apnea and stroke. *Curr Neurol Neurosci Rep*, *15*(1), 503. http://dx.doi.org/10.1007/s11910-014-0503-3.
60. Cumbler, E., & Simpson, J. (2015). Code Stroke: multicenter experience with in-hospital stroke alerts. *J Hosp Med*, *10*(3), 179–183.
61. Cumming, T. B., Marshall, R. S., & Lazar, R. M. (2013). Stroke, cognitive deficits, and rehabilitation: still an incomplete picture. *Int J Stroke*, *8*(1), 38–45.
62. Dabus, G., & Nogueira, R. G. (2013). Current options for the management of aneurysmal subarachnoid hemorrhage-induced cerebral vasospasm: a comprehensive review of the literature. *Int Neurol*, *2*, 30–51.
63. Daelen, S. V., Peetermans, M., Vanassche, T., Verhamme, P., & Vandermeulen, E. (2015). Monitoring and reversal strategies for new oral anticoagulants. *Expert Rev Cardiovasc Ther*, *13*(1), 95–103.
64. D'Amore, C., & Paciaron, M. (2012). Border-zone and watershed infarctions. *Front Neurol Neurosci*, *30*, 181–184.
65. Datar, S., & Rabinstein, A. A. (2014). Cerebellar infarction. *Neurol Clin*, *32*(4), 979–991.
66. Favaloro, E. J., & Lippi, G. (2015). Laboratory testing in the era of direct or non-vitamin K antagonist oral anticoagulants: a practical guide to measuring their activity and avoiding diagnostic errors. *Semin Thromb Hemost*, *41*(2), 208–227.
67. de Man-van Ginkel, J. M., Gooskens, F., Schepers, V. P. M., Schuumans, M. J., Lindeman, E., & Hafsteinsdóttir, T. B. (2012). Screening for post-stroke depression using the patient health questionnaire. *Nurs Res*, *61*(5), 333–341.
68. de Man-van Ginkel, J. M., Hafsteinsdóttir, T., Lindeman, E., Burger, H., Grobbee, D., & Schuurmans, M. (2012). An efficient way to detect post-

stroke depression by subsequent administration of a 9-item and 2-item patient health questionnaire. *Stroke, 43*(3), 854–856.
69. Diedler, J., Sykora, M., & Hacke, W. (2011). Critical care of the patient with acute stroke. In J. P. Mohr, et al. (Ed.), *Stroke: pathophysiology, diagnosis, and management* (5th ed.) (pp. 1008–1048). Philadelphia: Elsevier Saunders.
70. Diedler, J., Santos, E., Poli, S., & Sykora, M. (2014). Optimal cerebral perfusion pressure in patients with intracerebral hemorrhage: an observational case series. *Crit Care, 18*(2), R51. http://ccforum.com/content/18/2/R51.
71. Diringer, M. N., Bleck, T. P., Hemphill, J. C., et al. (2011). Critical care management of patients following aneurysmal subarachnoid hemorrhage: recommendation from the Neurocritical Care Society's multidisciplinary consensus conference. *Neurocrit Care, 15*(2), 211–240.
72. Dlamini, N., & Kirkham, F. J. (2009). Stroke and cerebrovascular disorders. *Curr Opin Pediatr, 21*(6), 751–761.
73. Dobkin, B. H. (2011). Rehabilitation and recovery of the patient with stroke. In J. P. Mohr, et al. (Ed.), *Stroke: pathophysiology, diagnosis, and management* (5th ed.) (pp. 1116–1133). Philadelphia: Elsevier Saunders.
74. Drake, C. G. (1998). Report of the World Federation of Neurological Surgeons Committee on a Universal Subarachnoid Hemorrhage Grading Scale. *J Neurosurg, 68*, 985–986.
75. Dupre, C. M., Libman, R., Dupre, S. I., Katz, J. M., Rybinnik, I., & Kwiatkowski, T. (2014). Stroke chameleons. *J Stroke Cerebrovasc Dis, 23*(2), 374–378.
76. Dyne, P. L., & Waxman, M. A. (2011). Comorbid diseases in pregnancy. In J. E. Tintinalli, et al. (Ed.), *Tintinalli's emergency medicine: a comprehensive study guide* (7th ed.) (pp. 684–690). New York: McGraw-Hill.
77. Easton, J. D., Saver, J. L., Alberts, G. W., et al. (2009). Definition and evaluation of transient ischemic attack. *Stroke, 40*(6), 2276–2293.
78. Eckerle, B. J., & Southerland, A. M. (2013). Bedside evaluation of the acute stroke patient. In K. M. Barrett, & J. F. Meschia (Eds.), *Stroke* (pp. 1–15). West Sussex UK: Wiley-Blackwell.
79. Edholm, K., Ragle, N., & Rondina, M. T. (2015). Antithrombotic management of atrial fibrillation in the elderly. *Med Clin North Am, 99*(2), 417–430.
80. Edlow, J. A., Samuels, O., Smith, W. S., & Weingart, S. D. (2012). Emergency neurological life support: subarachnoid hemorrhage. *Neurocrit Care, 17*(Suppl. 1), S47–S53.
81. Edlow, J. A., Figaji, A., & Samuels, O. (2015). Emergency neurologic life support: subarachnoid hemorrhage. *Neurocrit Care, 23*(Suppl. 2), S103–S109.
82. Edmonds, H. L., Isley, M. R., Sloan, T. B., Alexandrove, A. V., & Razumovsky, A. Y. (2011). American Society of Neurophysiologic Monitor and the American Society of Neuroimaging joint guidelines for transcranial doppler ultrasonic monitoring. *J Neuroimaging, 21*(2), 177–183.
83. Eerenberg, E. S., Kamphuisen, P. W., Sijpkens, M. K., Meijers, J. C., Buller, H. R., & Levi, M. (2011). Reversal of rivaroxaban and dabigatran by prothrombin complex concentrate: a randomized, placebo-controlled, crossover study in healthy subjects. *Circulation, 124*(14), 1573–1579.
84. Egashira, Y., Xi, G., Chaudhary, N., Hua, Y., & Pandey, A. S. (2015). Acute brain injury after subarachnoid hemorrhage. *World Neurosurg, 84*(1), 22–25.
85. Elhammady, M. S., Heros, R. C., & Morcos, J. J. (2011). Surgical management of asymptomatic carotid stenosis. In J. P. Mohr, P. A. Wolf, J. C. Grotta, M. A. Moskowitz, M. R. Mayberg, & R. von Kummer (Eds.), *Stroke: pathophysiology, diagnosis, and management* (5th ed.) (pp. 1403–1416). Philadelphia: Elsevier Saunders.
86. Eller, J. L., Snyder, K. V., Siddiqui, A. H., Levy, E. I., & Hopkins, L. N. (2014). Endovascular treatment of carotid stenosis. *Neurosurg Clin North Am, 25*(3), 565–582.
87. Epple, C., & Steiner, T. (2015). Acute stroke in patients on new direct oral anticoagulants: how to manage; how to treat? *Expert Opin Pharmacother, 15*(14), 1991–2001.
88. Fahy, B. G., & Sivaraman, V. (2002). Current concepts in neurocritical care. *Anesthesiol Clin North Am, 20*(2), 441–462.
89. Feoktistov, A., & Diamond, M. (2014). Diagnosing and understanding adult headache. *Otolaryngol Clin North Am, 47*(2), 175–185.
90. Ferro, J. M., & Canhão, P. (2011). Cerebral venous thrombosis. In J. P. Mohr, P. A. Wolf, J. C. Grotta, M. A. Moskowitz, M. R. Mayberg, & R. von Kummer (Eds.), *Stroke: pathophysiology, diagnosis, and management* (5th ed.) (pp. 516–530). Philadelphia: Elsevier Saunders.
91. Filippidis, A., Kapsalaki, E., Patramani, G., & Fountas, K. N. (2009). Cerebral venous sinus thrombosis: review of the demographics, pathophysiology, current diagnosis, and treatment. *Neurosurg Focus, 27*(5), E3. http://dx.doi.org/10.3171/2009.8.FOCUS09167.
92. Fink, M. E. (2012). Osmotherapy for intracranial hypertension: mannitol versus hypertonic saline. *Continuum (Minneapolis Minn), 18*(3), 640–654.
93. Fiorella, D., Zuckerman, S. L., Khan, I. S., Ganesh, N. K., & Mocco, J. (2015). Intracerebral hemorrhage: a common and devastating disease in need of better treatment. *World Neurosurg, 84*(4), 1136–1441.
94. Fischer, J., & Mathieson, C. (2001). The history of the Glasgow Coma Scale: implications for practice. *Crit Care Nurs Q, 23*(4), 52–58.
95. Reference was deleted in page proofs.
96. Fitzgerald, M. J. T., Gruener, G., & Mtui, E. (2012). Cerebrovascular disease. In *Clinical neuroanatomy and neuroscience* (6th ed.) (pp. 377–391). Philadelphia: Saunders Elsevier.
97. Flemming, K. D. (2013). Diagnosis of stroke mechanisms and secondary prevention. In K. M. Barrett, & J. F. Meschia (Eds.), *Stroke* (pp. 55–77). West Sussex UK: Wiley-Blackwell.
98. Flower, O., & Hellings, S. (2012). Sedation in traumatic brain injury. *Emerg Med Int*, 637171. http://dx.doi.org/10/1155/2012/637171.
99. Förster, A., Szabo, K., & Hennerici, M. G. (2008). Mechanisms of disease: pathophysiological concepts of stroke in hemodynamic risk zones-do hypoperfusion and embolism interact? *Nat Clin Pract Neurol, 4*(4), 216–225.
100. Frontera, J. A., & Ahmed, W. (2014). Neurocritical care complications of pregnancy and puerperium. *J Crit Care, 29*(6), 1069–1081.
101. Frontera, J. A., Lewin, J. J., Rabinstein, A. A., et al. (2015). Guideline for reversal of antithrombotics in intracranial hemorrhage. A statement for healthcare professionals from the Neurocritical Care Society and Society of Critical Care Medicine. *Neurocrit Care, 24*(1), 6–46.
102. Frontera, J., Ziai, W., O'Phelan, K., et al. (2015). Regional brain monitoring in the neurocritical care unit. *Neurocrit Care, 22*(3), 348–359.
103. Fugate, J. E., & Rabinstein, A. A. (2012). Intensive care unit management of aneurysmal subarachnoid hemorrhage. *Curr Neurol Neurosci Rep, 12*(1), 1–9.
104. Fugate, J. E., & Rabenstein, A. A. (2014). Update on intravenous recombinant tissue plasminogen activator for acute ischemic stroke. *Mayo Clin Proc, 89*(7), 960–972.
105. Gahart, B. L., & Nazareno, A. R. (2015). *2015 Intravenous medications* (31st ed.). St. Louis: Elsevier.
106. Galvin, R., Geraghty, C., Motterlini, N., Dimitrov, B. D., & Fahey, T. (2011). Prognostic value of the ABCD^2 clinical prediction rule: a systematic review and meta-analysis. *Fam Pract, 28*(4), 366–376.
107. Gebel, J. M. (2012). Neurocritical care of intracerebral hemorrhage. In E. M. Manno (Ed.), *Emergency management of neurocritical care* (pp. 55–62). West Sussex UK: Wiley-Blackwell.
108. George, P. M., & Steinberg, G. K. (2015). Novel stroke therapeutics: unraveling stroke pathophysiology and its impact on clinical treatments. *Neuron, 87*(2), 297–309.
109. Ghandehari, K. (2013). Challenging comparison of stroke scales. *J Res Med Sci, 18*(10), 906–910.
110. Gigante, P. R., Hwang, B. Y., & Connolly, E. S. (2012). External ventricular drain management and ventriculoperitoneal shunt. In K. Lee (Ed.), *The neuro ICU book* (pp. 411–426). New York: McGraw-Hill.
111. Giles, M. F., & Rothwell, P. M. (2008). Risk prediction after TIA: the ABCD system and other methods. *Geriatrics, 63*(10), 10–13, 16.
112. Gocan, S., & Fisher, A. (2008). Neurologic assessment by nurses using the National Institutes of Health Stroke Scale: implementation of best practice guidelines. *Can J Neurosci Nurs, 30*(3), 31–42.
113. Goldstein, L. B., & Sacco, R. L. (2011). Primary prevention of stroke. In J. P. Mohr (Ed.), *Stroke: pathophysiology, diagnosis, and management* (5th ed.) (pp. 242–251). Philadelphia: Elsevier Saunders.
114. Gomes, J. A., & Manno, E. (2013). New developments in the treatment of intracerebral hemorrhage. *Neurol Clin, 31*(3), 721–735.

115. Gonzales, N. R., & Grotta, J. C. (2011). Pharmacologic modification of acute cerebral ischemia. In J. P. Mohr, P. A. Wolf, J. C. Grotta, et al. (Eds.), *Stroke: pathophysiology, diagnosis, and management* (5th ed.) (pp. 1049–1083). Philadelphia: Elsevier Saunders.
116. Goralnick, E., & Bontempo, L. J. (2015). Atrial fibrillation. *Emerg Med Clin North Am, 33*(3), 597–612.
117. Gould, B., McCourt, R., Asdaghi, N., et al. (2013). Autoregulation of cerebral blood flow is preserved in primary intracerebral hemorrhage. *Stroke, 44*(6), 1726–1728.
118. Granger, C. V., Cotter, A. C., Hamilton, B. B., Fiedler, R. B., et al. (1993). Functional assessment scales: a study of persons with stroke. *Arch Phys Med Rehabil, 74*, 133–138.
119. Greer, D. M., Homma, S., & Furie, K. L. (2011). Cardiac diseases. In *Stroke: pathophysiology, diagnosis, and management*(5th ed.) (pp. 814–827). Philadelphia: Elsevier Saunders.
120. Grise, E. M., & Adeoye, O. (2012). Blood pressure control for acute ischemic and hemorrhagic stroke. *Curr Opin Crit Care, 18*(2), 132–138.
121. Grisold, W., Oberndorfer, S., & Struha, W. (2009). Stroke and cancer: a review. *Acta Neurol Scand, 119*(1), 1–16.
122. Gross, B. A., & Du, R. (2012). Vasospasm after arteriovenous malformation rupture. *World Neurosurg, 78*(3-4), 300–305.
123. Gross, H., et al. (2012). Emergency Neurologic Life Support: acute ischemic stroke. *Neurocrit Care, 17*(Suppl. 1), S29–S36.
124. Gross, H., Guilliams, K. P., & Sung, G. (2015). Emergency Neurologic Life Support: acute ischemic stroke. *Neurocrit Care, 23*(Suppl. 2), S94–S102.
125. Groysman, L., & Sung, G. (2012). Acute management of cerebral ischemia. In E. M. Manno (Ed.), *Emergency management of neurocritical care* (pp. 45–54). West Sussex UK: Wiley-Blackwell.
126. Guey, S., Tournier-Lasserve, E., Hervé, D., & Kossorotoff, M. (2015). Moyamoya disease and syndromes: from genetics to clinical management. *Appl Clin Genet, 8*, 49–68.
127. Gupta, R. (2012). Care of the interventional patient in the neurointensive care unit. In E. M. Manno (Ed.), *Emergency management of neurocritical care* (pp. 84–91). West Sussex UK: Wiley-Blackwell.
128. Hackett, M. L., & Pickles, K. (2014). Part I: Frequency of depression after stroke: an updated systematic review and meta-analysis of observational studies. *Int J Stroke, 9*(8), 1017–1025.
129. Hafez, S., Coucha, M., Bruno, A., Fagan, S. C., & Ergul, A. (2014). Hyperglycemia, acute ischemic stroke, and thrombolytic therapy. *Transl Stroke Res, 5*(4), 442–453.
130. Haque, R., Crisman, C., Hwang, B., Connolly, E. S., & Meyers, P. M. (2012). Endovascular surgical neuroradiology. In K. Lee (Ed.), *The neuro ICU book* (pp. 358–384). New York: McGraw-Hill.
131. Helal, I., Reed, B., Mettler, P., et al. (2012). Prevalence of cardiovascular events in patients with autosomal dominant polycystic kidney disease. *Am Nephrol, 36*(4), 362–370.
132. Helbok, R., Kurtz, P., & Claassen, J. (2012). Multimodality monitoring. In K. Lee (Ed.), *The neuro ICU book* (pp. 253–267). New York: McGraw-Hill.
133. Hemphill, J. C., Bonovich, D. C., Besmertis, L., Manley, G. T., & Johnston, S. C. (2001). The ICH score: a simple, reliable grading scale for intracerebral hemorrhage. *Stroke, 32*(4), 891–897.
134. Hemphill, J. C., Newman, J., Zhao, S., & Johnston, S. C. (2004). Hospital usage of early do-not- resuscitate orders and outcome after intracerebral hemorrhage. *Stroke, 35*(5), 1130–1134.
135. Hemphill, J. C., Greenberg, S. M., Anderson, C. S., et al. (2015). Guidelines for the management of spontaneous intracerebral hemorrhage. *Stroke, 46*(7), 2032–2060.
136. Holloway, R. G., Arnold, R. M., Creutzfeldt, C. J., et al. (2014). Palliative and end-of-life care in stroke. A statement for the health care professionals from the American Heart Association/American Stroke Association. *Stroke, 45*(6), 1887–1916.
137. Hunt, W. E., & Hess, R. M. (1968). Surgical risk as related to time of intervention in the repair of intracranial aneurysms. *J Neurosurg, 28*(1), 14–20.
138. Hurwitz, A., Massone, R., & Lopez, B. L. (2014). Acquired bleeding disorders. *Emerg Med Clin North Am, 32*(3), 691–713.
139. Hwang, B. Y., Appelboom, G., Kellner, C. P., et al. (2010). Clinical grading scales in intracerebral hemorrhage. *Neurocritical Care, 13*(1), 141–151.
140. Hwang, D. Y., Matouk, C. C., & Sheth, K. N. (2013). Management of the malignant middle cerebral artery syndrome. *Semin Neurol, 33*(5) 448–455.
141. Januszewich, L., & Buesch, B. (2014). Neurologic disorders and therapeutic management. In L. D. Urden, K. M. Stacy, & M. E. Lough (Eds.), *Critical care nursing: diagnosis and management* (7th ed.) (pp. 646–680). St. Louis: Elsevier.
142. Jauch, E. C., Saver, J. L., Adams, H. P., et al. (2013). Guidelines for the early management of patients with acute ischemic stroke: a guideline for healthcare professionals from the American Heart Association/American Stroke Association. *Stroke, 44*(3), 870–947.
143. Jauch, E. C., Pineda, J. A., & Hemphill, J. C. (2015). Emergency neurologic life support: intracerebral hemorrhage. *Neurocrit Care, 23*(Suppl. 2), S83–S93.
144. Jeon, S. B., Koh, Y., Choi, H. A., & Lee, K. (2014). Critical care for patients with massive ischemic stroke. *J Stroke, 16*(3), 146–160.
145. Johnston, S. C., Rothwell, P. M., Nguuyen-Huynh, M. N., et al. (2007). Validation and refinement of scores to predict very early stroke risk after transient ischaemic attack. *Lancet, 369*(9558), 283–292.
146. Jordan, J. D., & Powers, W. J. (2012). Cerebral autoregulation and acute ischemic stroke. *Am J Hypertens, 25*(9), 946–950.
147. Jordan, J. D., Mortbitzer, K. A., & Rhoney, D. H. (2015). Acute treatment of blood pressure after ischemic stroke and intracerebral hemorrhage. *Neurol Clin, 33*(2), 361–380.
148. Kalanuria, A., Armonda, R. A., & Razumovsky, A. (2013). Use of transcranial Doppler ultrasound in the neurocritical care unit. *Neurosurg Clin North Am, 24*(3), 441–456.
149. Kalaria, C., Nyquist, P. A., & Kittner, S. (2015). The therapeutic value of laboratory testing for hypercoagulable states in secondary stroke prevention. *Neurol Clin, 33*(2), 501–513.
150. Kallmünzer, B., & Kollmar, R. (2011). Temperature management in stroke: an unsolved, but important topic. *Cerebrovasc Dis, 31*(6), 532–543.
151. Kanal, E., Barkovich, A. J., Bell, C., et al. (2013). ACR guidance document on MR safe practices: 2013. *J Mag Res Imaging, 37*(3), 501–530.
152. Kapadia, A., Schweizer, T. A., Spears, J., Cusimano, M., & Macdonald, R. L. (2014). Nonaneurysmal perimesencephalic subarachnoid hemorrhage: Diagnosis, pathophysiology, clinical characteristics, and long-term outcome. *World Neurosurg, 82*(6), 1131–1143.
153. Kasner, S. E. (2006). Clinical interpretation and use of stroke scales. *Lancet Neurol, 5*(7), 603–612.
154. Kaste, M., & Roine, R. O. (2011). General stroke management and stroke units. In J. P. Mohr, P. A. Wolf, J. C. Grotta, M. A. Moskowitz, M. R. Mayberg, & R. von Kummer (Eds.), *Stroke: pathophysiology, diagnosis, and management* (5th ed.) (pp. 992–1007). Philadelphia: Elsevier Saunders.
155. Kellner, C., Piazza, M., Appelboom, G., & Connolly, E. S. (2012). Carotid revascularization and EC-IC Bypass. In K. Lee (Ed.), *The neuro ICU book* (pp. 427–437). New York: McGraw-Hill.
156. Kernan, W. N., Ovbiagele, B., Black, H. R., et al. (2014). Guidelines for the prevention of stroke in patients with stroke and transient ischemic attack. *Stroke, 45*(7), 2160–2236.
157. Khatri, P. (2014). Evaluation and management of the acute ischemic stroke. *Continuum (Minneap Minn), 20*(2), 283–295.
158. Kidwell, C. S., & Jahan, R. (2015). Endovascular treatment of acute ischemic stroke. *Neurol Clin, 33*(2), 401–420.
159. Kim, H., Pawlikowska, L., & Young, W. L. (2011). Genetics and vascular biology of brain vascular malformations. In J. P. Mohr, et al. (Ed.), *Stroke: pathophysiology, diagnosis, and management* (5th ed.) (pp. 169–186). Philadelphia: Elsevier Saunders.
160. Kim, A. S. (2014). Evaluation and prevention of cardioembolic stroke. *Continuum (Minneap Minn), 20*(2), 309–322.
161. Kirkman, M. A., Citerio, G., & Smith, M. (2014). The intensive care management of acute ischemic stroke: an overview. *Intensive Care Med, 40*(5), 640–655.

162. Kistka, H., Dewan, M. C., & Mocco, J. (2013). Evidence-based cerebral vasospasm surveillance. *Neurol Res Int,* 256713. http://dx.doi.org/10.1155/2013/256713.
163. Kizior, R. J., & Hodgson, B. B. (2015). *Saunders nursing drug handbook 2015.* St. Louis: Elsevier.
164. Kocak, Y., Ozturk, S., Ege, F., & Ekmekci, A. H. (2012). A useful new coma scale in acute stroke patients: FOUR Score. *Anaesth Intensive Care, 40*(1), 131–136.
165. Komar, M., Olszowska, M., Przewlocki, T., et al. (2014). Transcranial Doppler ultrasonography should it be the first choice for persistent foramen ovale screening. *Cardiovasc Ultrasound, 12*(16). http://www.cardiovascularultrasound.com/content/12/1/16.
166. Kornbluth, J., & Bhardwaj, A. (2011). Evaluation of coma: a critical appraisal of popular scoring systems. *Neurocrit Care, 14*(1), 134–143.
167. Kothari, R. U., Brott, T., Broderick, J. P., et al. (1996). The ABCs of measuring intracerebral hemorrhage volume. *Stroke, 27*(8), 1304–1305.
168. Kramer, A. H. (2013). Treatment of hemorrhagic stroke. In K. M. Barrett, & J. F. Meschia (Eds.), *Stroke* (pp. 78–102). West Sussex UK: Wiley-Blackwell.
169. Kroenke, K., Spitzer, R. L., Williams, J. B. W. (2001). The PHQ-9:validity of a brief depression severity measure. *J Gen Int Med,* 16(9), 606–613.
170. Kung, D. K., Chalouhi, N., Jabbour, P. M., et al. (2013). Cerebral blood flow dynamics and head-of-bed changes in the setting of subarachnoid hemorrhage. *Biomed Res Int.* http://dx.doi.org/10.1155/2013/640638.
171. Kunz, A., Dirnagl, U., & Mergenthaler, P. (2010). Acute pathophysiological processes after ischemia and traumatic brain injury. *Best Pract Res Clin Anesthesiol, 24*(4), 495–509.
172. Kutlubaev, M. A., & Hackett, M. L. (2014). Part II: predictors of depression after stroke and impact of depression on stroke outcome: an update systematic review of observational studies. *Int J Stroke, 9*(8), 1026–1036.
173. Lakhan, S. E., & Pamplona, F. (2012). Application of mild therapeutic hypothermia on stroke: a systematic review and meta-analysis. *Stroke Res Treat.* http://dx.doi.org/10.1155/2012/295906.
174. Lawton, M. T., Kim, H., McCulloch, C. E., Mikhak, B., & Young, W. L. (2010). A supplementary grading scale for selecting patients with brain arteriovenous malformations for surgery. *Neurosurgery, 66*(4), 702–713.
175. Lee, K. (2012). Subarachnoid hemorrhage. In K. Lee (Ed.), *The neuro ICU book* (pp. 1–34). New York: McGraw-Hill.
176. Leiva-Salinas, C., Smith, W., & Wintermark, M. (2012). Application of MR diffusion, CT angiography, and perfusion imaging in stroke neurocritical care. In E. M. Manno (Ed.), *Emergency management of neurocritical care* (pp. 207–213). West Sussex UK: Wiley Blackwell.
177. Lindgren, A. (2014). Stroke genetics: a review and update. *J Stroke, 16*(3), 114–123.
178. Lip, G. Y., & Halperin, J. L. (2010). Improving stroke risk stratification in atrial fibrillation. *Am J Med, 123*(6), 484–488.
179. Liu, Q., Ding, Y., Yan, P., Zhang, J. H., & Lei, H. (2011). Electrocardiographic abnormalities in patients with intracerebral hemorrhage. *Acta Neurochir Suppl, 111,* 353–356.
180. Long, X., Jingsheng, L., & Jizong, Z. (2013). Different grading scales for spontaneous subarachnoid hemorrhage and health-related quality evaluations. *World Neurosurg, 80*(6), 808–809.
181. Lyons, O. D., & Ryan, C. M. (2015). Sleep apnea and stroke. *Can J Cardiol, 31*(7), 981–927.
182. Maas, M. B., Berman, M. D., Guth, J. C., Liotta, E. M., Prabhakaran, S., & Naidech, A. M. (2015). Neurochecks as a biomarker of the temporal profile and clinical impact of neurologic changes after intracerebral hemorrhage. *J Stroke Cerebrovasc Dis, 24*(9), 2026–2031.
183. Macellari, F., Paciaron, M., Agnelli, G., & Caso, V. (2014). Neuroimaging in intracerebral hemorrhage. *Stroke, 45,* 903–908.
184. Malik, G. M., & Bhangoo, S. S. (2012). Vascular malformations (arteriovenous malformations) and dural arteriovenous fistulas. In R. G. Ellenbogen, S. I. Abdulrauf, & L. N. Sekhar (Eds.), *Principles of neurological surgery* (3rd ed.) (pp. 229–247). Philadelphia: Elsevier Saunders.
185. Mangla, R., Kolar, B., Almast, J., & Ekholm, S. E. (2011). Border zone infarcts: pathophysiologic and imaging characteristics. *Radiographics, 31,* 1201–1214.
186. Manno, E. M. (2012). Hypothermia: application and use in neurocritical care. In E. M. Manno (Ed.), *Emergency management in neurocritical care* (pp. 188–196). West Sussex UK: Wiley-Blackwell.
187. Manno, E. M. (2012). New treatment strategies in the management of large hemispheric strokes and intracerebral hemorrhages. In E. M. Manno (Ed.), *Emergency management in neurocritical care* (pp. 92–98). West Sussex UK: Wiley-Blackwell.
188. Manno, E. M. (2012). Update on intracerebral hemorrhage. *Continuum, (Minneap Minn), 18*(3), 598–610.
189. Mauldin, K. (2014). Nutrition alterations and management. In L. D. Urden, K. M. Stacy, & M. E. Lough (Eds.), *Critical care nursing: diagnosis and management* (7th ed.) (pp. 115–142). St. Louis: Elsevier.
190. Meader, N., Moe-Byrene, T., Llewellyn, A., & Mitchell, A. J. (2014). Screening for poststroke major depression: a meta-analysis of diagnostic validity studies. *J Neurol Neurosurg Psych, 85*(2), 198–206.
191. Meairs, S., Hennerici, M., & Mohr, J. P. (2011). Ultrasonography. In J. P. Mohr, et al. (Ed.), *Stroke: pathophysiology, diagnosis, and management* (5th ed.) (pp. 831–869). Philadelphia: Elsevier Saunders.
192. Mehdi, Z., Birns, J., & Bhalla, A. (2013). Post-stroke urinary incontinence. *Int J Clin Pract, 67*(11), 1126–1137.
193. Meschia, J. F., Bushnell, C., Boden-Albala, B., et al. (2014). Guidelines for the primary prevention of stroke. *Stroke, 45*(12), 3754–3832.
194. Metheny, N. A., & Frantz, R. A. (2013). Head-of-bed elevation in critically ill patients: a review. *Crit Care Nurs, 33*(31), 53–66.
195. Miller, E. L., Murray, L., Richards, L., et al. (2010). Comprehensive overview of nursing and interdisciplinary rehabilitation care of the stroke patient. *Stroke, 41*(10), 2402–2448.
196. Miller, B. A., Turan, N., Chau, M., & Pradilla, G. (2014). Inflammation, vasospasm, and brain injury after subarachnoid hemorrhage. *Biomed Res Int.* http://dx.doi.org/10.1155/2014/384342.
197. Miyamoto, S., Yoshimoto, T., Hashimoto, N., et al. (2014). Effects of extracranial-intracranial bypass for patients with hemorrhagic moyamoya disease. *Stroke, 45*(5), 1415–1421.
198. Moatti, Z., Gupta, M., Yadava, R., & Thamban, S. (2014). A review of stroke and pregnancy: incidence, management and prevention. *Eur J Obstet Gynecol Reproduct Biol, 181,* 20–27.
199. Mocco, J., Kim, S. H., Bendok, B. R., Boulos, A. S., Hopkins, L. N., & Levy, E. I. (2011). Interventional neuroradiology therapy of atherosclerotic disease and vascular formations. In J. P. Mohr, P. A. Wolf, J. C. Grotta, M. A. Moskowitz, M. R. Mayberg, & R. von Kummer (Eds.), *Stroke: pathophysiology, diagnosis, and management* (5th ed.) (pp. 1204–1225). Philadelphia: Elsevier Saunders.
200. Mohammed, I., Syed, W., & Kowey, P. R. (2013). Oral anticoagulants to reduce the risk of stroke in atrial fibrillation: how should a clinician choose? *Clin Cardiol, 38*(11), 663–670.
201. Mohr, J. P., Lazar, R. M., & Marshall, R. S. (2011). Middle cerebral artery disease. In J. P. Mohr, et al. (Ed.), *Stroke: pathophysiology, diagnosis, and management* (5th ed.) (pp. 382–424). Philadelphia: Elsevier Saunders.
202. Mok, V., & Kim, J. S. (2015). Prevention and management of cerebral small vessel disease. *J Stroke, 17*(2), 111–122.
203. Mokin, M., Khalessi, A. A., Mocco, J., et al. (2014). Endovascular treatment of acute ischemic stroke: the end or just the beginning? *Neurosurg Focus, 36*(1), E5.
204. Morr, S., Lin, N., & Siddiqui, A. H. (2014). Carotid artery stenting: current and emerging options. *Med Devices (Auckl), 7,* 343–355.
205. Mozaffarian, D., Benjamin, E. J., Go, A. S., et al. (2015). Heart disease and stroke statistics—2015 update: a report from the American Heart Association. *Circulation, 131*(4), 29–322.
206. Mozaffarian, D., Benjamin, E. J., Go, A. S., et al. (2016). Executive summary: heart disease and stroke statistics—2016 update: a report from the American Heart Association. *Circulation, 133,* 447–454.
207. Muzevich, K. M., & Voils, A. S. (2009). Role of vasopressor administration in patients with acute neurologic injury. *Neurocrit Care, 11*(1), 112–119.
208. Naqvi, J., Yap, K. H., Ahmad, G., & Ghosh, J. (2013). Transcranial Doppler ultrasound: a review of the physical principles and major applications in critical care. *Int J Vasc Med.* http://dx.doi.org/10.1155/2013/629378.
209. National Center for Chronic Disease Prevention and Health Promotion (/nccdphp). Division for Heart Disease and Stroke Prevention (/dhdsp).

(2015). *Stroke facts*. Atlanta, GA: Centers for Disease Control and Prevention. http://www.cdc.gov/stroke/facts.htm.
210. National Institute of Neurological Disorders and Stroke. (2003). *National institutes of health stroke scale*. Glenview, IL: U.S. Department of Health and Human Services.
211. National Institute of Neurological Disorders and Stroke. (2009). *Stroke: challenges, progress, and promise*. U.S.Department of Health and Human Services NIH Publication No. 09-6451. http://stroke.nih.gov/materials/strokechallenges.htm#Future3.
212. National Institute of Neurological Disorders and Stroke (NINDS). (2015). *Stroke: hope through research*. http://www.ninds.nih.gov/disorders/stroke/detail_stroke.htm.
213. Newell, D. W., & Vilela, M. D. (2011). Extracranial to intracranial bypass for cerebral ischemia. In J. P. Mohr, et al. (Ed.), *Stroke: pathophysiology, diagnosis, and management* (5th ed.) (pp. 1417–1425). Philadelphia: Elsevier Saunders.
214. Nguyen, P. L., & Chang, J. J. (2015). Stroke mimics and acute stroke evaluation: clinical evaluation and complications after intravenous tissue plasminogen activator. *J Emerg Med*, *49*(2), 244–252.
215. Normani, A. Z., Nabi, Z., Rashid, H., et al. (2014). Osmotic nephrosis with mannitol: review article. *Ren Fail*, *36*(7), 1169–1176.
216. Numis, A. L., & Fox, C. K. (2014). Arterial ischemic stroke in children: risk factors and etiologies. *Curr Neurol Neurosci Rep*, *14*(1), 422. http://dx.doi.org/10.1007/s11910-013-0422-8.
217. Nyquist, P., Bautista, C., Jichici, D., et al. (2015). Prophylaxis of venous thrombosis in neurocritical care patients: an evidence-based guideline: a statement for healthcare professionals from the Neurocritical Care Society. *Neurocrit Care*. http://dx.doi.org/10.10007/s12028-015-0221-y.
218. Oddo, M., Villa, F., & Citerio, G. (2012). Brain multimodality monitoring: an update. *Curr Opin Crit Care*, *18*(2), 111–118.
219. Oeinck, M., Neunhoeffer, F., Buttler, K. J., et al. (2013). Dynamic cerebral autoregulation in acute intracerebral hemorrhage. *Stroke*, *44*(10), 2722–2728.
220. Oh, H., & Seo, W. (2015). A comprehensive review of central post-stroke pain. *Pain Manag Nurs*, *16*(5), 804–818.
221. Oikarinen, A., Kääriäinen, M., & Kyngäs, H. (2014). A framework of counseling for patients with stroke in nursing: a narrative literature review. *J Neurosci Nurs*, *46*(5), E3–E14.
222. Ossi, R. G. (2013). Prevention and management of poststroke complications. In K. M. Barrett, & J. F. Meschia (Eds.), *Stroke* (pp. 103–118). West Sussex UK: Wiley-Blackwell.
223. Otite, F., Mink, S., Tan, C. O., et al. (2014). Impaired cerebral autoregulation is associated with vasospasm and delayed cerebral ischemia in subarachnoid hemorrhage. *Stroke*, *45*(3), 677–682.
224. Paciaroni, M., Caso, V., & Agnelli, G. (2009). The concept of ischemic penumbra in acute stroke and therapeutic opportunities. *Eur Neurol*, *61*(6), 321–330.
225. Pagana, K. D., & Pagana, T. J. (2014). *Mosby's manual of diagnostic and laboratory tests* (5th ed.). St. Louis: Elsevier.
226. Pamukcu, B., Lip, G. Y. H., & Lane, D. A. (2010). Simplifying stroke risk stratification in atrial fibrillation patients: implications of the CHA2DS2-VaSc risk stratification scores. *Age Ageing*, *39*(5), 533–535.
227. Perry, J. J., Sharma, M., Sivilotti, M. L. A., et al. (2011). Prospective validation of the ABCD2 score for patients in the emergency department with transient ischemic attack. *CMAJ*, *183*(10), 1137–1145.
228. Phipps, M. S., Desai, R. A., Wira, C., & Brava, D. M. (2011). Epidemiology and outcomes of fever burden among patients with acute ischemic stroke. *Stroke*, *42*(12), 3357–3362.
229. Pierot, L., Soize, S., Benaissa, A., & Wakhloo, A. K. (2015). Techniques for endovascular treatment of acute ischemic stroke: from intra-arterial fibrinolytics to stent-retrievers. *Stroke*, *46*(3), 909–914.
230. Pokorney, S. D., & Sherwood, M. W. (2013). Clinical strategies for selecting oral anticoagulants in patients with atrial fibrillation. *J Thromb Thrombolysis*, *36*(2), 163–174.
231. Pollack, C. V., Reilly, P. A., Eikelboom, J., et al. (2015). Idarucizumab for dabigatran reversal. *N Engl J Med*, *373*(6), 511–520.
232. Powers, W. J., Derdeyn, C. P., Biller, J., et al. (2015). AHA/ASA Focused update of the 2013 guidelines for the early management of patients with acute ischemic stroke regarding endovascular treatment: a guideline for health care professionals from the American Heart Association/American Stroke Association. *Stroke*, *46*(10), 3020–3025.
233. Prabhakaran, S., & Chong, J. Y. (2014). Risk factor management for stroke prevention. *Continuum (Minneap Minn)*, *20*(2) 296–208.
234. Prabhakaran, S., Ruff, I., & Berstein, R. A. (2015). Acute stroke intervention: a systematic review. *JAMA*, *313*(14), 1451–1462.
235. Quinn, T. J., & Langhorne, P. (2011). Barthel Index for stroke trials. *Stroke*, *42*, 1146–1151.
236. Rahme, R. J., Zammar, S. G., El Ahmadieh, T. Y., El Tecle, N. E., Ansari, S. A., & Bendok, B. R. (2014). The role of antiplatelet therapy in aneurysm coiling. *Neurol Res*, *36*(4), 383–388.
237. Raya, A. K., & Diringer, M. N. (2014). Treatment of subarachnoid hemorrhage. *Crit Care Clin*, *30*(4), 719–733.
238. Rodriguez-Hernández, A., Josephson, A. S., Langer, D., & Lawton, M. T. (2011). Bypass for the prevention of ischemic stroke. *World Neurosurg*, *76*(Suppl. 6), S72–S79.
239. Rosen, D. S., & Macdonald, R. L. (2005). Subarachnoid hemorrhage grading scales. *Neurocrit Care*, *2*(2), 110–118.
240. Rundek, T., & Sacco, R. L. (2011). Prognosis after stroke. In J. P. Mohr (Ed.), *Stroke: pathophysiology, diagnosis, and management* (5th ed.) (pp. 219–241). Philadelphia: Elsevier Saunders.
241. Sacco, R. L., Kasner, S. E., Broderick, J. P., et al. (2013). An updated definition of stroke for the 21st century. *Stroke*, *44*(7), 2064–2089.
242. Saccomano, S. J. (2012). Ischemic stroke: the first 24 hours. *Nurs Pract*, *37*(10), 12–18.
243. Saedon, M., Dilshad, A., Tiivas, C., et al. (2014). Prospective validation study of transorbital Doppler ultrasound imaging for the detection of transient cerebral microemboli. *Br J Surg*, *101*(12), 1551–1555.
244. Sampson, T. R., & Diringer, M. N. (2012). Post-procedural management of patients with aneurysmal subarachnoid hemorrhage. In E. M. Manno (Ed.), *Emergency management in neurocritical care* (pp. 73–83). West Sussex UK: Wiley-Blackwell.
245. Sattenberg, R. J., Saver, J. L., Gobin, Y. P., & Liebeskind, D. S. (2011). Cerebral angiography. In J. P. Mohr, P. A. Wolf, J. C. Grotta, M. A. Moskowitz, M. R. Mayberg, & R. von Kummer (Eds.), *Stroke: pathophysiology, diagnosis, and management* (5th ed.) (pp. 910–925). Philadelphia: Elsevier Saunders.
246. Sherzai, A. Z., & Elkind, M. S. V. (2015). Advances in stroke prevention. *Ann N Y Acad Sci*, *1338*, 1–15.
247. Skidmore-Roth, L. (2015). *Mosby's 2015 nursing drug reference* (28th ed.). St. Louis: Elsevier.
248. Spetzler, R. F., & Martin, N. A. (1986). A proposed grading system for arteriovenous malformations. *J Neurosurg*, *65*(4), 476–483.
249. Stapf, C., Mohr, J. P., Hartmann, A., et al. (2011). Arteriovenous malformations and other vascular anomalies. In J. P. Mohr, P. A. Wolf, J. C. Grotta, M. A. Moskowitz, M. R. Mayberg, & R. von Kummer (Eds.), *Stroke: pathophysiology, diagnosis, and management* (5th ed) (pp. 616–642). Philadelphia: Elsevier Saunders.
250. Stapleton, C. J., Walcott, B. P., Fusco, M. R., Butler, W. E., Thomas, A. J., & Ogilvy, C. S. (2015). Surgical management of ruptured middle cerebral artery aneurysms with large intraparenchymal or sylvian fissure hematomas. *Neurosurgery*, *76*(3), 258–264.
251. Starke, R. M., Komotar, R. J., & Connolly, E. S. (2011). Surgical decision making, techniques and periprocedural care of cerebral arteriovenous malformations. In J. P. Mohr, P. A. Wolf, J. C. Grotta, M. A. Moskowitz, M. R. Mayberg, & R. von Kummer (Eds.), *Stroke: pathophysiology, diagnosis, and management* (5th ed.) (pp. 1358–1365). Philadelphia: Elsevier Saunders.
252. Summers, D., Leonard, A., Wentworth, D., et al. (2009). Comprehensive overview of nursing and interdisciplinary care of the acute ischemic stroke patient. *Stroke*, *40*(8), 2911–2944.
253. Sureka, B., Bansal, K., Patidar, Y., Rajesh, S., Mukund, A., & Arora, A. (2015). Neurologic manifestations of chronic liver disease and liver cirrhosis. *Curr Probl Diagn Radiol*, *44*(5), 449–461.
254. Tai, Y. J., Weir, L., Hand, P., Davis, S., & Yan, B. (2011). Does a "code stroke" rapid access protocol decrease door-to-needle time for thrombolysis? *Intern Med J*, *42*(12), 1316–1324.

255. Taqi, M. A., & Torbey, M. T. (2012). Subarachnoid hemorrhage. In E. M. Manno (Ed.), *Emergency management in neurocritical care* (pp. 37–44). West Sussex UK: Wiley-Blackwell.
256. The Joint Commission. (2015). *Disease-specific care certification program: comprehensive stroke performance measurement implementation guide July 2015*. Chicago: The Joint Commission. http://www.jointcommission.org/assets/1/6/CSTKManual2015July.pdf.
257. Thrift, A. G., Cadilhac, D. A., Thayabaranathn, T., et al. (2014). Global stroke statistics. *Int J Stroke, 9*(1), 6–18.
258. Toni, D., Sacco, R. L., Brainin, M., & Mohr., J. P. (2011). Classification of ischemic stroke. In J. P. Mohr, P. A. Wolf, J. C. Grotta, M. A. Moskowitz, M. R. Mayberg, & R. von Kummer (Eds.), *Stroke: pathophysiology, diagnosis, and management* (5th ed.) (pp. 293–306). Philadelphia: Elsevier Saunders.
259. Torbey, M. T., Bösel, J., Rhoney, D. H., et al. (2015). Evidence-based guidelines for the management of large hemispheric infarction. A statement for health care professionals from the Neurocritical Care Society and the German Society for Neuro-Intensive Care and Emergency Medicine. *Neurocrit Care, 22*(1), 146–164.
260. Toyoda, K., & Ninomiya, T. (2014). Stroke and cerebrovascular disease in patients with chronic kidney disease. *Lancet Neurol, 13*(8), 823–833.
261. Toyoda, K. (2015). Cerebral small vessel disease and chronic kidney disease. *J Stroke, 17*(1), 31–37.
262. Treggiari, M. M. (2011). Hemodynamic management of subarachnoid hemorrhage. *Neurocrit Care, 15*, 329–335.
263. Tsze, D. S., & Valente, J. H. (2011). Pediatric stroke: a review. *Emergency Medicine International*. http://dx.doi.org/10.1155/2011/734506.
264. University of Washington Pharmacy Services. (2015). *General information: anticoagulation services*. Seattle WA: University of Washington. http://depts.washington.edu/anticoag/home/node.
265. van Bree, M. D., Roos, Y. B., van der Bilt, I. A., et al. (2010). Prevalence and characterization of ECG abnormalities after intracerebral hemorrhage. *Neurocrit Care, 12*(1), 50–56.
266. van Leeuwen, A. M., & Bladh, M. L. (2015). *Davis's comprehensive handbook of laboratory & diagnostic tests* (6th ed.). Philadelphia: F.A. Davis Company.
267. Vasudevan, J. M., & Browne, B. J. (2014). Hemiplegic shoulder pain: an approach to diagnosis and management. *Phys Med Rehabil Clin N Am, 25*(2), 411–437.
268. Veltkamp, R., & Horstmann, S. (2014). Treatment of intracerebral hemorrhage associated with new oral anticoagulant use: the neurologist's view. *Clin Lab Med, 34*, 587–594.
269. Verbalis, J. G., Goldsmith, S. R., Greenberg, A., et al. (2013). Diagnosis, evaluation, and treatment of hyponatremia: expert panel recommendations. *Am J Med, 126*(10, Suppl. 1), S1–S42.
270. Wakhloo, A. K., Gounis, M. J., & De Leo, M. J., III (2011). Endovascular treatment of cerebral aneurysms. In J. P. Mohr, P. A. Wolf, J. C. Grotta, M. A. Moskowitz, M. R. Mayberg, & R. von Kummer (Eds.), *Stroke: pathophysiology, diagnosis, and management* (5th ed.) (pp. 1241–1254). Philadelphia: Elsevier Saunders.
271. Wan, H., Alharbi, B. M., & Macdonald, R. L. (2014). Mechanisms, treatment, and prevention of cellular injury and death from delayed events after aneurysmal subarachnoid hemorrhage. *Expert Opin Pharmacother, 15*(2), 231–243.
272. Warlow, C., Sudlow, C., Dennis, M., Wardlaw, J., & Sandercock, P. (2003). Stroke. *Lancet, 362*(9391), 1211–1224.
273. Waxman, S. G. (2013). Vascular supply of the brain. In *Clinical neuroanatomy* (27th ed.) (pp. 163–181). New York: Lange Medical.
274. Webb, J., & Kwaitkowski, J. L. (2013). Stroke in patients with sickle cell disease. *Expert Rev Hematol, 6*(3), 301–316.
275. Weir, C. J., Bardford, A. P. J., & Lees, K. R. (2003). The prognostic value of the components of the Glasgow Coma Scale following acute stroke. *Q J Med, 96*(1), 67–74.
276. Wijdicks, E. F. M., & Rabinstein, A. A. (2002). Absolutely no hope? Some ambiguity of futility of care in devastating acute stroke. *Crit Care Med, 32*(11), 2332–2342.
277. Wijdicks, E. F. M., Bamlet, W. R., Maramottom, B. V., Manno, E. M., & McClelland, R. L. (2005). Validation of a new coma scale: the FOUR score. *Ann Neurol, 58*(4), 585–593.
278. Wijdicks, E. F. M., Sheth, K. N., Carter, B. S., et al. (2014). Recommendations for the management of cerebral and cerebellar infarction with swelling: a statement for healthcare professionals from the American Heart Association/American Stroke Association. *Stroke, 45*(4), 1222–1238.
279. Williams, L. S., Brizendine, E. J., Plue, L., et al. (2005). Performance of the PHQ-9 as a screening tool for depression after stroke. *Stroke, 36*(3), 635–638.
280. Wilson, D. A., Nakaji, P., Abia, A. A., et al. (2012). A simple and quantitative method to predict symptomatic vasospasm after subarachnoid hemorrhage based on computed tomography: beyond the Fisher scale. *Neurosurgery, 71*(4), 869–876.
281. Wojner-Alexandrov, A. W., & Alexandrov, A. V. (2011). Transcranial Doppler monitoring. In D. J. McHale-Wiegand, & K. K. Carlson (Eds.), *AACN procedure manual for critical care* (6th ed.) (pp. 849–860). St. Louis: Mosby.
282. Wroteck, S. E., Kozak, W. E., Hess, D. C., & Fagan, S. C. (2011). Treatment of fever after stroke: conflicting evidence. *Pharmacotherapy, 31*(11), 1085–1091.
283. Wu, C. C., Zheng, C. M., Lin, Y. F., Lo, L., Liao, M. T., & Lu, K. C. (2012). Role of homocysteine in end-stage renal disease. *Clin Biochem, 45*(16-17), 1286–1294.
284. Yazbeck, M. F., Rincon, F., & Mayer, S. A. (2012). Intracerebral hemorrhage. In K. Lee (Ed.), *The neuro ICU book* (pp. 35–51). New York: McGraw-Hill.
285. Yew, K. S., & Cheng, E. M. (2015). Diagnosis of acute stroke. *Am Fam Physician, 91*(8), 528–536.
286. Zhang, Y., & Rabenstein, A. A. (2011). Lower head of bed position does not change blood flow velocity in subarachnoid hemorrhage. *Neurocrit Care, 14*(1), 73–76.
287. Zuckerman, S. L., Eli, I. M., Morone, P. J., Dwann, M. C., & Mocco, M. (2014). Novel technologies in the treatment of intracranial aneurysms. *Neurol Res, 36*(4), 368–382.
288. Zweifler, R. W., & Silverboard, G. (2011). Arterial dissections and fibromuscular dysplasia. In J. P. Mohr, P. A. Wolf, J. C. Grotta, M. A. Moskowitz, M. R. Mayberg, & R. von Kummer (Eds.), *Stroke: pathophysiology, diagnosis, and management* (5th ed.) (pp. 661–686). Philadelphia: Elsevier Saunders.

14

Traumatic Spinal Cord Injury

Patricia A. Blissitt

TRAUMATIC SPINAL CORD INJURY

More than 12,500 new spinal cord injuries (SCIs) occur in the United States annually.[117] Whereas the international incidence of SCI varies widely, from 13 to 53 cases per million population,[80] the United States has one of the highest incidence rates at 40 cases per million. In addition, an unknown number of spinal cord injured are found dead at the scene.[3] Many, if not most of the estimated 276,000 individuals in the United States who survive the initial injury have physiologic and psychosocial needs that require the focused, detailed, and comprehensive approach attainable in a critical care environment.[117] Few injuries or illnesses present a bigger challenge to the critical care nurse and the interprofessional team than the patient with a traumatic SCI.

PATIENTS AT RISK

Nearly 50% of all traumatic SCI occurs in people age 16 to 30 years.[116] However, in the last 40 years, an upward trend in the mean age at injury has been noted from 28.7 to 42 years.[117] This may be a reflection of individuals living longer; improved prehospital resuscitation efforts increasing the survival of older persons with SCI at the scene; or an actual increased incidence of SCI among older persons.[83,117] Males have consistently been more likely to sustain traumatic SCI than females, at a ratio of 4:1, possibly related to greater risk-taking behavior among males.[117] With regard to ethnicity, in the United States, non-Hispanic whites continue to be the highest percentage of spinal cord–injured individuals, at approximately 64%, with non-Hispanic blacks at 23%, Hispanics at 10%, and the remaining racial/ethnic groups at 3%. The incidence of traumatic spinal cord injury in non-Hispanic white Americans is greater than the number of non-Hispanic blacks in the general population (12%).[117] The three leading causes of traumatic SCI are, in descending order: motor vehicle crashes, falls, and violence, especially gunshot wounds. Other significant causes of traumatic SCI include sports and work-related accidents.[117,168]

PREVENTION

Most traumatic spinal cord injuries are preventable.[167] Preventive strategies include avoiding alcohol intoxication when driving; wearing a seat belt; proper use of car seats; avoidance of distracted driving (e.g., cell phone use); and driving within speed limits congruent with legal restrictions, weather, and road conditions.[18] Several trauma prevention programs have been initiated in an attempt to modify the risk-taking behavior of young people. Some, such as Mothers Against Drunk Driving and Students Against Drunk Driving, are nonspecific to SCI, whereas others, such as the *Think First* program, specifically target brain and spinal cord injury. The *Think First* program, developed by the American Association of Neurological Surgeons in 1986, introduces students in elementary and high school to individuals with SCI, as well as members of the interprofessional teams who care for them.[128] The combined efforts of the spinal cord–injured individual and the healthcare provider give the young person a personal and professional perspective on living with SCI. Evaluations of the *Think First* program included efficacy studies that showed evidence of increased knowledge and changes in attitude and behavior as a result of attending a *Think First* program.[69,128,156] However, the success of prevention programs, defined as a decrease in the number of injuries, is unknown.[137] Furthermore, prevention programs must be tailored to the population at risk and the most likely etiologies to be effective.[38]

Efforts to prevent injuries in the home include having adequate lighting, particularly at steps, grab bars and other safety measures in the bathroom, and minimizing slippery floor surfaces. Properly worn protective sport gear, player and coach education, and appropriate training, such as physical conditioning and safe defensive strategies, may prevent some sport injuries.[18] Additional efforts include limiting sporting activities for those individuals with a previous SCI, degenerative spine disease, or congenital narrowing of the spinal canal.

DEFINITION

From a broader perspective, SCI may include nontraumatic etiologies, such as infection, tumors, and nontraumatic vascular events, but this chapter is limited to traumatic SCI. For a fortunate few, damage to the spine, vertebrae, or the supporting structures (the intervertebral disks and ligaments), does not necessarily result in an injury to the spinal cord. Conversely, an injury to the cord may occur in the absence of damage to the spine and its supporting structures. Spinal cord injury without radiographic abnormality (SCIWORA) is the term used to describe neurologic impairment in the absence of fracture or ligamentous injury on plain spine radiographs and computed tomography (CT) imaging.[151] As magnetic resonance imaging (MRI) may detect spinal cord injury not seen on plain radiographs or CT imaging, another term, spinal cord injury without computed tomography evidence of trauma (SCIWOCTET) for adults has emerged. These individuals may have neurologic deficits related to canal stenosis and degenerative changes (e.g., spondylosis).[39] SCIWORA has historically been primarily associated with pediatric SCI.[131] However, up to 14% of adults have been diagnosed with SCIWORA.[151] This percentage may change or SCIWORA may

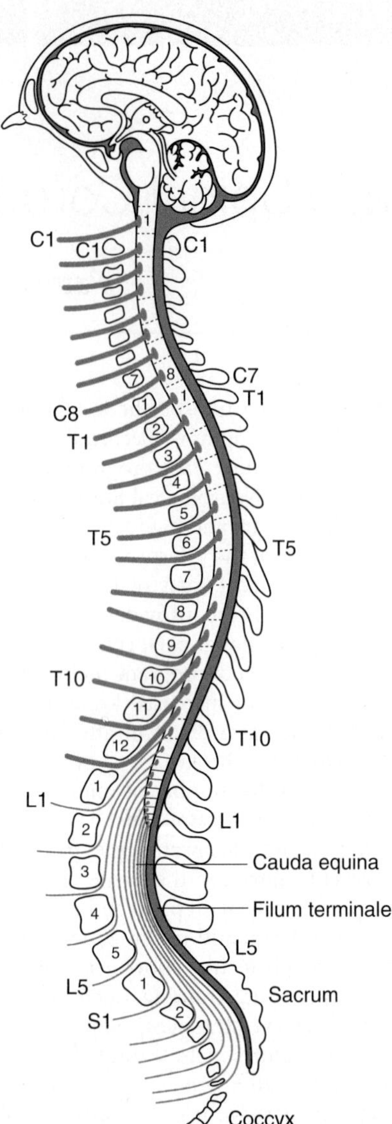

FIG. 14.1 Spinal nerves emerging from the spinal cord through the intervertebral foramina. (From Braddom, R. (2007). *Physical medicine and rehabilitation,* (3rd ed.). Philadelphia: Saunders.)

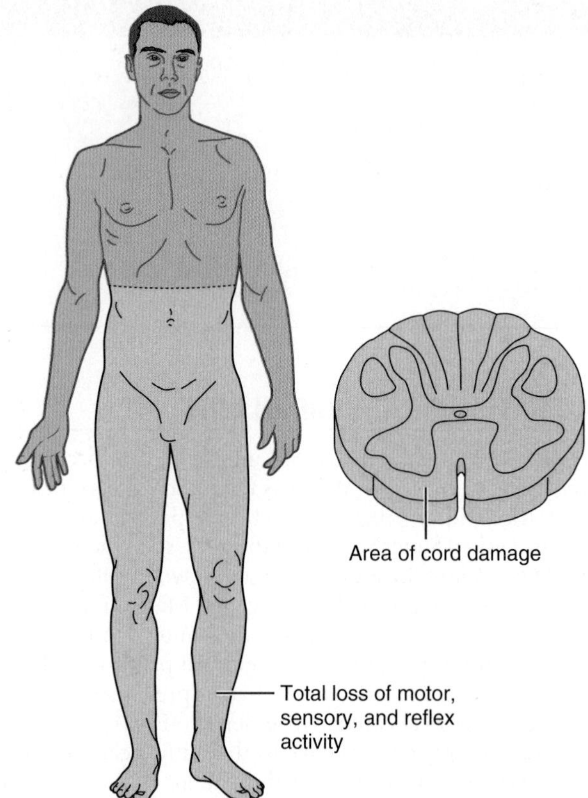

FIG. 14.2 Complete lesion.

be redefined to include MRI. MRI is increasingly being used to detect ligamentous/soft tissue injuries and may detect abnormalities not seen on CT or plain films.[151]

Traumatic SCI may be defined based on the level of injury: cervical, thoracic, lumbar, cervicothoracic, thoracolumbar, lumbosacral, sacral, and multilevel (not necessarily contiguous). The cervical spine and the thoracolumbar areas are most vulnerable to injury because they are the most mobile. The thoracic spine is supported by the anterior and posterior rib cage.[15] Cervical spinal cord injuries comprise approximately 55% of all spinal cord injuries, with thoracic, thoracolumbar, and lumbosacral or pure sacral spinal cord injuries at approximately 15% each.[7,9,168] Approximately 20% of all spinal cord-injured patients have injury at multiple noncontiguous vertebral levels.[153] The neurologic level, which may be different or the same as the level of spine injury, is the lowest level of the spinal cord with normal bilateral motor strength and sensation, as shown in Fig. 14.1. Tetraplegics, previously referred to as *quadriplegics,* are those with injuries at or above C7, and paraplegics are those with injuries below C7.[154]

In addition to level, SCI is classified as complete or incomplete. A complete injury occurs when all sensory and motor function below the level of spinal cord lesion is absent (Fig. 14.2).[15] An incomplete injury is defined as residual neurologic function, motor or sensory, below the level of neurologic injury. A number of incomplete syndromes with characteristic clinical findings exist, including anterior cord, posterior cord, Brown-Séquard, central cord, conus medullaris, and cauda equina.[19] These syndromes are summarized in Table 14.1.

Anterior cord syndrome results when the anterior motor and sensory pathways of the spinal cord are injured (Fig. 14.3). Voluntary movement, pain and temperature sensation, and light touch are impaired, while proprioception, vibration, and tactile discrimination are retained. In contrast, posterior cord injury (dorsal column syndrome) impairs proprioception, vibration, and tactile discrimination (Fig. 14.4).[28] Brown-Séquard syndrome is a physiologic hemi-transection of the spinal cord with (1) ipsilateral voluntary motor loss; (2) ipsilateral impairment of proprioception, vibration, and discriminatory touch; and (3) contralateral impairment of pain and temperature sensation (Fig. 14.5).[28] Central cord syndrome, an injury to the cervical region, is characterized by greater motor impairment and sensory deficits in the arms than the legs (Fig. 14.6). Central cord syndrome is associated with sacral sparing.[28] Sacral sparing refers to noninvolvement of the sacral nerve roots, which control bowel, bladder, and sexual function. Recovery from an incomplete injury is variable. However, the potential for a better outcome is greater with incomplete injury than with complete injury.[28]

In contrast, both conus medullaris syndrome and cauda equina syndrome result in loss of bowel and bladder function and sexual dysfunction (Fig. 14.7). Injury to the conus

TABLE 14.1 Spinal Cord Syndromes

Syndrome	Common Mechanisms of Injury	Features
Complete	Multiple	Disruption of all voluntary movement and sensory function below level of lesion Quadriplegia/tetraplegia: cervical spinal cord injury Paraplegia: thoracic spinal cord injury
Incomplete		Some movement or sensation below level of lesion
Anterior	Anterior cord compression/flexion Interruption of blood supply to anterior two thirds of spinal cord	Paralysis with loss of pain and temperature and light touch below injury
Posterior	Posterior cord compression/extension	Loss of vibration, proprioception, and tactile discrimination below injury
Central cord	Hyperextension to cervical spine	Motor loss greater in upper extremities than lower extremities; variable sensory and bladder function loss
Brown-Séquard	Penetrating injury; hemi-transection of spinal cord	1. Ipsilateral paralysis (lateral corticospinal tract disruption) 2. Ipsilateral loss of tactile discrimination, vibration, and proprioception (dorsal column disruption) 3. Contralateral loss of pain and temperature sensation (lateral spinothalamic tract)
Conus medullaris	Compression at distal end of spinal cord, approximately L1–L2	Bowel, bladder, sexual dysfunction; motor impairment variable, but may include flaccid paralysis
Cauda equina	Compression of lumbosacral nerve roots below L1	Areflexic bowel and bladder, radicular pain, variable (lower) motor and sensory loss

From References 20, 28, 88, 160, and 162.

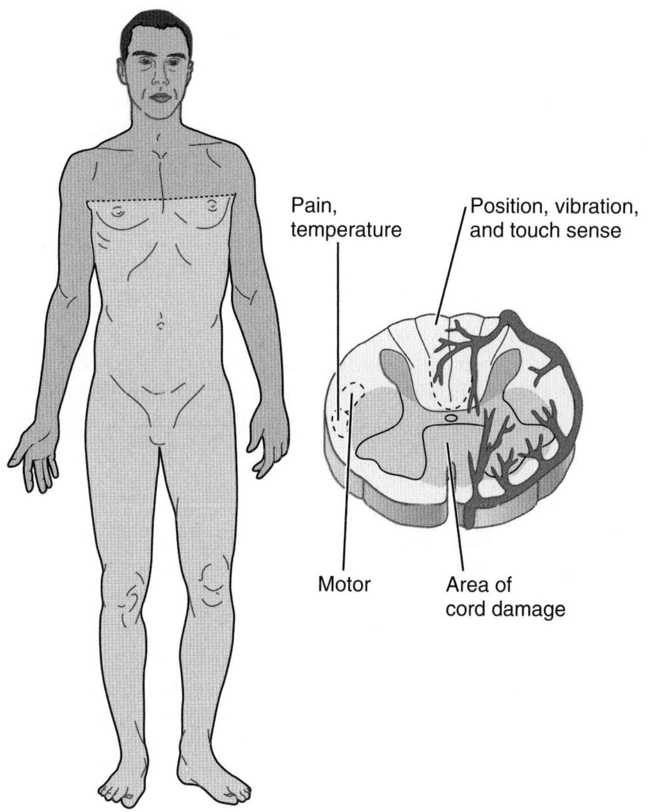

FIG. 14.3 Anterior cord syndrome.

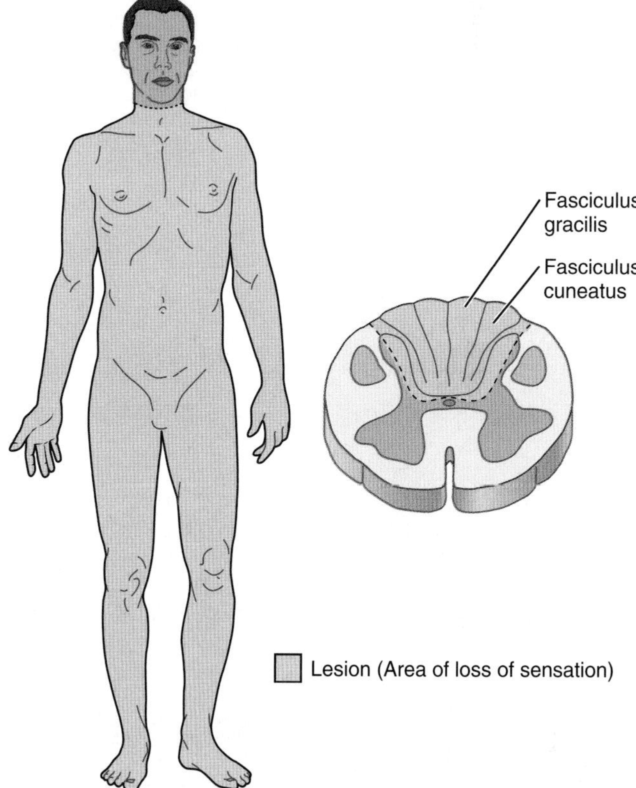

FIG. 14.4 Posterior cord syndrome.

medullaris, the cauda equina, and lumbar nerve roots may also impact lower limb movement to variable degrees. The cauda equina syndrome involves not only the lumbosacral nerve roots but also the peripheral nerve roots that extend beyond the conus medullaris at the end of the spinal cord.[28] In adults, the spinal cord ends at vertebral levels L1–L2.[168]

As with trauma in general, particular mechanisms of injury in spinal cord trauma are associated with and are predictive of specific clinical presentations. Typical mechanisms of injury in spinal cord trauma include hyperflexion, hyperextension, flexion-extension with rotation, distraction, compression, axial loading, or penetrating (Fig. 14.8).[7,15] The sudden stop of a moving vehicle may result in an acceleration-deceleration mechanism with resultant hyperflexion and hyperextension injuries.[7,15] Hyperflexion injuries fracture the vertebrae anteriorly, causing anterior cord injury and disruption of the posterior ligaments. Hyperflexion injuries are seen in diving accidents and front impact motor vehicle crashes. Hyperextension disrupts the anterior ligaments and may fracture the spinous processes, facets, or lamina. Falls and rear impact motor vehicle

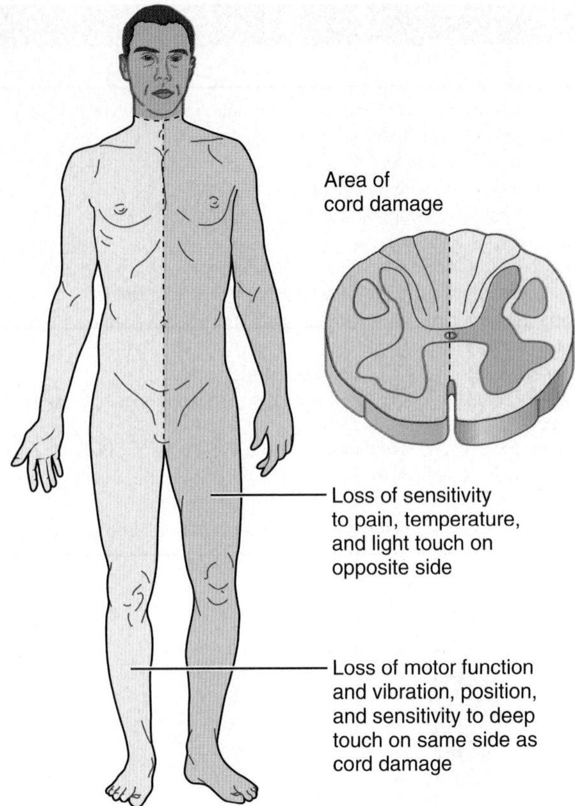

FIG. 14.5 Brown-Séquard syndrome.

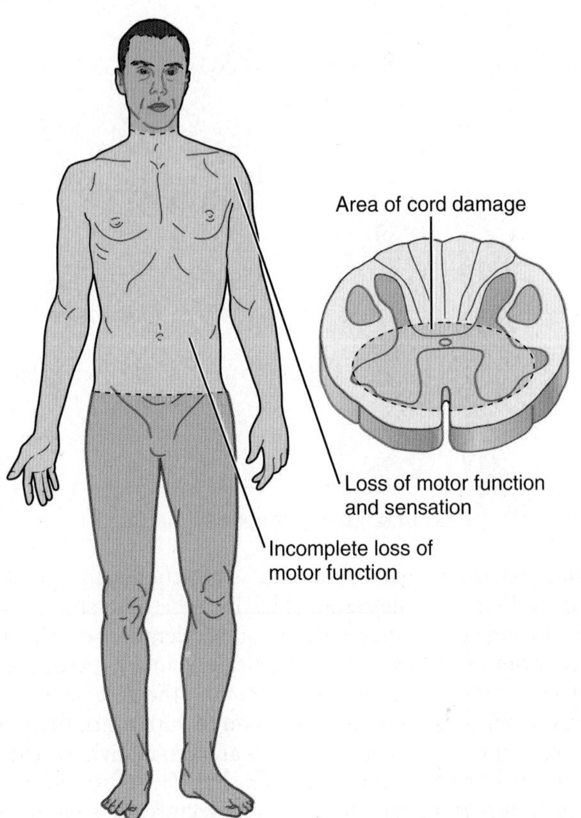

FIG. 14.6 Central cord syndrome.

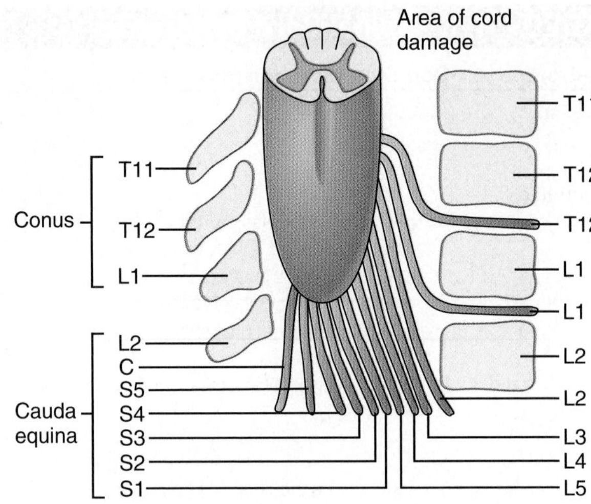

FIG. 14.7 Conus medullaris and cauda equina syndromes: motor and sensory function is lost in a variety of patterns. There is potential for recovery of function.

crashes result in hyperextension injury. Axial loading or vertical compression is associated with burst fractures from falls on the head or jumping. Rotation injuries tear the posterior ligaments.[7,16] Penetrating injuries such as stab wounds cause vascular injury and actual cutting of the spinal cord. Missiles cause injury at the point of impact but also cause additional trauma through kinetic energy, involving more than the area of direct impact.[7,15]

Injury to the vertebrae and ligaments may be classified as well. Vertebral fractures are described as simple, wedged or compressed, burst or comminuted, or teardrop. A simple fracture occurs at the spinous or transverse process without cord involvement. A wedge fracture results in anterior compression of the vertebral body. Burst or comminuted fractures frequently result in a shattered vertebral body with fragments compressing the spinal cord. A piece of the vertebra separates and lodges in the spinal canal in teardrop fractures. In teardrop fractures the vertebral body is displaced and the spinal cord is compressed. The vertebral injury may also be described as a dislocation, subluxation, or fracture-dislocation.[7,15] In a dislocation, one vertebra slides over another, one or both facets dislocate and lock, and the vertebrae are misaligned. Locked facets require traction or surgical reduction.[7,15] Subluxation is a partial dislocation of one vertebra. Subluxation or dislocation may result in an unstable injury. A fracture-dislocation is associated with cord and ligament injury. An unstable injury does not necessarily involve bony disruption, but refers to the integrity of the ligaments.[7,15] Vertebral facets may move out of alignment and become locked into position, requiring traction or surgical reduction.[7,15]

The first two cervical vertebrae are associated with specific bony injuries. C1 and C2 are referred to as the *atlas* and *axis*, respectively. Atlanto-occipital dislocation (AOD) refers to loss of stability in the area where the upper cervical spine (atlas, C1) joins with the cranium (occiput). AOD is often fatal as a result of brain stem injury and respiratory arrest.[89] A Jefferson fracture of C1 is a burst injury involving both the anterior and the posterior arches and may include a ligament tear (Fig. 14.9). This fracture sometimes results in death as well.[89] Injury to C2, or the axis, may present as an odontoid (dens) fracture of types I, II, or III (Fig. 14.10).[15] It may also present as a hangman's

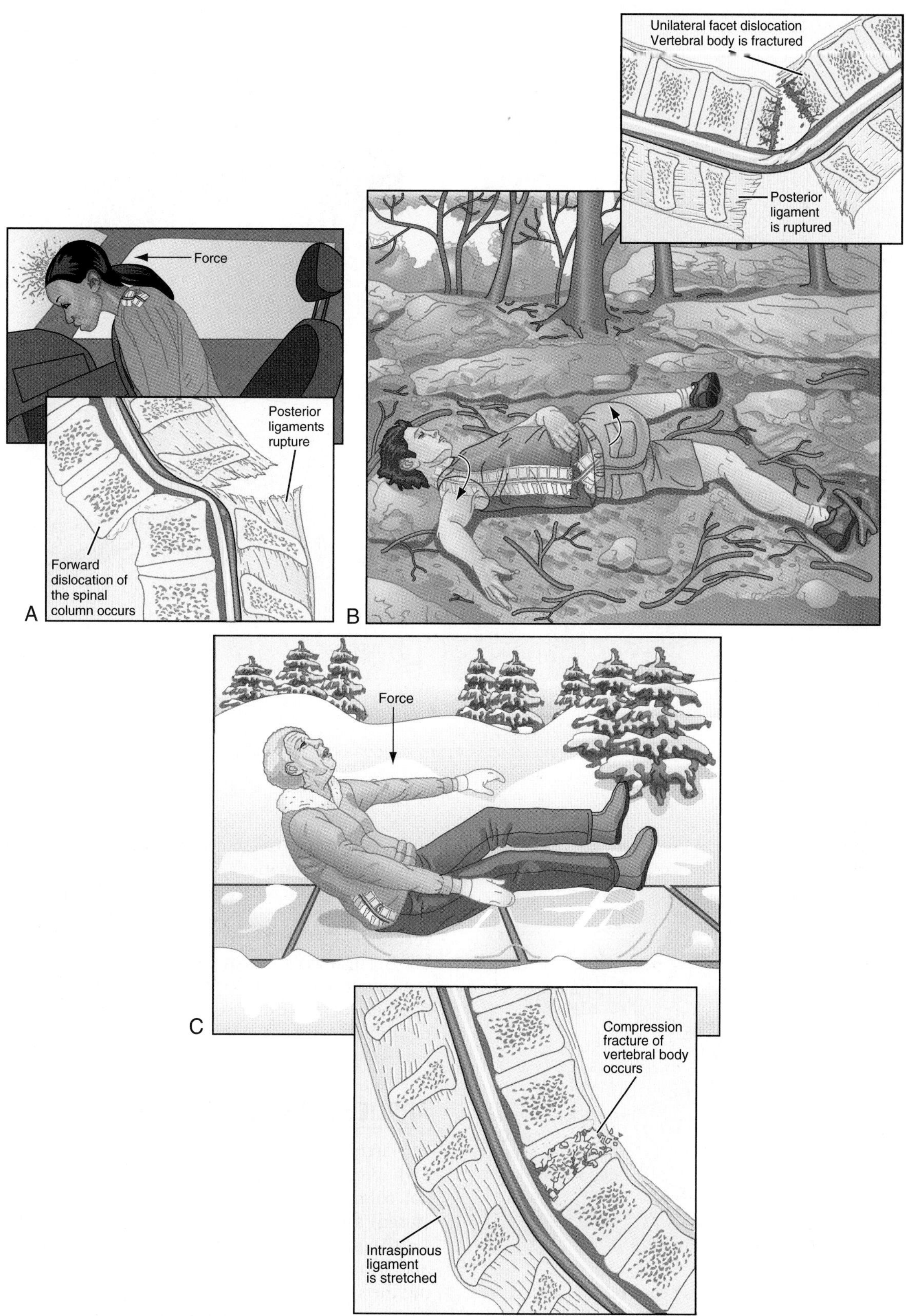

FIG. 14.8 Mechanisms of vertebral column injury. **A,** Flexion in a forward-moving victim. **B,** Flexion in a rotating victim. **C,** Flexion-axial compression.

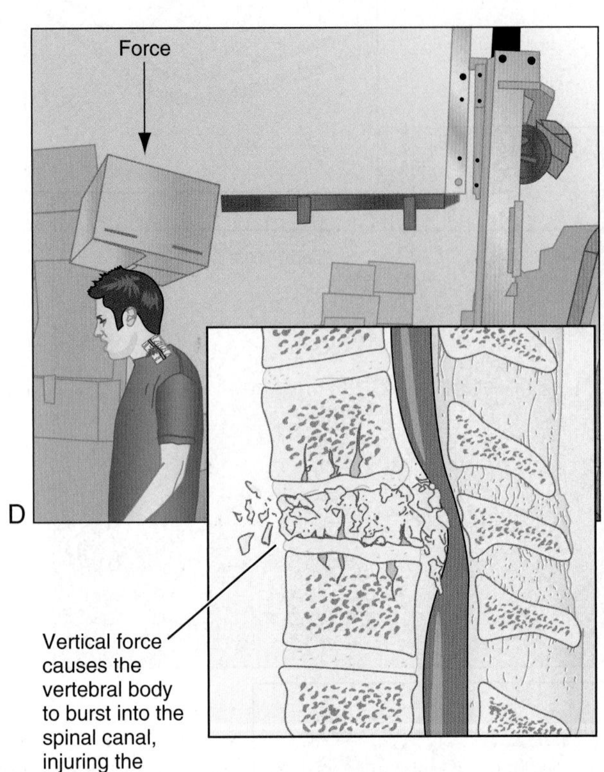

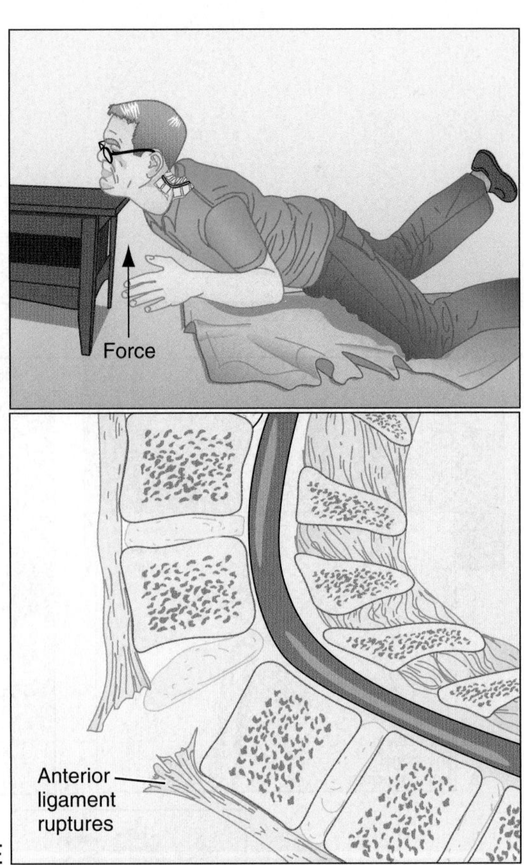

FIG. 14.8 cont'd D, Flexion-axial compression with vertical compression. E, Forced hyperextension.

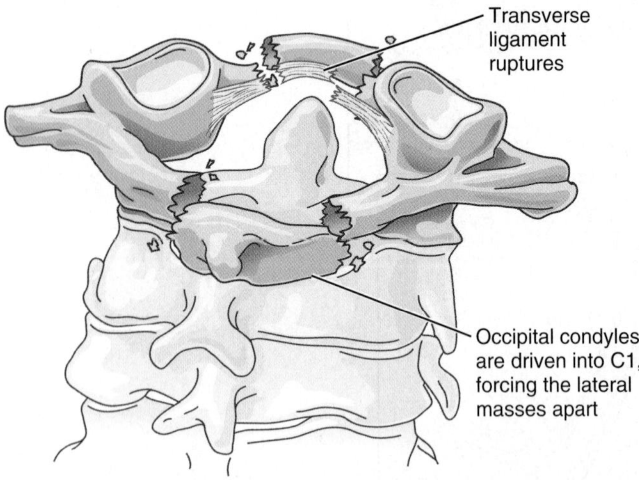

FIG. 14.9 Jefferson fracture.

fracture involving bilateral pedicles. A Type I odontoid fracture is an oblique fracture through the upper aspect of the odontoid. It is rare but usually stable. Type II occurs where the body of C2 meets the odontoid process. It is typically unstable and may not fuse. Type III involves the body of C2 but is typically more stable and fuses.[15] A hangman's fracture occurs at C2 as a result of axial loading and extension (Fig. 14.11). A hangman's fracture consists of bilateral fractures, ligamentous disruption, and subluxation. It is referred to as *traumatic spondylolisthesis* but may be asymptomatic.[89]

Anatomic differences associated with both ends of the life continuum, pediatric and geriatric, may contribute to SCI. Incomplete ossification of vertebrae, greater elasticity of the stabilizing ligaments, and the larger size of the head in relationship to the body contribute to SCI in children.[88,99] Osteoporosis and degenerative spine disease with narrowing of the spinal canal or deformation of the spine may increase the risk of SCI in older adults.[84]

APPLIED PATHOPHYSIOLOGY

The architecture of the spinal column affords the spinal cord and spinal nerves with some degree of protection. The spinal column consists of 7 cervical, 12 thoracic, 5 lumbar, 5 (fused) sacral, and 4 (fused) coccyx vertebrae (Fig. 14.12).[154] Cartilaginous intervertebral disks absorb some external loads, and ligaments assist in maintaining alignment and stabilizing the spine.[154] However, if the spinal column or its adjacent structures cannot withstand the imposed forces, these same structures may injure the spinal cord. The spinal cord has an H-shaped central core of gray matter that consists of neuronal cell bodies (Fig. 14.13). As shown in Table 14.2, the surrounding white matter is composed of ascending sensory (afferent) and descending motor (efferent) tracts. Some tracts cross; others do not.[130] The spinal cord at one or more levels may

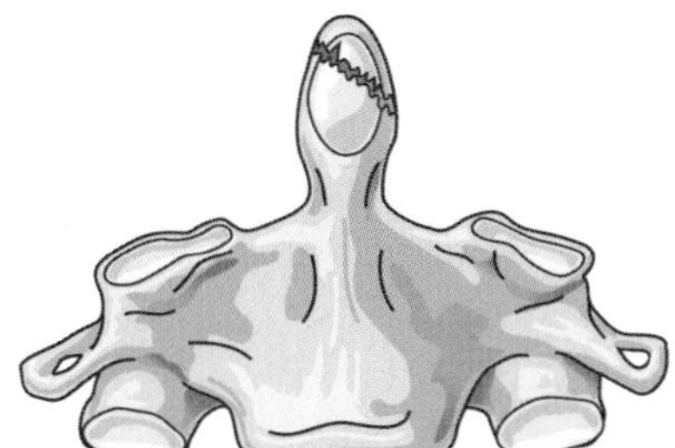
Type I
Located at superior tip of the odontoid process

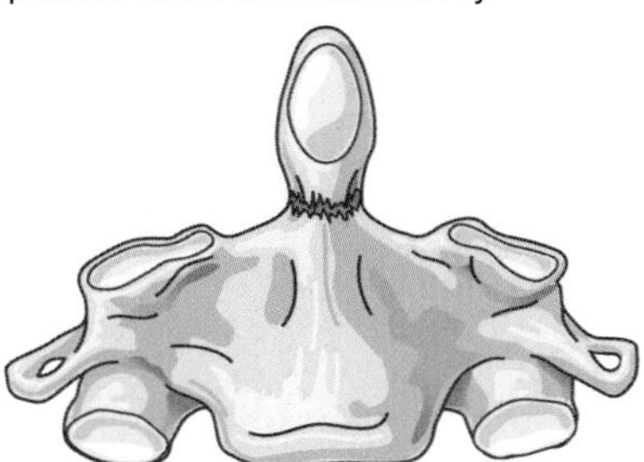
Type II
Occurs at the junction of the odontoid process and the vertebral body

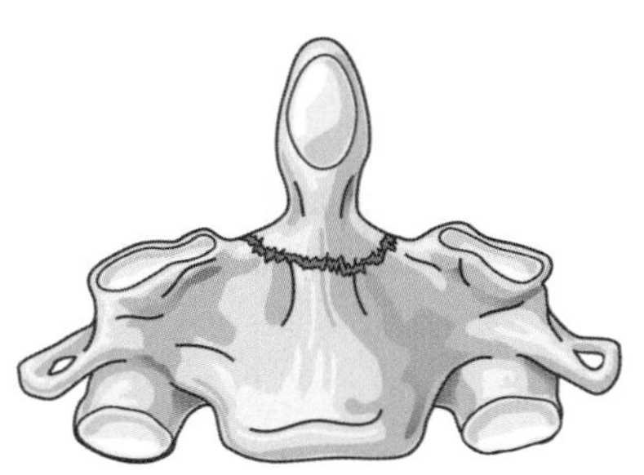
Type III
Extends into the body of the atlas

FIG. 14.10 Odontoid fractures. Type I: rare but usually stable. Type II: typically unstable and may not fuse. Type III: more stable and fuses.

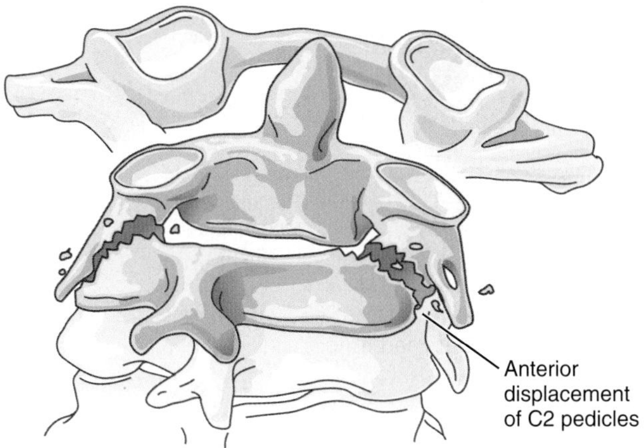
Anterior displacement of C2 pedicles

FIG. 14.11 Hangman's fracture.

be concussed (transient), contused with or without hematoma formation, lacerated, transected (rare), or compressed. All result in compromised blood flow.[143] The blood supply to the spinal cord consists of one anterior spinal artery and two posterior spinal arteries.[130] A single unilateral branch of the anterior spinal artery, the artery of Adamkiewicz, supplies up to two thirds of the anterior thoracolumbar (T5–L4) blood supply.[130] The spinal arteries arise from vertebral, deep cervical, intercostal, and iliac arteries and the aorta. The vertebral and deep cervical arteries supply the cervical cord, and the intercostals and aorta send blood to the thoracic level. The iliac vessels perfuse the lumbosacral region.[162]

Neurologic damage to the spinal cord is the result of both primary and secondary injury. Primary injury consists of the mechanical disruption that may occur as a result of contusion, compression, distraction, laceration, and transection. Secondary injury refers to the biological events that follow the primary injury, which further damage the spinal cord. Secondary injury occurs over minutes to weeks after the mechanical disruption.[31,143]

Similar in many aspects to the brain, injury to the spinal cord results in a sequence of events also referred to as *an ischemic cascade.* The spinal cord, like the brain, requires a near-constant source of oxygen and glucose for metabolism. When the metabolic needs of the cord are not met, secondary injury occurs as a result of calcium influx, the release of glutamate and other excitatory amino acids, free radical formation, inflammation, edema, and lipid peroxidation with disruption of the neuronal membrane and cell death.[9,31,129,143]

Within the first few minutes, the mechanical injury induces depolarization and opening of the potassium, sodium, and calcium channels. Depolarization releases glutamate and other neurotransmitters to open *N*-methyl-D-aspartate (NMDA) and α-amino-3-hydroxy-5-methyl-4-isoxazolepropionic acid (AMPA) channels, which also contribute to increased intracellular calcium. The influx of intracellular calcium is one of the more damaging aspects of the ischemic cascade. Calcium overload in the neuron causes mitochondrial damage that in turn halts aerobic metabolism and results in lactic acid accumulation, nitric oxide production, and the release of arachidonic acid (AA). AA is converted to deleterious vasoconstricting prostaglandins, such as $PGF_{2\alpha}$, and thromboxane A_2 (TXA_2), which results in additional vasoconstriction and platelet aggregation. Calcium-related mitochondrial dysfunction also contributes to free radical formation.[31,120,143]

Petechial hemorrhage, anaerobic metabolism, and free radical formation injure the lipid cell membranes and contribute to microvascular, axonal, and myelin damage and ischemia. Axons and myelin are further damaged by the activation of calpain, which results from the influx of calcium. Leukotrienes (LTs) induce polymorphonuclear leukocyte and macrophage influx, which causes inflammation and additional microvascular damage. Another contributor to secondary injury is the release of endogenous opiates associated with traumatic injury. Endorphins activate opiate receptors. The opiate receptors also contribute to ischemia by compromising vascular and metabolic function (Fig. 14.14).[31,120,143]

Also, like the brain, the spinal cord is thought to autoregulate to maintain adequate cord perfusion, with its vasculature constricting and dilating as needed. However the mean arterial pressure (MAP) range at which autoregulation is functional in the spinal cord is not known. As a result of impaired autoregulation, spinal cord blood flow passively follows increases and decreases in systemic blood pressure.[121]

Immediately following an injury, spinal shock occurs. Spinal shock is characterized as a flaccid paralysis with loss of sensation, autonomic dysfunction, areflexia, and bowel and bladder impairment below the level of the SCI. Spinal shock may resolve in 48 hours or persist as long as 6 weeks after the injury; shock is replaced with spasticity and hyperreflexia.[15] Spinal shock is *not* synonymous with neurogenic shock.[15,152] Neurogenic shock is the bradycardia, hypotension, and impaired thermoregulation that occurs secondary to the autonomic dysfunction of spinal shock. Neurogenic shock is the result of interrupted sympathetic outflow and subsequent unopposed vagal activity, venous

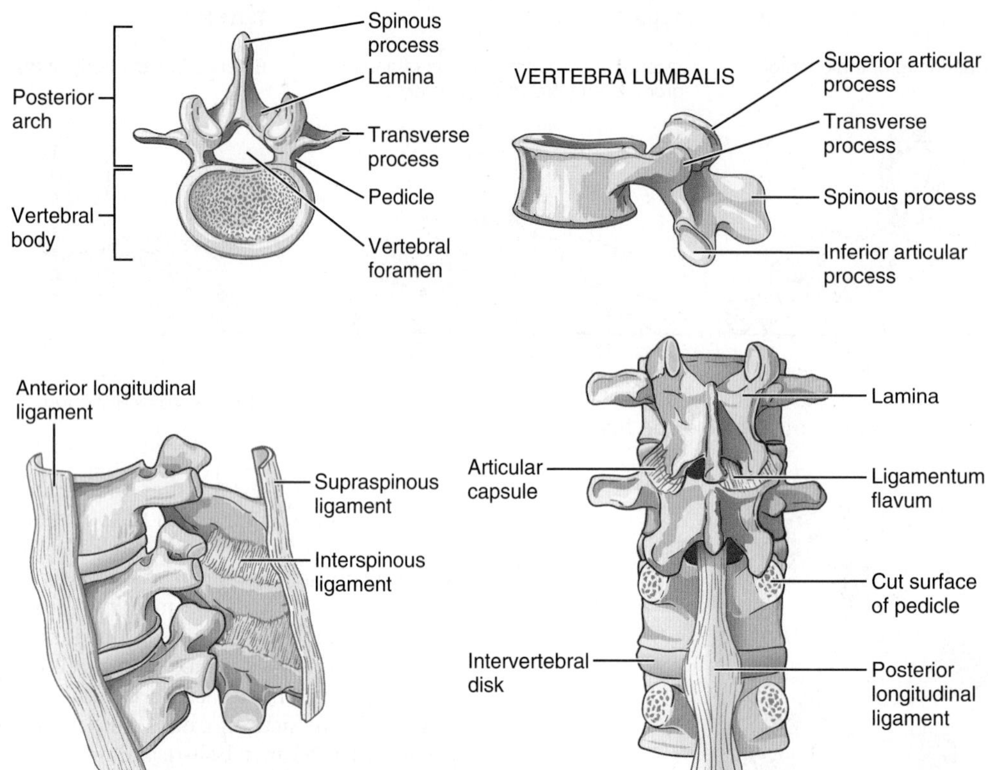

FIG. 14.12 Different views of the vertebrae and their chief ligaments.

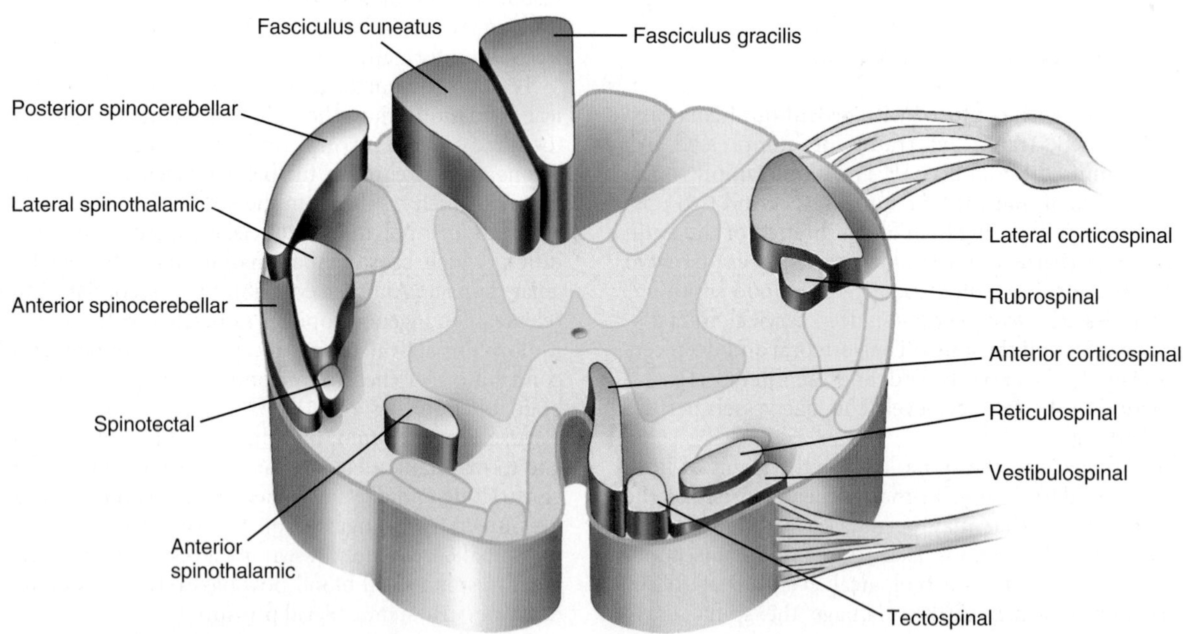

FIG. 14.13 Cross-section of the spinal cord. (From Thibodeau, G.A., Swisher, L. (2012). *Structure and function of the body* (14th ed.). St Louis: Mosby.)

pooling, decreased venous return, and decreased cardiac output with spinal cord injuries at T6 and above.[15] Interruption of input from the hypothalamus results in disturbances in temperature regulation, including the ability to shiver and sweat as needed to maintain a normal body temperature. A state of poikilothermy in which the systemic temperature changes with the ambient temperature may occur.[98]

Disruption of supraspinal input from above the level of the injury also results in autonomic dysreflexia/hyperreflexia (AD) (Box 14.1), a neurologic emergency usually occurring after the resolution of spinal and neurogenic shock. The clinical manifestations of hypertension, bradycardia, headache, facial flushing, piloerection, and sweating above (and possibly below) the lesion persist as long as the noxious peripheral stimulation continues.

TABLE 14.2 **Major Spinal Cord Tracts and Function**

Tract	Afferent/Efferent Origin/Destination Crossed/Uncrossed	Function
Motor		
Corticospinal tract	Efferent (descending) Origin: motor cortex Crosses where it terminates in spinal cord Destination: motor neurons in anterior horn	Voluntary movement
Lateral corticospinal tract	Efferent (descending) Origin: parietal lobe Crosses in medulla (decussation of pyramids) Destination: motor neurons in anterior horn	Voluntary movement
Rubrospinal tract	Efferent (descending) Origin: red nucleus in midbrain Crosses immediately Destination: motor neurons in anterior horn	Voluntary movement of upper extremities, especially distal musculature Inhibition of extensors and influence on muscle tone and posture
Vestibulospinal tract	Efferent (descending) Origin: vestibular nuclei Uncrossed Destination: motor neurons of cervical spine	Posture and balance in response to body position changes, especially head and neck
Lateral and medial reticulospinal tracts	Efferent (descending) Origin: reticular formation in brain stem Uncrossed Destination: motor neurons in posterior neuron	Posture, balance, and ambulation
Tectospinal tract	Efferent (descending) Origin: superior colliculus in midbrain Crosses soon after origin Destination: motor neurons in anterior horn of spinal cord	Coordination of head and eye movement in response to visual or auditory stimuli
Sensory		
Anterior spinothalamic tract	Afferent (ascending) Origin: posterior horn of spinal cord Crosses 1–2 segments above origin in spinal cord Destination: thalamus	Light touch
Lateral spinothalamic tract	Afferent (ascending) Origin: posterior horn of spinal cord Destination: thalamus	Pain and temperature
Posterior (dorsal) columns	Afferent (ascending)	Proprioception, vibration, tactile discrimination
Fasciculus gracilis	Origin: posterior lumbar and sacral spinal cord	Impulses from lower extremities
Fasciculus cuneatus	Origin: posterior cervical and thoracic spinal cord Both cross in medulla Destination: sensory strip of parietal lobe	Impulses from upper extremities
Posterior (dorsal) spinocerebellar tract (Clarke's column)	Afferent (ascending) Origin: posterior horn of spinal cord Uncrossed from sacrum and lower lumbar area Destination: cerebellum	Reflex proprioception, detailed control of movement and coordination; posture
Anterior spinocerebellar tract	Afferent (ascending) Origin: posterior horn of spinal cord Crossed and uncrossed Destination: cerebellum	Reflex proprioception, detailed control of movement and coordination; posture
Spinotectal tract	Afferent (ascending) Origin: posterior horn of spinal cord Crossed Destination: tectum of midbrain	Eye and head movement in response to visual stimuli

From References 130, 145, and 162.

More subtle increases in AD may occur with less dramatic increases in blood pressure. Nonetheless, AD is a neurologic emergency.[63] The noxious stimuli of AD are most often an overdistended bladder, a fecal impaction, uterine contractions, or a pressure ulcer. AD may result in a hypertensive crisis that causes an intracerebral hemorrhage, seizures, or a myocardial infarction.[63,102,103]

As with cerebral insults, spinal cord edema persists for several days following injury. Spinal cord edema may result in a neurologic deterioration for up to 1 week. Much later, the spinal cord may also develop a syrinx (a cystic cavity in the spinal cord), a tethered cord, or a surgical abscess, contributing to neurologic deterioration.[150] Syringomyelia may

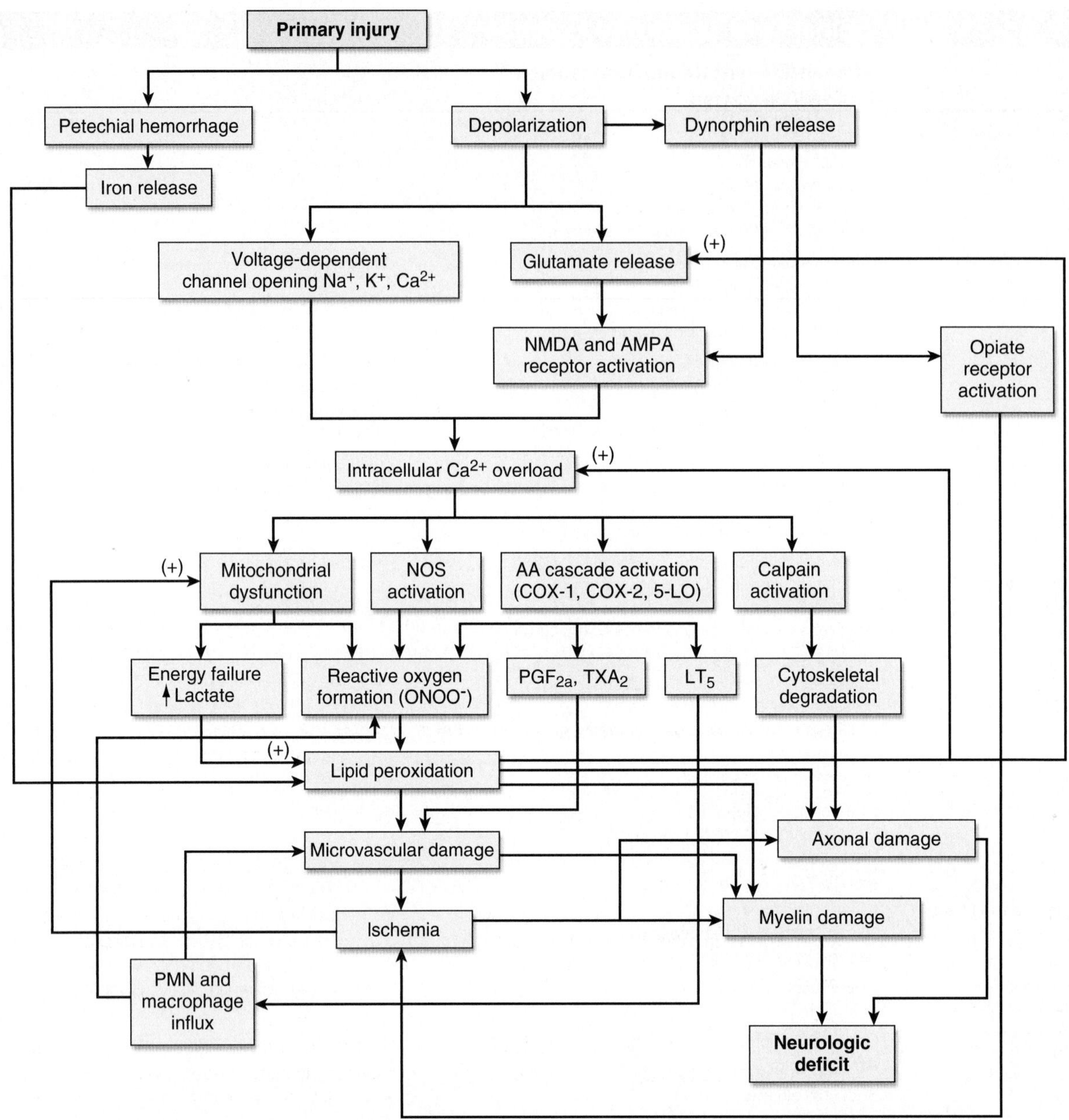

FIG. 14.14 Proposed pathophysiology of secondary neuronal injury following primary spinal cord injury. *AMPA,* α-Amino-3-hydroxy-5-methyl-4-isoxazolepropionic acid; Ca^{2+}, calcium; *COX,* cyclooxygenase; K^+, potassium; *5-LO,* 5-lipoxygenase; LT_5, leukotrienes; Na^+, sodium; *NMDA, N*-methyl-D-aspartate; *NOS* nitric oxide synthase; $ONOO^-$, peroxynitrite anion; PGF_{2a}, prostaglandin F_{2a}, *PMN,* polymorphonuclear leukocyte; TXA_2, thromboxane A_2. (From Hall, E.D., Springer, J.E. (2004). Neuroprotection and acute spinal cord injury: a reappraisal. *NeuroRX, 1*(1):80–100.)

present subtly with a change in sensory level, increased spasticity, or pain.[141]

Often of greater priority than the motor, sensory, and cardiovascular effects of traumatic SCI are the effects on the respiratory system. The phrenic nerve between C3 and C5 innervates the diaphragm. If input from the spinal cord to the diaphragmatic nerve is impaired, intubation and mechanical ventilation will be required. Many persons with spinal cord injuries found dead at the scene die from respiratory arrest. However, injuries as low as T6–T12 may be associated with pulmonary complications. T1 through T6 innervate the intercostal muscles required for deep breathing and coughing. T7 through T12 innervate the abdominal muscles used in expiration and coughing. Respiratory impairment results in hypoventilation, hypoxemia, hypercarbia, atelectasis, and pneumonia.[15,121] Pulmonary complications are the primary cause of mortality and morbidity in SCI.[157] Neurogenic pulmonary edema or pulmonary edema aggravated by volume resuscitation may compromise pulmonary status initially.[45] The mechanism is thought to be sudden, increased sympathetic activity resulting in pulmonary capillary leakage.[45] Other pulmonary complications include pulmonary emboli, adult respiratory distress syndrome, and sleep apnea. Venous stasis as a result of impaired mobility of the extremities places the SCI patient at greatest risk for deep vein thrombosis and pulmonary emboli.[140] Sleep apnea associated with SCI is obstructive or central and may be related to obesity or neurologic changes.[138,157]

BOX 14.1 Autonomic Dysreflexia

Pathophysiology

In autonomic dysreflexia (AD)/hyperreflexia, sensory nerves below a spinal cord injury from C1 to T6 transmit noxious ascending impulses to the spinal cord. Sympathetic neurons are stimulated. However, the usual inhibitory impulses above T6 are blocked by the SCI. As a result, sympathetic outflow from T6 to L2 is unopposed. Autonomic dysreflexia occurs after spinal shock resolves and reflexes become hyperreflexic.

Prevention

The best prevention for autonomic dysreflexia is compliance with bowel and bladder training and patient/family education.

Signs and Symptoms

Autonomic dysreflexia symptoms include the following:

1. Sudden large increase in systolic and diastolic blood pressures (e.g., systolic > 200 mm Hg) or an increase in blood pressure 20 to 40 mm Hg above baseline.
2. Pounding headache.
3. Bradycardia or a relative bradycardia compared to the patient's baseline heart rate.
4. Profuse perspiration, especially above the lesion, but also possible below the lesion.
5. Piloerection above or possibly below the level of the lesion.
6. Flushing, especially above the lesion, but also possible below the lesion.
7. Nasal congestion.
8. Visual changes.
9. Anxiety and apprehension.

Significance

AD is a true neurologic emergency. Failure to recognize and treat the symptoms of AD promptly, especially the hypertension, may result in myocardial infarction, seizures, or hemorrhagic stroke.

Causes

Autonomic dysreflexia may be caused by any noxious stimulus. Bowel and bladder problems are the most frequent causes, including bladder distention, an occluded catheter, urinary tract infection, catheterization, renal calculi, urologic or gastrointestinal instrumentation, fecal impaction, gastric ulcers, gallstones, and appendicitis. Pressure ulcers, blisters and burns, constrictive clothing, labor and delivery, sexual intercourse, deep vein thrombosis, pulmonary emboli, surgical and diagnostic procedures, and stimulants are other causes.

Treatment

Definitive treatment for AD is removing the noxious stimulation. However, while determining the noxious stimulation and continuing to monitor the patient's signs and symptoms, other interventions that may improve the clinical presentation temporarily include elevating the head of the bed unless contraindicated; loosening any constrictive clothing or devices; using a topical anesthetic such as 2% lidocaine lubricant when catheterizing the patient or removing a fecal impaction; and administering a short-acting antihypertensive, such as nitroglycerin or nifedipine to resolve hypertension.

From References 55, 63, 71, 98, 102, 140, and 159.

Immediately following SCI, the patient experiences gastric atony with hypoactive bowel sounds and delayed gastric emptying. This places the patient at risk for vomiting and aspiration. Within the first month, up to 4.2% of patients experience gastroduodenal ulceration and gastrointestinal hemorrhage.[76] Later, the patient will require a bowel training program to make elimination regular and predictable, and minimize the risk of ileus or AD.[76] Spinal cord patients are also at increased risk for acute acalculous cholecystitis, acute calculus cholecystitis, and pancreatitis.[24,36,53] The increased incidence of cholecystitis is thought to be related to decreased gastrointestinal motility, parenteral nutrition, mechanical ventilation with positive end-expiratory pressure, and the use of opiates.[24,36,53]

Urinary elimination is impaired as well. The flaccidity of the bladder requires the insertion of an indwelling catheter in the early stages of the injury. Once spinal shock has resolved, some SCI patients reflex void.[68] Loss of neural input, bone demineralization, and immobilization following SCI result in an increased risk of renal calculi.[140]

Following the resolution of spinal shock, spasticity of musculature below the level of the spinal cord lesion occurs. Reflexive movement, not under the patient's volition, may be mistaken as a sign of recovery by the patient and family. Spasticity is the result of an imbalance between excitatory and inhibitory impulses. The normal inhibitory input from the brain cannot modulate the excitatory impulses below the lesion to limit the spinal reflex movement.[44,76]

Immediately after traumatic spinal cord injury, patients experience acute pain for a number of reasons, including polytrauma and surgical incisions. However, the chronic pain that develops later in up to 80% of patients may be nociceptive or neuropathic or both.[140] The nociceptive pain is musculoskeletal or visceral in origin. Common etiologies of nociceptive pain are spasticity, abnormal posture, gait, and overuse of upper extremities. Neuropathic pain may result from spinal cord damage, or nerve root damage, or post-traumatic syringomyelia. Neuropathic pain at or below the level of the spinal cord injury is described as burning, aching, tingling, or stabbing.[140]

ASSESSMENT

As with other critically ill patients, airway, breathing, and circulation are of higher priority than the neurologic injury. However, all attempts must be made to prevent secondary injury while performing interventions to resolve cardiopulmonary compromise. Immobilization efforts, spine precautions, and a cervical collar are critical until the spine is cleared from injury.[7] Once the cardiopulmonary status of the patient is stabilized, serial bedside clinical assessment must take place in an organized and consistent manner. Up to 60% of all spinal cord-injured patients also experience TBI; therefore, the neurologic exam must be comprehensive, including mental status and cranial nerves, as well as attention to the spinal cord assessment.[106] Until proven otherwise, all trauma patients, especially those with TBI, are assumed to have an SCI.[7,120]

The spinal cord assessment is performed in a standardized and consistent format, making bilateral comparisons, moving down the body from head to toe. Muscle groups, dermatome level testing of sharp and dull sensation, and proprioception are included (Fig. 14.15). Superficial cutaneous reflexes and deep tendon reflexes, if included, will be hyporeflexic or areflexic. Priapism may be present initially, but usually resolves spontaneously. Tables 14.3 through 14.7 summarize assessment of the spinal cord.[28,95,113,154,162]

A standardized internationally recognized scoring system for delineating SCI is the American Spinal Cord Injury Association (ASIA) classification, shown in Fig. 14.16.[28] The ASIA score consists of a motor score composed of 10 muscle groups innervated from C5 through T1 and from L2 through S1 (the upper and lower extremities, respectively), as well as 28 dermatomes, as indicators of sensation. The ASIA Impairment Scale categorizes the injury as normal, complete, or variable

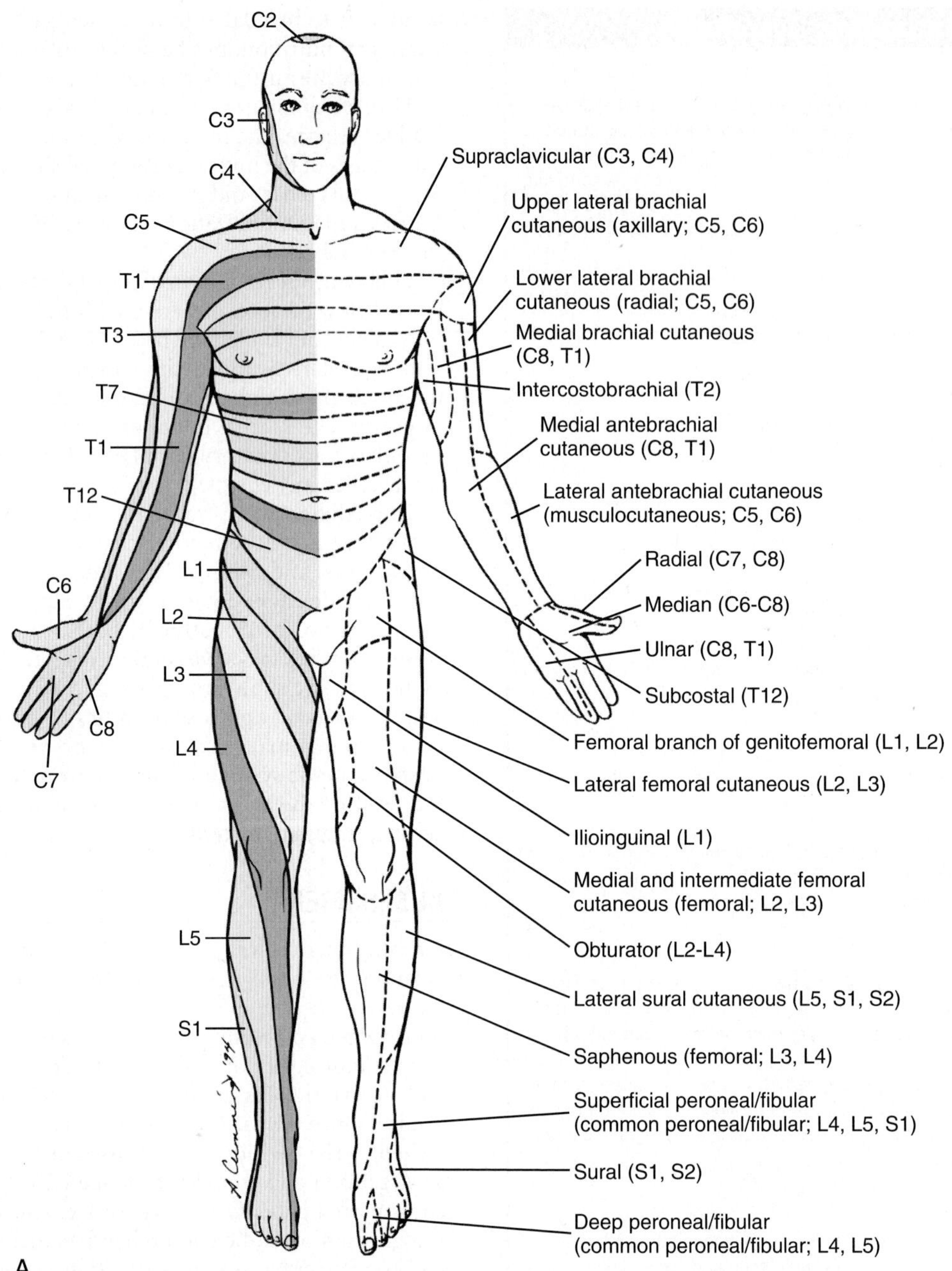

FIG. 14.15 Dermatomes. A, Anterior view.

degrees of incomplete.[28] The ASIA classification combines the severity (ASIA score) and the completeness of the injury (ASIA Impairment Scale) and has been found to correlate with outcome.[28] Use of the ASIA classification of spinal cord injury is a Level II recommendation from the Congress of Neurologic Surgeons (Box 14.2).[75]

Factors that may influence the patient's exam in addition to the SCI include TBI, alcohol or other drug use, pain, preexisting illness/injury, and other injuries, such as chest and abdominal injuries and long bone fractures.[7] A routine laboratory workup includes arterial blood gases, serum chemistries, complete blood count, coagulation studies, and urine/blood ethanol and drug screens.

The radiologic evaluation is of great priority for any patient with suspected spine or spinal cord injury. The patient with suspected spine or spinal cord injury might not be easily identified in every instance. In addition, the choice of imaging modality may not be easy to determine. Plain films are increasingly being supplemented or even replaced with CT and MRI. The American College of Surgeons now state that CT is recommended, while the cross-table lateral anterior-posterior and open-mouth odontoid views are described as alternative.[7] If plain cervical films are obtained, in addition to the lateral cross-table cervical spine view, the anteroposterior spine films and an open-mouth view of the cervical spine to visualize the odontoid process of C2 must be obtained. A complete cervical spine film series requires visualization of all seven cervical vertebrae, C1 through C7. To facilitate visualization of C7, a swimmer's view may be required. The swimmer's view requires the patient to be turned slightly more than laterally, with one arm extended toward the head and abducted 180 degrees while the other arm is extended posteriorly and toward the feet. This maneuver moves the shoulder away from the cervicothoracic junction exposing C7.[7]

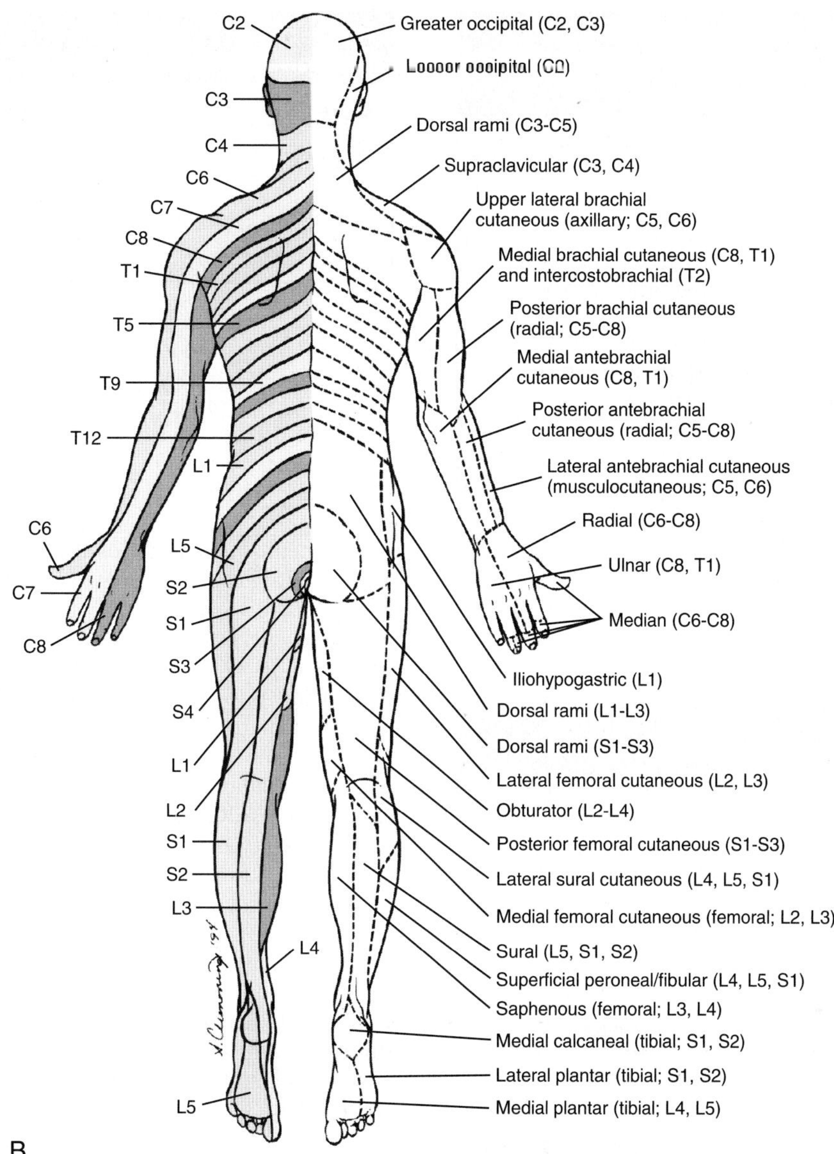

FIG. 14.15, cont'd **B,** Posterior view. (From AANN. (2004). AANN core curriculum for neuroscience nursing (4th ed.). St Louis: Saunders.)

TABLE 14.3 Cutaneous Reflexes, Level of Spinal Cord Innervation, and Method of Stimulation and Response

Reflex	Spinal Innervation	Stimulus	Response
Upper abdominal	T8-T9-T10	Stroke upper abdomen	Abdominal wall contraction causes umbilicus to move toward stimulus
Lower abdominal	T10-T11-T12	Stroke lower abdomen	Abdominal wall contraction causes umbilicus to move toward stimulus
Cremasteric	L1-L2	Stroke medial thigh	Testicular elevation
Bulbocavernosus	S3-S4	Pressure to glans penis	Contraction of anus
Anal wink	S2-S3-S4	Stroke perianal area	Contraction of external anal sphincter

From References 7, 113, 154, and 162.

TABLE 14.4 Muscle Groups and Associated Level of Spinal Cord Innervation and Method of Testing

Muscle Tested	Innervation	Method of Testing
Deltoids	C5	Raise arms
Biceps	C5	Flex elbow
Wrist extensors	C6	Extend wrist
Triceps	C7	Extend elbow
Hand intrinsics	C8-T1	Hand squeeze, flex finger, abduct finger
Iliopsoas	L2	Flex hips
Hip adductors	L2-L3-L4	Adduct hips (squeeze legs together)
Hip abductors	L4-L5-S1	Abduct hips (separate hips)
Quadriceps	L3-L4	Extend knee
Hamstrings	L4-L5-S1-S2	Flex knee
Tibialis anterior	L4	Dorsiflex foot
Extensor hallucis longus (EHL)	L5	Extend great toe
Gastrocnemius	S1	Plantar flex foot

From References 7, 113, 154, and 162.

TABLE 14.5 Muscle Strength Grading Scale

Score	Muscle Function
0	Absent; no muscular contraction detected
1	Flicker or palpable muscle contraction
2	Poor; active movement of muscle with gravity eliminated
3	Fair; active muscle movement against gravity
4	Good; muscle movement against some resistance (± may be used with this score to indicate degree of strength against resistance)
5	Normal strength; movement against resistance

From References 7 and 113.

TABLE 14.6 Deep Tendon Reflexes and the Associated Level of Spinal Cord Innervation

Reflex	Spinal Innervation
Brachioradialis (supinator)	C5-C6
Biceps	C5-C6
Triceps	C7-C8
Patellar (knee)	L2-L3-L4
Achilles (ankle)	S1-S2

From References 113 and 162.

If the patient is able to participate, flexion-extension films under the direction of a provider may aid in clearing the cervical spine. Flexion-extension films may assist in determination of the stability of the cervical fracture.[7] The patient's neck must not, under any circumstances, be forced into a pain-inducing position. Flexion-extension radiographic evaluation can also be performed under fluoroscopy.[7] If the patient is unable to cooperate in a bedside assessment to clear the spine, MRI will show ligamentous injury, epidural hematomas, and herniated disks. However, not every patient can undergo MRI imaging related to metallic fragments or clips, implanted devices, or hemodynamic instability.[7,33]

TABLE 14.7 Scoring Strength of Deep Tendon Reflexes

Score	Reflex Response
4+	Hyperreactive, clonus
3+	Very brisk
2+	Normal, average
1+	Diminished
0	No response, flaccid

From References 7 and 162.

Because of the devastating effects of SCI and the lack of well-designed prospective randomized controlled trials, clearance of the cervical spine was an area of great anxiety and debate without universally applied standards. As a result, some trauma patients have been subjected to additional x-ray exposure; transport out of the critical care unit to radiology with the increased possibility of disruption of life-sustaining interventions; and added discomfort and potential skin breakdown from wearing a cervical collar that may not have been necessary. Recommendations have recently been published to guide clinicians (see Box 14.2). In 2012, the American Association of Neurological Surgeons (AANS) and the Congress of Neurological Surgeons (CNS) made a Level I recommendation (based on 60 evidence-based publications, evidence Classes I through III) for radiographic examinations. Radiographic evaluation of the cervical spine is unnecessary in trauma patients who are awake, alert, not intoxicated, and asymptomatic, without neck pain or tenderness.[75,135] For symptomatic, obtunded, or unevaluable trauma patients, the AANS and CNS Level I recommendation states that high-quality CT imaging must be performed, utilizing plain films only if high-quality CT imaging is not available. Furthermore, MRI may be used if evidence for spinal cord injury is conflicting.[135]

Cervical spine immobilization for symptomatic awake trauma patients with neck pain or tenderness may be discontinued with normal CT and normal three-view cervical spine films (anteroposterior, lateral, and odontoid), and dynamic flexion-extension plain radiographs, or a normal MRI within 48 hours of injury (Level III recommendation; see Box 14.2). Discontinuation of cervical spine immobilization is also a AANS/CNS Level III recommendation (see Box 14.2) for obtunded patients with normal cervical spine CT imaging and at least one of the following: normal three-view cervical spine films (anteroposterior, lateral, and odontoid), normal MRI within 48 hours, or the experienced provider's discretion.[135]

Thoracic and lumbar radiographic evaluation is not addressed by AANS/CNS standards.[135] However, anteroposterior and lateral thoracic and lumbar radiographs are generally considered warranted in patients with neurologic deficits, pain, or a likely mechanism of injury. CT scans of the spine are generally more demonstrative in regard to bony abnormalities, whereas MRI is more likely to reveal soft tissue pathology or ligamentous injuries.[15]

Two organizations, the American College of Surgeons and the Neurocritical Care Society, have adopted the use of specific clinical assessment criteria for spine clearance without imaging, in the awake asymptomatic patient to lessen exposure to radiation, and the length of time a patient remains

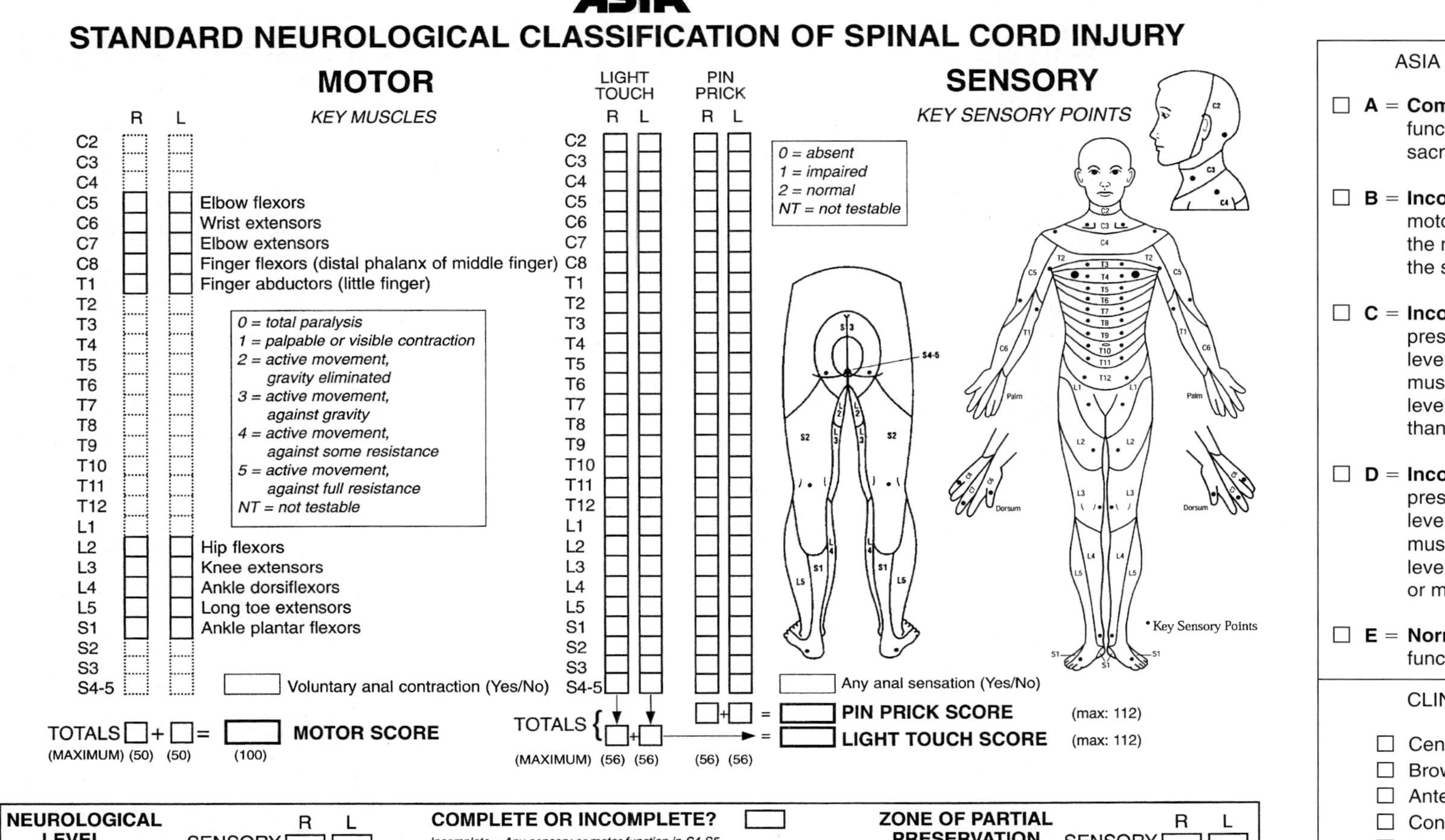

ASIA

STANDARD NEUROLOGICAL CLASSIFICATION OF SPINAL CORD INJURY

MOTOR

KEY MUSCLES

	R	L	
C2			
C3			
C4			
C5	☐	☐	Elbow flexors
C6	☐	☐	Wrist extensors
C7	☐	☐	Elbow extensors
C8	☐	☐	Finger flexors (distal phalanx of middle finger)
T1	☐	☐	Finger abductors (little finger)
T2			
T3			
T4			
T5			
T6			
T7			
T8			
T9			
T10			
T11			
T12			
L1			
L2	☐	☐	Hip flexors
L3	☐	☐	Knee extensors
L4	☐	☐	Ankle dorsiflexors
L5	☐	☐	Long toe extensors
S1	☐	☐	Ankle plantar flexors
S2			
S3			
S4-5			

0 = total paralysis
1 = palpable or visible contraction
2 = active movement, gravity eliminated
3 = active movement, against gravity
4 = active movement, against some resistance
5 = active movement, against full resistance
NT = not testable

☐ Voluntary anal contraction (Yes/No)

TOTALS ☐ + ☐ = ☐ **MOTOR SCORE**
(MAXIMUM) (50) (50) (100)

SENSORY

KEY SENSORY POINTS

	LIGHT TOUCH R	LIGHT TOUCH L	PIN PRICK R	PIN PRICK L
C2	☐	☐	☐	☐
C3	☐	☐	☐	☐
C4	☐	☐	☐	☐
C5	☐	☐	☐	☐
C6	☐	☐	☐	☐
C7	☐	☐	☐	☐
C8	☐	☐	☐	☐
T1	☐	☐	☐	☐
T2	☐	☐	☐	☐
T3	☐	☐	☐	☐
T4	☐	☐	☐	☐
T5	☐	☐	☐	☐
T6	☐	☐	☐	☐
T7	☐	☐	☐	☐
T8	☐	☐	☐	☐
T9	☐	☐	☐	☐
T10	☐	☐	☐	☐
T11	☐	☐	☐	☐
T12	☐	☐	☐	☐
L1	☐	☐	☐	☐
L2	☐	☐	☐	☐
L3	☐	☐	☐	☐
L4	☐	☐	☐	☐
L5	☐	☐	☐	☐
S1	☐	☐	☐	☐
S2	☐	☐	☐	☐
S3	☐	☐	☐	☐
S4-5	☐	☐	☐	☐
TOTALS (MAXIMUM)	(56)	(56)	(56)	(56)

0 = absent
1 = impaired
2 = normal
NT = not testable

☐ Any anal sensation (Yes/No)

☐ + ☐ = ☐ **PIN PRICK SCORE** (max: 112)
☐ + ☐ = ☐ **LIGHT TOUCH SCORE** (max: 112)

NEUROLOGICAL LEVEL *The most caudal segment with normal function*		R	L	**COMPLETE OR INCOMPLETE?** *Incomplete = Any sensory or motor function in S4-S5*	☐	**ZONE OF PARTIAL PRESERVATION** *Caudal extent of partially innervated segments*		R	L
	SENSORY	☐	☐				SENSORY	☐	☐
	MOTOR	☐	☐	**ASIA IMPAIRMENT SCALE**	☐		MOTOR	☐	☐

2000 Rev.

ASIA IMPAIRMENT SCALE

☐ A = **Complete:** No motor or sensory function is preserved in the sacral segments S4-S5.

☐ B = **Incomplete:** Sensory but not motor function is preserved below the neurological level and includes the sacral segments S4-S5.

☐ C = **Incomplete:** Motor function is preserved below the neurologic level, and more than half of key muscles below the neurological level have a muscle grade less than 3.

☐ D = **Incomplete:** Motor function is preserved below the neurologic level, and at least half of key muscles below the neurologic level have a muscle grade of 3 or more.

☐ E = **Normal:** Motor and sensory function are normal

CLINICAL SYNDROMES

☐ Central Cord
☐ Brown-Séquard
☐ Anterior Cord
☐ Conus Medullaris
☐ Cauda Equina

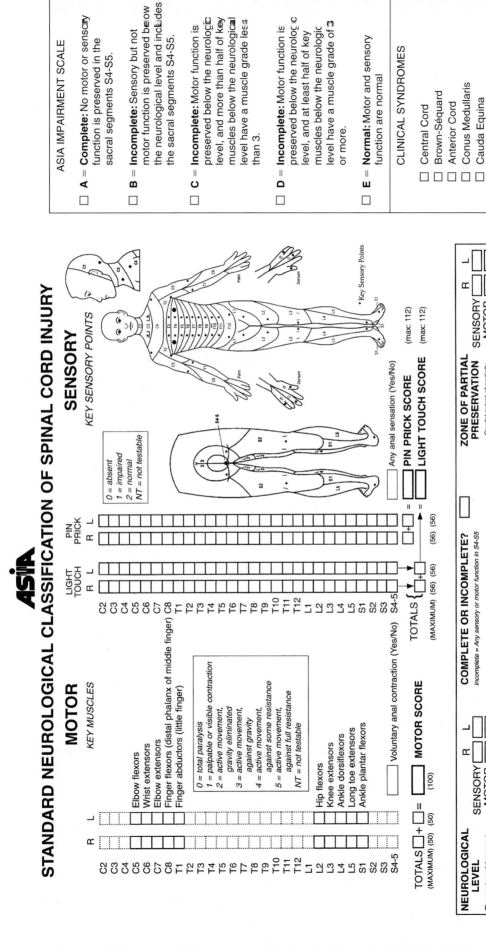

FIG. 14.16 American Spinal Injury Association (ASIA) scale. Standard neurologic classification of spinal cord injury: sensory and motor worksheet. (From Barker E. (2007). *Neuroscience nursing: a spectrum of care* (3rd ed.). St Louis: Mosby.)

BOX 14.2 Classification of Evidence*

Class I

- AANS/CNS: Evidence from at least one well-designed, randomized controlled clinical trial, including trial overviews. Class I evidence supports the strongest type of recommendations, Level I clinical practice guideline recommendations.
- CSCM: Evidence from large randomized trials with obvious results and low risk of error. Class I evidence supports *Grade A* clinical practice guideline recommendations, the strongest type.

Class II

- AANS/CNS: Evidence from at least one well-designed comparative clinical study, such as nonrandomized cohort studies, case-control studies, and less well-designed randomized controlled studies. Class II evidence supports Level II clinical practice guideline recommendations, which indicate a moderate degree of certainty.
- CSCM: Evidence from small-randomized trials with less certain results and moderate to high risk of error. Class II evidence supports *Grade B* clinical practice guideline recommendations, with an intermediate level of certainty.

Class III

- AANS/CNS: Evidence from case series; comparative studies using historical controls, case reports, and expert opinion; and significantly flawed randomized controlled trials. Class III evidence supports Level III clinical practice guideline recommendations that reflect a lack of clinical certainty.
- CSCM: Evidence from nonrandomized trials with concurrent controls. Class III evidence supports *Grade C* clinical practice guideline recommendations with the lowest degree of certainty.

Class IV and Class V (CSCM Only)

- CSCM: Evidence from nonrandomized trials with historical controls (Class IV) or case series with no controls (Class V). Class IV and V evidence supports *Grade C* clinical practice guideline recommendations, with the lowest degree of certainty.

*As defined by the American Association of Neurological Surgeons and Congress of Neurological Surgeons (AANS/CNS)[1,6,47,48,73-75,77,82,131-136] and the Consortium for Spinal Cord Medicine (CSCM)[23,40,64,94,103,104,111,119,164,166] guidelines.

on unnecessary spine precautions. The National Emergency X-Radiology Utilization Study (NEXUS) Criteria lists clinical criteria for patients who are at low risk for injury and imaging is not necessary (Table 14.8).[27] NEXUS is 100% sensitive for exclusion of cervical spinal cord injury. The Canadian Cervical Spine Rule includes both criteria for both low and high risk for cervical spinal cord injury, and has the greater specificity (Fig. 14.17).[7,81,147,149,150]

The spinal column stability of the thoracic and lumbar regions can be assessed using at least three different classification methods. One method is the Denis three-column injury model (Fig. 14.18). The damaged vertebra is divided vertically into anterior, middle, and posterior one-third. The anterior column consists of the anterior longitudinal ligament, anterior half of the vertebral body, and the intervertebral disk. The middle column includes the posterior longitudinal ligament, posterior half of the vertebral body, and the intervertebral disk. The posterior one-third is comprised of facet joints, the ligamentum flavum, and intraspinous and supraspinous ligaments. If two or more columns are damaged, the injury is classified as unstable.[15]

TABLE 14.8 National Emergency X-Radiography Utilization Study Criteria (NEXUS)

Study Criteria for Cervical Spine Imaging Is Unnecessary in Patients Meeting these Five Criteria
1. Absence of midline cervical tenderness
2. Normal level of alertness and consciousness
3. No evidence of intoxication
4. Absence of local neurologic deficit
5. Absence of painful distracting injury

From References 27 and 81.

MANAGEMENT

Before arrival in critical care, a number of interventions will have already taken place in the prehospital field and in the emergency department. Although basic and advanced measures to support the airway, breathing, and circulation take precedence over neurologic trauma, trauma resuscitation must be carried out with consideration for potential or actual SCI to minimize the risk of primary or secondary injury. Immobilization and stabilization of the spine is imperative and includes such maneuvers as modified jaw thrust to open and maintain the airway, application of a hard cervical collar, movement of the patient as a unit (log-roll technique), and placement on a backboard.[7]

In contrast to the past 25 years, the patient will not likely be placed on a methylprednisolone protocol. In 2013, the Congress of Neurological Surgeons and the American Association of Neurological Surgeons endorsed a Level I recommendation (see Box 14.2) that methylprednisolone is not recommended for acute spinal cord injury.[82] These organizations added that the use of methylprednisolone is not supported by either Class I (high-quality randomized controlled trials) or Class II (comparative studies, and nonrandomized cohort or case-control studies) evidence. Furthermore, they acknowledged that high-dose corticosteroids are associated with significant side effects.[82] Additionally, several other organizations, including the Neurocritical Care Society, American College of Surgeons, and the Consortium for Spinal Cord Medicine, previously denounced the use of corticosteroids.[7,147,165]

Corticosteroids have been contraindicated in TBI since 2000.[25] In 2000 the Brain Trauma Foundation and AANS published guidelines for the management and prognosis of severe TBI, including a standard regarding the role of steroids. Their review of multiple prospective randomized controlled clinical trials, Class I evidence, led them to conclude that the use of steroids in severe head injury does not reduce intracranial pressure or improve outcome and is therefore not recommended.[25] Previously however, methylprednisolone was an option (lowest level of evidence) in the management of SCI.[6,73] Acknowledged to be the most controversial recommendation, AANS/CNS classified methylprednisolone for 24 to 48 hours as an option (Class III evidence) that should be used only with the understanding that the detrimental effects may outweigh the benefits in acute cervical SCI. The methylprednisolone protocol was

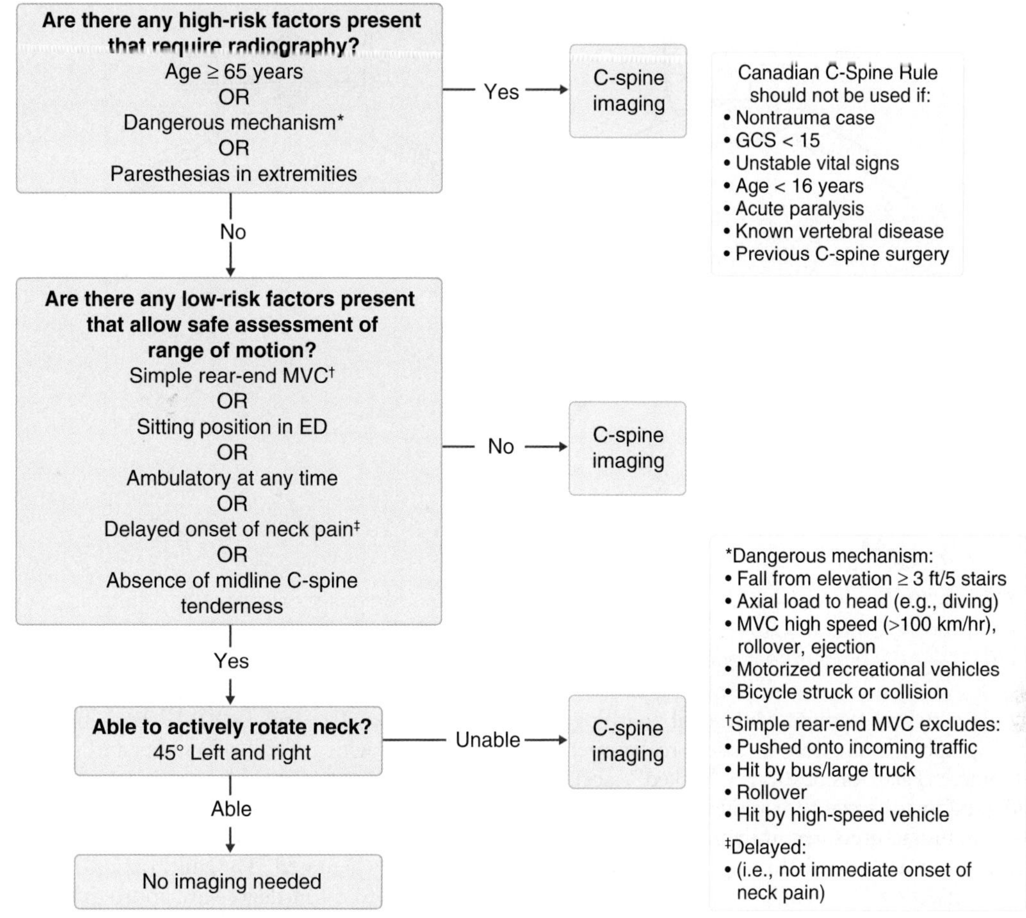
Are there any high-risk factors present that require radiography?
Age ≥ 65 years
OR
Dangerous mechanism*
OR
Paresthesias in extremities
Yes
C-spine imaging
No
Canadian C-Spine Rule should not be used if:
• Nontrauma case
• GCS < 15
• Unstable vital signs
• Age < 16 years
• Acute paralysis
• Known vertebral disease
• Previous C-spine surgery
Are there any low-risk factors present that allow safe assessment of range of motion?
Simple rear-end MVC†
OR
Sitting position in ED
OR
Ambulatory at any time
OR
Delayed onset of neck pain‡
OR
Absence of midline C-spine tenderness
No
C-spine imaging
Yes
Able to actively rotate neck?
45° Left and right
Unable
C-spine imaging
Able
No imaging needed
*Dangerous mechanism:
• Fall from elevation ≥ 3 ft/5 stairs
• Axial load to head (e.g., diving)
• MVC high speed (>100 km/hr), rollover, ejection
• Motorized recreational vehicles
• Bicycle struck or collision
†Simple rear-end MVC excludes:
• Pushed onto incoming traffic
• Hit by bus/large truck
• Rollover
• Hit by high-speed vehicle
‡Delayed:
• (i.e., not immediate onset of neck pain)

FIG. 14.17 Canadian Cervical Spine Rule for Radiography: cervical spine imaging unnecessary in patients meeting these criteria. (Modified from Stiell, I.G., Clement, C.M., McKnight, R.D., et al. Comparative validation of the Canadian C-Spine Rule and the NEXUS low-risk criteria in alert and stable patients. *N Engl J Med.* 2003; 349:2510–2518; and Stiell, I.G., Wells, G.A., Vandemheen, K.L., et al. The Canadian C-Spine Rule for radiography in alert and stable trauma patients. JAMA. 2001; 286:1841–1848.

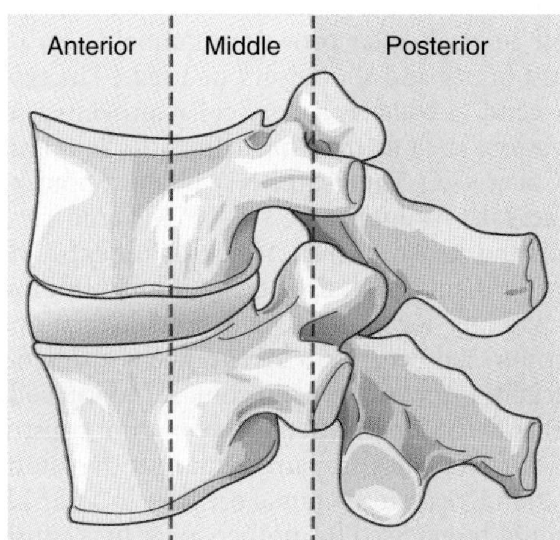
Anterior
Middle
Posterior

FIG. 14.18 Three-column theory of spinal stability. This theory is based on the overlap between columns, with the integrity of the middle column most important. If there is injury to the anterior and middle columns or to the posterior and middle columns, the resulting fracture is unstable.

weight-based and was to be initiated within 3 hours of injury for the 24-hour regimen or within 3 to 8 hours of injury for the 48-hour course of therapy. The methylprednisolone protocol was not indicated in penetrating SCI.[6,73,112,123]

Additional realignment of the spine and reduction of a fracture dislocation include the initiation of cervical traction or surgical decompression of the cervical, thoracic, or lumbar spine. These interventions may occur before or after admission to critical care. Tong traction for cervical spine injury consists of metal tongs with a weight and pulley system (Fig. 14.19). Gardner-Wells tongs are spring-loaded for ease of insertion and maintenance and do not require drilling of pin sites before insertion.[17,42] Crutchfield and Vinke tongs require drilling before pin insertion. The ring of the halo brace may be used instead of tongs. Gardner-Wells and Vinke tongs, as well as the halo ring, are available in nonferrous MRI-compatible styles.[42] The amount of weight used in cervical traction is controversial.[16] Some clinicians recommend the amount of weight to be used initially for traction is 5 pounds per vertebral level above and including the level of the fracture or dislocation. For example, a C5 fracture would have 25 pounds of traction initially. Others state that 10 pounds may be added for the head.[16] Up to 10 pounds or more per level may

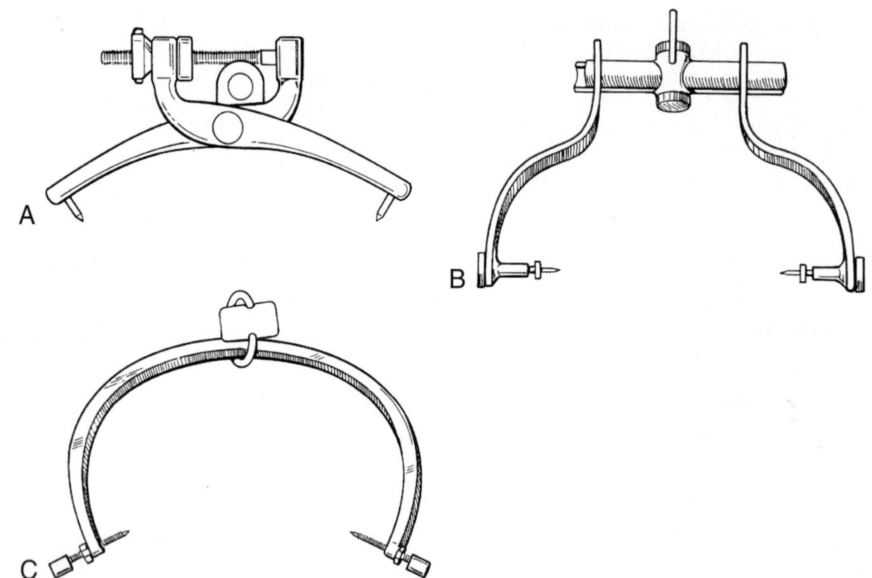

FIG. 14.19 Three types of cervical tongs. All types have a stainless-steel body with sharp tips at each end. **A,** Crutchfield tongs. **B,** Vinke tongs. **C,** Gardner-Wells tongs. (From Wiegand, D. J. L. M. (2011). *AACN procedure manual for critical care* (6th ed.). St Louis: Saunders.)

be added gradually per vertebral segment, with serial neurologic assessment and radiographic evaluation to assess realignment of the spinal vertebrae.[16] Facet dislocations ("locked" facets) may require considerably more weight for reduction, up to 140 pounds.[41] However, manufacturers recommend that traction be limited to 35 to 40 pounds with a halo ring. Gardner-Wells tongs are designed for insertion at an angle that allows the pins to support greater longitudinally applied forces.[42] However, MRI-compatible Gardner-Wells tongs consisting of titanium and carbon may only support 50 to 70 pounds of weight.[42] Manufacturers' directions should be followed for both the halo ring and Gardner-Wells tongs.[16,42] Pins are generally originally torqued at 6 to 8 pounds, but require being retorqued by the provider at 24 hours and halo pins again at 10 to 14 days.[16,42]

Tong traction is not without potential harm. Worsening of neurologic deficits may occur, particularly in people with distraction injuries and ankylosing spondylitis, a degenerative disease characterized by calcification of soft and ligamentous tissues. Other sequelae of tong traction include pin site infections, osteomyelitis, skull penetration, increased patient discomfort related to muscle spasms, and consequences of imposed bed rest, including aspiration. Inappropriate placement of the pins may result in cranial nerve damage and inability to completely close the eyelids with increased risk of corneal ulceration.[16,42] Analgesics and muscle relaxants may be of benefit immediately before, during, and after insertion.[42] To be effective, the weights must be hanging freely and the knot on the rope used to connect the weights to the tongs cannot be resting on the wheel of the pulley system. The use of tong traction is contraindicated in AOD because of the risk of medullary injury.[16,42,158] A 10% risk of neurologic deterioration with cervical tong traction in patients with AOD has been reported.[42,158]

Cervical traction may be placed on a regular hospital bed. However, a bed that allows greater turning of the patient is preferable. Two types of turning beds are an automatic rotating table, such as the RotoRest Delta Advanced Kinetic Therapy System (ArjoHuntleigh, San Antonio, TX),[8] and a manual wedge frame, such as the Stryker frame (Stryker Corp., Kalamazoo, MI) (Fig. 14.20).[121] Both beds have been studied extensively with regard to benefits and shortcomings. Patients on the manual turning frame may fall off the bed if the locking pin is not replaced securely after each turn, if the frames are not securely tight before turning prone or supine, or if the patient is restless or agitated. The automatic turning table will rotate the bed up to a 124-degree arc approximately every 5 minutes, which may aggravate the bradycardia and hypotension associated with neurogenic shock; result in respiratory compromise/desaturation; hamper incontinence and back care; shear the skin if the torso moves during rotation; and dislodge invasive monitoring and therapeutic devices. Turning with either bed may potentially allow an unstable fracture or dislocation to move out of alignment.[8]

For individuals not requiring the more stabilizing effect of cervical traction either because of early surgery or because of lack of indication, a number of hard cervical collars are available. A soft cervical collar provides minimal to no protection against cord injury and should not be used.[4] The typical first-responder cervical collar is a rigid collar providing maximum immobilization, such as the Philadelphia Collar (Philadelphia Cervical Collar Co., Thorofare, NJ) or the Stifneck Cervical Collar (Laerdal, Wappingers Falls, NY). Some cervical collars such as the Aspen (Aspen Medical Products, Irvine, CA) and Miami J (Ossur, Foothill Ranch, CA) have removable and cleanable padding for comfort and provide some protection against skin breakdown.[4] Skin breakdown is a significant concern, especially at the occiput and chin. A cervical collar is only as good as its fit, which must be secure but not constricting.[4] A tight cervical collar may impair jugular venous outflow from the brain and increase intracranial pressure in TBI.[4] Ideally, the patient should be assessed for proper collar fit according to the manufacturer's guidelines.

Spine precautions include not only the use of a cervical collar, but also proper movement of the patient as a unit (log-rolling), ideally with five people, two on each side and one at the head to stabilize the head and neck and direct the turn. A four-person logroll may be implemented if two perform the

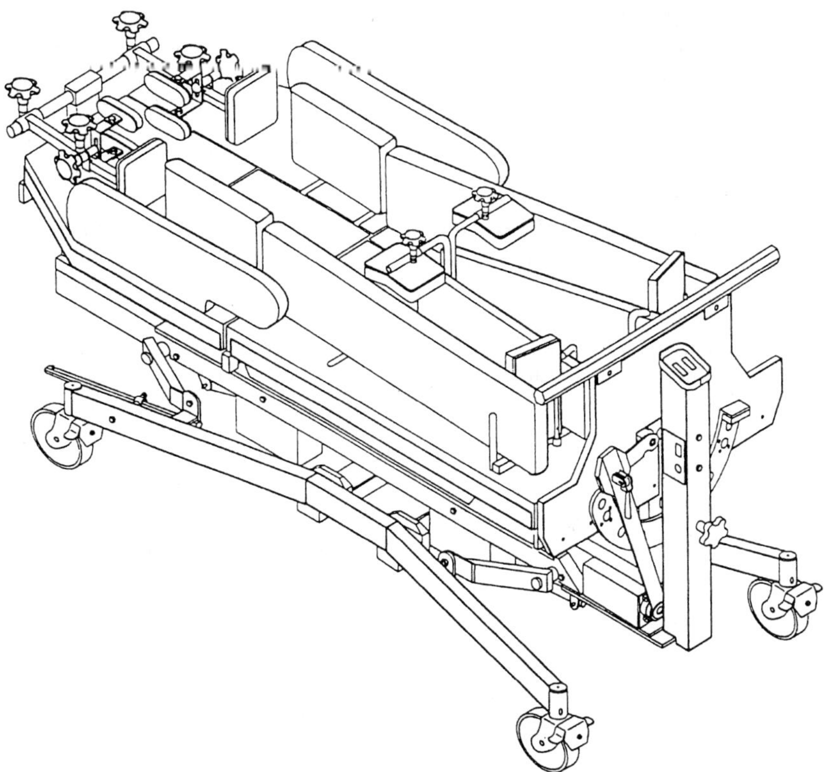

FIG. 14.20 Rotating kinetic treatment table. The table allows the patient to be rotated side to side, displacing weight to assist in pressure relief. It also facilitates pulmonary care. (From Wiegand, D. J. L. M. (2011). *AACN procedure manual for critical care* (6th ed.). St Louis: Saunders.)

logroll (toward them) with the leader manually stabilizing the head and the fourth person assessing the back and removing the spine board.[7] A brief neurologic assessment precedes and follows each turn.[60]

Mobilization of the spinal cord-injured patient as soon as possible is imperative to minimize the consequences of immobility. Whereas other injuries may also impact mobility, a decision regarding definitive treatment for the spine injury should be made as soon as possible. Long-term orthoses or surgery may be indicated in cervical and thoracolumbar spine injuries. The purpose of orthoses and surgery is realignment, decompression, and stabilization of the spine. A number of considerations and controversies exist in regard to surgery. The following questions should be asked: Is surgery indicated or will an orthotic device suffice? When is the best time for surgery? What is the best surgical approach/procedure? Will the patient need orthoses in addition to surgery? If closed reduction fails or neurologic deterioration occurs or worsens, open reduction and stabilization are indicated. Mounting evidence supports early decompression and stabilization (within 24 hours of injury) for the patient with spinal cord injury.[32,118]

Based on AANS/CNS guidelines, surgical fixation is recommended in: atlanto-occipital dislocations; some C1 (atlas) hangman's fractures; Types II and III odontoid (C2, axis) fractures with dens displacement greater than 5 mm, comminution of the dens fracture, and/or inability to achieve and maintain alignment; C3–C7 facet dislocations; and central cervical SCI.[1,158] Either internal or external fixation are options in C3–C7 fractures without facet dislocations. External fixation alone is recommended as an option in occipital condyle fractures, isolated atlas fractures with intact transverse ligaments, and isolated fractures of the axis body.[6,73] In penetrating SCI, surgery is indicated for incomplete injuries in the cervical spinal cord,

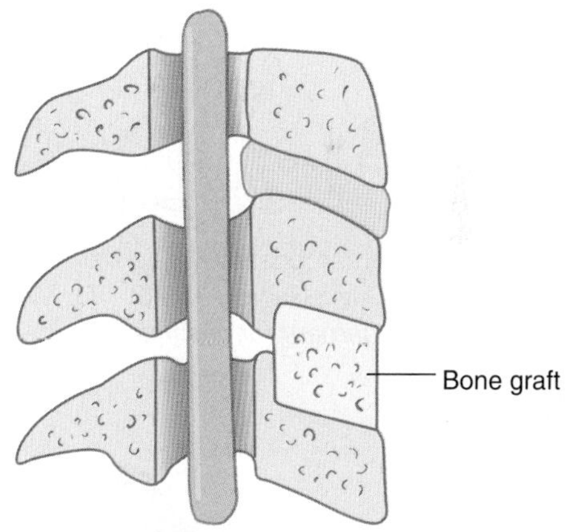

FIG. 14.21 Anterior corpectomy.

an expanding hematoma and radiographic evidence of compression, persistent cerebrospinal fluid (CSF) fistula, infection, and cauda equina injuries.[17,142] Surgery for bullet removal alone does not usually result in improved outcomes unless the injury involves the cauda equina.[142] While evidence-based recommendations regarding thoracolumbar injuries have not been published, indications for surgery include spine instability, neural compression, and risk of complications, such as neurologic deterioration, deformity, and pain.[13,37] A number of surgical procedures exist, including anterior and posterior approaches, corpectomy, decompressive laminectomy, and fusions using bone or instrumentation. Instrumentation consists of wiring, rods, rods and hooks, cages, plates, and screws.[127] An anterior corpectomy in which a bone graft is placed is shown in Fig. 14.21. A posterior approach using pedicle screws is illustrated in Fig. 14.22.

Locked facets that cannot be realigned with increasing traction and serial radiographic evaluations in association with neurologic deterioration require urgent surgery.[16] However, the optimal timing of other surgeries is less clear. One advantage of early surgery is prompt mobilization and initiation of aggressive occupational and physical therapy.[16,32] The urgency of surgery in the presence of a complete SCI is debated. Furthermore, because of an increased risk of secondary injury to the edematous spinal cord, surgery after the first 24 hours up to 8 days may be more harmful than postponement.[118] Possible complications of spine surgery include worsening of neurologic deficit related to additional surgical trauma and postoperative edema, cord compression with instrumentation, and interruption of vascular supply; worsening of pulmonary status related to anesthesia, an anterior thoracic approach, or postoperative immobilization and pain; CSF fistula; infection; hardware failure; and pseudarthrodesis, an abnormal fibrous fusion between bone.[16,142] Intraoperative monitoring of somatosensory-evoked potentials (SSEPs) and motor evoked potentials (MEPs) is used to alert the surgeon to potentially injurious changes during the surgical procedure. SSEPs measure electrical activity of the dorsal columns, and MEPs measure anterior and lateral corticospinal tract electrical activity. Decrements in evoked-potential amplitude are associated with spinal cord compromise.[58,109] Ultrasound is used during surgery to detect bone fragments in the spinal canal.[114]

Cervical orthoses are available in a number of styles, including collars, poster-type collars, and the halo. The halo is the gold standard, providing the most protection against motion from the occiput through C3.[16] Hard collars and poster collars are generally for nondisplaced C1–C2 fractures. The sterno-occipital mandibular immobilization (SOMI) brace provides three-point fixation and prohibits flexion-extension more effectively than a hard collar and it is less restrictive than a halo (Fig. 14.23 and Fig. 14.24).[4] A Minerva Cervicothoracic Orthotic (CTO) is available for middle to lower cervical spine injuries (Fig. 14.25).[4] Examples of thoracolumbosacral orthoses (TLSO) include the custom-made rigid plastic body jacket (clamshell) TLSO and the metal Jewett Brace (Florida Brace Corp., Winter Park, FL) (Fig. 14.26 and Fig. 14.27).[16] Complications from cervical orthoses range from skin breakdown to aspiration.[4] Additional complications of the halo orthoses include pin-site infection and osteomyelitis, penetration of the skull, subdural abscess, periorbital edema, scarring, cranial nerve palsies, fracture overdistraction, and persistent instability.[4]

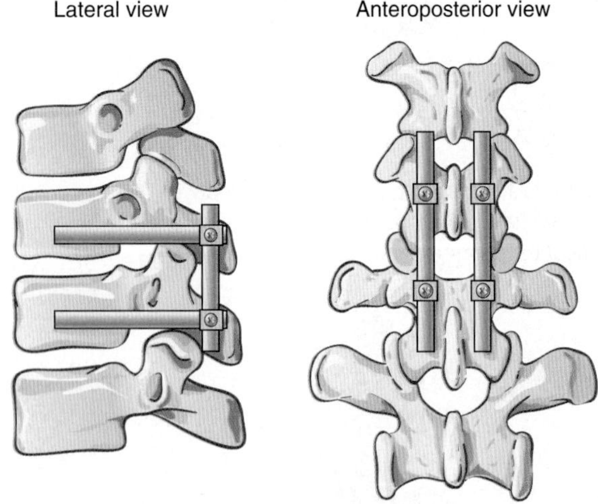

FIG. 14.22 Lateral and anteroposterior views of pedicle screw placement. (From Black, J.M., Hawks, J.H. (2005). *Medical-surgical nursing: clinical management for positive outcomes* (7th ed.). St Louis: Saunders.)

CRITICAL CARE MANAGEMENT

Critical care management of the spinal-cord injured patient requires attention to each and every system. The pulmonary, cardiac, and neurologic sequelae are the most immediately life-threatening, but each and every system can pose risk to the patient both acutely and chronically. The interprofessional care plan must include consideration for each system as well as a rehabilitation perspective on a consistent, ongoing basis from admission to discharge. An interprofessional clinical pathway may provide an efficient and effective framework for organizing care and goal-setting for the patient.

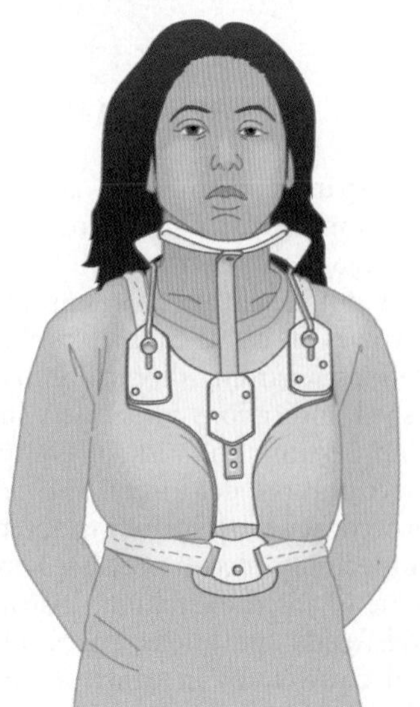
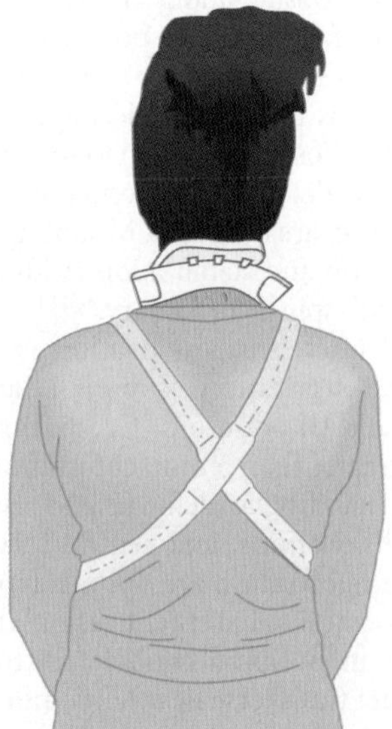

FIG. 14.23 SOMI brace. (From Lewis, S.L., Heitkemper, M.M., Dirksen, S.R., et al. (2007). *Medical-surgical nursing: assessment and management of clinical problems* (6th ed.). St Louis: Mosby.)

Neurologic

The continuum of care for SCI begins prehospital and continues in the emergency department (ED) and possibly into the operating room (OR) before the patient's admission to critical care. The care provided before the patient's arrival to the intensive care unit is the foundation from which the nurse and interprofessional team initiate their care. Continued consecutive monitoring of the patient's neurologic status by detailed clinical assessment is paramount.[15]

Unlike the brain, technology to measure spinal cord perfusion at the bedside is lacking. In addition to their application in surgery, somatosensory and motor-evoked potentials are sometimes used intermittently at the bedside in determination of a prognosis. Evoked potentials measure electrical activity, not blood flow.[58,109] By stimulating an extremity below the spinal cord lesion and recording the response from scalp electrodes, neuronal conduction can be assessed. However, evoked-potential monitoring presents too many technical difficulties to be conducted continuously and utilized in the day-to-day management of the patient.[58,109]

Neurologic deterioration may occur for a number of reasons, such as loss of alignment with or without surgery or traction; cord edema; and a change in the level of consciousness and mental status related to TBI, other injuries, a decline in oxygenation, medications, and sleep deprivation. Even subtle changes may warrant additional investigation.[15] Use of a detailed SCI flow sheet and a neurologic assessment performed jointly by both the on-coming nurse and the off-going nurse may facilitate prompt detection of neurologic deterioration. Spine precautions, such as maintaining the patient on a backboard; using a cervical collar; positioning the patient in reverse Trendelenburg to elevate the head of the bed; turning as a unit; and waiting to turn manually on a wedge turning frame or an automatic turning table bed, are to be maintained until prescribed otherwise.[44] In extremely unstable cervical spine injuries, such as an atlanto-occipital dissociation, head of bed elevation at zero degrees may be mandated until surgical stabilization. The provider who is maintaining stabilization of the cervical spine should direct all positioning of the patient.

Other neurologic injuries in addition to the SCI may be present. TBI and peripheral injuries complicate spinal cord assessment and management.[106] For example, Horner syndrome, which is sometimes seen with acute SCI, is related to disruption of the cervical sympathetic chain and presents with ptosis and miosis. These findings may be mistakenly interpreted as an indicator of intracranial pathology.[130]

By virtue of their close anatomic proximity, trauma to the cervical spine may also result in damage to the carotid and vertebral arteries.[20] Computed tomographic angiography (CTA) is recommended after blunt, nonpenetrating cervical trauma if the patient meets Denver Screening Criteria for (Assessment of) Blunt cerebrovascular injuries (BCVI) (Level I recommendation; Box 14.3). Conventional cerebral angiography is recommended if endovascular therapy is under consideration or if CTA is not available. MRI is recommended in complete spinal cord injury or vertebral subluxation injuries (Level III recommendation; see Box 14.2).[20,77] Vascular injury may result in transient ischemic stroke or a complete stroke if it is unrecognized and treatment with anticoagulation or repair of the vessel is delayed.[77]

Pulmonary

Hypoventilation as a direct result of the SCI is of major concern in cervical and thoracic cord injuries. Many if not most cervical cord-injured patients with or without other pulmonary injuries will be intubated before arrival to the critical

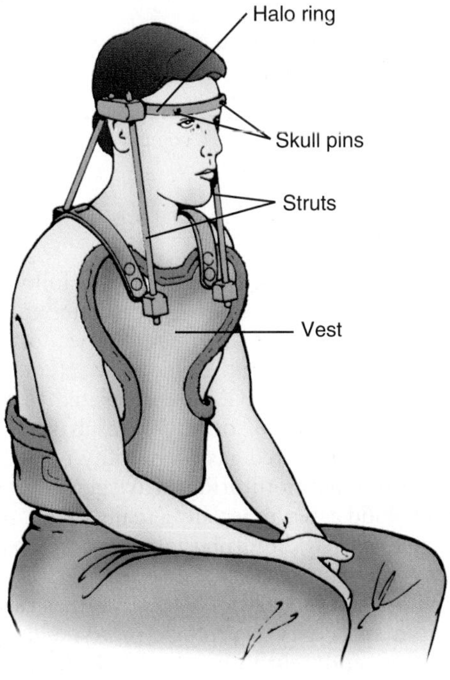

Halo ring
Skull pins
Struts
Vest

FIG. 14.24 Halo external fixator. (From Urden, L.D., Stacy, K.M., Lough, M.E. (2006). *Thelan's critical care nursing* (5th ed.). St Louis: Mosby.)

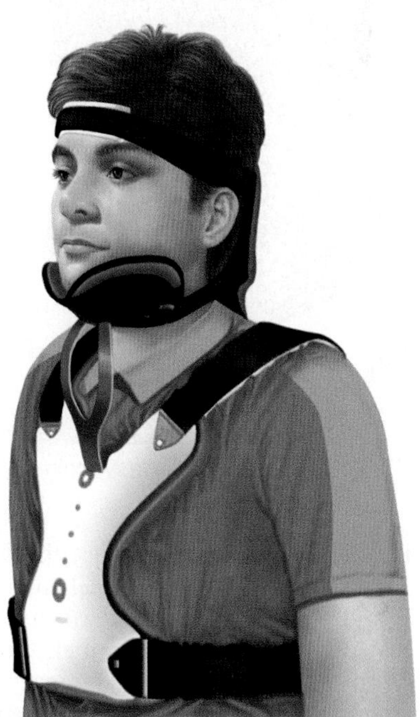

FIG. 14.25 Cervicothoracic orthotic. The Minerva brace is a custom-molded jacket that supports the chin and posterior skull. It encloses the pelvis or extends to the costal margins, depending on the stability required by the patient.

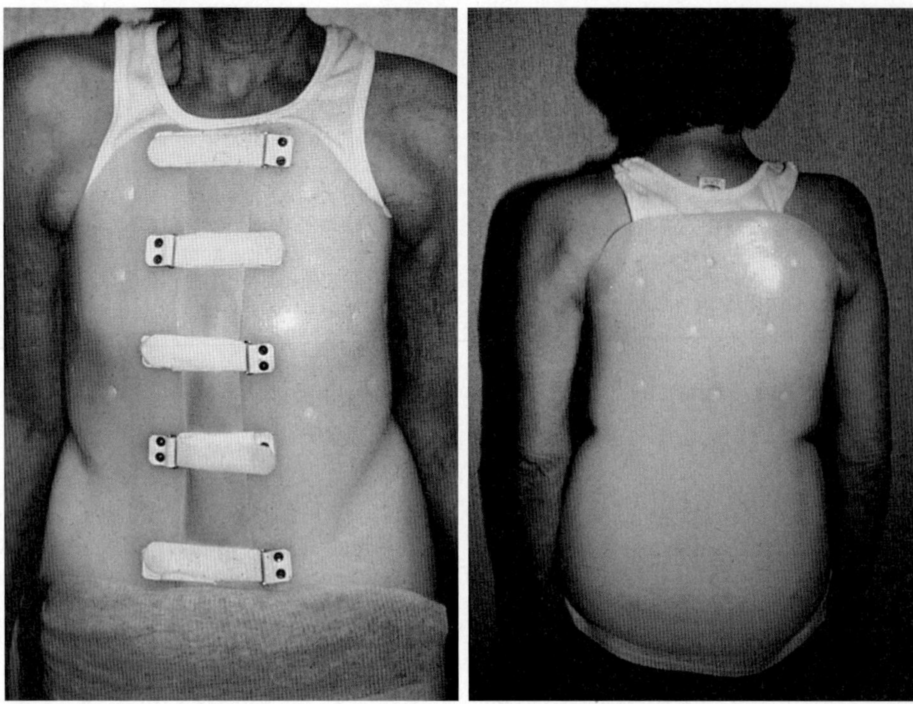

FIG. 14.26 Thoracic lumbar sacral orthotic (TLSO).

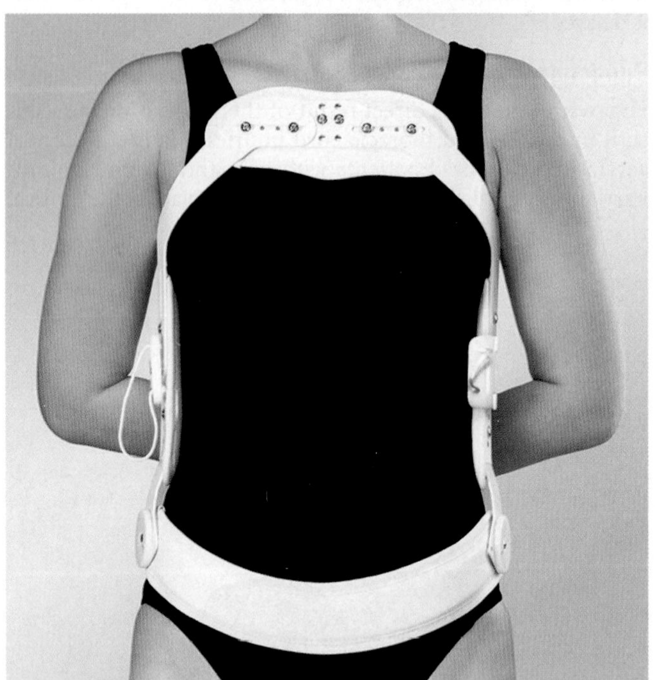

FIG. 14.27 Jewett brace. (Courtesy Orliman, 2016.)

care unit. With C3–C5 or higher injuries, the diaphragm is affected and apnea results. Lower cervical spinal cord injuries at C5–C7 and T1–T12 have impaired intercostal muscle function that may result in shallow, ineffective breathing (Table 14.9).[55,76,148,157] The forced vital capacity and maximum inspiratory and expiratory forces are reduced up to 70%.[55,121] Respirations are shallow and the patient exhibits decreased ability to cough and clear secretions. Some cervical and thoracic SCI patients will not require intubation immediately, but may within the first 24 hours, related to

BOX 14.3 Modified Denver Screening Criteria for BCVI

- Lateralizing neurologic deficit (not explained by CT)
- Infarct on head CT
- Nonexpanding cervical hematoma
- Massive epistaxis
- Anisocoria/Horner's syndrome
- GCS score < 8 without significant CT findings
- Cervical spine fracture
- Basilar skull fracture
- Severe facial fracture (LeForte II or III only)
- Seatbelt sign above clavicle
- Cervical bruit or thrill

BCVI, Blunt cerebrovascular injury; *CT,* computed tomography; *GCS,* Glasgow coma scale.
From References 20 and 77.

cord edema or neurogenic pulmonary edema following resuscitation.[19,148] Others will require immediate intubation at the scene related to their SCI, other injuries, or aspiration of gastric contents. Aspiration of gastric contents continues to be a risk factor for the SCI patient related to the supine position; cervical traction or orthotics, intubation, including tracheostomy; and impaired gastric motility related to spinal shock.[148] Continuous monitoring of oxygen saturation and serial arterial blood gases, especially a rising partial pressure of carbon dioxide ($Paco_2$), and physiologic parameters such as vital capacity will detect a gradual deterioration of pulmonary status. Nonemergent intubation is preferable, as care must be taken to avoid secondary neurologic injury. Sedation, analgesia, anesthetic, and neuromuscular blockade may facilitate oral intubation.[7,146] However, the paralytic medication succinylcholine is to be avoided following SCI. The massive denervation in SCI in combination with the depolarizing action of succinylcholine will result in a massive and potentially deadly

TABLE 14.9 Muscles of the Respiratory System

Muscle Group	Function	Innervation
Diaphragm	Major muscle of respiration During inhalation, the diaphragm contracts and moves downward During exhalation, the diaphragm relaxes, allowing for passive recoil	C3 to C5
Intercostal Muscles	During inhalation, the external intercostal muscles contract and elevate the rib cage During exhalation, the internal intercostal muscles contract and pull the ribs down	T1 to T11
Abdominal Muscles	Essential for an effective cough During exhalation, the abdominal muscles contract and compress the abdominal contents and push the diaphragm up	T6 to L1
Accessory Muscles	Elevate the rib cage and assist in deep ventilation Inadequate alone for effective ventilation	C1 to C3

From Stein, D.M., & Sheth K.N. (2015). Management of acute spinal cord injury. *Continuum* 21(1), 159–187:Table 10-3, p. 179.

release of potassium into the circulation.[55,110] Nasal intubation is contraindicated in the presence of basilar skull fractures and some facial trauma.[146]

Once intubated, mechanical ventilation simplifies maintenance of the airway and clearance of secretions. However, the patient is at increased risk for pneumonia. The leading cause of death for all SCI patients, intubated or not, is respiratory complications primarily resulting from pneumonia.[156,166] However, the risk of ventilator-associated pneumonia increases by 1% to 3% per day each day a patient is intubated.[55]

The ventilator mode utilized in management of respiratory dysfunction in acute spinal cord injury is somewhat controversial depending on the level of the spinal cord injury, pre-existing lung disease, concomitant chest trauma, and clinician preference. Tidal volumes may vary from 6 to 8 mL/kg to 20 mL/kg or greater as research is limited and results are inconclusive.[157] Larger tidal volumes recruit distal airways, stimulate the production of surfactant, increase oxygenation, and lessen the dyspnea experienced by patients receiving a smaller tidal volume. Smaller tidal volumes may reduce the risk of barotrauma.[26,166]

Regardless of the ventilator mode used, pulmonary status must be closely monitored, including chest auscultation, respiratory rate and character, arterial blood gases, oxygen saturation, end-tidal carbon dioxide monitoring, chest x-rays, sputum, white blood cell count, and temperature. Antibiotics should not be ordered prophylactically, but prescribed based on the culture and sensitivity of the sputum.[55,121] Pulmonary hygiene, including frequent turning and early mobilization, suctioning of secretions as needed, and assisted cough is critical and may decrease the need for prolonged mechanical ventilation, antibiotics, and repeated bronchoscopy to clear secretions.[26,121] Tetraplegics may have more effective breathing while lying supine or wearing an abdominal binder when the head is up. These interventions displace some of the weight of the abdomen away from the weakened diaphragm and chest muscles.[110,121,157] Assisted cough, also referred to as *quad coughing* or *quad-assisted coughing,* can be performed with a fist below the xiphoid process in a Heimlich-type maneuver or with open hands at the anterolateral base of each lung, pushing upward as the patient repeatedly coughs (Fig. 14.28).[119] Improper technique or placement of the hand may result in a rib or xiphoid process fracture. Migration and deformation of vena cava filters and small bowel perforation have been reported as well with assisted coughing. An adjunct or alterative to manually assisted coughing is mechanical assistance with the Mechanical Insufflator Exsufflator (MIE) (Cough-Assist, Philips-Respironics International Inc., Murrayville, PA). The MIE applies positive airway pressure followed by negative airway pressure through a tracheostomy, face mask, or mouthpiece to mimic a normal productive cough and facilitate secretion clearance.[10,157]

For patients with injuries at C4 or below, weaning from mechanical ventilation is a priority. Resolution of spinal shock with an associated increase in forced vital capacity, negative sputum cultures, fraction of inspired oxygen (FiO_2) requirement of 0.50 or less, and a minute ventilation of less than 10 liters may facilitate weaning 2 weeks or more after the injury.[55,121] A tracheostomy frequently improves pulmonary mechanics, eases suctioning, and is more comfortable than prolonged nasal or oral intubation. However, if an anterior surgical approach is taken to stabilize the cervical injury, the tracheostomy may be delayed to allow wound healing.[55,121,157] A number of weaning modalities are used, including pressure support, positive airway support, and increasingly longer T-piece or tracheostomy collar trials during the day while allowing the patient to rest on the ventilator at night. The best weaning method is not known.[121] The higher the level of injury, the longer the length of time to successfully wean from the ventilator and the greater likelihood of pulmonary complications.[55,121,157] Additionally, the more prolonged the length of time on the ventilator, the greater the amount of diaphragmatic atrophy and progressive reduction in function.[157] Respiratory muscle training (RMT) trials, utilizing a number of different methods, have also been conducted as an adjunct for ventilator weaning. However, the evidence for benefit is lacking.[157] Aggressive pulmonary hygiene remains a priority during and after successful ventilator weaning.

For patients with injuries at C4 and above, especially complete injuries, weaning from mechanical ventilation may not be possible and ventilator dependence will be permanent. However, DiMarco and others have experienced some success with combined intercostal and diaphragm pacing in tetraplegics.[157] Electrical stimulation of the phrenic nerve allows the diaphragm to contract and produce sufficient inspiratory volumes to potentially wean some patients from the ventilator. However, if the motor neurons in the spinal cord or either phrenic nerve are injured, pacing is ineffective. Pacing of a unilaterally functional phrenic nerve and intercostals may provide another alternative to ventilator dependence.[49] Traditionally, placement of these electrodes has required a thoracotomy, but they may now be placed laparoscopically.[49-51,148,157] More recently, diaphragmatic pacing has been accomplished by percutaneous stimulation of the diaphragm.[43]

In addition to hypoventilation, pulmonary edema, and pneumonia, venous thromboembolic (VTE) disease from impaired mobility of the extremities poses a constant threat to the lungs. Additional risk factors for VTE in acute spinal cord injury include Virchow's triad (stasis, hypercoagulability, and intimal injury) related to the abnormal platelet function and

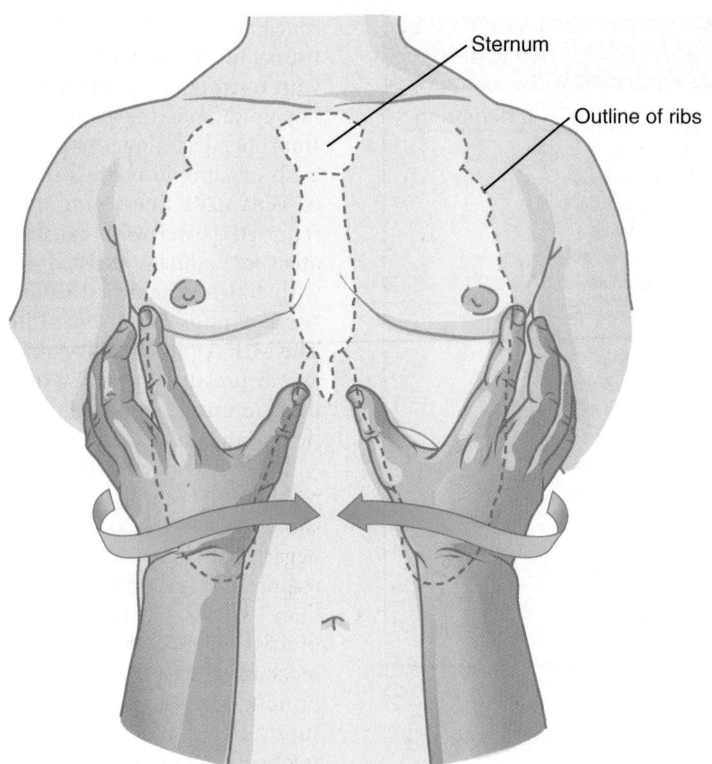

FIG. 14.28 Technique for quad-assisted coughing. Open hands at anterolateral base of each lung, pushing upward. (From Urden, L.D., Stacy, K.M., Lough, M.E. (2006). *Thelan's critical care nursing* (5th Ed.). St Louis: Mosby.)

alteration in fibrinolytic activity associated with spinal cord injury.[122] In the absence of prophylaxis or in inadequate prophylaxis, the incidence of VTE after spinal cord injury has been reported as high as 81%, with the greatest risk between 72 hours and 2 weeks after injury.[55] Among all hospitalized groups, patients with spinal cord injury have the highest risk of deep vein thrombosis without prophylaxis.[65] Deep vein thrombosis (DVT) prophylaxis includes mechanical devices and pharmacologic anticoagulation. Mechanical devices include sequential pneumatic compression devices, rotating beds, and electrical stimulation.[47,65] Elastic compression stockings are no longer recommended.[47,65] Limitations of elastic compression stockings for DVT prophylaxis include variation in fit, including equal pressure distribution at the ankle and calf, and the potential for vascular compromise and skin breakdown, particularly in the presence of lower extremity edema.[65] Pharmacologic anticoagulation includes low-dose heparin and low molecular weight heparinoids (enoxaparin [Lovenox], dalteparin [Fragmin]). A combination of mechanical and pharmacologic prophylaxis may provide more protection than either modality alone (Level I-II recommendation; see Box 14.2).[47,55,65]

Clinicians often delay anticoagulation because of concern for SCI or systemic hemorrhage or the need for surgery in the near future. Mechanical prophylaxis should be started as soon as possible and continued for at least 2 weeks. If no active bleeding or coagulopathy is present, subcutaneous unfractionated heparin or low molecular weight heparinoid should be delayed 24 to 48 hours after surgery, but started within 48 to 72 hours after spinal cord injury.[16,122]

Either low-dose subcutaneous unfractionated heparin or low molecular weight heparinoid, such as enoxaparin (Lovenox) or dalteparin (Fragmin), is safe and effective. A low-molecular-weight heparinoid may be preferable in spinal cord injury as it has been shown to be more effective in DVT prevention (but equivalent to unfractionated heparin in regard to pulmonary embolus prevention) and less likely to result in bleeding complications.[122] A 3-month course of prophylaxis is recommended (Level II recommendation; see Box 14.2). After 3 months, the risk of VTE lessens.[122] Intravenous heparin sufficient to increase the activated partial thromboplastin time (APTT) 1.5 to 2 times the control followed by oral warfarin with an international therapeutic ratio (INR) of 2.0 to 3.0 is also effective, but substantially increases the risk of bleeding and is usually reserved for patients with a confirmed VTE or pulmonary embolus.[55] Placement of a vena cava filter is no longer recommended for VTE prophylaxis but is recommended if anticoagulation has failed or if mechanical prophylaxis and/or anticoagulation are contraindicated.[47,65]

Diagnosis of DVT by physical assessment alone is difficult because of impaired sensation in SCI patients. However, the use of bedside ultrasound, including duplex Doppler, impedance plethysmography, and venous occlusion plethysmography is safe and reliable (Level III recommendation; see Box 14.2).[47] Venography is invasive and associated with increased risk of adverse events.[47] If pulmonary emboli are suspected, angiography remains the gold standard. However, limitations of pulmonary angiography include availability, expense, and complications. Ventilation perfusion scans and spiral CT of the chest are more widely used. The sensitivity and specificity of spiral CT, at 94% and 96%, respectively, are greater than those of ventilation-perfusion scans.[55,155]

Cardiac

At the time of injury, the loss of sympathetic input and subsequent unopposed parasympathetic (vagal) outflow place the cervical or thoracic spinal cord-injured patient at risk for hemodynamic instability manifested as cardiac dysrhythmias and systemic hypotension.[55] Continuous cardiac and arterial monitoring is prudent during the first 1 to 2 weeks following injury. Bradycardia is the most common dysrhythmia, and usually occurs within 2 weeks after injury.[55,98] Hypoxia or vagal stimulation by manipulation of a suction catheter or nasogastric/orogastric tube may induce a symptomatic bradycardia evidenced by a decrease in blood pressure or level of consciousness. Oxygenation and cessation of the vagal stimulation may be all that is required to increase the heart rate.[55] However, administration of intravenous atropine in symptomatic bradycardia may be necessary and is effective.[55] Occasionally a temporary pacemaker is needed until resolution of the neurogenic shock.[55,126]

The loss of tone in the peripheral vasculature and venous pooling as a result of cervical and thoracic SCI result in hypotension. Unlike hypovolemic shock, neurogenic shock is accompanied by bradycardia as described previously.[7] However, first-line treatment for both is fluid resuscitation. One to two liters of a nonglucose-containing intravenous solution is administered initially in an attempt to bring the blood pressure into the desired parameter. Too much fluid may aggravate cord edema and neurogenic pulmonary edema.[7] The desired blood pressure parameter is not known with certainty.[136]

Unlike traumatic brain injury, multimodality monitoring is not currently available for traumatic spinal cord injury. Any type of intraparenchymal probe or catheter placement to determine intraspinal/intrathecal pressure or spinal perfusion pressure may potentially increase the risk of secondary injury. However, the insertion of a lumbar subarachnoid catheter has been suggested.[121] Some clinicians advocate a spinal cord perfusion pressure greater than 60 mm Hg, but this is without substantial evidence.[12] The current recommendation based on available evidence is to attain and maintain a systolic blood pressure greater than 90 mm Hg and a MAP of 85 to 90 mm Hg in the first 7 days after injury (Level III recommendations; see Box 14.2).[121,136]

If the initial fluid is ineffective in raising the blood pressure, a vasopressor may be added. Ideally, vasopressors are added after the placement of a central venous catheter.[7] A pulmonary catheter may be helpful in selected cases in the hands of trained clinicians.[110] In neurogenic shock, the preload, heart rate, left ventricular end-diastolic pressure, stroke volume, systemic vascular resistance, and cardiac output are all decreased. Therefore, ideal vasopressors for SCI have chronotropic and alpha and beta properties.[55,121] Phenylephrine (Neo-Synephrine) should be used with caution. Because of its pure alpha-adrenergic action, phenylephrine may result in a reflex bradycardia.[55,121] Other effective choices in cervical and thoracic SCI include dopamine (Intropin) or norepinephrine (Levophed). Both agents have alpha- and beta-adrenergic effects and increase heart rate. Dobutamine (Dobutrex) can be used with dopamine or Levophed to increase cardiac output, but may cause hypotension. Therefore Dobutamine is not preferred and should not be used alone.[55,121]

Hemorrhagic shock in the presence of acute SCI often complicates the neurogenic picture, and the bradycardia may be masked by tachycardia related to actual exsanguination. However, in the case of neurogenic shock, the patient is usually warm and dry (unless the ambient temperature is low), in contrast to the patient who is hemorrhaging being cold and clammy. Both may be symptomatic hemodynamically as evidenced by impaired mentation and low urine output.[7,121]

The hypotension may persist with upright positioning long after the initial injury. The application of an abdominal binder, elastic leg wraps, or/and electrical stimulation of the lower extremities to promote lower extremity muscular contraction, after the patient has stopped receiving intravenous vasopressors may assist in maintaining the systemic blood pressure when mobilizing the patient.[55] Oral vasopressors, such as ephedrine or midodrine (Amatine, Proamatine) or fludrocortisone (Florinef), a mineralocorticoid that promotes sodium and water intravascular volume retention, are often administered approximately 45 minutes to 1 hour before raising the patient's head to assist in the maintenance of an adequate blood pressure while upright.[62,96,110,144]

Following resolution of neurogenic shock, the patient with spinal cord injury at T6 or higher is at risk for autonomic dysreflexia (AD). AD is also sometimes referred to as *autonomic hyperreflexia.* Prevention includes attention to bowel and bladder elimination and other less common precipitants. Prompt recognition and treatment of the classic paroxysmal hypertension or more subtle increase in blood pressure and other symptomatology associated with AD is critical to prevent severe disability or death from intracerebral hemorrhage, seizures, and myocardial infarction.[55,63,71,98,102,140,159] Initial management includes raising the head of the bed unless contraindicated and removing the noxious stimulation, such as alleviating a distended bladder or evacuating a rectal vault containing stool. Short-acting antihypertensives, such as nitroglycerin (Nitrol) and nifedipine (Procardia), may also be given to assist in lowering the blood pressure (Table 14.10).[55,63,71,98,102,140,159]

Pregnant patients with an injury at T6 or above who deliver after their spinal shock has resolved are at risk for AD related to uterine contractions. Regional anesthesia at the onset of labor may allow for a vaginal delivery without risk to the mother.[34,54,64] However, a cesarean section is indicated if the AD is uncontrollable.[54] The hypertension and subjective symptoms of AD may be mistakenly diagnosed as preeclampsia. With preeclampsia the systemic hypertension may persist while the blood pressure returns to baseline after the noxious stimuli is removed. Both preeclampsia and AD may exist at the same time.[34] Postpartum physiologic changes and the initiation of breastfeeding may provoke AD. Unless the AD is uncontrollable, breastfeeding is not strictly prohibited.[34]

Gastrointestinal

Following SCI, the gastrointestinal system is atonic. Bowel sounds may not be auscultated. Abdominal distention results from lack of motility and possibly from air swallowing or from attempts to provide supplemental oxygen and rescue breaths with a bag-valve-mask apparatus. The patient is at risk for emesis and aspiration.[53,76] An orogastric or nasogastric tube (in the absence of basilar skull fracture or other contraindication) is needed. After auscultation, aspiration, or radiographic exam to verify proper placement, the gastric tube is attached to low constant suction to minimize gastric content.[110] Gastric emptying time is directly related to the level of the spinal cord injury; the higher the level of spinal cord injury, the greater the impairment.[53] Intravenous metoclopramide (Reglan) may facilitate gastric motility.[53] If the impaired motility continues for 3 or more days, total parenteral nutrition is required to prevent malnutrition. Gradual introduction of enteral feedings at low

TABLE 14.10 Selected Medications for Patients with Traumatic Spinal Cord Injuries

Medication	Actions	Dosage	Special Considerations
Antispasticity			
Baclofen (Lioresal)	Skeletal muscle relaxant, antispasticity agent	5 mg PO/NG TID; can increase dose by 15 mg/day every 3 days as needed Maximum total daily dose is 80 mg	May cause drowsiness and hypotension; increase gradually; withdrawal seizures, hallucinations Use caution in renal impairment Do not discontinue abruptly; may result in rebound spasticity Also available as solution for intrathecal infusion
Dantrolene (Dantrium)	Skeletal muscle relaxant, antispasticity	25–400 mg PO/NG daily, given as divided doses TID May increase dose weekly if needed. Start with 25 mg daily for 7 days, followed by 25 mg TID for 7 days, 50 mg TID for 7 days, then 100 mg TID. Maximum dose is 400 mg/day, given as four divided doses	May cause drowsiness, weakness, fatigue, and seizures; increase gradually Monitor liver function tests closely; high risk of liver toxicity if hepatic impairment, age older than 35, and/or for female patients If no additional relief is obtained at higher doses, decrease dose to next lower dose
Tizanidine (Zanaflex)	Anti-spasticity deters the release of epinephrine and norepinephrine from spinal interneurons that relay signals between afferent and efferent tracts; may also inhibit the excitatory neurotransmitter glycine to decrease spasticity	From 8 to 36 mg/day in 3–4 divided doses; titrate slowly. Available as oral tablet and also immediate-release multi-particulate capsules	Monitor liver and renal function; may require dose adjustment
Gabapentin (Neurontin)	Decrease neuropathic pain May increase synthesis or accumulation of GABA in the brain by binding to an undefined receptor to decrease neuropathic pain.	100 mg TID; may increase by 300 mg weekly; maximum dose is 3600 mg/day in divided doses	Adverse effects include fatigue, drowsiness, dizziness, ataxia Contraindicated in severe renal impairment
Blood Pressure Control			
Ephedrine	Vasoconstriction; prevention of orthostatic hypotension	2.5 mg PO/NG daily	May cause tachycardia, hypertension, tremors, and anxiety Administer 45 min to 1 h before raising head
Midodrine (Amatine, ProAmatine)	Vasoconstriction; prevention of orthostatic hypotension	2.5–10 mg PO/NG TID	May cause hypertension, flushing, and restlessness Administer 45 min to 1 h before raising head May need to adjust dose for renal dysfunction
Nifedipine (Procardia)	Vasodilation; treatment of hypertension associated with AD	10–20 mg sublingual	Capsule must be opened and liquid contents (bite and chew) in contact with oral mucosa for rapid onset (1–5 min) May cause hypotension and headache
Nitroglycerin (Nitrostat, sublingual tablets)	Treatment of hypertension associated with AD	0.4% tablet sublingual	Onset is 1–3 min (sublingual)
Nitrol, Nitrobid (ointment)	Treatment of hypertension associated with AD	0.5-2 inches topical	Onset 15 min-1 h (topical)
Stool Softeners/ Stimulants	Soften stool and stimulate colon to facilitate bowel training		May cause diarrhea, abdominal cramping
Docusate (Colace)		100 mg PO/NG TID	
Senna-docusate (Senokot-S)		2 tablets PO/NG BID	
Bisacodyl (Dulcolax)		10 mg (1 suppository) per rectum daily after meal or bolus tube feeding	

AD, Autonomic dysreflexia/hyperreflexia; *BID,* two times a day; *GABA,* gamma-aminobutyric acid; *NG,* nasogastric tube; *PO,* per os; *TID,* three times a day.
From References 29, 72, 90, 96, 103, 104, 108, 144, and 165.

rates may be effective.[53] Withholding enteral feedings for high residuals is imperative to decrease the risk of aspiration.[110]

The sacral segments of the spinal cord innervate the bowel. Normal bowel function is preserved in incomplete spinal cord injuries with sacral sparing. At the time of a complete SCI, the bowel is flaccid. With the resolution of spinal shock, the bowel with an SCI above the sacrum, an upper motor neuron lesion, will become reflexic. This reflex activity may facilitate regular consistent bowel evacuation.[53] Initially, a suppository and digital evacuation will be required for bowel training. Digital stimulation is performed to further dilate the lower colon, reduce resistance to expulsion of stool, and facilitate peristalsis. Digital stimulation increases the efficacy of the bowel training.[53] With repeated consistent efforts at the same time each day, the bowel may eventually automatically expel stool at a predictable time or require only digital stimulation or a glycerin suppository. Bowel training is frequently begun with a bisacodyl (Dulcolax) suppository, a stool softener such as docusate (Colace) suppository, and digital stimulation.[29,53] Digital stimulation may induce AD after spinal shock resolves. A local anesthetic agent such as lidocaine ointment may prevent the onset of AD during bowel training. Bowel training is most effective if performed when the gastrocolic reflex is most active, immediately after a meal. Bowel care after the evening meal may be least disruptive in regard to interference with other rehabilitation efforts, including physical and occupational therapy in critical care. Supplemental fiber with adequate fluid intake and stool softeners may facilitate bowel training. Large-volume enemas are to be avoided.[29,53]

In a complete SCI at the sacral segments, a lower motor neuron lesion, the bowel remains areflexic after spinal shock is resolved. Bowel care with a lower motor neuron lesion may be more problematic than with an upper motor neuron lesion. Retention of formed stool with incontinence of liquid stool frequently occurs, with stool softeners and suppositories being less effective. Digital stimulation is ineffective and manual removal of stool may be necessary.[29,53]

With either a reflexic or an areflexic bowel, constipation in the spinal cord patient is a serious complication that is potentially life-threatening as it impairs gastrointestinal motility, increases the risk of aspiration with high gastric residuals, and is a frequent cause of autonomic dysreflexia with injuries above T6.[29,53]

Gastrointestinal complications of spinal cord injury include perforated gastric ulceration with hemorrhage, cholecystitis, appendicitis, bowel obstruction, and rectal bleeding from hemorrhoids. Colon cancer symptoms are often masked and often more advanced when discovered. For example, recognition of gastrointestinal complications may be delayed in spinal cord injury related to impaired or referred sensation or failure to attribute clinical presentation with acute pathology.[29]

Nutrition Support

No research has been published that firmly establishes the exact composite nutritional needs of the spinal cord patient.[2,48,93] Nutritional support should be started as soon as possible after spinal cord injury. Though initiation of nutrition within 72 hours is recommended and safe (Level III recommendation; see Box 14.2), early enteral nutrition has not been shown to impact neurologic outcome, length of stay, or incidence of complications.[47]

In general, patients with acute spinal cord injury have a 10% decrease in actual energy needs compared to predicted energy needs due to denervated muscle.[2] However, age, preexisting illness, other comorbidities, injuries, infection, wounds, or surgery will also affect requirements. Maintaining normoglycemia is essential for optimal neurologic outcome. Acute spinal cord injury is associated with obligatory large nitrogen losses for up to 2 months related to denervated musculature. Protein needs may be calculated at 2 grams per kilogram of ideal body weight per day to decrease the negative nitrogen balance.[2,22] A high fat diet is not recommended as it may contribute to obesity, metabolic syndrome, diabetes, and heart disease.[93] Fiber intake provides bulk and fluid retention in the colon to facilitate bowel elimination. However, excess fiber, particularly in the absence of adequate fluid intake, may contribute to constipation. A range of 15 to 30 grams is recommended daily.[2,29] Although spinal cord injury is associated with increased risk of osteoporosis, excess vitamin D and calcium are to be avoided as they may contribute to renal calculi. Daily calcium intake of 1 gram is reasonable.[29]

Normovolemia should be attained and maintained as soon as possible, with the avoidance of glucose-containing intravenous solutions. Early initiation of enteral fluids is recommended. Fluid needs are calculated based on the daily fluid requirements of the patient without spinal cord injury, at 30 to 40 mL/kg.[22] The Academy of Nutrition and Dietetics recommends 40 mL/kg plus an additional 500 mL daily.[2] One to two liters of fluid per day has been recommended in regard to promoting optimal stool consistency.[29]

Genitourinary

Like the gastrointestinal tract, the genitourinary system is flaccid immediately after the injury. Following the resolution of spinal shock, the upper motor neuron bladder, with injury above the sacral segments of the cord, will regain tone, which may facilitate reflex voiding.[76] Over time some patients will reflex void sufficiently to empty the bladder; others will require intermittent catheterization completely or for high residuals. Some patients are able to facilitate reflex voiding with the use of Credé, Valsalva, abdominal massage, or pubic hair pulling maneuvers.[29] As soon as fluid intake and output is stable, an effort to remove the indwelling catheter is prudent to minimize the risk of urinary tract infection and sepsis.[67] However, overdistention of the bladder is to be avoided. The normal adult bladder capacity is 400 mL to 500 mL.[29] To avoid overdistention, fluid intake may be limited or the frequency of intermittent catheterization increased. Prophylactic antibiotic therapy is not effective and may be detrimental. Urinalysis and culture and sensitivity should be obtained if the patient is symptomatic and antibiotics are prescribed based on those results only.[68] In the case of women who void incontinently, an indwelling catheter or urinary diversion procedure may continue to be necessary in critical care to avoid skin breakdown.[140]

Patients with a cauda equina injury, a lower motor neuron lesion, continue to have an areflexic bladder after the resolution of spinal shock and will not void.[76] An indwelling catheter with conversion to an intermittent catheterization regimen will be necessary.[68] With a lesion at the junction of the conus medullaris and the cauda equina, a mixed upper and lower neuron presentation also exists in which the patient may or may not void spontaneously. In incomplete injuries with sacral sparing, spontaneous voiding and urinary control are possible.[29,52]

Although removal of the indwelling urinary catheter as soon as possible is ideal, large-volume urinary retention is to be avoided because of the risk of autonomic dysreflexia in patients with SCI above T6. Urinary retention also increases the risk of infection and renal failure.[29] Other complications include renal calculi and an increased incidence of bladder cancer.[68,70,140,163]

Endocrine

Following SCI and the release of catecholamines, the patient is prone to hyperglycemia. Though less investigated than the negative effects of hyperglycemia in TBI, an elevated glucose in SCI is associated with secondary neuronal injury and poor neurologic outcomes.[66,125] Hyperglycemia may also increase the risk of infection. An intermittent subcutaneous insulin regimen or a continuous intravenous infusion may be needed initially to attain and maintain normoglycemia. Hypoglycemia may also be harmful to the injured spinal cord. The optimal blood glucose range is not currently known; research is lacking.[66,87,125]

Musculoskeletal

As soon as the patient is stable, physical and occupational therapy are consulted. Early mobilization is the goal. However, actual range of motion may be immediately contraindicated related to other injuries, such as extremity fractures or increased intracranial pressure. Nevertheless, a prompt consult with these therapies provides assistance with preventive positioning and the early minimization of contractures and deformities associated with SCI. During spinal shock the extremities are flaccid, with the resolution of spinal shock, spasticity occurs. Spasticity occurs in 66% to 80% of all spinal cord patients within the first 2 months to 1 year after injury.[29,76,140] Upper and lower extremity orthotics are frequently prescribed to promote normal alignment and minimize contractures.[23] Spasticity may actually assist in rehabilitation goals; however, spasticity and the pain associated with spasticity can also deter rehabilitation efforts. Spasticity also contributes to contractures and skin breakdown.[29,140] Enteral baclofen (Lioresal), dantrolene (Dantrium), and diazepam (Valium) have been found to be beneficial.[29,140] More recently, botulinum toxin (Botox), tizanidine (Zanaflex), an alpha-2-adrenergic agonist, and gabapentin (Neurontin), and pregabalin (Lyrica), both antiepileptic drugs, have been used in the management of spasticity.[29,140] Botulinum exerts its effect at the neuromuscular junction to temporarily inhibit acetylcholine release.[29,140] Tizanidine is thought to inhibit the release of epinephrine and norepinephrine from the spinal interneurons. In addition to the management of pain, gabapentin and pregabalin are thought to lessen excitatory neurotransmitters, thereby decreasing spasticity.[29,140]

Some patients may eventually require an intrathecal baclofen medication pump.[29] Pharmacologic treatment of spasticity and related problems are outlined in Table 14.10. Nonpharmacologic interventions for spasticity include range-of-motion exercise and functional electrical stimulation (FES).[23,41,139] Exercise may minimize long-term musculoskeletal complications of SCI, including osteoporosis, pathologic fractures, and heterotopic ossification–the abnormal deposition of bone around the joints of paralyzed extremities.[139] Fitting the patient with a wheelchair and mobilizing while in critical care provide benefits physiologically and psychosocially.[61,87,115]

Integumentary

The potential for skin breakdown starts from the time the patient is placed in a collar and on a backboard during prehospital care.[7] Although this does not preclude their use, every effort should be made to remove the patient from the backboard as soon as possible. Backboard time should not exceed 2 hours.[7] Once the spine has been stabilized, turning the patient in bed every 2 hours is a priority.[64] Pads that support and position the patient in a kinetic treatment table must be secure to preventing shearing with turning. With regard to sitting, an appropriate cushion and position changes every 15 to 30 minutes are essential.[22,64] Tilting the patient backward to alleviate pressure while up in a chair is facilitated with the use of a wheelchair rather than a cardiac chair or a regular chair. Turns and hygiene measures provide opportunities for skin assessment. Keeping the skin clean and dry and minimizing pressure are critical. Smoking and poor nutrition also contribute to pressure ulcer occurrence and impaired wound healing.[22] Skin under orthotic devices and at pin insertion sites needs serial assessment and preventative measures. Any evidence of skin breakdown must be treated aggressively.[22] Early collaboration with a skin and wound specialist is warranted. Pressure ulcers impede rehabilitation, lessen the quality of life, and potentially threaten survival as a result of osteomyelitis, musculoskeletal necrosis, erosion into vital structures, and sepsis.[100] Pressure ulcer prevention is a lifelong commitment.[64]

Pain

Though SCI patients may not be able to perceive touch, discriminate between sharp and dull, or demonstrate vibratory or proprioceptive ability, their pain is real. Pain may be nociceptive, associated with spasticity, visceral injury, musculoskeletal injury or fracture, acute illness, or neuropathic, at or below the level of the spinal cord injury, or both.[29,76] The relationship between spasticity and pain is not straightforward. Reduction of spasticity may or may not be effective in pain reduction.[139] Neuropathic pain may be characterized as paresthesias or dysesthesias and described by the patient as burning, stinging, tingling, piercing, stabbing, or cutting.[139] Neuropathic pain in spinal cord injury is not completely understood.[59] New onset neuropathic pain should raise suspicion for post-traumatic syringomyelia.[140] Antispasmodic medications, anticonvulsants, analgesics, and sedatives may be effective in the management of pain. Central-acting nonnarcotic agents such as phenytoin (Dilantin), carbamazepine (Tegretol), gabapentin (Neurontin), pregabalin (Lyrica), clonazepam (Klonopin), and amitriptyline (Elavil) have decreased discomfort for many patients. Gabapentin and pregabalin, in particular, have been shown to decrease neuropathic pain.[72] However, long-term use of sedation and medications that are psychologically and physiologically addicting interferes with rehabilitation efforts and eventually detracts from the patient's quality of life. These medications also complicate bowel and bladder elimination.[59] The AANS/CNS guidelines recommend the use of the International Spinal Cord Injury Basic Pain Data Set (ISCIBPDS) as the preferred instrument for the assessment of pain severity and physical and emotional functioning (Level I evidence).[75,86]

Pain is an important indicator of disease. However, pathology usually identifiable by the location and character of the pain may be misdiagnosed in patients with SCI. For example, gastrointestinal pathology related to hemorrhage may present as referred pain rather than abdominal discomfort. Alternatively, a patient with preexisting coronary artery disease may experience a myocardial infarction without the usual chest discomfort. Any hypotension and bradycardia may be mistakenly attributed only to neurogenic shock.[107]

Chronic pain after spinal cord injury is experienced by 25% to 96% of all individuals living with spinal cord injury.[107] A number of individual factors including psychologic, cognitive, and coping mechanisms contribute to the spinal cord patient's pain experience. A multimodal approach is optimal, including consideration for pharmacologic agents, physical modalities, psychologic interventions, and in even invasive procedures, such as rhizotomy and cordectomy, for selected patients.[107]

Psychosocial

The SCI patient faces a myriad of physical and psychosocial obstacles. They may vacillate among different stages of the grief process, denial, anger, bargaining, depression, and acceptance, in addition to disturbances in body image and self-concept. Because many SCI patients are young male teenagers and adults, they may be especially vulnerable to these psychosocial ramifications. Depression, anxiety, and stress may prevail for weeks to years.[92,111,124] Contributing factors may include concurrent traumatic brain injury, pre-existing alcohol and substance abuse, pain, lack of social support, feelings of sexual inadequacy, poor quality of life, and failure to adjust to the spinal cord injury.[91] Feelings of powerlessness may pervade as well.[14,111] This is frequently manifested by the patient repeatedly calling the nurse into the room in an attempt to control the environment. Even their ability to communicate their concerns is hampered by intubation and their inability to write messages. Initiation of a communication system as soon as possible is important. Collaboration with the speech therapist and the respiratory therapist in the initiation of a tracheostomy speaking valve may be a significant step in the patient's psychosocial well-being and rehabilitation.[11] One such valve, the Passy-Muir tracheostomy speaking valve, opens during inspiration, allowing air into the lungs, and closes during expiration, redirecting the exhaled air through the vocal cords, mouth, and nose to allow the patient to speak (Fig. 14.29).[78] The tracheostomy

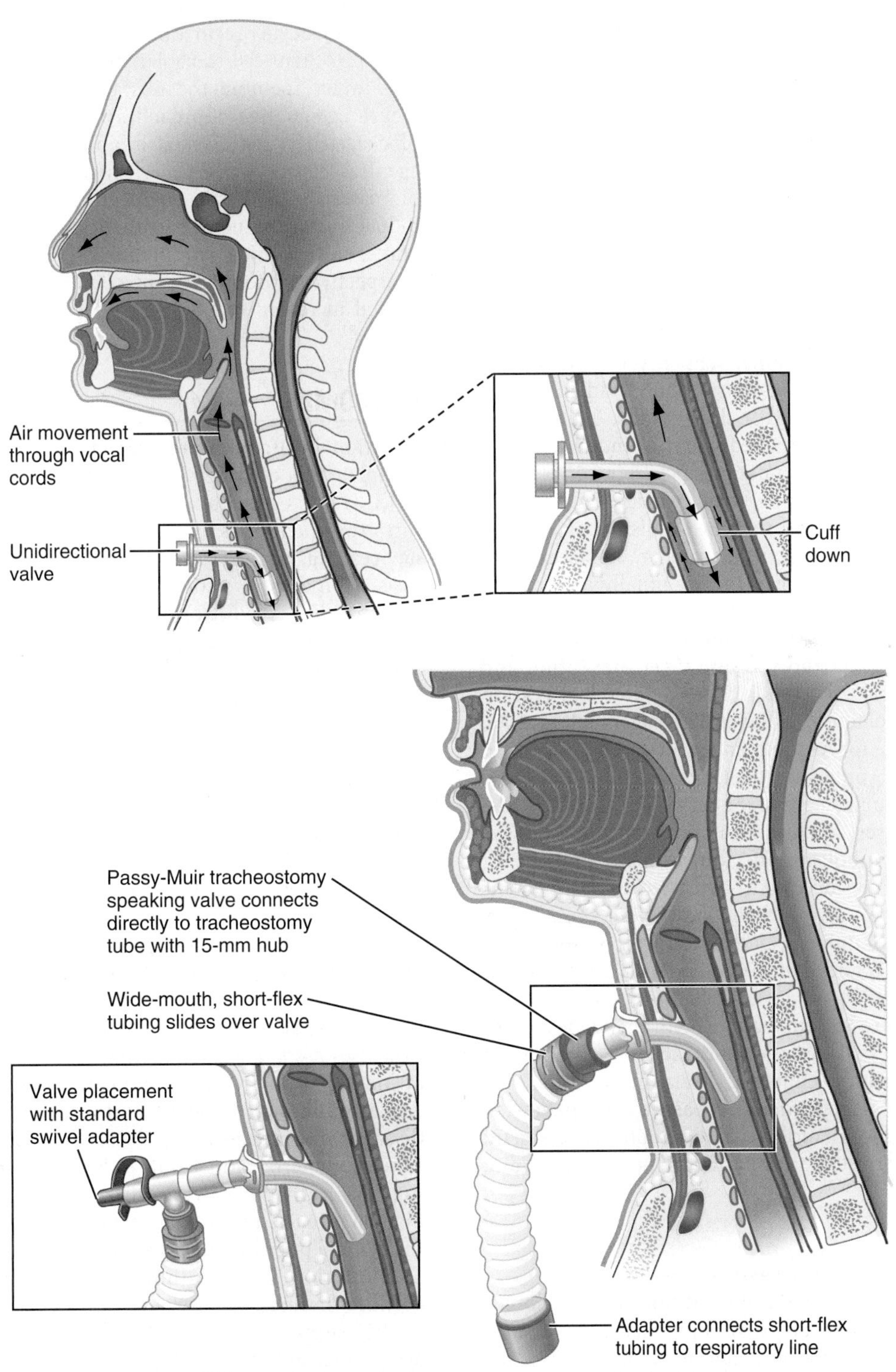

FIG. 14.29 Passy-Muir tracheostomy speaking valve.

cuff must be completely deflated and this may put the patient at increased risk for aspiration. Close monitoring of the patient's pulmonary status is necessary. The valve is not to remain in the airway when the patient is asleep. Vocal cord paralysis, excessive and thick pulmonary secretions, and tracheal or laryngeal obstructions are contraindications to its use.[78]

Research has demonstrated that acceptance and positive adaptation to the SCI may occur with some individuals.[105] However, life satisfaction studies are contradictory and inconclusive. The person's age at injury, level and duration of the injury, complications, activity limitations, and barriers to participation are factors that may influence their perception.[14,91] Cognitive behavioral therapy and goal planning may serve as therapeutic adjuncts in assisting the spinal cord patient to handle the physical limitations.[92,124]

EVIDENCE-BASED CARE

Major components of the care of the critically ill SCI patient have been addressed in evidence-based guidelines developed by the Consortium of Spinal Cord Medicine (CSCM), consisting of several interprofessional organizations that research and treat spinal cord patients and the AANS/CNS.[23,40,64,94,102-104,111,119] Many of the CSCM recommendations are Level II through V rather than Level I, the highest recommendations based on the most robust evidence, large randomized controlled trials with clear results. Much is yet to be substantiated by well-designed scientific inquiry. CSCM originally developed recommendations beginning in the late 1990s on the sequelae and long-term management of SCI, including respiratory, venous thromboembolism, bowel, pressure ulcers, autonomic dysreflexia, depression, upper extremity function, and outcome issues and eventually a summary guideline on early acute management.[23,40,94,103,111,119] The CSCM published second edition clinical practice guidelines on autonomic dysreflexia and pressure ulcer prevention and treatment in 2001 and 2014, respectively, and a first edition clinical practice guideline on bladder management in 2006 with similar criteria for recommendation levels.[64,102,104] In 2002, the AANS/CNS published the first guidelines that focus on the immediate management of the cervical spine injury and spinal cord injury itself in addition to some of the sequelae, including thromboembolism and nutritional concerns.[6,73] In 2013, the second edition of AANS/CNS *Guidelines for the Management of Acute Cervical Spine and Spinal Cord Injury* was published.[74,158] Standards, guidelines, and options were changed to Level I, II, and III recommendations, respectively (see Box 14.2). Many of the guidelines are Level II and III. Current AANS/CNS recommendations with the highest quality level of evidence, well-designed and executed randomized controlled trials, include clinical assessment of functional status (Spinal Cord Independence Measure III), pain (the ISCIBPDS), and symptomatology; radiographic assessment; and the evidence against the use of methylprednisolone and GM-1 ganglioside.[75,85,86,158]

RESEARCH

Research is ongoing in acute SCI. In addition to methylprednisolone, a number of other pharmacologic trials have demonstrated lack of clinical benefit or inconclusive results. Over the past 40 years, a number of clinical trials have been conducted with GM-1 gangliosides (Sygen), thyrotropin-releasing hormone (TRH), nimodipine, and autologous macrophages (ProCord), to name a few, without substantial evidence of their benefit.[5,57,101] Currently, spinal cord injury research focuses on neuroprotective and neuroregenerative approaches and functional restoration. Pharmacologic investigations include neuroprotective strategies to thwart cellular energy loss and release of intracellular glutamate, an excitotoxin, and the proinflammatory cytokine, tumor necrosis factor (TNFα).[17] Cell transplantation includes a variety of stem cells, including Schwann cells, olfactory ensheathing cells, neural stem/progenitor cells, oligodendrocyte precursors, and bone marrow-derived stromal cells.[57,129] Stem cell transplantation, including its use in spinal cord injury, is among the most debated clinical ethical issues.[129] Neuroregenerative approaches to spinal cord injury include blockage of growth (Rho) inhibitors through pharmacologic agents.[17] Restorative research focuses on the development of biomaterials for tissue engineering, operant conditioning to induce plasticity, neuroprosthetics, robotics, peripheral nerve grafts, and electrical stimulation.[41,129,143] No large multicenter prospective randomized controlled clinical trial has been conducted in regard to the use of hypothermia after spinal cord injury.[87]

OUTCOMES

Functional outcomes are predictable based on the level and completeness of injury (Table 14.11). A C5–C6 injury such as J.G.'s (see Case Study) would most likely allow him to perform some activities of daily living with assistance or orthotic devices. Aggressive rehabilitation beginning in critical care assists spinal cord patients to maximize their quality of life. The greatest amount of neurologic recovery occurs the first 6 to 9 months post injury. Improvement in motor function plateaus at 18 months to 2 years, after which there is little additional improvement.[56,91,161,164] However, the late complication of syringomyelia may result in further neurologic deterioration.[141]

Approximately 276,000 Americans are living with SCI.[116,117] Life expectancy is variable depending on the level (including ventilator dependency), the completeness of the injury, and the age at the time of injury.[116] High-level ventilator-dependent tetraplegics are likely to succumb to their injury within 10 to 15 years.[116] As a group, young paraplegics are expected to live up to 45 years after injury.[116] However, individuals 60 years and older who sustain SCI may only survive approximately 10 years post-injury.[116] The consequences of immobility secondary to the SCI dramatically impact the disease processes associated with aging, and spinal cord patients are at increased risk for ischemic cardiovascular disease, stroke, cancer, pulmonary disease, and infections.[10,22,84] Respiratory diseases and infection are the leading causes of death, with cancer, hypertension, and ischemic heart disease following.[35,116] Individuals living with SCI have an increased risk of bladder cancer, reportedly as much as 71 times higher than the general population, related to chronic indwelling catheters and infection.[70,79,163] Although longitudinal research is lacking, the findings of a review of studies published from 1982 to 2011 support that individuals living with spinal cord injury age prematurely.[85]

TABLE 14.11 Functional Goals for Spinal Cord-Injured Patients

Spinal Cord Level	Muscle Function	Functional Goals
C3-C4	Neck control Scapular elevators	Manipulate electric wheelchair with mouth stick Feed self with limitations using ball-bearing feeders Dress upper trunk Turn self in bed with arm slings Depend on others for bowel and bladder care
C5	Fair to good shoulder control Good elbow function	Propel wheelchair with hand rim projections Feed self with hand splint Require assistance getting to and from bed Depend on others for bowel and bladder care
C6	Good shoulder control Wrist extension Supinators	Transfer from wheelchair to bed and car with or without minimal assistance Feed self with tenodesis hands Assist getting to and from commode chair Require assistance with bladder care Drive with adapted van
C7	Weak shoulder depression Weak elbow extension Some hand function	Independently transfer to bed, car, and toilet Dress independently Propel wheelchair without hand rim projections Feed self without assistive devices Perform bowel and bladder care independently Drive car or adapted van with hand controls
C8-T4	Good to normal upper extremity muscle function	Transfer from chair or bed to wheelchair and return Maneuver wheelchair up and down curb Maneuver wheelchair to tub and return self to wheelchair
T5-L2	Partial to good trunk stability	Maneuver wheelchair independently Ambulate with limitations using long leg braces and crutches
L3-L4	All trunk-pelvic stabilizers intact Hip flexors Adductors Quadriceps	Ambulate with short leg braces with or without crutches, depending on level
L5	Hip extensors, abductors, knee flexors, ankle control	Do not require any equipment if plantar flexion is sufficiently strong to initiate steps after standing

From References 56 and 115.

ETHICAL CONSIDERATIONS

Acute SCI, particularly high-level complete cervical and ventilator-dependent tetraplegia, presents a number of ethical dilemmas, including the right to die, the right to refuse treatment, and the use of advance directives. Most acute SCI patients, in part because of their young age, will not have an advance directive already in place. Furthermore, the interprofessional team will be successful in stabilizing and maintaining the acute spinal cord-injured patient. However, long-term tetraplegia, ventilator dependence, and multiple complications may prolong the initial hospitalization, require frequent readmissions, delay rehabilitation, and require around-the-clock care by the family at home or in an assisted living facility. Pulmonary complications, such as pneumonia and pulmonary emboli, urinary tract infections, pressure ulcers, and sepsis are common reasons for readmission to acute or critical care.[46,116] SCI patient's quality of life is forever compromised.

Acute spinal cord-injured patients may experience profound depression and suicidal ideation; however, perceptions of their life may improve over time. As the patient's advocate, nurses have a responsibility to communicate the patient's stated wishes to the interprofessional team and to help the patient and family process their feelings.[97] Consultation with an ethics committee is recommended to assist the healthcare team, patient, and family members as they face ethical and legal decisions (Box 14.4).[132]

If the patient is competent and withdrawal of support is decided, but a member of the interprofessional team is uncomfortable participating in withdrawal of support, the environment must be conducive to the team member

BOX 14.4 Guidelines for Handling Ethical Dilemmas in Tetraplegia

1. Involve healthcare providers with neutral opinions regarding right to die/right to live issues.
2. Follow the patient's thoughts and decisions for consistency regarding wishes.
3. Introduce the patient to another spinal cord-injured patient to answer questions if possible.
4. Move the patient to less acute levels of care as soon as condition permits.
5. Evaluate congruence in the thoughts of the patient and the patient's family.
6. Establish the patient's competency.
7. Obtain informed consent for those who persist in their desire to withdraw life support.
8. Provide comfort measures and palliative care during the dying process while also attending to family.

From Reference 30.

expressing discomfort and being excused from the process. For SCI patients who choose life before leaving acute care, a discussion regarding advance directives is warranted with the SCI patient to ensure desired medical treatments are executed in the future.[21]

CONCLUSION

Care of the critically ill patient with SCI requires utmost attention to the neurologic injury to minimize secondary neuronal injury. However, once the neurologic injury is stabilized, the major causes of mortality and morbidity are rarely the SCI, but related to complications in other body systems. The time after the initial stabilization is just as challenging and critical to the spinal cord-injured patient's outcome as the first few days in the critical care environment. Much of the care is directed toward minimizing complications and assisting the patient to cope with the neurologic deficits remaining. Care of the critically ill traumatic SCI patient is truly the work of the critical care nurse.

CASE STUDY 14.1

J.G., a 22-year-old caucasian male, was an unrestrained driver involved in a rollover motor vehicle crash. The car broke the guardrail and rolled down a hill, and J.G. was found lying on the ground at the bottom of the embankment. His blood alcohol level was 0.15 mg%, consistent with intoxication and over the legal limit of 0.08 mg%. J.G. was complaining of neck pain and difficulty breathing, and his skin was cool and dry. He was confused but responsive. J.G. was able to follow commands with his face, shrug his shoulders, and move his arms weakly. He had no obvious signs of hemorrhage.

J.G.'s temperature was 35°C. He exhibited shallow respirations at 12 breaths/min with a blood pressure of 80/40 mm Hg and a heart rate of 45 beats/min. He could raise both arms, flex elbows, and extend wrists (functional deltoids, biceps, wrist extensors). He had bicep and brachioradialis deep tendon reflexes, but no triceps reflexes. J.G. was unable to extend his elbows or grip and could not move his lower extremities. He had a flaccid paralysis of his lower extremities without patellar or ankle deep tendon reflexes. He had no abdominal or bulbocavernous reflexes. Priapism was present initially. His sensory level was approximately C5–C6. C5–C6 fractures were visualized on spine films. His ASIA motor score was 16 and his ASIA sensory score was 28, for a total of 44. His ASIA Impairment Scale category was A, complete.

Decision Point:
What mechanisms of injury are likely to be associated with this injury?

Decision Point:
What associated injuries are likely?

Decision Point:
What are the initial priorities for his care?

REFERENCES

1. Aarabi, B., Hadley, M. N., Dhall, S. S., et al. (2013). Management of acute traumatic central cord syndrome (ATCCS). *Neurosurgery, 72*(Suppl. 2), S195–S204.
2. Academy of Nutrition and Dietetics. (2009). Spinal cord injury (SCI) evidence-based nutrition practice guideline: Executive summary of recommendations. http://www.andeal.org/topic.cfm?menu=5292&cat=3486.
3. Ackery, A., Tator, C., & Krassioukov, A. (2004). A global perspective on spinal cord injury epidemiology. *J Neurotrauma, 21*(10), 1355–1370.
4. Agabegi, S. S., Asghar, F. A., & Herkowitz, H. N. (2010). Spinal orthoses. *J Am Acad Orthop Surg, 18*(11), 657–667.
5 Amador, M. J., & Guest, J. D. (2005). An appraisal of experimental procedures in human spinal cord injury. *J Neurol Phys Ther, 29*(2), 70–86.
6. American Association of Neurological Surgeons and Congress of Neurological Surgeons. (2002). Guidelines for management of acute cervical spine and spinal cord injury. *Neurosurgery, 50*(Suppl. 3), S1–S178.
7. American College of Surgeons. (2012). Spine and spinal cord trauma. In *Advanced trauma life support student course manual* (9th ed.) (pp. 174–193). Chicago IL: American College of Surgeons.
8. ArjoHuntLeigh Getinge Group. (2014). *RotoRest Delta Advanced Kinetic Therapy System: User manual.* San Antonio: ArjoHuntleigh. P/N208137-AH RevD.
9. Austin, J. W., Rowland, J. W., & Fehlings, M. G. (2013). Pathophysiology of spinal cord injury. In M. G. Fehlings, A. R. Vaccaro, M. Boakye, S. Rossignol, J. F. Ditunno, & A. S. Burns (Eds.), *Essentials of spinal cord injury: basic research to clinical practice.* New York: Thieme.
10. Bach, J. R. (2012). Noninvasive respiratory management of high level spinal cord injury. *J Spinal Cord Med, 35*(2), 72–80.
11. Bach, J. R., Goncalves, M. R., Rodriguez, P. L., Saporito, L., & Soares, L. (2014). Cuff deflation: rehabilitation in critical care. *Am J Phys Med Rehabil, 93*(8), 719–723.
12. Badjatia, N. (2012). Neurotrauma. In K. Lee (Ed.), *The neuro ICU book* (pp. 77–90). New York: McGraw-Hill.
13. Bakhsheshian, J., Dahdaleh, N. S., Fakurnjad, S., Scheer, J. K., & Smith, Z. A. (2014). Evidence-based management of traumatic thoracolumbar burst fractures: a systematic review of nonoperative management. *Neurosurg Focus, 37*(1), E1. http://thejns.org/doi/abs/10.3171/2014.4.FOCUS14159.
14. Banko, L. (2005). Aging with spinal cord injury: a review of the literature. *SCI Nurs, 22*(3), 138–145.
15. Baron, B. J., McSherry, K. J., Larsons, J. L., & Scalea, T. M. (2011). Spine and spinal cord trauma. In J. E. Tintinalli, J. S. Stapczynski, O. H. Ma, D. M. Cline, R. K. Cydulka, & G. D. Meckler (Eds.), *Tintinalli's emergency medicine: a comprehensive study guide* (7th ed.) (pp. 1709–1730). New York: McGraw-Hill.
16. Bawa, M., & Fayssoux, R. (2013). Vertebrae and spinal cord. In K. L. Mattox, E. E. Moore, & D. V. Feliciano (Eds.), *Trauma* (7th ed.) (pp. 430–460). New York: McGraw-Hill.
17. Beattie, M. S., & Bresnahan, J. C. (2013). Promising preclinical pharmacological approaches to spinal cord injury. In M. G. Fehlings, A. R. Vaccaro, M. Boakye, S. Rossignol, J. F. Ditunno, & A. S. Burns (Eds.), *Essentials of spinal cord injury: basic research to clinical practice* (pp. 391–398). New York: Thieme.
18. Bellon, K., Kolakowsky-Hayner, S. A., Chen, D., McDowell, S., Bitterman, B., & Klaas, S. J. (2013). Evidence-based practice in primary prevention of spinal cord injury. *Top Spine Cord Inj Rehabil, 19*(1), 25–30.
19. Benour, M., Cenic, A., Hurlbert, R. J., & Tator, C. (2013). Evaluation of the patient with spinal cord injury. In M. G. Fehlings, A. R. Vaccaro, M. Boakye, S. Rossignol, J. F. Ditunno, & A. S. Burns (Eds.), *Essentials of spinal cord injury: basic research to clinical practice* (pp. 18–26). New York: Thieme.
20. Biffl, W. L., Moore, E. E., Offner, P. J., et al. (1999). Optimizing screening for blunt cerebrovascular injuries. *Am J. Surg, 178*(6), 517–521.
21. Blackmer, J., & Ross, L. (2002). Awareness and use of advance directives in the spinal cord injured population. *Spinal Cord, 40*(11), 581–594.
22. Bogie, K., Ho, C., Washington, M., et al. (2013). Interdisciplinary essentials in pressure ulcer management. In M. G. Fehlings, A. R. Vaccaro, M. Boakye, S. Rossignol, J. F. Ditunno, & A. S. Burns (Eds.), *Essentials of spinal cord injury: basic research to clinical practice* (pp. 158–180). New York: Thieme.
23. Boninger, M. L., Waters, R. L., Chase, T., Consortium for Spinal Cord Medicine et al. (2005). *Preservation of upper limb function following spinal cord injury: A clinical practice guideline for health-care professionals.* Washington, DC: Paralyzed Veterans of America.
24. Bosques, G., & Vogel, L. C. (2014). Medical complications and management. In L. C. Vogel, K. Zebracki, R. R. Betz, & M. J. Mulcahey (Eds.), *Spinal cord injury in the child and young adult* (pp. 197–208). London: Mac Keith Press.

25. Brain Trauma Foundation and the American Association of Neurological Surgeons. (2000). Role of steroids. *Management and prognosis of severe traumatic brain injury*. (pp. 131–138). New York: Brain Trauma Foundation.
26. Brown, R., DiMarco, A. F., Hoit, J. D., & Garshick, E. (2006). Respiratory dysfunction and management in spinal cord injury. *Respiratory Care, 51*(8), 853–870.
27. Brunett, P. H., & Cameron, P. A. (2011). Trauma in adults. In J. E. Tintinalli, J. S. Stapczynski, O. H. Ma, D. M. Cline, R. K. Cydulka, & G. D. Meckler (Eds.), *Tintinalli's emergency medicine: a comprehensive study guide* (7th ed.) (pp. 1671–1676). New York: McGraw-Hill.
28. Burns, S., Biering-Sorensen, F., Donovan, W., et al. (2012). International standards for neurological classification of spinal cord injury, revised 2011. *Top Spinal Cord Inj Rehabil, 18*(1), 85–99.
29. Burns, A. S., Wilson, J. R., & Craven, B. C. (2013). The management of secondary complications following spinal cord injury. In M. G. Fehlings, A. R. Vaccaro, M. Boakye, S. Rossignol, J. F. Ditunno, & A. S. Burns (Eds.), *Essentials of spinal cord injury: basic research to clinical practice* (pp. 244–262). New York: Thieme.
30. Butt, L., & Scofield, G. (1997). The bright line reconsidered: the issue of treatment discontinuation in patients with ventilator-dependent tetraplegia. *Top Spinal Cord Inj Rehabil, 2*(3), 85–94.
31. Cadotte, D. W., & Fehlings, M. G. (2012). Spinal cord injury. In R. G. Ellenbogen, S. L. Abdulrauf, & L. N. Sekhar (Eds.), *Principles of neurological surgery* (3rd ed.) (pp. 445–454). Philadelphia: Elsevier.
32. Cadotte, D. W., & Fehlings, M. G. (2013). Timing of surgery for acute spinal cord injury: from basic science to clinical application. In M. G. Fehlings, A. R. Vaccaro, M. Boakye, S. Rossignol, J. F. Ditunno, & A. S. Burns (Eds.), *Essentials of spinal cord injury: basic research to clinical practice* (pp. 265–290). New York: Thieme.
33. Cadotte, D. W., Mikulis, D. J., Stroman, P., & Fehlings, M. G. (2013). Imaging of acute spinal cord trauma and spinal cord injury. In M. G. Fehlings, A. R. Vaccaro, M. Boakye, S. Rossignol, J. F. Ditunno, & A. S. Burns (Eds.), *Essentials of spinal cord injury: basic research to clinical practice* (pp. 27–37). New York: Thieme.
34. Camune, B. D. (2013). Challenges in the management of the pregnant woman with spinal cord injury. *J Perinat Neonatal Nurs, 27*(3), 225–231.
35. Capoor, J., & Stein, A. B. (2005). Aging with spinal cord injury. *Phys Med Rehabil Clin N Am, 16*(1), 129–161.
36. Capps, E., Kinnau, K. F., & Crane, D. A. (2015). Beyond broken spines What the radiologist needs to know about late complications of spinal cord injury. *Insights Imaging, 6*(1), 111–122.
37. Charles, Y. P., & Steib, J. P. (2015). Management of thoracolumbar spine fractures with neurologic disorder. *Orthop Traumatol Surg Res 101*(Suppl. 1), S31–S40.
38. Chen, Y., Tang, Y., Vogel, L. C., & DeVivo, M. J. (2013). Cause of spinal cord injury. *Top Spinal Cord Inj Rehabil, 19*(1), 1–8.
39. Como, J. J., Samia, H., Nemunaitis, G. A., et al. (2012). The misapplication of the term spinal cord injury without radiographic abnormality (SCIWORA) in adults. *J Trauma Acute Care Surg, 73*(5), 1261–1266.
40. Consortium for Spinal Cord Medicine. (1999). *Prevention of thromboembolism in spinal cord injury* (2nd ed.). Washington, DC: Paralyzed Veterans of America.
41. Creasey, G. H. (2013). Electrical stimulation following spinal cord injury. In M. G. Fehlings, A. R. Vaccaro, M. Boakye, S. Rossignol, J. F. Ditunno, & A. S. Burns (Eds.), *Essentials of spinal cord injury: basic research to clinical practice* (pp. 538–544). New York: Thieme.
42. Daffner, S. D. (2013). Halo application and closed skeletal reduction of cervical dislocations. In M. G. Fehlings, A. R. Vaccaro, M. Boakye, S. Rossignol, J. F. Ditunno, & A. S. Burns (Eds.), *Essentials of spinal cord injury: basic research to clinical practice* (pp. 117–123). New York: Thieme.
43. Dalal, K., & DiMarco, A. F. (2014). Diaphragmatic pacing in spinal cord injury. *Phys Med Rehabil Clin N Am, 25*(3), 619–629.
44. Davidson, L. T., Middleton, J. W., & Oleszek, J. (2014). Spasticity. In L. C. Vogel, K. Zebracki, R. R. Betz, & M. J. Mulcahey (Eds.), *Spinal cord injury in the child and young adult* (pp. 167–181). London: Mac Keith Press.
45. Davison, D. L., Terek, M., & Chawla, L. S. (2012). Neurogenic pulmonary edema. *Crit Care, 16*(212). http://ccforum.com/content/16/2/212
46. DeJong, G., Tian, W., Hsieh, C.H., et al. (2013). Rehospitalization in the first year of traumatic spinal cord injury after discharge from medical rehabilitation. *Arch Phys Med Rehabil, 94*(Suppl. 4), S87–S97.
47. Dhall, S. S., Hadley, M. N., Aarabi, B., et al. (2013). Guidelines for the management of acute cervical spine and spinal cord injuries: deep venous thrombosis and thromboembolism in patients with cervical spinal cord injuries. *J Neurosurg, 72*(Suppl. 2), S244–S254.
48. Dhall, S. S., Hadley, M. N., Aarabi, B., et al. (2013). Guidelines for the management of acute cervical spine and spinal cord injuries: nutritional support after spinal cord injury. *J Neurosurg, 72*(Suppl. 2), S255–S259.
49. DiMarco, A. F. (2005). Restoration of respiratory muscle function following spinal cord injury: review of electrical and magnetic stimulation techniques. *Respir Phys Neurobiol, 147*(2–3), 273–287.
50. DiMarco, A. F., Onders, R. P., Ignagni, A., Kowalski, K. E., & Mortimer, J. T. (2005). Phrenic nerve pacing via intramuscular diaphragm electrodes in tetraplegic subjects. *Chest, 127*(2), 671–678.
51. DiMarco, A. F., Takaoka, Y., & Kowalski, K. E. (2005). Combined intercostal and diaphragm pacing to provide artificial ventilation in patients with tetraplegia. *Arch Phys Med Rehabil, 86*(6), 1200–1207.
52. Dvorak, M. F., & Lenehan, B. (2013). Management of acute spinal cord injury in thoracolumbar burst fractures including cauda equina syndrome. In M. G. Fehlings, A. R. Vaccaro, M. Boakye, S. Rossignol, J. F. Ditunno, & A. S. Burns (Eds.), *Essentials of spinal cord injury: basic research to clinical practice* (pp. 320–328). New York: Thieme.
53. Ebert, E. (2012). Gastrointestinal involvement in spinal cord injury: a clinical perspective. *J Gastrointestin Liver Dis, 21*(1), 75–82.
54. Elliot, S. L. (2013). Sexuality and fertility after spinal cord injury. In M. G. Fehlings, A. R. Vaccaro, M. Boakye, S. Rossignol, J. F. Ditunno, & A. S. Burns (Eds.), *Essentials of spinal cord injury: basic research to clinical practice* (pp. 143–157). New York: Thieme.
55. Evans, L. T., Lollis, S. S., & Ball, P. A. (2013). Management of acute spinal cord injury in the neurocritical care unit. *Neurosurg Clin N Am, 24*(3), 339–347.
56. Fallah, A., Dance, D., & Burns, A. S. (2013). Rehabilitation of the individual with spinal cord injury. In M. G. Fehlings, A. R. Vaccaro, M. Boakye, S. Rossignol, J. F. Ditunno, & A. S. Burns (Eds.), *Essentials of spinal cord injury: basic research to clinical practice* (pp. 235–243). New York: Thieme.
57. Fehlings, M. G., & Baptiste, D. C. (2005). Current status of clinical trials for acute spinal cord injury. *Injury, 36*(Suppl. 2), B113–B122.
58. Fehlings, M. G., Brodke, D. S., Norvell, D. C., & Dettori, J. R. (2010). The evidence for intraoperative neurophysiological monitoring in spine surgery. *Spine (Phila Pa 1976), 35*(Suppl. 9), S37–S46.
59. Finnerup, N. B. (2013). Pain in patients with spinal cord injury. *Pain, 154*(Suppl. 1), S71–S76.
60. Freeborn, K. (2005). The importance of maintaining spinal precautions. *Crit Care Nurs Q, 28*(2), 195–199.
61. Fries, J. M. (2005). Critical rehabilitation of the patient with spinal cord injury. *Crit Care Nurs Q, 28*(2), 179–187.
62. Furlan, J. C., & Fehlings, M. G. (2008). Cardiovascular complications after acute spinal cord injury: pathophysiology, diagnosis, and management. *Neurosurg Focus, 25*(5), E13. http://dx.doi.org/10.3171/FOC.2008.25.11.E13.
63. Furlan, J. C. (2013). Autonomic dysreflexia: a clinical emergency. *J Trauma Acute Care Surg, 75*(3), 496–500.
64. Garber, S. L., Bryce, T. N., Gregori-Torres, T. L., Ho, C., & Rader, C. (2014). *Pressure ulcer prevention and treatment following spinal cord injury: a clinical practice guideline for health-care professionals* (2nd ed.). Washington, DC: Paralyzed Veterans of America.
65. Geerts, W. H., Bergqvist, D., Pineo, G. F., et al. (2008). Prevention of venous thromboembolism: american College of Chest Physicians Evidence-Based Clinical Practice Guidelines (8th ed.). *Chest 133*(Suppl. 6), 381S–453S.

66. Godoy, D. A., Napoli, M. D., & Rabinstein, A. A. (2010). Treating hyperglycemia in neurocritical patients: benefits and perils. *Neurocrit Care, 13*(3), 425–438.
67. Goetz, L. L., & Klausner, A. P. (2014). Strategies for prevention of urinary tract infections in neurogenic bladder dysfunction. *Phy Med Rehabil Clin N Am, 25*(3), 605–618.
68. Goldmark, E., Niver, B., & Ginsberg, D. A. (2014). Neurogenic bladder: from diagnosis to management. *Curr Urol Rep, 15*(10), 448–455. http://dx.doi.org/10.1007/s11934-014-0448-8.
69. Greene, A., Barnett, P., Crossen, J., Sexton, G., Ruzicka, P., & Neuwelt, E. (2002). Evaluation of the THINK FIRST for KIDS injury prevention curriculum for primary students. *Inj Prev, 8*(3), 257–258.
70. Groah, S. L., Wietzenkamp, D. A., Lammertse, D. P., Whiteneck, G. G., Lezotte, D. C., & Hamman, R. F. (2002). Excess risk of bladder cancer in spinal cord injury: evidence for an association between indwelling catheter use and bladder cancer. *Arch Phys Med Rehabil, 83*(3), 346–351.
71. Gunduz, H., & Binak, D. F. (2012). Autonomic dysreflexia: an important cardiovascular complication in spinal cord injury patients. *Cardiology Journal, 19*(2), 215–219.
72. Guy, S., Mehta, S., Leff, L., Teasell, R., & Loh, E. (2014). Anticonvulsant medication use for the management of pain following spinal cord injury: Systematic review and effectiveness analysis. *Spinal Cord, 52*(2), 89–96.
73. Hadley, M. N., Walters, B. C., Grabb, P. A., et al. (2002). Guidelines for the management of acute cervical spine and spinal cord injuries. *Clin Neurosurg, 49*, 407–498.
74. Hadley, M. N., & Walters, B. C. (2013). Introduction to the guidelines for the management of acute cervical spine and spinal cord injuries. *J Neurosurg, 72*(Suppl. 2), S5–S16.
75. Hadley, M. N., Walters, B. C., Aarabi, A. B., et al. (2013). Guidelines for the management of acute cervical spine and spinal cord injuries: clinical assessment following cervical spinal cord injury. *J Neurosurg, 72*(Suppl. 2), S40–S53.
76. Hagen, E. M. (2015). Acute complications of spinal cord injuries. *World J Orthop, 6*(1), 17–23.
77. Harrigan, M. R., Hadley, M. N., Dhall, S. S., et al. (2013). Guidelines for the management of acute cervical spine and spinal cord injuries: management of vertebral artery injuries following non-penetrating cervical trauma. *J Neurosurg, 72*(Suppl. 2), S234–S243.
78. Hess, D. R., & Altobelli, N. P. (2014). Tracheostomy tubes. *Respir Care, 59*(6), 956–973.
79. Hess, M. J., Zhan, E. H., Foo, D. K., & Yalla, S. V. (2003). Bladder cancer in patients with spinal cord injury. *J Spinal Cord Med, 26*(4), 335–338.
80. International Spinal Cord Society. (2013). *International perspectives on spinal cord injury.* World Health Organization: Geneva Switzerland. http://www.who.int/disabilities/policies/spinal_cord_injury/en/.
81. Hoffman, J. R., Mower, W. R., Wolson, A. B., Todd, K. H., & Zucker, M. I. (2000). Validity of a set of clinical criteria to rule out injury to the cervical spine in patients with blunt trauma. National Emergency X-radiography Utilization Study Group. *N Engl J Med, 343*(2), 94–99.
82. Hurlbert, R. J., Hadley, M. N., Walters, B. C., et al. (2015). Pharmacological therapy for acute spinal cord injury. *J Neurosurg, 76*(Suppl. 1), S71–S83.
83. Jackson, A. B., Dijkers, M., Devivo, M. J., & Poczatek, R. B. (2004). A demographic profile of new traumatic spinal cord injuries: change and stability over 30 years. *Arch Phys Med Rehabil, 85*(11), 1740–1748.
84. Jagos, C. (2014). Special populations: the older adult trauma patient. In D. Gurney, J. Blackwell, J. S. Blansfield, M. Crowley, & D. McKeown (Eds.), *Trauma nurse core course provider manual* (7th ed.) (pp. 259–268). Des Plaines, IL: Emergency Nurses Association.
85. Jensen, M. P., Truitt, A. R., Schomer, K. G., Yorkston, K. M., Baylor, C., & Molton, I. R. (2013). Frequency and age effects of secondary health conditions in individuals with spinal cord injury: A scoping review. *Spinal Cord, 51*(12), 882–892.
86. Jensen, M. P., Wilderström-Noga, E., Richards, J. S., Finnerup, N. B., Biering-Sorensen, F., & Cardenas, D. D. (2010). Reliability and validity of the international spinal cord injury basic pain data set items as self-report measures. *Spinal Cord, 48*(3), 230–238.
87. Jia, X., Kowalski, R. G., Sciubba, D. M., & Geocadin, R. G. (2013). Critical care of traumatic spinal cord injury. *J Intensive Care Med, 28*(1), 12–23.
88. Jones, T. M., Anderson, P. A., & Noonan, K. J. (2011). Pediatric cervical spine trauma. *J Am Acad Orthop Surg, 19*(10), 600–611.
89. Kalani, M. Y. S., Filippidis, A. S., & Theodore, N. (2012). Injuries to the cervical spine. In R. G. Ellenbogen, S. I. Abdulrauf, & L. N. Sekhar (Eds.), *Principles of neurological surgery* (3rd ed.) (pp. 397–411). Philadelphia: Elsevier.
90. Kamen, L., Henney, H. R., III., & Runyan, J. D. (2008). A practical overview of tizanidine use for spasticity secondary to multiple sclerosis, stroke, and spinal cord injury. *Curr Med Res Opin, 24*(2), 425–439.
91. Kawanishi, C. Y., & Greguol, M. (2013). Physical activity, quality of life, and functional autonomy of adults with spinal cord injuries. *Adapt Phys Activ Q, 30*(4), 317–337.
92. Kennedy, P., & Smithson, E. F. (2013). Essential of spinal cord injury: Psychosocial aspects of spinal cord injury. In M. G. Fehlings, A. R. Vaccaro, M. Boakye, S. Rossignol, J. F. Ditunno, & A. S. Burns (Eds.), *Essentials of spinal cord injury: basic research to clinical practice* (pp. 205–212). New York: Thieme.
93. Khalil, R. E., Gorgey, A. S., Janisko, M., Dolbow, D. R., Moore, J. R., & Gater, D. R. (2013). The role of nutrition in health status after spinal cord injury. *Aging Dis, 4*(1), 14–22.
94. King, R. B., Biddle, A. K., Braunschweig, C., et al. (1998). *Neurogenic bowel management in adults with spinal cord injury.* Washington, DC: Paralyzed Veterans of America.
95. King, B. S., Gupta, R., & Narayan, R. K. (2000). The early assessment and intensive care management of patients with severe traumatic brain and spinal cord injuries. *Surg Clin North Am, 80*(3), 855–870.
96. Kizior, R. J., & Hodgson, B. B. (2015). *Saunders nursing drug handbook 2015.* St Louis: Saunders.
97. Kraft, M. R. (1999). Refusal of treatment: an ethical dilemma. *SCI Nurs, 16*(1), 9–13, 20.
98. Krassioukov, A. (2014). Autonomic dysfunction after spinal cord injury. In L. C. Vogel, K. Zebracki, R. R. Betz, & M. J. Mulcahey (Eds.), *Spinal cord injury in the child and young adult* (pp. 182–196). London: Mac Keith Press.
99. Kreykes, N. S., & Letton, R. W. (2010). Current issues in the diagnosis of pediatric cervical spine injury. *Sem Ped Surg, 19*(4), 257–264.
100. Kruger, E. A., Pires, M., Ngann, Y., Sterling, M., & Rubayi, S. (2013). Comprehensive management of pressure ulcers in spinal cord injury: Current concepts and future trends. *J Spinal Cord Med, 36*(6), 572–585.
101. Lammertse, D. P. (2004). Invited review: Update on pharmaceutical trials in acute spinal cord injury. *J Spinal Cord Med, 27*(4), 319–325.
102. Linsenmeyer, T. A., Baker, E. R., Cardenas, D. D., et al. (2001). *Acute management of autonomic dysreflexia: individuals with spinal cord injury presenting to health-care facilities* (2nd ed.). Washington, DC: Paralyzed Veterans of America.
103. Linsenmeyer, T. A., Bodner, D. R., Creasey, G. H., et al. (1998). *Neurogenic bowel management in adults with spinal cord injury.* Washington, DC: Paralyzed Veterans of America.
104. Linsenmeyer, T. A., Bodner, D. R., Creasey, G. H., et al. (2006). *Neurogenic bladder management for adults with spinal cord injury: a clinical practice guideline for health-care providers.* Washington, DC: Paralyzed Veterans of America.
105. Livneh, H., & Martz, E. (2005). Psychosocial adaptation to spinal cord injury: a dimensional perspective. *Psychol Rep, 97*(2), 577–586.
106. Lu, D. C., Phan, N., Beattie, M. S., & Manley, G. T. (2013). Concomitant traumatic brain injury and spinal cord injury. In M. G. Fehlings, A. R. Vaccaro, M. Boakye, S. Rossignol, J. F. Ditunno, & A. S. Burns (Eds.), *Essentials of spinal cord injury: basic research to clinical practice* (pp. 98–107). New York: Thieme.
107. Mailis, A., & Chapparro, L. E. (2013). Pain after spinal cord injury. In M. G. Fehlings, A. R. Vaccaro, M. Boakye, S. Rossignol, J. F. Ditunno, & A. S. Burns (Eds.), *Essentials of spinal cord injury: basic research to clinical practice* (pp. 195–204). New York: Thieme.
108. Malanga, G., Reiter, R. D., & Garay, E. (2008). Update on tizanidine for muscle spasticity and emerging indications. *Expert Opin Pharmacother, 9*(12), 2209–2215.

109. Malhotra, N. R., & Shaffrey, C. I. (2010). Intraoperative electrophysiological monitoring in spine surgery. *Spine (Phila PA 1976), 35*(25), 2167–2179.
110. Manno, E. M. (2012). Critical care management of acute spinal cord injury. In E. M. Manno (Ed.), *Emergency management in neurocritical care* (pp. 32–36). West Sussex, UK: Wiley-Blackwell.
111. Mask, J., Arlinghaus, K., Bosshart, H., et al. (1998). *Depression following spinal cord injury: a clinical practice guideline for primary care physicians.* Washington, DC: Paralyzed Veterans of America.
112. Matsumoto, T., Tamaki, T., Kawakami, M., Yoshida, M., Ando, M., & Yamada, H. (2001). Early complications of high-dose methylprednisolone sodium succinate treatment in the follow-up of acute cervical spinal cord injury. *Spine, 26*(4), 426–430.
113. McIlvoy, L., Meyer, K., Mahanes, D., Sachse, S., McQuillan, K. A., & Traumatic spine injuries. (2004). In K. A. McQuillan, M. K. Bader, & L. R. Littlejohns (Eds.), *AANN core curriculum for neuroscience nursing* (5th ed.). Chicago: American Association of Neuroscience Nurses.
114. Mueller, L. A., Degreif, J., Schmidt, R., et al. (2006). Ultrasound-guided spinal fracture repositioning, ligamentotaxis, and remodeling after thoracolumbar burst fractures. *Spine (Phila PA, 1976), 31*(20), E739–E746.
115. Nas, K., Yazmalar, L., Sah, V., A Aydin, & Önes, K. (2015). Rehabilitation of spinal cord injuries. *World J Orthop, 6*(1), 8–16.
116. National Spinal Cord Injury Statistical Center. (2014). *2014 Annual report: complete public version.* Birmingham, AL: University of Alabama. https://www.nscisc.uab.edu/reports.aspx.
117. National SCI Statistical Center. (2015). *Spinal cord injury (SCI) facts and figures at a glance.* Birmingham, AL: National SCI Statistical Center. https://www.nscisc.uab.edu/.
118. Niazi, T. N., Daubs, M., & Dailey, A. T. (2013). Principles of surgical management of spine trauma associated with spinal cord injury. In M. G. Fehlings, A. R. Vaccaro, M. Boakye, S. Rossignol, J. F. Ditunno, & A. S. Burns (Eds.), *Essentials of spinal cord injury: basic research to clinical practice* (pp. 124–134). New York: Thieme.
119. Parsons, K., Buhrer, R., Burns, S. P., et al. (2005). *Respiratory management following spinal cord injury: a clinical practice guideline for health-care professionals.* Washington, DC: Paralyzed Veterans of America.
120. Perry, E. C., Ahmed, H. M., & Origitano, T. C. (2014). Neurotraumatology. *2014 Handb Clin Neurol, 121*, 1751–1772.
121. Phan, N. (2013). Management of spinal cord injury in the intensive care unit. In M. G. Fehlings, A. R. Vaccaro, M. Boakye, S. Rossignol, J. F. Ditunno, & A. S. Burns (Eds.), *Essentials of spinal cord injury: basic research to clinical practice* (pp. 84–97). New York: Thieme.
122. Ploumis, A. (2013). Venous thromboembolism prophylaxis. In M. G. Fehlings, A. R. Vaccaro, M. Boakye, S. Rossignol, J. F. Ditunno, & A. S. Burns (Eds.), *Essentials of spinal cord injury: basic research to clinical practice* (pp. 135–142). New York: Thieme.
123. Pointillart, V., Petitjean, M. E., Wiart, L., et al. (2000). Pharmacological therapy of spinal cord injury during the acute phase. *Spinal Cord, 38*(2), 71–76.
124. Post, M. W. M., & van Leeuwen, C. M. C. (2012). Psychosocial issues in spinal cord injury: a review. *Spinal Cord, 50*(5), 382–389.
125. Prakash, A., & Matta, B. F. (2008). Hyperglycemia and neurological injury. *Curr Opin Anaesthesiol, 21*(5), 565–569.
126. Rangappa, P., Jeyadoss, J., Flabouris, A., Clark, J. M., & Marshall, R. (2010). Cardiac pacing in patients with a cervical spinal cord injury. *Spinal Cord, 48*(12), 867–871.
127. Raslan, A. M., & Nemecek, A. N. (2012). Controversies in the surgical management of spinal cord injuries. *Neurol Res Int,* Epub 2012 May 14. http://dx.doi.org/10.1155/2012/417834.
128. Rosenberg, R. I., Zirkle, D. L., & Neuwelt, E. A. (2005). Program self-evaluation: the evaluation of an injury prevention foundation. *J Neurosurg, 102*(5), 847–849.
129. Rosenfeld, J. V., Bandopadhayay, P., Goldschlager, T., & Brown, D. J. (2008). The ethics of the treatment of spinal cord injury: stem cell transplants, motor neuroprosthetics, and social equity. *Top Spinal Cord Inj Rehabil, 14*(1), 76–88.
130. Rossignol, S. (2013). Anatomy and physiology of the spinal cord. In M. G. Fehlings, A. R. Vaccaro, M. Boakye, S. Rossignol, J. F. Ditunno, & A. S. Burns (Eds.), *Essentials of spinal cord injury: basic research to clinical practice* (pp. 3–17). New York: Thieme.
131. Rozzelle, C. J., Aarabi, B., Dhall, S. S., et al. (2013). Guidelines for the management of acute cervical spine and spinal cord injuries: spinal cord injury without radiographic abnormality. *(SCIWORA) Neurosurgery, 72*(2), S227–S233.
132. Rundquist, J. (2002). The right to die—ethical dilemmas in persons with spinal cord injury. *SCI Nurs, 19*(1), 7–10.
133. Ryken, T. C., Aarabi, B., Dhall, S. S., et al. (2013). Guidelines for the management of acute cervical spine and spinal cord injuries: management of isolated fractures of the axis in adults. *Neurosurgery, 72*(2), S127–S131.
134. Ryken, T. C., Hadley, M. N., Aarabi, B., et al. (2013). Guidelines for the management of acute cervical spine and spinal cord injuries: management of acute combination fractures of the atlas and axis in adults. *Neurosurgery, 72*(2), S151–S158.
135. Ryken, T. C., Hadley, M. N., Walters, B. C., et al. (2013). Guidelines for the management of acute cervical and spinal cord injuries: radiographic assessment. *Neurosurgery, 72*(3), S54–S72.
136. Ryken, T. C., Hurlbert, R. J., Hadley, M. N., et al. (2013). Guidelines for the management of acute cervical spine and spinal cord injuries: the acute cardiopulmonary management of patients with cervical spinal cord injury. *Neurosurgery, 72*(2), S84–S92.
137. Sandlin, K. J., & Klaas, S. J. (2013). Assessment and evaluation of primary prevention in spinal cord injury. *Top Spinal Cord Inj Rehabil, 19*(1), 9–14.
138. Sankari, A., Martin, J. L., Bascom, A. T., Mitchell, M. N., & Badr, M. S. (2015). Identification and treatment of sleep-disordered breathing in chronic spinal cord injury. *Spinal Cord, 53*(2), 145–149.
139. Saulino, M. (2014). Spinal cord injury pain. *Phy Med Rehabil Clin N Am, 25*(2), 397–410.
140. Sezer, N., Akkus, S., & Uqurlu, F. G. (2015). Chronic complications of spinal cord injury. *World J Orthop, 6*(1), 24–33.
141. Shamji, M. F., Yuh, S.J., & Tsai, E. C. (2013). Posttraumatic syringomyelia: pathophysiology and management. In M. G. Fehlings, A. R. Vaccaro, M. Boakye, S. Rossignol, J. F. Ditunno, & A. S. Burns (Eds.), *Essentials of Spinal Cord Injury* (pp. 224–234). New York: Thieme.
142. Sidhu, G. S., Ghag, A., Prokuski, V., Vaccaro, A. R., & Radcliff, K. E. (2013). Civilian gunshot injuries of the spinal cord: a systematic review of the current literature. *Clin Orthop Related Research, 471*(12), 3945–3955.
143. Silva, N. A., Sousa, N., Reis, R. L., & Salgado, A. J. (2014). From basics to clinical: a comprehensive review on spinal cord injury. *Prog Neurobiol, 114*, 25–57.
144. Skidmore-Roth, L. (2015). *Mosby's 2015 nursing drug reference.* St Louis: Mosby.
145. Slazinski, T., & Littlejohns, L. R. (2010). Anatomy of the nervous system. In M. K. Bader, & L. R. Littlejohns (Eds.), *AANN core curriculum for neuroscience nursing* (5th ed.). Chicago IL: American Association of Neuroscience Nurses.
146. Souter, M. J. (2012). Airway management in the neurological and neurosurgical patient. In E. M. Manno (Ed.), *Emergency management in critical care* (pp. 12–20). Oxford, UK: Wiley-Blackwell.
147. Stein, D. M., Roddy, V., Marx, J., Smith, W. S., & Weingart, S. D. (2012). Emergency neurologic life support: traumatic spine injury. *Neurocrit Care, 17*(1), S102–S111.
148. Stein, D. M., & Sheth, K. N. (2015). Management of acute spinal cord injury. *Continnun (Minneap MN), 21*(1), 159–187.
149. Stiell, I. G., Clement, C. M., McKnight, R. D., et al. (2003). The Canadian C-spine rule versus the NEXUS low-risk criteria in patients with trauma. *N Engl J Med, 349*(26), 2510–2518.
150. Stiell, I. G., Wells, G. A., Vandenheem, K. I., et al. (2001). The Canadian C-Spine Rule for radiography in alert and stable trauma patients. *JAMA, 286*(15), 1841–1848.
151. Szwedowski, D., & Walecki, J. (2014). Spinal cord injury without radiographic abnormality (SCIWORA)-Clinical and radiologic aspects. *Pol J Radiol, 79*, 461–464.
152. Teufack, S., Harrop, J. S., & Sharan, A. D. (2013). Spinal cord injury classification. In M. G. Fehlings, A. R. Vaccaro, M. Boakye, S. Rossignol, J. F. Ditunno, & A. S. Burns (Eds.), *Essentials of spinal cord injury: basic research to clinical practice* (pp. 65–74). New York: Thieme.

153. Theodore, N., Hadley, M. N., Aarabi, B., et al. (2013). Prehospital cervical spine immobilization after trauma. *Neurosurgery, 72*(Suppl. 2), 22–34.
154. VanPutte, C., Regan, J., Russo, A., Seeley, R., Stephens, T., & Tate, P. (2014). Skeletal system. In *Seeley's anatomy and physiology* (10th ed.) (pp. 191–238). New York: McGraw-Hill.
155. Van Rossum, A. B., Pattynama, P. M., Ton, E. R., et al. (1996). Pulmonary embolism: validation of spiral CT angiography in 149 patients. *Radiology, 201*(2), 467–470.
156. Vassilyadi, M., Duquette, C., Shamji, M. F., Orders, S., & Dagenais, S. (2009). Evaluation of ThinkFirst for kids injury prevention curriculum for grades 7/8. *Can J Neurol Sci, 36*(6), 761–768.
157. Vázquez, R. G., Sedes, P. R., Fariña, M. M., Marqués, A. M., & Velasco, M. E. F. (2013). Respiratory management of the patient with spinal cord injury. *Biomed Res Inter.* Accessed at http://dx.doi.org/10.1155/2013/168757.
158. Walters, B. C., Hadley, M. N., Hurlbert, J., et al. (2013). Guidelines for the management of acute cervical spine and spinal cord injuries: 2013 update. *Neurosurgery, 60*(1), S82–S91.
159. Wan, D., & Krassioukov, A. V. (2014). Life-threatening outcomes associated with autonomic dysreflexia: a clinical review. *J Spin Cord Med, 37*(1). http://dx.doi.org/10.1179/2045772313Y.0000000098.
160. Wang, D., Bodley, R., Sett, P., Gardner, B., & Frankel, H. (1996). A clinical magnetic resonance imaging study of the traumatised spinal cord more than 20 years following injury. *Paraplegia, 34*(2), 65–81.
161. Waters, R. L., Adkins, R. H., Yakura, J. S., & Sie, I. (1994). Motor and sensory recovery following incomplete paraplegia. *Arch Phys Med Rehabil, 75*(1), 67–72.
162. Waxman, S. G. (2013). The vertebral column and other structures surrounding the spinal cord. In *Clinical neuroanatomy* (27th ed.) (pp. 67–77). New York: McGraw-Hill.
163. Welk, B., McIntyre, A., Teasell, R., Potter, P., & Loh, E. (2013). Bladder cancer in individuals with spinal cord injuries. *Spinal Cord, 51*(7), 516–521.
164. Whiteneck, G., Adler, C., Biddle, A. K., et al. (1999). *Outcomes following traumatic spinal cord injury: clinical practice guideline for health-care professionals.* Washington, DC: Paralyzed Veterans of America.
165. Wing, P. C., Dalsey, W. C., Alvarez, E., et al. (2008). *Early acute management in adults with spinal cord injury: a clinical practice guidelines for health-care professionals.* Washington, DC: Paralyzed Veterans of America.
166. Wong, S. L., Shem, K., & Crew, J. (2012). Specialized respiratory management of acute cervical spinal cord injury: a retrospective analysis. *Top Spinal Cord Inj Rehabil, 18*(4), 283–290.
167. World Health Organization. (2013). *Spinal cord injury fact sheet. N384.* Geneva, Switzerland: World Health Organization. Accessed at http://www.who.int/mediacentre/factsheets/fs384/en/.
168. Zhang, S., Wadhwa, R., Haydel, J., Torns, J., Johnson, K., & Guthikonda, B. (2013). Spine and spine trauma: Diagnosis and treatment. *Neurol Clin, 31*(1), 183–206.

15

Special Neurologic Patient Populations

Mary King

Patients with neurologic injuries or illnesses are the most vulnerable of all patients, and that vulnerability is magnified in critical care populations. Cognitive challenges, paresis or paralysis, and deficits with speech and comprehension require nurses to be strong patient advocates, while addressing the complexities of neurologic care to adequately meet the patients' needs. Basic nursing care does not change, but advances in technology for earlier diagnosis, management of disease states, surgical interventions, and rehabilitation compel the nurse to be an integral part of a interprofessional healthcare team to return the patient to an optimal state of recovery. This chapter will discuss neurologic disease states, diagnostic testing, and medications for special neuroscience patients (Table 15.1).

BRAIN TUMOR

The World Health Organization (WHO) classification system for nervous system tumors separates tumor types by the nerves or tissues from which the tumors arise, whether the tumor is primary or metastatic, and the location of the tumor. Brain tumors are further denoted by location as supratentorial (frontal, temporal, parietal, or occipital lobes) or infratentorial (cerebellum or brain stem); most tumors are supratentorial (Table 15.2).[26] The average age at diagnosis for all types of primary brain tumors is 57 years. In the United States, the overall lifetime risk of developing a brain tumor for all ethnicities and sexes is less than 1%, but high-grade malignant gliomas represent 2% of all cancer-related deaths in adults. However, the rate of brain and central nervous system (CNS) cancers is higher in children (newborn to age 19 years), and is the second most common cause of cancer deaths after leukemia. Why brain tumors occur is still under investigation, and much research has been compiled on genetic or viral factors, as well as cell phone use, electromagnetic fields, or other environmental sources (Box 15.1, Table 15.3).

A distinctive feature of brain tumors is they tend to remain within the CNS, and rarely metastasize to other areas of the body. The brain, however, is a common site for metastatic tumors originating from elsewhere in the body. Twenty to forty percent of cancer patients will suffer brain metastases or secondary brain tumors. The most common types of tumors that metastasize to the brain are lung (35%), breast (20%), skin/melanoma (10%), kidney (10%), and colon (5%). Metastatic brain tumors are generally not seen with an initial diagnosis of cancer (except lung cancer); thus routine screening for brain tumors at initial diagnosis is not recommended. The incidence of metastatic brain tumors has increased, as patients are surviving longer after cancer diagnosis and treatment. According to the Central Brain Tumor Registry of the United States (CBTRUS), overall survival rates for patients with brain tumors is 34% and 28% at 5 years and 10 years, respectively. However, survival rates differ with tumor histopathology. For example, glioblastoma survival rates are less than 5% at 5 years, and slightly greater than 2% at the 10-year mark; whereas the survival rates for a pilocytic astrocytoma at 5 years is 94% and 91% at 10 years.[26,27]

The most common indications of a brain tumor are progressive neurologic deficits such as headache (54%), motor weakness (45%), or seizure (26%). An important consideration for nurses to remember is the uniqueness of each person; a tumor in the same area of the brain may present with very different signs and symptoms, underscoring the importance of performing neurologic assessments tailored to the individual patient.[41]

Whether a tumor is metastatic or originated in the brain, the signs and symptoms of tumors vary depending on the size of tumor and the part of the brain affected (Table 15.4). For example, frontal tumors may cause changes in executive, or higher cognitive functions such as judgment, memory, personality, or behavior. A tumor located in the frontal lobe (inferior frontal gyrus), which is responsible for the motor control of speech, may result in a nonfluent aphasia, whereby the patient is unable to express thoughts.[18] Parietal tumors may affect contralateral sensory function, such as the inability to recognize common objects *(agnosia),* perform activities of daily living (ADLs), or wash one's face *(apraxia).* Agnosia can be further described according to the function affected. For example, a visual agnosia may relate to the inability to identify color (*color agnosia*) or the inability to recognize faces *(prosopagnosia),* whereas an auditory agnosia may result in the inability to recognize or identify sounds. Somatosensory agnosias are related to touch *(asterogonosis),* awareness of illness *(anosognosia),* or the ability to recognize or differentiate one's own body parts from those of another person *(autotopagnosia).* Temporal tumors may affect speech and language (if on the dominant side) or vision, as evidenced by visual field deficits or "field cut." Temporal tumors often present with new-onset seizures, especially in adults with no prior history of seizure activity. Occipital tumors may affect visual perception and fields. A tumor in the cerebellar region would yield complications with coordination and gait *(dysmetria* and *ataxia).*[14]

Dysmetria is the inability to "measure" a distance. Finger-to-nose testing (sometimes referred to as *past-pointing*) is one test that can be completed at the bedside to assess dysmetria. Often, the patient with dysmetria will have difficulty accurately reaching or grasping objects, such as reaching past objects or not far enough. Nursing considerations for patients with dysmetria may include strategies to ensure adequate nutrition, as spills are common, and the patient will have difficulty with getting food on a utensil and with utensil-to-mouth motions.

TABLE 15.1 Medications Frequently Used in the Care of the Critically Ill Neurologic Patients

Medication	Action	Indication and Usual Dosage	Special Considerations
Phenytoin (Dilantin)	Limit repetitive firing of action potentials through slowing of sodium channels	*Status epilepticus (SE) and maintenance therapy for seizure prophylaxis:* Loading dose 20 mg/kg IV at 50 mg/min Maintenance dose 1.5 mg/kg IV three times per day Therapeutic range 10–20 mcg/mL Many patients in SE may require serum levels of 25–30 mcg/mL to achieve seizure control	Risk of hypotension and cardiac dysrhythmias, especially with rapid infusion Risk of infusion site reactions and soft tissue injury, including "purple glove syndrome" Allergic reactions and side effects are not uncommon and can include confusion, diplopia, lymphadenopathy, rash, Stevens-Johnson syndrome, and toxic epidermal necrolysis
Fosphenytoin (Cerebyx)		Fosphenytoin ordered as "phenytoin equivalent" units	Water-soluble prodrug of phenytoin; less likely to cause infusion site reactions but much more expensive Anticonvulsant medications are not effective in preventing first seizures in patients with newly diagnosed brain tumors
Benzodiazepines			
Lorazepam (Ativan)	Acts at benzodiazepine binding sites near GABA receptors to decrease neuronal firing and transmission of impulses	*Status epilepticus:* Loading dose 0.1–0.15 mg/kg IV Follow with maintenance anti-epileptic drug	Slightly slower onset but longer acting than diazepam Needs refrigeration Can be administered rectally or sublingually, but these routes have not been extensively studied
Diazepam (Valium)		*Status epilepticus:* Loading dose 0.15 mg/kg IV Maintenance 4–8 mg/h IV Follow with maintenance anti-epileptic drug	Available as a rectal preparation when IV access is inadequate Not typically used as maintenance therapy
Midazolam (Versed)		*Status epilepticus:* Loading dose 0.2 mg/kg IV Maintenance 0.2–2.9 mg/kg/h IV	Unlike other benzodiazepines, is water soluble and therefore can be given intramuscularly; also available for intranasal, buccal, or rectal administration Rapid onset of action but short half-life requires frequent dosing
Barbiturates			
Phenobarbital (Luminal)	Acts on GABA receptor complex and limits synaptic transmission	*Status epilepticus:* Loading dose 20 mg/kg IV Maintenance 2–4 mg/kg/d IV	High risk of respiratory depression; higher doses result in stupor and coma Cardiovascular collapse can occur at high levels Long half-life of 90 hours prolongs effects of medication for days or weeks
Pentobarbital (Nembutal)		*Status epilepticus:* Loading dose 3–15 mg/kg IV over 1 h Maintenance 1–10 mg/kg/h IV to achieve desired effect on EEG Breakthrough seizures: Additional 3–5 mg/kg IV bolus	High risk of hypotension; long half-life of 10–20 hours Pentobarbital levels are not as helpful during treatment as EEG effect
Propofol (Diprivan)	General anesthetic; GABA receptor site agonist	*Status epilepticus:* Loading dose 1–5 mg/kg IV Maintenance 2–15 mg/kg/h IV	Rapid onset and offset of action High cost Significant lipid component in IV admixture; rarely, pancreatitis Rapid discontinuation of drug may precipitate seizures Risk for propofol infusion syndrome: profound hypotension, lipidemia, and metabolic acidosis
Corticosteroids			
Dexamethasone (Decadron)	Mode of action in reduction of peritumoral edema unclear: proposed mechanisms include inhibition of phospholipase A_2, stabilization of lysosomal membranes, and improvement of peritumoral microcirculation	*Treatment for peritumoral edema:* Loading dose 10 mg PO Maintenance 4 mg PO every 6 h Dosage varies between 4 and 100 mg/d *Treatment for bacterial meningitis (begin with first dose of antibiotics):* 10 mg IV every 6 h for 4 d *Myasthenia gravis (MG):* Steroid therapy reserved for patients with moderate or severe disease *Guillain-Barré (GBS):* Corticosteroids proved to be of no benefit	Dexamethasone is the preferred corticosteroid for treatment of brain tumors because of minimal mineralocorticoid effect and lower rates of infection and psychosis Side effects include immunosuppression, altered glucose metabolism, gastrointestinal irritation, mood swings, myopathy, fat redistribution, and peripheral edema Steroids for bacterial meningitis are contraindicated in septic shock, immunosuppression, and postneurosurgical meningitis

TABLE 15.1 Medications Frequently Used in the Care of the Critically Ill Neuroscience Patients—cont'd

Medication	Action	Indication and Usual Dosage	Special Considerations
Desmopressin acetate (DDAVP)	Form of vasopressin	*Diabetes insipidus:* 10–40 mcg (0.1–0.4 mL) intranasally once or twice daily *or* 2–4 mcg IV or subcutaneously once or twice daily *or* 0.1–0.8 mg/d divided into 2 or 3 doses in oral tablets	Side effects are uncommon and dose-related: headache, nausea, nasal congestion or rhinitis, flushing, and cramping In high doses, can cause hypertension
Intravenous immunoglobulin (IVIG)	Acts to modulate the immune system through multiple mechanisms involving immunoglobulin class G (IgG) and receptors on macrophages and B cells; enhances T cell function	*Myasthenia gravis:* 400 mg/kg IV for 5 d *Guillain-Barré syndrome:* 400 mg/kg IV daily for 5 d	IVIG and plasmapheresis are equally effective in treatment of MG and GBS When compared to plasmapheresis, IVIG has fewer complications and may be more comfortable for the patient Side effects of IVIG include expansion of plasma volume and self-limiting fever, myalgia, headache, nausea, and vomiting
Acyclovir (Zovirax)	Inhibits viral replication[42]	*Herpes simplex and varicella-zoster encephalitis:* 10 mg/kg three times daily for 14 d	Most effective when given early in course of encephalitis
Anthelminthics (Antiparasitics)			
Albendazole (Albenza)	Cysticidal drugs	*Neurocysticercosis:* 15 mg/kg/d for 1 week	Albendazole is superior to praziquantel in destroying brain cysts Adverse effects include headaches, increased seizure frequency, increased ICP, cerebral infarction, hyperthermia, hypotension, dysrhythmias, and death Antithelmintics should be given in conjunction with steroid/immunosuppressive therapy to decrease the inflammatory reaction to dying parasites Patients with calcified cysts do not require antihelmintics
Praziquantel (Biltricide)		*Neurocysticercosis:* 10–100 mg/kg administered every 8 h for 3–21 d *or* 25–30 mg/kg every 2 h for 3 doses	
Acetylcholinesterase Inhibitors			
Pyridostigmine (Mestinon)	Inhibits acetylcholinesterase and thus increases the availability of ACh to act on ACh receptors	*Myasthenia gravis:* Started at 30 mg 3 times per day Can be gradually increased to 60–90 mg four times per day based on response and tolerance Onset of action in 15–30 min with duration of approximately 4 h	Side effects include abdominal pain, diarrhea, and excessive salivation Cholinesterase crisis involving an excess of ACh at neuromuscular junction is characterized by worsening of weakness and abdominal pain, and hypersalivation Treatment involves reduction of dose

ACh, Acetylcholine; *EEG*, electroencephalography; *GABA*, gamma-aminobutyric acid; *ICP*, intracranial pressure; *IV*, intravenous; *PO*, per os.

Ataxia is a gait disturbance that is evidenced by a wide stance and a "wobbly" posture. Patients with ataxia are at high risk for falls and injury, requiring the nurse to be diligent with patient and family education and the initiation of fall prevention measures to keep the patient safe. A consult for physical and occupational therapy is essential and should be obtained as soon as the patient is stable and able to participate in treatments. Evidence has shown that early mobility is critical for the overall well-being of the patient, and to reduce length of stay and decrease the risk of complications. The American Association of Critical Care Nurses (AACN) has developed the "ABCDE Bundle" for critical care patients that provides criteria and a step-by-step assessment to assist the nurse in determining a patient's readiness for mobilization.[1] Recent updates to this bundle by the Society of Critical Care Medicine has expanded the initiative with "F" to include family, through open visitation, presence during critical events such as resuscitation efforts, participation in care, and shared decision-making with the patient and the healthcare team.[40]

Classifications of Brain Tumors

In addition to classifying brain tumors by origin, location, and primary versus metastatic types, the WHO classification system uses a grading scale to describe the tumor histopathology and to predict the biological "behavior" of the tumor cells (see

TABLE 15.2 Types of Tumors

Type of Tumor	Origin/Arises from
Meningioma	Meningeal cells; meninges are the tissue covering the brain and spinal cord
Glioblastoma	Astrocytic glial cells–supportive brain cells
Astrocytoma	Astrocytes–supportive brain cells
Oligodendrocytoma	Oligodendrocytes–supportive brain cells
Ependymoma	Ependymal cells–cells that line the ventricles
Neuroma/schwannoma	Schwann cells–peripheral nerve cells; form the myelin sheath around axons
Pituitary tumor	Pituitary epithelial cells in the adenohypophysis of the pituitary
Medulloblastoma/pediatric neuroendocrine tumor	Usually arises in the cerebellum; most frequently occurs between the ages of 5 and 9
Germinoma	Germ cells
Craniopharyngiomas, dermoids, and epidermoids	Embryonic remnants

From Reference 26.

Table 15.2).[26] WHO Grade I tumors are those that grow slowly (i.e., the cells have a low proliferative potential) and for which a cure may be possible with surgical resection. WHO Grade IV tumors are highly proliferative, hypercellular, and have a bizarre appearance; the presence of necrosis is a definitive finding. Surgical intervention for Grade IV brain tumors is palliative at best, and may not be appropriate, depending on the clinical picture of the patient. Brain tumors affect the brain directly by infiltrating or compressing cerebral tissue, or by eroding the bone. Clinical signs and symptoms are related to the location of the tumor within the brain, the growth rate, effects on brain structures, or side effects such as cerebral edema, obstructive hydrocephalus, and increased intracranial pressure (ICP).

Nurses should have an understanding of the grading scale as well as the origins of tumors to provide support and education to the patient and family. Knowing patients' presenting signs and symptoms and underlying pathology provides a baseline for the nurse to individualize assessments. An accurate baseline assessment provides a means for the nurse to communicate changes to the surgeon and to monitor the patient's progress during the recovery period. This is crucial for patients undergoing surgery for brain tumors, as deficits may worsen postoperatively due to cerebral edema related to the disruption of the blood-brain barrier (BBB).

Disruption of the BBB gives rise to increased vascular permeability, followed by a loss of the barrier effect, allowing plasma fluids to leak into the surrounding tissues. Cerebral edema around the tumor is a typical finding, and is usually seen in high-grade gliomas and metastatic tumors, but should not be considered a direct marker of malignancy. Treatment interventions such as chemotherapy, radiation therapy, and surgery can affect the development and severity of cerebral edema. The tumor itself is a space-occupying lesion that may cause a shift in cerebral structures, resulting in pressure and neurologic deficits; the addition of edema exacerbates this mass effect.[35]

Dexamethasone (Decadron), a synthetic adrenocortical steroid with rare/minimal mineralocorticoid effect, is the medication most commonly used for vasogenic cerebral edema. Vasogenic cerebral edema impairs cellular activity and is the result of increased permeability of capillary endothelial cells in the white matter of the brain, allowing plasma to seep into the extracellular space between myelin sheath layers. Once administered, there may be a rapid relief from neurologic signs or symptoms, with a subsequent decrease in cerebral edema. The effects of dexamethasone diminish within weeks or months, and the patient must be closely monitored for side effects. The most frequent side effects are hyperglycemia and hypertension.[35] Patients with diabetes may require increased insulin coverage; nondiabetic patients may require temporary dosing with insulin until the dexamethasone is tapered and discontinued. Dexamethasone treatment begins with a loading dose of 10 mg followed by 4 mg every 6 hours, but dosing can be as much as 100 mg per day. Dexamethasone is generally given by mouth (PO), but may be administered via intravenous (IV) injection.[35]

Brain tumors are diagnosed by a combination of patient presenting signs and symptoms and diagnostic exams that include computed tomography (CT) scan and magnetic resonance imaging (MRI). In general, there are no specific laboratory tests for brain tumors, with the exception of pituitary tumors,

BOX 15.1 World Health Organization Classification of Brain Tumors

Tumors of Neuroepithelial Tissue

- Astrocytic tumors (Grades I-IV)
- Oligodendroglial tumors
- Mixed gliomas
- Ependymal tumors
- Choroid plexus tumors
- Neuronal and mixed neuronal-glial tumors
- Neuroblastic tumors
- Pineal parenchymal tumors
- Embryonal tumors

Tumors of Peripheral Nerve

- Schwannomas (neuromas)
- Neurofibromas
- Perineuromas
- Malignant peripheral nerve sheath tumors

Tumors of the Meninges

- Tumors of meningothelial cells meningiomas
- Atypical meningiomas
- Anaplastic meningiomas
- Mesenchymal, nonmeningothelial tumors
- Primary melanocytic lesions

Lymphomas and Hematopoietic Neoplasms

- Malignant lymphomas
- Plasmacytomas
- Granulocytic sarcomas

Germ Cell Tumors

- Germinomas
- Embryonal carcinomas
- Yolk sac tumors
- Choriocarcinomas
- Teratomas
- Mixed germ cell tumors

Tumors of the Sellar Region

- Craniopharyngiomas
- Granular cell tumors

Metastatic Tumors

From Reference 34.

TABLE 15.3 **Commonly Occurring Primary Brain Tumors**

Tumor Type	Subtypes	Clinical Presentation	Comments/Treatment	Prognosis
Glioma	Grade I – Astrocytoma Cells are well-defined	Deficits related to location (supra- or infratentorial); new-onset seizure is the most common presentation; most often occurs between ages 20 and 40	Gross total removal is the treatment of choice; rarely possible to remove completely	Survival may range from 2 to 20 years, with an average of 5 to 6 years
	Grade II – Astrocytoma Cell differentiation less defined		Radiation and chemotherapy: overall controversial; not done for Grade I type	
	Grade III – Anaplastic astrocytoma Atypical cells; increased mitosis	Usually occurs in frontal lobe; diffuse cerebral symptoms and associated frontal lobe deficits; most common between ages 40 to 60; more common in males than in females	Surgery for resection and debulking of tumor; ease compression and ICP Radiation performed with concurrent temozolomide; adjuvant temozolomide	Average survival: 14–16 months
	Grade IV – Glioblastoma multiforme Rapidly growing cells; areas of necrosis/hemorrhage common within tumor	Usually occurs in frontal lobe; diffuse cerebral symptoms and associated frontal lobe deficits; most common between ages 40 to 60; more common in males than in females	Surgery for resection and debulking of tumor; ease compression and ICP Radiation is performed with concurrent temozolomide; adjuvant temozolomide	Average survival: 14–16 months
Meningioma	Less common, aggressive subtypes: Atypical meningioma Malignant meningioma	Related to compression of brain structures May cause headache, seizures Enhancing dural mass; may have calcification or edema	Slow growing; usually benign; attached to dura mater Falx cerebri most common location Amount of tumor resection related to favorable prognosis	"Cure" with total removal Many years with partial excision and radiation
Pituitary adenoma	Classified by hormonal content/structure	Visual loss Headache Cranial nerve deficits Symptoms related to imbalances of pituitary hormones	Benign Pharmacologic management of hormone imbalances Transsphenoidal hypophysectomy is usual surgical approach Radiation occasionally used for residual tumor tissue	Cure with complete resection; very good outcome in other cases
Schwannoma	Vestibular schwannoma is an "acoustic neuroma"	Often present with hearing loss or tinnitus Enhancing lesion	Slow growing; benign Surgically curable Cranial nerve deficits can result	Cure with total resection; tumor regrowth possible

ICP, Intracranial pressure.
From Reference 8.

TABLE 15.4 **Brain Tumor Location and Associated Signs And Symptoms**

Brain Tumor Location	Associated Neurologic Signs And Symptoms
Frontal lobe	Contralateral paresis/plegia; cognitive/behavioral/personality changes; emotional lability; memory deficits; loss of self-restraint
Temporal lobe	Seizures; aphasia; memory problems; visual field cut
Parietal lobe	Sensory deficits; visual field cut; language deficits; neglect syndromes; seizures
Occipital lobe	Visual loss or hallucinations
Cerebellum	Ipsilateral ataxia; nystagmus; vertigo; nausea
Brain stem	Dysphagia/gag reflex dysfunction; motor and sensory deficits; vertigo; hiccups; nystagmus; nausea and vomiting
Intraventricular	Symptoms related to obstruction of cerebrospinal fluid flow/hydrocephalus (gait disturbance, cognitive deficits, urinary incontinence); sudden death

which may result in hormone level derangements. In the event of seizure activity, electroencephalography (EEG) may be used to determine seizure focus and identify slowing of brain waves (Fig. 15.1).[16]

CT scans are helpful in identifying bony lesions in the brain or spine, or the presence of hemorrhage. CT scans may be used for those patients unable to undergo MRI scanning due to contraindications (i.e., cardiac pacemaker or claustrophobia). The use of MRI with or without contrast (gadolinium) is standard for diagnosis, as well as ongoing monitoring of primary and metastatic brain tumors. For the diagnostician, an MRI with contrast is able to distinguish small tumors situated near bone, and can provide an accurate picture of cerebral edema, as well as greater anatomic detail and visualization of the tumor and tumor characteristics. Low-grade tumors, in general, do not demonstrate enhancement around the tumor site, whereas high-grade tumors will demonstrate enhancement due to disruption of the BBB.[16]

Other exams may include magnetic resonance spectroscopy (MRS), which evaluates metabolic information about brain tumor composition to differentiate between malignant

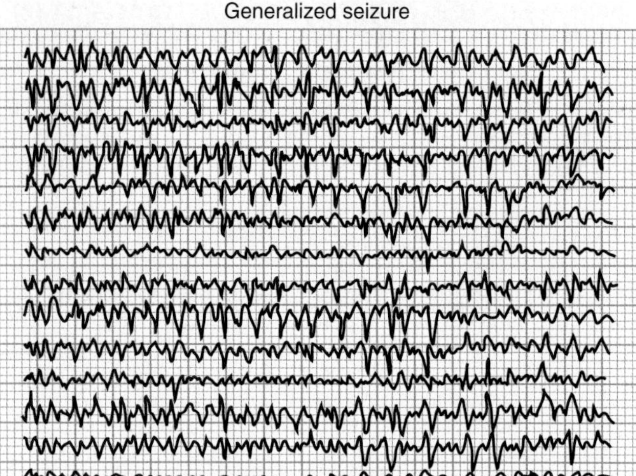

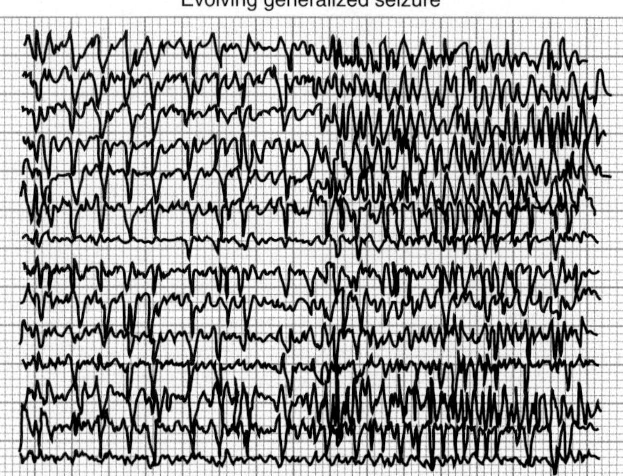

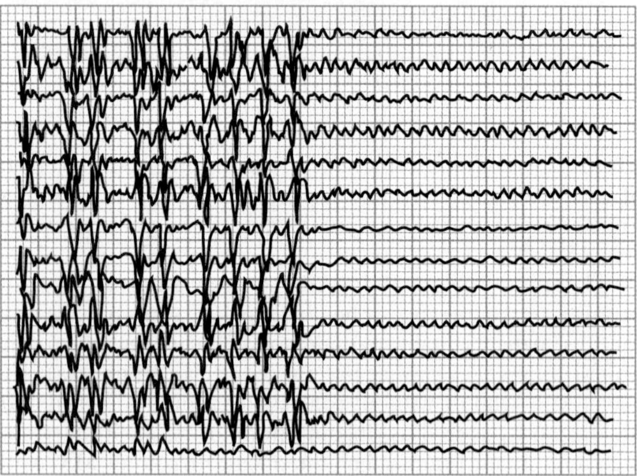

FIG. 15.1 EEG study of generalized electroencephalographically detected seizures that evolve over time.

versus nonmalignant or low- versus high-grade, or changes from low- to high-grade malignancy. Magnetic resonance angiography (MRA) can provide a noninvasive means to evaluate vascular structures, whereas thallium-201 single-photon emission CT may serve to differentiate radiation necrosis from tumor.[16]

Neuroepithelial Tissue Tumors

Astrocytic tumors arise from astrocytes, a type of glial cell. Glial cells (also called *neuroglia*) are the most common cells in the CNS, and support neuron function. In addition to the astroglial cells, oligodendroglia (oligodendrocytes) and microglial cells combine to perform critical functions in the CNS. The astrocytes work to maintain homeostasis, especially with regard to ion concentrations, and form scar tissue, or gliosis, when there is injury to the CNS. The oligodendrocytes form myelin sheaths, which are a type of electrical insulation for the CNS and are critical for neural conduction. Microglial cells act as phagocytes, and are activated during degenerative and inflammatory processes in the CNS.[2]

Astrocytic tumors range from a circumscribed astrocytoma (WHO Grade I) to the most common primary brain tumor, glioblastoma multiforme (GBM) (WHO Grade IV). GBM is a highly malignant, rapidly growing type of brain tumor that is found in the cerebral hemispheres in adults and in the brain stem in children. GBM rarely occurs in the cerebellum, and occurs in males more than females, with a peak incidence in people aged 50 to 70 years.[2]

Other types of neuroepithelial tumors include oligodendroglioma (WHO Grades II–IV), ependymoma, pineal tumor, and the embryonal tumors (i.e., primitive neuroectodermal tumor [PNET]), which are generally found in children under the age of 7, or medulloblastoma, which occurs in the cerebellum in children and young adults up to age 20. Oligodendrogliomas often present as new-onset seizures in adults, and may be calcified. As the ependymal cells lining the ventricular system and the central canal of the spinal cord are the source of ependymomas, there exists the potential for "seeding" of tumor cells throughout the cerebrospinal fluid (CSF) system. MRI of the brain and spinal cord is recommended to look for tumors elsewhere that may not be detected either by clinical symptoms or by limited (i.e., brain- or spine-only) imaging. Pineal tumors, by virtue of their location, cause obstruction of CSF flow (obstructive hydrocephalus) and create pressure on adjacent structures. Similarly, the medulloblastoma and PNET tumor types cause obstruction of the CSF flow and may seed throughout the CSF system.[2]

Peripheral Nerve Tumors

Patients with tumors arising from the cranial and spinal nerves present with deficits specific to particular nerves involved; depending on size and location, these tumors can cause mass effect and pressure on adjacent structures as well. A benign tumor arising from the Schwann cells (*schwannoma*) commonly occurs on cranial nerve (CN) VIII. In the past, this type of tumor was known as an *acoustic neuroma*; however, the term *vestibular schwannoma* is more accurate. A vestibular schwannoma causes compression of CN VIII, and patients present with tinnitus, disequilibrium, and unilateral hearing loss. As CN VII and CN VIII arise from the same embryologic tissue, and both leave the brainstem at the pontomedullary junction, the patient may also experience motor symptoms related to CN VII, such as ipsilateral facial weakness.[37] Facial weakness is associated with large tumors due to compression of the fourth ventricle in the brain, resulting in an obstructive hydrocephalus. Additionally, large tumors (average size > 27 mm) are associated with surgical complications. The surgeon will select a surgical approach that depends on the size of the tumor and degree of hearing loss. For example, a translabyrinthine approach will sacrifice hearing, whereas a retrosigmoid approach may preserve hearing. A middle fossa approach also tends to preserve hearing; however, the use of this approach is generally limited to small tumors in the internal auditory canal.[33]

Postoperative care of the patient with a vestibular schwannoma includes management of nausea/vomiting related to dizziness or vertigo. When vertigo is present, early mobility with physical therapy evaluations and treatments designed to help the patient to "reequilibrate" are key. Speech therapy may be needed in the event of CN VII deficits for swallow evaluation and aspiration precautions. Alterations in body image may be an important consideration when CN VII damage has occurred either as a result of tumor growth or surgical intervention. Patients may benefit from counseling or support groups, as available.[19]

Bilateral vestibular schwannoma is one of the main characteristics of neurofibromatosis Type II (NF II). Neurofibromatosis develops from a benign, peripheral nerve sheath tumor (neurofibroma). Whereas vestibular schwannomas are common in NF II, multiple lesions are the hallmark of neurofibromatosis Type I (NF I). NF I may also be referred to as von Recklinghausen's disease, von Recklinghausen neurofibromatosis, or peripheral neurofibromatosis. NF I subtypes include: cutaneous, subcutaneous, nodular, diffuse plexiform, and spinal. A large number of mast cells are associated with these tumors, resulting in local pruritus. Some patients afflicted with intracutaneous neurofibromas may have hundreds or thousands of these tumors, which can cause a great deal of disfigurement or discomfort, and require the skills of a plastic surgeon for removal. Spinal neurofibromas can occur at one or more locations along the nerve roots, and the patient may have sensory and motor deficits related to the tumor location.[19]

Neuroendocrine tumors (pituitary tumors) may arise from cells of the anterior pituitary gland, and are usually single tumors. Although these are considered benign tumors, they may cause endocrine dysfunction such as Cushing's disease, acromegaly, or prolactinoma. Pituitary tumors are classified by size and function: microadenoma (< 1 cm) versus macroadenoma (> 1 cm), and "functional" (secreting) versus "nonfunctional" (nonsecreting). Functional/secreting pituitary tumors may cause over- or under secretion of hormones, with resultant endocrine dysfunction. Nonfunctional/nonsecreting tumors generally are not evident until the tumor is of sufficient size to cause neurologic deficits due to pressure or mass effect on adjacent structures. The pituitary gland is located just above the optic chiasm; therefore, visual changes are often what prompt the patient to seek care. Bitemporal visual field deficits (a loss or decrease in peripheral vision) or cranial nerve palsy due to paralysis of extraocular muscles and headache may also be presenting symptoms. Pituitary tumors that occur before puberty or the closure of the epiphyses result in gigantism; after puberty or closure of the epiphyses, the patient will have acromegaly. Patients with acromegaly have distinctive features, including bony overgrowth of the forehead, jaw, and nose; enlarged tongue, hands, and feet; and thickened soft tissue of the face.[26]

Postoperative care of patients with pituitary tumors includes close monitoring of intake and output, urine and serum specific gravity, and serum cortisol related to possible disruption of pituitary-adrenal function. Assessment of the morning cortisol level on postoperative day 2 or 3 is the most common method used to ensure that the pituitary-adrenal axis is intact. The serum cortisol level is obtained at approximately 8:00 a.m., as the level varies throughout the day; the early morning measurement provides the most accurate picture of hypothalamus-pituitary-adrenal function. The nurse must ensure that the laboratory sample is obtained and processed accordingly, as the results will determine the next steps in medication therapy.[26]

Monitoring for diabetes insipidus (DI) through accurate measurement of intake and output with urine specific gravity and daily (or more frequent) measurements of serum electrolytes are vital. DI is evidenced by a massive volume of dilute urine with elevated serum sodium (hypernatremia). Patients with DI should not be fluid-restricted, but encouraged to drink fluids as desired. Most patients are able to maintain euvolemia and adequate fluid intake; however, desmopressin (DDAVP) may be required in some situations to mitigate the effects of DI.[26]

DDAVP is a synthetic equivalent of antidiuretic hormone (ADH) and is the treatment of choice for acute and chronic DI. DDAVP is given via subcutaneous (SC) or IV injection in a dose of 1–2 mcg, or 10 mcg intranasally after the nasal packing has been removed. DDAVP should be given only as needed in the early postoperative period (i.e., if urine output increases [polyuria] and increased thirst [polydipsia] returns), since DI may be transient, and hyponatremia may result with excess desmopressin.[26]

Pituitary Apoplexy

Pituitary apoplexy is an emergent situation that results from sudden hemorrhage or necrotic expansion of a pituitary tumor, resulting in neurologic and/or endocrine deterioration. An infarction may occur within the pituitary tumor or pituitary gland. The patient presentation is usually a sudden headache and/or a neurologic deficit such as ophthalmoplegia or a visual loss, mental status changes, or a loss of consciousness related to increased ICP and/or hypothalamic effects. Other clinical symptoms may result in pressure or compression in the cavernous sinus (proptosis, ptosis, or pressure on the carotid artery), stroke related to carotid artery compression, or a subarachnoid hemorrhage (SAH) as a result of the hemorrhage extending beyond the tumor and into the subarachnoid space.[14]

Nurses caring for patients with pituitary tumor (preoperatively and postoperatively) need to have an understanding of and ability to react promptly to signs and symptoms of pituitary apoplexy. Management of pituitary apoplexy requires prompt administration of corticosteroids, evaluation of endocrine function, and emergent decompression when there is a sudden loss of vision/visual fields or neurologic deterioration. Surgical intervention is aimed at decompression of adjacent structures, tissue retrieval for pathology, and ventricular drainage to relieve hydrocephalus. Complete resection or removal of the tumor is generally not required.[14]

Treatment Modalities

Surgery

Surgical intervention (craniotomy) to remove the tumor is a common first step in tumor management that provides a means of tissue removal for diagnosis, debulking of tumor mass, and management of mass effect (Fig. 15.2). Intraoperative exams may include MRI or stereotactic lasers; additionally, evoked potential electrophysiologic mapping of the brain may be employed to remove tumors while maintaining function for tumors near critical "real estate" such as the motor or speech areas. Collaboration with eye, ear, nose, and throat (EENT) specialists and plastic surgeons enables neurosurgeons to reach and resect skull base tumors. The primary goal for surgical

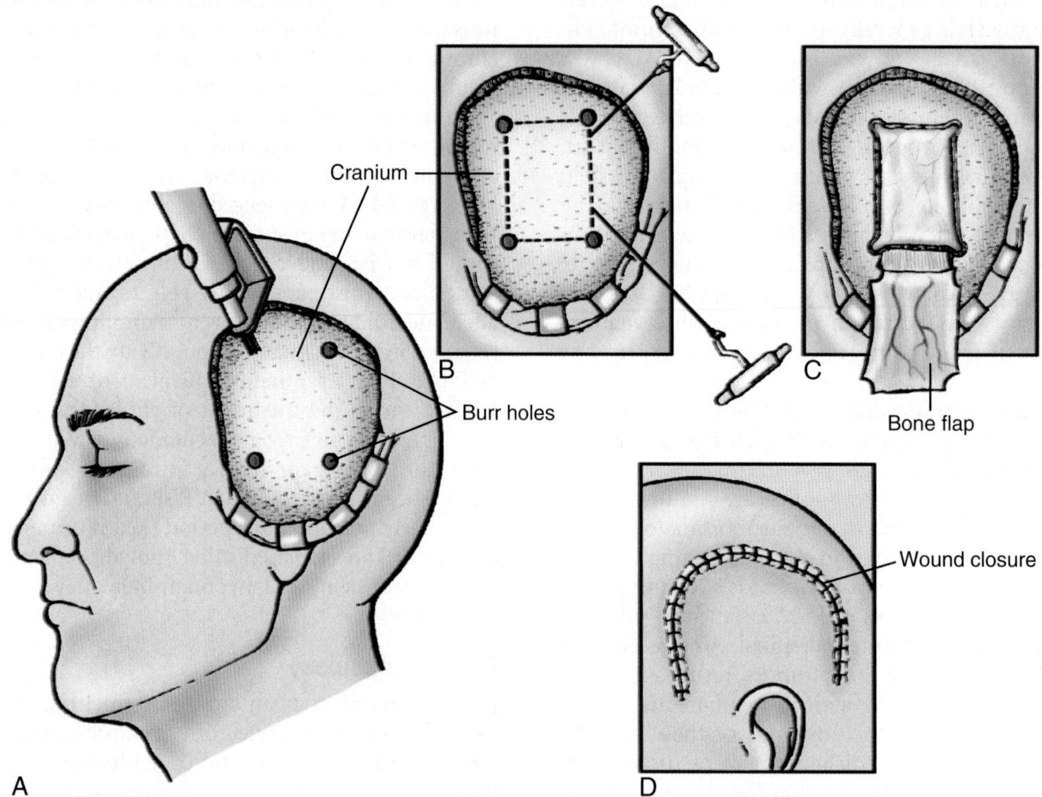

FIG. 15.2 Craniotomy procedure. **A,** Burr holes are drilled into the skull. **B,** A surgical saw is used to cut an aperture between the burr holes. **C,** The cranial contents are exposed. **D,** The bone is replaced and the wound is closed. (From Monahan, F., Sands, J., Neighbors, M., et al. (2007). *Phipps' medical-surgical nursing: health and illness perspectives* (9th ed.). St Louis: Mosby.)

intervention for malignant brain tumors is to obtain an accurate histopathologic diagnosis to direct treatments and debulk the tumor to relieve symptoms of mass effect; surgery in these cases is not curative.[8]

Radiation

Radiation therapy is often included as part of the treatment for benign or malignant brain tumors to stabilize or reduce the size of the tumor. Surgery may remove all visible signs of the tumor, but the microscopic cells that remain may seed into adjacent normal tissues; thus, radiation therapy is used to delay or prevent tumor recurrence. Because of their increased mitotic activity, tumor cells are more susceptible to radiation therapy, which destroys tumor cell DNA. However, the cores of malignant tumors have a large amount of hypoxic tumor cells that are more resistant to the DNA-destroying effects of radiation, thus creating a limited time in which radiation is beneficial.[8]

Several types of radiation therapy exist for the treatment of brain tumors. External beam radiation therapy (EBRT) is a conventional form of radiation used for tumors that are inoperable, after a diagnostic surgical procedure, or for those tumors that are sensitive to radiotherapy. EBRT can be delivered to the whole brain (whole brain EBRT) or only to the area with the tumor (focal EBRT). Intensity-modulated radiation therapy (IMRT) is a newer approach that uses a computer program to plan the distribution of the dose in order to provide differing doses to the tumor and the surrounding tissues. When the tumor borders are irregular, limiting the exposure of surrounding tissues to radiation aids in reducing associated tissue toxicity. Proton therapy uses proton particles instead of x-rays, and is similar to EBRT. This method limits exposure to normal brain tissues and delivers therapy with greater precision. Of note, this therapy is only available in a few centers in the United States.[8]

Stereotactic radiosurgery is a type of "conformal" radiation, meaning the high-dose external radiation beams are "conformed" or shaped to the tumor shape, thus limiting the exposure of surrounding brain tissues to radiation. Conformal therapy (radiosurgery) provides a highly focused dose of radiation and is beneficial for small lesions that are well-circumscribed. Radiosurgery is delivered by either a linear accelerator (LINAC) or gamma knife.[15]

Treatment with radiation does not always benefit the patient with brain tumor. Multiple factors determine the success or failure of radiation/radiotherapy. The presence of hypoxic cells contributes to a less than optimal result, since these cells are more resistant to radiation than are well-oxygenated cells. Hypoxic cells can remain viable after treatment. Side effects of radiation may be significant and cause much distress to the patient as well. Side effects are related to the radiation dose, location, and technique. The most common acute side effects include hair loss, fatigue, skin disorders, and somnolence; chronic side effects may include cerebral necrosis, a decrease in or loss of pituitary function, hydrocephalus, and impaired cognitive function. Several studies in recent years have examined the impact of cognitive impairments on the patient and on their family and caregivers as well.[8]

Chemotherapy

Chemotherapy is used as an adjunct to surgery and radiation treatment, and is the primary treatment for brain tumor recurrence. The most common chemotherapeutic agents used are alkylating agents, especially nitrosoureas: temozolomide (Temodar), carmustine (BCNU), lomustine (CCNU), Gliadel wafers (carmustine), procarbazine, or a combination of procarbazine, CCNU, and vincristine (PCV). Clinicians administer chemotherapeutic agents via a variety of routes, with oral and IV administration being the most common. Interstitial, intra-arterial, and intrathecal routes are options as well, depending on the tumor location and the medication. These routes provide the option to administer an increased dose that will mount a stronger attack on the tumor cells, while decreasing the side effects. For example, interstitial administration uses disc-shaped biodegradable medication wafers that are placed into the surgical bed after the tumor is removed. Intrathecal administration directs the chemo agent directly into the spinal fluid.[8]

Cytotoxic agents and cytostatic agents are broad categories of chemotherapy medications that cause cell death and cause cells to act more like normal cells, respectively. These categories are further divided by their mechanism of action, such as those agents that are only active during specific phases of the cell's life cycle (cycle-specific) or those that are active throughout the entire life cycle of the cell (cycle-nonspecific). These agents may be used alone or in combination for greater effectiveness against a maximum number of malignant cells.[8]

One of the main considerations and challenges in the development of chemotherapy agents used in brain tumors is the ability of the medications to pass through the BBB, while avoiding injury to normal neurologic cells. Even if a medication is able to penetrate the BBB to attack tumor cells, its ability to kill tumor cells is not guaranteed. Tumor cells can block or become resistant to the chemotherapeutic agent(s). Another factor affecting the efficacy of chemotherapy agents is somatic mutations of the tumor cells, which may enable them to use other pathways to continue growth.[26]

Care Considerations

Venous Thromboembolism

A common complication in patients with a malignant process is venous thromboembolism (VTE). Interestingly, the incidence of VTE in patients with cancer has been documented as far back as 1823. VTE is especially high in patients with malignant glioma, with an incidence of up to 30%, and overall incidence as high as 28%, making VTE the second leading cause of death in patients with cancer. In patients undergoing craniotomy for brain tumor, the risk of developing a symptomatic deep venous thrombosis (DVT) may be as high as 31%, with an associated risk of pulmonary embolism (PE) of approximately 5% and risk of mortality as high as 50%.[36] Multiple mechanisms activated by the tumor cells can result in blood coagulation, including the production of procoagulant, proaggregation, and fibrinolytic factors, as well as the release of proinflammatory and proangiogenic cytokines that interact with the patient's vascular and blood cells.[31] Despite knowledge of these facts, the mechanisms that lead the development of VTE are unclear; however, a histologic diagnosis of GBM, lengthy surgery, steroids, and chemotherapy (which decreases fibrinolytic activity) are thought to be among the risk factors. Additionally, large tumor size, leg paresis (which promotes venous stagnation), and older age are risk factors. Large tumors produce procoagulation factors; therefore, the larger the tumor, the greater the amount of procoagulation factors released. High-grade glial tumors have pathologic neovascularization, and an abundant vascular supply is found in brain metastases and meningiomas.[36]

Prevention of DVT/VTE is critical for all neurosurgical patients, and the National Institute for Health and Clinical Excellence (NICE) guidelines support the use of mechanical devices and pharmacologic prophylaxis in patients who are considered "low risk" for major bleeding. Mechanical methods of prevention include intermittent pneumatic compression (IPC) devices and graduated compression stockings (GCS). The IPC device has an air bladder within the "sleeve" that surrounds the leg and periodically inflates/deflates to promote emptying of the lower limb deep veins and prevent venous stasis. The mechanism of the GCS is not as clear; however, the device is thought to function by preventing distention of the veins.

Pharmacologic treatments, such as unfractionated heparin (UFH) or low-molecular-weight heparin (LMWH), are usually administered via the subcutaneous route. Patients undergoing surgery are at high risk for hemorrhagic complications. The neurosurgeon must consider each patient's situation and individualize the dosing, as well as when, and if, to begin these treatments in the postoperative period.[36]

Many organizations have developed nurse-driven protocols to apply an IPC device or GCS upon admission to the hospital. The protocols provide guidelines for nurses to begin preventative treatment without a specific provider order and within parameters that include contraindications for amputated limbs, burns, or other injuries to the lower extremities. The Centers for Medicare and Medicaid (CMS) have put forth requirements for provider documentation for prophylaxis, as well as when the patient is not a candidate for UFH or LMWH administration. Nurses must also provide documentation on mechanical interventions at prescribed intervals, including when the device is on or off.

Quality-of-Life Considerations

Disturbances in cerebral functioning are a major concern in patients with brain tumors. Members of the healthcare team must recognize that the tumor, treatment interventions, changes in metabolic functions, and psychological and social factors combine to determine the overall impact to quality of life (QOL). Seizures are the first symptom of an intracranial tumor in up to 90% of patients. Older antiepileptic medications are known to decrease cognitive functioning, affect memory, and slow overall cognition. Several tests are available to determine patients' cognitive abilities or impairments. The type of test chosen depends on the goal of the assessment: treatment outcome analysis, patient care, or rehabilitation. The Mini Mental Status Exam (MMSE), verbal fluency, or clock-drawing test (CDT) are among a variety of exams that can test neurocognitive functions and further assist the decision-making process for disease progression and QOL concerns.[21]

A brain tumor diagnosis is a life-changing event. Studies on patients and families have described a loss of stability in their lives after diagnosis. In addition to the diagnosis and coping with the side effects of the treatments, patients with brain tumors cite issues with depression and difficulty thinking and completing activities. Fatigue is a major factor that results from the illness and the patient's compensation for cognitive changes. Headaches; weakness; difficulty reading, writing, and speaking; and visual problems further add to the challenges faced by the patient and their loved ones. An inability to participate in favorite activities is felt by some to be worse than the diagnosis or treatment, leading to a profound sense of loss, including the loss of "self."[26]

Considerable research has been focused on caregivers and caregiver distress associated with the pressures of caring for loved ones with a cancer diagnosis. Many caregivers relate feeling inadequately prepared to cope with the demands of care; however, they report feeling better able to cope when the patient was accepting of their illness and showed appreciation for the work of the caregiver. A caregiver's ability to cope is influenced by a having supportive social network, having early access to information, and knowing that the home healthcare system was supportive when the situation became more difficult. Caregivers often describe a desire for more support to handle the stress of caregiving demands, but also find it difficult to set aside time to access available support systems such as support groups. Support systems are crucial when caregiving demands are the highest, and yet are most difficult to access at these times, due to limited time to attend. Caregivers also report their needs evolve over time. Although initially their needs are fulfilled by "just being there," the desire moves to a need to spend as much time as possible with their loved one, especially at the end of life. Caregivers are unable to or feel uncomfortable in asking for help throughout the disease process.[38]

Once the pathology has been confirmed and the provider/surgeon has delivered the cancer diagnosis to the patient, nurses have the challenge to meet the needs of the patient and family. Some patients or their family members may want to have as much information as possible from the outset; however, others may need time to adjust to the news and will seek information once a treatment plan has been discussed or implemented. The National Brain Tumor Foundation (NBT), the American Brain Tumor Association (ABTA), and the American Cancer Society (ACS) are resources to which the nurse may refer the patient and family for additional information and support.

A growing specialty is palliative care, and many hospitals have inpatient and outpatient palliative care providers; however, most hospitals require an order for a palliative care/end of life consult from the patient's attending provider. Palliative care may be excellent physical and psychological support for the patient and family as they make treatment decisions. The palliative care team supports the patient's decision-making, whether it is to continue aggressive therapies or to move toward more supportive care, such as hospice.

SEIZURES

Seizures are abnormal electrical discharges in the brain. The characteristics of the seizure are dependent on the location of the seizure (or *epileptiform foci*) in the brain. Epilepsy, which is one of the most common neurologic disorders, is defined as more than one seizure that is unprovoked and is caused by anatomic, biochemical, or physiologic changes. The causes of seizures range from idiopathic (unknown cause), cryptogenic (due to a presumed, but poorly defined cause), hypoxic acidosis, or a family history of seizures. Cerebral infections such as bacterial or viral meningitis, brain abscess, or encephalitis may be the source of seizures. In addition, seizures may be related to cerebral abnormalities, such as cerebral trauma with a loss of consciousness, brain tumors, arteriovenous malformations (AVMs), subdural hematoma, or neurofibromatosis. Children may have seizures associated with fever (febrile seizure) or an atypical type of seizure related to chromosomal abnormalities. Later in life, patients with Alzheimer's disease may have seizures as well. Approximately 10% of persons in the United States will have one unprovoked seizure in their lifetime; however, the overall prevalence of epilepsy in the United States is estimated at 6 per 1000 individuals. Up to 38% of children with epilepsy have mental retardation and developmental delays. Depression and mood disorders are found in approximately 20% of patients with epilepsy.[7]

Seizures occur when there is an imbalance in cerebral inhibition and excitation, leading to abnormal electrical activity (firing). Glutamate is one of the most important excitatory neurotransmitters of the CNS; N-methyl-D-aspartate is the receptor for glutamate, and is the target site for some antiepileptic drugs (AEDs). However, approximately 80% of epilepsy cases are the result of an insult to the brain; the exact type of insult is unknown in more than half of the patients afflicted. In the past, it was thought the incidence of seizures was highest in infants, and that the risk decreased over time. New evidence suggests that as the average age is increasing, so is the incidence of seizures and epilepsy. People are living longer, and thus experiencing increasing rates of neurologic illness and disease, particularly neurovascular/cerebrovascular and neurodegenerative diseases. In older persons, the presence of seizure activity should not be considered a diagnosis, but requires a prompt assessment and investigation to identify the underlying cause(s) and diagnosis. The majority of seizure activity in the elderly is the partial onset type, indicating a focal disturbance in brain function that is due to a specific and usually identifiable cause.[20]

Cerebrovascular disease is thought to be the major contributor to seizure onset and epilepsy in the elderly. Up to 4% of patients with stroke will have at least one seizure post-stroke; these seizures may occur early in the recovery period or up to 4 weeks or longer post-stroke, depending on the etiology. Early strokes are often related to a systemic problem (such as a metabolic imbalance), or a focal irritation (such as hemorrhage) on the cortex of the brain. Patients who experience late post-stroke seizures have a higher risk of developing epilepsy; the focal damage to the cerebral cortex is considered to be a pathologic development, as it results in irreversible injury to the brain.[20]

Sudden unexplained death in epilepsy (SUDEP) is defined as a "sudden, nontraumatic, nondrowning death in which no cause can be found in autopsy." The main risk factor for SUDEP is the presence of uncontrolled, generalized, tonic-clonic epilepsy. Measures to prevent SUDEP are not well defined.[7]

Seizure Classification

In 2010, the International League Against Epilepsy (ILAE) revised the classification of seizures to include two main categories: generalized and focal. Generalized seizures include the following subtypes: tonic-clonic, absence, clonic, tonic, atonic, and myoclonic. Generalized seizures begin in one area of the brain, rapidly extend bilaterally, and may involve the whole brain. Focal seizures originate and stay in one area of the brain. Focal seizures may be characterized by one or more subjective symptoms such as an aura or a disturbance in motor, sensory, autonomic, or cognition functions.[12]

The definition of epilepsy includes several symptoms that are associated with the seizure event, or occurred during the pre- or post-ictal phase (ictus meaning the seizure itself–the seizure may be referred to as an ictal event). Some patients experience an aura that occurs at the beginning of the seizure. The aura is a sensation or warning experienced by the person and may be a visual, auditory, or visceral experience; the aura is generally the same experience each time. Persons experiencing an aura may experience flashing lights, a metallic taste, or a foul odor. Prodromal symptoms also occur before a seizure, but these symptoms are usually in the form of depression or headache, and may precede a seizure by hours.[12]

Automatisms are more or less coordinated involuntary movements that occur as a result of stimulation of the autonomic nervous system (ANS) during impaired consciousness during or after seizure activity. The person may exhibit lip smacking or chewing (oral automatisms) or picking at clothing, pacing, or fidgeting (manual automatisms). These involuntary movements are generally associated with temporal lobe seizures, but may occur with other types of seizures as well. Automatisms should not be confused with autonomic symptoms such as pallor, sweating, flushing, piloerection, and pupil dilation.

To fully understand and explain seizure activity, the nurse must have an awareness of other terms and definitions associated with seizures and epilepsy. *Seizure semiology* is the term used to describe signs and symptoms during seizure activity. For example, *clonus* is used to describe spasms where the patient demonstrates continuous rigidity and relaxation. *Tonus* is the degree of tone or contraction evident in the muscle when the muscle is not shortening, as during contraction of the muscle.

Jacksonian march or Jacksonian seizure is noted when there is a spread of abnormal electrical activity from one area of the cerebral cortex to nearby areas of the brain. For example, the patient may start with twitching in the hand or arm, progressing to the whole arm, then to the face, on the same or opposite sides of the body.[12]

Todd's paralysis is a unique, yet confounding symptom of seizure activity that mimics other disease processes, particularly stroke. Todd's paralysis is a temporary condition that follows a partial or generalized seizure. The paralysis may last up to 24 hours before symptoms resolve; however, it is important for the clinician to note what side was involved, as this can be correlated with the epileptic focus on the motor strip of the brain. The effects of Todd's paralysis are thought to be due to neuronal exhaustion.[12]

Partial Seizures

Partial (also called *focal* or *local*) seizures begin in a localized (focal) area of the brain. There are three types of seizures that fall under the umbrella of partial seizures: simple, complex, and complex evolving into secondarily generalized. Simple partial seizures do not affect the person's level of consciousness, and are described by presenting symptoms: motor, sensory, autonomic, or psychic. Motor symptoms may include facial twitching or jerking motions of the hand. Sensory symptoms include sensations such as a metallic or unusual taste in the mouth. Autonomic symptoms may include epigastric discomfort, sweating, vomiting, or other sensations. Psychic symptoms may include hallucinations, illusions, or a sense of *déjà vu*. With a complex partial seizure, consciousness is impaired – the person may "stare off into space," speak nonsensically or not at all, or display automatisms. Partial seizures may deteriorate or evolve into secondarily generalized seizures. Partial seizures are more difficult to control and are likely to require treatment with more than one medication, or with a combination of medications.[7]

Generalized Seizures

Generalized seizures are divided into six categories: absence, myoclonic, clonic, tonic, tonic-clonic, and atonic. Of the generalized seizures, the tonic-clonic type is the most common, and was formerly referred to as a *grand mal seizure*. Tonic-clonic is a more descriptive and accurate depiction of the seizure experienced by the patient. A prodromal phase may precede the tonic-clonic seizure activity by hours or even days. The person may experience or exhibit irritability and tension, and some may have an aura, but others may have no warning at all. The tonic-clonic seizure usually begins with a sudden loss of consciousness, as the electrical discharges spread throughout the brain from the subcortex, thalamus, and the upper brainstem. The sudden and whole body contraction results in a stiffening of the muscles of the body with arms and legs extended in the tonic phase.[13]

Safety is the foremost concern for patients experiencing tonic-clonic seizures, as the onset of seizure activity may result in a fall and bodily injury. As the jaw tightens with the teeth clenched, the tongue or cheek may be injured (bitten). Attempting to place an object between the teeth or in the mouth should not be attempted, as this may cause further injury. In the past, it was thought that a bite block or other device should be placed between the patient's teeth to prevent them from "swallowing their tongue" during seizure activity. This is an intervention that is strongly discouraged, not to mention ineffective and dangerous. The patient should be turned to one side to allow secretions (saliva) to flow out of mouth, and objects should be moved away from the patient to prevent injury during the seizure. In the healthcare setting, padding for side rails of the bed is often standard. Additionally, suction should be operational and positioned at the bedside for immediate access.[25]

A distinctive cry is heard at the outset of the seizure, when air is forced through a contracted larynx with the tonic contraction. The patient may have apnea and appear cyanotic (dusky) during this phase. During this phase, which generally lasts less than 1 minute, the pupils dilate and are nonresponsive to light, and urinary incontinence is common. Bowel incontinence may occur, but is less frequent. The transition to the clonic phase is characterized by violent and rhythmic muscle contractions and hyperventilation, and periods of apnea may occur. During the clonic phase, there may be profuse diaphoresis, facial contortion with eye rolling, excessive salivation, and tachycardia. As the seizure subsides, there is a gradual decrease in the muscle contractions as the involved brain cells fatigue. The patient's extremities become limp, the pupils slowly become responsive to light (but may be unequal in size), and the patient often complains of fatigue, headache, and generalized muscle soreness. It is not uncommon for the patient to sleep for hours in the post-ictal phase. Other symptoms such as temporary aphasia or paralysis may be evident during this time, and up to 24 hours post-event. As dramatic as the tonic-clonic seizure appears, it is generally self-limiting and lasts on average 1 to 3 minutes.[11]

Other types of generalized seizures include absence, myoclonic, clonic, tonic, and atonic. Absence seizures are more common in children and are observed as "staring off into space." Generally, there is no loss of consciousness or postural control, but the patient may slow down or stop an activity during the seizure. Most absence seizures last less than 30 seconds and may be difficult to identify; however, absence seizures may occur up to hundreds of times per day, and the patient may be unaware of the seizures.

Myoclonic seizures are usually sudden symmetrical "jerks" that occur with sudden, brief muscle contractions. Clonic seizures are also symmetrical seizures that affect both sides of the body. Tonic seizures typically cause the entire body to stiffen, but may involve only the arms. Atonic seizures are an abrupt loss of postural muscle tone, also known as a *drop attack*. Atonic seizures are common in children, and last 1 to 2 seconds. Atonic seizures involve a high risk for injury; often children must wear protective headwear (helmet), as there is a very brief loss of consciousness (without post-ictal confusion).[11]

During seizure activity, the nurse's role is to maintain calm (in oneself and in others), maintain patient safety as much as possible, note the time of onset and end (duration), and observe the movements of the patient. If possible, patient activities prior to the event should be noted, as well as any complaints of aura or prodromal symptoms. If the patient is in bed or otherwise covered with a sheet/blanket, the nurse should remove the covering in order to be able to visualize the patient from "head-to-toe." The seizure duration, movements of the extremities and face, and any other distinguishing features (i.e., automatisms) should be communicated to the provider and documented in the patient record. The semiology of the seizure and patient assessment are key in the diagnosis of the seizure focus. The nurse should be aware of the differential diagnoses associated with seizures, as they may mimic other disease processes (i.e., the aforementioned Todd's paralysis). Among the differential diagnoses considered with seizure presentation are syncope (loss of consciousness and motor tone) or panic attacks (may have dizziness and feelings of fear or impending doom). In a transient ischemic attack (TIA), the clinical symptoms are dependent on the area of the brain affected (i.e., decreased perfusion), resulting in temporary weakness, alterations in speech, and numbness. The hallmark of a TIA is symptoms last for 24 hours or less (similar to Todd's paralysis) and a normal EEG.

Psychogenic Nonepileptic Seizures

Psychogenic nonepileptic seizures (PNES) often include a psychological component. Research has demonstrated that the incidence of PNES is higher in women than in men and is often correlated with a history of abuse (which is found in up to 86% of patients with PNES versus the less than 48% of patients with epilepsy). Of note, up to 20% of patients with PNES also have medically intractable seizures. These seizures have been referred to as *pseudoseizures*, but this connotation suggests that the seizures are fake; thus, the patients are presumed to be malingerers or using seizure activity for a secondary gain or attention. The term *pseudoseizure* is strongly discouraged, and this condition should be referred to as PNES. Clinical presentation may vary depending on the patient and patient's age, and the usual differential diagnoses should be considered as well. Psychological presentation also varies by patient, patient age, and history; however, head shaking, crying, pelvic thrusting, and asynchronized convulsions may be present. Treatment of the patient with PNES includes epilepsy monitoring, such as in a designated epilepsy monitoring unit, whereby their seizure activity can be correlated with video EEG (the gold standard of PNES diagnosis). Consultation with an epileptologist, as well as a psychologist, is crucial to the diagnosis and treatment of these challenging patients.[11]

Status Epilepticus

Status epilepticus (SE) is a neurologic emergency that entails high morbidity and mortality. The incidence of SE in the United States is 18 to 41 per 100,000 individuals, and there is presumed to be a higher rate among poorer populations. In approximately half of SE cases, the patient has no history of epilepsy. The main precipitating factor in children is some type of infection; in adults the main causes are stroke, hypoxia, alcohol intoxication/drug withdrawal, or a metabolic derangement. In patients with epilepsy, the onset of SE is more often as a result of drug withdrawal related to noncompliance with their AEDs. Males are affected at a higher rate than females, given the lower seizure threshold in men. Adults over age 60 are at highest risk, with an incidence of 86 per 100,000 individuals per year.[30]

Several definitions of SE have been proposed, and the ILAE have accepted that SE is "a seizure that persists for sufficient length of time or repeated frequently enough that recovery between attacks does not occur."[30] Researchers have attempted to place a time frame on seizure duration to define SE; the most commonly accepted time frame is 30 minutes, which is based on animal studies years ago that demonstrated significant brain damage after 30 minutes of seizure activity, even with blood pressure, temperature, and respiratory controls. Studies have shown that after 5 minutes, spontaneous cessation of generalized seizures is unlikely. It is thought that SE is a result of a breakdown of the mechanisms that would usually cause an isolated seizure to stop. The mechanisms of SE are thought to be related to a constant activation of the hippocampus, loss of gamma-aminobutyric acid (GABA)-mediated inhibitory synaptic transmission in the hippocampus, and the presence of glutaminergic excitatory synaptic transmission, which is important for maintaining the SE state.[30]

Physiologic and systemic changes brought about by SE are related to a massive release of catecholamines in the early stage, which causes tachycardia, cardiac arrhythmias, high pulmonary and left atrial pressures, and in some cases, pulmonary edema. Metabolic acidosis occurs as a result of lactic acidosis, respiratory failure, and elevated blood glucose. The patient's white blood cell (WBC) count rises with accompanying fever, which may be mistaken for an infectious process. After the initial catecholamine "rush," seizure activity continues for up to 30 minutes and the blood pressure (BP) decreases. After 2 hours of continuous seizure activity, the BP may be significantly low, and the patient may have low blood glucose and renal failure due to rhabdomyolysis and myoglobinuria. In the early stages of SE, which involves high pulmonary and blood pressures, there is an increase in cerebral blood flow, which in turn causes increased ICP. Cerebral edema may be present in later stages when compensatory mechanisms fail.[30]

Of note, not all patients in SE will have outward signs and symptoms of seizures. Nonconvulsive status epilepticus (NCSE) is a recognized condition in which the patient may not exhibit outward signs of seizure activity, or the seizure activity may be so subtle as to be missed; and in fact, may be missed for long periods, depending on other signs and symptoms. For example, a post-stroke patient who has an altered level of consciousness and a "wax and wane" neurologic assessment or mental status may present as sleepy, lethargic, confused, or slow to respond. With further examination and EEG testing, the presence of seizure activity may be diagnosed (Fig. 15.3). NCSE is characterized by prolonged seizure activity that is evident as epileptiform discharges on EEG. Refractory SE is a form of SE that cannot

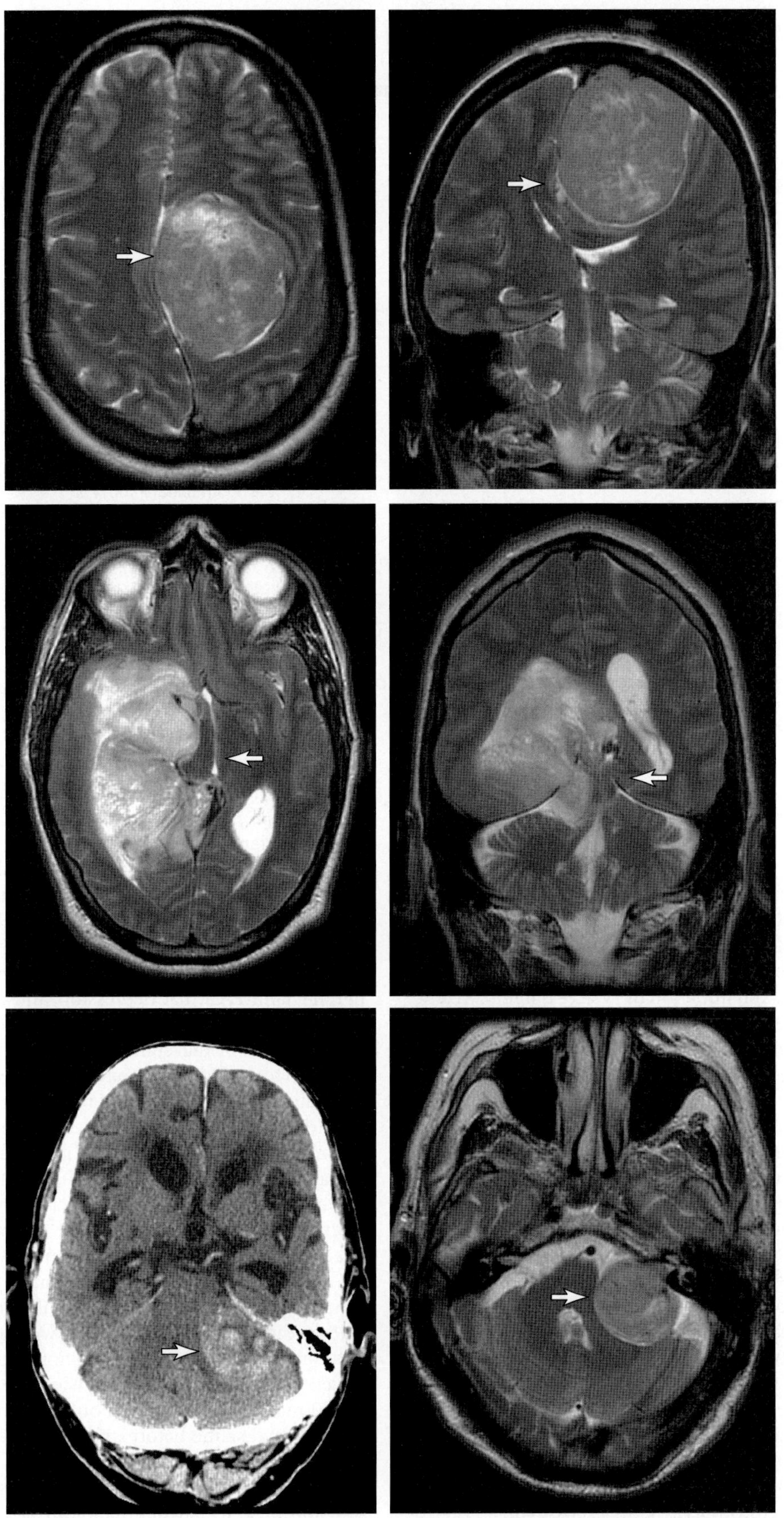

FIG. 15.3 Diagnostic imaging of brain tumors *(arrows)*.

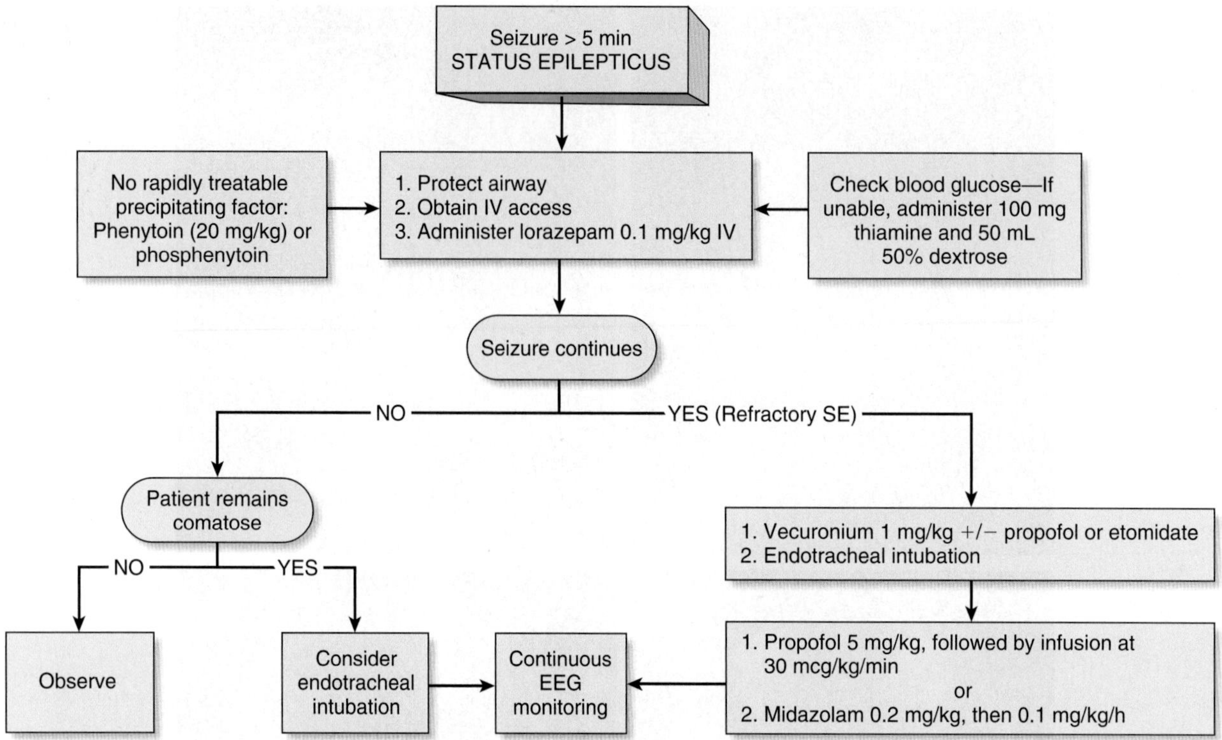

FIG. 15.4 Treatment algorithm for patient in status epilepticus.

be terminated with a first-line medication (such as benzodiazepines) or a second-line medication (phenytoin, valproic acid, levetiracetam, or phenobarbital). Nearly half of patients with SE will progress to refractory SE, which carries a nearly 40% mortality rate.[5]

Management of SE is aimed at stopping the SE, preventing seizure recurrence, investigating and managing the cause(s), and preventing complications (Fig. 15.4). The nurse should anticipate orders for toxin screening (blood and urine), blood counts and electrolytes, and initiation of IV access if not already present. Thiamine 100 mg IV is often given prophylactically for prevention of Wernicke's encephalopathy in susceptible patients. Arterial blood gas assessment should be completed to ensure adequate oxygenation; many patients may require intubation and mechanical ventilation for airway protection and ventilatory support. Once the patient is stabilized, a CT scan may be obtained to rule out an infectious process. Lumbar puncture may also be performed to aid in diagnosis and treatment, based on any findings.

Antiepileptic Medications

Medications to treat seizures and epilepsy have progressed rapidly in the past few years. Many of the newer medications do not require regular laboratory testing to ascertain therapeutic levels; most are at therapeutic levels after the first dose. The decision-making process of how and when to initiate pharmacologic support depends on seizure recurrence (often an isolated seizure/first seizure is not treated). Patients with abnormal tests (imaging or EEG) or a family history of seizures are initiated on antiepileptic medications as soon as possible.

Luminal sodium (phenobarbital) – not to be confused with pentobarbital (Nembutal) – is one of the oldest AEDs, and may be administered in a single or divided dose of 60–250 mg/day (oral) or 100–300 mg/day (IV). This medication is used in partial and generalized seizures. Patients may experience drowsiness initially, but this usually passes with tolerance. Children may experience hyperactivity. Patients may have difficulties with memory and cognition, and depression may be exacerbated in adults. Phenobarbital should not be stopped abruptly. High-dose IV administration of phenobarbital is sedating; therefore, caution should be taken to protect the patient's airway. The medication is diluted in polyethylene glycol, which may result in renal failure, cardiac depression, and seizures. Due to the side effects and the nature of phenobarbital, it is commonly used after other benzodiazepines and phenytoin have failed.[30]

Phenytoin (Dilantin) may be administered for partial and generalized seizures via the IV route. Phenytoin shows effectiveness for the treatment of SE. Phenytoin is given in doses of 300–600 mg/day; a loading dose of 1 g IV may be given to achieve a therapeutic level (10–20 mcg/mL) more rapidly. As phenytoin has an affinity for protein binding, monitoring free levels of phenytoin is the preferred method of laboratory monitoring. Side effects of phenytoin administration include: gingival hyperplasia, rash, nausea and vomiting, lethargy, nystagmus, and ataxia. IV phenytoin administration should not exceed 50 mg/min. The medication cannot be given with any other medications, and can only be given with 0.9% normal saline solution. Elderly patients' dosage must be given via a slow bolus infusion rate of 20–30 mg/min. The nurse should flush the IV line thoroughly with normal saline before and after phenytoin administration to avoid the development of precipitate in the IV line. "Purple glove syndrome" (PGS) is a rare complication of IV phenytoin administration resulting in purple discoloration, pain, and edema distal to the IV infusion site. The mechanisms of PGS are not clear, but may be related to higher than recommended doses, drug-induced vasculitis, or extravasation. Conservative treatment is usually sufficient to relieve the symptoms, but nurses should monitor for possible compartment syndrome as an extreme occurrence related to PGS.[9]

Fosphenytoin (Cerebyx) is often given as the loading bolus dose versus phenytoin, as fosphenytoin may be administered at a faster rate, but the clinician should be aware of the risks of arrhythmias and hypotension, which are the same as for phenytoin. Both medications are administered by weight-based dosing. Fosphenytoin is a phenytoin prodrug, and when administered IV, the medication is completely converted to phenytoin within 15 minutes.

Lorazepam (Ativan) administered IV has been favored as the first-line medication, with a rapid onset of action, a 2 to 3 hour half-life, and a long duration of action. Studies have shown lorazepam to stop seizures in up to 80% of cases. The usual dosing is 4–8 mg, and the anticonvulsant effects may last up to 12 hours. Doses may be repeated once, but tolerance for the medication develops quickly, and repeated doses may be much less effective. Therefore, lorazepam is not useful for long-term treatment. Caution should be taken, as lorazepam can cause a sudden drop in BP or severe respiratory suppression. Recent studies, such as the Rapid Anticonvulsant Medications Prior to Arrival Trial (RAMPART) favored intramuscular midazolam as the initial medication of choice as an alternative to IV lorazepam. Studies in the United States have shown that neurologists treating SE preferred lorazepam as the first-line medication, followed by fosphenytoin or phenytoin if patients do not respond, proceeding next to phenobarbital (luminal sodium). Benzodiazepines are the most effective AEDs for the treatment of SE, and diazepam (Valium) and midazolam (Versed) are frequently used for their ability to boost GABA and barbiturate receptor sites.

Levetiracetam (Keppra), which has been approved since 1999, is a first-line medication for the treatment of seizures. The medication is used to treat several types of seizures in children, adolescents, and adults, including partial-onset seizure, myoclonic seizures, and primarily generalized tonic-clonic seizures. In addition, levetiracetam has been used "off label" for the treatment of SE, as well as nonepileptic conditions such as neuropathic pain, headaches, movement disorders, and in some cases, for psychiatric conditions. The mechanism of action is thought to be binding to specific synaptic vesicle proteins on synaptic vesicles that occur throughout the CNS and on endocrine cells. The medication is eliminated through the kidneys (up to 66% is excreted unchanged in the urine); renal clearance is directly proportional to the patient's creatinine clearance. The elimination and half-life of the medication will be greatly prolonged in patients with impaired renal function or severe renal insufficiency. A key feature of levetiracetam is that it is not metabolized through the liver, and therefore avoids all pharmacokinetic drug-drug interactions.[11]

Anesthetic agents (i.e., midazolam and propofol) are used when SE is refractory to other medications. Midazolam has a short half-life, but as the duration of treatment increases, the half-life also increases. However, prolonged administration of midazolam is limited by the decrease in response to the drug over time. Propofol also has a short half-life, but should be administered with caution if infusing longer than 48 hours, due to the risk of *propofol infusion syndrome.* Propofol infusion syndrome presents with rhabdomyolysis, cardiac and renal failure, metabolic acidosis, and high serum triglyceride levels; the half-life is sustained, as the medication has an affinity for adipose tissue. Continuous EEG monitoring is required when using anesthetic agents in the treatment of SE, with a goal of electrographic seizure suppression. Often the goal is to attain an electrographic burst suppression pattern of 1–2 s bursts of cerebral activity within 10 s intervals of suppression. The provider may order this as a titration for the AEDs and anesthesia agents to achieve a level of "8 out of 10 suppressed".[5] Propofol should not be administered if the patient has an allergy to eggs, egg products, soy products, or soybeans. The medication is not recommended for use in obstetric patients, as it crosses the placental barrier and may cause neonatal respiratory depression; propofol also crosses into breast milk and should be avoided in nursing mothers, as the effects on the infant are unknown. Continuous infusions of propofol should not be administered unless the nurse has been specifically educated in the care of critically ill patients, airway management, and cardiovascular support.

Nursing Management

Nursing management of the patient with seizures and epilepsy requires a basic knowledge of types of seizures, clinical signs and symptoms of convulsive and nonconvulsive seizure types, and AEDs. Patients hospitalized for seizures require a comprehensive educational program to help them understand and manage their disease. Family members must be included in the education in order for them to be able to provide first aid when seizures occur outside of the healthcare facility. Patient/family teaching must include the importance of taking AEDs as prescribed and the risks of nonadherence to medication routines. Side effects of AEDs may be disturbing to the patient or interfere with body image and lifestyle, and are often a reason for noncompliance with medication regimens. For example, women of childbearing age must understand the interaction of AEDs with oral contraceptives; estrogen may increase the metabolism of the AED, thus lowering the AED level by as much as 50% and increasing the risk of breakthrough seizures.[12]

MENINGITIS

Meningitis is a life-threatening CNS infection, and in order to improve outcomes, early and accurate diagnosis and treatment are essential. Meningitis is an inflammation of the meninges surrounding the brain and spinal cord, and is usually the result of a bacterial or viral infection, but may also be caused by a fungus or parasite. Access to the brain and spinal cord by the infectious agent is usually via the blood-borne route, from an adjacent infection, or from pneumonia. Additional causes of meningitis may be related to neurosurgical procedures, penetrating head injuries, or other injuries, procedures, or congenital defects that create a pathway for bacteria or viruses to the CNS.

Bacterial Meningitis

Acute bacterial meningitis is an infectious, life-threatening disease that causes significant morbidity and mortality; at greatest risk are infants (< 2 months) and the elderly (Fig. 15.5). An important consideration for nurses caring for patients with bacterial meningitis is contagious disease prevention with appropriate isolation precautions to prevent the spread of this illness. Appropriate isolation is determined by the stage of the disease process. In the acute phase, the infection may be spread via droplets from the respiratory tract and secretions from the nasopharynx. Placing the patient in respiratory isolation until cultures are negative should protect staff, visitors, and other patients. This

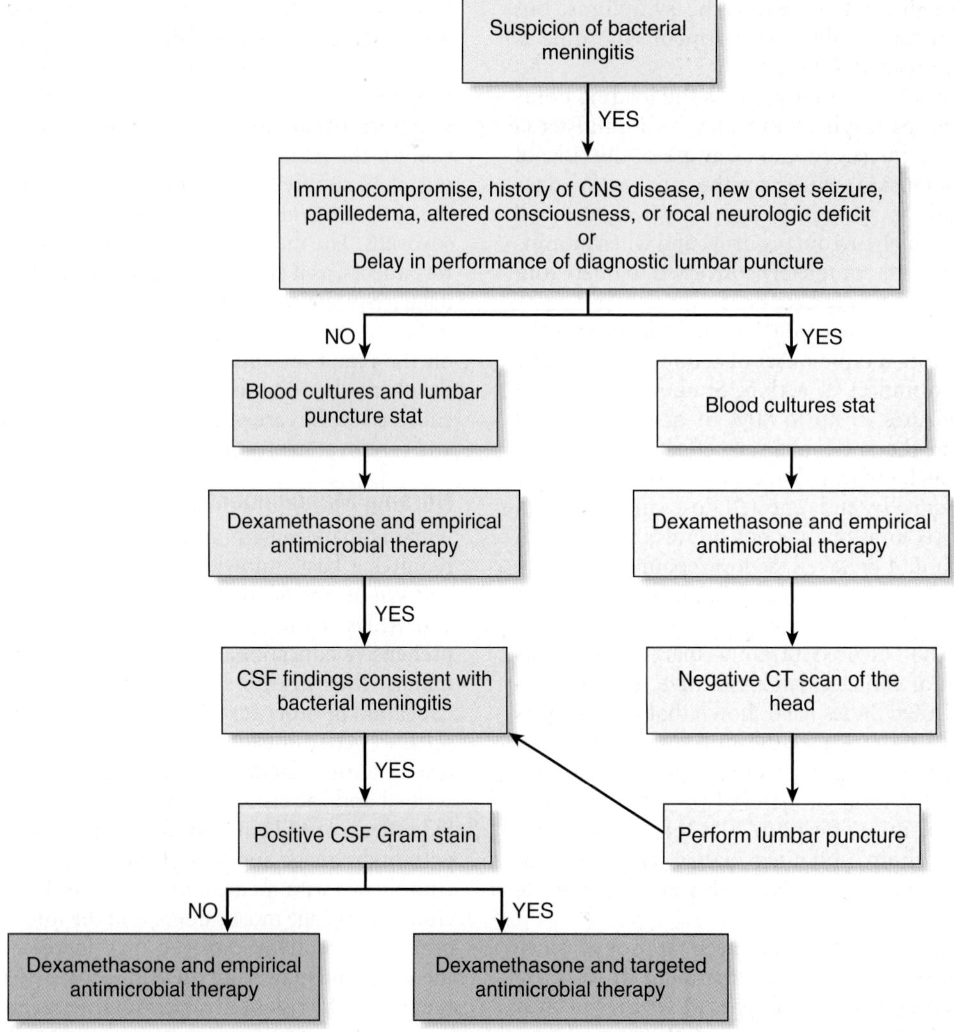

FIG. 15.5 Management algorithm for suspected bacterial meningitis. *CNS,* Central nervous system; *CSF,* cerebrospinal fluid; *CT,* computed tomography. (From Tunkel, A. R., Hartman, B. J., Kaplan, S. L., Kaufman, B. A., et al. (2004). Practice guidelines for the management of bacterial meningitis. *Clin Infect Dis, 39*(9), 1267-1284, doi:10.1086/425368.)

pyogenic infection affects the pia-arachnoid layers and SASs of the brain. Early diagnosis and treatment with antibiotics are crucial for saving lives; however, the emergence of multi-resistant strains of bacteria has made treatment a greater challenge.

Meningitis often presents with the classic symptoms of altered mental status, neck stiffness (nuchal rigidity), fever, and headache. Studies have shown that all classic symptoms were present in less than half of patients; the majority of patients presented with at least two of the four symptoms. Patients may also complain of photophobia (sensitivity to light) due to the presence of meningeal irritation. Kernig's sign and Brudzinski's sign are indicators of meningeal irritation associated with meningitis. Testing for the presence of Kernig's sign is performed with the patient lying supine; the examiner flexes the upper leg at the hip to a 90-degree angle, then attempts to extend the knee (Fig. 15.6). The presence of meningeal irritation will be evidenced by pain and spasm in the hamstring muscles and lower back with the knee extension. Passive flexion of the neck and head (toward the chest) causes a spontaneous and involuntary flexion of both hips and knees, indicating a positive Brudzinski's sign and meningeal irritation. Of note, both of these signs are meaningful when present; however, the absence of one or both signs does not indicate the absence of meningitis.[28] It is important for the provider to perform more than one diagnostic test, obtain a thorough patient medical history, and conduct a physical assessment and neurologic exam to determine the diagnosis. Information regarding the patient's recent travel, vaccination status, risk factors for HIV or other sexually transmitted diseases (STDs), and use of illicit drugs or immunosuppressive medications must be obtained. Consideration for the patient's location (i.e., local presence of microorganisms that may cause CNS infections, such as *Rickettsia*, *Trypanosome cruzi*, or *Leptospira* species) should be included in the patient's history. Often, patients with bacterial meningitis will have an illness that predisposes them to bacterial meningitis. For example, sinus infection, ear infection, lung infection, or septic shock may be seen prior to diagnosis in nearly half of patients with bacterial meningitis. Meningococcal patients with septic shock may not be diagnosed quickly, as the changes in mental status may be attributed to the shock state. Increased ICP may be present as a result of bacterial activity, which can cause purulent exudate, cerebral edema, hydrocephalus,

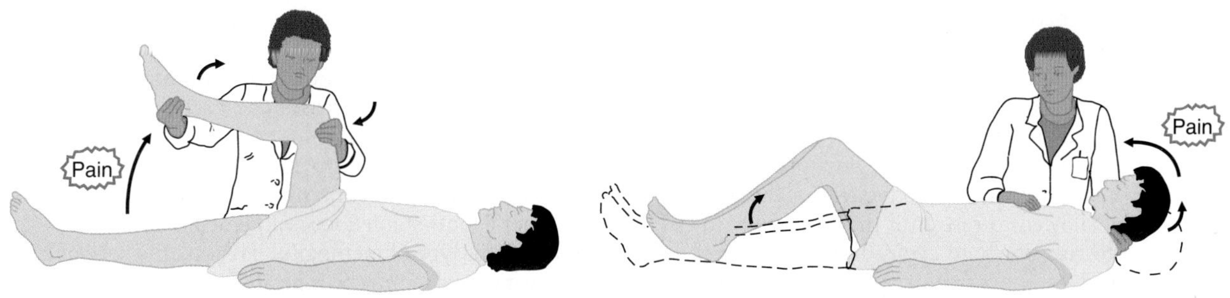

FIG. 15.6 Clinical assessment for neck pain in meningitis. (From Black, J. M., Hawks, J. H. (2009). *Medical-surgical nursing: clinical management for positive outcomes* (8th ed.). St Louis: Saunders.)

TABLE 15.5 Cerebrospinal Fluid Values Diagnostic for Meningitis

Parameter	Normal CSF	Bacterial Meningitis	Viral Meningitis	Fungal Meningitis
Opening pressure (mm H_2O)	100–180	200–500	≤ 250	> 200
Leukocyte count (white blood cells/mm^3)	0–5	Increased 1000–5000	Increased 50–1000	Increased >20
Neutrophils (%)	0	≥ 80	< 40	
Protein (mg/dL)	18–45	Elevated 100–500	Elevated <200	Elevated >45
Glucose (mg/dL)	45–80; 0.6 times blood glucose level	5–40; <0.3 times blood glucose level	> 45	< 40

CSF, Cerebrospinal fluid.
From Reference 44.

vomiting, and altered mental status. If neurologic symptoms are not treated aggressively and promptly, cerebral herniation is possible.[44]

Haemophilus influenzae and *Streptococcus pneumoniae* are gram-negative rod organisms that are primarily linked to the respiratory tract; these organisms, along with *Enterobacteriaceae* (which are associated with the enteric tract and the nasopharynx) are the main causes of bacterial meningitis. Once these bacteria attach to mucous membranes through the secretion of immunoglobin A (IgA) protease, they enter the bloodstream. Bacteria that are able to survive in the blood circulation despite attempts by neutrophils and phagocytosis to inactivate them enter the CSF system through the choroid plexus of the lateral ventricles, as well as other areas of the brain where the BBB has been compromised. There is little change in the cerebral cortex in the early stages of infection, other than inflammation. Diffuse degenerative changes may be evident in subacute cases, with associated tissue necrosis and glial propagation. Side effects of the infection may be related to scar tissue formation and fibrotic changes in the arachnoid layer; in the SAS, effusions and adhesions can interfere with normal CSF circulation, resulting in hydrocephalus. The duration of meningitis depends on how quickly treatment is started, the degree of infection present, and whether the infection can be quickly eliminated. Patient outcomes range from complete recovery to death.

Lumbar puncture (LP) may be one of the first tests performed in order to obtain CSF for diagnostic studies. The signs and symptoms of meningitis may mimic intracranial, space-occupying lesions; therefore, it is essential to determine if CT or other brain imaging should be completed prior to performing the LP. The presence of a space-occupying lesion versus an infectious process may place the patient at risk for herniation related to the shift in CSF when the LP is performed (Table 15.5).

Obtaining a CSF sample facilitates establishing a diagnosis of bacterial meningitis by identifying the microorganism and antibiotic susceptibility. Findings consistent with bacterial meningitis include CSF white count greater than 100 cells per μL and an elevated protein level. Gram staining provides a well-validated method to assess the presence of bacteria, and Gram stain of cultured CSF is the primary mechanism for diagnosis prior to the start of treatment.[6] In bacterial meningitis, the characteristic abnormalities that are present in addition to the elevated white count include: increased opening pressure with the LP, high protein count and concentration, polymorphonuclear leukocytic pleocytosis, and a decreased glucose concentration.

Preparing the patient for LP includes proper positioning, either lying on the side with head and knees flexed, or sitting up and using a table or similar item for the patient to lean on with the spine in a curved position. These positions provide widening of the spinal vertebrae and access to the lumbar intervertebral space at level L3-4/L4-5 (below the terminus of the spinal cord) for insertion of the needle. Pain or sedation medication may be administered for patient comfort pre- and post-procedure, but is not routinely needed. Once the intervertebral space is accessed, the nurse may be asked to ease the flexion of the legs in order to more accurately measure CSF pressure (sharply flexed legs may increase pressure on the intra-abdominal cavity, thus artificially increasing pressure). Normal pressure in adults (including the elderly) is between 10 and 20 cm; above 25 cm is considered pathologic. In children, values up to 28 cm are considered to be in the normal range. Post-procedure pain or some discomfort at the puncture site is normal, but more severe pain should be immediately investigated to rule out the presence of hematoma.

Some patients experience "shooting" or radicular pains in the legs during the procedure, which indicates the needle may be in a lateral position and should be readjusted by the practitioner. Radicular pain persisting after the procedure is rare.[4]

In the past, the patient was encouraged to lie flat following the procedure to avoid post-procedure low-pressure headache, but evidence suggests there is no benefit for this practice. Patients should be allowed to rest until they feel ready to rise, then encouraged to rise slowly to avoid dizziness and risk for falls. As CSF is produced at a rate of approximately 25 mL/h post-procedure, low-pressure headaches generally resolve quickly. Occasionally, the patient may experience a persistent low-pressure headache due to a spinal fluid leak that is at the same rate, or slightly higher than, the rate of CSF hourly replacement. In addition to a dull pain that involves the occipital region or the whole brain area, the patient may experience photophobia, nuchal rigidity, tinnitus, nausea, or hyperacusis (increased sensitivity to sound). The headache is worsened with the Valsalva maneuver or other activities that increase cranial pressure. Patients should remain flat and possibly in a slightly head-down position if tolerated; a small fluid bolus (500 mL) may be administered (large amounts of fluids have not been demonstrated to be effective). Additionally, caffeinated drinks and oral caffeine (300 mg) may provide relief due to caffeine's cerebral vasoconstrictive qualities.[4] A persistent headache may occur within 5 days post-procedure, and with supportive treatment, the headache generally resolves in approximately 1 week. For unresolved headache, a blood patch may be performed to relieve the headache quickly; resolution of headache generally occurs in less than 48 hours.

Once the meningitis diagnosis is confirmed, treatment can be started and directed to the disease-causing organism. *Streptococcus pneumonia* (pneumococcal meningitis) can be challenging to treat due to the rise of strains that are less susceptible to penicillin. Penicillin resistance is higher in some areas of the United States than others, but the rate is even higher in several other countries. Penicillin resistance is an indicator that there is decreased susceptibility to other antibiotics, thus leading to treatment failures. Where resistance to cephalosporins exists, empirical therapy should include vancomycin in combination with either ceftriaxone or cefotaxime, depending on the results of the susceptibility testing. Pneumococcal meningitis rates have decreased with the heptavalent pneumococcal conjugate vaccine; however, the number of cases that are caused by serotypes and resistant strains not covered by the vaccine have increased.

Neisseria meningitides and *Listeria monocytogenes* are treated with penicillin G, amoxicillin, or ampicillin. As with the pneumococcal strains, there is a reduced susceptibility to penicillin in many countries, leading to an increased risk of neurologic deficits or death in children with meningococcal meningitis. As a result, patients should be empirically treated with a third-generation cephalosporin (i.e., ceftriaxone or cefotaxime) until susceptibility testing is completed. Meningitis caused by group B streptococci is also treated with the aforementioned medications, in combination with an aminoglycoside. Alternatives to this therapy would be third-generation cephalosporins and vancomycin.[6]

The standard treatment for *H. influenzae* is third-generation cephalosporins, since the development of chloramphenicol-resistant and β-lactamase-producing resistant strains. These multidrug-resistant aerobic gram-negative bacilli are very concerning, especially among patients with healthcare-associated bacterial meningitis, as this microorganism is resistant to third- and fourth-generation cephalosporins and carbapenems, which significantly decreases the array of antibiotic options available for treatment.

Staphylococcus aureus meningitis occurs primarily after the placement of CSF shunts or other neurosurgical procedures. In general, anti-staphylococcal penicillins are more effective in treating this type of meningitis. Treating the patient empirically with vancomycin may be indicated until susceptibility testing is complete, but consideration should be given to the prevalence of methicillin-resistant *S. aureus*.[6]

Viral Meningitis

Viral meningitis is more common and less severe than bacterial meningitis, and is usually self-limiting. Viral meningitis is also referred to as *acute aseptic meningitis,* or *acute benign lymphocytic meningitis.* Aseptic meningitis results in a meningeal irritation, but no specific bacterial organism is identified. Enteroviruses (poliovirus, coxsackievirus, and echovirus) account for more than 80% of viral infections of the CNS. Multiple viruses are responsible for CNS infections including: arboviruses, herpesviruses, mumps, varicella-zoster, influenza, cytomegalovirus (CMV), Epstein-Barr virus (EBV), and West Nile virus (WNV). In the majority of viral meningitis cases, a specific organism cannot be identified as the causative agent. All ages may be affected, although children are the most susceptible to viral meningitis, and there exists a seasonal component to these infections; for example, arthropod-borne infections are more often seen in the summer or early fall.[44]

Although similarities exist between diagnosing bacterial and viral meningitis, presentation differs, as viral meningitis does not include altered level of consciousness or new-onset seizures. Viral meningitis begins with a headache, nuchal rigidity, low-grade fever, malaise, photophobia, and signs and symptoms of an upper respiratory viral infection. As with bacterial meningitis, a thorough health history is important–often the patient's pre-illness history will include a recent systemic viral infection. Diagnostic findings include clear CSF and negative cultures for bacteria, elevated WBC count with a majority of mononuclear cells, glucose within the normal range, and protein levels and a polymerase chain reaction (PCR) identifying enteroviruses (the main cause of aseptic meningitis cases) in the CSF.

Treatment of viral meningitis is based on the patient's symptoms and focuses on providing supportive care. Patients with severe pain or excessive vomiting may be hospitalized to better manage their symptoms, but mild cases are often well managed outside of the hospital setting. Supportive care may include bedrest with the head of bed elevated 30 degrees, fever management, a dark and quiet environment, analgesics for pain control, electrolyte monitoring, and fluid management. As with any CNS-affecting disease, close monitoring and accurate neurologic assessments are important, including monitoring for seizure activity and maintaining patient safety.[3]

ENCEPHALITIS

Encephalitis is an inflammation of the parenchyma, the functional brain tissue, versus the covering of the brain, as in bacterial and viral meningitis. The most common form of encephalitis is viral; however, encephalitis may be due to bacteria, fungi, or parasites. Although there are several specific causes of viral encephalitis, only a few are seen with any regularity in the United States. The same viruses that cause viral meningitis are the causative agents in viral encephalitis: enteroviruses (echovirus, poliovirus, and coxsackievirus), adenovirus, influenza-A, herpes simplex virus (HSV) Types 1 and 2, EBV, varicella-zoster, CMV, rabies, and arboviruses (Fig. 15.7). Arboviruses, such as the St. Louis equine encephalitis, WNV, or Western or Eastern equine encephalitis types, are transmitted by infected animals, ticks, or mosquitos. The time of year/seasons, geographic locations, and prevalence of local disease can assist the clinician in diagnosing and identifying the cause of encephalitis. Other nonviral toxic substances may cause encephalitis, such as arsenic, carbon monoxide, or lead.

The pathophysiology of encephalitis results in neurologic deficits related to neuronal cell damage as the virus enters the CNS. For example, HSV has a propensity to lodge in the temporal lobe. The presenting signs and symptoms are the same as for bacterial meningitis; patients who present with fever and an altered level of consciousness (ALOC) with or without a focal neurologic deficit should be worked up for encephalitis. Alterations in levels of consciousness may range from a short attention span to agitation/restlessness, disorientation, lethargy/drowsiness, and coma. Since encephalitis affects the brain tissues, the clinical symptoms seen will depend on the location of the inflammation in the brain, and can present in a wide variety from generalized seizures to aphasia, motor deficits (hemiparesis or paralysis), ataxia, nystagmus, facial weakness, and ocular paralysis.[44] Empirical treatment with acyclovir is recommended for suspected encephalitis or for patients presenting with symptoms including fever, ALOC, headache, and focal neurologic deficits.

Herpes Simplex Encephalitis

Herpes simplex encephalitis (HSE) is the most common, yet one of the more severe, life-threatening illnesses that results in an inflammation of the brain parenchyma. Two type of HSE exist: Type 1, which is the cause of the common "cold sore" and is dormant in most people; and Type 2, which is a sexually transmitted form and responsible for genital disease. Nearly all HSE infections are Type 1 (HSE-1), and although the exact mechanism that triggers the infection is unknown, infectious processes, fever, or emotional stress are thought to play a role in the development of HSE encephalitis.

Signs and symptoms are dependent on the area of the brain affected; however, HSE tends to migrate to the frontal and temporal lobes. In addition to the signs and symptoms common among all forms of meningitis/encephalitis, patients with HSE may exhibit bizarre behavior, memory loss, personality changes, seizures, or coma. Temporal lobe-generated deficits may be evident in the form of hallucinations involving taste and smell, anosmia, temporal lobe seizures, or aphasia. Hemorrhage and cerebral edema may cause increased ICP.[10]

In the early stages of HSE a definitive diagnosis may be difficult to establish. Unfortunately for the patient, this may result in lasting neurologic deficits, personality changes, seizures, post-infectious encephalomyelitis, or death. A mortality rate of up to 70% was associated with HSE prior to the use of acyclovir; this antiviral medication has positively impacted patient survival, and the mortality rate has declined to approximately 30%. Acyclovir (Zovirax) 10 mg/kg is given IV every 8 hours for 2 to 3 weeks. Other medications that may be used in the treatment of HSE include: dexamethasone (Decadron) for cerebral edema, administered as a starting bolus dose, then tapered; a proton-pump inhibitor (PPI) or an H2 blocker administered prophylactically for the prevention of stress ulcers and the gastric irritation associated with steroid use; a diuretic (furosemide, mannitol) for diuresis; acetaminophen for fever management; and AEDs (phenytoin, levetiracetam) for seizure prevention or control. Nurses should maintain routine supportive care for the critically ill patient and employ strategies for the prevention of hospital-acquired infections or complications such as catheter-associated urinary tract infections (CAUTI),

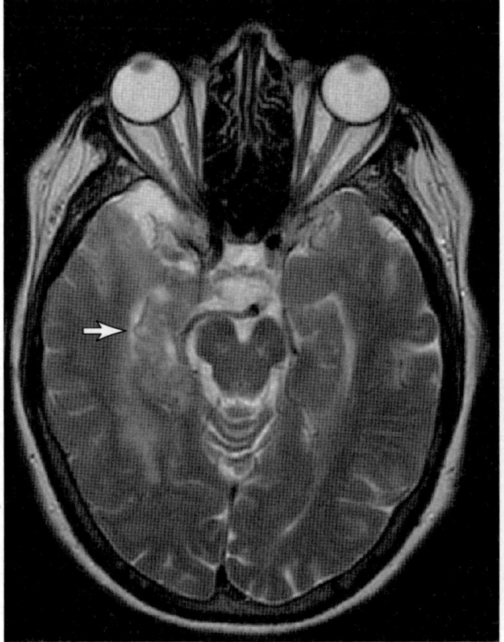

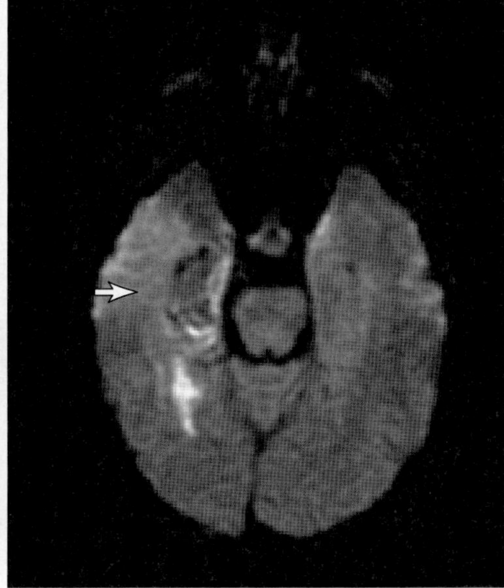

FIG. 15.7 MRI T_2 and diffusion-weighted images of herpes simplex encephalitis in the medial aspect of the right temporal lobe *(arrows)*.

hospital-acquired pressure ulcers (HAPU), central line-associated bloodstream infection (CLABSI), or sepsis.[3]

Anti-N-Methyl-D-Aspartate Receptor Antibody Encephalitis

Anti-N-methyl-D-aspartate receptor antibody encephalitis (anti-NMDAR encephalitis) has garnered attention in recent years as patients have come forward with their stories of illness and recovery. Additionally, providers and researchers have increased research and focus on this disease. Anti-NMDAR encephalitis is considered a limbic encephalitis. Typically, the onset of disease begins with a nonspecific fever, diarrhea, headache, or upper respiratory symptoms, followed by neurologic and psychiatric symptoms that progress in two stages.

Initial symptoms may be seen between 1 to 21 days after the prodromal symptoms occur. Nearly all patients present with psychiatric symptoms and seizures that are usually generalized or complex-partial. In the early stage, the patient may have amnesia, confusion, short-term memory loss, bizarre behavior, agitation, depression, paranoid thinking, and visual or auditory hallucinations. In the later stages, the patient may exhibit a decreased level of consciousness, lethargy, seizures, hypoventilation, autonomic instability, Parkinsonian rigidity, myoclonus, and other movement disorders. Patients are often admitted to a critical care unit for central hypotension and autonomic instability for respiratory support that may persist from 2 weeks to over 10 months.

This particular disorder is found primarily in women with an average age of 22 years, but may be seen in the elderly as well. Over half of these patients are found to have an ovarian teratoma, and removal of the tumor can be curative. The neuropsychiatric symptoms reverse within a few weeks after the tumor is removed, and IVIg or IV steroids are used as adjunctive therapy. Immune suppression is the main treatment for addressing the underlying autoimmune process (regardless of tumor presence). Treatment with IV steroids and either plasma exchange or IVIg should be implemented. For patients who are nonresponsive to these treatments, or whose condition deteriorates or relapses, the addition of rituximab, cyclophosphamide, or both is indicated. Early immunotherapy has been shown to promote better rates of recovery with fewer relapses; however, recovery is a slow process, due to the limitations of current treatment options to maintain control of the immune response within the CNS.

Anti-NMDAR encephalitis is a rare phenomenon, and although the likelihood is low for a critical care nurse to care for these challenging patients, awareness of the disease is essential. Research is increasing and more cases of this complicated, life-threatening disease process are more readily identified.[29]

OTHER NEUROLOGIC DISEASES

Patients with chronic neurologic diseases such as multiple sclerosis (MS), myasthenia gravis (MG), Parkinson's disease, and amyotrophic lateral sclerosis (ALS or "Lou Gehrig's disease") may be admitted to a critical care unit as a result of an exacerbation of their chronic disease process, or another illness or injury in which the chronic disease must be considered when determining treatments. Patients with MG may experience an exacerbation of their disease process and require intubation either as a temporary measure until the disease is more controlled, or as a step to protect their airway and respirations until a tracheostomy is performed for more definitive care. When patients with chronic disease processes deteriorate, the family may panic and summon assistance by calling emergency services, which may result in multiple invasive procedures that are ineffective and serve only to artificially prolong the patient's life. For this reason, patients with chronic, degenerative neurologic diseases should have advance directives and conduct difficult conversations with family and loved ones, as well as with their primary care provider and healthcare specialists.

Multiple Sclerosis

Multiple sclerosis (MS) is an inflammatory, demyelinating, autoimmune disease of the CNS that is a result of a combination of genetic and environmental factors. Environmental aspects include the place of residence in pre-adult years, age of exposure to EBV, and smoking. Patients who are seronegative for EBV are at low risk, whereas those who have been exposed later in life have a higher risk of developing the disease. MS affects women more than men, and onset is usually between ages 20 to 40. There are approximately 400,000 cases of MS in the United States.

The majority of cases of MS are *relapsing-remitting MS* (RRMS), whereby the acute attacks with neurologic impairment (relapse) are followed by periods of improvement (remittance). Eventually, RRMS will progress until patients do not have any periods of relapse, but experience a slow, progressive decline in their abilities. This is classified as *secondary progressive MS* (SPMS). Primary progressive MS has an older age of onset, affects men and women equally, and is evidenced by a slow, progressive myelopathy. A small portion of cases are of the progressive-relapsing form of MS. Other variants of MS include neuromyelitis optica and acute disseminated encephalomyelitis.

Over the past several years, clinicians have used MRI to help diagnose MS. However, it is important to obtain a thorough patient history to establish time and space in terms of dissemination, and to rule out other disease processes that may mimic MS. Signs and symptoms of demyelinating events such as optic neuritis or transverse myelitis should be used, as well as MRI, to establish the diagnosis. Standard MRI techniques such as fluid-attenuated inversion recovery (FLAIR) can detect areas of high signal in the white matter, the hallmark of the inflammatory demyelination of MS. Gadolinium contrast agents may show enhancement in new white matter lesions and is more specific and sensitive in diagnosing MS. Gadolinium may be useful to assess acute inflammation, as the lesions will enhance for a period of approximately 6 to 8 weeks. Two or more white matter lesions seen at the time of a clinically isolated event indicates a high risk of the patient having a diagnosis of MS.[39] Another diagnostic finding is the presence of oligoclonal bands in the CSF, which are seen in up to 95% of patients diagnosed with MS. Of note, this is not a definitive diagnosis, as oligoclonal bands are found in other neurologic disorders such as CNS infections; however, it is considered high risk for MS.[45]

Nearly 85% of people who develop MS will have a neurologic disturbance that may evolve over days or weeks – this is known as the *clinically isolated syndrome* or the *first demyelinating event*. The most common of these events involve the eyes, motor or sensory deficits, brainstem involvement, or a combination of abnormalities. Optic neuritis presents with pain in the eyes, blurred vision, decreased vision, and color desaturation. Cerebellar signs are evidenced by gait unsteadiness (ataxia of the limbs) or evoked nystagmus. Spinal cord involvement involves the long tracts, and the patient may have upper or lower extremity weakness, uni- or bilateral paresthesia, or numbness. A classic sign of MS related to spinal cord symptoms is Lhermitte's sign, which is characterized by an "electric shock-like" sensation down the back and extremities when the patient's head is flexed forward.[42] Brainstem involvement presents as blurred vision due to internuclear ophthalmoplegia. Bowel and bladder difficulties may occur, resulting in constipation, urinary frequency/incontinence, and erectile dysfunction.

Several medication regimens are available to treat MS. Most medications are very expensive, and maintaining compliance due to cost, presence of side effects, and route of administration (i.e., intramuscular [IM] injection) create challenges for the clinician as well as the patient.

Interferon-β-1a: an immunoregulatory medication that works as an antagonist of gamma interferon, interferon-β-1a (Avonex, Rebif) reduces the cytokine release while boosting suppressor T-cell function. This medication is aimed at reducing relapses in ambulatory RRMS. Avonex is administered via IM injection of 30 mcg once per week. Rebif is administered as an SC injection of 44 mcg three times per week.

Interferon-β-1b (Betaferon): has the same mechanisms of action as the interferon-β-1a-type medications previously described. This medication reduces relapses in ambulatory RRMS and SPMS, and is administered as an SC injection of 250 mcg every 2 days.

Glatiramer acetate (Copaxone): is a synthetic polypeptide that is believed to block myelin antigens from T lymphocytes and is used to reduce relapses in RRMS. This medication is given via an SC injection of 20 mg once per day.

Natalizumab (Tysabri): is a recombinant humanized monoclonal antibody to alpha-4 integrins that inhibits leucocyte movement from the blood to the CNS. It is used to reduce relapses in RRMS and is administered IV in a 300 mg dose over 1 hour once per month.

In the event of relapse, methylprednisolone IV (1 g/d for 3 days) is the treatment of choice, but is reserved for those relapses that significantly impact the patient's QOL. The treatment can speed the recovery from the relapse, but not the frequency of future relapses, and cannot prevent permanent disability that may result from the episode. Side effects of the medication may include psychosis, mood changes, aseptic hip necrosis, or elevated blood glucose. Plasma exchange may be performed in patients suffering a severe relapse who are unresponsive to steroids.[42]

Caring for patients with MS in the critical care setting encompasses not only the challenges presented by the disease and its treatments, but the addition of critical illness as well. As much as possible, adherence to the patients' usual routines, or resumption of their routines should begin as soon as possible to aid their recovery.

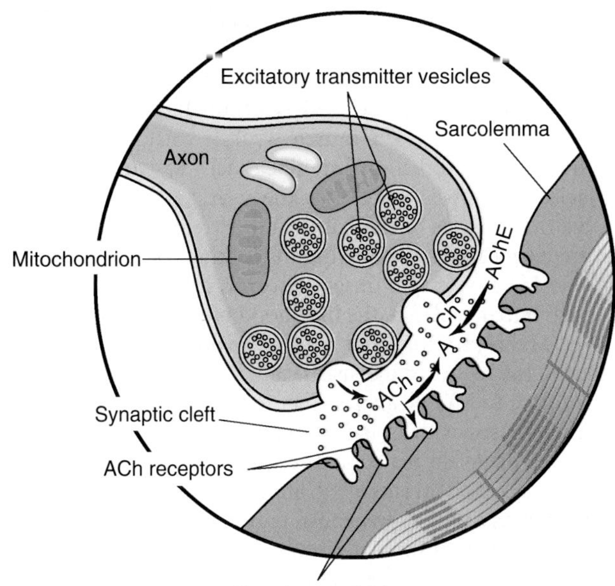

FIG. 15.8 Neuromuscular junction in myasthenia gravis. (From Monahan, F., Sands, J., Neighbors, M., et al. (2007). *Phipps' medical-surgical nursing: health and illness perspectives* (9th ed.). St Louis: Mosby.)

TABLE 15.6 Muscle Groups Affected in Myasthenia Gravis

Involved Muscle Group	Resultant Deficit
Facial	Facial droop Blank facial expression; inability to frown or smile; inability to tightly close eyelids or puff out cheeks; weakness in raising eyebrow, closing mouth
Extraocular	Diplopia; loss of conjugate gaze Asymmetric ptosis
Mastication	Difficulty chewing food Weak and slow tongue movements Fatigue during eating
Swallowing	Decreased pharyngeal and palatal weakness Dysphagia; regurgitation of liquid through nares; risk for aspiration
Speech	Dysarthria; poor articulation Dysphonia/altered voice quality; hypernasal speech
Musculoskeletal system	Altered muscle strength and functional ability in proximal upper and lower extremities Weakness of muscles of respiration; shortness of breath, shallow respirations, inability to cough effectively

Myasthenia Gravis

Myasthenia gravis (MG) is an autoimmune disease that affects the neuromuscular junction and is characterized by abnormal muscle weakness and fatigue. MG is a result of the action of autoantibodies on the acetylcholine receptors (AChRs) at the neuromuscular junction, causing alterations in nerve transmission (Fig. 15.8). The deficiency in AChRs is due to an antibody-mediated autoimmune attack; further failures in transmission desensitize any remaining AChRs, resulting in fatigability. MG is classified into five groups: ocular myasthenia; mild, moderate, and severe weakness with no ocular involvement; and very severe weakness, classified by intubation (with or without mechanical ventilation). A congenital MG syndrome has been identified that is present in children and does not have an autoimmune origin (Table 15.6).[17]

The initial patient presentation is often ocular in nature (ptosis and diplopia) or a bulbar weakness seen as slurred or nasal speech, voice alterations, or difficulties with chewing or swallowing. The degree of muscle weakness varies from day to day regardless of the muscles involved, and the weakness progresses as the day progresses with continued use of the affected muscles (fatigability). The muscle weakness usually progresses in a head-to-toe direction (craniocaudal), starting with ocular, facial, and lower bulbar weakness, and later progresses to involve the muscles of the trunk and extremities. In over half of patients with MG, the maximum weakness occurs within the first year after symptom onset; however, if the patient's symptoms are ocular-isolated, the likelihood of progressing to a generalized MG is minimal after a two-year duration of disease.[17]

Due to the nature of the disease and its fluctuating course, the average time to MG diagnosis is more than a year. Patients may be misdiagnosed with mood or anxiety disorders; the result of the delayed diagnosis may be a deterioration to myasthenia crisis. Myasthenia crisis is an emergent, life-threatening event that presents with severe muscle weakness, particularly of the respiratory muscles, and may necessitate intubation and mechanical ventilation. Characteristics of myasthenia crisis include ocular signs (weak eye movements and ptosis, but normal, reactive pupils) and facial and extremity weakness (with normal tendon and flexor/plantar reflexes). Infectious processes or medication withdrawal are risk factors for myasthenia crisis. Plasma exchange and IV immunoglobulin may be efficacious, but the response to plasma exchange is generally more predictable and preferable.[17]

Edrophonium chloride (Tensilon) is an acetylcholinesterase (AChE) inhibitor that has a rapid onset of action and allows acetylcholine (ACh) to interact longer with the decreased number of AChRs on the muscle endplate, resulting in a greater endplate depolarization. Muscle weakness will generally improve in over half of patients with ocular or generalized forms of MG who are treated with Tensilon. Side effects are uncommon and usually mild, but equipment and medications should be readily available in case of serious adverse effects such as bradycardia, asystole, or bronchoconstriction that would require emergent interventions.[25]

Treatment options include a variety of medications (AChE inhibitors, corticosteroids, immunosuppressants, immunotherapy) and thymectomy, depending on the patient's condition, the MG serologic status, and if thymoma is present. Individualized treatment regimens are crucial, and the patient is closely monitored with long-term follow-up. The goals of treatment are to control muscle weakness and achieve a remission of MG symptoms.

AChE inhibitors such as neostigmine (Bloxiverz, Prostigmin) and pyridostigmine (Mestinon) are the most commonly used treatments for MG. They can be used as monotherapy for symptomatic control, or as adjunctive therapy in patients with a more severe disease process. Common side effects are generally due to the cholinergic activity, and may include nausea, vomiting, abdominal cramps, diarrhea, and increased secretions (lacrimal, salivary, and bronchial). Anticholinergic medications can be used to mitigate the adverse effects, without compromising the nicotinic effects of the treatment drugs. Cholinergic crisis may occur due to high doses of AChE inhibitors, resulting in increased muscle weakness due to blocked depolarization at the neuromuscular junction.[17]

In terms of patient management, the nurse must have an understanding of the differences between myasthenia crisis and cholinergic crisis. Both situations can necessitate intubation/mechanical ventilation and critical care support. In patients with moderate to severe MG, a myasthenia crisis is a sudden relapse of the myasthenia symptoms that may be due to infection, surgery, or prednisone taper; for some patients, the cause is unknown. The anticholinergic medications may be discontinued during this time until the patient is stabilized. When the medications are reintroduced, the patient is reevaluated for response, and the medication regimen may need to be slowly reestablished. As motor strength and respiratory function improve, the patient is progressively weaned from mechanical ventilation.[23]

A cholinergic crisis is related to the toxic effects of AChE inhibitors, which have muscarinic and nicotinic effects. Muscarinic effects may include gastrointestinal symptoms (heartburn, abdominal cramps, diarrhea, nausea, and vomiting), cardiovascular symptoms (bradycardia), blurred vision, bronchoconstriction, increased bronchial secretions, and increased sweating and salivation. Nicotinic effects are evidenced by skeletal muscle twitching (fasciculations) and spasms that are followed by muscle fatigue and weakness. The former effects develop slowly and may be present for some time before the nicotinic effects, which are more rapid in onset, are seen. The patient will have profound generalized weakness, excessive pulmonary secretions, and impaired respiratory function. Management is similar to management of a myasthenia crisis and includes monitoring of respiratory function with possible intubation and mechanical ventilation, and temporarily stopping AChE inhibitors. The Tensilon test may be used to differentiate between the two situations: an improvement in muscle strength with injection of the drug indicates a myasthenia crisis, whereas deterioration or no improvement in muscle strength is indicative of a cholinergic crisis.[23] Nurses should be aware of the medications that may worsen MG, and patient teaching should stress the importance of checking with their healthcare provider before taking prescriptions or over the counter (OTC) medications. Examples of medications that worsen MG include: aminoglycoside antibiotics, fluoroquinolone antibiotics, macrolide antibiotics, calcium channel blockers, radiocontrast agents, and neuromuscular blockers.[24]

Patients with MG may be admitted for exacerbation of their disease process and are closely monitored for further deterioration of the respiratory status (rate, rhythm, labored/smooth, or abdominal breathing). In addition, the nurse should be aware of the patient's voice quality and assess for changes in intensity, tone, or fatigability. Assessment of the eyes (extraocular movements, diplopia, or ptosis) and the patient's ability to hold up his or her head are important aspects of the assessment as well. Patients with MG have progressive fatigue throughout the day, so the nurse should plan for activities such as physical/occupational therapy treatments early in the day in order to maximize patient participation. Key considerations include fall precautions due to an intolerance to activity, muscle weakness, and clumsiness.[23]

Amyotrophic Lateral Sclerosis

Amyotrophic lateral sclerosis (ALS) is an idiopathic progressive neurodegenerative disease that has no cure and results in death. Much research has been conducted on this devastating disease, which slowly and progressively robs the patient of muscle tone and control while keeping cognition intact until the end of life. Research goals have been aimed at slowing disease progression, as well as managing the secondary effects of respiratory failure and malnutrition. Currently, clinicians must rely on the patient's signs and symptoms and clinical criteria for diagnosis, as there are no biomarkers or other definitive tests for ALS.

In general, patients may present with a combination of upper and lower motor neuron signs in their extremities; bulbar signs (speech, swallowing difficulties presenting first, with limb involvement later); a "pure" upper motor neuron (UMN) involvement; or progressive muscular atrophy with pure lower motor neuron (LMN) involvement. The presence of UMN and LMN involving the brainstem and multiple spinal cord levels of innervation are the clinical hallmarks of the disease. The limb-onset form of the disease is present in approximately 70% of patients, followed by the bulbar-onset types in 25% of patients.[22]

UMN effects of the extremities are seen as spasticity, weakness, and brisk, deep tendon reflexes. The LMN effects are opposite, and include muscle fasciculation (twitching), muscle wasting, and weakness. Bulbar UMN creates difficulties for the patient in terms of a spastic dysarthria, causing slow, labored, and inarticulate speech. The gag reflex and jaw jerk may be pathologically brisk as well. Bulbar LMN involvement is seen as tongue wasting, weakness, flaccid dysarthria, and later dysphagia. The patient with flaccid dysarthria may have nasal speech due to weakness of the palate, hoarseness, and a weak cough.

Half of all ALS patients die within 30 months after symptom onset, and approximately 20% survive between 5 and 10 years. Initially, patients experience fatigue and a decreased capacity for exercise. Most will need assistance with ADLs. Dysphagia develops in most patients, resulting in weight loss and malnutrition. As the disease progresses, respiratory compromise is a common occurrence that leads to dyspnea and hypoventilation; once the patient develops dyspnea at rest, death is often imminent, as progressive weakening of the respiratory muscles leads to respiratory failure. Respiratory failure is complicated by pneumonia and the inability to breathe independently.[22]

Patients with ALS require supportive care for symptom management and a interprofessional approach to treatment. One medication, riluzole, is the first to slow the deterioration, and although it is known to act by inhibiting the presynaptic release of glutamate, the exact mechanisms of action are unknown. Discussions regarding advanced directives and end-of-life care should be addressed openly and with sensitivity during the early stages of the disease. Consultation with the palliative care specialists early in disease is encouraged to assist the patient and family with the decision-making process. Nursing care involves all of the usual routines, with special attention to the patient's potential or actual decline in pulmonary function and nutrition.[22]

Parkinson's Disease

Parkinson's disease (PD) is a progressive neurodegenerative disease that is incurable. The prevalence of PD increases with age. The cause of PD is thought to be environmental, and may be related to exposure to pesticides, herbicides, industrial chemicals, wood pulp mills, or farming, and to living in rural areas. Currently there is no strong or direct link to these factors, but they are thought to be contributing factors and thus should be a part of a thorough patient history. PD is not thought to be a genetic disease; however, genetic links have been documented. Therefore, it is believed that PD development may be caused by a combination of genetic and environmental factors.

Progressive development of tremor, rigidity, bradykinesia, and postural instability are the most common symptoms with an onset in middle age. The disease affects deep structures of the brain, in particular the neurons containing dopamine in the substantia nigra of the basal ganglia. Treatment is supportive, with the goal of symptom management through the utilization of medication regimens.[32]

Several medication classes are used for the treatment of symptoms of PD, including: monoamine oxidase B (MAO-B) inhibitors, levodopa, dopamine agonists, anticholinergic agents, catechol-O-methyltransferase (COMT) inhibitors, and amantadine. Levodopa is the most effective medication, and is the precursor to dopamine. Dopamine is metabolized before reaching the brain if given as an oral preparation, whereas levodopa crosses the BBB and is centrally converted to dopamine to restore the depleted stores in the basal ganglia in patients with PD. Carbidopa is used in conjunction with levodopa due to the conversion of the latter in the brain. Carbidopa is used to block the peripheral conversion of levodopa to dopamine to make more medication available to the brain. Carbidopa also reduces the side effects of levodopa, which may include nausea, vomiting, orthostatic hypotension, and cardiac arrhythmias. This medication combination is commercially available as levodopa/carbidopa (Sinemet). Long-term treatment with levodopa may involve rapid fluctuations in movement – the "on-off" picture that changes from normal ("on") to bradykinesia ("off").[32]

Dopamine agonists stimulate dopamine receptors in the brain and help to decrease the off periods. These agents, such as bromocriptine (Parlodel), pramipexole (Mirapex), or ropinirole (Requip), are given when patients are not able to tolerate higher doses of levodopa, when the patient's response to levodopa is declining, or when the patient's symptoms are not controlled with levodopa alone. The most common side effects are nausea and vomiting; the medications should be taken with food. Lightheadedness, constipation, hallucinations, or dyskinesias are among the other adverse effects.

Nursing considerations for patients with PD include diligent attention and adherence to their medication schedule and regimen. This is a challenge for patients in the hospital, particularly in the perioperative period as nothing by mouth, sedation, anesthesia, and other considerations may easily disrupt or delay needed PD medications. Patients and their family members should be encouraged to bring all medications (in the original bottles) with them to allow the healthcare provider(s) to ensure continuation of the appropriate medications and dosing schedule.

Patients who have become less responsive to medication treatments may be candidates for surgical intervention. Placement of a deep brain stimulator (DBS) has been demonstrated to be effective for the relief of tremors that greatly affect patients' QOL and ability to function from day to day. Patients whose symptoms are responsive to levodopa are considered to be candidates for DBS surgery; however, the risks versus benefits need to be considered. The surgeon must evaluate each individual patient before recommending surgical intervention. Deep brain stimulation involves implanting one or more electrodes in the subthalamic nucleus and the internal segment of the globus pallidus in the nuclei in the basal ganglia. The electrodes are then connected to a generator that delivers electrical stimuli to targeted areas in the brain. An external programmer turns the device on or off. Imaging (CT or MRI) is completed prior to the procedure to determine the target areas and is used as markers during surgery. All PD medications are stopped prior to surgery (on average, 12 hours prior) to minimize medication-induced dyskinesia that would interfere with the placement of the electrodes. Postoperative nursing care includes careful neurologic monitoring and assessments.[32]

Guillain-Barré Syndrome

Guillain-Barré syndrome (GBS) is a common cause of neuromuscular paralysis, with men more likely to be affected than women. GBS is not associated with systemic or autoimmune disorders, but more than half of the people afflicted have symptoms of an infection within 3 weeks of the onset of weakness. The most common signs of infection are fever, cough, sore throat, rhinorrhea, and diarrhea, and most studies cite the presence of an upper respiratory tract or gastrointestinal infection. Links between the onset of GBS with vaccinations, surgical procedures, or stressful events have been demonstrated, but no definitive relationships have been found (Box 15.2).[43]

LP is a key part of the diagnostic workup in patients suspected of GBS. CSF studies demonstrate an increase in protein, with normal CSF white cell count. Of note, CSF protein is often normal in the first week of diagnosis, but increases in nearly all patients by the end of the second week.[43]

The key feature of GBS is rapid, progressive, bilateral, and symmetric weakness of the extremities that may or may not involve the muscles used for respiration or cranial nerve–innervated muscles. Patients have decreased or absent deep-tendon reflexes in the affected limbs. Most patients reach maximal weakness within 2 weeks, but by definition of GBS, the maximal weakness is attained in 4 weeks. A plateau phase may last several days or months, followed by a slow recovery phase of varying duration. Approximately 25% of patients admitted to the hospital with GBS are unable to walk and will require intubation and mechanical ventilation for respiratory support. A small population of severely affected patients are unable to walk after 6 months despite treatments with IV-Ig or plasma exchange; others continue to have issues with severe fatigue and remain disabled. Patients with GBS may have difficulties completing ADLs and have notable weakness for 3 to 6 years after onset of the disease, impacting their social life.

A interprofessional team is needed to care for the patient with GBS. In addition to ongoing neurologic monitoring, pulmonary status/pulmonary function should be regularly monitored and interventions taken as necessary for patient support. Complications are related to weakness and immobility (i.e., DVT), other symptoms of autonomic dysfunction (ileus, pupils nonresponsive to light), or the recognition of pain. Therapies and mobilizing the patient should begin early (even if patients still require ventilator support, but are otherwise stable). Physical therapy and psychosocial support are crucial to the patient's recovery, well-being, and ability to handle the disease process. Patients and loved ones may be directed to national or local support groups for additional resources and assistance.[43]

BOX 15.2 Clinical Features of Guillain-Barré Syndrome

1. Progressive ascending symmetric weakness of the limbs
   - Involvement of proximal and distal muscles
   - Depressed or absent reflexes
   - Involvement of cranial nerves (facial nerves most commonly involved)
2. Numbness and tingling in the hands and feet
   - Mild sensory symptoms or signs
3. Respiratory failure
4. Pain
   - Back, shoulder girdle, and posterior thighs
5. Autonomic dysfunction
   - Cardiac dysrhythmias (tachycardia, bradycardia, asystole)
   - Orthostatic hypotension
   - Paralytic ileus
   - Bladder dysfunction
   - Abnormal sweating
6. Progression to peak disability in 4 weeks

CONCLUSION

The critical care nurse may encounter a wide variety of neurologic disease processes or injuries; this chapter has provided an overview of some of the common and not-so-common disease states. Often the patient with a chronic neurologic disorder is well-managed in the community, and events requiring hospitalization may not be directly related to their underlying disease process. Special consideration must be directed to these disorders, as the physical sequelae and/or medications required to keep the disease controlled may have significant impact on their treatment plan in the ICU and the overall ability for recovery. As these diseases are generally progressive neurodegenerative disorders, the nurse should develop a comfort level with providing education and support for the patient and their loved ones at the end of life. The knowledge of these disease processes and ability to work in collaboration with a interprofessional healthcare team will provide the patient and their family the greatest support during this crucial time of need.

REFERENCES

1. American Association of Critical Care Nurses (AACN). (2014). *Implementing the ABCDE Bundle at the bedside.* Retrieved from http://www.aacn.org/dm/practice/actionpakdetail.aspx?itemid=28328.
2. Baehr, M., & Frotscher, M. (2012). Elements of the nervous system. In *Duus' topical diagnosis in neurology* (5th ed.) (pp. 2–10). Stuttgart, Germany: Thieme.
3. Beckham, J. D., & Tyler, K. L. (2012). Neuro-intensive care of patients with acute CNS infections. *Neurotherapeutics, 9*(1), 124–138.
4. Ben, L. C., James, T. F., & Sinclair, A. J. (2012). Cerebrospinal fluid and lumbar puncture: a practical review. *J Neurol 259*, 1530–1545. http://dx.doi.org/10.1007/s00415-012-6413-x.
5. Betjemann, J. P., & Lowenstein, D. H. (2015). Status epilepticus in adults. *Lancet Neurol, 14*, 615–624. http://dx.doi.org.contentproxy.phoenix.edu/10.1016/S1474-4422(15)00042-3.
6. Brouwer, M. C., Thwaites, G. E., Tunkel, A. R., & Van de Beek, D. R. (2012). Dilemmas in the diagnosis of acute community-acquired bacterial meningitis. *Lancet, 380*(9854), 1684–1692. http://dx-.doi.org/. http://dx.doi.org.contentproxy.phoenix.edu/10.1016/S0140-6736(12)61185-4.
7. Buelow, J. M., Dean, P., Gilbert, K. L., Miller, W., & Plueger, M. (2010). *AANN core curriculum for neuroscience nursing* (5th ed.). Glenview, IL: American Association of Neuroscience Nurses.
8. Cahill, J. E., & Armstrong, T. S. (2014). *The clinical practice of neurological and neurosurgical nursing* (7th ed.). Philadelphia, PA: Lippincott, Williams, & Wilkins.
9. Chabra, P., Gupta, N., & Kaushik, A. (2013). Compartment syndrome as a spectrum of purple glove syndrome following intravenous phenytoin administration in a young male: a case report and review of the literature. *Neurol India, 61*(4), 419–420. http://dx.doi.org/10.4103/0028-3886.117611.
10. Chow, F. C., & Glaser, C. A. (2014). Emerging and reemerging neurologic infections. *Neurohospitalist, 4*(4), 173–184. http://dx.doi.org/10.1177/1941874414540685.

11. Crepeau, A. Z., & Treiman, D. M. (2010). Levetiracetam: a comprehensive review. *Expert Rev Neurother*, *10*(2), 159–171. http://dx.doi.org/10.1585/ERN.10.3.
12. England, K. M., & Plueger, M. D. (2014). *The practice of neurological and neurosurgical nursing*. (7th ed.). Philadelphia: Lippincott, Williams, and Wilkins.
13. Engel, J., Jr. (2013). Types of seizures. In *Seizures and epilepsy* (2nd ed.) (pp. 193–242). New York, NY: Oxford University Press.
14. Greenberg, M. S. (2010). *Handbook of neurosurgery* (7th ed.). New York: Thieme.
15. Heimans, J. J., & Reijneveld, J. C. (2012). Factors affecting the cerebral network in brain tumor patients. *J Neurooncol*, *108*, 231–237. http://dx-.doi.org/10.1007/s11060-012-0814-7.
16. Heiss, W. D., Raab, P., & Lanfermann, H. (2011). Multimodality assessment of brain tumors and tumor recurrence. *J Nucl Med*, *52*(10), 1585–1600. http://dx.doi.org/10.2967/jnumed.110.084210.
17. Herrington, J. B., Koopman, W. J., & Ricci, M. (2013). *Care of the patient with myasthenia gravis: AANN clinical practice guideline series*. Glenview, IL: American Association of Neuroscience Nurses.
18. Hickey, J. V., & Kanusky, J. T. (2014). Overview of neuroanatomy and neurophysiology. In *The clinical practice of neurological and neurosurgical nursing* (7th ed.) (pp. 48–93). Philadelphia: Lippincott Williams & Wilkins.
19. Hirbe, A. C., & Gutmann, D. H. (2014). Neurofibromatosis type 1: A multidisciplinary approach to care. *Lancet Neurol*, *13*(8), 834–843. http://dx.doi.org/10.1016/S1474-4422(14)70063-8.
20. Hoerth, M. T., & Drazkowski, J. F. (2010). Seizure emergencies in older adults. *Aging Health*, *6*(1), 97–110. http://dx.doi.org/10.2217/AHE.09.91.
21. Kehayov, I. I., Kitov, B. D., Zhelyazkov, C. B., Raykov, S. D., & Davarski, A. N. (2012). Neurocognitive impairments in brain tumor patients. *Folia Medica*, *54*(1), 14–21. http://dx.doi.org/10.2478/v10153-012-0001-9.
22. Kiernan, M. C., Vucic, S., Cheah, B. C., et al. (2011). Amyotrophic lateral sclerosis. *Lancet*, (377), 942–955.
23. Koopman, W. J., & Hickey, J. V. (2014). *The clinical practice of neurological and neurosurgical nursing* (7th ed.). Philadelphia: Lippincott, Wilkins, & Williams.
24. Lassiter, T. F., & Henkel, A. I. (2014). *The clinical practice of neurological and neurosurgical nursing*. (7th ed.). Philadelphia: Lippincott, Wilkins, & Williams.
25. Livesay, S. (2012). Neurologic problems. In J. G. Whetstone-Foster, & S. S. Prevost (Eds.), *Advanced practice nursing of adults in acute care* (pp. 184–238). Philadelphia: F. A. Davis Company.
26. Lovely, M. P., Stewart-Amidei, C., Arzbaecher, J., et al. (2014). *Care of the adult patient with brain tumor: AANN clinical guideline*. http://www.aann.org/apps/ws_downloads/download.php?task=submit.
27. Lovely, M. P., Stewart-Amidei, C., Page, M., et al. (2013). A new reality: long-term survivorship with a malignant brain tumor. *Oncol Nurs Forum*, *40*(3), 267–274. http://dx.doi.org/10.1188/13.ONF.267-274.
28. Magazzini, S., Nazerian, P., Vanni, S., et al. (2012). Clinical picture of meningitis in the adult patient and its relationship with age. *Intern Emerg Med*, *7*, 359–364. http://dx.doi.org/10.1007/s11739-012-0765-1.
29. Mann, A., Machado, N. M., Liu, N., Mazin, A., Silver, K., & Afzal, K. (2012). An Multidisciplinary Approach to the Treatment of Anti-NMDA-Receptor Antibody Encephalitis: a Case and Review of the Literature. *J Neuropsychiatry Clin Neurosci*, *24*(2), 247–254. http://search.proquest.com.contentproxy.phoenix.edu/docview/1315542055?accountid=35812.
30. Nair, P. P., Kalita, J., & Misra, U. K. (2010). Status epilepticus: why, what, and how. *J Postgrad Med*, 57(3), 242–252. http://dx.doi.org/10.4103/0022-3859.81807.
31. Noble, J., & Pasi, S. (2010). Epidemiology and pathophysiology of cancer-associated thrombosis. *Brit J Can*, *102*(Suppl. 1), S2–S9.
32. Nolden, L. F., Tartavoulle, T., & Porche, D. J. (2014). Parkinson's disease: Assessment, diagnosis, and management. *J Nurs Pract*, *10*(7), 500–506.
33. Olshan, M., Srinivasan, V., Landrum, T., & Sataloff, R. T. (2014). Acoustic neuroma: An investigation of associations between tumor size and diagnostic delays, facial weakness, and surgical complications. *Ear Nose Throat J*, *93*(8), 304–316. http://search.proquest.com.contentproxy.phoenix.edu/docview/1561358072?accountid=35812.
34. Piscatelli, N., Schill, D., & Batchelor, T. (2003). Classification of brain tumors. *UpToDate Online* 13.2. www.uptodate.com.
35. Roth, P., Regli, L., Tonder, M., & Weller, M. (2013). Tumor-associated edema in brain cancer patients: pathogenesis and management. *Expert Rev Anticancer Ther*, *13*, 1319–1325. http://dx.doi.org/10.1586/14737140.2013.852473.
36. Salmaggi, A., Simonetti, G., Trevisan, E., et al. (2013). Perioperative thromboprophylaxis in patients with craniotomy for brain tumors: a systematic review. *J Neurooncol*, *113*, 293–303. http://dx.doi.org/10.1007/s11060-013-1115-5.
37. Sanders, R. D. (2010). The trigeminal (V) and facial (VII) cranial nerves: head and face sensation and movement. *Psychiatry*, *7*(1), 13–16.
38. Sherwood, P., Hricik, A., Donovan, H., et al. (2011). Changes in caregiver perceptions over time in response to providing care for a loved one with a primary malignant brain tumor. *Oncol Nurs Forum*, *38*(2), 149–155. http://dx.doi.org/10.1188/11.ONF.149-155.
39. Sicotte, N. L. (2011). Neuroimaging in multiple sclerosis: neurotherapeutic implications. *Neurotherapeutics* *8*, 54–62. http://dx.doi.org/10.1007/s13311-010-0008-y.
40. Society of Critical Care Medicine. (2015). Family engagement and empowerment. http://www.iculiberation.org/SiteCollectionDocuments/ICU-Liberation-ABCDEF-Bundle-Implementation-Family-Engagement-Empowerment.pdf.
41. Stewart-Amidei, C., Arzbaecher, J., & Lupica, K. (2010). Nervous system tumors. In K. Mogensen (Ed.) *AANN core curriculum for neuroscience nursing* (5th ed.) (pp. 505–530). Glenview, IL: AANN.
42. Tsang, B. K., & Macdonall, R. (2011). Multiple sclerosis: diagnosis, management and prognosis. *Aust Fam Physician*, *40*(12), 948–955. http://search.proquest.com.contentproxy.phoenix.edu/docview/912383636?accountid=35812.
43. Van Doorn, P. A., Ruts, L., & Jacobs, B. C. (2008). Clinical features, pathogenesis, and treatment of Guillain-Barré syndrome. *Lancet Neurol*, *7*, 939–950. http://search.proquest.com.contentproxy.phoenix.edu/docview/201389747?accountid=35812.
44. VanDemark, M., & Hickey, J. V. (2014). *The clinical practice of neurological and neurosurgical nursing* (7th ed.). Philadelphia: Lippincott, Williams, & Wilkins.
45. Zipoli, V., Hakiki, B., Portaccio, E., et al. (2009). The contribution of cerebrospinal fluid oligoclonal bands to the early diagnosis of multiple sclerosis. *Mult Scler*, (15), 472–478. http://dx.doi.org/10.1177/1352458508100502.

16

Gastrointestinal Bleeding

Erica Deboer and Peggy L. Kirkwood

Bleeding into the gastrointestinal (GI) tract is a common problem found in critically ill patients and may have many sources. The bleeding may be caused by primary pathophysiology in the GI tract (e.g., gastric or peptic ulcers) or develop secondary to pathology outside of the GI tract (e.g., ovarian cancer perforating into the bowel). The source of the bleeding may be simple, short-term, and self-limiting, as with a Mallory-Weiss tear, or represent a life-threatening hemorrhage, as with a ruptured esophageal varix. Several different causes of GI bleeding may be found in the same patient. Whatever the cause, GI bleeding can have a negative impact on the patient's mortality and morbidity.

GI bleeding is rarely the cause for a hospitalization. However, patients hospitalized for treatment of GI bleeding have a mortality rate of approximately 10% to 13%.[24,48] Cause of death is usually a comorbidity, organ system dysfunction, or sepsis, rather than the GI bleed itself. The mortality rate associated with upper GI bleeding is approximately 4% in young adult patients, but may be as high as 15% in older patients.[24]

Sources of GI bleeding are characterized as either upper GI (i.e., esophagus, stomach, and duodenum) or lower GI (i.e., jejunum, ileum, colon, and rectum). The division between the upper and lower GI tract is considered the ligament of Treitz, which separates the duodenum and jejunum. Bleeding in the relatively short upper GI tract is more common and is usually caused by peptic ulcers or esophageal and gastric varices.[24,48] Bleeding from the much longer lower GI tract accounts for approximately 25% of GI bleeds.[25]

Patients at highest risk for GI bleeding usually have some pathology in the GI system. Some of these sources of bleeding may not cause large blood loss until they are significantly advanced (e.g., colon cancer). Other sources of bleeding, such as esophageal varices, are usually heralded by some identifiable history (i.e., chronic, excessive alcohol use) or symptoms (i.e., diarrhea with inflammatory bowel disease). In addition, it is estimated that more than 70% of US citizens are on aspirin therapy alone or in combination with an antiplatelet or anticoagulant agent, putting them at higher risk for GI bleeding.[1]

However, critically ill patients may also develop GI bleeding from a stress ulcer in response to their medical condition. Stress ulcer formation has been well documented in the critically ill. A number of methods have been used over the years to prevent its occurrence, including antacids and histamine H2-receptor blockade. Proton pump inhibitors (PPIs) are a significant tool in the prevention of stress ulcers and are more effective than histamine H2-receptor blockade.[2] In the absence of a hypersecretory state, the use of enteral nutrition (EN) may also be used as an effective method of stress ulcer prophylaxis in most critically ill patients.[20] Incorporating EN as a strategy for prophylaxis also decreases the incidence of *Clostridium difficile* colitis (also known as *pseudomembranous colitis*).[20]

APPLIED PHYSIOLOGY AND PATHOPHYSIOLOGY

The primary functions of the GI tract include absorbing nutrients (primarily from the small bowel) and water (from the large bowel), eliminating waste as stool, and providing immunity through gut-associated lymphatic tissue (GALT).[42] To support the multiple functions of the GI tract, there is a rich supply of blood vessels along its entire length, and it is therefore subject to many sources of bleeding.

Upper GI bleeding may be caused by a variety of disease processes. It may be as simple as a Mallory-Weiss tear of the esophagus, as complex as varices of the esophagus or stomach, or as devastating as cancer. However, upper GI bleeding is most often caused by peptic ulcer bleeding and acid disease processes occurring in the esophagus due to gastroesophageal reflux disease (GERD); in the stomach due to gastritis, erosions, and ulcer formation; or in the duodenum due to ulcer formation.[48]

A Mallory-Weiss tear is a laceration of the gastroesophageal junction mucosa that occurs with violent retching or vomiting. It is most often self-limiting, but occasionally requires intervention, such as endoscopy, for simple repair.

On the other hand, esophageal and gastric varices usually represent a complex life-threatening condition and carry a 15% to 20% mortality rate despite recent medical advances.[6,14] Esophageal and gastric varices are caused by liver disease, which increases the back pressure into the portal vein, resulting in dilation of the veins that drain from the esophagus, stomach, and the entire GI tract. Chapter 17 provides more comprehensive information about liver dysfunction and failure. When varices develop, they enlarge at a rate of 4% to 10% a year, increasing the likelihood that they will begin to bleed over time.[6,14,46] As with all veins, the veins from the esophagus and stomach are meant to be a low-pressure system, draining through the portal vein and into the liver. Damage to the liver's blood vessels by a

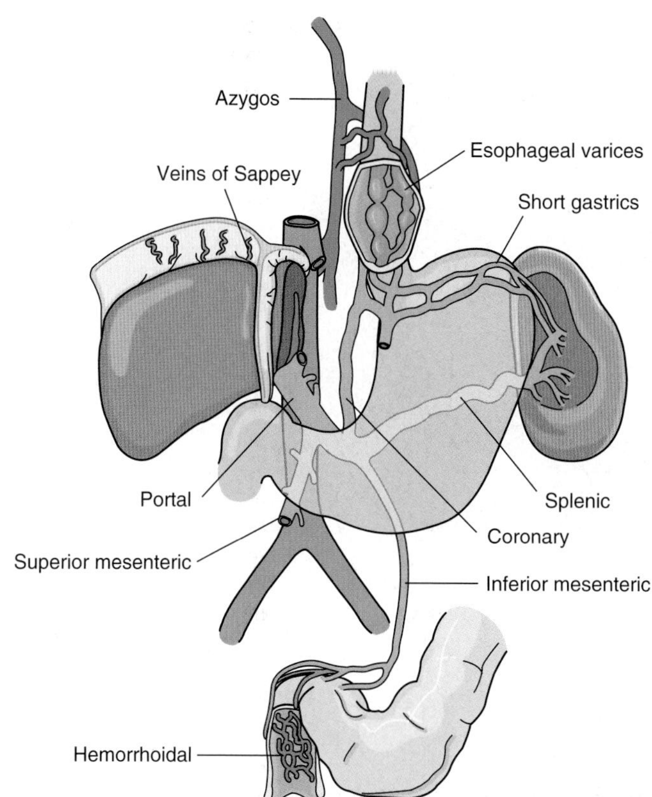

FIG. 16.1 Varices related to portal hypertension. (From Monahan, F., Sands, J., Neighbors, M., et al. (2007). *Phipps' medical-surgical nursing: health and illness perspectives* (9th ed.). St Louis: Mosby.)

variety of diseases, such as chronic alcohol ingestion, chemical exposure, and hepatitis, increases resistance to the flow of blood into the portal vein (Fig. 16.1). This increased resistance produces back pressure, which is transmitted into the esophagus and gastric veins and causes dilation. Over time, if the pressure becomes too great, the veins will leak or burst, dumping blood directly into the esophagus or stomach. Approximately 20% of patients with cirrhosis will develop bleeding varices.[6] The stomach usually reacts to large amounts of blood by reversing peristalsis, causing vomiting.

With acid disease processes, several types of injury may occur. Normally, the lower esophageal sphincter (LES) relaxes 1 to 2 hours after eating. Chyme, the semifluid mass of partially digested food, may occasionally be refluxed up into the esophagus by the peristalsis of the stomach. However, the acid in the chyme is usually neutralized by saliva and cleared back into the stomach by peristalsis, often within a couple of minutes. In the case of GERD, patients tend to have reduced LES pressures. Coupled with increased abdominal pressure (e.g., coughing, lifting, or bending forward) or a recumbent position after eating, it is much more likely the chyme will be refluxed into the esophagus. A number of structural abnormalities of the esophagogastric junction (e.g., hiatal hernia or incompetent esophagogastric sphincter) may also be present and contribute to the development of GERD.[30] Because the esophagus is subjected to repeated exposure to stomach acids, over time an erosive esophagitis may develop, which can progress to ulcers and bleeding.[35]

When food enters the stomach, it is exposed to acids and pepsin, converting it into the semifluid chyme by breaking down food fibers and protein, respectively. Secretion of the stomach acids is inhibited by prostaglandins. Normally, as the chyme is digested, the mucosal barrier of the stomach protects the gastric mucosa from the digestive actions of both pepsin and acid.

Gastritis is caused by any mechanism interfering with this normal process. One example of such a mechanism is seen with the ingestion of nonsteroidal antiinflammatory drugs (NSAIDs), which inhibit prostaglandins. This inhibition, in turn, allows for increased acid formation, gut inflammation, and an increased risk of bleeding.[26] Ethanol, or alcohol, may also cause chronic inflammation. As the gastritis continues, the disruption of normal processes that maintain the gastric mucosa may lead to gastric ulcer formation. The pathogen *Helicobacter pylori,* which adheres to the mucus-secreting cells in the stomach, may also cause a chronic gastritis that can lead to gastric mucosal atrophy.[19,44]

As seen with gastritis, *H. pylori* is also a major cause of duodenal ulcers further down the GI tract. A number of additional factors affecting acid and pepsin formation and control are also implicated in the formation of duodenal ulcers, which are actually more common than gastric ulcers. A duodenal ulcer may heal spontaneously, but will usually recur over time. If the ulcer is large enough to erode into the base of the duodenum, blood vessels are likely to be breached, allowing blood to enter the GI tract, where it may flow retrograde into the stomach to be vomited or passed in the stool (Fig. 16.2).

One type of ulcer that is common in critically ill patients is the stress ulcer. Stress ulcers are caused by hypoperfusion and ischemia of the GI tract (which are inherent with multisystem trauma), hemorrhage from a source other than the GI tract, and sepsis. See Fig. 16.3 for the pathophysiology of a stress ulcer.[3] In addition, stress ulcers have been related to emotional distress. Most stress ulcers form in the stomach or duodenum. Stress ulcers found in patients after brain surgery or with head trauma that causes increased intracranial pressure are called *Cushing's ulcers* and typically arise in the stomach, duodenum, or esophagus. The term *Curling's ulcer* has been applied to stress ulcers found in patients suffering from major burn injuries; these ulcers occur in the proximal duodenum.[3] These terms assist in classifying the more common stress ulcers. Regardless of the cause, the result is an ulcer eroding into the base of the GI tract, opening a blood vessel, and allowing free flow of blood into the gut (Fig. 16.4).[35]

Cancers of the upper GI tract may cause small amounts of blood loss, but usually present with other symptoms before significant blood loss occurs. Patients with cancers of the esophagus and stomach usually have symptoms that mimic GERD and ulcer disease, with an added feature of significantly rapid weight loss.

As with upper GI bleeding, blood loss in the lower GI tract may be caused by many disease processes. These include chronic diseases such as ulcerative colitis, as well as infection with *Escherichia coli* 0157:H7, which produces a potent cytotoxin that causes damage to the large intestine, leading to rapidly evolving bloody diarrhea.[11] Lower GI bleeding may also be caused by something as simple as internal hemorrhoids in the rectum from chronic straining to have a bowel movement, or as complex and lethal as colorectal cancer.

Mucosal angiodysplasia, a degenerative or congenital arteriovenous malformation of the GI vasculature, is the most common cause of lower GI bleeding, and may be confused with

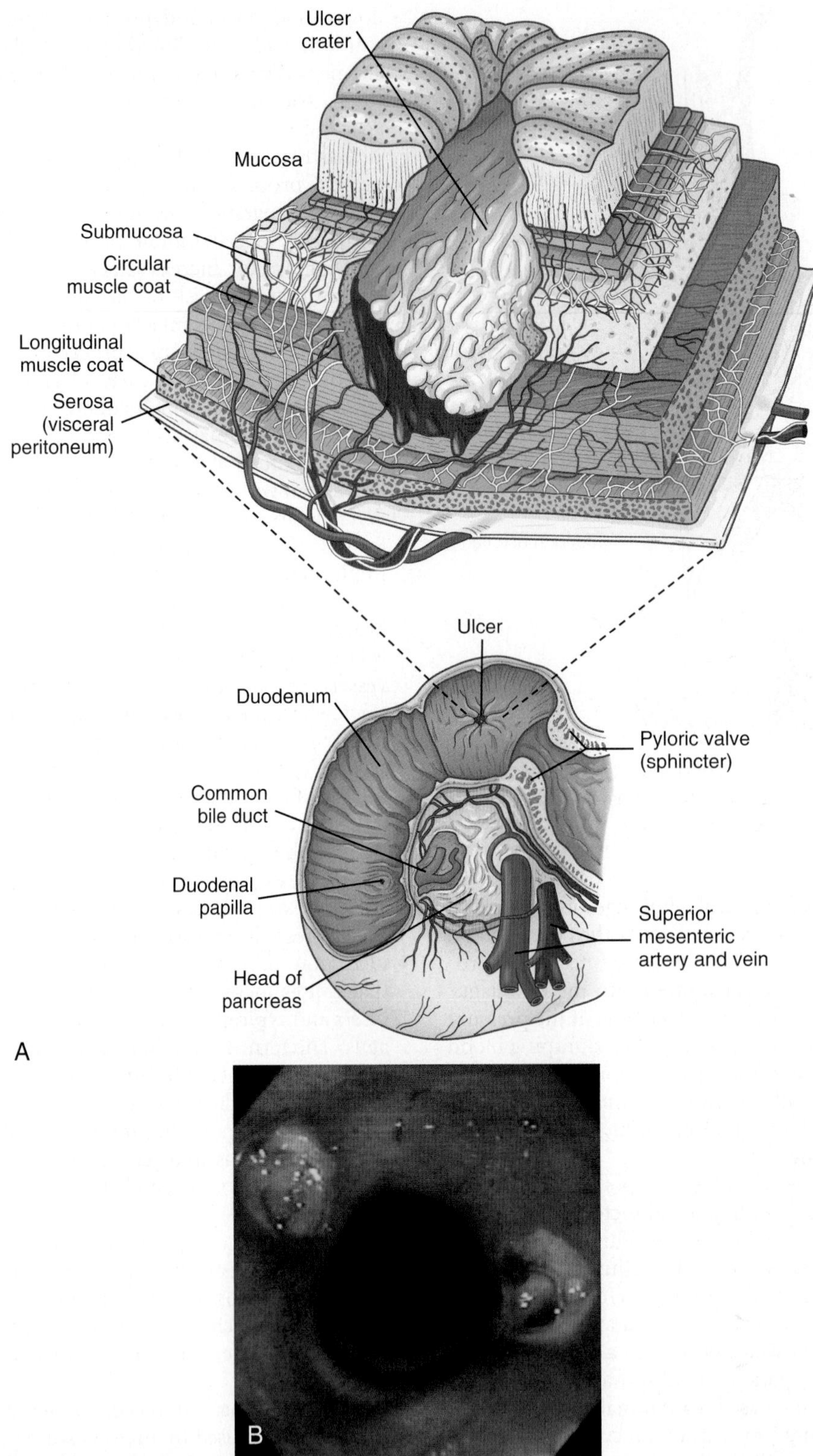

FIG. 16.2 Duodenal ulcer. **A,** Deep ulceration in the duodenal wall extending as a crater through the entire mucosa and into the muscle layers. **B,** Duodenal ulcer visualized by endoscopy. (From Phipps, W., Monahan, F., Sands, J., et al. (2007). *Medical-surgical nursing: health and illness perspectives* (8th ed.). St Louis: Mosby.)

Critical illness
Increased catecholamines
Shock or hypotension
Hypovolemia
↑ Vasoconstriction
↓ Cardiac output
Proinflammatory cytokine release
Splanchnic and mucosal hypoperfusion
↓ Bicarbonate secretion
↓ Mucosal blood flow
↓ Gastrointestinal motility
↓ Protective factors (e.g., HSP and TFF)
Acid back-diffusion
Acute stress-ulcer

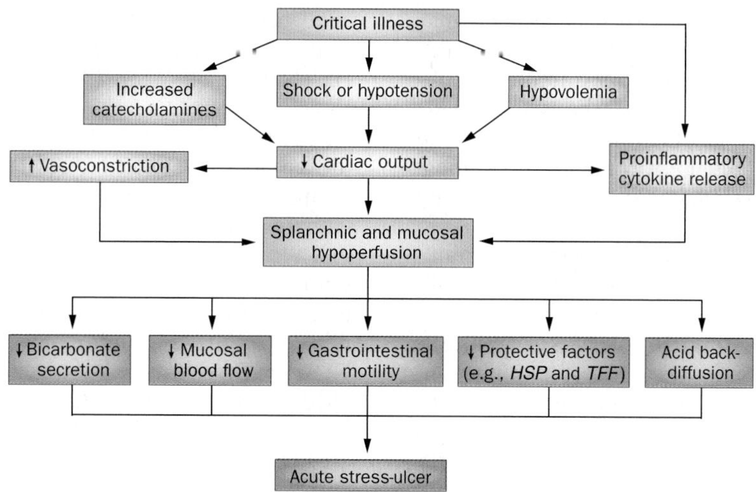

FIG. 16.3 Pathophysiology of stress ulcer formation. *HSP,* heat shock proteins; *TFF,* trefoil factor family. (Reprinted by permission from Macmillan Publishers Ltd. (2015). *Nature reviews gastroenterology & hepatology* 12, 98–107.)

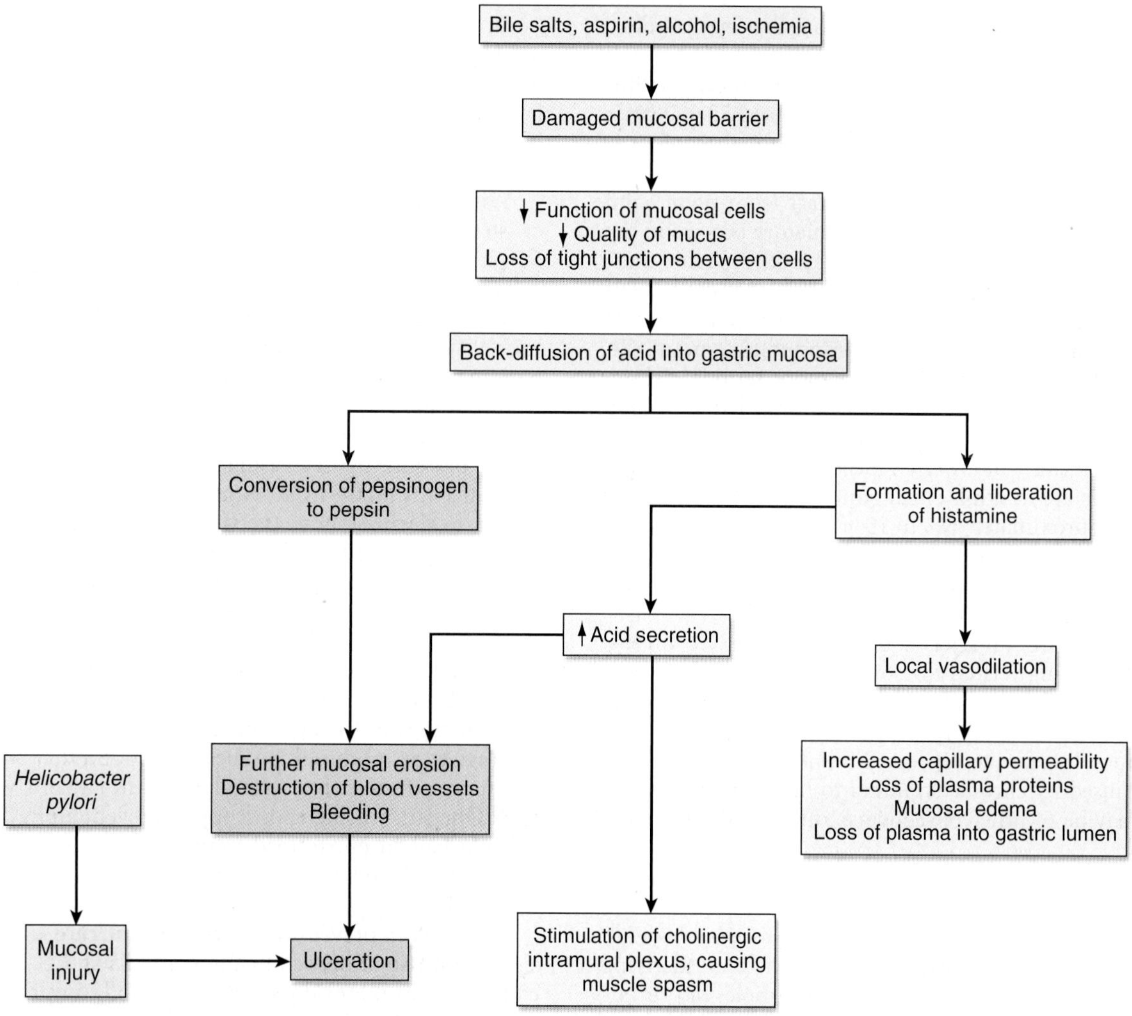

Bile salts, aspirin, alcohol, ischemia
Damaged mucosal barrier
↓ Function of mucosal cells
↓ Quality of mucus
Loss of tight junctions between cells
Back-diffusion of acid into gastric mucosa
Conversion of pepsinogen to pepsin
Formation and liberation of histamine
↑ Acid secretion
Local vasodilation
Helicobacter pylori
Further mucosal erosion
Destruction of blood vessels
Bleeding
Increased capillary permeability
Loss of plasma proteins
Mucosal edema
Loss of plasma into gastric lumen
Mucosal injury
Ulceration
Stimulation of cholinergic intramural plexus, causing muscle spasm

FIG. 16.4 Presentation of gastrointestinal bleeding.

bleeding from a diverticulum. The source of such bleeding may be very difficult to identify because of its location (i.e., middle of the jejunum), small size, and the small volume and subacute nature of the bleeding.[35,39] Patients may be asymptomatic or may present with GI bleeding, which may be chronic and well-compensated, or acute and life-threatening. Treatment of asymptomatic, nonbleeding angiodysplasia lesions is not recommended.[39]

In chronic diseases of the lower GI tract, such as Crohn's disease (also known as *regional enteritis*) and ulcerative colitis, the colon is the usual source of bleeding. Crohn's disease is caused by an idiopathic inflammatory process that affects the GI tract from the mouth to the anus. It is commonly confined to the ileocecal area (where the ileum merges into the colon) and the colon itself. The disease causes longitudinal and transverse fissures to develop and usually involves the entire intestinal wall. The fissures are caused by the continuing inflammation and create a "cobblestone" appearance with areas of edema.

Ulcerative colitis is another idiopathic inflammatory disease that is confined to the mucosal surface of the lower GI tract, usually the distal colon (sigmoid and rectum). The inflammation affects just the mucosal surface and usually does not penetrate through the intestinal wall. However, when severe, it can cause ulcerations, abscesses, and perforations that may produce large, bloody diarrheal stools.

E. coli 0157:H7 has been recognized as a significant pathogen since 1982, and still accounts for an estimated 73,000 cases of infection and 61 deaths per year in the United States.[11] It is typically associated with eating undercooked beef, but may also be spread by person-to-person contact from poor hand washing. The bacterium causes an inflammatory process in the colon that leads to sloughing of tissue in a bloody, mucoid diarrhea. The disease process is usually self-limiting if the patient is relatively healthy. However, patients younger than 5 years of age and older adults, or those with comorbidities, are at significantly greater risk for developing a more serious disease, hemolytic uremic syndrome, which causes massive red blood cell destruction and acute kidney injury.[11]

An additional cause of lower GI bleeding is diverticular disease. Diverticula are multiple small pouches in the colon. They are found in approximately 5% to 10% of the population, and are usually asymptomatic.[34] However, when the diverticula become filled with stool and develop inflammation, they may cause pain and bleeding, referred to as diverticulitis.

Hemorrhoids are another source of lower GI bleeds. Whereas GI bleeding related to esophageal and gastric varices is widely recognized, hemorrhoids may also be caused by portal hypertension (which causes dilation) and may leak or rupture, although much less frequently. In addition, hemorrhoids may simply be caused by chronic straining to have a bowel movement and may be of little consequence, other than the associated pain.

PREVENTION

Prevention of GI bleeding usually focuses on the underlying pathology, rather than the bleeding itself. Examples of prevention strategies include colorectal screening for occult blood and the use of PPIs in critically ill patients.[2,3] Additionally, patients with a known personal or family history or risk for a specific disease, such as colon cancer, may be routinely assessed with endoscopy to catch the disease state early. GERD may be prevented by several medications, such as antacids and histamine H2-receptor blockers; PPIs are currently the treatment of choice.[2,3]

The ubiquitous use of NSAIDs has had a major impact on the development of upper GI bleeding, and may be implicated in up to10% of upper GI bleeds.[26] NSAIDs are also associated with lower GI pathology, such as gut inflammation and bleeding. Whereas cyclooxygenase 2 (COX-2) inhibitors provide a significant decrease in the incidence of GI bleeding compared to NSAIDs; the increased number of cardiovascular deaths related to COX-2 inhibitors has tempered this advantage over NSAIDs. Even low-dose aspirin taken for its cardioprotective effect is associated with an increased incidence of GI bleeding. Ten to fifteen percent of hospital admissions for GI bleeding are associated with long-term, low-dose aspirin use.[26] Despite current recommendations to substitute clopidogrel (Plavix) for aspirin in patients with aspirin-induced gastric bleeding, clopidogrel had a higher bleeding rate when compared to aspirin with esomeprazole (Nexium), a PPI.[12] Goldstein, Huang, Amer et al. also found that adding a PPI for patients taking NSAIDs significantly decreased the incidence of bleeding episodes.[15] Medications used to treat GI bleeding are outlined in Table 16.1.

H. pylori is a significant cause of both gastric and duodenal ulcers, but because it is so prevalent, preventive therapy is not likely to have an effect on ulcer formation in the general population.[19] However, eradication of *H. pylori* should be provided if a patient has additional risk factors, such as chronic NSAID usage or a history of ulcers.[19]

With esophageal and gastric varices, prevention is focused on stopping both the initial and subsequent bleeding episodes. Surgical shunting of blood away from the liver with a portacaval shunt has been effective in preventing the initial bleeding episode, but this procedure is associated with greater operative mortality and increased encephalopathy.[6] Although endoscopic banding may prevent bleeding, there are not enough data to recommend this procedure for all patients.

Pharmacologic therapy consists of medications that reduce portal pressure by decreasing portal inflow or by decreasing resistance within the liver.[6] Nonselective beta blockade has been shown to decrease both the risk of bleeding and the number of bleeding-related deaths by allowing alpha-adrenergic constriction of the mesenteric arterioles, reducing portal venous flow.[6,48] However, beta blockers must be taken continually, or the varices will rebleed.[48] Long-acting nitrates, which cause systemic vasodilation, may be useful for those who are unable to tolerate beta blockage or who do not respond to it.[14,35] Various combinations of therapies have been studied, and a variety of findings were produced. Studies have found that band ligation was more effective than beta blockade in patients with cirrhosis.[28] One study using endoscopy to prevent an initial bleeding episode had to be stopped prematurely because of a significant (60%) bleeding rate, identified by the authors as being iatrogenic.[45]

Stress ulcer prevention in the critical care unit may pose significant risk of nosocomial pneumonia and *C. difficile*–associated diarrhea, and does not significantly improve mortality in critically ill patients.[9] Therefore, prevention strategies must be carefully considered and a treatment should be considered prior to initiation to evaluate the patient's comorbidities and potential for GI bleeding.[9]

TABLE 16.1 **Medications Used in Gastrointestinal Bleeding**

Medication	Actions	Dosage	Special Considerations
Esomeprazole (Nexium)	Proton pump inhibitor; reduces gastric acid secretion	20–40 mg/d PO for 4–8 weeks; maintenance dose of 20 mg/d PO	Should not be taken for more than 6 months No more than 20 mg/d in patients with severe hepatic failure Give 1 h before meals
Isosorbide mononitrate (Imdur)	Decreases blood pressure and subsequent gastrointestinal intravascular pressure	20 mg twice a day with approximately 7 h between doses; 30–120 mg of extended-release tablets once a day	*Significant* hypotension possible if used with sildenafil, tadalafil, or vardenafil May cause postural hypotension
Propranolol (Inderal)	Decreases blood pressure and subsequent gastrointestinal intravascular pressure	Initially, 80 mg PO divided into two doses or one extended-release form Maintenance dose of 120–240 mg daily or 120–160 mg of extended-release form	Use with caution in patients receiving calcium channel blockers or cardiac glycosides Avoid with haloperidol Contraindicated in patients with bronchial asthma, or with heart rates <60 beats/min
Omeprazole (Prilosec)	Proton pump inhibitor; blocks formation of gastric acid by competitive binding of secretory surface of gastric parietal cells	20–40 mg daily for most conditions; doses of 120 mg TID given in patients with pathologic hypersecretory conditions (e.g., Zollinger-Ellison syndrome)	Avoid giving with medications requiring low gastric pH (e.g., ampicillin, iron, ketoconazole), as poor absorption may occur
Octreotide (Sandostatin)	Decreases both splanchnic blood flow and portal vein pressure, allowing coagulation to take place	25–50 mcg/h continuous IV infusion for up to 5 days	May cause bradycardia; dysrhythmias; and glucose, fluid, and electrolyte imbalances
Vasopressin (Pitressin)	Decreases bleeding from varices by systemic vasoconstriction, which also decreases splanchnic blood flow and portal vein pressure	0.4 unit/min continuous IV infusion up to 1 unit/min	May cause hypertension and myocardial ischemia

PO, Per os (by mouth); *TID,* three times per day.

ASSESSMENT

Physical Assessment Findings

Patients with GI bleeding often present without pain. The initial assessment should focus on circulation, airway, and breathing. Establishing a baseline regarding hemodynamic stability, including the standard vital signs of heart rate, blood pressure, respiratory rate, pulse oximetry, temperature, and level of consciousness, must be accomplished as soon as possible, and may be helpful in determining the amount of blood lost.[41] If the patient is able to tolerate changes in position, orthostatic changes in blood pressure and heart rate may provide additional information. Frequent reassessments of these vital signs are important to determine significant changes and to establish a trend. Other assessments may provide additional information regarding the stability of the patient. As previously noted, pain is often not present with GI bleeding. However, if there is peritoneal irritation caused by a perforation of the GI tract, the abdomen may exhibit rigidity (increased abdominal wall muscle tone), guarding (spasm of abdominal wall muscles, detected on palpation), or both. Whereas both rigidity and guarding may indicate the need for immediate surgical evaluation, bleeding confined to the interior of the GI tract will not usually cause such symptoms. In addition, older adults are less likely to exhibit rigidity or guarding, as a result of the decreased muscle tone and changes in the sympathetic nervous system that occur with aging.

GI bleeding may initially present in many ways (Fig. 16.5). The bleeding may be found with a guaiac test of gastric contents or stool that reveals trace amounts of blood, as frank bright red vomitus, or the passage of bright red, bloody stool. Blood loss identified by guaiac testing requires a loss of more than 10 mL/day. Guaiac-positive stools may be found up to 2 weeks after the bleeding has stopped.[34] An underappreciated subtlety of guaiac testing is that the cards for testing vomitus and stool are separate and distinct, and cannot be used interchangeably. Bleeding from either the upper or the lower GI tract may also be significant and represent a life-threatening episode. Bright red blood in vomit is referred to as *hematemesis.* Hematemesis that is consistent in appearance with coffee grounds indicates that the blood has been in the stomach for a significant length of time, where the digestive enzymes have partially digested it. When hematemesis has occurred, placement of a nasogastric (NG) or orogastric (OG) tube for aspiration may be helpful in initially identifying the level of bleeding.[34]

When bright red blood comes from the rectum, it is referred to as *hematochezia.* Maroon, semi-liquid stools usually represent a bleeding site that is in the proximal colon (ascending or transverse). Blood loss may take the form of melena, which is stool that is black and tarry with a very distinct odor. Melena represents blood in the GI tract that has been altered by the intestinal juices, usually from the upper GI tract (Table 16.2).

Bleeding into and from the GI tract may be subtle and insidious, causing an iron deficiency anemia over time. Of greater concern is the rapid loss of significant amounts of blood from any source. Hypovolemia caused by the blood loss may be compensated for a time, but eventually, if the bleeding is not stopped, the patient will begin to display signs of hypovolemic shock.

An additional component of GI bleeding is the effect of the blood on the GI tract itself. Blood from the GI tract may range in color and consistency from bright red and liquid, to maroon

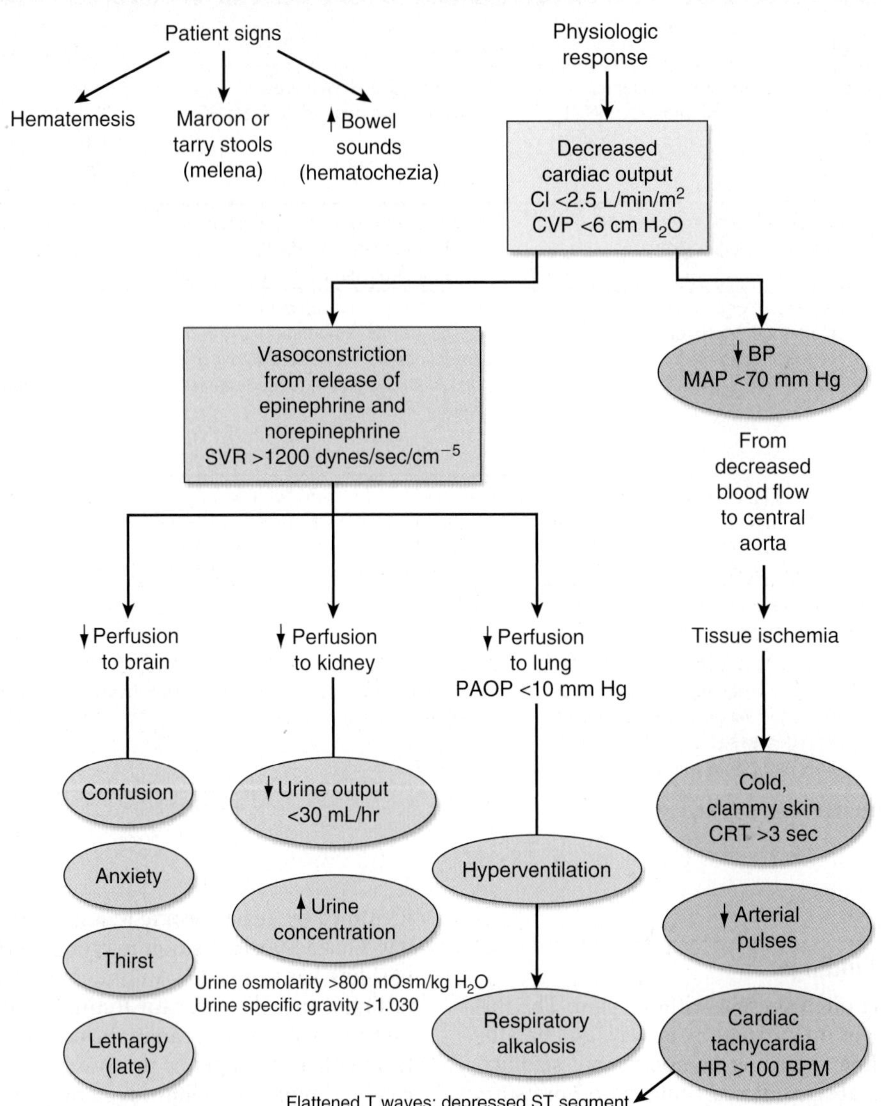

FIG. 16.5 Presentation of gastrointestinal bleeding. *BP,* Blood pressure; *BPM,* beats per minute; *CI,* cardiac index; *CRT,* capillary refill time; *CVP,* central venous pressure; *HR,* heart rate; *MAP,* mean arterial pressure; *PAOP,* pulmonary artery occlusion pressure; *SVR,* systemic vascular resistance.

TABLE 16.2 Presentations of Gastrointestinal Bleeding

Presentation	Definition
Acute bleeding	
Hematemesis	Bloody vomitus; either fresh, bright red blood or dark, grainy digested blood with "coffee grounds" appearance
Melena	Black, sticky, tarry, foul-smelling stools caused by digestion of blood in the gastrointestinal tract
Hematochezia	Fresh, bright red blood passed from rectum
Occult bleeding	Trace amounts of blood in normal-appearing stools or gastric secretions; detectable only with guaiac test

Data from Reference 41.

and semi-liquid, to black and tarry. The transitions in color and consistency are dictated by the length of time the blood is exposed to the digestive enzymes. In addition, the presence of blood within the GI tract will usually increase peristalsis, sometimes dramatically, resulting in diarrhea and incontinence of stool. If the source of the bleeding is in the upper GI tract, it will often cause vomiting. However, if the blood passes into, or originates in, the lower GI tract, its high osmotic load will cause its rapid passage, resulting in diarrhea or incontinence of stool.

The patient with GI bleeding may be completely asymptomatic or may be in hypovolemic shock from massive bleeding. Although the symptoms and physical assessment findings may suggest the type of disease process, they should always be confirmed with diagnostic studies. If pain is present, it is usually related to the underlying pathology. Upper GI bleeding caused by GERD or ulcers is often manifested by chronic indigestion, which usually increases in intensity over time before the initial bleeding episode. The upper abdominal pain associated with GERD typically occurs shortly after eating and may be increased by overeating, coughing, or assuming a recumbent position immediately after eating. The pain associated with gastric and duodenal ulcers is quite similar, as it is intermittent in nature, located in the upper abdomen, and relieved by antacids. However, pain from gastric ulcers may occur immediately after eating, whereas pain from duodenal ulcers usually begins when the stomach has emptied or at night, and then resolves by morning.

Patients with Crohn's disease typically have little pain, but the chronic inflammation of a section of the colon may produce some regional tenderness. The pain of ulcerative colitis, on the other hand, may range from vague discomfort to continuous cramping pain. Infections with *E. coli* 0157:H7 are not usually associated with pain, even though the patient may experience abdominal cramping. Patients with colorectal cancer may have pain, but it is usually a late sign. Hemorrhoids usually cause pain only during bowel movements with the passage of stool across the inflamed tissues.

If blood is deposited into the stomach from any source, it will usually result in nausea, retching, and vomiting. With varices, the bleeding may be insidious over a prolonged time, or the varix may rupture, causing a rapid loss of blood into the stomach, which represents a true emergency. Because the blood from a ruptured varix is venous, it is typically dark red. However, even though the source of the bleeding is venous, the back pressure from the portal hypertension may rapidly exsanguinate the patient. Bleeding from gastric or duodenal ulcers may be subtle and insidious as well, but may also become life-threatening if the ulcer penetrates into the blood vessels that are laced throughout the mucosal and muscular walls of stomach and duodenum.

As with bleeding from the upper GI tract, bleeding from the colon or rectum may be either subtle or massive. Minor bleeding may be found with Crohn's disease, but the seemingly small amounts of blood loss may lead to significant anemia over time. Bleeding is more prevalent in ulcerative colitis, especially with severe disease. Bleeding with colorectal cancer may also range from the subtle to the massive, especially in advanced cases. Bleeding from diverticulitis usually stops spontaneously, but the site may rebleed 20% to 30% of the time.[34] Blood from the ascending and transverse colon is usually dark red in color, whereas bleeding from the descending colon and rectum is bright red and usually on the surface of the stool, rather than mixed into it. Typically, the brighter red the blood, the more distal the bleeding source in the colon. Although hemorrhoids may cause bleeding, they usually do not represent a significant threat to the patient, unless they are caused by portal hypertension.

Laboratory Findings

The traditional use of measurement of hematocrit and hemoglobin levels may not provide an adequate evaluation of the scope of the blood loss because red blood cells (RBCs) and plasma are lost in equal proportion.[41] Additionally, with volume resuscitation, the hematocrit and hemoglobin levels will usually begin to decrease. On the complete blood count (CBC), the mean corpuscular volume (MCV) and the red blood cell distribution width (RDW) should also be noted. A low MCV and an elevated RDW suggest the presence of iron deficiency anemia and a chronic bleed or an acute-on-chronic GI bleed. A low platelet count may suggest the presence of portal hypertension.[41] Coagulation studies will allow the establishment of a baseline and provide data to track trends over time. Typing and cross-matching of the patient's blood to banked blood provides for the rapid transfusion of blood, should it be necessary.[34] Blood urea nitrogen (BUN) levels may be elevated because of the digestion and absorption of the protein in the blood as it passes through the small intestine, usually within 24 hours. However, this same phenomenon does not occur with bleeding originating in the colon, because digestion does not occur in the colon.[41]

Identification of an *H. pylori* infection can be determined either by invasive tests that sample the gut flora or by noninvasive tests (e.g., serologic, saliva, stool, or urine tests) to determine the presence of an IgG antibody specific to *H. pylori*. The most frequently used test is the rapid urea test (RUT), an invasive test performed during endoscopy. The RUT can determine the presence of *H. pylori* but is influenced by blood in the stomach, and caution must be taken to eliminate that factor. The noninvasive C-urea breath test (UBT) is the recommended test since it is not affected by blood in the stomach and can accurately diagnose *H. pylori*.[19]

Radiology Findings

Conventional radiographs are still relevant, but are generally less sensitive and specific for disease compared with more advanced cross-sectional imaging studies, such as ultrasonography, computed tomography (CT), and magnetic resonance imaging (MRI). Flat-plate abdominal x-rays may be used to identify the presence of as little as 5 mL of free air in the peritoneal space. Such a finding indicates that a perforation of the stomach or the small bowel has occurred. However, the flat-plate abdominal x-ray cannot detect or differentiate between blood and other types of fluid in the gut or in the peritoneal space.

Radiology studies using barium have a long history in identifying and quantifying GI disease. In the case of GI bleeding, such studies may be able to identify the source (such as a gastric or duodenal ulcer) and are safer and less invasive than endoscopy. Enteroclysis, sometimes referred to as small bowel follow through, is performed by filling the small bowel with contrast medium through a catheter advanced nasally or orally into the duodenum or jejunum; this procedure may provide an effective evaluation of bleeding in the small bowel, but has mostly been replaced by CT and MRI.[49]

CT and MRI are used with intravenous contrast (angiography) to identify sources of GI bleeding that may be difficult to identify by other means. This is particularly true with bleeding that has defied location by endoscopy. A unique aspect of CT is the use of digital reconstruction of the interior lumen of the GI tract. CT is more likely to be used because there are usually fewer restrictions associated with a CT compared to an MRI (i.e., scanning speed, issues with ferrous metals, and confined patient space).

Angiography, using radiopaque contrast media and fluoroscopy, may be very useful in identifying obscure or unknown sources of GI bleeding. However, a bleeding rate of greater than 0.5 mL/min must be present before an arterial bleeding site can be identified with angiography.[34] In addition to traditional fluoroscopy, both CT and MRI may also be used as platforms for angiography. Scintigraphy, the use of radionuclide contrast media and imagery, may also be used to identify a bleeding source and can identify bleeding sources with rates as low as 0.1 mL/min.[34]

Diagnostic Evaluations

Although contrast studies may find a bleeding lesion, some method of treatment must then be undertaken. Endoscopy is at the forefront of assessing and treating GI bleeding, as it offers the opportunity to directly visualize the lesion, remove samples for biopsy and study, and deliver therapy directly to the lesion.

Endoscopy is used when the patient presents with signs and symptoms indicating pathology that could be evaluated or treated, such as GI bleeding. It may also be used when other studies (e.g., contrast studies) are unable to identify the cause of the bleeding. The endoscope may be introduced into the upper GI tract through the mouth (esophagogastroduodenoscopy [EGD]) or into the colon (colonoscopy).

EGD provides rapid and effective assessment and treatment of upper GI bleeding sources in the vast majority of cases. An EGD should be performed within 24 hours of admission or earlier, depending on the hemodynamic stability.[4,32,36] EGD provides assessment and treatment, and may help predict the incidence of rebleeding. EGD should be considered whenever there is active upper GI bleeding. Although some clinicians prefer to perform gastric lavage (via an NG or OG tube) before the endoscopy to increase visibility, others believe that it may produce artifacts.[21] While gastric lavage may be helpful in clearing the stomach of blood, it has not been proven to stop bleeding; and iced gastric lavage may actually prolong bleeding and increase the clotting time.[34] Should lavage be considered, it is important to use warmed normal saline or lactated Ringer's solution to prevent hypothermia and the potentially significant loss of electrolytes in the lavage solution. Tap water may be used for the lavage, but its low osmolality may draw electrolytes out of the circulatory system into the stomach, where they are removed when the lavage solution is withdrawn from the stomach.

Care must be taken to ensure the patient's safety during the procedure. For patients who are actively bleeding, endoscopy should be completed in the critical care unit or the emergency department, where emergency intubation and respiratory management can be quickly accomplished, if needed. For those patients with relatively slow or inactive GI bleeding who are hemodynamically stable, the procedure may be performed in an endoscopy suite.

Endoscopy for lower GI bleeding is less straightforward. Patients with active bleeding and hematochezia or melena should have an EGD completed initially to eliminate the upper GI tract as the source of the bleeding. Traditionally, colonoscopy has been used only after adequate bowel preparation. However, some clinicians complete the test without bowel preparation in an early attempt to locate the source of active bleeding, often with guidance from angiography or scintigraphy, to approximate the bleeding location.[27]

A *capsule endoscopy*, in which a small video capsule is swallowed and passes through the entire GI tract, is an additional method that can be used to assess the distal small bowel, which is beyond the reach of endoscopes. As the capsule moves through the small bowel, the device transmits two images per second to a receiver carried by the patient. Whereas the quality of the video picture rivals that of traditional endoscopes, the passive images obtained may miss lesions due to obstructions from bile and mucus.[13,23] The process usually takes approximately 4 hours to complete, and is therefore not generally utilized in patients with acute GI bleeds.

PLAN OF CARE

The initial treatment of GI bleeding will depend on several factors, including the amount of blood loss, the time over which the blood was lost, the patient's response to the loss, and any underlying medical conditions, including comorbidities (Fig. 16.6). In addition, the risk of rebleeding should be assessed. Increased

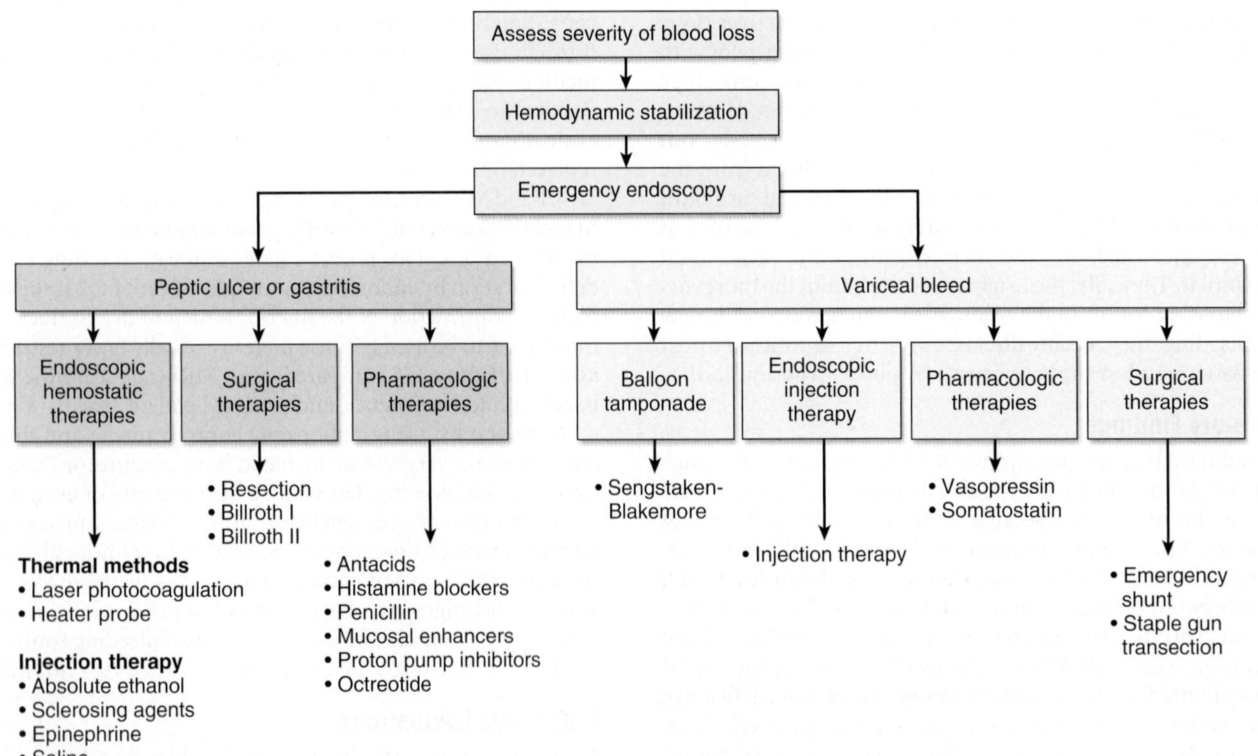

FIG. 16.6 Algorithm for guiding treatment of gastrointestinal bleeding.

risk is seen with older age, bleeding onset in the hospital, medical comorbidities, shock, coagulopathy, and the need for multiple blood transfusions.[22]

The prime consideration in an acutely ill patient with a GI bleed is to establish hemodynamic stability as quickly as possible.[36,41] Typically, significant blood loss will result in hypovolemic shock. Adequate fluid resuscitation should be provided using two large-bore (18-gauge or larger) peripheral IV catheters. Patients should receive rapidly infused crystalloid fluid to correct hypovolemia.[41] No more than 2 liters of crystalloid should be infused before switching to blood products at a 1:1:1 ratio of packed RBCs to fresh frozen plasma to units of platelets.[17] Blood transfusions may be required to assist with hemodynamic stability; however, the hemoglobin (Hgb) level threshold is controversial.[36] Some data indicate that a Hgb value of 7 g/dL produces improved results, and that overtransfusion may lead to rebound portal hypertension in patients with cirrhosis, causing further bleeding.[4,14,36,47] Although a Hgb value of 7 may be acceptable for most patients, patients with massive bleeding or ischemia may need a higher level. Caution must be taken when using Hgb levels to monitor patients with massive bleeding, due to the hemodilution that occurs when fluids are rapidly infused.[36] The use of recombinant clotting factor VIIa has also been shown to be effective in decreasing acute bleeding treatment failures in patients with significant liver disease.[5]

If massive hematemesis is present and the patient's airway is unable to be protected, endotracheal intubation should be rapidly accomplished.[36] When the bleeding is massive, a limited endoscopic evaluation may help pinpoint the source of the bleeding and facilitate further treatment, including surgical intervention. An NG or OG tube may be considered to clear blood from the bleeding site before endoscopy, but should not be used in an attempt to stop the bleeding by lavage.[4,41] Studies have failed to show a clear benefit on clinical outcomes for using an NG or OG tube, and NG tube insertion has been rated as the most painful commonly performed procedure.[41] Using IV erythromycin as an alternative to improving visibility has been found to be effective, as it appears to induce antral contractions and accelerate gastric emptying.[31] Once the patient has been stabilized, and the source of the bleeding has been identified, definitive treatment to stop the bleeding can be initiated.

Endoscopy, either as an EGD or as a colonoscopy, is the primary avenue for diagnosing and providing treatment options for GI bleeding in both the upper and the lower GI tract.[48] However, there are some differences in procedure based on the anatomy and the pathophysiology involved.

There are several endoscopic methods employed to stop bleeding. Injections of various substances (e.g., alcohol, epinephrine, saline, and various sclerosants) into the bleeding site will cause scarring or vasoconstriction and will stop the bleeding. Epinephrine is the most commonly used due to its low cost and wide availability. Injections are placed around and into the bleeding site and produce a local tamponade effect, as well as vasoconstriction.[8] Current clinical guidelines recommend using epinephrine in combination with another method due to its suboptimal efficacy.[4] Sclerosants, such as ethanol, produce local inflammation and subsequent fibrosis, but caution must be used to avoid tissue necrosis and perforation.[8]

Coagulation of the bleeding area or vessel with a laser or thermal probe is also effective. Isolation of the bleeding varix can be accomplished with various mechanical devices (i.e., clips or bands) that occlude the blood flow into the bleeding site.[48] Clips resemble simple staples, whereas bands resemble small rubber bands. Both types of devices are secured at the base of the varix, occluding its blood supply. Clinical guidelines recommend a combination of these methods.[4,7,48] Studies have shown that outcomes were not significantly different when bleeding varices were treated with epinephrine injection and thermal coagulation compared to ligation with clips.[38,47] Clips may be useful in patients who are on anticoagulants, and may produce more rapid healing then thermal methods.[7]

Adding omeprazole (Prilosec) to endoscopic therapy significantly decreases rebleeding episodes.[4,43] Bacterial infection can be a significant complication of endoscopy, and Hou et al. demonstrated that antibiotic prophylaxis significantly decreases both infection and rebleeding in patients with esophageal varices.[18]

Endoscopic procedures are both warranted and safe when performed on patients who are currently on antithrombotic regimens, provided that consideration is given to the risk of temporary interruption of the drugs.[1,4] In addition, medications should be promptly restarted when hemostasis is assured, or temporary bridge therapy should be provided if hemostasis is uncertain.[1] Novel oral anticoagulants (NOACs), such as dabigatran (Pradaxa), edoxaban (Savaysa), rivaroxaban (Xarelto), and apixaban (Eliquis), generally have a short half-life. Therefore, aggressive fluid resuscitation to allow for maximal renal excretion, holding the next dose, and use of coagulation factors (i.e., fresh frozen plasma or recombinant activated factor VII) may be helpful to decrease the risk of the procedure. Restarting the medication as soon as possible after hemostasis is achieved is recommended.[1,4] The Food and Drug Administration (FDA) has approved idarucizumab (Praxbind) as the first reversal agent specifically for dabigatran.[33]

Bleeding from a Mallory-Weiss tear is usually self-limiting and 80% to 90% of patients will stop bleeding spontaneously.[34] Occasionally, patients will require endoscopic procedures to stop the bleeding, using injection or coagulation therapies, with angiography and embolic therapy being reserved for those patients who rebleed.

Although esophageal and gastric varices may be treated endoscopically with both injection and coagulation therapies, medications such as octreotide (Sandostatin) and vasopressin (Pitressin) may be used systemically before the endoscopy in an attempt to slow the bleeding and allow endoscopic therapies to be pursued.[6,40] Octreotide decreases the amount of both splanchnic blood flow and portal vein pressure, allowing coagulation to take place. Octreotide is administered intravenously with an initial bolus of 25 to 100 mcg, followed by a continuous infusion of 25 to 50 mcg per hour. Because it controls bleeding in approximately 85% of bleeding varices, octreotide should be considered early in the course of treatment.[40] Vasopressin decreases bleeding from varices by systemic vasoconstriction, which also decreases splanchnic blood flow and portal vein pressure.[6] However, because it exerts its effects systematically, vasopressin can cause hypertension, and may induce myocardial ischemia and peripheral vasoconstriction. The hypertension associated with vasopressin may be treated with the addition of IV nitroglycerin to keep the systolic blood pressure between 90 and 100 mm Hg. Nitroglycerin decreases the systemic hypertension associated with vasopressin without affecting the splanchnic blood flow and pressure, and is more effective than vasopressin alone.[6]

Endoscopy has been established as the treatment of choice for bleeding esophageal varices, using both sclerosing agents (solutions injected into the bleeding sites that cause thrombosis and obliteration) and thermal coagulation modalities.[6] In addition, endoscopy allows the use of ligation or banding of the varices, which strangulates the defect, allowing it to slough off in time (Fig. 16.7). Banding with small "O" rings has evolved as the premier method for treating esophageal varices because of its quick application and lower complication rates compared to sclerotherapy, which may cause transmural damage to the esophagus.[6] Once the acute bleeding episode has been treated successfully, repeated endoscopy procedures are performed to obliterate all of the existing varices, significantly preventing rebleeding episodes. An additional benefit of banding is the rapidity with which the varices can be treated, limiting the number of procedures the patient must endure.[6]

Gastric varices usually bleed less often than esophageal varices, but the blood loss is often greater. Whereas banding and various modes of sclerotherapy are appropriate, use of a tissue adhesive (various forms of cyanoacrylate) that activates when it comes into contact with blood may be a safe alternative. However, there are multiple reports of significant adverse events associated with this therapy, including embolization and vessel wall ulceration.[8,37] Therefore, use of tissue adhesive should be limited to rescue therapy in selected patients with refractory nonvariceal bleeding who fail conventional endoscopic therapies.[8]

Because endoscopic treatment of gastric varices has a limited success rate and a significant rebleeding rate, other modes of therapy may be indicated to decrease the pressure being exerted on the gastric venous complex. One surgical option is the transjugular intrahepatic portosystemic shunt (TIPS) procedure. TIPS is the treatment of choice for patients who fail standard therapy with combination vasoactive drugs and endoscopic therapy, but carries risks of worsening liver function, encephalopathy, and 30% mortality at 30 days.[6,16]

A type of device that has become less common but still may have a place in caring for patients bleeding from esophageal or gastric varices is balloon tamponade (BT) therapy. This procedure may be used as a temporary bridge to TIPS, but is associated with serious complications in more than 20% of patients.[6] The devices, which consist of combinations of esophageal and gastric balloons (Sengstaken-Blakemore and Minnesota tubes), are also equipped with various suction ports to allow evacuation of blood from the esophagus or stomach (Fig. 16.8). The devices are effective in stopping bleeding, but rely on mechanical compression. Therefore, if the tubes are removed prematurely, the bleeding may resume. These devices are typically

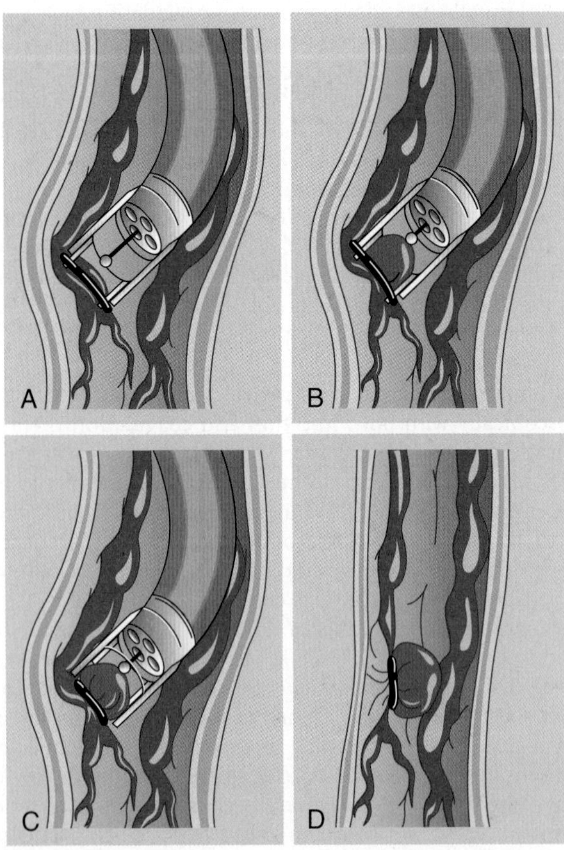

FIG. 16.7 Endoscopic variceal ligation technique. **A**, The endoscope, with an attached ligating device, is brought into contact with the varix just above the gastroesophageal junction. **B**, Suction is applied, pulling the varix-containing mucosa into the dead space created at the end of the endoscope. **C**, A tripwire is pulled, releasing the band around the aspirated tissue. **D**, Ligation is completed.

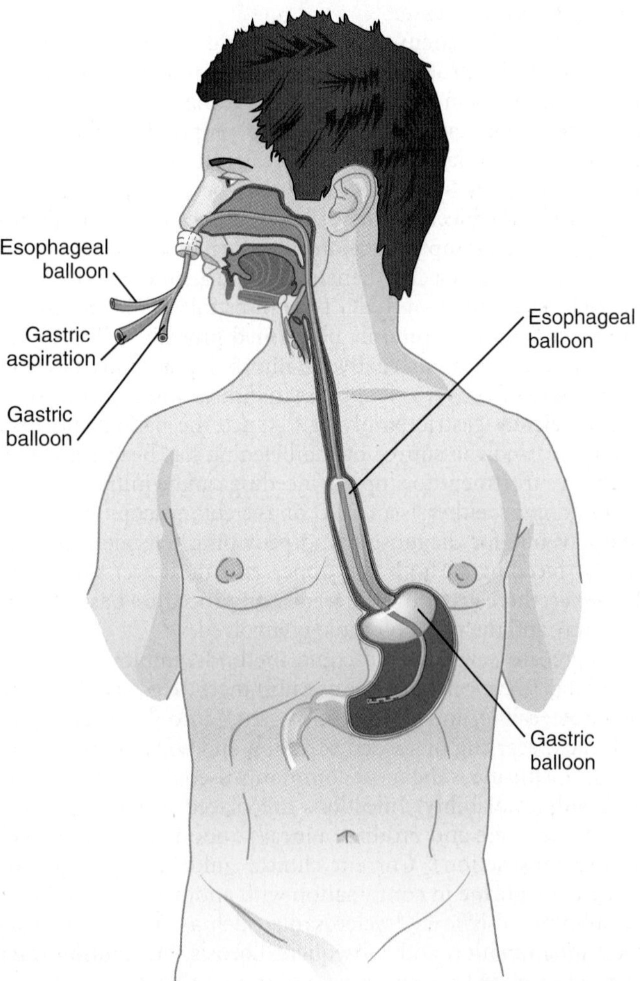

FIG. 16.8 Balloon tamponade therapy: Sengstaken-Blakemore tube in place, with both the esophageal and gastric balloons inflated.

employed when there are no readily available endoscopic therapies. In addition, they are technically difficult to maintain safely, and have the potential for many complications. A reference for using the device is found in the *AACN Procedure Manual for Critical Care.*[10]

Another emerging treatment option is a removable, covered, self-expanding metal stent that can be placed without the need for endoscopy.[16] The stent is placed at the gastroesophageal junction, and remains in place while the liver function recovers and secondary prophylaxis is initiated. A study that compared stent placement with BT reported that both methods achieve hemostasis, although the stent performed better in refractory bleeding.[16]

Gastric and duodenal ulcers are also typically treated with injection or coagulation endoscopy. Whereas ligation with a clip may be used for ulcers, Lin et al. found that injection sclerotherapy and thermal coagulation usually produce better outcomes.[29] Both techniques appear to be equally effective.[8] However, stress ulcers are much less likely to be successfully treated with endoscopy.[34]

Because of the impact of *H. pylori* on the formation of ulcers, the recommended treatment regimen is triple therapy, which includes a PPI to decrease acid production and two antibiotics to eliminate the pathogen. Alternatives may include sequential therapy, bismuth- or non-bismuth–based quadruple therapy, and levofloxacin-based regimens.[19] Selective therapy to eradicate *H. pylori* is more effective for duodenal ulcers than for gastric ulcers. Eradication of *H. pylori* is cost-effective for gastric ulcers, and can achieve a 91% eradication rate and a 97% ulcer healing rate in bleeding peptic ulcers.[19] Eradication treatment may decrease the likelihood of peptic ulcer rebleeding and associated complications.

Colonoscopy uses the same techniques to stop bleeding in the lower GI tract. Whereas hematochezia usually indicates bleeding from the lower GI tract, approximately 10% of the time the source is found in the upper GI tract, necessitating an endoscopic evaluation of the upper GI tract as well as the colon. Even if the bleeding site is not located and addressed during the colonoscopy, identifying the specific section of the colon that is the source of the bleeding will enable the surgeon to have a more focused surgical approach.[34]

Some bleeding sites (e.g., diverticula and angiodysplasia) may be more appropriately treated with angiotherapy, using intra-arterial vasopressin (usually in much smaller doses than are used systemically) to cause vasospasm. Additionally, angiography may be used to deploy coils or Gelfoam into the vessel at the bleeding site, causing thrombosis.[34]

Those patients who do not respond to medical, endoscopic, or radiologic invasive therapies may require surgical intervention. When a patient remains hemodynamically unstable, rapid surgical intervention may be the most effective treatment. As part of the surgical approach, endoscopy may also be used intraoperatively to assist in identifying the source of the bleed.[34] The surgical techniques will vary depending upon the source of the bleeding. A standard therapy is "oversewing" of various ulcers, often combined with selective vagotomy, removal of the offending portion, and anastomosis of the surgical wounds. A vagotomy will sever portions of the vagus nerve where it enters the stomach, decreasing acid production, which is partially controlled by the vagus nerve. One exception to the surgical approach is stress ulcers, because they are often scattered throughout the gastric mucosa and do not lend themselves to surgical removal. Stress ulcers will rebleed after surgery approximately 50% of the time. Therefore prevention is certainly the preferable alternative.

CONCLUSION

Gastrointestinal bleeding is a significant cause of both mortality and morbidity in the critical care setting. These are some of the most challenging patients, involving resuscitation, diagnostics, and therapy to stop the bleeding. Often, the bleeding pathology occurs due to preventable causes. Depending on the source of the bleeding, multiple modes of therapy are appropriate for stopping the source of the bleeding and preventing its recurrence. Understanding the pathophysiology and various treatments provides a more complete understanding of the nurse's role in providing care for these complex patients.

REFERENCES

1. Abraham, N. S. (2015). Management of antiplatelet agents and anticoagulants in patients with gastrointestinal bleeding. *Gastrointest Endoscopy Clin N Am, 25*, 449–462.
2. Alhazzani, W., et al. (2013). Proton pump inhibitors versus histamine 2 receptor antagonists for stress ulcer prophylaxis in critically ill patients: a systematic review and meta-analysis. *Crit Care Med J, 41*(3), 693–705.
3. Bardou, M., et al. (2015). Stress related mucosal disease in the critically ill. *Nat Rev Gastroenterol Hepatol, 12*, 98–107.
4. Barkun, A. N., Bardou, M., Kuipers, E. J., Sung, J., Hunt, R. H., et al. (2010). International consensus recommendations on the management of patients with nonvariceal upper gastrointestinal bleeding. *Ann Intern Med, 152*, 101–113.
5. Bendtsen, F., D'Amico, G., Rusch, E., de Franchis, R., Andersen, P. K., et al. (2014). Effect of recombinant factor VIIa on outcome of acute variceal bleeding: an individual patient based meta-analysis of two controlled trials. *J Hepatol, 61*(2), 252–259.
6. Bhutta, A. Q., & Garcia-Tsao, G. (2015). The role of medical therapy for variceal bleeding. *Gastrointest Endosc Clin N Am, 25*(3), 479–490.
7. Brock, A. S., & Rockey, D. C. (2015). Mechanical hemostasis techniques in nonvariceal upper gastrointestinal bleeding. *Gastrointest Endoscopy Clin N Am, 25*, 523–533.
8. Bucci, C., Rotondano, G., & Marmo, R. (2015). Injection and cautery methods for nonvariceal bleeding control. *Gastrointest Endoscopy Clin N Am, 25*, 509–522.
9. Buendgens, L., Koch, A., & Tacke, F. (2016). Prevention of stress-related ulcer bleeding at the intensive care unit: risks and benefits of stress ulcer prophylaxis. *World J Crit Care Med, 5*(1), 57–64.
10. Bunzli, K. (2011). Esophagogastric tamponade tube. D. L. McHale Wiegand (Ed.), *AACN procedure manual for critical care* (6th ed) (pp. 947–957). St Louis: Saunders.
11. Centers for Disease Control and Prevention (CDC). (2015). *Escherichia coli 0157:H7*. http://www.cdc.gov/ecoli/general/index.html/.
12. Chan, F. K., et al. (2005). Clopidogrel versus aspirin and esomeprazole to prevent recurrent ulcer bleeding. *N Engl J Med, 352*, 238–244.
13. Colli, A., Gana, J. C., Turner, D., Yap, J., Adams-Webber, T., et al. (2014). Capsule endoscopy for the diagnosis of oesophageal varices in people with chronic liver disease or portal vein thrombosis. *Cochrane Database Syst Rev, 10*:CD008760.
14. Garcia-Tsao, G., & Bosch, J. (2010). Management of varices and variceal hemorrhage in cirrhosis. *NEJM, 362*, 823–832.
15. Goldstein, J. L., Huang, B., Amer, F., et al. (2004). Ulcer recurrence in high-risk patients receiving nonsteroidal anti-inflammatory drugs plus low-dose aspirin: results of a post HOC subanalysis. *Clin Ther, 26*, 1637–1643.
16. Hogan, B. J., & O'Beirne, J. P. (2016). Role of self-explanding metal stents in the management of variceal haemorrhage: hype or hope? *World J Gastrointest Endosc, 8*(1), 23–29.

17. Holcomb, J. B., Tilley, B. C., Baraniuk, S., et al. (2015). Transfusion of plasma, platelets, and red blood cells in a 1:1:1 vs a 1:1:2 ratio and mortality in patients with severe trauma: the PROPPR randomized clinical trial. *JAMA. 313*(5), 471–482.
18. Hou, M. C., et al. (2004). Antibiotic prophylaxis after endoscopic therapy prevents rebleeding in acute variceal hemorrhage: a randomized trial. *Hepatology, 39*, 746–753.
19. Huang, T. C., & Lee, C. L. (2014). Diagnosis, treatment, and outcome in patients with bleeding peptic ulcers and *Helicobacter pylori* infections. *BioMed Res Int*, 658108. http://dx.doi.org/10.1155/2014/658108.
20. Hunt, R. T., et al. (2012). Stress prophylaxis in intensive care unit patients and the role of enteral nutrition. *J Parenter Enteral Nutr, 36*(6), 721–731.
21. Jairath, V., Kahan, B. C., Logan, R. F., et al. (2012). Outcomes following acute nonvariceal upper gastrointestinal bleeding in relation to time to endoscopy: results from a nationwide study. *Endoscopy, 44*, 723–730.
22. Kovacs, T. O., & Jensen, D. M. (2011). Endoscopic therapy for severe ulcer bleeding. *Gastrointest Endosc Clin N Am, 21*, 681–696.
23. Kwack, W. G., & Lim, Y. J. (2016). Current status and research into overcoming limitations of capsule endoscopy. *Clin Endosc, 49*, 8–15.
24. Laine, L., et al. (2012). Management of patients for ulcer bleeding. *Am J Gastroenterol, 107*, 345–360.
25. Laine, L., Yang, H., Chang, S. C., et al. (2012). Trends for incidence of hospitalization and death due to GI complications in the United States from 2001 to 2009. *Am J Gastroenterol, 107*, 1190–1195.
26. Lanas, A., Carrera-Lasfuentes, P., Arguedas, Y., Garcia, S., Bujanda, L., et al. (2015). Risk of upper and lower gastrointestinal bleeding in patients taking nonsteroidal anti-inflammatory drugs, antiplatelet agents, or anticoagulants. *Clin Gastroenterol Hepatol, 13*(5), 906–912 e2.
27. Leung, W. K., Ho, S. S., Suen, B. Y., et al. (2012). Capsule endoscopy or angiography in patients with acute overt obscure gastrointestinal bleeding: a prospective randomized study with long-term follow-up. *Am J Gastroenterol, 107*, 1370–1376.
28. Li, L., Yu, C., & Li, Y. (2011). Endoscopic band ligation versus pharmacology therapy for variceal bleeding in cirrhosis: a meta-analysis. *Can J Gastroenterol, 25*, 147.
29. Lin, H. J., Perng, C. L., Sun, I. C., et al. (2003). Endoscopic haemoclip versus heater probe thermocoagulation plus hypertonic saline-epinephrine injection for peptic ulcer bleeding. *Dig Liver Dis, 35*, 898–902.
30. Mikami, D. J., & Muryama, K. M. (2015). Physiology and pathogenesis of gastroesophageal reflux disease. *Surg Clin North Am, 95*(3), 515–525.
31. Pateron, D., Vicaut, E., Debuc, E., et al. (2011). Erythromycin infusion or gastric lavage for upper gastrointestinal bleeding: a multicenter randomized controlled trial. *Ann Emerg Med, 57*, 582–589.
32. Pennazio, M. (2004). Small-bowel endoscopy. *Endoscopy, 36*, 32–41.
33. Pollack, C. V., Reilly, P. A., Eikelboom, J., Glund, S., Verhamme, P., et al. (2015). Idarucizumab for Dabigatran reversal. *N Engl J Med, 373*(6), 511–520.
34. Porter, R. F., Zuckerman, G. R., & Gyawali, C. P. (2012). Upper and lower gastrointestinal bleeding: principles of diagnosis and management. In R. S. Irwin, & J. M. Rippe (Eds.), *Intensive care medicine* (7th ed). Philadelphia: Lippincott Williams & Wilkins.
35. Porth, C. M., & Grossman, S. (2014). *Pathophysiology: concepts of altered health states*. Philadelphia: Lippincott Williams & Wilkins.
36. Rajala, M. W., & Ginsberg, G. G. (2015). Tips and tricks on how to optimally manage patients with upper gastrointestinal bleeding. *Gastrointest Endoscopy Clin N Am, 25*, 607–617.
37. Rios Castellanos, E., Seron, P., Gisbert, J. P., et al. (2015). Endoscopic injection of cyanoacrylate glue versus other endoscopic procedures for acute bleeding gastric varices in people with portal hypertension. *Cochrane Database Syst Rev*, May 12; CD010180.
38. Saltzman, J. R., et al. (2005). Prospective trial of endoscopic clips versus combination therapy in upper GI bleeding (PROTECCT—UGI bleeding). *Am J Gastroenterol, 100*, 1503–1508.
39. Sami, S. S., Al-Arajo, A., & Ragunath, K. (2013). Review article: gastrointestinal angiodysplasia—pathogenesis, diagnosis and management. *Aliment Pharmacol Ther, 39*(1), 15–34.
40. Seo, Y. S., Park, S. Y., Kim, M. Y., Kim, J. H., Park, J. Y., et al. (2014). Lack of difference among terlipressin, somatostatin, and octreotide in the control of acute gastroesophageal variceal hemorrhage. *Hepatology, 60*, 954–963.
41. Simon, T. G., Travis, A. C., & Saltzman, J. R. (2015). Initial assessment and resuscitation in nonvariceal upper gastrointestinal bleeding. *Gastrointest Endoscopy Clin N Am, 25*, 429–442.
42. Spahn, T. W., & Kucharzik, T. (2004). Modulating the intestinal immune system: the role of lymphotoxin and GALT organs. *Gut, 53*, 456–465.
43. Sreedharan, A., Martin, J., Leontiadis, G. I., et al. (2010). Proton pump inhibitor treatment initiated prior to endoscopic diagnosis in upper gastrointestinal bleeding. *Cochrane Database Syst Rev*, (7), CD005415.
44. Tepes, B., O'Connor, A., et al. (2012). Treatment of *Helicobactor pylori* infection 2012. *Helicobacter 2012, 17*(Suppl. 1), 36.
45. Triantos, C., et al. (2005). Primary prophylaxis of variceal bleeding in cirrhotics unable to take beta-blockers: a randomized trial of ligation. *Aliment Pharmacol Ther, 15*, 1435–1443.
46. Tursi, T. (2010). Use of B-blocker therapy to prevent primary bleeding of esophageal varices. *J Am Acad Nurs Pract, 22*(12), 640–647.
47. Villanueva, C., Colomo, A., Bosch, A., Concepcion, M., Hernandes-Gea, V., et al. (2013). Transfusion strategies for acute upper gastrointestinal bleeding. *N Engl J Med, 368*, 11–21.
48. Wilkins, T., Khan, N., Nabh, A., & Schade, R. (2012). Diagnosis and management of upper gastrointestinal bleeding. *Am Fam Physician, 85*(5), 469–476.
49. Yeh, B. M., Carucci, L. R., Fidler, J. L., et al. (2011). Luminal imaging in the 21st century. *Am J Roentgenol, 197*, 28–29.

17

Liver Dysfunction and Failure

Rhonda K. Martin

INTRODUCTION

The liver is the largest internal organ of the human body, weighing 1200 to 1500 grams and performing more than 8000 defined functions.[5] The complexity of the liver's role means that alterations in function can cause a myriad of multisystem problems, whether the alteration is related to acute or chronic liver disease or to multisystem organ dysfunction.

Liver dysfunction is usually clinically defined by the presence of jaundice, ascites, or hepatic encephalopathy (HE), evident by an increase in the levels of liver injury enzymes (aspartate transaminase [AST]/alanine transaminase [ALT]), total or direct bilirubin, and the international normalized ratio (INR).[11,28]

ACUTE LIVER FAILURE

Acute liver failure, or ALF (formerly known as *fulminant liver failure*), is defined by the occurrence of jaundice and any degree of mental alteration (e.g., HE) in a patient without preexisting liver disease who has had an illness of less than 26-week duration.[51,73,84] It is a rapidly progressive clinical syndrome caused by massive hepatic necrosis leading to the development of severe hepatic failure. The onset of jaundice usually precedes the onset of encephalopathy in these cases. Paradoxically, the shorter the period from the onset of jaundice to hepatic coma, the better the prognosis.[84]

There are approximately 2000 cases of ALF in the United States each year, often affecting young adults and, more commonly, women (73%).[51,61] The most common cause of ALF has changed in recent years. In 1969, the most frequent cause of ALF was hepatitis B.[61] In 2013, the most common cause changed to drug-induced liver injury (DILI). DILI is divided into two categories: intrinsic, or drugs capable of liver injury in sufficiently high doses, and idiosyncratic, a less common form, where drugs cause ALF in susceptible individuals, and is less related to dose.[17] Common drugs involved in the intrinsic form include acetaminophen and organic solvents. For the idiosyncratic form, agents include isoniazid, fluoroquinolones, anticonvulsants, antidepressants, statins, ecstasy, cocaine, herbal supplements, and weight loss agents. The most common causes of DILI in the United States are acetaminophen toxicity (39%) and idiosyncratic hypersensitivity drug reactions (13%). Other ALF causes include hepatitis B, autoimmune liver disease, shock/hypoperfusion, Wilson's disease (a dysfunction of copper metabolism), and mushroom poisoning, usually with *Amanita phalloides*.[33,74]

Survival statistics for ALF have markedly improved in the last 3 decades. Hospital survival for ALF between 1973 and 1978 was between 15% to 17%; survival improved from 17% to 48% between 2004 and 2008.[85] The ALF Study group reported that of all ALF cases reviewed, 43% were spontaneous survivors without transplant, 23% died without transplant, and 69% of acetaminophen cases were spontaneous survivors. Of the 28% of patients who received a liver transplant for ALF, 84% had short-term survival.[50] Proposed reasons for these statistical changes are declines in hepatitis A and B due to vaccines and antivirals, increased awareness of proper acetaminophen dose, reduction in compounding acetaminophen in medications, and improvement in ALF management and referral to specialty centers.[85]

The most important factors in the treatment of ALF are to identify the cause, provide initial stabilization, early consultation, and referral to a liver tertiary or transplant center to evaluate overall prognosis for recovery and need for liver transplantation.[50,55] N-acetylcysteine (Mucomyst) is used in DILI. It rapidly restores the depleted glutathione stores in the liver that are used for drug metabolism, and supports hepatic mitochondrial function. It has been shown to be effective even when started late after drug ingestion.[17]

These cases are often devastating to patients and families because of the rapid onset, urgent need for liver transplantation, or progression to coma and death. Families need to be informed of the potential poor prognosis and possible need for transplant and kept involved in the decision-making process. A detailed history, including onset of symptoms, psychiatric history, and doses of all prescribed and over-the-counter medications, street drugs, and herbal and dietary supplements, is critical to diagnosis and management.[50,65] ALF patients should be referred and transferred to a transplant facility early in the presentation as they often deteriorate rapidly and require specialized intensive care, urgent transplant evaluation and listing, and possibly hepatic and renal extracorporeal support therapy.

ACUTE-ON-CHRONIC LIVER DYSFUNCTION AND FAILURE

Chronic liver disease is a disease state of greater than 6-month duration. Acute-on-chronic liver failure (ACLF) occurs in patients who have an underlying cirrhosis and experience an additional derangement (e.g., infection, bleeding, primary disease exacerbation, or secondary disease) causing acute liver decompensation.[5,85]

The risk factors for chronic liver disease vary according to the type and cause of disease. For instance, viral hepatitis and parasitic liver disease risk factors are related mostly to infectious exposure risks; nonalcoholic fatty liver disease and steatohepatitis are related to nutrition, obesity, and dyslipidemia.[19] Table 17.1 lists risk factors and acute treatment for the most common diseases associated with acute-on-chronic liver dysfunction/failure.

The incidence of liver disease in the United States is on the rise, but because the onset of many types of liver disease is

TABLE 17.1 Risk Factors and Acute Treatments for Common Liver Diseases

Liver Disease	Risk Factors	Acute Treatment
Alcoholic liver disease	Female, Hispanic, African-American, and Native American males, family history, obesity, iron overload, anxiety, depression	Abstinence, counseling, nutritional replacement, benzodiazepines, baclofen, prednisolone, pentoxifylline
Autoimmune hepatitis	Female, family history	Steroids, azathioprine
Budd-Chiari syndrome	Inherited and acquired clotting disorders, chronic infections and inflammatory disorders, tumors, trauma	Anticoagulation, TIPS/DIPS, listing for liver transplant
Drug-induced liver injury	Age, female, poor nutrition, underlying liver disease, obesity, diabetes, drug interactions, alcohol use	*Discontinue all but essential medications* Consider listing for liver transplant • Acetaminophen/paracetamol: • activated charcoal within 4 hours • N-acetylcysteine • Mushroom poisoning: penicillin G, N-acetylcysteine • Idiosyncratic hypersensitivity: • N-acetylcysteine • Supportive care
Fatty liver disease	Males, older adults, Hispanic, obesity, diabetes mellitus, lipid disorders	Dietary intake, Metformin, Pioglitazone, statins, insulin, vitamin E in nondiabetics, supportive therapy
HELLP (hemolysis, elevated liver enzymes, low platelets) syndrome	Pregnancy with: preeclampsia, caucasian, obesity, diabetes	Delivery of fetus, medical management
Hepatic abscess	Lower socioeconomic status in endemic areas, institutionalized patients, male-to-male sexual behavior, travelers	Antimicrobials, antiparasitics, abscess drainage
Hepatitis A	Fecal-oral transmission: daycare centers, contaminated food, infected mollusks; travel to endemic hepatitis A virus (HAV) areas; anal-oral sex	Supportive care, no effective antivirals
Hepatitis B	High-risk sexual behavior (unprotected sex, multiple partners, male-on-male partners), intravenous drug use, hemodialysis, healthcare workers, vertical transmission during pregnancy	Hepatitis B immune globulin, lamivudine, adefovir
Hepatitis C	Blood-borne transmission: transfusions, tattoos, intravenous drug use, multiple sex partners, infection with HIV	Antivirals, ribavirin
Hepatocellular carcinoma	Cirrhosis, chronic hepatitis B or C, α1-antitrypsin disease, exposure to carcinogens	Transarterial chemoembolization/bead embolization, ablative therapy, sorafenib, surgical resection, listing for transplant
Hereditary hemochromatosis	Family history of disease, caucasian, alcohol use	Therapeutic phlebotomy, iron chelating agents, listing for transplant
Primary biliary cirrhosis	Family history of disease	Ursodeoxycholic acid, bile acid sequestrants
Primary sclerosing cholangitis	Irritable bowel disease, male, age 40–60, family history of disease	Ursodeoxycholic acid, steroids, listing for transplant
Wilson's disease	Parents or siblings with the disease	Penicillamine, plasmapheresis, listing for transplant

DIPS, Direct intrahepatic portosystemic shunt; *TIPS,* transjugular intrahepatic portosystemic shunt.
From references 4, 9, 17, 20, 25, 34, 50, 71, 73, 74, 79, and 85.

insidious, with a latent period between onset and clinical detection, the true incidence and prevalence may not be known.[52] Chronic liver disease (CLD) and cirrhosis are the 12th leading cause of mortality in the United States, with a 3.2% increase from 2010 to 2011.[61] The most common cases of CLD are nonalcoholic fatty liver disease (20%), alcoholic liver disease (5%), chronic hepatitis C (5%), and chronic hepatitis B (0.5%–1%).[16] Hepatitis C virus (HCV) increased by 75% between 2010 and 2012, most likely related to illegal injection drug use, widespread HCV screening, and "peaking" of the epidemic patients who are showing symptoms of end-stage liver disease and hepatocellular carcinoma.[25] Chronic HCV is currently the leading cause of liver-related death and hepatocellular carcinoma in the Western world, with approximately 3.9 million people in the United States chronically infected, and those who are undiagnosed may be double that number.[25] Liver diseases can be classified into four major categories: hepatocellular diseases affecting the liver parenchyma, cholestatic diseases affecting the biliary ducts, metabolic diseases, and tumors (Box 17.1).

Disease prevention involves specific diagnoses and includes decreased alcohol intake, avoidance of hepatotoxic substances (including acetaminophen), weight control, limiting exposure to infectious diseases, and vaccination against hepatitis A and B. From 2000 to 2012, the incidence of hepatitis A and B markedly declined in the United States by 88% and 64%, respectively. This decrease is attributed to implementation of routine hepatitis A and B vaccines, universal precautions, and screening of the blood supply.[25,61] Currently, there is no vaccination available for hepatitis C. The recent release of N5SA and NS3/4 protease inhibitors and nucleotide inhibitors has shown remarkable promise, with effective cure rates of up to 96%, and reversal of hepatic inflammation and fibrosis in selected studies.[39] A vaccine has been developed for hepatitis E, and is awaiting widespread release.[79]

BOX 17.1 Classification of Hepatic Diseases

Cholestatic

- Primary
  - Primary biliary cirrhosis
- Secondary
  - Biliary cirrhosis
  - Congenital conditions (e.g., biliary atresia)
  - Drug-induced cholestasis
  - Sclerosing cholangitis

Hepatocellular

- Alcohol (Laënnec's cirrhosis)
- Autoimmune hepatitis
- Cryptogenic (cause unknown)
- Hepatitis
  - Infectious: bacterial, viral, parasitic
  - Drug-induced: NSAIDs, halothane, sulfonamides, ketoconazole, phenytoin, INH, rifampin, carbon tetrachloride, poisonous mushrooms
- Ischemia
- Vascular congestion (e.g., Budd-Chiari syndrome)

Metabolic

- Hemochromatosis
- Pregnancy (acute fatty liver; Hemolysis, Elevated Liver enzymes, and Low Platelet count [HELLP] syndrome)
- Wilson's disease

Tumors

- Hepatoblastoma
- Primary hepatocellular carcinoma
- Secondary tumors (e.g., lymphomas, metastasis)

INH, Isoniazid; *NSAID,* nonsteroidal anti-inflammatory drugs.

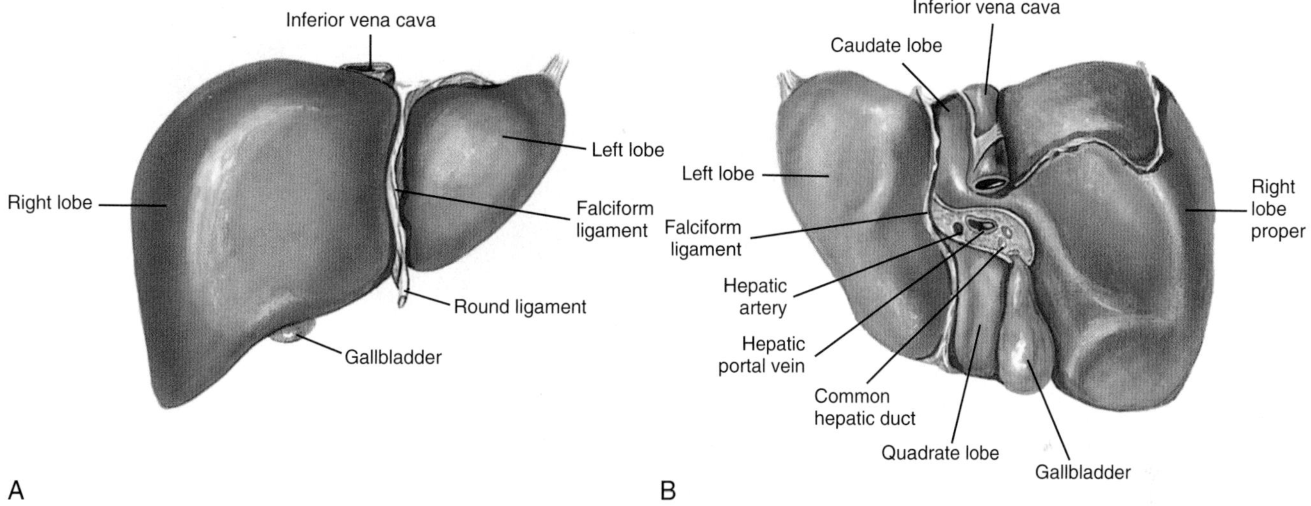

FIG. 17.1 Gross structure of the liver. **A,** Anterior view. **B,** Posterior view. (From Patton, K. T., Thibodeau, G. A. (2016). *Anatomy & physiology* (9th ed.). St Louis: Mosby.)

APPLIED PHYSIOLOGY

The liver is situated in the right upper quadrant of the abdomen, from the fifth rib to the manubrium. It is divided into two major lobes, which are further subdivided into eight functional segments (Fig. 17.1). The liver has a dual circulation much like that of the lungs. The portal vein brings blood directly from the mesenteric circulation to the parenchyma for processing, whereas the hepatic artery supplies the organ with oxygenated blood. Venous outflow is via the hepatic veins into the inferior vena cava.[5]

The functional unit of the liver is the lobule (Fig. 17.2). Blood enters the lobule via the portal tract, flowing over plates of hepatocytes for processing. It empties into the central vein, which progresses to the hepatic veins. Bile canaliculi run countercurrent to blood flow in the lobule, eventually gathering and forming the hepatic ducts and common bile duct. Bile moves to the gallbladder via the cystic duct for storage and concentration. The cystic duct branches off the common bile duct, which delivers bile to the duodenum through the sphincter of Oddi.[5,11]

The liver has tremendous functional reserve, maintaining homeostasis with only 20% of viable parenchyma. Its main functions are metabolic, excretory, detoxifying, and immunologic, and includes detoxification of toxins and drugs, breakdown of bilirubin, production of bile acids, production and deamination of proteins, fat metabolism, glucose and acid-base maintenance, excretion of drugs and hormones, and metabolism and storage of metals and vitamins.[5,16] Hepatic tests can be classified into four major groups (Table 17.2).

Cirrhosis

It has been said that if the patient lives long enough, all causes of chronic liver disease lead to cirrhosis.[38] Cirrhosis is the end result of chronic, ongoing liver disease. It begins with fibrosis, which is the healing process that mitigates with chronic liver injury.[18] The hepatic stellate cells, parenchymal liver cells thought to regulate intrahepatic blood flow, have been implicated in the formation of collagen and fibrin in the presence of liver damage. These fibrin fibers contract over time, causing shrinking and hardening of the liver, and distortion of the architecture of the lobules. This impairs blood flow through the liver, causing portal hypertension, splenomegaly, ascites, and variceal bleeding. Manifestations of cirrhosis can be detected by using abdominal ultrasound, computed tomography (CT), or magnetic resonance imaging (MRI). Early stages and progression of cirrhosis are confirmed by liver biopsy.[20,48]

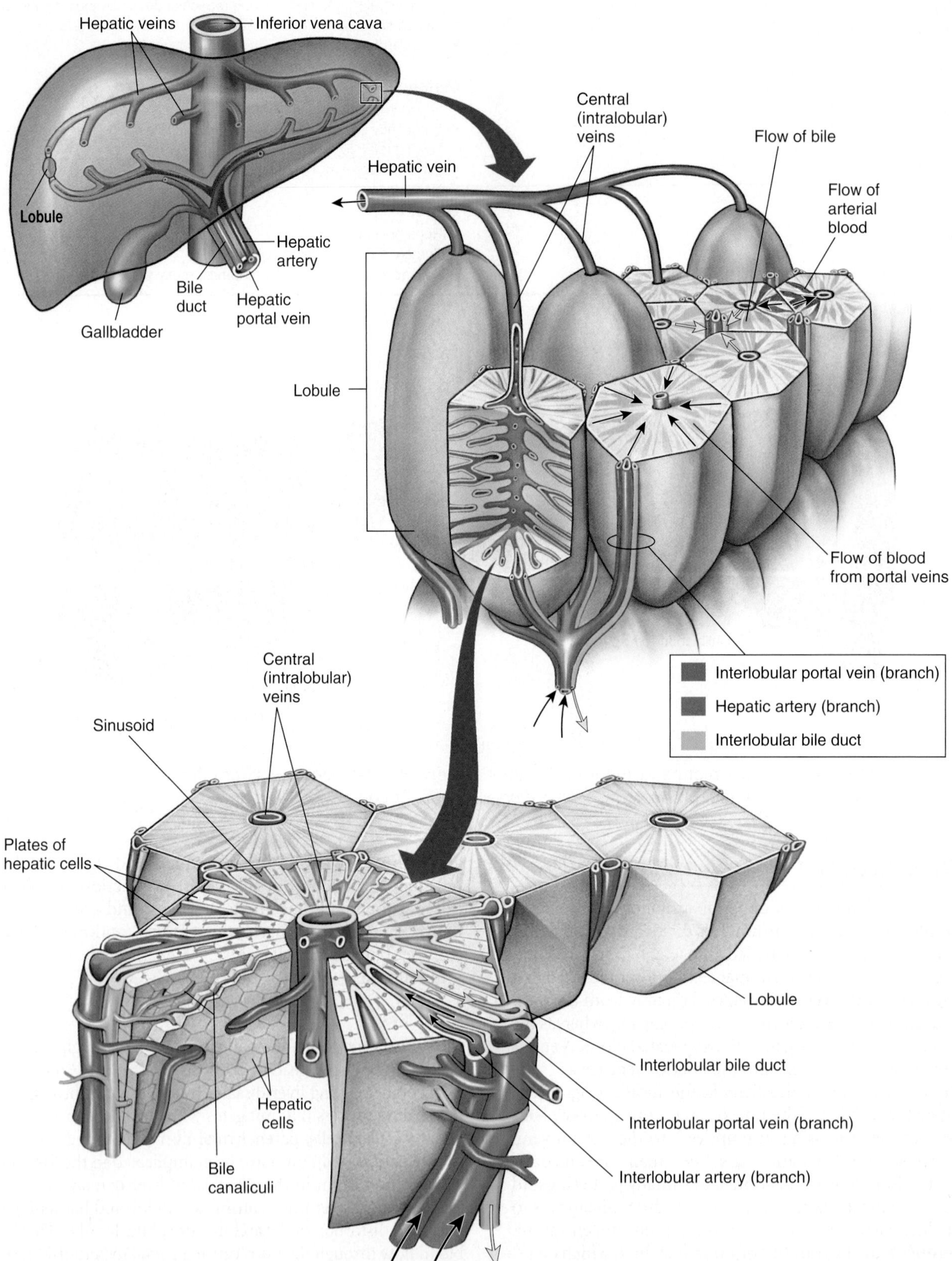

FIG. 17.2 Structure of the lobule, the functional unit of the liver. (From Patton, K. T., Thibodeau, G. A. (2016). *Anatomy & physiology* (9th ed.). St Louis: Mosby.)

TABLE 17.2 Liver Function Tests

	Normal Values	Clinical Implications
Clearance		
Ammonia	10–80 mcg/dL	Increases with hepatocellular dysfunction as ammonia metabolism is decreased
Galactose clearance		Decreased in diminished hepatic function
Lidocaine clearance to MEGX (monoethylglycinexylidide)	Decreased in diminished hepatic function, decreased hepatic perfusion	
Cholestasis		
Alkaline phosphatase	30–120 units/L	Increases in obstruction and cirrhosis
Bilirubin		
Indirect (unconjugated)	0.2–0.8 mg/dL	Increases with lysis of red blood cells
Direct (conjugated)	0.1–0.3 mg/dL	Increases with hepatocellular injury or obstruction
Total	0.3–1.0 mg/dL	Increases with biliary obstruction
γ-Glutamyltransferase (GGT)	8–38 units/L; females younger than 45: 5–27 units/L	Most sensitive liver enzyme in detecting obstruction, cholangitis, or cholecystitis Can be used to detect chronic alcohol ingestion
Liver Injury		
Alanine aminotransaminase (ALT)	4–36 units/L	Increases in hepatocellular injury
Aspartate aminotransaminase (AST)	0–35 units/L	Increases in hepatocellular injury May rise to 20 times normal in acute hepatitis In acute extrahepatic obstruction, quickly rises to 10 times normal; falls as swiftly In cirrhosis, degree of elevation correlated to degree of inflammation
Lactate dehydrogenase (LDH) LHD isoenzyme 4: most liver specific	100–190 units/L	Increases in hepatitis
Clotting Function Tests		
INR	1.0	
Prothrombin time	11–12.5 sec or 85%–100% of control	Increases with chronic liver disease, vitamin K deficiency
Partial thromboplastin time	25–40 sec	Increases with severe liver disease
Protein Studies		
Total serum protein	6.4–8.3 g/dL	Decreases with hepatocellular injury, cirrhosis
Serum albumin	3.5–5 g/dL	Decreases in cirrhosis, liver disease, viral hepatitis, ascites
Serum globulin	2.3–3.4 g/dL	Decreases in cirrhosis, liver disease, viral hepatitis; can increase in autoimmune hepatitis

The severity and prognosis of liver failure resulting from cirrhosis are assessed using the Child-Turcotte-Pugh scoring system (Table 17.3). Cirrhosis can be considered compensated or decompensated. Compensated, or stable, cirrhosis is defined by biopsy-proven cirrhosis in a patient who has never had signs of decompensation (e.g., variceal hemorrhage, ascites, encephalopathy). Conversely, cirrhotic patients who experience any of these complications are described as having decompensated cirrhosis. The onset of decompensation is associated with higher mortality.[55,71] Disease severity and mortality risk in patients with alcoholic hepatitis may be estimated by using a discriminant function formula (Maddrey score), calculated as follows:[4,50]

$$\text{Discriminant Function} = 4.6 \times \left(\left[\begin{array}{l}\text{prothrombin time} - \\ \text{prothrombin control}\end{array}\right] + [\text{serum bilirubin level}]\right)$$

A value greater than 32 mg/dL is associated with a high short-term mortality, and has been used to determine the need for specific treatment in patients with severe alcoholic hepatitis.

TABLE 17.3 Child-Turcotte-Pugh System for Scoring the Severity and Prognosis of Liver Failure Caused by Cirrhosis

	POINTS SCORED FOR INCREASING ABNORMALITY		
Clinical and Biochemical Measurements	**1**	**2**	**3**
Encephalopathy (grade)	None	1 and 2	3 and 4
Ascites	Absent	Slight	Moderate
Bilirubin (mg/dL)	1–1.9	2–2.9	>3
Albumin (g/dL)	>3.5	2.8–3.5	<2.8
Prothrombin time (sec prolonged)	1–4	4–6	>6
For primary biliary cirrhosis: bilirubin (mg/dL)	1–4	4–10	>10
Child Grade	**Total Score**		
A	5–6		
B	7–9		
C	≥10		

BOX 17.2 West Haven Criteria of Altered Mental State

Stage 0: Lack of detectable changes in personality or behavior; asterixis absent.
Stage 1: Trivial lack of awareness; shortened attention span; impaired addition or subtraction skills; hypersomnia, insomnia, or inversion of sleep pattern; euphoria or depression; asterixis is detectable.
Stage 2: Lethargy or apathy; disorientation; inappropriate behavior; slurred speech; obvious asterixis.
Stage 3: Gross disorientation; bizarre behavior; semistuporous to stupor; asterixis is generally absent.
Stage 4: Coma.

Hepatic Encephalopathy

Hepatic encephalopathy (HE) is defined as a disturbance in central nervous system function resulting from hepatic insufficiency. These disturbances are usually exhibited clinically as interruption of nerve impulse transmission, and cognitive and behavioral changes.[11,23,37] These changes are staged from 0 to 4 (Box 17.2). HE occurs in 30% to 40% of patients with cirrhosis. The pathophysiology of HE is incompletely understood. There is evidence that ammonia plays a key role in HE. Ammonia is produced in the gut by urease activity of bacteria on nitrogenous waste products, and from deamination of glutamine in the small bowel. Ammonia levels often do not correlate with levels of HE; patients with minimally elevated venous ammonia levels in ALF can be comatose, whereas patients with chronic liver disease and ammonia levels higher than 100 mg/dL will exhibit minimal signs of HE.[21] Serum ammonia levels are best measured in arterial blood samples, before passage through the liver.[5] Other substances recognized in the development of HE are octopamine, phenol, mercaptans, and intrinsic benzodiazepines.[13,47] It is believed that these substances in part induce gamma-aminobutyric acid (GABA) pathways, which downregulate nerve impulse transmission. This downregulation is characterized by altered nerve transmission, and is exhibited as asterixis, hippus (asterixis or jerking contraction of the pupils), decreased or absent deep tendon reflexes, or absent gag and corneal reflexes.[5,85] Deposition of manganese in the central nervous system has also been implicated in neurologic dysfunction in chronic liver disease, as it deposits in the basal ganglia and induces extrapyramidal symptoms.[35]

Patients with chronic liver disease can have induction or worsening of HE by precipitating factors. These factors include infection, bleeding, fluid and electrolyte imbalances, medications, hypoxia, portosystemic shunting, and primary or secondary disease exacerbation. Many medications are key factors in triggering HE, and include sedatives, narcotics, and diuretics. Alterations in hepatic, splanchnic, or systemic circulation can shunt blood from the hepatic parenchyma, bypassing the liver and preventing the processing of toxins, leading to HE.[5,14] Causes of this include portal vein thrombosis (PVT), spontaneous or surgical portosystemic shunt, and placement of a transjugular intrahepatic portosystemic shunt (TIPS).[15,22] The development of overt HE is usually seen in patients who are Child Class B or C, and carries an overall poor prognosis without transplantation.[37]

The role of nursing in detecting and managing HE cannot be overemphasized. Early detection and intervention will prevent worsening of encephalopathy and cerebral edema, and prevent aspiration. The nurse needs to be alert to changes in mental status and rapidly implement appropriate treatments, including administering medications, providing for patient safety and fall prevention, preventing aspiration, placing nasogastric or enteral feeding tubes, and preparing for elective intubation to protect the airway.[5] Patients with HE of 3 or 4 must be managed in the ICU setting. Mental status is assessed using the Glasgow Coma Scale and a HE scoring scale, such as the West Haven criteria, every 1 to 2 hours.[73] Patient and family education and support about HE and treatment are essential. Patients often become depressed, afraid, or confused with encephalopathy and require reorientation, assistance with activities of daily living (ADLs), and empathy.[65]

Treatment of HE is based on several areas. The most important aspect of management is to treat the precipitating factors or conditions. Dietary education is considered first-line management for HE. Protein converts to urea and ammonia, which can increase ammonia levels; however, the catabolic state of liver disease increases the need for protein for immune system and organ maintenance. Dietary protein is usually restricted for the first 24 hours and then reintroduced with moderate protein restriction, usually 1 to 1.5 grams of protein per kilogram per day, or 60 to 80 g/day.[41,56] Vegetable and dairy proteins are preferred to animal sources, as they provide a higher calorie-to-nitrogen ratio and more nonabsorbable fiber, increasing colonic acidification and decreasing ammonia-producing bacteria. Oral and enteral formulas that have high levels of branched-chain amino acids are also preferred, as higher serum levels of branched-chain amino acids to aromatic amino acids can improve HE.[56] Zinc is a cofactor for urea cycle enzymes and promotes clearance of ammonia. Oral zinc supplement is recommended in zinc-deficient or malnourished patients.[41]

The effects of sedatives and narcotics are prolonged in liver disease and can worsen HE. Sedation of these patients should be avoided; if agitation is unmanageable, short-acting benzodiazepines or propofol (Diprivan) should be used, and can be reversed with flumazenil (Romazicon), if necessary.[5,51] Naloxone (Narcan) should be given if narcotic use is suspected as a precipitator of HE.[5]

The mainstays of treating HE remain correction of the precipitating factors and use of nonabsorbable disaccharides and antibiotics. The most commonly used medication is lactulose, a nonabsorbable disaccharide. It works by acidifying the colon, encouraging diffusion of ammonia from the blood into the gut. The cathartic effect of lactulose also encourages expulsion of ammonia ions. It can be given orally or via nasogastric tube, or as a retention enema when diluted with water. The goal for dosing is to produce two to three bowel movements per day.[5,23] Use of lactulose can increase abdominal distention, fluid and electrolyte loss through diarrhea, and hypernatremia. If these occur, lactulose dosing should be decreased or discontinued. Polyethylene glycol (GoLYTELY) and oral mannitol (Osmitrol) are also used for bowel cleansing if lactulose is inadequate. It is important to monitor for systemic dehydration with all these therapies, as this can cause vascular shunting, decreased hepatic perfusion, and worsen HE.

Enteral antibiotics are used to treat HE in place of, or in conjunction with, lactulose. These work by decreasing the number of gut flora and reducing the activity of glutaminase in intestinal villi. Rifaximin (Xifaxan), a nonabsorbable antibiotic, is a safe and well-tolerated treatment.[57,58] It is often used in combination with lactulose in resistant cases. A 2015 study showed combination therapy did not reduce hospital length of stay for acute

HE, but did result in lower readmission rates.[23] Flumazenil and bromocriptine (Parlodel) exert their neurologic effects directly on the brain. Flumazenil is recommended for stage 3 or 4 encephalopathy, or suspected benzodiazepine use. A large, multicenter trial reported no incidence of seizures with flumazenil use in liver disease patients.[23,51] Bromocriptine can be used in cases unresponsive to other therapies.[14] Neomycin and metronidazole are used in some centers, but there is no clear efficacy data. Acarbose and sodium benzoate can be used for resistant HE. Although gastrointestinal (GI) absorption of neomycin is poor, it does occur, and the absorbed drug can be nephrotoxic and ototoxic.[5] If a spontaneous or surgical portosystemic shunt or TIPS is present, occlusion with placement of vascular coils can be considered when all other treatment options have failed and portal hypertension is controlled.[23,63]

Two recent randomized studies have been published on the use of probiotics to alter the gut microbiome and improve HE. Although the overall effect of probiotics was mild, there was significant improvement in the stage 1 patients over placebo.[51]

Portal Hypertension

Portal hypertension (PHTN) can be caused by any condition that impairs portal blood flow. The types of PHTN are classified in relation to where the cause of increased pressure occurs in relation to the sinusoids of the lobule.[71] Presinusoidal PHTN occurs before the sinusoids, usually in the portal vein and its branches, and includes PVT (usually from tumors or masses) and cavernous vein transformation. Sinusoidal PHTN occurs within the liver parenchyma, with increased intrahepatic resistance. This is seen with cirrhosis, schistosomiasis (a parasitic disease), and sarcoidosis. Postsinusoidal PHTN occurs primarily in the hepatic veins and branches and includes Budd-Chiari syndrome (a coagulopathic disorder causing hepatic vein thrombosis and resistance to blood outflow), veno-occlusive disease of the hepatic veins or inferior vena cava, and severe congestive heart failure.[5,71] PVT occurs due to sluggish portal vein flow from cirrhosis, hepatobiliary malignancy, abdominal infections, and myoproliferative disorders. PVT contributes to worsening portal hypertension. Prevalence of the disorder worldwide is increasing; it is estimated to be as high as 26% in high-risk groups.[53] It is treated with low-dose anticoagulation and embolectomy or venoplasty by interventional radiology.[53,55]

Progression of cirrhosis or severe necrosis promotes resistance to blood flow through the liver. In turn, the myelofibroblasts and stellate cells within the liver sinusoids cause vasoconstriction within the sinusoids in response to systemic vasoconstrictors, such as endothelin-1 and angiotensin II, leading to an increase in portal resistance. Blood backs up under pressure in the portal, splenic, and mesenteric circulation, causing portal hypertension.[5,35] This in turn results in portosystemic shunts, esophageal and gastric varices, hemorrhoids/rectal varicies, caput medusae (enlarged, engorged umbilical and abdominal veins), and ascites.[22,70]

As portal pressure builds, the spleen enlarges. Splenomegaly from portal hypertension causes sequestration of blood cells, particularly platelets, and leads to anemia, leukopenia, and thrombocytopenia.[5,70]

The effects of PHTN can be debilitating and life-threatening. The most severe complications of PHTN are ascites, spontaneous bacterial peritonitis, HE, hepatorenal syndrome, varices, and gastrointestinal (GI) bleeding.

Ascites

Ascites is the most common major complication of the three complications of cirrhosis, and is seen in some cases of ALF.[27,71] It is the accumulation of fluid and protein in the peritoneal space with resulting abdominal distention.[10,18] This maldistribution of fluid and oncotic molecules increases the amount of total body water, diluting the serum sodium and decreasing intravascular volume.[35,69,71]

Ascites is most commonly caused by PHTN, although up to 20% of cases can have nonhepatic causes (e.g., carcinoma, peritoneal tuberculosis, or heart failure).[22,35,44] Communication of fluid from the abdominal compartment into the negative pleural space via small defects in the diaphragm causes hepatic hydrothorax, with hypoxia, orthopnea, atelectasis, and possible pneumonia. Hepatic hydrothorax occurs in 5% of all patients with cirrhosis and 12% of all patients with decompensated cirrhosis. This is most commonly seen on the right side.[18,63] Treatment is the same for ascites, with serial thoracentesis as needed. Chest tube insertion is contraindicated, as it is associated with very high morbidity and mortality in cirrhotic patients.[69]

New onset ascites warrants a diagnostic paracentesis to a fluid cell count, total protein, and to calculate a serum-ascites albumin gradient (SAGG), which aides in pinpointing the origin of the ascites as cirrhotic, cardiac, or malignant.[35,71] SAAG is calculated by measuring the albumin concentration in ascites and serum specimens taken the same day, and subtracting the ascites value from the serum value. A SAAG of greater than or equal to 1.1 g/dL indicates portal hypertension.[18,69] Ascites fluid should be placed immediately in aerobic and anaerobic blood culture bottles to aide in organism identification.[71] A polymorphonuclear (PMN) count of greater than 250 cells/mm^3 is indicative of ascites infection. For recurrent infections, fungal cultures should be considered.[70] Repeat diagnostic paracentesis is recommended in hospitalized patients to track response to treatment (defined as a 25% or more decrease in the fluid PMN count) and detect changes in infectious agents.[5,18] Treatment is usually cephalosporins or fluoquinolones.[9,20]

The mainstay of treatment of ascites includes limiting sodium intake to 2 g/day taking diuretics, and educating the patient regarding compliance with restrictions and the plan of care.[2,69] Diuretics used should be potassium-sparing diuretics; such as aldosterone antagonists that exert their effect on the collecting tubules. This treatment is effective in liver disease because these patients do not completely metabolize intrinsic aldosterone, resulting in sodium and water retention. It is used in combination with loop diuretics, which help control the hyperkalemia seen with aldosterone antagonists and are synergistic in producing diuresis.[69,71] Diuretics are very effective when serum creatinine level is less than 1.5 mg/dL and renal function is intact. Monitor for hypotension, renal dysfunction, cramps, HE, and painful gynecomastia.[35] Because of underlying hypotension, fluid restriction is not necessary until the serum sodium is 125 mOsm or less. Beta blockers for portal hypertension must be monitored carefully, and discontinued for a decrease in mean arterial pressure (MAP) or increase in creatinine. Nonsteroidal antiinflammatory agents, angiotensin converting enzyme inhibitors, and angiotensin receptor blockers should be avoided to prevent acute kidney injury (AKI).[9,35,71] Large-volume paracentesis rapidly removes the abdominal fluid via a percutaneous needle or trocar and is used for patients with respiratory distress related to abdominal distention. Albumin 25% is used as a volume expander and infused at 6 to 8 g/L of fluid removed to prevent the hemodynamic and renal instability associated with large fluid shifts.[5,10,69,76,80] Albumin is usually given if more than 4 liters of ascites is removed. Albumin also increases vascular oncotic pressure, with improved diuresis with diuretics.[69,80] Additionally, positioning the patient in the supine position, with legs elevated, has been shown to decrease ascites and lower extremity edema.[35]

In cases of massive ascites resistant to diuretics, renal impairment, and hepatic hydrothorax, a TIPS is used to help control ascites and improve intravascular volume to promote kidney function (Fig. 17.3). The TIPS helps to reestablish a low-pressure channel for blood flow from the portal to the hepatic circulation by means of a vascular stent placed between branches of the portal and hepatic veins through the liver parenchyma. The stent is placed under fluoroscopy by the interventional radiologist.[15,24] Alternately, a direct intrahepatic portosystemic shunt (DIPS) can be placed, using intravascular ultrasound guidance, between a portal vein branch and the inferior vena cava with a polytetrafluoroethylene-covered stent to prevent bleeding into the intraabdominal space.[31] These stents can become occluded, initially by thrombus or over time by endothelialization of the

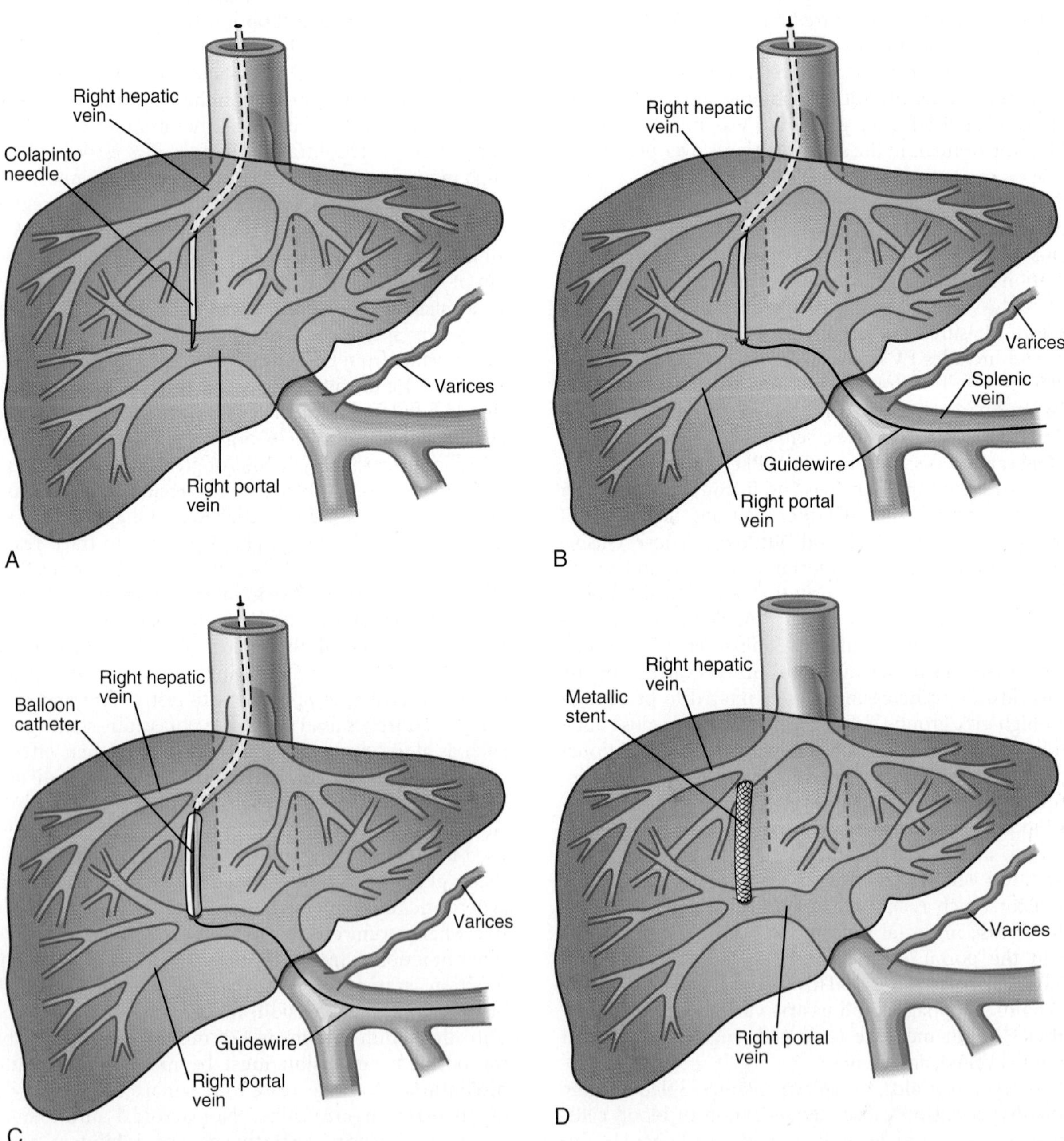

FIG. 17.3 Transjugular intrahepatic portosystemic shunt (TIPS) to help control ascites. **A,** A sheathed transjugular needle is advanced out of a hepatic vein into an intrahepatic branch of the portal vein. **B,** A guidewire is threaded through the needle into the splenic vein. **C,** The parenchymal liver tract between the hepatic and portal veins is ligated using a balloon angioplasty catheter. **D,** A metallic stent is deployed with the shunt tract.

lumen. TIPS patency is monitored by periodically performing abdominal Doppler ultrasonography. Immediate complications of TIPS placement include hemorrhage, infection, congestive heart failure from increased preload, renal dysfunction from contrast dye, and HE from increased shunting of blood past the liver parenchyma.[15] Nursing care post-TIPS includes frequent physical assessment for worsening HE (altered mental status, asterixis, increased serum ammonia concentration); bleeding (abdominal distention, tenderness or rebound tenderness indicative of intraabdominal bleeding and peritoneal irritation, increased heart rate with decreased blood pressure, increased pulse pressure, decreased hematocrit); fever; chills; signs and symptoms of congestive heart failure or renal failure (including shortness of breath, rales, decreased oxygen saturation, jugular venous distention, decreased urine output, increased creatinine level); and worsening hepatic function (increased INR, increased bilirubin level).[15] Surgical shunts are reserved for patients for whom TIPS/DIPS is not possible or available.[5]

For patients with persistent tense ascites or recurrent hepatic hydrothorax who are not liver transplant or TIPS candidates, placement of a peritoneovenous or pleurovenous (Denver) shunt should be considered. Implantable devices are preferred due to fewer complications by using minimally invasive techniques (usually interventional radiology placement) versus open surgical technique for placement. These shunts have either one or two one-way valves and a pump chamber incorporated into a length of tubing. The distal end is placed into the peritoneal or pleural cavity, and the venous return end is placed in the internal jugular or subclavian vein for fluid return. When the patient or caregiver compresses the subcutaneous pump chamber, fluid is pushed into the shunt and returns to the venous system, the one-way valve prevents reflux of blood and ascites into the shunt.[54] It should be pumped at least 20 times, twice daily, with the patient in the supine position. Nursing care includes teaching the patient and family the technique for pumping and shunt care. Postoperative gram-negative antibiotics should be continued for at least 7 days.[54,85] Complications include immediate postoperative disseminated coagulation (detected by monitoring INR, fibrinogen, and D-dimer levels), fluid leakage from the wound sites with delayed healing, shunt occlusion, venous thrombus, cardiac overload, variceal bleeding, and bacteremia.[86] Early placement has been shown in limited studies to improve patient's symptoms, but not survival, in end-stage liver disease.[7,64]

Systemic Hemodynamics

Patients with liver disease are in a constant state of systemic inflammatory response syndrome. This manifests with low MAP and peripheral vascular resistance. These systemic changes are related to a number of factors including accumulation of vasoactive peptides and cytokines, such as tumor necrosis factor-alpha (TNFα) and interleukins 1 and 6.[55] Hepatic necrosis in ALF and thrombotic or traumatic injury can trigger massive inflammation, driving the systemic inflammatory response syndrome (SIRS), and progressing to multisystem organ dysfunction syndrome (MODS).[85] The formation of ascites also creates fluid shifts with a decrease in intravascular volume, further lowering blood pressure and filling pressures.

It has long been recognized that patients with end-stage liver disease and cirrhosis tend to decompensate with minor physiologic stresses, particularly exhibiting signs of congestive heart failure, renal failure, and cardiovascular collapse. Although no formal definition for this phenomenon exists, it is termed *cirrhotic cardiomyopathy.* It is described as cardiac dysfunction in cirrhotic patients characterized by impaired contractile responsiveness to stress or altered diastolic relaxation. It can also include prolonged QT interval or other electrophysiologic abnormalities in the absence of known cardiac disease. Nursing care and treatment are the same for heart failure and are supportive in nature. Titrate vasoactive medications carefully, and observe for an atypical response.[5]

Patients with liver failure at times require hemodynamic monitoring with a central venous pressure (CVP) line. Pulmonary artery catheterization is rarely necessary in patients with ALF and is associated with significant morbidity.[50]

The target MAP is greater than or equal to 75 mm Hg, with patients with increased intracranial pressure (ICP) requiring a higher MAP to maintain cerebral perfusion pressure (CPP) at 60–80 mm Hg.[50] Fluid boluses with normal saline, albumin, or blood products help to normalize the CVP to 8 to 10 mm Hg. Norepinephrine is the first-line vasopressor for patients unresponsive to optimized fluid resuscitation. If there is not an adequate response to volume challenge and norepinephrine, vasopressin may potentiate the effects of norepinephrine. This may allow a decrease in norepinephrine infusion rate, which may avoid intense vasoconstriction in peripheral tissues that can lead to ischemia.[50] However, vasopressin can lead to an increase in ICP in severe HE, and should be used with caution in these patients. Patients with persistent hypotension after these treatments should be tested for a relative or absolute adrenal insufficiency, and considered for a trial of hydrocortisone.[50,73] Troponin levels may be persistently elevated in ALF or ACLF; the reasons are uncertain, but are believed to be related to metabolic stress rather than coronary ischemia.[84]

Glucose, Acid-Base, and Electrolyte Imbalances

Metabolic derangements are common in acute and chronic liver failure. Acidosis can be caused by an increase in serum lactate levels from reduced conversion in the diseased liver or by respiratory compromise from abdominal distention, ascites, hepatic hydrothorax, or depressed respiratory rate.[73] Respiratory alkalosis is associated with the tachypnea and hypocapnia of worsening encephalopathy. Metabolic alkalosis may develop following administration of citrated blood products, as the citrate converts in part to bicarbonate.[42] Serum glucose, magnesium, phosphorus, and potassium levels are frequently low from poor intake and the use of diuretics and may require replacement throughout the hospital course.[50] Hyponatremia is usually dilutional in nature and should **not** be corrected rapidly, as this can result in demyelinating syndromes (e.g., central pontine and oncotic myelinolysis, seizures). Because lactate conversion is impaired, the infusion of lactated Ringer's solution is discouraged in liver dysfunction.[5,84]

The first-line treatment for metabolic correction is adequate fluid resuscitation. High lactate levels often recover with adequate fluid administration; normal saline is the solution of choice in most cases.[50,84] Serum glucose levels tend to elevate in early ALF or in chronic liver failure patients who are in stressed states (e.g., infection, bleeding). Hypoglycemia is seen in severe liver failure, as glucose generation and regulation are lost.[5,42] Capillary glucose levels should be monitored frequently, usually every 1 to 4 hours. Dextrose 10% infusions or enteral feedings are given to maintain glucose levels. Magnesium replacements are considered to maintain normal levels and to prevent dysrhythmias, particularly torsade de pointes.

Malnutrition

Patients with hepatic disorders are prone to malnutrition, because of the key role of the liver in regulating the body's nutritional state and energy balance, and from being in a persistent hypercatabolic state.[60] Patients with chronic and acute liver disease have varying degrees of nutritional deficiencies, which are referred to as protein energy malnutrition (PEM). Traditionally, protein was restricted in patients with HE to prevent generation of ammonia. However, because of varying degrees of protein deficiency, hypermetabolism, and PEM, protein requirements may be high.[66] The highest protein and caloric requirements are for patients with acute alcoholic hepatitis, who conversely usually have the poorest baseline nutritional status. Malabsorption, particularly from medications causing high gut motility (e.g., lactulose, neomycin), can also increase malnutrition resulting in varying degrees of protein energy malnutrition.

Consultation with a nutritionist is imperative to improve and maintain nutritional balance, especially in the presence of renal dysfunction.[40] Enteral feedings should be initiated early to provide substrate, prevent stress ulcers, and maintain gut integrity. Special care must be exercised to prevent aspiration, including keeping the head of the bed elevated (>30 degrees), monitoring tube feeding residuals, observing for abdominal distention, and using duodenal or jejunal feeding tubes. Multivitamin, thiamine, and folate supplements are required to replenish depleted stores. If enteral feedings cannot be established, it is appropriate to start parenteral nutrition as soon as possible.[56] Thiamine 100 mg and folate 1 mg are given daily; all vitamins can be given enterally or intraveneously.[40,41] Patients with liver dysfunction have PEM until proven otherwise. The aim is for maximum tolerable protein intake, usually 1.2 g/day (range 1–1.5 g/d); protein restriction is considered only for severe (stage 3 or 4) encephalopathy, usually 60–80 g/day. Branched-chain amino acid formulas are reserved for patients with stage 3 or 4 HE. Enforcement of fluid restriction for patients with hyponatremia (1000–1500 mL/d) and ascites, maintenance of sodium restriction of 2 g/day for patients with ascites and edema are key nursing interventions. Glucose monitoring should be routinely performed and glucose and insulin administration provided as needed. Supplements such as zinc, folic acid, thiamine, multivitamins, and evaluation for fat-soluble vitamin deficiencies (A, D, E, K) should be considered for all patients.

Patients with cirrhosis have disruptions in the GI flora, with bacterial overgrowth that promotes increased intestinal wall permeability. Probiotics can assist in restoring normal bacterial strains and levels in the gut. Further study is needed to determine the most effective bacterial strains and proper dosing; in general, they are safe and well tolerated.[19]

Coagulopathy

Coagulopathy is common in ALF and ACLF. Causes are multifactorial, with derangements of both clot formation and degradation. Thrombocytopenia is due to splenic sequestration in portal hypertension and decrease in thrombopoietin. The liver synthesizes all clotting factors, except von Willebrand factor, tissue plasminogen activator, and plasminogen activator inhibitor type I, which are derived from endothelial tissue. Synthesis of clotting factors by the liver is decreased, along with decreased absorption and utilization of vitamin K. The decrease in hepatic production of antithrombotics and antithrombolytics can also result in accelerated clot formation and destruction. Additionally, GI bleeding accelerates the utilization of clotting factors.[26,73] Although liver failure patients do not meet the classic definition of disseminated intravascular coagulation (DIC), D-dimer levels are elevated in cirrhotic patients and some ALF patients. These levels are highest in patients with ascites and hepatocellular carcinoma.[72,77] Despite a deficiency of procoagulants (clotting factors, fibrinogen, and platelets) and anticoagulants (protein C and S, antithrombin III), it should be noted that spontaneous bleeding is infrequent in ALF.[73] The same can be noted in ACLF, despite low platelet levels and elevated INR values. Conversely, the incidence of PVT has been on the increase in recent years. These conditions are thought to be related to a global decrease in all coagulation factors, and a "rebalancing" of the coagulation system in liver disease, with increased von Willebrand factor, and decreased levels of the anticoagulants protein C and S, that favor portal vein and peripheral thrombosis.[26]

Vitamin K is routinely decreased in these patients, and should be replaced IV over 30 minutes to prevent hypotension, or given IM daily. Heparin in central lines for patency should be avoided in coagulopathic patients; sodium citrate 3% is recommended for line maintenance.[27,42] Transfusions are to be used only as needed, for active bleeding or prior to invasive procedure. An increase in pretransplant transfusions correlates with an increased incidence of AKI after transplantation.[43]

It is important not to overhydrate patients, maintain CVP at 8 to 10 mm Hg and MAP at 60 to 70 mm Hg, especially in those patients with varices.[16] Transfusion rates should be monitored carefully. Targeted blood replacement therapy involves replacing those factors that are proven deficient or needed to control bleeding.[21,29] Red blood cells are generally given to keep the hemoglobin between 7 and 8, but target values should be based on patient condition. Platelets are generally not transfused with no evidence of bleeding, or at or below 50,000/mm^3 if there is active bleeding or before invasive procedures.[32] Fresh frozen plasma (FFP) or frozen plasma (FP) is administered if the INR is greater than 1.5 in the presence of bleeding or before invasive procedures. Cryoprecipitate is given if the fibrinogen level is less than 100 mg/dL. If the INR is not corrected with 2 to 4 units of FFP, or if the patient is volume overloaded, procoagulant medications should be considered. Factor VIIa is a clotting factor that is poorly produced in liver failure, and is volatile and found in inadequate amounts in banked blood products.[68] Factor VIIa is given as slow IV bolus and can rapidly correct the INR to normal range without the fluid load of FFP. It can be given prior to placement of an ICP monitor or liver biopsy. However, the risk of thrombosis is high, dosing often requires repeating, it is expensive, and can induce antibody formation with repeated doses.[26,81] Prothrombin complex concentrate (Kcentra) contains the vitamin K–dependent factors II, VII, IX, and X, as well as antithrombotic protein C and S. It is used in reversing warfarin, and for urgent decrease (within 30 minutes) of the INR. It has a longer half-life than factor VIIa, is given as a one-time dose, and is more cost effective than factor VIIa. Monitor the patient for arteriovenous thrombosis. Side effects include nausea, headache, arthralgias, and hypotension.[81]

Gastrointestinal Bleeding

Bleeding from esophagogastric varices accounts for one third of all deaths of patients with cirrhosis. Up to 90% of all cirrhotic patients will experience a GI bleed. Indicators for a

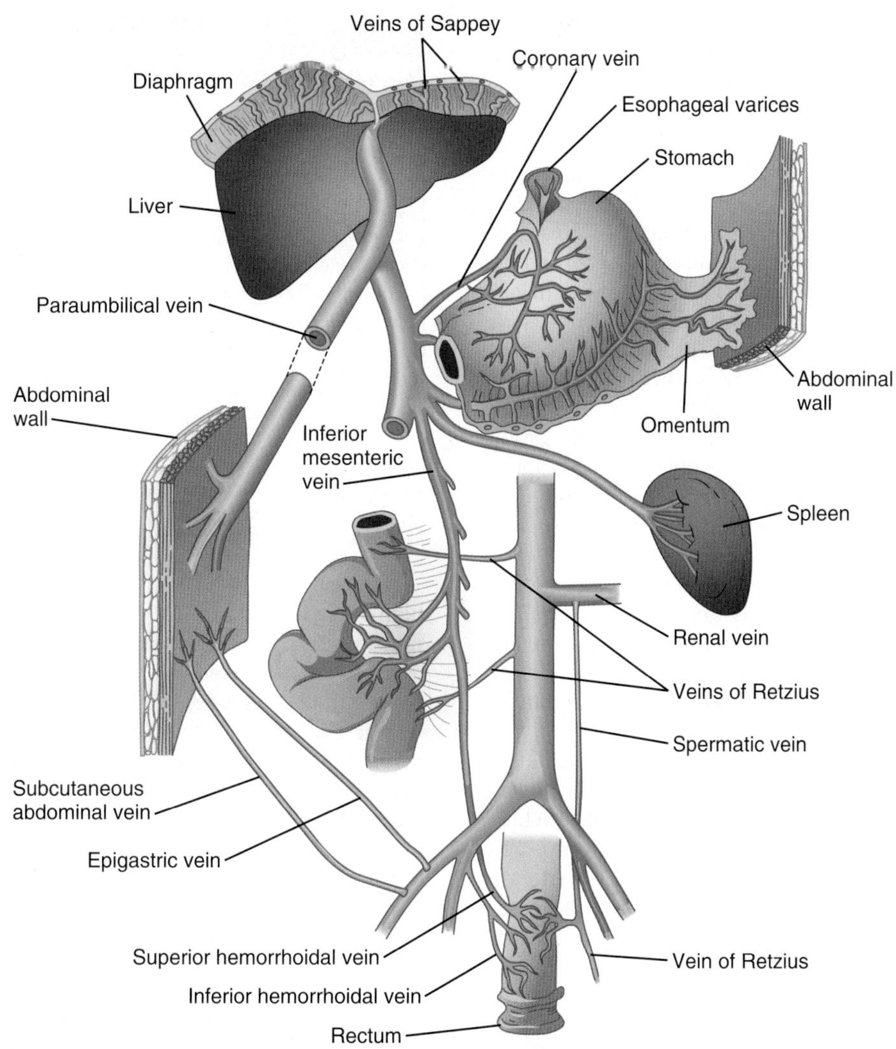

FIG. 17.4 Collateral circulation in the liver. (From UCSD–The Liver Center/Center for Transplantation.)

poor prognosis with high mortality include active bleeding at the time of endoscopy, decompensated cirrhosis (Child-Turcotte-Pugh [CTP] Grade C, or Model for End-Stage Liver Disease [MELD] of >20), the difference between the portal vein and right atrial pressure, or portosystemic gradient of greater than 20 mm Hg, and multisystem organ dysfunction.[5,36,82]

The formation of portal hypertension increases the pressure in the veins of the GI tract. As a result of this increased pressure, a system of collateral circulation develops (Fig. 17.4). This collateral circulation connects with systemic veins to shunt a portion of the portal venous blood back into systemic circulation, bypassing the liver and lowering portal pressure. Even with this shunting, under continued high pressures, the thin venous walls weaken and develop pouches with loss of competence of the venous valves, creating varices (particularly in the esophagus, stomach, and internal and external rectum). Varices can rupture, causing life-threatening GI bleeding. The veins of the gastric lining can also become engorged and friable, causing portal hypertensive gastropathy.[27]

Nonspecific beta antagonists or blockers (e.g., propranolol [Inderal], atenolol [Tenormin]) are used chronically to decrease portal pressure and prevent bleeding, and have been proven to prevent rebleeding.[1] Their use in critical care should be monitored closely; they can cause a decrease in MAP and prevent physiologic tachycardia. They should be stopped if the patient is actively bleeding or hemodynamically unstable.[36] Nitrates have been used with beta blockers to prevent variceal bleeding. This results in potent vasodilatation; the result of recent trials has not supported their continued use.[5,36]

Esophagogastroduodenoscopy (EGD) is performed to examine the upper GI tract and manage bleeding by variceal banding. This is accomplished by placing rubber bands at the base of the varix under direct endoscopic visualization. Endoscopic sclerotherapy, in which a sclerosing agent such as ethanol is injected directly into the varix to induce thrombosis, is also used to control bleeding.[6,24,25] Banding of esophageal varices is preferred over sclerotherapy because it results in less incidence of variceal ulceration and recurrent bleeding. Gastric varices tend to be more difficult to control and those along the lesser curvature of the stomach may be amenable to banding. Treatment of bleeding fundal varices includes EGD with application of tissue adhesive or thrombin. The patient should be electively intubated prior to EGD to control the airway and prevent aspiration. The TIPS is used as a second-line therapy in esophageal varices patients who have failed pharmacologic therapy and endoscopic intervention.[36] For fundal varices, urgent TIPS is recommended if endoscopic therapy is not possible, or after failure of a single EGD treatment. Once TIPS is placed, it often allows access to the gastric veins for direct embolization of the gastric varix[5,55]

A temporary method for a massive or continued GI bleed is the gastroesophageal compression tube. These tubes are more commonly known as *Sengstaken-Blakemore or Minnesota tubes,* and are most helpful in controlling bleeding gastric varices, which are not normally amenable to banding or sclerotherapy. These tubes should only be used for 24 hours.[36] Esophageal rupture, necrosis, and pneumomediastinum are the most serious complications from their use. If GI bleeding is recurrent after variceal banding/sclerotherapy or is uncontrolled, TIPS can be done emergently to decrease portal pressure.[5,36] A surgical portosystemic shunt should be reserved when band ligation fails, and TIPS is not available, or not possible due to portal or hepatic vein thrombosis.[5]

Rectal variceal rupture is less common than esophageal and gastric variceal bleeding, but more difficult to control. Medical treatment is the same as for esophageal varices. Colonoscopy can be performed to localize bleeding and allow for application of fibrin. For variceal bleeding uncontrolled by all conventional measures, selective embolization of the involved vessels via vascular catheters by the interventional radiologist can be considered.[36,73]

The nurse must be alert to signs and symptoms of GI bleeding, particularly in the 5 days after the initial incident, when the patient is most prone to rebleeding.[36,73] Symptoms include variations in pulse pressure, decreased blood pressure and CVP or pulmonary artery occlusive pressure, falling hematocrit, abdominal distention, blood or coffee ground material in the nasogastric tube, emesis, melena, or hematochezia. Nasogastric tubes should be inserted with minimal trauma and placed to low intermittent suction to prevent erosions to the gastric mucosa. Rectal tubes and trumpets should be avoided to prevent hemorrhoid or rectal variceal bleeding, which is difficult to control. Treatment includes octreotide (Sandostatin) infusion to decrease portal pressure, with gastric protective agents.[1] Lactulose or other cathartics and nonabsorbable antibiotics are used to decrease the protein load from breakdown of blood in the gut and prevent worsening of HE. Crystalloid therapy is not preferred over blood administration. Blood component therapy should be targeted to volume replacement without over hydration and distention of varices and rebleeding to a hemoglobin level of approximately 8 g/dL.[73] Factor VIIa or KCentra can be used to treat bleeding in patients with fluid overload. The usual target CVP range is 8 to 10 mm Hg. Antibiotics are used to prevent or treat gram-negative infection after GI bleeding and interventional procedures, and have been shown to decrease mortality.[5,36,73]

Infection

Infection is the most common precipitant of ACLF, and all patients with liver dysfunction are at risk for bacterial or fungal infection[73] (Box 17.3). This is due in part to the loss of Kupffer cell function within the hepatic sinusoids. These cells phagocytize gram-negative bacteria leaked from the gut; loss of Kupffer cell function results in gram-negative bacteremia.[45] Malnutrition and increase in toxins cause general immune system suppression, and increased gut permeability, increasing the likelihood of infection.[5,37] There is an immunoparesis as well, with monocyte deactivation, which is worse in the patient with

BOX 17.3 Infection Control in Liver Dysfunction

- Strict hand hygiene
- Central line site monitoring and care
- Evaluate gag reflex, and early intubation for stage 3 to 4 HE, or upper GI bleeding to prevent aspiration
- Meticulous oral care with antimicrobial solution
- Bathing with chlorhexidine solution
- Infection surveillance, with blood, urine, sputum, ascites cultures, chest radiograph
- Treat documented infections
- Antibiotics after GI bleeding
- Avoid steroid use
- Albumin replacement in sepsis and spontaneous bacterial peritonitis
- Prophylactic antimicrobials ONLY for resistant HE and pre-liver transplant
- External fecal incontinence device; avoid rectal tubes

GI, Gastrointestinal; *HE,* hepatic encephalopathy.
From References 50, 55, 73, and 84.

high bilirubin and mitochondrial dysfunction.[84] Bacterial infections occur in 34% of all cirrhotic patients admitted to the hospital.[73] A 2011 review of 178 studies showed development of an infection quadrupled mortality in ACLF.[5]

The presence of ascites predisposes the patient to spontaneous bacterial peritonitis. This is defined as a polymorphic neutrophil (PMN) count of greater than 250 mm^3 in ascitic fluid.[18,45] Treatment of spontaneous bacterial peritonitis includes intravenous antibiotics and albumin, which reduces the incidence of renal dysfunction. Massive hepatic necrosis occurs in ALF, which triggers release of proinflammatory cytokines, which in turn increases the incidence of multisystem organ dysfunction, infection, and sepsis.[73] Prophylactic antibiotics in the general ALF and ACLF patients have not been shown to decrease blood-borne infections or improve survival and may promote resistant pathogens.[46,50,73] Except for diagnosed infections, unexplained progression of HE, or pretransplant patients, infection surveillance and targeted antibiotic therapy are recommended.[32,45,50,73] Infections must be detected and treated aggressively, as they can cause ACLF, exacerbate HE, precipitate hepatorenal syndrome Type I, and prevent the patient from receiving a transplant or cause complications after transplant.[11] Prophylactic antibiotics and antifungals should be considered for pretransplant patients. Aminoglycosides are poorly metabolized in liver failure patients and are hepatotoxic and nephrotoxic; they should not be used in patients with liver failure.[50] Steroids are to be avoided, or dosing decreased, as they have been shown to increase the risk of infection in this population.[50,73] For spontaneous bacterial peritonitis, albumin must be given along with antibiotics, as a survival benefit has been shown.[3]

Hepatopulmonary Syndrome and Portopulmonary Hypertension

The lung vasculature is affected in liver disease, in that microdilation of capillary channels can occur, causing hepatopulmonary syndrome, or arterial constriction can result in portopulmonary hypertension.[19,30] Hepatopulmonary syndrome occurs in approximately 10% to 15% of patients with cirrhosis, and is defined by intrapulmonary capillary dilation, intrapulmonary shunting, and abnormal alveolar gas exchange with lowered oxygen saturation. Although the exact cause is not understood, nitric oxide overproduction has been implicated in animal models.[5] Symptoms include hypoxia that does not improve with oxygen administration, dyspnea, clubbing of digits, and cyanosis. Oxygenation sometimes improves with laying the patient flat to perfuse alveolar beds. Treatment is symptomatic. The syndrome often reverses over time after liver transplantation.[11]

Portopulmonary hypertension (PPH) is defined as a mean pulmonary artery pressure of greater than 25 mm Hg with a pulmonary artery occlusive pressure of less than 15 mm Hg. It is estimated to occur in 4% to 16% of all cirrhotic patients.[5] Right-side cardiac catheterization with vasoactive agents is sometimes required to confirm the diagnosis. Symptoms include fatigue, dyspnea, and peripheral edema. Treatment for PPH is the same as that for primary pulmonary hypertension: prostaglandins, epoprostenol (Flolan), and treprostinil (Remodulin) infusions, inhaled iloprost, or oral sildenafil or bosentan (Tracleer). The condition reverses over months to years after liver transplant. Liver transplantation is contraindicated in moderate to severe cases unresponsive to treatment because of high mortality from right ventricular dysfunction and graft venous congestion, particularly during anesthesia induction.[55,59]

BOX 17.4 Criteria for Diagnosing Hepatorenal Syndrome

Major criteria

- Chronic or acute liver disease with advanced hepatic failure and portal hypertension
- Low GFR: serum creatinine > 133 µmol/L or 24 h creatinine clearance < 40 mL/min
- Absence of shock, ongoing bacterial infection, or treatment with nephrotoxic drug
- Absence of gastrointestinal or renal fluid losses
- No sustained improvement in renal function following diuretic withdrawal and expansion of plasma volume with 1.5 L of isotonic saline
- Proteinuria < 0.5 g/d and no ultrasonographic evidence of obstructive uropathy or parenchymal renal disease

Additional criteria

- Urine volume < 0.5 L/d
- Urine sodium < 10 µmol/L
- Urine osmolality > plasma osmolality
- Urine red blood cells < 50 high power field
- Serum sodium concentration < 130 µmol/L

GFR, Glomerular filtration rate.
From Reference 9.

Acute Kidney Injury and Hepatorenal Syndrome

Acute kidney injury (AKI) is common in ALF, occurring in up to 70% of all cases. It is linked to an overall increase in mortality, and decreased graft survival after liver transplant.[43] The causes are multifactorial, and include prerenal hypovolemia, acute tubular necrosis, drug toxicity (especially acetaminophen), SIRS, use of vasopressors, and hepatorenal syndrome.[9,73,84] Liver patients with AKI have an acute reduction in their glomerular filtration rate, with creatinine clearance used as the usual biomarker. This marker is limited in liver disease, as it is based on muscle mass and liver patients tend to have muscle wasting, increased creatinine secretion, and increased distribution of total body creatinine, particularly in ascites, which dilutes the serum result. Therefore, serum creatinine results tend to overestimate renal function in liver patients.[8] Per the Acute Kidney Injury Network (AKIN), AKI is defined as an increase in serum creatinine by greater than or equal to 0.3 mg/dL within 48 hours; increase in serum creatinine greater than or equal to 1.5 times baseline within 48 hours; or urine volume of less than 0.5 mL/kg/hour for 6 hours.[8,59,73]

Abdominal hypertension is called the *hidden factor* in causing AKI. Ascites, hepatic enlargement, and tissue edema can markedly increase pressure in the abdominal compartment, inferior vena cava, and renal veins. This results in renal outflow obstruction and reduced renal perfusion pressure. If this is suspected, intraabdominal pressure should be measured and managed appropriately.[84]

Hepatorenal syndrome (HRS) occurs in acute and chronic liver disease. The prevalence in cirrhosis with ascites is 18% after 1 year, and 39% at 5 years.[9] It is characterized by splenic arterial vasodilation, reduced cardiac output, and alterations in intrinsic renal blood flow.[9] There are two types: Type I and Type II. Type I has a rapid onset and progression and is usually triggered by bacterial infections. Most patients die within 2 weeks of onset of Type I HRS if not treated. Type II is characterized by a slow, steady reduction in renal function with resistance to diuretics. The diagnosis of HRS is one of exclusion, focused on eliminating other causes of renal dysfunction or AKI[10] (Box 17.4). Liver failure patients, particularly with ascites, tend to have low intravascular volume and systemic vascular resistance (SVR), which promotes prerenal azotemia and lowered urine output. Fluid bolus with normal saline or albumin tends to restore urine output in these cases. Recommended albumin dosing is 1 g/kg followed by 20–40 g/day.[3,8,10,50,73] If the patient is fluid resuscitated, with adequate MAP and no evidence of renal disease, sepsis, or use of nephrotoxic medications, the patient is characterized as having HRS. HRS should be managed by monitoring urine output, weight, hemodynamic parameters, blood urea nitrogen levels, creatinine, serum electrolytes, and urine sodium and urea. Prevention of HRS includes avoidance of nephrotoxic agents, fluid resuscitation to euvolemia, paracentesis with albumin replacement, and splenic bed vasoconstriction.[5] Urinary neutrophil gelatinase-associated lipocalin (N-GAL) is being investigated as a biomarker for the diagnosis of HRS. New criteria have been proposed for diagnosing AKI and HRS in the setting of cirrhosis that take into account the changes in creatinine, fluid shifts, and timing of physiologic changes that occur in cirrhotic patients.[8,32] Prevention of HRS is imperative. Prevention includes avoiding spontaneous bacterial peritonitis with long-term oral norfloxacin, prompt treatment of spontaneous bacterial peritonitis, adequate albumin replacement with large volume paracentesis, and correct management of diuretic therapy, including stoppage when creatinine levels increase.[9]

Treatment of HRS focuses on redirecting internal and external renal blood flow. Diuretic dosing should be lowered, or discontinued.[7,8] Maneuvers that redirect ascites to peripheral circulation (TIPS, DIPS, and peritovenous shunt) have been shown to increase circulating volume and improve HRS.[9] The kidneys maintain intrinsic blood flow by producing prostaglandins, which cause renal vasodilation. Prostaglandin inhibitors, such as nonsteroidal antiinflammatory medications, should not be given to liver failure patients.[8,42] A combination of midodrine (a peripheral vasoconstrictor), octreotide (a splenic vasoconstrictor), and albumin (an oncotic agent) has been used to successfully treat HRS.[3,7] Vasoconstrictors can induce side effects in up to 40% of patients, namely, diarrhea, abdominal pain, myocardial stress and infarction, intestinal ischemia, and fluid overload.[9] Terlipressin (a potent splenic vasoconstrictor), and albumin infusions are currently the standard treatment for hepatorenal syndrome type I worldwide; however, terlipressin is not available in the United States.[39,59]

Dialytic therapy may be required as support until infection subsides or as a bridge to transplantation. The preferred mode of dialysis is continuous renal replacement therapy or extended daily dialysis rather than intermittent hemodialysis.[9,16] This prevents the hypotension and worsening cerebral edema seen with hemodialysis, and provides for real-time fluid and electrolyte regulation.[16,42,84] Continuous therapies also have the advantage of more aggressive bicarbonate administration for pH correction, and for removal of ammonia.[27,86] Studies have shown efficacy in extracorporeal albumin dialysis (ECAD) in improving patients with HRS type I.[9,47] HRS, if not severe or prolonged, usually reverses with liver transplantation.[10,11]

Cerebral Edema and Herniation

Cerebral edema is realized as the most serious complication of liver failure. Any patient with stage 3 or 4 HE should be treated as a cerebral edema patient. Approximately 20% of patients with ALF die from increased ICP and cerebral herniation. Treatment options for increased ICP in ALF are limited, and many patients have uncontrolled intracranial hypertension unresponsive to conventional therapy.

The pathologic mechanisms are not fully understood, but are believed to be cytotoxic and vasogenic in origin, and linked to edema of astrocytes in the brain and loss of cerebral blood flow autoregulation. Cerebral ammonia accumulates due to inadequate hepatic detoxification. It is enzymatically converted to osmotically active glutamine, which then accumulates in the astrocytes and causes swelling, particularly in the cerebral cortex. Studies have repeatedly shown that an arterial ammonia level of 150 to 200 mg/dL is associated with increased risk of cerebral herniation.[13,21,73] Herniation rarely occurs when serum ammonia levels are less than 100 mg/dL.[73] Noncontrast head CT scan usually shows a generalized tightness of the brain with no shift in the ventricles. ICP monitoring is performed in some centers, with a goal to keep it less than 20 to 25 mm Hg and a CPP of 50 to 60 mm Hg. ICP monitoring has not been shown to improve neurologic outcome or survival in ALF, although it may change neurologic and overall management, particularly for liver transplantation.[47,73]

Patients should be positioned with the head of bed elevated 30 degrees, with the patient's head midline.[65] The environment should be kept quiet and nonstimulating. The patient should be monitored hourly and as needed for clinical signs and symptoms of cerebral edema: Glasgow Coma Scale, systemic hypertension, bradycardia, papillary abnormalities, decerebrate posturing, and epileptiform activity.[65] A randomized, controlled study showed that hypernatremia induced with hypertonic saline to a serum sodium level of 145–155 mEq/L was more effective in preventing the development of cerebral edema than management at normal serum sodium levels. Serum sodium levels should be monitored judiciously before the start of and during therapy, as a rapid increase of serum sodium can result in demyelinating syndrome.[85] Mannitol is effective in reducing ICP in ALF and can be used if renal function is adequate and serum osmolality is less than 320 mOsm/L.[42,51] Recommended intravenous bolus is 0.5–1 g/kg body weight. Blood and urine osmolarity should be monitored after the second or third dose.[65] Hyperventilation to reduce partial pressure of arterial carbon dioxide ($Paco_2$) to 25 to 30 mm Hg has been shown to quickly lower ICP, but the effects are short-lived, and the treatment is not recommended.[32] Agents used in controlling HE are continued in cases of cerebral edema. An ammonia-scavenging agent, ornithine phenylacetate (OPA), provides for renal excretion of glutamine, and is in clinical trials.[78] Seizures can occur, especially in the presence of electrolyte derangements. Phenytoin is the drug of choice for seizures over other agents that are hepatically or renally excreted.[42] Cisatracurium besylate (Nimbex) is preferred if neuromuscular blockade and paralysis are required, as it is metabolized through an acid-base pathway that is independent of the kidneys and liver. Propofol is the preferred sedative agent as it is reversible with flumazenil and better tolerated hemodynamically. It should be used, along with intubation and ventilation, for HE of Stage 3 or 4.[9,50,74] Manual hyperinflation by bag ventilation decreases cerebral venous return and increases ICP, and should be avoided.[65] Continuous renal replacement therapy has been demonstrated to reduce serum levels of ammonia, and can assist in maintaining hypothermia and reducing ICP.[85] For persistent ICP elevations, barbiturates are used. In rare cases of severe ICP elevation, lactic acidosis, or hepatic necrosis, a hepatectomy is performed if the patient is listed and awaiting liver transplant.[85]

Previously, moderate therapeutic hypothermia (TH) (32°C to 33°C) was promoted for reducing ICP and stabilizing cerebral metabolism.[45] Studies have concluded there is no clinical advantage or survival benefit over mild hypothermia (36°C to 37°C).[46,50,77] A multicenter cohort analysis showed TH did not consistently affect 21-day survival, but was associated with clinical benefit in some patients, particularly for acetaminophen overdose, with no increase in bleeding or infections.[47] This treatment should be implemented for patients with ALF and stages 3 to 4 HE by using ice packs or cooling blankets, decreasing the room temperature, cooling the ventilator humidifier, or employing commercially available regional cooling systems. For refractory intracranial hypertension, short-acting barbiturates may be considered.[50]

INTERPROFESSIONAL PLAN OF CARE

The liver failure patient is one of the most complex and challenging patients seen in critical care. Meticulous care coordinated among many disciplines is required for a positive patient outcome. The critical care nurse is the key factor in providing empathetic and coordinated care.[75] The coordinated management of ALF patients in particular should be started at presentation at community hospitals and carried through to transfer to a tertiary liver center. This helps to ensure the patient's condition is optimized throughout the continuum of care. Box 17.5 is an example of a treatment protocol for referring hospitals and interfacility transport.

REFERRAL/LISTING FOR LIVER TRANSPLANTATION

Liver transplantation remains the mainstay of treatment for many patients with liver failure. Chronic liver disease patients should be referred for transplantation when exhibiting

BOX 17.5 Acute Liver Failure Transport Protocol Example

UCSD Medical Center

The Liver Center/Center for Transplantation, Treatment Protocol

Management of Acute Hepatic Failure for Outside Medical Facilities and for Interfacility Transport

Outside Medical Facility

1. Contact the hepatologist on call at UCSDMC by contacting the page operator at ________. After the case is reviewed and discussed with the referring provider, the hepatologist will contact the Hillcrest Transfer Center to initiate transfer to UCSDMC Hillcrest.
2. If drug overdose is suspected:
   - Contact the Poison Control Center
   - Draw acetaminophen levels
   - For acetaminophen toxicity, continue N-acetylcysteine PO or IV until AST/ALT are normalized.
3. Send the following tests: comprehensive drug screen, blood alcohol level, comprehensive metabolic panel (SMAC 22), magnesium, complete blood count with differential, PT/TTP, INR, fibrinogen, blood cultures, urinalysis, urine culture, chest x-ray, urine electrolytes, total protein, and urea.
4. Place 2 large-bore peripheral IV catheters, preferably in the antecubital space. AVOID CENTRAL LINE PLACEMENT. If a central line catheter is needed, correct the INR to 1.5 or less, and use the femoral or internal jugular veins. DO NOT use the subclavian sites, as this can result in a life-threatening pneumothorax or hemothorax.
5. IT IS VITAL THAT THESE PATIENTS BE COOLED TO A TEMPERATURE OF 34–35°C. This has been shown to decrease cerebral edema in liver failure. Treat the patient as you would a head injury patient:
   - Place cooling blankets above and below the patient.
   - Place ice packs over the liver, in the femoral and antecubital spaces, and over the internal jugular veins.
   - Keep the head of the bed elevated at a 45-degree angle. Do not flex the knees.
   - Keep the head midline.
   - Maintain a quiet, nonstimulating environment.
6. Sedate the patient with propofol as needed for agitation.
7. For stage 3 or 4 hepatic encephalopathy, intubate the patient.
8. Do not overhydrate the patient; use normal saline, blood products, or albumin for volume expansion. Do not use lactated Ringer's solution.

Interfacility Transportation

1. Maintain cerebral edema precautions and mild hypothermia throughout transport.
   - Place cooling blankets above and below the patient.
   - Place ice packs over the liver, in the femoral and antecubital spaces, and over the internal jugular veins.
   - Keep the head of the bed elevated at a 45-degree angle. Do not flex the knees.
   - Keep the head midline.
2. Do NOT use lactated Ringer's for fluid replacement. Do NOT overhydrate the patient.
3. Bring ALL test results, chart notes, and digitalized images with the patient.
4. Call the UCSD Hillcrest Transfer Center for any questions regarding transport or clinical management, at telephone ________. They will connect you with the hepatologist on call.

ALT, Alanine transaminase; *AST,* aspartate aminotransferase; *INR,* international normalized ratio; *PO,* per os; *PT,* prothrombin time; *TTP,* thrombotic thrombocytopenic purpura; *UCSD,* University of California, San Diego.

evidence of synthetic dysfunction (low albumin level, elevated PT/PTT), experiencing their first complication of decompensation (ascites, variceal bleeding, HE), worsening renal dysfunction, diagnosed with hepatocellular tumors, or developing malnutrition.[55] All cases of ALF should be considered for referral to a tertiary center for transplant evaluation and listing in an expedient manner. The ventilated ICU patient who is meticulously managed can be transplanted with acceptable long-term outcomes as long as the patient is in stable condition.[5,48]

The MELD score, originally used to predict 90-day mortality in patients with chronic liver disease, is now used by the United Network for Organ Sharing (UNOS) to prioritize and list patients with chronic liver disease for transplant in the United States. Implemented in 2002, the score is a logarithmic calculation based on three laboratory values: total bilirubin level, INR, and creatinine level. The calculation produces a numeric score. Patients with a MELD score greater than or equal to 15 should be considered for liver transplantation evaluation.[48,55] Patients with a MELD score of 30 or more have a higher risk of mortality. Status 1 (highest priority) on the UNOS transplant list is not associated with the MELD score and is reserved for patients with ALF with a predicted life expectancy of less than 7 days.[11,54] Status 1 patients have the highest priority for receiving organs due to the critical nature of the liver failure. Patients with concurrent renal failure may require simultaneous listing for liver and kidney transplant.[11,55,82]

LIVER SUPPORT DEVICES

There remains an obvious need to support liver disease patients with devices as a bridge to liver transplant, or ideally to regeneration and recovery of native organ function. The development and availability of liver support devices (LSDs), however, have lagged behind other artificial organ support devices, such as renal dialysis, ventilators, membrane oxygenators, and ventricular support devices. This is related to the complexity of liver functions and the difficulty in developing technology to mimic these functions. The ideal LSD must be able to regulate fluid, electrolyte, glucose, and acid-base balance, and provide clearance of circulating ammonia, false neurotransmitters (such as GABA), cytokines, and other hepatic toxins (particularly those that are protein-bound, such as bilirubin). The device should also synthesize critical molecules and orchestrate all these functions to preserve homeostasis and allow for hepatic regeneration and recovery while yielding no complications from the therapy.[28,62]

Depending on whether or not cellular components are used, LSDs are classified as nonbiologic or biologic. Nonbiologic support devices use noncellular technologies to mimic certain aspects of liver function. The technologies utilize special filter membranes and resins, charcoal, or albumin in the dialysate to remove larger-molecular-weight or protein-bound substances that are not removed by conventional dialysis methods.[18,69]

Conventional dialysis therapies are also used in part for liver support. These modalities are particularly useful in patients experiencing renal dysfunction often seen with liver disease. Continuous renal replacement therapies (CRRTs) are routinely used for fluid, glucose, electrolyte, acid-base regulation, and removal of small to middle weight molecules, including ammonia and some cytokines. Plasmapheresis and therapeutic plasma exchange (TPE) involves the removal of toxins and inflammatory mediators by plasma removal and replacement.[13] A recent longitudinal study demonstrated a modest increase in survival with TPE versus standard medical therapy.[83] Nonbiological liver support systems that use albumin dialysis target large molecule toxin removal, particularly bilirubin.[12,78] None of these nonbiologic methods provide synthesis of critical substances.

Biologic LSDs employ isolated liver cells in bioreactors to mimic liver function. Other detoxifying components, such as charcoal and resin columns, are sometimes added to the system. These devices have the advantage of providing some synthetic function and toxin clearance that is comparable to native liver function.[6] Several types are being developed worldwide; three are in active development in the United States with clinical trials in process. There are multiple case reports and small studies showing stabilization of condition and successful bridging to transplant using LSDs. A review and meta-analysis of three recent extracorporeal liver support (ELS) trials suggests improvement in HE, CPP, and survival in ALF. Another meta-analysis of 19 trials suggested that there is a reduction in mortality in ACLF patients, but not in ALF patients. Biologic LSDs with albumin infusion are in development in Europe.[49] These devices are being utilized as "bridging tools" to hepatic recovery or transplant.[62,67]

Controlled trials of devices are needed, but are difficult to design and fund. Safety remains a concern, particularly transmission of disease from bioreactor hepatocytes. The efficacy of therapeutic plasma exchange and ELS requires further investigation with larger, multifacility studies.[84] The profession needs to actively focus on specific areas of LSD development and research and sequence these activities logically to best utilize time and resources. As clinical trials are completed, it is anticipated that both modalities will have a place in treating liver failure, with the less expensive nonbiologic LSDs used for less sick patients, and the more costly and complicated biologic LSDs reserved for more critical patients.[84] Besides LSDs, other modalities in development include implantable, constructed livers of hepatocytes grown on an artificial matrix, hepatocyte transplantation, and transgenic xenografts harvested from genetically altered animals to resemble human livers.[84]

CONCLUSION

The complexity of liver dysfunction and disease and the multisystem effects it creates make the nursing management of these patients one of the most challenging in critical care. Interprofessional planning and care coordination and timely referral for transplant are essential in producing optimal patient outcomes. The increase in spontaneous survival for some causes of ALF and in ACLF overall can be attributed to judicious nursing and interprofessional care.

CASE STUDY 17.1

S.M. is a 19-year-old African American female who presented in the emergency department of a small community hospital with her mother. S.M. has complained of difficulty concentrating and tremors for 2 weeks. Three days ago she complained of nausea, vomiting, edema, and yellowed eyes. Her mother states that S.M. has been moody and depressed, and on the day of admission had hallucinations and became violent toward family members. Her physical findings included being responsive to commands, flailing all extremities, and yelling 1 or 2 incomprehensible words. There was no asterixis. Her deep tendon reflexes were reduced to + 1/4. She had a minimal gag reflex, and sluggish pupillary response at 4 mm bilaterally. Her skin was warm and flushed, with scleral icterus. Her abdomen was flat with minimal bowel sounds. Her liver border was palpated at 5 cm below costal margin. She was anuric. Her vital signs included a temperature of 99.2°F; pulse was 110 beats/min; respiratory rate was 34 breaths/min; and blood pressure was 125/80 mm Hg. Her laboratory values revealed glucose: 63 mg/dL; BUN: 76 mg/dL; creatinine: 3.6 mg/dL; sodium: 148 mEq/L; potassium: 5.0 mEq/L; bicarbonate: 13 mEq/L; magnesium: 1.5 mEq/L; ammonia: 145 mcg/dL; AST: 5400 u/L; ALT: 4900 mg/L; bilirubin: direct 2.1 mg/dL, total 4.5 mg/dL; white blood cell count: 10.0/mm^3; hemoglobin: 13.5 g%; hematocrit: 42%; platelets: 145,000/mm^3; and ratio INR 4.0.

Decision Point:

Based on the onset of symptoms and clinical data, what type of liver failure does the patient have?

Decision Point:

What is the initial treatment plan for this patient?

REFERENCES

1. Abba, M., El Damarawy, M., Seyam, M., et al. (2007). Denver peritoneovenous shunt in the management of refractory ascites due to chronic liver diseases: impact of patients' selection on its outcome. *J Egypt Soc Parasitol*, *37*(Suppl. 3), 1159–1174.
2. Abraldes, J. G., Dell'Era, A., & Bosch, J. (2004). Medical management of variceal bleeding in patients with cirrhosis. *Can J Gastroenterol*, *18*, 109–113.
3. Afinogenova, Y., & Tapper, E. (2015). The efficacy and safety profile of albumin administration for patients with cirrhosis at high risk of hepatorenal syndrome is dose dependent. *Gastroenterol Rep*, *3*(3), 216–221.
4. Akriviadis, E., et al. (2000). Pentoxifylline improves short-term survival in severe acute alcoholic hepatitis: a double-blind, placebo-controlled trial. *Gastroenterology*, *119*, 1637–1648.
5. Al-Khafaji, A., & Huang, D. (2011). Critical care management of patients with end-stage liver disease. *Crit Care Med*, *39*(5), 1157–1166.
6. Allen, J., Hassanein, T., & Bhatia, S. (2001). Advances in bioartificial liver devices. *Hepatology*, *34*(3), 447–455.
7. Angeli, P., et al. (1999). Reversal of type 1 hepatorenal syndrome with the administration of midodrine and octreotide. *Hepatology*, *29*, 1660–1670.
8. Angeli, P., Gines, P., Wong, F., et al. (2015). Diagnosis and management of acute kidney injury in patients with cirrhosis: revised consensus recommendations of the International Club of Ascites. *J Hepatol*, *62*(4), 968–974.
9. Angeli, P., & Morando, F. (2010). Optimal management of hepatorenal syndrome in patients with cirrhosis. *Hepat Med*, *2*, 87–98.
10. Arroyo, V., et al. (1996). Definition and diagnosis of refractory ascites and hepatorenal syndrome in cirrhosis. *Hepatology*, *23*(11), 164–176.
11. Bacon, B. R. (2000). Liver anatomy and physiology. In B. R. Bacon, & A. M. Bisceglie (Eds.), *Liver disease: diagnosis and management*. New York: Churchill Livingstone.
12. Banares, R., & Vaquero, J. (2014). Molecular adsorbent recirculating system and bioartificial devices for liver failure. *Cin Liver Dis*, *18*, 945–956.
13. Biancofiore, G., Bindi, L., et al. (2003). Combined twice-daily plasma exchange and continuous veno-venous hemodiafiltration for bridging severe acute liver failure. *Transpl Proc*, *35*(8), 3011–3014.

14. Blei, A. T., & Cordoba, J. (2005). Hepatic encephalopathy. *Am J Gastroenterol, 96*, 1868–1876.
15. Boyer, T., & Jaskal, Z. (2005). The role of transjugular intrahepatic protosystemic shunt in the management of portal hypertension. *Hepatology, 41*(2), 1–15.
16. Carithers, R. L. (2004). AASLD practice guideline: liver practice guideline: liver transplantation. *Liver Transplant, 1*, 122–135.
17. Chalasani, N., Hayashi, P., & Bonkovsky, H. (2014). ACG Clinical Guideline: the diagnosis and management of idiosyncratic drug-induced liver injury. *Am J Gastroenterol, 109*(7), 950–966.
18. Chaney, A. (2015). Cirrhosis complications: ascites and spontaneous bacterial peritonitis. *Clin Rev*, 33–37.
19. Cheung, K., Lee, S., & Raman, M. (2012). Prevalence and mechanisms of malnutrition in patients with advanced liver disease, and nutrition management strategies. *Clin Gastroenterol Hepatol, 10*, 117–125.
20. Choudhury, J., & Sanyal, A. (2003). Treatment of ascites. *Curr Treat Options Gastroenterol, 6*(6), 481–491.
21. Clemmesen, J. O., Larsen, F. S., Kondrup, J., et al. (1999). Cerebral herniation in patients with acute liver failure is correlated with arterial ammonia concentration. *Hepatology, 29*, 648–653.
22. Conn, H., Palmaz, J., et al. (2000). *TIPS: transjugular intrahepatic portosystemic shunts.* New York: Igaku-Shoin.
23. Courson, A., Jones, M., & Twilla, J. (2016). Treatment of acute hepatic encephalopathy: comparing the effects of adding rifaximin to lactulose on patient outcomes. *J Pharm Pract, 29*(3), 212–217.
24. D'Amico, G., et al. (2005). Uncovered transjugular intrahepatic portosystemic shunt for refractory ascites: a meta-analysis. *Gastroenterology, 129*, 1282–1293.
25. Dan, C., Moses-Einsenstein, M., & Valdiserri, R. (2015). Viral hepatitis: new U.S. screening recommendations, assessment tools, and treatments. *AJN, 115*(7), 26–35.
26. Dasher, K., & Trotter, J. (2012). Intensive care unit management of liver-related coagulation disorders. *Crit Care Clin, 28*, 389–398.
27. Davenport, A., Will, E. J., & Davidson, A. (1993). Improved cardiovascular stability during continuous modes of renal replacement therapy in critically ill patients with acute hepatic and renal failure. *Crit Care Med, 21*, 328–338.
28. Demetriou, A., et al. (2004). Prospective, randomized controlled trial of a bioartificial liver in treating acute liver failure. *Ann Surg, 239*(5), 667–670.
29. Dotter Interventional Institute. *IVUS guided DIPS.* http://www.ohsu.edu/dotter/dips.htm.
30. Fallon, M. (2001). *Hepatopulmonary and portopulmonary hypertension.* Dallas, TX: AASLD Annual Meeting.
31. Farsad, K., Fuss, C., Kolbeck, K., et al. (2012). Transjugular intrahepatic portosystemic shunt creation using intravascular ultrasound guidance. *J Vasc Interv Radiol, 23*(12), 1594–1602.
32. Francoz, C., & Durand, F. (2012). A new look at renal dysfunction in the cirrhotic patient. *Crit Care*, 2012.
33. Friedman, L. S., & Keefe, E. (1998). *Handbook of liver disease.* New York: Churchill Livingstone.
34. Frohlich, S., N, et al. (2014). Alcoholic liver disease in the intensive care unit: outcomes and predictors of prognosis. *J Crit Care, 29*, 1131e1–1131e3.
35. Fullwood, D., & Purushothaman, A. (2013). Managing ascites in patients with chronic liver disease. *CPD, 28*(23), 51–58.
36. Garcia-Tsao, G., Sanyal, A., Grace, N., et al. (2007). Practice guideline: prevention and management of gastroesophageal varicies and variceal hemorrhage in cirrhosis. *Am J Gastroenterol, 102*, 2086–2102.
37. Gines, P., Quintero, E., Arroyo, V., et al. (1987). Compensated cirrhosis: natural history and prognostic factors. *Hepatology, 7*, 12–18.
38. Hassanein, T. (1995). *Personal communication.*
39. Hassanein, T. (2004). *Personal communication.*
40. Haynes, G., et al. (2003). Albumin administration—what is the evidence of clinical benefit? A systematic review of randomized controlled trials. *Eur J Anaesthesiol, 20*(10), 771–793.
41. Hebuterne, X., & Vanbiervliet, G. (2011). Feeding the patient with upper gastrointestinal bleeding. *Curr Opin Clin Nutr Metab Care, 14*(2), 197–201.
42. Hermite, L., Quenot, J., Nadji, A., et al. (2012). Sodium citrate versus saline catheter locks for non-tunneled hemodialysis central venous catheters in critically ill adults: a randomized controlled trial. *Intensive Care Med, 38*(2), 279–285.
43. Hilmi, I., Damian, D., Al-Khafaji, A., et al. (2015). Acute kidney injury following orthotopic liver transplantation: incidence, risk factors, and effects on patient and graft outcomes. *Br J Anaesth, 114*(6), 919–926.
44. Iyamana, I., Anene, A., Reddick, M., et al. (2015). Clinical utility of intravascular ultrasound guided portal vein access during transjugular intrahepatic portosystemic shunt (TIPS) creation: comparison with conventional technique. *JIR, 26*(2), S94.
45. Jalan, R., et al. (2004). Moderate hypothermia in patients with acute liver failure and uncontrolled intracranial hypertension. *Gastroenterology, 127*, 1338–1346.
46. Karvellas, C., Stravitz, T., Battenhouse, J., Lee, W., et al. (2015). Therapeutic hypothermia in acute liver failure: a multicenter retrospective cohort analysis. *Liver Transpl, 21*(10), 4–12.
47. Karvellas, C., Fix, O., Battenhouse, H., et al. (2014). Outcomes and complications of intracranial pressure monitoring in acute liver failure: a retrospective cohort study. *Crit Care Med, 42*(5), 1157–1167.
48. Knaak, J., McVey, M., Bazerbachi, F., et al. (2015). Liver transplantation in patients with end-stage liver disease requiring intensive care unit admission and intubation. *Liver Transpl, 21*(6), 761–767.
49. Lee, K., Baker, L., Stanzani, G., et al. (2015). Extracorporeal liver assist device to exchange albumin and remove endotoxin in acute liver failure: results of a pivotal pre-clinical study. *J Hepatol, 63*(3), 634–642.
50. Lee, W., Larson, A., & Stravitz, R. (2011). AASLD position paper: the management of acute liver failure: update 2011. http://www.aasld.org/sites/default/files/guideline_documents/alfenhanced.pdf.
51. Lodono, M., Abraldes, J., Altamiran, J., et al. (2015). Clinical trial watch: report from the Liver Meeting (AASLD), Boston, November, 2014. *J Hepatol, 62*(5), 1196–1203.
52. Maddrey, W., Schiff, E., & Sorrell, M. (2001). *Transplantation of the liver.* Philadelphia: Lippincott Williams & Wilkins.
53. Manzano, M., Barranco-Fragoso, B., Uribe, M., et al. (2015). Portal vein thrombosis: what is new? *Ann Hepatology, 14*(1), 20–27.
54. Martin, L. (2012). Percutaneous placement and management of peritoneovenous shunts. *Sem Interventional Radiol, 29*(2), 129–134.
55. Martin, P., DiMartini, A., Fang, S., et al. (2013). Evaluation for liver transplantation in adults: 2013 practice guidelines by the AASLD and the American Society of Transplantation. *Hepatology 59*(3), 1144–1165.
56. Martindale, R., McClave, S., Vanek, V., et al. (2009). Guidelines for the provision and assessment of nutritional support therapy in the adult critically ill patient: Society of Critical Care Medicine (SCCM) and American Society for Parenteral and Enteral Nutrition (ASPEN). *J Parenter Enteral Nutr, 33*(3), 277–316.
57. Mas, A., Rodes, J., Sunyer, L., et al. (2003). Comparison of rifaximin and lactitol in the treatment of acute hepatic encephalopathy: results of a randomized, double-blind, double-dummy, controlled clinical trial. *J Hepatol, 38*, 51–58.
58. Massa, P., Vallerino, E., & Dodero, M. (1993). Treatment of hepatic encephalopathy with rifaximin: double-blind, double-dummy study versus lactulose. *Eur J Clin Res, 4*, 7–18.
59. Mehta, R., Kellum, J., Shah, S., et al. (2007). Acute Kidney Injury Network Group: report of an initiative to improve outcomes in acute kidney injury. *Crit Care, 11*, R31.
60. Montano-Loza, A. J., Duarte-Rojo, A., Meza-Junco, J., et al. (2015). Inclusion of sarcopenia within MELD (MELD Sarcopenia) and the prediction of mortality in patients with cirrhosis. *Clin Transl Gastroenterol. Jul 16*,(6), 102.
61. *National Vital Statistics.* (2013). http://www.cdc.gov/nchs/data/nvsr/nvsr64/nvsr64_02.pdf.
62. Nevens, F., & Laleman, W. (2012). Artificial liver support devices as treatment option for liver failure. *Best Pract Res Clin Gastroenterol, 26*, 17–26.
63. Ochs, A. (2005). Transjugular intrahepatic portosystemic shunt. *Dig Dis, 23*(1), 56–64.
64. Oida, T., Mimatsu, K., Kano, H., et al. (2011). Early implantation of Denver shunt. *Hepatogastroenterology, 58*(112), 2026–2028.
65. O'Neal, H., Olds, J., & Webster, N. (2006). Managing patients with acute liver failure: developing a tool for practitioners. *Brit Assoc Crit Care Nurs, 11*(2), 63–68.
66. Purnak, T., & Yilman, Y. (2013). Liver disease and malnutrition. *Best Prac Res Gastroenterol, 27*, 619–629.

67. Quin, G., Shao, J., Wang, B., et al. (2014). Artificial liver support system improves short- and long-term outcomes of patients with HBV-associated acute-on-chronic liver failure: a single center experience. *Medicine, 93*(28), e338.
68. Romero-Castro, R., et al. (2004). Recombinant-activated factor VII as hemostatic therapy in eight cases of severe hemorrhage from esophageal varices. *Clin Gastroenterol Hepatol, 2*(1), 78–84.
69. Rozga, J., Piatek, T., & Malkowski, P. (2013). Human albumin: old, new, and emerging applications. *Ann Transplant, 10*(18), 205–217.
70. Runyon, B. (2013). Introduction to the revised AASLD Practice Guidelines management of adult patients with ascites due to cirrhosis 2012. *Hepatology, 57*(4), 1651–1653 2013.
71. Runyoun, B. (2013). Management of adult patients with ascites due to cirrhosis: update 2012. *Hepatology, 57*(4), 1651–1653, 2013.
72. Saray, A., Mesihovic, R., Gornjakovic, S., et al. (2012). Association between high D-dimer plasma levels and ascites in patients with liver cirrhosis. *Med Arch, 6696*, 372–374.
73. Siddique, M., & Stravits, T. (2014). Intensive care unit management of patients with liver failure. *Clin Liver Dis, 18*, 957–978.
74. Singanayagam, A., & Bernal, W. (2015). Update on acute liver failure. *Curr Opin Crit Care, 21*, 134–141.
75. Slatore, C., Hansen, L., Ganzini, L., et al. (2012). Communication by nurses in the ICU: qualitative analysis of domains of patient-centered care. *Am J Crit Care, 21*(6), 410–418.
76. Sort, P., Navasa, M., Arroyao, V., et al. (1999). Effect of intravenous albumin on renal impairment and mortality in patient with cirrhosis and spontaneous bacterial peritonitis. *N Engl J Med, 34*, 403–409.
77. Spadaro, A., Tortorella, V., Morace, C., et al. (2008). High circulating D-dimers are associated with ascites and hepatocellular carcinoma in liver cirrhosis. *World J Gastroenterol, 14*(10), 1549–1552.
78. Stange, J., Hassanein, T., et al. (2002). The Molecular Adsorbent Recycling System as a liver support system based on albumin dialysis: a summary of preclinical investigations, prospective, randomized, controlled clinical trial and clinical experience from 19 centers. *Artif Organs, 26*(2), 1525–1594.
79. Thomas, E., Yoneda, M., & Shiff, E. (2015). Viral hepatitis: past and future of HBV and HDV. *Cold Springs Harb Perspect Med, 5*(2):a021345.
80. Trotter, J., Pieramici, E., & Everson, G. (2005). Chronic albumin infusions to achieve dieresis in patients with ascites who are not candidates for TIPS. *Dig Dis Sci, 50*(7), 1356–1360.
81. UC San Diego Health System. (August, 2015). *Prothrombin Complex Concentrate (4-component, human) (Kcentra) Monograph.*
82. Wedd, J., & Biggins, S. (2013). MELD Score, allocation, and distribution in the United States. *Clin Liver Dis, 2*(4), 148–151.
83. Wiersema, U., Kim, S., Roxby, D., et al. (2015). Therapeutic plasma exchange does not reduce vasopressor requirement in severe acute liver failure: a retrospective case series. *BMC Anesth, 8*(15), 15–30.
84. Wiesner, R. H. (2004). MELD/PELD and the allocation of deceased donor livers for Status 1 recipients with acute fulminant hepatic failure, primary nonfunction, hepatic artery thrombosis, and acute Wilson's disease. *Liver Transpl, 10*, S17–S22.
85. Willars, C. (2014). Update in intensive care medicine: acute liver failure. Initial management, supportive treatment, and who to transplant. *Curr Opin Crit Care, 20*(2), 202–209.
86. Won, J., Choi, S., Ko, H., et al. (2008). Percutaneous peritoneovenous shunt for treatment of refractory ascites. *J Vasc Radiol, 19*(17), 1717–1722.

18

Acute Pancreatitis

Eleanor Fitzpatrick

Acute pancreatitis is an acute inflammatory condition within the pancreas caused by premature activation of pancreatic enzymes and digestion of the gland by its own enzymes. In the normal pancreas, these enzymes are transported via the pancreatic duct into the duodenum, where they are activated and used for digestion of carbohydrates, fats, and proteins (Fig. 18.1). In acute pancreatitis, the intracellular proteases are activated before transport. Acute pancreatitis ranges in severity from a mild glandular form of edema to severe hemorrhagic or infected pancreatic necrosis with multiple organ dysfunction syndrome (MODS). The disease affects not only the pancreas, but also surrounding structures and remote organ systems, which are adversely affected due to the often severe systemic inflammatory response initiated by acute pancreatitis. The systemic inflammatory manifestations in acute pancreatitis are related to the host (bodily) response to the pancreatic injury with cytokine cascade and a compensatory antiinflammatory response that can predispose to infection. When this process is ongoing, the risk of organ failure is increased.[46] Acute pancreatitis is self-limiting in approximately 80% of cases; however, the fulminant (severe) form of the disorder results in high mortality rates and requires complex management techniques. Some of these strategies include interventional drainage procedures, minimally invasive or open surgical interventions, endoscopic or angiographic corrections, and clinical support for the failure of multiple organ dysfunction.[13,23,46] The two main types of acute pancreatitis (mild and severe) are classified as interstitial edematous pancreatitis and necrotizing pancreatitis. Interstitial pancreatitis affects the majority of patients in which there is a lack of pancreatic or peripancreatic parenchymal necrosis. In interstitial pancreatitis there is diffuse enlargement of the gland due to inflammatory edema.[46] In the more severe form, necrotizing pancreatitis, tissue necrosis is present in either the pancreatic parenchyma or in the peripancreatic tissue. Necrotizing pancreatitis can be sterile or infected and parenchyma involvement is a marker for more severe disease.[46]

DEFINITION

Acute pancreatitis is a disorder of the exocrine pancreas. The function of the exocrine pancreas consists of the synthesis and secretion of digestive enzymes into the small intestine to catalyze the hydrolysis and digestion of carbohydrates, proteins, and fats.[37] Many of the enzymes are proteases synthesized as proenzymes (zymogens) and require proteolytic activation by cleavage of their propeptides.[37] The enzymes amylase, trypsin, lipase, and others are secreted in their inactive form, becoming active upon entrance to the duodenum. Acute pancreatitis is an inflammatory condition of the pancreas initiated by injury to the acinar cells of the exocrine pancreas, resulting in premature activation and release of damaging enzymes.[37]

The mortality rate in pancreatitis is quite variable; the overall rate ranges from 3% for patients with interstitial edematous pancreatitis to 15% for those who develop the necrotizing form of the disease.[42,45] Severe acute pancreatitis is associated with a 20% mortality rate, and when infected necrosis ensues, the mortality rate increases to between 40% and 70%.[13]

The incidence of acute pancreatitis ranges from 13 to 45 cases per 100,000 per year, accounting for approximately 2% of all hospital admissions.[47] Acute pancreatitis is the leading cause of hospitalization for gastrointestinal diseases in the United States. There are more than 280,000 admissions for this disorder each year in the United States.[13,33] An increased incidence of acute pancreatitis has been shown since 2003, perhaps related to a higher sensitivity of diagnostic tests or to the advancing age of the population.[46]

PATIENTS AT RISK

Eighty percent of all episodes of acute pancreatitis are caused by gallstone disease (including biliary sludge and biliary microlithiasis) with migration of stones or excessive alcohol consumption.[23] The remaining 20% of cases are attributable to a multitude of causes, including hyperlipidemias, hypercalcemic states, a variety of medications, infections, trauma, endoscopic retrograde cholangiopancreatography (ERCP), and other etiologies (Box 18.1). In approximately 10% to 20% of those with pancreatitis, no cause is ever identified; this is termed *idiopathic disease*.[23,47]

Persons at risk of developing acute pancreatitis may be able to prevent its occurrence or recurrence. However, many etiologies of this disorder (e.g., gallstone formation and prescribed medication use) may impede implementing preventive strategies. Those who use alcohol in excess may prevent pancreatitis by limiting alcohol intake. Some lipid disorders may be controlled by diet and medications.[13] Prevention of pancreatitis in patients with gallstones involves cholecystectomy during current admission or within 6 weeks, depending on the degree of severity of the illness. Offending medications should be discontinued whenever implicated in medication-induced pancreatitis.[13] Prophylaxis or rapid treatment for some infections may prevent the subsequent development of acute pancreatitis. There are several lifestyle factors that also pose an increased risk of developing acute pancreatitis. Smoking and obesity are associated with an increased risk of contracting acute pancreatitis and controlling these factors may result in a decreased risk

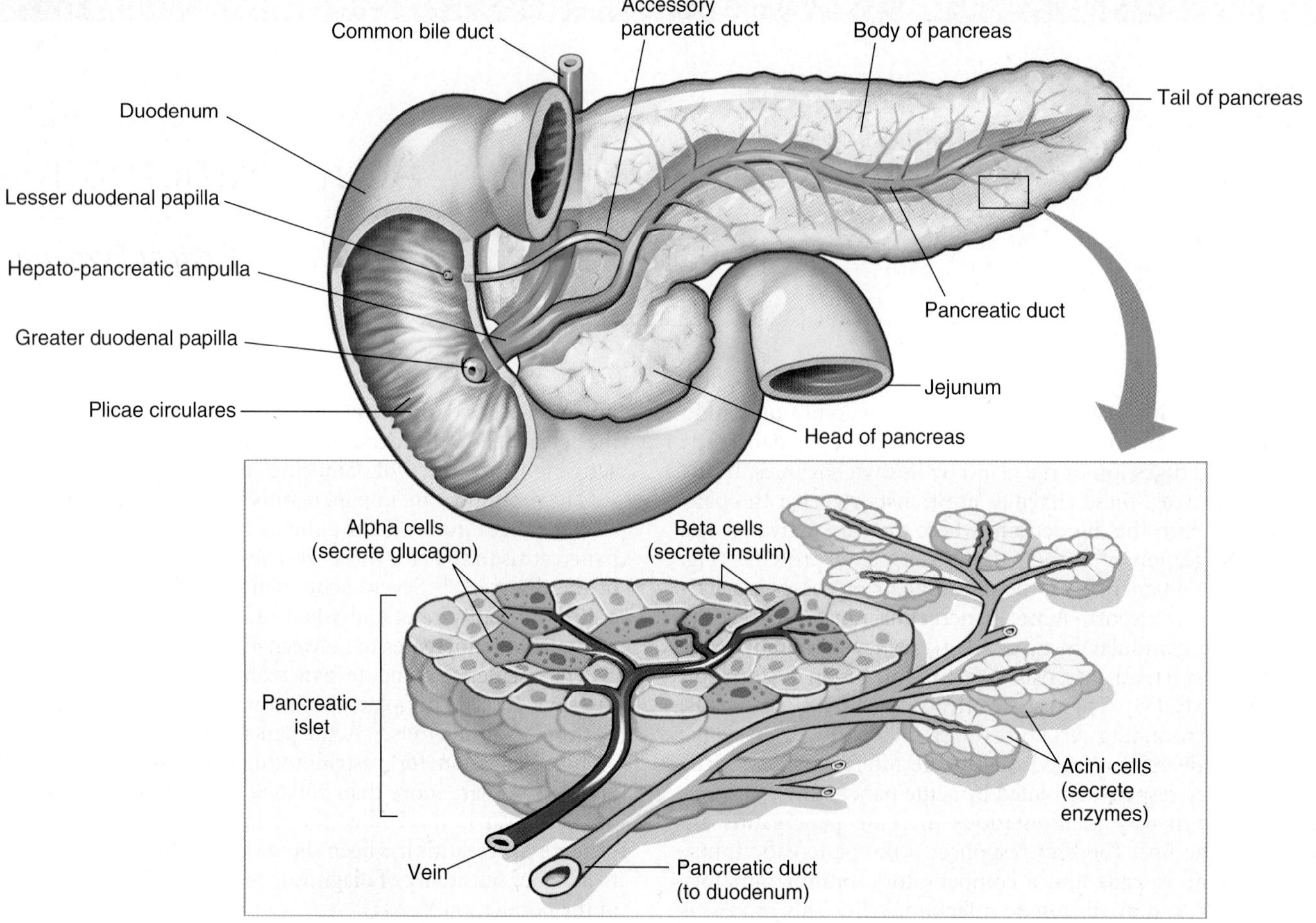

FIG. 18.1 The normal pancreas. (From Patton, K. T., Thibodeau, G. A. (2016). *Anatomy & physiology* (9th ed.). St Louis: Mosby.)

BOX 18.1 Etiologies of Acute Pancreatitis Biliary Disease

- Gallstones
- Biliary sludge
- Microlithiasis
- Alcohol
- Medications
  - Thiazide diuretics
  - Acetaminophen
  - Oral contraceptives
  - L-Asparaginase
  - Furosemide
  - Sulfonamides
  - Azathioprine
  - Tetracycline
- Lipid abnormalities
  - Hypertriglyceridemia
- Hypercalcemia
- Surgery (particularly gastric or biliary)
- Trauma
- Infectious agents
  - Viruses (hepatitis, mumps, coxsackie, rubella)
  - Bacteria *(Legionella, Mycoplasma pneumoniae, Campylobacter)*
- Pregnancy: second and third trimesters
- Hereditary
- Idiopathic

of the disease.[47] The degree to which prevention strategies are successful in limiting the occurrence and/or recurrence of acute pancreatitis is unknown.

APPLIED PHYSIOLOGY

Pancreatitis is a disorder of the exocrine pancreas in which the enzymes necessary for metabolism of carbohydrates, fats, and protein are prematurely activated by events within the acinar cells before their transport into the duodenum. In homeostasis, trypsinogen and other proteases remain in an inactive state during synthesis, transport, and storage within membrane-confined zymogen granules found in acinar cells and after secretion into the pancreatic duct.[7] Though the exact pathophysiology of this premature activation of the pancreatic proteases trypsin and phospholipase A is unknown, the likely cause remains related to events within the acinar cell after deleterious injury to this cell type.[7] Reduced blood flow to the organ may also play a role in pathogenesis by triggering activation of enzymes within the acinar cell. Once an inciting insult has occurred to the acinar cell, three pathologic responses follow (Fig. 18.2). In its normal state, the pancreas is protected from its proteolytic enzymes by secreting inactive proenzymes (zymogens) and also by producing trypsin inhibitor. Other protective mechanisms include an acidic pH within zymogen granules, preventing enzymatic

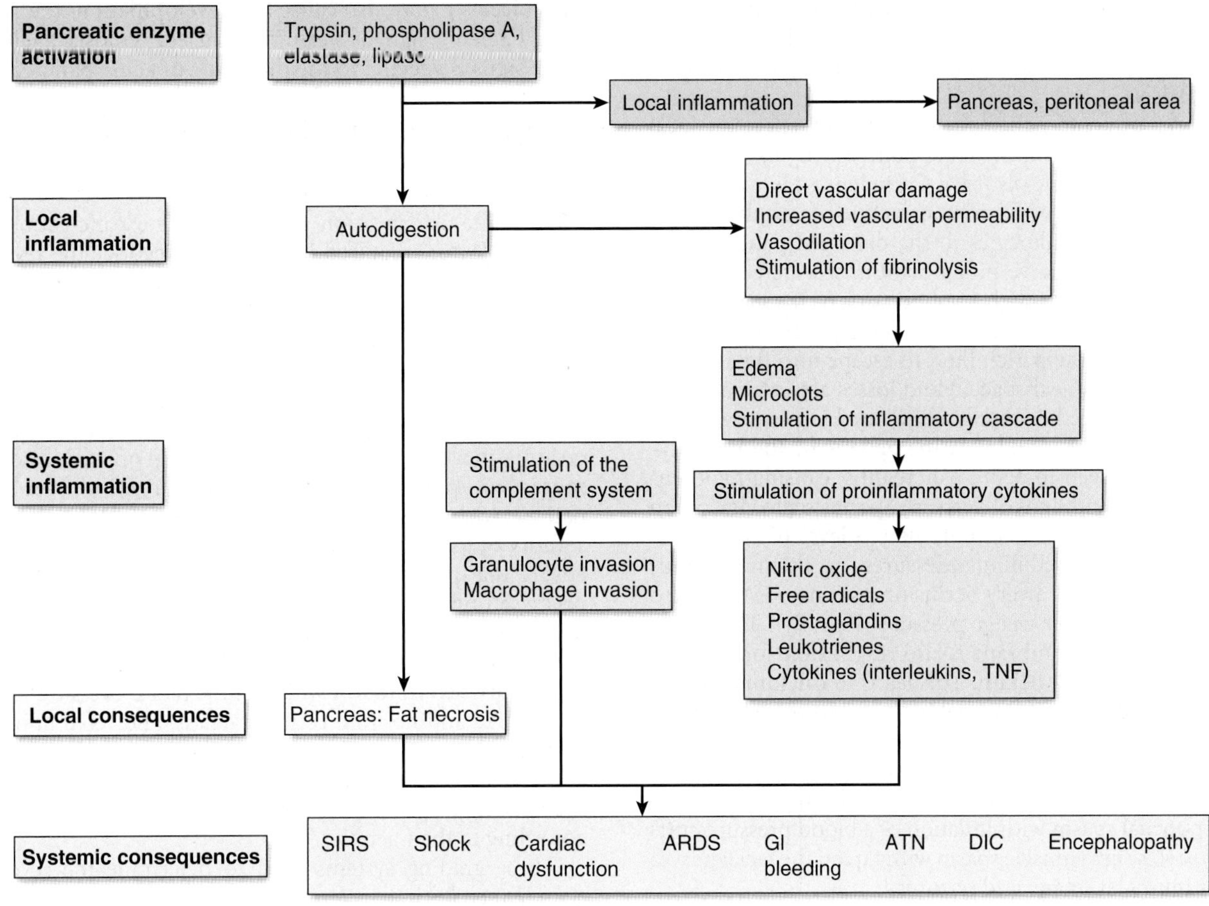

FIG. 18.2 Pancreatic acinar cell injury. *ARDS,* Acute respiratory distress syndrome; *ATN,* acute tubular necrosis; *DIC,* disseminated intravascular coagulation; *GI,* gastrointestinal; *SIRS,* systemic inflammatory response syndrome; *TNF,* tumor necrosis factor.

activity, and the presence of proteases that degrade other already active proteases. Theoretically, premature activation of trypsinogen when acinar cell homeostasis is disrupted could overwhelm protective mechanisms and lead to damage of the zymogen-confining membrane and the release of activated proteases.[7] When these inherent protective mechanisms are overwhelmed, the acute inflammatory process is initiated by enzyme-induced tissue destruction. Intracellular zymogens are activated, normal pancreatic secretion is inhibited, and proinflammatory and proapoptotic (causing cell death) mediators are released.[7,37] Once the acinar cell and proenzyme-containing zymogen granules are injured, trypsinogen is activated to trypsin and other pancreatic enzymes and cytokines are released from the damaged pancreatic cells; this begins the autodigestion of the gland and structures surrounding the pancreas within the pancreatic bed. This phenomenon is believed to be related to the acinar cell damage then affecting lysosomes and zymogen granules within the cell itself, causing inappropriate fusion of these two intracellular structures and the subsequent premature activation of trypsinogen.[7] This triggers a cascade effect, leading to the activation of other pancreatic enzymes, such as lipase, which begin to digest peripancreatic fat. Zymogen activation and autodigestion result in a local inflammatory response. The inflammatory mediators are released into the general circulation and result in cytokine-mediated systemic leukocyte activation.[7,37] The severe inflammation results in early glandular edema that may contribute to diminished blood flow to the organ. The vascular insult within the pancreas continues with the onset of vascular thrombosis and vasospasm, causing the release of oxygen-free radicals, contributing to further apoptosis (pancreatic cell death).[37] The inflammatory process may extend to peripancreatic tissues and to the systemic circulation. Another important mechanism in the pathogenesis of acute pancreatitis is obstruction of the pancreatic duct and impaired bile flow with interstitial collection of lipase, which can initiate local inflammation.[7,37]

The intense inflammation and edema caused by the release of activated enzymes and digestion of the pancreas by these enzymes are responsible for the primary symptom of pancreatitis—abdominal pain. Abdominal pain occurs as a presenting symptom in 95% of those with acute pancreatitis.[23] This pain is commonly described as midepigastric (due to sympathetic innervation from the celiac plexus), deep, constant, sharp, burning, excruciating, and may radiate to the dorsal regions of the back.[16,23] Pain receptors in the retroperitoneum are also stimulated by the resultant cell death and necrosis that ensues from the destructive active intracellular enzyme activity of trypsinogen, phospholipase A, and elastase. Finally, patients may present with pain related to the obstruction of the pancreatic duct from a migrating gallstone. Abdominal distention, nausea, vomiting, and paralytic ileus are seen in many patients with acute pancreatitis. This is related to the effects of the copious amounts of retroperitoneal fluid and the local inflammatory processes suppressing the action of intestinal peristalsis.

Hallmarks of acute pancreatitis include its effect on local as well as distant structures. Acute pancreatitis may progress from a local to a systemic disorder. Complement is activated in response to the action of trypsin, attracting macrophages and polymorphonuclear leukocytes to the damaged pancreas and pancreatic bed. Progressive inflammation and increasing vascular permeability result with local necrosis of the gland.[7] The damaged capillary membrane, now hyperpermeable, allows large amounts of protein-rich fluid to escape into the interstitium and retroperitoneal space. Fluid losses are extreme, with up to 6 liters or more becoming sequestered in pancreatic and peripancreatic edema.[7,37] This is the genesis of the hemodynamic instability seen in acute pancreatitis, causing hypotension, tachycardia, and signs of decreased perfusion to vital organ systems (decreasing urine output, altered level of consciousness) as well as decreased filling pressures (e.g., central venous pressure or pulmonary artery occlusion pressure [PAOP] also called pulmonary artery wedge pressure [PAWP]). The highly permeable capillary membrane is also responsible for losses of electrolytes, especially calcium. This leads to calcium combining with the free fatty acids present in the locale from fat necrosis. This process, known as *saponification,* causes the deposition of calcium soaps.[7] Hypocalcemia can be severe and is clinically identifiable by neuromuscular changes, including Trousseau's sign (carpopedal spasm with inflation of a blood pressure cuff) and Chvostek's sign (muscle spasm with tap on the facial nerve) as well as muscular tetany and seizures.[17]

Cardiovascular compromise may also result from the damaging effects of the enzymes, particularly elastase. This enzyme has a direct effect on the structural integrity of blood vessels, leaving patients at risk for developing thrombosis or, in rare cases, hemorrhage. Changes in the arterial wall are secondary to contact with proteolytic enzymes and other products of pancreatic injury. Arteries in close proximity to an inflamed or infected site may be the only risk factor for the formation of an arterial injury or pseudoaneurysm, which may rupture and cause spontaneous hemorrhage.[17]

Tachypnea and dyspnea are also seen in severe acute pancreatitis as a result of splinting from the presence of subdiaphragmatic inflammation. These symptoms arise when patients are experiencing pain and may be hypoventilating, thus precipitating the development of atelectasis and potentially pneumonia. Pleural effusions, especially on the left side, can develop with the migration of large amounts of retroperitoneal fluid into the thoracic cavity via lymphatic channels.[17] Patients with pleural effusions may present with basilar crackles.

Necrotic tissue and areas of hemorrhage within the pancreas and its surrounding tissue provide an excellent medium for bacterial infection, especially with organisms from an inflamed biliary tree and permeable colonic sources. Any infectious process in this area increases the morbidity and mortality associated with severe acute pancreatitis. These processes may also result in increased pain, development of fever, and an elevated white blood cell (WBC) count.

Rare physical findings include ecchymosis of the groin, flank, and thigh (Grey Turner's sign) related to retroperitoneal bleeding into the fascia in hemorrhagic acute pancreatitis. This bleeding may also cause the development of the uncommon Cullen's sign of periumbilical ecchymosis. Neither of these signs is specific to the diagnosis of acute pancreatitis.[17]

ASSESSMENT OF SEVERITY AND EARLY RISK STRATIFICATION

The Atlanta classification system for acute pancreatitis delineates the factors required in order to categorize the severity of the disease. According to this classification system, there are three levels of severity: mild, which is self-limiting and from which patients recover with supportive care within approximately 1 week; moderately severe, in which patients experience transient failure that resolves within 48 hours or a local complication not associated with organ failure; and severe acute pancreatitis, in which the hallmark is persistent organ failure lasting more than 48 hours. Mortality rates increase to over 30% in patients who develop persistent organ failure.[23,42] Assessing the severity of each case on an ongoing basis is critical in order to ensure that patients receive rapid interventions in the appropriate setting.[23] The Atlanta classification system defines organ failure as respiratory decompensation with arterial oxygen pressure/fractional inspired oxygen greater than or equal to 300, circulatory deterioration with systolic blood pressure less than 90 mm Hg and no fluid responsiveness, and renal injury with elevated plasma creatinine.[23] Using this information, clinicians guide the timing and aggressiveness of interventions as well as the most appropriate placement of patients within the hospital according to their acuity.

Three grading systems used to determine the severity of acute pancreatitis are: Ranson's criteria, the Modified Glasgow System (despite their limitations, including the inability to fully gauge severity until after 48 hours), and the Acute Physiology and Chronic Health Evaluation (APACHE) II system (Box 18.2). These risk stratification systems use clinical assessment parameters and biochemical measurements to determine the severity of acute pancreatitis.[17,42] The mortality rates associated

BOX 18.2 Ranson's Criteria for Predicting the Severity of Acute Pancreatitis at Admission or on Diagnosis

- Age >55 years (>70 years)*
- Leukocyte count >16,000/mm³ (>18,000/mm³)*
- Serum glucose level > 200 mg/dL (>220 mg/dL)*
- Serum LDH >350 units/L (>400 units/L)*
- Serum AST >250 units/L

During Initial 48 Hours

- Decrease in hematocrit >10%
- Increase in BUN >5 mg/dL (>2 mg/dL)*
- Total serum calcium level >8 mg/dL
- Base deficit >4 mEq/L (>5 mEq/L)*
- Estimated fluid sequestration >6 L (>4 L)*
- Partial pressure of arterial oxygen <60 mm Hg

*Criteria values for nonalcoholic acute pancreatitis differing from those in alcohol-related disease, which are in parentheses.

For correlation between number of positive criteria and related mortality, see Box 18.3.

AST, Aspartate transaminase; *BUN,* blood urea nitrogen; *LDH,* lactate dehydrogenase.

From Reference 5.

with the number of Ranson's criteria are presented in Box 18.3. It is important to quickly identify, on admission, those 20% of patients who will develop the most severe disease with complications, as these individuals may benefit most from early critical care management.[8,23]

The Acute Physiology and Chronic Health Evaluation (APACHE) III is an additional method for risk stratification. The computerized tomography (CT) grading system of Balthazar is also used (Table 18.1). All grading systems have limitations but can be used to aid the clinician in identifying severity and thus anticipating the course of the disease and its outcomes. Clinical criteria, serum markers, and radiographic features are several of the methods used for early risk stratification.[17]

A high index of suspicion by the clinician is vital when monitoring these patients in order to identify when changes may be heralding the onset of complications. The APACHE II score can be used at the 24-hour mark and daily thereafter and can be applied to predict the onset of complications and the potential for increased mortality. Those patients who develop extrapancreatic complications such as respiratory or renal dysfunction, or those who have pancreatic necrosis on contrast-enhanced CT, will likely experience the most severe course of the disease.[11,13]

Several new clinical scoring systems have been developed and have some clinical utility, but the search is still ongoing for even more timely and efficient risk stratification scoring mechanisms. The Bedside Index for Severity in Acute Pancreatitis (BISAP) and the Harmless Acute Pancreatitis Score (HAPS) are two of the most recently developed scoring systems. The BISAP score assigns points to each of these factors: blood urea nitrogen (BUN) greater than 25 mg/dL, impaired mental status, systemic inflammatory response syndrome, age greater than 60 years, and pleural effusion. The development of two or more of these criteria during the first 24 hours of hospitalization identifies patients at increased risk for morbidity and mortality. The HAPS score identifies those patients at low risk for severe acute pancreatitis by examining three parameters: absence of rebound tenderness and/or guarding, normal hematocrit level, and normal serum creatinine level. The Sequential Organ Failure Assessment (SOFA) score is used to determine injury to other organs in acute pancreatitis. Elevated BUN level within 24 hours of admission has also been associated with increased mortality.[14,42]

BOX 18.3 Ranson's Criteria and Related Mortality

Number of Positive Criteria	
0–2	<5% mortality
3 4	20% mortality
5–6	40% mortality
7 or more	100% mortality

From Reference 15.

TABLE 18.1 Computed Tomography Severity Index

Characteristic	CT Severity Index (CTSI)
Level of Inflammation	
Normal pancreas	0
Focal or diffuse enlargement	1
Peripancreatic inflammation	2
Single collection of fluid	3
Multiple fluid collections or gas	4
Pancreatic Necrosis	
None	0
Less than 30% necrosis	2
30%–50% necrosis	4
Greater than 50% necrosis	6

From Reference 4. Used with permission.

DIAGNOSIS OF ACUTE PANCREATITIS

Laboratory Findings

As the cells of the pancreas are destroyed, the enzymes amylase and lipase are released into the circulation during an acute attack. Measurement of amylase and lipase levels is used for the confirmation of the diagnosis of acute pancreatitis. Serum enzyme levels, typically three times greater than normal, are seen to increase within 6 to 12 hours. The half-life of elevated amylase is shorter than that of lipase, and clearance of amylase is affected by impaired renal function and intravascular fluid status. Because it persists longer after the onset of the attack and because the pancreas is the only source of lipase, estimation of serum lipase levels has somewhat more superior sensitivity and specificity and greater accuracy than lipase.[7,23,39] Isoamylase levels specific to pancreatic injury are measured in some laboratories and are more indicative of the disease. Urine amylase levels may also be elevated and remain so for several days. Serum lipase level is a reliable marker of acute pancreatitis. It remains elevated for a longer period and has a sensitivity and specificity for the disease that approaches 90%.[7,8] Neither serum amylase nor serum lipase levels correlate to the severity of the disease.

WBC count may be elevated because of the inflammatory process or resultant infection and the hematocrit level may provide information about hemoconcentration and correlate with severe disease.[8] Derangements in serum glucose levels are common as beta cells of the pancreas, which produce insulin, are also damaged by the inflammatory process. Liver function tests may be mildly elevated, especially bilirubin levels and transaminases, if the acute pancreatitis is related to a biliary cause such as gallstone disease.[8]

A history of fasting triglyceride levels higher than 1000 mg/dL or a persistent elevation after the acute inflammatory process has resolved may be seen if hypertriglyceridemia is the cause of acute pancreatitis.[14] Many enzymes and serum markers are released by damaged pancreatic cells when they are injured in severe acute pancreatitis. These levels have been tested for their ability to provide prognostic information in the setting of acute pancreatitis. Research is ongoing in an effort to identify a serum marker accurate in its predictive value for the severity of pancreatitis. Two promising laboratory tests are C-reactive protein (CRP) and urinary trypsinogen activation peptide (uTAP). CRP is a marker of inflammation and is elevated in acute pancreatitis. This test is readily available and inexpensive, with 86% sensitivity within 48 hours of presentation of symptoms. A CRP value of 150 mg/L may be the point of differentiation between mild and severe acute pancreatitis.[14] Pancreatic zymogen destruction and activation of trypsinogen are key occurrences in acute pancreatitis. In an effort to determine the severity of the disease, trypsinogen activation peptide (TAP) has been studied. uTAP concentrations have provided good prognostic information related to the severity of acute pancreatitis. This is a manual test with limited stability, thus preventing its widespread use. More clinically applicable testing of uTAP is in development.[14] Though not yet clinically applicable; several other serum markers may hold diagnostic promise including procalcitonin, interleukin-6, and neutrophilic elastase; these are all elevated in acute pancreatitis but are not specific for the disease.[7]

Radiology Findings

Though CT imaging is frequently not necessary for the diagnosis of acute pancreatitis, contrast-enhanced CT scanning (CECT) may be used for the identification of acute pancreatitis when the diagnosis is uncertain. CECT is also used for staging of the severity of acute pancreatitis, for detection of complications such as necrosis, and to evaluate patients whose condition is not improving despite therapy.[8,14,16] Dynamic CT carries an 87% sensitivity for diagnosis of this disorder.[7,8] This level of sensitivity allows for the differentiation of severe acute pancreatitis from many other conditions that may present with abdominal pain and elevated levels of pancreatic enzymes. Of note is the ability of this diagnostic modality to delineate local complications such as peripancreatic necrosis with or without infection.[14] Grading systems for the severity of acute pancreatitis have been developed using CT imaging alone to determine risk stratification of the disease.[14] The computed tomography severity index (CTSI) quantifies the presence and amount of pancreatic necrosis and extent of inflammation, and it has shown promise in predicting outcomes in acute pancreatitis (see Table 18.1).[7,8,14]

Plain radiographic films of the chest and abdomen are two initial diagnostic interventions used to identify abnormalities responsible for the onset of abdominal pain and other presenting symptoms. The chest x-ray may reveal the presence of pleural effusion, particularly left-sided, often associated with acute pancreatitis.[7,14]

Abdominal ultrasonography can be used to detect gallstones, although bowel gas from pancreatitis-related ileus may limit its accuracy. Ultrasound is, however, a routine element of the evaluation process for acute pancreatitis. It provides important information regarding the pancreas and biliary structures and does so quickly and efficiently as it is readily available.[7,8,14] Magnetic resonance imaging (MRI) and magnetic resonance cholangiopancreatography (MRCP) with gadolinium provide information about the pancreas similar to that obtained with CT scanning, but provide more valuable information regarding the biliary tree. This technology should be considered especially in cases of recurrent idiopathic acute pancreatitis.[14] MRI and MRCP as well as endoscopic ultrasound (EUS) have the capability of detecting small bile duct stones and sludge and are useful diagnostic tools.[8,14]

The many diagnostic interventions are important in identifying acute pancreatitis within the earliest possible timeframe in order to institute interventions quickly. The diagnosis of acute pancreatitis is generally straightforward. It involves a complete history and physical examination and laboratory and radiologic assessments. To determine a diagnosis of acute pancreatitis, two of three criteria must be present:

1. Central upper abdominal pain that occurs acutely and may radiate to the back.
2. Serum amylase or lipase levels that are greater than three times the upper limit of normal.
3. Characteristic features on abdominal imaging that are consistent with acute pancreatitis. According to the experts of the Atlanta Classification 2012, imaging studies are not required for all patients in order to make a diagnosis of acute pancreatitis.[38]

COMPLICATIONS OF ACUTE PANCREATITIS

Cardiac and Systemic Complications

The injury to the pancreas alone is not responsible for the morbidity and mortality of acute pancreatitis. It is in fact the systemic and local complications that ensue that can threaten the course and patient outcomes of this devastating disease entity (Fig. 18.3). In addition to the regional pancreatic inflammation related to the local complications, a systemic response to the activated neutrophils and complement products in the area occurs and is linked to distant organ dysfunction.[17] This response is in part related to the absorption of activated enzymes and inflammatory mediators from the retroperitoneum.

The first weeks after the onset of symptoms in acute pancreatitis are marked by systemic inflammatory response syndrome (SIRS).[7,17] Release of proinflammatory mediators is thought to contribute to the pathogenesis of SIRS-related multisystem complications involving injury to the heart, lungs, kidneys, and other organs.[7,17] See Chapter 31 for a comprehensive review of SIRS.

Microvascular endothelial cell injury with systemic capillary leak, which occurs in association with the release of inflammatory mediators, bradykinin, and histamine, places the patient at increased risk for MODS.[2] Cardiovascular complications of severe pancreatitis often mimic septic shock even though no infection is present; in fact, no organism exists. Hypovolemic shock is one complication caused by the capillary damage related to the action of enzymes and vasoactive substances. Bleeding, a rare complication, can develop as a consequence of the erosion of local blood vessels by elastase and other enzymes. Progressive and uncontrolled vasodilation occurs, prompted by the kinin released from damaged acinar cells; this contributes to the severity of the shock state. Those patients whose assessment and management include the use of a pulmonary artery catheter (PAC) or minimally invasive hemodynamic monitoring will exhibit a decreased systemic vascular resistance. Cardiac output will be increased in response to the massive fluid sequestration and other factors. Theorized myocardial depressant factors (MDFs) of tumor necrosis factor (TNF), interleukin-1B, and nitrous oxide released in sepsis may also contribute to the development of cardiovascular complications.[7] Dysrhythmias are also frequently seen. They may arise from the severe electrolyte abnormalities seen in acute pancreatitis, as well as to the presence of MDFs and the depressed contractile response of the myocardium in acute sepsis.

Pulmonary Complications

The pulmonary complications associated with acute pancreatitis are many, ranging from mild hypoxemia to life-threatening acute lung injury. Hypoxia can arise from atelectasis associated with the hypoventilation seen with abdominal pain and distention and from diaphragmatic elevation caused by the large amounts of retroperitoneal fluid. Pleural effusions, common on the left side, result from the movement of peripancreatic fluid through lymphatic channels into the pleural space. This

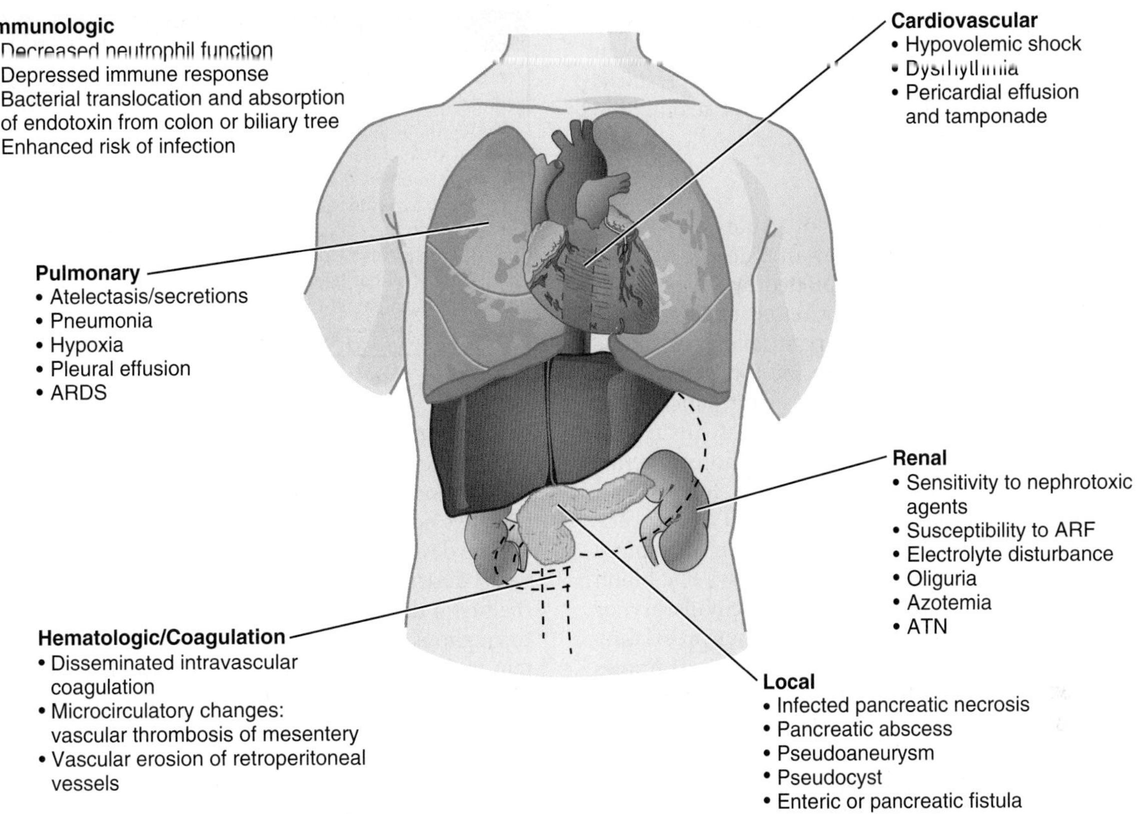

FIG. 18.3 Local and systemic complications of acute pancreatitis. *ARDS,* Acute respiratory distress syndrome; *ARF,* acute renal failure; *ATN,* acute tubular necrosis. (From Alspach, J. (2001). *AACN's instructor resource manual for the core curriculum* (handout 5–36). Philadelphia: Saunders. Used with permission.)

results in a reduced vital capacity, negatively impacting normal ventilation.

Pancreatitis-associated lung injury is complex and not fully understood. The underlying mechanisms associated with the development of acute lung injury (ALI) in pancreatitis include the release of inflammatory mediators (e.g., neutrophils, cytokines, chemokines, and adhesion molecules).[12,35] Vasoactive substances and cytokines absorbed at the site of pancreatic injury are transported to other organ systems. These biochemicals, including phospholipase A and free fatty acids, incite injury to the lung, disturbing and ultimately destroying the alveolar capillary membrane, increasing capillary permeability. Migrating neutrophils, implicated as mediators of ALI and acute respiratory distress syndrome (ARDS), release toxic products of elastase and collagenase at the site of the damaged alveoli.[12,13,35] Pancreatic elastase activates pulmonary TNF, which also contributes to neutrophil infiltration and pulmonary vascular leak. Activation of these processes results in interstitial fluid migration within the lungs and worsening, refractory hypoxemia, resulting in ARDS. Hypoxemia related to ARDS as well as to atelectasis, pneumonia, and pleural effusion must be readily identified and aggressively treated because these are all significant factors in patient outcomes. Up to 60% of deaths occurring within the first week after the onset of severe acute pancreatitis are caused by pulmonary complications.[12,35,48]

Renal Complications

The pathogenesis of the renal complications associated with acute pancreatitis is not fully understood but may be explained by the development of hypovolemia and hypotension with resultant decreased glomerular filtration rate (GFR). However, even patients without any history of hypovolemia, hypotension, or sepsis can develop membranous glomerulonephropathy and acute tubular necrosis (ATN).[17] Other nephrotoxic insults, such as myoglobin released from damaged pancreatic tissue, damage the distal renal tubules and may contribute to the onset of ATN and acute renal failure.[6,22] The development of acute kidney injury (AKI) occurs in approximately 20% of patients and is a poor prognostic indicator, increasing the mortality rate to more than 80%.[22,36]

Gastrointestinal Complications

Gastrointestinal complications may also arise from the inherent cardiovascular instability. Decreased perfusion to the gastrointestinal tract may contribute to adynamic ileus. The local inflammatory process in the retroperitoneum can have a direct negative impact on gastrointestinal structures. Patients can develop splenic vein thrombosis, which precipitates esophageal and gastric varices with the potential for rupture. Weakened mesenteric and splenic vessels, altered by damaging proteases, can form a pseudoaneurysm that also can rupture and cause dangerous hemorrhage.[14,17]

Hematologic and Coagulation Derangements

Pervasive microvascular endothelial cell injury impacts normal coagulation. Microcirculatory injury with vascular thrombosis can adversely affect the mesenteric circulation with resultant visceral ischemia. The onset of disseminated intravascular coagulation in acute pancreatitis may be in response to exaggerated microvascular clotting from enzyme-related injury or be caused by the development of severe sepsis. The result is uncontrolled microvascular clotting, depletion of coagulation proteins, and bleeding.

Organ Failure

Organ failure systemic complications of acute pancreatitis are defined as persistent organ failure or an exacerbation of a preexisting comorbidity which is precipitated by the development of acute pancreatitis.[2] The Atlanta Consensus Conference on Acute Pancreatitis, 2012, defined organ failure using the Modified Marshall System that evaluates the three organ systems most commonly affected by severe acute pancreatitis: respiratory, cardiovascular, and renal. Persistent organ failure is defined objectively as a score of two or more systemic abnormalities lasting for longer than 48 hours for one (or more) of the three organ systems.[4] The Marshall System utilizes the partial pressure of arterial oxygen/fraction of inspired oxygen (Pao_2/Fio_2) ratio, serum creatinine, and systolic blood pressure as measures of organ damage.[16] Renal, circulatory, or respiratory organ failure or exacerbation of serious preexisting comorbidities related directly to acute pancreatitis are examples of systemic complications caused by the SIRS that accompanies acute pancreatitis and, in turn, can lead to the onset of multiple organ dysfunction. Examples include exacerbation of underlying heart disease (coronary artery disease or congestive heart failure), chronic diabetes, obstructive lung disease, and chronic liver diseases.[4,38]

Local and Systemic Infectious Complications

Infectious complications are the most challenging complication to manage in acute pancreatitis, frequently worsening the clinical course.[2] Those with severe acute pancreatitis are at increased risk for infection because of the use of invasive venous and arterial catheters in the assessment and management of this disease. Episodic hyperglycemia associated with pancreatitis is also a risk factor for infection. Translocation of gut bacteria from an unused or underused intestinal mucosa can result in sepsis or abscess formation. Absorption of endotoxins from an inflamed adjacent colon or biliary system can also yield similar infectious sequelae. See Box 18.4 and Table 18.2 for recommendations for infection prevention in acute pancreatitis.

There are two phases in acute pancreatitis that relate to the development of local and systemic complications. The early phase, which occurs within 1 to 2 weeks after symptom onset, is characterized by the onset of a SIRS. Organ failure in this first phase results from severe systemic inflammation arising from the response to local pancreatic injury. This early phase is usually complete by the end of the first week but may extend into the second week. Cytokine cascades are activated by the pancreatic inflammation, which manifest as the SIRS. When SIRS is persistent, there is an increased risk of developing organ failure. The second phase, which occurs after the 1 to 2 week early period, is characterized by a counteractive, compensatory, antiinflammatory response syndrome (CARS) that may contribute to an increased risk of infection, which is not fully understood.[4,38] The late phase is characterized by persistence of systemic signs of inflammation, by the presence of local complications (e.g., parenchymal or peri-parenchymal necrosis, infection, pseudocyst), and by the development of sepsis.[22] The late phase occurs only in patients with moderately severe or severe acute pancreatitis. Organ failure in the CARS phase occurs due to infections, such as infected necrosis.[18] It is important to identify local complications by radiologic imaging in order to initiate evidence-based management strategies.[4,38]

BOX 18.4 Infection Prevention

Infection in acute pancreatitis is associated with increased morbidity and mortality. Preventing infections is of the utmost importance to nurses and the entire interprofessional team. It is believed that intestinal bacteria that cross a disrupted mucosal barrier are responsible for a majority of these infections. Enteral nutrition initiated early in the course of the disease may protect the intestinal mucosa from breakdown. There is no effect on the rate of infection with the routine use of systemic antibiotic prophylaxis or probiotics. Routine selective bowel decontamination (SBD) has not been shown to reduce the infectious complications of acute pancreatitis.[18] The routine standards of care regarding hand hygiene and universal precautions should be meticulously followed.

The development of pancreatic necrosis resulting from local vessel destruction and thrombosis may begin to develop within the first 4 days of the onset of symptoms. This process evolves throughout the first 4 weeks and the necrotic pancreas will contain variable amounts of fluid and solid material.[22] It is seen in 5% to 10% of patients with acute pancreatitis and is defined as nonenhancement of pancreatic parenchyma on CECT.[43] Once necrotic, this area can either be sterile or can become secondarily infected. Infection of this type is a potentially life-threatening cause of sepsis in acute pancreatitis.[22] Infected pancreatic necrosis is the development of a diffuse area of nonviable pancreatic parenchyma that is secondarily infected, most commonly with *Escherichia coli, Bacteroides, Staphylococcus,* or *Candida albicans.* Infected necrosis is diagnosed by the presence of one of the following three criteria: (1) ongoing signs of sepsis or the combination of clinical signs, or both, and the CT finding of gas within the areas of necrosis; (2) percutaneous image-guided fine-needle aspiration (FNA) with a culture positive for bacteria or fungi; or (3) secondary event after instrumentation.[22] Fever, leukocytosis, and abdominal pain are the hallmarks of the complication. The extensive tissue damage and loss associated with infected pancreatic necrosis also carry the potential of additional complications including intraabdominal abscess, intestinal or pancreatic fistula formation, and bleeding from other retroperitoneal structures.[22] The majority of patients with severe early organ dysfunction have been identified as also having pancreatic necrosis on CECT scan.[22]

Pancreatic abscess, a walled-off, intraabdominal collection of pus and debris, is a late local complication of acute pancreatitis, often taking 4 to 6 weeks to develop. Signs and symptoms include increased abdominal tenderness, fever, and leukocytosis. This abscess commonly develops following the infection of an area of pancreatic necrosis. With rapid intervention (i.e., percutaneous or endoscopic drainage or surgical excision and lavage), this complication can be controlled, limiting adverse patient outcomes.[2]

Pancreatic pseudocysts are collections of pancreatic secretions (fluid) enclosed by a wall of fibrous or granulation tissue that does not have a layer of epithelial cells in its lining. They develop as a result of an active protease-weakened capsular structure and persistent pancreatic ductal leak.[4] Pseudocysts are rare and form only in interstitial pancreatitis and are fluid-filled with no solid material.[4,22] They may take up to 6 weeks to become mature. Pseudocysts may cause increased

TABLE 18.2 **Infection Prevention Strategies**

Infection in Acute Pancreatitis	Assessment Parameters	Interventions	Desired Outcomes
Potential for infection related to bacterial or fungal invasion of retroperitoneal exudates and systemic absorption of these organisms and of inflammatory substances. When infection occurs it is frequently late in the course of the disease. Translocation of gut bacteria is the theorized cause of infection of pancreatic necrosis.	Monitor for fever Monitor WBC Abdominal assessment for increasing pain, which may indicate the onset of infection. Monitor for other signs of infection or inflammation.	Rapid identification of infectious source and source control. The use of antibiotics without source control is ineffective. One method of source control is percutaneous drainage of infected collections. If organism-specific antibiotics are deemed appropriate, they should be used with caution because the course of acute pancreatitis is often protracted and multiple antibiotic regimens may be required as multiple infections may develop. Unnecessary and prolonged use of antibiotics increases the risk of the development of resistant organisms.	No fever Absence of signs of infection Organisms eradicated.

WBC, White blood cell count.
From Reference 11.

abdominal discomfort, rupture, become infected, or become so large that they obstruct the intestine or genitourinary system; therefore, they must be monitored closely via ultrasound or CT scan to determine if and when an intervention is required.[4,22]

MANAGEMENT OF ACUTE PANCREATITIS

The clinical course of acute pancreatitis varies from mild disease to the severe, necrotizing form. Those patients with the mild form (80% of cases) will require intravenous therapy and optimal pain management.[22,39] Those with severe acute pancreatitis (20% of cases) may benefit from intensive monitoring given the potential for progressive organ dysfunction or local complication. Scoring systems are available to identify those who will progress to the severe form of the disease and are advantageous, but cannot replace the assessment and interventions of skilled clinicians. The supportive care provided in critical care is vital to improving patient outcomes as there is a dearth of evidence-based interventions and a lack of consensus to guide clinical practice in the management of severe acute pancreatitis.[19,39]

Fluid Management

Inflammation is the hallmark of severe acute pancreatitis. Early in the course of the disease, there is an extravasation of protein-rich intravascular fluid into the peritoneal cavity, resulting in hemoconcentration. Hematocrit (Hct) monitoring may be used to identify those at risk for hemoconcentration before altered perfusion becomes apparent, but is controversial due to the lack of high-quality evidence to support this practice.[19] Hct levels may provide a framework by which practitioners can assess the effectiveness of interventions aimed at restoring normal intravascular fluid status. Elevated Hct levels have been shown to have an association with the development of pancreatic necrosis.[19] Fluid sequestration, losses, and third-spacing results in hypovolemia. Fluid resuscitation counteracts this process and restores the microcirculation, supporting oxygenation of the pancreas and other organs. This may prevent further local injury to the pancreas.[9] Therefore, monitoring Hct levels has some value but should not be used as the sole marker of adequate fluid resuscitation; rather, other data should be evaluated, including heart rate, blood pressure, and BUN levels.[9,19]

Maintaining adequate intravascular volume may be considered the most essential therapeutic goal in the management of acute pancreatitis. Patients with acute pancreatitis can sequester enormous amounts of fluid not only into the retroperitoneal space, but also into the intraperitoneal cavity, the gut, and the pleural cavity.[19,39] It is critically important that the marked intravascular fluid losses be estimated and replenished aggressively.[19,21] Adequate fluid resuscitation may require many liters of crystalloid or colloidal fluids in 24 hours during the first days after admission.[19] Early and vigorous intravenous hydration via large-bore peripheral intravenous access is critical to restore circulating volume and is recommended by several observational studies.[10] The World Congress of Gastroenterology guidelines recommend a rapid initial crystalloid infusion to correct the initial deficit within the first few hours of presentation, guided by vital signs, oxygen saturation, and urine output. After this period, the recommendation is for 35 mL/kg/day and additional amounts to replete ongoing third space losses.[36,39]

Central venous access lines or the use of PACs not only provide access for rapid infusion of intravenous fluids and blood but also provide critical clinical data needed to manage the hemodynamically unstable patient or the patient with coexistent cardiopulmonary disease who requires aggressive volume resuscitation. To estimate the required fluid resuscitation requirements, central venous pressure (CVP) may be monitored closely together with hourly urine excretion. Goals for CVP should be based upon the most current evidence on end points of resuscitation in the range of approximately 8 to 12 mm Hg; urine output should be maintained at 0.5 mL/kg/hour and mean arterial pressure of greater than 65 mm Hg.[20] In those patients whose course is complicated by sepsis or the SIRS response, the resuscitation strategy may involve administration of intravenous fluid targeted to a specific PAOP. In addition, other end points of resuscitation are currently viewed as necessary when attempting to achieve hemodynamic stability and improve perfusion in acute pancreatitis. Stroke volume variation (SVV) or pulse pressure variation (PPV) are important parameters for assessment of the effectiveness of fluid resuscitation. These parameters are measured with the use of an arterial line and provide information on volume responsiveness in the critically ill. In an effort to meet these end points and provide the needed amount of fluid, the minimal requirements must be calculated and retroperitoneal losses estimated in the first 24 to 48 hours. The known or estimated retroperitoneal losses must be added to the maintenance fluid needs to correct potentially life-threatening deficits such as end-organ damage and especially renal failure, which can occur with underresuscitation. The adverse effects of overresuscitation include pulmonary edema, respiratory failure, and abdominal compartment syndrome (ACS).[13] To avoid these extremes in resuscitation, initial fluid therapy with crystalloid at 5 to 10 mL/kg/hour, as well as ongoing assessment with the clinical and invasive measurements mentioned, and with the biochemical parameters of lactate, as well as hematocrit, is recommended.[13]

Vigorous intravenous hydration may improve vascular supply and pancreatic perfusion and prevent the development of necrosis and other complications. The intravascular hypovolemia that accompanies acute pancreatitis subsequently leads to diminished pancreatic blood flow. Preventing further pancreatic ischemia by aggressive volume resuscitation may thwart further activation and release of inflammatory mediators.[2,9,13] Aggressive fluid resuscitation is also recommended to reduce the risk of developing acute renal failure and other organ failure and to decrease the rates of persistent SIRS.[21]

Percutaneous and Endoscopic Interventions

Patients with pancreatic necrosis of either the sterile or the infected variety are at risk for multiorgan complications. Patients with sterile necrosis may be managed medically with supportive care and the use of intravenous hydration and pain management.[22] Once infection develops, the therapeutic approach is directed toward removal of the infected necrotic tissue. Interventional, minimally invasive, or open surgical approaches (pancreatic necrosectomy) may be required.[9] Percutaneous or endoscopic catheter drainage is the first step of what is known as the *Step-Up Approach*. Catheters are placed via the left or right retroperitoneal approach in order to drain the infection. This intervention, coupled with appropriate, targeted antibiotic therapy, may be the only necessary treatment for some patients, but it is not known what subgroup of patients will require additional techniques.[9,27]

Another form of management of severe acute pancreatitis is endoscopic retrograde cholangiopancreatography (ERCP). ERCP may be used for those patients with evidence of biliary obstruction (e.g., jaundice) or cholangitis and a persistently elevated serum bilirubin level (> 5 mg/dL). In these patients, early ERCP with sphincterotomy and stone extraction is indicated. If ERCP is not available or cannot be performed because of extreme technical difficulty, alternative methods of biliary drainage should be considered. This procedure is not indicated for those with mild biliary pancreatitis without cholangitis.[2,21]

Surgical Treatment

Two minimally invasive surgical techniques are part of the next interventions in the Step-Up Approach. Minimal access retroperitoneal pancreatic necrosectomy (MARPN), also known as *sinus tract endoscopy* and *video-assisted retroperitoneal debridement (VARD)* are procedures that provide access to the necrotic pancreas through the tract of a radiologically placed drainage catheter. Debridement and lavage is performed via the catheters over three to five sessions. Endoscopic drainage and necrosectomy are carried out under direct vision or ultrasound guidance through the gastric or duodenal wall into the necrosis.[9,27,44] Some patients will require the next step: an open surgical necrosectomy, formerly the standard treatment of infected necrosis. Through a laparotomy incision, necrotic tissue is excised and healthy pancreatic tissue is preserved. Varied additional surgical techniques accompany the necrosectomy. These techniques include open or closed packing with planned reoperation with lavage and further debridement or postoperative continuous lavage to remove residual debris. Open surgical necrosectomy carries high rates of morbidity and mortality and is often performed on the most critically ill patients. This factor prompted the development of the less invasive techniques in the Step-Up Approach.[2,9,27,43] There is currently no evidence indicating the superiority of either of the techniques in this approach, but postponement of interventions is generally recommended after the fourth week from the onset of symptoms. This period allows the necrotic collections to become walled off and for the necrotic tissue to become liquefied.[2,27,43] Because of the massive inflammatory process, a right hemicolectomy may be necessary when the transverse colon is compromised.[2,9,27,43]

Continuous peritoneal lavage via indwelling catheters placed at the time of necrosectomy may also be implemented after the initial procedure. This lavage with closed suction allows for the continued removal of debris, devascularized tissue, and toxins, and minimizes systemic absorption of these local toxins.

Pain Management

Pain management for the patient with acute pancreatitis demands an interprofessional approach. This primary presenting symptom is most disconcerting to patients and their families. Controlling pain to within acceptable patient limits is perhaps the most important goal in the management of acute pancreatitis. The use of opiates for pain management is a common and effective modality. There is some thought that the pain associated with pancreatitis may be exacerbated by the use of morphine. Morphine does cause smooth muscle contraction around the sphincter of Oddi, but there is little evidence that this is a clinically significant development, though its use may result in pain. Morphine and other narcotics (e.g., fentanyl [Sublimaze], hydromorphone [Dilaudid]) have not been shown to adversely affect patient outcomes and are often recommended.[7,23] Opioids are more effective than nonsteroidal antiinflammatory medications in alleviating the pain associated with acute pancreatitis, but there is no evidence that one is superior for this purpose.[5] Patient-controlled analgesia may be appropriate for some patients, but not for the most critically ill. Patient positioning may alleviate pain when a semi-Fowler's position is used and the patient's legs are positioned toward the chest. Maintaining nothing by mouth (NPO) status is thought to prevent/decrease pain because of avoidance of pancreatic stimulation.[2,13,23] The presence of nausea, vomiting, abdominal distention, and ileus also contributes to the need for remaining NPO until the acute inflammatory process resolves.

Antibiotic Therapy

The treatment of acute pancreatitis remains symptom-focused and supportive, with no specific medications currently available.[2,7] Despite many prospective, randomized controlled studies, few medications have been shown to be effective in the management of this disease. One category of medications found to be effective in the management of some patients with pancreatitis is antibiotics. Antibiotics are not indicated for patients with a mild form of the disease. They have no benefit in preventing infection of a necrotic pancreas and have no effect on morbidity or mortality rates. Therefore, there is no indication for early antibiotic therapy to prevent infection (known or presumed) of pancreatic necrosis.[9,13,21,23] Antibiotics based upon culture and sensitivity are indicated for patients with documented infection, including cholangitis, infected pancreatic necrosis, or in cases of strong clinical suspicion of these conditions.[2]

Nutrition

Patients with acute pancreatitis are at nutritional risk because of protein losses, an extreme catabolic state, and lack of oral intake. Severe acute pancreatitis is associated with tryptic autodigestion of the pancreas, protein catabolism, metabolic instability, and increased nutritional requirements. Nutritional support is a required, therapeutic intervention for patients with severe acute pancreatitis. Enteral nutrition (EN) is the preferred route and has been shown to decrease the development of organ failure and infected pancreatic necrosis when compared to parenteral nutrition.[1,34] Because these complications are believed to occur due to translocation of gut bacteria from a disturbed intestinal mucosa, enteral feedings thwart this effect by stimulating intestinal motility and enhancing splanchnic blood flow, which may preserve the mucosa.[15,21,23,29] EN in acute pancreatitis can be administered via either the nasojejunal or nasogastric route.[21,22] The nasogastric route is equivalent to the nasojejunal route and can be the route for early, initial feeding.[13] Patients with severe acute pancreatitis complicated by organ failure, pancreatic necrosis, and/or fluid collections may benefit from placement of a nasojejunal feeding tube within the first week for sustained feeding.[29,40] The jejunal route can be achieved by the insertion of a nasojejunal tube beyond the ligament of Treitz or by surgical placement of a jejunal catheter. Parenteral nutrition can be administered in acute pancreatitis as second-line therapy if nasogastric or nasojejunal tube feeding is not tolerated and nutritional support is required.[21,22] As an example, the patient with an adynamic ileus would not be a candidate for EN. Though it is known that EN may not meet all of the nutritional requirements of patients with acute pancreatitis because of feeding interruptions for studies, positioning, diagnostic testing, and also because of high residuals in the stomach, as well as other causes, it is still the most effective nutritional intervention.[21,29,40] EN should be considered primary therapy in severe acute pancreatitis. It not only provides needed protein and calorie nutrition, but also limits increases in gut permeability, thus reducing the septic potential of bacterial translocation. Evidence-based data also exist indicating that EN, initiated early (within 48 hours of onset of the disease), can diminish disease severity in severe acute pancreatitis, reduce the incidence of complications (e.g., organ failure, central line sepsis), and shorten the length of hospitalization.[23,25,29,34] No specific formulation of immunonutrition has been shown to improve outcomes.[13] However, the International Association of Pancreatology/American Pancreatic Association (IAP/APA) Working Group Acute Pancreatitis Guidelines recommend the use of either elemental or polymeric enteral nutrition formulations because they are relatively inexpensive and provide similar feeding tolerance and benefits compared to more expensive feedings.[21] Small peptide medium-chain triglyceride semielemental formula, infused into the stomach or small bowel, is recommended by International Consensus Guidelines. These guidelines support the use of EN, even when complications such as pseudocysts or necrosis ensue.[31] The protein intake goal for any patient with acute pancreatitis is 1.2 to 2.0 g/kg/day. There is a nutritional requirement for essential fats, and some of the energy should be supplied enterally or parenterally as lipids. It is safe to provide lipids either enterally or parenterally in most patients if serum triglyceride levels remain less than 400 mg/dL.[29] Monitor patients during their nutritional therapy for acute-phase protein levels and quantitative urine urea nitrogen levels to assess the impact of either enteral or parenteral nutrition on preventing protein/calorie malnutrition. Patients with the mild form of the disease can resume oral feeding as soon as the abdominal pain and laboratory parameters begin to improve. There is no need to wait for complete resolution of pain or for normalization of laboratory studies to begin oral intake.[13,21]

Pseudocysts, Fistulas, and Abscesses

The development of a pancreatic pseudocyst, one of the local complications of acute pancreatitis, may resolve spontaneously but may also become infected, cause urinary or gastrointestinal obstruction, or rupture, releasing toxic enzymes and inflammatory cytokines. It may contain several liters of exudate. It is generally agreed that early in the development of the pseudocyst, manipulation or drainage should not be attempted unless complications ensue.[7,14,22] Once the encapsulation has matured, it can be drained endoscopically, percutaneously, or, in some cases, surgically.

A late complication of acute pancreatitis, which is also caused by disruption of the pancreatic duct due to destruction of the surrounding parenchyma, is a pancreatic fistula. Fistulas may occur due to the severe effects of pancreatic enzymes or may result as a complication of pancreatic debridement. One method to control this complication is the use of endoscopic debridement, which thwarts the development of an external fistula.[13,44]

Intraabdominal abscesses may occur late in the course of acute pancreatitis and be responsible for a delayed septic state. Such abscesses can be percutaneously drained and the infection treated with appropriate antibiotics. Surgical debridement and lavage may be required if the abscess is not amenable to percutaneous drainage.

Management of Systemic Complications

Systemic complications of acute pancreatitis include pulmonary, cardiovascular, renal, and gastrointestinal sequelae. Intensive assessment for early signs of the onset of these abnormalities is a critical part of the interprofessional plan of care.

Respiratory

Worsening hypoxemia and respiratory distress with radiographic changes may manifest pulmonary complications. The prevention and management of atelectasis and pneumonia include vigorous pulmonary hygiene, incentive spirometry, turning, positioning, and close scrutiny of continuous pulse oximetry and arterial blood gas results. The goal for these interventions is to maintain the Pao_2 greater than 70 mm Hg and arterial oxygen saturation greater than 93%. If severe, pleural effusion may be managed by thoracentesis or chest tube placement. The development of pulmonary emboli is thwarted by prophylaxis of deep vein thrombosis by the use of antithrombotic compression sleeves or stockings and subcutaneous heparin, unless the patient is actively bleeding. Noninvasive positive pressure ventilation may be used to treat some of the respiratory abnormalities associated with acute pancreatitis. Respiratory failure in severe acute pancreatitis may be related to the development of one or more of these complications or to the occurrence of ARDS. Respiratory failure associated with acute pancreatitis is managed with intubation and mechanical ventilation, often using the lung protective strategies of low tidal volume and high respiratory rate with permissive hypercapnia.[17,48] Other ventilatory interventions include positive end-expiratory pressure (PEEP) with levels of Fio_2 adequate to achieve a Pao_2 of greater than 60 mm Hg. Barotrauma and oxygen toxicity are always concerns in the management of pancreatitis-related ARDS. Placing the patient in the prone position has also shown some benefit, especially if initiated early in the course of the syndrome.[17,48]

Cardiovascular

Patients with acute pancreatitis are at risk for the onset of cardiovascular complications (e.g., dysrhythmias and hypovolemic or septic shock). Electrolyte (e.g., calcium, magnesium, and potassium) and glucose derangements also occur frequently and are problematic. Patients must be closely monitored for the early development of these potentially life-threatening disorders. Cardiac monitoring, careful control of intake and output, monitoring of CVP and pulmonary artery (PA) pressures and/or of SVV or PPV, and maintenance of aggressive volume resuscitation are all key in prevention of these complications. In addition, serum electrolytes and glucose levels must be frequently assessed in an effort to correct any deficiency. Low total levels of calcium (< 8 mg/dL) are not only a negative prognostic sign but also precipitate dysrhythmias and therefore must be effectively managed. It is most accurate, when evaluating for hypocalcemia, to measure the ionized or unbound level of calcium. This is the physiologically active form of calcium. Losses of potassium and magnesium into retroperitoneal exudates also mandate frequent serum determinations and replacement to maintain levels within the normal range. Members of the healthcare team also must monitor for the development of clinical signs and symptoms related to electrolyte abnormalities (e.g., cardiac abnormalities and muscular tetany). Chapter 22 provides detailed information on electrolyte abnormalities. Persistent dysrhythmias not eradicated by aggressive electrolyte replacement may require the use of dysrhythmia medications. The shock state may necessitate the use of vasoactive medications when volume resuscitation alone does not correct the hemodynamic instability. Overall, the use of inotropes and vasoactive substances should be considered only after intravascular volume has been optimized.[17]

Renal and Gastrointestinal Complications

The renal and gastrointestinal complications of acute pancreatitis may occur because of decreased blood flow to these organs related to hemodynamic instability. Local inflammation may also play a role in the onset of these disorders.[13,22,26,37]

Renal complications. When preventive measures such as aggressive volume resuscitation fail and acute renal failure develops, patients may require management with hemodialysis. Patients with persistent hemodynamic compromise are treated with renal replacement therapy, commonly in the form of continuous veno-venous hemodialysis (CVVHD). An adynamic ileus may develop related to decreased intestinal motility and is managed with nasogastric suction and continued NPO status.

Gastrointestinal complications. Patients with acute pancreatitis can develop gastrointestinal bleeding (Chapter 16) from many sources. Upper gastrointestinal bleeding related to peptic ulcer formation can be effectively prevented by the use of histamine antagonists or proton pump inhibitors.[7,14] Identification of the bleeding site and hemodynamic stabilization of the patient with a life-threatening hemorrhage of the gastrointestinal tract are of critical importance. Bleeding sites may be diagnosed and eradicated by endoscopic methods such as bipolar or laser coagulation. Angiography may be needed to identify a source of bleeding; it also facilitates interventions such as angiographic embolization of bleeding vessels due to a ruptured pseudoaneurysm caused by pancreatitis.[3] Surgery may be required to repair or remove a bleeding site if nonsurgical methods prove unsuccessful. While diagnosis and definitive management are underway, aggressive volume resuscitation continues. Recurrent gastrointestinal bleeding or gastrointestinal perforation will require surgical correction.

Glycemic Reactions

Hyperglycemia is a common condition in acute pancreatitis and demands close scrutiny and protocol-driven management based upon evidence-based criteria. The desired blood glucose range in adult hospitalized patients receiving nutrition support, such as those with severe acute pancreatitis, is between 140 and 180 mg/dL (7.8–10 μmol/L). This recommendation is based upon evidence that hyperglycemia is associated with increased morbidity and mortality in hospitalized patients, both in the ICU and the non-ICU setting.[24,28] There have been no clinical trials specifically designed to determine the effect of different blood glucose targets on clinical outcomes in acute pancreatitis. In critically ill patients, rigorous glucose control may lead to moderate and severe hypoglycemia, both of which are associated with an increased mortality.[30]

The strategy of glucose control without hypoglycemia may also be effective in the prevention and management of sepsis and septic shock. Hyperglycemia and its associated overproduction of oxygen-free radicals may worsen organ failure and should be controlled.[30] The cytokine-induced insulin-resistant state of tissues in acute pancreatitis may be causative of hyperglycemia, often requiring insulin administration via the intravenous route.

Bleeding

Bleeding, though a rare complication, must be closely monitored because of the potential for disruption in the gastrointestinal mucosa and for development of disseminated intravascular coagulation (DIC). Nurses should monitor for bruising and bleeding, especially at venipuncture sites and other breaks in skin integrity. Stools are assessed closely for the presence of gross or occult blood. Intravenous and arterial punctures should be minimized. Small-bore needles are used as necessary, and pressure is applied to the site to prevent bleeding. Coagulation studies are monitored closely for abnormalities, and coagulation proteins are replaced as needed. Shock caused by a hemorrhagic event, whatever its cause, is treated aggressively with intravenous fluids, blood, and blood products as necessary (see Chapter 26). The end points of resuscitation may include normalization of the patient's blood pressure, pulse, and indices of end-organ perfusion (e.g., mentation, urine output, skin perfusion) but should also include an assessment of SVV and continued volume responsiveness. If central access is in place or inserted, filling pressures and minimally invasive determinants of cardiac output and SVV or PPV are monitored with the goal of volume resuscitation to normalize these parameters.

Inflammation

There have been attempts to control the inflammatory response in patients with severe acute pancreatitis. This uncontrolled inflammation is believed to be responsible for the massive physiologic response and the multitude of complications. The role of many inflammatory mediators in acute pancreatitis has been investigated in hopes of identifying an antiinflammatory therapy, but there has been limited success and few human studies.[22] Intravenous protease inhibitors have no effect on mortality, pain, infection, or other complications of acute pancreatitis and are not recommended.[2,41] There is no compelling evidence to support the use of immune-modulating therapies such as anti-TNF or lexipafant, a platelet-activating factor (PAF) antagonist. Other medications trialed, but without evidence of effectiveness in the treatment of severe acute pancreatitis, include somatostatin and octreotide.[22]

SUPPORTIVE CARE

Though most tactics in the management strategy for acute pancreatitis are aimed at supportive interventions, perhaps the most vital tactic in caring for the patient with severe acute pancreatitis is to effectively eliminate the cause whenever possible. In the case where alcohol is the inciting agent in acute pancreatitis, nurses, case managers, and social workers are key in providing resources for post-acute counseling to the patient and family. The management of this disease and the myriad of complications with which it presents are quite complex. An interprofessional approach is critical for successful treatment and optimal patient outcomes.

Patient and family support and education are of the utmost importance throughout all phases of this often life-changing and frequently life-threatening disease. Providing education regarding diagnostic testing, plan of care, and pain management interventions can reduce the stress and anxiety brought on by an acute hospitalization, which may also include a prolonged stay in a critical care unit. Early and progressive mobility should be undertaken on patients with acute pancreatitis, even if they require prolonged ventilatory management. Physical and occupational therapists play an important role in the recovery phase as they, along with the nursing staff, focus on range of motion, tactics to prevent pressure ulcers, and the prevention of functional loss.[22]

CONCLUSION

Once the diagnosis of severe acute pancreatitis has been made, thus begins the need for expert, evidence-based management in an effort to reduce organ involvement and potential dysfunction. Intensive assessment and monitoring are necessary for the identification of complications so that interventions might commence rapidly.

It is necessary to keep in mind that there are few effective remedies for the physiologic impact acute pancreatitis brings to bear on the human host. Further research is required to explore new medications, new management strategies for the complications, and new methods to improve patient outcomes.

CASE STUDY18.1

J.D. is a 44-year-old male who developed severe, sharp, excruciating midepigastric pain radiating to his mid back. He also began vomiting large amounts of bilious fluid. He was taken to the emergency department (ED) where he was still in severe pain, rating it at a level 8 on a numeric pain scale of 0 to 10. J.D.'s medical history is significant for hypertension controlled with hydrochlorothiazide (Microzide). J.D.'s heart rate was regular at 138 beats/min, blood pressure was 80/44 mm Hg, respiratory rate was regular at 32 breaths/min, and he had a temperature of 100°F.

J.D. was noted to have abdominal tenderness, distention, and decreased bowel sounds. He remained hypotensive; lactated Ringer's solution was administered at 150 mL/h. His respiratory status was monitored closely as his breath sounds were somewhat decreased with few bibasilar crackles. His oxygen saturation by pulse oximetry (Spo_2) was 90%, and he was administered oxygen at 2 L/min. STAT laboratory results showed an elevated serum amylase level of 775 units/L, a lipase level of 1290 units/L, a WBC count of 18,000/mm^3, an ionized calcium level of 3.2 mg/dL, and a potassium level of 3.0 mEq/L. He was given 9.3 mEq of intravenous calcium gluconate over 1 hour and 40 mEq of potassium chloride over 4 hours. An ultrasound of the abdomen was performed, revealing two large gallstones and retroperitoneal fluid. The diagnosis of acute pancreatitis was made and was thought to be due to gallstones. A CECT study was not performed at this time. Given his hemodynamic and pulmonary status, he was admitted to the critical care unit.

J.D. was admitted to surgical critical care. He rapidly decompensated with unstable vital signs and became hypotensive and tachycardic; his urine output was less than 30 mL/h. A CECT scan revealed pancreatic necrosis and retroperitoneal inflammation with large retroperitoneal fluid sequestration. His Spo_2 was 88% on supplemental oxygen; arterial blood gas showed a Pao_2 of 54 mm Hg. He was tachypneic and complained of shortness of breath. His chest x-ray continued to show pleural effusion and atelectasis.

Decision Point:
What complication(s) is J.D. likely experiencing?

Decision Point:
What interventions are required for J.D.?

REFERENCES

1. Al-Omran, M., Albalawi, Z. H., Tashkandi, M. F., & Al-Ansary, L. A. (2010). Enteral versus parenteral nutrition for acute pancreatitis. *Cochrane Database Syst Rev* (1), CD002837. http://dx.doi.org/10.1002/14651858.CD002837.pub2.
2. Bakker, O. J., van Santvort, H. C., Besselink, M. G., Schepers, N. J., Bruno, M. J., Boermeester, M. A., et al. (2014). Treatment options for acute pancreatitis. *J Gastroenterol Hepatol, 11*(9), 462–469.
3. Balanchandra, S., & Siriwardena, A. K. (2005). Systematic appraisal of the management of major vascular complications of acute pancreatitis. *Am J Surg, 190*(3), 489–495.
4. Banks, P. A., Bollen, T. L., Dervenis, C., et al. (2012). Acute Pancreatitis Classification Working Group. Classification of acute pancreatitis–2012: revision of the Atlanta classification and definitions by international consensus. *Gut, 62*(1), 102–111.
5. Basurto, O. X., Rigau, C. D., & Urrutia, G. (2013). *Opioids for acute pancreatitis pain (Review)*. The Cochrane Collaboration. Hoboken, NJ: John Wiley & Sons, Ltd.
6. Bosch, K., Poch, E., & Grau, J. M. (2009). Rhabdomyolysis and acute kidney injury. *N Engl J Med, 361*(3), 62–72.
7. Conwell, D. L., Banks, P., & Greenberger, N. J. (2015). Acute and chronic pancreatitis. In D. Kasper (Ed.), *Harrison's principles of internal medicine* (19th ed.). New York: McGraw-Hill.
8. Cucher, D., Kulvatunyou, N., Green, D. J., & Ong, E. S. (2014). Gallstone pancreatitis: a review. *Surg Clin North Am, 94*, 257–280.

9. da Costa, D. W., Boerma, D., van Santvoort, H. C., Horvath, K. D., Werner, J., Carter, C. R., et al. (2014). Staged multidisciplinary step-up management for necrotizing pancreatitis. *Br J Surg, 10*(1), e65–e79.
10. De-Madaria, E., Soler-Sala, M. G., Sanchez-Paya, J., et al. (2011). Influence of fluid therapy on the prognosis of acute pancreatitis: a prospective cohort study. *Am J Gastroenterol, 106*(10), 1843–1850.
11. De Waele, J. J. (2014). Acute pancreatitis. *Curr Opin Crit Care, 20*(2), 189–195.
12. Elder, A. S., Saccone, G. T., & Dixon, D. L. (2012). Lung injury in acute pancreatitis: mechanisms underlying augmented secondary injury. *Pancreatology, 12*(1), 49–56.
13. Fagenholz, P. J., & de Moya, M. A. (2013). Acute inflammatory surgical disease. *Surg Clin N Am, 24*(2014), 1–30.
14. Friedman, L. S. (2015). Liver, biliary tract and pancreas disorders. In M. A. Papadakis, & S. J. McPhee (Eds.), *Current medical diagnosis & treatment*. New York: McGraw-Hill, Lange.
15. Fritz, S., Hackert, T., Hartwig, W., Rossmanith, F., et al. (2010). Bacterial translocation and infected pancreatic necrosis in acute necrotizing pancreatitis derives from small bowel. *Am J Surg, 200*(1), 111–117.
16. Goldenberg, D. E., Gordon, S. R., & Gardner, T. B. (2014). Management of acute pancreatitis. *Expert Rev Gastroenterol Hepatol, 8*(5), 687–694.
17. Goldman, L., & Schafer, A. I. (2015). *Goldman-Cecil medicine* (25th ed.). Philadelphia: Elsevier.
18. Gooszen, H. G., Besselink, M. G. H., van Santvoort, H. C., & Bollen, T. L. (2013). Surgical treatment of acute pancreatitis. *Langenbeck's Arch Surg, 398*(6), 799–806.
19. Haydock, M. D., Mittal, A., Wilms, H. R., Phillips, A., Petrov, M. S., & Windsor, J. A. (2013). Fluid therapy in acute pancreatitis: anybody's guess. *Ann Surg, 257*(2), 182–188.
20. Hirota, M., Takada, T., Kitamura, N., et al. (2010). Fundamental and intensive care of acute pancreatitis. *J Hepatobiliary Pancreat Sci, 17*(6), 45–52.
21. International Association of Pancreatology. (2015). IAP/APA evidence-based guidelines for the management of acute pancreatitis. *Pancreatology, 13*(Suppl 2), e1–e15.
22. Jeyarajah, D. R. (2014). Advances in the management of pancreatic necrosis. *Curr Probl Surg, 51*(9), 374–408.
23. Johnson, C. D., & Besselink, M. G. (2014). Acute pancreatitis. *BMJ, 349*, g4859.
24. Krinsley, J. S. (2003). Association between hyperglycemia and increased hospital mortality in a heterogeneous population of critically ill patients. *Mayo Clin Proc, 78*(12), 1471–1478.
25. Li, J. Y., Yu, T., Chen, G.C., et al. (2013). Enteral nutrition within 48 hours of admission improves clinical outcomes of acute pancreatitis by reducing complications: a meta-analysis. *PLoS ONE, 8*(6), e64926.
26. Maksimov, M., Kyhala, L., Nieminem, A., et al. (2014). Early prediction of persistent organ failure by soluble CD73 in patients with acute pancreatitis. *Crit Care Med, 42*(12), 2556–2564.
27. Martin, R. F., & Hein, A. R. (2013). Operative management of acute pancreatitis. *Surg Clin North Am, 93*(2013), 595–610.
28. McAlister, F. A., Majumdar, S. R., Blitz, S., Rowe, B. H., Romney, J., & Marrie, T. J. (2005). The relation between hyperglycemia and outcomes in 2,471 patients admitted to the hospital with community-acquired pneumonia. *Diabetes Care, 28*(4), 810–815.
29. McClave, S. A. (2013). Nutrition in pancreatitis. *World Rev Nutr Diet, 105*, 160–168.
30. McMahon, M., Nystrom, E., Braunschweig, C., Miles, J., & Compher, C. (2013). ASPEN Guidelines: nutrition support of adult patients with hyperglycemia. *J Parenter Enteral Nutr, 37*(1), 23–36.
31. Mirtallo, J., Forbes, A., McClave, S. A., & Jensen, G. I. (2012). International consensus guidelines for nutrition therapy in pancreatitis. *J Parenter Enteral Nutr, 36*(3), 284–291.
32. Reference deleted in page proof.
33. Peery, A. F., Dellon, E. S., Lund, J., et al. (2012). Burden of gastrointestinal disease in the United States: 2012 update. *Gastroenterology, 143*(5), 1179–1187.
34. Petrov, M. S., Pylypchuk, R. D., & Uchugina, A. F. (2009). A systematic review on the timing of artificial nutrition in acute pancreatitis. *Br J Nutr, 101*(6), 787–793.
35. Pezzilli, R., Bellacosa, L., & Felicani, C. (2009). Lung injury in acute pancreatitis. *J Pancreas, 10*(5), 481–484.
36. Pezzilli, R., Zerbi, A., Di Carlo, V., Bassi, C., & Delle Fave, G. F. (2010). Practical guidelines for acute pancreatitis. *Pancreatology, 10*(5), 523–535.
37. Sah, R. P., Dawra, R. K., & Saluja, A. K. (2013). New insights into the pathogenesis of pancreatitis. *Curr Opin Gastroenterol, 29*(5), 523–530.
38. Sarr, M. G., Banks, P. A., Bollen, T. L., Dervenis, C., Gooszen, H. G., et al. (2013). The new revised classification of acute pancreatitis 2012. *Surg Clin North Am, 93*(3), 549–562.
39. Schepers, N. J. (2013). Early management of acute pancreatitis. *Best Pract Res Clin Gastroenterol, 27*(5), 727–743.
40. Seminerio, J., & O'Keefe, S. J. (2014). Jejunal feeding in patients with pancreatitis. *Nutr Clin Pract, 29*(3), 283–286.
41. Seta, T., Noguchi, Y., Shikata, S., & Nakayama, T. (2014). Treatment of acute pancreatitis with protease inhibitors administered through intravenous infusion: an updated systematic review and meta-analysis. *BMC Gastroenterol, 14*(102), 1–11.
42. Singh, V. K., Bollen, T. L., Wu, B. U., et al. (2011). An assessment of the severity of interstitial pancreatitis. *Clin Gastroenterol Hepatol, 9*(12), 1098–1103.
43. Trikudanathan, G., Attam, R., Arain, M. A., Mallery, S., & Freeman, M. L. (2014). Endoscopic interventions for necrotizing pancreatitis. *Am J Gastroenterol, 109*(7), 969–981.
44. Van Brunschot, S., Fockens, P., Bakker, O. J., Besselink, M. G., Voermans, R. P., Poley, J. W., et al. (2014). Endoscopic transluminal necrosectomy in necrotizing pancreatitis: a systematic review. *Surg Endosc, 28*(5), 1425–1438.
45. Van Santvoort, H. C., Bakker, O. J., Bollen, T. L., et al. (2011). A conservative and minimally invasive approach to necrotizing pancreatitis improves outcome. *Gastroenterology, 141*(4), 1254–1263.
46. Wu, B., & Banks, P. A. (2013). Clinical management of patients with acute pancreatitis. *Gastroenterology, 144*, 1272–1281.
47. Yadev, D., & Lowenfels, A. B. (2013). The epidemiology of pancreatitis and pancreatic cancer. *Gastroenterology, 144*(6), 1252–1261.
48. Zhou, M. T., Chen, C.S., Chen, B.C., Zhang, Q.Y., & Andersson, R. (2010). Acute lung injury in acute pancreatitis: mechanisms and potential intervention. *World J Gastroenterol, 16*(17), 2094–2099.

SUGGESTED READINGS

Baron, T. H. (2014). Endoscopic management of biliary disorders. *Surg Clin N Am, 94*, 395–411.

de C Ferreira, L. E., & Baron, T. H. (2013). Acute biliary conditions. *Best Pract Res Clin Gastroenterol, 27*(5), 745–756.

Guo, Z. Z., Wang, P., Huang, Z.Y., & Tang, C.W. (2014). The crosstalk between gut inflammation and gastrointestinal disorders during acute pancreatitis. *Curr Pharm Des, 20*, 1051–1062.

Mounzer, R., Langmead, C. J., Wu, B. U., et al. (2012). Comparison of existing clinical scoring systems to predict persistent organ failure in patients with acute pancreatitis. *Gastroenterology, 142*(7), 1476–1482.

Vidarsdottir, H., Moller, P. H., Vidarsdottir, H., et al. (2013). Acute pancreatitis: a prospective study on incidence, etiology, and outcome. *Eur J Gastroenterol Hepatol, 25*, 1068–1075.

The Gut in Critical Illness

Michelle A. McKay

During episodes of critical illness, the gastrointestinal (GI) system often becomes compromised. Physiologic changes (e.g., the shunting of blood from the GI tract to the vital organs) result in hypoperfusion and decreased tissue oxygenation and function. Consequently, changes to normal gut physiology (e.g., digestion, absorption, immunity, and protection) may occur; this may further compromise the critically ill patient. Assessment of GI perfusion in the critically ill patient is a useful strategy to monitor for signs of hypoperfusion or adequacy of resuscitation.

This chapter will explore three key issues related to the gut in critical illness: assessment of the adequacy of gut perfusion using gastric tonometry; prevention of stress-related mucosal disease; and the assessment and management of intra-abdominal hypertension and abdominal compartment syndrome.

NORMAL GASTROINTESTINAL PHYSIOLOGY

The physiology of the GI system is most commonly associated with its role in digestion and absorption of nutrients (e.g., amino acids, lipids, vitamins, minerals, and water). However, during critical illness, normal GI physiology responsible for digestion and absorption of nutrients may be altered. For example, the primary function of the stomach is to produce gastric acid and pepsin. Whereas gastric acid production is commonly thought to increase in critical illness, most critically ill patients do not hypersecrete gastric acid.[28] Rather, gastric acid secretion is often diminished in the critically ill, with an increase in gastric pH observed even when gastric acid secretion is not pharmacologically inhibited.[41,77]

The small bowel also plays an important part in the digestion and absorption of nutrients. Mechanical digestion, together with the chemical digestion of carbohydrates, amino acids, lipids, and nucleic acids, is essential for breaking down the nutrients into a form absorbable by the small intestine.[80] The processes of diffusion, facilitated diffusion, osmosis, and active transport in the small intestine are responsible for the absorption of 90% of all nutrients.[80] The remaining 10% of nutrients are absorbed in the stomach and large intestine. The ability of the small intestine to absorb these nutrients can be impaired during critical illness[16]; however, the cause of this malabsorption remains unclear.

Whereas the digestion and absorption of nutrients is an important aspect of normal GI physiology, the GI tract's role in immunity and protection is of equal importance to the critically ill patient. The GI tract has a variety of protective mechanisms in place that prevent the movement of substances (other than nutrients, water, and electrolytes) across the gut wall (Table 19.1). In the setting of critical illness, where GI hypoperfusion may be present, these mechanisms that normally protect the body against movement of bacteria across the gut wall may be diminished.

ALTERATIONS TO NORMAL GASTROINTESTINAL PHYSIOLOGY IN CRITICAL ILLNESS

Alterations to normal GI physiology in critical illness are primarily related to hypoperfusion and decreased oxygenation in this highly metabolic area. Previously, GI dysfunction in critical illness was described in relation to clinical presentations that became symptomatic as a result of well-established GI ischemia[42] (Box 19.1). Consequently, a focus on the prevention and early detection of GI ischemia has become vital in minimizing ischemia-related gut dysfunction in the critically ill.

Gastrointestinal Mucosal Hypoperfusion

Adequate oxygenation is necessary to maintain normal structure and function in all body tissues. Regional oxygen delivery is influenced by alterations in global oxygen delivery and oxygen consumption; however, GI hypoxia may also be present despite normal oxygen delivery and consumption.[10,20]

The GI system is particularly susceptible to alterations in regional blood flow and oxygen delivery (Box 19.2). The ability of the GI system to undergo intense vasoconstriction and to shunt blood to the central circulation results in a regional decrease in blood flow and oxygen delivery, while nonspecific measurements of total body oxygen delivery remain unchanged.[29] During shock states, decreased blood flow because of vasoconstriction occurs in this region first and is restored last, following successful resuscitation.[81] In shock states, the gut attempts to maintain adequate cellular oxygenation by increasing the amount of oxygen extracted from the blood. This increase in oxygen extraction may prevent serious compromise of tissue oxygenation even in the presence of reduced oxygen delivery.[3] Despite the ability of the gut to increase oxygen extraction in the setting of reduced oxygen delivery, the GI system remains susceptible to hypoxia, particularly if oxygen consumption is limited by oxygen delivery.[37]

The anatomic arrangement of the GI blood supply may also contribute to mucosal hypoxia (Fig. 19.1). Within the mucosa a series of finger-like projections called *villi* are formed. These villi vastly increase the epithelial surface area available for digestion and absorption. The blood vessel arrangement in each villus consists of a central arteriole and venous capillaries. Blood flows through these vessels in opposite directions and, coupled with their close proximity, facilitates the diffusion of oxygen and other small molecules between the blood vessels, resulting in a decrease in oxygen delivery to the villus tip.[80]

TABLE 19.1 Protective Mechanisms of the Gastrointestinal System

Mechanism	Protective Action
Epithelial cell shedding	Limits bacterial adhesion
Gut-associated lymphoid tissue	Provides immune tolerance against food antigens and normal intestinal flora
Hydrochloric acid secretion	Increases gastric acidity and destroys bacteria
Kupffer cells	Liver tissue macrophages that destroy foreign substances
Motility	Propels bacteria through GI tract
Mucin production	Prevents adhesion of bacteria to wall of GI tract
Zona occludens	Prevents bacteria from moving across wall of GI tract

GI, Gastrointestinal.

BOX 19.1 Gastrointestinal Dysfunction in Critical Illness

- Acalculous cholecystitis
- Gallbladder perforation
- Gastrointestinal perforation
- Gastrointestinal stress bleeding
- Intolerance of enteral feeds
- Ileus
- Ischemic enterocolitis
- Mechanical obstruction
- Pancreatitis

Data from Reference 42.

BOX 19.2 Causes of Tissue Hypoxia Within the Gastrointestinal System

- Countercurrent oxygen exchange from vessels within the villi with decreasing blood supply.
- Redistribution of blood to vital organs may persist even when normal systemic hemodynamics have been reestablished.
- Splanchnic vasoconstriction is proportionally greater than other vascular beds.

From References 71 and 72.

In low-flow states, the slow transit time leads to stasis and competitive extraction of oxygen at lower levels of the villus, producing hypoxia at the villus tip. Furthermore, reductions in arterial blood pressure cause the precapillary sphincters to relax. The relaxation of these sphincters promotes blood flow to more capillaries, increasing the number of perfused capillaries and the size of the vascular bed. The combination of low blood pressure and a larger vascular bed slows blood flow through the villi, ultimately contributing to hypoxia and ischemia at the villus tip.[38]

During the period of ischemia and hypoxia, by-products of anaerobic metabolism, known as *oxygen free radicals,* are generated. With successful resuscitation of the GI tract, blood flow and oxygen delivery are restored to the area; simultaneously, oxygen free radicals are liberated. These oxygen free radicals contribute to microvascular and mucosal changes characteristic of ischemia and reperfusion of the gut mucosa.[8,44]

Consequences of Gastrointestinal Hypoperfusion

The consequences of GI hypoperfusion are significant and include the following:

- Disruption of the physical barrier to pathogens.
- Disruption of chemical control of bacterial overgrowth.
- Decreased peristalsis.
- Reduced immunologic activities of gut-associated lymphoid tissue.

In healthy individuals, all of these mechanisms work efficiently to contain bacteria within the GI tract. However, during critical illness, reduced oxygenation may contribute to decreased cellular function and failure of these protective mechanisms. Consequently, bacterial proliferation and translocation from the GI tract to the systemic circulation may occur, resulting in a systemic inflammatory response or SIRS.[33,71,72]

Disruption of the physical barrier to pathogens. The mucosal lining of the entire GI tract creates a physical barrier to bacterial invasion. The mucosa is composed of epithelial cells produced and replaced approximately every 3 to 5 days.[73] This constant shedding means that pathogens have little chance to colonize and invade the GI tract because they are shed simultaneously

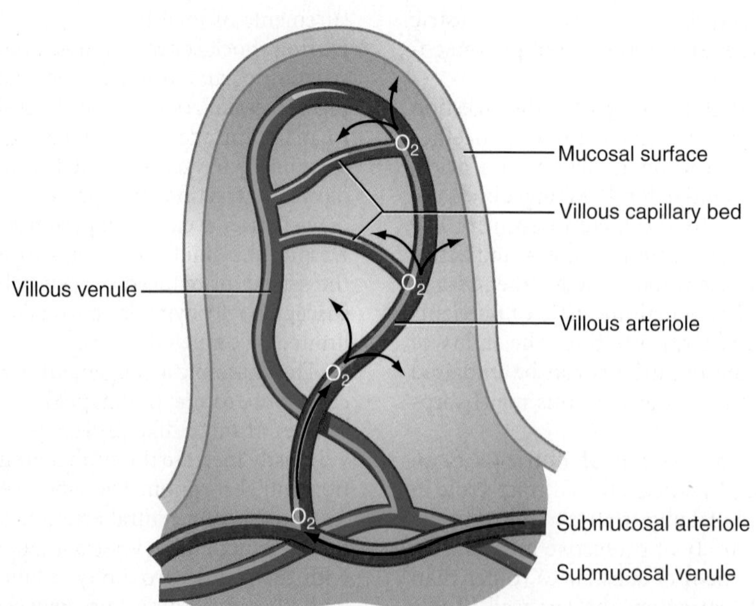

FIG. 19.1 Blood supply to the gastrointestinal (GI) mucosa villus.

with the epithelial cells. The epithelial cells are highly metabolic, consuming large amounts of oxygen, and consequently are susceptible to reduced oxygen delivery and changes in vascular flow.[75] Reductions in mucosal oxygen delivery may lead to mucosal atrophy and epithelial cell death, reducing the ability of the epithelial cells to provide a mechanical barrier to pathogens.

The junctions between epithelial cells also provide a barrier to microorganisms. Intermediate junctions (zonula adherens) function primarily in cell-cell adhesion,[69] whereas the tight junctions (zonula occludens) limit the movement of bacteria and toxins across the gut wall.[53] The impaired mucosal perfusion and mucosal atrophy associated with critical illness may increase the permeability of the tight junctions and permit the movement of pathogens across the mucosal barrier.[72,78]

Mucus cells also line the surface of the GI mucosa, and, when stimulated by food or irritation, secrete large quantities of very thick, alkaline mucus. In the stomach, a mucus layer approximately 1 mm thick is formed, coating the wall of the stomach and protecting it against autodigestion.[80] Further protection is provided by the glycoproteins contained within the mucus that prevent bacteria from adhering to and colonizing the mucosal wall.[23]

When hypoperfusion occurs, blood is shunted away from the splanchnic circulation to more vital organs, but returns after hemodynamic resuscitation.[72] In an ischemia/reperfusion injury where the villi are damaged, proinflammatory factors are released, and there is an increased intestinal permeability with mucosal disruption, which allows for bacterial translocation.[72]

Disruption of chemical control of bacterial overgrowth. Parietal cells in the stomach produce hydrochloric acid and keep the intragastric environment relatively acidic, with a pH of approximately 3.0. Acidic pH has both bactericidal and bacteriostatic properties,[76] thus limiting overgrowth in the stomach. The effectiveness of this inhibition of bacterial growth by hydrochloric acid production may be reduced in the critically ill because hydrochloric acid production within the stomach has been noted to decrease as a consequence of critical illness.[15,36] Changes in gastric pH associated with critical illness may facilitate bacterial proliferation within the stomach.

The secretion of bicarbonate in the small intestine provides further protection for the epithelium. The binding of bicarbonate ions with hydrogen ions to form water and carbon dioxide (CO_2) prevents hydrogen ions from damaging the duodenal wall.[51] Although this is a relatively efficient system, some hydrogen ions still reach the mucosal layer and the bicarbonate in the microvasculature is needed to neutralize them. In normal physiologic states, as the number of hydrogen ions increases, there is a proportional increase in mucosal blood flow, supplying more bicarbonate ions.[51] However, in critical illness, often associated with a low-flow state within the gut, bicarbonate ion production may be limited, reducing the effectiveness of this protective mechanism and allowing damage to the gut mucosa to occur.

Further down the GI tract, normal gut flora, capable of surviving in the more alkaline environment of the lower gut, attach to the mucosal cells of the colon, preventing colonization of unwanted pathogens.[69] Antibiotic therapy, commonly used in the management of critical illness, may reduce the population of normal gut flora and provide opportunities for pathogenic overgrowth.[39,72]

Bile salts may also provide protection against bacteria by breaking down the liposaccharide portion of the endotoxin and thereby detoxifying gram-negative bacteria in the gut.[55] The deconjugation of bile salts into secondary bile acids also inhibits the proliferation of pathogens and may destroy their cell walls.[30] However, normal gut flora is required for the deconjugation of bile acids to secondary bile acids; therefore, a reduction in the number of normal gut flora, such as may occur secondary to antibiotic therapy, may inhibit this protective mechanism. Bile salts are commonly thought to reflux in critical illness thereby injuring the mucosal tissue and causing damage.[76]

Reduced immunologic activities of gut-associated lymphoid tissue. Protection against bacterial invasion is also provided by gut-associated lymphoid tissue,[63] one of the largest immune organs in the body.[69] When this lymphoid tissue is exposed to antigens, it has the ability to mount cell-mediated and humoral-mediated immune responses,[69] which have a cytotoxic effect on the bacteria.[23] Thus the immunologic function of the GI system is important in maintaining regional and global protection against the invasion of bacteria. However, in critical illness, reduced oxygen and nutrient supply could impede the ability of the gut to function as an immunologic organ, and thus the GI system's ability to protect the body against bacteria is diminished.

The GI tract's various physical, chemical, and immunologic barriers provide the initial defense against bacterial invasion. Should bacteria and their by-products cross the gut barrier and enter the systemic circulation, the reticuloendothelial system, made up of Kupffer cells in the liver and spleen, provides a back-up defense. In the event that pathogens cross the gut barrier and enter the systemic circulation, they will drain from the extensive vasculature supplying the GI tract and into the portal vein.[80] The blood is then directed to the liver. As blood enters the liver, it comes into contact with the extensive reticuloendothelial system, where the pathogens are destroyed through phagocytosis by the Kupffer cells.[62] However, alterations in regional blood flow in critical illness result in a shunting of blood into the central circulation and a simultaneous decrease in hepatic blood flow. Consequently, pathogens and debris that enter the intestinal circulation may not reach the Kupffer cells and systemic bacteremia may result.

The blood vessels of the GI system are part of an extensive system called the splanchnic circulation, which includes blood flow through the liver, spleen, and pancreas. The structure of the splanchnic circulation is such that blood passes through the gut, spleen, and pancreas before entering the liver by way of the portal vein. Consequently, the changes in GI perfusion have the capacity to impact hepatic perfusion, oxygenation, and function. In approximately 10% to 22% of critically ill patients, ischemic hepatitis or "shock liver" occurs in times of cardiac, circulatory, or respiratory failure. The patient will have a sharp but transient increase in serum aminotransferase level up to 20 times the normal level without any other known reason, such as hepatitis.[43] Ischemic hepatic injury influences morbidity and mortality and therefore must be considered a priority in the critically ill patient.[32] Physiologic changes contributing to ischemic hepatitis include alterations to the portal and arterial blood supply, as well as the hepatic microcirculation.[43] The degree to which the liver is damaged is directly related to the severity and duration of hypoperfusion; both anoxic and reperfusion injury can damage hepatocytes and the vascular endothelium.

The liver plays an important role in the inflammatory process. Kupffer cells, tissue macrophages in the liver, normally detoxify substances that may trigger systemic inflammation and produce proteins and antiproteases that control the inflammatory response. However, in the setting of splanchnic hypoperfusion, liver dysfunction may occur and these processes may be inhibited.

Interprofessional Plan of Care

The interprofessional team must work together to ensure accurate assessment and early intervention of GI mucosal hypoperfusion. Strategies should be implemented to improve tissue oxygenation that are appropriate to the patient's clinical presentation, such as fluid resuscitation, inotropic or vasoactive agents, and blood products. Adequate resuscitation strategies should be assessed, including blood pressure (BP), mean arterial pressure (MAP), heart rate (HR), urine output, and neurologic status. These global assessments are important and can clearly indicate the need for more direct and aggressive resuscitation. However, these parameters do not reflect regional perfusion and may be within acceptable limits even with mucosal hypoperfusion. If mucosal hypoperfusion is noted early, circulatory compromise will be identified earlier, allowing for appropriate treatment and improvement in end-organ perfusion.

GASTRIC TONOMETRY

The GI system is complex in its structure and function. Its role in the digestion and absorption of nutrients is well understood, and its ability to protect the body against the invasion of organisms is increasingly being appreciated. In the critically ill, the role of the gut has become an area of interest because of its susceptibility to ischemia and hypoxia that may be linked to alterations in its structure and function, which in turn contributes to the development of multiple organ dysfunction syndrome (MODS).

Gastric tonometry has been developed as a minimally invasive method of monitoring perfusion, and possibly oxygenation, of the GI tract and splanchnic organs. Monitoring of perfusion and oxygenation in the GI region is important because changes in GI blood flow may occur in the absence of systemic hemodynamic disturbances.[40,47] Such changes can provide an earlier warning of hypoperfusion than conventional assessments of perfusion (e.g., arterial blood pressure). Hypoperfusion contributes to decreased oxygen delivery within the highly metabolic splanchnic region, with longer-term consequences being the development of GI dysfunction and MODS.[72] The ability of gastric tonometry to provide real-time and specific monitoring of gastric perfusion makes it a possible tool for monitoring patients at risk of splanchnic hypoperfusion,[26,40] although more recent studies have not supported this concept.[66] Early attention to gastric hypoperfusion may prevent the development of MODS and improve outcomes for critically ill patients,[34] although data suggesting an improvement in outcomes based on treatment guided by tonometrically derived variables are lacking.[34,67,82]

Principles of Gastric Tonometry

Gastric tonometry is designed to monitor splanchnic perfusion because a reduction in blood flow to this area is thought to be an *early* indicator of the development of shock. The ability to monitor the adequacy of splanchnic perfusion allows clinicians to observe the early development of shock that would otherwise be undetected by monitoring global measurements of perfusion and oxygenation (e.g., hypotension, decreased cardiac output, and increased lactate levels).[12] The physiologic underpinnings of gastric tonometry include the links between tissue oxygen delivery, cellular utilization of oxygen, and CO_2 production described earlier in this chapter.

During periods of decreased gastric blood flow, anaerobic metabolism occurs where lactic acid is generated causing an accumulation of CO_2.[65] Theoretically, the CO_2 produced by the GI mucosa during cellular activity should move from an area of higher partial pressure (mucosa) to an area of lower partial pressure (gastric lumen). Because the tonometer balloon is permeable to CO_2 and is situated in the gastric lumen, the gas diffuses from the gastric lumen into the balloon until equilibrium is reached.[61] Simply, the measurement of gastric intramucosal CO_2 concentration is achieved by the sampling of fluid or air from a CO_2-permeable balloon, which forms part of the gastric tonometer (Fig. 19.2). Whereas gastric tonometry was utilized in the 1990s as a clinical monitor,[65] its widespread adoption in the current time period has not occurred. This may be due in part to the technical limitations and potential for procedural error associated with using this device. Zhang et al.[82] published a meta-analysis exploring whether gastric tonometry–guided therapy had any effect on measureable outcomes. After analyzing six relevant randomized controlled trials, gastric tonometry showed no significant effect on hospital mortality, intensive care unit (ICU) mortality, or ICU and hospital length of stay. When compared with control groups, gastric tonometry–guided therapy significantly reduced total mortality of critical care patients[82]; however, limitations to the meta-analysis could have made the study grossly underpowered.[65]

The use of gastric tonometry in the assessment of the critically ill patient will likely be debated for some time, contributing to the slow incorporation of this technology in clinical practice. Nevertheless, the physiologic underpinnings of this technology are valuable to consider within the context of any critically ill patient, and provide nurses with a sound foundation for considering the role of oxygen delivery and the effect of shock on the GI tract during episodes of critical illness.

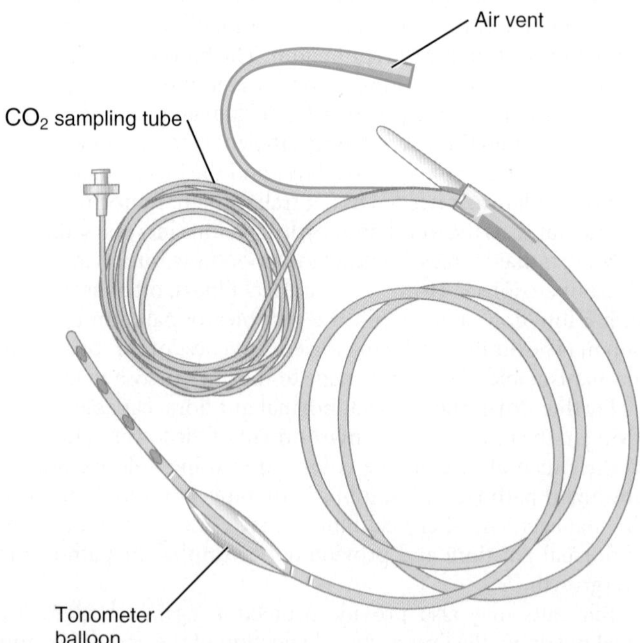

FIG. 19.2 The gastric tonometer. *CO_2*, Carbon dioxide.

STRESS-RELATED MUCOSAL DISEASE IN CRITICALLY ILL PATIENTS

In the early 1930s an association between central nervous system injury and gastroduodenal disease became apparent.[21] Some years later, endoscopic studies in patients with severe cutaneous burns[22] showed similar results. It is now commonly accepted that the physiologic stress associated with critical illness contributes to the development of stress-related mucosal disease.

Prevalence

Stress-related mucosal disease is common in the critically ill and is associated with an increase in morbidity and mortality.[6,27,54] The prevalence of this problem in the critically ill depends on how stress-related mucosal disease is defined. The definition is an important consideration when evaluating research in this area. Endoscopic studies suggest that this injury occurs rapidly and the prevalence of mucosal injury is between 75% and 100%.[6,22] Occult bleeding is defined as a positive guaiac test of stool or gastric aspirate. When this clinical end point is used, the prevalence of stress-related mucosal disease is estimated to be 15% to 50%.[31] Clinically, overt bleeding is defined as clinical evidence of bleeding and occurs in approximately 5% of critically ill patients.[27] Clinically significant bleeding is defined as overt bleeding accompanied by hemodynamic changes (e.g., hypotension, tachycardia, or a drop in hemoglobin level)[79] and is estimated to occur in 1% to 4% of patients.[1,7]

Pathophysiology

Diffuse superficial erosions or deeper, more focal lesions that are more likely to result in clinically important bleeding characterize stress-related mucosal injury. A strong association between physiologic stress and mucosal injury has been identified, although the pathophysiology of this clinically important problem is not fully understood.[27] It is thought the factors contributing to stress-related mucosal disease in the critically ill are related to a number of factors and result from an imbalance between protective mechanisms that promotes mucosal injury (Table 19.2).

Risk Factors

The risk of developing stress-related mucosal disease is not the same for all critically ill patients. A number of factors are associated with the risk of stress-related mucosal disease (Box 19.3). Patients with multiple risk factors are particularly susceptible.

Two independent risk factors have been identified and include mechanical ventilation for longer than 48 hours and coagulopathy. In a landmark prospective multicenter study, risk factors for clinically significant bleeding associated with stress-related mucosal disease were examined in patients admitted to intensive care. Patients with respiratory failure who required mechanical ventilation for longer than 48 hours were 16 times more likely to develop stress-related mucosal disease (odds ratio 15.6) while patients with a coagulopathy, demonstrated by a platelet count of less than 50,000/mm^3, an international normalized ratio of greater than 1.5, or a partial thromboplastin time of greater than 2.0 times the control value, were four times more likely (odds ratio 4.3).[18] Interestingly, the data in this study showed that of the 847 patients with risk factors, only 31 (3.7%) experienced clinically significant bleeding, and of the 1405 patients without risk factors, only 2 (0.1%) experienced clinically significant bleeding.

Although the prevalence of clinically significant bleeding is low for critically ill patients, even for those with risk factors, it remains a clinical concern because of the associated increased mortality rate. Peura and Johnson[68] found that patients with stress-related mucosal bleeding had a mortality rate of 57% compared to those without risk factors who had a mortality rate of 24%. Similarly, Cook et al.[18] found increased mortality

TABLE 19.2 Factors Contributing to Stress-Related Mucosal Disease

Protective mechanisms	Mucosal prostaglandins	Protect mucosa by stimulating blood flow, mucus, and bicarbonate production Stimulate epithelial cell growth and repair
	Mucosal bicarbonate barrier	Forms a physical barrier to acid and pepsin, preventing injury to epithelium
	Epithelial restitution and regeneration	Epithelial cells rapidly regenerate, but process is highly metabolic and may be impaired by physiologic stress
	Mucosal blood flow	Helps remove acid from mucosa, supplies bicarbonate and oxygen to mucosal epithelial cells
	Cell membrane and tight junctions	Tight junctions between mucosal epithelial cells prevent back-diffusion of hydrogen ions
Factors promoting injury	Acid	Acid is a key issue in pathogenesis of stress-related mucosal injury; however, not all critically ill patients hypersecrete acid; however, small amounts of acid may still cause injury; prevention of acid secretion has led to a reduction in injury
	Pepsin	May cause direct injury to mucosa
	Mucosal hypoperfusion	Reduced mucosal blood flow results in reduced oxygen and nutrient delivery, making epithelial cells susceptible to injury Contributes to mucosal acid-base imbalances Results in formation of free radicals
	Reperfusion injury	Nitric oxide, which causes vasodilation and hyperemia, is released during hypoperfusion and results in an increase in cell-damaging cytokines
	Intramucosal acid-base balance	Mucus layer protects epithelium and traps bicarbonate ions that neutralize acid; thus decrease in bicarbonate secretion results in intramucosal acidosis and local injury
	Systemic acidosis	Results in increased intramucosal acidity
	Free oxygen radicals	Generated as a result of tissue hypoxia, free oxygen radicals cause oxidative injury to mucosa
	Bile salts	Bile salts reflux from duodenum into stomach and may have a role in stress-related damage although exact mechanism is uncertain
	Helicobacter pylori	Conflicting results about role of *Helicobacter pylori* as a cause of stress-induced mucosal disease in critically ill

From References 7, 8, 9, 17, 35, 44, 73, 76, and 78.

BOX 19.3 Risk Factors Associated with the Development of Stress-Related Mucosal Bleeding

- Coagulopathy
- CNS injury/surgery
- Hepatic failure
- Multiple organ dysfunction syndrome
- Mechanical ventilation longer than 48 hours
- Multiple trauma
- Organ transplantation
- Shock
- Severe sepsis
- Severe burns (> 30% of body surface area)
- Renal failure
- History of peptic ulcer disease/upper GI bleed
- Intensive care admission longer than 1 week

CNS, Central nervous system; *GI*, gastrointestinal.
Data from References 13, 35, and 79.

associated with stress-related mucosal disease (48.5% versus 9.1%). Clearly, it is important to identify patients at risk for the development of stress-related mucosal bleeding so appropriate treatment strategies can be initiated as well as ensuring those with low or no risk are not given unnecessary prophylaxis.

STRESS-RELATED MUCOSAL DISEASE: PROPHYLAXIS

When considering the pathophysiology of stress-related mucosal disease, it is clear that GI ischemia contributes to the development of injury. Adequate regional resuscitation plays an important role in preventing this complication of critical illness. Likewise, acid secretion is an important factor, even though many critically ill patients hyposecrete gastric acid.[27] Consequently, therapy is often initiated to maintain the gastric pH greater than 4.0. Medications used in the prophylaxis of stress-related mucosal disease are shown in Table 19.3.

TABLE 19.3 Medications Used to Minimize Stress-Related Mucosal Injury

Medication	Action	Dosage	Special Considerations
Antacids	Weak bases that readily combine with hydrochloric acid, neutralizing it	Aluminum hydroxide magnesium carbonate (Maalox): 10–20 mL PO 3–4 times daily between meals and at bedtime	Aluminum-containing antacids may bind with other drugs (e.g., warfarin, digoxin); not utilized frequently in the intensive care setting
Histamine-2 Receptor Blockers			
Cimetidine (Tagamet)	Inhibits action of histamine at H_2 receptor site located primarily in gastric parietal cells, resulting in inhibition of gastric acid secretion	800 mg PO at bedtime, or 400 mg PO morning and at bedtime, or 300 mg PO 3 times daily and 400 mg PO at bedtime; 300 mg IV every 6–8 h; should not exceed 2400 mg/d	Cimetidine may slow metabolism of other drugs, thereby enhancing their effects
Ranitidine (Zantac)	Inhibits action of histamine at H_2 receptor site located primarily in gastric parietal cells, resulting in inhibition of gastric acid secretion	300 mg PO taken as single dose or 150 mg taken twice daily; 50 mg IV (e.g., 2 mL diluted in 20 mL of 0.9% sodium chloride and given as slow injection over not less than 5 min), may be repeated every 6–8 h; or as IV infusion of 25 mg/h for 2 h; infusion may be repeated at 6–8 h intervals Can give as continuous infusion at 6.25 mg/h	Dosage should be reduced if renal failure is present
Famotidine (Pepcid)	Inhibits action of histamine at H_2 receptor site located primarily in gastric parietal cells, resulting in inhibition of gastric acid secretion	20 mg dose IV over period of no less than 2 min or by infusion of 20 mg over a 30-min period every 12 h	
Proton Pump Inhibitors			
Lansoprazole (Prevacid)	Inhibit production of hydrogen ions in parietal cells, thereby blocking hydrochloric acid secretion	15–30 mg PO daily	
Omeprazole (Prilosec)	Inhibit production of hydrogen ions in parietal cells, thereby blocking hydrochloric acid secretion	20–40 mg PO daily	
Pantoprazole (Protonix)	Inhibit production of hydrogen ions in parietal cells, thereby blocking hydrochloric acid secretion	40 mg PO daily; IV 20–40 mg daily	
Esomeprazole (Nexium)	Inhibit production of hydrogen ions in parietal cells, thereby blocking hydrochloric acid secretion	20–40 mg PO daily 20–40 mg IV daily	
Sucralfate (Carafate)	In presence of acid, sucralfate polymerizes to form thick paste-like substance that adheres to gastric mucosa, protecting it from acid	1 g PO 4 times daily (before meals and bedtime) for up to 8 weeks	Sucralfate needs an acidic environment to work so should not be taken with meals or antacids Use caution in renal impairment due to risk of aluminum accumulation and toxicity Can reduce bioavailability of common medications

IV, Intravenous; *PO*, per os.

Antacids

Antacids directly neutralize gastric acid and have been shown to be effective in reducing significant stress-related bleeding.[60] One of the disadvantages of this therapy is the time-intensive nature of administering antacids every 1 to 2 hours. Furthermore, antacids can contribute to further complications (e.g., aluminum toxicity, hypophosphatemia, diarrhea, or hypermagnesemia). These factors have led to their infrequent use within the critical care setting.

Histamine-2 Receptor Antagonists and Proton Pump Inhibitors

Histamine-2 receptor antagonists (H2RAs) are commonly used in the critically ill to inhibit the production of gastric acid, which is achieved by the medication's binding to the histamine-2 receptor on the basement membrane of the parietal cell.[10] A limitation of histamine-2 receptor antagonists is the development of tolerance that may occur within 72 hours of administration.[35] Nevertheless, this pharmacologic strategy to prevent stress-related mucosal disease remains commonplace in critical care.[1,7,48] Proton pump inhibitors (PPIs) work by irreversibly binding to the proton pump, effectively blocking all three receptors responsible for gastric acid secretion by the parietal cell.[76] Available PPIs include omeprazole (Prilosec), lansoprazole (Prevacid), esomeprazole (Nexium), and pantoprazole (Protonix).

Many recent studies have focused on the use of H2RAs and PPIs in the critical care population due to the widespread use of these medications. The Surviving Sepsis Campaign guidelines recommend the use of PPIs over H2RAs in patients with severe sepsis or septic shock.[24] Multiple meta-analyses have been published in the past five years regarding the use of H2RAs and PPIs in the critically ill population in an attempt to decide which medication is superior to the other. In 2012, Barkun et al.[7] performed a meta-analysis of 13 studies with 1587 patients from 1993 to 2010 to determine rates of clinically significant upper GI bleeding, nosocomial pneumonia, all-cause mortality, and ICU days. Regardless of the definition of bleeding, Barkun et al.[7] found that prophylactic PPIs significantly decreased the incidence of upper GI bleeding. Both PPIs and H2RAs were found to have no significant association with nosocomial pneumonia, no statistical difference in mortality, and no significant reduction in ICU length of stay.

Alhazzani et al.[1] performed a meta-analysis on 14 randomized trials with a total of 1720 patients. PPIs were associated with lower risk of clinically important bleeding and overt bleeding than H2RAs. There was no statistical difference related to mortality, nosocomial pneumonia, and ICU length of stay. Krag et al.[48] (2014) completed a meta-analysis of 20 trials with 1971 adult ICU patients regarding use of H2RAs and PPIs versus placebo or no prophylaxis. Krag et al.[48] found that H2RAs were superior to PPIs; however, there was a high risk of bias and sparse data when adequately analyzed. Concern has been discussed regarding PPIs and H2RAs and development of nosocomial pneumonia; however, the previously mentioned meta-analyses were unable to identify any association.[1,7,48] New data is emerging related to the use of PPIs and the development of *Clostridium difficile* infection. Buendgens et al.[14] found the use of PPIs as a strong risk factor for the development of *C. difficile* infection in ICU patients due to the altered acid secretion along with the loss of the physiologic barrier to bacterial overgrowth. More research in this area needs to be executed to confirm these findings. Both PPIs and H2RAs are widely used in ICUs for the prevention of stress-related mucosal disease. The risk versus benefit is likely an ongoing debate that will be played out in the literature.

Sucralfate

Sucralfate (Carafate) offers protection against stress-related mucosal disease by providing a protective barrier on the surface gastric epithelium, stimulating mucus and bicarbonate secretion and epithelial renewal, improving mucosal blood flow, and enhancing prostaglandin release.[35] Given orally or via a nasogastric tube, sucralfate is well tolerated, but appears to be less effective than H2RAs in decreasing clinically significant bleeding.[17] Previous reports comparing sucralfate with ranitidine showed a decrease in the development of pneumonia in those patients receiving sucralfate; however, these findings were not supported in a subsequent Level I randomized controlled trial.[17]

Enteral Nutrition

Enteral nutrition has been shown to prevent mucosal ischemia by increasing splanchnic blood flow and increasing intragastric pH; therefore, it is considered a stress ulcer prevention mechanism.[44] Several studies have demonstrated a lower incidence of stress-related bleeding in mechanically ventilated[70] and burn patients,[64] whereas others were unable to show a significant effect on increasing gastric pH.[11] It has been suggested that stress ulcer prevention medications are not necessary when enteral nutrition is tolerated.[59] However, further research is needed before it is considered common practice in critical care.

Critical illness and the associated hypoperfusion can contribute to the development of stress-related mucosal disease. Consequently, monitoring and prophylactic treatment are important in minimizing the clinically important bleeding associated with an increased mortality rate.

Interprofessional Plan of Care

With the exception of providing nutritional support, the primary goal of GI management in the critically ill centers on ensuring adequate GI perfusion and minimizing the physiologic consequences of hypoperfusion, such as the development of stress-related mucosal disease. The interprofessional team must ensure adequacy of resuscitation by assessing BP, MAP, urine output, and neurologic status due to the inherent risk for development of stress-related mucosal disease due to mucosal hypoperfusion. All risk factors for stress-related mucosal disease should be assessed to ensure early prophylactic treatment is instituted, thereby avoiding clinically significant bleeding.

ABDOMINAL COMPARTMENT SYNDROME

Abdominal compartment syndrome (ACS) is recognized frequently in critically ill patients. The torso is considered a single compartment with rigid sides (spine, pelvis, and coastal arches) and partially flexible sides (abdominal wall and diaphragm).[58] When the intra-abdominal pressure (IAP) rises in this closed anatomic space, blood flow may be reduced and tissue viability threatened.[58] When a persistently high IAP is observed, the term *intra-abdominal hypertension* (IAH) is used. The term *ACS* is used to describe a combination of increased intra-abdominal pressure and organ dysfunction.[58]

Due to increasing awareness of this important topic by intensive care specialists, the World Society of the Abdominal Compartment Syndrome (WSACS) was created in 2004 to develop consensus definitions and statements as well as an organized approach to the management of IAH and ACS (Box 19.2).[46] WSACS has updated definitions due to the increasing literature support regarding ACS, as well as agreed upon an abdominal compartment grading system (Table 19.4). IAH is defined as a sustained or repeated elevation in IAP greater than or equal to 12 mm Hg.[46] ACS is a sustained IAP greater than 20 mm Hg associated with a new organ dysfunction or failure.[46] Timely intervention and treatment are necessary; failure to recognize ACS is most often fatal.[58]

ACS is further delineated into classifications of primary, secondary, and recurrent related to the pathology of the disease or specific injury. Primary ACS refers to a disease process or injury occurring in the actual abdominopelvic region that may require early surgical intervention or interventional radiology.[46] Secondary ACS develops due to sepsis, capillary leak, massive fluid resuscitation, or burns; it does not originate from the abdominopelvic region.[25] Secondary ACS is considered an avoidable condition since it most often occurs in relation to the treatment of injury or illness.[58] Recurrent ACS happens after resolution of primary or secondary IAH/ACS. Recurrent ACS is associated with a higher mortality.[58] Consequently, it is imperative that all clinicians be aware of the underlying physiologic changes, assessment, and management in at-risk patients (Table 19.5).

TABLE 19.4 Abdominal Compartment Grading System

Grade	Bladder Pressure (mm Hg)
I	12–15
II	16–20
III	21–25
IV	Greater than 25

From Reference 46.

Etiology

For some time, many clinicians have come to associate the development of ACS with surgical patients; however, it is evident ACS can and does occur in a variety of patient populations.[4] Possible risk factors associated with increased IAH are related to four major crises within the abdominal compartment: diminished abdominal wall compliance, increased intraluminal contents, increased intra-abdominal contents, and capillary leakage/fluid resuscitation. Refer to Box 19.4 to see a complete list of updated risk factors delineated by WSACS in 2013. Independent risk factors for the development of ACS include body mass index (BMI) greater than 30, acidosis with a pH less than 7.20, hypothermia, infusion of greater than 5 L of crystalloid within 24 hours, and transfusion of more than 10 units of packed red blood cells within a 24-hour period.[25]

Pathophysiology

In the spontaneously breathing patient, normal IAP is atmospheric or subatmospheric, but IAPs of 5–7 mm Hg have been noted as well.[58] Increased IAP results from an increase in pressure within the confined anatomic space of the abdominal cavity. Asymptomatic elevations in IAP have been seen in the morbidly obese as well as during pregnancy; therefore, elevation of IAP must always be considered related to the patient's baseline IAP.[58] Clinical data show that increases in IAP result in physiologic changes in vital organ function due to inadequate perfusion and oxygenation.[5] Once perfusion is compromised, a vicious cycle of hypoxia, anaerobic metabolism, edema, decreased capillary flow, and increasing pressure ensues.[5] If left untreated, an elevation in IAP can lead to SIRS or even MODS.[72] IAH may be a key factor in developing MODS due to the prevalence of increased IAP in patients who develop organ

TABLE 19.5 Physiologic Changes Associated with Abdominal Compartment Syndrome

System	Physiologic Effects
Respiratory	Cephalad deviation of diaphragm leads to decreased lung and chest wall compliance Peak inspiratory pressures increase Functional residual volume and lung capacity are reduced, resulting in ventilation/perfusion mismatching Hypoxia and hypercarbia may result, necessitating mechanical ventilation Pulmonary vascular resistance increases Lung edema due to leaky capillaries
Cardiovascular	Inferior vena cava and portal vein compression results in decreased venous return Decreased left ventricular compliance Artificially increased right atrial pressure, pulmonary artery occlusion pressure Decreased cardiac index Elevated systemic vascular resistance from arteriolar vasoconstriction and increased IAP
Renal	Oliguria (IAP 15 – 20 mm Hg); may be the first visible sign of IAH Anuria (IAP > 25 mm Hg) May be a consequence of decreased cardiac output, compression of renal vessels, increased renal vascular resistance, or redistribution of blood flow to renal medulla
Gastrointestinal	Decreased splanchnic perfusion and tissue hypoxia Increased gastrointestinal mucosal acidosis Reduced hepatic blood flow Abnormalities in normal gut mucosal barrier function, which may permit bacterial translocation Decreased abdominal wall blood flow Increased pressure on esophageal varices may result in bleeding
Neurologic	Increased intracranial pressure because of impaired venous return

IAH, Intra-abdominal hypertension; *IAP*, intra-abdominal pressure.
From References 2, 5, 52, and 58.

failure.[5,50] It is critical to remember that due to the abdominal compartment's location within the human body, an elevation in IAP can affect the pathophysiology of all organ systems.[19] A summary of the physiologic changes associated with ACS is provided in Table 19.5.

Because IAP is variable among patients, it has been suggested that abdominal perfusion pressure (APP) be calculated by subtracting IAP from MAP. An APP greater than or equal to 60 mm Hg has been stated as the appropriate target for perfusion end points.[58] It appears that the calculation of APP may be a more clinically useful resuscitation end point and is statistically superior in predicting survival from IAH and ACS than either MAP or IAP; however, further well-designed research is needed in this area.[58]

Measurement of Intra-Abdominal Pressure

Clinical assessment of the abdomen is not a sensitive or accurate technique for detecting increased IAP.[45,46,52] A variety of techniques for measuring IAP are described in the literature, including bladder measurement techniques and manometry.[57] Manometry techniques are rapid and cost-effective; however, they have not been validated and are consequently not used routinely in clinical assessment.[57] Measurement of pressure within the bladder has been validated as closely approximating IAP and has evolved as the gold standard for IAP measurement.[46]

Bladder Measurement of Intra-Abdominal Pressure

The original technique described by Kron et al.[49] involves disrupting the sterile closed urinary drainage system. Under sterile conditions, the indwelling urinary catheter is disconnected and 50 to 100 mL of normal saline solution (NSS) injected. The bladder is then clamped distal to the collection port. A manometer or transducer is connected using a 16-gauge needle for each individual measurement. This technique is time consuming and involves multiple manipulations of a normally closed, sterile system.

Refinements of this technique have been implemented to simplify the procedure, limit the number of manipulations, and maintain the closed sterile urinary catheter system. The revised closed system utilizes equipment easily obtainable in the critical care environment although commercially prepared kits designed for IAP measurement are also available. A standard pressure transducer system (pressure tubing, a flush device, transducer, and two stopcocks) with a 500-mL or 1000-mL intravenous bag of NSS is necessary, as well as a 25-mL Luer-Lock syringe.[56] Bladder pressure measurement is always performed at end expiration while the patient is in the supine position with the transducer zeroed at the level of the mid axillary line at the iliac crest.[58] The urinary bladder must be completely emptied prior to the measurement, followed by clamping the bladder drainage system just distal to the catheter and connection of the drainage bag tubing.[56,58] The pressure monitoring system is connected to the sampling port on the urinary drainage system after being cleansed with a chlorhexidine swab. The syringe is connected to the stopcock of the pressure system and filled with 25 mL of NSS, which is the standard amount of fluid utilized to measure bladder pressure due to higher amounts possibly causing an elevated result.[46] After instillation of the 25 mL of NSS into the bladder, the pressure is read via the monitor at end expiration. Once a reliable reading has been obtained, the catheter drainage system is unclamped, and the 25 mL is allowed to drain. WSACS recommends bladder pressure measurements be performed when one risk factor for IAH/ACS is present.[46] These measurements should be performed every 4 to 6 hours until the risk factors are resolved or the increased IAP has returned to normal for 24 to 48 hours (Fig. 19.3).[58]

BOX 19.4 Risk Factors Associated with Abdominal Compartment Syndrome

Primary	Secondary
Abdominal trauma	Ischemia/reperfusion injury
Abdominal aortic aneurysm rupture/ abdominal aortic cross clamp	Septic shock
Intestinal obstruction or ileus	Major burns
Severe constipation	Always associated with shock and massive resuscitation, regardless of etiology
Major abdominal surgery	
Abdominal sepsis	
Large abdominal tumors	
Pancreatitis	
Liver dysfunction/cirrhosis/ascites/ transplantation	
Need for mechanical ventilation with PEEP greater than 10 cm H_2O	
Pneumonia	
Age	
BMI	

BMI, Body mass index; *PEEP,* positive end-expiratory pressure.
From References 5, 46, and 58.

Management of Abdominal Compartment Syndrome

Surveillance for IAH and ACS requires close observation of the patient to identify potential risk factors and relevant changes to physiologic parameters. For those patients who are at risk, close monitoring of IAP is required and preemptive measures instituted. Decompressive laparotomy (DL) is the definitive treatment for severe ACS due to the resulting immediate decrease in IAP and improvements in organ function once DL is performed.[46] However, DL is associated with multiple complications and the mortality rate is as high as 50%.[46] Therefore, recommendations have been made regarding appropriate management of increasing IAP in an effort to decrease the need for DL. These suggestions include appropriate sedation and analgesia, neuromuscular blockade, nasogastric/colonic decompression, body positioning, promotility agents, such as neostigmine, and fluid resuscitation protocols. Although most of this is standard care of the critically ill patient, it deserves mention as a less invasive treatment option.[46] When all medical interventions fail to decrease IAP, and ACS continues, DL is the necessary treatment.

Abdominal Decompression

Clinicians assess the patient for signs of physiologic deterioration (e.g., oliguria, hypotension, and acidosis) along with an IAP in excess of 25 mm Hg and use these clinical assessment findings to determine the optimal timing for abdominal decompression.[58] Early decompression has been associated with reversal of abnormal function (e.g., improvement in peak airway pressures, cardiac output, and urinary output). Unfortunately, despite these dramatic improvements in physiologic function, a 50% mortality rate may remain in patients who undergo abdominal decompression.[58]

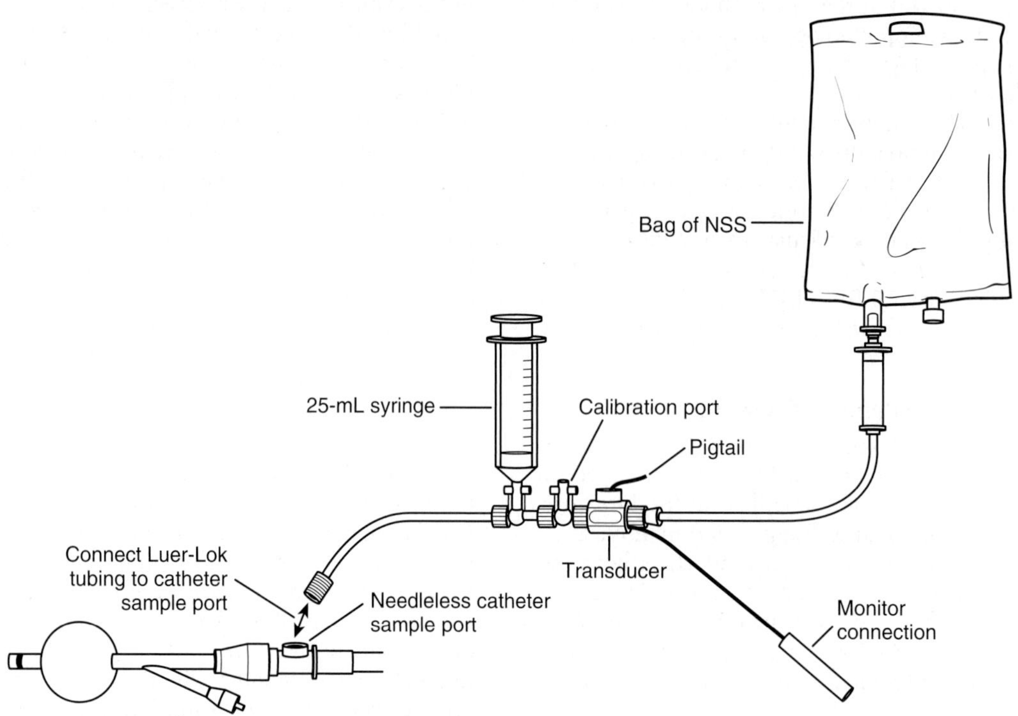

FIG. 19.3 The closed-system single-measurement technique. *NSS,* Normal saline solution.

Temporary Abdominal Closure

In surgical patients at risk of developing IAH, primary fascial closure may result in tamponade, IAH, and recurrent ACS. For this reason, a number of alternatives to primary fascial closure have been investigated. General principles of this strategy include providing a tension-free and watertight coverage of the abdominal contents to prevent fluid loss and evisceration.[25] Delayed closure of the abdomen presents a number of challenges for the clinician, including mechanical containment of the abdominal contents, removal of exudate, the measurement of third-space fluid losses, and infection control. Other challenges include protein loss and malnutrition concerns, as well as the development of enteroatmospheric fistulas and incisional hernias.[25]

Prosthetic mesh. Temporary closure of the abdomen can be achieved in a variety of ways. Nonabsorbable prosthetic mesh may be used. Prosthetic mesh allows the wound to granulate and reduce in size. The fascia is allowed to approximate at a gradual rate as bowel edema subsides. However, the use of mesh closure is associated with an increased rate of enterocutaneous fistula formation.[25]

The Bogota bag. The Bogota bag, constructed from a sterilized 3-L genitourinary irrigation bag, is another alternative method of temporary closure and protection of the abdominal contents. The use of this bag provides a transparent, watertight seal, allowing the underlying bowel to be regularly assessed.[25] Limitations of this device include trauma to the abdominal wall when securing the bag and the inability to actively remove exudate. Although this is still utilized in some areas due to being readily available and cheap, most US trauma centers have abandoned this technique because of the development of new and more effective treatments for the open abdomen.[25]

The Wittmann patch. The Wittmann patch is an artificial burr closure of the abdomen and uses a Velcro-like device to reduce the gap between the wound edges. The device is sutured to the free fascial edges, allowing two prosthetic sheets to be joined along the midline, achieving wound closure.[25] Like the Bogota bag, this technique exposes the fascial edges to further trauma. The Wittmann patch does not allow for effective drainage of intra-abdominal infected fluid, which is contraindicated in sepsis.[25]

Topical negative pressure. Topical negative pressure is a newer technique that avoids trauma to the fascia or skin. This technique is described in Fig. 19.4. The use of topical negative pressure allows for multiple procedures; control of exudate, and a decrease in intra-abdominal pressure; minimizes fascial trauma; and reduces the frequency of dressing changes.[25] The negative pressure created by this device is useful in reducing IAP by decreasing edema and facilitating evacuation of intra-abdominal fluid. Roberts et al.[74] performed a systematic comparative review of 11 studies with a total of 1018 patients to determine if negative pressure wound therapy (NPWT) was superior to alternative types of temporary abdominal closure methods. Roberts et al.[74] found NPWT may be associated with improved patient-centered outcomes, such as in-hospital mortality, fascial closure rate, and hospital and ICU length of stay. Whichever technique is used to manage the open abdomen, the key issues in patient management include infection control, fluid balance, and minimization of iatrogenic tissue injury.

Many critically ill patients are at risk for the development of increased IAP and ACS. The increase in mortality associated with the development of ACS warrants close monitoring of IAP, particularly in at-risk patients, so that early intervention can be instituted and complications associated with ACS minimized.

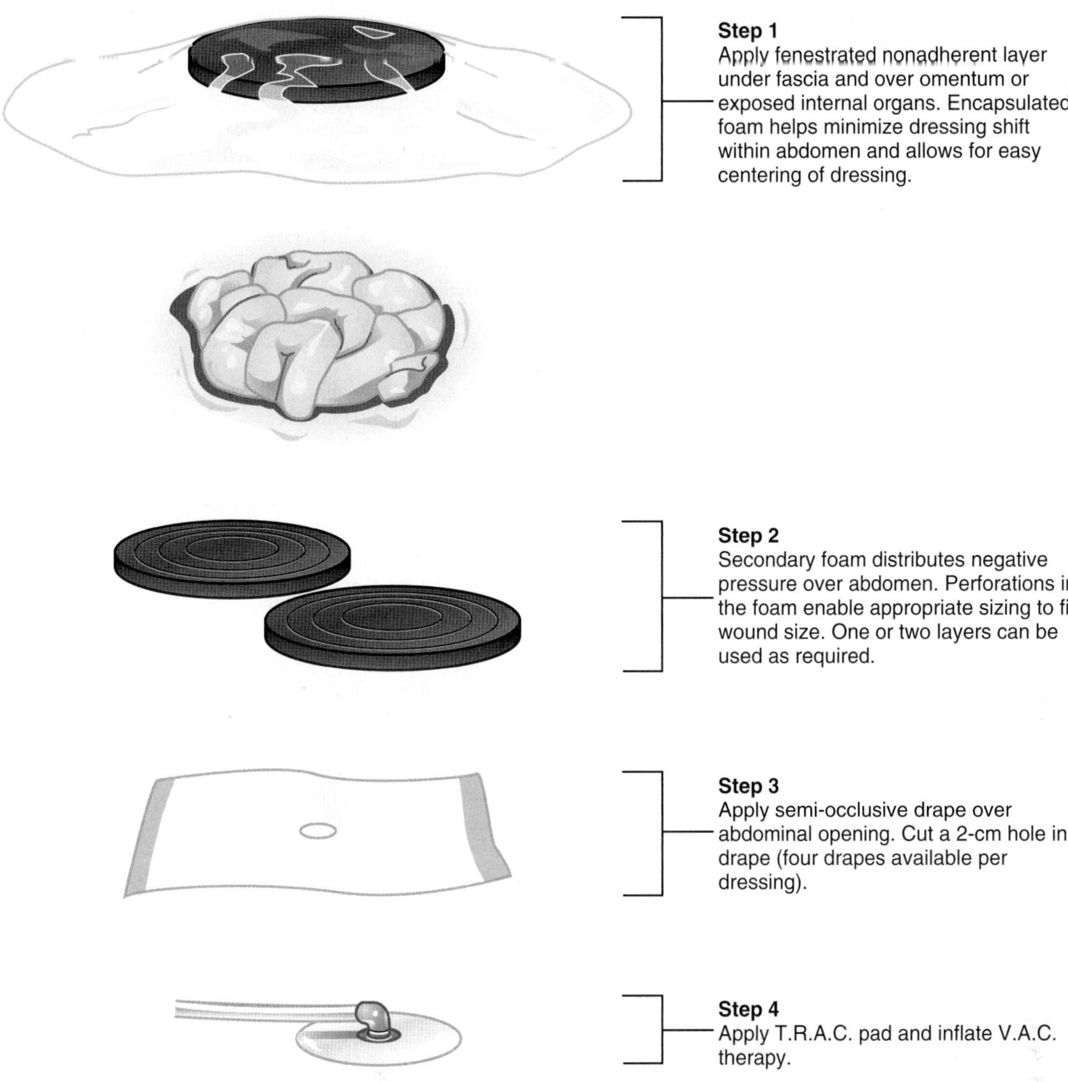

Step 1
Apply fenestrated nonadherent layer under fascia and over omentum or exposed internal organs. Encapsulated foam helps minimize dressing shift within abdomen and allows for easy centering of dressing.
Step 2
Secondary foam distributes negative pressure over abdomen. Perforations in the foam enable appropriate sizing to fit wound size. One or two layers can be used as required.
Step 3
Apply semi-occlusive drape over abdominal opening. Cut a 2-cm hole in drape (four drapes available per dressing).
Step 4
Apply T.R.A.C. pad and inflate V.A.C. therapy.

FIG. 19.4 Applying topical negative pressure using the vacuum-assisted closure abdominal dressing system.

CONCLUSION

Critically ill patients at risk for increased intra-abdominal pressure will benefit from monitoring, and in some cases abdominal decompression may be warranted. Patients should be monitored for elevated IAP based on present risk factors. The identification of persistently increased IAP will result in timely treatment and prevention of further complications. If abdominal decompression is required, the interprofessional team should visually monitor the bowel and assess for changes in perfusion if possible to allow for early identification of compromised blood flow to the gut.

REFERENCES

1. Alhazzani, W., Alenezi, F., Jaeschke, R. Z., Moayyedi, P., & Cook, D. J. (2013). Proton pump inhibitors versus histamine 2 receptor antagonists for stress ulcer prophylaxis in critically ill patients: a systematic review and meta-analysis. *Crit Care Med*, *41*(3), 693–705. http://doi.org/10.1097/CCM.0b013e3182758734.
2. Ameloot, K., Gillebert, C., Desie, N., & Malbrain, M. L. N. G. (2012). Hypoperfusion, shock states, and abdominal compartment syndrome (ACS). *Surg Clin North Am*, *92*(2), 207–220. http://doi.org/10.1016/j.suc.2012.01.009.
3. Antonsson, J. B., et al. (1995). Changes in gut intramucosal pH and gut oxygen extraction ratio in a porcine model of peritonitis and hemorrhage. *Crit Care Med*, *23*(11), 1872–1881.
4. Atema, J. J., van Buijtenen, J. M., Lamme, B., & Boermeester, M. A. (2014). Clinical studies on intra-abdominal hypertension and abdominal compartment syndrome. *J Trauma Acute Care Surg*, *76*(1), 234–240. http://doi.org/10.1097/TA.0b013e3182a85f59.
5. Balogh, Z. J., & Butcher, N. E. (2010). Compartment syndromes from head to toe. *Crit Care Med*, *38*(Suppl. 9), S445–S451. http://doi.org/10.1097/CCM.0b013e3181ec5d09.
6. Bardou, M., & Barkun, A. N. (2013). Stress ulcer prophylaxis in the ICU: who, when, and how? *Crit Care Med*, *41*(3), 906–907. http://doi.org/10.1097/CCM.0b013e31827c02a4.
7. Barkun, A. N., Bardou, M., Pham, C. Q. D., & Martel, M. (2012). Proton pump inhibitors vs. histamine 2 receptor antagonists for stress-related mucosal bleeding prophylaxis in critically ill patients: a meta-analysis. *Am J Gastroenterol*, *107*(4), 507–521. http://doi.org/10.1038/ajg.2011.474.
8. Beltran, N. E., Ceron, U., Sanchez-Miranda, G., et al. (2012). Incidence of gastric mucosal injury as measured by reactance in critically ill patients. *J Intensive Care Med*, *28*(4), 230–236. http://doi.org/10.1177/0885066612450415.
9. Beltran, N. E., & Sacristan, E. (2015). Gastrointestinal ischemia monitoring through impedance spectroscopy as a tool for the management of the critically ill. *Exp Biol Med*, 1–11. http://doi.org/10.1177/1535370215571876.
10. Bersten, A., & Soni, N. (2009). *Oh's intensive care manual* (6th ed.). Philadelphia, PA: Butterworth-Heinemann Elsevier.

11. Bonten, M. J. M., et al. (1996). Intermittent enteral feeding: the influence on respiratory and digestive tract colonization in mechanically ventilated intensive-care-unit patients. *Am J Resp Crit Care Med, 154*, 394–399.
12. Boyd, O., et al. (1993). Comparison of clinical information gained from routine blood-gas analysis and from gastric tonometry for intramural pH. *Lancet, 341*, 142–145.
13. Brophy, G. M., Brackbill, M. L., Bidwell, K. L., & Brophy, D. F. (2010). Prospective, randomized comparison of lansoprazole suspension, and intermittent intravenous famotidine on gastric ph and acid production in critically ill neurosurgical patients. *Neurocrit Care, 13*(2), 176–181. http://doi.org/10.1007/s12028-010-9397-3.
14. Buendgens, L., Bruensing, J., Matthes, M., et al. (2014). Administration of proton pump inhibitors in critically ill medical patients is associated with increased risk of developing Clostridium difficile-associated diarrhea. *J Crit Care, 29*(4), 696.e11–696.e15. http://doi.org/10.1016/j.jcrc.2014.03.002.
15. Calvet, X., et al. (1995). Effect of ranitidine in gastric intramucosal pH determinations in critically ill patients. *Am J Resp Crit Care Med, 151*(4), A334.
16. Chapman, M. J., & Deane, A. M. (2015). Gastrointestinal dysfunction relating to the provision of nutrition in the critically ill. *Curr Opin Clin Nutr Metab Care, 18*(2), 207–212. http://doi.org/10.1097/MCO.0000000000000149.
17. Cook, D., et al. (1998). A comparison of sucralfate and ranitidine for the prevention of upper gastrointestinal bleeding in patients requiring mechanical ventilation. *N Engl J Med, 338*, 791–797.
18. Cook, D. J., Fuller, H. D., & Guyatt, G. H. (1994). Risk factors for gastrointestinal bleeding in critically ill patients. *N Engl J Med, 330*, 377–381.
19. Correa-Martín, L., Castellanos, G., García-Lindo, M., Díaz-Güemes, I., & Sánchez-Margallo, F. M. (2013). Tonometry as a predictor of inadequate splanchnic perfusion in an intra-abdominal hypertension animal model. *J Surg Res, 184*(2), 1028–1034. http://doi.org/10.1016/j.jss.2013.04.041.
20. Cruz, R. J., Garrido, A. G., De Natale Caly, D., & Rocha-E-Silva, M. (2011). Hepatosplanchnic vasoregulation and oxygen consumption during selective aortic blood flow reduction and reperfusion. *J Surg Res, 171*(2), 532–539. http://doi.org/10.1016/j.jss.2010.05.037.
21. Cushing, H. (1932). Peptic ulcers and the interbrain. *Surg Gynecol Obstet, 55*, 1–34.
22. Czaja, A. J., McAlhany, J. C., & Pruitt, B.-A. J. (1974). Acute gastroduodenal disease after thermal injury. An endoscopic evaluation of incidence and natural history. *N Engl J Med, 291*, 925–929.
23. Dark, D. S., & Pingleton, S. K. (1993). Nutrition and nutritional support in critically ill patients. *J Intensive Care Med, 8*, 16–33.
24. Dellinger, R. P., Levy, M. M., Rhodes, A., et al. (2013). Surviving sepsis campaign: international guidelines for management of severe sepsis and septic shock, 2012. *Intensive Care Med, 39*(2), 165–228. http://doi.org/10.1007/s00134-012-2769-8.
25. Demetriades, D., & Salim, A. (2014). Management of the open abdomen. *Surg Clin North Am, 94*(1), 131–153. http://doi.org/10.1016/j.suc.2013.10.010.
26. DeSouza, R. L., et al. (2001). Assessment of splanchnic perfusion with gastric tonometry in the immediate postoperative period of cardiac surgery in children. *Arq Bras Cardiol, 77*(6), 509–519.
27. Fennerty, M. B. (2002). Pathophysiology of the upper gastrointestinal tract in the critically ill patient: rationale of the therapeutic benefits of acid suppression. *Crit Care Med, 30*(Suppl. 6), S351–S355.
28. Fennerty, M. B. (2004). Rationale for the therapeutic benefits of acid-suppression therapy in the critically ill patient. *Medscape Gastroenterol, 6*(3).
29. Fiddian-Green, R. G. (1993). Associations between intramucosal acidosis in the gut and organ failure. *Crit Care Med, 21*(2), S103–S107.
30. Flock, M. H., et al. (1972). The effect of bile acids on intestinal microflora. *Am J Clin Nutr, 25*, 1418–1426.
31. Frandah, W., Colmer-Hamood, J., Nugent, K., & Raj, R. (2012). Patterns of use of prophylaxis for stress-related mucosal disease in patients admitted to the intensive care unit. *J Intensive Care Med, 29*(2), 96–103. http://doi.org/10.1177/0885066612453542.
32. Fuhrmann, V., Kneidinger, N., Herkner, H., et al. (2011). Impact of hypoxic hepatitis on mortality in the intensive care unit. *Intensive Care Med, 37*(8), 1302–1310. http://doi.org/10.1007/s00134-011-2248-7.
33. Gabrielli, A., Layon, A. J., & Yu, M. (2012). *Civetta, Taylor, & Kirby's manual of critical care (electronic resource)*. Philadelphia: Wolters Kluwer Health/Lippincott Williams & Wilkins.
34. Gomersall, C. D. E., et al. (2000). Resuscitation of critically ill patients based on the results of gastric tonometry. *Crit Care Med, 28*, 607–614.
35. Goodwin, C. M., & Hoffman, J. A. (2011). Deep vein thrombosis and stress ulcer prophylaxis in the intensive care unit. *J Pharm Pract, 24*(1), 78–88. http://doi.org/10.1177/0897190010393851.
36. Groeneveld, A. B. J. (1996). Gastrointestinal exocrine failure in critical illness. In J. L. Rombeau, & J. Takala (Eds.), *Gut dysfunction in critical illness*. Berlin: Springer.
37. Haglund, U. (1993). Intestinal mucosal blood flow and oxygenation in sepsis. *Br J Intensive Care*, 49–54.
38. Haglund, U. (1994). Gut ischaemia. *Gut* (Suppl. 1), S73–S76.
39. Hajela, N., Ramakrishna, B. S., Nair, G. B., Abraham, P., Gopalan, S., & Ganguly, N. K. (2015). Gut microbiome, gut function, and probiotics: implications for health. *Indian J Gastroenterol, 34*, 93–107. http://doi.org/10.1007/s12664-015-0547-6.
40. Heard, S. O. (2003). Gastric tonometry: the hemodynamic monitor of choice (Pro). *Chest, 123*(Suppl. 5), 469S–474S.
41. Higgins, D., Mythen, M. G., & Webb, A. R. (1994). Low intramucosal pH is associated with failure to acidify the gastric lumen in response to pentagastrin. *Intensive Care Med, 20*, 105–108.
42. Hinds, C. J., & Watson, D. (2008). *Intensive care, a concise textbook* (3rd ed.). Philadelphia, PA: Elsevier Saunders.
43. Horvatits, T., Trauner, M., & Fuhrmann, V. (2013). Hypoxic liver injury and cholestasis in critically ill patients. *Curr Opin Crit Care, 19*(2), 128–132. http://doi.org/10.1097/MCC.0b013e32835ec9e6.
44. Hurt, R. T., Frazier, T. H., McClave, S. A., et al. (2012). Stress prophylaxis in intensive care unit patients and the role of enteral nutrition. *JPEN J Parenter Enteral Nutr, 36*(6), 721–731. http://doi.org/10.1177/0148607112436978.
45. Katsios, C., Ye, C., Hoad, N., Piraino, T., Soth, M., & Cook, D. (2013). Intra-abdominal hypertension in the critically ill: interrater reliability of bladder pressure measurement. *J Crit Care, 28*(5), 886.e1–886.e6. http://doi.org/10.1016/j.jcrc.2013.04.003.
46. Kirkpatrick, A. W., Roberts, D. J., De Waele, J., et al. (2013). Intra-abdominal hypertension and the abdominal compartment syndrome: updated consensus definitions and clinical practice guidelines from the World Society of the Abdominal Compartment Syndrome. *Intensive Care Med, 39*(7), 1190–1206. http://doi.org/10.1007/s00134-013-2906-z.
47. Koivisto, T., et al. (2001). Gastric tonometry after subarachnoid haemorrhage. *Intensive Care Med, 27*(10), 1614–1621.
48. Krag, M., Perner, A., Wetterslev, J., Wise, M. P., & Hylander Møller, M. (2014). Stress ulcer prophylaxis versus placebo or no prophylaxis in critically ill patients: a systematic review of randomised clinical trials with meta-analysis and trial sequential analysis. *Intensive Care Med, 40*(1), 11–22. http://doi.org/10.1007/s00134-013-3125-3.
49. Kron, I. L., Harman, P. K., & Nolan, S. P. (1984). The measurement of intra-abdominal pressure as a criterion for abdominal re-exploration. *Ann Surg, 199*, 28–30.
50. Kyoung, K.H., & Hong, S.K. (2015). The duration of intra-abdominal hypertension strongly predicts outcomes for the critically ill surgical patients: a prospective observational study. *World J Emerg Surg, 10*(1), 22. http://doi.org/10.1186/s13017-015-0016-7.
51. Lash O'Neill, P. (1996). Gastrointestinal system: target organ and source of multiple organ dysfunction syndrome. In V. Huddleston Secor (Ed.), *Multiple organ dysfunction and failure: pathophysiology and clinical implications*. St Louis: Mosby.
52. Lee, R. K. (2012). Intra-abdominal hypertension and abdominal compartment syndrome a comprehensive overview. *Crit Care Nurse, 32*(1), 19–31. http://doi.org/10.4037/ccn2012662.
53. Li, X., Hammer, A. M., Rendon, J. L., & Choudhry, M. a. (2015). Intestine Immune Homeostasis after Alcohol and Burn Injury. *Shock, 43*(6), 1. http://doi.org/10.1097/SHK.0000000000000353.
54. Lin, P.C., Chang, C.H., Hsu, P.I., Tseng, P.L., & Huang, Y.B. (2010). The efficacy and safety of proton pump inhibitors vs histamine-2 receptor antagonists for stress ulcer bleeding prophylaxis among critical care patients: a meta-analysis. *Crit Care Med, 38*(4), 1197–1205. http://doi.org/10.1097/CCM.0b013e3181d69ccf.

55. Lord, L. M., & Sax, H. C. (1994). The role of the gut in critical illness. *AACN Clin Issues, 5*(4), 450–458.
56. Lynn-McHale Weigand, D. (2011). *AACN procedure manual for critical care* (6th ed.). St Louis: Elsevier Saunders.
57. Malbrain, M. L. N. G. (2004). Different techniques to measure intra-abdominal pressure (IAP): time for critical re-appraisal. *Intensive Care Med, 30*, 357–371.
58. Malbrain, M. L. N. G., De Laet, I. E., De Waele, J. J., & Kirkpatrick, A. W. (2013). Intra-abdominal hypertension: definitions, monitoring, interpretation and management. *Best Pract Res Clin Anaesthesio, 27*(2), 249–270. http://doi.org/10.1016/j.bpa.2013.06.009.
59. Marik, P. E., Vasu, T., Hirani, A., & Pachinburavan, M. (2010). Stress ulcer prophylaxis in the new millennium: a systematic review and meta-analysis. *Crit Care Med, 38*(11), 2222–2228. http://doi.org/10.1097/CCM.0b013e3181f17adf.
60. Marini, J. J., & Wheeler, A. P. (2010). *Critical care medicine: the essentials* (4th ed.). Philadelphia: Wolters Kluwer Lippincott Williams & Wilkins.
61. Marshall, A. P., & West, S. H. (2004). Gastric tonometry and monitoring gastrointestinal perfusion: using research to support nursing practice. *Nurs Crit Care, 9*(3), 123–133.
62. Maynard, N. D. (1993). *Splanchnic ischaemia in the critically ill*. London: London University Press.
63. McVay, L. D. (1996). Immunology of the gut. In J. L. Rombeau, & J. Takala (Eds.), *Gut dysfunction in critical illness*. Berlin: Springer.
64. Moscona, R., et al. (1985). Prevention of gastrointestinal bleeding in burns: the effects of cimetidine or antacids combined with early enteral feeding. *Burns Incl Therm Inj, 12*, 65–67.
65. Mythen, M. G. (2015). Does gastric tonometry-guided therapy reduce total mortality in critically ill patients? *Crit Care, 19*, 172.
66. Öz, B., Akyüz, M., Emek, E., et al. (2015). The effectiveness of gastric tonometry in the diagnosis of acute mesenteric ischemia in cases where a contrast-enhanced computed tomography cannot be obtained. *Ulus Cerrahi Derg, 31*(1), 26–29. http://doi.org/10.5152/UCD.2014.2725.
67. Palizas, F., Dubin, A., Regueira, T., et al. (2009). Gastric tonometry versus cardiac index as resuscitation goals in septic shock: a multicenter, randomized, controlled trial. *Crit Care, 13*(2), R44. http://doi.org/10.1186/cc7767.
68. Peura, D. A., & Johnson, L. F. (1985). Cimetidine for prevention and treatment of gastroduodenal mucosal lesions in patients in an intensive care unit. *Ann Intern Med, 103*, 173–177.
69. Phillips, M. C. L. R., & Olson (1993). The immunologic role of the gastrointestinal tract. *Crit Care Nurs Clin North Am, 5*(1), 107–120.
70. Pingleton, S., & Hadzima, S. K. (1983). Enteral alimentation and gastrointestinal bleeding in mechanically ventilated patients. *Crit Care Med, 11*(1), 13–16.
71. Piton, G., Manzon, C., Cypriani, B., Carbonnel, F., & Capellier, G. (2011). Acute intestinal failure in critically ill patients: is plasma citrulline the right marker? *Intensive Care Med, 37*(6), 911–917. http://doi.org/10.1007/s00134-011-2172-x.
72. Puleo, F., Arvanitakis, M., Van Gossum, A., & Preiser, J. C. (2011). Gut failure in the ICU. *Semin Respir Crit Care Med, 32*(5), 626–638. http://doi.org/10.1055/s-0031-1287871.
73. Quenot, J.P., Thiery, N., & Barbar, S. (2009). When should stress ulcer prophylaxis be used in the ICU? *Curr Opin Crit Care, 15*(2), 139–143. http://doi.org/10.1097/MCC.0b013e32832978e0.
74. Roberts, D. J., Zygun, D. A., Grendar, J., et al. (2012). Negative-pressure wound therapy for critically ill adults with open abdominal wounds. *J Trauma Acute Care Surg, 73*(3), 629–639. http://doi.org/10.1097/TA.0b013e31825c130e.
75. Romito, R. A. (1995). Early administration of enteral nutrients in critically ill patients. *AACN Clin Issues, 6*(2), 242–256.
76. Schirmer, C. M., Kornbluth, J., Heilman, C. B., & Bhardwaj, A. (2012). Gastrointestinal prophylaxis in neurocritical care. *Neurocrit Care, 16*(1), 184–193. http://doi.org/10.1007/s12028-011-9580-1.
77. Stannard, V. A., et al. (1988). Gastric exocrine "failure" in critically ill patients: incidence and associated features. *Br Med J, 296*, 155–156.
78. Syam, A. F., Simadibrata, M., Wanandi, S. I., Hernowo, B. S., Sadikin, M., & Rani, A. A. (2011). Gastric ulcers induced by systemic hypoxia. *Acta Med Indones, 43*(4), 243–248.
79. Tasaka, C. L., Burg, C., Vanosdol, S. J., et al. (2014). An interprofessional approach to reducing the overutilization of stress ulcer prophylaxis in adult medical and surgical intensive care units. *Ann Pharmacother, 48*(4), 462–469. http://doi.org/10.1177/1060028013517088.
80. Tortora, G., & Derrickson, B. (2012). *Principles of anatomy & physiology* (13th ed.). Hoboken, NJ: Wiley.
81. Vallet, B., Neviere, R., & Chagnon, J.L. (1996). Gastrointestinal mucosal ischaemia. In J. L. Rombeau, & J. Takala (Eds.). *Gut dysfunction in critical illness*. Berlin: Springer.
82. Zhang, X., Xuan, W., Yin, P., Wang, L., Wu, X., & Wu, Q. (2015). Gastric tonometry guided therapy in critical care patients: a systematic review and meta-analysis. *Crit Care, 19*(1), 22.

20

Liver, Kidney, and Pancreas Transplantation

Patricia Radovich

INTRODUCTION

Currently there are more than 123,000 people awaiting organ transplantation; 101,000 are awaiting a kidney transplant, over 3100 are awaiting a pancreas or kidney-pancreas transplant, and more than 15,000 individuals await liver transplantation. Transplantation has come a long way since the first organ transplant in 1963, and is a dynamic and continually evolving area of practice.[55]

Patients wait from 2 to 4 years for a liver, kidney, or pancreas transplant, unless they are diagnosed with acute liver failure. The current wait for patients with acute liver failure is approximately 7 days.[59] Since 2000, the number of liver and kidney recipients has increased more than 80%.[13] Patients with end-stage disease awaiting transplantation present the clinical challenge of maintaining a patient with multisystem organ dysfunction until transplantation. The process is a complex intermixture of the patient disease, the timing of transplantation, and the quality of organ received. Increasing recipient demand and increases in deaths on the waiting lists have resulted in changes to the organ selection criteria and an increase in the use of expanded or marginal donors.[13] Wait times for organ transplantation are further impacted by the organ, blood type, acuity scores, such as the Model for End Stage Liver Disease (MELD), and the United Network for Organ Sharing (UNOS) region. These factors result in some patients being dual-listed within the UNOS network in hopes of receiving an organ(s) sooner in another region. In the immediate posttransplantation setting, the resumption of organ function and recognition of delayed graft function or ischemia dominate the nursing care of the transplant patient. After the early postoperative hours, the focus of nursing care turns to prevention of complications secondary to pretransplant organ damage and prevention of infection. This includes the regulation of immunosuppression (through trough levels, kidney function, and liver function tests), monitoring the patient for immunosuppression-related toxicities (such as acute kidney injury from calcineurin immunosuppressant use), and drug-drug interactions or allergies due to all the new medications being administered simultaneously.

LIVER TRANSPLANTATION

Liver Recipient Prior to Transplantation

Liver transplantation has become a routine procedure with excellent outcomes.[59] One year survival has improved from 25% in the 1980s to over 83%, with a 5-year survival rate of approximately 80%.[55] Liver recipients before transplantation are usually in the hospital, either in acute care or critical care, although in some circumstances, patients are at home. Patients on the UNOS waiting list for liver transplant receive organs based upon the MELD score, except in the case of acute liver failure. Patients with acute liver failure receive a listing status of 1, the highest listing, due to the estimated life span of less than 72 hours. In patients with chronic liver disease, the MELD score is determined by a logarithmic calculation based on three laboratory values: total bilirubin level, international normalized ratio (INR), and creatinine level.[59] The MELD score has been shown to be an accurate predictor of survival after liver transplantation. A comparison of pretransplant and posttransplantation outcomes has shown that, in patients who undergo liver transplantation due to chronic liver disease, survival is improved only in those with a MELD score of greater than 15 at the time of the transplant.[55,59] Today, patients must have a minimum score of 15 before they can receive a transplant. Some of the reasons for patients' failure to qualify for consideration of a transplant are ongoing destructive behaviors (drug or alcohol abuse), inability to comply with the preoperative or postoperative treatment regimen, severe cardiovascular disease, morbid obesity, pulmonary hypertension, or complete occlusion of the splanchnic venous circulation.[55] The etiology of liver recipients' liver disease is varied, and recipients may suffer from a variety of organ system dysfunctions as a result of their liver failure before transplantation that will carry over into their postoperative course and influence their progress to recovery (Box 20.1).[42]

The recurrence of liver disease after transplantation can be immediate, or can occur after several years, as in the patient with biliary liver disease.[42] Patients awaiting liver transplant may suffer from encephalopathy; as their condition worsens, this alteration in consciousness may progress from personality changes and lethargy to coma, potentially refractory to medical management. In addition, the development of hepatorenal syndrome affects both the fluid balance and the ability to eliminate toxins cleared by the renal system. As liver dysfunction worsens, a systemic problem with coagulopathy occurs, making the patient susceptible to bleeding and therefore at an increased risk of intracranial hemorrhage. The portal hypertension causes engorged veins, which, coupled with increasing INR and decreasing platelets, increases the risk of gastrointestinal (GI) hemorrhage from varices. These complications, together with the severe malnutrition that accompanies liver disease, create a complex patient with neurologic, cardiovascular, pulmonary, GI, gastrourinary, and immune system dysfunction. It is this complex patient who proceeds to the operating room and returns to the critical care unit. Chapter 17 provides a comprehensive overview of liver failure.

Psychologically, patients may have very different perspectives as a result of the diverse etiologies of acute liver failure. Some patients with acute hepatic failure may progress to

BOX 20.1 Etiologies of Liver Disease

Acute
- Drug-induced (acetaminophen, herbal supplements, prescription medication)
- Viral hepatitis (hepatitis A or B)
- Viral hepatitis D in the presence of existing hepatitis B infection and cirrhosis
- Viral hepatitis E in pregnant females
- Autoimmune disease
- Iatrogenic

Cirrhosis
- Alcoholic liver disease
- Autoimmune disease
- Viral hepatitis (hepatitis B and C)
- Biliary atresia
- Primary biliary cirrhosis
- Primary sclerosing cholangitis
- Nonalcoholic fatty liver disease
- Acute on chronic liver disease
- Cryptogenic
- Hepatic veno-occlusive disease (Budd-Chiari syndrome)
- Wilson's disease
- Hemochromatosis
- Glycogen storage disease
- α_1-Antitrypsin deficiency
- Urea cycle defects
- Primary hereditary oxalosis

transplant with an awareness of the changes in their condition, whereas others may find their postoperative course a more difficult experience, for example, if they lapsed into coma before transplantation occurred. Patients with chronic liver failure experience both elation and guilt after transplantation, as they recall their extreme disability before the transplant but also handle the emotional impact that in most cases, someone died for their transplantation.[3,42] Many transplant programs have transplant psychiatrists and counselors on staff to assist with patients' posttransplant recovery.

Types of Liver Donors

In the past, liver transplantation was only performed using organs from donors after brain death. With the increase in individuals awaiting liver transplantation and the rising number of deaths while waiting, today's liver transplants may come from two additional sources: living donors (partial liver transplant) and organs recovered after the donor experiences cardiac death. Organ donation after the determination of brain death remains the most common method of donation.[13]

Living liver donation was initially developed for pediatric recipients, but is now offered in most adult liver transplant programs. The Adult-to-Adult Living Donor Liver Transplantation Cohort Study (A2ALL) identified risk factors for mortality after living donor liver transplant (LDLT). Medical records of transplant recipients who had a living and deceased donor were evaluated at the nine A2ALL centers between 1998 and 2003. There were more complications leading to retransplantation or death after LDLT versus Deceased Donor Liver Transplant (DDLT) (15.9% vs. 9.3%, $p = 0.023$). Complication rates were higher after LDLT versus DDLT, but declined with center experience to levels comparable to DDLT.[18] In 2011, Olthoff et al. examined the US national experience and defined risk factors for patient mortality and graft loss in LDLT.[43] LDLT procedures at nine A2ALL centers ($n = 702$) and 67 non-A2ALL centers ($n = 1664$) from January 1998 through December 2007 again found that center experience was a significant factor in graft outcome. However, researchers did not find any significant difference in overall mortality between A2ALL and non-A2ALL centers. Except for center experience, risk factor effects between A2ALL and non-A2ALL centers were not significantly different. Mortality and graft loss risk factors were similar in A2ALL and non-A2ALL centers.[18,43] A recipient's MELD score must be greater than 12 but less than 25 to receive an LDLT. This procedure is considered a low-risk operation in the pediatric population, and is a more complex procedure in the adult population. In some cases, the donor is more susceptible to complications than the recipient, because the donor is losing 60% of a functioning liver, whereas the recipient is gaining 60% of a fully functional liver in place of a dysfunctional liver. Ideally, a donor larger than the recipient is sought so less liver volume can be taken from the donor.[42,54] Partial liver transplantation is considered by some to be an underutilized resource, given the increasing demand for transplantation.[54] The recipient of a partial liver transplant may have postoperative complications that are different than those experienced by a patient who has received a whole organ, due to the arterial anastomosis, biliary anastomosis, and, in some cases, hepatic vein reconstruction required. Additionally, the recipient is receiving a liver that is less than 100% in volume and must be in a condition where the volume of liver received will support the patient's needs. Patients receiving a whole organ may be considerably more ill at the time of surgery, because of progressive liver dysfunction and the severity of their disease process (Fig. 20.1).[13,54]

The deceased donor process can involve the use of a whole organ or a split liver. In a split liver transplant, the donated organ is divided into two grafts. One portion of the split liver (usually the left lobe) goes to a child, and the right lobe goes to an adult; however, it is also possible a small adult may benefit from a left lobe procedure.[13] The whole-organ donation provides an entire liver to a patient awaiting liver transplantation. Those receiving a whole organ are more severely ill (i.e., have a high MELD score), and often have decompensated disease and multisystem dysfunction. Upon arrival in the critical care unit, these patients can present a challenge to the critical care nurse. The transplant team, including the surgeon, social workers, psychiatrists, and the family, determine which procedure is best for the recipient by using the MELD score along with the patient's anatomic structure (Fig. 20.2).

Preoperative Care

Preoperative care is focused on keeping the patient as healthy as possible. The hospitalized liver failure patient may be malnourished require close neurologic observation for progressive encephalopathy and coagulopathies. These patients may require mechanical ventilation, monitoring and correction of fluid and electrolyte imbalances due to progressive renal dysfunction, and advanced neurologic monitoring, including placement of a subarachnoid screw or bolt. Patients are at increased risk for the development of infections with prolonged hospitalization; therefore, impeccable aseptic technique is critical.[6,8,40]

Postoperative Considerations

Individual variability characterizes the immediate postoperative care of the liver recipient. In many units, the length of

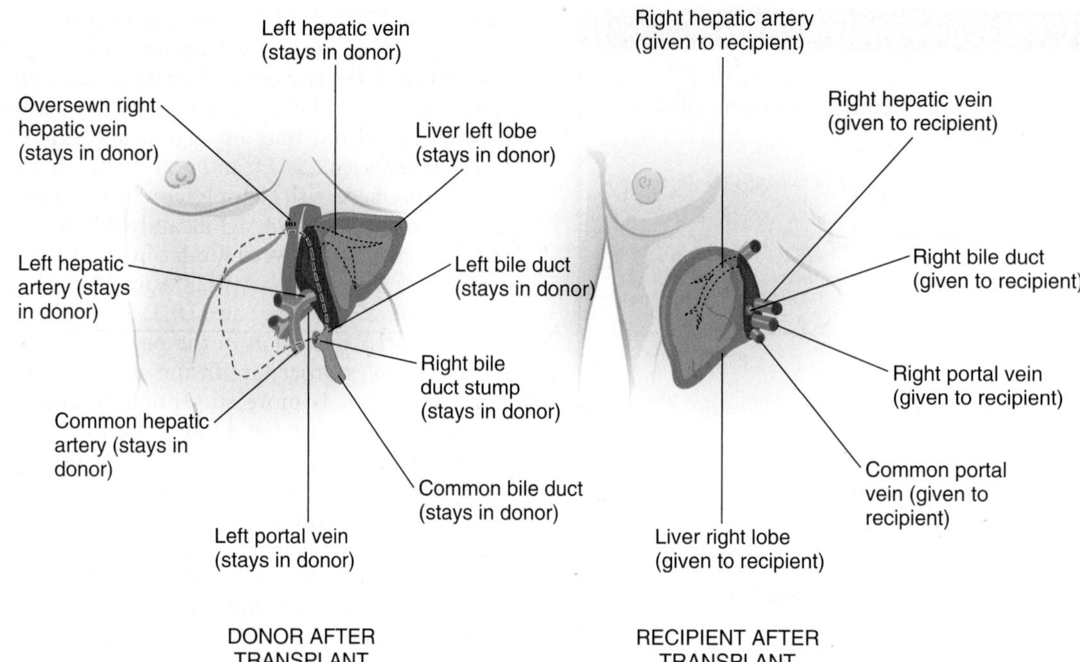

FIG. 20.1 Liver transplantation—portion taken from donor and portion transplanted to recipient.

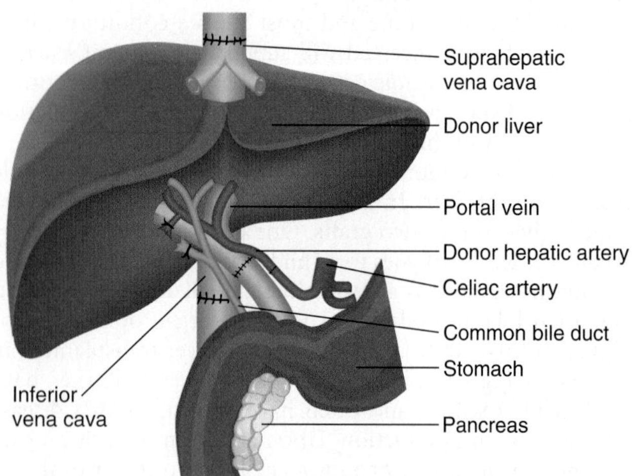

FIG. 20.2 Suture lines following liver transplantation.

stay in the intensive care unit (ICU) is less than 24 hours.[40,48] Some patients may have a more difficult course, with prolonged surgery times and multiple transfusions. These circumstances may lead to prolonged stay in critical or acute care, transfer to rehabilitation, close outpatient supervision, or frequent readmissions for complications.[48,52] Although there have been numerous improvements in the preoperative workup, surgical techniques, and intraoperative care, liver transplantation remains an arduous surgery. Depending upon the facility, patients may be transferred from the operating room to the postanesthesia care unit (PACU) for recovery and extubation, or may be transferred directly to the surgical intensive care or designated transplant unit for recovery and postoperative care.[6]

Mayo Clinic has published on the use of "fast-tracking" of the liver transplant patient. In a fast-track program, the patient is extubated early, recovers from anesthesia in the PACU, and is then transferred to the acute care unit. The attending surgeon and the anesthesiologist determine the disposition of each patient. Bulatao et al. examined fast-tracked patients from 2003 to 2010 in order to develop a reliable method of determining which patients were suitable for fast-tracking.[6] Of 1296 liver transplant recipients included in the study, 704 (54.3%) were successfully fast-tracked, and 592 (45.7%) were directly admitted to the ICU after transplantation. Using nine variables, the researchers created a scoring system that classified patients according to the likelihood of being successfully fast-tracked to the acute care surgical unit. The variables included: age, BMI, male gender, MELD score, pretransplant length of stay, number of previous transplants, volume of packed cells transfused, operative time, and use of vasopressors during the last hour of surgery. The recipient's preoperative cardiopulmonary function, previous upper abdominal surgical operations, and any history of significant levels of encephalopathy were also considered. The scoring system was validated in an independent group of 372 liver transplant recipients.[6] The study findings are limited, due to the inability to randomize patients, the inability to control for potential clinical factors affecting the postoperative outcomes, and the fact that they represent the experience of a single large-volume center. The potential for the use of a framework to enhance patient flow, such as that described in this study, is an area for more research, as it may provide an innovative, cost-effective, efficient, high-quality method of delivering individualized care in the postoperative setting.

The postoperative patient arriving in critical care will have a pulmonary artery catheter (PAC) and an arterial line, and may often have another central venous access or dialysis catheter on the opposite side from the PAC. Additionally, the patient will have abdominal drains, a nasogastric tube, a Foley catheter, and possibly a T-tube. Upon arrival to the unit, the clinical status must be assessed with vital signs, urine output, drain output, arterial blood gas, and laboratory testing including a comprehensive metabolic panel, lactate, complete blood count, prothrombin time (PT), and INR. Admission assessment includes

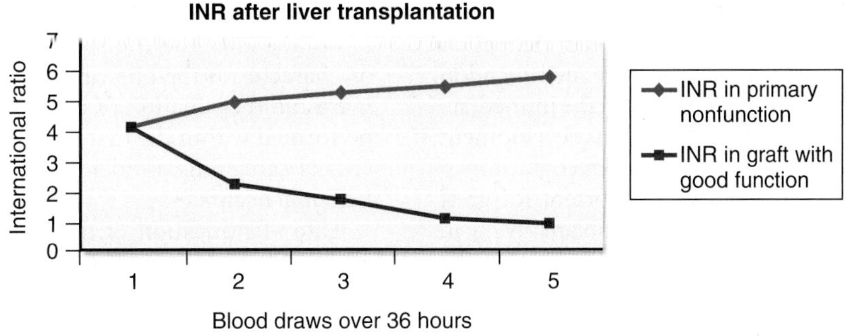

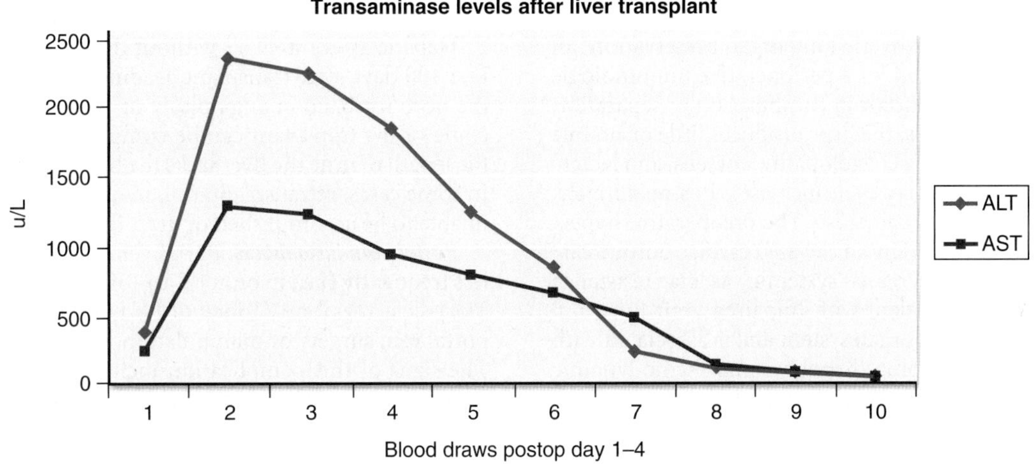

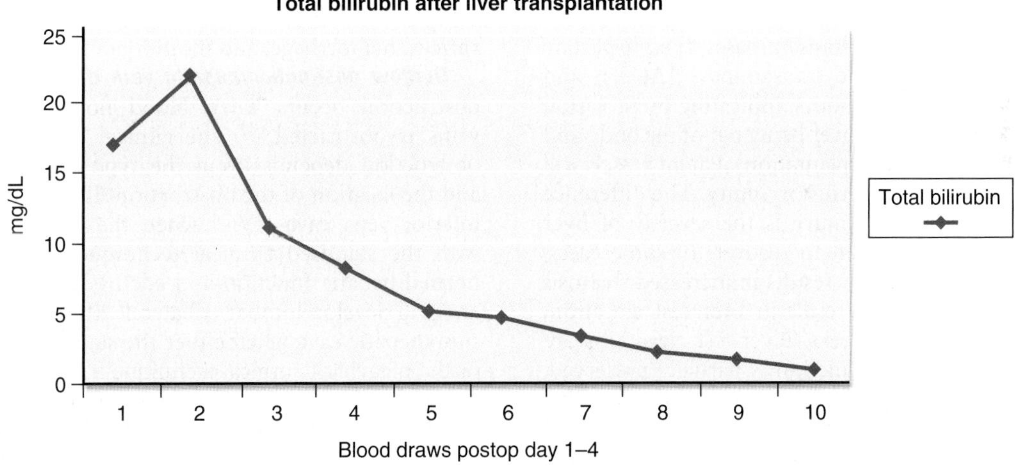

FIG. 20.3 Laboratory value testing after liver transplantation. *ALT,* Alanine transaminase; *AST,* aspartate transaminase; *INR,* international normalized ratio.

assessing ventilation and neurologic function, and determining if the drains are working correctly and are connected to suction or a bulb, based on surgical orders.[42,52] If the patient is not extubated prior to or upon arrival to the critical care unit, the patient will usually be weaned and extubated within 24 hours.[42,48,52] Key assessment activities of the critical care nurse include monitoring graft function and identifying subtle early findings of graft dysfunction, such as acute rejection or hepatic artery thrombosis, which is a serious problem that will typically occur within the first week of transplant. A Doppler ultrasound should be ordered by the transplant team to be performed usually within 12 hours of the transplant procedure. Improving bilirubin, normalization of INR, resolving acidosis, normalizing of liver tests, stabilization of serum glucose levels, adequate urine output, and increased biliary drainage along with increasing mental status are indicative of good graft function.[40,52] Critically ill patients with severe elevation of liver tests prior to transplantation may exhibit a slow progressive decrease in their total bilirubin level after transplantation over several weeks before complete normalization. The PT and INR should begin to normalize within the first few hours after transplantation, and the patient's level of consciousness should improve over the 12 hours following surgery.[13,42,55] If the laboratory tests do not show normalization, there is concern for primary graft nonfunction (PNF) (Fig. 20.3).

Postoperative Complications

Primary graft nonfunction. Survival of the liver transplant patient depends upon early graft function, early identification of dysfunction, and appropriate interventions. In the immediate postoperative period, graft function is a concern, as development of PNF occurs in up to 3% of grafts.[52] Early recognition of PNF as compared to reperfusion injury is important for graft survival. Ideally, transplant teams like to transplant livers in under 12 hours from the time they are procured to lessen the chance of PNF, preservation injury, and ischemic reperfusion injury.

Graft injury (where the liver is damaged) within the first 3 days is most often caused by PNF or hepatic artery thrombosis.[39] PNF can result from an unstable donor, preexisting disease in the donor, inadequate or overly long organ preservation, an imperfect recipient operation, or a perioperative immunologic reaction. These factors can occur in combination or separately. In the majority of PNF cases, the liver produces little or no bile after reperfusion, preexisting coagulopathy worsens, and lactate levels fail to decrease (or may even increase). Postoperatively, the patient usually remains comatose. The preoperative hyperdynamic state, demonstrated by an elevated cardiac output/cardiac index (CO/CI) and decreased systemic vascular resistance (SVR), continues in the patient with impaired graft function. PNF adversely affects every organ system and is associated with coagulopathy, persistent coma, hypoglycemia, hemodynamic instability, and acidosis. If the situation does not improve within 24 to 36 hours, the patient's only chance for survival is retransplantation. Overall, this is the most lethal complication of liver transplantation.[13,23,42]

Ischemic reperfusion injury. Ischemic reperfusion injury can be seen in the first 72 hours. Signs are similar to PNF, with liver function tests—specifically the transaminases (i.e., aspartate transaminase [AST] and alanine transaminase [ALT]), and bilirubin—elevated for 24 to 48 hours, indicating preservation injury (injury resulting from the liver being out of the body and stored in cold solution until transplantation). Patent vessels will be present on ultrasound in reperfusion injury. The difference between PNF and reperfusion injury is the severity of liver injury and the ability of the graft to recover. In some cases, the severity of preservation injury results in increased steatosis (fat) in the new liver; this can result in liver test elevation, which may persist for several weeks. Liver test elevations are usually lower, as the synthetic function is partially preserved. These patients may continue to have some coagulopathy, but it is less severe. Because of the poor liver function, portal hypertension may continue, resulting in postoperative ascites. The treatment of this condition is mainly supportive; most grafts will eventually recover, although some patients may require retransplantation.[42,48,56]

Hepatic artery thrombosis. Although hepatic artery thrombosis (HAT) can occur early or late in the recovery period, this complication occurs in 3% of patients, and can be due to technical issues such as cold ischemia, anastomotic problems, or rejection.[42,55] This condition usually occurs when there is a size discrepancy between the donor and recipient vessels. HAT is seen more often in LDLTs. HAT results in ischemia, and is the second leading cause of graft failure in the immediate postoperative period.[13,42] The patient will present with rapid dysfunction in the early postoperative period. Because the hepatic artery is the sole blood supply for the bile ducts, HAT may cause necrosis of the bile ducts and the operative anastomosis, leading to delayed bile leak in 7 days to 2 months after the transplant. Changes in the volume, color, or character of the bile can indicate a hepatic artery problem. Ultrasound evaluation of liver anastomosis and flow is usually performed within the first few hours after the patient arrives in critical care, and can identify this condition before significant ischemia occurs.[42]

Late identification of thrombosis of the hepatic artery can lead to bilomas (i.e., the collection of bile outside the bile ducts) and bacteremia, which results from abscess formation and may lead to sepsis. Often these patients will respond to antibiotics. Delayed diagnosis can result in biliary dehiscence with peritonitis, or loss of portions or the entire liver graft because of necrosis in the first few days to 2 weeks after transplantation.[8,42]

Hepatic artery stenosis without thrombosis can occur in the first 100 days after transplant, leading to graft dysfunction and the need for balloon angioplasty or surgical revision. The outcome of the transplant can be compromised, depending upon the length of time the liver lacks the hepatic artery blood supply. In some cases, retransplantation may be necessary, if revision is unable to be accomplished or graft failure continues.[13,23,42,48]

Portal vein thrombosis. Portal vein thrombosis (PVT) occurs less frequently (i.e., in only 1% to 13% of recipients) than HAT. The risk factors for PVT include PVT before transplant, previous portal vein surgery or manipulation, or a hypercoagulable state. The signs of this complication include development of portal hypertension, ascites, edema, encephalopathy, and elevated liver function tests. This complication is seen most commonly in the first month after transplantation. An ultrasound in the first few hours of transplant can diagnose reduced flow in the portal vein. If the thrombus develops after the first month, complications including portal hypertension, encephalopathy, variceal hemorrhage, and multiorgan failure will be seen.[8,40,48]

Outflow obstruction/hepatic vein thrombosis. Outflow tract obstruction occurs when blood flow through the hepatic veins is obstructed.[3,42] The clinical presentation of outflow obstruction depends upon the type of outflow anastomosis and the location of the obstruction. If the obstruction is at the inferior vena cava (IVC) when the transplant is performed with the standard surgical technique, the patient will have normal hepatic function and edema of the lower extremities, and will develop lumbar collaterals. If the obstruction is at the suprahepatic cava when either the standard surgical technique or the piggyback surgical technique is performed, the recipient can have the full manifestation of Budd-Chiari syndrome. Budd-Chiari syndrome occurs with obstruction of the hepatic vein, which prevents blood from leaving the liver and returning to the heart. The symptoms include ascites, abdominal pain, and elevation of liver function tests. Outflow tract obstruction can lead to hemorrhage because of an anastomotic leak or bleeding from collateral vessels. This is usually recognized within 24 hours of the initial surgery. Venous congestion or Budd-Chiari syndrome occurs in 1% to 3% of transplants, and may present up to 1 month posttransplant with jaundice, ascites, GI bleeding, hepatomegaly, and coagulopathy.[42,48,52]

Inferior vena cava injury. Obstruction of or damage to the IVC is a rare complication of liver transplantation that has significant consequences, including intractable ascites and hepatic dysfunction. Although venoplasty and stenting are effective in many cases, patients who fail first-line treatment may require surgical intervention or retransplantation. Damage to the IVC can occur as the result of unexpected dense adhesions between the liver and the retrohepatic vena cava or the presence of a liver tumor near the vena cava. Another type of injury is stenosis; this is another uncommon complication that may present with lower extremity edema or ascites. Angioplasty and stenting offer a rapid, minimally invasive therapy for inferior vena caval stenosis.[26,45]

Postoperative bleeding. Postoperative bleeding is a potential early complication following liver transplantation. The literature suggests that 10% to 15% of patients require reoperation for intraabdominal hemorrhage.[40] The effects of chronic liver disease, severity of portal hypertension, quantity of transfusions, and preexisting coagulopathy contribute to the risk of postoperative bleeding. Any preexisting coagulopathy should be corrected by the time the patient reaches critical care postoperatively.[13] Patients who receive living donor or split livers are at increased risk for this condition. Patients will present with tachycardia, hypotension, increased intraabdominal distention, oliguria, increased peak airway pressures, and elevated drain output.

Hemodynamic instability. Hemodynamic instability may exist before the transplant and continue in the early postoperative period because of the hyperdynamic circulatory status of these patients. Patients undergoing liver transplantation may sustain large-volume fluid or blood losses. Even without these losses, there is often fluid sequestration as the result of hypoalbuminemia, alterations in sodium metabolism (e.g., hyponatremia from too much intravascular water), and intestinal ileus caused by general anesthesia, manipulation of the intestinal tract during surgery, and the extent of the surgery. These patients require monitoring via a PAC. Initially, patients may present with a cardiac output (CO) greater than 12 L/min and an SVR below 400 dynes. An intraoperative course that involves large volume losses, transfusion requirements, and long operative times, in addition to preoperative malnutrition, abnormal renal function, and ascites, increases the risk for the development of inadequate vascular volume. Low filling pressures, falling CO, and increasing SVR will reflect the volume and cardiac status of these patients. The less complicated cases will respond to fluid infusion, similar to other surgical patients. The patient who is critically ill with multisystem dysfunction and a long, difficult intraoperative course will require a more careful approach to volume replacement. Overuse of crystalloid infusions may worsen the hyponatremia and increase the accumulation of total body water. The infusion of large volumes of albumin or plasma fractions may result in the overcorrection of the hyponatremia and a significant risk of central pontine myelinolysis.[23,46,48,52]

Pulmonary dysfunction. Prior to transplantation, some patients will present with hepatopulmonary syndrome (HPS). HPS is a pulmonary vascular disorder characterized by chronic liver disease, intrapulmonary vascular dilation, and arterial hypoxemia. The degree of hypoxemia varies with each patient, with little correlation to either the severity or the cause of the underlying liver disease. Patients will have resolution of this condition after transplantation, usually over days to months.[42]

Liver transplant patients are at increased risk of additional pulmonary complications in the postoperative period. The severity of the liver disease, comorbidities (diabetes, atelectasis, or acute renal injury), and preoperative procedures can escalate the risk of the patient developing pulmonary complications. Postoperatively, this risk is increased with graft dysfunction, the number of transfusions, duration of mechanical ventilation, and the immunosuppression status. The patient without HPS and with an uncomplicated liver transplant requiring few transfusions and a shorter surgical time will usually be extubated within 12 to 24 hours of the surgical procedure. Patients with more complicated surgeries, or with preexisting pulmonary conditions such as atelectasis, severe malnutrition, or pulmonary edema, may have a more complicated pulmonary course and remain intubated for 3 to 4 days. These patients require close monitoring of their oxygen saturation and ventilatory status.[11]

Infection. Infection is a major concern, as it is a significant cause of complications, increased length of hospital stay, increase hospital costs, and mortality.[10] Many transplant candidates are at an increased risk for developing an infection due to their end-stage disease processes, and many require critical care while waiting for their transplant. Aspiration pneumonia, intraabdominal infections, or catheter-related (central line or urinary) infections are the most common infections.[10]

Before transplant, factors such as age (> 65 years old), the inability to vaccinate prior to transplant due to end-stage organ disease, or lack of attention to updating vaccinations prior to transplant increase the risk for infection.[22] Intraoperative factors that can predispose a patient to infection include surgical technique (duct-to-duct or Roux-en-Y); injury to vagal, phrenic, or laryngeal nerves during surgery; ischemic injury to the graft; prolonged surgical time; and increased bleeding. Postoperative factors that increase the risk of infection include immunosuppression, vascular complications, bleeding, reexploration, central venous lines, and urinary catheters. Surgical site infection is the most common infection during the first 30 days.[22]

It is estimated that 80% of all transplant recipients will have at least one significant infection during the first year.[25,26,31] Postoperative infections have a variety of etiologies. They may occur because of nosocomial pathogens, as a result of reactivation of latent infections, or from opportunistic infections. Early infections are primarily bacterial. Common organisms include *Clostridium difficile,* vancomycin-resistant *Enterococcus,* methicillin-resistant *Staphylococcus aureus,* and extended spectrum β-lactamase gram-negative bacilli.[51] Bacterial infections may arise as a result of indwelling catheters; catheters should be removed as soon as possible or, for patients in whom catheter removal is not possible, changed on a regular basis. Other sources of bacterial infection are pneumonia, abdominal or biliary infections, and wound infections. Bacteremia is more common in patients with underlying diabetes mellitus and malnutrition.[10,22] Late-occurring infections are generally fungal or viral.[10,51] Liver transplant recipients are at increased risk for fungal infections such as mucormycosis or aspergillosis.[5] Exposure to fungi usually occurs by direct contact or inhalation from environmental sources. Rates and types of infections vary with geographic locale and the intensity of the environmental exposure. Most infections start in the respiratory tract or skin, but can disseminate to other organs. The major host factors include prolonged and profound immunodeficiency, breaks in skin integrity, and chronic respiratory disease (cystic fibrosis, asthma, bronchiectasis, and a history of smoking). Less commonly, infection can be transmitted as a result of contamination of the preservation fluid, or from the donated organ.[4,27]

Opportunistic infections are rare in the first week after transplantation. These infections tend to appear after the first month. Frequent and thorough hand hygiene by the healthcare team, patients, and visitors may minimize the occurrence of these infections. Tissue-invasive or systemic viral infections usually occur within the first month and include cytomegalovirus (CMV), Epstein-Barr virus (EBV), herpes simplex virus (HSV), varicella-zoster virus (VZV), and adenovirus. These may present as fever, malaise, nausea, vomiting, diarrhea, leukopenia, and failure to thrive. VZV emerges primarily as shingles. Other opportunistic infections include *Nocardia asteroides, Clostridium difficile, Candida* species, *Listeria monocytogenes, Mycobacterium tuberculosis, Pneumocystis jirovecii, Aspergillus* species, or *Mucor*.[5,20,22,42]

Recurrence of hepatitis B or C can occur within the first week, causing inflammation and elevation of transaminase levels. Immediate postoperative treatment with entecavir may prevent the recurrence of hepatitis B. Treatment of recurrent hepatitis C with the advent of direct-acting antivirals (DAAs) is becoming more commonplace, with minimal side effects. Some transplant programs are choosing to treat patients with DAAs while on the list awaiting transplant.

Biliary complications. Biliary complications following liver transplantation are a major complication of liver transplantation, with an incidence of 5% to 32%. Biliary complications include biliary strictures, leaks, and stones.[16] When seen in the early postoperative period, they can be secondary to necrosis of HAT surgical anastomosis. The early complications are seen more frequently in LDLT or split liver transplants, with an incidence as high as 30%. These complications occur secondary to the size discrepancy of the vessels between donor and recipient.[40,42,52] Recipients of split livers (partial grafts or reduced-size grafts) can have bile leakage from the cut surface, the cystic duct remnant, unrecognized accessory ducts, or choledochoenteric anastomoses. Eighty percent of all biliary complications occur within the first 6 months after transplantation, and the majority occur within the first 3 months.[42] Late bile leaks are usually due to ischemic injury or removal of T-tubes. With the reduction in use of T-tubes, this complication is seen less frequently.[42] Clinical presentation of this complication may be subtle. Patients commonly present with fever, leukocytosis, jaundice, shoulder pain, right upper quadrant pain, and increased drainage with a bilious appearance. Noninvasive examinations may not detect small obstructions or leaks.[8,40,42,48] Complications of the biliary system can be due to technical complications of the anastomosis or ischemic injury related to compromised arterial blood supply, preservation injury, rejection, or ascending infection, where microorganisms from the duodenum translocate into the bile ducts because of obstruction and bile stasis.[19,42]

In addition to biliary leaks, patients can develop biliary strictures. These strictures may be anastomotic or ischemic; the mechanism of injury is the same as that for a biliary leak. Biliary strictures evolve over time and present after the first month posttransplantation. The patient may present with jaundice, cholangitis, or asymptomatic elevation of liver function tests, specifically the alkaline phosphatase and bilirubin levels.[42] Ultrasound may not identify the biliary tract problem, and an endoscopic retrograde cholangiopancreatography (ERCP) can be successful in identification and placement of internal biliary stents that bypass the biliary stricture or leak, decompress biliary blockages, and remove stones. Biliary complications after liver transplantation are common, and continue to be a challenge. The successful use of ERCP has resulted in decreased utilization of surgical revision and percutaneous transhepatic cholangiography (PTC) management. Surgical approaches and PTC are usually reserved for when endoscopic therapy is unsuccessful or not feasible, resulting in the return to the operating room for a revision and choledochojejunostomy to Roux limb (Roux-en-Y).[2,16]

Renal failure and electrolyte abnormalities. Prior to transplantation, patients with advanced liver disease can develop hepatorenal syndrome (HRS). There are two types of HRS. In some patients, the renal failure is not an acute injury, but is determined to be chronic kidney disease; these patients may receive a kidney transplant simultaneously with their liver transplant. The second type of HRS is characterized by acute renal failure, increased urine, plasma osmolality, low urinary sodium level, and the absence of pathologic changes in the kidney (i.e., the tubular function remains intact).[12] The acute renal failure seen in HRS should resolve after liver transplantation. Intraoperative factors that can impact acute kidney injury include hypotension and a large number of transfusions. Postoperative hyperglycemia, poor graft function, increased intraabdominal pressure, and nephrotoxicity increase the risk of renal dysfunction. Patients at increased risk for delayed return of renal function and the resulting fluid and electrolyte imbalances may require the use of renal replacement therapy until renal function returns.[44,48] The use of calcineurin inhibitors for immunosuppression should be adjusted during this time to prevent worsening of the renal function due to nephrotoxicity.[5] Other nephrotoxic medications such as aminoglycosides should be avoided. Some recipients may receive renal replacement therapy (RRT) before, during, or after transplantation. This is a clinical decision based upon biochemical and clinical indications. Biochemical indicators include sustained refractory hyperkalemia, hyponatremia or hypernatremia, hypercalcemia, and metabolic acidosis in the presence of serum urea levels greater than 30 μmol/L. The clinical indications for RRT are a urine output of less than 0.3 mL/kg for 24 hours or anuria for 12 hours, PNF or multiple organ dysfunction, refractory volume overload, and a need for the creation of intravascular space for blood transfusions or nutrition.[1,21,44,48,56] The RRT modality may be intermittent hemodialysis, prolonged intermittent RRT, continuous renal replacement therapy (CRRT), continuous venovenous hemofiltration (CVVH), continuous venovenous hemodialysis (CVVHD), or continuous venovenous hemodiafiltration (CVVHDF).[1,21,56] With the introduction of the MELD score, more patients are receiving RRT before transplantation; the national average is approximately 11%, but can reach levels of as high as 33% of patients at some transplantation centers.[31] Agopian et al. examined the medical records of 1517 adults who underwent orthotopic liver transplantation (OLT), 500 (33%) of whom received pretransplant RRT.[1] Of these 500 patients, 99 (20%) required intraoperative renal replacement therapy (IORRT), which was planned in 70 patients (71%) and emergent in 29 (29%). The recipients receiving planned IORRT had significantly longer pretransplant ICU hospitalization; higher pretransplant potassium, MELD scores, and total bilirubin levels; lower blood urea nitrogen (BUN); and received preoperative CRRT, mechanical ventilation, and vasopressors.[31] Overall, approximately 14% of liver recipients may develop chronic renal failure.[1,13,56] Many of those who develop chronic kidney disease had chronic renal dysfunction prior to transplantation.[46,58]

Postoperative Interventions

Nutrition. Pretransplant nutrition is challenging in patients with liver failure. Protein-energy malnutrition is frequently seen in patients who undergo liver transplantation, and can affect their survival.[41] Most transplant programs have a dedicated transplant dietician who evaluates each patient and coordinates the patient's nutritional goals to optimize the patients prior to transplant. Because anthropometrics may underestimate the level of malnutrition, dieticians may use the Controlling Nutritional Status (CONUT), Spanish Society of Parenteral and Enteral Nutrition (SENPE) criteria, and Nutritional Risk Index (NRI) assessment measures.[33] These indices are calculated based on analytical parameters that examine albumin, lymphocytes, and cholesterol in combination with weight or body mass index (BMI).[33] Preoperatively, it is important that accurate assessment of the nutritional status and early intervention occur. However, the metabolic abnormalities induced by liver failure make traditional assessment of the nutritional status difficult.[41] Some studies have examined the use of bioelectrical impedance to assess nutritional status in the critically ill patient, and have shown benefit in pretransplant management.[24,37,41] Because preoperative malnutrition and the loss of skeletal muscle mass, called *sarcopenia,* have a significant negative impact on the posttransplantation outcome, it is essential to provide adequate nutritional support during all phases of liver transplantation. Oral nutrition is preferred, but enteral nutrition may be required to provide the necessary caloric intake. Some of the current perioperative nutritional interventions in liver transplant patients include the use of synbiotics, micronutrients, and branched-chain amino acid supplementation. Immune system–modulating formulas, fluid balance, and nocturnal meals are also utilized. More than 80% of liver transplant patients exhibit moderate to severe malnutrition in the face of enteral and parenteral supplementation.[41,48] Very low protein intake is associated with malnutrition and mortality. It is the patient's liver function in the postoperative period that determines the level of metabolic stress and nutritional needs. In some centers, initiation of enteral feeding is instituted preoperatively through the placement of nasal jejunal tubes.[40] When the allograft function is stable, the immediate postoperative hypermetabolism is short. However, if the postoperative course includes delayed graft function, the patient may be volume-overloaded and intolerant of enteral feedings. These patients may require parenteral nutrition to provide adequate calories and protein, and to correct metabolic abnormalities while minimizing sodium and water accumulation.[42] The combined efforts of an interprofessional team to ensure early assessment and adequate intervention preoperatively and during the acute posttransplantation period are crucial to help prevent infection, promote wound healing, support metabolic demands, replenish lost stores, and mediate the immune response.[19]

Glycemic control. Posttransplant glucose control is important for solid organ transplant patient survival.[50] Studies have shown that uncontrolled hyperglycemia is associated with graft dysfunction and failure, as well as increased complications.[7,50] Many factors contribute to elevated postoperative glucose levels. The body is under a significant stress related to the transplant surgery. The elevated physiologic stress results in an endocrine response with activation of the adrenal cortex. The adrenal cortex activation stimulates the release of corticosteroids, which results in the development of hyperglycemia and insulin resistance. In addition, the patient is given intravenous glucocorticoids preoperatively to prevent graft reject, resulting in hyperglycemia, decreased insulin uptake, and increased hepatic glucose production. Postoperatively, the use of calcineurin inhibitors may also cause elevated blood glucose levels.[49,50]

Glucose monitoring should be started upon arrival in the acute or critical care unit. Glucose management should be a high priority, as hyperglycemia during the immediate post-operative period is an independent predictor of morbidity and mortality in patients with and without a diagnosis of diabetes.[32] Continuous insulin infusion should be the preferred method of insulin administration, maintaining glucose levels between 100 mg/dL and 150 mg/dL.[29]

Diagnostic testing. Evaluation of the patient for vascular or biliary complications requires that the patient undergo ultrasound within the first 12 hours of the postoperative period. This test is usually done at the patient's bedside. If there is persistent dysfunction, magnetic resonance imaging (MRI) can be performed in conjunction with magnetic resonance angiography (MRA) and magnetic resonance cholangiopancreatography (MRCP) to evaluate the vessels and bile ducts. A liver biopsy may also be performed, either percutaneously at the bedside or by the transjugular method in interventional radiology, to provide histologic information on inflammation caused by rejection, recurrent disease, reperfusion injury, or outflow obstruction.[13,19,42,48] In the event of biliary stricture or obstruction, an ERCP may be performed to remove stones or place stents.

Transplant immunology and rejection. The suppression of the body's immune system, which enables it to distinguish self from nonself, is important to the survival of the transplanted organ. Rejection in the liver transplant patient can occur in the early days to weeks after transplantation. Hyperacute rejection occurs within minutes to days posttransplant, and is extremely rare. Acute cellular rejection following liver transplantation has decreased in incidence, but it still affects up to a quarter of liver transplantation recipients.[42] Most episodes occur within 1 month posttransplantation, although acute cellular rejection may present later.[3] The incidence of late acute cellular rejection (> 90 days posttransplantation) can be associated with recent changes in and lower levels of immunosuppression.[36,52,55,57] In addition to the type and level of immunosuppression, certain transplantation-related characteristics may influence the risk of rejection. As an example, patients who receive an organ from a LDLT may have a lower rate of acute cellular rejection compared with DDLT recipients.[13] Graft injury, evidenced by elevated liver function tests between 3 and 14 days after transplantation, can be due to acute cellular rejection. This form of rejection is T-cell mediated, and causes tissue destruction. In chronic rejection, there is intimal hyperplasia of small- and medium-sized arteries, resulting in progressive ischemia in the transplanted organ. This leads to loss of the bile ducts, ductopenic rejection, and cholestasis, which over time may lead to retransplantation.[4,36,42] Although patients with both acute and chronic rejection may remain asymptomatic, some patients may present with symptoms of a nonspecific nature, with complaints of malaise, decreased appetite, right upper quadrant pain, jaundice, and low-grade fever. The first laboratory tests that will show elevations identifying rejection are the alkaline phosphatase and gamma-glutamyltransferase (GGT) levels, followed by an elevation of the remainder of the liver function tests.[23]

The consequences of acute cellular rejection are variable. Although it can predispose to steroid-resistant rejection and graft loss, most episodes do not have long-term adverse effects, except in hepatitis C virus (HCV)–positive patients.[4,9,34] The diagnosis of acute cellular rejection is usually suspected by elevations in serum aminotransferase and alkaline phosphatase levels, which typically precede the clinical symptoms of jaundice and fever. However, biochemical parameters are not sensitive or specific for detecting acute cellular rejection, and do not correlate with its severity.[5,9,34,42] Thus, the diagnosis should be confirmed by liver biopsy before initiating treatment for rejection. Histologic features include endotheliitis, nonsuppurative cholangitis, and mixed mononuclear cell portal inflammation.[42]

High-dose corticosteroids are usually first-line therapy for acute cellular rejection. Methylprednisolone doses vary among centers, ranging from 500-mg to 1000-mg boluses given daily for 1 to 3 days. A gradual corticosteroid taper is provided at some centers following bolus methylprednisolone. The addition of mycophenolate mofetil (CellCept) to the medication regimen and changing to tacrolimus (Prograf) from cyclosporine (Gengraf) have also been recommended.[4,13,42] A small percentage of acute rejection episodes will not respond to steroids; antilymphocytic agents (muromonab-CD3 [OKT3], antilymphocyte globulin [ALG] [Atgam], antithymocyte globulin [ATG] [Thymoglobulin]), or anti-interleukin-2 receptor antibodies are used to address rejection in these cases.[4,13,42] Whereas ATG is more commonly used and may cause fever and chills, OKT3 is a monoclonal antibody that can cause patients to develop pulmonary edema and severe flulike symptoms. Patients receiving this medication should have a chest radiograph immediately before drug administration and should be premedicated with medications such as methylprednisolone (Medrol), acetaminophen (Tylenol), and an antihistamine.[4,13,42] Commonly used immunosuppressant medications are shown in Table 20.1.

Medication Metabolism

The metabolism of medications during recovery from liver transplantation depends upon the degree to which the new liver functions normally. If the new liver is significantly compromised by ischemia, infection, recurrent disease, or rejection, more complex management is required. Medication toxicities may develop in the early postoperative period in the patient with delayed return of liver function and ongoing or developing renal impairment. Cyclosporine and tacrolimus may cause dose-related cholestasis and nephrotoxicity, which are readily reversed with dose reduction. In addition, tacrolimus or cyclosporine activity may be inhibited by or may inhibit the metabolism of other medications. Some medications (e.g., aminoglycosides, erythromycin, and ketoconazole) work synergistically with tacrolimus, everolimus (Afinitor), and cyclosporine to cause nephrotoxicity. Other medications (e.g., azithromycin [Zithromax], verapamil [Calan], fluconazole [Diflucan], erythromycin, and cimetidine [Tagamet]) increase tacrolimus or cyclosporine levels, resulting in toxicity.[16,33] Some medications (e.g., phenytoin [Dilantin], rifampin [Rifadin], and certain herbs) decrease tacrolimus or cyclosporine efficacy and have the potential to increase the risk of rejection.[42] Posttransplant impairment of bile acid synthesis, reduced biliary secretion, and altered intestinal absorption may all predispose the recipient to total parenteral nutrition (TPN) cholestasis. In the immediate postoperative period, reduced hepatic function can also result in altered metabolism of narcotics and sedatives. The dosing of these medications needs to be carefully monitored to prevent alterations in mentation.

Assessment of the Liver Transplant Patient

Initial postoperative assessments completed upon arrival of the patient in the critical care unit are similar to other postoperative patients, with evaluation of airway, breathing, and circulation. Evaluation of endotracheal tube placement, ventilator settings and alarms, breath sounds, and pulse oximetry are completed. Hemodynamic lines are connected, and initial measurements are taken to assess the stability of the patient. Drains, tubes, and dressings are assessed for patency, color, and amount of drainage. Initial blood samples are sent to the laboratory for evaluation of liver function, electrolytes, blood counts, and coagulation studies.[23]

After this initial assessment, specific assessments are completed for baseline comparison. Assessment of the neurologic system is a priority as the liver transplant recipient is prone to neurologic abnormalities. These abnormalities can range from profound coma to transient peripheral neuropathy. Initially, the assessment is focused upon recovery from anesthesia.[23] Alterations in mental status occur in 10% to 30% of recipients.[52] Persistent coma may be symptomatic of primary nonfunction of the graft. Patients who are alert after surgery may still demonstrate the effects of pretransplant encephalopathy, sleep deprivation and disorientation, or posttransplant immunosuppression (induced by steroids or calcineurin inhibitors). Steroids can cause psychosis, mood swings, increased irritability, and severe depression. Tacrolimus can cause headaches, peripheral neuropathy, paresthesia, and tremors.[52] Seizures occurring posttransplantation are due to metabolic and electrolyte anomalies such as hyponatremia or toxicity from calcineurin inhibitors, and require monitoring of complete metabolic panels and medication levels. Seizures may be the result of an intracranial event (e.g., stroke).[23,52]

A head computed tomography (CT) or MRI should evaluate any change in level of consciousness. Treatment of seizures is complicated by the fact that most antiseizure medications interfere with the metabolism of many immunosuppressive medications, such as cyclosporine, tacrolimus, everolimus, and sirolimus (Rapamune). Gabapentin (Neurontin) and levetiracetam (Keppra) are the only antiseizure medications that do not require hepatic metabolism and do not influence the plasma levels of immunosuppressive medications. Intracranial hemorrhage can occur spontaneously in the setting of coagulopathies, thrombocytopenia, and hypertension. Cerebral edema is common in patients who have undergone liver transplant for acute hepatic failure. The hyperammonemia caused by acute hepatic failure leads to swelling of the astrocytes and increased water content in the brain. This leads to increased cerebral edema and intracranial pressure, and in some cases, herniation.[52] A very rare complication called *central pontine myelinolysis*, which results when hypernatremia exists prior to transplant and is then rapidly corrected during surgery, may cause significant central nervous system injury.[42,52]

It is important to assess drains for types and amounts of drainage to ensure that postoperative bleeding, reduced bile production, and biliary leaks are identified early.[15,42] Monitoring of liver function tests, coagulation studies, and acid-base balance is also important. If the graft is not functioning (PNF), coagulopathies will persist, lactic acid will accumulate (leading to metabolic acidosis), and liver function tests will not begin

TABLE 20.1 **Immunosuppressant Medications Used after Liver, Kidney, or Pancreas Transplant**

Medication	Actions	Dosage	Special Considerations
Cyclosporine (Neoral, Gengraf, Sandimmune)	Inhibition of T lymphocytes through suppression of IL-2 production and release	IV: 5–6 mg/kg 12 h before transplant Maintenance: 2–10 mg/kg/d in divided doses PO: 10–18 mg/kg 4–12 h before transplant Maintenance: 5–15 mg/kg/d in divided doses, tapered to 3–10 mg/kg/d	Monitor serum concentrations Monitor for nephrotoxicity (25%–37% incidence); hepatotoxicity (4%–7% incidence); usually responsive to dose reduction May cause hypertension, tremors, confusion, seizures, hyperkalemia, hypomagnesemia, hemolytic-uremic syndrome, hyperlipidemia Multiple drug, food, and herbal interactions Brands are not bioequivalent and should not be used interchangeably. Oral dose will depend on formulation
Tacrolimus (Prograf)	Inhibition of T lymphocytes through suppression of IL-2 production	Liver transplant: PO: 0.1–0.15 mg/kg/d divided into two doses given every 12 h IV: 0.03–0.05 mg/kg/d as continuous infusion Renal transplant: PO: 0.2 mg/kg/d in 2 divided doses 12 h apart IV: 0.03–0.05 mg/kg/d as continuous infusion	Monitor serum concentrations Monitor for nephrotoxicity and glucose intolerance May cause hypertension, tremors, confusion, seizures, hyperkalemia, hemolytic-uremic syndrome, and hyperlipidemia
Sirolimus (Rapamycin)	Inhibition of activation and proliferation of T lymphocytes by IL-2, IL-4, and IL-5	PO: 6 mg loading dose Maintenance: 2–5 mg/d Doses adjusted based on 24-h trough levels.	Black box warning: Not recommended for use in first 30 days post liver transplant due to hepatic artery thrombosis Monitor serum concentrations Monitor CBC, renal function tests, and lipids May cause hypertension, hyperlipidemia, bone marrow suppression, and hemolytic-uremic syndrome
Everolimus (Zortress, Certican)	Inhibiting the proliferation, and thus clonal expansion, of antigen-activated T lymphocytes, which is driven by T lymphocytes–specific interleukins, (e.g., IL-2 and IL-15).	Dose: 1.0 mg twice per day is recommended for the hepatic transplant population, with the initial dose administered approximately 4 weeks after transplantation	The daily dose of Certican should always be given orally in two divided doses, consistently either with or without food and at the same time as cyclosporin microemulsion or tacrolimus; certican tablets should be taken whole and not crushed before use. Monitor CBC and LFTs Blood levels may be monitored
Mycophenolate mofetil (CellCept)	Inhibits inosine monophosphate dehydrogenase in the purine synthesis pathway, thereby inhibiting T and B lymphocytes	Renal: 1 g twice daily IV/PO Liver: 1 g twice daily IV; 1.5 g twice daily PO	Compatible only with D_5W infusions May cause bone marrow suppression, diarrhea, and vomiting Monitor CBC and LFTs Blood levels may be monitored
Azathioprine (Imuran)	Interferes with DNA and RNA synthesis, and inhibition, differentiation, and proliferation of both T and B lymphocytes	Renal transplant: IV/PO: 2–5 mg/kg/d on day of transplant; 1–3 mg/kg/d as maintenance	May cause bone marrow suppression, hepatotoxicity, nausea, and vomiting Monitor CBC and LFTs
Methylprednisolone (Solu-Medrol)	Suppresses leukocyte migration; inhibits lymphokine-mediated amplification of macrophages and lymphocytes	PO: 4–100 mg/d Dose will depend on degree of immunosuppression required IV: 100–250 mg intraoperative, then dose tapered per provider order until PO initiated Liver: bolus of 250–500 mg IV q 24 h for 3 doses for rejection	Monitor for hyperglycemia, hypokalemia, fluid retention, hypertension, impaired wound healing, myopathy, osteoporosis, gastric ulcers, sleep disturbances, and psychosis
Prednisone	Suppresses leukocyte migration; inhibits lymphokine-mediated amplification of macrophages and lymphocytes	PO: 4–48 mg/d Dose will depend on degree of immunosuppression required Dose will depend on time since transplant, rejection history, and infection history	Monitor for same adverse effects as for methylprednisolone

CBC, Complete blood cell count; *D_5W*, 5% dextrose in water; *IL*, interleukin; *IV*, intravenous; *LFTs*, liver function tests; *PO*, *per os* (orally); *q*, every.

to normalize. Liver function tests will be increased in the first few hours after transplantation, but after the first 24 hours they should begin progressing toward normal. The liver function stabilization process will take several days, with the bilirubin lagging behind the AST and ALT.[13]

Liver transplant recipients frequently have renal dysfunction along with electrolyte and acid-base disturbances before transplantation. After transplantation, they have significant increases in total body sodium and water content; these patients receive high doses of corticosteroids during the procedure, along with large volumes of blood products and crystalloid solutions. Many of the patients will have a mild metabolic acidosis on arrival to the critical care unit due to lactic acid accumulation, which results from decreased tissue perfusion during the procedure, as well as the large volume of blood transfusions.[13,23] This period of acidosis is transient; the patients develop metabolic alkalosis from corticosteroids and the use of diuretics, producing a hypochloremic and hypokalemic alkalosis. In addition, nasogastric hydrogen ion losses and citrate in blood products contribute to alkalosis. In the immediate postoperative period, the development of alkalosis and hypocalcemia can occur secondary to blood component therapy and the conversion of the citrate anticoagulant in the new liver to bicarbonate. Once the allograft begins to function well, electrolyte replacement can begin.[23] The use of histamine H_2 receptor agonists (H_2 blockers) and the resumption of gastric function will reduce the hydrogen ion loss. The critical care nurse must monitor the comprehensive metabolic panels for alterations in liver function tests, electrolyte abnormalities, and renal function. The metabolic imbalance can cause cardiac dysfunction and arrhythmias.[13,23]

Patients are usually extubated within the first 24 hours after surgery. Atelectasis, pleural effusions, metabolic alkalosis, and the abdominal incision may affect pulmonary function. Arterial blood gas analysis, assessment of breath sounds, oral hygiene, and management of secretions are important in preventing complications. Early mobilization along with positioning and good pulmonary toilet can also aid in reducing the risk of infection.[22,23,52]

Early initiation of nutrition is important, as these patients are significantly nutritionally compromised preoperatively. If early extubation is not possible, or if neurologic conditions prevent oral intake, enteral nutritional support should be initiated as soon as possible. Although infrequent, it is important to monitor the patient for complications such as bowel perforation, biliary or vascular anastomotic leaks, or stenosis. Other conditions, which are uncommon but can occur, include pancreatitis and intraabdominal infections.[23,52] Output from surgical drains can be an early indicator of complications or graft dysfunction. If the patient has a T-tube, the drainage should be golden brown or dark green. If there is no output, or if the output is a different color, the surgeon should be notified to assist with further assessment. The drainage from the Jackson-Pratt (JP) drains should be serosanguineous. Bloody or cloudy drainage from JP drains can indicate bleeding or infection.[23,42]

Oliguria is common in the early recovery phase and usually resolves within 24 hours. Many patients will have abnormal renal function preoperatively because of low serum albumin levels, diuretic use, and paracentesis, resulting in low intravascular volumes and decreased renal perfusion. Patients may also suffer from HRS, which will not resolve spontaneously posttransplantation, but will resolve more gradually as the liver function improves. Postoperative oliguria may develop as a result of intraoperative blood and body fluid losses. Fluid administration and fluid shifts occurring postoperatively will resolve oliguria. Immunosuppression medication doses are adjusted based upon serum creatinine levels. Accurate intake and output in conjunction with hemodynamic monitoring via a PAC are important for maintaining the patient's fluid balance.[42]

The assessment of the liver transplant patient focuses on a systemic evaluation of each organ system with integration of the laboratory values, preexisting conditions, and effects of interventions. The integration of organ systems and the effects of dysfunction on other body systems are also key to optimal patient outcomes in transplantation. Any malaise, pain, or tenderness over the liver area, development of jaundice, or elevation of liver function tests are of concern.

The care of the liver transplant patient presents the critical care team with one of the more complex and challenging endeavors. Early recognition of complications and communication of these findings allow for prompt intervention and progress toward optimal outcomes for these patients.

RENAL TRANSPLANTATION

Recipients

Renal transplantation offers a potential to return to a healthy life. It has many advantages over dialysis, the primary advantage being an improved quality of life. With improvements in tissue typing, immunosuppression, and postoperative treatment, patient and graft survival rates continue to increase.[59] The main causes of renal failure leading to transplantation are diabetes mellitus, hypertension, and glomerulonephritis. Patients awaiting kidney transplantation are at increased risk for cardiovascular, pulmonary, and neurologic complications, in addition to an increased risk of infection because of their immunocompromised state.[14,46,53] Currently, most patients undergoing kidney transplantation do not require admission to critical care, unless they have comorbidities that increase their postoperative risk or develop intraoperative complications that require close monitoring. The most common complication requiring a kidney transplant patient to be admitted to critical care is respiratory distress.[14,43]

Kidney transplant patients may receive their organs from non–heart-beating donors (the heart has arrested, and the donor is declared deceased according to circulatory-respiratory criteria), from deceased donors (brain death determination has been made), or from living donors.[52] The surgery is approximately 3 hours in duration. The donated kidney is implanted in the right or left lower quadrant of the recipient, as determined by the anatomy of the donated kidney, through a hockey stick–shaped incision extending from the iliac crest to the symphysis pubis (Fig. 20.4).

Postoperative Complications

The complications occurring most often following kidney transplantation are urologic complications; hemodynamic instability; hypertension; fluid, electrolyte, or acid-base imbalances; and ongoing renal dysfunction. Infection, pancytopenia, recurrent renal disease, and hyperlipidemia may also develop weeks to months after the transplant.[43]

Urologic

Urologic complications are more common (1% to 3%) when wound healing is impaired.[14,43,46,58] These complications can

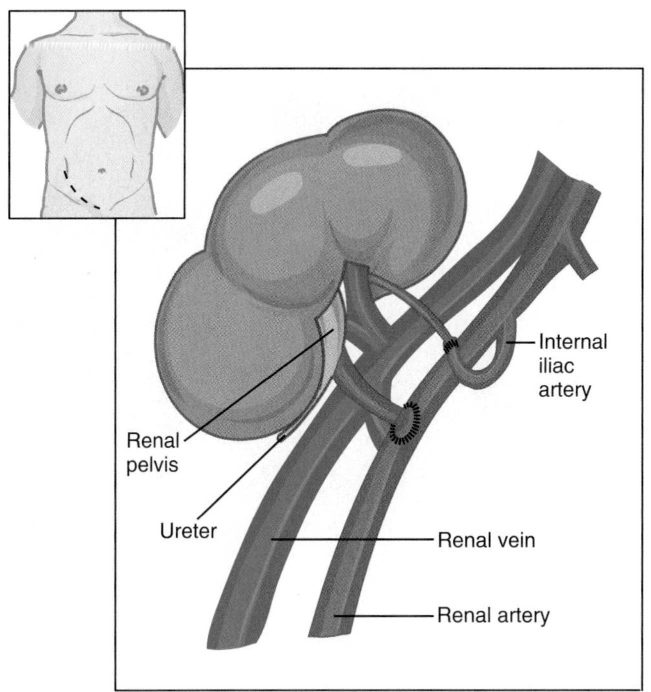

FIG. 20.4 Standard lower-quadrant incision and suture lines for renal allograft.

include the development of a lymphocele (a pocket of lymph accumulation); compression of the iliac vein, causing ipsilateral leg swelling; hematoma, leading to pain; infection; and ureteral stenosis or occlusion. Ureteral obstruction can be diagnosed by hydronephrosis, as visualized by ultrasound. It may develop as the result of blood clots, poor implantation, ureteral sloughing, or ureteral kinking. Symptoms may include pain over the transplanted kidney or lower abdominal pain, decreased urine output, and increased BUN and serum creatinine levels.[43] Stenting or surgical repair may be required to reduce the obstruction.

Urine leaks from the anastomotic site may occur in the early postoperative period or at the onset of posttransplant diuresis. They may be the result of technical problems (e.g., a non-watertight reimplantation of the ureter), or may develop from ureteral sloughing secondary to disruption of ureteral blood flow or a tight ureteral stenosis. Urine leaks are characterized by decreased urine output with increasing serum creatinine level and severe pain. This can also be indicative of rejection. An ultrasound should be performed to determine if there is a surgical problem and if a biopsy is necessary. If the symptoms are due to a urologic complication, reinsertion of the Foley catheter is required, and the patient is returned to the operating room for reexploration.[43,58]

Vascular

Pseudoaneurysms secondary to infection, arterial thrombus, or venous thrombosis require early identification in order to preserve the organ. Arterial or venous thrombus can occur as early as the first 2 to 3 days after transplantation, and are characterized by decreased urine output, swelling, and pain. Late renal arterial stenosis leading to hypertension and graft dysfunction may require dilation and stenting or surgical intervention.[43]

Postoperative bleeding may occur when the small vessels in the renal hilum have increased perfusion. The bleeding of these vessels may not have been apparent intraoperatively secondary to vasospasm of these small vessels. Renal ultrasound with Doppler is performed in the first 24 hours postoperatively to provide early identification of these problems.[43]

Hemodynamic Instability

Prolonged cold ischemic time can result in delayed function of the transplanted kidney, leading to intravascular volume problems. These patients can be volume-overloaded before dialysis has been restarted postoperatively, if oliguria or anuria is present. Volume depletion may occur in the patient with high-output renal failure, requiring close monitoring of central venous pressure (CVP), blood pressure (BP), and heart rate.[43]

Approximately 60% to 80% of kidney transplant recipients have multifactorial etiology of their hypertension.[43] Some of the etiologies include the effects of retained native kidneys, parenchymal disease of the transplanted organ, effects of immunotherapy, renal artery stenosis, and weight gain.[35] Preoperative hypertension is rarely cured by kidney transplantation, and may continue to be a problem in the postoperative care of the kidney transplant patient. Cardiovascular death, as a result of myocardial infarction, stroke, or complications of peripheral vascular disease, is the most common type of death in renal transplant patients.[39]

Electrolyte and Acid-Base Imbalances

Electrolyte imbalances, including hyperkalemia, hyperphosphatemia, and hyponatremia, exist before kidney transplantation. Patients are dialyzed before surgery to minimize the impact of these imbalances during the intraoperative period. In the postoperative period, these electrolyte imbalances may continue, or can be exacerbated by the transplant. Surgical tissue destruction coupled with the impaired renal function leads to further hyperkalemia, a frequent postoperative complication. Hyponatremia can also occur with excessive administration of hypotonic fluids in the presence of renal impairment. Hypomagnesemia is a manifestation of high-output acute tubular necrosis, and hypophosphatemia results when the glomerular filtration rate (GFR) suddenly normalizes in patients with preexisting hyperparathyroidism, which is common in patients with renal disease. In addition to these imbalances, the impaired renal excretion of hydrogen ions after surgery can lead to metabolic acidosis. Close monitoring of electrolytes and the acid-base balance is essential in the early postoperative days.[39]

Renal Dysfunction

Patients receiving deceased donor kidneys with preservation times of greater than 24 hours may experience delayed graft function. Renal dysfunction in the postoperative period is characterized as anuria (< 50 mL/24 h) or oliguria (< 400 mL/24 h), and is the result of acute tubular necrosis (ATN). However, urine leak, ureteral obstruction, and vascular thrombosis must be ruled out. The period of ATN can last from several days to weeks, with gradually improving kidney function (Box 20.2). These patients are at high risk for developing fluid overload in the immediate postoperative period. Most patients can be supported by dialysis until urine output increases and serum creatinine and BUN levels begin to normalize.[39]

Polyuria is commonly observed after living related kidney donation, and is the result of osmotic diuresis in the face of rapidly normalizing GFR. In some renal transplant patients, the development of ATN creates a renal concentration deficit that results in increased urine output with azotemia. These patients

BOX 20.2 Etiologies of Renal Failure After Initial Graft Function

- Volume depletion
- Arterial thrombosis
- Venous thrombosis
- Anastomotic stricture
- Obstruction by perinephric fluid (hematoma or lymphocele)
- Drug-induced nephrotoxicity
- Allergic interstitial nephritis
- Hemolytic-uremic syndrome

are at high risk of dehydration unless their volume status is carefully monitored and maintained.

Delayed graft function can result in the need for dialysis in the first few weeks after transplantation. Ischemic ATN occurs in 10% to 40% of patients, and carries with it the increased risk of acute rejection.[39]

Rejection

Hyperacute rejection is mediated by preformed antibodies, and can occur immediately following the vascular anastomosis or days later (i.e., delayed hyperacute rejection). This condition is characterized by necrosis of parenchymal tissue, which results in a toxic state that progresses to disseminated intravascular coagulation. There is an abrupt decrease in renal function, with rapidly increasing serum creatinine level, fever, malaise, graft tenderness, and oliguria. This condition often leads to graft loss even with antirejection treatment.[28,39] Today, with the use of induction treatment with polyclonal immunoglobulin G (IgG) antibodies or monoclonal antibodies and glucocorticoids, it is uncommon for patients to experience hyperacute rejection.[28]

Acute cellular rejection can occur within the first 6 months after transplantation, and may not be manifested as an elevated serum creatinine level.[28,39] It is instead characterized by fever, chills, myalgia, and arthralgia, and can be reversed with immunosuppressive treatment. In other cases, the patient may have an unexplained rise in serum creatinine of more than 20% with various degrees of reduced urine output, weight gain, and edema.[28]

Chronic rejection, or chronic allograft nephropathy, occurs most commonly after the first 6 months posttransplant. This condition is characterized by a slow decrease in the GFR with a slow increase in the serum creatinine level, accompanied by proteinuria and a worsening of the patient's systemic hypertension. It can be due to inadequate immunosuppression or nonimmunosuppressive factors, including hypertension, hyperlipidemia, nephrotoxicity, viral infections, ischemia, reperfusion injury, or the use of herbal supplements. Some patients may develop frank nephrotic syndrome (massive proteinuria) with edema, hypoalbuminemia, and hyperlipidemia.[38]

Infection

Infection in the kidney transplant patient is a significant concern because of the higher amounts of immunosuppression received, the alteration in the body's normal defenses due to surgery, and the impact of end-stage renal disease. Comorbidities of diabetes mellitus, lupus, malnutrition, and increased age may compound the effects of the immune response.[28,39] Common infections in the first month include bacterial and fungal wound infections, urinary tract infections, nosocomial pneumonitis, and line-associated bacteremias and fungemias.[39] Viral infections, especially those caused by CMV, EBV, HSV, and VZV, may be reactivated in the transplant patient due to pharmacologic immunosuppression and donor-recipient mismatching.[17] Infection with parvovirus or human polyomavirus (BK virus [BKV]) may also occur and can lead to graft dysfunction and potential graft loss.[39]

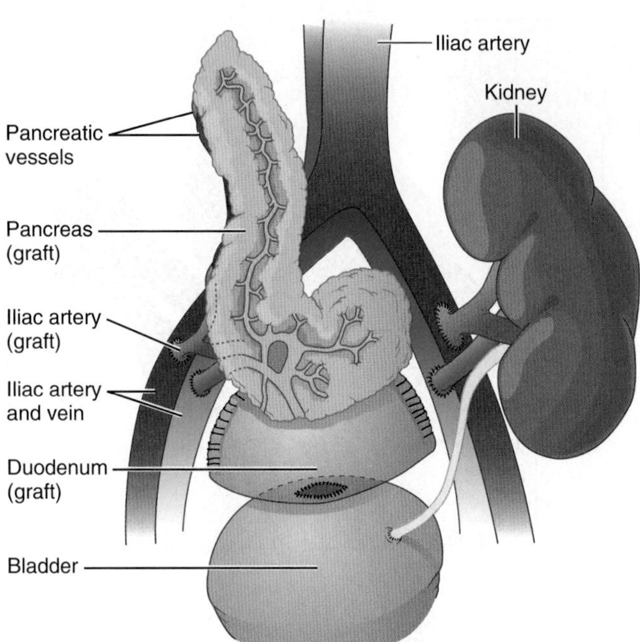

FIG. 20.5 Simultaneous kidney-pancreas transplant.

KIDNEY-PANCREAS OR PANCREAS-ONLY TRANSPLANTATION

Recipients

Pancreatic transplantation is a method of physiologically controlling glucose metabolism. As of 2015, there are a little over 1000 patients awaiting pancreas-only transplants. In 2014, there were 245 pancreas-only transplants performed.[59] Pancreas transplants are performed to achieve a euglycemic state. Pancreatic transplantation can be performed in three ways: pancreas alone; pancreas simultaneously transplanted with a kidney; or pancreas transplanted after an earlier kidney transplant. The majority of recipients for a pancreatic transplant have type 1 diabetes mellitus. Select type 2 diabetes patients who are insulin-dependent and have diabetic nephropathy may be considered. Recipients of a pancreatic transplant are admitted to critical care for 24 hours to ensure glycemic control and to monitor for the development of pancreatitis or rejection. The pancreas is a very immunogenic organ; the risk of rejection is higher than that for other organs.[30]

The pancreas transplant can be performed with either bowel (enteric) or bladder drainage (Fig. 20.5). Enteric drainage has distinct advantages over bladder drainage, and is more frequently used today. The use of enteric drainage has eliminated the complications of acidosis and dehydration, as well as many of the urologic complications. There are increased risks for abdominal complications with enteric drainage, such as peritonitis. In patients receiving a pancreas transplant after a kidney transplant, enteric drainage is preferred because it allows for better monitoring of the pancreas graft independent of the kidney transplant.[30,38]

Postoperative Complications and Considerations

Postoperative complications of pancreatic transplantation include vascular complications, acidosis, dehydration, rejection infection, hematuria, glycemic control, pancreatitis, and urethritis.[38]

Vascular

Vascular thrombosis occurs in 3% to 10% of transplanted organs.[38] It is a very early complication, occurring within 48 hours of transplantation. The thrombosis usually occurs in the pancreas portal vein. The cause is believed to be associated with reperfusion pancreatitis and the relatively low-flow state of the transplanted pancreas. Anticoagulation is the treatment for this condition. In patients who receive a simultaneous kidney-pancreas transplant, splenic vein thrombosis can occur if the anticoagulation is ineffective. Recipients who receive a pancreas alone are at risk for thrombosis of the transplanted organ, and necrosis if the anticoagulation is ineffective.[30,38]

Acidosis and Dehydration

In patients with a bladder-drained pancreas, bicarbonate and water secretions are not reabsorbed in the distal intestine, but instead are washed out of the bladder with the urine. Without replacement of the lost water and bicarbonate, these patients develop severe metabolic acidosis and dehydration with orthostatic hypotension. In addition, dehydration combined with hypotension and hypercoagulability causes thrombosis, which can lead to graft loss.[47] Intravascular volume must be maintained, and assessments of vital signs with CVP and urine output are key to maintaining blood flow. Serum bicarbonate levels less than 10 μmol/L and potassium levels greater than 6 μmol/L can develop. As a result of these conditions, patients are at an increased risk for electrocardiographic changes and dysrhythmias. Intravenous fluids often contain bicarbonate replacement, and oral supplementation is needed once the diet is advanced. These conditions do not occur in patients with enteric drainage.[30,38]

Immunosuppression

Management of immunosuppression is critical to long-term outcomes after transplantation. Intense immunosuppression prevents rejection, but increases the risk of infection and malignancy and may contribute to dysfunction of other organ systems. Weak immunosuppression decreases the risk of infection and malignancy, but increases the risk of rejection and subsequent transplanted organ dysfunction. Consequently, appropriate immunosuppression requires careful attention and close monitoring, and is always individualized (seeTable 20.1).[38]

Rejection

Early detection of graft rejection is a challenge. In recipients with simultaneous kidney-pancreas transplant, kidney dysfunction has been used to monitor both kidney and pancreas rejection. In bladder-drained pancreas transplants, monitoring the urinary amylase level provides information on the function of the pancreatic graft. With more enteric drainage transplants being performed, hyperglycemia can be a sign of rejection. The use of radionuclide pancreas examinations, and in some cases pancreatic biopsies, can provide information for timely diagnosis and treatment of rejection.[38]

Infection

The most common type of infection in the pancreas transplant patient with bladder drainage is urinary tract infections, which occur in more than 35% of patients.[30,38] The risk of infection is increased because of diabetes, recent urinary tract surgery, indwelling Foley catheters, immunosuppression therapy, and an increase in the urine pH from the pancreatic bicarbonate secretions. Recurrent urinary tract infections may also develop. Common organisms are *Staphylococcus, Enterococcus, Pseudomonas,* and *Candida;* thus, the risk for septicemia is high.[38]

Hematuria

Hematuria occurs in a small number of bladder-drained pancreatic recipients.[38] It is usually a result of ischemia-reperfusion injury to the duodenal mucosa or to a bleeding vessel on the suture line. The condition is aggravated by the anticoagulation protocols, but is self-limiting, lasting on average 1 to 2 weeks. The main concern is prevention of urethral obstruction from blood clots.

Glycemic Control

In the first few days to weeks after pancreatic transplantation, there is dramatic improvement in glucose control; however, hyperglycemia may occur as a result of the steroids used for immunosuppression. This usually responds to dose reduction. Occasionally, the hyperglycemia is due to delayed graft function. When hyperglycemia presents suddenly, it may be the result of pancreas graft thrombosis, and requires an ultrasound evaluation. If the thrombosis occurs early, or there is associated graft pain and fever, the patient may return to the operating room for reexploration.[30,38]

Pancreatitis

Almost all patients will have some degree of pancreatitis. Temporary elevation of serum amylase levels for 48 to 96 hours after transplantation is common. These episodes are usually transient and mild.[30,38] Allograft pancreatitis may be caused by reperfusion injury, donor instability, increased age of the donor, increased ischemic time, or rejection. In patients with enteric drainage, the development of a bowel obstruction may lead to pancreatitis. Patients with bladder drainage may develop reflux pancreatitis. This may be the result of urinary retention and reflux to the pancreas via the duodenal cuff, as a result of diabetic bladder dysfunction, bladder outlet obstruction, or a urinary tract infection (UTI). Reflux pancreatitis results in loss of bladder tone, reflux, and microbial irrigation. In the absence of retention, obstruction, or UTI, it may be caused by disruption of bladder filling pressures (bladder nerves sense when the bladder is full, which usually correlates with approximately 300 to 500 mL of urine).[38]

Urethritis

Many patients who receive bladder-drained grafts suffer from urologic complications secondary to pancreatic digestive enzymes and altered urinary pH. They are at increased risk for developing urethral strictures and cystitis with inflammation and hemorrhage. In worse cases, they may develop ureteral disruption. Female recipients are at risk for developing excoriating lesions of the perineum after a vaginal yeast infection, gross hematuria, anastomotic leaks, graft pancreatitis, rejection, thrombosis, or CMV duodenitis. Approximately 20% of bladder drainage recipients will require enteric conversion.[38]

Assessment

Nursing assessment of the kidney or kidney-pancreas transplant patient focuses on fluid and electrolyte management and prevention of infection. In addition, for those patients who received a pancreas transplant, glycemic monitoring is crucial. Accurate intake and output measurement and CVP pressure monitoring are key to maintaining fluid hemostasis. Evaluation and notification of the healthcare team of any electrolyte or glucose abnormalities and attention to electrolyte balance correction will minimize these patients' risk of complications. Assessment of vital signs, skin temperature, and wound integrity for early signs of infection can prevent the development of more serious infections and sepsis.

CONCLUSION

With the number of transplants being performed annually in the United States increasing, and the survival rates continuing to increase, critical care teams are more likely to see patients admitted with complications from their transplant or for non–transplant-related causes such as motor vehicle accidents or myocardial infarctions. Transplant patients take some form of immunosuppressive medication for the rest of their lives. Inadequate immunosuppression can lead to rejection, whereas too much immunosuppression can lead to increased risk of infection. Immunosuppressive regimens also put patients at increased risk for the development of malignant disease, including cancer of the skin, lips, colon, breast, and cervix, along with lymphomas. Transplant recipients can become pregnant and require the care of a high-risk obstetrician. It is important to note that, regardless of the reason the patient is admitted, the transplant team should be notified to evaluate the current condition and the immunosuppression regimen, and to provide consultation during the hospitalization.

The complexity of postoperative care is increased in transplant patients. Their special needs require attention to detail and identification of the nuances that can indicate the development of a complication that would place both the patient and the transplanted organ at risk.

REFERENCES

1. Agopian, G., Dhillon, A., Baber, J., et al. (2014). Liver transplantation in recipients receiving renal replacement therapy outcomes analysis and the role of intraoperative hemodialysis. *Am J Transplant, 14*, 1638–166.
2. Ayoub, W. S., Esquivel, C. O., & Martin, F. (2010). Biliary complications following liver transplantation. *Digestive Disease Science, 55*(6), 1540–1546. http://dx.doi.org/10.1007/s10620-010-1217-2.
3. Baranyi, A., Krauseneck, T., & Rothenhausler, H. B. (2013). Posttraumatic stress symptoms after solid organ transplantation: preoperative risk factors and the impact on health related quality of life and life satisfaction. *Health Qual Life Outcomes, 11*, 1111–121.
4. Bertuzzo, V.R., Ercolani, G., Cescon, M., Pinna, A.D. Retransplantation. In A.D. Pinna, & G. Ercolani (Eds.), *Abdominal solid organ transplantation: immunology, indications, techniques and early complications*. Gewerbestrasse, Switzerland: Springer International Publishing.
5. Bhat, M., Al-Busafi, S. A., Deschênes, M., & Ghali, P. (2014). Care of the liver transplant patient. *Can J Gastroenterol, 28*, 213–219.
6. Bulatao, I. G., Heckman, M. G., Rawal, B., et al. (2014). Avoiding stay in the intensive care unit after liver transplantation: a score to assign location of care. *Am J Transplant* (9), 2088–2096. http://dx.doi.org/10.1111/ajt.12796.
7. Chakkera, H. A., Knowler, W. C., Devanapalli, Y., et al. (2010). Relationship between inpatient hyperglycemia and insulin treatment after kidney transplantation and future new onset diabetes mellitus. *Clin J Am Soc Nephrol, 5*, 1669–1675.
8. Chaney, A. (2014). Primary care management of the liver transplant patient. *Nurse Pract, 39*(12), 26–33.
9. Cotler, S. J., Brown, R. S., & Travis, A. C. (2013). Treatment of acute cellular rejection in liver transplantation. *UpToDate*. http://www.uptodate.com/contents/treatment-of-acute-cellular-rejection-in-liver-transplantation?source=see_link.
10. Cupples, S. A. (2011). Transplant infectious disease: implications for critical care nurses. *Crit Care Nurs Clin North Am, 23*, 519–537.
11. De Gaspen, A., Feltracco, P., Ceravola, E., & Mazza, E. (2014). Pulmonary complications in patients receiving a solid organ transplant. *Curr Opin Crit Care, 20*, 411–419.
12. De Luca, L., Westbrook, R., & Tsochatzis, E. A. (2015). Metabolic and cardiovascular complications in the liver transplant recipient. *Ann Gastroenterol, 28*, 1–11.
13. Diaz, G. C., Wagener, G., & Renz, J. F. (2013). Postoperative care/critical care of the transplant patient. *Anesthesiol Clin, 31*, 723–735.
14. Douthitt, L., Bezinover, D., Yemura, T., et al. (2012). Perioperative use of continuous renal replacement therapy for orthotopic liver transplantation. *Transplant Proc, 44*, 1314–1317.
15. Ercolani, G., Cescon, M., Pinna, A.D. Postoperative Technical Complications. In A.D. Pinna, & G. Ercolani (Eds.), *Abdominal solid organ transplantation: immunology, indications, techniques and early complications*. Gewerbestrasse, Switzerland: Springer International Publishing.
16. Fabrizi, F., Dixit, V., Martin, P., & Messa, P. (2010). Chronic kidney disease after liver transplantation: recent evidence. *Int J Artif Organs, 33*, 803–811.
17. Fortun, J., Martin-Davila, P., Pascual, J., et al. (2010). Immunosuppressive therapy and infection after kidney transplantation. *Transpl Infect Dis, 12*(5), 397–405. http://dx.doi.org/10.1111/j.1399-3062.2010.00526.x.
18. Freise, C. E., Gillespie, B. W., Koffron, A. J., & A2ALL Study Group, et al. (2008). Recipient morbidity after living and deceased donor liver transplantation: findings from the A2ALL Retrospective Cohort Study. *Am J Transplant, 12*, 2569–2579.
19. García-Rodríguez, M., Piñón-Villar, Mdel, C., Lopez-Calvino, B., et al. (2015). Assessment of nutritional status and health-related quality of life before and after liver transplantation. *BMC Gastroenterol, 15*, 6. http://dx.doi.org/10.1186/s12876-015-0232-3.
20. Giannelli, M., Bartoletti, M., & Viale, P. (2015). Infection complications after abdominal organ transplant. In A. D. Pinna, & G. Ercolani (Eds.), *Abdominal solid organ transplantation: immunology, indications, techniques and early complications*. Gewerbestrasse, Switzerland: Springer International Publishing.
21. Gonwa, T. A., McBride, M. A., Anderson, K., Mai, M. L., Wadei, H., & Ahsan, N. (2006). Continued influence of preoperative renal function on outcome of orthotopic liver transplant (OLTX) in the US: where will MELD lead us? *Am J Transplant, 6*, 2651–2659.
22. Green, M. (2013). Introduction: infections in solid organ transplantation. *Am J Transplant, 13*, 3–8.
23. Grogan, T. A. (2011). Liver transplantation: issues and nursing care requirements. *Crit Care Nurs Clin North Am, 23*, 443–456.
24. Hammad, A., Kaido, T., & Uemoto, S. (2015). Perioperative nutritional therapy in liver transplantation. *Surg Today, 45*, 271–283.
25. Hernandez, M. D. P., Martin, P., & Simkins, J. (2015). Infectious Complications After Liver Transplantation. *Gastroenterol Hepatol, 11*, 742–753.
26. Hsu, S. C., Jeng, L. B., Thorat, A., et al. (2014). Management of extensive retrohepatic vena cava defect in recipients of living donor liver transplantation. *Transplant Proceedings, 46*, 699–704. http://dx.doi.org/10.1016/j.transproceed.2013.11.118.
27. Hupriker, S., & Shoham, S. (2013). Emerging fungal infections in solid organ transplantation. *Am J Transplant, 13*, 262–271.
28. Issa, N., & Braun, W. E. (2010). Immunosuppression for renal transplant patients and common medical problems in renal transplantation. *Disease Management*, *Cleveland Clinic*.

29. Jacobi, J., Bircher, N., Krinsley, J., et al. (2012). Guidelines for the use of an insulin infusion for the management of hyperglycemia in critically ill patients. *Crit Care Med, 40*, 3251–3276.
30. James, M. M. (2011). Nursing care of the pancreas transplant recipient. *Crit Care Nurs Clin North Am, 23*, 425–441.
31. Kawecki, D., Pacholczyk, M., Lagiewska, B., et al. (2014). Bacterial and fungal infections in the early post-transplantation period after liver transplantation: etiologic agents and their susceptibility. *Transplant Proceedings, 46*, 2777–2781.
32. Lazar, H. L., McDonnell, M., Chipkin, S. R., et al. (2008). The society of thoracic surgeons practice guideline series: blood glucose management during adult cardiac surgery. *Ann Thorac Surg, 87*, 663–669.
33. Lee, Y., Kwon, O., Shin, C. S., & Lee, S. M. (2015). Use of bioelectrical impedance analysis for the assessment of nutritional status in critically ill patients. *Clin Nutr Res, 4*, 32–40. http://dx.doi.org/10.7762/cnr.2015.4.1.32.
34. Lucey, M. R., Terrault, N., Ojo, L., et al. (2013). Long-term management of the successful adult liver transplant: 2012 practice guideline by AASLD and the American Society of Transplantation. *Liver Transpl, 19*(1), 3–26. http://dx.doi.org/10.1002/lt.23566.
35. Mangray, M., & Vella, J. (2011). Hypertension after kidney transplant. *Am J Kidney Dis, 57*(2), 331–341. 11p. http://dx.doi.org/10.1053/j.ajkd.2010.10.048.
36. McCaffery, D. A. (2011). Crit Care Nurs Clin North Am. *Crit Care Nurs Clin of North Am, 23*, 393–404.
37. Meireles, M. S., Wazlawik, E., Bastos, J. L., & Garcia, M. F. (2012). Comparison between nutritional risk tools and parameters derived from bioelectrical impedance analysis with subjective global assessment. *J Acad Nutr Diet, 112*(10), 1543–1549. http://dx.doi.org/10.1016/j.jand.2012.07.005.
38. Molmenti, E. P., & Dowling, M. J. (2015). *Kidney and Pancreas Transplantation*. New Deli, India: 2015 Dowling Jaypee Brothers Medical Pub.
39. Morris, P., & Knechtle, S. J. (2013). *Kidney Transplantation - Principles and Practice: expert Consult 7e (Morris, Kidney Transplantation)*. Philadelphia, Publisher: Saunders.
40. Murthy, T. V. S.P. (2008). Critical care issues in liver transplantation: a review. *Indian J Anaesth, 52*, 705–712.
41. Ney, M., Abraldes, J. G., Ma, M., et al. (2015). Insufficient protein intake is associated with increased mortality in 630 patients with cirrhosis awaiting liver transplantation. *Nutr Clin Pract, 30*, 530–536.
42. O'Leary, J. G., & Trotter, J. F. (2015). Late complications and recurrence of disease after transplant. In R. W. Busuttil, & G. B. Klintmalm (Eds.), *Transplantation of the liver: expert consult* (pp. 1051–1061). Philadelphia: Saunders.
43. Olthoff, K. M., Abecassis, M. M., Emond, J. C., & Adult-to-Adult Living Donor Liver Transplantation Cohort Study Group, et al. (2011). Outcomes of adult living donor liver transplantation: comparison of the Adult-to-Adult Living Donor Liver Transplantation Cohort Study and the national experience. *Liver Transplant, 17*, 789–797. http://dx.doi.org/10.1002/lt.22288.
44. Parikh, A., & Shaw, A. (2012). The economics of renal failure and kidney disease in critically ill patients. *Crit Care Clin, 28*, 99–111.
45. Parvinian, A., & Gaba, R. C. (2014). Sequential Venoplasty for Treatment of Inferior Vena Cava Stenosis Following Liver Transplant. *J Clin Imaging Sci, 4*, 50.
46. Petrowsky, H., Rana, A., Kaldas, F. M., et al. (2014). Liver transplantation in highest-acuity recipients: identifying factors to avoid futility. *Ann Surg, 259*, 1186–1194.
47. Ponticelli, C., Moia, M., & Montagnino, G. (2009). Renal allograft thrombosis. *Nephrol Dial Transplant, 24*, 1388–1393. http://dx.doi.org/10.1093/ndt/gfp003.
48. Razonable, R. R., Findlay, J. Y., O'Riodan, A., et al. (2011). Critical care issues in patients after liver transplantation. *Liver Transplant, 17*(5), 511–527.
49. Rehman, A., Setter, S. M., & Vue, M. H. (2011). Drug-Induced Glucose Alterations Part 2: Drug-Induced Hyperglycemia. *Diabetes Spectr, 24*, 234–238. http://dx.doi.org/10.2337/diaspect.24.4.234.
50. Rollins, J. L. (2013). Hyperglycemic management after solid organ transplantation. *Crit Care Nurs Clin North Am, 25*, 31–38.
51. Romero, F. A., & Razonable, R. R. (2011). Infections in liver transplant recipients. *World J Hepatol, 3*(4), 83–92. http://doi.org/10.4254/wjh.v3.i4.83.
52. Rudow, D. L., & Goldstein, M. J. (2008). Critical Care Management of the Liver Transplant Recipient. *Crit Care Nurs Q, 31*, 237–243.
53. Russell, C. L. (2013). Optimal care for kidney transplant recipients. *OR Nurse, 7*, 36–40.
54. Saidi, R. F., Jabbour, N., Li, Y., Shah, S. A., & Bozorgzadeh, A. (2011). Outcomes in partial liver transplantation: deceased donor split-liver vs. live donor liver transplantation. *HPB (Oxford), 13*, 797–801. http://dx.doi.org/10.1111/j.1477-2574.2011.00360.x.
55. Thompson, J. A., & Kukla, A. (2015). Liver and pancreas transplantation. In S. W. Ashley (Ed.), *Scientific American Surgery*. Philadelphia: Decker Intellectual Properties.
56. Thuluvath, P. J., Guidinger, M. K., Fung, J. J., Johnson, L. B., Rayhill, S. C., & Pelletier, S. J. (2010). Liver transplantation in the United States, 1999–2008. *Am J Transplant, 10*, 1003–1019.
57. Thurairajah, P. H., Carbone, M., Bridgestock, H., et al. (2013). Late acute liver allograft rejection; a study of its natural history and graft survival in the current era. *Transplantation, 95*, 955–959.
58. Tinti, F., Umbro, I., Giannelli, V., et al. (2011). Acute renal failure in liver transplant recipients: role of pretransplantation renal function and 1-year follow-up. *Transplant Proceedings, 43*, 1136–1138. http://dx.doi.org/10.1016/j.transproceed.2011.02.042.
59. United Network for Organ Sharing (UNOS) Statistics. (2015). *Organ procurement and transplantation network (OPTN). Liver Transpl.* 17(7):789–797, 2011. http://www.unos.org.

21

Electrolyte Emergencies

Nicole Kupchik

Electrolyte imbalances impact both the mortality and morbidity of critically ill patients and can present a range of issues that often require the efforts of an interprofessional team. Typically, electrolyte imbalances are the result of an underlying disease, but may also be caused by a patient's behaviors (e.g., a patient with a psychiatric disorder who drinks 10 gallons of water in less than 24 hours). They may be iatrogenic, as seen with the excessive use of diuretics or prolonged bedrest. Electrolyte imbalances may present as a minor problem or represent a life-threatening emergency requiring immediate treatment.

The electrolyte imbalances most commonly seen in the critical care setting are those involving potassium, sodium, and calcium. Phosphorus and magnesium imbalances are less commonly discussed in nursing literature. As a result, there may be less general knowledge regarding the importance of these electrolytes in bodily functions, the assessment and cause of their abnormalities, and an understanding of the appropriate therapy.

Laboratory-derived serum electrolyte values are usually used as the reference points for these imbalances. However, these values must be assessed in the context of the patient's disease process, a physical examination, and an understanding of the patient's comorbidities and current treatments. Electrolyte reference values will differ from reference to reference and from institution to institution, depending upon the method of analysis used.[34] In the clinical setting, it is important to understand and have access to the specific institution's reference values.

An additional issue for consideration is that different parts of the world use different units of measurement. Countries that use Système Internationale (SI) units of measurement convey electrolyte concentrations in terms of a millimole (mmol), which is equal to one thousandth of the molecular weight of the electrolyte in question. Healthcare institutions in the United States typically report some electrolyte concentrations (potassium and sodium) in terms of milliequivalents per liter (mEq/L). Calcium, magnesium, and phosphorus are usually reported in milligrams per deciliter (mg/dL). For those electrolytes that are measured in mEq/L, a simple conversion to mmol/L units is found by dividing the mEq/L by the chemical's valence (mmol/L equals mEq/L divided by the valence). However, a significant amount of confusion exists when comparing the remaining electrolytes (calcium, magnesium, and phosphorus) because they are measured in milligrams per deciliter (mg/dL) in the United States and millimoles per liter (mmol/L) with the SI system.[26] For clarity, it must be noted not only that the reference measurement is different (mg vs. mmol) but also that the reference volumes for each are different (mg/dL vs. mmol/L). For ease of reference and to avoid confusion, both measurement systems will be displayed when discussing the various electrolyte levels. The electrolyte levels used as both "normal" and excessively high and low "critical" levels in this chapter are derived from Jacobs, DeMott, and Oxley and are specific to the adult patient (Table 21.1).[15] It is important to note that the critical levels from this source are often significantly beyond the normal upper and lower limits. If an electrolyte level is outside the normal range but has not reached the critical limit, it needs to be thoroughly evaluated in the context of the patient's condition and may require emergency treatment to prevent patient harm.

The most effective prevention for electrolyte imbalances is to maintain adequate nutrition. In a normal, healthy state, adults seldom need any electrolyte supplementation. However, as previously noted, electrolyte abnormalities in a healthy patient may be caused by patient behaviors or by therapies designed to treat a specific disease.

APPLIED PHYSIOLOGY

Electrolytes are found throughout the body in bone, muscle, and cartilage; bound to protein; and in intracellular and extracellular fluid as free or ionized electrolytes in the blood's serum. Electrolytes are either positively charged ions, referred to as cations, or negatively charge ions, referred to as anions. Each electrolyte charge is shown by a superscript "+" or "–" after the chemical symbol (e.g., K^+ for potassium and Na^+ for sodium).[14] Serum electrolyte measurements are the basis for diagnosing and treating electrolyte imbalances. Electrolytes are actively shifted back and forth between the intracellular fluid (ICF) and extracellular fluid (ECF) by the various mechanisms of the cellular membrane. The shifting of electrolytes creates electrical potentials that occur at the cellular level, allowing each cell to complete its specific function. The relative distribution of the various electrolytes in both intracellular and extracellular fluids is displayed in Table 21.2. Electrolyte concentrations are also affected by the acid-base balance (see Chapter 22). Each electrolyte is regulated by specific pathways within the body and each has specific roles in maintaining homeostasis.[26]

TABLE 21.1 Normal Adult Serum Levels of Electrolytes

Electrolyte	US Units	Système Internationale (SI) Units
Potassium	3.5-5.5 mEq/L	3.5-5.5 mmol/L
Sodium	135-145 mEq/L	135-145 mmol/L
Calcium		
Serum	8.6-10 mg/dL	2.15-2.50 mmol/L
Ionized	4.64-5.28 mg/dL	1.16-1.32 mmol/L
Magnesium	1.5-2.3 mg/dL	0.62-0.95 mmol/L
Phosphorus	2.5-4.5 mg/dL	0.81-1.45 mmol/L

Data from Reference 15.

TABLE 21.2 Distribution of Electrolytes in Body Compartments

	Extracellular Fluid (ECF)	Intracellular Fluid (ICF)
Potassium	5 mEq/L	156 mEq/L
Sodium	142 mEq/L or mmol/L	10 mEq/L or mmol/L
Calcium	5 mg/dL	4 mg/dL
Magnesium	2 mg/dl or mEq/L	26 mg/dL or mEq/L
Phosphate	2 mg/dL	40-95 mg/dL

Modified from Reference 14.

POTASSIUM

Applied Physiology

Potassium (K^+) is the major intracellular electrolyte. Approximately 98% of the body's total potassium is normally stored inside the cells (in the ICF), and the other 2% is maintained in the ECF. This is referred to as the potassium gradient.[5] This gradient regulates the electrical membrane potential of both muscle and nerve cells, affecting the excitability of both types of cells, and contributes to contractions of skeletal, smooth, and cardiac muscles.[14] The most life-threatening issue related to potassium imbalance occurs in cardiac conduction and contraction. Extremes of potassium cause significant conduction defects and dysrhythmias. A high serum potassium level will decrease the resting potential of a cell; thus the cell will require a greater stimulus to reach the threshold potential. This will result in decreased contractile force of the heart and delayed conduction, causing widened QRS complexes and bradycardia. With a decreased serum potassium level, the resting potential of a cell will be increased, requiring less stimulus to reach the threshold potential of the cell, and making it more likely the patient will develop ventricular dysrhythmias. In addition, the rate of repolarization is increased with high serum potassium levels and decreased with low serum potassium levels. Because of its importance in a variety of systems, even small changes in serum potassium concentrations may produce significant changes in cellular functioning.[5,20,34]

Potassium is important for maintenance of the osmotic gradient within cells, maintenance of acid-base balance, and concentration of urine by the kidney. Potassium is an important component in energy metabolism, including the conversion of carbohydrates to energy, amino acids into protein, and glucose into glycogen.[34]

Since most potassium comes from the diet, this can be problematic in a hospitalized patient receiving nothing by mouth (NPO). Potassium's excretion is primarily regulated by the kidneys. However, because the kidneys may take several hours to excrete a significant load of potassium, it can shift back and forth between the ECF and ICF quite rapidly, temporarily normalizing serum potassium levels.

In the kidney, potassium is initially freely filtered out of the blood as it passes through the glomerulus. Potassium is selectively reabsorbed from the filtrate in the proximal tubule and loop of Henle. Then, depending on serum levels, potassium may be secreted into the filtrate in the distal and collecting tubules and eliminated in the urine. This mechanism allows the body to closely regulate potassium levels based on the ECF concentration. Aldosterone plays an important role in regulating both potassium and sodium concentrations. Aldosterone causes the kidneys to retain sodium at the expense of potassium, which is then lost into the urine. Renal regulation of potassium is also significantly affected by the hydrogen ion concentration (acid).[34]

Shifts of potassium between the ICF and ECF are caused by a number of factors. Endogenous and exogenous sources of epinephrine and insulin cause a shift of potassium from the ECF to the ICF. Epinephrine causes the shift to occur as a response to stress, pain, or any process stimulating the sympathetic nervous system—the fight or flight response. Insulin causes the shift of potassium into the cells to sequester the high potassium loads that may occur with the ingestion of a meal. Conditions that cause an increased extracellular osmolality, such as diabetic ketoacidosis (DKA), will cause water to shift out of the cells, creating an artificial increase in the ICF potassium level, which then moves into the ECF by diffusion. In an acidotic state, excess hydrogen ions (H^+) enter the cells and force the potassium into the ECF, increasing the serum levels of potassium. In an alkalotic state, this process is reversed, pulling potassium into the cells and decreasing the serum levels. Both of these processes are in response to the cell's attempt to maintain electrical neutrality. The body has a tremendous ability to adapt to increased intake of potassium over time. This process, known as *potassium adaption,* occurs as the potassium intake increases, causing an increase in renal excretion of potassium.[14] However, in certain clinical situations, especially when the shifts occur rapidly, the increased intake of potassium can produce changes in the potassium levels that are lethal.[34]

Laboratory Findings

As noted in Table 21.1, a normal potassium value is 3.5 to 5.5 mEq/L (3.5 to 5.5 mmol/L). The correct technique in drawing the potassium blood sample is important to ensure accurate results. If the patient squeezes the fist during a venous blood draw, the muscular contraction may release potassium from the muscles, falsely elevating the potassium level. In addition, the use of a tourniquet should be avoided if possible.[15] Because hemolysis of red blood cells will liberate potassium and falsely elevate the serum level, it is imperative to make every effort to prevent hemolysis from occurring. Hemolysis can occur with something as simple as shaking the blood-filled tube or sending the sample through a pneumatic tube system.[26]

Hyperkalemia

Fig. 21.1 provides an algorithm for diagnosing the cause of hyperkalemia. Because potassium is efficiently excreted by the kidneys, it is unusual for hyperkalemia to occur when renal

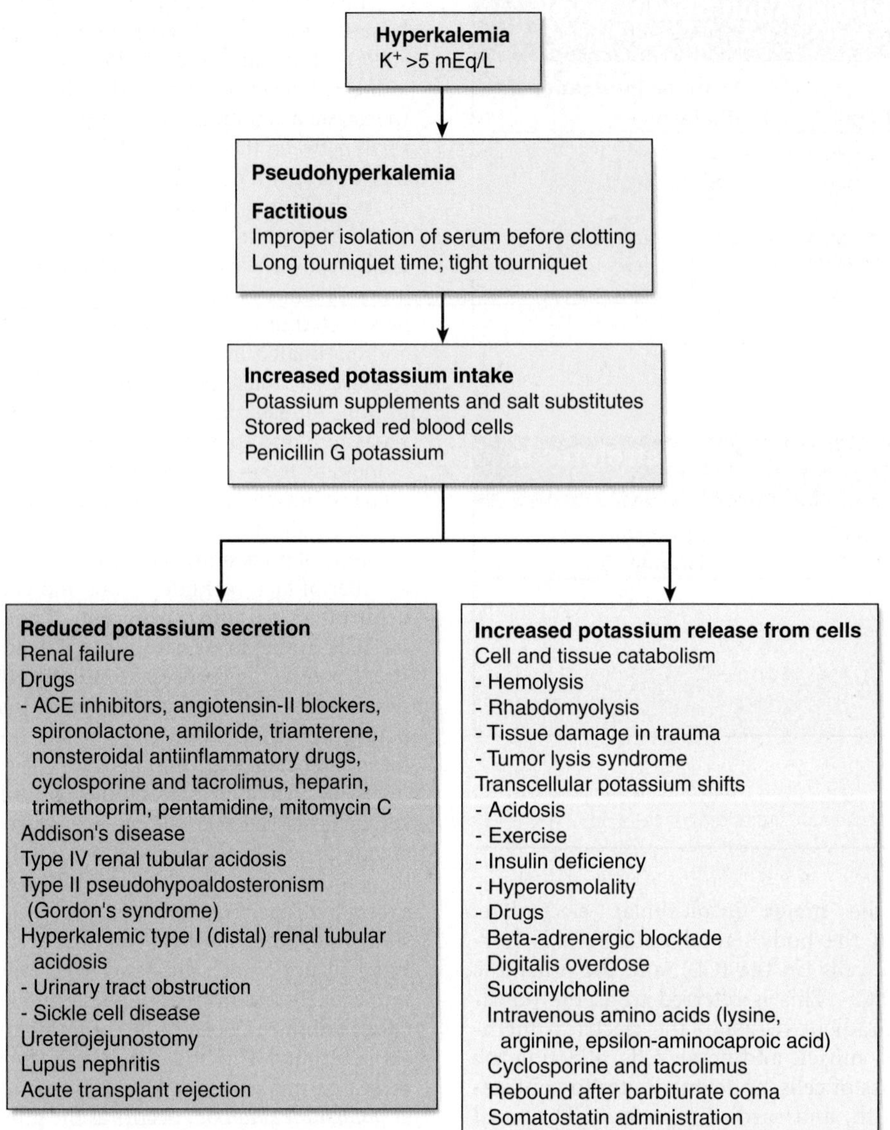

FIG. 21.1 Algorithm for diagnosing the cause of hyperkalemia. *K^+*, Potassium.

function is normal. When the kidneys are damaged, as in acute tubular necrosis (ATN), or in a more chronic condition such as chronic renal failure, there is a loss of ability to filter and excrete potassium and hyperkalemia occurs, with the level increasing above 5.5 mEq/L (5.5 mmol/L). If renal function is even partially compromised from a variety of sources (e.g., nonsteroidal antiinflammatory drugs [NSAIDs], hypotension, hypoxia, hypovolemia, sepsis, advanced age), the patient is at an increased risk for hyperkalemia, especially when supplemental potassium is given. Close observation of laboratory results is necessary to identify problems early.

A number of medications can cause an elevated potassium level. Two common classes of drugs given to patients with hypertension or heart disease are angiotensin-converting enzyme (ACE) inhibitors and angiotensin receptor blockers (ARBs). Both classes are implicated in hyperkalemia, especially when diabetes, heart failure, or decreased renal function is also present.[30,32] The use of spironolactone (Aldactone), a potassium-sparing diuretic used in the treatment of hypertension and heart failure, inhibits potassium secretion into the filtrate of the distal renal tubule.[26] Subcutaneous heparin, 5000 units twice a day, can increase potassium levels by up to 1.7 mEq/L (1.7 mmol/L) over a period of 3 days.[32] There are also a number of herbal supplements that have substantial amounts of potassium (noni juice, alfalfa, dandelion, horsetail, and nettle). Digitalis-like substances that may exacerbate hyperkalemia are found in such herbal remedies as chan su, milkweed, lily of the valley, Siberian ginseng, and hawthorn berries.[30] The risk factors for hyperkalemia tend to be cumulative, increasing the likelihood for hyperkalemia when more factors are present. Within the critical care setting, renal insufficiency or failure, coupled with the delivery of exogenous potassium, is a common cause of hyperkalemia.[5,14,34]

Elevated potassium levels are also seen in a state of acidosis. This can be caused by a variety of respiratory or metabolic sources (e.g., hypoventilation, lactic acid accumulation, certain drug overdoses, or DKA). As the pH decreases, the accumulating hydrogen ions are shifted into the ICF, driving the potassium into the ECF and increasing serum levels.

Since potassium is available mostly in the ICF, any mechanism that causes significant muscle damage (e.g., crush injuries, burns, damage to large muscle groups) will cause the release of potassium from the damaged tissue.[14] In addition, such injuries also release excessive amounts of myoglobin, which can obstruct the glomerulus, preventing potassium from being filtered from the blood. This process is referred to as rhabdomyolysis and, even in the face of normal baseline renal function, these sudden increases in potassium levels may drive the ECF level into the abnormally high range.[26]

Additional causes of hyperkalemia include excessive use of potassium-containing salt substitutes, a common dietary recommendation for cardiac patients to decrease sodium consumption, especially if large amounts are consumed quickly.[15,32] Addison's disease, and the resultant decrease in aldosterone production, can cause a decrease in the amount of potassium excreted by the kidney, raising the potassium level. Again, it must be noted that significant increases in potassium levels are usually the result of some decrease in renal function with a concomitant increase of potassium in the ECF.

As noted previously, potassium has a significant impact on the action potential of cells. This is especially important in the cardiac system, where both the conduction system and the myocardium itself rely on potassium. As the potassium level increases, the cells will depolarize more rapidly from their resting potential. If the potassium continues to increase, the resting potential will exceed the threshold potential and the cells will not be able to repolarize. This phenomenon is frequently seen in the characteristic electrocardiogram (ECG) changes that reflect both hyperkalemia and hypokalemia (Fig. 21.2 and Table 21.3). As the potassium level increases, the T wave becomes tall and peaked, with a shortened QT interval. If the potassium level continues to increase, the PR interval will become prolonged, the QRS complex will widen, and the ST segment will become depressed, often with bradycardia.[5,34] Because of the importance of potassium in neuromuscular conduction and contraction, elevated potassium levels will interfere with these functions within the heart and can be lethal if not quickly corrected.

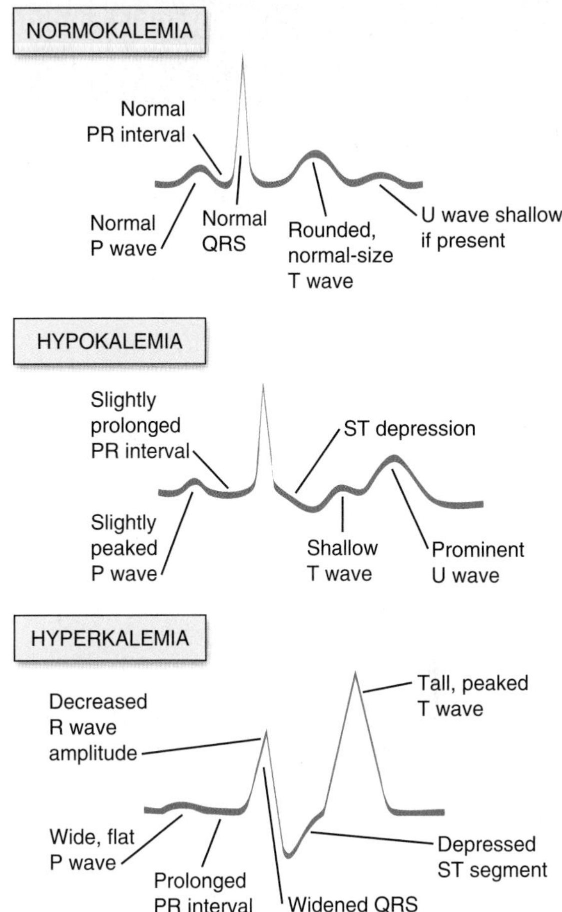

FIG. 21.2 ECG changes with potassium imbalances.

Physical Assessment Findings

In hyperkalemia, commonly seen symptoms include paresthesias (typically the first sign), nausea, vomiting, abdominal cramps, diarrhea, weakness, dizziness, muscle cramps, hypotension,[14,26] and ascending paralysis. In addition, the ECG changes described previously may be the first indication of the abnormality.[5,20,34]

Laboratory Findings

When potassium levels increase to greater than 5.5 mEq/L (> 5.5 mmol/L), the nurse will need to assess for contributing factors such as the presence of potassium in IV solutions, parenteral nutrition (PN), and medications; the existence of acidosis; decreasing renal function; and the use of medications that could increase potassium levels.[15] The patient's condition will also need to be assessed to determine if they are exhibiting signs and symptoms of hyperkalemia with the potassium level likely to continuing to rise. If the patient is exhibiting signs and symptoms of hyperkalemia, immediate treatment will need to be initiated. A potassium level of greater than 6.5 mEq/L (> 6.5 mmol/L) is considered a critical level and medical emergency.[15,16]

Treatment

When hyperkalemia is noted, the first steps are to reduce potassium intake, by eliminating any potassium supplementation, and any medication that potentially increases potassium levels (e.g., spironolactone, ACE inhibitors, ARBs).[5,20]

The American Heart Association's Advanced Cardiac Life Support for Experienced Providers (ACLS-EP) uses a staggered approach to treating hyperkalemia. Mild hyperkalemia (5 to 6 mEq/L [5 to 6 mmol/L]) is treated by removing potassium from the body by a number of means, including furosemide (Lasix), 1 mg/kg (40–80 mg) slow IV push; sodium polystyrene sulfonate (Kayexalate), 15 to 50 g, per mouth, nasogastric tube or per rectum (PR) via retention enema; or dialysis, depending upon the patient's history and condition.[5] Sodium polystyrene sulfonate is a resin that exchanges sodium for potassium in the gut, increasing the sodium concentration in the ECF. It should be used with caution in patients with heart failure, concurrent hypernatremia, or new onset gastrointestinal issues (obstruction). In addition, if given per rectum, it must be retained for more than 30 to 60 minutes to create effective ion exchange, which can be a challenge for the patient.[26,39]

New agents to treat mild, nonemergency hyperkalemia work by binding free potassium ions in the gastrointestinal tract and releasing either sodium and/or calcium ions for exchange. Sodium zirconium cyclosilicate (ZS-9), which is an inorganic, nonabsorbable crystalline compound that exchanges both sodium and hydrogen ions for potassium, is currently under investigation. The efficacy of ZS-9 in hyperkalemic outpatients

TABLE 21.3 Electrocardiographic Findings Associated with Disturbances in Serum Electrolyte Levels

Electrolyte Abnormality	Electrocardiographic Findings
Hypokalemia	Decreased T-wave amplitude T-wave inversion ST segment depression Prominent U wave Prolongation of QT (U) interval Ventricular tachycardia Torsades de pointes
Hyperkalemia	
Mild	Large-amplitude T waves "Peaked" or "tented" T waves
Moderate	PR interval prolongation Decreased P-wave amplitude, disappearance QRS complex widening Conduction blocks with escape beats
Severe	Sine wave pattern Ventricular fibrillation Asystole
Hypocalcemia	Prolongation of QTc interval Ventricular dysrhythmias Torsades de pointes
Hypercalcemia	Shortening of QTc interval Bradydysrhythmias
Hypomagnesemia or hypermagnesemia	No unique ECG abnormalities, but often associated with calcium abnormalities

was evaluated in randomized placebo-controlled trials, which found the mean serum potassium was significantly lower with ZS-9 as compared with placebo. Similarly, the proportion of normokalemic patients was significantly greater with ZS-9 and serious adverse events were uncommon. It is suggested that ZS-9 has an acute effect on intestinal potassium secretion, rather than simply a reduction in potassium absorption.[19] Patiromer (Veltassa) is a newly released agent that works by binding potassium in the colon in exchange for calcium. In the OPAL-HK study, 76% of participants who were hyperkalemic and receiving RAAS inhibitor therapy reached normal serum potassium levels within 4 weeks.[29,49] These agents are effective over days to weeks. Therefore, they are not indicated for emergency treatment of hyperkalemia, but for use in mild hyperkalemia.

ACLS-EP defines moderate hyperkalemia as potassium levels from 6 to 7 mEq/L (6 to 7 mmol/L) and recommends therapies that are designed to create a temporary shift of potassium from the ECF into the ICF, thus temporarily decreasing the serum potassium levels. This shift may be accomplished by one of three different medications. Sodium bicarbonate, up to 1 mEq/kg, is given over 5 minutes, creating a temporary alkalosis. A combination of glucose (25 g of a 50% solution) and regular insulin (10 units) given over 15 to 30 minutes drives potassium into the ICF. Nebulized albuterol, 5 to 20 mg, may be given over 15 minutes.[5]

With a severe potassium elevation (> 6.5 mEq/L [> 6.5 mmol/L]) or when a widened QRS complex or other potassium-induced ECG changes are found, immediate steps must be taken to counteract the effects of potassium on the cardiac conduction system. The initial emergency treatment is to give 5 to 10 mL of 10% calcium chloride over 2 to 5 minutes. Calcium chloride is then followed by sodium bicarbonate or IV insulin and glucose, as noted previously, to shift the potassium from the ECF to the ICF. Follow-up treatment removes potassium from the body and includes diuretics, exchange resins, or renal replacement therapy (dialysis). Dialysis is the treatment of choice with hyperkalemia associated with renal failure.[5,26] Table 21.4 summarizes the treatments for hyperkalemia.

Hypokalemia

Applied Physiology and Pathophysiology

Hypokalemia (< 3.5 mEq/L [< 3.5 mmol/L]) may be caused by a number of problems. Fig. 21.3 provides an algorithm to use in diagnosing the causes of hypokalemia. Whereas a lack of dietary intake is a possible source of the problem, hypokalemia is typically confined to those patients who do not consume adequate amounts of protein, fruits, and vegetables.[50] The groups at risk for inadequate intake include older adults, patients with chronic alcohol abuse, patients with eating disorders, and patients receiving loop diuretics.[14] In addition, though it is not clear how the relationship occurs, hypokalemia can also be caused by hypomagnesemia.[26]

A change in the blood pH can have a profound effect on potassium levels. A decrease in the hydrogen ion concentration will cause an increase in the pH, a state of alkalosis, that drives the potassium into the intracellular fluid, decreasing the serum potassium levels.[14]

The body may lose potassium from both the gastrointestinal (GI) and renal systems. Vomiting, diarrhea, and GI suctioning will cause a loss of potassium but, more importantly, sodium, chloride, and hydrogen ions are also lost. The loss of both fluid and sodium further activates the renin-angiotensin-aldosterone system, which causes the kidneys to increase potassium excretion because of sodium retention, decreasing the serum potassium levels. The loss of hydrogen ions may create an alkalotic state, driving the potassium from the ECF to the ICF. Diarrhea may also cause significant losses of potassium because the considerable amounts of potassium in the intestinal contents will not be absorbed as a result of its rapid transit through the gut.[14,26] Potassium is reabsorbed in the distal tubules of the kidneys. Common diuretics (thiazides, furosemide, bumetanide [Bumex], osmotic diuretics) cause an increase in secretion of sodium, which in turn increases the tubular urine flow. This increased tubular urine flow then inhibits potassium reabsorption, causing hypokalemia as potassium is lost in the urine. This is the rationale for potassium supplementation in many patients taking diuretics. The use of loop and osmotic diuretics is the most common cause of hypokalemia.[34] Hypokalemia is found in more than 20% of hospitalized patients and may be present in 40% of patients taking thiazide diuretics.[11] Another medication implicated in hypokalemia is the common bronchodilation agent albuterol. Two treatments within 1 hour can decrease the serum potassium level by up to 1 mEq/L (1 mmol/L).[11]

When a diabetic patient experiences DKA or hyperosmolar hyperglycemic state (HHS), the excess hydrogen ions cause a significant shift of potassium from the ICF to the ECF, increasing the serum potassium level. Potassium is lost in the significant diuresis that occurs early with hyperglycemia. This is one of the hallmarks of DKA and HHS. When DKA and HHS are treated with fluids, the acidosis is reversed and the potassium in the ECF shifts into the ICF, causing a clinically significant

TABLE 21.4 Treatments For Hyperkalemia

Treatment	Dose	Route	Time to Onset	Duration of Effect	Mechanism of Action and Effects
Calcium chloride, calcium gluconate*†	1-2 g (10-20 mL of 10% solution)	Intravenous over 5-10 min	1-2 min	10-30 min	Antagonizes cardiac conduction abnormalities
Sodium bicarbonate*	50-100 mEq	Intravenous over 2-5 min	30 min	2-6 h	Increases serum pH; redistributes potassium into cells
Insulin (regular)* (with dextrose)	5-10 units	Intravenous with 50 mL of 50% dextrose injection	15-45 min	2-6 h	Redistributes potassium into cells
Dextrose 50%	50 mL (25 g)	Intravenous over 5 min	30 min	2-6 h	Increases insulin release; redistributes potassium into cells; prevents hypoglycemia when insulin is given
Dextrose 10%	1000 mL (100 g)	Intravenous over 1-2 h	30 min	2-6 h	Increases insulin release; redistributes potassium into cells; prevents hypoglycemia when given with insulin
Furosemide	20-40 mg	Intravenous	5-15 min	4-6 h	Increases renal potassium loss
Sodium polystyrene sulfonate‡	15-60 g	Oral or rectal	1 h	4-6 h	Resin exchanges sodium for potassium; increases fecal potassium elimination
Albuterol	10-20 mg	Nebulized over 10 min	30 min	1-2 h	Stimulates sodium-potassium pump; redistributes potassium into cells
Hemodialysis	2-4 h	Not applicable	Immediate	Variable	Removes potassium from plasma
Patiromer (Veltassa)	8.4 g daily	Oral	7 hours	Days	Binds potassium in GI tract
ZS-9 (not approved)	10 g	Oral	Hours	Days	Binds potassium in GI tract

*First-line therapies in hyperkalemic emergencies.
†Repeat dose in 5 minutes if abnormal electrocardiogram persists. Calcium chloride may also be used, but calcium gluconate is preferred over calcium chloride for peripheral venous administration because it causes less venous irritation. Calcium chloride (1000 mg = 13.6 mEq calcium) provides three times more calcium than calcium gluconate (1 g = 4.56 mEq calcium).
‡Can be used to treat acute hyperkalemia, but the effects may not be seen for several hours. Removes 0.5-1 mEq of potassium per 1 g of sodium polystyrene sulfonate.
GI, Gastrointestinal.

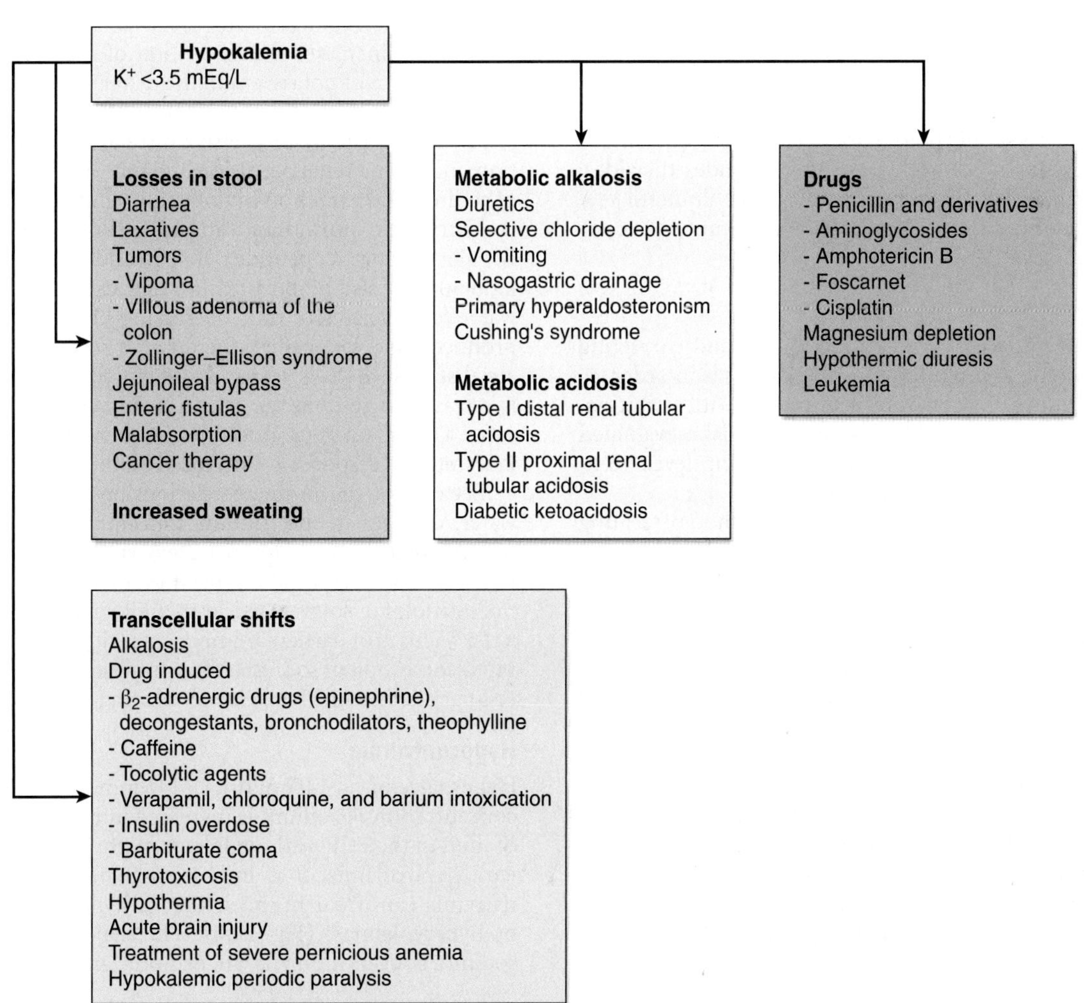

FIG. 21.3 Algorithm for diagnosing the causes of hypokalemia.

lowering of the ECF potassium level. Insulin exacerbates this process because it facilitates the passage of both glucose and potassium into the ICF.[4]

When the potassium level in the ECF is low, the ECG is adversely affected. The PR interval becomes prolonged and the ST segment depressed. The T wave becomes flattened and the U wave may become noticeable. Whereas ECG changes associated with hypokalemia are not usually life-threatening, when associated with digitalis toxicity they can cause lethal ventricular dysrhythmias, particularly in patients with preexisting cardiac dysfunction.[11] Potassium and digitalis compete for the same binding sites of the sodium-potassium pump on the cellular membrane. If there is less potassium to bind to the sites, digitalis will bind to the sites and exert an exaggerated effect, such as profound bradycardia.[14]

Physical Assessment Findings

The symptoms related to hypokalemia include neuromuscular irritability, with muscular weakness or fatigue (usually of the large muscle groups of the legs or arms), muscle cramps or tenderness, paresthesias, and paralysis (seen with severe hypokalemia). The patient may have GI symptoms such as anorexia, nausea (with or without vomiting), abdominal distention, and paralytic ileus (seen with severe hypokalemia).[14,34] The abdominal complaints may hinder the patient from consuming normal nutrition, causing a further decrease in potassium levels.[34] In addition, the ECG changes may be the first indication of the abnormality (see Table 21.3).[5,11,34]

Laboratory Findings

When the potassium level decreases below 3.5 mEq/L (< 3.5 mmol/L), the reasons for the losses must be investigated. GI losses include vomiting, diarrhea, and GI suctioning, and the presence of alkalosis should be assessed. A careful review of medications that could cause the hypokalemia includes thiazides, furosemide, bumetanide, osmotic diuretics, and albuterol.[14] A potassium level of less than 2.5 mEq/L (< 2.5 mmol/L) is considered a critical level.[15]

Treatment

Hypokalemia is initially treated by identifying and correcting losses of potassium. A careful review of GI losses is in order, as significant amounts of potassium may be lost with vomiting, GI suctioning, or diarrhea. Medications should be evaluated for their potential for decreasing serum potassium levels (e.g., diuretics, insulin, albuterol, amphotericin B).

Oral replacement therapy is the preferred method of treating hypokalemia; however, when the patient's condition is unstable, IV replacement may be needed.[26] When using the oral route to replace potassium, 40 to 100 mEq may be given daily. It is preferably given with meals and usually not more than 20 mEq at any one time to prevent nausea and vomiting.[26,40] When delivering IV potassium for replacement in a stable patient, the usual dose is no more than 10 to 20 mEq per hour. If the potassium concentration is greater than 20 mEq/L, use a central IV line to prevent burning of peripheral veins. When a patient is suffering from life-threatening hypokalemia (paralysis, impaired respiratory function, or unstable cardiac dysrhythmias), a rapid central IV infusion of potassium chloride (2 mEq/min over 10 minutes) followed by a slower infusion of 1 mEq/min over 10 minutes, for a total dose of 30 mEq, may be considered.[5] Institution protocols may vary and the nurse needs to review these protocols.

SODIUM

Applied Physiology and Pathophysiology

As noted in Table 21.2, sodium is the most abundant cation in the ECF, accounting for approximately 90% to 95% of the total ECF cation load. Because it is the most abundant electrolyte in the ECF, it has a major impact on water balance by its influence on osmolarity, the concentration of an osmotically active substance within a solution. Simply put, where sodium goes, water tends to follow, helping to maintain the water balance in the various compartments of the body. Sodium also interacts with both potassium and calcium to regulate the propagation of nerve impulses and muscular contractions. Sodium is involved in transportation of materials across the cellular membranes, various cellular functions, cellular metabolism, and acid-base balance.[1,14]

The normal serum sodium concentration is 135 to 145 mEq/L (135 to 145 mmol/L) and is maintained by renal function, which, in turn, is influenced by multiple factors. The average Western diet is very high in sodium, usually 5 to 6 grams per day, much more than the modest 500 mg/day the body requires.[14] Sodium is freely filtered from the blood in the glomerulus of the kidney, with the resultant renal filtrate being exceptionally high in sodium. As the filtrate travels through the distal tubules of the kidney, sodium is selectively reabsorbed, depending on the sodium concentration in the blood, as regulated by the macula densa of the glomerulus. The resorption of sodium is significantly impacted by activation of the renin-angiotensin-aldosterone system. When the ECF sodium level or renal perfusion is decreased or the potassium level increases, aldosterone increases the resorption of sodium and decreases the resorption of potassium in the distal tubules. In addition to the effects of aldosterone, angiotensin II, the end product of the renin-angiotensin system, also causes a systemic vasoconstriction, increasing renal perfusion and increasing the reabsorption of sodium and excretion of potassium in the urine.

Natriuretic hormones (atrial natriuretic peptide [ANP], B-type natriuretic peptide [BNP], and urodilatin from the kidney) decrease blood pressure and cause both sodium and water to be excreted, thus decreasing blood pressure.[14] ANP, produced and secreted in the atria, is released with increased atrial stretch. BNP is secreted and stored in the ventricles and is released in response to increases in ventricular filling pressures. Urodilatin is produced in the tubules of the kidneys and is secreted in response to increased blood pressure.

Because of the intimate relationship between sodium and water, changes in the sodium concentration (the amount of sodium for a given amount of water) will also result in changes in the serum osmolality (concentration of a solution expressed in milliosmoles of solute particles per kilogram of solute [mOsm/kg]).[34] This is of particular importance during treatment, as too rapid correction of sodium concentrations may cause increased cellular edema, which can be devastating within the brain.

Hypernatremia

Hypernatremia (>145 mEq/L [> 145 mmol/L]) occurs when the concentration of sodium is increased in relation to the amount of fluid in the ECF. Although hypernatremia is often associated with hypovolemia, it is important to remember that hypernatremia can occur in the setting of hypovolemia, euvolemia, or hypervolemia[50] (Fig. 21.4). The major effect of increased sodium concentration is an osmotic gradient, pulling water

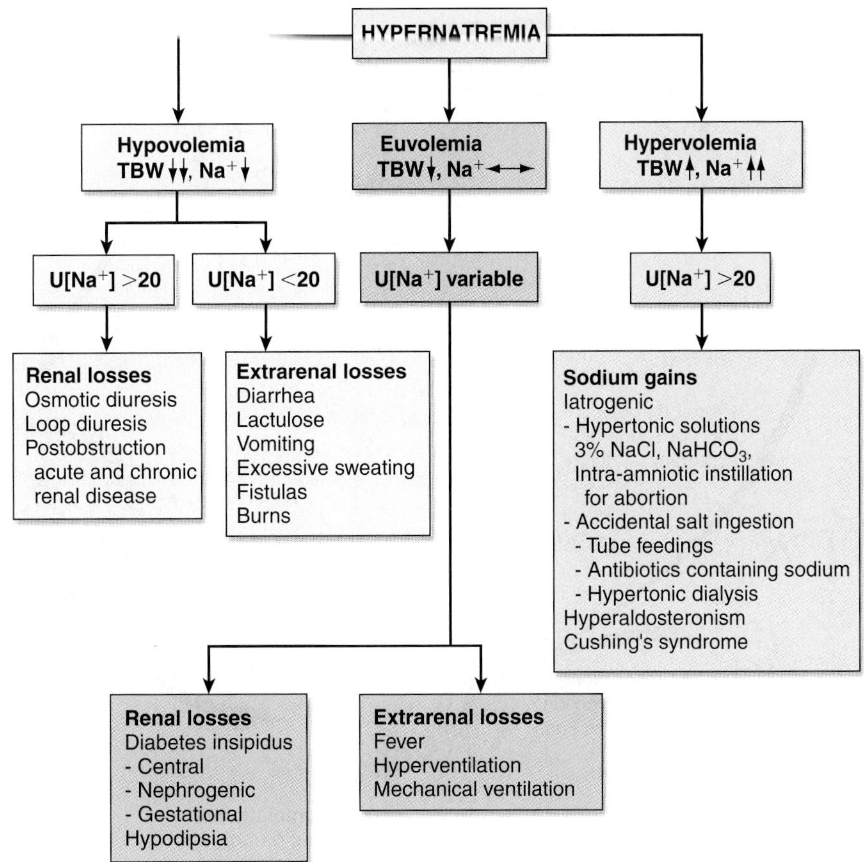

FIG. 21.4 Algorithm for diagnosing the causes of hypernatremia. *Na^+*, Sodium; *NaCl*, sodium chloride; *$NaHCO_3$*, sodium bicarbonate; *TBW*, total body water; *U*, urinary.

from the ICF into the ECF, a process that may create significant cellular dehydration, and subsequent dysfunction of individual cells, organs, and systems. Hypernatremia is caused by two processes: (1) net water loss or (2) net sodium gain.[1]

Net water losses are further divided into "pure" water losses and losses of hypotonic fluid. With pure water losses, the body loses significant amounts of free water and insignificant amounts of sodium. Examples of this type of loss include large insensible losses over a short period of time, such as that which is seen with high body temperatures, unconditioned exercise, or inadequate water intake (hypodipsia). Pure water losses may also be caused by diabetes insipidus.

Hypernatremia is also caused by hypotonic fluid loss; whereas both sodium and water are lost, the proportion of water loss is greater, creating a net loss of water. Most commonly, this process occurs via the kidneys, often with the use of various diuretics. Another renal cause of hypotonic fluid loss is the osmotic diuresis that occurs with mannitol administration or hyperglycemia. Serum osmotic pressure draws fluid from the ICF into the ECF. As the blood volume increases, filtration pressure increases and sodium is resorbed. The net result is the loss of more water than sodium into the urine, creating hypernatremia. Hypotonic fluid loss also occurs in the GI tract with vomiting, diarrhea, GI suctioning, enterocutaneous fistulas, or with the use of osmotic agents in the GI tract, such as lactulose. Significant burns can also cause hypotonic fluid loss.[1]

Hypernatremia may be caused by a net gain of sodium. Whereas this can be seen with seawater ingestion and the administration of excessive amounts of sodium chloride, it is much more commonly associated with iatrogenic causes. Such causes include hypertonic enteral or parenteral nutrition and hypertonic solutions delivered to the patient in the form of IV solutions, enemas, emetics, or dialysis. Hypernatremia may also be caused by primary hyperaldosteronism, which increases the release of aldosterone, causing the kidneys to reabsorb more sodium than water. Cushing's syndrome, a condition of excessive glucocorticoid steroid production, also causes the retention of sodium, leading to hypernatremia.[1]

Physical Assessment Findings

The physical assessment of a patient with sodium imbalances may yield conflicting findings. Often similar findings occur with both hypernatremia and hyponatremia. It is imperative that the physical assessment findings be correlated with both various laboratory tests and the patient's history.

The signs and symptoms associated with hypernatremia are more commonly seen with sudden or large shifts in the sodium concentration and are manifested by the loss of fluid from the ICF to the ECF as the body attempts to decrease sodium concentration in the ECF. The dehydration will cause weight loss, requiring significant attention to daily weights. Thirst, if the patient can express it, is often the first sign of hypernatremia. Older, bed-bound, and mentally challenged patients are at increased risk because of their inability to express thirst or

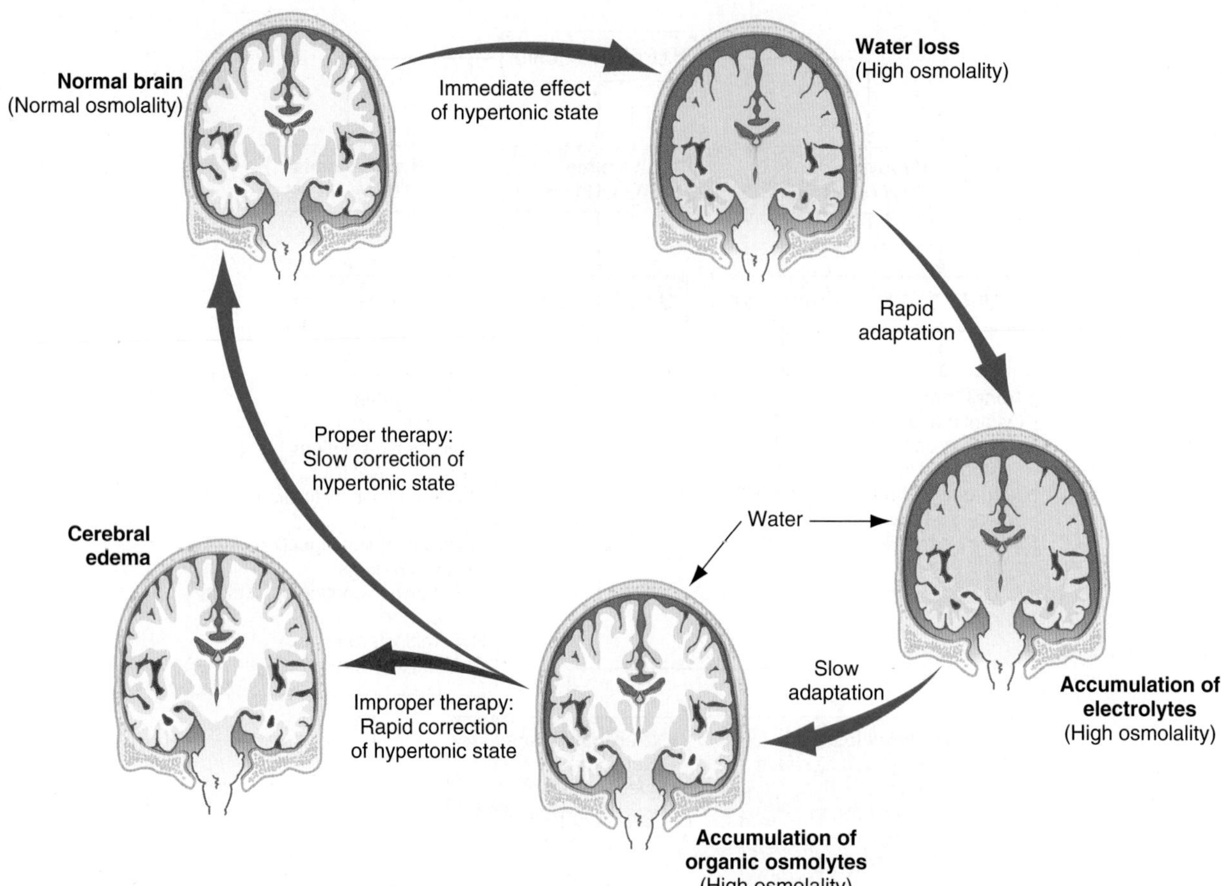

FIG. 21.5 Impact of hypernatremia on the brain.

acquire fluids in response to thirst. Dehydration becomes more clinically evident, with dry mucous membranes and sclera. Salivation decreases, making it difficult to swallow. As the central nervous system (CNS) cells become dehydrated, the patient may complain of headache or exhibit restlessness and agitation. If the hypernatremia occurs quickly, the cell crenation and brain shrinkage can cause rupture of blood vessels and hemorrhage.[1] Reflexes will be decreased, and as the hypernatremia worsens, the patient may slip into a coma or develop seizures.[34]

Laboratory Findings

When the serum sodium concentration is greater than 145 mEq/L (>145 mmol/L), there should be an investigation of why it is elevated to possibly prevent further increase. A serum sodium concentration of greater than 150 mEq/L (> 150 mmol/L) is considered a critical level.[15]

Treatment

A thorough evaluation of the patient is mandatory before elevated serum sodium concentration is treated, in order to ensure appropriate treatment of the cause. The cause of the sodium imbalance must be addressed while treating the hypernatremia.[1] If the patient is hemodynamically unstable, fluid resuscitation with an isotonic fluid is appropriate until the patient is stable. At this point, the sodium imbalance may be addressed. If the issue is water loss, then "free water" is delivered to the patient in the form of 5% dextrose (D_5W), often in combination with hypotonic sodium chloride (0.2% to 0.45% NaCl).[1] The treatment course is usually extended over 48 hours to prevent too rapid a correction of the serum sodium level. If the sodium level is corrected too quickly with rapid administration of free water, the blood-brain barrier will prevent the equalization of fluid in cerebral tissue, which may cause significant cerebral edema (Fig. 21.5).[26] If hypernatremia is being caused by excess sodium being delivered to the patient, in the form of IV fluids, medications, or enteral or parenteral nutrition feedings, they must be stopped and modified to decrease the sodium loads.

Hyponatremia

Hyponatremia (< 135 mEq/L [< 135 mmol/L]) occurs when the concentration of sodium is decreased in relation to the amount of fluid in the ECF. It is a common finding and present in 15% to 20% of admissions in patients presenting to the emergency department.[44] It represents one of the most confusing of the electrolyte disorders, because a patient with hyponatremia may present with a low, normal, or even elevated intravascular or extracellular volume (Fig. 21.6). Indeed, some of the same pathologies that cause hypernatremia can also cause hyponatremia, such as vomiting, diarrhea, or diuretic use.[1,2] Hyponatremia may be caused by mechanisms that cause the body to lose more sodium than water. Examples include renal losses, such as seen with diuretics, osmotic diuresis (e.g., mannitol, hyperglycemia, or the presence of ketones), and the effects of Addison's disease (adrenocortical insufficiency). The loss of more sodium than water can also occur with vomiting, diarrhea, excessive sweating, or when fluid is sequestered in the ECF away from the vascular system ("third spaced"), as found in burns, pancreatitis, or muscle trauma.[2]

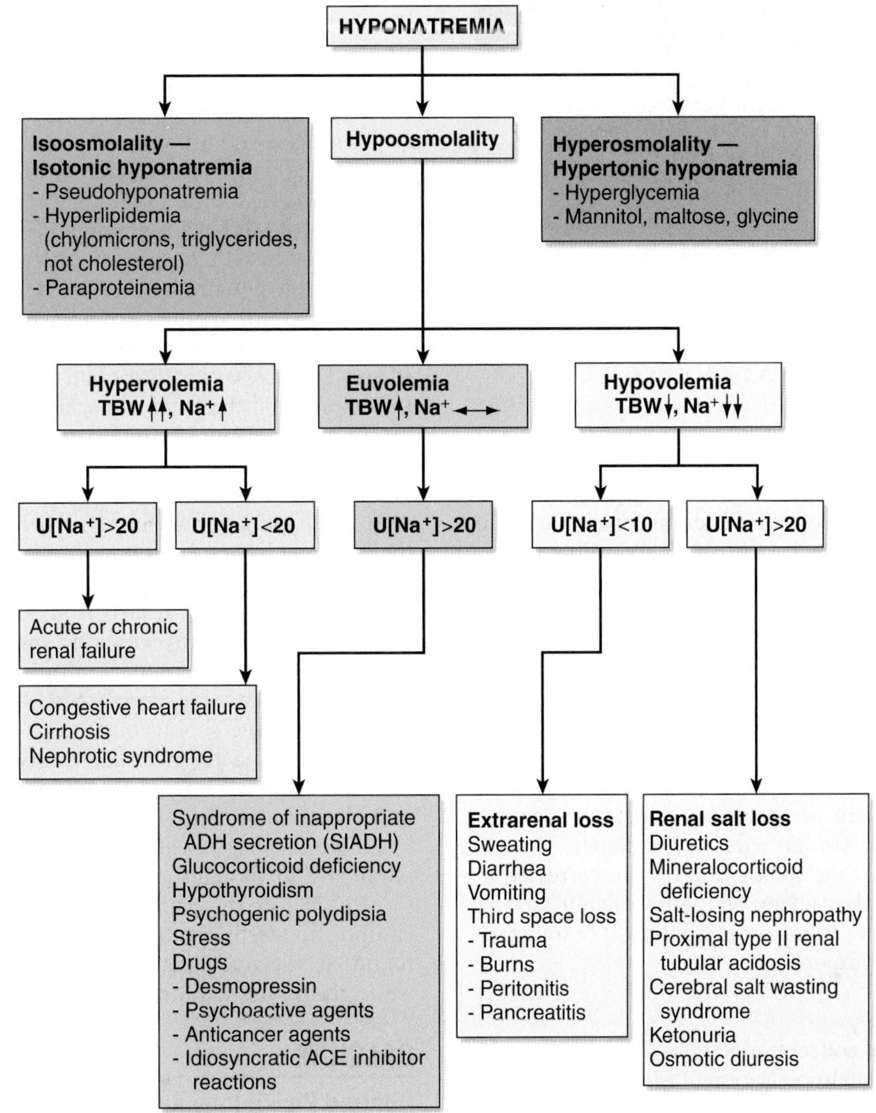

FIG. 21.6 Algorithm for diagnosing the causes of hyponatremia. *Na^+*, Sodium; *TBW*, total body water; *U*, urinary.

Hyponatremia may also be caused by processes that increase the amount of water in the ECF. If the ECF water volume increases without a concomitant increase in the sodium levels, the sodium concentration will decrease, causing hyponatremia. This is sometimes referred to as a *dilutional* or hypovolemic hyponatremia. Examples include decompensated heart failure, liver disease, acute or chronic renal failure, or even pregnancy.[2]

A patient with normal circulating fluid volumes may also have hyponatremia. For example, thiazide diuretics tend to cause the excretion of more sodium than water. Over time, this can create a hyponatremic state. Hypothyroidism and adrenocortical insufficiency cause more sodium than water to be excreted by the kidneys.[2]

Syndrome of inappropriate antidiuretic hormone (SIADH) may also cause hyponatremia. Antidiuretic hormone (ADH) is normally released from the posterior pituitary gland in response to decreased circulating blood volume, causing the kidneys to reabsorb water and increasing the ECF. In SIADH, the normal negative feedback system is disrupted and ADH continues to be secreted. As water is continually reabsorbed, a dilutional hyponatremia develops. SIADH is caused by stress, pain, lung cancers, head trauma, or multiple medications.[7,26,34]

It is worth mentioning that a patient suffering from DKA or HHS may have a relative hyponatremia that may actually mask normal or even high sodium levels.[2,15] As blood glucose elevates osmotic pressure in the intravascular spaces, the high glucose levels seen in both DKA and HHS exert an osmotic effect, diluting the sodium. In order to maintain normal osmotic pressure, sodium is secreted by the tubules in an effort to decrease osmotic pressure. This dilution of the ECF and secretion of sodium may cause an artificial hyponatremia, when, in fact, the sodium level may be normal or even elevated. A simple formula can provide accurate information regarding the true serum sodium level. For every 100 mg/dL the blood glucose level is above 100, add 1.6 mEq or mmol to the measured sodium level

BOX 21.1 Sample Serum Sodium Level Calculation

For example, if the glucose level was 924 mg/dL and the measured serum sodium level was 128 mEq/L (128 mmol/L), the *corrected* sodium level would be 140.8 mEq/L (140.8 mmol/L), a normal sodium level.
924-100 = 824 (difference for glucose above 100)
8 per 100
8 × 1.6 = 12.8
128 + 12.8 = 140.8 (corrected sodium)

to obtain the *corrected* sodium level (Box 21.1). The corrected sodium calculation is required to deliver the appropriate fluid for resuscitation of patients in both DKA and HHS.[2]

Physical Assessment Findings

As with hypernatremia, the signs and symptoms of hyponatremia are more commonly seen with sudden or large shifts in the sodium concentration. The decreased sodium concentration in the ECF will cause water to collect in the ICF, leading to cellular edema. The patient will exhibit significant pitting edema, in the legs or on the sternum. The early signs of fatigue, muscle cramps, and weakness are often seen in patients who are excessively exercising. Coexisting nausea, vomiting, abdominal cramps, and diarrhea may also be present. As the water content of the CNS cells increases, dysfunction becomes more evident; signs include headache and lethargy. If the hyponatremia continues, the CNS edema will continue to increase and symptoms will evolve to gross motor weakness, disorientation, confusion, and decreased deep tendon reflexes. Ultimately, seizures and coma may occur.[34] If the sodium level is not corrected in a timely manner, the cerebral edema will cause a significant rise in the intracranial pressure and may cause an uncal or transtentorial herniation of the temporal lobe.[15]

Laboratory Findings

When the serum sodium concentration is decreased below 135 mEq/L (< 135 mmol/L), an investigation of why it is low should be instituted, which may prevent its further decline. A serum sodium concentration of less than 125 mEq/L (< 125 mmol/L) is considered a critical level.[15]

Additional laboratory tests that are helpful with a differential diagnosis in hyponatremia include urine sodium and blood urea nitrogen (BUN). A random urine sodium level of less than 10 mmol/L, coupled with a low serum sodium level, indicates that the kidneys are attempting to compensate for hyponatremia by reabsorbing sodium. A urine sodium level greater than 10 mmol/L, coupled with a low serum sodium level, indicates that some pathology (e.g., diuretics) is causing the kidneys to lose sodium inappropriately. In SIADH, the urine sodium level may be greater than 20 to 40 mmol/L, whereas with hypothyroidism the urine sodium level may be greater than 40 mmol/L. Calculating the fractional excretion of sodium (FENa) assists the nurse in assessing the cause of sodium loss. The fractional excretion of sodium is expressed by the formula:

$$\text{FENa} = [(\text{urine NA} \div \text{urine Cr}) \times (\text{serum Cr} \div \text{serum Na})] \times 100$$

with the result being a percentage. A FENa of less than 1%, coupled with hyponatremia, usually indicates that the kidneys are attempting to compensate for hyponatremia by reabsorbing sodium.[15]

Treatment

The initial treatment for hyponatremia in a patient with normal or increased ECF volume is almost always water restriction. Loop diuretics (e.g., furosemide) may be added to the treatment to increase the amount of ECF volume excreted in the urine. Replacing lost sodium may also be a key component of treatment. If the patient can tolerate oral intake, replacement may be accomplished with a diet high in sodium. If the patient is unable to eat but has a functioning GI system, the sodium may be delivered by GI tubes (nasal, oral, or percutaneous). When a patient has hyponatremia associated with hypovolemia or cannot take sodium via the GI tract, parenteral replacement with normal saline (NS) or lactated Ringer's solution is appropriate. It may be necessary to use small amounts of hypertonic (3% to 5%) saline if the patient is symptomatic and is normovolemic or hypervolemic. Extreme caution must be exercised using hypertonic saline, as sodium concentration may be corrected too quickly.[2,26]

If the hyponatremia has existed for more than 48 hours, the CNS will have had an opportunity to accommodate to the low sodium concentration. If the sodium level is corrected too quickly, water will be drawn from the brain, creating dehydration, osmotic demyelination, and cerebral damage (Fig. 21.7).[2,34] Whereas there are multiple formulas for correcting sodium levels and appropriate time frames to be used,[2,26] the guiding principle should be to treat the patient's symptoms rather than to reach a given laboratory value.

When hyponatremia is caused by SIADH, treatment of the underlying cause must also be addressed. The treatment of hyponatremia begins with water restriction and loop diuretics, advancing to thoughtful administration of hypertonic saline (3% to 5%) as the patient's condition dictates.[26] The use of vasopressin receptor antagonists (tolvaptan [Samsca]) has been found to selectively increase water excretion by the kidneys while promoting sodium retention.[12,54]

CALCIUM

Applied Physiology and Pathophysiology

Most of the calcium in the body (99%) is stored in the bones and teeth; serum calcium (also referred to as *total* calcium) represents the remaining 1% and is divided into three distinct components. Approximately 10% of serum calcium is in a "complexed" form bound to another electrolyte and not available for the cells to use as an electrolyte. Another 47% is bound to protein, but this amount may vary with both the amount of protein in the blood and the blood's pH. Like complexed calcium, protein-bound calcium does not function as an electrolyte but is readily available to influence the ionized calcium level. The remaining 43% of serum calcium is free or ionized calcium that does act as an electrolyte. However, the levels of protein-bound calcium may fluctuate with the pH, which in turn will affect the ionized calcium level. If the pH is increased (alkalosis), the increase in protein-bound calcium will cause a decrease in ionized calcium and vice versa. It is therefore important, when caring for a hypoalbuminemic patient, to make a correction to the calcium level to account for the additional calcium that will be unbound to protein. This correction can be made using the following formula:

$$\text{Serum calcium concentration} + [0.8 \times (4 - \text{serum albumin concentration})]$$

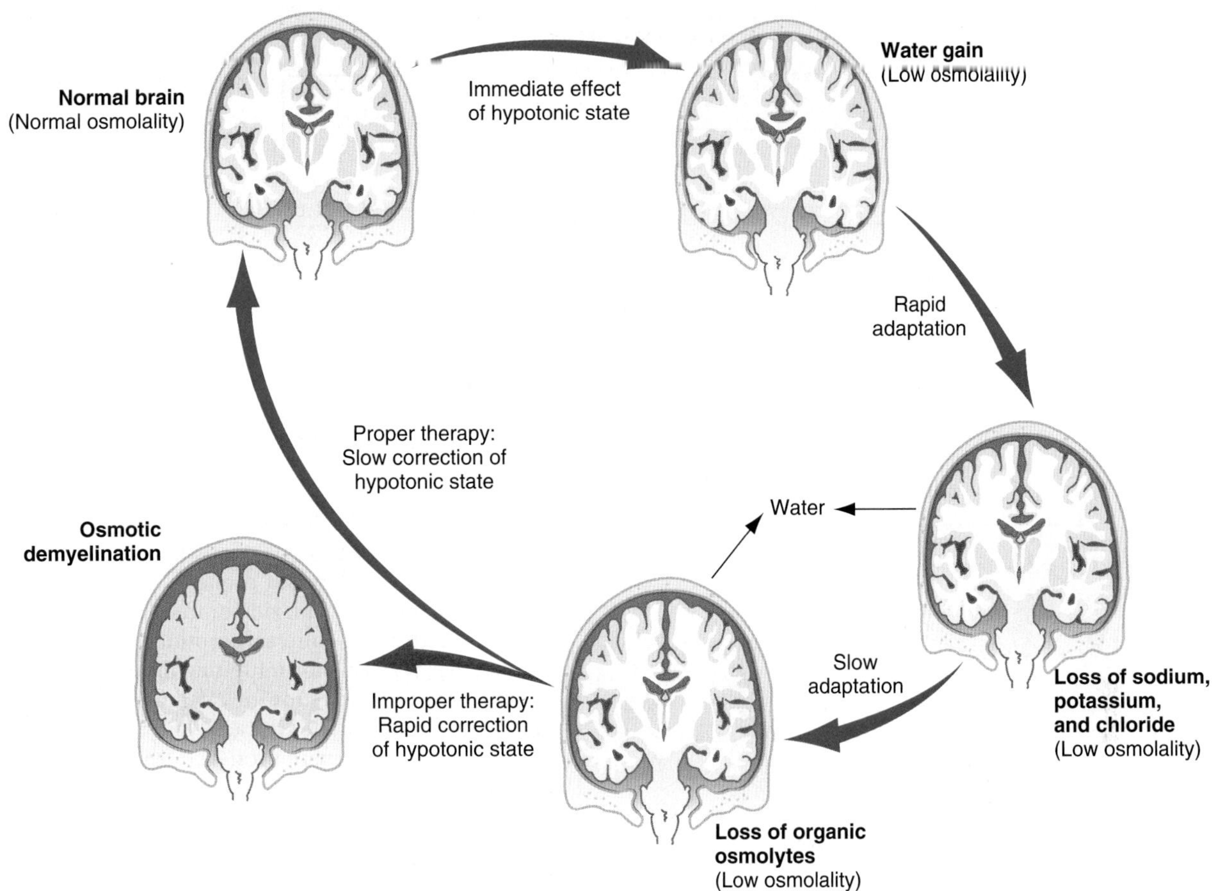

FIG. 21.7 Impact of hyponatremia on the brain.

Even though the proportions of protein-bound and ionized calcium may change with the pH, the total serum calcium concentration does not change.[8,15,26,55]

A large variety of body functions are dependent upon calcium, including muscle contraction, contractility of the heart and blood vessels, platelet aggregation, and coagulation.[6] Calcium is important in nerve transmission and cardiac contraction, relaxation, and automaticity.[8,26] As it is a major extracellular cation, it is usually actively pumped out of the cells, along with sodium. Calcium also makes the cellular membrane more impervious to elevated potassium and magnesium levels.[6]

Calcium levels in the body are regulated by the parathyroid glands (Fig. 21.8). There are usually four parathyroid glands, which are located on the posterior aspect of the thyroid gland (Fig. 21.9). The number of parathyroid glands may vary quite normally from as few as two to as many as six. The parathyroid gland manufactures and secretes parathyroid hormone (PTH), in response to the ionized calcium level. When the ionized calcium level decreases, PTH is released, causing the ionized calcium levels to increase by several mechanisms. As calcium is stored primarily in bone, PTH will cause the release of calcium from bone and reabsorption of calcium into the ionized form by decreasing the calcitonin level. Calcitonin, a hormone secreted by the thyroid gland, is responsible for the deposition of calcium in bone; a decrease in its concentration will liberate calcium from bone, increasing the ionized calcium level.[6] In the kidneys, PTH increases the amount of calcium reabsorbed from filtrate in the proximal and distal tubules, while at the same time decreasing the amount of phosphorus reabsorbed. This selective resorption of calcium and excretion of phosphorus allows for an increase in the ionized calcium level, without increasing the phosphorus levels. When the phosphorus is reabsorbed at the same rate as calcium, chelation of calcium and phosphorus will occur and it may be deposited in soft tissue.[33,34] PTH also will stimulate the kidneys to synthesize 1,25-dihydroxyvitamin D (vitamin D_3, the active form, also known as *calcitriol*), which, in turn, increases calcium uptake from the GI tract.[6,8,33,34,55] Increases in the ionized calcium levels will create negative feedback to the parathyroid gland, which will decrease the secretion of PTH.[34,55]

Hypercalcemia

The most common causes of hypercalcemia are cancers and hyperparathyroidism, both of which liberate calcium from bone.[6,26] As many as 20% of patients with cancer have hypercalcemia.[55] Although the mechanism is not entirely clear, it is known that some cancers secrete a parathyroid-like substance that would cause hypercalcemia. Hypercalcemia is also caused by prolonged immobilization, muscle weakness, or paralysis preventing weight bearing. Excessive ingestion of milk products or calcium-containing antacids may also cause hypercalcemia. Women who ingest large amounts of calcium in an effort to prevent osteoporosis may develop hypercalcemia.[8,34,55]

Physical Assessment Findings

Calcium is important in neuromuscular and cardiovascular activity; signs and symptoms will typically be seen in these areas.[34] Hypercalcemia (> 10 mg/dL [> 2.50 mmol/L]) will

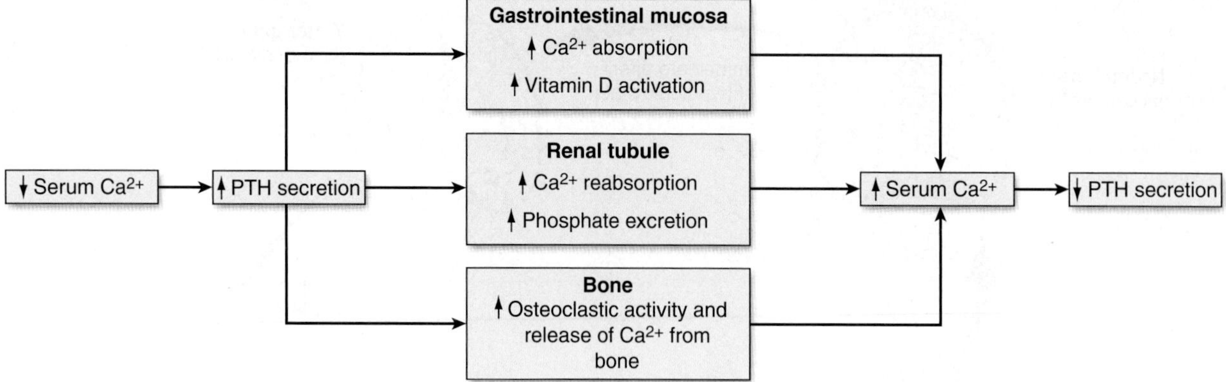

FIG. 21.8 Calcium homeostasis. *Ca^{2+}*, Calcium; *PTH*, parathyroid hormone.

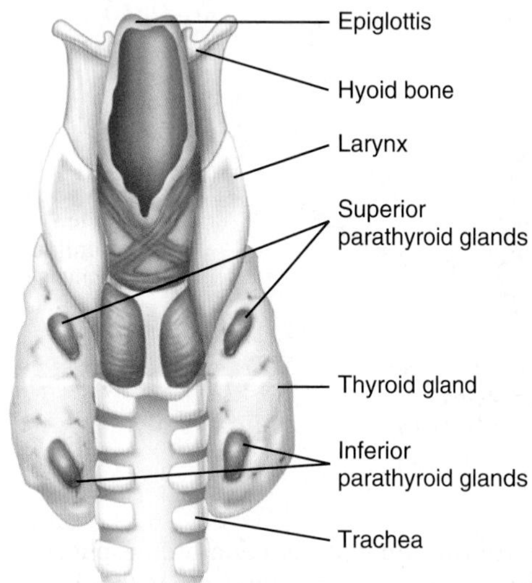

FIG. 21.9 Thyroid and parathyroid glands.

usually result in decreased neuromuscular activity, resulting in muscular weakness, loss of muscle tone, and lethargy. Hypercalcemia may cause changes in behavior ranging from subtle changes in personality to stupor or coma. The patient may experience nausea, vomiting, anorexia, and constipation. Cardiovascular effects include shortening of the QTc interval, hypertension, and atrioventricular (AV) blocks, all of which may be potentiated by digitalis toxicity and can lead to cardiac arrest (see Table 21.3).[6,26] High levels of calcium in the urinary filtrate may interfere with the ability of ADH to cause the kidneys to concentrate urine, leading to a significant diuresis. Chronic, excessive calcium in the urine may cause the deposition of renal calculi in the tubules or collecting system.[34,55]

Laboratory Findings

Hypercalcemia is defined as a serum calcium level greater than 10 mg/dL (> 2.50 mmol/L). Critical levels are considered greater than 14 mg/dL (> 3.50 mmol/L).[16] A prolonged blood draw with an excessively tight tourniquet can falsely elevate the calcium levels, as can elevated levels of protein or albumin.[33]

Treatment

Hypercalcemia is initially treated with rehydration and increased urinary loss of calcium through forced diuresis with fluids and loop diuretics. Typically, 500 mL of NS is bolused and then the patient is assessed for response. This pattern is repeated until the patient is stable. The fluid challenge may be coupled with furosemide (1 mg/kg).[6] Thiazide diuretics are contraindicated as they may increase calcium reabsorption. Steroids are effective in treating hypercalcemia by inhibiting the effects of vitamin D, increasing the renal excretion of calcium, and decreasing the uptake of calcium from the GI tract.[6]

Bisphosphonates (pamidronate [Aredia], etidronate [Didronel]) help lower calcium levels and have been used extensively in various types of cancers[8,27] and chronic renal disease patients. Researchers have recently begun to use this class of drugs to increase bone density and decrease serum calcium levels in hemiplegic stroke patients[42] and patients immobilized with hip fractures.[43] If a patient does not tolerate the bisphosphonates, plicamycin (an antibiotic used in oncology) may be considered, but it has significant side effects and is less effective.[27] Other drugs that are sometimes used to decrease liberation of calcium from bones include calcitonin (Miacalcin) and glucocorticoids.[6,33] If the patient has preexisting heart failure or renal failure, renal replacement is needed to remove the excess calcium.[6] If the patient is suffering from primary hyperparathyroidism, surgical excision of the glands is indicated.[8]

Hypocalcemia

Hypocalcemia is much less common than hypercalcemia[6] and is the result of one of three different mechanisms: increased renal losses, binding of ionized calcium to protein, or decreased PTH. Phosphate and calcium maintain an inverse relationship (when one increases, the other decreases, and vice versa). Elevated phosphate levels are often found in patients with renal insufficiency and failure. When phosphate levels increase because of renal failure, calcium levels are often decreased. Other factors influencing calcium balance include magnesium, vitamin D, and inflammatory mediators. As magnesium levels decrease, the release of PTH and its action on bone, liberating calcium, are suppressed. Magnesium deficiency needs to be corrected before the calcium levels can be normalized. Excessive vitamin D will also suppress the secretion of PTH.[9,33,55] There are increasing data to suggest that inflammatory mediators may down regulate PTH, decreasing the calcium level.[9] Another author suggests that hospitalized older adults are at risk for vitamin D deficiency, which can also cause hypocalcemia.[22]

Hypocalcemia may be incorrectly identified when the total serum calcium level is found to be low (< 8.6 mg/dL [< 2.15

mmol/L]) in combination with hypoproteinemia. Because of the amount of calcium that is protein-bound (47%), the amount of protein (primarily albumin) in the serum will impact the total serum calcium level. If the total calcium level is determined to be below normal limits, an ionized calcium level must be measured to determine the true amount of the active calcium electrolyte. Various references use a variety of formulas to calculate the effect of low protein (or albumin) levels on the amount of ionized calcium. However, the only truly effective way to determine the amount of ionized calcium is to actually measure it.[22,26] Hypocalcemia may also be caused by acute pancreatitis; the saponification of fats and calcium in the retroperitoneum effectively removes the calcium from the circulation.[26,34] The delivery of large amounts of banked blood, especially over a short time, may cause hypocalcemia because the citrate used to preserve banked blood combines with the ionized calcium and eliminates it from the stores of active electrolytes. Citrate is metabolized by the liver, so any disease process (e.g., shock, liver disease, sepsis) that decreases liver function may increase the levels of citrate,[14,55] which will combine with more calcium. Data from 2004 indicate that propofol (Diprivan) decreases calcium levels and increases PTH levels, but it is unclear if there is any clinical relevance to these changes.[6]

Physical Assessment Findings

Hypocalcemia typically causes increased neuromuscular activity and negative effects on the cardiovascular system. Increased neuromuscular activity causes a decrease in the excitation threshold and is characterized by numbness and tingling, particularly around the mouth and in the hands and feet. Muscle spasms and tetany of the hands, feet, and face may be seen or elicited during an assessment. Chvostek's sign (twitching of the lip, nose, or face in response to a repeated tapping of the facial nerve just below the zygomatic arch, anterior to the ear) or Trousseau's sign (a forceful flexion of the fingers and hand when a blood pressure cuff is inflated above the systolic pressure and held for 3 minutes) are both indicators of tetany (Figs. 21.10 and 21.11).[8,55] Hyperreflexia is also found.[14] The cardiovascular effects of hypocalcemia are significant and can include hypotension, increased QT interval (which may lead to ventricular dysrhythmias, including ventricular tachycardia and Torsades de pointes [TdP]),[6] decreased cardiac output, and decreased response to medications that utilize calcium, including digitalis, dopamine (Intropin), and norepinephrine (Levophed) (see Table 21.3).[33]

Laboratory Findings

Hypocalcemia is defined as a serum calcium level less than 8.6 mg/dL (< 2.50 mmol/L). Critical levels are equal to or less than 6 mg/dL (≤1.50 mmol/L).[15] When low serum calcium levels are found, an ionized calcium MUST be measured before the delivery of calcium (gluconate or chloride). The normal range of ionized calcium is 4.64 to 5.28 mg/dL (1.16 to 1.32 mmol/L), with a critical value of less than 2.8 mg/dL (< 0.7 mmol/L).[15]

Treatment

The treatment for hypocalcemia is relatively straightforward: administer calcium. However, different calcium preparations supply different amounts of calcium (Table 21.5). Calcium chloride has three times as much elemental calcium as calcium gluconate. Calcium chloride is 27% elemental calcium, calcium gluconate only 9%. If the patient is relatively stable and able to tolerate oral intake, calcium in the form of either citrate or carbonate can be given.[8] When treating hypocalcemia in the critical care setting, IV calcium, in the form of calcium gluconate or chloride, is given slowly when the patient is symptomatic or has significantly low calcium levels.[8,34,55] Whereas some authorities recommend calcium gluconate

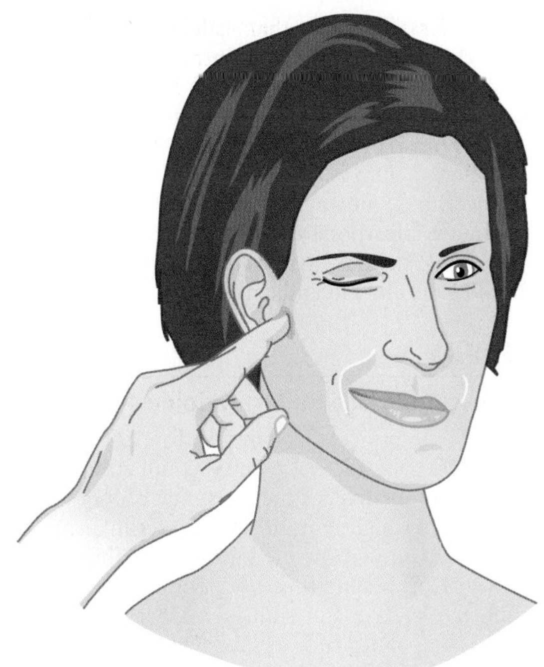

FIG. 21.10 Chvostek's sign.

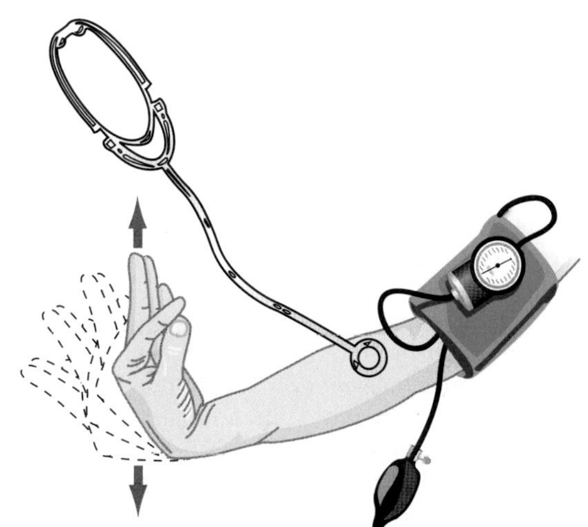

FIG. 21.11 Trousseau's sign.

TABLE 21.5 Calcium Supplements

Calcium Salt	Elemental Calcium (mEq/g)	Elemental Calcium (%)	Elemental Calcium Provided by 1 g of Salt (mg)
Calcium chloride	13.6	27	270
Calcium gluconate	4.56	9	90

because it is less irritating than calcium chloride,[6,26] it is approximately one third the concentration of calcium chloride (0.465 mEq/L vs. 1.4 mEq/L).[37,38] If calcium chloride is given, it should be delivered into the largest available vein and via a central vein, if possible. If the patient's condition allows the extra fluid, calcium is ideally mixed with a compatible IV solution and should not be delivered in the same IV line at the same time as bicarbonate or phosphorus, as it will form a precipitate.[26,55] Whenever hypocalcemia is found, magnesium levels should be evaluated and corrected if low.[8]

MAGNESIUM

Applied Physiology and Pathophysiology

Magnesium is necessary for multiple functions essential to maintain life. Among these are nerve conduction; membrane stabilization; cardiovascular tone; movement of sodium, potassium, and calcium in and out of cells; and cellular metabolism of energy.[34,46] Magnesium is the fourth most abundant cation in the body and the second most abundant intracellular cation. Approximately 50% of magnesium is stored in bone and 39% to 49% is stored in the intracellular space.[34] Only about 1% to 2% of body magnesium is available in the ECF and approximately 0.3% is available in serum. One third to one half of serum magnesium is bound to protein or chelated to salts, and approximately one half is ionized.[3,24]

Magnesium is absorbed mostly in the jejunum and ileum. The kidneys play the largest role in maintaining magnesium balance. Renal excretion drops to very low levels when magnesium needs to be conserved and increases tremendously when serum magnesium levels rise, thus maintaining a strict balance. The thick, ascending loop of Henle is where most of the magnesium filtered by the glomeruli is reabsorbed. Loop diuretics and thiazides impede reabsorption, causing increased urinary magnesium losses.[16,35]

Whereas magnesium concentration in the serum is very low, it is important in more than 300 enzyme reactions. It is required for the metabolism of carbohydrates, protein, and fat; for genetic transcription and replication; and for all reactions involving adenosine triphosphate (ATP), including the functioning of the sodium-potassium pump, membrane stabilization, nerve conduction, and neuromuscular function.[46]

Laboratory Values

Normal ranges for magnesium are 1.5 to 2.3 mg/dL (0.62 to 0.95 mmol/L), as shown in Table 21.3. Serum magnesium levels are poor indicators of the overall body magnesium status. Like potassium, hemolysis will elevate serum magnesium levels as intracellular levels are more than 16 times higher than ECF levels.[24] In addition, any other process that results in cell breakdown and release of intracellular contents will raise serum magnesium levels, possibly masking a deficiency. Examples of this are catabolism and rhabdomyolysis. Acidemia results in redistribution of magnesium from ICF to ECF, raising serum magnesium levels.[41] Alkalosis has the opposite effect, lowering serum magnesium levels.[24]

Hypermagnesemia

Serum magnesium levels above the normal range occur in 5.7% to 9.3% of hospitalized patients.[51-53] However, because magnesium levels are not part of most routine laboratory panels, hypermagnesemia is often missed. In one study, researchers assessed the magnesium levels of all of the blood samples delivered to a laboratory for routine electrolyte analysis (n = 1033) and found magnesium abnormalities in 546 of the samples. They also found that 87% (52/59) of patients with hypermagnesemia did not have a request for a magnesium level by the provider.[51]

The patients at greatest risk for hypermagnesemia are those with renal insufficiency or failure, especially with iatrogenic magnesium supplementation. As creatinine clearance falls below 30 mL/min, slightly increased magnesium levels are commonly seen and patients are usually asymptomatic. Symptomatic hypermagnesemia rarely occurs without magnesium supplementation.[13] Even with good renal function, excessive magnesium supplementation can be life-threatening. Case reports have demonstrated hypermagnesemia in patients with normal renal function from oral or rectal Epsom salts;[28,46] medication errors in IV repletion of magnesium deficiency;[47] oral intake of magnesium hydroxide, magnesium carbonate, or magnesium citrate from common antacid or laxative formulas;[24,25,48] and the use of magnesium to decrease labor contractions.

Physical Assessment Findings

Hypermagnesemia primarily affects the central nervous and cardiovascular systems.[24] Mild hypermagnesemia is usually asymptomatic. Signs and symptoms of hypermagnesemia begin as levels rise above 4.9 mg/dL (> 2 mmol/L) when deep tendon reflexes become diminished. As magnesium levels further increase, severe vasodilation and hypotension may be seen. When magnesium levels rise above 9.7 mg/dL (> 4 mmol/L), changes in the cardiac conduction system and neuromuscular paralysis may lead to respiratory failure and cardiac arrest.[5] As long as deep tendon reflexes are present, respiratory paralysis is not likely.[24] ECG changes may include increased PR and QT intervals, increased QRS duration, and complete AV block, and may progress to asystole (see Table 21.3).[20] Hypocalcemia often accompanies high magnesium levels and worsens symptoms.[20]

Laboratory Findings

Mild hypermagnesemia is usually asymptomatic. Early signs do not usually appear until magnesium levels rise above 4.9 mg/dL (> 2.01 mmol/L). However, there is considerable variability in the literature regarding the relationship between elevated magnesium levels and the onset of signs and symptoms.

Treatment

Since most cases of life-threatening hypermagnesemia are iatrogenic, prevention is key. Generally, avoid giving any medication containing magnesium to patients with renal failure. If magnesium must be given, the patient should be closely monitored for hypermagnesemia and the supplementation stopped, as needed.[5,20]

If hypermagnesemia is identified, the first step in treatment is to discontinue any magnesium supplementation. Often, this is all that is required to correct mild to moderate hypermagnesemia in patients with good renal function. In more severely hypermagnesemic patients, there are two additional mainstays of treatment. The first is to remove magnesium from the body. When renal function is sufficient, renal magnesium excretion can be induced by giving normal saline and furosemide. Monitor for potassium and calcium deficits and correct as needed. Renal replacement therapy must be used to remove magnesium when renal function is impaired. The second mainstay of treatment for moderate to severe hypomagnesemia is to antagonize the effect of magnesium by giving intravenous calcium as chloride or gluconate.[5,20]

Hypomagnesemia

Hypomagnesemia is clinically much more common than hypermagnesemia. Magnesium depletion may have severe consequences for patients and often goes unrecognized.[52] The incidence of hypomagnesemia in hospitalized patients is 11% to 26% in the general medical population,[21,51] 61% in postoperative patients admitted to critical care,[10] and 20% in general medical patients admitted to critical care.[35] Patients with other electrolyte disturbances, such as low potassium, sodium, phosphorus, and calcium levels, are at higher risk of hypomagnesemia, because of the interactions of magnesium with other electrolytes.[3,36,51,52]

Low magnesium levels are usually caused by poor intake, increased renal or GI excretion, or acute shifts between the ICF and ECF. Hypomagnesemia from poor intake is seen in alcoholism, in protein-calorie malnutrition, and in patients receiving magnesium-free parenteral nutrition. Excess GI magnesium losses occur in short-bowel syndrome, steatorrhea, chronic diarrhea, and GI suctioning. Increased renal magnesium losses are commonly seen in patients with uncontrolled diabetes and patients with renal tubular disorders. Ketoacidosis from starvation or diabetes increases renal magnesium loss.[3] Multiple medications may lead to hypomagnesemia, including thiazides, loop diuretics, aminoglycosides, cyclosporine, cisplatin, and amphotericin B. Magnesium may shift from the ECF to the ICF when insulin and dextrose are given, especially in the presence of metabolic alkalosis. Hungry bone syndrome following parathyroidectomy may cause low serum levels as the magnesium is deposited in newly formed bone.[45]

Hypocalcemia and hypokalemia typically accompany magnesium deficiency. Renal potassium conservation is impaired in hypomagnesemia, resulting in refractory hypokalemia. Thus magnesium deficiency must be suspected when hypokalemia does not correct despite supplementation.[24,35]

Physical Assessment Findings

Low magnesium levels often cause no symptoms. When symptoms are present, they mainly involve the neurologic and cardiovascular systems. Hypocalcemia, hypokalemia, and metabolic alkalosis often accompany magnesium deficiency, so signs and symptoms may overlap.[16] The most common symptoms include muscle twitches, cramps, hyperactive deep tendon reflexes, vertigo, or ataxia. Chvostek's sign or Trousseau's sign or paresthesias may be present. Other symptoms may include mental status changes, dysphagia, nystagmus, tetany, new-onset hyperglycemia, or seizures (see Figs. 21.10 and 21.11).[6,24,35] The clinician may suspect hypomagnesemia when low potassium levels do not respond to supplementation and when other electrolyte abnormalities such as hyponatremia and hypocalcemia are present.[20]

Cardiovascular symptoms include tachycardia, ventricular dysrhythmias, especially TdP, and worsening signs of digitalis toxicity. ECG changes that occur include ST depression, T-wave inversion, prolonged QT interval, widened QRS complex, shortened PR interval, and flattening or inversion of P waves in the precordial leads (see Table 21.3). Treatment-resistant ventricular fibrillation or other dysrhythmias suggest magnesium deficiency.[5,20,35]

Laboratory Findings

Low serum magnesium levels indicate a deficiency. However, normal levels do not rule out deficiency. Low magnesium levels may be seen in hypoproteinemia because 20% of serum magnesium is protein-bound.[3] Even when serum magnesium levels are normal, a high index of suspicion for deficiency should be maintained for patients with high risk.

Treatment

Treatment of magnesium deficiency depends on whether symptoms are present and, if so, how severe they are. Mild or asymptomatic hypomagnesemia may be treated with oral or enteral magnesium salts such as magnesium sulfate or magnesium oxide. Keep in mind that the major side effect of oral or enteral magnesium salts is diarrhea.

Moderate to severe symptomatic hypomagnesemia is treated with intravenous magnesium sulfate (1 to 2 g).[5] Additional doses may be needed in patients with severe hypomagnesemia manifesting as seizures or TdP.

Calcium salts (gluconate and chloride), usually 1 gram of gluconate, are also given because hypomagnesemic patients are also hypocalcemic.[20] Because correction of a total body magnesium deficiency may take days to weeks of therapy,[5] additional magnesium to replace the total body deficit can be given as 6 g in daily intravenous fluid over 3 to 7 days.[5]

In patients with renal insufficiency, magnesium must be given cautiously. If, during infusion, deep tendon reflexes decrease or disappear, or if hypotension develops, stop the infusion and measure the magnesium level.[24]

PHOSPHORUS

Applied Physiology and Pathophysiology

Phosphorus, a nonmetallic chemical element, is crucial to all body functions. In any discussion of how phosphorus functions in the body, it is important to have an understanding of terms to prevent misconceptions or confusion. Phosphorus, the chemical element, is never found alone in the body; it is always combined with other elements, usually in the form of inorganic phosphates (abbreviated as HPO_4^{2-} and $H_2PO_4^{-}$).[50] Although some authorities may use the terms interchangeably, in the context of this chapter, the word *phosphorus* will be used when discussing the laboratory value and the word *phosphate* will be used when discussing how phosphorus is utilized in body functions.

Phosphate is the essential energy source for cellular function in the body and the maintenance of life. When ATP is cleaved to adenosine diphosphate (ADP), a phosphate molecule is liberated, creating energy for the cell. This process is crucial to electrolyte transport (sodium, potassium, calcium) across cellular membranes; nerve conduction; red blood cell function; muscular contractions; metabolism of carbohydrates, protein, and fats;[26,31] and in virtually every enzyme system.[50] Phosphate is important as a building block of cellular membranes and is responsible for many intracellular functions, including mitochondrial function[26,31,55] and leukocytosis.[31]

The vast majority of phosphate is found in the bone and is inextricably linked with calcium metabolism; phosphorus and calcium are inversely related to each other (if one increases, the other decreases).[14] Phosphates in the blood circulate either protein-bound (12%), complexed with other minerals (33%), or in an ionized form. A normal diet provides more than adequate amounts of phosphate. The kidneys are responsible for elimination of 90% of phosphate and will retain phosphate as needed by the body, by reabsorbing it in the renal tubules in response to plasma phosphate levels.[26,31,50]

Phosphate (and calcium) levels are regulated by PTH, vitamin D, and calcitonin. These three substances interact to control absorption from the GI tract, deposition and resorption from bone, and excretion and resorption by the kidneys. PTH, secreted in response to hypocalcemia, decreases the circulating or serum phosphate level by increasing its excretion from the kidneys. Vitamin D increases phosphate uptake from the GI tract, and calcitonin decreases phosphate excretion from the kidneys.[14,31,55]

Hyperphosphatemia

The incidence of hyperphosphatemia is most commonly seen in the setting of renal insufficiency and failure. Because the kidneys are efficient in eliminating phosphate, levels do not usually increase until the kidneys have lost more than 75% of their function.[15] Phosphate levels may also increase because of tumor lysis (resulting from chemotherapy for cancer), large muscle trauma (crush injuries), and heatstroke. Hyperphosphatemia may also be caused by the excessive use of phosphate-containing enemas or laxatives, even with normal kidney function. If a renal failure patient ingests excessive amounts of vitamin D, hyperphosphatemia may occur. Excessive phosphate combines with calcium to form an insoluble compound called calcium phosphate, which may be deposited throughout the body, especially the kidneys, heart, lungs, cornea, and skin. While rare, it is a serious complication in patients suffering from end-stage renal failure and inadequate control of their phosphate levels.[9,26,55]

Physical Assessment Findings

Elevated phosphate combines with ionized calcium and decreases the calcium level, with the major signs and symptoms seen with hyperphosphatemia related to the low calcium concentration. Hypocalcemia typically causes increased neuromuscular activity and negative effects on the cardiovascular system. The increased neuromuscular activity is caused by the decrease in the excitation threshold and is exhibited by numbness and tingling, particularly around the mouth and in the hands and feet. Muscle spasm, to the point of tetany, of the hands, feet, and face may be seen or even elicited during an assessment. Chvostek's sign and Trousseau's sign are both indicators of tetany. Hyperreflexia is also found (see Figs. 21.10 and 21.11).[26] The cardiovascular effects of hypocalcemia are significant and can include hypotension, increased QT interval (which may lead to ventricular dysrhythmias, including ventricular tachycardia and TdP),[5] decreased cardiac output, and decreased response to medications that act through calcium, including digitalis, dopamine, and norepinephrine.[34,55]

Laboratory Findings

Phosphates are the chemically active forms of phosphorus that the body uses for energy. However, laboratory values are expressed in terms of phosphorus.[26]

Hyperphosphatemia is defined as phosphorus levels greater than 4.5 mg/dL (> 1.45 mmol/L). Because the effects of hyperphosphatemia are long term and do not have a significant impact on patient survival, there is no critical level.[15]

Treatment

The main treatments of hyperphosphatemia are decreasing the intake of phosphates and binding phosphates in the gut using a variety of agents (aluminum hydroxide, calcium acetate, lanthanum, sevelamer). All of these agents work in the GI tract and are not available in an IV. If a patient has reasonable renal function, a saline IV may increase phosphate excretion.[26]

Hypophosphatemia

Hypophosphatemia is a significant issue for critically ill patients. Hypophosphatemia can occur because of a depletion of body stores or a shift of phosphates from the ECF into the ICF.[26] Depletion of body stores occurs with excessive alcohol use. Whereas there is some relation to the inadequate diets of most patients with chronic alcoholism, hypophosphatemia has been found in chronic alcoholism patients with normal diets, leading to speculation that some other mechanism is also involved. Medications used to bind phosphorus in the GI tract can cause significant hypophosphatemia when used to excess. Extensive thermal burns may cause hypophosphatemia. It usually occurs a number of days after the initial injury and is thought to be related to the forced diuresis that results from fluid resuscitation.[26,31,55] In addition, hypophosphatemia is a common occurrence in patients receiving continuous renal-replacement therapy.[50] Hospitalized older adults are at risk for vitamin D deficiency, which can also cause hypophosphatemia.[22]

A shift of phosphate from the ECF to the ICF is a significant cause of hypophosphatemia and can occur in a variety of settings. Patients may have several of these causes simultaneously in the critical care setting. Epinephrine has been implicated in causing a decrease in phosphate levels in patients,[17,18] but its mechanism is unclear. Respiratory alkalosis, caused by overventilation, can cause a shift of phosphorus into the cells with a resultant decrease in the phosphorus level by up to 0.5 mg/dL (0.16 mmol/L). Patients suffering from DKA and HHS can excrete significant amounts of phosphate in the urine and still have normal serum phosphorus levels. The treatment of both of these diabetic emergencies with insulin and fluids will drive phosphate from the ECF into the ICF, potentially creating a significant hypophosphatemia.[26]

A significant cause of hypophosphatemia is known as *refeeding syndrome*, which occurs when a malnourished patient is started on either parenteral or enteral nutrition. A malnourished patient will have a depleted ICF phosphate level, whereas the ECF level will remain relatively normal. When the patient begins to receive nutrition, even in modest amounts, the increased levels of glucose and insulin, from either the parenteral formula or the patient's pancreas, cause a significant shift of phosphates from the ECF into the ICF. This shift dramatically decreases the ECF phosphate level and puts the patient at risk for hypophosphatemia. This usually occurs from 24 to 72 hours after the feedings start, and is more common in parenteral than enteral nutrition.[23,26,31]

The effects of hypophosphatemia are significant and wide ranging and are the result of a decrease in the levels of ATP and 2,3-diphosphoglycerate (2,3-DPG), an enzyme that is necessary for the release of oxygen from red blood cells. Low ATP and 2,3-DPG levels cause red blood cells to be more fragile, more likely to hemolyze, and less able to release oxygen to peripheral tissues.[31] Both factors are implicated in significant tissue hypoxia. Because of the low phosphate levels, muscular strength will decrease and the muscles may even begin to disintegrate, causing an increase in creatinine phosphokinase (CPK) level and rhabdomyolysis. This muscle weakness and destruction is also implicated in respiratory failure, and especially in the failure of mechanically ventilated patients who are unable to be weaned because of muscle fatigue. The respiratory muscle failure, coupled with the tissue hypoxia, can have a profoundly negative effect on the patient who is being weaned. The heart is also susceptible to hypophosphatemia-induced decreases in contractility. Hypophosphatemia may even cause a cardiomyopathy that can be reversed with phosphate repletion. In addition, hypophosphatemia is associated with a decreased response to both inotropic and vasoactive medications.[26,31]

Physical Assessment Findings

The major assessment findings in hypophosphatemia are seen as muscular weakness, changes in mental status (increased irritability, weakness, numbness, lack of coordination, confusion, seizures, coma), hypoxia, and potential difficulty in maintaining cardiac output or blood pressure, even with supportive medications.[16,17,26]

Laboratory Findings

When the phosphorus level drops below 2.5 mg/dL (< 0.81 mmol/L) hypophosphatemia exists. When the phosphorus level drops below 1.5 mg/dL (< 0.49 mmol/L), severe hypophosphatemia exists. A critical level is considered below 1 mg/dL (< 0.32 mmol/L).[15]

Treatment

The initial treatment of hypophosphatemia is to treat the causes, if possible. If the patient has a functioning GI tract, oral or enteral replacement with a variety of phosphate products is appropriate. The ability of the patient to tolerate such products may be limited by nausea or diarrhea. If the patient is unable to tolerate the oral or enteral replacement, or if the hypophosphatemia is significant (< 1 mg/dL [< 0.32 mmol/L]), slow replenishment via IV may be utilized, using any number of published dosing schemes. If the replenishment is too rapid, hypocalcemia may occur. The key to replenishment of phosphates is that it must be done over a period of days to allow equilibrium to occur between the ECF and the ICF.[26,50]

CONCLUSION

Electrolyte imbalances represent some of the most complex medical emergencies faced by critical care nurses. The physiologic processes of potassium, sodium, calcium, magnesium, and phosphorus are interlinked and may present a confusing picture. However, an in-depth knowledge of the pathophysiology can prepare the critical care nurse with the methods of assessment, identification, and treatment that can sometimes dramatically influence their patients' lives.

REFERENCES

1. Adrogué, H. J., & Madias, N. E. (2000). Hypernatremia. *N Engl J Med, 342*, 1493–1499.
2. Adrogué, H. J., & Madias, N. E. (2000). Hyponatremia. *N Engl J Med, 342*, 1581–1589.
3. Alfrey, A. C. (2003). Normal and abnormal magnesium metabolism. In R. W. Schrier (Ed.), *Renal and electrolyte disorders* (6th ed.). Philadelphia: Lippincott Williams & Wilkins.
4. American Diabetes Association. (2004). Hyperglycemic crises in diabetes. *Diab Care, 27*(Suppl. 1), S94–S102.
5. Sinz, E., Navarro, K., & Soderberg, E. S. (Eds.). (2015). *ACLS for experienced providers: manual and resource text* (1st ed.). American Heart Association.
6. Ariyan, C. E., & Sosa, J. A. (2004). Assessment and management of patients with abnormal calcium. *Crit Care Med, 34*(Suppl), S146–S154.
7. Batcheller, J. (1994). Syndrome of inappropriate antidiuretic hormone secretion. *Crit Care Nurs Clin North Am, 6*, 687–692.
8. Bushinsky, D. A., & Monk, R. D. (1998). Calcium. *Lancet, 352*, 306–311.
9. Carlstedt, F., & Lind, L. (2001). Hypocalcemic syndromes. *Crit Care Clin, 17*, 139–153.
10. Chernow, B., et al. (1989). Hypomagnesemia in patients in postoperative intensive care. *Chest, 95*, 391–397.
11. Cohn, J. N., et al. (2000). New guidelines for potassium replacement in clinical practice. *Arch Intern Med, 160*, 2429–2436.
12. Gheorghiade, M., et al. (2003). Vasopressin V2-receptor blockade with tolvaptan in patients with chronic heart failure: results from a double-blind, randomized trial. *Circulation, 107*, 2690–2696.
13. Gibbs, M. A., Wolfson, A. B., & Tayal, V. S. (2002). Electrolyte disturbances. In J. A. Marx (Ed.), *Rosen's emergency medicine: concepts and clinical practice* (vol. 2). St Louis: Mosby.
14. Huether, S. E. (2002). The cellular environment: fluids and electrolytes, acids and bases. In K. L. McCance, & S. E. Huether (Eds.), *Pathophysiology: the biological basis for disease in adults and children* (4th ed.). St Louis: Mosby.
15. Jacobs, D. S., DeMott, W. R., & Oxley, D. K. (2004). *Lexi-Comp's laboratory test handbook* (3rd ed.). Cleveland, OH: Lexi-Comp.
16. Kapoor, M., & Chan, G. Z. (2001). Fluid and electrolyte abnormalities. *Crit Care Clin, 17*, 503–529.
17. Kjeldsen, S. E., et al. (1988). Decreased serum phosphate in essential hypertension: related to increased sympathetic tone. *Am J Hypertens, 1*(4 Pt 1), 403–409.
18. Kjeldsen, S. E., et al. (1986). Serum phosphate and sympathetic tone in mild essential hypertension. *Acta Med Scand Suppl, 714*, 119–123.
19. Kosiborod, M., Rasmussen, H. S., Lavin, P., Qunibi, W. Y., Spinowitz, B., et al. (2014). Effect of sodium zirconium cyclosilicate on potassium lowering for 28 days among outpatients with hyperkalemia: the HARMONIZE randomized clinical trial. *JAMA, 312*(21), 2223.
20. Lavonas, E. J., Drennan, A. G., Heffner, A. C., et al. (2010). American Heart Association ACLS guidelines update 2015 part 10: special circumstances of resuscitation. *Circulation, 132*(Suppl. 2), S501–S518.
21. Lum, G. (1992). Hypomagnesemia in acute and chronic care patient populations. *Am J Clin Pathol, 97*, 827–830.
22. Lyman, D. (2005). Undiagnosed vitamin D deficiency in the hospitalized patient. *Am Fam Pract, 71*, 299–304.
23. Marinella, M. A. (2003). The refeeding syndrome and hypophosphatemia. *Nutr Rev, 61*, 320–323.
24. Matz, R. (1993). Magnesium: deficiencies and therapeutic uses. *Hosp Pract (Off Ed), 28*(4A), 79–82, 85–87, 91–92.
25. McLaughlin, S. A., & McKinney, P. E. (1998). Antacid-induced hypermagnesemia in a patient with normal renal function and bowel obstruction. *Ann Pharmacother, 32*, 312–315.
26. Metheny, N. M. (2010). *Fluid and electrolyte balance: nursing considerations* (5th ed.). Philadelphia: Lippincott Williams & Wilkins.
27. Myers, J. S. (2001). Oncologic emergencies. In S. E. Otto (Ed.), *Oncology nursing* (pp. 498–581). St Louis: Mosby.
28. Nordt, S. P., et al. (1996). Hypermagnesemia following an acute ingestion of Epsom salt in a patient with normal renal function. *J Toxicol Clin Toxicol, 34*, 735–739.
29. Packham, D. K., Rasmussen, H. S., Lavin, P. T., et al. (2015). Sodium zirconium cyclosilicate in hyperkalemia. *N Engl J Med, 372*(3), 222–231.
30. Palmer, B. F. (2004). Managing hyperkalemia caused by inhibitors of the renin-angiotensin-aldosterone system. *N Engl J Med, 351*, 585–592.
31. Peppers, M. P., Geheb, M., & Desai, T. (1991). Hypophosphatemia and hyperphosphatemia. *Crit Care Clin, 7*, 201–214.
32. Perazella, M. A. (2000). Drug-induced hyperkalemia: old culprits and new offenders. *Am J Med, 109*, 307–314.

33. Piano, M. R., & Huether, S. E. (2002). Mechanisms of hormonal regulation. In K. L. McCance, & S. E. Huether (Eds.), *Pathophysiology: the biological basis for disease in adults and children* (4th ed.). St Louis: Mosby.
34. Porth, C. M. (2004). *Essentials of pathophysiology*. Philadelphia: Lippincott Williams & Wilkins.
35. Reinhart, R. A., & Desbiens, N. A. (1985). Hypomagnesemia in patients entering the ICU. *Crit Care Med, 13*, 506–507.
36. Rubeiz, G. J., Thill-Baharozian, M., Hardie, D., et al. (1993). Association of hypomagnesemia and mortality in acutely ill medical patients. *Crit Care Med, 21*, 203–209.
37. RXlist.com. (2015). *Calcium chloride*. http://www.rxlist.com/calcium-chloride-drug.htm.
38. RXlist.com. (2015). *Calcium gluconate*. http://www.rxlist.com/calcium-gluconate-drug.htm.
39. RXlist.com. (2015). *Kayexelate*. http://www.rxlist.com/kayexalate-drug.htm.
40. Rxlist.com. (2015). *Potassium extended release*. http://www.rxlist.com/potassium-chloride-extended-release-tablets-drug.htm.
41. Salem, M., Munoz, R., & Chernow, B. (1991). Hypomagnesemia in critical illness: a common and clinically important problem. *Crit Care Clin, 7*, 225–252.
42. Sato, Y., et al. (2000). Beneficial effect of intermittent cyclical etidronate therapy in hemiplegic patients following an acute stroke. *J Bone Miner Res, 15*, 2487–2494.
43. Sato, Y., et al. (2004). Beneficial effect of etidronate therapy in immobilized hip fracture patients. *Am J Phys Med Rehabil, 83*, 298–303.
44. Spasovski, G., Vanholder, R., Allolio, B., et al. (2014). Clinical practice guideline on diagnosis and treatment of hyponatremia. *Eur J Endocrinol, 170*, G1–G47.
45. Stern, J. M. (2005). Oncology fluid and electrolyte disorders. *Support Line, 27*(3), 19–27.
46. Tofil, N. M., Benner, K. W., & Winkler, M. K. (2005). Fatal hypermagnesemia caused by an Epsom salt enema: a case illustration. *South Med J, 98*, 253–256.
47. Toto, K. H., & Yucha, C. B. (1994). Magnesium: homeostasis, imbalances and therapeutic uses. *Crit Care Nurs Clin North Am, 6*, 767–783.
48. Vissers, R. J., & Purssell, R. (1996). Iatrogenic magnesium overdose: two case reports. *J Emerg Med, 14*, 187–191.
49. Weir, M. R., Bakris, G. L., Bushinshy, D. A., Mayo, M. R., Garza, D., et al. (2015). Patiromer in patients with kidney disease and hyperkalemia receiving RAAS inhibitors. *N Engl J Med 372(3)*, 211–221.
50. Weiss-Guillet, E., Takala, J., & Jakob, S. (2003). Diagnosis and management of electrolyte emergencies. *Best Pract Res Clin Endocrinol Metab, 17*, 623–651.
51. Whang, R., & Ryder, K. W. (1990). Frequency of hypomagnesemia and hypermagnesemia: requested vs. routine. *JAMA, 263*, 3063–3064.
52. Whitemire, S. J. (2003). Fluids, electrolytes and acid-base balance. In L. E. Matarese, & M. M. Gottschlich (Eds.), *Contemporary nutrition support practice* (2nd ed.). Philadelphia: Saunders.
53. Wong, E. T., et al. (1983). A high prevalence of hypomagnesemia and hypermagnesemia in hospitalized patients. *Am J Clin Pathol, 79*, 348–352.
54. Wong, F., et al. (2003). A vasopressin receptor antagonist (VPA-985) improves serum sodium concentration in patients with hyponatremia: a multicenter, randomized, placebo-controlled trial. *Hepatology, 37*, 182–191.
55. Yucha, C. B., & Toto, K. H. (1994). Calcium and phosphorus derangements. *Crit Care Nurs Clin North Am, 6*, 747–766.

Complex Acid-Base Disorders and Associated Electrolyte Imbalances

Paula McCauley

Acid-base and electrolyte imbalances are common in acutely ill patients. They frequently complicate critical illness and are often the central focus of urgent or emergent therapy. Those affected by acute and chronic kidney disease, volume depletion, acute respiratory distress, chronic obstructive pulmonary disease (COPD), and shock have increased risk for these disorders.

In the acutely ill adult, mixed acid-base disorders are common. Differentiating between a compensated acid-base disorder and a mixed disorder can be challenging. Additionally, acid-base disorders are often accompanied by electrolyte imbalances, complicating both the clinical presentation and the treatment. This chapter will review acid-base physiology and discuss a systematic approach to diagnosing acid-base disturbances utilizing arterial blood gas (ABG) interpretation methods. The etiology, clinical manifestations, associated electrolyte imbalances, and treatment of primary disorders will be reviewed. A case study will be utilized to illustrate the salient aspects of caring for acutely ill patients with acid-base and electrolyte emergencies.

ACID-BASE PHYSIOLOGY

Acid-base balance is maintained through complex, bidirectional interactions mainly regulated between the cellular, renal, and pulmonary systems. The cardiovascular, gastrointestinal (GI), and hepatic systems also play important roles. Disruptions in any one of these systems can result in an acid-base imbalance with severe adverse consequences.

The arterial pH is the primary indicator of acid-base balance and is a reflection of hydrogen ion (H^+) concentration in the blood. Under normal circumstances, the pH is maintained within the range of 7.35 to 7.45. The arterial pH is affected by the interplay of acids (substances able to give up H^+ ions) and bases (substances able to accept H^+ ions). As the H^+ concentration in the blood increases, the pH decreases. Conversely, as the H^+ concentration in the blood decreases, the pH increases. Maintaining the H^+ concentration and pH within normal limits is, in part, controlled by the carbonic-acid-bicarbonate buffer system. The buffer systems work to maintain the ratio of acid to bicarbonate at 20:1. As long as this ratio is maintained, the pH will remain within normal limits.

The principal function of the lungs in acid-base homeostasis is to regulate $Paco_2$. An alteration in pH, Pao_2, or $Paco_2$ triggers chemoreceptor stimulation, causing an increase or decrease in rate and depth of ventilation. Hypo- or hyperventilation will occur in an attempt to return the pH to normal. CO_2 can be converted to carbonic acid (gas) and excreted via the lungs. The lungs respond within minutes of the derangement.

The role of the kidney in acid base homeostasis is to maintain balance through reabsorption or excretion of bicarbonate, and generation of ammonium NH_4 in the distal tubules, which facilitates H^+ secretion. Renal compensation happens hours after the derangement begins and may take 3 to 5 days for full compensation.

Sodium phosphate ($NaHPO_4$), hemoglobin (Hgb), and serum proteins (albumin) also function as buffers. Serum proteins can act by releasing or binding H^+ as needed to maintain homeostasis. Hgb, a protein in red blood cells, buffers acids in a similar fashion to serum proteins and can carry CO_2.[1-3,7,17,19,22]

Definitions and Normal Values

The primary parameters important in acid-base assessment include the acids; H^+ and partial pressure of arterial carbon dioxide ($Paco_2$); and the base HCO_3^-. Diagnosing acid-base imbalances at the bedside begins with assessing serum chemistries and the ABG (Table 22.1).

Acidemia is defined as a decrease in the blood pH below 7.35, whereas acidosis is a physiologic process characterized by a primary decrease in HCO_3^- level (metabolic acidosis) or a primary increase in $Paco_2$ (respiratory acidosis). Conversely, alkalemia is defined as an increase in the blood pH above 7.45, whereas alkalosis is a physiologic process characterized by a primary increase in the HCO_3^- level (metabolic alkalosis) or a primary decrease in the $Paco_2$ (respiratory alkalosis).[3,7,17,22]

Understanding Compensation

Acid-base disorders are caused by primary changes in the excretion of $Paco_2$ (respiratory disorders) or changes in the plasma HCO_3^- level (metabolic disorders). Under normal circumstances, all deviations from normal in acid-base balance trigger compensatory mechanisms that tend to return blood pH toward the normal level. It is important to emphasize that the H^+ ion concentration is determined by the ratio of the $Paco_2$ to HCO_3^- concentration. Metabolic acid-base disorders result in deviations in HCO_3^- from normal, whereas respiratory acid-base disorders are due to deviations in $Paco_2$ from normal.

In metabolic acidosis, the H^+ concentration is increased because the bicarbonate concentration is reduced. As the acidosis develops, causing the $Paco_2$ to fall, the H^+ concentration returns toward normal because the ratio is partially restored to the normal level. Compensation will occur, stimulating an increase in minute ventilation, resulting in a decrease in $Paco_2$ to 22 mm Hg.

Conversely for a metabolic alkalosis, a primary increase in HCO_3^- plasma concentration, the compensatory mechanism is a decrease in minute ventilation, resulting in an increase in $Paco_2$. This increase in $Paco_2$ acts to move the blood pH toward normal. It is important to remember that these compensatory mechanisms do not return the blood pH completely to the normal range of 7.35 to 7.45, but rather toward the normal range.[4,8,9,12,18]

TABLE 22.1 Labs Used in Acid-Base Assessment: Normal Values

Arterial Blood Gas	
pH	7.35–7.45
$Paco_2$	35–45 mm Hg
HCO_3^-	24–28 mEq/L
Serum Chemistries	
Na^+	135–145 mEq/L
K^+	3.5–5.5 mEq/L
Cl^-	95–105 mEq/L
CO_2	26–32 mEq/L

Cl^-, Chloride bicarbonate; *K^+*, potassium; *Na^+*, sodium; *$Paco_2$*, partial pressure of arterial carbon dioxide.

Application of Acid-Base Principles

The assessment and diagnosis of acid-base disorders require a systematic approach beginning with interpretation of the ABG in conjunction with evaluation of serum chemistries and calculation of the anion gap. Evaluation of the anion gap is critical in acid-base assessment because it will aide in identification of the underlying differential of many causes of metabolic acidosis. An elevated gap may be the only clue to the presence of a metabolic acidosis in the setting of a mixed acid-base disorder where the pH is normal (two or more primary disorders occurring simultaneously). For example, a patient with a respiratory alkalosis and a metabolic acidosis may have a normal arterial pH despite a low HCO_3^- level and a low $Paco_2$ (lower than that which would occur with compensation for the metabolic acidosis). Systematic assessment of the ABG and the anion gap will allow for the diagnosis and treatment of these complex acid-base disorders, and is outlined in Box 22.1.

BOX 22.1 Systematic Approach to Diagnosing Simple and Mixed Acid-Base Disorders

STEP 1: Using the Arterial Blood Gas, Identify the Most Apparent Disorder

A. Evaluate the pH.
- If the pH is less than 7.35, acidemia is present and may be due to a metabolic or respiratory disorder.
- If the pH is greater than 7.45, alkalemia is present and may be due to either a metabolic or a respiratory disorder.

B. Determine the primary disorder. If the measured pH and $Paco_2$ are both abnormal, assess the direction of change.
- If both values change in the same direction, the primary acid base abnormality is metabolic.
- If they change in opposite directions, the primary acid base abnormality is respiratory.

STEP 2: Determine If Compensation Is Present or If There Is a Mixed Acid-Base Disorder

Determine if the pH is normal and either the HCO_3^- or the $Paco_2$ (or both) is abnormal: a mixed acid-base disorder. This situation should not be misinterpreted as compensation of a primary disorder because the pH is not normalized even with full compensation. To identify one of the acid-base disturbances present, start by picking the HCO_3^- or $Paco_2$ value that is most abnormal.

A. If a metabolic acidosis is present, use the following formula to calculate what the predicted $Paco_2$ would be if compensated:

$Paco_2 = 1.5 \times (HCO_3^-) + 8\ (\pm 2)$.

Example: pH = 7:30; $Paco_2$ = 30 mm Hg; HCO_3^- = 14 mEq/L

Predicted $Paco_2 = 1.5 \times 14 + 8$
$= 21 + 8$
$= 29$ mm Hg

When fully compensated, the $Paco_2$ closely approximates the last two digits of the blood pH within the range of 7.10 to 7.40. This rule-of-thumb applies only to metabolic acidosis and does not apply for a pH outside of this range. If the $Paco_2$ does not approximate the last two digits of the pH, a mixed acid-base disturbance should be considered. In the example given, you can quickly interpret this as a compensated metabolic acidosis because the digits to the right of the pH decimal point = 30 and the $Paco_2$ = 30 mm Hg.

B. If there is a *metabolic alkalosis,* use the following formula to calculate what the predicted $Paco_2$ would be if compensated:

$Paco_2 = 40 + 0.7 \times (\text{measured } HCO_3^- - \text{normal } HCO_3^-)$

Example: pH = 7.49; $Paco_2$ = 48 mm Hg; HCO_3^- = 36 mEq/L

Predicted $Paco_2 = 40 + 0.7\ (36 - 26)$
$= 40 + 0.7\ (10)$
$= 40 + 7$
$= 47$ mm Hg

Interpretation: Compensated metabolic alkalosis. The calculated predicted $Paco_2$ of 47 mm Hg approximates the measured $Paco_2$ of 48 mm Hg.

C. If a respiratory acidosis is present, use the following rules to determine what the predicted concentration would be if compensated.

Acute respiratory acidosis:
HCO_3^- concentration increases by up to 1 mEq for every 10 mm Hg increase in $Paco_2$

Chronic respiratory acidosis:
HCO_3^- concentration increases by up to 3.5 mEq for every 10 mm Hg increase in $Paco_2$

D. If there is a respiratory alkalosis, use the following rules to determine what the predicted concentration would be if compensated.

Acute respiratory alkalosis:
HCO_3^- concentration decreases by up to 2 mEq for every 10 mm Hg decrease in $Paco_2$

Chronic respiratory alkalosis:
HCO_3^- concentration decreases by up to 5 mEq for every 10 mm Hg decrease in $Paco_2$

If the measured values do not approximate the predicted values using the formulas and rules in Step 2, a mixed acid-base balance is present.

STEP 3: Calculate the Anion Gap

Calculation of the anion gap is the third step in diagnosing an acid-base disorder and is important in determining the presence of mixed imbalances as well as differentiating an elevated anion gap metabolic acidosis from a nonelevated anion gap metabolic acidosis (see Fig. 22.2).

When calculating the anion gap using the serum chemistry panel, it is important to remember that the concentration on the chemistry panel is represented as total CO_2 concentration. The normal range for the anion gap is approximately 9 to 16 mEq/L.

From References 3, 4, 8, 13, 17, 19, and 20.

The Anion Gap

The extracellular fluid is normally electroneutral, meaning that the sum of anions (negative ions) is equal to the sum of cations (positive ions) (Fig. 22.1). The primary measured anions in the plasma include chloride (Cl^-) and the primary cation is sodium (Na^+). Potassium (K^+) may or may not be included in the calculation and so it is imperative that the provider refer to their laboratory procedure when calculating. The ions not included in the anion gap formula are termed *unmeasured ions.*

The smaller quantities of anions not included in the anion gap formula include albumin, sulfate, phosphate, and others. The smaller quantities of cations not included in the formula include calcium (Ca^{2+}), magnesium (Mg^{2+}), and others. Because the unmeasured ions are not all included in the formula, there is a normal variance or "gap" ranging from approximately 9 to 16 mEq/L; the normal range may vary depending on the individual laboratory. If this gap is increased, it signifies the presence of additional unmeasured ions in the plasma. The addition of H^+, an acid, is buffered by a base, causing an increase in the anion gap and signifying the presence of a metabolic acidosis. When calculating the anion gap using the serum chemistry panel, it is important to remember that the HCO_3^- concentration is represented as total CO_2 concentration on the chemistry panel. The total CO_2 concentration is a combination of HCO_3^- concentration, dissolved CO_2 concentration, and H_2CO_3 concentration, the most predominant of which is HCO_3^- concentration. Typically, the plasma total CO_2 concentration is approximately 1 mEq greater than the arterial concentration in the anion gap formula.

Box 22.2 demonstrates calculation of the anion gap. In the example, the anion gap of 25 mEq/L is greater than the expected gap of 9 to 16 mEq/L and signifies the presence of a metabolic acidosis. If the anion gap is greater than 20 mEq/L, a metabolic acidosis is present.

In a metabolic acidosis caused by the addition or accumulation of acid in the plasma (e.g., lactic acidosis, ketoacidosis, renal failure), there will be an increase in the anion gap. If the metabolic acidosis is due to the loss of bicarbonate (e.g., diarrhea, GI fistula), the anion gap will remain within normal limits despite the presence of a metabolic acidosis.[14,21,22]

Box 22.3 lists causes of metabolic acidosis differentiated by the anion gap.

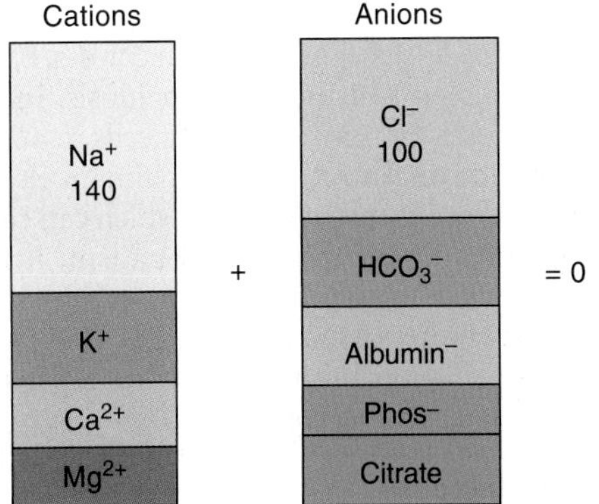

FIG. 22.1 The anion gap. *Ca^{2+}*, Calcium; *Cl^-*, chloride; *HCO_3^-*, bicarbonate; *K^+*, potassium; *Mg^{2+}*, magnesium; *Na^+*, sodium; *Phos*, phosphate.

PRIMARY ACID-BASE DISORDERS

Metabolic Acidosis

Metabolic acidosis is characterized by physiologic processes resulting in a decrease in the plasma bicarbonate concentration, whereas acidemia is defined as an arterial pH of less than 7.35. There are three general mechanisms responsible for a metabolic acidosis:

- Increased acid production (e.g., ketoacidosis, lactic acidosis)
- Decreased acid excretion (e.g., renal failure)
- Bicarbonate loss (e.g., diarrhea, GI fistula)

Causes of Metabolic Acidosis

Causes of metabolic acidosis are differentiated by those disorders associated with an elevated anion gap (> 20 mEq/L) and those associated with no significant elevation in the anion gap (< 20 mEq/L) (Fig. 22.2). In the critical care setting, there are four common causes of an elevated anion gap metabolic acidosis: lactic acidosis, ketoacidosis, renal failure (uremia), and ingestion of

BOX 22.2 Calculation of the Anion Gap

Cl^- = Chloride, Na^+ = sodium, K^+ = potassium.
Anion Gap = $Na^+ - (Cl^- + HCO_3^-)$
Given the following Serum Chemistries
Na^+ = 140 mEq/L
K^+ = 5 mEq/L
Cl^- = 100 mEq/L
CO_2 = 15 mEq/L
Anion gap calculation: $Na^+ - (Cl^- + HCO_3^-)$
= 140 − (100 + 15)
= 140 − 115
= 25 mEq/L

BOX 22.3 Causes of Metabolic Acidosis

Elevated Anion Gap*	Non–Anion Gap
Ketoacidosis	Gastrointestinal bicarbonate loss
Uremia (renal failure)	Diarrhea
Salicylate intoxication	Pancreatic or biliary fistula
Starvation ketosis	Ileostomy
Methanol	Small bowel drains
Alcoholic ketosis	Ureterosigmoidostomy
Unmeasured osmoles: ethylene glycol, paraldehyde	Anion exchange resin: cholestyramine
Lactic acidosis	Renal tubular acidosis

*The mnemonic KUSSMAUL can be used to help remember the causes of a metabolic acidosis associated with an elevated anion gap.

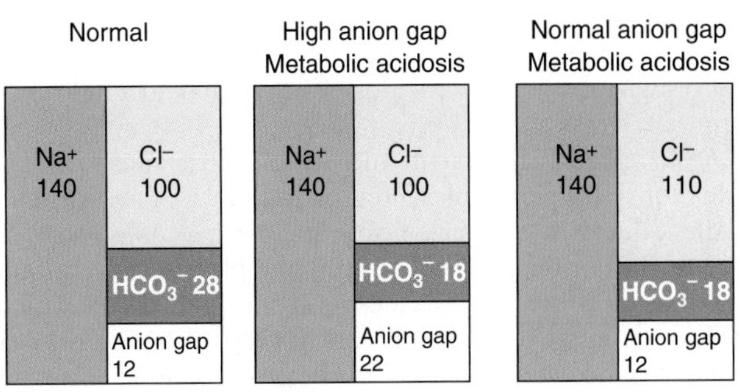

FIG. 22.2 Metabolic acidosis: high vs. normal anion gap. *Cl^-*, Chloride; *HCO_3^-*, bicarbonate; *Na^+*, sodium.

toxins. The most common cause of a non–anion gap metabolic acidosis is GI bicarbonate loss from diarrhea (see Box 22.3).[16]

A mnemonic device used to remember these factors is MUDPILES: Methanol, Uremia, Diabetic ketoacidosis (DKA), Paraldehyde, Isoniazid (INH) and Iron, Lactic acid, Ethylene glycol and Ethanol and Salicylates. An additional mnemonic is KUSSMAUL: Ketoacidosis, Uremia, Salicylates, Starvation ketosis, Methanol, Alcoholic ketosis, Unmeasured osmoles, and Lactate.[4,7,8]

Elevated Anion Gap Metabolic Acidosis

Lactic acidosis. Lactic acidosis is a common cause of metabolic acidosis in the critically ill patient. Lactic acidosis is typically the result of tissue hypoxia associated with inadequate perfusion or severe hypoxia. When tissues receive inadequate blood flow or oxygen delivery, they convert from aerobic to anaerobic metabolism, resulting in the production of lactic acid. Common causes of lactic acidosis include shock states, mesenteric ischemia, acute respiratory failure, severe anemia, carbon monoxide poisoning, and metformin.[20] In the critically ill patient, lactic acidosis is often accompanied by acute renal failure caused by renal hypoperfusion. The metabolic acidosis in this situation can be quite severe and is compounded by reduced renal clearance of lactic acid as well as other acids.[14,15]

Ketoacidosis. Ketoacidosis occurs when cells are unable to use glucose as an energy source for metabolism and convert to the metabolism of fatty acids, which produces ketoacids (beta-hydroxybutyrate and acetoacetate). There are three causes of ketoacidosis: DKA, alcohol ingestion, and starvation. DKA typically occurs in the type 1 diabetes patient who has inadequate insulin for a given level of physiologic stress, resulting in hyperglycemia with a blood glucose level that is typically greater than 300 mg/dL.[9] DKA can occur from omission of insulin therapy, new-onset type 1 diabetes, or a physiologic stress raising the blood glucose level (e.g., infection, acute myocardial infarction, trauma, surgery, pregnancy). When there is inadequate insulin in the setting of hyperglycemia, cellular starvation occurs and metabolism converts from utilization of glucose to the breakdown of fatty acids; the end products of fatty acid metabolism are ketoacids.[11]

Alcoholic ketoacidosis is due to excessive alcohol ingestion and is often associated with starvation. Both alcoholic and starvation ketoacidosis are associated with hypoglycemia and decreased hepatic production of glucose. In this state of hypoglycemia, the pancreas releases less insulin and cells must convert to metabolism of fatty acids for energy. As in DKA, the metabolism of these fatty acids produces ketoacids. Unlike DKA, starvation and alcoholic ketoacidosis are characterized by blood glucose levels less than 150 mg/dL.[9] In all three states of ketoacidosis (DKA, alcoholic, and starvation), the buildup of ketoacids in the plasma reduces the plasma bicarbonate level and results in a metabolic acidosis associated with a high anion gap.

Renal failure. In both acute and chronic renal failure, there is a reduction in the glomerular filtration rate and a decreased ability of the kidneys to clear acids from the plasma. As a result, H^+ accumulates in the plasma, lowering the plasma concentration and causing a metabolic acidosis. In the critically ill patient, the presence of renal failure often perpetuates or worsens other causes of metabolic acidosis because of limited clearance of acids in the setting of overproduction of acids. Examples of concomitant causes of metabolic acidosis in a critically ill patient include septic shock with ischemic acute tubular necrosis, DKA with dehydration and prerenal acute renal failure, and trauma with rhabdomyolysis and nephrotoxic acute tubular necrosis.[6,15]

Ingestion of toxins. The ingestion of various acid-producing substances can cause a metabolic acidosis. These substances include salicylate (aspirin), ethylene glycol (antifreeze and organic solvents), methanol (wood alcohol), and paraldehyde (sedative). Typically, the ingested substance is not an acid but is metabolized into an acid (methanol, ethylene glycol). The increase in acid production lowers the plasma bicarbonate level and results in a high anion gap metabolic acidosis. Additionally, concurrent tissue hypoperfusion and lactic acidosis often contribute to metabolic acidosis in these patients.[17,21]

Non–Anion Gap Metabolic Acidosis

A non–anion gap metabolic acidosis is due to a loss of bicarbonate from either the kidneys or the GI tract. The most common cause of this type of metabolic acidosis in the acutely ill patient is diarrhea. Diarrhea causes a loss of bicarbonate and an increase in chloride concentration, leading to metabolic acidosis with a normal anion gap. A less common cause of a non–anion gap metabolic acidosis is renal tubular acidosis (RTA).

Gastrointestinal bicarbonate loss. The loss of bicarbonate from the GI tract results in an increase in H^+ and chloride concentrations. Moderate to severe diarrhea is the most common cause of a non–anion gap metabolic acidosis and is often associated with volume depletion that may cause a concomitant lactic acidosis if volume depletion is severe.[21] Other causes of GI bicarbonate loss that can cause a non–anion gap metabolic acidosis include ileostomies, small bowel drains, and pancreatic drains or fistulas.

Renal tubular acidosis. RTA is characterized by an impairment of the renal tubules' ability to reabsorb and excrete H^+, resulting in a metabolic acidosis not associated with an increase in the anion gap.[21]

Manifestations of Metabolic Acidosis

Metabolic acidosis affects many organ systems and is often associated with electrolyte imbalances. The life-threatening effects of a severe metabolic acidosis, a pH less than 7.2, are manifested in many body systems and are most prominent in the cardiovascular, metabolic, and neurologic systems (Box 22.4).[8,10,15]

Electrolyte Imbalances Associated with Metabolic Acidosis

Hyperkalemia

Defined as a serum K^+ level greater than 5 mEq/L, hyperkalemia is commonly seen with metabolic acidosis. In the setting of metabolic acidosis, H^+ moves into the cells in an attempt to reduce plasma acid concentrations. To maintain electrical neutrality, potassium moves out of the cell, which can cause hyperkalemia (Fig. 22.3). In the critically ill patient, hyperkalemia and metabolic acidosis are often compounded by comorbidities (e.g., acute renal failure, tissue catabolism). These factors play an important role in contributing to the ongoing hyperkalemia associated with metabolic acidosis.[7]

Ionized Calcium Increase

Defined as calcium greater than 5 mg/dL or 1.32 mmol/L, an increase in the ionized calcium level can occur in the

BOX 22.4 Manifestations of Severe Metabolic Acidosis (pH < 7.2)

Cardiovascular
- Decreased cardiac contractility
- Increased pulmonary vascular resistance leading to pulmonary edema
- Arteriolar vasodilation (hypotension and decreased systemic vascular resistance)
- Decreased responsiveness to catecholamines (endogenous and exogenous)
- Decreased ventricular fibrillation threshold

Neurologic
- Altered mental status
- Increased intracranial pressure (cerebral vasodilation)

Respiratory
- Hyperventilation

Metabolic
- Catabolism
- Insulin resistance

Electrolyte Imbalances
- Hyperkalemia
- Increased ionized calcium level

Abdominal
- Nausea, vomiting, abdominal pain

From References 1 and 12.

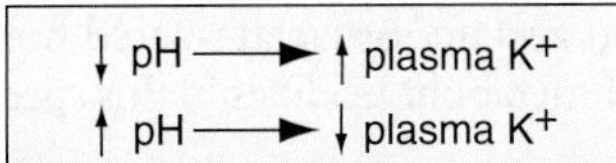

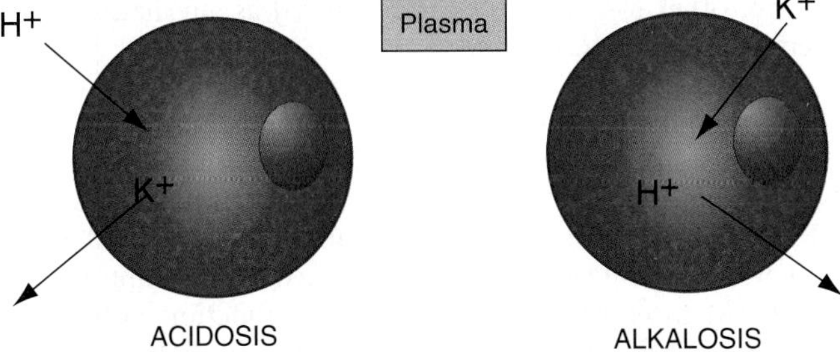

FIG. 22.3 Effect of pH on transcellular shifting of K^+ and hydrogen. *H^+*, Hydrogen; *K^+*, potassium.

setting of a metabolic acidosis. Calcium circulates in the plasma in three forms: free or unbound (ionized); protein bound; and complexed to anions such as phosphate, lactate, citrate, and bicarbonate. Although the total calcium level is more commonly measured, the ionized calcium level is the physiologically active form of calcium in the body and a more important indicator of the clinical severity of calcium imbalances. Changes in plasma H^+ concentration will affect the ionized calcium level through a change in protein binding. The pH and ionized calcium concentration tend to be inversely related. In the setting of a metabolic acidosis, proteins act as a buffer by binding H^+ and maintain electrical

TABLE 22.2 Treatment of the Underlying Cause of Elevated Anion Gap Acidosis

Disorder	Treatment
Diabetic ketoacidosis	Insulin, saline
Acute renal failure	Dialysis
Salicylate intoxication	Diuresis, alkalinization of urine, dialysis
Starvation ketosis	Refeeding (glucose and thiamine), electrolyte replacement
Methanol	Ethanol infusion, dialysis
Alcoholic ketoacidosis	Glucose, thiamine, saline, electrolyte replacement
Ethylene glycol	Ethanol infusion, dialysis
Lactic acidosis	Correct underlying cause

neutrality by releasing calcium, thereby increasing ionized calcium levels. Conversely, in the setting of a metabolic alkalosis, proteins release H^+ and bind calcium, resulting in a decrease in ionized calcium levels. It is important to remember that the total calcium concentration will not be affected by these shifts; the patient may develop signs and symptoms of hypocalcemia in the setting of a normal total calcium concentration. An ionized calcium level must be obtained to more accurately assess the effect of pH on changes in the ionized calcium level. For each 0.1 unit decrease in the pH, the ionized calcium level will increase by 0.2 mg/dL.[5]

Treatment of Metabolic Acidosis

There are three steps in the management of metabolic acidosis. These include the identification of the cause, determination of compensation, and implementation of appropriate interventions. The first priority should always be aimed at identifying and correcting the primary disorder (Table 22.2).

In DKA, the metabolic acidosis is corrected by the administration of intravenous insulin. Providing insulin to these patients converts metabolism from fatty acids back to glucose, thereby stopping ketoacid production. Treatment must also include adequate hydration in order to improve renal perfusion and promote excretion of ketoacids.[11]

In patients with acute renal failure, treating metabolic acidosis can be challenging, especially if the patient is volume expanded. Administration of sodium bicarbonate to the oliguric, volume-overloaded patient with acute renal failure can be catastrophic because of the high sodium load that could result in pulmonary edema. In these patients, metabolic acidosis may be best treated with renal replacement therapy (RRT).[12]

The metabolic acidosis associated with salicylate intoxication is treated with alkalinization of the blood and the urine, using intravenous sodium bicarbonate. Increasing the blood pH in this setting reduces the diffusion of salicylate into the central nervous system (CNS), where it is toxic; additionally, alkalinization of the urine improves renal excretion of salicylate. However, fluid overload can occur with sodium bicarbonate; therefore, it should be administered cautiously to those at risk (patients with underlying heart or renal disease and advanced age). For these patients, salicylate intoxication can be treated with RRT.[12,15]

Starvation and alcoholic ketosis are characterized by hypoglycemia and low insulin levels. These disorders are treated by restoring caloric intake with glucose, which stimulates insulin release and suppresses ketogenesis.[9] It is also important to replace thiamine, electrolytes, and volume in these malnourished patients, which will aid in prevention of Wernicke's encephalopathy.[17]

Methanol and ethylene glycol poisonings often occur as a result of a suicide attempt or accidental ingestion. Ethylene glycol is the organic solvent in antifreeze. Ingestions of both of these poisons are associated with CNS disturbances and severe anion gap metabolic acidosis. Both methanol and ethylene glycol intoxication are treated by inhibiting the generation of toxic metabolites that occurs as alcohol dehydrogenase metabolizes these poisons. This is accomplished by administering intravenous or oral ethanol. Ethanol has a greater affinity for alcohol dehydrogenase than methanol and ethylene glycol. When ethanol is administered in the setting of methanol or ethylene glycol poisoning, alcohol dehydrogenase will preferentially metabolize ethanol, thereby decreasing generation of toxic metabolites from methanol and ethylene glycol. RRT is also an effective treatment for clearing methanol and ethylene glycol from the blood in patients with large ingestions or severe metabolic acidosis.[1]

Lactic acidosis is probably one of the most challenging types of metabolic acidosis to treat in the acutely ill adult. It typically occurs with septic, cardiogenic, or hypovolemic shock and is associated with hemodynamic compromise, hypoperfusion, and tissue hypoxia. To stop the production of lactic acid, perfusion to tissues must be restored by treating the underlying cause. If the metabolic acidosis is severe (pH < 7.20), there is decreased responsiveness to both endogenous and exogenous catecholamines, which means that vasopressors and positive inotropes are not effective at improving hemodynamics and restoring perfusion in these patients. Additionally, acute renal failure often accompanies these various types of shock, complicating the metabolic acidosis by reducing renal acid clearance. RRT may be needed to correct metabolic acidosis in patients with severe lactic acidosis and renal failure.[14]

After treating the underlying cause, the second step in treating a metabolic acidosis is to confirm the presence of respiratory compensation. If the $Paco_2$ is higher than that predicted using the formulas previously discussed (see Box 22.1), a respiratory acidosis is also present. In the setting of a metabolic acidosis combined with a respiratory acidosis (mixed disorder), there is compensation failure and the acidemia can be severe. In this situation, the pH can be improved by supporting ventilation. Increasing the minute ventilation (increased tidal volume or respiratory rate) will create an artificial respiratory compensatory response by decreasing the $Paco_2$ and raising blood pH. If the patient is not on a ventilator and is demonstrating signs of respiratory fatigue (i.e., restlessness, tachypnea, shallow respirations), intubation should be considered to support ventilation and decrease the $Paco_2$.[12]

Bicarbonate Therapy

The third consideration in the treatment of a metabolic acidosis is administration of sodium bicarbonate. The administration of bicarbonate to correct metabolic acidosis is controversial. Before giving bicarbonate, every effort should be made to correct the underlying process causing the acidosis and support ventilation and respiratory compensation. In the setting of a severe metabolic acidosis (pH < 6.90 to 7.10 and HCO_3^- level < 8 to 10 mEq/L), and in the setting of acute kidney injury or chronic kidney disease, bicarbonate may be administered. The goal of administering bicarbonate in metabolic acidosis is to prevent or reverse the detrimental consequences of severe acidemia on the cardiovascular system, restore hemodynamic stability, and allow for additional time to treat the underlying cause. Additionally, there are many detrimental side effects of bicarbonate, including volume overload, hyperosmolality, "overshoot" metabolic alkalosis, and a decrease in oxygen release from Hgb.[15]

Sodium bicarbonate. Intravenous sodium bicarbonate is most commonly used for the treatment of a severe metabolic acidosis when indicated. It should be administered via a continuous intravenous infusion. Bolus dosing should be avoided except in emergent situations.[1] The bicarbonate infusion should be continued until the pH reaches approximately 7.20. The appropriate dose of sodium bicarbonate required to correct a patient's serum level can be estimated using the base deficit formula, shown hereafter. An example is illustrated in Box 22.5. In critically ill patients, many ongoing processes will perpetuate or compensate for the metabolic acidosis and can make it difficult to predict the base deficit accurately. Trending repeated measurements of the ABG and serum electrolytes (to calculate the anion gap) must be performed in order to guide therapy.[14]

Side effects of sodium bicarbonate. Side effects of sodium bicarbonate are serious and include hypernatremia, hyperosmolality, alkalosis, volume overload, and a rapid drop in the ionized calcium level. Sodium bicarbonate should be administered very cautiously in patients with heart failure and renal failure because of a limited ability to excrete sodium and the potential to worsen volume overload. Intermittent dialysis or continuous renal replacement therapy using a bicarbonate-based buffer, versus an acetate- or lactate-based buffer, can be used in the treatment of metabolic acidosis in this specialized population.

Alternative Treatments of Metabolic Acidosis

Because of the adverse effects of sodium bicarbonate administration, other forms of base have evolved as alternative treatments for metabolic acidosis.

THAM (tris[hydroxymethyl]aminomethane) is a sodium free compound that buffers protons. Administration of THAM does not result in CO_2 generation, as seen with sodium bicarbonate, and therefore THAM does not lower intracellular pH. THAM has not been widely used because it is eliminated by the kidneys and is only effective if it is excreted.[14] This limits the use of THAM to patients with normal renal function. Additional side effects of THAM include hyperkalemia, hepatotoxicity, and respiratory depression.

BOX 22.5 Calculating the Base Deficit

Base deficit formula:

HCO_3^- deficit = 0.5 × body weight (kg) × (desired HCO_3^- − measured HCO_3^-)

Example: Calculating the base deficit

Patient weight = 70 kg

Measured HCO_3^- = 12 mEq/L

Desired HCO_3^- = 26 mEq/L

HCO_3^- deficit = 0.5 × 70 × (26−12)

= 0.5 × 70 × 14

= 0.5 × 980

490 mEq/L $NaHCO_3$

RRT is an effective treatment for metabolic acidosis, especially in patients with renal failure or certain intoxications (e.g., ethylene glycol, salicylate). Clinically, it is difficult and may be deleterious to administer large quantities of bicarbonate by bolus or continuous infusion because of the risk of volume overload, pulmonary edema, hypernatremia, and hyperosmolality. However, with RRT, large quantities of base can be delivered, volume status can be normalized, and electrolyte imbalances can be treated. Various types of RRT can be used to treat acid-base and electrolyte disorders in the acutely ill adult, including hemodialysis and continuous renal replacement therapies (CRRT). For treating metabolic acidosis, the use of bicarbonate as a source of base in the dialysate is recommended over the other bicarbonate precursors (lactate or acetate) because of the potential detrimental effects if these acids accumulate before being metabolized.[6]

METABOLIC ALKALOSIS

Metabolic alkalosis is a common acid-base disorder seen in the critical care setting.[23] It can be defined as a physiologic process that can cause alkalemia if not corrected, whereas alkalemia is defined as an increase in the blood pH greater than 7.45. Metabolic alkalosis is due to a primary increase in plasma bicarbonate concentrations, resulting in an increase in blood pH. Severe alkalemia (blood pH > 7.60) can be life-threatening because of its effect on cerebral and myocardial perfusion.

Causes of Metabolic Alkalosis

Metabolic alkalosis is usually due to loss of acid combined with chloride loss. In the hospitalized patient, metabolic alkalosis most commonly results from either diuretics causing renal loss of acid (ammonium chloride), prolonged nasogastric (NG) suctioning, or vomiting causing GI loss of acid (hydrochloric acid).[10] In these situations, metabolic alkalosis is typically associated with hypochloremia and volume depletion, also termed a *contraction alkalosis* (Box 22.6).

In states of volume depletion, the kidney will respond by reabsorbing sodium and water. Renal reabsorption of sodium can occur as either sodium chloride or sodium bicarbonate. In most states of metabolic alkalosis, there is a preexisting chloride deficiency, so the kidney must reabsorb sodium bicarbonate instead of sodium chloride, thus maintaining and perpetuating the metabolic alkalosis that was originally due to acid loss. This type of metabolic alkalosis usually responds to chloride administration (sodium chloride or potassium chloride) and is referred to as *chloride-responsive* metabolic alkalosis.[3,13]

A less common cause of metabolic alkalosis is termed *chloride-resistant* metabolic alkalosis. In the acutely ill patient, this can occur with administration of substrates such as lactate, citrate, or acetate. Lactate is a component in the intravenous lactated Ringer's solution and in dialysate solutions. Citrate is an anticoagulant and preservative used in the preparation of packed red blood cell transfusions and RRT. Acetate is a component commonly added to parenteral nutrition and dialysate. When given in sufficient quantities, these substrates can generate or perpetuate a metabolic alkalosis as the liver converts them to bicarbonate.[3,13]

Manifestations of Metabolic Alkalosis

Metabolic alkalosis can compromise myocardial and cerebral perfusion by causing arteriolar constriction. Additionally, metabolic alkalosis causes respiratory depression and decreased tissue oxygenation and is associated with numerous electrolyte imbalances (Box 22.7).

Electrolyte Imbalances Associated with Metabolic Alkalosis

Electrolyte imbalances are common with metabolic alkalosis. In part, this is due to the volume and electrolyte depletion occurring with diuretics and vomiting or with NG suctioning. Additionally, metabolic alkalosis causes electrolyte imbalances because of transcellular shifts of electrolytes and changes in protein binding of some electrolytes, especially calcium.[7,8,10]

Hypokalemia

Defined as a serum potassium level less than 3.5 mEq/L, hypokalemia is common in metabolic alkalosis because of renal and GI losses of potassium (diuretics, vomiting, or diarrhea).

BOX 22.6 Causes of Metabolic Alkalosis

Chloride Responsive	Chloride Resistant
Vomiting	Administration of bicarbonate precursors
Nasogastric suction	Lactate
Diuretic therapy	Citrate
Loop diuretics	Acetate
Thiazides	Potassium depletion
	Hyperreninemic states
	Primary hyperaldosteronism

BOX 22.7 Manifestations of Severe Metabolic Alkalosis (pH >7.6)

Cardiovascular
- Arteriolar constriction
- Decreased coronary blood flow, leading to angina, acute myocardial infarction (MI) in patients with coronary artery disease
- Predisposition to refractory supraventricular dysrhythmias

Neurologic
- Decreased cerebral blood flow
- Paresthesias, tetany, seizures (secondary to decreased ionized calcium)
- Lethargy, delirium, stupor

Respiratory
- Hypoventilation leading to hypercapnia and hypoxemia
- Failure to wean from ventilator

Electrolyte Imbalances
- Hypokalemia
- Decreased ionized calcium
- Hypomagnesemia (associated imbalance)
- Hypophosphatemia (associated imbalance)

Metabolic
- Decreased oxygen delivery at tissue level
- Stimulation of organic acid production

Hypokalemia also occurs as a result of transcellular shifts of extracellular potassium into the cell in exchange for hydrogen. H^+ moves out of the cell in an attempt to correct the alkalosis and potassium moves into the cell to maintain electrical neutrality.

Low-Ionized Calcium

Low-ionized calcium is defined as an ionized calcium level less than 4 mg/dL or 1.16 mmol/L. Calcium-protein binding is influenced by plasma pH. In alkalemic states, H^+ ions are released from protein. This exposes negatively charged sites that bind ionized calcium, thus reducing the plasma ionized calcium concentration (Fig. 22.4). The clinical significance of this phenomenon is that in an alkalemic state, there is a reduction in the ionized calcium level and the patient may develop manifestations of hypocalcemia such as paresthesias, tetany, and seizures, despite a normal total calcium level.

Hypophosphatemia and Hypomagnesemia

Hypophosphatemia is defined as serum phosphorus level less than 2.8 mg/dL and hypomagnesemia is defined as serum magnesium level less than 1.5 mEq/L. Low phosphorus and low magnesium levels typically accompany metabolic alkalosis. However, metabolic alkalosis is not a primary cause of these electrolyte imbalances as it is with hypokalemia and low ionized calcium concentration. Because metabolic alkalosis is commonly associated with diuresis or vomiting/NG suction, there can be excessive renal or GI losses of both phosphorus and magnesium. Hypomagnesemia potentiates the neuromuscular manifestations of low ionized calcium level, including tetany and seizures. Additionally, hypomagnesemia in the setting of metabolic alkalosis potentiates the arrhythmogenic effects of hypokalemia, including both supraventricular and ventricular dysrhythmias.

Treatment of metabolic alkalosis. In the volume-depleted patient with chloride-responsive metabolic alkalosis, every effort should be made to stop the processes responsible for causing the metabolic alkalosis. The cause of vomiting should be determined and treated, NG suctioning should be discontinued if possible, and the diuretic dose should be decreased or withheld or a potassium-sparing diuretic should be considered.

These patients need replacement of volume with normal saline. Additionally, chloride must be replaced in the form of sodium chloride or potassium chloride. Remember that the most common causes of metabolic alkalosis in the acutely ill adult are vomiting or NG suctioning with loss of hydrochloric acid and diuresis with loss of ammonium chloride. In these volume-depleted, chloride-deficient patients, the kidney is reabsorbing sodium, but because there is a chloride deficiency, sodium is reabsorbed as sodium bicarbonate. This renal reabsorption of sodium bicarbonate perpetuates the existing metabolic alkalosis. Replacing chloride is a critical part of correcting metabolic alkalosis. As chloride stores are replenished, the kidney will reabsorb sodium chloride and excrete bicarbonate.

Concurrent electrolyte imbalances are common in the setting of a metabolic alkalosis and treatment often includes replacement of chloride, potassium, phosphate, and magnesium. Patients with cardiac and renal dysfunction present challenges to correcting metabolic alkalosis because administration of sodium chloride may cause volume overload and administration of potassium chloride may result in hyperkalemia.

Special Patient Populations Requiring Aggressive Treatment of Metabolic Alkalosis

Alkalemia reduces respiratory drive. Patients with COPD pending intubation or failure to wean and extubate should be closely monitored for respiratory failure. Aggressive treatment of metabolic alkalosis in these patients will improve respiratory drive.[4,17]

Alkalemia causes arteriolar vasoconstriction. Patients with coronary artery disease and acute myocardial infarction should be closely monitored for the development of ischemia. Aggressive correction of metabolic alkalosis will improve coronary blood flow by promoting arteriolar vasodilation. In the patient with cerebral dysfunction, aggressive correction of metabolic alkalosis will improve cerebral blood flow by promoting arteriolar vasodilation.

If alkalemia is still severe despite attempts to correct the underlying disorder, the diuretic acetazolamide (Diamox), 250 to 375 mg once or twice a day, may be administered to enhance renal excretion.[2] This may be useful in the patient who is volume overloaded and cannot tolerate a saline infusion to correct alkalosis. Infusion of intravenous hydrochloric acid as a 0.1 to 0.2 N solution (100 to 200 mmol of hydrogen/L) at a rate of 0.1 to 0.2 mmol/kg/hour has been used for many years to aggressively treat severe metabolic alkalosis.[2] However, a serious side effect of hydrochloric acid administration is tissue necrosis should extravasation occur. Precursors of hydrochloric acid, such as ammonium chloride, may be considered for

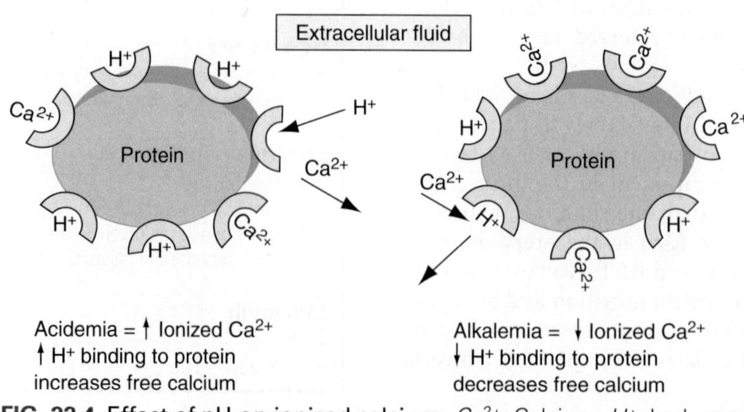

FIG. 22.4 Effect of pH on ionized calcium. *Ca^{2+}*, Calcium; *H^+*, hydrogen.

treatment of a metabolic alkalosis but also have deleterious side effects including elevation of serum ammonia levels and tissue necrosis.[2]

The treatment of chloride-resistant metabolic alkalosis and volume expansion is focused on removal of the underlying cause of the persistent mineralocorticoid activity. If this is not possible, administration of potassium-sparing diuretics (amiloride or spironolactone) to block the action of mineralocorticoids in the kidneys that are promoting renal H^+ loss may be effective in these patients.[7,17]

RESPIRATORY ACIDOSIS

Respiratory acidosis is a clinical disorder characterized by alveolar hypoventilation resulting in hypercapnia ($Paco_2$ > 45 mm Hg) and acidemia (arterial pH < 7.35). CO_2 is a metabolic waste product eliminated by the lungs. If the lungs fail to eliminate CO_2, it will accumulate in the blood, causing acidemia. Hypercapnia is the result of inadequate ventilation. Hypoxemia typically accompanies respiratory acidosis because of hypoventilation.[4,7,17]

Causes of Respiratory Acidosis

Respiratory acidosis should be differentiated between acute and chronic causes of hypoventilation (Box 22.8).

Compensation in Respiratory Acidosis

The initial clinical approach to the patient with a respiratory acidosis is to determine whether the disorder is acute or chronic, or if it is acute-on-chronic. For example, a patient with stable chronic COPD or asthma can have an acute exacerbation with an increase in $Paco_2$ above the baseline. The compensatory mechanism for an increase in $Paco_2$ is to increase the plasma bicarbonate concentration. In an acute respiratory acidosis, the carbonic-acid- bicarbonate buffer system is ineffective because the CO_2 produced in the buffering reaction cannot be eliminated as a result of the existing respiratory disorder.[9] However, nonbicarbonate buffers (e.g., protein, phosphate, Hgb) can effectively absorb the excess H^+. This response occurs within hours of the onset of an acute respiratory acidosis but produces only minimal compensation.

The definitive compensatory response for a persistent respiratory acidosis is in the kidneys but will take 3 to 5 days to complete.[9,12] The renal response to a respiratory acidosis is to increase the production and reabsorption of bicarbonate and to increase the production and excretion of the acid ammonium.[12] In an acute respiratory acidosis, the compensatory response will only increase the HCO_3^- level by up to 1 mEq for every 10 mm Hg increase in the $Paco_2$.[18] Renal compensation to a chronic respiratory acidosis will increase the HCO_3^- level by up to 3.5 mEq for every 10 mm Hg increase in the $Paco_2$.[18]

Manifestations of Respiratory Acidosis

The clinical manifestations of an acute respiratory acidosis are seen primarily in the neurologic system and can be attributed to vasodilation causing an increase in cerebral blood flow and also to a decrease in the pH of the cerebral spinal fluid. Hypoxemia invariably accompanies an acute respiratory acidosis and may dominate the clinical presentation with signs and symptoms of acute respiratory distress (e.g., tachypnea, restlessness).[12] With chronic respiratory acidosis, symptoms are less common, since renal compensation has had time to return the pH toward normal (Box 22.9).

Treatment of Respiratory Acidosis

The most important aspect of treating respiratory acidosis, as with all acid-base disorders, is to diagnose and treat the underlying cause. Initially, supplemental oxygen should be administered to treat accompanying hypoxemia. In patients with COPD exacerbation, supplemental oxygen should be administered cautiously because hypoxemia, versus hypercapnia, stimulates their respiratory drive.

Reversal of a high $Paco_2$ will always require an increase in alveolar ventilation. This is accomplished by controlling the underlying disease. For example, asthma should be treated with bronchodilators and steroids, narcotic oversedation can be reversed with naloxone (Narcan), pneumonia with severe

BOX 22.8 Causes of Respiratory Acidosis

Disorders Affecting Gas Exchange

Pneumothorax or hemothorax	Asthma/COPD
Acute lung injury	Interstitial lung disease
Pulmonary emboli	Pulmonary fibrosis
Asthma/COPD exacerbation	Pulmonary edema

Respiratory Muscle Weakness

Neuromuscular blockade	Neuromuscular disorders
Hypophosphatemia and hypokalemia	Multiple sclerosis
Acute spinal cord injury: C3, C4, C5	Guillain-Barré
Diaphragmatic paralysis secondary to trauma	Amyotrophic lateral sclerosis

Decreased Respiratory Drive

Narcotics	Pickwickian syndrome
Anesthetics	Primary hypoventilation
Sedatives	Central sleep apnea
Cerebral trauma	Myxedema coma (hypothyroidism)

Airway Obstruction

Foreign body
Laryngospasm

COPD, chronic obstructive pulmonary disease.

BOX 22.9 Manifestations of Acute Respiratory Acidosis

Neurologic

- Increased cerebral blood flow
- Headache, blurred vision
- Restlessness, anxiety
- Tremors, asterixis
- Somnolence
- Stupor, coma

Cardiovascular

- Peripheral vasodilation and hypotension
- Dysrhythmias

Pulmonary

- Accompanying hypoxemia

hypoxemia and hypercapnia will require treatment with antibiotics, treatment of pulmonary edema will include aggressive diuresis. In some instances, endotracheal intubation and mechanical ventilation will be necessary for management of symptomatic or progressive hypercapnia, severe hypoxemia, or depression of the respiratory center. The decision to intubate and mechanically ventilate the patient is based on clinical judgment and is dependent on many factors such as reversibility of illness, severity of illness, and patient fatigue.[9]

RESPIRATORY ALKALOSIS

Respiratory alkalosis is a clinical disorder characterized by hypocapnia ($Paco_2$ < 35 mm Hg) and alkalemia (pH > 7.45). Respiratory alkalosis occurs as a result of increased elimination of CO_2 beyond what would normally be produced as a metabolic waste product. Respiratory alkalosis is due to hyperventilation.[8,10,19]

Causes of Respiratory Alkalosis

Respiration is regulated by two sets of chemoreceptors: central chemoreceptors located in the respiratory center in the brain stem, and peripheral chemoreceptors located in the carotid and aortic arteries. The central chemoreceptors are stimulated by a drop in the cerebrospinal fluid pH, which typically occurs from an increase in $Paco_2$ or metabolic acidosis. The peripheral chemoreceptors are stimulated primarily by hypoxemia. When the Pao_2 falls below 60 mm Hg, the peripheral chemoreceptors signal an increase in ventilation to improve hypoxemia; this results in a drop in the $Paco_2$.[9] Many nonphysiologic stimuli can also cause hyperventilation, including direct stimulation of the respiratory center, mechanical ventilation, and pulmonary disease (Box 22.10).

BOX 22.10 Causes of Respiratory Alkalosis

Hypoxemia (Pao_2 < 60 mm Hg)
- Asthma
- Chronic obstructive pulmonary disease
- Heart failure
- High-altitude residence
- Hypotension
- Pneumonia
- Pulmonary edema
- Pulmonary emboli
- Severe anemia

Cardiopulmonary Disease (Independent of Hypoxemia)
- Heart failure
- Mitral valve disease
- Pulmonary hypertension

Direct Stimulation of Respiratory Center
- Anxiety or pain
- Hepatic failure
- Neurologic disorders (stroke, tumors)
- Pregnancy (caused by progesterone)
- Rapid correction of metabolic acidosis with sodium bicarbonate
- Salicylate intoxication

Hyperventilation
- Anxiety attacks, psychogenic conditions
- Mechanical ventilation (high rate or tidal volume settings)

From References 9 and 12.

Compensation in Respiratory Alkalosis

There are two components in the compensatory response to a respiratory alkalosis: an acute response and a chronic response. The initial buffering response to an acute respiratory alkalosis is to move H^+ ions out of the cell (proteins, phosphate, and hemoglobin) into the extracellular space. This cellular response occurs within minutes of the onset of an acute respiratory alkalosis but does not dramatically increase the pH. The compensatory response to an acute respiratory alkalosis will only decrease plasma HCO_3^- levels by up to 2 mEq for every 10 mm Hg rise in the $Paco_2$.[18]

In the presence of a persistent or chronic respiratory alkalosis, a more powerful renal compensatory response will take 2 to 3 days to achieve maximum compensation. The kidneys decrease renal H^+ ion and ammonium excretion, thereby retaining more acid, reducing plasma HCO_3^- levels and lowering the pH toward normal. In a chronic respiratory alkalosis, the plasma HCO_3^- will decrease by up to 5 mEq for every 10 mm Hg decrease in the $Paco_2$.[18] The renal response to persistent respiratory alkalosis is much greater than the cellular compensatory response seen with an acute respiratory alkalosis.

Manifestations of Respiratory Alkalosis

The symptoms of an acute respiratory alkalosis are primarily due to increased irritability of the central and peripheral nervous systems. Alkalosis impairs cerebral function, increases membrane excitability, and reduces cerebral and coronary blood flow by causing arteriolar vasoconstriction. Similar to metabolic alkalosis, there are many electrolyte imbalances associated with respiratory alkalosis, including a low ionized calcium level, hypokalemia, and hypophosphatemia (Box 22.11).

Electrolyte imbalances associated with acute respiratory alkalosis can occur rapidly in response to an increased pH and are due to transcellular electrolyte shifts. As hydrogen moves out of the cell to lower the pH, potassium will move into the cell, resulting in hypokalemia. Additionally, phosphate moves

BOX 22.11 Manifestations of Acute Respiratory Alkalosis

Neurologic
- Reduced cerebral blood flow
- Light-headedness
- Altered level of consciousness
- Paresthesias (circumoral and peripheral)
- Hyperreflexia and tetany
- Seizures

Cardiovascular
- Reduced coronary artery blood flow
- Refractory supraventricular and ventricular dysrhythmias

Pulmonary
- Pulmonary vasculature vasodilation

Electrolyte Imbalances
- Low ionized calcium
- Hypokalemia
- Hypophosphatemia (rapid onset)
- Low serum bicarbonate (compensatory)

rapidly into the cell and can reduce the serum phosphate levels to as low as 0.5 to 1.5 mg/dL.[9] The ionized calcium level also falls, as free calcium binds to proteins in exchange for hydrogen release.

Treatment of Respiratory Alkalosis

The treatment of respiratory alkalosis, similar to the treatment of the previously discussed acid-base disorders, should be directed at correction of the underlying disorder causing the hyperventilation. For example, a patient being mechanically ventilated with high minute volumes should have the tidal volume or the rate settings reduced. In conscious patients with symptomatic alkalemia, rebreathing into a paper bag will increase the pH by increasing the $Paco_2$ in the inspired air.[12,17]

MIXED ACID-BASE DISORDERS

A mixed acid-base disorder is defined as two or more primary acid-base disorders that occur simultaneously. These disorders may mask each other and can be diagnosed only with a thorough evaluation of acid-base status. For example, a patient with acute decompensated heart failure, hypotension, and pulmonary edema who is receiving high-dose diuretics can have a triple acid-base disorder: metabolic acidosis secondary to hypotension causing hypoperfusion, resulting in a lactic acidosis; metabolic alkalosis secondary to diuretics causing renal acid loss; and respiratory acidosis resulting from pulmonary edema with $Paco_2$ retention. In this scenario, it is possible that the patient could have a relatively normal pH because of the offsetting effects of alkalosis and acidosis.[12]

Mixed acid-base disorders can also present with grossly abnormal changes in pH when the primary disorders block compensation for each other.[12] For example, a patient with a respiratory acidosis caused by acute respiratory distress *and* a metabolic acidosis caused by acute renal failure could present with a life-threatening acidemia. In this example, the presence of a primary respiratory acidosis prevents a compensatory hypocapnia in the setting of a primary metabolic acidosis. Additionally, the presence of a primary metabolic acidosis caused by renal failure renders the kidneys unable to generate a compensatory increase in the plasma bicarbonate level in the setting of a primary respiratory acidosis.

A systematic approach to diagnosing simple and mixed acid-base disorders (see Box 22.1) is critical to identifying the presence of mixed imbalances. Table 22.3 provides examples of common mixed acid-base disorders seen in the critical care setting. There are many possibilities and combinations of mixed acid-base disorders; however, the two primary acute respiratory acid-base disorders, respiratory acidosis and respiratory alkalosis, cannot coexist.[12]

CONCLUSION

Acid-base and electrolyte imbalances are extremely common in the acutely ill adult. Extreme aberrations in the blood pH can cause life-threatening hemodynamic derangements and organ dysfunction, especially when the acid-base derangement is acute. Successful treatment of acid-base imbalances is contingent upon an accurate diagnosis, which becomes challenging in the setting of mixed acid-base disorders. It is critically important to assess acid-base status with a systematic approach to ensure recognition of all acid-base disorders that may be present, even in the setting of a normal pH.

TABLE 22.3 Common Causes of Mixed Acid-Base Disorders in the Acutely Ill Adult

Acid-Base Disorders	Example	Clinical Features
Metabolic acidosis and respiratory acidosis	Acute renal failure with pulmonary edema	High anion gap acidosis and hypoventilation with $Paco_2$ retention
Metabolic acidosis and respiratory alkalosis	Salicylate intoxication	High anion gap acidosis with respiratory stimulation and hyperventilation with $Paco_2$ loss
	Sepsis with severe liver disease	
Metabolic acidosis and metabolic alkalosis	Diabetic ketoacidosis with vomiting	Ketoacidosis with gastrointestinal hydrochloric acid loss
	Heart failure patient receiving high-dose loop diuretics	Lactic acidosis with high anion gap and excessive renal acid loss secondary to diuretics
Respiratory acidosis and metabolic alkalosis	ARDS with permissive hypercapnia and gastric suction	Hypoventilation with retention of $Paco_2$ and gastrointestinal hydrochloric acid loss
	COPD patient receiving high-dose loop diuretics	
Respiratory alkalosis and metabolic alkalosis	Hyperventilation in neurosurgical patient receiving loop diuretics	High minute volume settings on ventilator with $Paco_2$ loss and excessive renal acid loss secondary to diuretics
Metabolic alkalosis, metabolic acidosis, and respiratory alkalosis	Protracted vomiting with hypovolemic shock in patient with a neurologic disorder causing hyperventilation	Loss of hydrochloric acid with vomiting, high lactic acid level from shock causing drop in HCO_3^-, low $Paco_2$ from hyperventilation
		Patient could present with normal pH despite triple acid-base disorder
Metabolic acidosis, metabolic alkalosis, and respiratory acidosis	Cardiogenic shock with pulmonary edema in patient receiving high-dose diuretics	Lactic acidosis caused by shock, retention of $Paco_2$ because of pulmonary edema and poor gas exchange, renal acid loss secondary to diuretics

ARDS, Acute respiratory distress syndrome; *COPD,* chronic obstructive pulmonary disease; *$Paco_2$,* partial pressure of arterial carbon dioxide.
From Reference 12.

CASE STUDY 22.1

C.S. is a 27-year-old male admitted to the emergency department (ED) after a motor vehicle collision. He had been trapped in his vehicle for over 6 hours before being extricated. He sustained crush injuries to his upper and lower extremities as well as blunt abdominal trauma. His vital signs include blood pressure (BP): 80/palpable, heart rate (HR): 138 beats/min, and respirations: 34 breaths/min. Physical exam revealed that pupils were equal and reactive to light and difficult to arouse. He was in a sinus tachycardia; S_1, S_2 were heard. His lungs were clear and his abdomen was distended and diffusely tender with decreased bowel sounds. His upper and lower extremities were lacerated, discolored, and edematous.

Laboratory Values:

Serum Chemistries	Arterial Blood Gas
Na^+: 140 mEq/L	pH: 7.15
K^+: 6.9 mEq/L	$Paco_2$: 16 mm Hg
Cl^-: 100 mEq/L	Pao_2: 90 mm Hg
CO_2: 8 mEq/L	HCO_3^-: 16 mEq/L
Creatinine: 2.5 mg/dL	Saturation: 97%
BUN (blood urine nitrogen): 16 mg/dL	
Glucose: 140 mg/dL	

A 12-lead electrocardiogram (ECG) is obtained and shows sinus tachycardia with PR = 0.22 ms, flattened P waves, QRS = 0.14 ms, tall peaked T waves.

The patient is intubated, put on a ventilator, and hyperventilated. A urinary catheter and NGT is placed to low wall suction and two central lines are placed. The following medications are administered: sodium bicarbonate 2 vials IV, insulin 10 units IV, D_{50} 1 ampule IV, calcium gluconate 10% 10 mL IV. The central venous pressure (CVP) is measured at 2 cm H_2O. IV normal saline (NS) is administered "wide open," and despite volume replacement, the CVP does not increase. A bicarbonate infusion was ordered. Nephrology is consulted for emergency dialysis.

12 hours after admission:

Temperature is 38.4°C. Vital signs HR 114, RR 24, BP 102/56. He remains intubated and sedated, his NGT has drained 1 L of bilious secretions. His urine out is 30 mL/kg, skin is warm and dry. Vent settings are fraction of inspired oxygen (Fio_2) 0.6 A/C 12 TV 600 positive end-expiratory pressure (PEEP) 5 cm. His follow-up labs:

Laboratory Values:

Serum Chemistries	Arterial Blood Gas
Na^+: 131 mEq/L	pH: 7.41
K^+: 2.7 mEq/L	$Paco_2$: 55 mm Hg
Cl^-: 70 mEq/L	Pao_2: 58 mm Hg
CO_2: 28 mEq/L	HCO_3^-: 26 mEq/L
Glucose: 196 mg/dL	Saturation: 93%
Creatinine: 2.4 mg/dL	
BUN: 42 mg/dL	
Mg^{2+}: 1.6 mEq/L	

Decision Point:
Determine the etiology of the acid-base disorder from the original admission data.

Decision Point:
What are the manifestations of metabolic acidosis?

Decision Point:
Was it appropriate to treat the metabolic acidosis with $NaHCO_3$?

Decision Point:
What is the acid-base disorder 12 hours after admission?

Decision Point:
How should the acid-base disorders be treated?

REFERENCES

1. Androgue, H. J., & Madias, N. E. (1998). Management of life-threatening acid-base disorders, Pt 1. *N Engl J Med, 338*(1), 26–34.
2. Androgue, H. J., & Madias, N. E. (1998). Management of life-threatening acid-base disorders, Pt 2. *N Engl J Med, 338*(2), 107–111.
3. Ayers, P., Dixon, C., & Mays, A. (2015). Acid-base disorders: learning the basics. *Nutr Clin Pract, 30*(1), 14–20.
4. Berend, K., de Vries, A. P. J., & Gans, R. O. B. (2014). Physiological approach to assessment of acid–base disturbances. *N Engl J Med, 371*, 1434–1445.
5. Bushinsky, D., & Monk, R. (1998). Calcium. *Lancet, 352*, 306–311.
6. Cerdá, J., Tolwani, A., & Warnock, D. (2012). Critical care nephrology: management of acid-base disorders with CRRT. *Kidney Int, 82*(1), 9–18.
7. Cho, K. C. (2014). Electrolyte & acid-base disorders. In M. A. Papadakis, S. J. McPhee, & M. W. Rabow (Eds.), *Current medical diagnosis & treatment 2015*. New York: McGraw Hill Education.
8. Dzierba, A. L., & Abraham, P. (2011). A practical approach to understanding acid-base abnormalities in critical illness. *J Pharm Pract, 24*(1), 17–26.
9. Faubel, S., & Topf, J. (1999). *The fluid, electrolyte and acid-base companion*. San Diego: Alert and Oriented Publishing.
10. Halperin, M., & Goldstein, M. (1999). *Fluid, electrolyte, and acid-base physiology; a problem-based approach* (3rd ed.). Philadelphia: Saunders.
11. Hardern, R. D., & Quinn, N. (2003). Emergency management of diabetic ketoacidosis in adults. *Emerg Med J, 20*, 210–213.
12. Kaehny, W. D. (2003). Pathogenesis and management of respiratory and mixed acid-base disorders. In R. W. Schrier (Ed.), *Renal and electrolyte disorders* (6th ed.). Philadelphia: Lippincott Williams & Wilkins.
13. Kaufman, D. C., Kitching, A. J., & Kellum, J. A. (2015). Acid-base balance. In J. B. Hall, G. A. Schmidt, & J. P. Kress (Eds.), *Principles of critical care* (4th ed.). New York: McGraw Hill.
14. Kraut, J. A., & Madias, N. E. (2014). Lactic acidosis. *N Engl J Med, 371*(24), 2309–2319.
15. Kraut, J., & Kurtz, I. (2006). Controversies in the treatment of acute metabolic acidosis. *Nephrol Self Assess Program, 5*(1), 1–9.
16. Kraut, J., & Madias, D. (2012). Differential diagnosis of nongap metabolic acidosis: value of a systematic approach. *Clin J Am Soc Nephrol, 7*(4), 671–679.
17. Mount, D. B., & DuBose, T. D., Jr. (2015). Fluid and electrolyte imbalances and acid-base disturbances: case examples. In D. Kasper, A. Fauci, S. Hauser, D. Longo, J. Jameson, & J. Loscalzo (Eds.), *Harrison's principles of internal medicine* (19th ed.). New York: McGraw Hill.
18. Preston, R. A. (2002). *Acid-base, fluids, and electrolytes; made ridiculously simple*. Miami: MedMaster.
19. Rogers, A., & McCutcheon, K. (2013). Understanding arterial blood gases. *J Perioper Pract, 23*(9), 191–197.
20. Sterns, R., & Palmer, B. (2006). Fluid, electrolyte, and acid-base disturbances. *Nephrol Self Assess Program, 5*(1), 10–54.
21. Szaflarski, N. L., & Hanson, W. (1997). Metabolic acidosis. *AACN Clin Issues, 8*(3), 481–496.
22. Vichot, A., & Rastegar, A. (2014). Use of anion gap in the evaluation of a patient with metabolic acidosis. *Am J Kidney Dis, 64*(4), 653–657.
23. Woodrow, P. (2010). Essential principles: blood gas analysis. *Nurs Crit Care, 15*(3), 152–156.

Acute Kidney Injury

Mary Jo Kelly and Lisa Carriger

Acute kidney injury (AKI) is the most common renal syndrome seen in critically ill patients, and has the potential to negatively impact all other body systems. By definition, AKI is an abrupt decrease in kidney function, encompassing a wide spectrum of severity from risk of injury to kidney failure.[4,24,25,29] Between 20% and 50% of critically ill patients will develop AKI, often accompanied by multiple organ dysfunction syndrome (MODS).[6,29] The incidence of AKI is highest in sepsis patients at 68.4%, followed by mechanically ventilated patients at 63.9%, and surgical patients at 50% to 52%.[53] Despite many advances in care and outcomes of critically ill patients, mortality in patients with AKI remains near 50%.[6] Patients at risk for developing AKI during hospitalization have one year mortality rates of 34% to 39%.[44] Patients that require renal replacement therapy (RRT) have an in-hospital mortality rate of 60%.[30]

Given the negative impact of renal insufficiency on mortality, even in its mild forms, efforts to prevent AKI are imperative. Although AKI is not always preventable, patients who present with increased risk and who require additional prophylactic attention have been well described in the literature.[45] Advanced age, preexisting renal insufficiency (even mild elevation in creatinine level), diabetes, hypertension, and heart failure have long been recognized as increased risk factors for the development of AKI in patients admitted to critical care. Risk also increases with pathologic stressors such as hypotension or sepsis,[39] or when the patient's plan of care requires diagnostic procedures or certain treatment modalities, such as medications, surgery, nonsurgical interventions, and cardiopulmonary resuscitation (CPR). Studies show that the incidence of AKI in surgical patients is dependent on the type of surgical procedure performed, as well as the intraoperative and postoperative care that is provided.[13,16] These studies found that many of the existing risk factors for developing AKI postsurgery are similar to the risk factors that many critically ill patients face.

Critically ill patients often have a host of conditions that increase their risk for developing AKI. Vulnerable patients are those who are older, have lower renal reserves, and may have hypertension, diabetes, cardiac disease, hepatitis C, or human immunodeficiency virus.[15,22,41] Additionally, as patients age, those with chronic renal failure (CRF) who are maintained on dialysis as part of their lifestyle may be admitted with an acute, nonrenal crisis that requires continued RRT during their critical care stay.

In summary, whereas advanced age, diabetes, and elevated preoperative creatinine levels appear to be the best predictors of the development of postoperative/postprocedural AKI, and a consequent increase in length of stay and mortality, many other factors play a role. All patients admitted to critical care should be assessed for their risk of developing renal dysfunction.

PREVENTION OF ACUTE KIDNEY INJURY

Whenever possible, prophylactic interventions should be instituted in patients identified to be at risk for the development of AKI. Prevention begins with identifying patients at risk, avoiding nephrotoxic substances, and providing careful assessment and monitoring of the following:[21,25]

- Serum creatinine and urine output volumes/measurements
- Possible risk factors for AKI
- Fluid balance: if no bleeding is present, use isotonic fluids initially to expand the intravascular volume, rather than colloids
- Diuretics: NOT recommended to prevent AKI; however, they may be used to manage fluid overload
- Hemodynamics: in patients with septic shock or high-risk patients in the perioperative setting, use protocol-based management of hemodynamic and oxygenation parameters to avoid development or worsening of AKI
- Nutritional support: avoid restricting protein, as the aim is to avoid or delay RRT initiation; aim for a total energy intake of 20–30 kcals/kg/day
- Low-dose dopamine is no longer recommended to prevent or treat AKI
- Fenoldopam (Corlopam) and nesiritide (Natrecor) are NOT recommended to prevent or treat AKI
- Avoid the use of intravenous (IV) aminoglycosides to treat infections, unless no other less nephrotoxic agent is available

The target outcomes for intervention include preservation of existing renal function, prevention of the complications associated with AKI, and avoidance of the need for chronic RRT.

DEFINITION

AKI is commonly described as an abrupt reduction in renal function. The glomerular filtration rate (GFR), a clinical assessment tool used to measure renal function, is the volume of plasma cleared of a given substance in a minute. A normal GFR in adults is 100–125 mL/min/1.73 m^2).[40] Any decrease in GFR leads to the retention of nitrogenous waste products (azotemia) and the associated inability of the body to maintain normal fluid and electrolyte homeostasis.[20] In 2012, the Kidney Disease: Improving Global Outcomes (KDIGO) guidelines for AKI combined the 2004 Risk/Injury/Failure/Loss/End-stage (RIFLE) criteria and the 2005 Acute Kidney Injury criteria to provide one clinically relevant and universally accepted definition for AKI: "AKI is defined as an increase in serum creatinine by greater than or equal to 0.03 mg/dL within 48 hours; or increase of serum creatinine level greater than or equal to 1.5 times above baseline; which is known or presumed to have

BOX 23.1 Stages of Acute Kidney Injury

Stage	Serum Creatinine	Urine Output
1	1.5 times baseline OR ≥ 0.3 mg/dL (≥ 26.5 mmol/L) increase	< 0.5 mL/kg/h for 6–12 h
2	2.0–2.9 times baseline	< 0.5 mL/kg/h for 12 h
3	3.0 times baseline OR Increase in serum creatinine to ≥ 4.0 mg/dL (≥ 353.6 mmol/L) OR Initiation of renal replacement therapy	< 0.3 mL/kg/h for ≥ 24 h OR Anuria for ≥ 12 h

risen in the last 7 days; or an absolute increase in creatinine level of 0.5 mg/dL or greater above a certain cutoff point (e.g., 2 to 3.5 mg/dL)."[25,39] The risk classification tool provides a staging for AKI, with stage 1 being initial injury and stage 3 requiring intervention with RRT (Box 23.1).

APPLIED PATHOPHYSIOLOGY

Types of Acute Kidney Injury

The etiologies of AKI are commonly classified into three broad categories, each of which is associated with the location of the dysfunction. Physiologically, normal renal function is the sum of adequate filtration of the blood, renal tubule processing of the filtrate, and elimination of the final urine product. Therefore, kidney injury (dysfunction) can occur secondary to a reduction in renal blood flow that prohibits adequate filtration (i.e., prerenal or transient); secondary to an inflammatory, ischemic, or nephrotoxic injury to the tubules (i.e., intrarenal or persistent); or from obstruction of ultrafiltrate or urine elimination (i.e., postrenal). The multiple causes of each type of AKI are most easily understood when related to the underlying pathophysiology. Diagnosis of the type of kidney injury is imperative so that appropriate interventions can be instituted without delay. The diagnosis will be made using patient history and physical assessment findings, along with pertinent laboratory and radiologic findings.

Prerenal Acute Kidney Injury

Prerenal AKI is caused by any clinical condition resulting in inadequate or decreased renal perfusion. Common etiologies of prerenal AKI in the critically ill are listed in Box 23.2. No matter which clinical situation is responsible for the decrease in renal blood flow, the pathophysiologic consequences are the same. The decrease in renal perfusion decreases afferent arteriole pressure, leading to a decreased GFR. In response to this decreased GFR, although there is no actual damage to the glomerular filtration or nephron function, the kidney is unable to function normally.

The kidneys normally receive 25% of the cardiac output (CO), called the *renal fraction,* which is approximately 1200 mL/min.[5] Whereas renal oxygen consumption is high, normal renal blood flow is in excess of that required for simple renal metabolic requirements, reinforcing that high flow is necessary for urine formation and other renal functions. Likewise, the interrelatedness of the renal vasculature and renal tubules is reflective of the interdependence between blood supply and renal function (Fig. 23.1).

BOX 23.2 Causes of Prerenal Acute Kidney Injury

Hypovolemia
- Hemorrhage
- Gastrointestinal losses: vomiting, diarrhea, nasogastric loss
- Burns
- Diaphoresis
- Overdiuresis
- Movement into interstitial space (edema, ascites)
- Hypovolemic shock

Decreased Cardiac Output
- Myocardial infarction
- Tamponade
- Cardiac dysrhythmias
- Heart failure
- Pulmonary embolism
- Tension pneumothorax

Decreased Effective Circulating Volume
- Anaphylaxis
- Severe sepsis/septic shock
- Multiple organ dysfunction syndrome
- Neurogenic shock
- End-stage liver disease

Other/Alteration in Renal Perfusion
- Intraabdominal compartment syndrome
- Renal vascular thrombosis or stenosis
- Medications

Medications
- Loop diuretics
- Angiotensin-converting enzyme inhibitors
- Prostaglandin inhibitors
- Chemotherapeutic agents
- Vasoactive medications (e.g., epinephrine, norepinephrine)

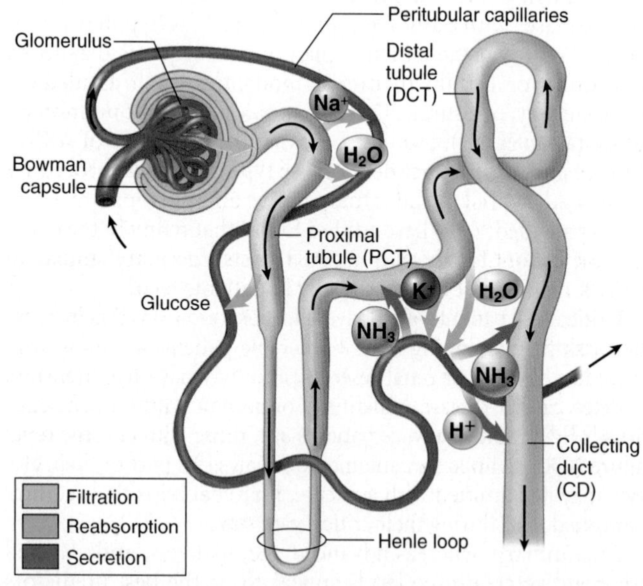

FIG. 23.1 Components of the nephron. *Arrows* indicate either blood or urine flow. (From Patton, K. T., Thibodeau, G.A. (2016). *Anatomy & physiology* (9th ed.). St Louis: Mosby.)

TABLE 23.1 Differential Laboratory Diagnosis of Renal Dysfunction

	Normal	Prerenal	Intrarenal	Postrenal
Urine volume	1–1.5 L/d	< 400 mL/d	< 400 mL/d	Variable
Urine specific gravity	1.010–1.020	≥1.020	Fixed (≤1.010)	Fixed (≤1.010)
Urine osmolality	500–850 mOsm/L	> 500 mOsm/L	< 350 mOsm/L	≤ 350 mOsm/L
Serum BUN	10–20 mg/dL	> 25 mg/dL	> 25 mg/dL	< 25 mg/dL
Serum creatinine	0.6–1.2 mg/dL	Normal to slightly elevated	> 1.2 mg/dL	> 1.2 mg/dL
Serum BUN:creatinine ratio	10:1	≥20:1	(10–15):1; both elevated, but ratio remains constant	(10–15):1; both elevated, but ratio remains constant
Urine sodium		< 20 mEq/L	> 40 mEq/L	> 40 mEq/L
FENa		< 1%	> 1%*	> 1%

*When the patient is not under the influence of diuretics.
BUN, Blood urea nitrogen; *FENa*, fractional excretion of sodium.

Blood flow to the kidneys and the GFR is normally protected through renal autoregulation. The primary purpose of autoregulation is to maintain constant renal blood flow, which provides for precise control of renal excretion of water and other solutes.[5] Autoregulation occurs in both the efferent and afferent arterioles by influencing the degree of vascular tone through vasoconstriction or vasodilation in response to changes in arterial pressure or renal tubular flow to maintain normal renal blood flow. The renal autoregulation mechanism is able to accommodate fluctuations in the systolic blood pressure (SBP) from 70 mm Hg to 180 mm Hg, while maintaining a minimal change of 10% in the GFR.[12]

In addition, normal compensatory mechanisms are stimulated whenever low pressure or perfusion is sensed by the kidney. Activation of the renin-angiotensin-aldosterone system (RAAS) results in peripheral and glomerular vasoconstriction via adrenergic stimulation by angiotensin II (further decreasing renal perfusion) and an increase in sodium and water reabsorption, as the manifestation of the activity of both angiotensin II and aldosterone. The aldosterone-induced sodium reabsorption results in a low urine sodium level and low fractional excretion of sodium (FENa) (Table 23.1).

Urine sodium values less than 20 mEq/L are most often associated with volume depletion severe enough to compromise renal blood flow. This suggests that tubular function is still intact, conserving sodium appropriately. A urine sodium value greater than 40 mEq/L suggests that tubular function is impaired, as seen in intrarenal AKI and CRF. FENa can be a useful measurement to evaluate renal tubular function. It assesses the ratio of the amount of sodium in the urine to the amount of sodium filtered by the kidney. Normally, less than 1% of sodium is excreted because kidneys with normal function reabsorb 99% of all filtered sodium. When the FENa is greater than 1%, it is suggestive of tubular dysfunction.

Under the influence of antidiuretic hormone (ADH)—which is also stimulated by low renal perfusion—and aldosterone, more water is reabsorbed, leading to decreased urine production (oliguria) and increased urine concentration (increased urine specific gravity and osmolality).

Urea is easily filtered and actively reabsorbed much more readily than creatinine, primarily because of the smaller molecular size of urea and its affinity to movement with water. Serum blood urea nitrogen (BUN) levels elevate while, for a time, serum creatinine levels remain relatively normal. This is demonstrated by one of the hallmark signs of prerenal AKI, which is a BUN:creatinine ratio of 20:1 or greater.

Renal blood flow is also influenced by the sympathetic nervous system (SNS), hormones, and medications. Anything that stimulates the SNS (e.g., hypotension) will cause renal vasculature vasoconstriction. Hormonal influences include the RAAS and ADH, which have been already discussed. Renal prostaglandins (i.e., PGE_2 and PGI_2) modulate the impact of vasoactive substances on the kidney. Whereas renal prostaglandins do not have a major influence on the GFR in normal circumstances, they are thought to temper the renal vasoconstriction effects of the SNS, especially on the afferent arterioles. This opposition to vasoconstriction helps prevent excess reduction of renal blood flow.

Certain pharmacologic interventions (e.g., epinephrine and norepinephrine) cause renal vasoconstriction. Prostaglandin inhibitors (e.g., aspirin and other nonsteroidal antiinflammatory drugs) may cause significant reductions in renal blood flow under stressful situations, such as volume depletion or surgery.[12]

Intrarenal Acute Kidney Injury

AKI is classified as intrarenal (intrinsic) when there is inflammatory, nephrotoxic, or ischemic injury directly to the nephron. Intrinsic insults to the kidneys result in renal cellular damage to the vasculature, glomerulus, tubules, or interstitium, ultimately leading to decreased function. A healthy glomerulus prevents filtration of plasma proteins and cellular elements. However, when the glomerulus has been damaged, proteins and cellular debris can enter the renal tubules and lead to obstruction of the lumen. Common causes of intrarenal AKI are listed in Box 23.3.

The major cause of intrarenal AKI is acute tubular necrosis (ATN), which is caused by ischemic or nephrotoxic insults to the kidney.[37] In critical care, greater than 50% of all ATN is associated with sepsis.[52,53] Postoperative ATN is responsible for approximately 16.7% to 30% of all nosocomial AKI.[15]

Inflammatory (e.g., glomerulonephritis) and immune disorders (e.g., systemic lupus erythematosus and poststreptococcal infections) can also cause intrarenal injury. With these disorders, the GFR is decreased because of immune-related hemodynamic changes, as well as physical structural damage. Intrarenal AKI may be the sequela of infectious or infiltrative diseases (e.g., sarcoidosis and cancers such as lymphoma or leukemia), as well as some medications. Whereas there is neither tubule nor glomerular damage, interstitial nephritis is characterized by inflammatory cell infiltrates in the renal interstitium and a decrease in the GFR.

As discussed earlier, the kidneys are highly metabolic and receive a large portion of the CO, and are therefore extremely vulnerable to ischemic or toxic injury. In ischemic or nephrotoxic injury, there is damage to both the vasculature and the tubules. Tubular injury is most common. Nephrotic ischemic injury is the most common cause of intrarenal AKI, and presents as ATN. With less oxygen available, there is decreased adenosine triphosphate (ATP) production, and therefore wastes and toxins accumulate in the cells. In the tubules, an increase in intracellular calcium level leads to necrosis and apoptosis, with relocation of the sodium, potassium, and adenosinetriphosphatase (ATPase) from the basement membrane. This relocation interferes with normal sodium transport, which increases distal delivery of sodium chloride, causing swelling of cells and activation of tubular glomerular feedback, ultimately decreasing GFR. If ischemia worsens, nitric oxide is produced, causing cellular damage and lysis of tubular cells. Cast formation, tubular obstruction, and tubular destruction result, causing backleak of the glomerular filtrate, which leads to interstitial edema and further decreases GFR. Cumulatively, these mechanisms contribute to the decreased renal function observed in ATN.

ATN also results in vascular endothelium injury. The damaged endothelium responds in an exaggerated fashion to vasodilators released as part of the stress response (e.g., bradykinin and acetylcholine). This response, along with the loss of autoregulation, exacerbates the effects of the ischemia.

Given the significant blood flow through the kidney, it is by nature susceptible to damage as toxic substances are filtered. The kidney's great reabsorptive and concentrating abilities lead to the delivery of large amounts of toxins to the tubular epithelial cells. When presented with a nephrotoxin, the generation of toxic metabolites, high energy consumption requirement, and marginal oxygen delivery further increase the susceptibility of the kidney to damage.

Contrast-induced nephropathy (CIN) is the third leading cause of AKI in hospitalized patients.[23] Although CIN has less than a 10% occurrence rate, it is associated with increased morbidity, mortality, and medical costs.[23,27] Both nonmodifiable and modifiable risk factors for developing CIN have been identified. The most important nonmodifiable risk factors are diabetes and preexisting renal impairment, defined as patients with a GFR of less than 90 mL/min per 1.73 m^2 in the diabetic patient or a GFR of less than 60 mL/min per 1.73 m^2 in the nondiabetic patient.[19] Additional nonmodifiable risks include age greater than 75, hypercholesterolemia, and a ventricular ejection fraction of less than 40%. Modifiable risks for CIN include recent exposure to contrast, dehydration, hypotension, anemia, shock, sepsis, administration of nephrotoxic agents, and the use of an intraaortic balloon pump.[19] Although the pathophysiology is not fully understood, the insult is thought to be multifactorial. Contrast agents may produce renal hemodynamic impairment, renal tubular cell toxicity, and AKI secondary to increased levels of adenosine, endothelin, and free radicals and a reduction in the levels of prostaglandins and nitric oxide.[23] Other sources cite oxidative stress and uricemia as contributing to the pathophysiology of CIN.[27] All of these factors contribute to prolonged vasoconstriction of the arteriole, stasis of contrast material in the renal vasculature (resulting in reduced blood flow), decreased GFR, and ischemia from vasoconstriction.

The risk of CIN may be decreased by avoiding medications that increase vasoconstriction of the arterioles, reduce volume, or are nephrotoxic. CIN is a growing concern in the medical field, and prevention relies on addressing the side effects of contrast media. Many prevention strategies for CIN have been proposed over the years, but only two have been shown to be effective: hydrating the patient with isotonic crystalloids pre- and postprocedure to optimize intravascular volume and enhance clearance of contrast, and administering a second agent to prevent cytotoxic injury.[19,23,27] Studies have shown that including secondary agents, such as N-acetylcysteine (NAC; Mucomyst) and allopurinol (Zyloprim) can help reduce the risk of developing CIN. These medications may contribute to the reduction of CIN by acting as an antioxidant agent to bind free radicals released during the use of contrast, as with NAC; or by acting as an oxidase inhibitor to reduce uricemia for the prevention of renal hypertrophy, proteinuria, hypertension, and renal scarring, as with allopurinol.[23,27]

BOX 23.3 Etiologies of Intrarenal AKI

Inflammatory
- Poststreptococcal glomerulonephritis
- Membranous glomerulonephritis
- Membranoproliferative glomerulonephritis (from antigen-antibody complexes, cryoglobulins)
- Interstitial nephritis
- Acute pyelonephritis
- Allergic nephritis
- Hypercalcemia
- Uric acid nephropathy
- Myeloma of the kidney
- Rhabdomyolysis (trauma, seizures, prolonged coma, muscle disease)
- Myoglobin
- Transfusion reaction

Ischemic
- Prolonged hypoperfusion
- Renal artery thrombosis
- Shock

Nephrotoxic
- Medications: aminoglycoside antibiotics, anesthetic agents
- Radiographic contrast dyes
- Pesticides
- Fungicides
- Heavy metals
- Organic solvents

Obstructive
- Renal thrombosis
- Nephrolithiasis
- Sickle cell disease
- Trauma/crush injuries

Postrenal Acute Kidney Injury

If the dysfunction of the kidney is related to obstruction of the renal flow structures beyond the nephron, it is termed postrenal AKI. In response to the obstruction of urine flow, the ureters and renal pelvis dilate (visible on ultrasound or computed tomography [CT] scan), and intratubular pressure may increase until it exceeds glomerular filtration pressure, causing the GFR to decrease. A complete obstruction will cause the filtration to cease entirely, while a partial obstruction will decrease filtration. As with any decrease to the GFR, initially the tubules will respond by increasing reabsorption of sodium and water, leaving the urine volume low, the urine sodium level high, and the urine concentration high. Over time, as the tubules become damaged, sodium and water reabsorption decreases. Permanent renal damage can occur if the obstruction is not addressed. The extent of that damage is determined by the location, duration, and degree of obstruction. Common etiologies of postrenal AKI in the critically ill are listed in Box 23.4.

ASSESSMENT

Assessment findings of the prerenal AKI patient correlate with the cause of the decreased blood flow to the kidneys. If the underlying problem is hypovolemia or decreased systemic vascular resistance, the patient will present with symptoms such as hypotension and tachycardia. If hypovolemia is serious, the patient may manifest signs of hypovolemic shock (see Chapter 28). In septic shock, massive vascular dilation leads to a relative hypovolemia which decreases perfusion to the kidneys. If the decreased perfusion is secondary to decreased CO, the patient's presentation will be different (Table 23.2). Pertinent laboratory findings seen in AKI, including the laboratory differentiation between prerenal and intrarenal AKI etiologies, are outlined in Table 23.1. Application of assessment findings aids in accurate diagnosis of the cause of decreased renal blood flow, and will therefore aid in appropriate treatment.

The physical assessment findings in the intrarenal AKI patient differ depending on the underlying cause of the problem. When the injury is ischemic in nature secondary to prolonged decreased perfusion, the patient may initially present with hypovolemia or decreased CO. As renal dysfunction progresses, patient presentation will include manifestations of the lack of renal function.

Renal tubular dysfunction leads to hindered sodium reabsorption, increased urine sodium levels, and an FENa greater than 1%. The concentrating ability of the kidney is impaired, resulting in lower urine osmolality and specific gravity.

BOX 23.4 Etiologies of Postrenal AKI

Tubular Obstruction

- Polycystic kidney
- Uric acid crystals

Ureteral Obstruction

- Tumors
- Strictures
- Fibrosis

Bladder Obstruction

- Prostatic hypertrophy
- Tumors
- Calculi
- Blood clots
- Neurogenic causes
- Anticholinergic medications

Urethral Obstruction

- Calculi
- Strictures
- Stenosis
- Catheter obstruction

TABLE 23.2 Assessment Findings in Prerenal Acute Kidney Injury

Fluid Deficit/Ineffective Circulating Volume	Decreased Cardiac Output
Oliguria	Oliguria
Tachycardia	Tachycardia
Hypotension	Hypotension
Dry mucous membranes	
Decreased PAP, PAOP, RAP	Elevated PAP, PAOP, RAP
Flat neck veins	Distended neck veins
Lethargy	
Coma	

PAP, Pulmonary artery pressure; *PAOP*, pulmonary artery occlusion pressure; *RAP*, right atrial pressure.

Uremic Complications

The impact of the accumulation of uremic waste products in the CRF patient is well known. There continues to be limited information regarding the complications of uremic retention compounds in AKI. The studies that do exist point to the inflammatory response of uremic toxins within the body, which present themselves in many areas of multiorgan dysfunction.[33] Some studies show that uremic toxicity is dependent on the rate of progression of renal injury. During the acute phase, uremic compounds increase the inflammatory response and decrease the kidney's ability to filter antioxidants' antiinflammatory and vasodilating substances through the glomeruli.[33] Whereas some of the compounds found in CRF and AKI are comparable, many of the effects found in AKI are due to inflammatory responses rather than long-term accumulation.[14] Additional studies must be completed to determine the full effects of uremic toxins in AKI.

Cardiovascular Manifestations

The cardiovascular manifestations of AKI can almost all be linked to the volume status of the patient. For example, hypertension is a common finding in these patients, due to volume overload and increased peripheral vascular resistance. Since renal perfusion is often low, the RAAS system is activated, which increases angiotensin II, thereby increasing sodium and water retention and peripheral vasoconstriction. CO is often high for similar reasons but may decrease over time as fluid shifts to the interstitial space, which may cause peripheral or pulmonary edema, ascites, or intraabdominal hypertension. In addition, CO may be compromised by the metabolic acidosis, hypertension, anemia, and electrolyte abnormalities seen in AKI.

Patients may develop heart failure or have preexisting heart failure exacerbated by AKI. Dysrhythmias are common, and may be related to acidosis, hyperkalemia, hypermagnesemia, and hypocalcemia. Hyperkalemia results in prolonged PR intervals, peaked T waves, widened QRS complexes, and cardiac arrest if left untreated. Continuous electrocardiogram (ECG) monitoring is indicated to assess for life-threatening dysrhythmias and ECG changes.

Over time, uremic pericarditis may develop. The pericardial sac, which is usually aseptic, becomes inflamed, and fluid accumulates in response to the uremic toxins. Clinically, patients may present with pain, fever, and pericardial friction rub. The rub may occur before the pain, and may disappear with the accumulation of fluid. These patients may be tachycardic, hypotensive, have a narrowed pulse pressure, and have a paradoxical pulse. Both uremic pericarditis and pericardial effusions may result in cardiac tamponade. Cardiac tamponade is a medical emergency as ventricular filling is reduced, and emergent drain placement is indicated.

Respiratory Manifestations

For an already ischemic kidney, hypoxemia presents an added renal risk. Fluid volume overload can lead to pulmonary congestion, pleural effusions, or intraabdominal hypertension, all of which may decrease gas exchange. The patient with AKI also experiences interstitial edema caused by dysregulation of the inflammatory cascade, and increased vascular permeability (capillary leak), which can lead to lung perfusion dysregulation, fluid shifts, and pulmonary edema. Urea retention products contribute to oxidative stress, which in turn increases inflammation and leads to additional capillary leak in the pulmonary bed.[31] Urea products may also contribute to the development of pulmonary edema, causing the patient to present with shortness of breath and frothy sputum, along with rales and rhonchi. These patients may have normal cardiac filling pressures related to the previously described loss of capillary integrity and fluid leak. Commonly, these patients have hypoalbuminemia, which decreases colloid oncotic pressure, allowing fluid to move interstitially more easily.

The kidney is a highly metabolic organ. In addition to the constant vigilance of the critical care nurse, current monitoring and therapeutic technology make hypoxemia easy to anticipate but not always easy to treat. Even brief interruptions in oxygenation can worsen any ischemic intrarenal damage. Using arterial and venous oxygen saturations (Sao_2 and Svo_2, respectively) to monitor oxygen extraction by vital organs can provide data regarding oxygen consumption (Vo_2) and oxygen delivery (Do_2) to the kidneys.[9] Since organ perfusion is reliant on a combination of Vo_2 and Do_2, small changes in either component can lead to a consequential hypoxemic event. Evaluating the cause for changes to Sao_2 and Svo_2 can provide data for interventions to minimize the repercussions of decreased CO, decreased oxygen-carrying capacity, and abnormal oxygen extraction. These emergent situations must be responded to quickly in order to preserve oxygen delivery to the kidneys and prevent further intrarenal damage and worsening metabolic acidosis (lactic acidosis).

Hematologic Manifestations

Anemia will be seen as early as 10 days after the onset of renal dysfunction. Anemia decreases the blood's oxygen-carrying capacity, which may further compromise cardiac and pulmonary stability.

Critically ill patients have a number of factors that contribute to bone marrow suppression, and they may experience bleeding, hemodilution, decreased red blood cell survival, gastrointestinal (GI) bleeding, perioperative blood loss, and intravascular hemolysis, all of which contribute to an anemic state. Anemia is worsened by acidosis, uremic toxins, and decreased or absent erythropoietin production. Without adequate erythropoietin, there is decreased synthesis and increased breakdown of the red blood cell membrane, decreasing the cell's half-life. The subsequent anemia, specifically the decrease in erythrocytes, interferes with platelet interaction with the endothelial walls of the vessels. Uremic coagulopathies, such as excessive bleeding and thrombosis, are related to uremic toxins that disturb platelet production, aggregation, and adhesion. Additional factors that are related to coagulation abnormalities include inflammation, endothelial changes, abnormal activation of the clotting cascade, and abnormal activation of the fibrinolytic system.[35]

Uremic anemia decreases platelet activation by inactivating prostacyclin. The decrease in platelet activation reduces adenosine diphosphate (ADP) release from the platelets. Normally, when ADP is released from the platelets, it binds to the P2Y1, P2Y12, and P2X1 receptors on other platelets in order to increase platelet activation. When platelet activation is no longer needed, the free ADP in the blood is normally converted to adenosine, which is a platelet activation inhibitor. The disruption of the platelet activation system may lead to an increased bleeding risk.[35]

Because many critical care patients have concomitant cardiac and pulmonary disease, anemia and coagulopathies may be catastrophic. Attending to the dysfunction of the hematologic system by providing support through blood product transfusions and the administration of other medications can decrease the risk of such complications.

The risk of infection is increased because of leukocyte dysfunction. The leukocyte count may rise, but the ability of the leukocyte to combat infection is impaired. Normal inflammatory responses are also blunted. Therefore, the nurse should continually assess for signs of infection. Infection prevention interventions include using strict aseptic technique, minimizing invasive line manipulation, providing frequent mouth and pulmonary care, minimizing use of vascular catheters, removing indwelling catheters when possible, and monitoring the white blood cell count, vital signs, and signs of infection.

Gastrointestinal Manifestations

The patient's nutrition will be affected as a result of uremia-mediated gastritis, which may result in anorexia, nausea, dyspepsia, vomiting, diarrhea, constipation, and gastric ulceration. There is evidence that AKI itself may be caused by the inflammatory cascade. Since the inflammatory response is seldom localized to one organ system, the kidney is caught up in the flood of inflammatory mediators. Unable to excrete these factors, the kidney cannot compensate for the resultant acidosis, contributing to the inflammatory response. Acidosis leads to increased levels of nitric oxide (NO; a vasodilator) and lowers blood pressure (BP), or may lead to shock. NO exacerbates lung and GI injury, hindering the natural GI barrier function of preventing bacterial translocation.[34]

AKI patients have a tendency toward GI bleeding. The kidney plays a role in the inactivation and removal of GI hormones. As renal function is lost, plasma gastrin and gastric ammonia levels rise. This may lead to gastritis and the development of ulcerations. With the development of acute, erosive ulcerations, both the upper and lower GI tract may be affected. The risk for GI bleeding may be exacerbated once RRT is begun, as a consequence of the anticoagulation that may be used.

Neurologic Manifestations

Uremic encephalopathy occurs secondary to the saturation of uremic toxins in the blood and, subsequently, the saturation of the blood-brain barrier. The increased levels of uremic toxins in the blood saturate and overwhelm the organic anion transporter, OAT3, at the blood-brain barrier. The oversaturation of this efflux transporter allows the uremic toxins to enter the brain and alter the metabolism of neurotransmitters, causing alterations in cognitive function.[17] Neurologic changes observed in the AKI patient are directly related to the rate at which renal dysfunction develops; however, these patients usually respond favorably to RRT. Mental status abnormalities should be considered warning signs indicating that the patient needs to be started on RRT. The patient may become depressed, apathetic, and obtunded. These patients may manifest changes in consciousness, showing alterations in psychomotor skills, thinking, memory, speech, perception, and emotion. Signs of neurologic alteration often proceed more rapidly in the AKI patient than in the CRF patient.

INTERVENTIONS

Patients with AKI must be managed collaboratively by the entire healthcare team. This collaboration must begin with the early recognition of those patients who might be at risk for the development of AKI. Unfortunately, much of the care available for the patient with AKI is supportive, rather than curative. However, whereas the interventions used have changed over the past few years, there remains a focus on early recognition of the risk for AKI, as well as the early institution of RRT to prevent complications.

In prerenal AKI, target outcomes include accurate cause identification and intervention, restoration of renal blood flow, preservation of existing renal function, prevention of the complications associated with AKI (and the associated prolonged length of stay), and avoidance of the need for chronic RRT.[8] Interventions should focus on identifying the cause of the hypoperfusion and treating accordingly. If the problem is volume-related, then volume should be aggressively replaced. If the patient is in heart failure, interventions may include antidysrhythmic medications, positive inotropic agents, preload and afterload manipulations, and, in some situations, advanced therapies such as an intraaortic balloon pump or mechanical circulatory support. If the problem is decreased systemic vascular resistance, vasoconstrictors should be administered. Because of the widespread systemic effects of AKI, there are a variety of clinical challenges for the critical care team, including maintaining fluid, electrolyte, and acid-base balances; preventing and treating infection; preventing further kidney damage; minimizing the effects of the developing uremia; and establishing adequate nutrition.

Because prevention of AKI is of utmost importance, the restoration of adequate circulating blood volume takes precedence over other interventions in the oliguric patient. Anticipatory interventions, such as additional fluid, should also be implemented.

In the situation of exposure to radiocontrast dyes, if the patient has diabetes, is elderly or dehydrated, or has even slight elevation in creatinine level, periprocedural IV fluid should be administered to prevent CIN. The team pharmacist should also be consulted for modifying drug doses and anticipating the effects of radiocontrast dye. These steps are crucial in preventing CIN in many critically ill patients.

Fluid Balance

Fluid balance in the patient with compromised renal function is a challenge. Renal perfusion must be maintained, while not placing the patient at risk for the complications of fluid overload. Initially, patients may present with a fluid volume deficit. Any patient who has experienced a fluid loss and is at risk for fluid volume deficit is also a candidate for the development of prerenal AKI. If the insult is too great or the healthcare team is unable to adequately intervene, renal dysfunction may progress.

Typically, patients with renal dysfunction will not have maintenance IV fluids infusing. Efforts to manage fluid balance often begin with monitoring cardiac filling pressures in order to establish a clear picture of the patient's fluid status. If the patient demonstrates orthostatic hypotension, has a central venous pressure (CVP) less than 4 mm Hg, has a decreased urine output (UOP), or demonstrates decreased cardiac filling pressures on an echocardiogram, a crystalloid fluid challenge may be considered, using normal saline (NS) as a 1000 mL bolus over 30 minutes. NS is the fluid of choice, as it is the most isotonic fluid that can be used without adding potentially dangerous electrolytes (e.g., potassium and calcium, which are found in lactated Ringer's [LR]) to the vascular space.[41] Hypotonic IV solutions, such as D_5W (5% dextrose in water) or half NS, can redistribute quickly into the intracellular space, and therefore will not increase the intravascular volume to support perfusion of the kidney.

The only colloid that should be considered is albumin, and it should be used cautiously while monitoring fluid status, signs of fluid overload, and cardiac filling pressures, when available. Colloids may redistribute and take additional water from the circulatory space into the interstitial space, thus worsening pulmonary edema.

If there is no response to the fluid challenge (i.e., improvement of cardiac filling pressures or the presence of urine within 30 minutes), additional fluid may be administered until the CVP reaches 6 to 8 mm Hg. If there is no urine response, and symptoms of intravascular depletion have not improved, fluids may be given to reach a CVP goal of 10 to 12 mm Hg. If signs of intravascular volume depletion and hypoperfusion persist, a vasoactive medication may be indicated. A continued lack of UOP may indicate that the cause is intrarenal rather than prerenal.

As described previously, intrarenal AKI results in the loss of the kidneys' ability to form and concentrate urine. Management of this stage of AKI becomes critical as the patient will likely become oliguric. As renal function deteriorates, fluid overload often becomes more of an issue. Whereas there is no evidence that diuretics decrease the incidence of AKI, decrease morbidity and mortality, decrease the length of hospital stay, or alter the need for dialysis, diuretics may convert oliguric AKI to nonoliguric AKI, which, although comforting to clinicians, does little for the patient.[1,28] The diuretics chosen should be planned to present as little risk to the fragile patient as possible. If they are ineffective, residual problems may develop.

Fluid overload is a common finding in AKI as the kidneys are incapable of excreting fluids. This may manifest in heart failure, pulmonary edema, and cerebral edema. The occurrence of these disorders in the patient with AKI strongly suggests a fluid volume excess and needs to be treated aggressively. If fluid overload does not respond to diuretics, uncontrollable fluid overload is generally the determining factor that RRT is necessary. Whereas AKI patients may show normal cardiac filling pressures with a modest weight gain, they may still develop pulmonary edema. This may occur as a result of inadequately treated uremia, which, although previously thought to cause a capillary leak syndrome, has more recently been demonstrated to represent an imbalance in hydrostatic and oncotic fluid pressures, leading to pulmonary infiltrates.

Caution should be applied to the use of daily weights as the gold standard of fluid balance. The catabolic AKI patient not receiving an adequate daily diet, whether enteral or parenteral, may lose weight at the rate of a half-pound per day. The critical care nurse, in collaboration with the nutritionist, should estimate daily visceral weight loss in the patient who is receiving inadequate daily calories.

Although less likely to occur before the institution of RRT, the patient may develop a fluid volume deficit despite the reduced excretion during AKI. This can occur due to GI bleeding, diarrhea, or vomiting. In these cases, the sodium level will likely be unchanged; fluid replacement is required and should match the composition of the fluid lost.[16]

Alterations in Electrolyte Balance

Hypernatremia frequently occurs as a result of loss of excretion capability. Hyponatremia can also develop as a result of fluid repletion with hypotonic solutions.[41] Hyponatremia is exacerbated by impaired free water clearance and causes cellular edema, including cerebral edema, which may lead to hyponatremic encephalopathy. Neurologic symptoms range from headache to confusion to coma.[50] The more acute the onset of hyponatremia, the more likely the patient will experience serious signs and symptoms, including seizures.

Hyperkalemia is also a common complication of AKI, and clinicians should be well informed in its management. Monitoring potassium levels and ECG tracings should be priority assessments in the treatment of an AKI patient. Potassium levels should be maintained at less than or equal to 6.5 mEq/L to avoid the risk of cardiac arrhythmias, which may range from peaked T waves to cardiac arrest.[41] Refer to Chapter 21 for additional information on hyperkalemia. If there are changes to the patient's ECG, or the potassium level is higher than 6.5 mEq/L and cannot be lowered using conservative interventions, RRT should be considered.

A key to solving these recurrent problems is to make serial assessments and evaluations in patients at risk for AKI, which includes those critically ill patients with risk factors. Routine evaluations of electrolyte values will guide replacement at correct rates, thus avoiding iatrogenic electrolyte imbalance. It is also important to remember that cardiac stability in AKI patients may be enhanced by addressing their electrolyte abnormalities aggressively.

Metabolic Acidosis

The kidneys play a key role in the preservation of acid-base balance. When renal function is decreased, the kidneys are unable to excrete anions such as chloride and phosphate.[54] Therefore, metabolic acids accumulate in the serum and create a metabolic acidosis. There is also decreased production of bicarbonate due to the decreased proximal tubule reabsorption and regeneration. Because these patients are also hypoalbuminemic, they have a reduced protein buffering capacity. All these factors lead to metabolic acidosis. Additionally, many patients have other etiologies of acidosis that are coexistent with the renal-mediated acidosis. These might include lactic acidosis or shock, respiratory acidosis induced by permissive hypercapnia ventilation in acute lung injury, or, less frequently, ketoacidosis.

The first defense against metabolic acidosis is dietary restriction of protein, liberalized as soon as the patient is started on RRT. The acidosis can be moderated with bicarbonate (HCO_3^-) infusion as needed, but if the HCO_3^- concentration is less than 15 mEq/L and is refractory to other interventions, RRT should be initiated.[41] As with electrolyte abnormalities, it is important to remember that aggressively treating acidosis may be part of the key to addressing cardiac instability.

RENAL REPLACEMENT THERAPY

RRT, delivered through a variety of means, is a process by which fluid and waste products are filtered through a semipermeable membrane to assist in elimination from the body. RRT may be performed with or without the addition of a dialysate solution (patient-specific and prepared by prescription to include fluid, glucose, and electrolytes). The decision to implement RRT is usually based on one of the following issues: volume overload that is unresponsive to diuretics or fluid restriction, symptomatic hyperkalemia, severe metabolic acidosis, or symptomatic or rapidly progressing uremia (i.e., altered mental status, GI bleeding, or pericarditis with pericardial effusion).

Although there have been recommendations in the literature as early as 1960 that RRT be started earlier rather than later, there is no clear consensus on the best method; an optimal, clearly defined starting point; or an optimal dose of RRT. Studies conducted decades ago showed reduced morbidity and mortality with early initiation of RRT.[26,38,46] More current studies have not shown similar results, which is perhaps a reflection of the more complex contemporary patient.[18,32] The therapy chosen and dose prescribed must be individually tailored to the patient's clinical condition.

RRT is classified as either intermittent or continuous (Fig. 23.2). Most commonly, one of four types of RRT is employed for critically ill patients: peritoneal dialysis (PD), hemodialysis (HD), sustained low-efficiency dialysis (SLED)/extended daily dialysis (EDD), or continuous renal replacement therapy (CRRT), of which there are a number of variations. The four types have advantages and disadvantages and vary in their effectiveness, need for anticoagulation, complications, and the time, access, and technical support required. The latter three types are used most frequently in critical care. Multiple clinical trials have been performed to identify the best treatment out of these three modalities; all three have proven to be effective for volume and solute removal, and none has stood out in terms of impacting patient mortality rates.[42]

Peritoneal Dialysis

Utilizing the peritoneal membrane as the semipermeable membrane, PD is the least frequently used type of RRT in critical care. The dialysate fluid is infused through a catheter into the peritoneal cavity, where it dwells for a prescribed period of time (1 to 6 hours) and is then drained. Through osmosis, diffusion, and filtration via the concentration gradients established by the composition of the dialysate (e.g., a higher glucose concentration, which enhances water elimination), excess water, electrolytes, and waste products move into the peritoneal cavity/compartment and are removed from the body when the effluent (dialysate plus ultrafiltrate) is drained. This process is repeated throughout treatment. Patients are at risk for the development of peritonitis, protein loss into the dialysate, and hyperglycemia.

Whereas PD may be effective, the process of fluid and waste elimination is not as efficient as with other types of RRT. Therefore, PD is rarely the first choice for renal replacement in critical care. However, it does offer several advantages over other methods. Because fluid movement is slower, patients with cardiovascular instability are not subject to the effects of rapid fluid shifts, making PD more tolerable. PD is also considered a safer option in patients with cerebral edema. As an additional benefit, patients undergoing PD do not require anticoagulation,

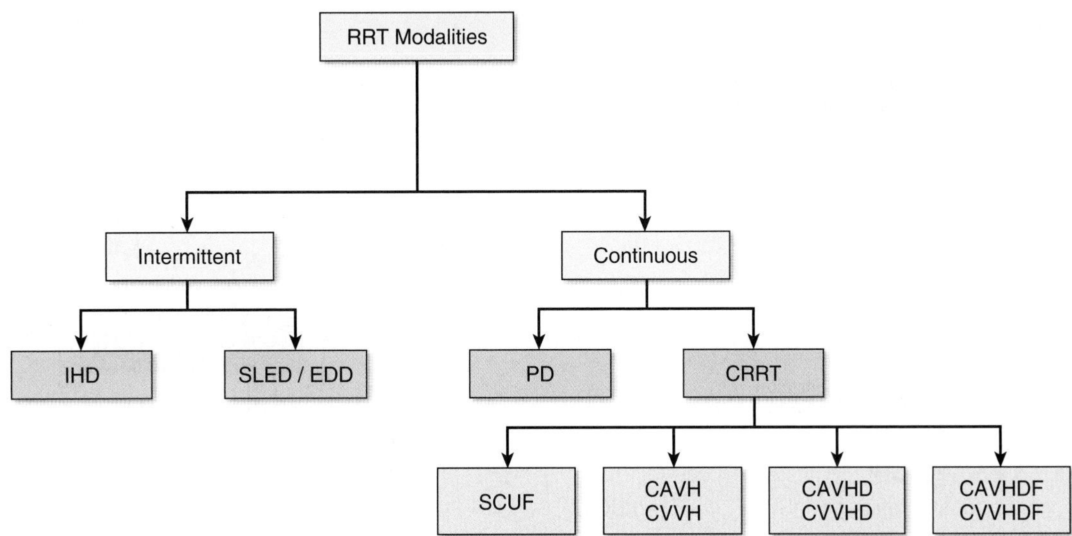

FIG. 23.2 Modalities of renal replacement therapy (RRT). *CAVH,* Continuous arteriovenous hemofiltration; *CAVHD,* continuous arteriovenous hemodialysis; *CAVHDF,* continuous arteriovenous hemodiafiltration; *CRRT,* continuous renal replacement therapy; *CVVH,* continuous venovenous hemofiltration; *CVVHD,* continuous venovenous hemodialysis; *CVVHDF,* continuous venovenous hemodiafiltration; *EDD,* extended daily dialysis; *IHD,* intermittent hemodialysis; *PD,* peritoneal dialysis; *SCUF,* slow continuous ultrafiltration; *SLED,* sustained low-efficiency dialysis.

so those at risk for bleeding may be candidates. It may also be used in selected healthcare facilities, such as those without access to advanced technology, and in certain patient populations, such as pediatric patients. Patients with CRF who have been on PD at home may be maintained on PD while in the critical care area.

Hemodialysis

HD is an extremely effective method of removing fluid and waste products. It involves the movement of the patient's blood through a hemofilter with a semipermeable membrane that separates the blood compartment from the effluent compartment. HD requires a dual lumen hemodialysis central venous access catheter to be in place. Once the dialysis circuit is primed with the patient's blood, the dialysate fluid is infused into the effluent compartment of the hemofilter in the opposite direction of the blood flow. This countercurrent flow produces an increased concentration gradient, making the filter more efficient in solute removal. The positive hydrostatic pressure in the blood compartment and the negative hydrostatic pressure in the effluent compartment create a transmembrane pressure gradient that determines the amount of fluid removal (ultrafiltration).

Possibly the greatest advantage of HD is its efficiency. Fluids, wastes, and electrolytes can be effectively removed within a 3- to 4-hour window of time on a daily or every other day schedule. This may be especially important in patients with toxic potassium levels or fluid overload progressing to pulmonary edema. However, large fluid shifts can make HD unsuitable for some critically ill patients.

Because HD can cause rapid fluid shifts, hypotension, and dysrhythmias, the patient must be monitored carefully, especially during the initiation of treatment. This is crucial in the critically ill adult with comorbidities complicating their ATN, such as recent myocardial infarction, septic shock, or adult respiratory distress syndrome. If the HD filter is anticoagulated, this may increase the potential for bleeding in these patients.

HD is a technical and complex procedure that is generally performed by specially trained HD nurses, and generally not the critical care nurse. The *AACN Procedure Manual for Critical Care* is an excellent reference for those seeking more information about the details of the dialysis procedure itself.[2] Even so, the critical care nurse does remain responsible for ongoing nursing care. During HD, the nurse must be prepared to quickly intervene with ordered fluid and/or medication administration if the patient becomes hemodynamically unstable. The patient may begin bleeding from surgical sites, sites of skin breakdown, the oral cavity, or airways. If anticoagulants are used, frequent coagulation studies are monitored to identify inadvertent systemic anticoagulation.

A hybrid of traditional HD is currently being employed by some institutions. SLED and EDD are both slower dialysis therapies provided over 6 to 12 hours. The patient is dialyzed using a conventional dialysis machine utilizing modified blood and dialysate flow speeds.[7] These methods combine the advantages of both HD and CRRT, providing for hemodynamic stability but achieving enhanced water and solute removal.

Continuous Renal Replacement Therapies

CRRT is an additional means by which fluids, wastes, and electrolytes, as well as other small to medium size solutes, can be removed from the body via ultrafiltration and dialysis. There are a number of different procedures available, including the following options: slow, continuous ultrafiltration (SCUF) (Fig. 23.3); continuous arteriovenous hemofiltration (CAVH)—fluid removal and convective solute removal using replacement fluid (Fig. 23.4); continuous arteriovenous hemodialysis (CAVHD)—fluid removal and diffusive solute removal with dialysate (Fig. 23.5); continuous arteriovenous hemodiafiltration (CAVHDF)—fluid removal and convective and diffusive solute removal using dialysate and replacement fluid (Fig. 23.6); continuous venovenous hemofiltration (CVVH)—fluid removal and convective solute removal using replacement fluid (Fig. 23.7); continuous

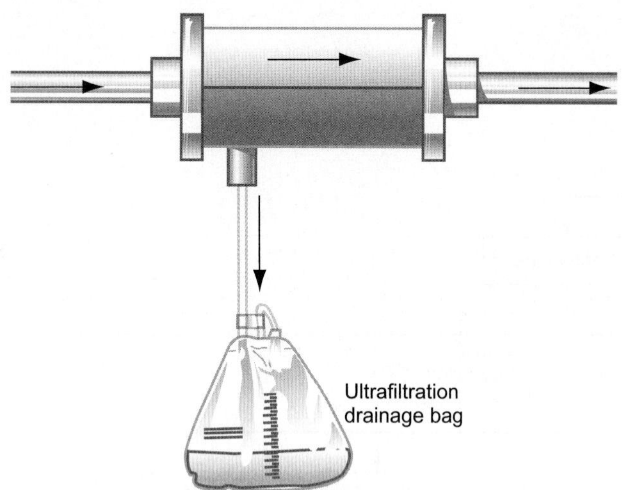

FIG. 23.3 Slow, continuous ultrafiltration (SCUF): fluid removal, no fluid replacement.

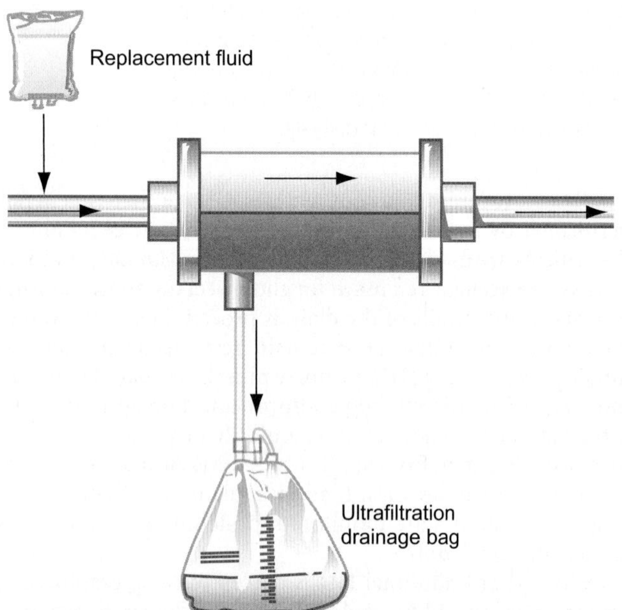

FIG. 23.4 Continuous arteriovenous hemofiltration (CAVH): fluid removal and fluid replacement.

venovenous hemodialysis (CVVHD)—fluid removal and diffusive solute removal with dialysate (Fig. 23.8); and continuous venovenous hemodiafiltration (CVVHDF)—fluid removal and convective and diffusive solute removal using dialysate and replacement fluid (Fig. 23.9). Table 23.3 provides information about the CRRT modalities, including the principles of solute removal, vascular access needed, indications for use, advantages and disadvantages, and complications.

CRRT offers many of the same benefits of hemofiltration as HD, including the ability to control acid-base status and manage electrolyte imbalances, uremic control, and biocompatibility. In addition, CRRT provides hemodynamic stability through the slow continuous fluid removal rate. Fluid removal is continuous and slow as compared to the 1- to 4-L removal during a 3- to 4-hour HD treatment. Because fluid removal is slower, the change in serum osmolality seen with HD that creates a fluid shift into the extracellular space does not occur. A recent survey reported that 52% of nephrologists used CRRT for non-AKI

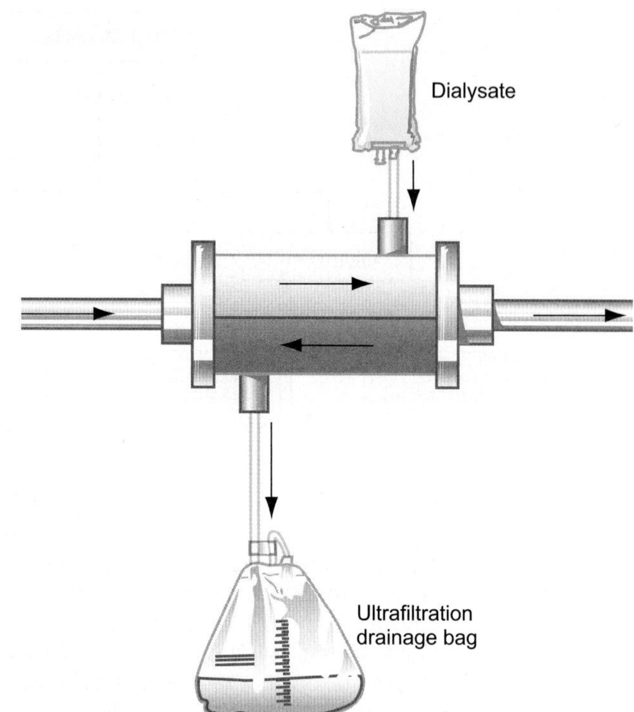

FIG. 23.5 Continuous arteriovenous hemodialysis (CAVHD): fluid and solute removal with dialysate.

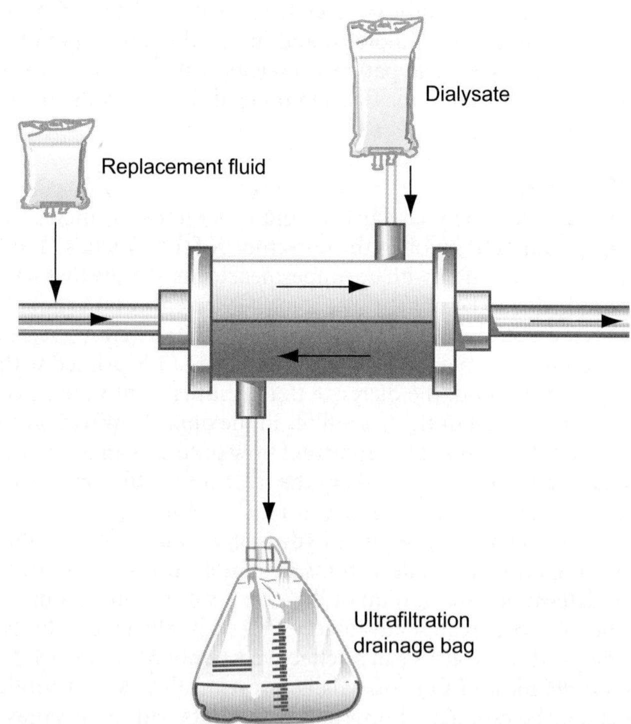

FIG. 23.6 Continuous arteriovenous hemodiafiltration (CAVHDF): fluid replacement with dialysate.

reasons, such as fluid control, heart failure, acute respiratory distress syndrome, and sepsis.[42]

All CRRT machines use a highly permeable biocompatible hemofilter similar to those used in HD. These consist of hollow fibers or sheets of biofilter in a plastic case. The filter material, pore size, and affinity to water/solute removal determine the efficiency of the filter and the amount/rate of solute removal/clearance.

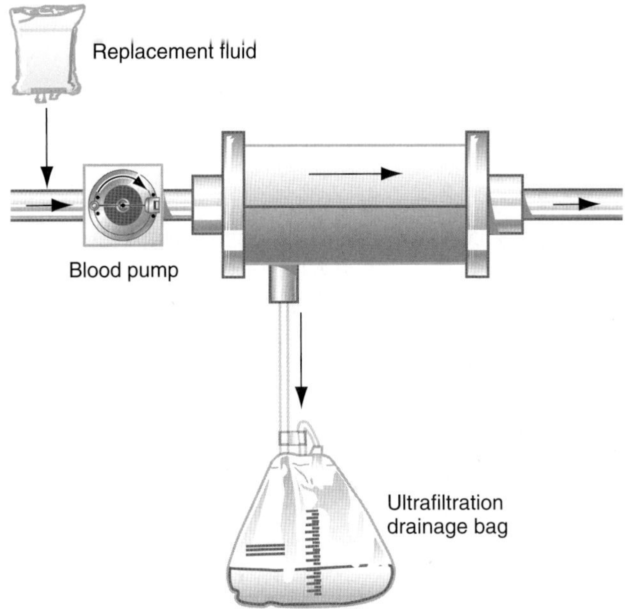

FIG. 23.7 Continuous venovenous hemofiltration (CVVH): fluid removal with fluid replacement.

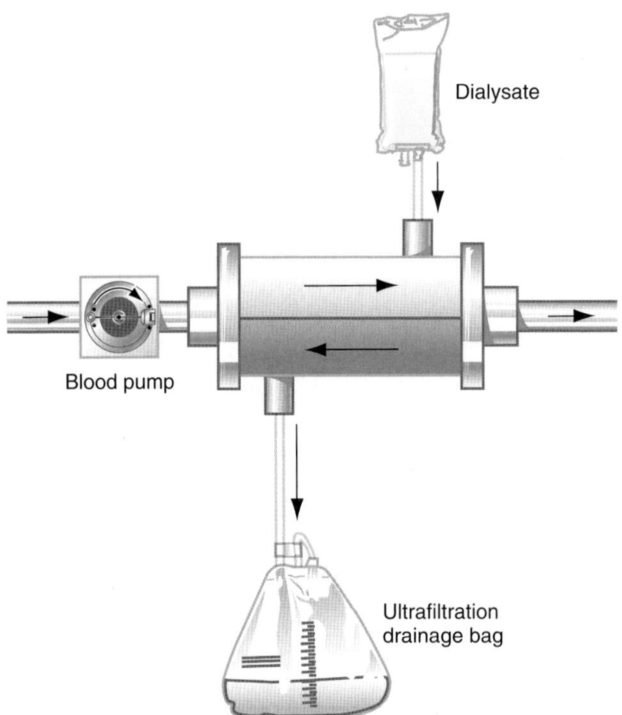

FIG. 23.8 Continuous venovenous hemodialysis (CVVHD): fluid and solute removal with dialysate.

Whereas the various CRRT methods are described as simplistic, automatic, or integrated, CRRT machines contain all the necessary pumps and scales or flow monitors to measure effluent amounts, with a computerized control module to monitor and coordinate operations. With venovenous therapies, the blood is pumped from the venous vascular access through the hemofilter circuit. The vascular access required for renal replacement is a dual-lumen vascular access catheter designed for RRT that is inserted in the central vein. A functioning vascular access catheter is critical to the success of any mode of CRRT. The catheter lumen size, catheter patency, and catheter positioning must be adequate to ensure that adequate blood flow rates can be achieved. Placement should be checked to ensure that there is no overlap with any other vascular access catheter. Infection prevention standards should be maintained to prevent catheter-associated infection.

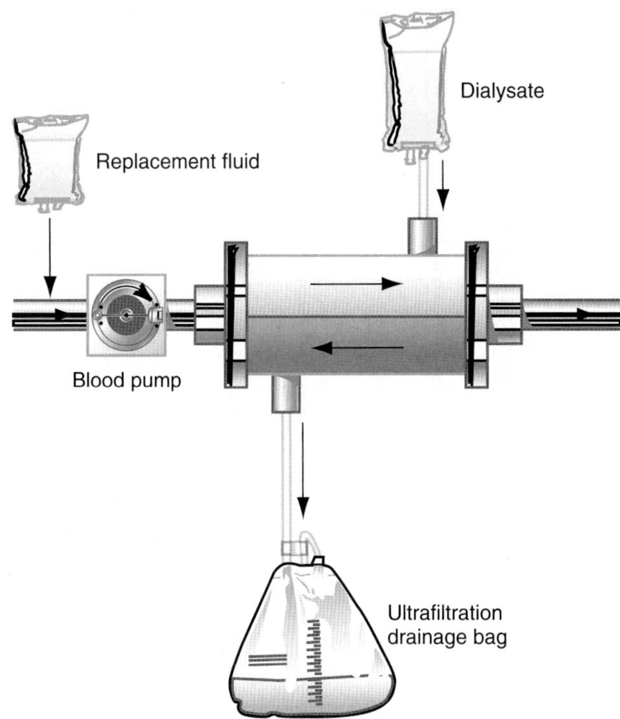

FIG. 23.9 Continuous venovenous hemodiafiltration (CVVHDF): fluid replacement with dialysate.

As the blood flows through the hemofilter (at a typical rate of 150–250 mL/min in adult patients), anticoagulation or dilution may be required to minimize premature clotting of the circuit. There are additional pumps that provide heparin, citrate, or other anticoagulants to prevent clotting of the hemofilter circuit. The hemofilters are highly permeable to water and electrolytes and other small solutes such as bicarbonate, creatinine, and urea nitrogen, but are relatively impermeable to plasma proteins and blood cellular components. The potential for loss of large amounts of fluid exists, and serum osmolality can greatly increase, placing the patient at risk for dehydration. Therefore, replacement IV solutions are used in varying amounts, depending upon the patient's net hourly fluid loss. The effluent also contains large amounts of bicarbonate. Losing large amounts of bicarbonate can worsen the patient's metabolic acidosis. Consequently, the replacement fluid often has a high bicarbonate content, and is not merely a maintenance fluid such as NS or LR, which contain only the precursor to bicarbonate.

Many critical care patients in the United States receive the CVVHD mode of CRRT.[42] This involves infusing a dialysate solution into the effluent compartment of the hemofilter, countercurrent to the flow of blood. As in HD, concentration gradients are established to enhance or prevent removal of solutes, while helping avoid acid-base and electrolyte imbalance. The concentration gradient allows more efficient

TABLE 23.3 Continuous Renal Replacement Therapies

Mode	Principles Involved	Vascular Access	Pump Assisted	Indications	Advantages	Complications and Disadvantages*
Ultrafiltration therapies						
SCUF (slow, continuous ultrafiltration)	Convection	Arteriovenous Venovenous	No Yes	Diuretic-resistant, volume-overloaded, hemodynamically unstable patient or patient with elevated ICP who cannot tolerate rapid fluid shifts	Continuous, gradual treatment	**Anticoagulation, bleeding** **Hypotension** **Hypothermia** **Access catheter complications (bleeding, clotting, infection)** **Requires strict monitoring of fluid and electrolyte replacement to avoid deficits or overload** **Air embolism** **ICU setting only** **Requires 1:1 nurse-to-patient ratio** Large-bore arterial cannulation required Ideally need MAP of 60 mm Hg to drive extracorporeal circuit Poor control of azotemia, may need dialysis Minimal solute clearance Poor emergent treatment of hyperkalemia/acidosis Loss of limb (distal arterial ischemia)
CAVH (continuous arteriovenous hemofiltration)	Convection	Arteriovenous	No	Diuretic-resistant, volume-overloaded, hemodynamically unstable patient who cannot tolerate rapid fluid shifts Parenteral or enteral alimentation in volume-overloaded patient	Continuous, gradual treatment (fewer high and low extremes) High rate of fluid removal/replacement allows flexibility in fluid balance	**Anticoagulation, bleeding** **Hypotension** **Hypothermia** **Access complications (bleeding, clotting, infection)** **Requires strict monitoring of fluid and electrolyte replacement to avoid deficits or overload** **Air embolism** **ICU setting only** **Requires 1:1 nurse-to-patient ratio** Prolonged, large-bore arterial cannulation required Ideally need MAP of 60 mm Hg to drive extracorporeal circuit Poor control of azotemia, may need dialysis Poor emergent treatment of hyperkalemia/acidosis Loss of limb (distal arterial ischemia)
CVVH (continuous venovenous hemofiltration)	Convection	Venovenous	Yes	Diuretic-resistant, hemodynamically unstable, volume-overloaded patient who cannot tolerate rapid fluid shifts Parenteral or enteral alimentation in volume-overloaded patient	Precise fluid control Can be used in patients with low MAP Ease of initiation Large volume of fluid, including parenteral nutrition, may be administered No arterial cannulation Better solute clearance than CAVH	**Anticoagulation, bleeding** **Hypotension** **Hypothermia** **Access complications (bleeding, clotting, infection)** **Requires strict monitoring of fluid and electrolyte replacement to avoid deficits or overload** **Air embolism** **ICU setting only** **Requires 1:1 nurse-to-patient ratio** Requires special pump to augment blood flow through extracorporeal circuit Requires training of ICU nurses in management of patients receiving CRRT

Dialysis therapies						
CAVHD (continuous arteriovenous hemodialysis) CAVHDF (continuous arteriovenous hemodiafiltration)	Diffusion Diffusion and convection	Arteriovenous	No	Volume-overloaded, hemodynamically unstable patient with azotemia or uremia Catabolic acute kidney injury Electrolyte imbalances and acidosis Parenteral and enteral alimentation in volume-overloaded, catabolic patient	Continuous fluid balance control Large fluid volumes, including parenteral nutrition, may be administered	**Same as CAVH** Hypernatremia Hypophosphatemia
CVVHD (continuous venovenous hemodialysis) CVVHDF (continuous venovenous hemodiafiltration)	Diffusion Diffusion and convection	Venovenous	Yes	Volume-overloaded, hemodynamically unstable patient with azotemia or uremia Catabolic acute kidney injury Electrolyte imbalances and acidosis Parenteral and enteral alimentation in volume-overloaded, catabolic patient	No arterial cannulation Continuous fluid balance control Large volume of parenteral nutrition may be administered Better solute clearance than CAVHDF Tolerated by patients with low MAP	**Same as CVVH** Hypophosphatemia

*Complications and disadvantages appearing in boldface are common to CAVH, CAVHD, CVVH, and CVVHDF.

ICU, Intensive care unit; *ICP,* intracranial pressure; *MAP,* mean arterial pressure.

Modified from Giuliano, K., & Pysznik, E. (1998). Renal replacement therapy in critical care: implementation of a unit-based CVVH program. *Crit Care Nurs,* 18, 40–45.

removal of solutes, without high volume ultrafiltration volumes. In addition, some institutions are using hybrid RRT in place of CRRT setups. These include SLED and EDD and use standard HD machines. The nursing model of care is usually shared and collaborative between nephrology and critical care nurses.

The KDIGO clinical practice guidelines for AKI released in 2012 showed no benefits of CRRT over intermittent hemodialysis (IHD) in clinical outcomes. Yet CRRT remains a frequently used RRT modality in the critically ill. A recent study followed admissions to critical care units and assessed the RRT modality used in patients who developed AKI over a 7-year period.[47] CRRT was utilized 52% of the time, and IHD 47% of the time.[47] The modality utilized leaned towards CRRT when the patient required vasopressors, possibly highlighting the physiologic benefits of CRRT.

CRRT requires the involvement of trained nursing and medical staff 24 hours a day. Maintaining competency can be a challenge if the modality is underutilized and requires review to ensure safe CRRT care.[3] In order for a CRRT team to be successful, care must be collaborative between the critical care nurses, nephrology nurses, nephrologists, critical care providers, pharmacists, nutritionists, and material services/clinical engineering staff.

Drug Therapy During Renal Replacement

Consultation with the team pharmacist is necessary throughout the care of the AKI patient. Before RRT, medication dosing must be tailored to the patient's renal function. During RRT, the pharmacist is key to making necessary adjustments in drug therapy. Many drugs that clear through the kidneys are even more greatly affected by renal replacement. There are few studies of the actual percentages of drug removal during CRRT, so the nurse will have to estimate, with the pharmacist's help, which drugs are more greatly affected and thus need to have either a substitute drug administered or an increase in dosage provided. For example, if midazolam (Versed) is being used for sedation and the patient wakens or becomes agitated during filtration, propofol (Diprivan) could be substituted. The GFR is more important than the absolute serum creatinine level in adjusting dosages. These data should be monitored by the nurse so that the team can track drug dosing and effects between and during RRT. The intrinsic renal function, including the phase of the function, must be considered when making medication decisions regarding patient care.

During CRRT, the clearance rate of medications may be altered due to the continual filtration process. The use of vasoactive medications, sedation, analgesics, and neuromuscular blockade agents must be closely monitored by nursing staff to ensure adequate dosing and positive patient outcomes. Many times, the clearance rate of medications is increased during CRRT, and higher dosages are required to achieve the same effect.

NUTRITION IN ACUTE KIDNEY INJURY WITH RENAL REPLACEMENT THERAPY

In the AKI patient, the goal of nutrition is to prevent protein energy wasting (PEW), reduce the inflammatory response and oxidative stress, support immune function, and reestablish electrolyte balances.[36] In the critical care unit, approximately 40% of patients with AKI will experience PEW.[10] Patients with AKI are at risk for undernutrition and increased protein loss due to the physiologic demands of critical illness, such as metabolic acidosis, inflammation, and other effects of catabolism.[36] These dietary needs are increased in the patient on RRT due to protein loss from ultrafiltration.[36] Meeting the nutritional needs of the patient with hypermetabolic demands is an urgent process.

Studies show that patients with AKI and a poor nutritional status are at risk for increased morbidity and mortality.[10,36] The current standard is to start nutrition as early as possible. If the patient is unable to eat, the nurse should recommend feeding tube placement, unless contraindicated. If the patient cannot be fed by enteral means, then parenteral feeding should be started as soon as possible, again to maintain the patient in an anabolic state, maximize tissue healing, and stop tissue breakdown.

Once on RRT, the patient has more specific nutritional needs resulting from the increased loss of proteins, decreased serum phosphorous, and hidden calorie sources during the filtration process.[10] The critical care nurse should be aware of these unique nutritional requirements and ensure that the patient's nutritional needs during RRT are met. The AKI patient is acutely hypermetabolic and catabolic, with worsening azotemia from tissue breakdown. The team dietitian will recommend either enteral or parenteral nutrition that contains adequate protein, carbohydrates, and fats to provide an energy source that will spare tissue breakdown. Enteral nutrition is preferable. However, if using the gut is contraindicated by GI dysfunction or hemodynamic instability, then parenteral nutrition is indicated.[10]

It is essential to provide adequate protein with all the essential amino acids in order to preserve the body's visceral protein stores. CRF patients require special protein-limited diets to decrease the rate of accumulation of waste products that must be cleared by dialysis. Typically, patients can receive hemodialysis no more than two to three times weekly, whereas in critical care, the patient may be maintained on CRRT or have daily HD. Thus there is no need to limit protein intake in these patients because the patient can be dialyzed or hemofiltered easily in critical care. AKI patients become rapidly and deeply catabolic if undernourished. Indirect calorimetry is recommended to identify caloric needs.[36] Caloric delivery should provide 100% to 130% of resting energy expenditure. Vitamin and electrolyte supplements should be provided as needed.

Critically ill patients with AKI are at an increased risk for hypo- and hyperglycemia. The metabolic disruptions that occur as a result of the "kidney-centered" systemic inflammatory syndrome experienced by AKI patients cause endocrine dysfunction that results in insulin resistance.[10,36] Insulin resistance is related to an increased risk of mortality.[11] Insulin resistance results from uremia and metabolic dysfunction created by renal dysfunction. Other notable causes for hyperglycemia include stress hyperglycemia in the critically ill patient and critical-illness associated hyperglycemia (CIAH). The insulin resistance leads to a state of hyperinsulinemia, thus the risk for hypoglycemia from the impending need for RRT.[11] In addition, the kidney is responsible for 50% of insulin clearance. The decreased rate of GFR in AKI reduces the clearance of insulin, resulting in hyperglycemia and increasing the potential for hypoglycemia. The original call by the Surviving Sepsis Campaign was for tight glycemic control of blood sugars near 110 mg/dL;[48] however, new studies call for less stringent control, with blood sugar levels of less than 180 mg/dL.[11] The critical care nurse must be mindful of the metabolic changes that occur with AKI and monitor and control blood sugars carefully to avoid the adverse complications of hyper- and hypoglycemia. Frequent measurement of blood glucose levels and treatment with insulin are necessary. The recommendation is for continuous serum blood glucose monitoring and insulin infusion to manage glycemic variability.[11]

INTERPROFESSIONAL PLAN OF CARE

Once a patient develops any type of AKI, the primary goal is to reestablish homeostasis as quickly as possible. The underlying cause should be identified and eliminated if possible. In addition to the provider, advanced practice nurse, and critical care staff nurse team, the pharmacist and dietitian are crucial to the development and implementation of a plan of care.

Prevention of AKI must be a priority and begins with early identification of those patients at risk. When patients are identified as at risk for AKI, the critical care nurse should institute interventions as needed to ameliorate the risk of AKI. In prerenal situations, every effort should be made to promptly restore adequate perfusion so that the renal function does not become further impaired. If the insult is intrarenal, interventions should be instituted to address the patient's fluid overload and electrolyte imbalances, including the following: ensuring adequate oxygenation; preventing or treating infection; providing adequate, early nutrition; preventing further nephrotoxicity by monitoring and modifying medication administration; and treating the patient's acid-base abnormalities. When appropriate, RRT should be instituted. Although the critical care nurse is usually not directly responsible for RRT, the nurse will maintain responsibility for the overall care of these patients, including any complications that arise during therapy.

ON THE HORIZON

The hallmark in AKI prevention is early recognition and prevention. Researchers have been working to identify more sensitive and specific biomarkers to identify AKI. As of 2015, we have GFR, serum creatinine, and UOP, but the changes seen using these criteria occur hours after the injury occurs.[43,49,51] Both serum and urine biomarkers are being studied for their potential to provide an early identification tool to determine when a patient is at risk for AKI.[43,49,51]

The literature suggests that biomarkers are currently used clinically to identify patients who are at risk for developing AKI, but cannot determine when to begin RRT.[43,49,51]

CONCLUSION

Caring for patients with AKI is challenging for the critical care team and must begin with a focus on prevention. Because of their position at the bedside, the role of the critical care nurses to identify patients at risk, as well as recognize and treat the common causes of AKI, cannot be overstated. There is much controversy over best practice in the care of these patients and the long-term effects of AKI are unclear. As with other organs, progressive renal disease after severe AKI is common.

CASE STUDY 23.1

Risk Factors for Developing Acute Kidney Injury

While working in his garden, 75-year-old R.F. complained to his wife about increasing back pain. He was encouraged by his wife to rest. Several hours later when she tried to wake him, he was unarousable. She called 911 and he was taken to the emergency department. His vital signs on admission were blood pressure (BP) 70/52 mm Hg, mean arterial pressure (MAP) (56), and heart rate (HR): 136 beats per minute with frequent premature ventricular contractions. His skin was pale, cool, and clammy, and neck veins were flat. His medical history was unremarkable. A central line was placed and normal saline (NS) run wide open. He was sent for an urgent CT scan, where it was revealed that he had a leaking abdominal aneurysm. He was taken to the operating room, where he had a successful resection of his aneurysm. After surgery, R.F. was admitted to critical care with an arterial pressure of 94/42 mm Hg, MAP (59), central venous pressure (CVP) 3 mm Hg, and he remains responsive to fluid boluses. Urine output is 5 mL/h with blood urea nitrogen (BUN) 45 mg/dL and creatinine 1.7 mg/dL, despite running fluids. The anesthetist reports that the aortic cross-clamp time was prolonged. Despite fluid resuscitation, his renal function continues to deteriorate. Eight hours later, his creatinine was 2.5 mg/dL, BUN 65 mg/dL, and he was anuric. Furosemide (Lasix) 40 mg IV was given, but there was no response to the diuretics.

Despite all efforts, R.F. was diagnosed with acute tubular necrosis (ATN). He has been fluid resuscitated to CVP 14 mm Hg and he was no longer fluid responsive. His BP remains low 100s/60s with vasoactive medication support. He remains anuric. Creatinine continues to increase. Electrolyte levels require intervention.

Decision Point:

What was the original insult that most likely led to R.F.'s developing acute kidney injury?

Decision Point:

What measure would you expect to carry out in the immediate postoperative period to help minimize risk of developing acute kidney injury?

Decision Point:

What are your treatment options for dialyzing this patient?

REFERENCES

1. Ahmed, U., Iqbal, H., & Akbar, S. (2014). Furosemide in acute kidney injury-A vexed issue. *Austin J Nephrol Hypertens*, *1*(5), 1025.
2. Astle, S. (2013). Continuous renal replacement therapies. In D. L. M. Wiegand (Ed.), *AACN procedure manual for critical care* (6th ed.). Philadelphia: Saunders.
3. Bellomo, R., D'Intini, V., & Ronco, C. (2005). Renal replacement therapy in the ICU. In M. P. Fink, et al. (Ed.), *Textbook of critical care* (5th ed.) (pp. 1151–1158). Philadelphia: Saunders.
4. Bellomo, R., Kellum, J., & Ronco, C. (2012). Acute kidney injury. *Lancet*, *380*, 756–766.
5. Carlstrom, M., Wilcox, C., & Arendshorst, W. (2015). Renal autoregulation in health and disease. *Physiol Rev*, *95*(2), 405–511. http://dx.doi.org/10.1152/physrev.00042.2012.
6. Case, J., Khan, S., Khalid, R., & Khan, A. (2013). Epidemiology of acute kidney injury in the intensive care unit. *Crit Care Res Pract*, 2013. http://dx.doi.org/10.1155/2013/479730.
7. Depner, T., & Craig, M. (2012). Slow extended daily dialysis for critically ill patients. In T. Ing, M. Rahman, & C. Kjellstrand (Eds.), *Dialysis: history, development, and promise* (pp. 457–470). Hackensack, NJ: World Scientific Publishing CO.
8. Dirkes, S. (2011). Acute kidney injury: not just renal failure anymore? *Crit Care nurse*, *31*(1), 37–50.

9. Evans, R., Goddard, D., Eppel, G., & O'Connor, P. (2011). Factors that render the kidney susceptible to tissue hypoxia in hypoxemia. *Am J Physiol, 300*, 931–940.
10. Fiaccadori, E., Regolisti, G., & Maggiore, U. (2013). Specialized nutritional support interventions in critically ill patients on renal replacement therapy. *Curr Opin Clin Nutr Metab Care, 16*(2), 217–224.
11. Fiaccadori, E., Sabatino, A., Morabito, S., Bozzoli, L., Donadio, C., et al. (2016). Hyper/hypoglycemia and acute kidney injury in critically ill patients. *Clin Nutr, 35*(2), 317–321.
12. Hall, J., & Guyton, H. (2015). *Textbook of medical physiology* (13th ed.; pp. 305–323, 427–445). Philadelphia, PA: Elsevier.
13. Harris, D., McCrone, M., Koo, G., Weltz, A., Chiu, W., et al. (2015). Epidemiology and outcomes of acute kidney injury in critically ill surgical patients. *J Crit Care, 30*(1), 102–106.
14. Herget-Rosenthal, S., Glorieux, G., Jankowski, J., & Jankowski, V. (2009). Uremic toxicity in acute kidney injury. *Semin Dial, 22*(4), 445–448.
15. Heung, M., & Koyner, J. (2015). Entanglement of sepsis, chronic kidney disease, and other comorbidities in patients who develop acute kidney injury. *Semin Nephrol, 35*(1), 23–37. http://dx.doi.org/10.1016/j.semnephrol.2015.01.004.
16. Hobson, C., Singhania, G., & Bihorac, A. (2015). Acute kidney injury in the surgical patient. *Crit Care Clin, 31*(4), 705–723.
17. Hosoya, K., & Tachikawa, M. (2011). Roles of organic anion/cation transporters at the blood-brain and blood-cerebrospinal fluid barriers involving uremic toxins. *Clin Exp Nephrol, 15*(4), 478–485. http://dx.doi.org/10.1007/s10157-011-0460-y.
18. Jamale, T., Hase, N., Kulkarni, M., Pradeep, K., Keskar, V., et al. (2013). Earlier-start versus usual-start dialysis in patients with community-acquired acute kidney injury: a randomized controlled trial. *Am J Kidney Dis, 62*(6), 1116–1121.
19. Jorgensen, A. (2013). Contrast-induced nephropathy: pathophysiology and preventive strategies. *Crit Care Nurse, 33*(1), 37–46.
20. Juncos, L., & Juncos, L. (2012). Prerenal azotemia. In E. Lerma, & M. Rosner (Eds.), *Clinical decisions in nephrology, hypertension, and kidney transplantation* (pp. 175–182). New York, NY: Springer.
21. Kellum, J., & Lamiere, N. (2013). Diagnosis, evaluation, and management of acute kidney injury: a KDIGO summary (Part 1). *Crit Care, 17*(204), 1–15.
22. Kellum, J. A. (2015). Persistent acute kidney injury. *Crit Care Med, 43*(8), 1785–1786.
23. Khaledifar, A., Ebrahimi, A., Kheiri, S., & Mokhtari, A. (2015). Comparison of N-acetylcysteine, ascorbic acid, and normal saline effect in prevention of contrast-induced nephropathy. *ARYA Atheroscler, 11*(4), 1–5.
24. Khwaja, A. (2012). KDIGO clinical practice guidelines for acute kidney injury. *Nephron Clin Pract, 2012*(120), c179–c184.
25. KDIGO clinical practice guideline for acute kidney injury. (2012). Kidney Int Suppl 2, 1–138. http://www.kdigo.org/clinical_practice_guidelines/pdf/KDIGO%20AKI%20Guideline.pdf.
26. Kleinknecht, D., et al. (1972). Uremic and non-uremic complications in acute renal failure: evaluation of early and frequent dialysis on prognosis. *Kidney Int, 1*, 190–196.
27. Kumar, A., Bhawani, G., Kumari, N., Murthy, K., Lalwani, V., & Raju, C. (2014). Comparative study of renal protective effects of allopurinol and N-acetyl-cysteine on contrast induced nephropathy in patients undergoing cardiac catheterization. *J Clin Diagn Res, 8*(12), 3–7. http://dx.doi.org/10.7860/JCDR/2014/9638.5255.
28. Labib, M., Khalid, R., Khan, A., & Khan, S. (2013). Volume management in the critically ill patient with acute kidney injury. *Crit Care Res Pract.* http://dx.doi.org/10.1155/2013/792830 Epub 2013 Feb7.
29. Lamiere, N., Bagga, A., Cruz, D., De Maeseneer, J., Endre, Z., et al. (2013). Acute kidney injury: An increasing global concern. *Lancet, 382*(9887), 170–179.
30. Li, P., Burdmann, E., & Mehta, R. (2013). Acute kidney injury: global health alert. *Arab J Nephrol Transplant, 6*(2), 75–81.
31. Libetta, C., Sepe, V., Esposito, P., Galli, F., & Dal Canton, A. (2011). Oxidative stress and inflammation: implications in uremia and hemodialysis. *Clin Biochem, 44*(2011), 1189–1198. http://dx.doi.org/10.1016/j.clinbiochem.2011.06.988.
32. Lim, C., Tan, C., Kaushik, M., & Tan, H. (2015). Initiating acute dialysis at earlier Acute Kidney Injury Network stage in critically ill patients without traditional indications does not improve outcome: a prospective cohort study. *Nephrology (Carlton), 20*, 148–154.
33. Lisowska-Myjak, B. (2014). Uremic toxins and their effects on multiple organ systems. *Nephron Clin Pract, 128*(3-4), 303–311.
34. Lundberg, J., & Weitzbera, E. (2013). Biology of nitrogen oxides in the gastrointestinal tract. *Gut, 62*(4), 616–629.
35. Lutz, J., Menke, J., Sollinger, D., Schinzel, H., & Thurmel, K. (2014). Haemostasis in chronic kidney disease. *Nephrol Dial Transplant, 29*, 29–40. http://dx.doi.org/10.1093/ndt/gft209.
36. McCarthy, M., & Phipps, S. (2014). Special nutrition challenges: current approach to acute kidney injury. *Nutr Clin Pract, 29*(1), 56–62.
37. Obermuller, N., Geiger, H., Weipert, C., & Urbchat, A. (2014). Current developments in early diagnosis of acute kidney injury. *Int Urol Nephrol, 46*(1), 1–7.
38. Parsons, F. M., et al. (1961). Optimum time for dialysis in acute reversible renal failure: description and value of improved dialyzer with large surface area. *Lancet, 1*, 129–134.
39. Patschan, D., & Muller, G. (2015). Acute kidney injury. *J Inj Violence Res, 7*(1), 19–26. http://dx.doi.org/10.5249/jivr.v7i1.604.
40. Quigley, R. (2012). Developmental changes in renal function. *Curr Opin Pediatr, 24*(2), 184–190.
41. Rahman, M., Shad, F., & Smith, M. (2012). Acute kidney injury: a guide to diagnosis and management. *Am Fam Physician, 86*(7), 631–639.
42. Ronco, C., Ricci, Z., De Backer, D., Kellum, J., Taccone, F., et al. (2015). Renal replacement therapy in acute kidney injury: controversy and consensus. *Crit Care, 19*(146), 1–11.
43. Schiffl, H., & Lang, S. M. (2012). Update on biomarkers of acute kidney injury. Moving closer to clinical impact? *Mol Diagn Ther, 16*(40), 199–207.
44. Sileanu, F., Murungan, R., Lucko, N., Clermont, G., Kane-Gill, S., Handler, S., & Kellum, J. (2014). AKI in low-risk versus high-risk patients in intensive care. *Clin J Am Soc Nephrol, 10*(2), 187–196.
45. Singbartl, K., & Kellum, J. (2012). AKI in the ICU: Definition, epidemiology, risk stratification, and outcomes. *Kidney Int, 81*(9), 819–825.
46. Teschan, P. E., et al. (1960). Prophylactic hemodialysis in the treatment of acute renal failure. *Ann Intern Med, 53*, 992–1016.
47. Thongprayoon, C., Cheungpasitporn, W., & Ahmed, A. (2015). Trends in the use of renal replacement therapy modality in intensive care unit: a 7-year study. *Ren Fail, 37*(9), 1444–1447.
48. Van den Berghe, G., Wouters, P., Weekers, F., et al. (2001). Intensive insulin therapy in critically ill patients. *N Engl J Med, 345*, 1359–1367.
49. Vanmassenhove, J., et al. (2015). Urinary and serum biomarkers for the diagnosis of acute kidney injury: an in-depth review of the literature. *Nephrol Dial Transplant, 28*, 254–273.
50. Verbalis, J., Goldsmith, S., Greenburg, A., Korzelius, C., Schrier, R., et al. (2013). Diagnosis, evaluation, and treatment of hyponatremia: expert panel recommendations. *Am J Med, 126*(10), s1–s42.
51. Wasung, M. E., Chawla, L. S., & Madero, M. (2015). Biomarkers of renal function, which and when? *Clin Chim Acta, 438*, 350–357.
52. Zarjou, A., & Agarwal, A. (2011). Sepsis and acute kidney injury. *J Am Soc Nephrol, 22*(6), 999–1006. http://dx.doi.org/10.1681/ASN.2010050484.
53. Zeng, X., McMahon, G., Brunelli, S., Bates, D., & Waikar, S. (2014). Incidence, outcomes, and comparisons across definitions of AKI in hospitalized individuals. *Clin J Am Soc Nephrol, 9*, 12–20.
54. Zheng, C., Liu, W., Zheng, J., Liao, M., Ma, W., et al. (2014). Metabolic acidosis and strong anion gap in critically ill patients with acute kidney injury. *Biomed Res Int.* http://dx.doi.org/10.1155/2014/819528. Epub 2014 Aug 5.

24

Glycemic Control

Mary Fran Tracy

Diabetes mellitus (DM) is a chronic disorder of metabolism characterized by hyperglycemia. The disease state is associated with major abnormalities in the metabolism of carbohydrates, proteins, and fats. With increasing duration and severity of hyperglycemia, specific complications develop. These include microvascular, macrovascular, neurologic, and physiologic alterations, which ultimately affect many organ systems.

Recently, the US Centers for Disease Control and Prevention released new statistics describing diabetes in America, which estimate that 29.1 million Americans, or 9.3% of the US population, have this disease. Of those, 21 million people are diagnosed and 8.1 million people remain undiagnosed.[6,15] An estimated 86 million Americans have prediabetes, which is defined as having an impaired fasting glucose (IFG) level or impaired glucose tolerance (IGT). Diabetes is the seventh leading cause of death, with a mortality rate 1.7 times higher in adults with DM than adults without DM.[15,44] The incidence of cerebrovascular accidents (CVAs) is 1.5 times greater in persons with diabetes. Seventy-one percent of adults with diabetes have hypertension, and it is the leading cause of new cases of blindness, kidney failure, and nontraumatic lower extremity amputations. Approximately 60% to 70% of people with diabetes have mild to severe peripheral or autonomic neuropathies.[6] Dental disease, complications of pregnancy, and susceptibility to infection are all sequelae of hyperglycemia.[6,15] The total cost of diabetes care in the United States in 2012 was $245 billion. Of this, $176 billion was spent on direct medical costs and $69 billion was spent on indirect costs, such as disability, work loss, and premature mortality.[4,15]

For years, attention to diabetes management has centered on ambulatory care. The reports of the Diabetes Control and Complications Trial (DCCT)[24] and the United Kingdom Prospective Study Group (UKPDS)[66,67] demonstrated that glycemic control does, in fact, reduce the risks and complications of retinopathy, neuropathy, and nephropathy in this population. These results provided the impetus for enhanced glycemic control and diabetes self-management after their publication. However, evidence that glycemic control was of value in the acute care setting was essentially nonexistent until 1999.[19,33,34,65,70] In 2004, the American College of Endocrinology[2] released a position statement on inpatient diabetes and metabolic control stating, "As the result of recent clinical trials and focused research efforts, it is now apparent that new approaches and intensified efforts at metabolic regulation may improve short-, intermediate-, and long-term outcomes in patients with diabetes in the hospital for therapeutic procedures and for treatment of the complications of this illness." Whereas newer data have been generated that raise questions about the tightness of glycemic control that is appropriate for differing critical care populations, experts continue to believe that glycemic control itself is in the best interest of the critically ill.[5,13,29,40,46,53,68]

When the acute complications of diabetes, including diabetic ketoacidosis (DKA), hyperosmolar hyperglycemic state (HHS), and moderate to severe hypoglycemia, occur, they usually result in a hospital admission. It is estimated that individuals with hyperglycemia have a 50% increased risk of hospitalization within their lifetime and a 20% increased risk of postoperative complications, including myocardial infarctions (MI) and CVAs.[19,70] The incidence of hospitalization increases with age, duration of diabetes, and the presence of diabetes-related complications. The actual prevalence of diabetes in hospitalized patients is not known because diabetes is not typically the principal diagnosis.[16]

In acute and critical care, hyperglycemia has become a key variable in the quest to understand and enhance quality care and clinical outcomes. An elevation in blood glucose level, altered peripheral uptake, and utilization of insulin are well documented in critically ill patients.[69] Several sentinel research studies have been key to initiating the dialogue regarding glycemic control in the critically ill. Van den Berghe[69,70] reported that intensive insulin therapy via intravenous (IV) insulin infusion to maintain a blood glucose level at less than or equal to 110 mg/dL substantially reduced in-hospital mortality and morbidity among critically ill patients in surgical critical care.[69] Malmberg et al. reported that intensive insulin treatment reduced long-term mortality in diabetic patients with an acute MI, despite significantly high admission levels of blood glucose and hemoglobin A_{1c} (HbA_{1c}).[50] Subsequent studies have shown that there may be issues with aggressive glucose control. In particular, investigators of the Normoglycemia in Intensive Care Evaluation-Survival Using Glucose Algorithm Regulation (NICE-SUGAR) study reported an increase in patient mortality when glycemic control targets were less than 140 mg/dL.[31] Setting a glycemic target slightly higher, at less than 180 mg/dL, showed a lower mortality rate than when targeting glucose values of 81–108 mg/dL.[30] Whereas this has resulted in some debate regarding exactly what glycemic value targets should be in different populations, these studies have also motivated clinicians in direct hospital care to shift the paradigm from focusing only on prevention of hypoglycemia (while treating the chief complaint and disorder) to providing actual glycemic management.

PATIENTS AT RISK

Individuals at risk in the acute care environment include patients diagnosed with DM; patients with stress-induced hyperglycemia, sepsis, multisystem failure, or obesity; and patients administered large doses of exogenous steroids or other pharmacologic agents that alter glucose metabolism. This accounts for a large percentage of critically ill patients. Risk of complications while hospitalized is determined by the diagnosis of DM before admission, the age at diagnosis and duration of the disease, the presence and severity of secondary complications of diabetes, and the degree of glycemic control achieved before admission as demonstrated by the HbA_{1c} value. Typically, individuals who have had DM for more than 10 years, who were diagnosed as a child, or who have an HbA_{1c} level greater than 7% are at increased risk. Additionally, all critically ill patients are at risk from lack of detection and management of hyperglycemia.

DEFINITION

DM is "a group of metabolic diseases characterized by hyperglycemia resulting from defects in insulin secretion, insulin action, or both."[8] Hyperglycemia can be related to DM or can exist independently of the presence of the disease. The following criteria are included in the diagnosis of DM: an HbA_{1c} greater than or equal to 6.5%; a fasting plasma glucose level greater than or equal to 126 mg/dL; symptoms of diabetes plus a random plasma glucose measurement greater than or equal to 200 mg/dL; or a 2-hour postload (75 g of anhydrous glucose dissolved in water) glucose level greater than or equal to 200 mg/dL during an oral glucose tolerance test.[8] Hyperglycemia in the absence of diabetes can be determined by any elevation of plasma glucose level above the normal range of 70 to 100 mg/dL. Prediabetes, a name that encompasses IGT and IFG, is now diagnosed as a fasting plasma glucose value of 100 to 125 mg/dL and an HbA_{1c} of 5.7% to 6.4%.[8]

CLASSIFICATION OF DIABETES MELLITUS

There are several types of DM and hyperglycemia. Type 1 diabetes is an autoimmune disease resulting in an absolute deficiency of insulin. The hormone insulin is produced by the beta cells located within the islets of Langerhans in the pancreas. These cells are destroyed over a variable period of time. Type 1 DM comprises 5% to 10% of those with the diagnosis of diabetes.[8] In type 1, it is possible for an individual to have additional autoimmune disorders, including Graves' disease, Hashimoto's thyroiditis, Addison's disease, celiac sprue, vitiligo, autoimmune hepatitis, myasthenia gravis, and pernicious anemia.[8,63] The autoimmune destruction of beta cells can be determined by the presence of specific antibodies such as insulin autoantibodies, islet cell antibodies, autoantibodies to islet tyrosine phosphatase markers, and glutamic acid decarboxylase autoantibodies.[8] Type 1 diabetes can present as DKA. It occurs primarily in children and youth, yet it can also occur in adulthood and is life-threatening if untreated. Latent autoimmune diabetes, or type 1½, is a category of diabetes currently being researched and explored.[17,36]

Type 2 DM accounts for 90% of all individuals with this disease.[8] Of the individuals with type 2, 80% have *diabesity*.[55] This is representative of the dual epidemic in the United States of type 2 diabetes and obesity. A state of insulin resistance, type 2 diabetes is hallmarked by a defect of the peripheral receptors and altered insulin secretory function.[8] Individuals with type 2 DM frequently have normal to elevated insulin levels initially, but over time will have diminished insulin secretion. Initially, fasting blood glucose levels may be within normal range, but postprandial levels are elevated. Metabolic acidosis is not commonly associated with this form of diabetes, although it can occur. Type 2 diabetes occurs more commonly in the adult, yet the incidence of the disease in children has been shown to have increased since 2002 with the rise of childhood obesity and sedentary lifestyles in today's youth.[22] The focus in type 2 diabetes today is prevention and delay of onset of the disease.[9]

Gestational diabetes mellitus (GDM) occurs during pregnancy. It is defined as "any degree of glucose intolerance with onset or first recognition during pregnancy."[8] The prevalence of GDM is estimated at up to 14% of all pregnancies in the United States. Of all pregnancies complicated by diabetes, 90% are attributed to GDM and only 10% are attributed to preexisting primary DM in the patient.

Prediabetes is a condition in which the fasting plasma glucose level is between 100 and 125 mg/dL.[8] Individuals falling into this category are at high risk for developing type 2 DM. Typically, individuals demonstrate characteristics of the metabolic syndrome such as central adiposity, hyperglycemia, hyperlipidemia, hypertension, and, in females, polycystic ovary syndrome. It is estimated that 50% of all individuals with prediabetes will develop type 2 diabetes in their lifetime.

The last classification of DM encompasses all other reasons and causes of hyperglycemia. Included in this category are those with genetic defects, diseases of the exocrine pancreas (e.g., pancreatitis, neoplasia, cystic fibrosis, hemochromatosis), endocrinopathies (e.g., acromegaly, Cushing's disease, somatostatinoma), chemically induced hyperglycemia (secondary to glucocorticoids, immunosuppressants, estrogens, loop diuretics), and stress-induced hyperglycemia (e.g., surgery, trauma, infection).[8] Hyperglycemia in acute care in the nondiabetic individual falls into this category.

PHYSIOLOGY OF GLUCOSE METABOLISM

Euglycemia is achieved through the actions of pancreatic islet cell hormones. Glucagon, the antagonist to insulin, is produced by the alpha cells within the islets of Langerhans. Insulin and amylin are produced by the beta cells, and somatostatin is produced by the delta cells. It is the careful balance of glucose entering and leaving the bloodstream related to the action of these hormones that maintains glucose homeostasis[12] (Fig. 24.1).

Regulation of insulin begins with the autonomic nervous system. Pancreatic islet cells are innervated with parasympathetic and sympathetic nerves. The parasympathetic nerves extend via the vagus nerve. It is thought that these nerves play a significant role in insulin secretion that occurs at the sight and smell of food. Sympathetic nerves are employed and stimulated at times of acute stress. Thus, stress-induced hyperglycemia is a phase of inhibited insulin secretion and stimulated glucagon secretion,

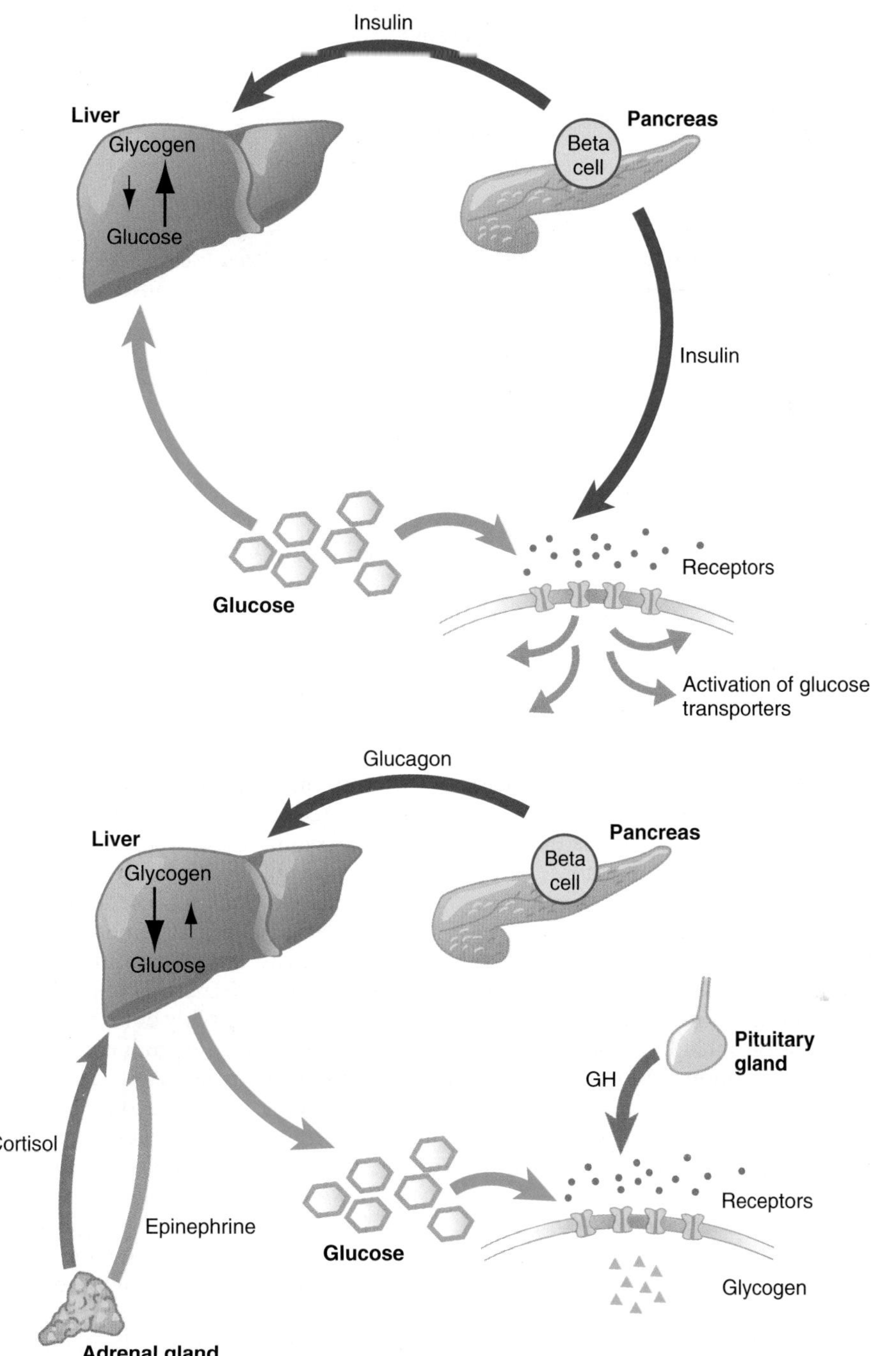

FIG. 24.1 Regulation of serum glucose concentration.

resulting in a state of insulin resistance and a rise in blood glucose level. There are also neuropeptides that are located within the islet nerve terminals. Vasoactive intestinal peptide, cholecystokinin, galanin, and neuropeptide Y have been identified as playing a role in the transfer of glucose from the intestines, kidneys, and liver to insulin-dependent tissues or insulin-independent tissues.

Functions of the Pancreatic Hormones

Insulin's chief role is to allow glucose to move from the blood into insulin-sensitive tissues (muscle and fat) to provide fuel and allow for the storage of energy. Insulin promotes glycogenesis while inhibiting lipolysis, ketogenesis, gluconeogenesis, glycogenolysis, and glycemia. Thus the storage of proteins and fats is also promoted because glucose is utilized for energy rather than proteins or fats. This is depicted in Fig. 24.2. Identified in 1987, amylin is a second beta cell hormone that assists in the regulation of blood glucose level.[12] Amylin is released along with insulin, but functions differently. The main role of amylin is to alter the flow of glucose into the bloodstream during the postprandial phase by delaying gastric emptying, decreasing glucagon secretion from the alpha cells, and minimizing the post meal glucose spike.[12] Glucagon increases blood glucose concentrations. This is accomplished by promoting gluconeogenesis, glycogenolysis in the liver and skeletal muscle, lipolysis, and

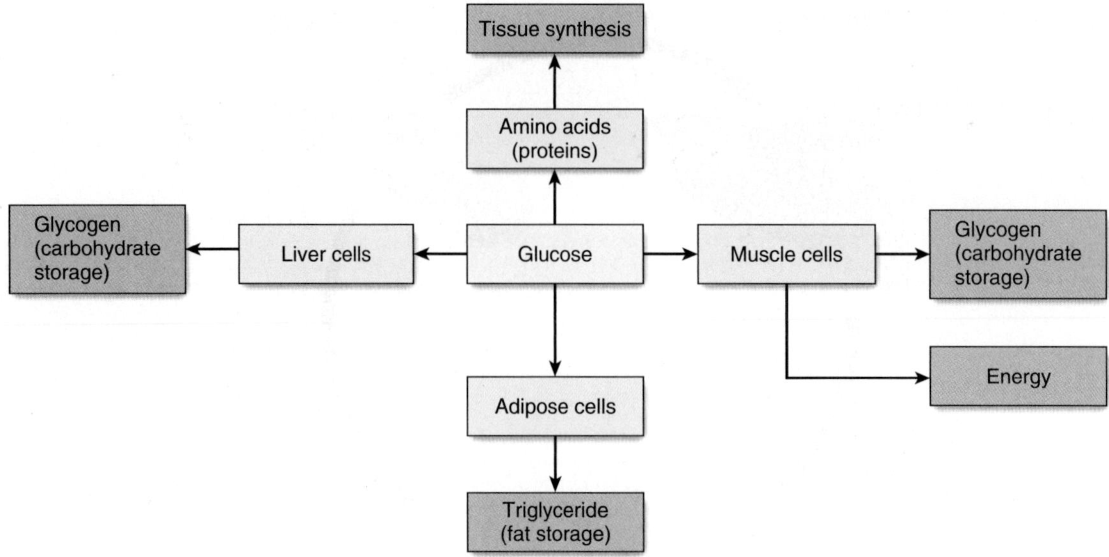

FIG. 24.2 Normal metabolism of glucose in the presence of sufficient insulin.

proteolysis. Somatostatin acts as an inhibitor to the secretion of both insulin and glucagon.

The hormones cannot function properly without cell receptors. Insulin and glucagon must be able to bind to the receptor in order for glucose to be transported. Specific glucose transporters have been identified and are named GLUT-1 through GLUT-5. GLUT-4 is specific to muscle and fat, and it is this transporter that allows for glucose transport after insulin has bound to the receptor.[71]

Under normal conditions, the pancreatic islets secrete insulin continuously to maintain euglycemia. This continuous insulin secretion regulates glucose levels through gluconeogenesis and glycogenolysis in the liver and kidney. It also regulates elevations in blood glucose concentration that are the result of counterregulatory hormone release, including glucagon, cortisol, catecholamines, and growth hormone. Additional boluses or bursts of insulin are secreted in response to meals in order to prevent postprandial glucose excursions. The amount of insulin secreted is regulated by arterial glucose concentrations, which are maintained between 70 and 100 mg/dL.

From a study conducted in 2011, incretin hormones, or glucagon-like peptide-1 (GLP-1), have been determined to be naturally occurring, insulin-releasing hormonal factors secreted by the intestine to facilitate metabolic homeostasis in response to food ingestion.[35,71] For further information, see Table 24.1. GLP-1 receptor (GLP-1R) agonists activate the beta cell GLP-1R, increasing the ability of the pancreas to release insulin in response to ingested glucose. GLP-1 inhibits excessive postprandial glucagon release, and it assists in regulating nutrient absorption. Gastric peristalsis is slowed, increasing digestion and facilitating nutrient absorption as the food moves from the stomach into the small intestine. This action helps reduce or avoid gastric dumping. All of this contributes to a decrease in postprandial glucose peaks.

PATHOPHYSIOLOGY OF DIABETES MELLITUS AND HYPERGLYCEMIA

Glucose homeostasis requires an individual to have normal insulin secretion and normal sensitivity to insulin. Regardless of the cause of hyperglycemia, altered insulin secretion or altered insulin sensitivity leading to insulin resistance results in pathogenesis.

Historically it was believed that at least 80% to 90% of the beta cells needed to be destroyed by an autoimmune process by the time metabolic decompensation occurred in type I diabetes. However, a meta-analysis suggests that the appearance of type 1 symptoms can vary significantly with age, so that as little as a 40% reduction in beta cells in a young adult can precipitate clinical symptoms of type 1 DM.[43] Regardless, at the time symptoms present, the insulin secretion is insufficient at this point to regulate hepatic glucose production. Initially, postprandial hyperglycemia occurs, demonstrating the inability of the body to suppress hepatic glucose production during meal absorption, as well as some decreased peripheral glucose uptake and utilization. As the availability of insulin further diminishes, increased basal hepatic glucose production and decreased glucose uptake by peripheral tissues cause fasting hyperglycemia. This can cause glucose toxicity, a state of hyperglycemia in which the glucose transporters available on both insulin-dependent (muscle, fat) and non–insulin-dependent tissues (brain, red blood cells, wounds) are severely reduced or inactivated (Fig. 24.3).

The renal threshold of glucose is approximately 180 mg/dL.[37] When blood glucose reaches this value, the kidney begins the process of osmotic diuresis, and glucosuria results. It is important to note that the normal aging process actually increases renal threshold and pregnancy decreases renal threshold. Thus an older adult may not display glucosuria until the blood glucose level reaches 300 mg/dL, and, in a pregnant woman, glucosuria may occur at 120 mg/dL.[37] Polyuria and polydipsia are the classic symptoms of hyperglycemia. Without available insulin, the cells are effectively starving and not being nourished. To compensate, lipolysis and proteolysis occur, resulting in weight loss, and polyphagia develops. DKA, which is life-threatening, begins when glucagon, growth hormone, epinephrine, and cortisol levels increase, contributing to hepatic glucose production, lipolysis, ketogenesis, and proteolysis. With osmotic diuresis, the skin becomes warm and dry, rubor can be detected on the cheeks, and changes occur in vision. This is secondary to the volume depletion of the vitreous humor and the accumulation of sorbitol behind the lens of the eye, causing the lens to temporarily change shape. If this state persists

TABLE 24.1 Injectable Incretin Hormones

Medication	Actions	Dosage	Special Considerations
Pramlintide (Symlin)	Adjunct therapy in type 1 and type 2 patients who have less than optimal postprandial glycemic control.	Type 1: initial dose 15 mcg; titrate by 15 mcg up to 30–60 mcg as needed. Type 2: initial dose 60 mcg; can use up to 120 mcg as needed Subcutaneous administration concurrent with mealtime insulin as a separate injection; 2 inches away from insulin injection.	Dose must be held if NPO or eating less than 30 g of CHO. Contraindicated in gastroparesis. Nausea is a common side effect. Do not titrate until nausea has been absent for 3 days. Decrease insulin (preprandial, short, or rapid-acting) by 50% during start of pramlintide. If $HbA_{1c} > 9\%$, pramlintide should not be used.
Exenatide (Byetta)	Adjunct therapy to improve glycemic control in type 2 patients on metformin, a sulfonylurea, or a combination of both. Contraindicated in type 1 DM, severe renal impairment, severe gastrointestinal disease.	Initiate at 5 mcg subcutaneously twice daily: after 1 month, can titrate to 10 mcg twice daily if needed. Administer with meals.	Contraceptives and antibiotics should be taken 1 h before injection. Dose must be held if NPO or eating less than 30 g of CHO.
Liraglutide (Victoza)	Adjunct therapy to diet and exercise in patients with type 2 DM Contraindicated in patients with personal or family history of medullary thyroid cancer or multiple endocrine neoplasia syndrome type 2.	Initiate at 0.6 mg daily; after 1 week may increase to 1.2 mg daily with a maximum dose of 1.8 mg daily. Subcutaneous administration once daily without regard to meals. Administer as separate injection from insulin. If > 3 days since last dose, reinitiate at 0.6 mg to decrease GI intolerance.	Not indicated for use in type 1 DM or in DKA. Use with caution when initiating or escalating dose in patients with renal failure. Delays gastric emptying so can experience GI intolerance.
Albiglutide (Tanzeum)	Adjunct therapy to diet and exercise in patients with type 2 DM. Contraindicated in patients with personal or family history of medullary thyroid cancer or multiple endocrine neoplasia syndrome type 2. Not recommended in patients at risk for acute pancreatitis or those with severe GI disease.	Initiate at 30 mg every week with maximum dose of 50 mg every week. Subcutaneous administration weekly, same day every week without regard to meals.	Not indicated for use in type 1 DM or in DKA. Use with caution when initiating or escalating dose in patients with renal failure.
Dulaglutide (Trulicity)	Adjunct therapy to diet and exercise in patients with type 2 DM. Contraindicated in patients with personal or family history of medullary thyroid cancer or multiple endocrine neoplasia syndrome type 2. Not recommended in patients at risk for acute pancreatitis or those with severe GI disease.	Initiate at 0.75 mg every week with a maximum dose of 1.5 mg every week. Subcutaneous administration weekly, same day every week without regard to meals.	Not indicated for use in type 1 DM or in DKA. Use with caution when initiating or escalating dose in patients with renal failure.

CHO, Carbohydrate; *DKA*, diabetic ketoacidosis; *DM*, diabetes mellitus; *GI*, gastrointestinal; *HbA_{1c}*, hemoglobin *A_{1c}*; *NPO*, nothing by mouth.
From Reference 11.

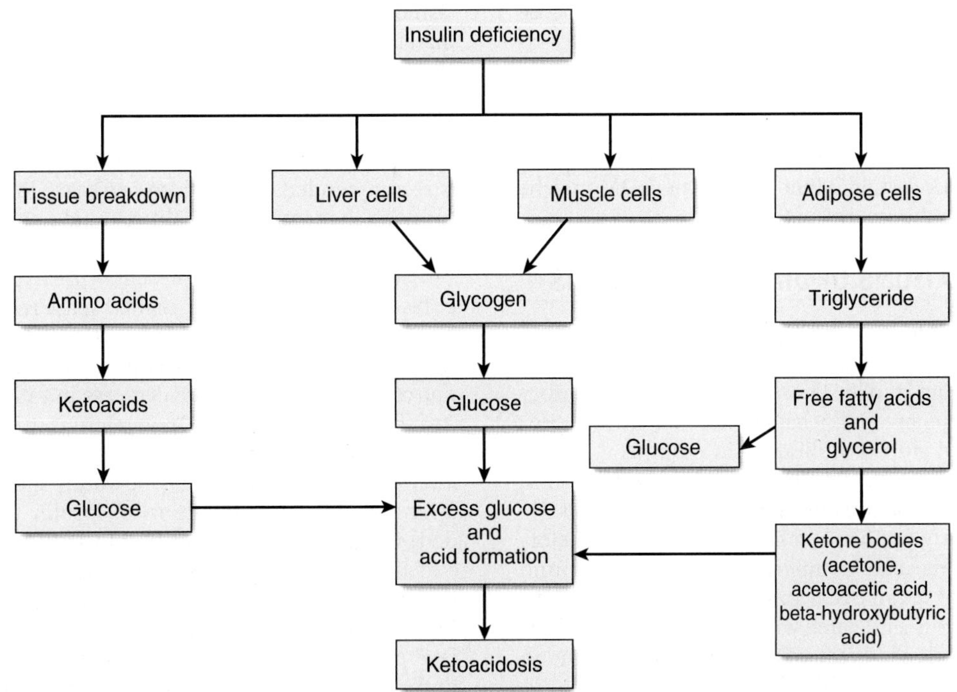

FIG. 24.3 Untreated diabetic ketoacidosis.

TABLE 24.2 Laboratory Values for DKA and HHS

Laboratory Values	Mild DKA	Moderate DKA	Severe DKA	HHS
Glucose	>250 mg/dL	>250 mg/dL	>250 mg/dL	>600 mg/dL
Sodium	Variable	Variable	Variable	Normal or high
Potassium	Variable	Variable	Variable	Variable
Venous pH	7.25–7.30	7–7.24	<7	>7.3
Bicarbonate	15–18 mEq/L	10 to <15 mEq/L	<10 mEq/L	>15 mEq/L
Serum beta-hydroxybutyric acid	Positive	Positive	Positive	Small
Serum osmolality	Variable	Variable	Variable	>320 mOsm/kg
Anion gap	>10	>12	>12	Variable
BUN/creatinine	Elevated	Elevated	Elevated	Elevated
Amylase	Increased	Increased	Increased	May increase
Hematocrit	Increased	Increased	Increased	Increased
Liver functions	May increase	May increase	May increase	May increase

BUN, Blood urea nitrogen; *DKA,* diabetic ketoacidosis; *HHS,* hyperosmolar hyperglycemic state.

without adequate intervention, nausea, vomiting, weakness, anorexia, and eventual abdominal pain and cramping develop secondary to the presence of ketone bodies, specifically, acetone, acetoacetic acid, and beta-hydroxybutyric acid. Kussmaul respirations develop when the metabolic acidosis is severe. In some individuals, a fruity odor to the breath can be detected.

In type 2 DM, dysfunction of insulin secretion and of the peripheral receptors occurs. Individuals secrete insulin at low, normal, or high rates, but the secretion of the hormone may be delayed or altered in response to a glucose load. This typically results in postprandial hyperglycemia. The receptors resist, allowing insulin to bind to the site, and do not allow glucose to enter the cell for utilization or storage. Glycogenolysis occurs, further raising the blood glucose concentrations, and peripheral uptake of glucose is diminished.

A less common form of type 2 DM in children is called *maturity-onset diabetes of the young.* This is actually an autosomal dominant form of DM in which a mutation of the hepatocyte nuclear factor (HNF) or glucokinase genes occurs, resulting in lowered insulin production by the pancreas (HNF) or abnormal glucose sensing by the beta cells and impaired insulin secretion (glucokinase).[25] Symptoms of this form of type 2 DM include fatigue, dry skin, and a wound that will not heal. Frequently, individuals with this disease remain undiagnosed until an event occurs, such as cellulitis, MI, or cholecystitis, causing the need for one to seek medical attention. However, all symptoms of type 1 DM may be present, depending on the severity of the disease.

ACUTE COMPLICATIONS OF DIABETES MELLITUS

Diabetic Ketoacidosis

DKA is a serious, life-threatening condition caused by a profound insulin deficiency and an elevation of counterregulatory hormones, leading to increased hepatic and renal glucose production and impaired glucose utilization in peripheral tissues. As a result, free fatty acids and ketone bodies are released into the bloodstream, causing ketonemia and metabolic acidosis[42,65] characterized by hyperglycemia, ketosis, dehydration, and electrolyte imbalance. This acute complication is primarily found in type 1 patients, but it can occur in patients with type 2 DM as well. DKA in adults is associated with a mortality rate of less than 1%, but can increase to greater than 5% in the aged and in those with concomitant critical illness.[42]

Causes or Precipitating Factors of Diabetic Ketoacidosis

The onset of type 1 DM can present as DKA simultaneously when an individual is discovering the presence of an illness. Infection is the most common trigger for DKA.[42] Other triggers include stress, CVA, MI, alcohol abuse, pancreatitis, trauma, drugs, anorexia or bulimia, the deliberate or inadvertent omission of insulin, mismanagement of glucose levels when ill, pregnancy, and ambulatory continuous subcutaneous insulin infusion pump malfunction.

The signs and symptoms of DKA occur within a short period of time, often within 24 hours. Excess caloric intake over the amount of insulin available (either omission of insulin, undertreatment, or an absolute lack of produced usable insulin) or excess production from counterregulatory sources can result in DKA. The signs and symptoms previously stated for hyperglycemia apply to DKA. If left untreated, altered mental status or sensorium and coma are signs of ensuing death. Table 24.2 identifies laboratory values seen in DKA.

The treatment of DKA is focused on fluid replacement, continuous IV insulin therapy, and electrolyte stabilization. Osmotic diuresis occurs when the glucose level remains greater than the renal threshold and the body compensates to clear glucose and ketones. This can result in profound fluid loss. For hypovolemic shock, administer normal saline (NS) and/or plasma expanders. For mild hypotension with a high or normal sodium level, the use of 0.45% NS at 15–20 mL/kg/hour is recommended.[42] If sodium levels are low, 0.9% NS is used. Induced changes in osmolality should not exceed 3 mOsm/kg/hour.

Patients in DKA can present with hyperkalemia due to a potassium shift to the extracellular space resulting from acidosis and insulin insufficiency. Alternatively, patients can also present with low or normal potassium levels due to the significant diuresis, signifying a severe decrease in total body potassium.[42] As insulin is administered, potassium is driven from the bloodstream into the cell. This results in a drop in serum potassium level. Therefore, the initial potassium should be greater than 3.3 mEq/L prior to initiation of insulin to prevent a further detrimental decrease in potassium levels. As fluid is replaced and the amount of insulin administered plateaus, potassium will reenter the blood space and can result in hyperkalemia. Electrocardiogram monitoring is necessary in moderate to severe DKA to monitor for peaked T waves with hyperkalemia or the appearance of a U wave due to hypokalemia, alerting staff

TABLE 24.3 Insulin Preparations: Onset, Peak, And Duration*

Insulin Preparation	Onset of Action	Peak Duration	Effective Duration	Maximum Duration
Human				
Rapid-Acting Insulin Analogs				
Lispro (Humalog)	15–30 min	0.5–1.5 h	3–4 h	4–6 h
Aspart (NovoLog)	15–30 min	0.5–1.5 h	3–4 h	4–6 h
Glulisine (Apidra)	15–30 min	0.5–1.5 h	3–4 h	4–6 h
Short-Acting Insulin				
(Regular)	0.5–1 h	2–3 h	3–6 h	6–8 h
Intermediate-Acting Insulin				
(NPH)	2–4 h	6–10 h	10–16 h	14–18 h
Long-Acting Insulin Analogs				
Glargine (Lantus)	1.1 h	None	24 h	24 h
Detemir (Levemir)	3–4 h	6–8 h	6–23 h	23 h
Premixed Fixed Combinations				
Humulin and Novolin 70/30; Humulin 50/50	Peak as NPH and regular			
Humalog mix 75/25	15–30 min	Dual peak	10–16 h	14–18 h
NovoLog mix 70/30	15–30 min	Dual peak	10–16 h	14–18 h
Animal				
Short-Acting Insulin				
(Regular)	0.5–2 h	3–4 h	4–6 h	6–10 h
Intermediate-Acting Insulin				
(NPH)	4–6 h	8–14 h	16–20 h	20–24 h

*There are many variables that can affect the absorption rates of subcutaneous insulin injections. This timetable is a guideline to aid in predicting an individual's response to insulin.
NPH, Neutral protamine Hagedorn.
From Reference 11.

to cardiac irritability in either case. Bicarbonate use in DKA to treat metabolic acidosis is discouraged unless the pH is less than 6.9.[42] Intubation may be required with severe metabolic acidosis. Electrolyte levels should be monitored every 2 hours in DKA until they reach normal levels, at which time they can be checked every 4 hours, then daily as the DKA resolves.

The administration of IV insulin allows peripheral receptors to become saturated with insulin, eventually achieving a level at which the glucose is allowed to enter the cell. IV insulin infusion requires hourly blood glucose monitoring until stable, which is defined as within the target range for 4 consecutive hours.[2] When the blood glucose level stabilizes, monitoring every 2 hours is appropriate. A return to hourly testing is indicated if the glucose concentration fluctuates outside of the designated target range. The titration of insulin can be done using standardized protocols[26,27,41,45,49,56,60] or by 0.5-unit increments to maintain blood glucose levels within a specified target range. The goal is to have the glucose level decrease by 50 to 70 mg/dL/hour.[42] When the blood glucose level reaches 200 mg/dL, IV fluids should be changed to D5W (5% dextrose in water) 0.45% NS at 150–250 mL/h to provide a dextrose source.[42] Glycemic targets for individuals being treated for DKA are individually established on the basis of the patient's insulin sensitivity factor, age, and weight, and may range from as high as 200 mg/dL for a neonate to as low as 80 to 110 mg/dL for an intensely managed individual.[2,13]

As the glycemic target is achieved and the ketosis cleared, usually over a 24-hour time period, the insulin regimen must shift from IV insulin to basal/bolus subcutaneous management, which mimics normal pancreatic function.[42] As ketosis clears, the patient's nausea, vomiting, and abdominal cramping will subside and they can begin a clear liquid intake, eventually starting a consistent carbohydrate (CHO) meal plan. Basal insulin is the insulin delivered that will stabilize blood glucose levels for 24 hours. Thus intermediate- and long-acting insulins noted in Table 24.3 are basal insulins. Neutral protamine Hagedorn (NPH), given twice daily (in the morning and at bedtime) for true basal coverage, is the only intermediate-acting insulin available in the United States. Glargine, a long-acting insulin, is peakless and is administered once a day. On occasion, it is given twice a day if a large volume of the drug (> 100 units) is being given at one time. Detemir, a twice-a-day insulin with long action, has special properties in that it binds to albumin, increasing the predictability of action. However, in patients with renal or hepatic impairment, a decreased clearance of the insulin is seen as the impairment worsens. In general, the total daily dose of subcutaneous insulin in transitioning from IV infusion to subcutaneous dosing is based on a range of 0.4–1 unit/kg/24 hours. The total amount of IV insulin used in the last 24 hours can be used to predict the total amount of subcutaneous (SQ) insulin required. Fifty percent of the total daily dose should be given as basal insulin and the remaining 50% should be provided as bolus or prandial insulin.[48] The first SQ injection of basal insulin as the patient is transitioned from IV to SQ administration must be administered 2 hours before the discontinuation of the infusion.[42] Monitor the blood glucose at the time of the first SQ injection, 2 hours later at the time of the IV infusion discontinuation, and then 2 hours later. At this point, glucose monitoring can be transitioned to the routine of fasting, preprandial, and bedtime glucose levels.

Bolus insulin includes rapid- and short-acting insulin. Rapid-acting insulin is used for prandial coverage and correction of abnormally elevated blood glucose levels. Because the duration of rapid-acting insulin is 3 to 4 hours, this type of insulin medication works extremely well for CHO counting, for adjustment of insulin-to-CHO ratios, and for the purpose of correcting an abnormally elevated blood glucose level. Aspart, lispro, and glulisine are the available rapid-acting analogs. Regular insulin is short-acting insulin. Because it can be given every 6 hours, regular insulin is appropriate for glucose level correction when an individual is receiving nothing by mouth (NPO), is receiving continuous total parenteral nutrition, or is receiving a continuous enteral feed. It is also beneficial, in combination with the intermediate-acting insulin NPH, to maintain euglycemia overnight when the patient is receiving cycled nocturnal feedings and steroid bursts, because this insulin combination peaks simultaneously with peak corticosteroid levels in the bloodstream. Regular insulin should not be utilized in the fed state for correction. The action time of regular insulin is 4 to 6 hours, which is beyond the administration times of regular insulin before meals and at bedtime. Therefore, it can accumulate or "stack," creating the potential for hypoglycemia later in the day. The exception to this rule is the individual who is termed a *grazer*, a person who nibbles and eats throughout the day without actual meal patterns. There is a peak onset of action with regular insulin, making it necessary to administer 30 minutes prior to meals, which is not practical in the inpatient setting.

In the fed state, the consistent CHO meal plan is the standard diabetes diet. CHOs are the chief source of immediate fuel and are responsible for the postload peak glucose spike, typically at the 2-hour postprandial mark. By providing consistent amounts of CHOs throughout the day at meals, and snacks only if desired, wide glycemic excursions are reduced and targets can be achieved. In patients with type 1 DM and many with type 2 DM, it is beneficial to match rapid-acting insulin to CHO intake, to maintain targets. As previously mentioned, this is accomplished by providing an insulin-to-CHO ratio that is a set number of units of rapid-acting insulin for a set number of CHO grams or units. In the hospital setting, insulin is given immediately during or after the meal to ensure that the patient will indeed consume the CHO units provided on the meal tray. Because no one eating pattern is appropriate for all patients, it is important to utilize a collaborative approach between the patient, dietitian, and provider to set and achieve mutual goals, particularly in the hospital setting where glycemic control can be a challenge.[28]

The identification of precipitating factors is critical to the successful treatment of DKA, as interventions must be initiated to treat underlying infections or comorbid conditions. Ongoing assessment, intervention, and monitoring are critical. Observing and assessing for indications of fluid overload secondary to the fluid replacement, respiratory distress secondary to the metabolic acidosis, cerebral edema secondary to the rapidity of glucose level decrease and rehydration, and hypoglycemia must be the standard of practice.

Patient and family education is extremely important following an acute DKA event. Preventing future episodes can occur only if the individual understands the reasons for the DKA event and is instructed in its management, including how to appropriately manage and problem solve changes in glucose level related to illness; how to compensate for increased insulin requirements with the utilization of a SQ insulin correction scale with rapid-acting insulin; and when it is necessary to call for assistance. Also, the availability of medications and tools for self-management, including a glucose meter, test strips, lancets, ketone sticks, and adequate nutritional supplements, is crucial. Follow-up care and education should be established before discharge.

HYPEROSMOLAR HYPERGLYCEMIC STATE

HHS is a syndrome manifested by severe hyperglycemia, absence of ketosis, profound dehydration, and neurologic manifestations with high osmolality (Fig. 24.4).[57] HHS evolves over several days to several weeks, occurring most often in type 2 DM patients and in older adults, though 20% of patients with HHS do not have a previous diagnosis of DM.[57] In HHS, insulin availability is insufficient to facilitate glucose utilization and uptake at peripheral sites, resulting in hyperglycemia. In addition to insulin insufficiency, there are also increased levels of counterregulatory hormones.[57] Although it may occur, there is limited lipolysis and ketogenesis. Massive osmotic diuresis is the hallmark of HHS, with significant volume depletion and electrolyte loss. If this is untreated, death may occur.[42] Mortality rates are higher than with DKA; they are reported to be between 10% and 20% with HHS.[57]

The chief precipitating factors for HHS are infection, especially pneumonia and urinary tract infections; myocardial ischemia; stroke, trauma and medications such as glucocorticoids, thiazide diuretics, phenytoin, beta blockers, and atypical antipsychotics. Because HHS is more commonly associated with older adults, many individuals who develop HHS have dementia or altered mentation. There may be a delay in the identification of HHS as the abnormal mental state masks the neurologic changes associated with the syndrome. Residents of long-term care facilities are at increased risk for the development of HHS.[42] A contributing factor may also be the altered thirst response of the elderly, leading to inadequate oral intake.[57]

The symptoms associated with HHS are polydipsia, polyuria, polyphagia, weakness, dehydration, weight loss, and blurred vision. Gastrointestinal symptoms, such as nausea, vomiting, abdominal pain, and cramping, are much milder in HHS compared to DKA. Physical findings include altered skin turgor, tachycardia, hypotension, alteration in mental status, focal neurologic signs (e.g., hemisensory deficits, hemiparesis, aphasia), and seizures. See Table 24.2 for a list of laboratory values common in HHS and how those values compare to what is typically seen in DKA.

As in DKA, the primary treatment for HHS is fluid replacement, insulin therapy, correcting hyperosmolality, and electrolyte replacement. Initial treatment of fluid therapy is for intravascular and extravascular volume expansion, and increasing renal perfusion. Hemodynamic monitoring, measurement of intake and output, and physical examination are measures to determine adequacy of fluid replacement.[42] Individuals who have cardiac or renal comorbidities must be monitored carefully during fluid resuscitation to

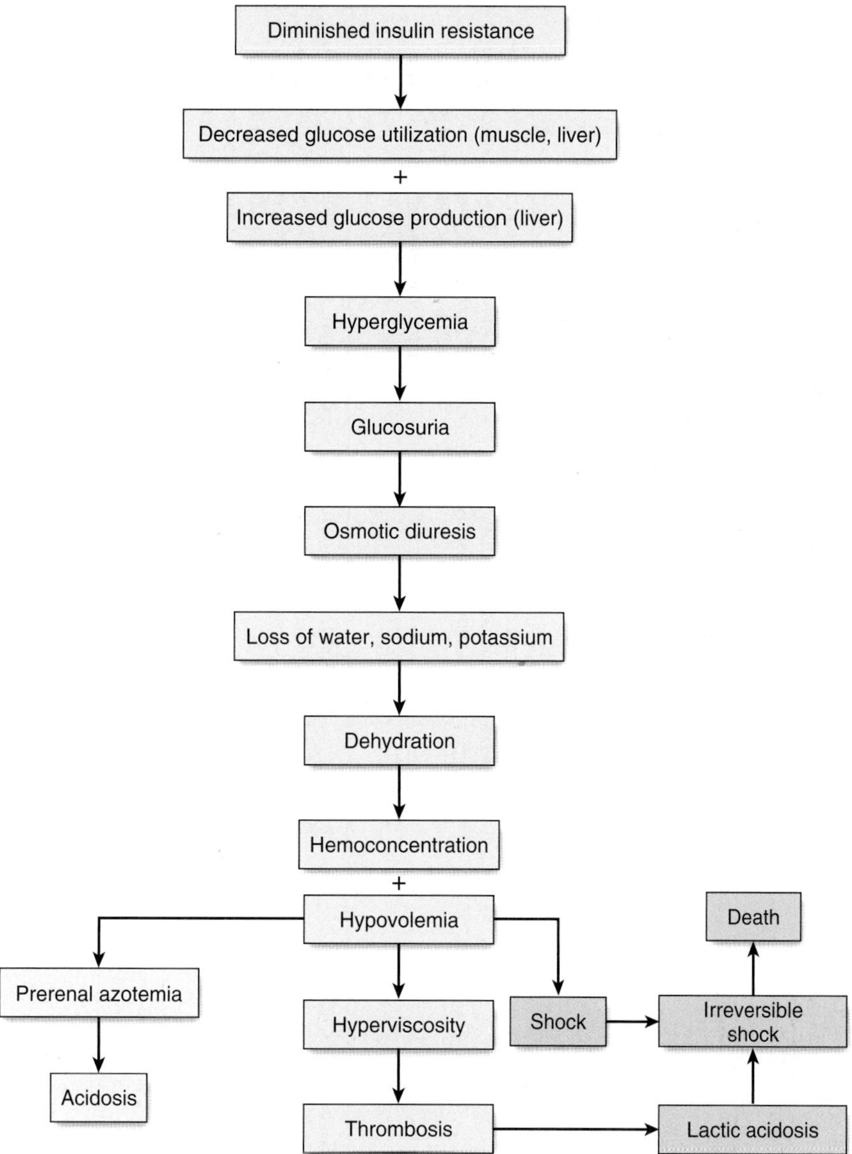

FIG. 24.4 Pathophysiology of hyperosmolar hyperglycemic state.

avoid overload. Electrolytes, particularly potassium, magnesium, and phosphorus, are replaced as necessary, and monitoring is done every 2 hours until electrolyte levels are stable. When the blood glucose level reaches 300 mg/dL, it is important that some dextrose (typically as dextrose 5% with 0.45% NaCl) be administered to offer some caloric source and to avoid hypoglycemia.[42] The amount is dependent on the patient's age and comorbid conditions.

As in DKA, IV insulin infusions are the standard of practice. IV insulin is given as regular insulin in a 1:1 concentration (1 unit of U-100 regular human insulin to 1 mL of NS). IV insulin should be continued until the HHS is resolved, as demonstrated by corrected laboratory values and the individual's ability to tolerate oral food and fluids. Once this occurs, insulin should be transitioned to basal/bolus SQ management. The first dose of basal insulin should be administered 2 hours before the discontinuation of the insulin infusion.[42] Rapid-acting insulin (such as aspart, lispro, or glulisine) should be administered to cover prandial intake or as correction. Oral diabetes agents are not able to maintain euglycemia in an acute crisis. If appropriate, they can be reinstituted closer to discharge to determine effectiveness. A list of oral diabetes agents is provided in (Table 24.4).

Nutrition goals include provision of energy for basic metabolic requirements, calories for reasonable weight, maintenance of euglycemia, maintenance of normal blood pressure, and maintenance of lipid profile within normal limits. Individualizing the plan to encourage compliance and satisfaction by the client is also important. A consistent CHO meal plan is standard. However, because 80% of individuals with type 2 DM are obese,[55] counting fat grams to achieve overall caloric reduction has been successful. Within the hospital setting, it is important to note that multiple nutrition-related issues affect glycemic control and can result in hypoglycemia. People who are ill frequently have a decreased appetite; meal trays may be delayed from the kitchen; the timing of meals is inconsistent because of tests, procedures, and rounds; inconsistent CHO content alters glycemia; physical activity is decreased from the well state; and glucose monitoring may not be timely.[61] Thus the nurse must work

TABLE 24.4 Oral Diabetes Agents

Class/Action	Generic (Trade Name)	Dose Size (in mg)	Dose/Day (in mg)	Dose Interval	Peak (h) / Duration (h)	Side Effects	Contraindications
Sulfonylurea/secretagogue; beta cell	Glyburide (Micronase, DiaBeta, Glycon, Glynase)	1.25,2.5, 5	1.25–20	1–2 times daily with meals	4 / 12–24	Weight gain, hypoglycemia, gastrointestinal (GI) upset, photosensitivity	Use caution in older adults with decreased renal function
Sulfonylurea/secretagogue; beta cell	Micronized glyburide (Glynase PresTab)	1.5, 3, 4.5, 6	0.75–12	1–2 times daily with meals	2 / 12–24	Weight gain, hypoglycemia, GI upset, photosensitivity	Use caution in older adults with decreased renal function
Sulfonylurea/secretagogue; beta cell	Glipizide (Glucotrol)	5, 10	2.5–40	1–3 times daily, 30 min before meals	1–3 / 12–24	Weight gain, hypoglycemia, GI upset, photosensitivity	Use caution in older adults with decreased renal function
Sulfonylurea/secretagogue; beta cell	Glipizide-GITS (Glucotrol XL)	2.5, 5, 10	2.5–20	Once daily with meal	6–12 / 24	Weight gain, hypoglycemia, GI upset, photosensitivity	Use caution in older adults with decreased renal function
Sulfonylurea/secretagogue; beta cell	Glimepiride (Amaryl)	1, 2, 4	1–8	Once daily with meal	2–3 / 24	Weight gain, hypoglycemia, GI upset, photosensitivity	Use caution in older adults with decreased renal function
Meglitinide/secretagogue; beta cell	Repaglinide (Prandin)	0.5, 1, 2	0.5–16	1–4 times daily, 1–30 min before meals	1 / 4-6	Weight gain, hypoglycemia, GI upset, photosensitivity	Sole therapy in type 1 diabetes DKA
Meglitinide/secretagogue; beta cell	Nateglinide (Starlix)	60, 120	180–360	1–3 times daily, 1–30 minutes before meals	1 / 4	Weight gain, hypoglycemia	Type 1 diabetes DKA
Thiazolidinedione/sensitizer; receptor	Rosiglitazone (Avandia)	2, 4, 8	4–8	1–2 times daily	n/a / Days–weeks	Edema, weight gain, increased ovulation in premenopausal women	Do not give if ALT is greater than 2.5 times ULN. Monitor LFTs every 2 months for first 12 months of therapy. Evaluate for previous MI, CAD, HF, aortic or mitral valve disease. Use cautiously in Class I or II NYHA HF; do not use in Class III or IV NYHA HF. Monitor weight.
Thiazolidinedione/sensitizer; receptor	Pioglitazone (Actos)	15, 30, 45	15–45	Once daily	n/a / Days–weeks	Edema, weight gain, increased ovulation in premenopausal women	Do not give if ALT is greater than 2.5 times ULN. Monitor LFTs every 2 months for first 12 months of therapy. Evaluate for previous MI, CAD, HF, aortic or mitral valve disease. Use cautiously in Class I or II NYHA HF; do not use in Class III or IV NYHA HF. Monitor weight.
Biguanide/sensitizer; liver, receptor	Metformin (Glucophage; Riomet oral solution 100 mg/mL)	500, 625, 750, 850, 1000	1000–2550	1–3 times daily with meals	2–3 / 12–18	Nausea, diarrhea, abdominal pain, possible resumption of ovulation in premenopausal anovulatory women	Lactic acidosis is a rare side effect if renal, hepatic, or cardiac disease or dysfunction is present, particularly with advanced age. Caution patients against excessive alcohol intake with hepatic impairment. Discontinue metformin at time of or before radiologic studies involving IV iodinated contrast materials. Withhold metformin for 48 h after procedure and restart only after renal function has been reevaluated and determined to be normal. Do not give if creatinine greater than 1.4 mg/dL in females; greater than 1.5 mg/dL in males.

Biguanide/sensitizer; liver, receptor	Metformin extended release (Glucophage XR)	500, 750, 1000	1000–2000	Once daily with evening meal	4–8/24	Nausea, diarrhea, abdominal pain, possible resumption of ovulation in premenopausal anovulatory women	Lactic acidosis is a rare side effect if renal, hepatic, or cardiac disease or dysfunction is present particularly with advanced age. Caution patients against excessive alcohol intake with hepatic impairment. **Discontinue metformin at time of or before radiologic studies involving IV iodinated contrast materials. Withhold metformin for 48 h after procedure and restart only after renal function has been reevaluated and determined to be normal.** **Do not give if creatinine greater than 1.4 mg/dL in females; greater than 1.5 mg/ dL in males.**
Alpha-glucosidase inhibitor/ delays digestion and absorption of CHO; small intestine	Acarbose (Precose)	25, 50, 100	150–300	1–3 times daily at the start of each meal	n/a/2–3	Diarrhea, flatulence, abdominal discomfort	**Do not give if creatinine greater than 2 mg/dL or creatinine clearance less than 25 mL/min.** Use cautiously with inflammatory bowel disease, colonic ulceration, or obstructive bowel disorders. Do not give if cirrhosis of the liver is present.
Alpha-glucosidase inhibitor/ delays digestion and absorption of CHO; small intestine	Miglitol (Glyset)	25, 50, 100	150–300	1–3 times daily at the start of each meal	n/a/2–3	Diarrhea, flatulence, abdominal discomfort	**Do not give if creatinine greater than 2 mg/dL or creatinine clearance less than 25 mL/min.** Use cautiously with inflammatory bowel disease, colonic ulceration, or obstructive bowel disorders. Do not give if cirrhosis of the liver is present.
SGLT-2 inhibitor; Increases urinary glucose excretion and delays glucose absorption in GI tract	Cangliflozin (Invokana)	100, 300	100–300	Once daily; recommended to take with first meal of day	1–2	Hypotension, hyperkalemia, genital mycotic infections, UTIs, constipation, nausea	May lead to DKA Contraindicated in severe renal impairment Not recommended for use in severe liver disease
SLGT-2 inhibitor; Increases urinary secretion of glucose; improves muscle insulin sensitivity	Dapagliflozin (Farxiga)	5, 10	5–10	Once daily with or without food	2	Hypotension, genital mycotic infections, UTIs, nausea, constipation	Contraindicated in severe renal impairment Do not use in patients with active bladder cancer
DDP-4 inhibitor; Stimulates insulin synthesis and release from pancreatic beta cells	Sitagliptin (Januvia)	25, 50, 100	100	Once daily with or without food	<3	Severe and potentially disabling joint pain, nausea, vomiting, abdominal pain, peripheral edema	Use decreased dose in severe renal impairment Monitor for development of acute pancreatitis

Continued

TABLE 24.4 Oral Diabetes Agents—cont'd

Class/Action	Generic (Trade Name)	Dose Size (in mg)	Dose/Day (in mg)	Dose Interval	Peak (h) / Duration (h)	Side Effects	Contraindications
DDP-4 inhibitor; Stimulates insulin synthesis and release from pancreatic beta cells	Saxagliptin (Onglyza)	2.5, 5	2.5–5	Once daily without regard to meals	2	Severe and potentially disabling joint pain, nausea, vomiting, abdominal pain	Use decreased dose in severe renal impairment Monitor for development of acute pancreatitis Limit dose to 2.5 mg when used concurrently with potent CYP3A4/5 inhibitor
DDP-4 inhibitor; Stimulates insulin synthesis and release from pancreatic beta cells	Linagliptin (Tradjenta)	5	5	Once daily without regard to meals	1.5	Severe and potentially disabling joint pain, nausea, vomiting, abdominal pain	Monitor for development of acute pancreatitis Do not use if patient requires potent glycoprotein inducers (e.g., rifampin)
Fixed combinations	Glyburide and metformin (Glucovance)	1.25/250, 2.5/500, 5/500	2.5/500–20/2000	1–2 times daily with meals	See above	See above	See above
Fixed combinations	Glipizide and metformin (Metaglip)	2.5/250, 2.5/500, 5/500	2.5/500–10/2000	1–2 times daily with meals	See above	See above	See above
Fixed combinations	Rosiglitazone and metformin (Avandamet)	1/500, 2/250, 2/500, 4/500, 2/1000, 4/1000	1/500–8/2000	1–2 times daily with meals	See above	See above	See above
Fixed combinations	Sitagliptin and metformin (Janumet)	50/500, 50/1000	50/500–100/2000	2 times daily with meals	See above	See above	See above
Fixed combinations	Saxagliptin and metformin (Kombiglyze XR)	2.5/1000, 5/500, 5/1000	5/500–5/1000	Once daily with evening meal	See above	See above	See above
Fixed combinations	Pioglitazone and metformin (ActoPlus Met)	15/500, 15/850	15/500–30/1700	1–2 times daily with meals	See above	See above	See above
Fixed combinations	Pioglitazone and metformin (ActoPlus Met XR [extended release])	15/1000, 30/1000	15/1000–30/1000	Once daily with evening meal	See above	See above	See above
Fixed combinations	Pioglitazone and glimepiride (Duetact)	30/2, 30/4	30/2–30/4	Once daily with main meal	See above	See above	See above
Fixed combinations	Repaglinide and metformin (Prandimet)	1/500, 2/500	1/500–6/1500	Within 15 minutes before meals; omit dose for any meal that is skipped	See above	See above	See above

NOTE: Development and information on oral agents is rapidly changing. Please refer to package insert for full medication information.

ALT, Alanine aminotransferase; *CHO,* carbohydrate; *CAD,* coronary artery disease; *DKA,* diabetic ketoacidosis; *GI,* gastrointestinal; *HF,* heart failure; *LFT,* liver function test; *MI,* myocardial infarction; *NYHA,* New York Heart Association; *ULN,* upper limits of normal; *UTI,* urinary tract infection.

From Reference 11.

closely with the patient and the dietitian to optimize consistency and stabilize glucose level.

Blood glucose monitoring is routinely done at the bedside. Point-of-care testing is critical and should be done every 4 or every 6 hours when the patient is NPO and hourly when the patient is receiving an IV infusion of insulin;[53] fasting, preprandial, and bedtime glucose monitoring should occur when the patient is being fed. Obtaining 2-hour postprandial blood glucose levels may be required to determine the adequacy of the insulin-to-CHO ratio prescribed. Nocturnal values are also helpful between 2 a.m. and 3 a.m. to identify hypoglycemia.

All precipitating factors must be identified and treated. Ongoing observation and assessment of mentation and neurologic checks are necessary. Obtaining information from a relative or care facility regarding baseline mental status can be quite helpful in determining any alterations the patient is experiencing.

In an effort to prevent a recurrence of HHS, patient, family, and staff education might be indicated. Adjustment of the patient's medical regimen as indicated and follow-up care are extremely important.

HYPERGLYCEMIA

Hyperglycemia in the inpatient setting can be a result of several factors: stress decompensation of type 1, type 2, or other forms of DM; withholding of antihyperglycemia medications or administration of medications that provoke hyperglycemia, such as glucocorticoids and vasopressors; or provision of nutrition enterally or parenterally.[5] Regardless of whether an individual is known to have diabetes, hyperglycemia has been associated with poor clinical outcomes and increased mortality and morbidity.[2,19,20,32,52,58,62,70] The connection between hyperglycemia and less than optimal clinical outcomes has been studied extensively. Findings have demonstrated associations with immune function, the inflammatory process, vascular alterations, and neuronal damage.[14,19,21,23,54]

Individuals with hyperglycemia have decreased host resistance and immunosuppression.[20] Hyperglycemia leads to impaired leukocyte function and the resulting diminished phagocytosis leads to impaired bacterial killing.[51] A reduction in T-cell populations for both CD-4 and CD-8 subsets has also been reported. Bacterial, viral, and fungal growth have increased in clients with blood glucose levels greater than 200 mg/dL.[20] It appears that any patient with an elevated blood glucose level is at increased risk for infection. Elevated glucose levels impair collagen synthesis and wound healing.[51] This holds particular importance for postoperative patients and those with nonhealing or deep wounds.

The largest volume of research has been conducted in the cardiovascular population. In this population, it is apparent that elevated blood glucose levels are associated with ischemia, infarction, and reduced coronary collateral blood flow.[19] Platelet aggregation and "sticky" red blood cells increase thrombus formation. This increases the risk of a pulmonary embolism, a deep vein thrombosis, a clotted IV access line, or a major thrombotic event. Catecholamine alterations and elevations in blood pressure are also found in hyperglycemia.[18] Inflammatory markers such as free radicals, cytokines, and nitric oxide can be found in the presence of hyperglycemia.[58] These are associated with acute MI and the severity of resultant cardiac dysfunction. Endothelial cell dysfunction is linked to increased cellular adhesion, increased cell permeability, inflammation, and thrombosis.[58,64] It is thought that hyperglycemia has a direct effect on endothelial cell function by causing chemical inactivation of nitric oxide.[23] This information explains why 50% of individuals with known DM have cardiovascular disease.[15]

Cerebral ischemia also can occur from hyperglycemia. Clement et al. [19] summarize findings associated with increased mortality, length of stay, and severity in acute stroke. These outcomes are the result of increased tissue acidosis and lactate levels found with increased blood glucose concentrations, the effects of stress, and the release of insulin counterregulatory hormones.[14,19]

Stress-induced hyperglycemia is the result of an increased release of counterregulatory hormones. When these are released, catabolism is increased, hepatic gluconeogenesis occurs, and lipolysis begins. Serum glucose, free fatty acids, ketones, and lactate are byproducts of this cycle. As the glucose concentration rises, insulin secretion is hindered by glucose toxicity. This cycle cannot be stopped without treatment interventions to achieve euglycemia.

The treatment for acute hyperglycemia includes all modalities that assist in maintaining near-euglycemia. Continuous IV insulin infusion is the best method for treatment of persistent hyperglycemia in critically ill patients. Treatment should begin minimally if blood glucose is greater than or equal to 180 mg/dL, with a target range of 140–180 mg/dL. Tighter control may be necessary for select patients but with vigilant monitoring for hypoglycemia.[53] Use of sliding scale insulin is strongly discouraged in the inpatient setting but rather use of basal/bolus insulin is recommended.[53] Selection of appropriate fluids, nutrition, insulin (or incretins and orals), and concomitant pharmacologic agents, and also treatment for comorbid conditions, are essential to achieve good outcomes. The provider, advanced practice nurse, staff nurse, pharmacist, dietitian, social worker, care coordinator, and educator should work together to create a coordinated plan of care in order to achieve optimal outcomes.

HYPOGLYCEMIA

Iatrogenic hypoglycemia occurs in people with type 1 and advanced type 2 diabetes who are treated with insulins or sulfonylureas and in those who are taking incretin hormones in combination with insulin or a sulfonylurea. Hypoglycemia is a limiting factor in glycemic control as it can result in severe injury and even death.[47,59] This was evident in the DCCT,[24] which found that intensive glycemic management to target glucose levels reduced long-term sequelae of DM, such as microvascular and neuropathic complications, with one risk: the frequency of hypoglycemia increased.

Hypoglycemia is a low plasma glucose concentration below or equal to 70 mg/dL.[59] It is accompanied by symptoms that are relieved when the plasma glucose level is raised. Inpatients may experience hypoglycemia due to altered nutritional state or patterns, heart failure, renal or liver impairment, malignancy, sepsis, or infection. In addition, there can be iatrogenic causes of hypoglycemia, such as altered ability to self report symptoms, decreased nutritional intake, changes in NPO status, inappropriate timing of insulin in relation to intake, changes in dextrose infusions, and interruptions in enteral and parenteral nutrition without replacement in dextrose intake.[5] In the past, hypoglycemia has been categorized as mild (60 to 70 mg/dL), moderate (46 to 59 mg/dL), and severe (≤ 45 mg/dL). In 2013, the American Diabetes Association Workgroup on Hypoglycemia identified severe hypoglycemia as "an event requiring assistance of another person to actively administer CHO, glucagons, or other corrective actions."[59] They also documented symptomatic hypoglycemia as an event during which typical symptoms of hypoglycemia are accompanied by a glucose level less than or equal to 70 mg/dL, and asymptomatic hypoglycemia as an event not accompanied by typical symptoms of hypoglycemia but with a glucose level less than or equal to 70 mg/dL.[59] Whereas a cutoff glucose of 69 mg/dL may seem high to deem as hypoglycemia, recommending this level allows for varied accuracies of glucometers and provides time to prevent severe hypoglycemia episodes through repeat testing, a change in regimen, or a change in behavior to prevent a further decline in glucose levels.[59] The problem is compounded by excess insulin or a secretagogue (a beta cell stimulating oral hypoglycemia agent) available in the bloodstream, physical activity, caloric intake,[7] drug interactions, alcohol, altered insulin sensitivity, gastroparesis, and renal insufficiency.

When hypoglycemia occurs in diabetes, the physiologic mechanism of counterregulation (regulation of plasma glucose levels) is impaired. Insulin levels do not decrease, glucagon levels do not increase, and epinephrine levels are increased because of a lower glycemic threshold for epinephrine secretion.[10] Hypoglycemic unawareness, or a loss of the warning symptoms of hypoglycemia, can develop in people who have frequent episodes of hypoglycemia and often in those with longstanding diabetes.[59]

The signs and symptoms of hypoglycemia can be divided into two categories, adrenergic and neuroglycopenic symptoms. Adrenergic symptoms are seen from excessive secretion of counterregulatory hormones, such as epinephrine, which increases the liver's glucose production and inhibits glucose utilization, and glucagon, which stimulates the release of glycogen from the liver. Growth hormone and cortisol have minimal action in an acute hypoglycemic event. Diaphoresis, tremors, tachycardia, hypotension, anxiety, hunger, pallor, circumoral tingling, and increased respirations are early warning signs of a low blood glucose level. Neuroglycopenic symptoms develop when there is an inadequate supply of glucose to the central nervous system. Dizziness, headache, clouding of vision, blunted mental activity, loss of fine motor skills, confusion, slurred speech, irritability, abnormal behavior, numbness, fatigue, seizures, and loss of consciousness are associated with severe hypoglycemia, which may be fatal.

The treatment of hypoglycemia in acute care needs to be consistent. Standardized protocols or order sets enable the care provider to respond in a timely manner with appropriate intervention. Oral CHOs should be the first choice for treatment in an alert patient who is able to swallow and eat. One CHO unit or 15 g of CHO will raise blood glucose concentration 30 to 45 mg/dL. The rule of 15 is often instituted and also taught to patients: administer 15 g of CHO and recheck blood glucose level in 15 minutes. Administer an additional 15 g of CHO and recheck every 15 minutes until the glucose level is greater than 100 mg/dL.[7] When a patient is semiconscious or unconscious, glucagon can be administered subcutaneously or intramuscularly, or 50% dextrose can be given IV. It is important to note that glucagon can cause severe nausea and vomiting. Therefore, the patient should be placed in the side-lying position so that aspiration does not occur during administration. Prevention of hypoglycemia and its severity is warranted. However, it must not be achieved at the expense of glycemic control. Vigilance and consistent monitoring of patients on glycemic control protocols is important to reduce the risks of severe hypoglycemia while still avoiding uncontrolled hyperglycemia.[47] Thus careful management of insulin, oral agents, nutrition, IV fluids, pharmacologic therapy, and conditions that can predispose an individual to hypoglycemia must be assessed and evaluated regularly.

PATIENT AND FAMILY EDUCATION

Diabetes self-management knowledge and behaviors are essential to prevent hospital readmissions, including all cause admissions,[39] and to improve outcomes and quality of life.[38] Ideally education for patients and families starts on hospital admission, continuing through to discharge instructions and a follow-up plan.[5] Providing education in the hospital is a challenge at best, with a patient who is experiencing stress from hospitalization and who is not feeling well in a busy environment that is not necessarily conducive to learning.[5] The goal in these situations is to ensure the patient and family comprehend essential survival skills, including understanding the disease, healthy eating patterns, how to safely take their glycemic control medications, and how to manage glucose when ill.[5] The focus of this education should be to serve as a bridge to more in-depth, ongoing outpatient education where the patient and family can attain all needed knowledge and skills.[3]

Diabetes self-management education begins as all education does, with a minimal learning needs assessment that includes current knowledge, health literacy, cognitive and visual ability, dexterity, coping skills, and problem-solving ability.[1,3,38] Inpatient education sessions should stay patient and family-centered, optimize active participation, utilize teach back methods, and be conducted in focused, short sessions.[1,3] As the patient moves through the inpatient setting, from critical care to acute care to discharge, it is important to pay particular attention to handoffs in terms of education completed and education still needing to be imparted. Patients with diabetes who are being discharged need to be able to demonstrate an understanding of the disease, informed decision-making particularly related to hyper/hypoglycemia recognition and treatment, adequate self-care behaviors, and informed problem-solving in order to perform safe self-care until they can be followed up with outpatient care, education, and resources.[38,53]

CONCLUSION

Glycemic management in the hospitalized patient directly impacts the clinical outcomes of patients with DM or hyperglycemia. It is imperative that members of the healthcare team are diligent in the assessment, intervention, and evaluation of all variables that affect serum glucose concentrations in an effort to achieve optimal glycemic control.

ACKNOWLEDGMENT

The author gratefully acknowledges Joseph Barrera, MD, for his thoughtful review of this chapter.

CASE STUDY 24.1

M.E. is a 24-year-old female admitted to the intensive care unit (ICU) for DKA. Her past medical history is significant for type I diabetes, severe diabetic gastroparesis requiring intermittent use of tube feedings at home via a gastrojejunostomy (GJ) tube, and hypothyroidism. On arrival in the ICU, M.E. is tachypneic, pale, clammy, and complaining of nausea and severe abdominal pain.

Admission Assessment and Lab Values

Blood pressure (BP): 88/57 mm Hg, heart rate (HR): 141 beats per minute (bpm), respiratory rate (RR): 34, temperature: 98.5°F, arterial oxygen saturation (Spo_2): 99%, blood glucose: 596 mg/dL, ketones: 1.7 mg/dL, potassium (K): 3.3 mEq/L, blood urea nitrogen (BUN): 17 mg/dL, creatinine: 1.55 mg/dL, arterial blood gases: pH: 6.93, partial pressure of carbon dioxide (Pco_2): <10, partial pressure of oxygen (Po_2): 120, bicarbonate (HCO_3^-): 4.

M.E. was immediately intubated. A fluid bolus of 0.9% NS IV was initiated as well as fentanyl 50 mcg/kg/h and midazolam at 2 mg/h. Norepinephrine IV was initiated at 0.08 mcg/kg/min and titrated to maintain an adequate BP in addition to continuation of the fluid resuscitation. A continuous insulin infusion was initiated and maintained at 12 units/h with hourly glucoses decreasing from 596 to 239 over 5 hours. The insulin infusion was then titrated hourly between 1–3 units/h to achieve and maintain blood glucoses between 110s and 140s. As the patient stabilized, the norepinephrine infusion was discontinued and fluid boluses continued to a total of 7 L of 0.9% NS infused. Arterial blood gases slowly started to normalize: pH: 7.39, Pco_2: 21, Po_2: 192, HCO_3^-: 13, as did the patient's other lab values (e.g., K^+ = 3.9 mEq/L).

The following morning (ICU Day #2), the patient tolerated a pressure support trial and was successfully extubated. The serum ketone value had decreased to 1.0 mg/dL. The patient started to slowly initiate oral intake in addition to receiving tube feeding via GJ tube. ICU Day #3, M.E.'s serum ketones were 0.1 mg/dL, oral intake was improving, and the IV insulin infusion was stable between 1–2 units/h with blood glucoses continuing to range from 110s to 130s. The patient was transferred out of the ICU to the medical surgical floor with the plan to transition to basal/bolus dosing of insulin, monitoring of lab values and intake/output, and planned discharge the following day.

Decision Point:

How quickly should the patient's blood glucose be corrected and what is the risk associated with correcting the blood glucose value too quickly?

Decision Point:

What changes in potassium level should be anticipated with initiation of the insulin infusion?

Decision Point:

What are key interventions to avoid hypoglycemia when administering a continuous insulin infusion?

Decision Point:

What are the hallmark treatments of DKA?

Decision Point:

Briefly describe how to transition from IV administration to an SQ basal/bolus regimen.

REFERENCES

1. American Association of Diabetes Educators. (2013). Communicating effectively with patients: the importance of addressing health literacy and numeracy. http://www.diabeteseducator.org/docs/default-source/legacy-docs/_resources/pdf/research/aade_health_literacy_and_numeracy_white_paper_final.pdf?sfvrsm=2.
2. American College of Endocrinology. (2004). Position statement on inpatient diabetes and metabolic control. *Endocr Pract*, *10*(1), 77–82.
3. American Diabetes Association. (2012). Diabetes inpatient management. *Diabetes Educ*, *38*, 142–146.
4. American Diabetes Association. (2012). Economic costs of diabetes in the U.S. in 2012. *Diabetes Care*, *36*, 1033–1046.
5. American Diabetes Association. (2015). Diabetes care in the hospital, nursing home, and skilled nursing facilities. Sec. 13 in Standards of Medical Care in Diabetes. *Diabetes Care*, *38*(Suppl. 1), S80–S85.
6. American Diabetes Association. (2015). Fast facts, data and statistics about diabetes. http://professional.diabetes.org/content/fast-facts-data-and-statistics-about-diabetes.
7. American Diabetes Association. (2015). Glycemic targets. Sec 6. in Standards of Medical Care in Diabetes 2015. *Diabetes Care*, *38*(Suppl. 1), S33–S40.
8. American Diabetes Association. (2010). Diagnosis and classification of diabetes mellitus. *Diabetes Care*, *33*(Suppl. 1), S62–S69.
9. American Diabetes Association. (2015). Prevention or delay of type 2 diabetes. *Diabetes Care*, *38*(Suppl. 1), S31–S32.
10. American Diabetes Association Workgroup on Hypoglycemia. (2005). Defining and reporting hypoglycemia in diabetes. *Diabetes Care*, *28*(5), 1245–1249.
11. American Society of Health-System Pharmacists. (2015). *AHFS drug information*. Bethesda, MD.
12. Aronoff, S. L., et al. (2004). Glucose metabolism and regulation: beyond insulin and glucagon. *Diabetes Spectr*, *17*, 183–190.
13. Bruno, A., et al. (2010). Diabetes mellitus, acute hyperglycemia, and ischemic stroke. *Curr Treat Options Neurol*, *12*(6), 492–503.
14. Capes, S. E., et al. (2001). Stress hyperglycemia and prognosis of stroke in nondiabetic and diabetic patients: a systematic overview. *Stroke*, *32*, 2426–2432.
15. Centers for Disease Prevention and Control. (2014). *National diabetes statistics report, 2014*. http://www.cdc.gov/diabetes/pubs/statsreport14/national-diabetes-report-web.pdf.
16. Centers for Disease Prevention and Control. (2010). National Hospital Discharge Survey: 2010 table. Average length of stay and days of care – number and rate of discharges by first-labeled diagnostic categories. http://www.cdc.gov/nchs/data/nhds/2average/2010ave2_firstlist.pdf#x2013;%20Number%20and%20rate%20of%20discharges%20by%20first-listed%20diagnostic%20categories%20[PDF%20-%2058%20kB.
17. Chaillou, S. L., et al. (2010). Clinical and metabolic characteristics of patients with latent autoimmune diabetes in adults (LADA): absence of rapid beta-cell loss in patient with tight metabolic control. *Diabetes Metab*, *36*, 64–70.
18. Chaudhuri, A. (2002). Vascular reactivity in diabetes mellitus. *Curr Diab Rep*, *2*, 305–310.
19. Clement, S., et al. (2004). Management of diabetes and hyperglycemia in hospitals. *Diabetes Care*, *27*(2), 553–591.
20. Coursin, D. B. (2004). Perioperative diabetic and hyperglycemic management issues. *Crit Care Med*, *32*(Suppl. 1), S116–S125.
21. CREATE-ECLA Trial Group Investigators. (2005). Effect of glucose-insulin-potassium infusion on mortality in patients with acute ST-segment elevation myocardial infarction. *JAMA*, *293*(4), 437–446.
22. Dabelea, D., et al. (2014). Prevalence of type I and type 2 diabetes among children and adolescents from 2001 to 2009. *JAMA*, *311*, 1778–1786.
23. Dandona, P. (2002). Endothelium, inflammation, and diabetes. *Curr Diab Rep*, *2*, 311–315.
24. Diabetes Control and Complications Trial Research Group. (1993). The effect of intensive treatment of diabetes on the development and progression of long-term complications in insulin-dependent diabetes mellitus. *N Engl J Med*, *329*, 977–986.

25. Diabetes, U. K. Maturity onset diabetes of the young (MODY). https://www.diabetes.org.uk/Guide-to-diabetes/What-is-diabetes/Other-types-of-diabetes/MODY/.
26. Dortch, M. J., et al. (2008). A computerized insulin infusion titration protocol improves glucose control with less hypoglycemia compared to a manual titration protocol in a trauma intensive care unit. *JPEN J Parenter Enteral Nutr*, *32*, 18–27.
27. Dumont, C., & Bourguignon, C. (2012). Computerized insulin dose calculator and the process of glycemic control. *AJCC*, *21*(2), 106–114.
28. Evert, A. B., et al. (2103). Nutrition therapy recommendations for the management of adults with diabetes. *Diabetes Care*, 36(11), 3821-3842
29. Falciglia, M., et al. (2009). Hypoglycemia-related mortality in critically ill patients varies with admission diagnosis. *Crit Care Med*, *37*(12), 3001.
30. Finfer, S., & NICE-SUGAR Study Investigators, et al. (2009). Intensive versus conventional glucose control in critically ill patients. *N Engl J Med*, *360*, 1283–1297.
31. Finfer, S., & NICE-SUGAR Study Investigators, et al. (2012). Hypoglycemia and risk of death in critically ill patients. *N Engl J Med*, *367*, 1108–1118.
32. Finney, S. J. (2003). Glucose control and mortality in critically ill patients. *JAMA*, *290*, 2041–2047.
33. Furnary, A. P. (1999). Continuous intravenous insulin infusion reduces the incidence of deep sternal wound infection in diabetic patients after cardiac surgical procedures. *Ann Thorac Surg*, *67*, 353–362.
34. Furnary, A. P., et al. (2003). Continuous insulin infusion reduces mortality in patients with diabetes undergoing coronary artery bypass grafting. *J Thorac Cardiovasc Surg*, *125*, 1007–1021.
35. Garber, A. J. (2011). Long-acting glucagon-like peptide 1 receptor agonists. A review of their efficacy and tolerability. *Diabetes Care*, *34*, S279–S284.
36. Gebel, E. (2010). The other diabetes: LADA or type 1.5. *Diabetes Forecast*. http://www.diabetesforecast.org/2010/may/the-other-diabetes-lada-or-type-1-5.html#.V_EWM7CnDM0.email.
37. Goldstein, D. E., et al. (2004). Tests of glycemia in diabetes. *Diabetes Care*, *27*, 1761–1773.
38. Haas, L., et al. (2012). National standards for diabetes self-management education and support. *Diabetes Educ*, *38*, 619.
39. Healy, S. J., et al. (2013). Inpatient diabetes education is associated with less frequent hospital readmission among patients with poor glycemic control. *Diabetes Care*, *36*, 2960–2967.
40. Jauch, E. C., et al. (2013). Guidelines for the early management of patients with acute ischemic stroke: a guideline for health professionals from American Heart Association/American Stroke Association. *Stroke*, *44*, 870–947.
41. Juneja, R., et al. (2009). Computerized intensive insulin dosing can mitigate hypoglycemia and achieve tight glycemic control when glucose measurement is performed frequently and on time. *Crit Care*, *13*, R163.
42. Kitabchi, A. E., et al. (2009). Hyperglycemic crises in adult patients with diabetes mellitus. *Diabetes Care*, *32*, 1335–1343.
43. Klinke, D. J., II. (2008). Extent of beta cell destruction is important but insufficient to predict the onset of type 1 diabetes mellitus. *PLoS One*.
44. Kochanek, K. D., et al. (2014). Mortality in the U.S., 2013. *NCHS Data Brief*, *168*, 1–8.
45. Krikorian, A., Ismail-Beigi, F., & Moghissi, E. S. (2010). Comparisons of different insulin infusion protocols: a review of recent literature. *Curr Opin Clin Nutr Metab Care*, *13*(2), 198–204.
46. Krinsley, J. S. (2003). Association between hyperglycemia and increased hospital mortality in a heterogeneous population of critically ill patients. *Mayo Clin Proc*, *78*(12), 1471.
47. Krinsley, J. S., & Grover, A. (2007). Severe hypoglycemia in critically ill patients: risk factors and outcomes. *Crit Care Med*, *35*, 2262–2267.
48. Magaji, V., & Johnston, J. M. (2011). Inpatient management of hyperglycemia and diabetes. *Clin Diabetes*, *29*, 3–9.
49. Magaji, V., et al. (2012). Comparison of insulin infusion protocols targeting 110–140 mg/dL in patients after cardiac surgery. *Diabetes Technol Ther*, *14*(11), 1013–1017.
50. Malmberg, K., et al. (1997). Prospective randomized study of intensive insulin treatment on long-term survival after acute myocardial infarction in patients with diabetes (DIGAMI study). *BMJ*, *314*, 1512–1515.
51. McDonnell, M. E., & Umpierrez, G. E. (2012). Insulin therapy for the management of hyperglycemia in hospitalized patients. *Endocrinol Metab Clin North Am*, *41*(1), 175–201.
52. McGuire, D., et al. (2004). Association of diabetes mellitus and glycemic control strategies with clinical outcomes after acute coronary syndromes. *Am Heart J*, *147*(2), 246–252.
53. Moghissi, E. S., & American Association of Clinical Endocrinologists/American Diabetes Association, et al. (2009). Consensus statement on inpatient glycemic control. *Endocr Pract*, *15*(4), 1–17.
54. Najarian, J., et al. (2005). Improving outcomes for diabetic patients undergoing vascular surgery. *Diabetes Spectr*, *18*(1), 53–60.
55. National Institute of Diabetes and Digestive and Kidney Diseases. (2012). Do you know some of the health risks of being overweight? https://www.niddk.nih.gov/health-information/health-topics/weight-control/health_risks_being_overweight/Pages/health-risks-being-overweight.aspx.
56. Nerenberg, K. A., et al. (2012). Piloting a novel algorithm for glucose control in the coronary care unit. *Diabetes Care*, *35*, 19–24.
57. Pasquel, F. J., & Umpierrez, G. E. (2014). Hyperosmolar hyperglycemic state: a historic review of the clinical presentation, diagnosis, and treatment. *Diabetes Care*, *37*, 3124–3131.
58. Port, S., et al. (2005). Blood glucose: a strong risk factor for mortality in nondiabetic patients with cardiovascular disease. *Am Heart J*, *149*(8), 209–214.
59. Seaquist, E. R., et al. (2013). Hypoglycemia and diabetes: a report of a workshop of the American Diabetes Association and the Endocrine Society. *Diabetes Care*, *36*, 1384–1395.
60. Shetty, S., et al. (2012). Adapting to the new consensus guidelines for managing hyperglycemia during critical illness: the updated Yale Insulin Infusion Protocol. *Endocr Practice*, *18*, 363–370.
61. Swift, C., & Boucher, J. (2005). Nutrition care for hospitalized individuals with diabetes. *Diabetes Spectr*, *18*(1), 31–38.
62. Trence, D. L. (2003). The rationale and management of hyperglycemia for inpatients with cardiovascular disease: time for change. *J Clin Endocrinol Metab*, *88*, 2430–2437.
63. Triolo, T. M., et al. (2011). Additional autoimmune diseases found in 33% of patients at Type 1 diabetes onset. *Diabetes Care*, *34*, 1211–1213.
64. Trovati, M., & Anfossi, G. (2002). Mechanisms involved in platelet hyperactivation and platelet-endothelium interrelationships in diabetes mellitus. *Curr Diab Rep*, *2*, 316–322.
65. Umpierrez, G., et al. (2002). Hyperglycemia: an independent marker of in-hospital mortality in patients with undiagnosed diabetes. *J Clin Endocrinol Metab*, *87*(3), 978–982.
66. United Kingdom Prospective Diabetes Study Group (UKPDS). (1998). Intensive blood glucose control with sulfonylureas or insulin compared with conventional treatment and risk of complications in patients with type 2 diabetes. *Lancet*, *352*, 837–853.
67. United Kingdom Prospective Diabetes Study Group (UKPDS). (1998). Intensive blood glucose control with metformin on complications in overweight patients with type 2 diabetes. *Lancet*, *352*, 854–865.
68. UpToDate. (2015). Glycemic control and intensive insulin therapy in critical illness. http://www.uptodate.com/contents/glycemic-control–and-intensive-therapy-in-critical-illness?source=preview&language=en-US&anchor=H10&selectedTitle=20~150#H10.
69. Van den Berghe, G., et al. (2001). Intensive insulin therapy in critically ill patients. *N Engl J Med*, *345*, 1359–1367.
70. Van den Berghe, G., et al. (2003). Outcome benefit of intensive insulin therapy in the critically ill: insulin dose versus glycemic control. *Crit Care Med*, *31*(2), 359–366.
71. Wilcox, G. (2005). Insulin and insulin resistance. *Clin Biochem Rev*, *26*, 19–39.

Pituitary, Thyroid, and Adrenal Disorders

Diane Byrum

Almost every cell and organ in the body is influenced by the endocrine system, which plays a vital role in maintaining homeostasis. Hormones are chemical substances released from endocrine glands that transfer information and instructions regulating the function of the specific target gland or tissue. Hormones are secreted in minimal amounts in response to a need, producing either a local or a global effect (e.g., cortisol affects every cell in the body).[3,5,15] To serve as a reservoir for acute changes, many hormones are transported in the vascular system bound to plasma proteins. Although many different hormones circulate throughout the bloodstream, each one affects only the cells that are genetically programmed to receive and respond to its message. Hormone levels are influenced by factors such as stress, infection, and changes in fluid balance.[3,5,15]

The endocrine system is regulated by feedback in much the same way that a thermostat regulates the temperature in a room. For instance, when a signal is sent from the hypothalamus to the pituitary gland in the form of a "releasing hormone," the pituitary gland secretes a "stimulating (or tropic) hormone" into the circulation. The tropic hormone signals the target gland to secrete its own specific hormone. As the level of hormone rises in circulation, the hypothalamus and pituitary gland stop the secretion of releasing and stimulating hormones. This slows secretion from the target gland. Hormones maintain homeostatic balance as a result of this interactive negative feedback system, which utilizes other hormones, blood, chemicals, and the nervous system (Fig. 25.1).[3,5,15]

When the endocrine system is out of control, many local and systemic responses can be manifested as changes in energy metabolism, fluid and electrolyte imbalances, and disruption of homeostasis. Many common disorders are either deficiencies or excesses of hormones. Excesses or deficiencies are either primary (related to the target gland or organ response to the hormone) or secondary (related to defects in secretion of the releasing/inhibiting hormone or tropic hormone).[3,5] However, hormone-resistant states and iatrogenic causes also play a role in endocrine disorders.[5] Additionally, aging can lead to endocrine function abnormalities, including changes in levels of hormones secreted, response by the target gland or organ, metabolism of the hormone, or decreased biological activity (Fig. 25.2).[18,27] Understanding and integrating knowledge of the endocrine system's intricate relationship to all cells will help critical care nurses make clinical decisions related to the care of patients with endocrine disorders.[3,5,13,23,30]

APPLIED PATHOPHYSIOLOGY

Via the autonomic nervous system, the sympathetic nervous system and endocrine system are coordinated through activities of the anterior hypothalamus, the anterior and posterior pituitary glands, the thyroid gland, and the adrenal medulla and cortex (Fig. 25.3). As a starting place to understand the outcomes of stimulation of these various organs, the hypothalamus is connected to the posterior pituitary via nerve tracts. Of interest to critical care clinicians, antidiuretic hormone (ADH), which is also known as arginine vasopressin (AVP), is produced and stored in the hypothalamus. However, it is released by the posterior pituitary in response to either increases in serum osmolality (> 290 mOsm/L), thirst, or decreases in the circulating volume.[3,5,6,15] ADH regulates the amount of body water through its action on the distal tubules and collecting ducts of the nephron, normally impermeable to water.[1,5,10,12] The actions of ADH occur in the cortical and medullary collecting ducts of the kidney through the vasopressin receptor V2. ADH binds to V2 receptors and mediates the antidiuretic response by activating aquaporin 2 (AQP2) water channels. Activation of AQP2 results in increased permeability of this normally water-tight membrane. Driven by the osmotic gradient of sodium, water is reabsorbed into the vascular bed, producing concentrated urine. In response to decreasing osmolality (< 275 mOsm/L), via the negative feedback loop, the release of ADH is inhibited.[12] In addition, stimulation or inhibition of ADH is impacted by a number of medications and situations commonly seen in critical care.[28]

The hypothalamus is connected to the anterior pituitary through a capillary system that allows secretion of thyrotropin-releasing hormone (TRH) directly into the blood supply to the anterior pituitary. TRH, a releasing factor, is synthesized and stored in the hypothalamus and is secreted in response to decreased levels of T_4 (thyroxine) or T_3 (triiodothyronine), exposure to cold, catecholamines, and arginine vasopressin release. The response to TRH release is bimodal: first, it stimulates the anterior pituitary gland to release thyrotropin-stimulating hormone (TSH); and second, it increases hormone synthesis. TRH and TSH release is inhibited by increased T_3 and T_4 levels, glucocorticoids, chronic illness, somatostatin, and pituitary tumors.[5,10,11,15]

Both T_3 and T_4 contain 59% to 65% of the iodine in the body.[5,10,15] In order for T_3 and T_4 to be synthesized by the follicular cells of the thyroid gland, iodide must be oxidized into iodine; therefore, the ability of the thyroid gland to autoregulate is directly influenced by the availability of iodide.[24] Ninety percent of total thyroid hormone (TH) is the physiologically inactive form T_4 and 10% is the physiologically active form T_3. Once secreted into the bloodstream, T_3 and T_4 are bound to proteins and T_4 is converted to the physiologically active form T_3 as needed.[5,10,11] Low albumin and protein levels can affect the availability of both T_4 and T_3 since 99% of all TH is bound to protein in the plasma.[5,10]

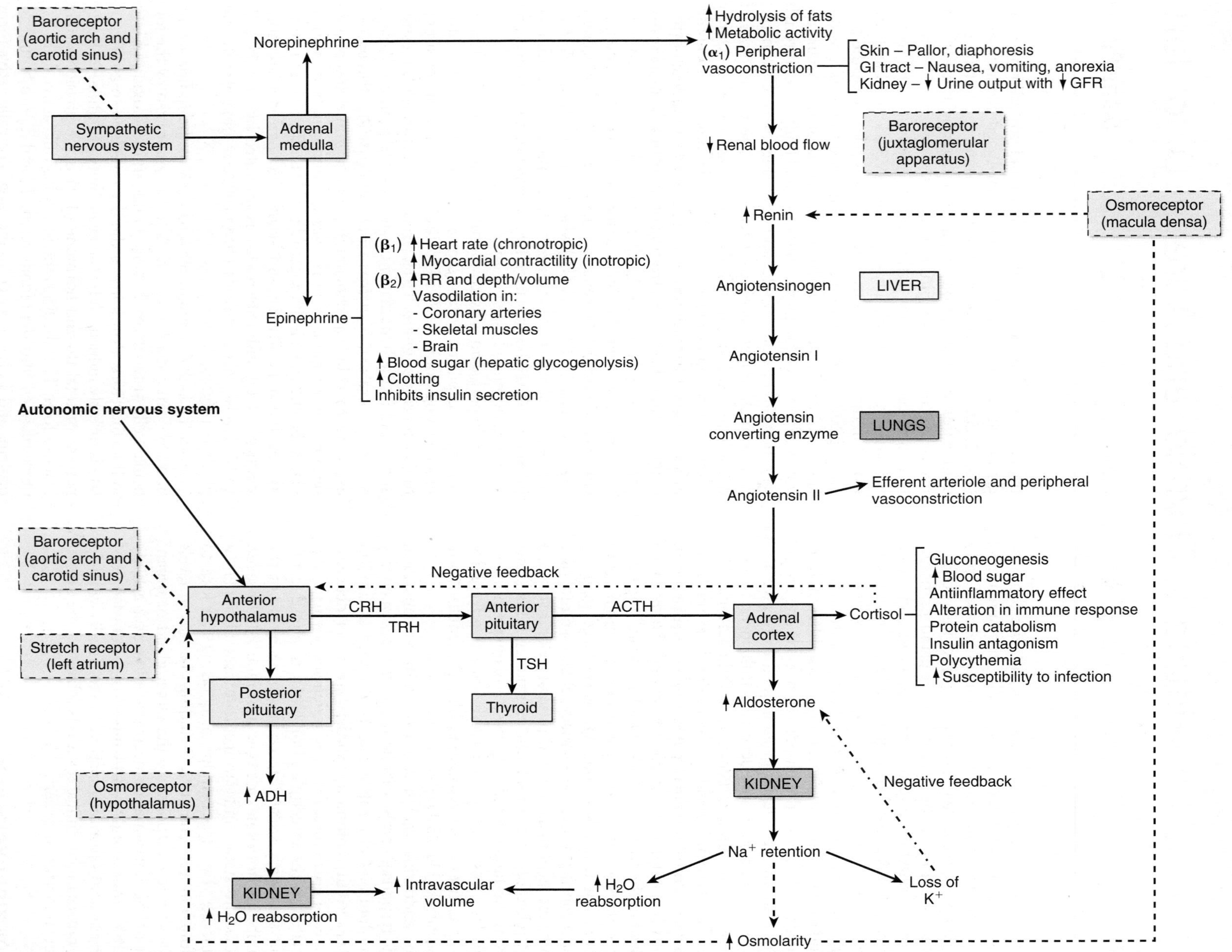

FIG. 25.1 Hormonal maintenance of homeostasis. *ACTH,* Adrenocorticotropic hormone; *ADH,* antidiuretic hormone; *CRH,* corticotropin-releasing hormone; *GFR,* glomerular filtration rate; *GI,* gastrointestinal; *K+,* potassium; *Na+,* sodium; *RR,* respiratory rate; *TRH,* thyroid-releasing hormone; *TSH,* thyroid-stimulating hormone. (Modified from and used with permission of Louis R. Stout.)

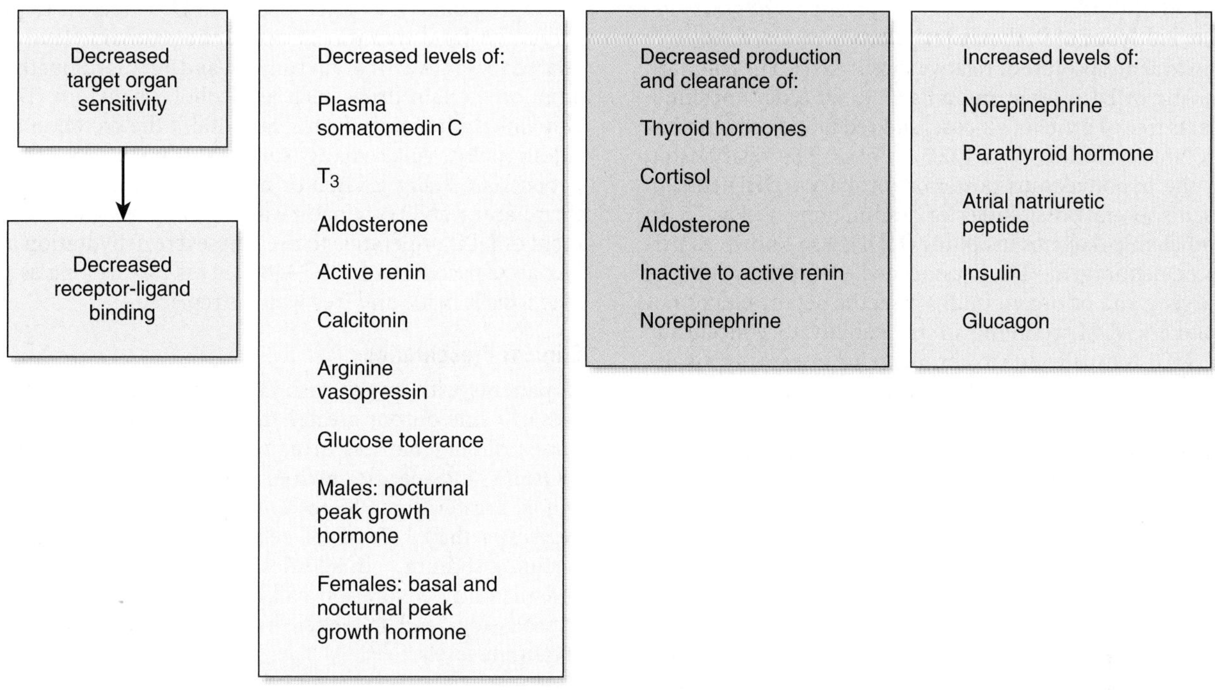

FIG. 25.2 Changes in the endocrine system associated with aging. (From Porterfield, S. (2001). *Endocrine physiology*. St Louis: Mosby.)

As described previously, TH secretion is under the control of the hypothalamus-anterior pituitary-thyroid gland axis and is regulated through a negative feedback system. TH affects most body systems and cells. Effects of TH include the following: regulation of basal metabolic rate and temperature by increasing beta-adrenergic receptors in cardiac muscle (positive inotropic and chronotropic effects on the heart), skeletal muscle, adipose tissue, and lymphocytes; regulation of catecholamine sensitivity; regulation of hypoxic and hypercapnic drives; regulation of the 2,3-diphosphoglycerate content in red blood cells, which assists with release of oxygen to the tissues; regulation of gut motility; regulation of bone turnover; regulation of muscle contraction and relaxation; regulation of cholesterol synthesis; and regulation of hormone and pharmacologic agent turnover.[1,3,5]

The two adrenal glands sit atop each kidney. Each gland consists of two distinct areas: the cortex, or outer layer, and the medulla, or inner layer. The adrenal medulla secretes catecholamines (epinephrine and norepinephrine), which stimulate the sympathetic nervous system alpha and beta receptors. The adrenal cortex secretes glucocorticoids, such as cortisol, in response to adrenocorticotropic hormone (ACTH). In addition, mineralocorticoids (e.g., aldosterone) are also secreted indirectly from the adrenal cortex in response to increased potassium levels, activation of the renin-angiotensin system, or decreased plasma volume.[3,5,8,10,12]

The adrenal glands are under the control of the hypothalamus-anterior pituitary axis and the sympathetic nervous system. The body sends a signal to the hypothalamus via the central nervous system in response to a stressor such as pain, hypotension, hypoglycemia, hypoxemia, trauma, or cytokine discharge. Based on the interpretation of this message by the hypothalamus, corticotropin-releasing hormone (CRH) is either secreted or inhibited. If secreted, CRH travels to the anterior pituitary via the rich blood supply connection, where ACTH is secreted. ACTH travels to the adrenal gland, where it acts to secrete cortisol directly or aldosterone indirectly. When glucocorticoids are released from the cortex, the following actions occur:

- Increased sodium/water retention with potassium excretion
- Synthesis of sodium-potassium-adenosine triphosphatase, which effects synthesis of catecholamines and catecholamine receptors, producing a positive inotropic effect
- Decreased nitric oxide production, affecting vascular permeability
- Increased breakdown of protein while inhibiting protein synthesis
- Increased gluconeogenesis with decreased glucose uptake
- Enhanced fat deposits on the face, neck, abdomen, and supraclavicular area
- Suppression of immune-inflammatory responses by decreasing the function and accumulation of lymphocytes, monocytes, macrophages, eosinophils, mast cells, and basophils.[3,5,10,15]

The hormones associated with fight or flight (epinephrine and norepinephrine) are stored in the adrenal medulla and released in response to stress, pain, hypoxia, hypoglycemia, hypotension, fluid loss, anxiety, surgery, or trauma. These catecholamines produce alpha-adrenergic activity, which increases heart rate, oxygen consumption, and carbon dioxide production; dilates bronchioles; slows digestion; and stimulates gluconeogenesis and lipolysis as energy sources.[3,5,10,15] In response to increased serum cortisol levels, the hypothalamus inhibits CRH from being released and the negative feedback mechanism is able to keep cortisol levels within a narrow range[10]

DISORDERS OF ANTIDIURETIC HORMONE

There are two disorders of ADH: diabetes insipidus (DI) and syndrome of inappropriate ADH (SIADH). DI is caused by a *lack* of ADH whereas SIADH is caused by an *excess* of ADH.

Diabetes Insipidus

Definition and Types of Diabetes Insipidus

DI is defined as an absolute or relative lack of ADH. The hallmark characteristic of DI is large amounts (2 to 20 L/day) of dilute urine that is free of protein, glucose, and red blood cells and has a specific gravity of less than 1.005.[1,8,10,12,29] The relationship between the hypothalamus-posterior pituitary-ADH-nephron axis presents several possibilities for dysfunction (see Fig. 25.3):

- Hypothalamic diabetes insipidus (HDI), also known as primary or nephrogenic DI, is associated with dysfunction of the target gland or organ. In this case, the nephron does not respond to ADH, resulting in an inability to concentrate urine. HDI is usually due to chronic renal disease, hypokalemia, hypercalcemia, medications such as lithium and demeclocycline (Declomycin), and disease processes that damage the interstitium of the nephron.[5,12,26] In nephrogenic DI, levels of circulating ADH can be either normal or increased.
- Neurogenic diabetes insipidus (NDI), or secondary DI, results from a lack of production of ADH in the hypothalamus, an inability to store ADH in the pituitary, or a malfunction of the osmoreceptors. NDI is distinguished from other causes of DI by decreased levels of plasma AVP.[12]
- Dipsogenic diabetes insipidus (DDI), or psychogenic DI, is an obsessive-compulsive disorder in which the patient ingests large amounts of water, thereby essentially turning off ADH secretion.[12]
- Gestagenic DI occurs during pregnancy. This form of DI leads to an increased breakdown of ADH related to increased levels of circulating vasopressinase, an enzyme responsible for the breakdown of AVP.[12,22]

Patients at Risk

Neurogenic DI is the most common dysfunction seen in patients with damage to the hypothalamus/posterior pituitary area as a result of head trauma or neurosurgery. If only the posterior pituitary is damaged, ADH can still be manufactured and secreted from the hypothalamus.[8,9,12,22]

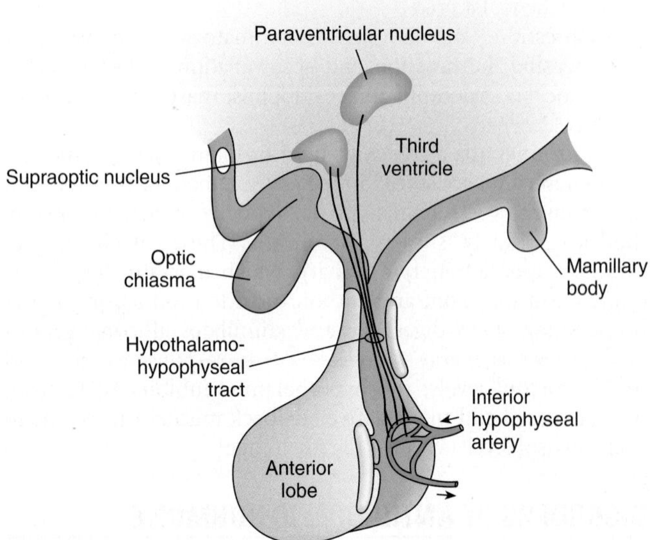

FIG. 25.3 Mechanisms of endocrine control: hypothalamus connection and influence of posterior pituitary.

Approximately 20% to 30% of all DI is related to pituitary surgery or head trauma impacting the pituitary gland,[9] 25% is related to removal of brain tumors, and 30% is idiopathic.[8,12] In addition, certain drugs such as alcohol, phenytoin (Dilantin), and alpha-adrenergic agents can inhibit the secretion of ADH. Additionally, since many surgical, trauma, or critically ill patients are being sedated or mechanically ventilated, limiting their natural ability to ingest water, prompt diagnosis and treatment of DI is imperative to prevent severe dehydration and cardiovascular collapse.[1,8,10,12] Mortality is rare as long as prompt diagnosis is made and free water is replaced.

Clinical Presentation

In patients with known risk factors for DI, presentation consists of urine output greater than 200 mL/h for 2 consecutive hours; dilute, colorless urine with urine osmolality 50 to 150 mOsm/L, and specific gravity 1.005 or less.[23] Plasma osmolality will be greater than 285 mOsm/L and serum sodium level will be greater than 147 mEq/L related to loss of free water, while retaining sodium.[23] In addition, signs and symptoms of hypovolemia and dehydration will be present, such as tachycardia, hypotension, and increased blood urea nitrogen (BUN) and creatinine levels.[6,13,23]

Diagnostic Evaluation

To diagnose DI, specific laboratory tests should include serum and urine osmolality, serum ADH levels, serum sodium level, and urine specific gravity. There are two diagnostic tests that differentiate HDI from NDI.[13] The water deprivation test can be used in a noncritically ill patient to differentiate ADH deficiency from other types of polyuria. However, because this test can take up to 18 hours to complete, it is rarely used for critically ill patients.[1,12,13]

The most definitive test is a vasopressin replacement test, which replaces aqueous vasopressin 5 U IV (5 units intravenous). Measurements of urinary output and urine osmolality are collected before exogenous vasopressin replacement. The urinary output and urine osmolality are measured every 30 minutes for 2 hours. HDI is diagnosed if urine output and osmolality decrease after administration of exogenous vasopressin, signaling a problem with the hypothalamus-pituitary axis (HPA). NDI is diagnosed when there is no decrease in urine output and osmolality following administration of exogenous vasopressin, signaling a decreased response in the collecting duct of the kidney tubules.[12,13,23]

Interprofessional Plan of Care

Collaborative management of the patient with DI should include rehydration with hypotonic (0.45% normal saline) solutions to replace free water. Exogenous vasopressin replacement should be administered to prevent dehydration and hypovolemic shock. Patients with DI should have continuous monitoring of intake and output, weight, and vital signs, as well as monitoring of laboratory values such as serum sodium, serum osmolality, and urine specific gravity. Close attention must be paid to provide adequate nutrition with either parenteral hyperalimentation or enteral tube feedings. If hyperalimentation is required, the patient must be closely monitored for increased glucose to prevent additional free water loss. Because enteral feedings may pull water into the gastrointestinal tract, free water may be added to hypertonic tube feedings to prevent diarrhea.[1,8,12] DI can transiently resolve only to reappear or become permanent.[1,12,13,23,29] See Table 25.1 for information on medications used to treat DI.

Syndrome of Inappropriate Antidiuretic Hormone

Definition and Types of Syndrome of Inappropriate Antidiuretic Hormone

SIADH is the most common cause of hyponatremia.[1,12,21,29] SIADH is defined as inappropriate retention of free water leading to dilutional hyponatremia related to excess ADH.[12,29] The patient retains excess water in relation to sodium. Serum sodium level is less than 134 mEq/L, and serum osmolality is less than 280 mOsm/L. Urine osmolality increases, with urine sodium levels greater than 40 mmol/L and urine specific gravity 1.030.[1,23] The increased intravascular fluid leads to an increase in the glomerular filtration rate and increased atrial natriuretic peptide release, contributing to the excretion of sodium. Occasionally, the excess water accumulates in the intracellular space rather than the intravascular space, causing some patients to remain euvolemic or become only slightly volume-overloaded.[1,10,12]

Other underlying disease processes causing hyponatremia must be ruled out before SIADH can be confirmed. Adrenal insufficiency and hypothyroidism should be assessed with measurements of random serum cortisol and TSH levels.[1,6,12] In addition, nephrotic syndrome, acute renal failure, hepatic failure, and cardiac failure should be eliminated as possible diagnoses; all of these can lead to hyponatremia and increased extracellular fluid volume.[12]

SIADH can manifest as four osmoregulatory defects:

- Type A SIADH (approximately 40% of all cases) is caused by a (malignant or nonmalignant) tumor that secretes erratic amounts of ADH-like substances.[6,12]
- Type B SIADH (approximately 35% of all cases) results from reset osmostat occurring in chronic debilitating illness, such as encephalitis, HIV, malnutrition, quadriplegia, and psychosis, as well as in pregnancy.[6,12,23] The osmoreceptors are reset to secrete ADH at lower serum osmolalities (250 to 260 mOsm/L)[12] or the osmoreceptors are overly sensitive to serum osmolality changes.[6,12]
- Type C SIADH (approximately 25% of all cases) is rare and is associated with temporary dysfunction of the osmoreceptors, which causes ADH to leak, and selective loss of suppression causes continued secretion even though osmolality is low.[6,12,23]
- Type D SIADH (approximately 10% of all cases) is related to increased sensitivity of ADH in the nephron.[1,12]

Patients at Risk

Patients presenting with neurologic trauma, hemorrhage, meningitis, encephalitis, and neurologic effects of alcohol withdrawal are at risk for the development of SIADH.[6,10,12,13,23] In

TABLE 25.1 Medications Used in Diabetes Insipidus and Syndrome of Inappropriate Antidiuretic Hormone

Medications	Actions	Dosages	Special Considerations
Diabetes Insipidus (DI)			
Desmopressin (DDAVP) (Neurogenic DI)	Acts on renal tubules to promote sodium and water reabsorption	Nasal: (100 mcg/mL) 10–20 mcg daily Oral: 100–1000 mcg daily in 2–3 divided dose Subcutaneous: 0.1–2 mcg daily in 2 divided doses Intravenous: 0.1–2 mcg daily in 2 divided doses	Lithium and demeclocycline diminish ADH effects while fludrocortisone and glucocorticoid steroids enhance ADH response
Vasopressin (Neurogenic DI)	Acts on renal tubules to promote sodium and water reabsorption	Subcutaneous: 5–10 units every 4–6 h Intramuscular: 5–60 units daily given in 2–4 divided doses	Hypersensitivity Anaphylaxis Mainly used to diagnose
SIADH			
Demeclocycline (Declomycin) (Nephrogenic)	Interferes with action of ADH renal collecting duct	150 mg PO 4 times a day or 300 mg twice a day	Effect may take 1 week (not indicated in emergency management) Hypersensitivity to tetracyclines Nephrotoxic: monitor BUN/creatinine May cause photosensitivity
Furosemide (Lasix) (Nephrogenic)	Elicits a loss of free water by inhibition of sodium and chloride reabsorption in ascending loop of Henle and distal tubule	40 mg IV initially—may increase to 80 mg IV if insufficient response	Ototoxicity, photosensitivity
Conivaptan (Vaprisol)	Vasopressin-receptor antagonist (vaptan) blocks the V2 vasopressin receptors that leads to increased free water excretion thus serum sodium levels	Load: 20 mg IV infusion over 30 minutes; and THEN 20 mg IV as continuous infusion over 24-hour period for 2-4 days After initial day of treatment, may increase to 40 mg/day if necessary	Monitor serum sodium and volume status frequently; a significant increase in serum sodium (>12 mEq/L/24 hours) may result in serious neurologic effects
Tolvaptan (Samsca)	Vasopressin-receptor antagonist (vaptan) blocks the V2 vasopressin receptors that leads to increased free water excretion thus serum sodium levels	Initial: 15 mg PO daily Maintenance: Increase PRN after >24 h to 30 mg/day; may increase further, not to exceed 60 mg/day Not to exceed 30 days of treatment	Monitor serum sodium

ADH, Antidiuretic hormone; *BUN,* blood urea nitrogen; *DI,* diabetes insipidus; *SIADH,* syndrome of inappropriate antidiuretic hormone.
Data from References 1, 3, 5, 8, 9, 12, 13, 14, 21, 22, 23, 26, and 29.

addition, oat cell or small cell carcinomas of the lung produce a paraneoplastic syndrome in which ADH-like substances are found in the tumor cells. These ADH-like substances have the ability to synthesize, store, and secrete ADH and are found in 60% of patients with small cell carcinomas.[3] Slow tumor growth over time can lead to a gradual increase in water retention and hyponatremia.[3] In addition, other tumors of the duodenum, pancreas, brain, prostate, and thymus, as well as leukemia, lymphoma, and Hodgkin's disease, can produce ADH-like substances.[3,6,12] Nonmalignant pulmonary disease processes that may lead to SIADH hyponatremia include viral/bacterial pneumonias and tuberculosis.[3,12] Medications associated with SIADH include: desmopressin (DDAVP), dopamine antagonist, opiates, chlorpropamide (Diabinese), chemotherapeutic agents, nonsteroidal antiinflammatory drugs (NSAIDs), thiazide diuretics, angiotensin-converting enzyme inhibitors, angiotensin receptor blockers, narcotics, and selective serotonin reuptake inhibitors (SSRIs).[1,14,23] Other common causes include anesthesia, pain, anxiety, alcohol withdrawal, stress response (from trauma, surgery, burns, or sepsis), hypoxemia, hypotension, and positive-pressure ventilation.[12,14]

Clinical Presentation

SIADH presentation is dependent on how quickly hyponatremia occurred and its duration. The clinical presentation of SIADH relates to hyponatremia and relative water intoxication, as well as neurologic and gastrointestinal manifestations such as personality changes, headache, confusion, abdominal cramps, nausea, and vomiting.[1,14] Subtle signs and symptoms include inability to concentrate, weakness, fatigue, dyspnea on exertion, anorexia, loss of taste, and increased thirst.[1,12,14] SIADH can occur slowly over time, allowing the brain cells to adjust, masking the neurologic symptoms.[1,3,12,14] If hyponatremia occurs rapidly, it can lead to seizures, coma, and a 50% chance of death.[1,12,14]

Diagnostic Evaluation

Hyponatremia can be caused by many underlying disease processes. Therefore, differential diagnoses should be considered and ruled out before a diagnosis of SIADH is made. A series of preliminary lab studies would include serum and urine osmolality, urine specific gravity, urine sodium calculation of fractional excretion of sodium, serum electrolytes, urea, creatinine, BUN, triglycerides, uric acid, and ADH levels.[1,14] Hyponatremia is a common finding in SIADH, hypothyroidism, adrenal insufficiency, and liver disease. SIADH is ruled in as the cause for hyponatremia when the following specific laboratory values are normal: TSH, cortisol, potassium, glucose, and protein levels.[1,14] Chest x-ray and head computed tomography (CT) scan may be helpful to rule out carcinomas, lung disease, or cerebral edema.[1]

Interprofessional Plan of Care

Collaborative management of the patient with mild SIADH should include restriction of fluids to 1000 to 1500 mL/day and institution of measures to alleviate thirst/dry mouth by providing oral care, chilled beverages, and hard candy (if conscious).[23] Patients who have severe hyponatremia (< 115 mEq/L) should be treated with 3% sodium chloride by calculating the deficit (Chapter 21) and replacing sodium to increase the serum sodium level no more than 1 to 2 mEq/L/hour over the first 2 to 4 hours, decreasing to 0.5 to 1.9 mEq/L/hour as the serum sodium level approaches 120 mEq/L. Sodium must be replaced slowly to prevent the brain cells from shrinking, which could lead to a complication known as osmotic demyelination syndrome or central pontine myelinolysis.[1,14,23]

In addition, medications can be used to reduce the secretion of ADH or block the effects.[1,12,14,29] Demeclocycline can decrease the kidneys' response to ADH, whereas the loop diuretic, furosemide (Lasix), helps to diurese excess water and raise the serum sodium level.[12,14,29] Potassium, magnesium, and phosphorus levels need to be monitored to prevent electrolyte imbalances.[12,14,29] Conivaptan (Vaprisol) and tolvaptan (Samsca) are vasopressin receptor antagonists also used to treat hyponatremia (see Table 25.1).[1,21]

Conclusion

Early recognition of SIADH can be difficult, as the major presenting symptom is hyponatremia. Hyponatremia has a myriad of causes, which must be ruled out before making the diagnosis of SIADH. Once the diagnosis is made, early treatment focused on slowly replacing sodium and reducing intravascular volume should be instituted.

THYROID GLAND DISORDERS

The conditions associated with thyroid dysfunction include hyperthyroidism, which can lead to the life-threatening disorder thyroid storm (thyrotoxicosis); and hypothyroidism, which can lead to the life-threatening disorder myxedema coma.

Hyperthyroidism (Thyrotoxicosis/Thyroid Storm)

Hyperthyroidism results from increased levels of circulating T_3 and T_4. The major systemic effects associated with hyperthyroidism are increased metabolic activity, intolerance to heat, and stimulation of the sympathetic nervous system.[6,17,32] The most common causes of hyperthyroidism are Graves' disease, resulting from an autoimmune toxic goiter, and multinodular goiter, seen commonly in the older adult population. Other causes include an inappropriate secretion of TSH from pituitary neoplasms secreting TSH-like substances, as well as nonneoplastic pituitary secretion of TSH.[32] As with all disorders of HPA relationships there are two distinct mechanisms of thyroid dysfunction. Primary disorders, in which TSH levels are increased, are related to the thyroid gland-target organ/tissue response, and secondary disorders, in which TSH levels are decreased, are associated with problems in the axis.[3,6,30]

Although hyperthyroidism is a relatively common disorder, thyroid storm, a life-threatening exacerbation of hyperthyroidism, is rare (10%). Thyroid storm has a 20% to 30% mortality rate even with prompt treatment and is more common in women (10%) than men (2%), with a peak age of occurrence at 20 to 49 years.[11,17,29,30] Because of the long half-lives of T_3 (22 hours) and T_4 (approximately 7 days), a thyroid storm can last for a considerable period of time.[11,17,30]

Patients at Risk

Any patient with preexisting hyperthyroidism or undiagnosed hyperthyroidism is at risk. In older adults, hyperthyroidism can be mimicked by other underlying disease processes or expected age-related changes.[9,27] Often the elderly patient will present with nervousness, palpitations, tremors, fatigue, and depression. Many older patients are already being treated with beta-adrenergic blockers for hypertension, medications that can effectively conceal any tachycardia and tremors.[11,17] Older adult patients are at increased risk whenever their thyroid hormone replacement medication is increased or changed. This is related to decreased metabolism of the drug and increased half-life of the drug in older people; in addition, different brands may have different levels of thyroid hormone.[11,17]

Thyroid storm is an exaggerated form of hyperthyroidism and has a variety of triggers. Medications placing the patient at risk include NSAIDs, salicylates, tricyclic antidepressants, insulin, thiazide diuretics, amiodarone (Cordarone), chronic steroid therapy, and fludrocortisone agents.[11,17,28] Additional triggers that pose a risk include nonadherence with antithyroid medications, infection, trauma, surgical procedures (Table 25.2),[10] alcohol abuse, pregnancy, radioactive iodine therapy, diabetic ketoacidosis, and both physical and emotional stress.[1,11,17,25,32]

Clinical Presentation

The hallmark signs of thyroid storm are fever, tachycardia, tremors, intolerance to heat, sweating, nausea, vomiting, and diarrhea.[1,11,13,17,32] Less common findings include weight loss with increased appetite, emotional lability, pulmonary edema, and congestive heart failure. The most common dysrhythmias associated with thyroid storm are supraventricular tachycardias, most commonly atrial fibrillation.[11,17] Often in undiagnosed hyperthyroidism, thyroid storm may present as a cerebrovascular accident (CVA), other dysrhythmias (ventricular tachycardia or third-degree block), adrenal insufficiency, coma, jaundice, rhabdomyolysis, acute renal failure, shock, or status epilepticus.[11,17] Sepsis, pheochromocytoma, and malignant hyperthermia have a similar clinical presentation to thyroid storm.[1,32]

Diagnostic Evaluation

Diagnosis of thyroid storm is based primarily on the presenting clinical assessment and not diagnostic tests. Results of measurements of thyroid levels are useful to differentiate primary disease from secondary disease.[3,5,11,13] Thyroid function tests include T_3, T_4, free T_4, T_3 resin uptake, and TSH levels. TSH level is the gold standard used to differentiate primary from secondary thyrotoxicosis.[1,11,17,30] TSH level is decreased in primary disease and increased in secondary disease.[11] T_3 and T_4 levels will be elevated in primary disease, as well as in thyroid storm, because of the increased hypermetabolic state requiring physiologically active T_3. This is a direct result of the amount of T_4 available, as well as what is being synthesized.[1,11]

Interprofessional Plan of Care

Collaborative management of the patient with thyroid storm should include early recognition of the condition based on

TABLE 25.2 Surgical Considerations for Endocrine Disorders

Endocrine Disorder	Preoperative Considerations	Postoperative Considerations
Hyperthyroidism (thyroid storm)	Establish euthyroid if possible If euthyroid not possible: beta blocker to decrease SNS response to surgery, block conversion to T_3 • Propylthiouracil: blocks TH synthesis • Glucocorticoids: block release and conversion of TH • Drugs have shortened half-life related to hypermetabolic state	Related to compromised airway with removal of thyroid gland: Hematoma, edema, fludrocortisone (obstruction or stridor) • Hypocalcemia (vocal cord tetany, paralysis) • Laryngeal nerve injury (stridor)
Hypothyroidism (myxedema coma)	Assess fluid/electrolyte/hormone status TSH, T_3, T_4 (replace) Cortisol (adrenal insufficiency) Treat hypoglycemia Treat hyponatremia	Hypoventilation: • Blunted baroreceptor responses to hypercarbia and hypoxemia • Muscle weakness • Compromised airway related to large tongue, goiter, obesity Cardiac considerations: • Decreased CO and SV, bradycardia, HF, ECG changes (long QT, T wave inversion) Gastrointestinal considerations: • Delayed gastric emptying (may need NG tube) • Drugs have increased half-lives • Sedatives should be used in small amounts with caution and close observation Emergent surgery considerations: • Aggressive supportive care post-op • Judicious monitoring of response to treatment • T_4 dose daily • Stress-dose steroids every 8 h • PA catheter Fluids: • Avoid HF and further hyponatremia
Adrenal insufficiency	Assess for hypoglycemia and treat Assess for hyperkalemia and treat Steroid coverage is related to operation duration and complexity (lower doses for hernia and higher doses for CABG) Hydrocortisone steroid of choice related to 1:1 glucocorticoid/mineralocorticoid	Monitor for hypoglycemia and treat Monitor for hypotension and treat with fluids (such as NS) Replace steroids as needed

CABG, Coronary artery bypass graft; *CO*, cardiac output; *ECG*, electrocardiogram; *HF*, heart failure; *NG*, nasogastric tube; *NS*, normal saline; *PA*, pulmonary artery; *SNS*, sympathetic nervous system; *SV*, stroke volume; *TH*, thyroid hormone; *TSH*, thyroid-stimulating hormone; T_3, triiodothyronine; T_4, thyroxine.
Data from Reference 10.

the patient's clinical presentation.[11,17,32] Treatment should include first-line medications such as propylthiouracil (PTU) to block peripheral effects of TH and propranolol (Inderal) which blocks conversion of T_4 to T_3.[1,23,32] Medications such as iodides and lithium can also be used to inhibit TH release. Propranolol is the first-line drug for the treatment of the beta-adrenergic effects such as tachycardia, hypertension, and tremors.[11,17] Dexamethasone (Decadron) can be used as a T_4 to T_3 conversion blocker and to assist with stabilization of the cell membrane; however, it may worsen hyperglycemia.[11,17,23] Supplemental oxygen should be given to support the increased oxygen demands of the hypermetabolic state, and hydration is a concern as it relates to loss of fluid from diaphoresis and insensible losses.[13,25] During the acute phase, nutrition must be supported to prevent loss of lean body mass and protein.[23,] For patients with exophthalmos, protrusion of the eye related to swelling, lubricating drops can be administered along with eye shields to protect the eyes.[1] For a more in-depth look at thyroid storm medications, see Table 25.3.

Conclusion

Rapid recognition of patients presenting with thyroid storm is the key to decreasing mortality. If the patient's clinical presentation is consistent with thyroid storm, do not delay treatment to await confirmation of thyroid function tests.[1,11,17] Treatment focuses on decreasing thyroid hormone synthesis and secretion, blocking sympathetic nervous system stimulation, and supporting circulation.

Hypothyroidism and Myxedema Coma

Hypothyroidism is the most common thyroid dysfunction. The different types of hypothyroidism can range from subclinical asymptomatic to severe forms of hypothyroidism with multiple system effects. Hypothyroidism occurs more commonly in older adults, with a 14% to 18% occurrence.[11] As with all other HPA dysfunctions, there is a primary and a secondary cause. Primary disorders (95% of all cases) are thyroid gland dysfunction, which occurs commonly in Hashimoto's thyroiditis or in response to antithyroid treatment.[1] The decreased function of the thyroid gland leads to decreased production of TH and an increase in TSH secretion, leading to formation of a goiter.[11,17,30,32] Secondary causes from dysfunction in the hypothalamus or pituitary are less common and result from failure of the pituitary to produce TSH. In addition to primary and secondary causes, there are iatrogenic causes that include treatment for Graves' disease, thyroidectomy, external iodine ingestion, amiodarone lithium, interferon, and interleukin-2.[11,17,30,32]

Myxedema coma is an uncommon but life-threatening disorder in which profound hypothyroidism occurs.[11] This causes an inability to regulate temperature, altered mental status, and impaired respiratory function, which eventually leads to a coma.[1,11] It occurs most commonly in older women who have undiagnosed or subclinical hypothyroidism with exposure to cold, infection, stress of illness, or medications.[17]

Patients at Risk

Patients at risk for the development of hypothyroidism and possible myxedema coma are older, female, hospitalized patients, and Caucasians with preexisting hypothyroidism.[1,11] The incidence of hypothyroidism ranges from 0.5% to 6% in younger patients and up to 14% to 18% in older adult patients, with a fivefold to tenfold increased incidence in women more than men.[1,32] If not promptly treated, myxedema coma carries a 30% to 60% mortality rate.[1] Even with immediate recognition and treatment, mortality rates are 45%.[1,32]

Precipitating factors for patients at risk include an infection, exposure to cold, heart failure, trauma, surgical procedures, CVA, gastrointestinal bleed, and carbon dioxide retention. Common medication causes include sedatives, tranquilizers, narcotics, diuretics, amiodarone, lithium, and phenytoin as well as nonadherence with thyroid replacement.[1,11,17,30,32]

Clinical Presentation

Confusion with decreased level of consciousness related to reduced blood flow, reduced oxygen delivery, and decreased glucose levels; hypothermia; and unique thick skin changes are present in most patients with hypothyroidism. The thick skin is a result of accumulation of a mucopolysaccharide substance consisting of hyaluronic acid and chondroitin sulfate bound to protein to form a sticky gel in the interstitial spaces. Water and sodium are drawn into the interstitial space, which leads to nonpitting edema and intravascular volume loss.[1,11,17] Other

TABLE 25.3 Medications Used in Thyroid Storm

Medications	Actions	Dosages	Special Considerations
Propylthiouracil (PTU) Methimazole (Tapazole)	Inhibits synthesis of TH (organification of iodine) Inhibits peripheral conversion of T_4 to T_3	600 mg loading, then 300–400 mg PO/NG/PR every 6 h	Comatose patients will need NG tube for instillation; only dispensed in an oral preparation
Potassium iodide	Iodides inhibit release of TH by accumulation of colloids and decrease vascularity of gland	5 drops every 6 h PO	Precede administration with thioamides (PTU) to prevent thyroid storm Administer 1 h after thiomide
Propranolol (Inderal)	Beta blocker reduces symptoms of increased thyroid hormone: tachycardia, increased BP and blocks conversion of T_4 to T_3	40–80 mg PO every 4 h; 2 mg IV slow every 4 h	First-line drug and may be only drug needed to control thyroid storm Avoid in decompensated HF
Dexamethasone or Hydrocortisone (Solu-Cortef)	Blocks peripheral conversion of T_4 to T_3; antipyretic	Dexamethasone 2 mg every 6 h, × 48 h, then taper Hydrocortisone 100 mg IV every 8 h	Use of steroids in thyroid storm has been associated with increased survival

BP, Blood pressure; *HF,* heart failure; *HR,* heart rate; *MVo₂* → MVO_2, myocardial oxygen consumption; *NG,* nasogastric; *PO,* per os; *TH,* thyroid hormone; T_3, triiodothyronine; T_4, thyroxine.
Data from References 1, 6, 11, 13, 17, 25, 30, and 32.

common physical findings related to this accumulation of substance in the interstitial spaces are hoarseness and periorbital edema.[1,11,32]

Decreased intravascular volume, decreased metabolism, and peripheral vasoconstriction lead to decreased blood flow to the extremities. This inhibits the generation of heat to the hands and feet.[11,17] Physiologic changes related to the cardiac system include decreased blood pressure, heart rate, contractility, and cardiac output as well as slowed conductivity.[11,17,32] Nonspecific ST changes and T wave inversion are common. Low-voltage and ventricular dysrhythmias may be noted.[1,11,17] Pulmonary changes occur as a result of a blunted response in the chemoreceptors that detect hypercarbia and hypoxemia. Hypoventilation is related to muscle weakness. Pleural effusions are common because of sodium and water drawn into the intravascular spaces.[1,11,17,32] Hypoglycemia is common and related to the inability to break down carbohydrates, lipids, and protein as an energy source. CVA must be ruled out because patients often present as unconscious or obtunded.[11,17]

Diagnostic Evaluation

There are several tests that can be ordered to assess thyroid function. As the most sensitive indicator, TSH level will be elevated in primary disease states when the thyroid is dysfunctional. In secondary disease states TSH level is decreased, representing a dysfunction in the HPA. T_4 and T_3 levels are decreased and unreliable measurements in myxedema coma because most T_4 and T_3 are bound to protein. Reliable assessments are free T_4 (FT_4) and free T_3 (FT_3). Additional lab values include electrolytes (primarily serum sodium), serum glucose, serum osmolality, and arterial blood gases to assess hypoxia and hypercarbia.[1]

Interprofessional Plan of Care

Initial priorities for the patient with myxedema coma should include intubation and mechanical ventilation for correction of hypercapnia and hypoxia. IV thyroid hormone replacement should be started while awaiting confirmation of myxedema from laboratory tests. A serum cortisol should be drawn to rule out adrenal insufficiency and cortisol replacement should be done based on the cortisol level along with the thyroid hormone replacement. Correction of hypothermia should be done with passive rewarming blankets and increased room temperature. In addition, hyponatremia of sodium levels less than 120 mEq/L should be corrected with hypertonic (3%) saline in small doses to avoid volume overload. These patients are at increased risk for myocardial ischemia and infarction, therefore close cardiac monitoring is imperative.[11,17,32] Because gastric motility decreases, food should be withheld early until severe hypothyroidism reversal has been established.

Conclusion

Early recognition of patients presenting with myxedema coma is the key to decreasing mortality as this dysfunction affects every body system. Immediate and aggressive management consisting of multiple treatments is imperative to survival. The plan of care should focus on replacing thyroid hormone, restoring sympathetic nervous system stimulation, and supporting circulation and oxygenation.

ADRENAL INSUFFIENCY IN CRITICAL ILLNESS

Definition of Adrenal Insufficiency

Addison's disease is defined as hypofunction of the adrenal gland, whereas adrenal insufficiency (AI) is defined as an absolute lack of cortisol or relative lack of cortisol that occurs in critical illness.[1,5,9,30] The normal stress response is activated in the face of pain, hypotension, hypoglycemia, hypoxemia, trauma, or cytokine discharge.[1,9] Normal cortisol levels are diurnal, peaking at approximately 8:00 a.m. with the lowest levels occurring at 4:00 p.m.[1,9] Critically ill patients in stressed states can have consistently high levels of serum cortisol, from 2 to 10 times normal, with loss of diurnal differences.[1,9,24]

In an acute illness functional AI can occur without warning. There is no structural abnormality in the pituitary or adrenal gland; the problem is one of down regulation of the cortisol receptors related to proinflammatory cytokines competing with glucocorticoid, which can lead to a diminished response to exogenous replacement of ACTH or cortisol. Down regulation, along with diminished cortisol breakdown, can result in misleading normal cortisol levels.[2,7,9]

Patients at Risk

The incidence of AI in general is less than 0.01%. However, the incidence increases up to 30% overall in all critically ill patients, and with patients in septic shock the incidence may be as high as 50% to 60%. It is difficult to determine the exact percentage as the underlying disease processes, as well as the severity of illness, vary widely. Patients with sepsis, systemic inflammatory response syndrome (SIRS), and multiple traumas, as well as complicated surgical patients, are at the greatest risk for AI[1,2,9,10] (Table 25.4). In addition, medications used in the treatment of critically ill patients can lead to secondary AI (e.g., corticosteroids); or increased cortisol metabolism, such as with ketoconazole (Nizoral), etomidate (Amidate), rifampin (Xifaxan), and phenytoin (Dilantin). Furthermore, there are many other etiologies for AI: history of Addison's disease, patients who have recently received glucocorticoids or may be withdrawing from glucocorticoids, HIV infection; carcinoma of breast, lung, or liver; fungal infections; tuberculosis; acute hemorrhage; and pituitary removal.[1,2,9]

Clinical Presentation

The hallmark of AI in the critically ill is refractory, vasopressor-dependent hypotension with increased cardiac output and decreased systemic vascular resistance.[9,13,26,30] The alpha and beta receptors develop SIRS-induced catecholamine insensitivity[16,19] and become less responsive to cortisol even if the serum cortisol level is normal. These desensitized alpha and beta receptors may lead to decreased vascular responsiveness and myocardial depression.[19] Early recognition of AI in these patients can eliminate the need for high doses of vasopressors with possible harmful effects.[1,4,9,24,30] Other signs and symptoms of AI in critically ill patients include hyponatremia, hyperkalemia, hypercalcemia, hypoglycemia, metabolic acidosis, and eosinophilia. Nonspecific signs include weakness, fatigue, weight loss, unexplained fever, and hyperdynamic circulation, which is usually associated with SIRS or septic shock.[1,9,16,19]

TABLE 25.4 Pituitary, Adrenals, and Thyroid During Sepsis

Gland/Hormone	Effects of Sepsis	Effects of Hormone Replacement	Current Evidence-Based Management
Pituitary/ADH	Endotoxins in sepsis diminish catecholamine receptor response Vasopressors use catecholamine receptors to stimulate constriction	Vasopressin: • Can reverse diminished response of catecholamine receptors • Causes pulmonary vasoconstriction • Lowers heart rate via baroceptor mediation • Stimulates ACTH release, leading to increased serum cortisol levels	Vasopressin administration 0.04 unit/min IV infusion can reduce or eliminate need for vasopressors
Adrenal/cortisol	Inactivation of fludrocortisol Decreased number of or response to fludrocortisol receptors "Catecholamine insensitivity" receptors become less responsive to catecholamines (alpha and beta)	Cortisol can reverse diminished response of catecholamine receptors	Hydrocortisone replacement should be considered for all critically ill patients based on patient response Future research is needed to determine the appropriate hydrocortisone replacement dose
Thyroid/T_3, T_4	Decreased conversion of T_4 to T_3 Dysfunction of protein binding to TH	Hypothyroxinemia is a strong predictor of mortality; 84% mortality rate noted for an initial T_4 value <3 mg/dL	No substantial evidence to show T_4 replacement improves outcomes

ACTH, Adrenocorticotropic hormone; *ADH*, antidiuretic hormone, *TH*, thyroid hormone; *T_3*, triiodothyronine; *T_4*, thyroxine.
Data from References 2, 4, 8, 16, and 19.

Diagnostic Evaluation

Adrenal insufficiency in critically ill patients has been the focus of numerous studies over the last decade. The commonly used term is *relative adrenal insufficiency* in critical illness. The ACTH adrenal pathway is producing a maximal amount of cortisol; however, it remains insufficient to meet the demand. The mechanism is related to reduced cortisol breakdown, which suppresses ACTH plasma levels, thus reducing cortisol production. Cortisol responses to the ACTH stimulation test show a positive correlation between cortisol production and clearance.[2] The ACTH stimulation test measuring cortisol response continues to be an option to address adrenal insufficiency. Additionally, a random total cortisol of less than 10 mc/dL is also an indicator. Either an ACTH stimulation test or random cortisol should be performed early on all patients with a diagnosis of septic shock to recognize those patients in which cortisol replacement could be beneficial.[1,2,4,7,9,20,31] If the presumed diagnosis is AI, treatment should begin as soon as the test is completed, before results are reported. However, dexamethasone 2 mg IV can be administered before the corticotropin stimulation test because it does not interfere with the test.[1,4,9,24] A study by Vassiladi et al. evaluated adrenal dysfunction over time of a disease process and found that long-stay critically ill patients were at the greatest risk to develop AI.[31]

Jong et al. studied the response of the adrenal gland as a function of the endogenous cortisol-to-ACTH ratio to exogenous ACTH. The cortisol-to-ACTH ratio is used to measure adrenal sensitivity and can be followed over time from the acute critically ill phase through recovery. The study concluded that in critical illness-related corticosteroid insufficiency (AIRCI), decreased adrenal sensitivity to endogenous ACTH can predict a diminished response to exogenous ACTH, revealing adrenal dysfunction in any stage of the disease process.[7]

Other laboratory values should be followed closely, including complete blood count (CBC), electrolytes (sodium, potassium, calcium), BUN, serum creatinine, and serum glucose. Hypoglycemia should be treated with dextrose IV. Thyroid function tests should be performed to rule out thyroid dysfunction or assess concomitant thyroid disorder.[1,4,9,24] If AI is suspected or diagnosed and the patient has untreated hyperthyroidism, the glucocorticoid replacement dose should be doubled or tripled to compensate for increased cortisol breakdown and clearance.[4]

Interprofessional Plan of Care

If there is a high suspicion of adrenal insufficiency in the critically ill patient and a random serum cortisol measurement is less than 25 mcg/dL, hydrocortisone to 300 mg IV, given in divided doses, should be administered. The response to this treatment should be assessed. If there is clinical improvement, subsequent IV hydrocortisone doses should be considered.[1,4,9,24] Other treatments of AI focus on treatment of hypotension using fluids and vasopressors. In critical illness, ADH stores can become depleted, adding to the hypovolemia. Therefore, a continuous drip of arginine vasopressin (0.04 mg/min) may be used to treat hypotension.[4,9] Serum sodium depletion and serum potassium excess can be normalized by adding an aldosterone replacement, fludrocortisone.[4] In addition, hypoglycemia should be treated with 50% dextrose IV to normalize blood glucose level. A continuous infusion of 2 to 4 mg/kg of 25% dextrose in D_5W (5% dextrose in water) may be used to prevent further hypoglycemia.[1,4,13]

Conclusion

Adrenal insufficiency in the critically ill patient is an emergent situation superimposed on an already stressed patient. Adrenal insufficiency as a result of critical illness, especially sepsis and septic shock, requires early identification and management to prevent morbidity and mortality related to persistent catecholamine-resistant shock. The care of the patient focuses on replacing cortisol and correcting hypotension, hyponatremia, and hypoglycemia.

CASE STUDY 25.1

Adrenal Insufficiency

J.W. is a 24-year-old male with bilateral lower extremity (BLE) crush injuries. He was taken to a local hospital for stabilization and prepared for transfer to a trauma center. During the 75-minute ambulance transport, J.W. had several episodes of hypotension and hypoxemia. He was unconscious upon admission to the trauma center and was taken to the OR immediately for vascular repair of the popliteal and femoral arteries, debridement of BLE, and external fixation.

On day 3, J.W. spiked a fever of 103°F. He developed poor vascular supply and areas of necrosis, and he was returned to the OR for debridement. After surgery, he was hypotensive (65–70 mm Hg systolic) despite 2 L of normal saline (NS) and three boluses of 250 mL of 3% sodium chloride for hypotension and hyponatremia. He was started on norepinephrine (Levophed) drip for blood pressure support. Later that same afternoon, he returned to the OR for bilateral above-the-knee (AK) amputation. He was mechanically ventilated with fraction of inspired oxygen (Fio_2) 60% and continued to be hemodynamically unstable.

Assessment: central venous pressure (CVP) = 3 mm Hg; heart rate (HR) = 136 beats/min. Ventilator settings are as follows: assist control, rate = 16, Fio_2 = 60%, tidal volume (V_T) = 900, positive end-expiratory pressure (PEEP) = 15 mm Hg. Laboratory values: arterial blood gases (ABGs), pH = 7.27, partial pressure of arterial carbon dioxide ($Paco_2$) = 50 mm Hg, partial pressure of arterial oxygen (Pao_2) = 71 mm Hg; HCO_3^- = 17 mEq/L, O_2 saturation = 82%, Na^+ = 129 mEq/L, K^+ = 5.8 mEq/L, Ca^{2+} = 12 mg/dL, serum glucose = 84 mg/dL; Hgb = 10 g/dL, Hct = 30%, white blood count (WBC) = 2000/mm^3, platelets = 75,000/mm^3; creatinine = 2.8 mg/dL, BUN = 30 mg/dL, serum cortisol = 22 mcg/dL (6 p.m.). He remains hypotensive and unresponsive to fluids. The provider orders vasopressin drip at a continuous rate of 0.04 unit/min.

On day 5, J.W. was placed on high-frequency oscillating ventilation for worsening respiratory failure related to ventilator-associated pneumonia. On day 7, J.W. expired.

Decision Point:

Discuss events of day 3 that place J.W. at risk for adrenal insufficiency.

Decision Point:

Discuss hemodynamic parameters as they relate to the diagnosis of adrenal insufficiency.

Decision Point:

Discuss ABGs and ventilator settings and what ventilator setting changes are needed.

Decision Point:

Discuss lab values as they pertain to adrenal insufficiency.

Decision Point:

Discuss the serum cortisol level.

Decision Point:

Discuss why the provider ordered a vasopressin drip.

Decision Point:

Why did the provider order dexamethasone before a corticotropin stimulation test?

Decision Point:

Explain how a corticotropin stimulation test is performed and why the test was ordered.

Decision Point:

What would you expect the provider to order for the diagnosis of adrenal insufficiency?

REFERENCES

1. Baird, M. S., & Bethel, S. (2011). Endocrinologic disorders. In M. S. Baird, & S. Bethel (Eds.), *Manual of critical care nursing* (6th ed., pp. 695–749). St. Louis: Elsevier/Mosby.
2. Boonen, E., & Van den Berghe, G. (2014). Endocrine response to critical illness: novel insights and therapeutic implications. *J Clin Endocrinol Metab*, *99*(5), 1569–1582.
3. Brown, T. A. (2012). Endocrine physiology. In T. A. Brown (Ed.), *Rapid review physiology* (2nd ed., pp. 65–101). Philadelphia: Elsevier/Saunders.
4. Charmandari, E., et al. (2014). Adrenal insufficiency. *Lancet*, *38*, 2152–2167.
5. Costanza, L. S. (2014). Endocrine physiology. In L. S. Costanza (Ed.), *Physiology* (5th ed., pp. 383–446). Philadelphia: Saunders/Elsevier.
6. Daniels, G. H. (2011). Clinical endocrinology: a retrospective. In M. Shlomo (Ed.), *Williams textbook of endocrinology* (12th ed., pp. 13–29). Philadelphia: Saunders/Elsevier.
7. De Jong, M. F. C. (2015). Diminished adrenal sensitivity to endogenous and exogenous adrenocorticotropic hormone in critical illness: a prospective cohort study. *Crit Care*, *19*, 1. http://dx.doi.org/10.1186/s13054-014-0721-8.
8. Fenske, W., & Alloio, B. (2012). Current state and future perspectives in the diagnosis and management of diabetes insipidus: a clinical review. *J Clin Endocrionol Metab*, *97*(10), 3426–3437.
9. Gerlach, H. (2011). Adrenal insufficiency. In J. L. Vincent, E. Abraham, F. Moore, P. M. Kockanek, & M. P. Fink (Eds.), *Textbook of critical care* (6th ed., pp. 1215–1254). Philadelphia: Elsevier/Saunders.
10. Gibbison, B., Angelini, G. D., & Lightman, S. L. (2013). Dynamic output and control of the hypothalamic-pituitary-adrenal axis in critical illness and major surgery. *BMJ*, *111*(3), 347–360.
11. Hampton, J. (2013). Thyroid gland disorder emergencies. *AACN Adv Crit Care*, *24*(3), 325–332.
12. Hannon, M. J., & Thompson, C. J. (2016). In J. L. Jameson (Ed.), *Endocrinology: adult and pediatric* (7th ed., pp. 298–311). Philadelphia: Elsevier/Saunders.
13. Hassan-Smith, Z., et al. (2011). Overview of the endocrine response to critical illness: how to measure it and when to treat. *Best Pract Res Clin Endocrinol Metab*, *25*(2011), 705–717.
14. Hong, L. (2014). Management of hyponatremia associated with syndrome of inappropriate antidiuretic hormone secretion. *Top Clin Nutr*, *29*(2), 187–196.
15. Huffmyer, J. L., & Nmeergut, E. C. (2013). In H. C. Hemmings, & T. D. Egan (Eds.), *Pharmacology and physiology for anesthesia: foundations and clinical application* (pp. 523–535). Philadelphia: Elsevier/Saunders.
16. Khardori, R., & Castillo, D. (2012). Endocrine and metabolic changes during sepsis: an update. *Med Clin N Am*, *96*(2012), 1095–1105.
17. Klubo-Giezdzinska, J., & Wartofsky, L. (2012). Thyroid emergencies. *Med Clin North Am*, *96*(2012), 385–403.
18. Lamberts, S. W. J. (2011). Endocrinology and aging. In M. Shlomo (Ed.), *Williams textbook of endocrinology* (12th ed., pp. 1219–1233). Philadelphia: Saunders/Elsevier.
19. Milas, Z., Naylor, D. F., & Milas, K. (2014). Endocrine changes in critical illness K. In J. L. Cameron, & A. M. Cameron (Eds.), *Current surgical therapy* (11th ed., pp. 1279–1284). Philadelphia: Elsevier/Saunders.
20. Obini, J. B., et al. (2013). Predictive factors of adrenal insufficiency in patients admitted to acute medical wards: a case control study. *BMC Endocrine Disorders 13*(3). http://www.biomedicalcentral.com/1472-6823/13/3.
21. Peri, A., & Combe, C. (2012). Considerations regarding the management of hyponatremia secondary to SIADH. *Best Pract Res Clin Endocrinol Metab*, *26*, S16–S26 Suppl.
22. Saifan, C., et al. (2013). Diabetes insipidus: a challenging diagnosis with new drug therapies. *ISRN Nephrol*, 797620.
23. Sanborn, M. R., & Sims, C. A. (2013). Endocrine evaluation. In L. E. Le Roux, J. M. Levine, & A. Kofke (Eds.), *Monitoring in neurocritical care* (pp. 200–208). Philadelphia: Elsevier/Saunders.
24. Schroeder, E., & Low Wang, C. C. (2013). Adrenal insufficiency. In M. McDermott (Ed.), *Endocrine secrets* (6th ed., pp. 254–260). Philadelphia: Elsevier/Saunders.

25. Siegel, S. C., & Hodak, S. P. (2012). Thyrotoxicosis. *Med Clin North Am, 96*(2012), 175–201.
26. Sims, C. (2010). How do I diagnose and manage acute endocrine emergencies in the ICU? In C. S. Deutschman, & P. J. Neiglan (Eds.), *Evidence-based practice of critical care* (pp. 525–541). Philadelphia: Elsevier/Saunders.
27. Sobel, S. I., et al. (2014). Aging and endocrinology. In M. McDermott (Ed.), *Endocrine secrets* (6th ed., pp. 453–465). Philadelphia: Elsevier/Saunders.
28. Thomas, Z., et al. (2010). Drug induced endocrine disorders in the intensive care unit. *Crit Care Med, 38*(Suppl. 6), S219–S230.
29. Todd, S. R. (2014). Disorders of water balance. In J. E. Prillo, & P. R. Dellinger (Eds.), *Critical care medicine: principles of diagnosis and management* (4th ed., pp. 841–849). Philadelphia, PA: Saunders.
30. Van Den Berghe, G. (2016). Endocrine aspects of critical care medicine. In J. L. Jameson (Ed.), *Endocrinology: adult and pediatric* (7th ed., pp. 2084–2095). Philadelphia, PA: Saunders.
31. Vassiliadi, D. A., et al. (2014). Longitudinal assessment of adrenal function in the early and prolonged phases of critical illness in septic patients: relations to cytokine levels and outcomes. *J Endocrinol Metab, 991*(12), 4471–4480.
32. Wiersinga, W. M. (2015). Hypothyroidism and myxedema coma. In J. L. Jameson (Ed.), *Endocrinology: adult and pediatric* (6th ed., pp. 1540–1556). Philadelphia: Elsevier/Saunders.

26

Blood Conservation and Blood Component Replacement

Dana M. Kyles

Transfusion practices continue to evolve with rapid progression seen over the past several decades. While there is a belief that poorer outcomes are associated with higher rates of blood administration, and that many blood transfusions are unnecessarily utilized, approximately 14 million blood transfusions occur in the United States annually.[62] Blood transfusion was the most frequently performed procedure in 2009, occurring in more than 10% of all hospitalizations that included a procedure.[38,54] In addition, these patients may also receive other blood components to manage coagulopathy or active bleeding. Although blood transfusions can be life-saving, they can also be associated with risks ranging from poorer patient outcomes, such as a transfusion reaction, to death. Several large randomized clinical trials[7,22,23,34] and prospective observational studies[10,61] have assessed the efficacy of allogeneic red blood cell (RBC) transfusions. The trials indicated that restricting RBC transfusions in nonhemorrhaging patients showed no significant negative effect on patient outcomes, and may improve outcomes in some patient populations.

Anemia is a common problem in critically ill patients and is often associated with poor outcomes. The causes are multifactorial and thought to be a result of frequent iatrogenic phlebotomy, coagulation disorders, sepsis, nutritional deficiencies (i.e., iron, vitamin B_{12}, folic acid), bone marrow suppression, renal failure, impaired erythropoietin response and production, hemodilution, inflammation, abnormalities in iron metabolism, and other severe illnesses (Table 26.1). The primary causes of anemia are blood loss and abnormal or inadequate production of RBCs. Acute anemia, the consequence of an abrupt reduction in the number of RBCs, may be due to hemolysis or acute frank hemorrhage as a result of surgical procedures, gastrointestinal (GI) bleeding, or trauma. An additional cause of anemia in critically ill patients is blunted production of endogenous erythropoietin, consistent with anemia related to chronic inflammation.[8,9] While mean serum erythropoietin concentrations are much lower in critically ill patients compared to patients with iron-deficiency anemia, there does not appear to be an association between erythropoietin and hemoglobin (Hgb) levels.[55]

Rapid alterations of serum iron metabolism can contribute to critical care–associated anemia. This is thought to be a result of the heightened inflammatory process, disturbance in iron circulation, decreased serum iron levels, and increased iron storage. Minimum information exists about the reason for altered iron metabolism in the development of iron anemia in critically ill patients.[45] Transferrin, serum iron, and total iron-binding capacity are low in critically ill patients.[9] Serum ferritin levels are normal or elevated. Iron deficiency is a potential cause of blood loss because RBCs require iron for production, growth, and maturation. When there is insufficient iron, less Hgb is produced in the RBCs, resulting in decreased oxygen delivery to the tissues.

Approximately 63% of critically ill patients have Hgb levels below 12 g/dL on admission to critical care.[39] By day 3 in critical care, the percentage of patients with a Hgb level of less than 12 g/dL increases to 95%.[9] Clinical manifestations of mild to moderate anemia are tachycardia, exertional dyspnea, fatigue, and weakness. Severe anemia can cause decreased oxygen delivery to tissues, resulting in anaerobic metabolism and lactate production, myocardial infarction, and ischemic stroke.

To restore and maintain hemostasis, oxygen-carrying capacity, and quality of life for the patient, clinicians must be knowledgeable about component therapy, blood component modifications, adverse effects, blood conservation techniques, and alternatives to transfusion.

CONTROVERSIES IN TRANSFUSION

An RBC transfusion provides immediate improvement of low Hgb levels resulting from deficient RBC production or blood loss. Normal Hgb levels are between 12 and 16 g/dL in women and 13.5 and 18 g/dL in men.[6] The optimal Hgb level in critically ill patients has not been determined. When Hgb levels are reduced, the oxygen-carrying capacity and total oxygen content in the blood decrease. Hgb is intended to rapidly bind oxygen in the lungs and unload it in the tissues.

The normal relationship between Hgb and oxygen unloading is illustrated by the oxyhemoglobin dissociation curve (Fig. 26.1). Oxygen's capability to bind to Hgb is affected by several factors that result in a shifting or reshaping the curve. Hgb function may be altered by a variety of reasons (e.g., pH or 2,3-diphosphoglycerate [DPG] levels). When pH is decreased or DPG levels are increased, oxygen affinity for Hgb decreases, shifting the dissociation curve to the right thereby increasing the delivery of oxygen to tissues. The standard curve is also shifted to the right by an increase in temperature or partial pressure

TABLE 26.1 Selected Types of Anemia

Type of Anemia	Definition/Pathophysiology
Anemia of chronic inflammatory disease	Chronic disorders with an inflammatory component, such as infection, leading to anemia
Aplastic anemia	Potentially fatal, caused by destruction of bone marrow stem cells and inhibited RBC production; results in pancytopenia and bone marrow hypoplasia
Iron deficiency anemia	Inadequate supply of iron; need for iron is greater than absorption because of impaired gastrointestinal absorption or blood loss from trauma, severe menorrhagia, or gross hematuria
Pregnancy	During pregnancy, plasma volume increases while RBC mass decreases
Sickle cell anemia	Congenital disease causing hemolysis and vascular occlusion because of an abnormal Hgb molecule causing RBC destruction and a sickled shape
Thalassemias	Hereditary hemolytic anemia characterized by defective and impaired Hgb production and impaired RBC synthesis

Hgb; Hemoglobin; *RBC,* red blood cell.

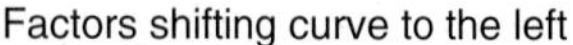

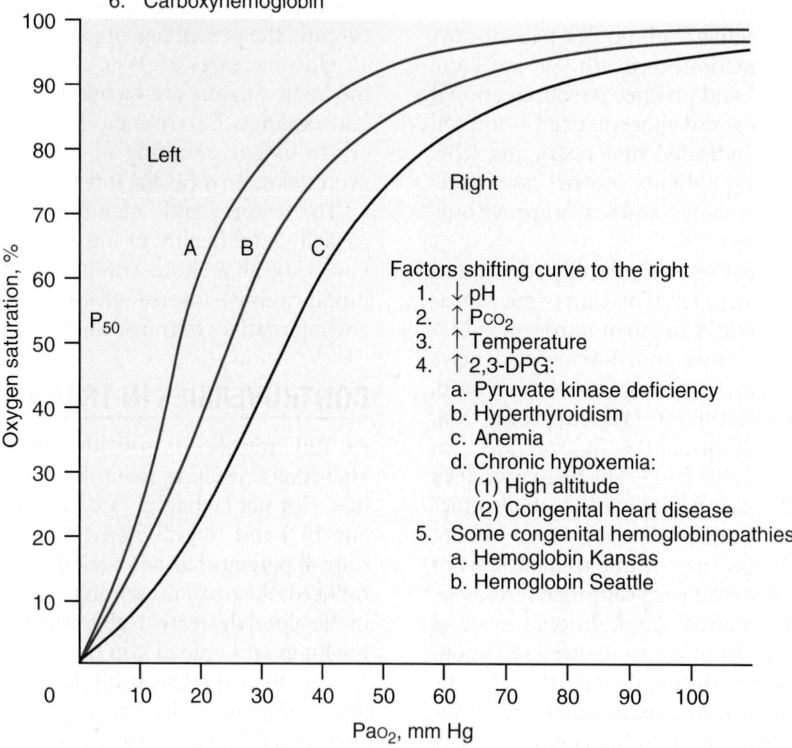

FIG. 26.1 Oxyhemoglobin dissociation curve. *A,* The curve is shifted to the left because of hemoglobin's increased affinity for oxygen. *B,* The standard oxyhemoglobin dissociation curve. *C,* The curve is shifted to the right because of hemoglobin's decreased affinity for oxygen. *2,3-DPG,* 2,3-diphosphoglycerate; *Pao_2,* partial pressure of arterial oxygen; *Pco_2,* partial pressure of carbon dioxide. (Modified from Kinney M.R., et al. (Eds.), (1998). *AACN's clinical reference for critical care nursing* (4th ed.). St. Louis: Mosby. In L.D. Urden, K.M. Stacy, & M.E. Lough, (2014). *Critical care nursing* (7th ed.). St. Louis: Mosby.)

of arterial carbon dioxide ($Paco_2$).[41] Alternatively, the curve is shifted to the left by an increased pH or by decreased DPG levels, temperature, or $Paco_2$. A leftward shift increases the affinity of the oxygen for the Hgb, simplifying the mechanism in which Hgb adheres to oxygen, while making it more difficult for oxygen to be released.[41]

Historically, both the literature and clinical practice supported the notion that an RBC transfusion is necessary when the Hgb level is less than 10 g/dL. Such recommendations are based more on tradition than clinical trials and do not take into account the patient's clinical scenario (e.g., whether the patient is experiencing symptoms, the patient's tolerance to the anemia, the underlying pathophysiology).

In 1999, the results of the Transfusion Requirements in Critical Care (TRICC) study were published, recommending the use of restrictive transfusion thresholds in the critically ill patient, suggesting that anemia does not negatively affect short-term mortality[23,27,35] A randomized, controlled clinical trial by Hebert et al. suggests a restrictive transfusion threshold appears to be safe in critically ill patients with cardiovascular disease.[23] Currently, the typical transfusion threshold is a Hgb level of 7 to 8 g/dL, equivalent to a hematocrit (Hct) of 21% to 24%.[59] However, Hgb or Hct levels should not be the only transfusion triggers because this may result in unnecessary administration of blood components.[25]

A large number of patients are anemic on admission to critical care or become anemic during their critical care stay.[53] A lack of compelling data has resulted in variable transfusion practices and helps to explain the frequency of transfusion in critical care. A Canadian multicentered, randomized, controlled clinical study by Hebert et al. discovered that transfusion practices vary significantly among physicians and institutions.[22] A European prospective, observational, cross-sectional study of 3534 patients demonstrated that anemia was common in critically ill patients and that 37% of subjects with a Hgb concentration of less than 10 g/dL received a transfusion during their critical care admission.[61]

On the other hand, studies have revealed worse outcomes in critical care patients with anemia. The anemia and blood transfusion in the critically ill (CRIT) study demonstrated that a hemoglobin concentration of less than 9 g/dL during the critical care stay was a predictor of increased mortality and length of stay.[10] In patients undergoing cardiac surgery, preoperative anemia was associated with the development of infection, prolonged ventilation time, prolonged ICU stay, and death.[28,31]

Blood components continue to be transfused in critical care despite increasing evidence that blood transfusions may contribute to adverse outcomes (e.g., immunosuppression, transfusion-related acute lung injury [TRALI], organ dysfunction, transmission of infectious diseases [i.e., hepatitis B or West Nile virus], hemolytic and nonhemolytic transfusion reactions, and alloimmunization).

BLOOD CONSERVATION

At the present time, healthcare professionals are pursuing new alternatives to blood transfusions as many patients are disinclined to receive blood because of religious convictions, medical concerns, or personal preference. There are a growing number of alternatives already being instituted to decrease the need for a blood transfusion (e.g., bloodless surgery programs, the use of pharmacologic agents, laser technology or cauterization, and volume expansion). Another important alternative modification would include a universally acceptable, lower transfusion threshold, except in patients with ongoing hemorrhage.

Blood conservation requires vigilant preparation, proactive strategies involving interprofessional teams to prevent complications, and careful monitoring of the patient. The primary principles of blood conservation include increasing erythropoiesis, minimizing perioperative and iatrogenic blood loss, and optimizing hemostasis and blood transfusion practices.

Increasing Erythropoiesis

To maintain adequate oxygen delivery to tissues, there must be an adequate number of circulating RBCs. When tissues experience hypoxia, the kidneys and liver respond by producing erythropoietin. Nutrients that play an important role in erythropoiesis include iron, vitamin B_{12}, and folate. Euvolemic anemic patients with adequate tissue perfusion may benefit from the administration of these nutrients. Others may require pharmacologic intervention with agents such as recombinant human erythropoietin (rHuEPO) to increase erythropoiesis (Table 26.2).

Minimizing Perioperative and Iatrogenic Blood Loss

Various techniques can be used during surgery to minimize bleeding and decrease the need for transfusion. Hypotensive anesthesia, also known as controlled hypotension, involves intentionally lowering the patient's blood pressure below normal throughout surgery. This is performed while maintaining perfusion to the heart, lungs, and other organs and tissues. Blood loss is thought to decrease when the patient's blood pressure is low. Other techniques for minimizing blood loss associated with surgery are listed in Table 26.3.

Optimizing Hemostasis and Blood Transfusion Practices

Hemostasis is the method of fibrin formation at the site of vascular injury. This includes the formation of the platelet plug, coagulation activation, and cessation of antithrombotic control mechanisms and fibrin clot degradation, also known as fibrinolysis.

Traditionally, the clotting cascade was described as consisting of an intrinsic and extrinsic pathway. While this classical view of the clotting cascade has been valuable in the interpretation of clotting times, it is considered an in vitro model and may not be physiologically accurate. It has been established that the exposure of tissue factor at the site of injury is the primary physiologic event initiating clotting whereas subsequent coagulation response occurs on the platelet surface and is regulated by specific receptors.[36]

The critical care nurse caring for a patient undergoing bloodless treatment should be knowledgeable of pharmacologic means and other alternatives to transfusion to prevent and treat anemia.

ALTERNATIVES TO TRANSFUSION

Recombinant Human Erythropoietin

Recombinant human erythropoietin (rHuEpo) is a synthetic growth factor used to supplement the intrinsic hormone normally produced by the kidneys that promotes the formation of RBCs by the bone marrow. Erythropoietin regulates the production of RBCs and initiates the production of Hgb. In the setting of anemia or anticipated anemia, administering erythropoietin prophylactically may decrease the need for blood transfusions.

TABLE 26.2 Pharmacologic Means to Prevent and Treat Anemia in Critical Care

Medication	Action	Dose	Special Considerations
Aprotinin (Trasylol)	Inhibits fibrinolysis by attaching to plasminogen; prevents it from attaching to the fibrin clot	Cardiopulmonary bypass surgery: 10,000 units IV over 10 min, then loading dose of 1–2 million units over 20–30 min, followed by infusion of 250,000–500,000 units/h until surgery is complete 1–2 million units are typically added to pump priming fluid as well	Often given during cardiac surgery procedures requiring cardiopulmonary bypass to prevent platelet dysfunction. Potent hemostatic agent that prevents blood loss and preserves platelet function. Naturally occurring serine protease inhibitor Risk of anaphylaxis if patient exposed to products containing aprotinin within previous 12 months
Conjugated estrogens	Exact mechanism unknown although it may include reactivation of platelets and elevated factor VIII and vWF coagulation factors	Abnormal uterine bleeding; 25 mg IV; repeat in 6–12 h if needed	
Epsilon aminocaproic acid (Amicar)	Inhibits fibrinolysis by attaching to plasminogen; prevents it from attaching to the fibrin clot	Hemorrhage: 4–5 g IV over 1 h, then 1 g/h for 8 h or until hemostasis achieved Can also give 5 g PO, then 1 g/h PO for 8 h or until hemostasis achieved	Promotes clot stability and is useful as adjunctive therapy in hemophilia and some other bleeding disorders
Ferrous sulfate (especially if ferritin levels are decreased)	Hematopoietic agent	Dose depends upon formulation	
Fibrin sealants	The fibrinogen and thrombin in the fibrin sealant combines in the presence of factor XIII and calcium chloride to create a seal or glue	Used in a variety of surgical settings including trauma, neurosurgery, and cardiovascular	Tissue adhesive consisting of human fibrinogen and usually bovine thrombin Before commercial products available, used "fibrin glue" made in the blood bank from fibrinogen concentrations found in cryoprecipitate
Folate	Assists in RBC production	400 mcg daily	Nutritional support Megaloblastic anemia is caused by deficiencies in the B vitamins such as folate, vitamin B_{12}, or both
Recombinant human erythropoietin (rHuEpo)	Regulates erythropoiesis, resulting in higher hemoglobin/hematocrit levels Reduces the need for RBC transfusion	Dosing dependent on indication	Erythropoietin is released into the plasma and binds to the surface of RBCs located in the bone marrow in response to a decrease in tissue oxygenation
Recombinant activated factor VII (rFVIIa) (Novoseven)	Activates coagulation independent of factors VIII and IX Initiates generation of thrombin and fibrin formation Coagulation is activated locally at the site of vascular injury RFVIIa binds with tissue factor and activates factors IX and X to their active forms, such as IXa and Xa	IV bolus only; give over 2–5 min Hemophilia A or B patients with inhibitors: 90 mcg/kg given every 2 h until hemostasis is achieved or the treatment has been determined inadequate 35 to 120 mcg/kg in clinical trials For factor VII deficiency, use 15–30 mcg/kg every 4–6 h until adequate hemostasis is achieved Depending on severity of bleeding, dose and interval may be adjusted	Hemostatic agent used to treat hemophilia A or B patients with or without inhibitors in the United States. Also FDA-approved for treatment of factor VII deficiency Hypersensitivity to mouse, hamster, or bovine protein products
Tranexamic acid	Antifibrinolytic agent that inhibits the activation of plasminogen to plasmin, preventing it from attaching to the fibrin clot	Postoperative hemostasis: 0.5–1 g IV given 2–3 times daily for several days after surgery; if further dosing is needed, can use 1–1.5 g PO 3–4 times daily	Promotes clot stability and is useful as adjunctive therapy in hemophilia and some other bleeding disorders[27]
Vitamin B_{12}	Hematopoietic agent	Pernicious anemia: 100 mcg IM daily for 1 week, followed by 100 mcg IM every other day for 7 doses, then every 3–4 days for 2–3 weeks, then monthly	Megaloblastic anemia is caused by deficiencies in the B vitamins such as folate, vitamin B_{12}, or both
Vitamin C	Hematopoietic agent Enhances iron absorption	Dose ranges from 100 mg to 2 g daily depending upon severity of vitamin C deficiency	
Vitamin K (Phytonadione)	Required for the production of specific coagulation factors (factors II, VII, IX, and X) in the liver	Hypoprothrombinemia: 2.5–25 mg IV or subcutaneously, repeat in 6–8 h if needed Can also use 2.5–25 mg PO, repeat in 12–48 h if needed	Useful as adjunct therapy in the management of hemorrhage Causes of vitamin K deficiency include inadequate dietary intake, poor absorption, and drug interactions (e.g., antibiotics, stroke medications)

FDA, Food and Drug Administration; *IM,* intramuscular; *PO,* per os; *RBC,* red blood cell; *vWF,* von Willebrand's factor.
Data from References 16, 22, 27, 34, 35, 46, 50, and 51.

TABLE 26.3 Optimizing Hemostasis and Minimizing Blood Loss

Increasing Erythropoiesis	Minimizing Perioperative and Latrogenic Blood Loss	Optimizing Hemostasis and Blood Transfusion Practices
Discontinue medications known to inhibit platelet function (e.g., aspirin, corticosteroids, naproxen [Aleve], clopidogrel [Plavix], ticlopidine [Ticlid], and heparin) Discontinue herbal replacements that may predispose to bleeding (e.g., garlic, ginkgo, ginseng) Administer iron, vitamin B_{12}, and folate	Minimize blood draws by using micro- or pediatric-size blood specimen tubes for laboratory testing Use group blood draws to minimize discard volumes Use smallest recommended discard when drawing samples from lines Apply digital pressure to bleeding sites and institute mechanical occlusion of bleeding vessels by using hemostatic clips or clamps to obstruct blood vessels to minimize bleeding at site of surgery Consider preoperative autologous donation Consider autologous blood cell salvage (autotransfusion) Use controlled hypotension: intentionally lowers blood pressure to decrease pressure on blood vessels to minimize bleeding Consider acute normovolemic hemodilution Consider surgical technique (e.g., staged surgeries)	For external bleeding, consider use of topical hemostatic agents (e.g., thrombin) Discontinue medications that may alter coagulation factor activity Avoid hypothermia (keep patient's temperature > 35°C) Apply ice pack after phlebotomy to limit hematoma formation

Data from Reference 16.

RHuEpo requires adequate iron stores in order to work effectively. Oral iron will not be sufficient if there is ongoing blood loss. Intravenous (IV) iron supplements, therefore, may be more advantageous. Response to rHuEpo may not be seen until day 3 after therapy begins in iron-depleted patients. Currently, the use of erythropoiesis-stimulating agents in critical care units is off-label unless the patient has an approved clinical indication.[1,11,49]

Vitamin K

Bleeding can occur from vitamin K deficiency resulting from poor nutritional status, antibiotic use, infections, or anticoagulants (e.g., warfarin [Coumadin]). Vitamin K assists in the production of calcium-binding coagulation factors II, VII, IX, and X. Although plasma and plasma products can correct factor deficiencies associated with vitamin K deficiency, they should be used only when there is a risk of life-threatening bleeding. According to the *Circular of Information for the Use of Human Blood and Blood Components*, plasma is contraindicated when coagulopathy can be corrected more effectively with specific therapy, such as vitamin K.[4]

BLOOD COMPONENT REVIEW

The fundamental objective in transfusion therapy is to assist with oxygen delivery to tissues by maintaining the Hgb concentration. The second objective is to maintain hemostatic factor levels to prevent or control bleeding.

Whole blood (WB) is living tissue able to transport electrolytes, proteins, hormones, vitamins, antibodies, heat, and oxygen to the tissues of the body. It can be transfused as WB or as one of its components (Fig. 26.2). Up to four blood components can be processed from 1 unit of WB through a series of centrifugation methods. These components include RBCs, plasma, platelets, and cryoprecipitated antihemophilic factor, also known as cryoprecipitate. The plasma can be made into several blood derivatives (e.g., volume expanders, coagulation factor concentrates, and immune globulins).

Blood components may be administered through peripheral IV catheters, intraosseous catheters, portacaths, and most central lines, including peripherally inserted central catheter (PICC) lines. The size of the catheter lumen should be large enough to allow appropriate flow rates to occur and the component to be transfused within a 4-hour period. Blood components ideally should be transfused through an 18-gauge IV catheter with a standard 170- to 260-micrometer filter to remove clots and debris. Blood components may be transfused through a smaller gauge IV catheter without a pressure device. If the component is rapidly transfused using a pressure device, hemolysis may occur. To ease the flow of the blood component through the smaller size IV catheter, the component may be diluted with compatible IV fluid if the patient can tolerate the additional volume.

Only IV solutions approved by the US Food and Drug Administration (FDA) (e.g., 0.9% normal saline [NS]) may be administered with blood components. Other compatible FDA-approved solutions include Normosol and Plasmalyte. Lactated Ringer's and other solutions that contain calcium should never be infused through the same tubing as blood components. Calcium adheres to citrate (the anticoagulant mixed with the blood components to inhibit clotting during storage) and this leads to hypocalcemia.

Patients rarely need all of the components of WB. Therefore, only the necessary portions of WB are transfused to the patient. This treatment is referred to as blood component therapy, allowing several patients to benefit from 1 unit of WB. Exceptional patient and blood management is achieved by giving only the desired or essential components.

Whole Blood

Description

WB contains all blood elements (RBCs, white blood cells [WBCs], platelets, and plasma). Each unit of WB contains approximately 500 mL of WB and 70 mL of preservative-anticoagulant. The Hct of a typical unit is 33%.[12] This component is not ordinarily used because it is not as readily available

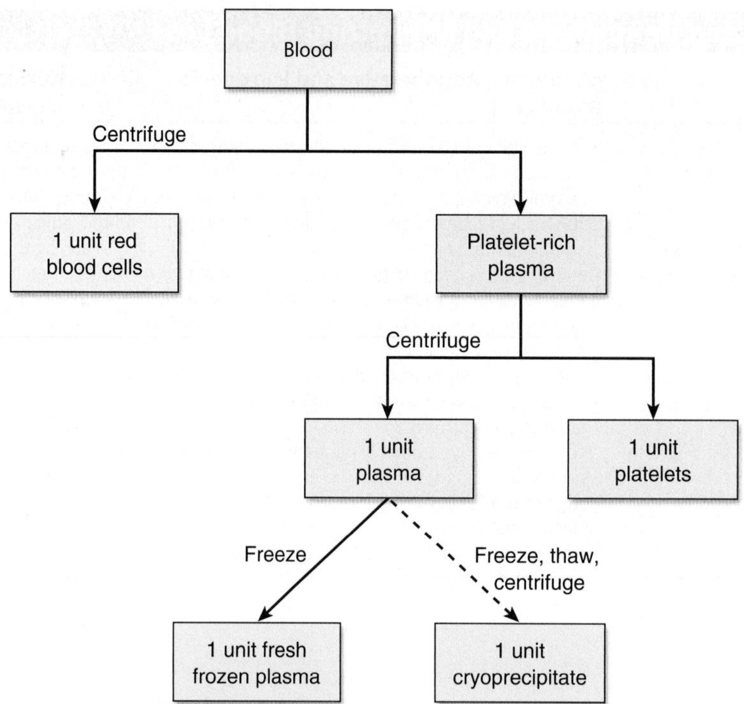

FIG. 26.2 Components made from whole blood.

TABLE 26.4 Compatibility Chart of ABO Antigens-Antibodies

Recipient's Blood Type	Antigens on Red Blood Cell	Antibodies in Plasma/Serum
O	Neither A nor B	Anti-A and anti-B
A	A	Anti-B
B	B	Anti-A
AB	A and B	Neither anti-A nor anti-B

TABLE 26.5 Proper Storage Temperatures for Blood Components

Component	Storage Temperature
Whole blood	1°–6°C
Red blood cells	1°–6°C
Fresh frozen plasma, liquid plasma, thawed plasma	1°–6°C
Platelets	20°–24°C
Cryoprecipitate	20°–24°C

Data from Reference 43.

as RBCs and other blood components. WB is generally used for autologous transfusion or collected to extract the blood components. It is uncommon to transfuse WB to the general patient population.

Once WB is placed in refrigeration, the platelets are no longer viable. During storage, therapeutic levels of coagulation factors V and VII decrease. A unit of WB must be ABO identical to the recipient (Table 26.4). Table 26.5 lists the proper storage temperature for blood components.

Indications

WB supplies oxygen-carrying capacity and restores blood volume expansion. It may be useful in bleeding patients with symptomatic anemia and a volume deficit in excess of 20% to 30% of their total blood volume. It may be administered to patients who require plasma for clotting factors and have symptomatic anemia or acute bleeding. For most purposes, a unit of WB is therapeutically equivalent to a unit of RBCs and a unit of plasma. WB is transfused regularly during open-heart surgery on adult and pediatric patients, and exchange transfusions in newborn babies with hemolytic disease.

Red Blood Cells

Description

Each year in the United States, approximately 15 million units of RBCs are transfused.[62] RBCs continually transport oxygen from the lungs to the tissues and are responsible for removing waste (i.e., carbon dioxide [CO_2]). As the blood passes through the body's tissue, Hgb, a protein that binds to oxygen, carries and releases the oxygen to the cells. Hgb contains iron, making it an excellent vehicle for transporting oxygen and CO_2.

RBCs account for approximately 40% of the blood volume. This ratio of RBCs to overall fluid volume is a frequently measured number—the Hct. Bone marrow is continually producing new blood cells. The average life cycle of an RBC is 120 days. After this length of time, RBCs are removed by both the liver and the spleen. The blood itself, however, is recirculated throughout the body. One unit of RBCs is prepared from WB. One unit of RBCs increases the Hgb by 1 g/dL and the Hct by 3% in a nonbleeding, 70-kg patient with an average blood volume.

Once RBCs are separated from a unit of WB, an anticoagulant preservative solution is added to prolong cell life. There are several types of anticoagulant solutions. Optisol, also known as AS-5, is one type of anticoagulant containing mannitol, sodium, adenine, and dextrose. Optisol extends the shelf life of

TABLE 26.6 **Component Compatibility Chart**

Recipient's Blood Type	COMPONENT TO BE TRANSFUSED AND PERMISSIBLE DONOR TYPE				
	Whole Blood	**Red Blood Cells**	**Plasma**	**Platelets**	**Cryoprecipitate**
O	O	O	Any type	Any type	Any type
A	A	A or O	A or AB	A or AB	A or AB
B	B	B or O	B or AB	B or AB	B or AB
AB	AB	Any type	AB	AB	AB

the unit to 42 days.[12] Most units of RBCs have a Hct between 55% and 80%, depending on the anticoagulant used. The average total volume of an RBC unit is 350 mL. One unit of RBCs contains close to 200 mL of RBCs, 100 mL of preservative solution, and approximately 50 mL of plasma. Components should not be placed in staff or patient refrigerators or refrigerators intended for medications. All RBC transfusions must be ABO/Rh compatible with the recipient (Tables 26.4 and 26.6). RBCs do not provide viable platelets, neutrophils, or clinically significant amounts of plasma containing coagulation factors. RBCs should be transfused within 4 hours once transfusion is started.

Improvements in cell preservative solutions over the past 15 years have increased the shelf life of RBCs from 21 to 42 days. Rare RBCs (i.e., ones lacking particular antigens) may be stored frozen for up to 10 years. When verifying the RBC label before transfusion, it is important to ensure that the date and time of the unit and the compatibility testing have not expired. If the compatibility testing has expired, the component is considered uncrossmatched and requires a justification form by the primary care provider.

Indications

The major indication for RBC transfusion is symptomatic anemia that has not or will not respond to treatment involving vitamin B_{12}, folic acid, or iron. Transfusion of RBCs should be contingent on clinical presentation rather than arbitrary Hct or Hgb values. Hebert et al. showed that a restrictive RBC transfusion strategy in critically ill patients, maintaining Hgb levels between 7 and 9 g/dL in patients who are not actively bleeding, appeared to be safe in patients with cardiovascular disease.[23] The possible exception to this was patients with acute myocardial infarction and unstable angina.[22] Other considerations include the duration of the anemia, intravascular volume of the recipient, any planned procedures, impending major blood loss, and any preexisting or coexisting medical conditions.

Fresh Frozen Plasma

Description

Fresh frozen plasma (FFP) is prepared from 1 unit of WB by centrifugation or by apheresis collection. It is then frozen and stored at a temperature less than −30°C for up to 1 year. FFP contains normal levels of all clotting factors except platelets. One unit of FFP has a volume of approximately 200 mL. Table 26.6 describes which blood types of FFP can be transfused with other blood types.

Indications

FFP is indicated when there is a need to replace coagulation factors in association with massive transfusion or disseminated intravascular coagulation (DIC), and for the treatment of thrombotic thrombocytopenic purpura. It is also indicated for reversal of warfarin anticoagulation or when high risk for bleeding is present (e.g., patients with documented coagulation factor deficiencies [i.e., liver dysfunction]) undergoing an invasive procedure. It should not be transfused as a colloid replacement or a primary volume expander, for nutritional support or replacement, or to promote wound healing. In the absence of an inhibitor (e.g., heparin), hemostasis can be achieved when coagulation factor (e.g., factors VII, X, V) levels are at least 30% of normal and the fibrinogen level is greater than 100 mg/dL.[3] The typical initial dose of FFP is 10 to 20 mL/kg but is dependent upon the patient's clinical response.

Thawed Plasma

Thawed plasma is derived from FFP, thawed at 30°C to 37°C, and maintained for up to 5 days. Thawed plasma differs from FFP because the factor V and factor VIII levels continue to decrease and, therefore, should not be transfused for replacement of these specific coagulation factors. Some institutions will relabel a unit of FFP as thawed plasma if the component is not transfused within 24 hours of being thawed. Others will label all thawed units of FFP as thawed plasma and store them at the appropriate temperature with a 5-day outdate. Thawed plasma should not be transfused in patients requiring replacement of factor V or factor VIII clotting factors. In addition, some facilities may have different or additional criteria used to determine whether patients may receive thawed plasma.

Cryoprecipitate

Description

Cryoprecipitate is obtained when a unit of FFP is slowly thawed at 4°C and centrifuged, producing a component rich in fibrinogen, fibronectin, factor VIII, von Willebrand's factor, and factor XIII. It is available in individual or pooled concentrates and should be considered if the patient is bleeding and the fibrinogen level is less than 100 mg/dL. Jointly, the American Association of Blood Banks (AABB), the American Red Cross, America's Blood Centers, and the Armed Services Blood Program's *Circular of Information for the Use of Human Blood and Blood Components*[4] require each pool of cryoprecipitate to contain a minimum of 150 mg of fibrinogen and 80 units of factor VIII in approximately 5 to 20 mL of plasma. Cryoprecipitate should be ABO compatible if suspended in plasma during preparation. One unit of cryoprecipitate contains a volume of 10 to 20 mL. Once collected, it can be stored at −18°C for a maximum of 1 year. Cryoprecipitate is later thawed in a 37°C water bath and prepared in individual bags or as a pooled component. Once thawed, it must be kept at room temperature and has an expiration time of 4 hours.[40]

Indications

Cryoprecipitate is indicated for bleeding patients with significant hypofibrinogenemia (< 100 mg/dL) or those who require an invasive procedure. The primary indications for cryoprecipitate are the treatment of fibrinogen dysfunction (e.g., patients with DIC) and fibrinogen deficiency (e.g., acute blood loss or liver disease). Effectiveness of cryoprecipitate transfusions is monitored by serum fibrinogen levels and assessment of clinical bleeding.

Platelets

Description

More than 2 million apheresis platelets are transfused each year in the United States.[62] Platelets are transfused for thrombocytopenia in patients with trauma, major surgical bleeding, platelet dysfunction, and hematologic malignancies. Platelet transfusions should be based on the patient's individual requirements and the cause of the platelet dysfunction or thrombocytopenia. Platelet transfusion practices remain controversial despite studies showing that a threshold of 10,000/μL for prophylactic platelet transfusion is effective in uncomplicated thrombocytopenic patients.[15] To reduce the formation of platelet alloantibodies, it is important to limit the platelet exposure to the recipient.

The plasma of a platelet component should be ABO compatible with the recipient's RBCs wherever possible. Multiple platelet transfusions can cause platelet refractoriness as a result of platelet alloimmunization—the formation of antibodies usually directed against human leukocyte antigens (HLAs) destroying randomly chosen donor platelets. Table 26.7 compares apheresis platelets with pooled platelets. HLA and platelet-specific alloantibodies are not naturally occurring. The most common causes of HLA alloimmunization are previous blood transfusions and pregnancy. WBCs express HLA Class I antigens and may stimulate HLA antibodies in some patients. For most patients, HLA alloimmunization is not associated with clinical problems. However, it can be associated with platelet transfusion refractoriness. Platelets express HLA Class I antigens. Therefore, patients who are HLA alloimmunized may rapidly clear transfused platelets, reflective of immune destruction, resulting in an inadequate platelet response called platelet refractoriness.[16] Refractoriness is defined as a consistent failure to achieve expected posttransfusion platelet counts. Refractoriness may be a result of multiple nonimmune conditions often existing in patients who require long-term platelet therapy. To assess the effectiveness, a platelet count should be performed 10 to 60 minutes after the transfusion.[57]

Apheresis Platelets

Apheresis platelets are obtained from a single donor with the use of an apheresis machine. Centrifugation techniques separate the platelets from the RBCs, WBCs, and most of the plasma. The platelets are kept in a collection bag for later transfusion to a patient. Apheresis platelets generally contain 3×10^{11} platelets or more, depending on collection practices. Apheresis platelets are advantageous due to a number of reasons: the need to pool multiple platelet concentrates is eliminated, which decreases donor exposures and risk of bacterial contamination; ease of handling; and quicker process due to requirements to test platelets for bacteria. Apheresis platelets are typically transfused to alloimmunized patients experiencing refractory thrombocytopenia. Platelets not yet pooled may be stored for up to 5 days; once platelets are pooled, they must be transfused within 4 hours.

TABLE 26.7 Comparison of Apheresis Platelets with Pooled Platelets

Apheresis Platelets	Pooled Platelets
Reduced donor exposure per transfusion	Less risk to donor
Reduced turnaround time and wastage	Lower preparation costs
Lower WBC content	Reduced plasma exposure to donor
HLA-matched platelets	Increased donor exposure to recipient
Five-day shelf life	Four-hour expiration once pooled

WBC, White blood cell.

Pooled Platelets

Pooled platelets are from multiple donors and are often ordered as a six-pack of platelets, indicating six pooled units of WB platelet concentrates from six separate donors. Platelet concentrates are prepared from 1 unit of WB by centrifugation and are resuspended in 60 mL of residual plasma. Each unit contains an average of more than 5.5×10^{11} platelets per unit. Platelets that have not been pooled or combined may be stored at room temperature for up to 5 days.

Indications

Indications for platelet transfusions are thrombocytopenia, treatment of bleeding, or abnormal platelet function. The etiology of the patient's thrombocytopenia and platelet function should be considered when determining a transfusion threshold. Abnormal platelet function and the cause or severity of bleeding may lower the transfusion threshold. Prophylactic platelet transfusions may be given when the platelet count falls below 10,000/μL in oncology patients with acute leukemia, in hematopoietic stem cell transplant recipients, and in other uncomplicated thrombocytopenic patients. A platelet count greater than 10,000/μL is usually sufficient to prevent spontaneous hemorrhage.

Actively bleeding patients, or those who are undergoing a major invasive procedure, usually require a platelet count between 50,000 and 100,000/μL to avoid severe bleeding complications. Effectiveness of platelet transfusion is monitored by the serum platelet count.

Platelets contain WBCs and plasma. They are available as pooled platelet concentrates from multiple units of WB platelets or by a single-donor procedure known as platelet pheresis. Platelet concentrates are combined from 4 to 10 donors. A unit of single-donor platelets is usually equivalent to six or more platelet concentrates, the dose commonly ordered for a single platelet transfusion in an adult. Platelet storage is limited to 5 days. A standard size apheresis unit is equivalent to a pool of approximately 4 to 8 single-donor units. The typical dose for an adult recipient is 1 unit of WB platelets/kg. As an example, a 70-kg patient would receive 7 units of WB platelets.

Granulocytes

Description

Granulocytes are essential for destruction of bacteria and fungi and are one of several types of white blood cells that are administered rarely during specialized transfusion therapy. Granulocytes are collected using an apheresis machine from an ABO-compatible and Rh-compatible donor and should be infused soon after collection because their viability quickly diminishes over time. If this is not possible, storage should be at room temperature for no longer than 24 hours after collection. Granulocytes should not be transfused using a microaggregate or leukocyte reduction filter. Granulocytes should be irradiated to prevent graft-versus-host disease (GVHD) when administered to allogeneic bone marrow transplant (BMT) recipients.

Indications

According to the *AABB Technical Manual*,[18] granulocyte transfusion is controversial but typically administered to patients with the following conditions:

- Severe neutropenia
- Documented infection for 24 to 48 hours not responsive to antibiotics or other therapies
- Bone marrow showing myeloid hypoplasia
- Probable bone marrow function recovery

BLOOD COMPONENT MODIFICATION

Leukocyte Reduction

Leukocyte reduction (LR), also known as leukoreduction, is indicated to decrease occurrence of recurrent febrile nonhemolytic transfusion reactions, to decrease incidence of HLA alloimmunization, and to reduce risk of cytomegalovirus (CMV) infection. LR does not prevent GVHD, nor does it replace the need for irradiation or use of CMV-seronegative components. Most states in this country do not mandate LR of blood components as standard practice. Washing of RBCs and platelets is not considered a substitute for LR because washing does not remove enough leukocytes to prevent alloimmunization. The majority of WBCs have been removed, eliminating undesirable effects caused by WBCs and their by-products. Components that can be leukocyte-reduced include platelets, RBCs, and WB.

Leukocyte filtration may occur in three scenarios: prestorage, when the component is collected; poststorage, when the component is in the laboratory; or at the bedside, when the unit is transfused. Prestorage LR seems to have several advantages over bedside LR. These advantages include a lower incidence of febrile reactions and alloimmunization.[56,58] Leukocyte reduction filters allow RBCs and platelets to pass through the filter while leukocytes are trapped. Manufacturers have modified apheresis machinery to collect platelets with low levels of leukocytes. Additional filtration is unnecessary if this collection method is used.

Indications for Washed Red Blood Cells or Platelets

Before LR filters, washing RBCs was considered the best way to prepare a leukocyte-reduced unit. Today, washing RBCs is not cost-effective, is less efficient, and shortens the availability of units because of an abbreviated shelf life once the component is washed. Washed components are prepared by washing RBCs or platelets with 1 to 2 L of 0.9% NS in an automated cell washer. Washed components remove all but traces of plasma, decrease leukocytes, and remove debris and platelets. Washed RBCs can be considered for patients who have had repeated hypersensitivity reactions to blood components despite prophylactic administration of antihistamines. Washing RBCs or platelets may not reduce the proteins enough to prevent hypersensitivity reactions (e.g., immunoglobulin A [IgA]-deficient patients).[13] After the components are washed with saline, they are centrifuged and the supernatant removed. Washed RBCs are indicated if the plasma in the component contains antibodies known to be harmful to the recipient or to remove constituents for which the intended recipient is known to have severe side effects. Recipients who are IgA deficient require washed units. RBCs must be transfused within 24 hours of washing because the hermetic seal of the component has been broken. Platelets must be transfused within 4 hours of washing.[14]

Volume Reduction

Volume reduction occurs when the majority of plasma is removed from platelets and granulocytes after centrifugation. As a result, plasma proteins and cytokines are removed. Volume reduction decreases the component to approximately 100 mL or a specified amount. Plasma volume reduction is indicated in patients who cannot tolerate the full volume of a component or when ABO-incompatible WB platelets are transfused.

Cytomegalovirus-Negative Components

CMV resides on the leukocytes of individuals who have been infected with the virus. The purpose of CMV-negative components is to prevent primary CMV infection in immunocompromised CMV-negative patients at risk of developing serious complications from a primary CMV infection. CMV-negative blood components are indicated for many reasons including CMV-negative bone marrow or organ transplant recipients, even if the marrow or organ donor is also CMV negative; AIDS- or HIV-infected patients; pregnant women; or patients with a congenital immune deficiency. CMV transmission can be prevented by administering CMV-seronegative blood components or LR components. Components that may be CMV negative include RBCs, platelets, WB, and granulocytes. Worldwide, there are a substantial number of CMV-positive carriers with no history of exhibiting the illness. This virus is known to cause CMV-associated pneumonia, myocarditis, retinitis, hepatitis, and gastroenteritis.

Gamma Irradiation

The purpose of irradiating blood components is to prevent transfusion-associated GVHD. Irradiation of WB, granulocytes, RBCs, and platelets inactivates T lymphocytes and prevents them from proliferating and attacking the recipient's tissues as well as altering the genetic material. Irradiated components are indicated for immunocompromised patients (e.g., allogeneic BMT patients). Bone marrow or stem cell transplant candidates requiring transfusion before completing the harvest and patients with congenital or acquired cellular immune deficiencies should also receive irradiated components.[37] Failure to irradiate blood components in these populations can result in transfusion-associated GVHD.

CONSIDERATIONS IN BLOOD TRANSFUSION

ABO/Rh Compatibility

Blood is typed according to the presence or absence of antigens on the surface of the RBC and antibodies in the plasma. Plasma contains antibodies to antigens that are not present on the RBC. For example, if the RBC has the A antigen, the plasma will contain the B antibody. Transfusion of ABO-incompatible blood may cause severe intravascular hemolysis.

Rhesus (Rh) System

RBCs contain hundreds of antigens on their surface in addition to the ABO antigen blood group. The Rhesus (Rh) system is the most clinically significant non-ABO RBC blood group system (Table 26.8). Approximately 85% of the population is Rh positive and 15% of the population is Rh negative. It is extremely immunogenic and can cause hemolytic disease of the newborn and transfusion reactions if the wrong Rh type product is infused. The Rh (also known as the D antigen) is present if the D antigen is on the RBC. Uncrossmatched group O RBCs are often used during emergencies until the patient's ABO and Rh type have been determined. Rh-negative RBCs are used for females of childbearing age and pediatric patients, and Rh-positive group O RBCs are transfused to males and females of nonchildbearing age. When group O RBCs are transfused, it is imperative that a pretransfusion specimen be drawn. Rho(D) immune globulin (RhoGAM) should be given within 48 hours of giving Rh-positive blood to an Rh-negative woman of childbearing age. Natural occurring D antibodies (anti-D) do not exist unless the patient has been exposed during prior transfusions or pregnancy.

Group O RBCs are not without risk. Unanticipated blood group antibodies can cause fatal transfusion reactions. Many facilities require a provider to complete a justification form documenting the need for the uncrossmatched RBC transfusion.

Autologous Transfusion

There are several categories of autologous transfusion available. These include preoperative (blood that is collected and stored until needed), perioperative (acute normovolemic hemodilution [ANH] and cell saver), and postoperative (autotransfusion devices).

Preoperative Autologous Donation

Autologous blood donation is the process of collection, storage, and transfusion of a patient's own blood. There are risks and benefits of preoperative autologous donation. Benefits include preventing some adverse effects (e.g., febrile or allergic transfusion reactions) and providing compatible blood for patients with alloantibodies. Risks include bacterial contamination at the time of donation, potential clerical errors during the collection of the pretransfusion (type and crossmatch) specimen, or possible transfusion of the wrong unit of blood.

These potential complications make it imperative that autologous blood be transfused astutely and only when specifically indicated. It is never reasonable to transfuse an autologous unit simply because it is available or would otherwise be discarded. Similarly, autologous blood should not be transfused to replace iron, to promote wound healing or general well-being, or to normalize the Hgb level.

Perioperative Blood Salvage

In blood salvage techniques, blood shed in the perioperative or postoperative period is collected, processed, and reinfused into the patient. Processing includes filtration or centrifugation and washing before reinfusion.

Acute Normovolemic Hemodilution

ANH is the removal of WB from a patient before a surgical procedure. The WB is replaced with crystalloid IV fluid (e.g., NS) as a substitute to the WB removed. The blood is collected in a standard blood bag containing an anticoagulant and reinfused during surgery, if indicated. The patient must be stable enough to accommodate any potential anemia that the procedure may cause. Collection devices are frequently used to collect the shed blood during surgery and then wash the cells before retransfusion. This procedure is widely used for cardiac, orthopedic, trauma, transplant, and other surgical procedures.

Postoperative Blood Collection

In postoperative blood collection, washed or unwashed blood is collected from a surgical drain and reinfused to the patient within 6 hours of the collection.[21] Forty-micrometer microaggregate filters are used to filter the shed blood before transfusion.

Directed Donor Transfusion

Directed donation is blood that has been donated by a person specified by the patient. Many people elect to have specific individuals (e.g., family members) donate blood for them because they feel that blood from designated individuals is safer than blood donated by anonymous volunteers. However, there is no established medical or scientific evidence that blood from directed donors is advantageous. Therefore, the same rigorous donor screening criteria are followed as for regular volunteer blood donors.

Directed donations between blood relatives are gamma-irradiated to prevent transfusion-induced GVHD. Donors must be ABO/Rh compatible with the patient.

Generally, directed donation is discouraged, as there are many risks. For example, blood should not be transfused to a female of childbearing age by her partner, as it may increase the risk for hemolytic disease of the newborn. Blood donated by a blood relative to another (e.g., between siblings) may cause alloimmunization of potential transplant recipients. Requesting directed donations from family and friends may place the potential donor in an uncomfortable situation, especially if the person does not qualify to donate blood. To prevent being excluded, the potential donor may answer questions untruthfully, unintentionally compromising the safety of the recipient.

Massive Transfusions

Substantial bleeding requiring massive transfusion can occur in a variety of clinical scenarios and is associated with substantial mortality and morbidity. Multiple definitions for

TABLE 26.8 Rh Considerations for Blood Components

	RH CONSIDERATIONS FOR BLOOD COMPONENTS				
Patient's Rh Type	**Whole Blood**	**Red Blood Cells**	**Plasma**	**Platelets**	**Cryoprecipitate**
Rh positive	Positive or negative	Positive or negative	Positive or negative	Positive or negative	Irrelevant
Rh negative	Negative	Negative	Positive or negative	Negative	Irrelevant

massive transfusion exist; however, historically, massive transfusion has been defined as receiving 10 RBC units in 24 hours or the replacement of one or more blood volumes within 24 hours.[23,24,29,50,61] Blood volume is estimated as 70 mL/kg, or approximately 5000 mL, equivalent to 10 or more units of WB in a 70-kg adult.

Early in the new millennium, historical transfusion paradigms were challenged mainly based on the results from the US Military in Iraq, where thawed AB FFP was administered together with RBCs, as well as platelets from the start of resuscitation.[26] This regimen was based on the notion that it was problematic to dilute the concentration of platelets and coagulation factors by RBCs before administering platelets and plasma to massively bleeding patients.[30] Since then, a new approach has emerged aimed at avoiding coagulopathy by proactive resuscitation with blood components in a balanced ratio of RBC:plasma:platelets. The benefits of rapid, balanced blood component resuscitation were studied in the Pragmatic, Randomized Optimal Platelets and Plasma Ratios (PROPPR) trial, which was a partially blinded, prospective, randomized study comparing resuscitation with units of plasma, platelets, and RBCs in either 1:1:1 or 1:1:2 ratios.[26] This has been reported to be associated with reduced mortality. Additionally, a change toward applying the rate of transfusion in a shorter time frame such as 2 or 6 hours has been broadly accepted.[47,58]

The availability and prompt transfusion of RBCs and blood components are essential to the successful resuscitation of patients who experience acute, massive blood loss. Many institutions have a massive transfusion protocol to ensure prompt availability of blood components and provide guidelines for facilitating timely and adequate replacement of massive blood loss with appropriate blood components. Indications for a massive transfusion include, but are not limited to, the following:

- Significant hemorrhage (e.g., massive upper GI hemorrhage, ruptured aortic aneurysms, and equivalent clinical scenarios)
- Continual hypotension resulting from blood loss exceeding 1500 mL
- Both considerable blood loss and a likelihood that additional considerable blood loss will continue over a short time
- Ongoing blood loss requiring at least 10 units of RBC replacement within 2 hours

The challenge of massive transfusion is that patients may already be in the resuscitation phase before any components besides RBCs are ordered. For some patients, the fibrinogen level is extremely low or becomes low within 30 minutes of arrival into critical care or the emergency department. The purpose of implementing a massive transfusion protocol is to obtain blood components for the patient in a timely manner, to stabilize the coagulation parameters, and to use fewer components before the patient becomes hypothermic or acidotic. Many institutions do use protocols for massive transfusions that incorporate use of a massive transfusion pack (MTP). An MTP may consist of a variety of components that include a balanced transfusion therapy regimen with blood components aiming for a balanced plasma:platelets:RBC ratio starting immediately when the massive bleeding is encountered and until surgical hemostasis is achieved. Furthermore, many hospitals administer tranexamic acid in patients with massive hemorrhage where increased fibrinolysis is prevalent, such as obstetric bleeding emergencies, trauma, vascular surgery with reperfusion injuries, pelvic surgery, and intracranial hemorrhage.

Another concern regarding the transfusion guidelines was that conventional coagulation tests, like prothrombin time (PT) and activated partial thromboplastin time (aPTT), were applied to identify patients in need of plasma substitution. It is important to note that plasma-based coagulation tests are thought to be inappropriate for monitoring coagulopathy and guide therapy in trauma patients. According to the cell-based model, hemostasis occurs in three phases: initiation, amplification, and propagation, with the magnitude of the thrombin generation, the *thrombin burst,* finally determining the hemostatic capability of the formed clot.[2] Therefore, tests that reflect this new understanding of hemostasis, such as viscoelastical hemostatic assays (VHAs), thrombelastography (TEG), and rotational thrombelastometry (ROTEM) should be used to accurately monitor hemostasis.[30] Timelines of an optimal transfusion strategy and VHA results are critical to improved survival in the massively bleeding patient. Once bleeding has subsided, all subsequent blood orders should be based on results of coagulation tests. Randomized controlled studies evaluating different hemostatic resuscitation regimens in patients with massive hemorrhage are needed.

Use of Blood Warmers

To minimize the occurrence of dysrhythmias and prevent cardiac arrest associated with massive transfusion, blood warmers are often used for patients who are receiving several rapid transfusions. Blood warmers are not indicated in routine transfusions, but should be used when transfusing blood to patients who have cold agglutinins, which are antibodies that react at cold temperatures. Several types of blood warmers are available on the market, including radiant plate and coil warmers and water bath devices.

Some blood warmers have an external pressure device allowing a unit of blood to be transfused within a few minutes. External pressure devices should not exceed 300 mm Hg of pressure and must apply pressure evenly over the entire component bag. These should only be used with a large-gauge catheter to prevent hemolysis. Manufacturer instructions should be followed.

ADVERSE EFFECTS RELATED TO TRANSFUSION OF BLOOD COMPONENTS

Transfusion of blood components is considered transplantation of foreign cells and exposes the patient to multiple hazards, including a variety of transfusion reactions, diseases, and inflammatory complications. Transfusions are associated with the potential for negative impact on patient outcomes and are thought to increase infections and hospital length of stay.[60] It is important that clinicians be able to recognize complications and implement immediate interventions, as well as explain the reactions and adverse effects to the patient or the family.

Transfusion of blood components does not come without risk and should not be taken lightly. Any component can cause a reaction. Manifestations of transfusion reactions vary depending on the type of blood component transfused and the clinical condition of the patient receiving the transfusion. Until proven otherwise, any adverse reaction occurring at the time of the transfusion should be considered a transfusion reaction.

Any suspected transfusion reaction or adverse reaction should be reported to the blood bank because it may be involved in the patient's workup and evaluation. There may also be a reason to quarantine other components donated by the donor in question or other components associated with the unit in question.

Bacterial Contamination

Bacterial contamination of blood components is one cause of transfusion-associated morbidity and mortality. Most deaths[32] related to bacterial contamination of blood components that are reported to the FDA are associated with the transfusion of platelets.[17] Bacterial contamination occurs more often in platelet components, occurring in an estimated 1:1000 to 1:3000 platelet units transfused.[4] The risks increase when platelets are pooled. Bacteria proliferate depending on the type of component and how it is stored. RBCs have been known to contain *Acinetobacter, Escherichia, Staphylococcus,* and *Pseudomonas* species.[19] Platelets have contained such organisms as *Staphylococcus, Streptococcus, Acinetobacter, Klebsiella,* and *Serratia.*[20] In 2004 the AABB required blood banks to implement strategies to limit bacterial contamination in platelet concentrates and detect growth of bacteria during storage.

Bacteria can be introduced into a donated unit of blood during collection, processing, or pooling, causing sepsis or life-threatening septic shock to the recipient. If the patient experiences severe rigors and high fever (> 2°C increase), and severe hypotension, it is important to consider bacterial contamination. Other signs and symptoms include abdominal pain, vomiting, hemoglobinuria, DIC, renal failure, and circulatory collapse, which can occur within minutes of starting the transfusion. Symptoms may occur during or shortly after completion of the transfusion.

Treatment of bacterial contamination includes broad-spectrum antibiotics, vasopressor support in the event of septic shock, and acetaminophen (Tylenol). The implicated unit should be returned to the blood bank so that a Gram stain and culture of the unit can occur. The recipient should also have a Gram stain and culture performed (Table 26.9).

Transfusion-Associated Graft-Versus-Host Disease

GVHD is a rare complication of a blood transfusion and is associated with greater than 90% mortality rate.[37] GVHD is also associated with other transplantations (e.g., BMT). However, its mortality rate associated with BMT is much lower, at 20% to 25%.[21]

The recognition and proliferation of viable donor T lymphocytes present in cellular blood components, called *engraftment,* can result in transfusion-associated GVHD (TA-GVHD), which is seen in a susceptible recipient unable to recognize or destroy the lymphocytes. This generates an immune response against the recipient's antigens. The donor lymphocytes proliferate and injure organs, such as bone marrow, skin, liver, and the gastrointestinal tract. Severely immunocompromised patients (e.g., BMT recipients, Hodgkin's disease) or recipients of directed donations from first-degree relatives are at risk for TA-GVHD. Blood components that contain T cells (e.g., RBCs, WB, platelets, granulocytes) can cause TA-GVHD. Fortunately, TA-GVHD can be prevented by gamma irradiation of cellular blood components.

TA-GVHD usually manifests 3 to 30 days after a transfusion.[37] Signs and symptoms include diarrhea, rash, fever, pancytopenia, elevated levels of hepatic enzymes, and elevated bilirubin levels. Patients have died from overwhelming infection and hematopoietic failure, resulting in more than 90% mortality rate from TA-GVHD.[37]

The diagnosis of TA-GVHD is frequently delayed because symptoms are mild or are attributed to the primary illness. Laboratory tests may show pancytopenia, abnormal liver function tests, and electrolyte abnormalities induced by diarrhea.[37] If TA-GVHD is suspected, a biopsy will be taken from the affected skin. A definitive diagnosis is made only if the circulating lymphocytes have a different HLA phenotype from the patient's tissue cells, proving that the circulating lymphocytes came from the donor.[37]

Delayed Hemolytic Transfusion Reaction

A delayed hemolytic transfusion reaction (DHTR) is caused by minor blood group incompatibility, such as Rh incompatibility. This anamnestic response, which is the heightened level of the immune response that occurs with the second exposure to an antigen, occurs in patients who have been exposed and sensitized to an antigen during a prior transfusion (Rh-positive RBCs transfused to an Rh-negative recipient) or pregnancy. After the exposure occurs, an antibody develops.

DHTRs can take as long as a week or more to present. Signs include extravascular hemolysis, fever, hyperbilirubinemia, decrease in Hct/Hgb levels 3 to 7 days posttransfusion, jaundice, and hemoglobinuria.

A delayed response does not generally activate an acute response, and the patient may be asymptomatic. These reactions may be overlooked because they are usually less severe than an acute hemolytic transfusion reaction. Future transfusions should be avoided until the antibody that caused the reaction can be identified and antigen-negative components become available. Diagnosis is confirmed by a positive indirect antiglobulin test (Coombs' test).

Febrile Nonhemolytic Transfusion Reaction

A febrile nonhemolytic transfusion reaction (FNHTR) is a common reaction, believed to be due to patient antibodies to leukocyte antigens contained in the donor component. Another theory is that cytokines created during storage of the blood component cause fever and chills in the transfused patients. This type of reaction is more common in patients who have a history of transfusion or pregnancy.[37] A pretransfusion temperature should be assessed to establish a baseline and allow for evaluation of whether the patient became febrile during or following a transfusion. This will help determine whether the fever was caused by the transfusion or by an underlying condition (e.g., infection or the disease process). If the temperature increases greater than 1°C above baseline early in the transfusion or several hours, typically 1 to 2 hours, after the conclusion of the transfusion, an FNHTR should be considered. Fever is often seen in more life-threatening reactions (e.g., bacterial contamination or acute hemolytic transfusion reactions). Therefore it is important to evaluate the patient and notify the blood bank of such occurrences. The fever will usually respond to antipyretics, and meperidine (Demerol) may be useful in treating the rigors. Depending on the severity of the symptoms, the practitioner may request to restart the transfusion at a slower rate. Subsequent transfusions may require premedication with acetaminophen or diphenhydramine (Benadryl). Febrile reactions may be prevented if leukocyte-reduced components are transfused. A patient can still have an FNHTR in the absence of fever if the patient has received prophylactic

TABLE 26.9 **Adverse Reactions Related to Transfusion of Blood Components**

Type of Reaction	Clinical Presentation	Treatment And Management	Prevention
Acute hemolytic transfusion reaction	Hemoglobinuria Renal failure Dyspnea, tachypnea, hypoxemia Fever (1°C increase in body temperature above baseline) with or without chills Rigors with or without fever Hypotension or hypertension Coagulopathy: diffuse bleeding Severe chest, abdomen, or flank pain Generalized bleeding, DIC Pain at infusion site Urticaria, pruritus, localized edema Hemoglobinuria or anuria Nausea and vomiting Sense of impending doom or anxiety Diaphoresis	Diuretics and additional IV fluids may be administered to increase renal perfusion. Use laboratory tests in investigation. Determine renal function (blood urea nitrogen, creatinine levels). Determine bleeding status (platelet count, PT/INR, aPTT, Hgb/Hct). Determine need for subsequent blood component transfusions. Stop transfusion and send blood bag, administration set, and IV solutions to blood bank.	Rule out clerical error at the time of drawing the blood bank specimen or identifying patient at the time of transfusion. To prevent nonimmune hemolysis, infuse compatible, FDA-approved IV fluids and medications. Pressure devices should not exceed 300 mm Hg. Transfusion through small-bore IV catheters should be avoided when administered via a pressure device.
Febrile nonhemolytic transfusion reactions	Fever Possible rigors Headache Vomiting	To reduce patient's temperature, administer an antipyretic. Provider may request restarting the transfusion at a slower rate. Otherwise, the transfusion may need to be stopped if patient continues to have symptoms. Signs and symptoms may mimic more severe reactions, such as AHTR. Use meperidine to prevent or treat rigors. Other medications that may be used are antihistamines and corticosteroids.	Leukoreduced components may be warranted. Premedicate with an antipyretic. Administer meperidine to prevent rigors.
Allergic reaction (mild)	Hives Urticaria Pruritus Flushing of skin	Symptoms may subside by slowing rate of transfusion. Administer antihistamine to relieve patient's symptoms or prophylactically if patient experiences recurrent urticarial reactions. Use volume expansion for hypotension or epinephrine (5 mL of a 1:10,000 solution).	Premedicate with antihistamine.
Allergic reaction (moderate)	Periorbital or perioral edema Wheezes Possible hypotension	Stop the transfusion. Epinephrine may be indicated for severe, persistent urticaria associated with bronchospasm.	When allergic reactions occur despite pretransfusion antihistamine, washed cells may be indicated. Rule out IgA deficiency. If negative, transfuse washed RBCs or platelets.
Allergic reaction (severe), anaphylaxis	Hypotension Respiratory distress Bronchospasms Cough Shock Facial edema Nausea and emesis Absence of fever	May be necessary to administer epinephrine (0.4 mL of 1:1000 solution subcutaneous), steroids, or oxygen as appropriate. Never restart a transfusion when an anaphylactic reaction is suspected or has occurred. Subsequent transfusions may require 0.9% normal saline washed RBCs.	When allergic reactions occur despite pretransfusion antihistamine, washed cells may be indicated. Rule out IgA deficiency. If negative, transfuse washed RBCs or platelets.
Transfusion-related acute lung injury	Severe, progressive dyspnea and decrease in Sao_2 Bilateral pulmonary infiltrates (white-out) on chest x-rays Noncardiogenic, bilateral pulmonary edema Hypertension or hypotension Tachycardia Chills Wheezes Bronchospasm Cough Dyspnea Cyanosis Fever (1°C to 2°C increase in temperature)	Provide supportive care with administration of oxygen, intubation with mechanical ventilation, and blood pressure support. Corticosteroids and diuretics are not indicated. Notify blood bank immediately if TRALI is suspected. WBC antibody studies may need to be performed on both patient and blood donor(s).	Institute permanent deferral of donors implicated in TRALI reactions.

Continued

TABLE 26.9 Adverse Reactions Related to Transfusion of Blood Components—cont'd

Type of Reaction	Clinical Presentation	Treatment And Management	Prevention
Bacterial contamination	Fever increase greater than 2°C (3.5°F) Nausea or vomiting Abdominal cramping Chills, rigors Sudden and severe hypotension Generalized bleeding, DIC Shock Hemoglobinuria Renal failure Dryness and flushing	Inspect component for abnormal color, clotting, or hemolysis. Perform a Gram stain and culture of both patient and implicated unit. Broad-spectrum antibiotics may be indicated.	Inspect unit before administration for discoloration. Blood banks have several methods to detect bacteria (e.g., Gram stain) or to prevent bacterial contamination (e.g., extensive donor screening).

AHTR, Acute hemolytic transfusion reaction; *aPTT*, activated partial thromboplastin time; *DIC*, disseminated intravascular coagulation; *FDA*, Food and Drug Administration; *Hct*, hematocrit; *Hgb*, hemoglobin; *INR*, international normalized ratio; *PT*, prothrombin time; *RBC*, red blood cell; *Sao_2*, arterial oxygen saturation; *TRALI*, transfusion-related acute lung injury; *WBC*, white blood cell.
Data from References 5, 6, 40, and 50.

antipyretics, because these will not suppress the shaking, chills, and discomfort (see Table 26.9).

Allergic Transfusion Reactions

Interaction of a preexisting antibody to a protein or allergen in donor blood may cause an allergic reaction, ranging from mild, to moderate, to severe. This antibody-allergen reaction triggers a cascade of chemical events that affect the respiratory, cardiovascular, and gastrointestinal systems.

Mild Allergic

Mild allergic transfusion reactions are common during and after transfusion. Symptoms include urticaria (hives), pruritus (itching), erythema, and flushing of the skin. Mild reactions respond to IV antihistamines.

Moderate Allergic

Symptoms of moderate allergic reactions include the upper airway and involve laryngeal edema. Wheezing, cyanosis, anxiety, dyspnea, nausea, vomiting, and diarrhea are all signs of moderate allergic reactions. Moderate reactions may respond to IV antihistamines or may require epinephrine (0.4 mL of a 1:1000 solution subcutaneously). Washed RBCs and platelets may be necessary to prevent future allergic reactions.

Severe Allergic

Severe allergic reactions or anaphylactic reactions can cause hypotension, tachycardia, shock, dysrhythmias, and cardiac arrest. Administration of epinephrine (0.4 mL of a 1:1000 solution subcutaneously) and steroids may be necessary. Supportive care with intubation, mechanical ventilation, oxygen, and IV fluids may be indicated. The transfusion should not be restarted if an anaphylactic reaction is suspected or confirmed. Anaphylactic reactions may be associated with anti-IgA antibodies in individuals with IgA deficiency.

Nonimmune-Related Hemolysis Transfusion Reaction

Bacterial contamination, accidental freezing of donor units, infusion of incompatible IV fluids either in the donor bag or in the infusion line, incompatible medication administration (no medications should be infused through the same tubing with blood components unless they have been FDA approved), excessive heating (> 42°C) of donor units, and pressure devices used for rapid administration can result in nonimmune hemolysis. Nonimmune hemolysis presents with symptoms of hemolysis, yet an antibody screen and direct antiglobulin test (DAT) performed in the laboratory are negative. New-onset hemolysis with a negative DAT fits best with physical/mechanical hemolysis of RBCs. Treatment is focused on the cause of the hemolysis. If physical hemolysis is suspected, a careful analysis of conditions associated with transfusion must be done.

Some patients may tolerate a transfusion with lysed cells without difficulty. Others may experience renal failure, hemoglobinemia, hemoglobinuria, hyperkalemia, hypotension, and other signs of shock. This is usually a diagnosis of exclusion because it mimics hemolytic transfusion reactions, bacterial contamination, and sepsis.

Whenever a transfusion reaction is suspected, the blood bag, tubing, and IV fluids should be sent to the blood bank for evaluation. Care is supportive and may require monitoring of serum potassium level and electrocardiogram signs of hyperkalemia. The patient's kidneys should be well hydrated, yet fluid overload, particularly in patients with impaired renal or cardiac function, should be avoided.

To prevent lysis, it is important to infuse compatible, FDA-approved IV fluids or medications with blood components. IV pumps, warmers, and pressure devices (not to exceed 300 mm Hg) should be well maintained. Transfusion through small-bore catheters should be avoided, especially with pressure devices for infusion. An 18-gauge needle is recommended for adults. Smaller gauge needles (23 gauge or larger) can be used for transfusion in adults but may restrict the flow rate of the transfusion and lengthen the time to infuse a unit (see Table 26.9).

Acute Hemolytic Transfusion Reaction

A hemolytic transfusion reaction is an immunologic or nonimmunologic destruction or rupture of transfused RBCs with the release of intracellular hemoglobin (Fig. 26.3). It occurs most commonly from an incompatibility of antigen on the transfused cells with an antibody in the recipient's circulation. Severe hemolytic reactions may occur when as little as 10 mL of ABO-incompatible RBCs are transfused to a recipient. The blood reacts with the antibodies that exist in the recipient. The antibody and antigen interaction initiates complement activation, coagulation activation, and an inflammatory response related to cytokines.[37] The primary concerns during treatment are optimizing renal perfusion and hemodynamic support with

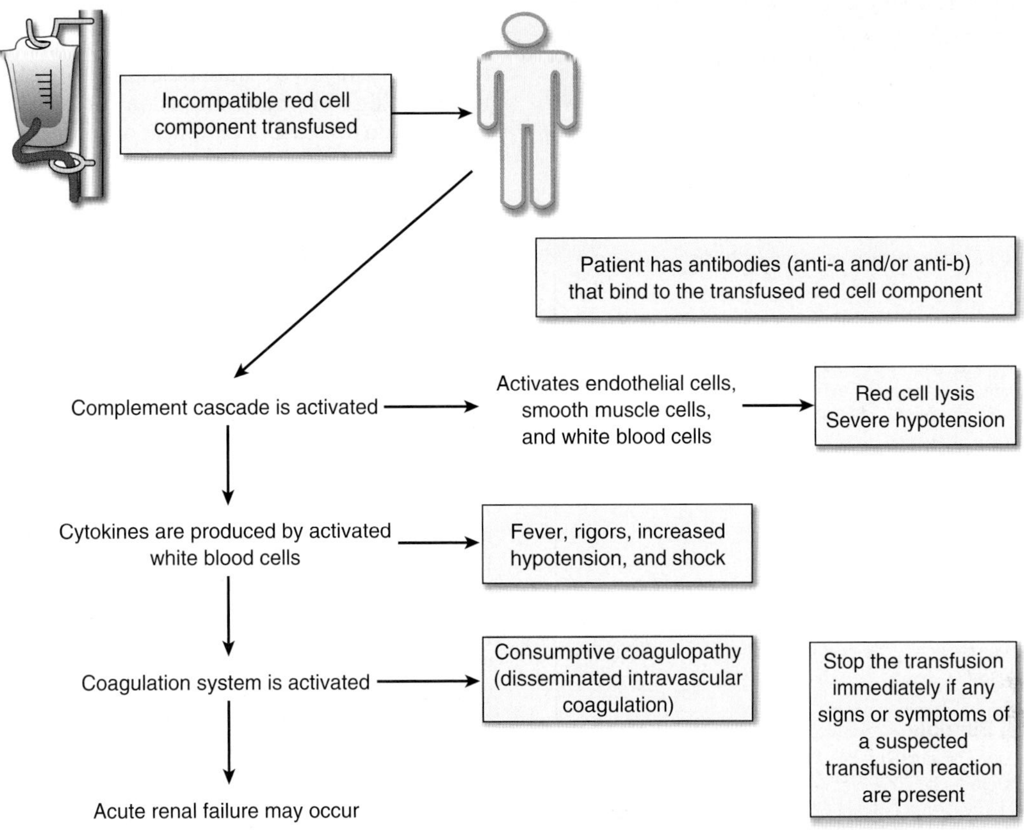

FIG. 26.3 Pathophysiology of an acute hemolytic transfusion reaction (AHTR).

vasopressor agents if the patient becomes hypotensive. If the patient develops coagulopathy, blood component administration may be necessary.

Acute hemolytic transfusion reaction signs and symptoms usually appear within the first 5 to 15 minutes after the transfusion is started, but can happen anytime during the transfusion or afterward, depending on the patient's response. Additional blood components should be avoided until the transfusion reaction investigation is complete. If the reaction is thought to be caused by the wrong blood type, O-negative RBCs should be transfused if necessary. Diuretics and additional fluids may be administered to increase renal perfusion. Lab testing (blood urea nitrogen, creatinine, platelet count, prothrombin time/international normalized ratio [PT/INR], aPTT, and Hgb/Hct) may be ordered to determine renal function, bleeding status, and need for subsequent blood component transfusions.

Clerical errors (e.g., not accurately identifying the patient during collection of the pretransfusion specimen or at the time of administration) are the most common cause of ABO-incompatible transfusions. Vigilance in performing the pretransfusion/compatibility testing (type and crossmatch) and verification by transfusing clinicians according to hospital policies is necessary to prevent a mismatched transfusion. Box 26.1 lists the laboratory tests performed to evaluate for most suspected hemolytic transfusion reactions.

Transfusion-Associated Circulatory Overload

Transfusion-associated circulatory overload (TACO) is the second leading cause of reported transfusion-related fatalities in the United States.[48] It is an adverse event that results in hydrostatic pulmonary edema due to overwhelming a transfused patient's circulatory system.[37] The clinical findings associated with TACO include the acute onset of respiratory dysfunction, demonstrated by cough, dyspnea, tachypnea, rales/rhonchi/wheezing on auscultation and desaturations requiring supplemental oxygen; hypertension; tachycardia; jugular venous distention; profuse diaphoresis; and response to diuretic therapy.[37] Once symptoms suggest TACO, the transfusion should be discontinued. If symptoms continue, it may be necessary to administer diuretics or perform therapeutic phlebotomy.[37] Further transfusions should be administered slowly.

Transfusion-Related Immune Modulation

Since the early 1970s, transfusion of blood components has been associated with immune suppression.[5,45] Allogeneic transfusions have been associated with poor patient outcomes. Immunomodulatory effects may perhaps be related to the WBCs in blood or storage time of the transfused blood.

Effects of transfusion-related immune modulation (TRIM) include increased postoperative infections, increased tumor recurrence, increased critical care morbidity and mortality, and increased multiple organ dysfunction syndrome (MODS). LR will not eliminate TRIM but might diminish its occurrence. Transfusion of allogeneic blood can induce a complex set of effects on the immune system. Prospective clinical studies are required to determine whether leukoreduced blood components are helpful in decreasing the occurrence of TRIM. Some clinical studies suggest that the risk of postoperative infection complications has declined in patients that receive nonleukoreduced components.

BOX 26.1 Laboratory Investigation Assessment After an Acute Hemolytic Transfusion Reaction

Laboratory testing following an acute hemolytic transfusion reaction (AHTR) will frequently indicate hemoglobinemia or hemoglobinuria (result of free hemoglobin clearance by the kidneys), elevated serum bilirubin levels (total and indirect), and a positive direct antiglobulin test (DAT). Additional tests performed are lactate dehydrogenase (LDH) (elevated in AHTR) and haptoglobin (decreased if intravascular hemolysis present).

Haptoglobin

Haptoglobin is a protein that is produced in the liver and binds to free hemoglobin (Hgb) (that is, Hgb not contained within red blood cells [RBCs]) in an attempt to remove it. When RBCs are actively being destroyed, the rate of haptoglobin destruction by the liver will exceed the rate at which new haptoglobin is created. Thus the levels of haptoglobin in the blood will decrease, which is what occurs if intravascular or extravascular hemolysis is present.[51] Haptoglobin measures the rate at which RBCs are being destroyed.

Lactate Dehydrogenase

LDH exists in RBCs and is released from damaged cells. LDH is in several tissues such as the heart, liver, and lungs. LDH is an indicator of acute or chronic tissue damage. LDH level is elevated in intravascular or extravascular hemolysis.[52]

Indirect and Total Bilirubin

Bilirubin is a breakdown product of Hgb. When the liver breaks down old RBCs, bilirubin is produced. The liver cannot clear bilirubin from the circulation. The bilirubin is either indirect bilirubin or direct bilirubin. The levels of bilirubin in the blood will be elevated in both intravascular and extravascular hemolysis.[52]

Direct Antiglobulin Test or Direct Coombs' Test

The direct Coombs' test measures the presence of antibodies on the surface of RBCs. It is used to detect autoantibodies and alloantibodies against RBCs. Many diseases and drugs (e.g., penicillin, cephalosporins, streptomycin) can lead to production of these antibodies. These antibodies sometimes destroy RBCs and cause anemia.

Transfusion-Related Acute Lung Injury

TRALI has been recognized as a significant classification of lung injury with an immunologic, noncardiogenic basis for many years. In 1983, Popovsky et al. first described noncardiogenic pulmonary edema as a complication related to transfusion treatment.[43] TRALI is defined as noncardiogenic pulmonary edema related to the transfusion of all plasma-containing blood components, including WB, RBCs, plasma, platelets, and cryoprecipitate. It has also occurred after administration of IV immune globulin (IVIg). Before the mid-1980s, the only recognized transfusion reactions involving pulmonary complications included anaphylactic reactions and volume overload. Since 2007, TRALI has been recognized as the leading cause of death related to transfusion in the United States.[33,42] The majority of TRALI cases have been related to passive infusion of HLA and human neutrophil antigen (HNA) antibodies. The mortality from TRALI is 5% to 25%, with the lower rates being more common.[45] TRALI is an underdiagnosed and underreported complication of transfusion. TRALI is often not diagnosed correctly, leading to inappropriate patient treatment.

There are two theories as to the cause of TRALI. The first theory involves donor WBC antibodies, such as Class I and Class II anti-HLA, human leukocyte antigen (HLA) and/or human neutrophil antigens (HNAs) being formed through exposure to foreign antigens through pregnancy or transfusion to a recipient.[37] WBC antibodies can form from exposure to foreign WBCs in prior transfusions or pregnancies. Antibody strength can decrease or disappear over time. Some patients will continue to make strong antibodies years after their last pregnancy or transfusion. Either these WBC antibodies direct themselves against the recipient's antigens or the recipient's WBC antibodies direct themselves against the donor's WBC antigens. However, this scenario does not consistently cause TRALI.[59] The second theory involves two events. The first event involves pulmonary endothelial activation in the recipient causing pulmonary sequestration of neutrophils. Following this, a second event occurs causing specific HLA- and HNA-antibodies to be directed against recipient neutrophils in the lungs, resulting in endothelial damage, capillary leak, and TRALI.[59]

Symptoms occur within 6 hours from the start of the transfusion and may include cough, dyspnea, tachycardia, cyanosis, hypotension, hypertension, chills, fever (1°C to 2°C increase in temperature), and bilateral pulmonary edema without other signs of volume overload (see Table 26.9).[37,46] Intubated patients with TRALI have copious secretions that collect in the endotracheal tube. TRALI should be considered in all cases of respiratory distress with significant hypoxemia related to a transfusion and should meet the criteria of acute lung injury (ALI). TRALI may at first be confined to the lower lung fields. After several hours, it usually involves the entire lung (i.e., white-out on chest radiograph by interstitial and alveolar infiltrates). While TRALI resolves within 48 to 96 hours from onset, lung injury is often irreversible.[44]

Treatment for TRALI is supportive with administration of oxygen, intubation with mechanical ventilation, and blood pressure support. Corticosteroids and diuretics are not indicated.[37] Diuretics are not indicated because TRALI is not related to volume overload. The blood bank should be notified immediately if TRALI is suspected. Single donors have been traced as the cause of multiple incidents of TRALI and transfusion reactions, so it is critical that such information is communicated to the laboratory. Failure to report to the hospital transfusion service and the blood collection facility may present risk to future recipients. Permanent deferral of donors implicated in TRALI reactions may be necessary.

Post-Transfusion Purpura

Post-transfusion purpura is similar to DHTR except it involves a patient developing an alloantibody in response to a platelet antigen. Recipients will become thrombocytopenic within 5 to 10 days after transfusion. Treatment may include plasmapheresis, used to help decrease the circulating platelet antibody. Intravenous immunoglobulin (IVIG), a mixture of proteins containing antibodies, predominantly IgG, has also been proven to be effective as it provides passive, temporary immunity for the body.[37]

Disease Transmission

Risks of Transmission of Transfusion-Related Diseases

Multiple methods have been utilized to decrease the risk of the transmission of infectious diseases associated with transfusion. Even with strict donor deferral methods, there are many risks associated with transfusion when selecting potential blood donors. The following risks should be considered: hepatitis B and C, HIV and AIDS, human T-cell lymphotropic virus, and other viruses and parasites including *Babesia,* parvovirus, malaria, Chagas' disease, Lyme disease, and West Nile virus. Because of these risks, it is important to transfuse only when necessary and attempt to limit donor exposure.

CONCLUSION

Caring for critically ill patients who require transfusion is challenging and multifaceted. Current transfusion practice guidelines and thresholds are controversial. Strategies should be directed toward reducing the transfusion threshold and minimizing blood loss. Concerns about complications related to transfusion have resulted in close examination of conventional transfusion practices in critical care. Future research should be directed toward determining optimal transfusion strategies in a variety of patient populations when blood conservation techniques are not possible.

CASE STUDY 26.1

D.A., a 19-year-old female, was a restrained driver involved in a high-speed motor vehicle crash. She was intubated at the scene and transported to the local trauma hospital with right torso trauma. Her systolic blood pressure was 94 mm Hg and her heart rate was 142 beats/min. Her abdomen was large and distended. She had a prolonged capillary refill time, was cold to touch, and appeared pale and mottled. Once admitted, she was taken directly to the operating room (OR). A 12-gauge French central line catheter was inserted and she was typed and cross-matched and coagulation studies, arterial blood gas (ABG), and blood chemistry labs were drawn. Her temperature was 35.0°C. Rewarming was initiated by using warm IV fluids to 39.0°C and warm humidified oxygen through the ventilator to keep her core body temperature greater than 35.0°C. A urine catheter was inserted and an exploratory laparotomy was performed, indicating both liver and splenic lacerations. A splenectomy was performed; the Grade IV and V liver lacerations to the right liver lobe were packed using a damage control technique, known as peri-hepatic packing, to control hepatic hemorrhage. Her Hgb level declined to 7 g/dL, equivalent to a Hct of 21%. Her INR was 2.6, PT 28.5, fibrinogen level 86 mg/dL, and platelet count was 50,000 cells/mm^3. During surgery, D.A. received a total of 10 units of RBCs, 6 units of plasma, and 1 L of IV crystalloid through a blood warmer/rapid infuser. She also received a unit of apheresis platelets. Her urine output was minimal throughout the case. She was transferred to critical care.

After 36 hours in critical care, D.A. developed several complications, including liver and renal failure, sepsis, heparin-induced thrombocytopenia, and necrosis of her abdominal wall. She grew increasingly hypoxemic, requiring increased amounts of oxygen and positive end-expiratory pressure. Her renal function decreased (creatinine level was 3.6 mg/dL). She developed increasing intra-abdominal pressures, was hypotensive, and was difficult to ventilate. She was taken immediately to the OR for a second exploratory laparotomy with drainage of the liver laceration and decompression of her abdominal compartment syndrome. During the unpacking of her abdomen, the surgeons noted a severe liver laceration with leakage of bile. A total of 2–2.5 L of old blood, serum, and bile was removed from her abdominal cavity. The surgeons proceeded with the surgery and obtained swabs of the peritoneal fluid for Gram stain and culture. She required 3 units of RBCs perioperatively for a Hct of 23%.

Decision Point:

What laboratory studies should be obtained at this time? What investigations should be done to assist in determining the cause of her hemolysis?

Decision Point:

What blood components are indicated?

Decision Point:

What is the nurse's role in assessing for an incompatible blood transfusion?

REFERENCES

1. Afshar, M., & Netzer, G. (2013). Updates in critical care for the nephrologist: transfusion in nonhemorrhaging critically ill patients. *Adv Chronic Kidney Dis, 20*, 30–38.
2. Allen, G. A., Wolberg, A. S., Oliver, J. A., Hoffman, M., Roberts, H. R., & Monroe, D. M. (2004). Impact of procoagulant concentration on rate, peak and total thrombin generation in a model system. *J Thromb Haemost, 2*(3), 402–413.
3. American Association of Blood Banks. (2003). *Further guidance on methods to detect bacterial contamination of platelet concentrates*. Bethesda, MD: Association Bulletin #03–12.
4. American Red Cross. America's Blood Centers, American Association of Blood Banks (2013). *Circular of information for the use of human blood and blood components*, Bethesda, MD: American Association of Blood Banks.
5. Bordim, J. O., & Blajchman, M. A. (2002). Transfusion-associated immunomodulation. In T. L. Simon, et al. (Ed.), *Rossi's principles of transfusion medicine* (3rd ed.). Philadelphia: Lippincott Williams & Wilkins.
6. Bufford, K. D., et al. (2005). Recombinant factor VIIa as adjunctive therapy for bleeding control in severely injured trauma patients: two parallel randomized, placebo-controlled, double blind clinical trials. *J Trauma, 59*(1), 8–15.
7. Carson, J. L., Terrin, M. L., Magaziner, J., et al. (2006). Transfusion trigger trial for functional outcomes in cardiovascular patients undergoing surgical hip fracture repair (FOCUS): the principal results. *Blood* (ASH Annual Meeting Abstracts), *114*: LBA-6.
8. Corwin, H. L. (1999). Blood transfusions in the critically ill patient. *Dis Mon, 45*, 409–426.
9. Corwin, H. L. (2001). Anemia in the critically ill: the role of erythropoietin. *Semin Hematol, 38*(Suppl. 7), 24–32.
10. Corwin, H. L., Gettinger, A., Pearl, R. G., et al. (2004). The CRIT study: anemia and blood transfusion in the critically ill—current clinical practice in the United States. *Crit Care Med, 32*, 39–52.
11. Corwin, H. L. (2002). Efficacy of recombinant human erythropoietin in critically ill patients; a randomized controlled trial. *JAMA, 288*, 2827–2835.
12. Dumont, L. J., Papari, M., Aronson, C. A., & Dumont, D. F. (2014). Whole-blood collection and component processing. In M. K. Fung, B. J. Grossman, C. Hillyer, & C. M. Westhoff (Eds.), *AABB technical manual* (18th ed., pp. 138–148). Bethesda, MD: American Association of Blood Banks.
13. Dunbar, N. M. (2014). Hospital storage, monitoring, pretransfusion processing, distribution, and inventory management of blood components. In M. K. Fung, B. J. Grossman, C. Hillyer, & C. M. Westhoff (Eds.), *AABB technical manual* (18th ed., pp. 215–223). Bethesda, MD: American Association of Blood Banks.
14. Dunbar, N. M. (2014). The positive direct antiglobulin test and immune-mediated hemolysis. In M. K. Fung, B. J. Grossman, C. Hillyer, & C. M. Westhoff (Eds.), *AABB technical manual* (18th ed., pp. 425–426). Bethesda, MD: American Association of Blood Banks.
15. Estcourt, L., et al. (2012). Prophylactic platelet transfusion for prevention of bleeding in patients with haematological disorders after chemotherapy and stem cell transplantation. *Cochrane Database Syst Rev. May, 16*, 5, CD004269.
16. Forest, S. K., & Hod, E. A. (2016). Management of the platelet refractory patient. *Hematol Oncol Clin North Am, 30*(3), 665–677.
17. Galel, S. A. (2014). Infectious disease screening. In M. K. Fung, B. J. Grossman, C. Hillyer, & C. M. Westhoff (Eds.), *AABB technical manual* (18th ed.). Bethesda, MD: American Association of Blood Banks.
18. Ghiglione, M., & Puca, K. E. (2014). Patient blood management. In M. K. Fung, B. J. Grossman, C. Hillyer, & C. M. Westhoff (Eds.), *AABB technical manual* (18th ed.). Bethesda, MD: American Association of Blood Banks.
19. Goldman, M., & Blajchman, M. A. (1991). Blood product-associated bacterial sepsis. *Transfus Med Rev, 5*, 73–83.
20. Goodnough, L. T. (2005). Alternatives to allogeneic transfusion. In P. L. Mintz (Ed.), *Transfusion therapy: clinical principles and practices* (2nd ed.). Bethesda, MD: AABB Press.

21. Heaton, A., et al. (1989). In vivo regeneration of red cell 2,3–diphosphoglyceric following transfusion of DPG-depleted AS-1, AS-3 and CPDA-1 red cells. *Br J Haematol, 71*(4), 131–136.
22. Hebert, P. C., et al. (2001). Is a low transfusion threshold safe in critically ill patients with cardiovascular diseases? *Crit Care Med, 29*(2), 227–234.
23. Hebert, P. C., Wells, G., Blajchman, M. A., et al. (1999). A multicenter, randomized, controlled clinical trial of transfusion requirements in critical care. Transfusion Requirements in Critical Care Investigators, Canadian Critical Care Trials Group. *N Engl J Med, 340*, 409–417.
24. Hess, J. R., & Hiippala, S. (2005). Optimizing the use of blood products in trauma care. *Crit Care, 9*(Suppl. 5), S10–S14.
25. Hill, S., et al. (2002). Transfusion thresholds and other strategies for guiding allogeneic red blood cell transfusion (Cochrane Review). *The Cochrane Library*. Update Software: Oxford, Issue 2.
26. Holcomb, J. B., Tilley, B. C., Baraniuk, S., et al. (PROPPR Study Group. 2015). Transfusion of plasma, platelets, and red blood cells in a 1:1:1 vs a 1:1:2 ratio and mortality in patients with severe trauma: the PROPPR randomized clinical trial. *JAMA, 313*(5), 471–482.
27. Humphries, J. E., & Ortel, T. L. (2005). Treatment of acquired disorders of hemostasis. In P. L. Mintz (Ed.), *Transfusion therapy: clinical principles and practices* (2nd ed.). Bethesda, MD: AABB Press.
28. Hung, M., Besser, M., Sharples, L. D., et al. (2011). The prevalence and association with transfusion, intensive care unit stay and mortality of pre-operative anaemia in a cohort of cardiac surgery patients. *Anaesthesia, 66*, 812–818.
29. Johansson, P. I. (2012). Coagulation monitoring of the bleeding traumatized patient. *Curr Opin Anaesthesiol, 25*(2), 235–241.
30. Johansson, P. I., Hansen, M. B., & Sorensen, H. (2005). Transfusion practice in massively bleeding patients: time for a change? *Vox Sang, 89*(2), 92–96.
31. Kim, C., Connell, H., McGeorge, A., et al. (2015). Prevalence of preoperative anaemia in patients having first-time cardiac surgery and its impact on clinical outcome. A retrospective observational study. *Perfusion, 30*, 277–283.
32. Kopko, P. M., et al. (2002). Transfusion-related acute lung injury: report of a clinical look-back investigation. *JAMA, 287*, 1968–1971.
33. Kopko, P. M., & Popovsky, M. A. (2012). Transfusion-related acute lung injury. In M. A. Popovsky (Ed.), *Transfusion reactions* (4th ed., pp. 191–215). Bethesda, MD: AABB Press.
34. Lacroix, J., Hebert, P. C., Hutchison, J. S., et al. (2007). Transfusion strategies for patients in pediatric intensive care units. *N Engl J Med, 356*, 1609–1619.
35. LaMuraglia, G. M., et al. (2000). The reduction of the allogeneic transfusion requirement in aortic surgery with a hemoglobin-based solution. *J Vasc Surg, 31*, 299.
36. Linden, J. V., & Pisciotto, P. T. (1992). Transfusion-associated graft-versus-host disease and blood irradiation. *Transfus Med Rev, 6*, 116.
37. Mazzei, C. A., Popovsky, M. A., & Kopko, P. M. (2014). Noninfectious complications of blood transfusion. In M. K. Fung, B. J. Grossman, C. Hillyer, & C. M. Westhoff (Eds.), *AABB technical manual* (18th ed., pp. 688–690). Bethesda, MD: American Association of Blood Banks. 677.
38. Morton, J., Anastassopoulos, K. P., Patel, S. T., et al. (2010). Frequency and outcomes of blood products transfusion across procedures and clinical conditions warranting inpatient care: an analysis of the 2004 healthcare cost and utilization project nationwide inpatient sample database. *Am J Med Qual, 25*, 289–296.
39. National Blood Data Resource Center. (2001). *Comprehensive report on blood collection and transfusion in the United States*. Bethesda, MD: National Data Resource Center.
40. Nester, T., Jain, S., & Poisson, J. (2014). Hemotherapy decisions and their outcome. In M. K. Fung, B. J. Grossman, C. Hillyer, & C. M. Westhoff (Eds.), *AABB technical manual* (18th ed., p. 510, 672). Bethesda, MD: American Association of Blood Banks.
41. Perez, P. et al, for the BACTHEM group and the French Haemovigilance Network (2001). Determinants of transfusion-associated bacterial contamination: results of the French BACTHEM case-control study. *Transfusion, 41*, 862–872.
42. Peters, A. L., Van Stein, D., & Vlaar, A. P. (2015). Antibody-mediated transfusion-related acute lung injury; from discovery to prevention. *Br J Haematol, 170*(5), 597–614.
43. Popovsky, M. A., et al. (1983). Transfusion-related acute lung injury associated with passive transfer of antileukocyte antibodies. *Am Rev Respir Dis, 128*, 185–189.
44. Popovsky, M. A., et al. (1992). Transfusion-related acute lung injury: a neglected, serious complication of hemotherapy. *Transfusion, 32*, 589–592.
45. Popovsky, M. A. (2001). Hemolytic transfusion reactions. In M. A. Popovsky (Ed.), *Transfusion reactions*. Bethesda, MD: AABB Press.
46. Popovsky, M. A., & Haley, N. R. (2000). Further characterization of transfusion-related acute lung injury: demographics, clinical and laboratory features and morbidity. *Immunohematology, 16*, 157–159.
47. Rahbar, E., Fox, E. E., del Junco, D. J., et al. (2013). Early resuscitation intensity as a surrogate for bleeding severity and early mortality in the PROMMTT study. *J Trauma Acute Care Surg, 75*(1 Suppl. 1), S16–S23.
48. Raval, J. S., et al. (2015). Passive reporting greatly underestimates the rate of transfusion-associated circulatory overload after platelet transfusion. *Vox Sang, 108*, 387–392.
49. Rogiers, P., et al. (1997). Erythropoietin response is blunted in critically ill patients. *Intensive Care Med, 23*, 159–162.
50. Savage, S. A., Zarzaur, B. L., Croce, M. A., & Fabian, T. C. (2013). Redefining massive transfusion when every second counts. *J Trauma Acute Care Surg, 74*(2), 396–400.
51. Schiffer, C. A., et al. (2001). Platelet transfusion for patients with cancer: clinical practice guidelines of the American Society of Oncology. *J Clin Oncol, 19*, 1519.
52. Silvergleid, A. J. (2005). *Transfusion-associated graft-versus-host disease*. UpToDate http://www.uptodate.com.
53. Sirchia, G., Rebulla, P., & Sabbioneda, L. (1995). Preparation of white cell-reduced red cells by filtration: comparison of a bedside filter and two blood bank filter systems. *Transfusion, 35*, 421–426.
54. Spence, R. K., & Mintz, P. L. (2005). Transfusion in surgery, trauma, and critical care. In P. L. Mintz (Ed.), *Transfusion therapy: clinical principles and practices* (2nd ed.). AABB Press: Agency for Healthcare Research and Quality: HCUP facts and figures: statistics on hospital-based care in the United States, 2007, Rockville, MD, Agency for Healthcare Research and Quality; 2010 Bethesda, MD.
55. Spotnitz, W. D., et al. (2005). Clinical uses of fibrin sealant. In P. L. Mintz (Ed.), *Transfusion therapy: clinical principles and practices* (2nd ed.). Bethesda, MD: AABB Press.
56. Staudinger, T., Locker, G. J., & Frass, M. (1996). Management of acquired coagulation disorders in emergency and intensive-care medicine. *Semin Thromb Hemost, 22*, 93–104.
57. Suzuki, K., et al. (1992). Transfusion-associated graft-versus-host disease in a presumably immunocompetent patient after transfusion of stored packed red cells. *Transfusion, 32*, 358–360.
58. Taylor, R. W., et al. (2002). Impact of allogenic packed red blood cell transfusion on nosocomial infection rates in the critically ill patient. *Crit Care Med, 30*, 102249–102254.
59. Toy, P., et al. (2005). Transfusion-related acute lung injury: definition and review. *Crit Care Med, 33*, 721–726.
60. Vamvakas, E. C., & Blajchman, M. A. (2009). Transfusion-related mortality: the ongoing risks of allogeneic blood transfusion and the available strategies for their prevention. *Blood, 113*, 3406–3417.
61. Vincent, J. L., Baron, J. F., Reinhart, K., et al. (2002). Anemia and blood transfusion in critically ill patients. *JAMA, 288*, 1499–1507.
62. Whitaker, B. I., & Hinkins, S. (2011). The 2011 national blood collection and utilization survey report. US Department of Health and Human Services. http://www.hhs.gov/ash/bloodsafety/2011-nbcus.pdf.

27

Coagulopathies

Diane K. Dressler

Dramatic events in critical care often involve coagulopathies, which are disorders of blood coagulation. The term coagulopathy refers to any condition in which the blood's ability to clot is impaired.[22] This includes hemostasis disorders, which cause excessive bleeding, and also hypercoagulable states, which result in inappropriate clotting. Coagulopathy is a threat to every critically ill patient, particularly those with sepsis and those who have undergone trauma or extensive surgery.[22,25] Although some patients have inherited disorders of coagulation such as hemophilia, acquired disorders such as disseminated intravascular coagulation (DIC) are most likely to complicate critical illness. This chapter will describe normal hemostasis and the multiple disease processes that lead to coagulation abnormalities, as well as how to recognize and manage these disorders. Disorders of coagulation that are commonly seen in critically ill patients include trauma-induced coagulopathy, postoperative coagulopathy, medication-induced coagulopathy, thrombocytopenia, excessive fibrinolysis, bleeding associated with failure of specific organ systems, and common thrombotic disorders.

NORMAL HEMOSTASIS AND THE PATHWAYS TO A CLOT

Following an injury, hemostasis is accomplished by the harmonious interaction of three components: the injured blood vessel wall, platelets, and the plasma coagulation factors. The multiple events involved in blood clotting begin with spasm of the injured vessel wall and progress through a series of steps that result in clot formation. Vascular spasm is initiated by nerves in the vessel wall, and slows the loss of blood. The spasm is enhanced by the release of thromboxane A_2 from circulating platelets, and by the release of other potent vasoconstrictors, including endothelin.[19] The degree of spasm is proportional to the amount of trauma, with more spasm occurring with greater injury.

The subsequent hemostatic process entails two major steps. During the first step, platelet adhesion and aggregation occurs, resulting in formation of a platelet plug at the site of blood vessel injury. The second step involves the formation of a fibrin clot (Fig. 27.1).[19,28]

Hemostasis is initiated when the injured vessel lining and exposed collagen activate the blood platelets, beginning the processes of platelet adhesion and aggregation. When stimulated, the platelets change in shape from disks to spheres, exposing receptors that enable the platelets to stick to the surface of the damaged vessel.[45] These glycoprotein IIb/IIIa receptors are essential for binding platelets to each other and to fibrinogen during clot formation.[19] Platelet adhesion also depends on a protein produced by the vascular endothelium and bone marrow called von Willebrand factor (vWF). When endothelial cells are damaged, collagen is exposed, and vWF attaches to factor VIII, and which then binds to collagen. Platelet receptors then bind to vWF to enhance adhesion.[19] Platelets contain mitochondria and enzyme systems that enable them to release adenosine diphosphate (ADP) and synthesize prostaglandins—substances that are essential for stimulating the accumulation of more platelets.[28] The continued release of ADP and thromboxane A_2 results in self-perpetuating platelet aggregation.[45] Platelet plugs form, stopping the flow of blood from small tears in the vessel. These tiny platelet plugs are important for sealing injured capillaries and preventing petechiae from forming following minor bumps and slight trauma associated with normal activities. In addition to their role in clot formation, platelets help maintain vascular endothelium integrity by nurturing the tissue.

Although platelet plugs can stop the flow of blood from tiny injuries, when a larger clot is needed, the aggregation of platelets is only the beginning of the process. As platelet plugs form, tissue factor is released from the injured tissue, and the attraction and activation of other plasma coagulation factors begins. The fibrin complex that eventually makes up the clot is assembled on the platelet surfaces, where glycoprotein IIb/IIIa receptors and platelet phospholipids combine to form a mesh that traps red blood cells and enables hemostasis.

Two traditional pathways have been used to outline the process of fibrin clot formation: the extrinsic and intrinsic pathways.[15,19,45] In this model, blood clotting is initiated by the extrinsic pathway, in response to injury, and is augmented by the intrinsic (or contact activation) pathway.[43] Currently a more physiologically accurate interaction of the clotting components is used, which recognizes an earlier and more extensive relationship between the various factors[28] (Fig. 27.2).

The overall process of hemostasis involves a series of linked reactions, beginning with the activation of inactive procoagulant proteins and leading to the subsequent stimulation of a series of active proteins, culminating in the formation of a fibrin clot. This process is often referred to as the coagulation cascade. The major procoagulant factors involved in this process are listed in Table 27.1. The liver produces most of the plasma coagulation factors, including the procoagulant proteins known as fibrinogen, prothrombin, and factors V, VII, IX, X, and XI. These factors circulate through the blood in an inactive form until needed for hemostasis. Some of these factors are referred to by their common names (e.g., prothrombin), whereas other factors are referred to by Roman numerals followed by an "a" once they are activated (e.g., factor VII becomes VIIa). Although there are many factors involved in the coagulation process, it is most important to understand that without

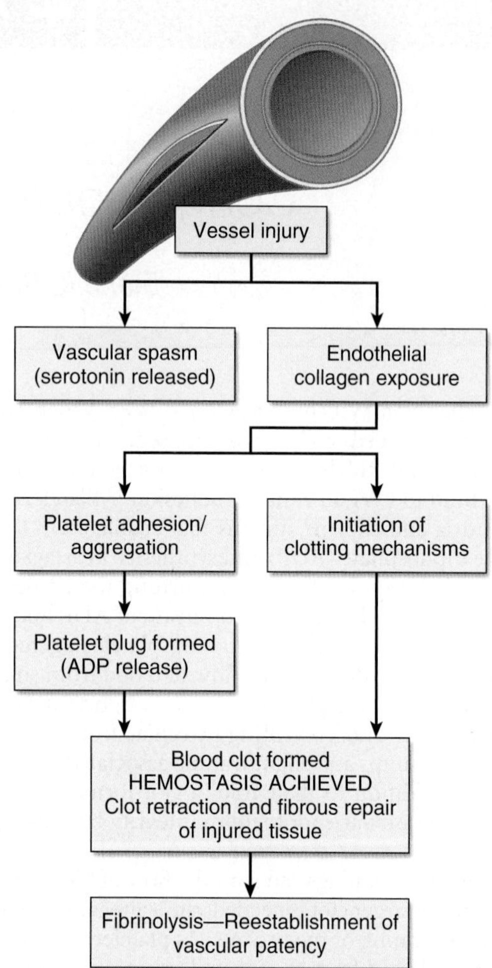

FIG. 27.1 The physiology of blood coagulation. *ADP,* Adenosine diphosphate.

adequate factor levels, platelet phospholipids, and calcium, the cascade is unable to generate an effective clot.

Clot formation begins when tissues and blood vessels are traumatized (see Fig. 27.2).[21,45] The process may also be activated within blood vessels due to damaged endothelium, exposed collagen, injured blood cells, endotoxins, and immune reactions. Tissue trauma results in the release of tissue factor from injured endothelial cells. The subsequent interaction of tissue factor with activated factor VII, platelets, and calcium activates factor X, advancing the process to the point where thrombin is generated. Simultaneously, tissue factor and VIIa activate factor IX and other factors that make up the traditional intrinsic pathway, leading to the activation of more factor X. The activation of factor IX through these mechanisms greatly amplifies the generation of thrombin.[28]

In the next phase of the sequence, Xa forms a complex with factor Va and calcium.[21] Prothrombin is then cleaved to generate thrombin, a powerful procoagulant that is considered to be the major enzyme responsible for blood clotting, as it cleaves fibrinogen into fibrin, which forms the fibrin clot.[28] This process is dramatically amplified as thrombin initiates feedback loops that activate factors XI and VIII, dramatically increasing clot formation.[21]

Finally, through a series of events involving factor XIII (the fibrin stabilizing factor), fibrin monomers become fibrin polymers, which become stable fibrin, forming the actual blood clot. The mesh-like clot consists of fibrin strands, red blood cells, and platelets. Clot formation usually occurs within minutes, and rapid clot formation is necessary to prevent the platelet plug and clot from washing away from the shear forces of blood flow.[28] After the clot is formed, the mesh retracts, squeezing out the serum and further stabilizing the cross-linked fibrin.

Following the clotting of a blood vessel, the fibrinolytic system is activated. The purpose of the fibrinolytic system is to gradually break down the clot and reestablish flow through the vessel. As a clot forms, plasminogen, the proenzyme for fibrinolysis, is incorporated into the clot. Naturally occurring plasminogen activators in the vascular endothelium begin the process, and ultimately plasminogen becomes plasmin, a substance capable of lysing the clot.[19] This mechanism is essentially the same as that involved in the fibrinolysis that is achieved when thrombolytic agents are used to treat acute myocardial infarction (AMI), but it occurs at a slow rate, allowing the torn vessel to repair itself. As clots dissolve, fibrin degradation products (FDPs), also known as fibrin split products (FSP), are released into the circulation. If present in large amounts, FDPs can act as anticoagulants.

Under normal conditions, there is an intricate balance between procoagulants and anticoagulants. Natural inhibitors of coagulation (e.g., antithrombin III, protein C, protein S, and tissue factor pathway inhibitor [TFPI]) oppose blood clotting and maintain the blood in a fluid state. If an injury occurs, clotting is initiated and should remain localized to the site of injury.[29] Any extra circulating activated factors (e.g., thrombin) are cleared from the circulation by substances such as antithrombin III. Plasmin breaks down fibrin clots; however, even plasmin is inactivated by antiplasmin, preventing excessive fibrinolysis.[12,19] This intricate balance may be upset by critical illness, which can destroy or inappropriately stimulate the processes of clotting and fibrinolysis, resulting in coagulopathy.

DISSEMINATED INTRAVASCULAR COAGULATION

DIC is a common disorder of coagulation in the critical care population. Always a secondary process or complication of another disorder, DIC may occur in acute or chronic forms; the acute process is seen most often in the critically ill. The process of DIC is unique because the patient experiences hemorrhage and thrombosis simultaneously. The International Society on Thrombosis and Hemostasis has defined DIC as an acquired syndrome characterized by the intravascular activation of coagulation.[22] The process is systemic rather than localized, and causes damage to the microvasculature that usually leads to organ dysfunction.[31]

Pathophysiology of DIC

The main feature of DIC is intravascular clotting. Multiple tiny clots form and are deposited in the microcirculation, where they block perfusion and contribute to multiple organ failure.[31] This extensive clotting is sometimes referred to as a *consumptive coagulopathy* because it depletes the blood of platelets and coagulation factors. Clotting components are utilized much more quickly than the liver and bone marrow can replace them.[21] The overall result is that clots are deposited where they are not needed (in the microvasculature), yet a stable clot cannot form at an injury

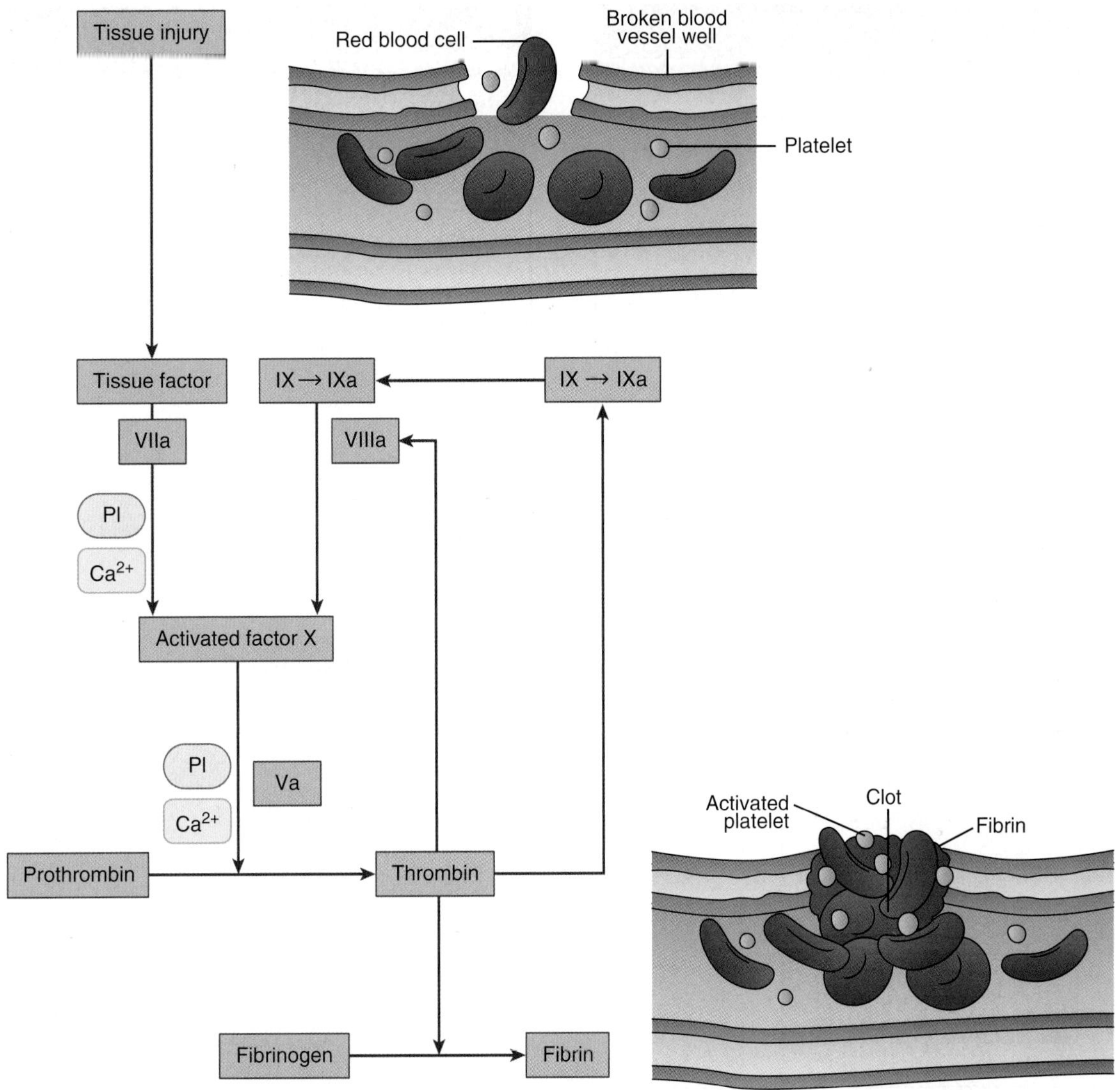

FIG. 27.2 Coagulation cascade. The revised model of blood coagulation is initiated by tissue injury. The generation of thrombin is followed by amplification through feedback loops that activate additional factors.

site. As the process continues, the patient often begins to bleed and may exhibit continuous oozing or frank hemorrhage.[29]

The type of intravascular clotting that occurs in DIC differs significantly from physiologic clotting. Clots form in the bloodstream in response to a thrombogenic stimulus that triggers the generation of thrombin and the coagulation cascade (Fig. 27.3). The underlying disorder results in damage to body tissues and endothelial injury. This injury triggers systemic activation of coagulation, resulting in unregulated thrombin activity, the formation of microvascular thrombi, consumption of platelets and coagulation factors, and abnormal fibrinolysis.[19,31] Initially, fibrinolysis may be suppressed, but later, the activation of fibrinolysis in turn leads to release of FDPs and D-dimers, a process that may lyse microthrombi while also contributing to more bleeding.

The pathophysiology of DIC is thought to be a physiologic response to the patient's underlying disorder and stimulation of the inflammatory response. Many of the known triggers for DIC involve damage to the vascular endothelium and subsequent activation of inflammation.[31] In addition to initiating hemostasis, the cellular elements of the blood, including leukocytes and platelets, are activated, and the anticoagulant substances produced by the vascular endothelium are altered. Inflammatory cytokines (e.g., interleukins 1 and 6 [IL-1, IL-6], and tumor necrosis factor-alpha [TNFα]) are released, leading to the generation of thrombin and subsequent clot formation. In addition, these cytokines can disable antithrombin III, protein C, and other natural anticoagulants.[31] As the inflammatory response is activated in addition to hemostasis, there can be inappropriate stimulation of clotting, fibrinolysis, or both.

Predisposing clinical conditions associated with DIC are multiple, ranging from shock to snakebite (Box 27.1). In critically ill patients, sepsis is the most common trigger for DIC.[21,22] The organisms involved may be gram-negative or gram-positive.[21] The most well-studied pathophysiology associated with DIC is that of gram-negative bacteremia, which leads to endotoxin release and the subsequent activation of inflammation and hemostasis.[18] The invading pathogens activate the inflammatory system, leading to the release of proinflammatory cytokines, which in turn stimulate procoagulants like tissue factor,

TABLE 27.1 Coagulation Factors and Common Names

Factor	Common Name
I	Fibrinogen
II	Prothrombin
III	Tissue factor
IV	Calcium
V	Proaccelerin
VI	Accelerin
VII	Proconvertin
VIII	Antihemophilic factor
IX	Christmas factor
X	Stuart factor
XI	Plasma thromboplastin antecedent
XII	Hageman factor
XIII	Fibrin-stabilizing factor
Von Willebrand Factor (vWF)	Factor VIII-related antigen

Modified from Reference 48a.

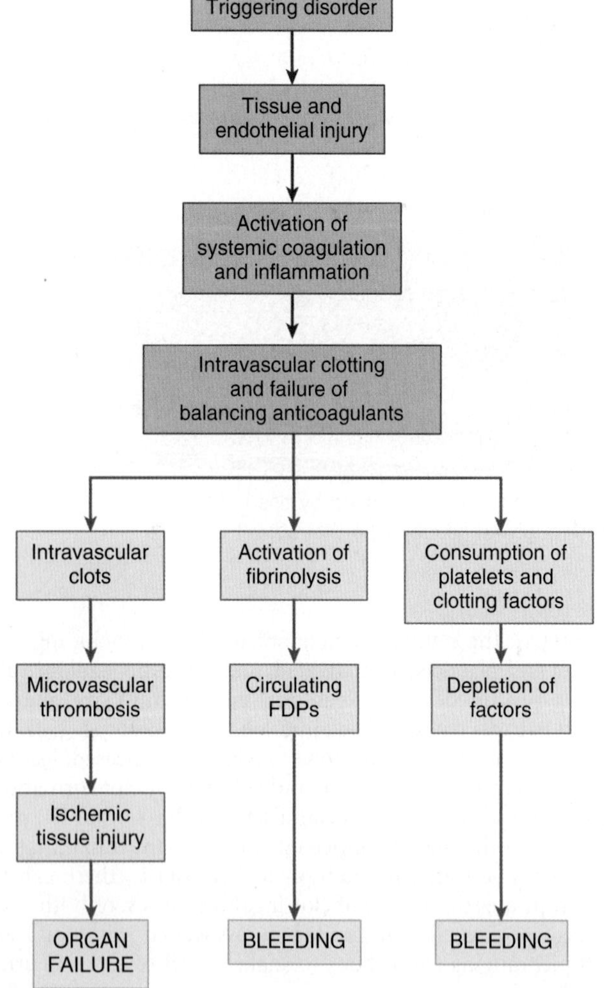

FIG. 27.3 The pathophysiology of disseminated intravascular coagulation.

impairing natural anticoagulants and the fibrinolytic process.[22] Sepsis from other organisms (e.g., viruses, protozoa, and fungi) is also associated with DIC.

Extensive trauma, including the trauma from extensive surgery, may also trigger DIC. The mechanisms involved include endothelial damage, release of tissue factor, and the release of tissue breakdown products (e.g., fat and phospholipids) that can activate clotting.[31] Systemic cytokine release is also thought to play a major role in trauma patients, as well as patients with sepsis.[22] Cytokines damage the vascular endothelium, activating the coagulation pathway and resulting in the deposition of clots in the microcirculation of major organs.

Complications of trauma, sepsis, and shock constitute additional triggering factors. DIC is further stimulated by hypothermia, hypotension, and acidosis.[18] There is a well-established relationship between the degree of hypothermia and coagulopathy due to blood clotting mechanisms being impaired at low body temperatures. Hypotension and poor perfusion damage the vascular endothelium and lead to metabolic acidosis, which may further alter blood coagulation and trigger clotting.

DIC has long been associated with obstetric problems. Obstetric complications that cause leakage of amniotic fluid, including placenta damage, may result in the release of tissue factors into the blood, triggering systemic clotting and activation of DIC.[31]

Other diagnoses associated with DIC include immunologic conditions (e.g., transfusion reactions) and other diverse disorders (e.g., heatstroke). Patients with cancer may also develop DIC because both solid tumors and hematologic malignancies

BOX 27.1 Clinical Conditions Associated with Disseminated Intravascular Coagulation

Infection and Sepsis
- Gram-negative sepsis
- Gram-positive sepsis
- Viral, protozoal, and fungal sepsis

Trauma
- Extensive traumatic injury
- Thoracic surgery
- Burns
- Snakebite
- Heatstroke

Shock
- Septic shock
- Hypovolemic shock

Malignancy
- Leukemia
- Solid tumors
- Metastatic cancer

Obstetric Complications
- Amniotic fluid embolus
- Abruptio placentae
- Preeclampsia
- Dead fetus syndrome

Vascular Abnormalities
- Aortic aneurysm
- Vascular malformation

Immunologic Reactions
- Blood transfusion reactions
- Immune complex disorders

Data from References 18, 19, and 30.

are known to release cytokines, which may precipitate coagulation problems.[31] Metastatic cancer is commonly associated with the chronic form of DIC.

Although there are many disorders and conditions that may trigger DIC, prompt identification and management of the disorder is important, because ongoing coagulopathy is a predictor of outcome in the critically ill. DIC has been identified as an independent predictor of mortality, especially in patients with sepsis and trauma, adding incentive to timely identification of the clinical and laboratory features of this syndrome.[31]

Clinical Manifestations of DIC

The clinical picture of DIC is quite variable, and can be dramatic, often presenting with bleeding.[16,22] The bleeding is caused by the continuous consumption of coagulation factors and the fibrinolysis of existing clots. The patient may develop oozing of blood from multiple sites, including incisions and puncture sites. Even sites that are partially healed may begin to bleed as fibrinolysis dissolves preexisting clots. Significant hemorrhagic events such as bleeding from the gastrointestinal (GI) tract and central nervous system are possible.

Patients may develop petechiae, purpura, and large areas of ecchymosis.[19] A peculiar type of skin ischemia, called purpura fulminans, may develop as capillaries become clotted.[31] Purpura fulminans is characterized by gray to purple discoloration of the skin on the lips, nose, ears, fingers, and toes.[45] There are sharp irregular areas of demarcation from normal areas of the skin, and the patient is at risk for necrosis in the affected areas. The deposition of fibrin in the microvasculature can also lead to multiple organ dysfunction syndrome. Major organ systems may be affected by microcirculatory clotting, increasing the risk of acute renal failure, acute lung injury, hepatic failure, gut failure, and brain dysfunction.[47]

Bleeding and thrombotic/ischemic problems may occur in different tissues and with varying intensity. Clinical manifestations of thrombosis typically result from microcirculatory occlusion. However, in chronic DIC, large thrombi may dominate the clinical picture.[18] DIC may also be detected on an abnormal coagulation panel, but without any clinical signs of bleeding or thrombosis.[31]

Laboratory Features of DIC

Unlike inherited coagulation disorders, acquired disorders may not be diagnosed by a single lab value. DIC is associated with multiple abnormalities in the coagulation mechanism and multiple laboratory indicators of coagulopathy. Table 27.2 lists normal coagulation test values on the panel of tests used to screen for DIC. Rapidly developing thrombocytopenia typically occurs early in DIC, and increases the risk of hemorrhage.[29] Both platelets and fibrinogen levels are low because these factors have been consumed during extensive and inappropriate clotting. The general coagulation tests are usually elevated in DIC. The prothrombin time/international normalized ratio (PT/INR) measures the integrity of the traditional extrinsic and common pathways.[15,42] The activated partial thromboplastin time (aPTT) measures the integrity of the traditional intrinsic and common pathways.[15,42] Thrombin time is another general test of coagulation. Whereas all of these values may show prolonged clotting times in DIC, none of them are diagnostic of the disorder.

There are a number of tests for fibrinolysis that are positive, but not specific, for DIC. FDPs will be elevated. The newer D-dimer test is an accurate enzyme-linked immunosorbent assay (ELISA) that is a more specific indicator of fibrinolysis than other tests, as D-dimers result only from dissolving clots.[45] FDPs and D-dimers are also elevated in response to trauma, recent surgery, inflammatory conditions, and thromboembolism.[29] Low levels of plasminogen and α_2-antiplasmin are also indicative of excessive fibrinolysis.[29]

TABLE 27.2 Coagulation Panel Results in Disseminated Intravascular Coagulation

Test	Normal Value*
Activated partial thromboplastin time	21–35 sec
D-dimer assay	< 0.0–0.6 mg/L FEU
Fibrin degradation products	Less than 10 mcg/mL
Fibrinogen	200–400 mg/dL
Hemoglobin	14–17.4 g/dL for males 12–16 g/dL for females
INR	0.8–1.2: normal 2.0–3.0: moderate-level anticoagulation 2.5–3.5: high-level anticoagulation
Prothrombin time	11–13 s
Thrombin time	7–12 s
Platelet count	150,000–400,000/μL

*Values may differ depending on the source.
FEU, Fibrinogen equivalent units; *INR*, international normalized ratio.
Data from References 15 and 30.

Thromboelastography (TEG) may also be used in the diagnosis of DIC to assess platelet function and fibrinolytic activity. Whereas standard coagulation tests are designed to monitor anticoagulation, this test can be performed rapidly at the bedside and provides information on clot formation, strength, and breakdown during coagulopathy.[43]

Individual factors such as factor V are known to be consumed in DIC, and factor assays may be performed to distinguish DIC from other coagulopathies.[29] Normally, the levels of these factors are approximately 100%, and depletion is indicative of consumption. The complete blood count (CBC) will show a drop in hemoglobin (Hgb) and hematocrit (Hct), reflecting the extent of bleeding. The peripheral blood smear may also show the presence of schistocytes, which are distorted and fragmented red cells that were sheared by circulating through partially clotted vessels.[18]

Because there is no single test that is specific for DIC, the International Society of Thrombosis and Hemostasis has proposed a scoring system for the diagnosis.[31] In patients with a condition known to be associated with DIC, the following indicators are scored: platelet count, fibrin-related markers, PT/INR, and fibrinogen level. A calculation is performed to determine the probability of DIC. Box 27.2 illustrates this calculation using laboratory tests that are generally available in most facilities.

When analyzing the results of a coagulation panel, there are additional, important considerations. Preexisting conditions (e.g., liver disease, surgery, or cancer) may affect factor levels. Monitoring trends in the values may be most important as they indicate whether the coagulopathy is improving or worsening. Diagnosing DIC and other acquired coagulation disorders may be difficult, and sometimes a definitive diagnosis cannot be determined.

Management of DIC

In the critically ill patient, DIC can quickly become a life-threatening situation. Currently, there is no definitive treatment for DIC. Instead, identification and treatment of the patient's

BOX 27.2 A Scoring System for the Diagnosis of Disseminated Intravascular Coagulation

Step 1: Presence of a disorder associated with DIC.
- No = 0
- Yes = 2

Step 2: Perform screening tests.
- Platelet count (>100 = 0, <100 = 1, <50 = 2)
- Fibrin-related marker (no increase = 0, moderate increase = 2, strong increase = 3)
- PT/INR (normal = 0, above normal = 1, 2 × normal = 2)
- Fibrinogen (normal = 0, less than normal = 1)

Step 3: Calculate score.
- If greater than or equal to 5, score is compatible with diagnosis of DIC.
- If less than 5, score is suggestive but not affirmative of DIC.

DIC, Disseminated intravascular coagulation; *INR,* international normalized ratio; *PT,* prothrombin time.
Data from Reference 30.

primary disorder is considered to be the most important goal.[16] DIC is always a complication of another disorder, and if that process can be stopped, it may also be possible to control the coagulopathy. For example, if the patient is septic, removing the source of infection and starting antimicrobial treatment may slow or stop the coagulopathic process. For some patients, treatment of the underlying problem can lead to improvement within hours; for others, DIC may progress in spite of treatment.

Effective management can be challenging in a patient with both bleeding and thrombosis. Providing general critical care support with fluid management, hemodynamic management, and support of ventilation and oxygenation is important. These interventions are key because hypoxia, hypotension, and acidosis contribute to continuing coagulopathy.[17,25]

Additional interventions may include the administration of blood products and pharmacologic therapy. Transfusion of blood and blood products is prescribed for patients with active hemorrhage or those who require surgery or invasive procedures.[29] Choosing the product for each patient is key to supporting good patient outcomes. Administration of packed red blood cells (PRBCs) maintains oxygen-carrying capacity, and is necessary for optimizing and maintaining oxygen delivery and utilization. Platelet concentrate (PC) may be given for bleeding caused by thrombocytopenia. Fresh frozen plasma (FFP) provides fibrinogen, prothrombin, and many other plasma coagulation factors. Cryoprecipitate is administrated to patients with DIC specifically to replace fibrinogen, as well as factor VIII and vWF. Vitamin K may be administered to enhance production of clotting components.[19] In addition to the standard blood components, administration of recombinant activated factor VIIa (rFVIIa) is reported to reduce hemorrhage in trauma patients. However, rFVIIa is not recommended for DIC at time of printing because there is insufficient evidence of its safety and efficacy.[21]

There are always concerns pertaining to blood administration. Known potential adverse effects include transfusion-associated acute lung injury (TRALI), circulatory overload, transmission of infection, immune system modulation, alloimmunization with the development of reactive antibodies, acute febrile reactions, and other reactions.[5,43]

In patients with DIC, there has historically been additional concern that transfusion of components may add "fuel to the fire" as the transfused platelets and fibrinogen may be used for more inappropriate clotting, although this has never been proven in clinical studies.[45] Regardless of these potential concerns, patients who have severe hemorrhage require transfusion to support end-organ perfusion, maintain oxygen-carrying capacity, and replace lost components. For the actively bleeding patient, a laboratory-guided transfusion protocol provides a guide to therapy.[49] General management guidelines advise close monitoring of Hgb, platelet counts, INR, aPTT, and fibrinogen levels.[22] The administration of blood and blood components in DIC is based on expert opinion more than on specific guidelines. PRBCs are given for a low Hgb levels in patients who are actively bleeding. An INR greater than 1.5 may be considered an indication for FFP. For patients with a fibrinogen level less than 100 mg/dL, 10 units of cryoprecipitate are given. A platelet transfusion may be indicated for a patient with a platelet count of less than 50,000/μL.[22] Chapter 26 provides more comprehensive information on blood transfusion therapy.

Patients with abnormal lab results but no clinical evidence of bleeding are generally not prescribed blood and blood components.[31] Patients requiring an invasive procedure may need transfusion to correct laboratory defects.

Pharmacologic therapy may also be used to treat DIC, especially when thrombosis is the dominant clinical problem. Although controversial, heparin may be administered with the goal of interrupting the intravascular generation of thrombin and preventing further clotting of the microvasculature.[31] Heparin is most often prescribed for patients with evidence of thromboembolism and extensive fibrin deposition (e.g., purpura fulminans). However, the risk of further bleeding from heparin is a consideration and patients must be closely monitored. The efficacy of heparin in DIC has not been supported in clinical trials.[22,31]

Work continues on trials of new agents that may be useful in the treatment of DIC. Administration of TFPI aims to inhibit the excessive activation of tissue factor in order to limit clotting.[21] Antithrombin III is a natural regulator of thrombin, but may be overwhelmed in the presence of DIC, causing excessive clotting. Administration of antithrombin III (AT III) may inhibit clotting, but there are concerns regarding the risk of bleeding.[44] For patients in whom fibrinolysis dominates the clinical picture, fibrinolytic inhibitors such as tranexamic acid may be used.[31] However, anti-fibrinolytic agents are generally contraindicated in DIC.[22] Additional trials are planned to determine the efficacy of all of these agents in DIC.

In patients fortunate enough to survive DIC, physiologic processes aid in recovery. Plasmin eventually breaks down the fibrin in the microvasculature, restoring circulation. Leukocytes remove fibrin deposits and complexes, further enhancing the circulation. Over time, the liver and bone marrow replace depleted plasma coagulation factors, platelets, and red blood cells. These processes can enable patients to recover from this serious complication.

TRAUMA-INDUCED COAGULOPATHY

Many trauma patients present with severe coagulopathy and require rapid intervention, including the transfusion of blood products. Early control of coagulopathy is correlated with improved survival in this population.[8] Bleeding occurs from traumatic injuries, but the development of coagulopathy is a more complex process that involves depletion, dilution, and inactivation of clotting factors.[25] In addition to hypovolemia, traumatic shock leads to an intense inflammatory response, which is followed by the release of proinflammatory mediators such as IL-1 and TNFα. As the systemic inflammatory response syndrome (SIRS) continues, the process can lead to acute respiratory distress syndrome (ARDS) and multiple organ failure.[1] During acute SIRS, procoagulant factors are produced, which results in a coagulopathy similar to DIC.

A number of factors increase the risk of coagulopathy associated with trauma. Patients may have comorbid conditions that increase the risk of bleeding. In addition, taking antithrombotic medications may increase risk of bleeding.[17] Patients may also experience hypothermia and acidosis after an injury. Hypothermia can occur due to environmental exposure during prehospital care or in the emergency department or operating room (OR). Hemostasis functions best at normal body temperature, and a body temperature less than 36°C may lead to coagulopathy as platelet function and coagulation enzyme function are inhibited.[8,43] Hypothermia may also activate fibrinolysis, which can destroy needed clots.[17] Metabolic acidosis develops from hypotension, poor perfusion, and decreased oxygen delivery to tissues, resulting in anaerobic metabolism and the production of lactic acid. Excessive use of crystalloids and respiratory acidosis may also contribute to an acidotic state. Severe acidosis impairs coagulation, worsening bleeding problems. Hypothermia, acidosis, and coagulopathy constitute a *lethal triad* of problems that has long been associated with increased mortality.[8,17,25]

Managing patients with trauma-induced coagulopathy includes prevention and treatment of hypothermia and acidosis, as well as early recognition and treatment of coagulopathy. Hypothermia can be minimized by controlling the patient's environment. This includes avoiding cold room temperatures and removing wet clothes and dressings from the patient.[25] The patient's core temperature should be monitored, and the patient should be warmed by warm blankets or with a forced air warming system. Blood products and intravenous (IV) fluids may also be warmed through an infusion system.

Metabolic acidosis can be minimized by maintaining hemodynamic stability and adequate ventilation and oxygenation.[17,25] Patient vital signs, hemodynamic parameters, level of consciousness, and urine output should be assessed frequently.

The routine infusion of large volumes of crystalloid IV fluids is no longer recommended for trauma patients. Crystalloids can worsen coagulopathy by causing dilution of essential clotting components.[8,25] Care is now focused on early recognition of coagulopathy, which requires massive transfusion and the availability of an institutional transfusion protocol to facilitate rapid access to essential blood products.[48a] The term *massive transfusion* refers to the administration of more than 10 units of PRBCs in a 24-hour period.[8,48a] Although massive blood transfusion may lead to TRALI and other complications, it may be lifesaving in severely injured patients.[5,8] The preferential use of blood products over crystalloids began in military settings, and has now transitioned to civilian settings. Protocols include administration of a 1:1 ratio of FFP to PRBCs, a strategy that has been called *damage control resuscitation.*[35] Additional protocols include PC at a ratio of 1:1:1 of FFP:PRBC:PC.[8,25,48a]

Trauma-induced coagulopathy may not always result in obvious hemorrhage; evidence-based triggers for massive transfusion include combinations of the following indicators:[8]

- Acidosis evidenced by a base deficit of > 6
- Hgb < 11 g/dL
- Hypothermia < 36°C
- INR > 1.5
- SBP < 90 mm Hg

Additional clinical indicators include physical assessment parameters such as mental status and peripheral pulses.[8] TEG may also be used by trauma teams to monitor coagulation abnormalities and direct treatment.[1,25] Obtaining coagulation panel results may take excessive time and the values may be inadequate for the diagnosis and treatment of patients with trauma.[2,3] TEG can rapidly provide clinically useful information at the point of care.

In addition to the use of PRBCs, FFP, and PC in a massive transfusion protocol, patients with ongoing coagulopathy and low fibrinogen levels may receive cryoprecipitate.[49] rFVIIa may also be used for ongoing coagulopathy. In patients with suspected excessive fibrinolysis, tranexamic acid (TXA) may be administered to inhibit plasminogen activation and subsequent fibrinolysis.[25]

POSTOPERATIVE COAGULOPATHY

Postoperative bleeding can occur after any surgery. Patients at particular risk include those with presurgical conditions such as hepatic insufficiency, an inherited disorder of coagulation, or preoperative anticoagulation. However, even with preoperative screening of coagulation parameters, it is not always possible to predict which patients will have bleeding problems.[42] This section focuses on bleeding complications following cardiac surgery,[11] which are common.

Postoperative coagulopathy is a serious complication. Moderate to severe bleeding is associated with increased mortality and an increased need for blood products, placing the patient at risk for transfusion-related complications.[11,49] Patients with excessive bleeding may also need to return to the OR for additional surgery.

A universal definition of what constitutes perioperative bleeding has been proposed by the International Initiative on Haemostasis Management in Cardiac Surgery.[11] Five classes of bleeding are determined by clinical indicators, including the amount of chest tube drainage, the number of blood transfusions, the need for surgical reexploration or delayed sternal closure, and the use of rFVIIa.[11]

There are a number of factors that put patients at risk, beginning with the use of cardiopulmonary bypass (CPB).[49] As blood passes through the bypass circuit, contact between blood components and the oxygenator activate both coagulation and fibrinolysis.[39] Bleeding may result from excessive fibrinolysis as tissue plasminogen activator is released from endothelial cells.[49] The inflammatory process is activated and leads to cytokine release and the stimulation of neutrophils, thereby increasing the risk of coagulopathy. Both the number and the function of platelets are decreased during CPB.[49] Hypothermia (used to decrease oxygen requirements during surgery) contributes to impaired platelet function and postoperative coagulopathy.[39] Heparin is used to prevent clotting in the bypass circuit, and is reversed with protamine at the end of the surgery.[39]

Other risk factors include the use of preoperative anticoagulation medications, previous cardiac surgeries, and complex procedures. Patients are instructed to discontinue anticoagulant medications before a planned surgery. However, stopping platelet inhibitors, glycoprotein inhibitors, and other anticoagulants before urgent procedures may not be possible. Previous thoracic operations produce adhesions that must be dissected during surgery, significantly increasing the procedural trauma.[49] Complex surgeries such as implantation of left ventricular assist devices (LVADs) or cardiac transplantation also pose an increased risk of bleeding.[49]

Most postoperative bleeding occurs within the first 4–6 hours after surgery. It is important to distinguish between coagulopathy and bleeding caused by inadequate hemostasis at the surgical site. Patients with coagulopathy will usually have bleeding from multiple sites, in addition to excessive chest tube drainage. Patients with inadequate hemostasis will generally have excessive chest tube drainage (>150–200 mL/h) without bleeding from other sites.[49] In the latter case, reoperation may be necessary to identify the site of bleeding and stop the hemorrhage.

A coagulation panel is drawn on patients who have clinical signs of bleeding. The panel may include a CBC with platelet count, PT/INR, aPTT, fibrinogen, D-dimer, and measurement of additional factor levels. The use of TEG is supported by guidelines from the National Institute for Health and Care Excellence (NICE), as it compares favorably with standard lab testing.[40] In cardiac surgery patients, TEG is associated with decreased mortality, fewer complications, a lower transfusion rate, and decreased cost.[40]

Although blood conservation always remains a goal, postoperative bleeding is treated with administration of PRBCs and FFP. Administration of apheresed platelets may also be indicated due to platelet dysfunction in postoperative coagulopathy.[49] Serial coagulation panels should be performed to determine whether additional blood products are needed. A coagulation-based hemotherapy service has been shown to facilitate the management of perioperative bleeding in high-risk cardiac surgical patients.[49] A pathologist specializing in hemotherapy coordinates the diagnosis and treatment through a lab in close proximity to the OR and critical care unit. Transfusion algorithms are used to guide the administration of blood products. For example, if chest tube drainage is 1000 mL, then 2 units of PRBCs, 1 unit of FFP, and 1 unit of PC should be administered.[49] Welsh et al. report a decrease in the number of blood products used and better outcomes with this type of support.[49]

Pharmacologic therapy may be used to prevent or treat postoperative coagulopathy. Protamine may be administered to reverse heparin. Currently, the lysine analogs TXA (Cyklokapron and Transamin) and epsilon aminocaproic acid (Amicar) are recommended by the Society of Thoracic Surgeons and the Society of Cardiovascular Anesthesiologists.[14] The efficacy of these drugs to control bleeding and limit the need for blood products in the perioperative period are still under investigation. Another agent used to treat postoperative coagulopathy is desmopressin acetate (DDAVP),[14] which acts by stimulating the release of vWF by endothelial cells, enhancing platelet aggregation.[22] rFVIIa is a more expensive alternative, and is generally reserved for patients who continue to bleed despite routine interventions.[11]

Blood conservation guidelines from the Society of Thoracic Surgeons and the Cardiovascular Anesthesiologists provide interventions that can minimize postoperative coagulopathy and the need for blood products. Preoperative recommendations include discontinuing antithrombotic and antiplatelet agents, administration of recombinant erythropoietin in patients with preoperative anemia, and reversal of warfarin (Coumadin) with FFP or prothrombin complex concentrate (PCC).[14]

MEDICATION-INDUCED COAGULOPATHY

Prevention of venous thromboembolism (VTE) is an important focus of care, as it is well-documented that deep venous thrombosis (DVT) and pulmonary embolism (PE) lead to increased morbidity, mortality, and healthcare costs.[9] There are many indications for anticoagulation in current clinical practice, and these include patients with conditions commonly seen in critical care.[27] For example, anticoagulants are an important part of the treatment regimen for patients with acute coronary syndromes, valvular heart disease, atrial fibrillation, and other cardiovascular conditions. However, suppression of the normal coagulation system carries with it the risk of bleeding.[33] Bleeding may be provoked by tissue trauma or may be spontaneous, and can include bleeding from procedure sites, retroperitoneal hemorrhage, GI bleeding, and intracranial bleeding.

Risks and benefits of anticoagulation therapy must be carefully assessed due to the risk of bleeding problems. For patients in atrial fibrillation, various versions of the CHA_2DS_2-VASc scoring system (congestive heart failure, hypertension, age >75 years, diabetes mellitus, stroke, vascular disease, age 65-74, gender) are used to determine whether anticoagulation is needed. Other scoring systems, including the HAS-BLED and $HEMORR_2HAGES$ scoring systems, identify patients at high risk of bleeding from comorbid conditions such as liver disease and stroke.[41] There are also guidelines for the discontinuation of anticoagulant medications prior to surgery and invasive procedures.[10,33]

The use of anticoagulants has increased in current clinical practice, particularly in hospitalized patients. Recommendations on VTE prophylaxis from the Institute for Healthcare Improvement include evaluation of all hospitalized patients for risk of VTE and use of pharmacologic thromboprophylaxis for high-risk patients, unless there are contraindications.[24] Many new antithrombotic medications have been added to the list of conventional agents. Commonly used anticoagulants, their major mechanisms of action, and interventions needed to reverse their effects are listed in Table 27.3. The classes of antithrombotic agents will be discussed briefly, along with the implications for potential bleeding problems.

Platelet Inhibitors

Drugs that inhibit platelet activity include aspirin, nonsteroidal antiinflammatory drugs (NSAIDs), $P2Y_{12}$ adenosine diphosphate receptor antagonists, and glycoprotein IIb/IIIa antagonists. Aspirin and NSAIDs inhibit cyclooxygenase and the subsequent production of thromboxane A_2, a necessary step for platelet aggregation (Fig. 27.4).[4] Aspirin is the most potent NSAID, with effects that occur within 1 hour and last for the duration of the platelet's life span (5 to 7 days). Aspirin is used to prevent thromboemboli from forming in the arterial system, thereby lowering the risk of cardiovascular events. Patients who have taken aspirin may have postoperative and postprocedure oozing and bleeding. These patients may be treated with platelet transfusion or DDAVP.[23]

Clopidogrel (Plavix) is the most commonly used ADP-$P2Y_{12}$ inhibitor.[4] This oral agent inhibits ADP-induced

TABLE 27.3 **Anti-Thrombotic Medications**

Medication	Mechanism of Action	Reversal
Abciximab (Reopro)	Glycoprotein IIb/IIIa receptor blocker	Platelet transfusion
Alteplase (tPA)	Thrombolytic (fibrinolytic)	No specific reversal agent
Apixaban (Eliquis)	Direct Xa inhibitor	No specific reversal agent
Argatroban	Direct thrombin inhibitor	No specific reversal agent
Aspirin	Irreversible inhibitor of cyclooxygenase	Platelets, consider use of desmopressin
Bivalirudin (Angiomax)	Direct thrombin inhibitor	FFP, cryoprecipitate, FVIIa
Clopidogrel (Plavix)	Inhibits ADP-P2Y12 receptors on platelets	Platelet transfusion
Dabigatran (Pradaxa)	Direct thrombin inhibitor	Idarucizumab (Praxbind)
Eptifibatide (Integrilin)	Glycoprotein IIb/IIIa receptor blocker	Platelets
Fondaparinux (Arixtra)	Inhibits Xa	No specific reversal agent
Heparin (unfractionated)	Xa and thrombin inhibition	Protamine
Low molecular weight heparin	Same as unfractionated heparin; mainly Xa effect	Protamine
Rivaroxaban (Xarelto)	Direct anti-Xa inhibitor	No specific reversal agent
Warfarin (Coumadin)	Vitamin K antagonist	IV vitamin K, PCC, FFP

IV, Intravenous; FFP, fresh frozen plasma; PCC, prothrombin complex concentrate; tPA, tissue plasminogen activator.
Data from References 3, 22, 25, and 48.

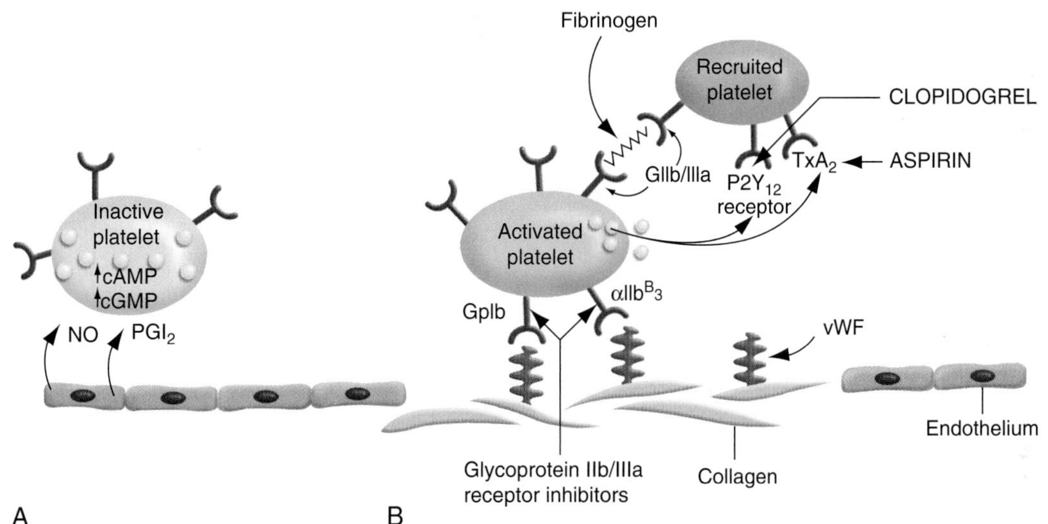

FIG. 27.4 Platelet activation sequence, including site of action for platelet-inhibiting medications. **A,** The inactive, circulating platelet. **B,** The activated platelet releases mediators such as TxA_2 and exposes glycoprotein receptors. Platelet-inhibiting medications act at different places in the activation sequence to inhibit platelet aggregation and clot formation. *ADP,* Adenosine diphosphate; *cAMP,* cyclic adenosine monophosphate; *cGMP,* cyclic guanosine monophosphate; *GpIb,* glycoprotein Ib; *NO,* nitric oxide; *PGI_2,* prostacyclin; *TxA_2,* tranexamic acid; *vWF,* von Willebrand factor.

platelet aggregation, decreasing the risk of cardiovascular events. Clopidogrel inhibits platelet aggregation for approximately 1 week, and when combined with aspirin, the risk of a bleeding complication increases.[33] Treatment for bleeding problems includes platelet transfusion.

The glycoprotein IIb/IIIa inhibitors include IV preparations of abciximab (ReoPro), eptifibatide (Integrilin), and tirofiban (Aggrastat). These agents act on the platelet membrane glycoproteins, where they inhibit the final phase of platelet aggregation, preventing the platelets from combining with fibrinogen.[4] Glycoprotein inhibitors are used during percutaneous coronary interventions, and pose a higher risk of postprocedure bleeding. Treatment for bleeding complications may include transfusion of platelets or blood components containing fibrinogen, depending on the specific glycoprotein inhibitor.[33]

Warfarin

Warfarin is a commonly used oral anticoagulant that is associated with major bleeding complications.[38] This agent inhibits the production of the vitamin K–dependent coagulation factors in the liver, including prothrombin; factors VII, IX, and X; and the anticoagulants protein C and S.[4,23] As shown in Fig. 27.5, warfarin inhibits the hemostatic system at multiple sites. The clinical goal is to achieve an INR of 2.0 to 3.0, depending on the indication for anticoagulation.[20] Warfarin acts slowly and takes days to achieve peak effectiveness, as the body must clear itself of the vitamin K–dependent clotting factors. Unfortunately, it also takes days to reverse the effects. This can become an important issue when patients are injured or when they require emergency surgery or invasive procedures. The risk of bleeding from warfarin increases with an

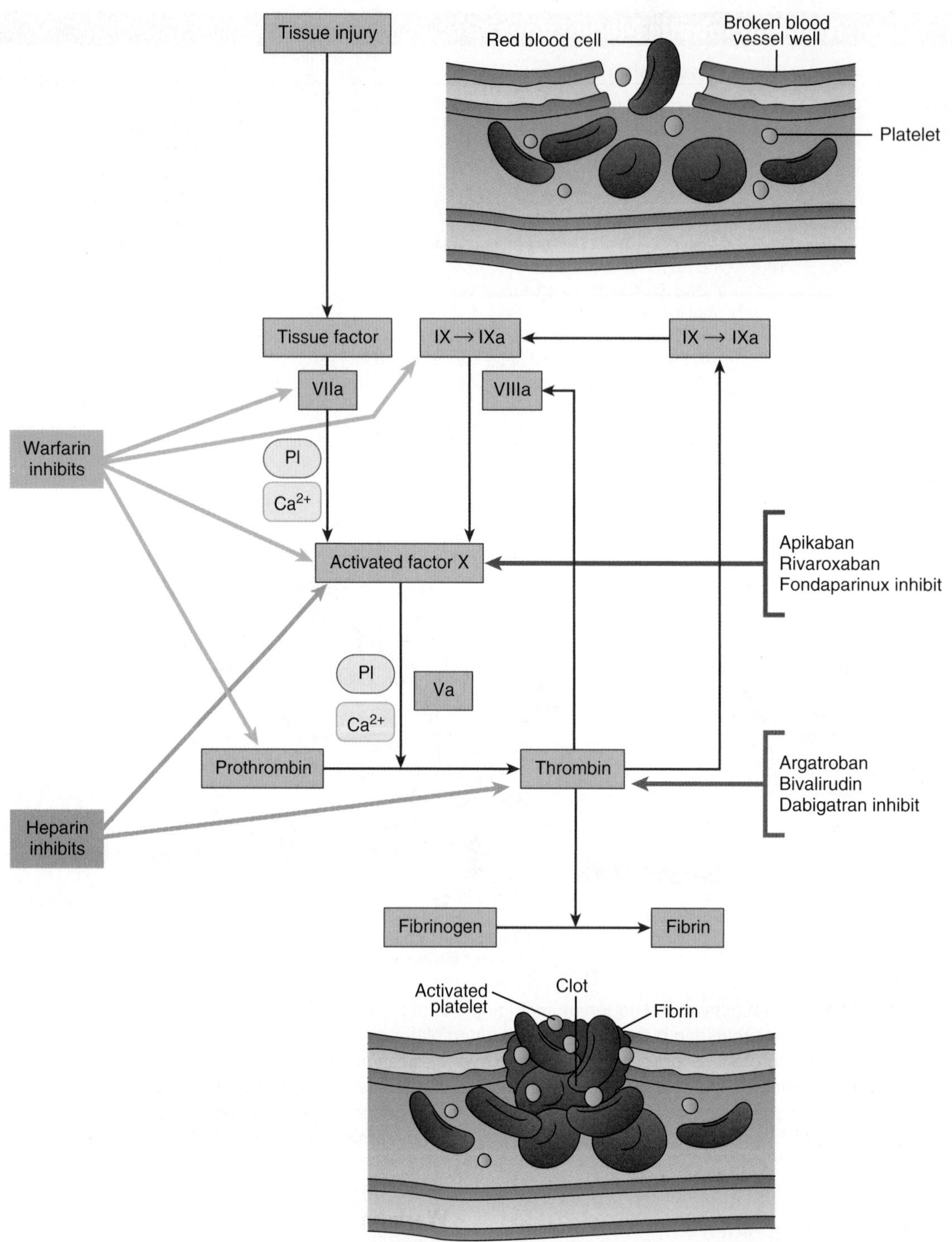

FIG. 27.5 Coagulation cascade and sites of action of anticoagulant medications.

INR greater than 4.5.[20] Bleeding complications from warfarin are particularly common in the elderly, and often lead to emergency hospitalization.[41] Other risk factors for bleeding complications include fluctuating INR levels, and a history of GI bleeding, cerebrovascular disease, and malignancy. In the event of bleeding complications believed to be associated with warfarin, the American College of Chest Physician guidelines on evidence-based management of anticoagulant therapy have specific recommendations for rapid reversal of warfarin. Vitamin K may be administered (up to 10 mg IV), along with PCC (preferred) or FFP.[20] PCC contains factors II, VII, IX, and X.[35] The benefits of PCC include the ability to provide rapid factor replacement using a small volume.

New Oral Anticoagulants

New oral anticoagulants include direct factor Xa inhibitors (apixaban [Eliquis], rivaroxaban [Xarelto]) and direct thrombin inhibitors (dabigatran [Pradaxa]).[27] Indications for these drugs includes prevention of stroke in atrial fibrillation, prevention of VTE, and treatment of VTE not related to orthopedic surgery.[4] These agents have some distinct advantages when compared to warfarin, as they do not have dietary restrictions and do not require routine blood testing, because of their wide therapeutic windows.[23] In clinical trials, these drugs have been shown to be safe and effective for the prevention and treatment of thromboembolism when compared with warfarin and other anticoagulants.[9,41] In general, the new anticoagulants carry a similar risk of bleeding as compared to warfarin. Doses may be reduced to decrease the risk of bleeding in patients with renal impairment.[41] Of concern is the reversal of bleeding in patients receiving the new oral anticoagulants. To date, the only reversal agent available is idarucizumab (Praxbind) specifically to reverse the effects of dabigatran. Trials on the use of blood products such as PCC, as well as other reversal agents, are in process.[23]

Heparin

Unfractionated heparin (UFH) binds to antithrombin III, inhibiting both thrombin and factor Xa.[23] The result is inhibition in the final steps of the coagulation pathway, preventing the formation of new clots (see Fig. 27.5). Heparin has a rapid onset and a short half-life, and is used to produce immediate anticoagulation in patients with acute thrombosis.[20] Heparin is also used extensively during hemodialysis and cardiac procedures. Because of patients' unpredictable responses to heparin, laboratory testing with aPTT or heparin assays is required, and doses may need frequent adjustment.[33] Complications of heparin therapy include bleeding and heparin-induced thrombocytopenia (HIT).

Low molecular weight heparin (LMWH) is derived from unfractionated heparin through a manufacturing process that alters the molecular structure leading to smaller molecules. LMWH mainly inactivates factor Xa, and has been shown to be as effective as full-dose UFH for all types of venous thrombosis, prompting recent shifts in treatment protocols. Advantages of LMWH include a more predictable response in comparison to UFH. Weight-based dosing is used, and routine laboratory monitoring is not considered necessary, because of the predictable response.[4] When indicated, LMWH activity can be measured by anti-factor Xa assay.[23] Caution must be used for patients with renal insufficiency, because LMWH is excreted by the kidneys.[24]

Fondaparinux (Arixtra) is a synthetic anticoagulant that selectively inhibits factor Xa.[23] It is administered subcutaneously and is used as an alternative to LMWH to prevent DVT. No laboratory monitoring is required, and there is no risk of HIT.[4]

Bleeding is a potential major complication with all forms of heparin and synthetic heparins, and the GI tract is a common site of life-threatening bleeding. Both types of heparin can be reversed by stopping the drug and administering protamine.

Direct Thrombin Inhibitors

The direct thrombin inhibitors are a class of drugs that inhibit thrombin-mediated fibrin formation.[4] These agents include the IV preparations of argatroban and bivalirudin (Angiomax), and the oral agent dabigatran.

Argatroban is a synthetic direct thrombin inhibitor used for the treatment and prevention of thromboembolic disorders in patients with HIT.[7] Patients receiving argatroban are monitored by aPTT testing, with a goal of 1.5–3.0 times the normal control value.[4] Bivalirudin is a synthetic agent similar to hirudin, an anticoagulant isolated from the saliva in leeches,[4] and may be used during percutaneous interventional cardiac procedures because of its short half-life.

Thrombolytic Agents

Thrombolytic agents such as alteplase (Activase) are used in AMI, stroke, and other thromboembolic events. Alteplase is identical to natural tissue plasminogen activator (tPA), and binds with plasminogen, converting it into plasmin, which lyses fibrin clots.[4] Patients should be evaluated for contraindications before these medications are prescribed because they pose a significant risk of bleeding due to lysis of hemostatic plugs at the site of vascular procedures (e.g., femoral site), and may cause serious problems, including intracranial hemorrhage.[4] If bleeding occurs, the drug is stopped, and reversal may require blood products.

THROMBOCYTOPENIA

Thrombocytopenia is a common disorder seen in critically ill patients.[23] Causes may include increased destruction of platelets (associated with sepsis), autoimmune disorders (such as immune thrombocytopenia purpura), diseases of the liver and spleen, and use of intravascular devices (e.g., intraaortic balloon pump).[23] Decreased production of thrombocytes by the bone marrow may occur in patients receiving cytotoxic drugs or those with bone marrow depression from neoplastic disorders.[13] Thrombocytopenia is also a feature of consumptive coagulopathies (i.e., DIC) and other disorders associated with hemorrhage. Regardless of the cause, thrombocytopenia is associated with increased mortality in the critically ill.[31] This is particularly true if it persists for more than 4 days after admission to the critical care unit, or if the patient's platelet count drops by more than 50% while in the critical care unit.[29]

Thrombocytopenia is defined as a platelet count of less than 150,000/μL.[44] A low platelet count does not always lead to bleeding; however, patients with a platelet count of less than 20,000/μL to 50,000/μL are considered at risk of spontaneous bleeding.[44] At these low levels, patients may also develop petechiae, ecchymosis, and bleeding from mucous membranes or injury sites. These clinical signs are related to the capillary fragility that occurs in thrombocytopenia, as well as a low platelet count.[23] There is significant variation, however, in how low the platelet count can drop before a patient develops signs of bleeding. Regardless of the platelet count, another consideration is whether the platelets are functional. Platelet function can be inhibited by drugs, hypothermia, acidosis, and uremia. Poor quality platelets can lead to bleeding problems.

Treatment of thrombocytopenia involves identifying and treating the underlying cause. In patients with active bleeding or the potential for hemorrhage, platelet transfusions may be given to maintain a platelet count greater than 50,000/μL.[22] The expected rise in the platelet count depends on platelet consumption, as well as the number of units transfused. Patients may form human leukocyte antigen (HLA) antibodies, become refractory to platelet transfusion, and require HLA-matched platelets.[13,22] Desmopressin may be administered to patients to enhance vWF release and restore platelet function.

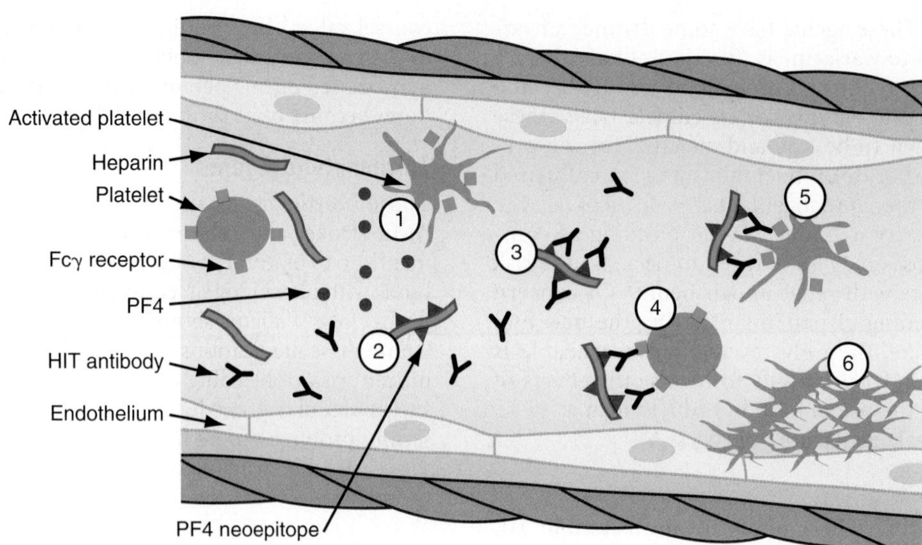

FIG. 27.6 The pathophysiology of heparin-induced thrombocytopenia (HIT). *(1)* Activated platelets release PF4. *(2)* Heparin binds to PF4, generating an antigen that leads to production of antibodies in susceptible individuals. *(3)* Antibodies combine with PF4 to form immune complexes. *(4)* Platelet receptors react with the complexes. *(5)* Activation of more platelets and the coagulation cascade. *(6)* Clots form, platelets are consumed. *PF4,* Platelet factor 4. (From McCance, K. L., & Huether, S. E. (2014). *Pathophysiology: the biologic basis for disease in adults and children* (7th ed.). St. Louis: Mosby.)

HEPARIN-INDUCED THROMBOCYTOPENIA (HIT)

HIT is a rare but serious complication associated with heparin that is characterized by a drop in platelet count and the clinical appearance of thromboembolic events. There are two types of HIT.[6] Type I HIT affects approximately 10% of patients receiving heparin, and involves a mild reduction in the platelet count 1 to 4 days after starting heparin.[19] It is thought to be a direct effect of heparin, and is considered benign.[6] Type II HIT affects up to 5% of patients exposed to heparin, and is a much more serious condition. This type is characterized by a 30% to 50% reduction in platelets and typically occurs 5 to 10 days after heparin is started, but can occur earlier if the patient has been previously exposed. Type II HIT is an immune-mediated process that is mediated by antibodies to platelet factor 4 (PF4).[6] HIT autoantibodies bind to heparin-PF4 complexes on the surface of platelets, activating the platelets (Fig. 27.6). The resulting clotting abnormality may induce venous or arterial thromboembolism, including pulmonary emboli and thrombosis affecting the upper or lower extremities. As clots form, the platelet complexes are consumed by macrophages and used up in the formation of thrombi, causing thrombocytopenia.[6] Patients with confirmed HIT have up to a 50% risk of experiencing a thrombotic event within 30 days after diagnosis.[6] However, not all patients who develop antibodies will have clinical manifestations of the disorder.[30] Complications of thrombi induced by HIT include skin necrosis, limb gangrene, and organ infarction.

A diagnosis of HIT is suspected when the platelet count drops dramatically in a patient who is receiving heparin, or who received heparin within the past few weeks. The drop in platelet count generally occurs before thrombosis. HIT should be suspected in a patient with a 50% drop in platelet count, even if the count is still within the normal range.[6] The "4 Ts" score can be used to identify clinical indicators of HIT.[7] These include the degree of *T*hrombocytopenia, *T*iming in relation to heparin administration, *T*hrombotic events, and al*T*ernative causes of thrombocytopenia. Although no test is 100% specific for HIT, confirmation is made through HIT antibody testing.[7] These tests are complex and may take time, so interventions should be started before confirmatory testing results are known.

When HIT is suspected, all forms of heparin should be stopped. Because HIT is an immune reaction, the amount of heparin is not relevant, so even the heparin in IV flushing solutions or priming solutions for blood circuits must be discontinued.[7] A direct thrombin inhibitor (e.g., IV argatroban) is started to disrupt the generation of thrombi and prevent further compromise to the circulation.[7,30] Warfarin is not prescribed during the acute phase because it can lead to decreased levels of protein C and exacerbate thrombosis.[30] Those diagnosed with HIT should avoid heparin for life.[7]

The potential for HIT has important implications for clinical practice. Heparin should be used only when truly needed, and is now avoided for some previously routine uses (e.g., capping peripheral IV lines). When heparin is indicated, LMWH may be prescribed because it is less likely to cause HIT.[6] Also, patients receiving heparin should be monitored for drops in their platelet count and any clinical indicators of thrombosis. It should be noted that, whereas thrombocytopenia is common in critically ill patients, only a small number are diagnosed with HIT.

EXCESSIVE FIBRINOLYSIS

Excessive fibrinolysis (also called hyperfibrinolysis) is an acute, severe bleeding disorder that can resemble DIC. Disorders and procedures including liver disease, trauma, cardiothoracic

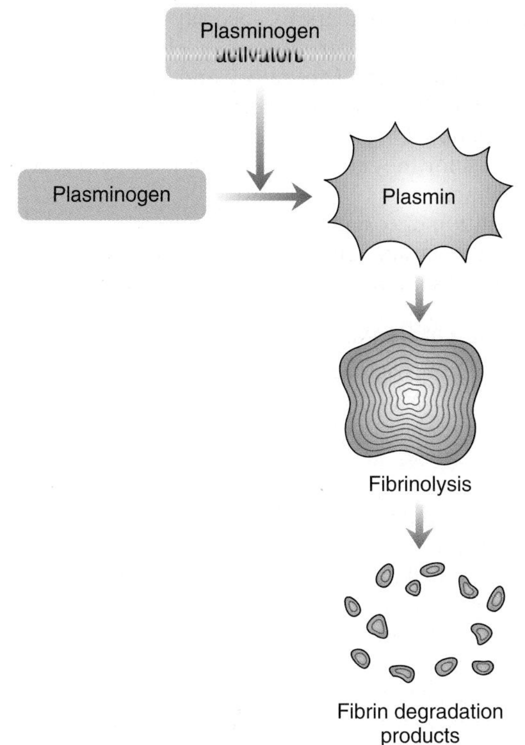

FIG. 27.7 Fibrinolysis. (From Copstead, L. C. & Banasik, J. L. (2013.). *Pathophysiology* (5th ed.). St. Louis: Saunders.)

surgery, and disseminated cancer may precipitate hyperfibrinolysis.[12,22] Extensive tissue damage releases naturally occurring tPA. This triggers plasminogen to become plasmin, the substance that lyses fibrin clots (Fig. 27.7). When the activation of this system is excessive, a fibrinolytic state similar to that induced by fibrinolytic drugs develops. In a patient with surgical wounds or trauma, excessive bleeding can result, because the patient is unable to form stable clots.[12]

The coagulation panel will show elevated PT/INR and aPTT. Other testing includes the use of TEG to evaluate for fibrinolysis.[12] However, other indicators of fibrinolysis such as FDPs and D-dimer are of limited value, as they are known to be elevated in trauma, surgery, DIC, or other situations in which clotting and subsequent fibrinolysis occur. The patient's response to an antifibrinolytic drug may confirm the diagnosis.

Treatment of excessive fibrinolysis initially aims to correct the underlying cause.[12] The antifibrinolytic agents TXA and epsilon-aminocaproic acid can be administered to inhibit fibrinolysis.[12,22]

BLEEDING ASSOCIATED WITH LIVER DISEASE

Coagulopathy is commonly associated with both acute and chronic liver disease. The liver synthesizes many key procoagulant proteins, including fibrinogen, factor V, and the vitamin K–dependent factors.[22] In addition, the liver clears substances that participate in feedback loops that control circulating active factors. Because the liver also produces thrombopoietin to stimulate platelet production and plasminogen for fibrinolysis, patients with liver disease may also have problems with thrombocytopenia and enhanced fibrinolysis.[46] The result is that these patients are at risk for bleeding, and some can be considered to be *autoanticoagulated.* Serious bleeding may follow any trauma or surgery, and local lesions in the GI tract, such as ulcers or varices, may bleed spontaneously.[34,46]

The coagulation panel may show many abnormalities in the patient with liver failure. Typically, the INR is elevated and the platelet count is decreased, but routine tests of coagulation do not reliably predict bleeding.[47] Some patients may have laboratory values similar to those seen in DIC.[46] Treating liver-associated coagulopathy involves interventions to treat the underlying disease. Other interventions are indicated in patients who are actively bleeding or who require surgery or invasive procedures. Transfusion with FFP, PCC, and platelets helps temporarily.[34] Desmopressin may also be helpful because it raises the levels of factor VIII and vWF.[46]

BLEEDING ASSOCIATED WITH UREMIA

Patients with renal disease often develop ecchymosis, purpura, epistaxis, and excess bleeding at injury sites. Uremia and the associated metabolic abnormalities have an adverse effect on platelet function, which places the patient at risk of bleeding. The changes to platelets include vWF dysfunction and decreased production of thromboxane A_2, resulting in the inability to form a platelet plug.[22] This is a qualitative problem, so whereas the platelet count may be normal, the bleeding time will be prolonged. The bleeding tendency is first treated by interventions that reduce uremia, such as dialysis.[46] Patients also benefit from cryoprecipitate and desmopressin to raise plasma levels of vWF and enhance platelet function.[22,23]

There are additional concerns when heparin is used in patients with renal problems. Because the half-lives of both UFH and LMWH are increased in patients with renal insufficiency, the dose is adjusted to avoid bleeding problems.[4]

BLEEDING ASSOCIATED WITH HEAD INJURY

Bleeding problems are a threat to patients with head injuries. Trauma to the brain leads to the release of a large amount of tissue factor, triggering the coagulation system soon after the primary injury.[36] In addition, brain injury can lead to platelet dysfunction. Together, these two changes augment trauma-related coagulopathy, which may require transfusion of blood products and other interventions to treat.[36]

HYPERCOAGULBILITY STATES

Critically ill patients are known to be at high risk for excessive hemostasis, which increases the risk for VTE. Some patients have a primary hypercoagulable condition because of a genetic mutation that affects the production of coagulation factors. For example, 2% to 15% of Caucasians carry the factor V Leiden gene. The mutant factor Va they produce cannot be inactivated by activated protein C (APC), so inappropriate clotting can result in VTE.[19] However, it is more common for critically ill patients to exhibit secondary thrombotic problems as a complication of their diseases and disorders. Patients with many conditions may develop a *hypercoagulable state* that results in the formation of inappropriate blood clots (Box 27.3). Patients at risk for thromboembolic events include those with venous stasis and conditions that alter blood composition to favor coagulation, which includes patients with a malignancy,

BOX 27.3 Clinical Conditions Associated with Thromboembolism

- Trauma
- Postoperative state
- Malignancy
- Pregnancy
- Bedrest and immobility
- Diabetes mellitus
- Atherosclerosis and myocardial infarction
- Heparin-induced thrombocytopenia
- Hyperviscosity
- Obesity
- Oral contraceptives
- Thrombotic thrombocytopenia purpura

Data from References 18, 19, and 42.

pregnant patients, and patients in postoperative or posttraumatic states.[18,42]

Malignancy has long been recognized as a risk factor for thromboembolism, and in some patients, a thrombotic event is the first sign of cancer.[32] A number of mechanisms are involved in the relationship between cancer and blood clots.[42] Solid tumors produce procoagulants such as tissue factor and a substance called cancer procoagulant.[32] Both of these mediators can activate platelets, enhance blood coagulation, and interfere with natural anticoagulants. Mediators are also known to damage the endothelium of blood vessels and interfere with fibrinolysis, impairing the body's natural ability to dissolve clots.[32] Subacute, chronic DIC also occurs in cancer patients, including those with adenocarcinoma and leukemia, and is most likely to cause thromboembolic problems.[32]

Pregnancy is associated with an increased risk for thrombi, for a number of reasons. The placenta releases factors that have procoagulant effects, leading to a hypercoagulable state that peaks in the postpartum period.[19] Venous stasis is increased by pressure on the pelvic veins during pregnancy, and tissue trauma occurs during delivery, adding to the risk.

Patients are also at risk of thromboembolism following surgery or trauma.[26] Tissue factor is released from injured tissue to promote clotting during the acute period, but the activated factors can lead to systemic changes that have procoagulant effects during the recovery period. When this hypercoagulable state is added to endothelial injury and venous stasis, the normal hemostasis process is amplified to include inappropriate clotting, in addition to the appropriate clotting at the injury site.

DVT and pulmonary emboli are the most common thromboembolic events in clinical practice. Anticoagulant therapy should be started in patients when there is a high clinical suspicion of acute VTE.[26] Guidelines from the American College of Chest Physicians provide details on recommended anticoagulant agents and length of therapy.[26]

INTERPROFESSIONAL PLAN OF CARE

The care of patients with coagulopathy requires intensive management by a interprofessional team. When coagulopathy is recognized, the team must intervene quickly to prevent hemorrhage, which can lead to hypovolemic shock, acute anemia, and tissue hypoxia. The team routinely consists of a number of providers in specialty practice, including a hematologist, critical care nurses, a pharmacist, respiratory therapists, and others. Laboratory and blood bank personnel are also important team members who support clinical care for these patients.

Priorities for the care of patients with coagulopathy include the following:

- Recognition of coagulopathy
- Early intervention and control of bleeding
- Emotional support of the patient and family

Recognition of Coagulopathy

Management of coagulopathy depends on a timely and accurate diagnosis.[22] All critically ill patients are considered to be at risk for bleeding problems, and evaluation for occult bleeding facilitates early diagnosis and intervention.[37] Identification of patients at risk begins with a patient and family history of bleeding problems. This includes bleeding after dental procedures, injury, surgery, or other procedures.[42] Easy bruising, heavy menses, or bleeding after childbirth can also suggest a problem. Knowledge of conditions that can trigger coagulopathy (such as sepsis) can help clinicians focus on patients at risk. It is important to know the pathophysiology of the various types of coagulopathies in order to understand how the pathophysiology leads to particular clinical signs. In addition, a detailed medication list should be obtained, including herbals and over-the-counter medication, as well as when anticoagulants were started and stopped.

A comprehensive assessment should be carried out to identify signs of bleeding or thrombosis. Identifying the type of signs (such as purpura), the sites of bleeding or thrombosis (such as the skin and GI tract), and the pattern of onset will assist with a prompt diagnosis. The patient's skin, mucous membranes, and all incisions and puncture sites should be observed.[42] Surgical drains and x-rays are checked for unexpected fluid collection. Patients are also assessed for abnormal swelling of the extremities or abdomen, as well as pain indicative of tissue trauma. Hemodynamics are monitored for early signs of hypovolemia, such as tachycardia, labile blood pressure, low central venous pressure (CVP), and low urine output. Core body temperature should be checked frequently for hypothermia.

Laboratory indicators are a very important part of the diagnostic process, and an understanding of coagulation parameters is essential for patient management. Serial lab testing should be performed to detect trends in the CBC and coagulation studies. If there is a clinical suspicion of coagulopathy, PT/INR, aPTT, and platelet count should be evaluated. Serum bicarbonate and lactic acid levels should be monitored for metabolic acidosis.

Early Intervention and Control of Bleeding

Interventions are initiated to control bleeding and restore hemostasis. Local measures such as application of pressure and hemostatic agents should be used. All anticoagulant medications should be stopped and reversed through the use of pharmacological agents or transfusion, if applicable. In an actively bleeding patient, PRBCs are administered to restore blood volume and maintain oxygen-carrying capacity.[43] Blood products such as FFP and platelets are used as indicated by the patient's clinical status and lab results. Patients should be observed for febrile reactions and other types of transfusion reactions.[13] Patients who receive massive transfusion should be monitored for fluid overload, hypothermia, hypocalcemia, and depletion of clotting factors.[43]

Bleeding precautions are instituted for patients at risk. This includes alerting team members when invasive procedures are considered and postponing nonemergency procedures.[42] A hematologist may be consulted as part of the preoperative or preprocedure evaluation for patients with conditions that increase the risk of bleeding. Blood pressure readings (especially automatic cuffs) should be performed with minimal pressure, as cuff pressure can cause petechiae and ecchymosis. Pressure should be applied to any puncture site for an extended period of time, followed by application of a pressure dressing.[18] Gentle mouth care and suction strength should be used to avoid trauma to mucous membranes.[45] Specialty mattresses and beds can help avoid skin trauma. Patients should be moved and turned gently. Prophylaxis for GI ulceration should be prescribed.

Prevention of hypothermia, hypotension, and acidosis is another important goal.[17,18] Prevention of hypothermia is carried out by removal of wet dressings and clothing and by preventing exposure. Warmed blankets, forced air warming devices, and warmed IV fluids and blood may be used. Maintenance of adequate blood pressure, ventilation, oxygenation, and tissue perfusion help prevent acidosis.

Emotional Support of the Patient and Family

Coagulopathy provokes great anxiety in patients and their families. It is important to provide clear, concise explanations of the problem, probable cause, and diagnostic evidence, including basic lab results. The plan of care, including massive transfusion and other interventions, should be explained, along with a discussion of the benefits and risks. Frequent updates on the patient's condition are essential, and it is important to include data that may not be obvious, such as a rising platelet count.

CONCLUSION

Critically ill individuals may have multiple risk factors for life-threatening complications such as coagulopathy. They need constant monitoring for indicators of bleeding problems, so that the signs are recognized early and interventions are prompt and successful. Critical care nurses play a key role in the assessment and recognition of coagulopathy and in the initiation of appropriate interventions. Prevention of bleeding problems continues to be a priority, and is a combined medical and nursing responsibility. Future advances in knowledge of the complexities of blood coagulation will improve the ability to predict and treat coagulation problems, decreasing the incidence of coagulopathy.

CASE STUDY 27.1

Tom is a 55-year-old man who was diagnosed with dilated cardiomyopathy 3 years ago. He had an implantable cardioverter defibrillator (ICD) placed 2 years ago due to his high risk of sudden cardiac death. In spite of maximal medical therapy, his heart failure progressed. Eight months ago, he had a ventricular assist device (VAD) implanted as a bridge to cardiac transplantation. He was anticoagulated with warfarin and discharged from the hospital to wait for a donor heart.

Tom was readmitted to the hospital when a suitable donor heart became available. On admission, his hemoglobin was 10.5 g/dL, his platelet count was 210,000/μL, and he had an aPTT of 40 seconds. The INR was 2.5, indicating full therapeutic anticoagulation. A warfarin reversal protocol was used, and Tom received 5 mg IV vitamin K, 1000 units of PCC, and 4 units of fresh frozen plasma (FFP). A repeat INR was 1.7, and he was then taken to surgery. The surgery consisted of explant of the ICD, explant of the VAD, and orthotopic cardiac transplantation. During surgery, Tom received 4 more units of FFP and 2 units of apheresed platelets.

During the first few hours postoperatively in the critical care unit, chest tube drainage averaged 300 mL/h. A coagulation panel was sent to the lab, with the following results:

- Hgb 6.9 g/dL
- Hct 20%
- Platelet count 75,000/μL
- INR 1.5
- Fibrinogen 90 mg/dL

Tom was hypotensive, with a blood pressure of 72/46 mm Hg. The bedside nurse called the surgeon, who ordered a STAT chest x-ray, DDAVP 0.3 units/kg, 10 units of cryoprecipitate, 2 units of PRBCs, and 2 units of apheresed platelets. The chest x-ray did not reveal blood accumulating in the chest. Following these interventions, the chest tube drainage slowed down, and his blood pressure improved. A repeat coagulation panel revealed the following:

- Hgb 9.6 g/dL
- Hct 30.4%
- Platelet count 90,000/μL
- INR 1.3
- Fibrinogen 105 mg/dL

Tom's chest tube output and hemodynamics were watched closely over the next several hours. His chest tube output slowed down to 30 mL/h, and he continued to oxygenate well on the ventilator. The surgeon then felt comfortable weaning Tom off the ventilator and extubating.

Decision Point:

What were this patient's risk factors for coagulopathy?

Decision Point:

What were his clinical indicators of postoperative coagulopathy?

Decision Point:

Explain the rationale and expected outcomes for the following interventions: DDAVP, PRBCs, cryoprecipitate, FFP, and platelets.

REFERENCES

1. Axnderson, M. W., & Watson, G. A. (2013). Traumatic shock: the fifth shock. *J Trauma Nurs*, *20*, 37–43.
2. Benson, G. (2014). Rotational thromboelastometry and its use in directing the management of coagulopathy in the battle injured trauma patient. *J Perioper Pract*, *24*, 25–28.
3. Brazzel, C. (2013). Thromboelastography-guided transfusion therapy in the trauma patient. *AANA J*, *81*, 127–132.
4. Burchum, J. R., & Rosenthal, L. D. (2016). *Lehne's pharmacology for nursing care* (9th ed.). St. Louis: Elsevier.
5. Collins, T. A. (2011). Packed red blood cell transfusions in critically ill patients. *Crit Care Nurse*, *31*, 25–34.
6. Coutre, S. (2015). Clinical presentation and diagnosis of heparin-induced thrombocytopenia. In L.L.K. Leung (Ed.), *UpToDate*, Waltham, MA.
7. Coutre, S. (2015). Management of heparin-induced thrombocytopenia. In L.L.K. Leung (Ed.), *UpToDate*, Waltham, MA.
8. Davis, D., Johannigman, J. A., & Pritts, T. A. (2012). New strategies for massive transfusion in the bleeding trauma patient. *J Trauma Nurs*, *19*, 69–75.
9. Dobesh, P. P., & Fanikos, J. (2014). New oral anticoagulants for the treatment of venous thromboembolism: understanding differences and similarities. *Drugs*, *74*, 2015–2032.
10. Douketis, J. D., et al. (2012). Perioperative management of antithrombotic therapy: antithrombotic therapy and prevention of thrombosis (9th ed.). American College of Chest Physicians evidence-based clinical practice guidelines. *Chest*, 141(Suppl. 2), e326S-e350S.
11. Dyke, C., Aronson, S., Dietrich, W., et al. (2014). Universal definition of perioperative bleeding in adult cardiac surgery. *J Thorac Cardiovasc Surg*, *147*, 1458–1463.

12. Fay, W. P. (2015). Thrombotic and hemorrhagic disorders due to abnormal fibrinolysis. In L.L.K. Leung (Ed.), *UpToDate*, Waltham, MA.
13. Federici, A. B., Intini, D., Lattuada, A., et al. (2014). Supportive transfusion therapy in cancer patients with acquired defects of hemostasis. *Thromb Res*, *133*(S2), S56–S62.
14. Ferraris, V. A., Brown, J. R., Despotis, G. J., et al. (2011). 2011 update to the Society of Thoracic Surgeons and the Society of Cardiovascular Anesthesiologists blood conservation clinical practice guidelines. *Ann Thorac Surg*, *91*, 944–982.
15. Fischbach, F., & Dunning, M. B. (2015). *A manual of laboratory and diagnostic tests* (9th ed.). Philadelphia: Wolters Kluwer.
16. Frazier, T. (2012). Disseminated intravascular coagulation and implications for medical-surgical nurses. *Med Surg Matters*, *21*, 8–11.
17. Gerecht, R. (2014). The lethal triad: hypothermia, acidosis & coagulopathy create a deadly cycle for trauma patients. *JEMS*, *39*, 56–60.
18. Greenlaw, D. (2013). Common hematologic disorders. In P. G. Morton, & D. K. Fontaine (Eds.), *Critical care nursing: a holistic approach* (10th ed.). Philadelphia: Wolters Kluwer.
19. Grossman, S. (2014). Disorders of hemostasis. In S. C. Grossman, & C. M. Porth (Eds.), *Porth's pathophysiology* (9th ed.). Philadelphia: Wolters Kluwer.
20. Holbrook, A., Shulman, S., Witt, D. M., et al. (2012). Evidence-based management of anticoagulant therapy and prevention of thrombosis (9th ed.). American College of Chest Physicians evidence-based clinical practice guidelines. *Chest*, *141*(Suppl. 2), e152S–e184S.
21. Hook, K. M., & Abrams, C. S. (2012). The loss of homeostasis in hemostasis: new approaches in treating and understanding acute disseminated intravascular coagulation in critically ill patients. *Clin Trans Sci*, *5*, 85–92.
22. Hunt, B. J. (2014). Bleeding and coagulopathies in critical care. *N Engl J Med*, *370*, 847–859.
23. Hurwitz, A., Massone, R., & Lopez, B. L. (2014). Acquired bleeding disorders. *Emerg Med Clin North Am*, *32*, 691–713.
24. Jobin, S., Kalliainen, L., Adebayo, L., et al. (2012). *Venous thromboembolism prophylaxis*. Bloomington, MN: Institute for Clinical Systems Improvement (ICSI). http://www.guideline.gov.
25. Katrancha, E. D., & Gonzalez, L. S. (2014). Trauma-induced coagulopathy. *Crit Care Nurse*, *34*, 54–63.
26. Kearon, C., et al. (2012). Antithrombotic therapy for VTE disease: antithrombotic therapy and prevention of thrombosis (9th ed.). American College of Chest Physicians. *Chest*, *141*(Supp. 2), e419S–e494S.
27. Leung, L. L. K. (2015). Anticoagulation with direct thrombin inhibitors and direct factor Xa inhibitors. In P. M. Mannucci (Ed.), *UpToDate*, Waltham, MA.
28. Leung, L. L. K. (2015). Overview of hemostasis. In P. M. Mannucci (Ed.), *UpToDate*, Waltham, MA.
29. Levi, M., & van der Poll, T. (2013). Disseminated intravascular coagulation: a review for the internist. *Intern Emerg Med*, *8*, 23–32.
30. Levi, M. (2014). Cancer-related coagulopathies. *Thromb Res*, *133*(S2), S70–S75.
31. Levi, M. (2014). Diagnosis and treatment of disseminated intravascular coagulation. *Int J Lab Hematol*, *36*, 228–236.
32. Linkins, L. A., et al. (2012). Treatment and prevention of heparin-induced thrombocytopenia: antithrombotic therapy and prevention of thrombosis (9th ed.). American College of Chest Physicians evidence-based clinical practice guidelines. *Chest*, *141*, e4955–e5305.
33. Maddali, S., Biring, T., Kopecky, S., et al. (2013). *Antithrombotic therapy supplement*. Bloomington, MN: Institute for Clinical Systems Improvement (ICSI). http://www.guideline.gov.
34. Mannucci, P. M., & Tripodi, A. (2013). Liver disease, coagulopathies and transfusion therapy. *Blood Transfus*, *11*, 32–36.
35. Matsushima, K., Benjamin, E., & Demetriades, D. (2015). Prothrombin complex concentrate in trauma patients. *Am J Surg*, *209*, 413–417.
36. McCully, S. P., & Schreiber, M. A. (2013). Traumatic brain injury and its effect on coagulopathy. *Semin Thromb Hemost*, *39*, 896–901.
37. McEvoy, M. T., & Shander, A. (2013). Anemia, bleeding, and blood transfusion in the intensive care unit: causes, risks, costs, and new strategies. *Am J Crit Care*, *22*, eS1–eS13.
38. Menzin, J., Sussman, M., Nichols, C., et al. (2014). Use of blood products in patients with anticoagulant-related major bleeding: an analysis of inhospital outcomes. *Am J Health Syst Pharm*, *71*, 1635–1645.
39. Munro, N. (2013). Cardiac surgery. In P. G. Morton, & D. K. Fontaine (Eds.), *Critical care nursing: a holistic approach* (10th ed.). Philadelphia: Wolters Kluwer.
40. National Institute for Health and Care Excellence (NICE). (2014). Detecting, managing and monitoring haemostasis: viscoelastometric point-of-care testing (ROTEM, TEG and Sonoclot systems. http://www.guidelines.gov.
41. Nutescu, E. (2013). Oral anticoagulant therapies: balancing the risks. *Am J Health Syst Pharm*, *70*(S1), S3–S11.
42. Orfanakis, A., & DeLoughery, T. (2013). Patients with disorders of thrombosis and hemostasis. *Med Clin North Am*, *97*, 1161–1180.
43. Paterson, T. P., & Stein, D. M. (2014). Hemorrhage and coagulopathy in the critically ill. *Emerg Med Clin North Am*, *32*, 797–810.
44. Rome, S. I. (2014). Hematologic problems. In S. L. Lewis, et al. (Ed.), *Medical-surgical nursing* (9th ed.). St. Louis: Elsevier.
45. Russell, M., & Suarez, C. (2014). Hematologic disorders and oncologic emergencies. In L. D. Urden, et al. (Ed.), *Critical care nursing: diagnosis and management* (7th ed.). St. Louis: Elsevier.
46. Shah, N. L., Northup, P. G., & Caldwell, S. H. (2015). Coagulation abnormalities in patients with liver disease. In L. L. K. Leung (Ed.), *UpToDate*, Waltham, MA.
47. Tripodi, A., & Mannucci, P. M. (2011). The coagulopathy of chronic liver disease. *N Engl J Med*, *365*, 147–156.
48. Tune, B. (2012). Utilization of a massive transfusion protocol during liver lobe resection: a case report. *AANA J*, *80*, 174–176.
48a. Urden, L. D., Stacy, K. M., & Lough, M. E. (2018). *Critical care nursing* (8th ed.). St. Louis: Mosby.
49. Welsh, K. J., Nedelcu, E., Bai, Y., et al. (2014). How do we manage cardiopulmonary bypass coagulopathy? *Transfusion*, *54*, 2158–2166.

28

Shock and End Points of Resuscitation

Daria C. Ruffolo

INTRODUCTION

Shock is one of the most frequently encountered, yet perhaps most poorly understood, clinical finding in critical care today. It can be a challenge to the most seasoned nurse. By definition shock is a clinical expression of circulatory failure that results in inadequate tissue perfusion.[7,109] As a result there is an alteration of cellular energy production from the normal and efficient aerobic pathway to the less efficient anaerobic pathway. This results in cellular acidosis and the accumulation of the cellular waste product, lactic acid.[13,109] The inability to correct or reverse shock results in increasing oxygen debt, worsening tissue acidosis, organ system dysfunction, and eventually, death.[7,39,109] Key to preventing this fatal cascade is the ability to rapidly recognize and treat the patient before a refractory shock state is established (Table 28.1).

Shock arises from multiple causes: hypovolemia, cardiac pump dysfunction, sepsis, and anaphylaxis, to name a few. These vast forms of shock make the diagnosis of the syndrome yet even more elusive. What remains clear is that there is a great toll taken in the loss of human life. Cardiogenic shock, related to pump failure from cardiovascular disease, remains the leading cause of death in the United States with greater than 800,000 deaths annually.[109] Similarly, hypovolemic shock remains a major contributor to death from injury to those ages 1 to 44.[50] Death from septic shock is the 10th leading cause of death in the United States at a rate of over 200,000 deaths per year and a cost of nearly 17 billion dollars.[52]

The purpose of this chapter is to provide the nurse caring for patients with an advanced working knowledge of shock and its treatment through detailed discussion of the pathophysiology associated with various shock types, resuscitation strategies, as well as evidence-based global and regional end points utilized to guide the resuscitation process.

HISTORY OF SHOCK

Early descriptions of the abnormality of circulation and its impact on survival date back to Greek and Roman times when Galen, as a surgeon to the gladiators, wrote of suturing tendons and ligation of vessels to control bleeding.[63] Little advance was made over the years; in the 18th century Dr. Benjamin Rush treated George Washington for acute laryngitis by draining 1 liter of blood in less than 24 hours and the president died shortly thereafter.[63] There still remained no concept of the need for adequate circulation to sustain tissue perfusion and organ function. Throughout the Revolutionary and Civil wars there were clinical observations of the impact of blood loss and the physical appearance of the "sudden vital depression," or "final sinking of vitality."[9,40] It was with World War I and Dr. Walter Cannon's treatise on shock that there came the understanding of tissue perfusion and its impact on maintaining a normal acid-base balance. It was identified that during shock states there is shunting of blood away from the skin capillaries and it was also his work that brought early awareness of the potential complication associated with excessive fluid resuscitation.[40,71] In the 1940s, Dr. Alfred Blalock continued the work on tissue bed dysfunction during hypotension and early on identified that there were vital organ beds that are left wanting in early phases of shock, such as the splanchnic and the peripheral circulations. We owe Blalock for our modern typology of the syndrome as it was he who identified that shock is manifested by means beyond blood loss and named different types of shock that included hypovolemic, cardiogenic, vasogenic, and anaphylactic.[40,97]

Even with the advantages we have today with modern science, shock remains a clinical enigma. We continue to attempt to understand and define this state of disordered perfusion and many definitions from our predecessors still seem applicable (Box 28.1). However, and perhaps more practical to our patients, it is not our attempts at perfecting the definition of shock, but rather the focusing of our energies on identifying the clinical manifestation of the syndrome and subsequently reversing the potential ravaging effects it can have on their health and lives which is important.

CELLULAR METABOLISM AND DYSFUNCTION DURING SHOCK

Normal cellular function is dependent on sufficient amounts of oxygen reaching the cell mitochondria for use in the production of adenosine triphosphate (ATP).[7,32] This requires a four step process. First, oxygen is taken into the lungs to the pulmonary capillaries. Second, oxygen must diffuse into the blood. Third, oxygen must be transported through blood flow to the tissues and cells, and, finally, it must diffuse into the cell and mitochondria to be utilized.[7,32] Under normal circumstances, through the aerobic metabolic pathway, oxygen, along with

TABLE 28.1 Clinical Features of Shock

Organ System	Sign or Symptoms	Causes
CNS	Mental status changes	↓ Cerebral perfusion
Circulatory		
Cardiac	Tachycardia	Adrenergic stimulation
	Dysrhythmias	Coronary ischemia
	New murmurs	Valvular dysfunction/VSD
Systemic	Hypotension	↓ SVR, ↓ venous return
	↑ JVD	Right heart failure
Respiratory	Tachypnea	Pulmonary edema, muscle fatigue, acidosis, sepsis
	Cyanosis	Hypoxemia
Renal	Oliguria	↓ Perfusion, vasoconstriction, volume loss
Skin	Cool, clammy	Sympathetic stimulation, vasoconstriction
Other	Lactic acidosis	Anaerobic metabolism, hepatic dysfunction

CNS, Central nervous system; *JVD*, jugular vein distention; *SVR*, systemic vascular resistance; *VSD*, ventricular septal defect.
From Reference 7.

BOX 28.1 Definitions of Shock Over the Ages

"Shock is a momentary pause in the act of death."
John Collins Warren 1816

"It is not necessary to describe the minute symptoms of shock, apparent at first sight from excessive pallor of the countenance, the weakened or absent pulse, the confused state of mind, the nausea and vomiting, and the excessive bodily prostration with the rude unhinging of the machinery of life."
Samuel Gross 1870s

"Shock is a peripheral circulatory failure resulting from a discrepancy in the size of the vascular bed and the volume of intravascular fluid."
Alfred Blalock 1940s

"Shock is a syndrome that results from a depression of many functions in which there is reduction of effective circulatory volume and in which impairment of the circulation failure progresses until it eventuates in a state of irreversible circulatory failure."
Carl Wiggers 1950s

"State in which profound and widespread reduction in effective tissue perfusion leads first to reversible and if prolonged to irreversible cellular injury."
Kumar and Parrillo 1990s

"Clinical expression of circulatory failure that results in inadequate cellular oxygen utilization."
DeBacker and J-L Vincent 2013

From References 63, 71, and 109.

nutrient substrates, is converted through glycolysis to pyruvate. Pyruvate is, in turn, converted to acetyl coenzyme A (CoA). Through the tricarboxylic acid (Krebs) cycle, CoA is converted to hydrogen and then oxidized to water, generating 38 moles of high-energy ATP that serves as the power source to sustain normal cellular function.[7,8,32]

During shock states, the reduced delivery of oxygen to the cell, or the inability of the mitochondria to use the oxygen delivered, results in the less efficient anaerobic pathway. In the absence of adequate oxygen, pyruvate is converted to lactic acid rather than CoA, generating only 2 moles of ATP (Fig. 28.1).[7,32] This amount of ATP is insufficient to support

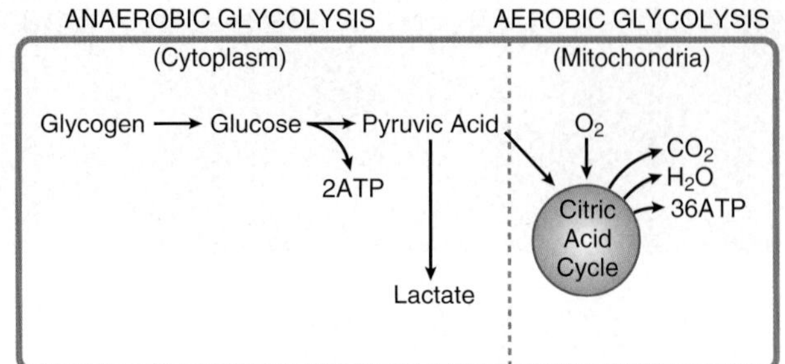

FIG. 28.1 Anaerobic and aerobic metabolism. (From Parillo, J. E. & Dellinger, R.P. (2014). *Critical care medicine: principles of diagnosis and management in the adult* (4th ed.). St Louis: Mosby.)

normal cellular metabolism and results in potentially dangerous cellular acidosis. As the cell succumbs to hypoxia, this results in ion pump dysfunction, intracellular edema, and leakage of cellular contents into the extracellular spaces. If this process is left unchecked, it progresses to a systemic level and endothelial dysfunction with activation of the inflammatory and antiinflammatory cascades. This in turn compounds the already compromised tissue perfusion and regional blood flow, leading to a deadly circuit of impaired circulation and acidosis. The key to preventing or reversing this undesirable event is optimization of cellular oxygen delivery and consumption.

OXYGEN DELIVERY, CONSUMPTION, AND DEBT

Oxygen Delivery

The delivery of oxygen to the cells and tissues is a complex and multifactorial process. Normal oxygen delivery (Do_2) is approximately 1000 mL/min; when indexed to body surface area, it is 600 mL/min. Oxygen delivery index (Do_2I) is determined by the product of the cardiac index (CI) and the arterial oxygen content (Cao_2). Common tissue oxygen indices are listed in Table 28.2.

Cardiac output (CO) is the product of the heart rate (HR) and stroke volume (SV). The SV is further determined by the preload, afterload, and contractility of the ventricle.[24,33] Cao_2 is primarily a product of the hemoglobin (Hgb) concentration and arterial oxygen saturation (Sao_2). Do_2 may be compromised if one or more of these components is negatively affected and will result in a reduction of oxygen delivery to the cells below the critical threshold required for normal cellular oxygen consumption (Fig. 28.2). For example, any reduction in CO, seen with alterations in HR, myocardial damage (contractility), hypovolemia (preload), or vascular outflow obstruction (afterload), will compromise oxygen delivery.[24,32,33,59] Pulmonary injury or pathology may affect delivery of oxygen to the blood, whereas conditions reducing Hgb concentration, as seen in hemorrhagic shock, will negatively affect Cao_2. There are many pathophysiological states associated with shock that can lead to compromised delivery of oxygen.

Oxygen Consumption

Under normal conditions, Do_2 to the tissues far exceeds the oxygen consumption (Vo_2) requirements of the cells. Cellular oxygen consumption requirements are approximately 250 mL/min, or 125 mL/min/m^2 when indexed to body surface area (Vo_2I). This translates into an oxygen extraction rate of 25%, or one-quarter of the Do_2I. The approximate 75% difference between Do_2I and

TABLE 28.2 Normal Values and Formulas for Tissue Oxygenation Indices

Tissue Oxygen Variable-Normal Values	Formula
Arterial oxygen content (17-20 mL/dL)	$Cao_2 = (0.0031 \times Pao_2) + (1.34\ Hgb \times [Sao_2/100])$
Venous oxygen content (12-15 mL/dL)	$Cvo_2 = (0.0031 \times Pvo_2) + 91.34\ Hgb \times [Svo_2/100])$
Arterial oxygen saturation (95%-100%)	$Sao_2 = 9\ Hbo_2/[Hgb + Hbo_2]) \times 100$
Oxygen delivery (950-1150 mL/min)	$Do_2 = CO \times Cao_2 \times 10$
Oxygen delivery index (550-600 mL/min/m^2)	$Do_2I = Do_2/BSA$
Oxygen consumption (195-285 mL/min)	$Vo_2 = CO \times (Cao_2 - Cvo_2) \times 10$
Oxygen consumption index (120-140 mL/min/m^2)	$Vo_2I = Vo_2/BSA$
Mixed venous oxygen saturation (65%-80%)	$Svo_2 = Sao_2 - (Vo_2/[CO \times 1.34\ Hgb \times 10])$
Central venous oxygen saturation (60%-80%)	$Scvo_2$

BSA, Body surface area; *Cao_2*, arterial oxygen content, *CO*, cardiac output, *Cvo_2*, venous oxygen content; *Do_2*, oxygen delivery; *Do_2I*, oxygen delivery index; *Hgb*, hemoglobin; *Hbo_2*, deoxyhemoglobin; *Pao_2*, partial pressure of arterial oxygen tension; *Pvo_2*, partial pressure of venous oxygen; *Sao_2*, arterial oxygen saturation; *$Scvo_2$*, central venous oxygen saturation; *Svo_2*, mixed venous oxygen saturation; *Vo_2*, oxygen consumption; *Vo_2I*, oxygen consumption index.
From Reference 33.

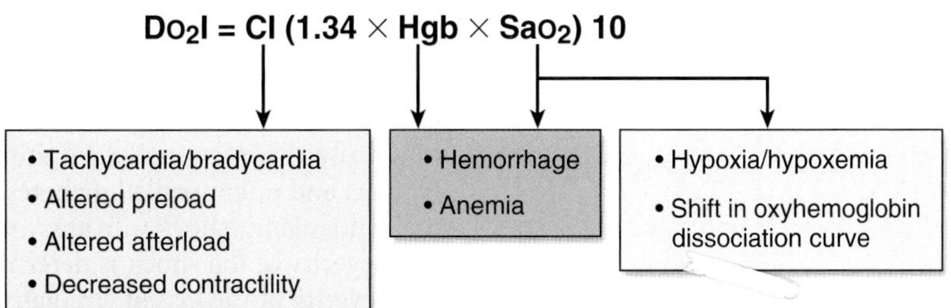

FIG. 28.2 Factors affecting oxygen delivery. *Do_2I*, Oxygen delivery index; *CI*, cardiac index; *Hgb*, hemoglobin; *Sao_2*, arterial oxygen saturation.

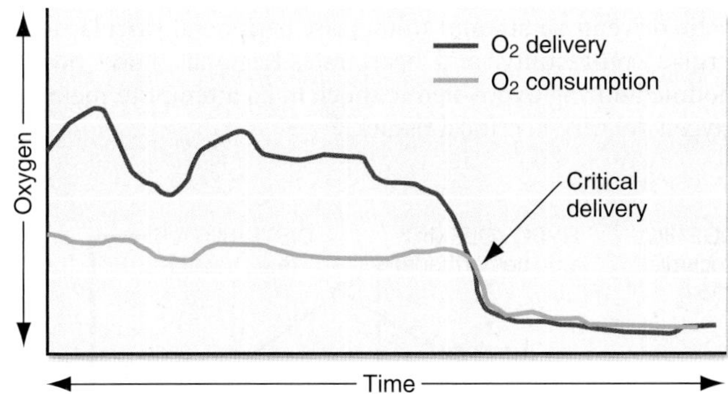

FIG. 28.3 Onset of oxygen delivery dependency: In circumstances where delivery is severely compromised (i.e., shock), delivery of oxygen to the tissues may fall below a critical threshold. Below this critical delivery threshold, oxygen consumption becomes dependent on oxygen delivery.

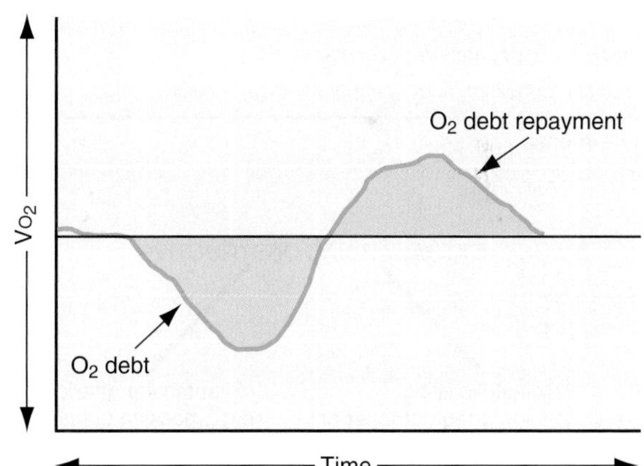

FIG. 28.4 Oxygen debt: The condition of supply dependency, if persistent, will result in conversion to anaerobic metabolism and a state of oxygen debt at the cellular level. Additional cellular compromise may occur when the cell is unable to utilize available oxygen. *Vo_2*, Oxygen consumption.

Vo_2I is a buffer, allowing for modest decreases in Do_2, as well as increases in cellular consumption based on changing metabolic needs. Conditions increasing cellular metabolism (e.g., fever, pain, agitation, shivering) will increase the Vo_2I, requiring a higher percentage of oxygen extraction. Conversely, alleviation of these conditions may reduce cellular oxygen requirements.[24,33,61]

Oxygen Delivery Dependence and Oxygen Debt

When delivery is severely compromised (i.e., shock), oxygen getting to the tissues may fall below a critical threshold (Fig. 28.3). Below this critical delivery (Do_2I) threshold, Vo_2I becomes "dependent" on oxygen delivery. Consequently, the cell cannot compensate for the decrease in oxygen delivery by extracting more oxygen to meet its metabolic needs; additional oxygen is not available.[33,61,73,103] If persistent, this condition of supply dependent will result in conversion to anaerobic metabolism and a state of oxygen debt at the cellular level (Fig. 28.4).[24,33,61] Additional cellular compromise may result when the cell is unable to use available oxygen (e.g., mitochondrial dysfunction associated with sepsis). The duration of the underlying conditions and extent to which the oxygen debt increases negatively affect organ function and mortality. Restoration of optimal oxygen delivery to the tissues in an effort to reverse this process is the primary goal of any resuscitation efforts.

BOX 28.2 Categories of Shock

Hypovolemic Shock
Hemorrhagic
Trauma, gastrointestinal bleeding, aortic disruption

Nonhemorrhagic
Dehydration, emesis, diarrhea, large open wounds

Cardiogenic Shock
Myocardial
Infarction, contusion, myocarditis, cardiomyopathies

Mechanical
Valvular failure, ventricular septal defect

Arrhythmias

Distributive Shock
Sepsis
Systemic inflammatory response syndrome, infection, pancreatitis, burns, trauma

Neurogenic
Spinal cord injury, peptic ulcer perforation

Anaphylaxis
Insect bites, allergen exposure

Obstructive Shock
Impairment of diastolic filling
Tension pneumothorax, cardiac tamponade, positive pressure ventilation

Impairment of systolic contraction
Pulmonary embolism, acute pulmonary hypertension

From Reference 7.

CLASSIFICATIONS OF SHOCK

As shock can be a complex syndrome to diagnose and treat, the clinical team caring for these patients is best served by utilizing the well-established typology and conceptual framework put forward by Hinshaw and Cox in the 1970s.[42] The four classifications of shock include hypovolemic, cardiogenic, obstructive, and distributive. Distributive shock may be further subdivided into septic, neurogenic, and anaphylactic shock (Box 28.2). It is important to note that most shock states incorporate different components of each of the shock categories and that the patient's clinical symptoms can be very diverse. Fig. 28.5 depicts the interrelationships of shock states.

Hypovolemic Shock

Hypovolemic shock, the most prevalent form of hypoperfusion, occurs when the vascular system loses blood or fluid either through hemorrhagic or nonhemorrhagic causes. This leads to a fall in preload and subsequent perfusion pressure. The most common form of hypovolemic shock is blood loss through traumatic injury, major surgery, ruptured aortic aneurysm, or gastrointestinal bleeding. Other, nonblood loss causes, include fluid losses from excessive vomiting, diarrhea, large wounds or fistulae, and uncontrolled diabetes.[13,50,73]

Hypovolemic shock warrants an accurate and early diagnosis. The severity of the shock is determined by the speed, duration, and severity of the loss of circulating volume. Hypotension and other clinical signs are often not apparent from small volume losses, but there is a progressive hemodynamic deterioration as losses increase that are described in four stages summarized in Table 28.3.[50,73,87] During this time there is an increase in sympathetic drive in an attempt to increase peripheral vascular tone, cardiac contractility, and heart rate. Regional blood flow is modified during hypovolemic shock in an attempt to maintain oxygen delivery to critical tissues.[59,73,87]

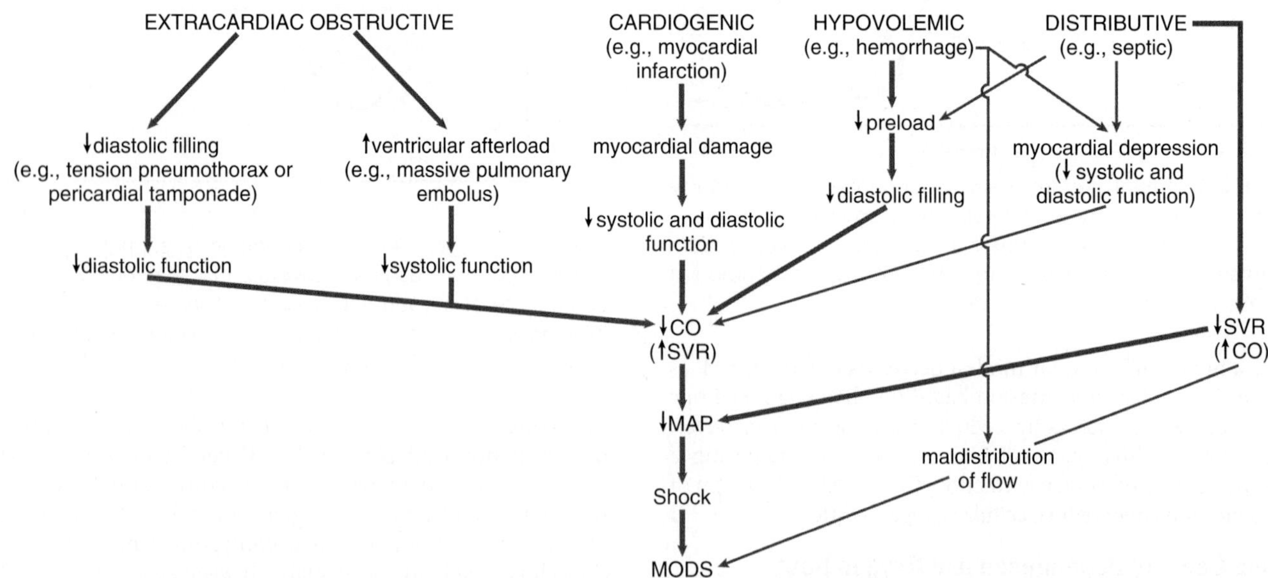

FIG. 28.5 The interrelationship of shock states. *CO*, Cardiac output; *MAP*, mean arterial pressure; *MODS*, multiple organ dysfunction syndrome; *SVR*, systemic vascular resistance. (From Parillo, J. E. & Dellinger, R. P. (2014). *Critical care medicine: principles of diagnosis and management in the adult* (4th ed.). St Louis: Mosby.)

A cascade of metabolic, hormonal, and inflammatory mediators is activated in attempts to maintain homeostasis. These initial beneficial responses can become detrimental to the patient as this persistent state can lead to local tissue hypoperfusion and subsequent organ dysfunction. These secondary mechanisms evoked to compensate for volume loss impact all vital organs and must be addressed as part of the resuscitative maneuvers.[50,87]

Cardiogenic Shock

Cardiogenic shock occurs when the heart is unable to pump enough blood to meet the body's demand for oxygen. The number one cause of cardiogenic shock is myocardial infarction. This condition may result from significant muscle ischemia associated with acute coronary syndrome, as well as structural damage from traumatic injury to the heart muscle, valves, or coronary arteries. Chronic conditions (e.g., heart failure, valvular pathology) may also result in cardiogenic shock. These inciting events lead to increased ventricular filling pressures, cardiac chamber dilation, ventricular failure, subsequent systemic hypotension, and its associated sequelae.[16,83] See Fig. 28.6 for a review of the pathophysiological sequence of cardiogenic shock.

Obstructive Shock

Obstructive shock results from a mechanical obstruction of blood flow and a subsequent reduction in CO. Even when the intravascular volume is sufficient, there are conditions that prevent normal circulation of this blood volume. These conditions

TABLE 28.3 Classification of Hemorrhagic Shock

	Compensated	Mild	Moderate	Severe
Blood Loss (mL)	≤1000	1000-1500	1500-2000	>2000
Heart rate (bpm)	<100	>100	>120	>140
Blood pressure	Normal	Orthostatic change	Marked fall	Profound fall
Capillary refill	Normal	May be delayed	Usually delayed	Always delayed
Respiration	Normal	Mild increase	Moderate tachypnea	Marked tachypnea: respiratory collapse
Urinary output (mL/h)	>30	20-30	5-20	Anuria
Mental status	Normal or agitated	Agitated	Confused	Lethargic, obtunded

From Reference 66a.

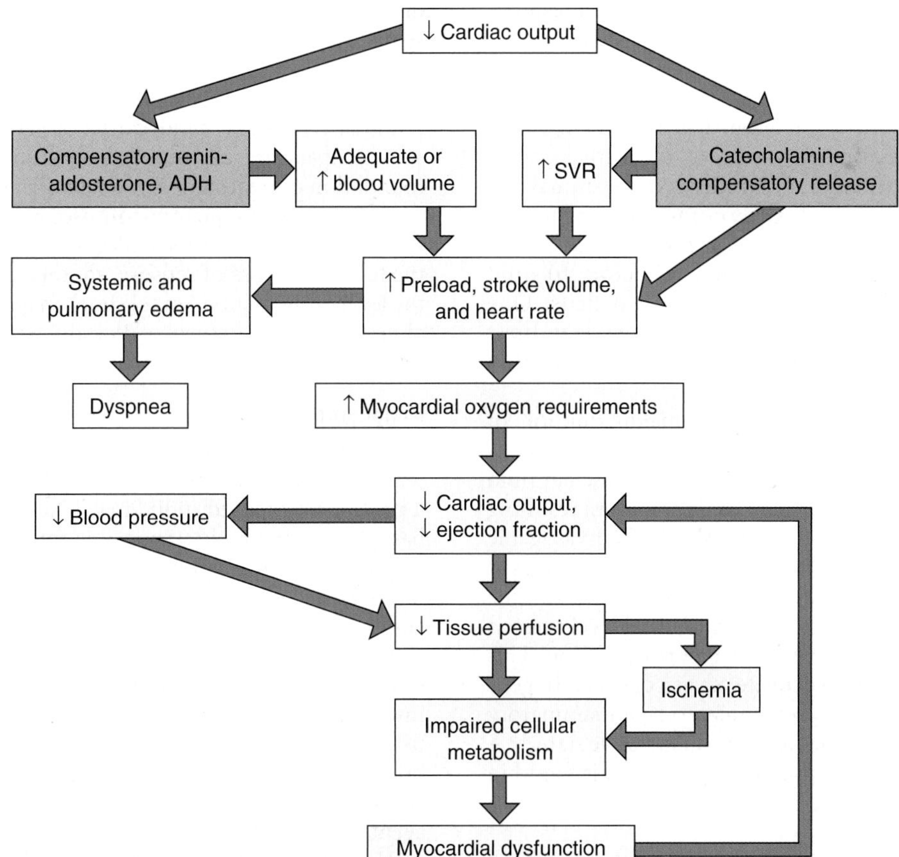

FIG. 28.6 The pathophysiological sequence of cardiogenic shock. *ADH*, Antidiuretic hormone; *SVR*, systemic vascular resistance. (From McCance, K.L. & Huether, S.E. (2014). *Pathophysiology: the biologic basis for disease in adults and children* (7th ed.). St Louis: Mosby.)

include tension pneumothorax, pericardial tamponade, pulmonary embolus, and abdominal compartment syndrome.[7,32] A tension pneumothorax causes an increase in intrathoracic pressure, resulting in compression of the heart and vena cava. Venous return to the heart is compromised, reducing preload and CO.

In cardiac tamponade, a collection of fluid within the unyielding pericardial sac compresses the myocardium, preventing adequate filling of the heart chambers. These events result in reduced CO through compromised preload, a reduction in coronary artery perfusion as aortic pressure falls, and progression to myocardial ischemia.

Pulmonary embolism causes outflow obstruction from the right ventricle through the pulmonary artery, resulting in compromised blood flow through the lungs, as well as into the left side of the heart. Normal gas exchange is compromised as "dead space" ventilation is increased in nonperfused portions of lung.

In abdominal compartment syndrome, increasing intraabdominal pressures compress the inferior vena cava and reduce venous return to the right ventricle, compromising preload. Compression of the descending aorta increases afterload and left ventricular workload, further compromising CO.

Distributive Shock

Though significantly different in etiology, the distributive types of shock similarly result in impaired or reduced systemic vascular resistance (SVR) with maldistribution of blood flow and altered organ perfusion. Although intravascular volume remains normal, a functional hypovolemia occurs as a result of increased vascular capacitance from reduction in SVR.

Septic Shock

Septic shock is the result of infection that overwhelms host defenses. Sepsis is the number one cause of death in critical care units, with approximately 1 million cases annually.[52] The critically ill and injured, as well as immunocompromised patients, are most at risk. Septic shock results from severe sepsis and is manifested by hypotension refractory to fluid resuscitation with associated tissue perfusion deficits. One of the approaches to treat patients in septic shock is to limit the infectious process and control the source of infection (Box 28.3).

These perfusion deficits are related to maldistribution of blood flow, vasodilation, and depression of myocardial contractility.[5,27,39] In addition, there is leakage of intravascular fluid volume as the result of mediator-damaged capillaries, resulting in a hypovolemic component to septic shock. The vasogenic effect on smooth muscle results in venodilation and decreased venous return, which compounds the intravascular volume deficit and vascular leak.[5,31] At the mitochondrial level there is an inability to extract and use oxygen in a normal fashion. This is seen even in the presence of adequate oxygen delivery. In general, patients transition from a predominately proinflammatory state to an antiinflammatory and immunosuppressive state.[4,5] A more detailed description of sepsis and septic shock is found in Chapter 31.

Neurogenic Shock

Neurogenic shock is a vasodilatory distributive shock from autonomic disturbance with interruption of the sympathetic pathways. This is most often the result of spinal cord injury (SCI) within the thoracic vertebral level, or peripheral nerve disease such as Guillain-Barre syndrome. The unopposed parasympathetic innervations cause profound vasodilation and hypotension.[20,62] Unlike other types of shock, compensatory tachycardia does not occur because of parasympathetic predominance. Rather, bradycardia is present, along with warm skin temperature and normal or flushed skin color.[20,62] The foundation of treatment is to maintain euvolemia.

A condition frequently confused with neurogenic shock is spinal shock. Spinal shock, also associated with SCI, results in the temporary loss of sensory, motor, or reflex function below the level of the injury. Spinal shock may last from days to weeks after the injury. Return of key reflexes (i.e., bulbocavernous reflex, deep tendon reflexes) signifies the end of spinal shock.[20]

BOX 28.3 Controlling Infection for the Patient in Shock: Source Control

- Specific anatomical diagnosis of infection for emergent source control should be sought and diagnosed
- In the septic shock patient, the effective intervention associated with the least physiologic insult should be utilized (i.e., percutaneous rather than surgical drainage)
- Remove and replace as needed any devices or vascular access that may be a source of infection

Common Sources of Infection

Suspected Site	Symptoms/Signs
Respiratory Tract	Pharyngeal inflammation, purulent secretions, coarse breath sounds
Urinary tract	Pyuria, hematuria
Vascular catheters	Redness, drainage at insertion site
Wound, skin, soft tissue	Inflammation, edema, erythema, pus, warmth
Gastrointestinal	Pain, distention, diarrhea, vomiting
Peritoneal dialysis (PD) catheter	Cloudy PD fluid, pain, fever
Indwelling pleural catheter	Redness, drainage from insertion site
Genital tract	Vaginal, penile discharge
Joint	Pain, warmth, redness, tenderness, decreased range of motion

From References 27 and 83a.

Anaphylactic Shock

Anaphylaxis is a clinical syndrome representing a severe systemic allergic reaction after exposure to a specific antigen in a previously exposed individual. The release of mast cells and basophil mediators is responsible for the systemic physiologic response seen in anaphylaxis. Anaphylactic shock is defined by the presence of cardiovascular collapse and associated airway compromise as the result of anaphylaxis.[7,114]

Causative agents of anaphylactic reactions that may lead to shock are mediated by immunoglobulin E (IgE). These include insect stings, medications, peanuts, tree nuts, latex, shellfish, fish, milk, eggs, and wheat. Anaphylactoid reactions related to nonIgE-mediated responses are associated with triggers such as nonsteroidal antiinflammatory drugs, diagnostic contrast agents, and opiates.[17,57]

Hemodynamic instability differentiates anaphylactic shock from anaphylaxis. This instability is caused by antigen-antibody–mediated vasodilation and redistribution of blood volume, as well as capillary permeability and loss of fluid volume into the interstitial space (angioedema). Although symptoms

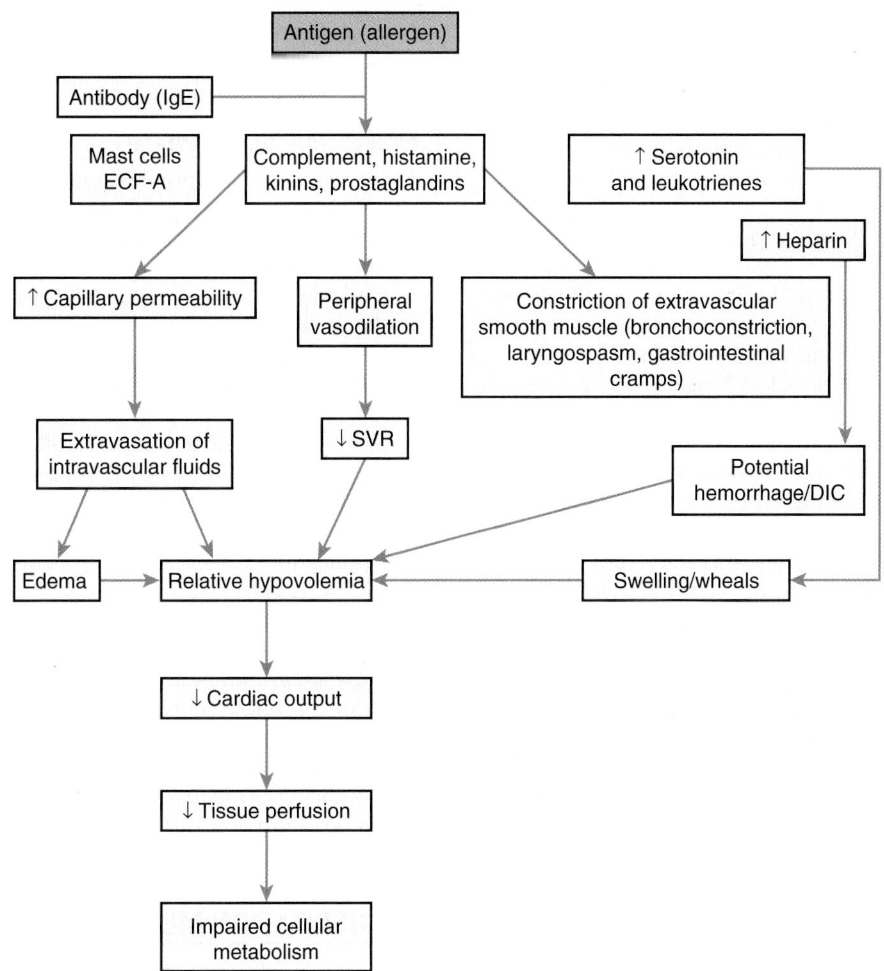

FIG. 28.7 The pathophysiological sequence of anaphylactic shock. *DIC*, Disseminated intravascular coagulation; *SVR*, systemic vascular resistance. (From McCance, K.L. & Huether, S.E. (2014). *Pathophysiology: the biologic basis for disease in adults and children* (7th ed.). St Louis: Mosby.)

usually present rapidly, onset may be delayed for as long as 1 hour after exposure. Resolution may begin as treatment is instituted, but can take up to 24 hours. An important and problematic aspect of these reactions is the potential for a second-phase reaction between 1 and 38 hours after the first (10 hours on average). This biphasic reaction pattern may be less severe, equally severe, or more severe than the first (Fig. 28.7).[57,93,114]

GENERAL PHASES OF SHOCK

The initial onset of shock is a cellular phenomenon; therefore, detection through traditional clinical assessment may be difficult, especially when strong compensatory mechanisms are intact. Uninterrupted shock occurs in a predictable pattern, moving from an initial compensatory stage through progressive or uncompensated shock and eventually to a refractory stage and death. Although overlap exists between the stages, defined pathophysiologic findings are attributed to each stage as shock progresses. Within all classifications of shock, each of these stages exists. However, the phases are most often associated with the model of hypovolemic shock. No matter what the precipitating event, the initial pathophysiology of all types of shock is similar.[7,32]

Compensatory Phase

The initial, or compensatory, phase is characterized by mechanisms designed to restore homeostasis. Compensatory mechanisms are aimed at preserving vital organ perfusion at the expense of integumentary and splanchnic perfusion. Whether the inciting event is a problem with volume (hypovolemic), the pump (cardiogenic), or resistance (distributive), perceived loss of vascular volume inhibits afferent discharge of baroreceptors in the aortic arch and carotid sinus, stimulating sympathetic nervous system output, causing the release of catecholamines to increase HR, contractility, and ultimately CO.

Patients enter the compensatory phase of shock after the initial insult. These compensatory changes are activated by the sympathetic nervous system and occur in an effort to maintain homeostasis. These initial responses primarily affect the cardiovascular system and are under neurohumoral control. This is mediated through stimulation of hormones from the adrenal cortex and medulla (i.e., norepinephrine, epinephrine).[7,39,75]

Activation of the anterior pituitary occurs with release of adrenocorticotropic hormone as well as endorphins, thyroid-stimulating hormone, and growth hormone. The posterior pituitary secretes antidiuretic hormone (ADH), stimulating the reabsorption of water from the kidneys. Activation of the renin-angiotensin-aldosterone system stimulates the release of aldosterone from the adrenal cortex, increasing sodium and water reabsorption. Cortisol is also secreted to increase mobilization of glucose and stimulate protein catabolism.[7,103,113]

The overall purpose of this response is to improve tissue perfusion and support cellular metabolism through four mechanisms. First, CO is improved via the increases in HR and contractility. Second, blood flow is increased to central, essential organs as the result of the peripheral vasoconstriction. Third, plasma volume is increased by the retention of sodium and water and the shifting fluid from the interstitium into the vascular space where leukocyte aggregation and the initiation of endothelial dysfunction takes place. Finally, glyconeogenesis and increased catabolism are designed to provide substrate availability for cell metabolism.[32,103,113]

Early clinical findings in the compensatory phase of shock are subtle and may be easily missed by the clinical team without methodic and intentional assessment. It is because of this lack of demonstrative signs this phase is referred to as *cryptic shock*. Early findings associated with the initial release of epinephrine and norepinephrine includes the onset of anxiety and restlessness along with pallor and a decrease in peripheral skin temperature. A hallmark sign of tissue hypoperfusion is a slight increase in HR, progressing to tachycardia, which is designed to compensate for initial reductions in SV in order to preserve CO. Therefore, normal blood pressure (BP) may be maintained for some time and is not a reliable indicator of shock in this phase. Later, arterial pulse pressure narrows as diastolic pressure increases in the face of reduced systolic pressure. Additionally, increases in HR and contractility will increase myocardial oxygen consumption.[32,113]

Efforts to restore vascular volume mediated through aldosterone and ADH result in renal conservation of water and reduction in urinary output (UO) to less than 0.5 to 1.0 mL/kg. Hypoperfusion of the splanchnic organs in this phase of shock may result in organ dysfunction and subsequent injury to the mucosal layer of the intestine.[7,103,113]

Reversal of shock in this phase usually results in favorable outcomes. Therefore, it is imperative that the nurses caring for patients at risk are aware of the subtle signs of shock and are instrumental in efforts to mobilize the care team to prevent the progression and subsequent harmful effects it can have on patients. The primary intervention for any shock state is the identification and reversal of the primary inciting cause.

Decompensated Phase

Progression of shock beyond the compensatory phase results in exhaustion of compensatory mechanisms. Worsening signs and symptoms associated with hypoperfusion manifest, along with hypotension. Hypotension is a hallmark clinical finding signaling the transition from the compensatory to decompensated shock phase. Impaired mitochondrial function occurs on the cellular level. Metabolic acidosis, reflecting onset of anaerobic metabolism, is clinically detectable through serum lactate and base deficit (BD). In addition, failure of the sodium-potassium pump results in cellular swelling with impairment of substrate diffusion necessary for normal function.[7,32,103,113]

During the compensatory phase of shock, perfusion to integumentary and splanchnic organs is initially shunted to preserve core organ function, resulting in ischemia of the intestinal mucosal layer. As shock progresses, perfusion to core organs such as the brain, heart, kidneys, and liver becomes significantly compromised. Clinical manifestations include altered level of consciousness, progressive hypotension, hypothermia, coagulopathy, and severe oliguria.[7,32,103]

Irreversible Shock Phase

Failure to reverse the progression of shock through either physiologic compensatory mechanisms or resuscitative measures results in further deterioration to irreversible or refractory shock. During this phase, ongoing hypoperfusion results in irreversible cellular and organ damage and patients transition to the "point of no return." Arterioles and venules passively dilate, and cellular and capillary permeability results in fluid shift to the interstitial space with impairment of oxygen delivery to the cell. Adrenal insufficiency and low cortisol levels have been linked to the cell membrane destabilization.[7,113] Mitochondrial dysfunction and failure of the sodium-potassium pump result in osmotic cellular swelling and death. Increasing lactate levels and worsening BD mark organ dysfunction and failure.[7,10,32]

Application of vasopressor agents may be necessary as endogenous catecholamine stores are exhausted. These measures may result in artificial improvement of hemodynamic values, but they do little to improve perfusion or function of organ systems suffering irreversible damage and necrosis. The hallmark of this phase is progression of organ system dysfunction, and eventually death. It is important for the healthcare team to identify patients that are transitioning to refractory shock and make every effort to involve the family in decision-making with the opportunity for open discussions regarding end of life care as appropriate.[7,32,103]

RESUSCITATION MEASURES IN SHOCK

Regardless of the type of shock, the overall goal of treatment is the restoration and maintenance of oxygen delivery to the tissues. Key to this process is a systematic and multiprofessional approach to patient assessment and care. This assessment is accompanied by priority-based therapeutic interventions. These interventions are all aimed at providing patients with the most effective care and ultimately maximizing the likelihood of recovery followed by a good quality of life. These therapies may have differing approaches based on the classification of shock and the venue of the resuscitation. With continual research and practice changes, it is important for the healthcare team to be vigilant in keeping abreast of the most current and evidence-based practices in caring for this challenging population.

Initial Evaluation

Initial priorities in the management of shock are guided by a primary assessment to detect immediate life-threatening issues with interventions based on these findings. This process should be employed regardless of the type of shock or the setting. A modified application of the ABC (airway, breathing, circulation) approach to assessment and intervention advocated in the instructional programs is applicable to all types of shock. All strategies are aimed at improving Do_2, as is illustrated in Fig. 28.8.

Airway and Breathing

Initial evaluation in shock requires priority evaluation of the airway with intervention, as necessary. Although not all patients require airway intervention, close assessment for progressive changes in level of consciousness and inability to maintain a

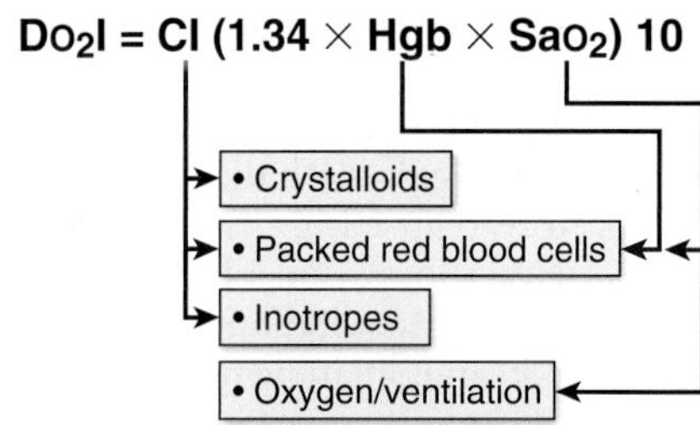

FIG. 28.8 Interventions augmenting oxygen delivery. *DO_2I,* Oxygen delivery index, *CI,* cardiac index; *Hgb,* hemoglobin; *SaO_2,* arterial oxygen saturation.

natural airway must be monitored. However, in the case of progressing shock, a proactive approach to gaining airway control is preferred over waiting until the patient has decompensated and can no longer protect their airway or breathe effectively to provide adequate oxygenation and ventilation. Definitive airway control is best accomplished by insertion of an endotracheal tube and providing mechanical ventilation if needed.[3,39] When anatomic or situational conditions (e.g., facial trauma) prevent intubation, insertion of a surgical airway is the preferable alternative.

Initial assessment of adequate respiratory function involves standard physical assessment principles. In addition to observation of respiratory rate and pattern and the presence and quality of breath sounds, adjuncts such as pulse oximetry and end-tidal carbon dioxide ($PETCO_2$) monitoring may be used.[36,49] $PETCO_2$ can be measured noninvasively by capnography and can reflect derangements in perfusion, metabolism, or gas exchange. Normally the partial pressure of carbon dioxide ($PaCO_2$)-$PETCO_2$ gradient is less than 5 mm Hg. In conditions of reduced or absent pulmonary blood flow, such as shock, $PETCO_2$ is also reduced or absent.[46,49] Arterial blood gases (ABGs) should be obtained to provide initial information about pulmonary gas exchange as well as information related to presence of acid-base abnormalities. All patients should receive high-flow oxygen (100%) initially, whether or not airway management is required. Oxygen therapy may be adjusted once adequate tissue oxygenation has been established.[3,39]

In patients requiring airway support, mechanical ventilation may also be required. The duration of mechanical ventilation and the ventilation strategies employed are determined by a number of patient-specific factors. Patients in whom shock may be rapidly reversed (e.g., operative repair of traumatic injury) may require mechanical ventilation only for a short time. Conversely, the need for ongoing resuscitation or the presence of complications (e.g., pneumonia or sepsis) may prolong the need for ventilation. Additionally, the application of specialized lung-protective ventilation modes and strategies may be indicated based on the patient's needs.

Circulation

The goal of this portion of intervention is the restoration and augmentation of intravascular volume (preload), as well as optimizing systemic vascular resistance (afterload) and myocardial contractility. When feasible, a multidisciplinary, team-based approach is preferred as it allows the simultaneous evaluation and administration of therapy to the patient. Before undertaking fluid resuscitative strategies to augment circulation there must be efforts made to obtain hemostasis in patients with uncontrolled hemorrhage. Thereafter, the therapies entertained to stabilize circulation encompass various strategies based on the type of shock and the individual needs of the patient.[3,39,98]

Fluid Resuscitation

Fluid Delivery and Warming Mechanisms

Patients in need of resuscitation in shock require reliable vascular access to deliver large volumes of fluid, blood, or medications quickly. In initial resuscitation, large-bore (14–18 gauge) peripheral venous access is sufficient. Central access may be reserved for those patients with anticipated ongoing resuscitation and monitoring needs, as well as those situations in which peripheral access is unobtainable.[3,50] An alternative means of vascular access is the intraosseous route and has been utilized successfully for fluid and medication administration during resuscitation. The intraosseous cavity is a noncollapsible space that contains a readily recruitable venous plexus that can be used for fluid and medication delivery. [55]

Equally important is the need to maintain normothermia in shock. Resuscitation with large quantities of fluid and banked blood products places the patient at risk for the development of hypothermia and associated coagulopathy. The presence of preexisting acidosis along with these factors has been well described in hemorrhagic shock patients as the "triad of death." Prevention, rather than treatment, is essential in reducing complications and associated mortality.[3,72,98]

All shock states, no matter what their etiology, result in a decreased venous return, or a decreased preload. Regardless of whether fluid is lost in the form of hemorrhage, as fluid shifts, or expansion of the intravascular capacity, because of vasodilation, preload augmentation with fluids must precede the use of vasopressor agents to increase vascular tone.

Isotonic Crystalloids

Isotonic crystalloid solutions are the mainstay of shock resuscitation today. There are a number of solutions from which the practitioners can chose. The most notable issues with isotonic solutions are that only approximately 25% remain in the intravascular space, whereas 75% will accumulate in the interstitial spaces. These solutions include isotonic saline solution (0.9% normal saline [NS]), balanced salt solutions (i.e., lactated Ringer's [LR]) and calcium-free, balanced salt solutions (i.e., PlasmaLyte). Crystalloid solutions have the advantage of being inexpensive and readily available in the clinical setting while providing adequate volume expansion in most situations.[15,84]

There are a number of concerns with any large volume resuscitation of isotonic solutions that include the potential for hyperchloremic acidosis from excessive 0.9% NS administration, whereas LR has alternative ions added to the solution such as lactate and acetate that can contribute to hyperlactatemia and metabolic alkalosis.[34,79,84] Additionally, there has been a change in practice away from the use of an aggressive fluid resuscitation in the face of shock from acute blood loss (i.e., penetrating injury). The approach is referred to as *delayed fluid resuscitation* or *controlled hypotensive resuscitation.* This is seen primarily in penetrating trauma cases where little to no fluid is given to the patient with mild hypotension as the patient is quickly moved to the surgical suite where there is operative control of bleeding. The foundation of this practice is that aggressive return of vigorous circulation with large volumes of crystalloid can result in increased blood loss from disruption of stabilized clot, hemodilution of clotting factors, and hypothermia before there is a surgeon poised to control bleeding.[1,84,100]

The volume of crystalloid required depends on the type of shock state. In hypovolemic shock related to hemorrhage, each milliliter of blood loss may require up to 3 mL of crystalloid solution to replace blood volume (3:1 ratio).[3,94] Although this may be effective in early compensatory shock, it is of limited value in ongoing hemorrhage because crystalloid solutions have no ability to carry oxygen. In such situations, administration of packed red blood cells (PRBCs) is required and should be considered after the administration of approximately 2 liters (L) of crystalloid without improvement in hemodynamic stability.[3,39,98]

In septic shock, capillary permeability and fluid shifts from intravascular to interstitial space create a relative hypovolemia. Although the patient appears edematous and volume overloaded, there is inadequate vascular volume, further compounding the problem of maldistribution of blood flow common in septic shock. The current Surviving Sepsis Campaign guidelines advocate for crystalloid fluid resuscitation to adequately restore the vascular volume.[5,7,27] If the patient does not respond to initial volume loading with isotonic fluids, the secondary suggestion is to use albumin.[27]

Similar capillary permeability may occur in anaphylactic shock as a result of histamine release with massive fluid shifts that can transfer up to 35% of the intravascular volume into the extravascular space within minutes. Short-term volume resuscitation may be necessary to compensate for this fluid shift that occurs along with the coexisting vasodilation.[23,79,100]

Two shock types in which volume resuscitation is not routinely indicated are cardiogenic and neurogenic shock. However, if there is suspicion that there is "mixed-shock" component and the patient may be hypovolemic on top of the aforementioned shock states, then traditional fluid resuscitation should be entertained. In cardiogenic shock, myocardial contractility is compromised and strategies are aimed at preload and afterload reduction to reduce unnecessary cardiac workload and oxygen requirements. The goal of treatment in cardiogenic shock is a rapid revascularization. Administration of fluid could be harmful unless cardiogenic shock is caused by right ventricular infarction and failure.[79,83] In neurogenic shock, vasodilation is responsible for a condition of relative hypovolemia. The use of alpha-adrenergic agents (e.g., phenylephrine) is aimed at restoring vascular tone and is the preferred treatment. Care must be taken to observe for and treat concomitant bradycardia.[20,62]

Isotonic crystalloid solutions continue to be the foundation of resuscitation in shock. No currently available isotonic crystalloid solution is ideal. Just as with any medication, fluid selection should be based on patient need, timing, and dosing in every effort to optimize effectiveness and minimize injury.

Hypertonic Crystalloids

Initially, hypertonic saline solution (HSS) was thought to have a number of desirable characteristics. First, the administration of HSS is associated with an immediate mobilization of fluids from the intracellular space to the extracellular compartments, specifically the intravascular space. Second, in animal models it has been shown to be associated with down regulation of neutrophil activation, proinflammatory mediators, and oxidative stress when compared to LR.[6,79,84]

HSS is most often defined as a concentration of 7.5%, either alone or in combination with synthetic colloids. In hypovolemic shock, it is clear that use of HSS results in lower fluid volume requirements.[6,84]

It is important to recognize that although theoretic and some physiologic benefits exist with the use of HHS, a survival benefit has not been recognized in the majority of studies. In 2009 the National Heart Lung and Blood Institute (NHLBI) halted the study by the Resuscitation Outcome Consortium (ROC) comparing HSS and NS in hemorrhagic shock patients as there was no significant difference in 28-day survival with a trend to earlier death with the HSS patients.[82] Other potential disadvantages to HSS include fluid volume overload associated with fluid shifts from the intracellular and interstitial space and hypernatremia.[34,84]

Colloid Solutions

Colloids consist of plasma protein fractions as well as synthetic solutions including hydroxyethyl starch (HES or hetastarch), dextran, and combination solutions of colloids and crystalloids.[41,84] Proponents of colloid solutions argue that they are more effective in expanding the intravascular volume because they are retained within the intravascular space and maintain colloid oncotic pressure that has the benefit of pulling volume from the interstitial and intracellular spaces.[1,100]

Theoretically, these qualities should make colloid solutions a desirable alternative to crystalloid solutions in shock resuscitation. The randomized, multicenter Colloid versus Crystalloid for the Resuscitation of the Critically Ill (CRISTAL) trial found that the use of colloids rather than crystalloids in resuscitation of the hypovolemic patient did not impact 28-day mortality.[6] Though a number of colloid solutions are available, for the purpose of clinical relevance, only albumin and HES solutions are further discussed.

Albumin

Albumin has been available for use in resuscitation since World War II. Five percent (5%) albumin solution is the most commonly used albumin concentration for fluid volume resuscitation. Infusion of 1 L of 5% albumin will increase the intravascular volume by approximately the same volume administered, 1 L.[7,30] Though impressive, the use of albumin as a resuscitation solution has failed to show outcome benefit over less expensive and more readily available crystalloid solutions.[30,95]

A publication of a meta-analysis by the Cochrane Injuries Group Albumin Review in 1998 reported a 6% increase in absolute risk of death with albumin use over crystalloid, and the use of albumin fell out of favor.[21] In contrast, in 2004, a multicenter, randomized control Saline versus Albumin Fluid Evaluation (SAFE) reported that a 4% albumin solution was compared with NS for fluid resuscitation; 28-day mortality was measured in patients admitted to critical care who required volume resuscitation. Although there was no increased mortality risk for patients treated with albumin, there was no reported clinical advantage to the routine use of albumin over crystalloid. This study did report that patients with traumatic brain injury resuscitated with albumin had nearly twice the mortality rates.[95]

Analysis of current research data does not support the routine use of colloids over crystalloid solutions as a resuscitation fluid in shock.[30,95] Although data suggest that albumin use may not be harmful as once believed, it is hard to justify utilizing it given the significant expense of albumin compared with readily available crystalloid solutions.

Hydroxyethyl Starch Solutions

HES solution is a synthetic colloid composed of 6% HES and sodium chloride. The theoretic benefits of using HES are similar to those associated with albumin.[41,78,84] Although beneficial in sustaining intravascular volume, HES solutions possess several undesirable characteristics, most notably the potential for acute renal failure and coagulopathy through inhibition of fibrin clot formation. Later generation HES solutions that are primarily utilized in Europe are seemingly less likely to cause coagulopathy.[41,78,80]

There are several large randomized trials looking at the impact on HES and resuscitation. One such study, Crystalloid versus Hydroxyethyl Starch Trial (CHEST), evaluated the general critical care population in need of fluid therapy and reported a 21% relative increase in the rate of renal replacement therapy with the HES group.[78] Another study, called the 6S trial, looked specifically at the use of HES in the septic patient population and determined that the use of HES with patient in septic shock had a higher mortality and renal failure rate.[80] The lack of proven benefit and potential for significant morbidity has left the use of HES out of the shock resuscitation armamentarium.

Blood Transfusion Therapy and Adjuncts

A large element of shock and effective resuscitation includes a discussion on transfusion therapy. Although crystalloid and colloid solutions are key components of fluid resuscitation, they lack the ability to carry oxygen and provide components necessary to support normal coagulation function.

The most common type of shock that will involve transfusion therapy is hypovolemic shock from blood loss. In the trauma population, approximately 11% of patients will require transfusion; of those 3% will require massive transfusion as defined by greater than 10 blood products within a 24-hour period.[1,109] Nurses caring for patients in need of transfusion therapy to reverse the impact of shock should have a good understanding of the potential complications associated with transfusion. See Chapter 26 for a comprehensive analysis of blood component therapy.

An effective resuscitative approach to the hemorrhaging patient is with the use of Damage Control Resuscitation (DCR). The tenets of DCR include permissive hypotension, as discussed previously, early and aggressive transfusion of blood products at a 1:1:1 ratio of packed red blood cells to platelets to fresh frozen plasma, and selective use of hemostatic adjuncts. The goal of this therapy is to minimize bleeding, increase end organ perfusion, prevent coagulopathy, and to minimize the complications associated with shock.[1,43,44,70]

The use of fresh whole blood (FWB) for resuscitations during military campaigns resulted in improved outcomes and gained the attention of the civilian medical community. It was apparent that infusing blood products at a ratio that most represented whole blood could simulate FWB. A number of observational studies supported this finding. The Pragmatic, Randomized Optimal Platelet and Plasma Ratios (PROPPR) looked at ratio therapy through a phase 3, multisite, randomized trial.[43,44] The findings did not reveal significant 30-day mortality when comparing 1:1:1 and 1:1:2 ratios. However, they did find that the 1:1:1 group had fewer deaths from exsanguination, no significant inflammatory-mediated complications such as acute respiratory distress syndrome (ARDS), or multiple organ failure, and it was determined this ratio was a safe therapy. Additionally, they determined that the use of ratio therapy resulted in rapid and more effective use of institutional massive transfusion protocols (MTP).[43,44,89]

Perhaps one of the most challenging patients to care for is the bleeding patient. The healthcare team must act quickly and effectively, and a key to the management of the bleeding patient is the cessation of blood loss and an accurate understanding the patient's coagulation profile.

Clinical measures of coagulopathy such as prothrombin time (PT), international normalized ratio (INR), and activated partial prothrombin time (aPTT) are what most clinicians are accustomed to monitoring when determining if a patient is coagulopathic. What is not generally known is that the patient's blood sample is warmed to standard body temperature (37°C) before analysis; this may falsely normalize the results. Additionally, these tests do not address platelet dysfunction caused by medications or hypothermia and most conventional coagulation values require dissemination to a core lab that can cause further delay of therapy.[7,45,100]

These limitations of traditional measures have brought into play the use of alternative measures of monitoring clotting and clot strength, thromboelastography (TEG), and rotational thromboelastometry (ROTEM). These are point of care (POC) tests that provide a rapid and personalized graphic coagulation profile of the patient. The use of TEG/ROTEM provides more effective and rapid initiation of MTP, more therapeutically directed transfusion of products, and improvement in 30-day and 90-day mortality in the trauma population.[44,45,100]

An additional therapy when caring for the bleeding patient is the use of hemostatic adjuncts such as tranexamic acid (TXA). This is a synthetic derivative of lysine that competitively inhibits the activation of plasminogen to plasmin; its effect is the prevention of fibrinolysis and thus halts bleeding.[99,105] The CRASH-2 trial was a large prospective, randomized trial that showed the use of TXA had a decrease in all-cause mortality, as well as death from bleeding alone. The impact was only seen when the medication was given within 3 hours of injury and in fact had higher morality when given after the 3-hour window.[92,99]

END POINTS OF RESUSCITATION

The resuscitation process is a continuum across the phases of care that can begin in the prehospital environment, onto admission, through surgery, and into critical care. Throughout this process, the nurse should be continually vigilant for changes in patient status and responses from interventions and observing clinical parameters that indicate resolution or worsening shock. Developing an understanding of these parameters, or "end points of resuscitation," is essential to effectively monitor the critically ill or injured patient in shock.

The goal of shock resuscitation is to restore oxygen delivery to the cells to support normal metabolic function. Determining when resuscitation is complete requires ongoing evaluation of physiologic markers or end points of resuscitation. These are clinical measures reflecting either global and/or regional changes or improvements in tissue perfusion and oxygenation. A clear understanding of the benefits and limitations of these end points is essential to improve clinical utility during resuscitation. Regardless of the type of shock, resuscitation efforts are guided by end points which help to determine the success of therapeutic interventions.[103,113]

In this section, specific end points are discussed, proceeding from basic clinical assessment to more complex laboratory data and information obtained from physiologic monitoring devices.

Global End Points of Resuscitation

Heart Rate

As noted, the assessment of routine vital signs provides an initial indication of physiologic improvement during resuscitation efforts. Increase in HR is an early compensatory effort to improve CO as part of the stress response mediated by the catecholamine release from the adrenal glands. Further efforts to increase CO by improving SV are achieved through renal conservation of fluid under the influence of ADH and aldosterone.[32,58]

Under many circumstances, tachycardia may be a reliable indicator to the onset of a compensatory response to shock. However, there are several disadvantages to using this parameter. Patients may be unable to develop a tachycardic compensatory response, or may develop tachycardia for reasons other than a compensatory response to shock.[32,58,75]

Those in the first category include patients with cardiac conduction disturbances, history of heart transplant, older adult patients, and those on medications (e.g., beta blockers) that preclude compensatory increases in HR. Patients in neurogenic shock from high SCI present with bradycardia as a result of lost sympathetic control and unopposed parasympathetic influence. This occurs even in the presence of coexisting hypovolemia that would normally trigger a tachycardic response in a patient without an SCI. Additionally, well-conditioned patients (i.e., athletes or young adults) with lower resting HRs may not become profoundly tachycardic, because they are able to compensate by increasing SV to improve CO.[54,58,75]

Patients in the second category may be tachycardic as a result of conditions other than shock. These include hypoxia as well as other physiologic triggers of the stress response, including pain, anxiety, and delirium. Damage to the myocardium in blunt cardiac injury or the presence of preexisting conduction disturbances may also preclude the usefulness of HR as a resuscitation end point. Finally, the presence of fever and influence of cytokines released as a result of systemic inflammatory response and sepsis result in persistent tachycardia independent of a compensatory response.[18,58]

Blood Pressure

BP, similar to HR, is a common parameter used to gauge hemodynamic stability and guide resuscitative efforts. In shock states, change in BP is a late finding, reflecting that compensatory mechanisms are already beginning to fail. For instance, a hemorrhaging patient would require a 30% to 40% volume loss or stage III shock before there is a drop in blood pressure (see Table 28.3). Consequently, BP is not a useful parameter for early detection of shock.[8,37,60]

Despite these issues, resuscitation efforts aimed at restoring adequate BP are appropriate as long as these limitations are considered. Initial efforts to improve BP may include administration of volume expanders in the face of suspected hypovolemia and the use of vasodilatory or vasopressor agents as indicated.[3,8,60] The BP end points for resuscitation must be individualized for each patient, type of shock, and determined in conjunction with other parameters more fully reflective of improved function at the end-organ level. A systolic BP of 100 mm Hg may be adequate to achieve organ perfusion in a healthy individual, whereas a higher pressure may be necessary in those with preexisting hypertension. Emphasis on maintaining improvements in mean arterial pressure (MAP), to greater than 60 mm Hg, may be more appropriate than a target systolic pressure.[8,60] Most importantly, it must be remembered that BP is a measurement of vascular tone, not perfusion. Inadequate organ perfusion may exist even in the presence of what has been traditionally thought to be a normal BP.[28,60,103]

An important aspect of using BP as an end point is the method by which it is measured. These may be grouped into two types. The first measurement of arterial pressure is accomplished through placement of a radial or femoral arterial catheter and allows for assessment of pressure on a continuous, real-time basis. The second method determines BP through the measurement of arterial blood flow. This is accomplished manually through direct auscultation of Korotkoff sounds by use of a stethoscope/Doppler, or through the use of an automated noninvasive oscillometric device. Although both methods measure BP, measurement is accomplished in different ways. Arterial lines directly measure pressure; auscultatory methods determine pressure through the measurement of flow. Because of this difference, comparative BPs evaluated via the two methods in the same patient may yield different results.[8,28,60,103]

Urine Output

The use of UO as an end point of resuscitation is based on the assumption that reductions or improvements in renal perfusion will subsequently result in similar changes in UO. In adults, the production of 1 to 2 mL/kg of urine per hour has been the accepted end point to reflect adequate end-organ perfusion. The renal blood flow and glomerular filtration rate (GFR) autoregulate so that there are not continually shifts in renal blood flow with variations of BP. This autoregulatory mechanism shuts down when the MAP is below 80 mm Hg, causing subsequent loss of flow to the renal bed, and UO may be reduced.[56,88]

The presence or absence of urine does not directly reflect shock states. For instance, in patients in whom normal renal function is reduced or even absent, this end point is not reliable. Such conditions may result in the presence of preexisting oliguria or anuria (i.e., chronic renal failure). Conversely, adequate UO despite perfusion abnormalities may exist when the kidneys are unable to concentrate urine. This may be observed in older adult populations as well as in the presence of renal failure or conditions such as diabetes insipidus. Further, the influence of medications affecting renal blood flow or those that induce artificial diuresis must be considered when using UO as a parameter to evaluate the adequacy of resuscitation.[88,96]

In uncompensated shock, the use of HR, BP, and UO may be appropriate end points in light of the limitations discussed. However, further evaluation of additional end points reflective of global tissue oxygenation is critical to determine if adequate tissue perfusion is present.[88,96]

Serum Lactate Levels

Lactic acid is a byproduct of anaerobic metabolism and has been recognized as a measurement of shock for over 45 years.[112] In normal conditions, lactate levels are less than 2 mmol/L. However, in the presence of shock, lactic acid levels rise.[10,112] As a resuscitation end point, Jansen et al. found that elevated lactate levels correlate with mortality in shock states.[47] A lactate level of more than 3 mmol/L that was decreased by at least 20% over 2 hours was associated with reduced morality.[47]

Lactate is efficiently metabolized in the patients with normal liver function. Therefore, in patients with liver disease in which lactate clearance may be impaired, elevated lactate levels may not always reflect hypoperfusion.[112] There are insufficient data to support the use of an absolute lactate value or range of values as an end point of resuscitation in isolation. However, the use of trended lactate levels used with other end points may be most helpful in guiding the need for more aggressive resuscitation measures.[10,47]

Arterial Base Deficit

Arterial BD is another indicator of anaerobic metabolism that may be used to guide resuscitation. Obtained as part of the ABG panel, arterial BD is reflective of serum bicarbonate utilization in an attempt to buffer acidosis. The BD has more predictive capacity of the state of shock than the pH, as the pH is impacted by attempts at acid-base compensatory mechanisms.[15,25,32,111]

Resuscitation measures used in successful restoration of tissue perfusion and cellular oxygenation should produce a reduction in BD as acidosis resolves. In the 1990s, Davis et al. classified base deficit abnormalities into mild, moderate, and severe. A mild BD is defined as levels between 2 and 5 mmol/L, moderate between 6 and 14 mmol/L, and severe BD at greater than 14 mmol/L. Worsening or failure of improving BD represents continued shock.[15,25]

A more recent large, multicenter looking at nearly 17,000 trauma patients suggested a reclassification of the BD.[76] The new grouping is classified into four strata of worsening BD: Class I = BD less than or equal to 2 mmol/L, Class II = BD greater than 2.0 to 6.0 mmol/L, Class III = BD greater than 6.0 to 10 mmol/L, and Class IV = BD greater than 10 mmol/L. The study assessed for demographics, injury characteristics, transfusion requirements, and fluid resuscitation. They found that those patients in Class III BD needed transfusions at a rate of approximately 50% and those in Class IV required massive transfusion greater than 50% of the time.[76]

In trauma patients, increasing BD is associated with ongoing blood loss. Significant BDs were also associated with lower BPs on admission and significant resuscitation fluid volume requirements.[114] Similar to other end points, trending BD is most helpful in determining the effectiveness of resuscitation measures. Patients who fail to improve their levels were found to have impaired oxygen consumption and extraction profiles as well as a greater tendency to develop multiorgan dysfunction syndrome and death.[1,15,77]

As with any end point, caution must be used in interpreting values in light of preexisting patient conditions and disease states. Elevations in BD unrelated to shock may be found. These include alcohol intoxication, hyperchloremic acidosis, and preexisting renal failure. Hyperchloremic acidosis is associated with the administration of large volumes of resuscitation fluids. This phenomenon occurs as the chloride portion of these balanced salt solutions raises serum chloride more rapidly than serum sodium concentrations. This results in hyperchloremia, favoring a shift toward hydrochloric acid in the balance with sodium hydroxide, causing pH to fall.[1,7,77]

Shock Index

Although POC testing can provide BD within minutes, not all facilities are equipped with such technology. The shock index (SI) is defined as a ratio of HR to systolic blood pressure (SBP) and calculated by dividing the HR by the SBP.[7,53] As HR and SBP alone have been shown to be unreliable in determining shock due to volume deficit, their ratio has been previously determined to be a more reliable measure for hemodynamic instability. The use of the SI has been utilized to assist in decision-making in the resuscitation of patients with shock. The classification for SI is divided into four groups: Group I = SI less than 0.6 indicates no shock, Group II = SI greater than 0.6 to less than 1 indicates mild shock, Group III = SI greater than 1 to less than 1.4 indicates moderate shock, and Group IV = SI greater than 1.4 indicates severe shock.[7,53,77]

Monitoring Technology

Hemodynamic Indices

To achieve desired end points of resuscitation, hemodynamic parameters (targets) contributing to DO_2I must be optimized. These targets must be individualized for each patient, but are primarily focused on improving the CO/CI component of the oxygen delivery equation, specifically HR and SV. Efforts to improve SV are more complex. They include the manipulation of cardiac preload, afterload, and contractility. The relationship among these parameters is illustrated in Fig. 28.9.

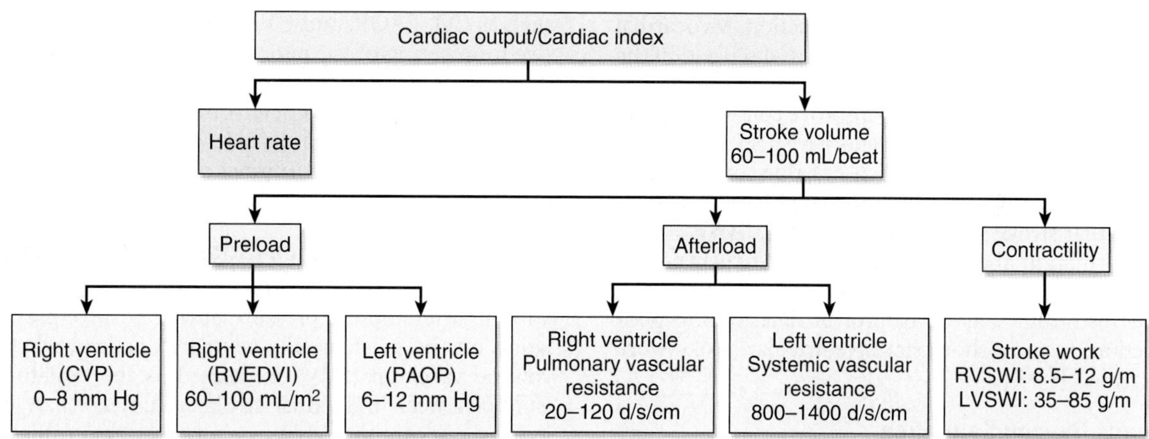

FIG. 28.9 Relationship of hemodynamic parameters. *CVP,* Central venous pressure; *RVEDVI,* right ventricular end-diastolic volume index; *PAOP,* pulmonary artery occlusion pressure; *RVSWI,* right ventricular stroke work index; *LVSWI,* left ventricular stroke work index.

Preload

Preload is blood volume in the ventricles prior to systole. Based on the principles of Starling's law, preload may be manipulated by increasing the volume into the ventricle to increase stretch of the myocardial fibers. This will result in increased recoil of these fibers during systole, increasing SV.[24,33] Limitation to this approach occurs with overstretch of the myocardial fibers, resulting in a decreasing SV and CO. This is represented by the plateau portion of the Starling curve. Traditional markers to evaluate preload include central venous pressure (CVP), pulmonary artery pressure (PAP), and pulmonary artery occlusion pressure (PAOP) also called pulmonary artery wedge pressure (PAWP). The main limitation of these parameters is that they are measurements of pressure rather than actual volume.[24,33,59]

Measurements of pressure have traditionally been used as a surrogate for volume, which is not feasible through standard hemodynamic monitoring devices at the bedside. The assumed relationship is that increasing pressures are reflective of increased preload volume. Conversely, low pressures reflect low volume. This relationship does not exist in the presence of certain cardiovascular pathology or other circumstances adversely affecting intrathoracic pressure. Such things may include valvular disease, decreased myocardial compliance, changes in chest wall compliance, abdominal compartment syndrome, and therapeutic strategies such as positive-pressure ventilation and positive end-expiratory pressure (PEEP). These conditions may result in hemodynamic pressure changes that are not necessarily reflective of volume.[33,59,66]

Afterload

Defined as resistance to blood-volume ejection from the ventricle, afterload is calculated as SVR for the left side of the heart and pulmonary vascular resistance (PVR) for the right side.[24,33] Manipulation of afterload in shock is dependent on the type of shock and characteristics. For example, in conditions of abnormally low afterload that result from the vasodilation of neurogenic shock or septic shock, the use of vasopressor agents may be necessary. Conversely, the patient in cardiogenic shock may require afterload-reduction measures such as vasodilators and balloon counterpulsation to improve CO.[33,59,83]

Contractility

Contractility is the force of myocardial contraction. Myocardial contractility is somewhat affected by preload as discussed in the context of Starling's law.[24,33] In addition to the manipulation of preload, the use of inotropic agents to improve contractility will improve SV and CO. Some of these agents have associated afterload-reducing properties as well, which must be considered in the face of preexisting hypotension. Calculated indices of right and left ventricular stroke work indices (RVSWI, LVSWI) provide some information about the degree of ventricular energy output. Stroke work indices describe the work the respective ventricles perform and may be helpful in determining poor cardiac function. In most shock states ventricular stroke work index is decreased.[2,7,24,33]

Mixed Venous Oxygen Saturation

The aforementioned assessment of the balance between Do_2 and Vo_2 is accomplished in the acute care setting by measurement of Svo_2 and more recently, measurement of central venous oxygen saturation ($Scvo_2$). Svo_2 is measured in the pulmonary artery through the use of a fiberoptic pulmonary artery catheter (PAC) and recorded in percentage of Hgb saturated with oxygen. Normal Svo_2 is between 60% and 80%, reflecting the saturation of mixed arterial blood after tissue extraction of oxygen from the blood when it has circulated through the body.[24,33,38,61] $Scvo_2$ measurement has been used in the early goal directed therapy and to guide resuscitation in the septic patient. $Scvo_2$ is approximately 5% higher than Svo_2, owing to the fact it is measured proximal to the right heart, where maximal extraction of oxygen from the blood has yet to occur. $Scvo_2$ is measured through the use of an oximetric multilumen catheter placed into the superior vena cava.[2,27,85]

Regardless of method, the measurement of Svo_2 or $Scvo_2$ provides information about the balance between oxygen delivered and consumed. A change in Svo_2 or $Scvo_2$ of 10% or more warrants closer evaluation. Assessment as to whether the change is related to an alteration in Do_2I or in Vo_2I is necessary.[38,61,81] Once cause is established, efforts aimed at improving supply and limiting unnecessary demand may be targeted.

Hemodynamic Monitoring

Patients who fail to respond in a predictable fashion to resuscitation measures may require additional monitoring to guide therapy. For decades this was in the form of a PAC. Traditionally this device provided information thought to be helpful in resuscitation, such as right-sided heart pressures, SV, mixed venous saturation, and intracardiac pressure.

The PAC was to be utilized as a diagnostic tool, but in and of itself was not therapeutic. It relied on the provider's skill at interpretation and intervention to best serve the patient. The use of the catheter carried with it inherent drawbacks such as the need for specially trained personnel and equipment, risks associated with central line placement such as pneumothorax or infection, potential for delay in therapy while awaiting insertion, and data acquisition before treatment and possibility of misinterpretation of complex data.[22,23,65,81] The Cochrane Collaboration on the use of PAC was published in 2013 and had been referred to as the "obituary" of the catheter. The final analysis concluded that the use of the PAC did not alter mortality, length of stay (LOS), or cost.[65,91]

In the newer age of hemodynamic monitoring in the patient in shock there has been a move from static indices such as CO, PAOP, and CVP to more dynamic and less invasive monitoring of the patient in shock. The primary goals of the management of shock are to obtain euvolemia and optimize CO. The ability to determine if the patient requires further fluid administration is referred to as *fluid responsiveness* and can be assessed in a number of minimally invasive bedside procedures.[2,11,64,85]

Pulse Pressure Variation /Stroke Volume Variation

Pulse pressure variation (PPV) is defined as the dynamic variation in arterial pulse pressure during positive pressure ventilation on the mechanically ventilated patient, whereas stroke volume variation (SVV) is defined as the beat-to-beat variability between individual stroke volumes. Analysis of these indices is accomplished by way of an arterial catheter and the use of a proprietary bedside monitoring system. The pressure changes are based on the heart-lung interaction during inspiration. Increased intrathoracic pressure changes the diameter of the vena cava, increases right atrial pressure and decreases venous return. After several heartbeats, the bedside monitor calculates the dynamic changes associated with fluid administration and are reviewed for determining the patient's response to fluid administration and for guiding further management of the patient.[2,11,64,102]

These therapies offer an alternative noninvasive means to assist in the management of resuscitation in shock. As the initiation of therapy only requires insertion of an arterial line, at many institutions the nurse can insert the required catheter needed to start assessment and intervention. Limitations to the use of PVV/SVV are that they cannot be utilized on patients with tidal volumes less than 8 mL/kg, those with open chest cavity, intraabdominal hypertension, or persistent cardiac arrhythmias.[11,22,102]

Passive Leg Raising

Many patients in shock are not utilizing mechanical ventilation or may have contraindications and therefore the PVV/SVV dynamic monitoring of fluid responsiveness cannot be utilized. In cases of circulatory failure, a passive leg raising (PLR) maneuver may be entertained to determine if the patient is in need of additional fluid. By transferring a volume of approximately 500 mL of venous blood from the lower body to the right heart, PLR mimics a fluid challenge.[66,74,85]

The advantage of the PLR is that no fluid has been given to the patient and if not tolerated, is reversible by lowering the legs. The maneuver entails a 45-degree leg elevation while at the same time placing the head of the bed from semi-recumbent to a flat position. Initiating from the semi-recumbent position adds the splanchnic circulation to the venous return and the interpretation of the PLR is more accurate. The CO response should be assessed within 1 to 2 minutes of elevation and can be measured by PVV/SVV in appropriate patients, echocardiogram, esophageal Doppler, or ultrasound (US).[66,74]

Esophageal Doppler

The esophageal Doppler offers the advantage of being less invasive than a PAC. When placed in the esophagus, information is obtained about descending aortic blood flow (Fig. 28.10). Hemodynamic variables (CO, preload, afterload, and contractility) can be calculated by interpreting the Doppler waveforms and assist in guiding therapy with data to support a reduction in complications and hospital stays. Disadvantages to this approach are the need for continual esophageal placement for ongoing monitoring and, because probe position is crucial to accurate information, it adds the element of operator dependency.[51,85]

Point of Care Ultrasonography

US is a safe and effective means to provide a rapid, portable, and focused diagnostic tool for use on the undifferentiated shock and/or cause of hypotension. US is typically utilized as a diagnostic tool in patients where a definitive cause of shock has not been determined based on clinical and laboratory evaluation or on those who are too unstable to be moved to imaging suites. There are a number of algorithmic approaches to US based on presumptive causes of shock; these assessments look at images of the heart, chest and abdominal cavities, aorta, and major vessels.[48,98,110]

The major advantage of US is the ability for rapid examination of vital structures that could be harbingers of the shock state. Other advantages are that it is portable, inexpensive, easily reproducible to guide effectiveness of intervention and therapy, and does not expose the patient to radiation. The major disadvantage to the use of US is that the interpretation and subsequent diagnosis and interventions are based on the skill of the provider.[48,110]

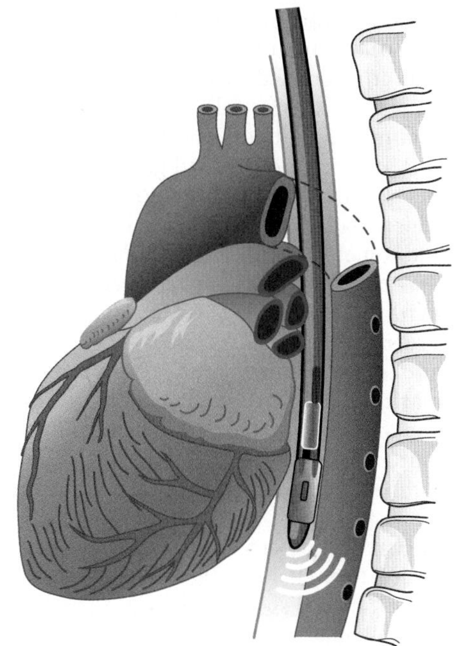

FIG. 28.10 Esophageal Doppler monitor probe.

REGIONAL RESUSCITATION END POINTS

Global resuscitation end points reflect a general picture of tissue oxygenation commonly referred to as *macrocirculation.* Over the decades there has been vast amount of research and clinical exploration to find physiologic markers that can provide an early indication of occult hypoperfusion. The regional tissue perfusion model is based on the concept that under physiologic stress the body will preferentially shunt blood from the peripheral and splanchnic tissues to augment perfusion of vital organs, primary the heart and brain. The ideal regional marker will be able to safely and accurately demonstrate the perfusion and oxygenation abnormalities earlier in shock state and can be rapidly and continuously monitored.[73,94,113]

The gastrointestinal (GI) system has been just such an area of research. The gut is highly susceptible to hypoperfusion in the compensatory stages of shock. The innermost layer of the intestine is most susceptible because it receives oxygen and nutrients by diffusion from the intestinal villi.[26,69,73] Deprivation of adequate perfusion for as little as 1 hour may result in mucosal damage and intestinal permeability. These circumstances can occur despite the presence of normal global parameters, and the condition has been termed *covert compensated shock.* The GI tract and integument beds have been much sought after as the potential link in the search for the "Holy Grail" of end points of resuscitation.

Regional Tissue Perfusion

The use of intestinal pH has been studied clinically since the 1980s. It is calculated using the partial pressure of CO_2

from the intestinal lumen measured through the use of device called a tonometer, placed in the stomach or intestine. Fiddian-Green et al. looked at the pH of the stomach utilizing a tonometry. This was followed by a number of small studies that found that patients that had normal global indices such as BP, lactate, and BD, had gastric tissue dysoxia in the stomach.[29] In subsequent lower-powered studies, intramucosal acidosis was consistently associated with poor outcome. Despite some promising early clinical findings, gastric tonometry has never been widely adopted. The technology was found to be too challenging and findings were not reproducible in larger studies.[69]

The tongue is the most proximal portion of the GI tract, sharing similar circulation and neuronal control as the esophagus and stomach. It was theorized that measurement of the partial pressure of sublingual CO_2 ($Pslco_2$) could provide the similar clinical value to pH obtained through gastric tonometry.[14,94]

The sublingual capnometry device consists of an electronic computer device that analyzes the concentration of CO_2, a fiberoptic probe, and a disposable sensor. The probe/sensor is placed in the sublingual pocket in contact with the sublingual mucosa. Although technically simpler to perform than gastric tonometry, some limitations of the device still exist. Most sublingual capnometry devices are designed for intermittent measurements of $Pslco_2$; therefore, repeat measures must be taken over time to trend changes in patient condition. In addition, any conditions limiting access to the oral cavity may prevent use of the device. These include oral trauma, surgical fixation of the jaw, and patient combativeness.[14,28,94]

Several research studies revealed some promising support for the use of sublingual capnometry; however, further research with larger sample sizes in homogeneous clinical conditions is still needed to confirm predictive ability and to determine its clinical usefulness in guiding resuscitation efforts.

Tissue oxygenation (Sto_2) can be obtained by way of several noninvasive techniques and has given hope to becoming an ideal resuscitation end point that can continuously measure the adequacy of oxygenation at the cellular level. Near-infrared spectroscopy (NIS) looks at light transmission through spectra that change when dysoxia is present in skin beds and is reflective of mitochondrial dysfunction that can lead to cellular damage and organ failure.[26,28,68,86]

Operationally, the device is noninvasive, consisting of the spectroscopy measurement device and sensors. The sensors are applied to the skin over the tissue area to be monitored and light is passed through the tissue between the probes. There have been a number of studies looking at the predictability of NIS measurement of Sto_2 and the accurate relationship to $Scvo_2$/Svo_2 and 28-day mortality. To date, they have been promising but still require a move to larger, more highly powered studies for clinical application.[12,28,106]

Another means to measure Sto_2 is through the use of sidestream dark field (SDF) imagery, which is done noninvasively through sublingual photometry. Stroboscopic light is absorbed by hemoglobin and as a result the handheld device makes is possible to visualize blood vessels. This provides a means of assessing microcirculation through an objective read out based on a scale called the microvascular flow index (MFI).[35,68] This has been studied by looking at patients in hemorrhagic shock, septic shock, and post cardiac arrest.[86,101,107] This has been proven to have some promising insight into early tissue warning by one of the largest, regional resuscitation, multicenter trials called the International Study on Microcirculatory Shock Occurrence in Acutely Ill Patients (microSOAP).[108]

NUTRITIONAL SUPPORT IN SHOCK

Critically ill patients in the ICU often require support for multiple dysfunctional organs. In addition, they often suffer from anorexia that prevents them from meeting their nutritional needs by oral intake alone. The considerations for nutritional support for patients in shock is multifactorial and includes the underlying cause of shock, organs which are dysfunctional, and the catabolic state related to their underlying illness.[19,104] Current high-powered studies suggest that no feeding or hypocaloric enteral feedings in the acute phase of critical illness is well tolerated for up to 7 days in the previously well-nourished patient. The traditional mindset of increasing infections associated with parenteral nutrition was not borne out in the Early Parenteral Nutrition and Supplemental Parenteral Nutrition (EPaNIC) trial.[19]

As important as how much and what to feed is when can the patient be safely fed. Patients in shock undergoing active resuscitation should have nutritional support measures delayed until hemodynamic stability has been achieved. During shock, compensatory redistribution of blood flow is away from the intestine and is shunted to the central organs. Additionally, the use of vasopressor agents further decreases already compromised tissue perfusion and requires the care provider to use scientific evidence to guide nutritional supplements during this therapy.[90,104]

The most current guidelines published by the American Society for Parenteral and Enteral Nutrition (ASPEN) and the Society of Critical Care Medicine (SCCM) suggest in the setting of significant hemodynamic instability (MAP < 60 mm Hg) where there are high or escalating dosage of catecholamine agents alone or in combination with active fluid or blood resuscitation, enteral nutrition should be withheld. Although enteral nutrition may be beneficial in maintaining intestinal mucosal integrity, the intestinal shock state may result in inadequate perfusion to accommodate normal digestive function and may further stress already compromised tissue oxygenation at the gut level. Additionally, although ischemic bowel injury is a rare complication of enteral nutrition, occurring less than 1% of the time, efforts to provide nutrition during shock offer potentially more risk of injury than benefit. Furthermore, no data can be found to support the use of parenteral nutrition in patients who are in shock.[67,90,104]

In the presence of adequate gut function, enteral feeding is preferred over parenteral nutrition. Enteral feeding helps to maintain the intestinal mucosal barrier, is associated with better wound healing, and is less costly than parenteral nutrition. If not contraindicated, enteral nutrition should begin within 24 hours. When enteral nutrition is contraindicated, parenteral nutrition may be considered.[67]

COMPLICATIONS OF SHOCK

The complications associated with shock are related to either hypoxic organ system injury from perfusion deficits or the side effects of resuscitation efforts. The degree of organ system dysfunction and failure is directly related to the duration and severity of shock. Inability to reverse the shock state in a timely manner will result in organ failure, even in systems unrelated to the initial insult. This includes neurologic injury, myocardial ischemia, acute respiratory distress syndrome, acute tubular necrosis/renal failure, hepatic failure, hematologic failure (such as disseminated intravascular coagulation), and intestinal ischemia.

Treatment-related complications include those of volume resuscitation, use of vasopressors, and reperfusion injury as circulation is restored. Intraabdominal hypertension and secondary abdominal compartment syndrome, for example, result as crystalloid solutions shift from the intravascular to interstitial space, increasing intestinal edema within the peritoneal cavity.[23,31,32] This results in pressure on pulmonary, cardiovascular, and renal structures, impairing normal function. Vasopressors employed to improve vascular tone and organ perfusion may ultimately reduce end-organ perfusion as blood is shunted away from some tissue beds. Ischemic injury and necrotic limbs may be an unintentional but realistic effect of these agents.[28]

Infections associated with preexisting patient medical conditions, current illness, and iatrogenesis are all too common occurrences in critical care. These include ventilator-associated pneumonia, catheter-related bloodstream infection, urinary tract infections, and wound infections. Reductions in tissue perfusion related to shock, medications, and nutritional deficit place the patient at risk for developing nosocomial pressure ulcers. Active effort to reduce potentially preventable complications through application of evidence-based guidelines is the role of the advanced practice nurse. These efforts help to achieve the ultimate goal of creating "safe passage" for the patient through the critical care environment.

CONCLUSION

The process of shock resuscitation is complex. All efforts are aimed at reversing tissue hypoxia and preserving organ function to optimize chances of patient survival. It requires a team approach in which each member contributes unique knowledge and skill. Monitoring the progression of resuscitation requires continual evaluation of multiple end points. Progression of monitoring from simple to complex parameters, some requiring invasive monitoring devices, has been the current practice in critical care. As technology and knowledge advance, there is hope that more sensitive end points will emerge, requiring less-invasive technology. As the main coordinator of patient care, clinical expert, consultant, educator, and researcher, the experienced nurse is in a key position to advance knowledge, influence care, and, most important, contribute to a positive outcome for the patient in shock.

CASE STUDY 28.1

J.T. is a 32-year-old male unrestrained driver who struck a cement bridge support at high speed. On arrival of EMS, he was unresponsive with a Glasgow Coma Score (GCS) score of 6, labored respirations at 30 per minute, weak radial pulses of 130 beats per minute (bpm), and a palpable BP of 84 mm Hg. He had sustained a large laceration to the forehead, crepitus was noted over the left chest, and also deformity of the left femur. On arrival to hospital he was intubated, underwent needle decompression of the left chest for a suspected tension pneumothorax, and received 2 L of lactated Ringer's (LR). HR was 140 bpm and BP had not improved. During primary assessment and intervention, his airway placement was reconfirmed by measurement of end-tidal CO_2 and auscultation of breath sounds. A 36 French chest tube was placed and 500 mL of blood removed. He received continued infusion of warmed LR and PRBCs. An arterial blood gas and lactate were drawn. Abdominal sonogram revealed large amounts of fluid in the pelvis and around the liver. Based on these findings, and continued hemodynamic instability, the massive transfusion protocol was started and J.T. was taken to the operating room for emergent laparotomy.

Two hours later, he arrived at the critical care unit. His injuries included ruptured spleen, multiple liver lacerations, and transection of the colon. He received 4 L of LR, 10 units of PRBCs, 9 units of fresh frozen plasma, and 9 units of platelets. His estimated blood loss was 4 L. His UO during the case was only 100 mL. Intraoperatively, a specimen was sent to thromboelastometry and an arterial line was placed. His data are outlined as follows:

Arterial blood gases: pH 7.20, $Paco_2$ 36, Pao_2 90, HCO_3^- 12, BD 11, Sao_2 93%.

Laboratory tests: Hgb 9, Hct 28, platelets 200, PT 16, WBC 18, lactate 8 mg/dL, TEG sent, glucose 180 mg/dL, BUN 20 mg/dL, Cr 0.8 mg/dL, Na^+ 136 mg/dL, K^+ 3.7 mg/dL, Cl^- 118 mg/dL, CO_2 26 mg/dL, Ca^{2+} 7 mg/dL.

Vital signs: T 35°C, HR 122, BP 100/50 mm Hg. CXR: large left pulmonary contusion and multiple left rib fractures.

As the critical care team takes over the care of this patient, the priority of care must focus on the continued resuscitation from shock that began in the prehospital phase of care.

Forty-eight hours later, J.T. is noted to be febrile (temp 39.5°C), HR 128, BP 102/60, with a WBC count of 24,000. Blood and urine cultures have been sent along with bronchoalveolar lavage fluid for culture and broad spectrum antibiotics are initiated. He has been taken back to the operating room twice for abdominal washout. His abdomen remains "open" with a vacuum closure system in place. He is noted to have a worsening oxygenation profile (Pao_2/Fio_2 ratio), decreased static lung compliance, worsening renal function (Cr 2.1 mg/dL, BUN 30 mg/dL), elevated liver profile, and climbing glucose levels (220 mg/dL). ABGs pH 7.32, $Paco_2$ 34, Pao_2 75, HCO_2 20. CXR shows bilateral white infiltrates. Over the past 24 hours he has required 6 L of LR and 2 additional units of blood and has persistent drops in MAP to less than 60mm Hg. A right heart catheter is placed with an initial CVP of 4 mm Hg and $Scvo_2$ of 53%. An additional liter of LR is given along with albumin 5% infusion. Despite fluid administration his MAP and $Scvo_2$ remain low. The decision was made to initiate norepinephrine at 2 mcg/min and titrate to achieve a MAP greater than 65 mm Hg. After 1 hour, norepinephrine was titrated to 10 mcg/min with minor improvement to MAP and a decision was made to add epinephrine titrated to 5 mcg/min.

Decision Point:

What parameters indicated incomplete resuscitation?

Decision Point:

What physiologic and global parameters suggest that this patient is in septic shock?

Decision Point:

What are the priorities of care for this patient?

BD, Base deficit; *BUN*, blood urea nitrogen; *Ca^{2+}*, calcium; *Cl*, chloride; *Cr*, creatinine; *CXR*, chest x-ray; *Hct*, hematocrit; *K^+*, potassium; *Na^+*, sodium; *Pao_2*, partial pressure of oxygen; *PT*, prothrombin time; *T*, temperature; *TEG*, thromboelastography; *UO*, urine output; *WBC*, white blood cell.

REFERENCES

1. Alam, H. B. (2011). New trends in resuscitation. *Curr Probl Surg, 48*(8), 531–564.
2. Alhashemi, J. A., Cecconi, M., & Hofer, C. K. (2011). Cardiac output monitoring: an integrative approach. *Crit Care, 15*, 1–9.
3. American College of Surgeons Committee on Trauma. (2008). *Advanced trauma life support for doctors (ATLS)* (8th ed.). Chicago: The American College of Surgeons.
4. Angus, D. C. (2011). The search for the effective therapy for sepsis. *JAMA, 306*, 2614–2615.
5. Angus, D. C., & van der Poll, T. (2013). Severe sepsis and septic shock. *N Engl J Med, 369*(9), 840–851.
6. Annane, D., Siami, S., Jaber, S., et al. (2013). Effects of fluid resuscitation with colloid vs. crystalloid on mortality in critically ill patients presenting with hypovolemic shock. *JAMA, 310*(17), 1809:1817.
7. Astiz, M. E. (2011). Pathophysiology and classifications of shock states. In J. L. Vincent, et al., *Textbook of critical care* (6th ed.). Philadelphia: Elsevier.
8. Augusto, J. F., Teboul, J. L., Radermakker, P., & Asfar, P. (2011). Interpretation of blood pressure signal: physiological bases, clinical relevance, and objectives during shock states. *Intensive Care Med, 11*, 411–419.
9. Bagwell, C. E. (2005). Respectful image, revenge of the barber surgeon. *Ann Surg, 241*, 872–878.
10. Bakker, J., Nijsten, M. W. N., & Jansen, T. C. (2013). Clinical use of lactate in monitoring critically ill patients. *Ann Intensive Care, 3*, 1–8.
11. Benes, J., Giglio, M., Brienza, N., et al. (2014). The effect of goal-directed fluid therapy based on dynamic parameters on post-surgical outcomes: a meta-analysis of randomized controlled trials. *Crit Care, 18*, 1–11.
12. Bezemer, R., Bartels, S. A., Bakker, J., et al. (2012). Clinical review: clinical imaging of the sublingual microcirculation in the critically ill. *Crit Care Med, 16*, 224–229.
13. Bonanno, F. G. (2011). Hemorrhagic shock: the "physiology approach." *J Emerg Trauma Shock, 4*(2), 233–243.
14. Boswell, S. A., & Scalea, T. M. (2003). Sublingual capnometry: an alternative to gastric tonometry for the management of shock resuscitation. *AACN Clin Issues, 14*(2), 176–184.
15. Bougle, A., Harrois, A., & Duranteau, J. (2013). Resuscitative strategies in hemorrhagic shock. *Ann Intensive Care, 3*, 1–9.
16. Burke, M., Lemm, H., Dietz, S., & Werdan, K. (2011). Pathophysiology, diagnosis and treatment of infarction related cardiogenic shock. *Cardiovasc Dis, 36*(2), 73–83.
17. Campbell, R. L., Hagan, J. B., Manivannan, V., et al. (2012). Evaluation of national institute of allergy and infectious disease and anaphylaxis network criteria for the diagnosis of anaphylaxis in emergency department patients. *J Allergy Clin Immunol, 129*, 748–752.
18. Caputo, N., Fraser, R., Paliga, A., et al. (2013). Triage vital signs do not correlate with serum lactate or base deficit and are less predictive of operative intervention. *Emerg Med J, 30*(7), 546–550.
19. Casaer, M. P., & Van den Berghe, G. (2014). Nutrition in acute phase of critical illness. *JAMA, 370*(13), 1227–1236.
20. Casha, S., & Christie, A. (2010). A systematic review of intensive cardiopulmonary management after spinal cord injury. *J Neurotrauma, 27*, 1–17.
21. The Cochrane Injuries Group Albumin Reviewers. (1998). Human albumin administration in critically ill patients: systematic review of randomized controlled studies. *Br Med J, 317*, 235–240.
22. Cooper, H. A., Najafi, A. H., Ghafourain, K., et al. (2014). Diagnosis of cardiogenic shock without the use of a pulmonary artery catheter. *Eur Heart J Acute Cardiovasc Care, 4*(1), 88–95.
23. Cordemans, C., DeLaet, I., Van Regenmortel, N., et al. (2012). Fluid management in critically ill patients: role of extravascular lung fluid, abdominal hypertension, capillary leak and fluid balance. *Ann Intensive Care, 2*(Suppl. 1), 1–12.
24. Darovic, G. O. (2002). *Hemodynamic monitoring: invasive and noninvasive clinical applications* (3rd ed.). Philadelphia: Saunders.
25. Davis, J. W. (1998). Base deficit in the elderly: a marker of severe injury and death. *J Trauma, 45*, 873–877.
26. Debacker, D., Ospina-Tascon, G., Salgado, D., et al. (2010). Monitoring the microcirculation in the critically ill. *Intensive Care Med, 36*, 1813–1825.
27. Dellinger, R. P., Levy, M. M., Rhodes, A., et al. (2013). Surviving Sepsis Campaign: international guidelines for management of severe sepsis and septic shock, 2012. *Intensive Care Med, 39*, 165–228.
28. Donati, A., Tibboel, D., & Ince, C. (2013). Towards integrative physiological monitoring of the critically ill. *Crit Care, 17*(Suppl. 5), 1–7.
29. Fiddian-Green, R. C. (1987). Predictive value of stomach wall pH for complications after cardiac operations: comparison with other monitoring. *Crit Care Med, 15*, 153–156.
30. Finfer, S. (2013). Reappraising the role of albumin for resuscitation. *Curr Opin Crit Care, 19*, 315–320.
31. Funk, D. J., Parillo, J. E., & Kumar, A. (2009). Sepsis and septic shock: a history. *Crit Care Clin, 25*, 83–101.
32. Gabrielli, A., Layon, A. J., & Yu, M. (2012). Shock states. In *Civetta, Taylor and Kirby's manual of critical care*, Philadelphia: Lippincott.
33. Gabrielli, A., Layon, A. J., & Yu, M. (2012). Hemodynamic monitoring and oxygenation. In *Civetta, Taylor and Kirby's manual of critical care* Philadephia: Lippincott.
34. Gheorghe, C., Dadu, R., Blot, C., et al. (2010). Hyperchloremic metabolic acidosis following resuscitation of shock. *Chest, 138*, 1521–1523.
35. Goedhardt, P. T., Khalizada, M., Bezemer, R., et al. (2007). Dark side field (DSF) imaging: a novel stroboscopic LED ring-based imaging modality. *Optical Expression, 15*, 15101–15114.
36. Gurigis, F. W., Williams, D. J., Kalynych, C. J., et al. (2014). End-tidal carbon dioxide as a goal of early sepsis therapy. *Am J Emerg Med, 32*, 1351–1356.
37. Guy, H. R., Bouamra, O., Spiers, M., et al. (2011). Vital signs and estimated blood loss in patient with major trauma: testing the validity of ATLS. *Resuscitation, 82*, 556–559.
38. Hameed, S. D. M., Aird, W. C., & Cohn, S. M. (2003). Oxygen delivery. *Crit Care Med, 31*(Suppl. 12), 658–667.
39. Harbrecht, B. C., Forsythe, R. M., & Peitzman, A. B. (2008). Management of shock. In D. V. Feliciano, et al. *Trauma* (6th ed.). New York: McGraw Hill.
40. Hardaway, R. (2003). A brief review of traumatic shock leading to a new theory and new treatment. *J Appl Res, 3*, 464–468.
41. Hartog, C. S., Kohl, M., & Reinhart, K. (2011). A systemic review of third generation hydroxyethyl starch. *Anesth Analg, 112*, 635–645.
42. Hinshaw, L. B., & Cox, B. G. (1972). *The fundamental mechanism of shock*. New York: Plenum.
43. Holcomb, J. B., Tilley, B. C., Baraniuk, S., et al. (2015). Transfusion of plasma, platelets, and red blood cells in a 1:1:1 vs. a 1:1:2 ratio and mortality with severe trauma. The PROPPR randomized clinical trial. *JAMA, 313*(5), 471–482.
44. Holcomb, J. B., Zarazabal, L. A., Michalek, J. E., et al. (2011). Increased platelet: RBC ratios are associated with improved survival after massive transfusion. *J Trauma, 71*, S318–S328.
45. Hunt, H., Stanworth, S., Curry, N., et al. (2015). Thromboelastography (TEG) and rotational thromboelastometry (ROTEM) for trauma induced coagulopathy in adult trauma patients with bleeding. *Cochrane Database Syst Rev, 2* Article # CD101438.
46. Hunter, C. L., Silvestri, S., Ralls, G., et al. (2014). The sixth vital sign: prehospital end-tidal carbon dioxide predicts in-hospital mortality and metabolic disturbances. *Am J Emerg Med, 32*, 160–165.
47. Jansen, T. C., van Bommel, J., & Bakker, J. (2009). Blood lactate monitoring in critically ill patients: a systemic health technology assessment. *Crit Care Med, 37*(10), 2827–2839.
48. Kanji, H. D., McCallum, J., Sirounis, D., et al. (2014). Limited echocardiography-guided therapy in subacute shock is associated in change of management and improved outcomes. *J Crit Care, 29*, 700–709.
49. Kheng, C. P., & Rahman, N. H. (2012). The use of end-tidal carbon dioxide monitoring in patients with hypotension in the emergency department. *Int J Emerg Med, 5*, 1–7.
50. Kobayashi, L., & Costantini, T. W. (2012). Hypovolemic shock resuscitation. *Surg Clin North Am, 92*, 1403–1423.
51. Labovitz, A. J., Noble, V. E., Bierig, M., et al. (2010). Focused cardiac ultrasound in the emergent setting. A consensus statement of the American Society of Echocardiography and American College of Emergency Physicians. *J Am Soc Echocardiogr, 23*, 1225–1235.

52. Lagu, T., Rothberg, M. B., Shieh, M. S., et al. (2012). Hospitalizations, costs and outcomes of severe sepsis in the United States. *Crit Care Med, 40*, 754–756.
53. Lanspa, M. J., Brown, S. M., Hirshberg, E. L., et al. (2012). Central venous pressure and shock index predict lack of hemodynamic response to volume expansion in septic shock. *J Crit Care, 27*, 609–615.
54. Larson, C. R., White, C. E., Spinella, P. C., et al. (2010). Association of shock, coagulopathy and initial vital signs with massive transfusion in combat casualty. *J Trauma, 69*, S26–S32.
55. Lee, P. M. J., Lee, C., Rattner, P., et al. (2014). Intraosseous versus central catheter utilization and performance during inpatient medical emergencies. *Crit Care Med, 43*(6), 1233–1238.
56. Legrand, M., & Payen, D. (2011). Understanding urine output in critically ill patients. *Ann Intensive Care, 1*(13), 1–8.
57. Leiberman, P., et al. (2010). The diagnosis and management of anaphylaxis parameter update: 2010. *J Allergy Clin Immunol, 126*, 477–483.
58. Magder, S. A. (2012). The ups and downs of heart rate. *Crit Care Med, 40*, 239–245.
59. Madger, S. A. (2012). Bench-to-bedside review: an approach to hemodynamic monitoring. *Crit Care Med, 16*, 236–242.
60. Madger, S. A. (2014). The highs and lows of blood pressure: toward meaningful clinical targets in patients with shock. *Crit Care Med, 42*(5), 1241–1251.
61. Maizes, J. S., Murtuza, M., & Kvetan, V. (2000). Oxygen transportation and utilization. *Respir Care Clin N Am, 6*(4), 473–500.
62. Mallek, J. T., et al. (2012). The incidence of neurogenic shock and spinal cord injury admitted to a high volume level one trauma center. *Am Surg, 78*(5), 623–626.
63. Manji, R. A., Wood, K. E., & Kumar, A. (2008). The history and evolution of circulatory shock. *Crit Care Clin, 25*, 1–29.
64. Marik, P. (2013). Non-invasive cardiac output monitoring: a state of the art review. *J Cardiothorac Vasc Anesth, 27*(1), 121–134.
65. Marik, P. (2013). Obituary: pulmonary artery catheter 1970-2013. *Ann Intensive Care, 3*(38), 1–6.
66. Marik, P. E., & Cavallazzi, R. (2013). Does the central venous pressure predict fluid responsiveness? An updated meta-analysis and a plea for some common sense. *Crit Care Med, 41*(7), 1774–1781.
66a. Martel, M. J. (2002). Hemorrhagic shock. In Society of Obstetricians and Gynecologists of Canada: *SOGC Clinical Practice Guidelines,* No. 115, 1-8.
67. McClave, S. A., Maindale, R. G., Vanek, V. W., et al. (2009). Guidelines for the provision and assessment of nutrition support therapy in the adult critically ill patient: Society of Critical Care Medicine (SCCM) and American Society for Parenteral and Enteral Nutrition (ASPEN). *JPEN J Parenter Enteral Nutr, 33*(3), 277–315.
68. Medina, E. R., Milstein, D. M. J., & Ince, C. (2013). *Monitoring technologies*. Philadelphia: Lippincott.
69. Miami Trauma Clinical Trials Group. (2005). Splanchnic hypoperfusion-directed therapies in trauma: a prospective, randomized control trial. *Am Surg, 71*, 252–260.
70. Miller, T. E. (2013). New evidence in trauma resuscitation-is 1:1:1 the answer? *Perioper Med, 2*, 1–9.
71. Millham, F. H. (2010). Historical paper in surgery: a brief history of shock. *Surgery, 148*, 1026–1037.
72. Mitra, B., Tullio, F., Cameron, P. A., & Fitzgerald, M. (2012). Trauma patients with the "triad of death." *Emerg Med J, 29*(8), 622–625.
73. Moore, K. (2014). The physiologic response to hemorrhagic shock. *J Emerg Nurs, 40*, 629–631.
74. Monnet, X., & Teboul, J.-L. (2015). Passive leg raising: five rules, not a drop of fluid. *Crit Care, 19*, 18–21.
75. Mutschler, M., Nienaber, U., Munzberg, M., et al. (2014). Assessment of hypovolemic shock at scene: is PHTLS classification of hypovolemic shock valid? *Emerg Med J, 31*(1), 35–40.
76. Mutschler, M., Nienaber, U., Brockanp, T., et al. (2013). Renaissance of base deficit for the initial assessment of trauma patients: a base deficit-based classification for hypovolemic shock developed on data from 16,305 patients. *Crit Care, 17*, 1–11.
77. Mutschler, M., Nienaber, U., Munzberg, M., et al. (2013). The shock index revisited. *Crit Care, 17*, 1–9.
78. Myburgh, J. A., Finfer, S., Bellomo, R., et al. (2012). Hydroxyethyl starch (HES) or saline for fluid resuscitation in intensive care. *N Engl J Med, 367*(20), 1901–1911.
79. Myburgh, J. A., & Mythen, M. G. (2013). Resuscitation fluid. *N Engl J Med, 369*(13), 1243–1251.
80. Mutter, T. C., Ruth, C. A., & Dart, A. B. (2013). Hydroxyethyl starch versus other fluid therapies: effects on kidney function. *Cochrane Database Syst Rev, 7*, CD007594.
81. Nebout, S., & Pirracchio, R. (2012). Should we monitor Scvo2 in critically ill patients? *Cardiol Res Pract, 2012*, 1–7.
82. NHLBI Stops Enrollment in Study of Concentrated Saline for Patients with Traumatic Brain Injury. (2009). NIH News. www.nhlbi.nih.gov.
83. O'Gara, P. T., Kuschner, F. G., Ascheim, D. D., et al. (2013). ACCF/AHA Guidelines for management of ST-elevation myocardial infarction: a report of the American College of Cardiology Foundation/American Heart Association. *J Am Coll Cardiol, 61*(4), e78–e140.
83a. Osman, O. F., & Askarai, R. (2014). Infection control in the intensive care unit. *Surg Clin North Am, 94*(6), 1175–1194.
84. Perel, K. J., Simons, F. E., & Ker, K. (2013). Colloid versus crystalloids for fluid resuscitation in critically ill patients. *Cochrane Database Syst Rev, 2*, CD000567.
85. Pincky, M. R. (2014). Functional hemodynamic monitoring. *Curr Opin Crit Care, 20*, 288–293.
86. Pranskunas, A., Koopmans, M., Koetsier, P. M., et al. (2013). Microcirculatory blood flow as a tool to select ICU patients eligible for fluid therapy. *Intensive Care Med, 39*, 612–619.
87. Privette, A. R., & Dicker, R. A. (2013). Recognition of hypovolemic shock. *Crit Care, 17*, 124–126.
88. Prowle, J. R., Ishikawa, K., May, C. N., & Bellomo, R. (2010). Renal plasma flow and glomerular filtration rate during acute kidney injury. *Ren Fail, 32*, 349–355.
89. Rahbar, M. H., Fox, E. E., Junco, D. J., et al. (2012). Coordination and management of multi-center clinical studies in trauma: experience from the prospective observational multi-center major trauma transfusion (PROMITT) study. *Resuscitation, 83*, 459–464.
90. Rai, S. S., O'Connor, S., Lange, K., et al. (2010). Enteral nutrition for patients in septic shock. *Crit Care Resusc, 12*(3), 177–181.
91. Rajaram, S. S., Desai, N. K., Kalra, A., et al. (2013). Pulmonary artery catheters for adult patients in the intensive care unit. *Cochrane Database Syst Rev, 2*, CD003408.
92. Roberts, I., Shakur, H., Afolabi, A., et al. (2011). The importance of early treatment with tranexamic acid in bleeding trauma patients (CRASH-2). *Lancet, 377*(9771), 1096–1101.
93. Rohacek, M., Edenhofer, H., Bircher, A., & Bingisser, R. (2014). Biphasic anaphylactic reactions: occurrence and mortality. *Allergy, 69*, 791–799.
94. Ruffolo, D. C., & Headley, J. M. (2003). Regional carbon dioxide monitoring. *AACN Clin Issues, 14*(2), 168–175.
95. The SAFE Study Investigators. (2004). A comparison of albumin and saline for fluid resuscitation in the intensive care unit. *N Engl J Med, 350*, 2247–2256.
96. Saotome, T., Ishikawa, K., May, C. N., et al. (2010). The impact on hypoperfusion on subsequent kidney function. *Intensive Care Med, 36*, 533–540.
97. Sethi, A. K., Sharma, P., & Mohta, M. (2003). Shock: a short review. *Indian J Anaesth, 47*, 345–359.
98. Shackelford, S. A., Colton, K., Stansbury, L. G., et al. (2013). Early identification of uncontrolled hemorrhage after trauma. Current status and future direction. *J Trauma Acute Care Surg, 77*(2), S222–S227 suppl.
99. Shakur, H., Roberts, I., Bautists, R., et al. (2010). Effects of tranexamic acid on death, vascular occlusive event and blood transfusion in trauma patients with significant hemorrhage (CRASH-2). *Lancet, 376*(9743), 23–32.
100. Shere-Wolfe, R. F., Galvagno, S. M., & Grissom, T. E. (2012). Critical care considerations in management of trauma patients following initial resuscitation. *Scand J Trauma Resusc Emerg Med, 20*(68), 1–15.
101. Spanos, A., Jhanji, S., Vivian-Smith, A., et al. (2010). Early microvascular changes in sepsis and severe sepsis. *Shock, 33*, 387–391.
102. Stoneking, L., DeLuca, L. A., Fiorello, A. B., et al. (2014). Alternative methods to central venous pressure for assessing volume status in critically ill patients. *J Emerg Nurs, 40*(2), 115–123.

103. Strehlow, M. C. (2010). Early identification of shock in critically ill patients. *Emerg Med Clin North Am, 28*(1), 57–66.
104. Thibault, R., Pichard, C., Wernerman, J., & Bendjelid, K. (2010). Cardiac shock and nutrition: safe? *Intensive Care Med, 37*, 261–268.
105. Valle, E. J., Allen, C. J., Van Haren, R. M., et al. (2013). Do all trauma patients benefit from tranexamic acid? *J Trauma Acute Care Surg, 76*(6), 1373–1378.
106. van Genderson, M. E., Klijn, E., Lima, A., et al. (2014). Microvascular perfusion as a target for fluid resuscitation in experimental circulatory shock. *Crit Care Med, 14*, e96–e105.
107. van Genderson, M. E., Lima, A., Akkerhuis, M., et al. (2012). Persistent peripheral and microcirculatory perfusion alterations after out of hospital cardiac arrest associated with poor survival. *Critical Care Med, 40*, 2287–2294.
108. Vellinga, N. A. R., Boerma, E. C., Koopmans, M., et al. (2014). International Study on Microcirculatory Occurrence in Acutely Ill Patients (microSOAP). *Crit Care Med, 43*(1), 43–56.
109. Vincent, J. L., & DeBacker, D. (2013). Circulatory shock. *N Engl J Med, 369*(18), 1726–1734.
110. Volpicelli, G., Lemorte, A., & Tullio, M. (2013). Point of care multi-organ ultrasonography for the evaluation of undifferentiated hypotension in the emergency department. *Intensive Care Med, 39*, 1290–1299.
111. Ward, K. R., Tiba, M. H., Ryan, K. L., et al. (2010). Oxygen transport characterization in human model of progressive hemorrhage. *Resuscitation, 81*(8), 987–993.
112. Weil, M. H., & Tang, W. (2009). Forty-five-year evolution of stat blood and plasma lactate measurement to guide critical care. *Clin Chem, 55*(11), 2053–2054.
113. Wilmont, L. A. (2010). Shock: early recognition and management. *J Emerg Nurs, 36*, 134–139.
114. Wood, R. A., Camargo, C. A., Lieberman, P., et al. (2014). Anaphylaxis in America: the prevalence and characteristics of anaphylaxis. *J Allergy Clin Immunol, 133*, 461–467.

29

Optimizing Hemodynamics: Strategies for Fluid and Medication Titration in Hypoperfusion States

Maria Fe White

Hemodynamics is defined as the forces involved in circulating blood throughout the body. The primary purpose of blood circulation is to deliver oxygen, the most vital of cellular nutrients. Without optimal hemodynamics, cellular hypoxia, organ failure, and patient mortality inevitably follow. However, very few evidence-based guidelines for the management of hemodynamics in hypoperfusion states are available. In recent years, disease-specific guidelines have emerged, such as those related to sepsis and hypovolemia associated with surgery and trauma. But in general, confusion and controversy prevail over how to best manage fluids and drug therapies to maximize organ perfusion.[32] As a result, critical care nurses often find themselves being guided by clinical tradition, expert opinion, or medical hearsay. This chapter is intended to assist nurses to gain a better understanding of hemodynamic pathologies, optimization strategies, and best practices in perfusion support. Physiologic concepts pertinent to this topic and employed in this chapter can be found in numerous textbooks and articles written for the bedside practitioner.[18,35,63]

HYPOPERFUSION STATES AND SYSTEMIC RESPONSES

Severe hypoperfusion is generally referred to as shock, and is characterized by tissue hypoxia and anoxia leading to hemodynamic compromise or collapse. A review of the general classifications of, phases of, and resuscitative measures for each of the shock states is found in Chapter 28. The main hemodynamic characteristics of hypovolemic, cardiogenic, and distributive shock are briefly reviewed here. Many patients with circulatory failure have characteristics of more than one of these types of shock. Threats can be attributed to one of the three components of the cardiovascular system: the heart (pump), the blood (volume), or the vessels (resistance).

Cardiogenic shock occurs when the heart (pump) is unable to pump enough blood to meet the body's demand for oxygen. The leading cause of cardiogenic shock is myocardial infarction (Box 29.1).

Hypovolemic shock, the most prevalent form of hypoperfusion, occurs when the vascular system loses blood or fluid either externally or internally, leading to a fall in perfusion pressure (Box 29.2).

Distributive shock occurs when blood vessels dilate inappropriately, and may be accompanied by capillary leakage (Box 29.3). Septic shock is the predominant form of distributive shock seen in critical care.

Neurohormonal Regulation

Regardless of the origin of hypoperfusion, the body's response is patterned and nonspecific. The physiologic response to hypoperfusion is the same as the reaction to any number of real, imagined, physical, or emotional perceived threats; the body does not differentiate.

The two most potent systems activated in a crisis include the sympathetic nervous system (SNS) and the renin-angiotensin-aldosterone system (RAAS). Although SNS activation involves multiple and complex processes affecting the entire body, this chapter will only cover the cardiovascular effects. When the SNS is stimulated, catecholamines are released into the circulation from the adrenal medulla and at synaptic interfaces from systemic nerve endings. Release of epinephrine and norepinephrine leads to the following changes: increased heart rate (HR), increased cardiac contractility, and increased vascular tone (Fig. 29.1). Vital organ vessels actually receive augmented flow via vasodilation, but the net effect is one of vasoconstriction and shunting of blood away from nonvital organs and toward vital organs (brain, heart, and skeletal muscle). These receptors have been labeled as alpha-adrenergic and beta-adrenergic. The heart is driven by beta-adrenergic receptors, whereas the vasculature has both alpha- and beta-adrenergic receptors. Vascular vital organ beds primarily have beta-2 receptors. Nonvital organ vascular beds primarily have alpha-receptors. The vascular response to alpha stimulation is constriction, and the response to beta-2 stimulation is dilation. Thus, during the stress response, both receptors are stimulated to maintain adequate perfusion.

The RAAS's primary purpose is to support blood pressure (BP) for efficient renal filtration and waste removal. With any fall in BP, the kidney secretes a tissue hormone called renin. Renin initiates a cascade of interactions that ultimately results in the release of aldosterone from the adrenal cortex and the production of angiotensin II from vessel linings (see Fig. 29.1). Aldosterone induces the nephron to retain sodium and water, and angiotensin II causes vessels to constrict.

In summary, hypoperfusion states activate the stress response mediated primarily by the SNS and RAAS. Together,

BOX 29.1 Causes of Cardiogenic Shock

- Acute coronary syndromes
    - ST elevation myocardial infarction (STEMI)
    - Non-ST elevation myocardial infarction (non-STEMI)
- Reperfusion injury states (stunned myocardium)
- Exacerbated chronic heart failure
- Cardiomyopathy
- Infectious or inflammatory processes
- Traumatic chest contusion
- Cardiotoxic drug exposure
- Negative inotropic excess (beta-blockers, calcium channel blockers)
- Structural abnormalities (valvular dysfunction, septal disruptions)
- Obstructive pathologies (cardiac tamponade, pulmonary emboli, tension pneumothorax)

BOX 29.2 Causes of Hypovolemic Shock

External Losses

- Decreased fluid intake
- Vomiting and diarrhea
- Diaphoresis
- Polyuria
- Hemorrhage
- Burns and wound exudate

Internal Losses

- Interstitial shifting (third spacing)
- Bowel sequestration
- Internal hemorrhage
- Ascites

these two systems elicit an upsurge in HR, contractility, vessel tone (afterload), and vascular volume (preload). For example, hypovolemic shock is appropriately managed by the body's stress reaction; increasing HR and contractility improves cardiac output (CO). Retaining sodium and water also addresses the issue of hypovolemia, whereas vascular constriction creates a more balanced relationship between the volume and the vascular bed, improving perfusion pressure. Distributive shock, however, is not supported as efficiently by this response because of the inability of the vasculature to respond with increased tone. Nevertheless, fluid reabsorption, increased HR, and increased contractility are able to maintain perfusion to some extent.

In the case of cardiogenic shock, the body's response appears to be more life-threatening than life-supporting. First, there is no significant improvement in contractility because patients are already at maximum endogenous catecholamine levels and are incapable of contributing much more without external stimulation. In addition, forcing a failing heart to beat faster and to circulate greater venous volume against higher arterial resistance is counterproductive. This is why, in cases of pump failure, the fight-or-flight system is termed the *vicious cycle* (Fig. 29.2). When a patient shows signs of hypoperfusion, whether the threat is to the pump, volume, or resistance, it is vital to determine the underlying cause to tailor therapeutic intervention to the source of the problem. In some clinical scenarios, the cause and treatment are evident. However, in cases in which it is less discernible, or when the patient is unstable enough to warrant continual assessment, invasive hemodynamic monitoring is useful.

BOX 29.3 Causes of Distributive Shock

- Sepsis
- Anaphylaxis
- Systemic inflammation of multiple causes (e.g., pancreatitis, fulminant hepatitis)
- Drug overdose
- Neurogenic insults (e.g., spinal cord injury, epidural drugs)

MONITORING HEMODYNAMIC MEASURES

The interpretation of hemodynamic values and measures from the pulmonary artery catheter (PAC) as they relate to the evaluation and management of hypoperfusion states is reviewed in this chapter. Intermittent thermodilution obtained through the PAC has been considered the gold standard for CO monitoring in the clinical setting since the late 1960s. This system was widely used until the 1990s, when a notable decline in its use was attributed to a shift in philosophy and replacement by newer technologies.[53] Some experts have proposed that this is more the fault of clinicians than the catheter.[9,38] Recent studies focusing on the PAC and outcomes have shown no positive association between PAC use for fluid management, survival in the intensive care unit (ICU), or survival in high-risk surgical patients. In critically ill patients, use of the PAC did not increase overall mortality or days in hospital, nor did it confer any benefit.[60] This conclusion, combined with the extreme level of invasiveness, the advanced training needed for placement, and incorrect parameter interpretation, have led to declining use of this system. However, the PAC is still useful for preload measurements in a variety of clinical settings.[53]

Whereas flow-dependent hemodynamic measures from the PAC (CO, mean arterial pressure [MAP], venous oxygen saturation [Svo_2], central venous pressure [CVP], and pulmonary artery occlusion pressure [PAOP] also known as pulmonary artery wedge pressure [PAWP]) have been the standard practice in critical care, technological advances in functional measures to evaluate fluid responsiveness have emerged. Measures like passive leg raising (PLR), transthoracic echocardiography (TTE), pulse pressure variation (PPV), end tidal CO_2 ($Etco_2$), and microcirculation and tissue perfusion monitoring are emerging technologies.

The use of PLR and PPV were investigated to evaluate preload response to fluid challenge. In contrast to saline fluid challenge, PLR can be used as a simple and reversible fluid volume challenge by translocating blood from lower extremities to central circulation, thus increasing the right ventricular preload. In a 70 kg man, PLR causes an approximate 300-mL blood bolus that persists for approximately 2 to 3 minutes before resulting in intravascular volume redistribution. Measurements of physiologic responses to fluid challenge, which may include CVP dynamic changes, peripheral PPV, or echocardiography, should be performed first with the patient in a supine position, and then remeasured when both legs are elevated at 45 degrees for 2 minutes.[8] A cohort study found that a stroke volume (SV) increase of 15% or higher induced by PLR predicted a volume response with a sensitivity of 81%, specificity of 93%, positive predictive value of 91%, and a negative predictive value of 85%.[65] Because the PLR maneuver requires manipulation of patient position, measurements may be inaccurate in abdominal compartment syndrome or when leg compression devices are present.[37]

TTE to assess fluid responsiveness has also been investigated as an alternative noninvasive bedside evaluation for fluid

Responder: Sympathetic nervous system

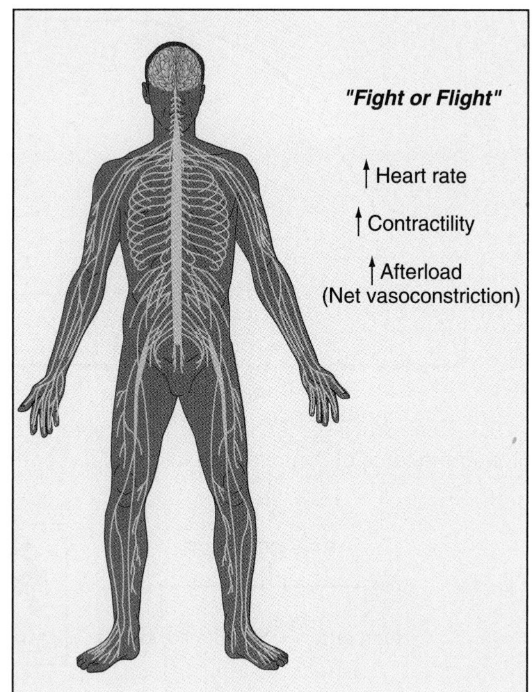

Responder: Renin-angiotensin-aldosterone system

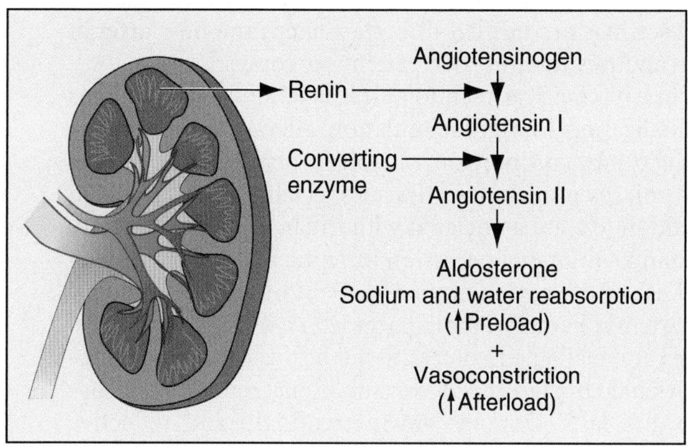

FIG. 29.1 Primary shock responders and their effects.

Do the Responders Work?

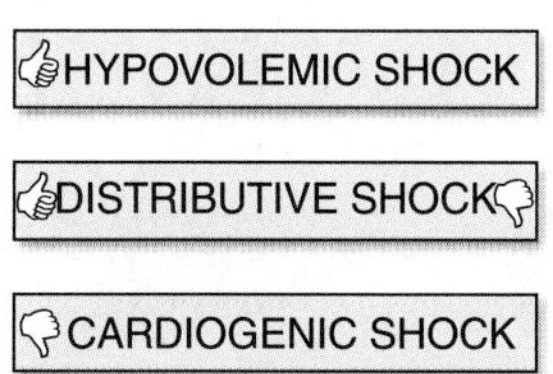

FIG. 29.2 The response to shock is the same regardless of the type. The stress responses that are typically helpful in hypovolemic shock have a minimal effect with distributive shock, and are harmful with cardiogenic shock.

responsiveness. The utility of measuring respiratory variations in inferior vena cava (IVC) size and SV is well-established and of proven accuracy, but requires training and skill. Measuring the collapsibility index is based on the appearance of the IVC or the superior vena cava (SVC). If a slight increase in CVP induces a marked increase in IVC diameter, this reflects a compliant vessel, and therefore a patient with a preload reserve.[42]

Conversely, if a marked increase in CVP is unable to dilate the vessel further, this reflects a poorly compliant vessel, and therefore a patient without any preload reserve.[13] TTE technology is now available in portable and hand-held devices. Right atrial (RA) pressure may be elevated with dampening of respiratory variations in IVC in patients with right ventricular (RV) failure or pulmonary hypertension due to left ventricular (LV) dysfunction or pulmonary thromboembolic disease.[42] In these situations, IVC size may be discordant with the RA pressure, and therefore not a reliable measure.

$Etco_2$ monitoring may be used as a surrogate for CO changes in response to fluid challenge in mechanically ventilated patients.[42] $Etco_2$ is determined by three factors: the production of CO_2 by cell metabolism, the pulmonary blood flow (i.e., CO) that drives CO_2 from the periphery to the lungs, and alveolar ventilation. Thus, if two of the three factors are constant (CO_2 production and alveolar ventilation), at least during a short period, changes in $Etco_2$ reflect changes in CO. Monge et al.[43] demonstrated that changes in $Etco_2$ correlated closely with changes in CO (as measured by the aortic blood flow velocity using an esophageal Doppler ultrasound) after a PLR fluid volume challenge maneuver in 35 mechanically ventilated critically ill patients with acute circulatory failure.

Recent technological advances in arterial waveform analysis have led to the widespread use of PPV monitoring systems to derive CO calculations. Pulse pressure (PP) arises because of the episodic nature of cardiac contraction and the properties of arterial circulation, which can be measured over time to derive a waveform; this information can then be used to calculate cardiac performance. The SV ejected into the aorta can be computed by measuring the associated increase in pressure. For instance, if the arterial compliance is 2 mL per 1 mm Hg pressure increment, then a pressure rise of 40 mm Hg would correspond to a SV of $40 \times 2 = 80$ mL.[44]

Current arterial PP monitoring systems include Lithium indicator Dilution Cardiac Output (LiDCO), Pulse indicator Continuous Cardiac Output (PiCCO), Flo-Trac, and MostCare. Most of them have been validated using comparisons to the gold standard CO thermodilution method. A peripheral arterial line is used for continuous PP monitoring; however, each system has its own limitations and should be interpreted in the context of the patient's clinical status, for example, spontaneous vs. mechanical ventilation, presence of cardiac arrhythmias, or depressed ventricular function. These proprietary systems have developed algorithms for obtaining CO as well as requirements for invasive line placement and calibration.[40] Although small-scale clinical trials using these monitors show promising data, large-scale multicenter trials in different patient populations and settings are needed to better determine how arterial waveform analysis can improve patient outcomes.[30]

Advances in imaging technologies have allowed clinicians direct visualization of microcirculation alterations, including vessel density and proportion of poorly perfused capillaries. Persistent microvascular alterations, especially in sepsis and in cardiogenic shock, are associated with organ failure and death. Poor skin and sublingual perfusion in septic patients have been identified as sensitive predictors of patient outcome, independent of systemic hemodynamic parameters. Currently, several techniques are available to assess tissue perfusion such as sidestream dark filed imaging (SDF) for sublingual microcirculatory perfusion and laser Doppler flowmetry (LDF) and reflective spectroscopy (RS) for perfusion and oxygenation of the skin. Low skin perfusion and oxygenation are associated with relatively low SV and CO in patients responding to fluid infusion. These noninvasive tissue perfusion and oxygenation techniques are not inferior to invasive hemodynamic measurements.[33]

For purposes of this discussion, it is assumed that the nurse understands proper techniques for deriving accurate hemodynamic measures. For more information, readers are referred to the American Association of Critical-Care Nurses Pulmonary Artery/Central Venous Presure Monitoring in Adults[2] at http://www.aacn.org/WD/Practice/Content/practicealerts.content?menu=Practice and to a textbook by M.E. Lough entitled *Hemodynamic Monitoring: Evolving Technologies and Clinical Practice.*[35]

IDENTIFYING AND INTERPRETING HEMODYNAMIC MEASURES

Direct and calculated hemodynamic measurements are physiologic indicators of preload, afterload, and contractility.[23,35] *Preload* is the blood volume in the ventricle that is to be ejected. It is delivered to the heart by veins. Any manipulation of vascular volume or venous return affects preload. *Afterload* is the resistance to moving the preload. It is primarily determined by arterial vascular tone. Any manipulation of arterial caliber affects afterload. *Contractility* is the cardiac muscle's strength that is used to move preload against afterload. It is a complex and difficult parameter to measure, as it is affected by both preload and afterload. Preload affects contractility via the Frank-Starling mechanism, with greater ventricular stretch resulting in greater cardiac contraction (Fig. 29.3). This effect is limited, however, and beyond a certain point, there is no increase in contractility, even with preload augmentation. Afterload can also impact contractility. With less resistance to flow (vasodilation), the myocardium ejects with less force. With greater resistance (vasoconstriction), the heart contracts with more force. However, if the heart has diminished muscle reserves, it will resort to tachycardia as a means of maintaining SV, CO, and BP.

Blood Pressure

BP measurement is commonly used to evaluate the adequacy of perfusion and overall cardiovascular function. The most accurate measurement of BP is made via functional arterial lines. In a hypoperfused state, the arterial line has become the gold standard, as opposed to noninvasive BP cuff instruments. With the move from mercury to aneroid devices, cuff BP may be more questionable, even in normal pressure ranges.[4,66]

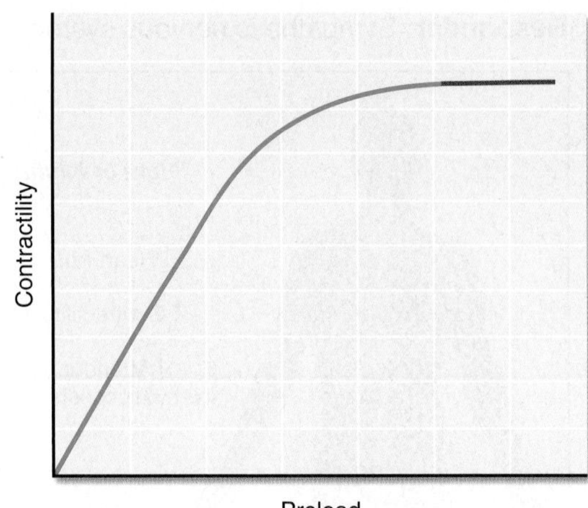

FIG. 29.3 Frank-Starling mechanism: the greater the stretch, the greater the force of contraction, but only up a certain extent.

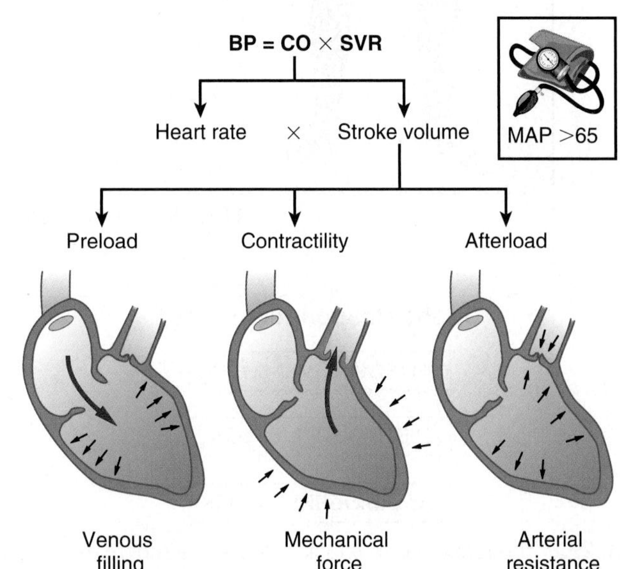

FIG. 29.4 Blood pressure is a function of cardiac output and systemic vascular resistance. *BP,* Blood pressure; *CO,* cardiac output; *MAP,* mean arterial pressure; *SVR,* systemic vascular resistance.

BP alone cannot assess perfusion. The level most commonly equated with adequate perfusion is a MAP of greater than 60 mm Hg (or a systolic pressure of > 90 mm Hg).[4,36] Symptomatic hypotension is one of the recognized precursors to cardiac arrest, and should be aggressively managed, as survival from arrest averages only 15% to 17%.[7] BP is the product of CO and systemic vascular resistance (SVR). CO primarily creates systolic pressure, and vascular resistance primarily determines diastolic pressure:

$$BP = CO \times SVR$$

CO is a product of HR and SV, the amount of blood ejected with each beat:

$$CO = HR \times SV$$

This formula is a function of preload, afterload, and contractility (Fig. 29.4).

TROUBLESHOOTING THE ETIOLOGY OF HYPOTENSION

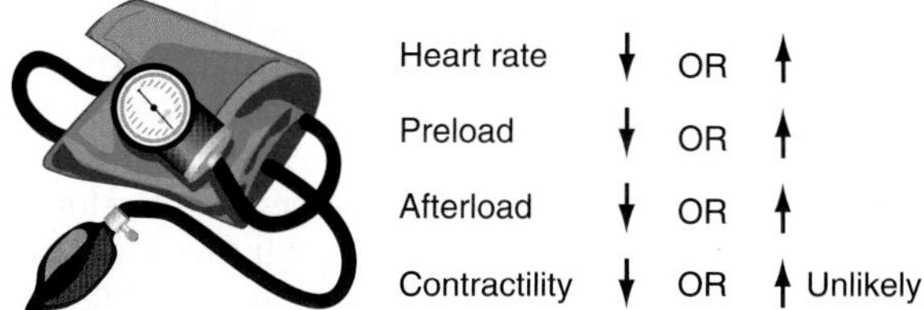

FIG. 29.5 Hypotensive states should not be oversimplified, because any of the parameters that contribute to blood pressure can be a factor in shock. In addition, both highs and lows can cause hemodynamic instability.

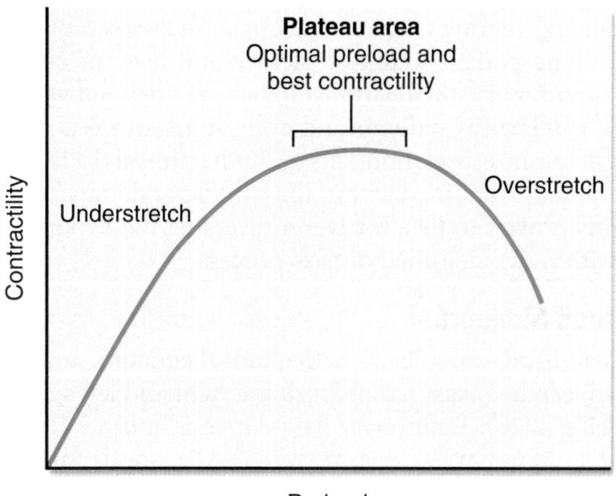

FIG. 29.6 The law of optimal stretch. This curve illustrates the limits of the Frank-Starling mechanism. Both understretching and overstretching of the ventricle can lead to a decrease in contractility and, therefore, a fall in blood pressure.

Any imbalance in HR, preload, afterload, or contractility can provoke hypoperfusion (Fig. 29.5). Likewise, regaining balance by addressing the cause and returning these parameters to their optimal levels can resolve hypoperfusion. For example, hypotension could be generated by either a high or a low HR. All patients have an optimal pace for achieving their best CO. Whether a patient experiences ventricular tachycardia at 160 beats/min or third-degree heart block at a rate of 30 beats/min, there can be hypotension and a decrease in perfusion.

As illustrated by the Frank-Starling curve in Fig. 29.6, myocardium that is either understretched or overstretched can lose contractility, resulting in a decline in pump function. Preload excesses can be systemic, as in hypervolemia, or isolated to the heart chamber alone, as in early pump failure. There is an optimal level of preload for maintaining the best hemodynamic balance. High preload gives the heart more volume to pump, and low preload forces the heart to pump faster to maintain BP. Both high and low preloads burden the heart with additional work and a higher oxygen demand.

In an effort to reduce cardiac workload, clinicians may want to decrease preload. However, the reflex tachycardia and vasoconstriction stimulated by an underfilled vascular system can sabotage this strategy. Although diuretics may lower BP, the patient's BP response to diuretics depends on the location on the Frank-Starling curve. When patients are hypovolemic (understretched) or even euvolemic (optimally stretched), diuretics may lower BP. However, if patients are hypervolemic or in heart failure (overstretched), diuretics may reduce ventricular volume, optimize stretch, maximize contractility, and even elevate BP.

Afterload also has variable effects on BP. In vasodilated states, BP is difficult to maintain, and perfusion declines. However, if arterial beds are constricted to improve BP, a critical point can be reached, beyond which the heart can no longer overcome resistance and fails to maintain CO. This is most likely to occur in patients with myocardial depression, and indicates the need for a vasodilator (such as nitroglycerin). Although vasodilators are appropriate for the treatment of hypertension, they also can be employed to reduce vascular tone and resistance to cardiac emptying. As with the other hemodynamic variables, there is an optimal level of afterload. An afterload that is too high or too low is detrimental to the maintenance of normal hemodynamics and effective tissue perfusion.

Contractility is low in hypotension and all states of hypoperfusion. For instance, in cardiogenic shock, contractility is diminished secondary to a direct myocardial insult. In hypovolemic shock, contractility is low as a consequence of poor stretch and inadequate stimulation of Frank-Starling mechanisms, all of which are reversed once preload is restored. In distributive shock, low contractility occurs as the result of vascular volume pooling in the periphery, as well as capillary leakage. In addition, distributive shock states lower afterload to levels that may inadequately stimulate the heart to respond with increased contractility. In the septic form of distributive shock, chemical mediators directly depress muscle function. Although rare, elevated contractility can also affect BP.

In summary, there are many factors that affect BP. Increased or decreased HR, preload, afterload, and contractility can all cause BP abnormalities. Identifying the problem is imperative to provide appropriate interventions.

Preload Measures

Preload can be assessed clinically by considering history, weight, intake and output, neck vein status, and other physical findings. In patients with heart failure, preload can be appraised by the level of B-type natriuretic peptide (BNP) in the blood. This neurohormone is secreted into the bloodstream by the ventricles when they are overly stretched. Serum levels greater than the normal upper limit of 100 pg/mL imply heart failure, but are only considered to be reliable in the absence of renal failure.[39] Preload can also be estimated invasively via central venous lines or the PAC. CVP is used as a measure of right ventricular preload, and PAOP as a measure of left ventricular preload. However, there are concerns related to these measures particularly PAOP, due to its indirect nature and reliance on the state of the pulmonary vascular bed for proper evaluation of the left heart. Pressure changes may not reflect volume changes alone, but also ventricular compliance and pleural and intraabdominal pressure (Fig. 29.7). Obtaining accurate CVP and PAOP data is dependent on precise bedside monitoring techniques.

The normal preload ranges may vary slightly depending on the reference source. Refer to Fig. 28.9 for the normal reference ranges for preload parameters (CVP and PAOP). Treatment decisions should be made based on data trends with clinical correlation, and not on one single reading. Interpretation of readings should be individualized so that therapy can be directed to the unique needs of each patient and the clinical pathway the clinician is trying to achieve.

Some experts in hemodynamics have dismissed pressure-based preload measures in favor of more sophisticated technologies. For example, the volumetric PAC can compute RV end-diastolic volume, which is a superior measure of preload.[6]

Secondary to the cardiac stiffening that is common in critical illness, CVP tends to reflect euvolemia in the typical critical care patient at higher than normal ranges. In the landmark study on early goal-directed therapy (EGDT) in severe sepsis conducted by Rivers and associates,[54] a CVP range of 8 to 12 mm Hg was used. With mechanical ventilation, RV compliance was found to be further diminished, and a CVP of 12 to 15 mm Hg was targeted. Using these CVP ranges for preload goals, a reduction in mortality of 34% was shown.[54]

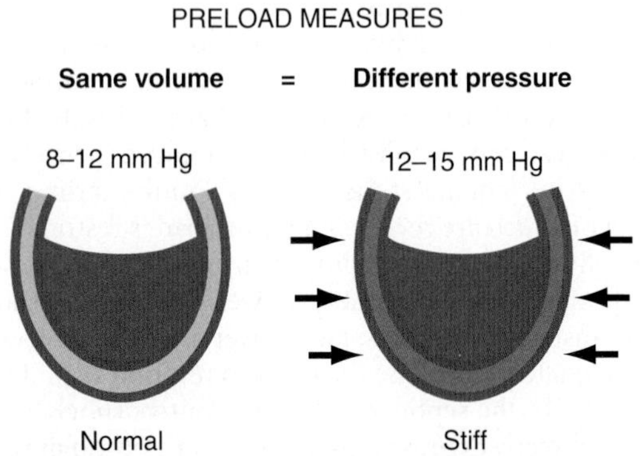

PRELOAD MEASURES

Same volume = Different pressure

8–12 mm Hg

12–15 mm Hg

Normal

Stiff

FIG. 29.7 Preload is a volume concept, yet it is traditionally measured as a pressure. Pressure does not equal volume; therefore, normal ranges for central venous pressure and pulmonary artery occlusion pressure do not apply to the critically ill.

Research has long shown that the majority of patients will develop pulmonary edema at PAOP levels of 18 mm Hg or more.[31,50] Therefore, the most accepted guideline for PAOP has been to maintain levels lower than this point. Young and previously healthy patients may do well at slightly lower PAOP levels, and older clients with myocardial ischemia or infarction may require somewhat higher levels. The best method for determining optimal preload may be to evaluate the response to fluid administration. Whenever a patient has symptomatic hypotension of uncertain pathology, fluid administration should be the first consideration. If a favorable response is observed, then fluid therapy should continue until an optimal response is sustained. Measures of a favorable response to fluid therapy beyond actual filling pressures include increasing BP, increasing CO, increasing urinary output (UO), decreasing HR, and normalizing venous saturation, along with an overall improvement in the patient's clinical picture and level of consciousness. In summary, the relationship between preload variables is complex in healthy patients and even more complex in disease states. Their interpretation and utility in clinical decision making should be examined within the context of therapeutic interventions proven to be effective in reversing the hypoperfusion state within the identified disease process.[22]

Afterload Measures

Afterload is measured by a mathematical equation and, as with preload, can be measured on both the right and left sides of the heart (Fig. 29.8). Pulmonary vascular resistance (PVR) closely parallels pulmonary artery pressure (PAP), and is thus of limited interest in most clinical situations. SVR is useful when accurately computed and coupled with clinical assessment.

SVR values higher than 1200 dynes imply vasoconstriction, and readings lower than 900 dynes imply vasodilation. Indexed

Afterload Measures

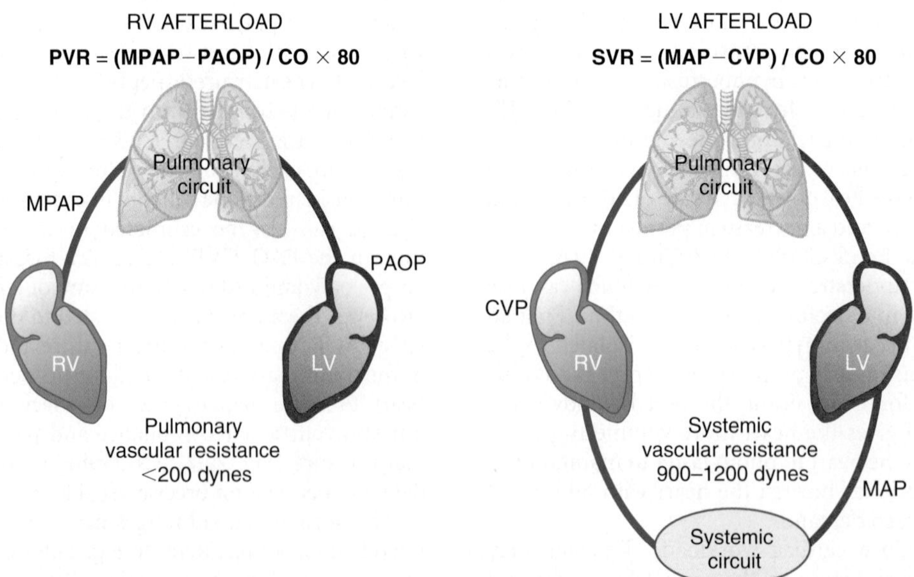

FIG. 29.8 Afterload measures for the right and left ventricles. The number 80 in the formulas is a constant that converts resistance into a unit of measure known as dynes. *CO,* Cardiac output; *CVP,* central venous pressure; *LV,* left ventricle; *MAP,* mean arterial pressure; *MPAP,* mean pulmonary artery pressure; *PAOP* pulmonary artery occlusion pressure; *PVR,* pulmonary vascular resistance; *RV,* right ventricle; *SVR,* systemic vascular resistance.

ranges of SVR (resistance divided by body surface area to correct for patient size), though more discriminating, are not widely used.

Because SVR is computed rather than directly measured, it may be dismissed from consideration of the hemodynamic profile. However, clinical findings for the evaluation of afterload are limited to skin characteristics alone, and tend to be subjective and unreliable. Hypovolemic and cardiogenic problems result in SNS- and RAAS-mediated vasoconstriction, causing patients to develop the classic cool and clammy appearance. Distributive shock, on the other hand, evokes vasodilation, and the skin is generally flushed, even warm, early in the physiologic process. Though imperfect, afterload computations can be an important safety check when using vasopressor agents for the treatment of hypotension. Vasoconstriction can improve BP, but if excessive, can decrease CO and organ perfusion, which is contradictory to the intent of the treatment.

Contractility Measures

Of all the variables affecting BP and hemodynamics, contractility is the most difficult to measure. As reviewed previously, contractility is affected by preload via the Frank-Starling curve. Although less emphasized, contractility is also influenced by afterload. When vessels constrict and afterload rises, normal hearts are stimulated to raise contractility to overcome resistance and maintain SV. Likewise, when vascular beds dilate and afterload declines, cardiac muscle is less stimulated, and contractility will decline. There are several measures used to evaluate contractility, but the most common is CO (Table 29.1). If a patient has a low CO, it may indicate actual myocardial depression (contractility). However, it may instead indicate inadequate myocardial stretch (low preload), excessive myocardial stretch (high preload), poor myocardial stimulation (low afterload), or excessive myocardial resistance (high afterload). Thus, measures of contractility are meaningful reflections of actual muscle function and the need for inotropic support only when preload, afterload, and even HR are in their optimal ranges (Fig. 29.9).

Measures other than CO are also equivocal. Stroke work index (SWI) may also be used to reflect cardiac strength, and as always, calculations are available to assess both right and left ventricular performance. Work relates to the mass moved, and assesses cardiac strength using a formula that computes how many grams of blood the heart moves with every beat to each squared meter of the body. A rise in SWI means that the heart is moving more blood, not that it is necessarily working harder. The measure would be better termed *stroke productivity index*, and should be viewed as a reflection of cardiac efficiency.

Despite being an imperfect measure of contractility, CO is still a useful criterion for assessing hemodynamics. Knowing how much blood the heart is pumping each minute does not explain the source of hypoperfusion, but only how critical the threat may be to the patient. Cardiac index (CI) is a measure of CO that corrects for body size, and is therefore helpful in setting a single normal range for patients of variable height and weight. Normal CI ranges are generally quoted as 2.5 to 3.5 L/min/m^2. Stroke volume index (SVI), a derivation of CI, is an even better parameter because it corrects for HR as well, typically averaging 40 to 50 mL/m^2 per beat. Still, SVI does not pinpoint contractility, but includes preload and afterload. When a patient is deemed to have adequate vascular volume (preload) and relatively normal vascular tone (afterload), then SVI can be utilized to guide inotropic therapy.

Overall Cardiovascular Performance and Perfusion Indicators

Of all the information gleaned from hemodynamic monitoring, the most meaningful is Svo_2. This value is derived from the pulmonary artery via the distal port of the PAC, and is used as a reflection of the balance between oxygen supply and demand. The normal range for Svo_2 is generally 70% to 80%, and indicates a stable oxygen balance. Neither a high nor a low Svo_2 is desirable; both imply oxygen imbalance and serve as a warning to clinicians to evaluate the patient. When the Svo_2 falls, it is secondary to either abatement of oxygen delivery or escalation of oxygen consumption. Likewise, when the Svo_2 rises, it is related to either escalation of oxygen delivery or abatement of oxygen consumption. Oxygen delivery is determined by three factors: arterial oxygen saturation (Sao_2)—the lung's ability to bring in oxygen; hemoglobin (Hgb)—the blood's ability to carry oxygen; and CO—the heart's ability to transport oxygen.

TABLE 29.1 Pulmonary Artery Catheter Measures Reflecting Contractility

Contractility Measures	Expected Ranges
Cardiac output	Different normal range for every body size Average 5–6 L/min
Cardiac index Controls for body size CO ÷ BSA	Average 2.5–3.5 L/min/m^2
Stroke volume index Controls for rate CI ÷ HR	Average 40–50 mL/m^2/beat
Ejection fraction Special equipment; not readily available	Average 50%–70%
Stroke work index A mathematical calculation; one each for the left and right ventricles:	
LVSWI = (MAP − PAOP) × SVI × 1000 × 0.0136	Average 40–80 g/m^2/beat
RVSWI = (MPAP − CVP) × SVI × 1000 × 0.0136	Average 7–12 g/m^2/beat

BSA, Body surface area; *CI*, cardiac index; *CO*, cardiac output; *CVP*, central venous pressure; *HR*, heart rate; *LVSWI*, left ventricular stroke work index; *MAP*, mean arterial pressure; *MPAP*, mean pulmonary artery pressure; *PAOP*, pulmonary artery occlusion pressure; *RVSWI*, right ventricular stroke work index.

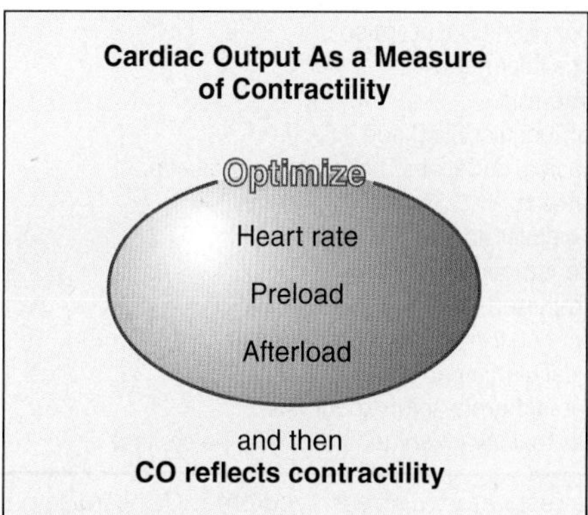

FIG. 29.9 Cardiac output (CO) can only be considered a measure of contractility when the other factors affecting it are in the optimal range.

Oxygen consumption is determined by cellular extraction (Box 29.4).

To troubleshoot a rise or fall in Svo_2, the three oxygen delivery factors (Sao_2, Hgb, and CO), along with oxygen consumption, must be considered. Unless there is an acute bleed, Hgb levels are stable in most critically ill patients. Likewise, unless there is a sudden temperature spike, seizure activity, or acute agitation, most patients have high, but stable, oxygen consumption. Thus, Sao_2 and CO are the remaining factors most likely to alter Svo_2. Sao_2 can be continuously measured via pulse oximetry (Spo_2) and rapidly ruled in or out as the cause of a change in Svo_2. If Sao_2, Hgb, and oxygen consumption are deemed stable, then Svo_2 becomes a reflection of CO. Thus, a fall in Svo_2 would be subsequent to a fall in CO. This may not appear to be a useful addition to the hemodynamic profile because it is already possible to measure CO *quantitatively*. However, Svo_2 monitoring is capable of assessing CO *qualitatively*, addressing the more important question of whether blood oxygen supply is adequate to meet cellular oxygen demands.

BOX 29.4 Clinical Conditions Associated with Changes in Venous Oxygen Saturation

Causes of Decreased Venous Saturation (Svo_2/$Scvo_2$)

Decreased oxygen delivery

Decreased oxygen saturation

- Decrease in inspired oxygen
- Respiratory diseases (pneumonia, pulmonary edema, COPD, ARDS)
- Pulmonary emboli
- Any alveolar ventilation or perfusion mismatch

Decreased hemoglobin

- Hemorrhage anemia (decreased erythropoietin, as in renal failure; B_{12} deficiency; decreased iron intake)
- Dysfunctional hemoglobin (sickle cell)

Decreased cardiac output

- Dysrhythmias
- Cardiogenic, hypovolemic, or vasogenic shock
- Obstructive states (tamponade, tension pneumothorax, pulmonary emboli)
- Excessive levels of PEEP

Increased oxygen consumption

- Increased activity (positioning, suctioning)
- Anxiety, pain, agitation, or restlessness
- High metabolic states (burns, trauma, fever, shivering)
- Hyperthermia

Causes of Increased Venous Saturation (Svo_2/$Scvo_2$)

Increased oxygen delivery

Increased Sao_2

- Supplemental oxygen therapy
- PEEP therapy
- Pulmonary disease resolution

Increased hemoglobin

- Blood transfusion
- Polycythemia (physiologic, as in COPD; pathologic)

Increased cardiac output

- Pacing therapy (HR)
- Fluid therapy (preload)
- Inotropic augmentation (contractility)
- Vasodilator therapy (afterload)

Decreased oxygen consumption

Decreased cellular need

- Hypothermia
- Neuromuscular blockade
- Analgesics, sedatives, anesthetic medications
- Antipyretics

Decreased cellular access

- Vasoconstriction
- Disseminated intravascular coagulation
- Microcirculatory inflammatory debris

Decreased cellular capability

- Cellular ischemia, injury, necrosis
- Cellular toxicity (cyanide, endotoxin, poisoning)

ARDS, Acute respiratory distress syndrome; *CO*, cardiac output; *COPD*, chronic obstructive pulmonary disease; *HR*, heart rate; *PEEP*, positive end-expiratory pressure; *Sao_2*, arterial oxygen saturation; *$Scvo_2$*, central venous oxygen saturation; *Svo_2*, mixed venous oxygen saturation.

If low Svo_2 implies low CO, then it would seem reasonable to assume that high Svo_2 implies high CO. However, a rise in Svo_2 is not often related to a rise in CO in the typical critical care patient. More likely, higher than normal Svo_2 readings are caused by an inability of cells to either access or extract oxygen. Limited cellular access to oxygen can be subsequent to excessive administration of vasopressors, disseminated intravascular coagulation (DIC), microcirculatory obstruction caused by inflammatory debris, and other shock-related pathologies. Cellular extraction defects can result from extended periods of hypoperfusion followed by tissue hypoxia. Svo_2 monitoring is the gold standard for evaluating cardiovascular performance and determining global perfusion. One advantage of using Svo_2 to guide therapy in shock is its reliability. The information it provides is not as dependent on proper technique as pressure transducer systems (CVP, PAP, and PAOP), making it more efficacious and less prone to human error.

Another site for sampling Svo_2 is from the vena cava. Measures can be taken intermittently or continuously using a specialized CVP catheter with oximetric capability.[8] Central venous oxygen saturation ($Scvo_2$) is generally approximately 10% higher than Svo_2 due to its location before the coronary sinus and the effect of venous admixture on Svo_2. Because of this, it is judicious to follow trends rather than individual values.[15] Although it is not a *mixed* venous specimen, $Scvo_2$-guided therapy may reduce mortality in hypoperfused septic patients.[8] The primary advantages of this catheter are the ease of insertion and the ability to collect data without traversing the heart. Newer catheters are available that can be inserted peripherally, which would avoid the complications of subclavian artery cannulation.

Regardless of how or where venous oxygen is measured, it reflects the final balance between oxygen delivery and uptake, which is the best appraisal of hemodynamic status. In order to recognize hypoperfusion, Svo_2/$Scvo_2$, blood lactate, and base deficit may be more meaningful than BP or Spo_2. Some have proposed using Svo_2 data as the cornerstone for directing therapy for all types of hypoperfusion states (Fig. 29.10).[50]

Putting It Together: Differentiating Hypoperfusion States

It is important to establish what is causing hypoperfusion so that therapy can be directed promptly and appropriately. Much of the hemodynamic information obtained in a hypoperfusion state will trend in the same direction. For example, all hypoperfusion states decrease BP and Svo_2. These measures do not distinguish between the source of the issue, but serve as a warning that perfusion is threatened. Hypovolemic shock and cardiogenic shock can be differentiated by preload analysis. Hypovolemic shock has low filling pressures (CVP and/or PAOP), reflecting depleted vascular volume, whereas cardiogenic shock has high filling pressures, indicating poor ventricular emptying. Both have low CO secondary to either a lack of preload (hypovolemic) or a lack of contractility (cardiogenic). In addition, both have SNS- and RAAS-mediated vasoconstriction and high SVR. Distributive shock has low filling pressures, but because of inappropriate vasodilation, the SVR is also low instead of high, as might be expected. In addition, CO may be elevated in distributive shock. In sepsis, the elevated CO is due to tachycardia, less resistance to flow (vasodilation), and shunting of blood from the microcirculation due to immune system cellular debris and DIC. In today's era of beta-blocker use, however, this pathognomonic finding may be less common with hypotension accompanied by a normal CO (Table 29.2).

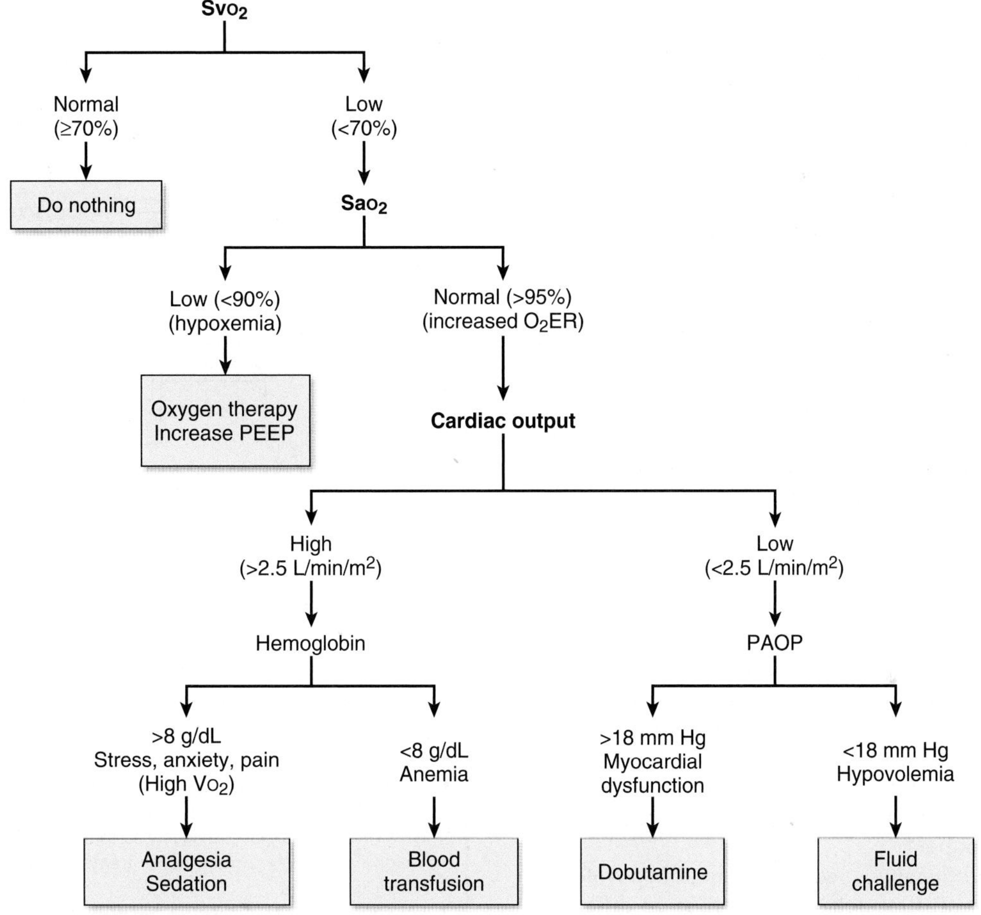

FIG. 29.10 Diagnostic and therapeutic algorithm based on mixed venous oxygen saturation. *O_2ER,* Oxygen extraction ratio; *PAOP,* pulmonary artery occlusion pressure; *PEEP,* positive end-expiratory pressure; *SaO_2,* arterial oxygen saturation; *SvO_2,* venous oxygen saturation; *VO_2,* oxygen consumption. (From Pinsky, M. R., & Vincent, J. L. (2005). Let us use the pulmonary artery catheter correctly and only when we need it. *Crit Care Med* 33(5), 1123-1124.)

TABLE 29.2 Hemodynamic Trends for Shock Differentiation

	Hypovolemic	LV Cardiogenic	RV Cardiogenic	Distributive
Blood pressure	↓	↓	↓	↓
Cardiac index	↓	↓	↓	↓↔
Central venous pressure	↓	↑↔	↑	↓
Pulmonary artery occlusion pressure	(↓)	(↑)	↑↔	↓
Systemic vascular resistance	↑	↑	↑	(↓)
Venous oxygen saturation	↑	↓	↓	↓

↑, Increased; ↓, decreased; ↔, no change; ◯, indicates most discriminating value for shock differentiation; *LV,* left ventricle; *RV,* right ventricle

SHOCK-SPECIFIC THERAPY

Traditional approaches to shock therapy include methodologies such as the titration of fluids and drugs to a target BP level. Pressure does not guarantee perfusion, and BP has not been shown to be a valid measure of hemodynamic adequacy. Successful reversal of cardiovascular collapse must focus on the cause and on improving cellular perfusion. A summary of the basic interventions for each of the shock states is given in Box 29.5.

Hypovolemic Shock

The treatment for hypovolemic shock is to replace preload. The type of replacement fluid used depends on what is lost. If the patient is hypovolemic secondary to hemorrhage, blood transfusion may be the fluid of choice. The best Hgb level for the critically ill is controversial, and has not been determined (see Chapter 26). For maximal oxygen-carrying capacity, a normal Hgb level seems desirable. To obtain the best cost-benefit ratio for patients, transfusions may be considered for Hgb levels lower than 7 to 8 g/dL. For patients with cardiopulmonary compromise, a Hgb of 9 g/dL might be the safest target. In patients with myocardial ischemia, anemia is poorly tolerated, and should be treated to maintain Hgb levels of greater than 11 g/dL.[57]

Severely injured patients experiencing hemorrhagic shock often require massive transfusion, defined as damage control resuscitation. The massive transfusion modality has been associated with improved outcomes.[25] In 2013, Holcomb et al. conducted the Pragmatic Randomized Optimal Platelet and Plasma Rations (PROPPR) trial to evaluate the effectiveness of transfusing patients with severe trauma and major bleeding using plasma, platelets, and red blood cells in a 1:1:1 ratio compared with a 1:1:2 ratio. The trial did not show significant differences in mortality at 24 hours or at 30 days between the two groups. More patients in the 1:1:1 group achieved hemostasis, and fewer experienced death due to exsanguination by 24 hours. Even though there was an increased use of plasma and platelets in the 1:1:1 group, no other safety differences were identified between the two groups.[24]

Intravenous fluid therapy is required to treat hypovolemia, regardless of the cause. Research shows there is no difference in outcome using crystalloids or colloids; therefore, normal saline (NS), lactated Ringer's (LR), albumin, and plasmanate are options for fluid resuscitation.[59] The challenge is not *what* to give, but *how much*. When there is a need for less volume, colloids can replace preload losses faster than crystalloids, but they cost more and have no mortality benefit. Some studies have shown a trend toward less inflammation, less incidence of renal failure in sepsis, and better myocyte function with albumin administration.[59] There is a trend toward a worse outcome in trauma with albumin, especially with brain injury. However, none of these findings are statistically significant.[59]

Hypertonic solutions like 3% or 5% sodium chloride and 25% (salt poor) albumin actually draw fluid from the cells and interstitial spaces to augment preload beyond what the solution itself could achieve. Because of this, hypertonic fluids may be of value when managing trauma patients with head injury.[62] When hypertonic solutions are used in place of NS, mannitol administration may not be necessary. Hypertonic sodium chloride solutions must be used with caution, especially in situations of normal intracranial pressure. Rapid elevation of serum sodium

BOX 29.5 Overview of Shock-Specific Strategies

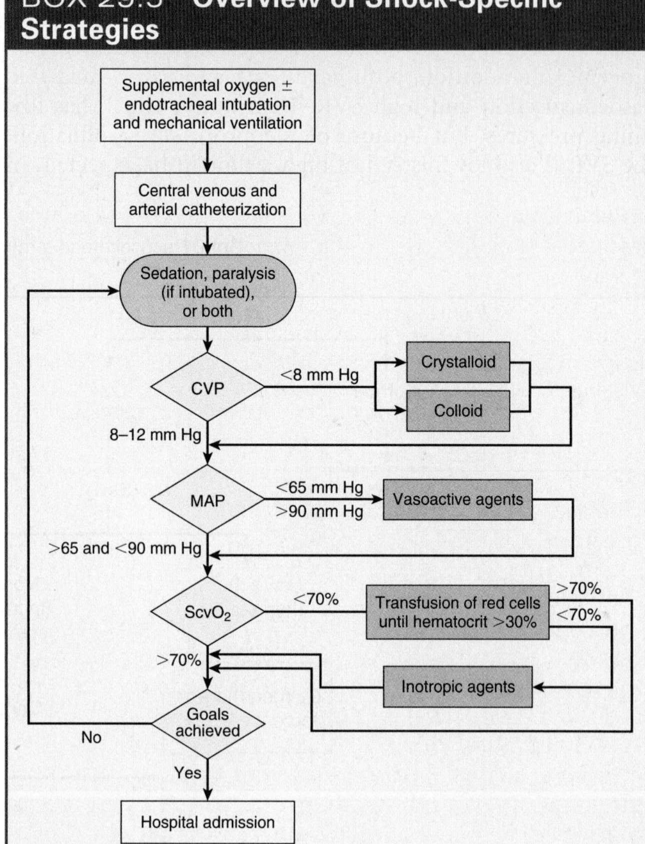

Hypovolemic Shock

- Locate and resolve source of fluid loss
- Fluid resuscitation: normal saline, albumin, or both to maintain PAOP 10–17 mm Hg
- Blood transfusion: as needed to maintain Hgb 7–9 g/dL

Distributive Shock

- Establish and address underlying cause
- Etiology-specific interventions (naloxone, airway support, antibiotics)
- Fluid resuscitation (as previously stated)
- Vasopressors to maintain MAP greater than 65 mm Hg and SVR 900–1200 dynes
- For sepsis: early goal-directed therapy

Cardiogenic Shock

- Emergent revascularization (for myocardial infarctions)
- Inotropes
- To maintain cardiac index greater than 2.2 L/min/m^2
- Intraaortic balloon counterpulsation
- Vasodilators
  To reduce preload and afterload if warranted
- Vasopressors
  For cardiogenic shock accompanied by inflammation (SVR <900 dynes)
  For right ventricular cardiogenic shock
- Fluid therapy for preload augmentation
- Pacer therapy for bradycardia
- Pulmonary vasodilators, if indicated

CVP, Central venous pressure; *Hgb,* hemoglobin; *MAP,* mean arterial pressure; *PAOP,* pulmonary artery occlusion pressure; *Scvo$_2$,* central venous oxygen saturation; *SVR,* systemic vascular resistance.

levels can result in cerebral dehydration, cellular shrinkage, and even herniation. It is important to monitor serum sodium levels and administer isotonic solutions with hypertonic sodium chloride so that fluid movement from the intracellular to extracellular space is moderated.

In some situations, vasopressor agents may be used to maintain BP until vascular volume is restored. However, excessive use of these drugs may enhance hydrostatic forces inside the vessel and push the infusing fluid into the interstitium *(third spacing)*. These patients are often thought to be refractory to therapy.[10] More fluid is administered, but using high-dose vasopressors for BP control thwarts any actual improvement in vascular volume. As a result, perfusion may never be reestablished. Measures for fluid resuscitation were also discussed in detail in Chapter 28.

Cardiogenic Shock

The heart plays a key role in hemodynamic stability and tissue oxygenation. Ventricular dysfunction is common, and if refractory to treatment, can also be lethal. The leading cause of cardiogenic shock is acute coronary syndrome (ACS) with myocardial infarction (MI), resulting in the loss of more than 40% of functional muscle.[5,26,31] Without adequate coronary flow, even powerful inotropes will be futile in improving hypotension. Therefore, the most effective treatment of pump shock is coronary artery reperfusion.[47] In 2013, a task force of the American College of Cardiology and the American Heart Association (ACC/AHA) gave a Class I recommendation to primary percutaneous coronary intervention or emergent coronary artery bypass grafting in patients with ST elevation MI (STEMI).[47] In addition, the SHOCK (*SH*ould we emergently revascularize *O*ccluded *C*oronaries in cardiogenic shoc*K*?) trial showed an absolute difference in survival of 13.2% in favor of early revascularization.[16] In the absence of aggressive treatment, mortality rates for cardiogenic shock are 70% to 80%.[34]

Evidence from the SHOCK trial also uncovered a previously unrecognized systemic inflammatory response during cardiogenic shock involving complement activation, nitric oxide (NO) release, and the evolution of inflammatory cytokines.[16] These findings imply that cardiogenic shock may be more than reduced ventricular performance. An inappropriate vasodilatory reaction may complicate the clinical picture. It may be useful to monitor SVR to identify this phenomenon so treatment can be directed appropriately.

Drug therapy for the support of patients in cardiogenic shock is generally necessary. Until definite therapy (coronary revascularization, mechanical support, or transplantation) is provided or the acute precipitation problem is resolved, temporary intravenous inotropic support is recommended to maintain perfusion and preserve end-organ function. However, long-term use of intermittent or continuous intravenous inotropes in patients with hypoperfusion due to end-stage heart disease are considered harmful in the absence of a specific indication or for reasons other than palliative care.[69]

Hypotension is addressed through the augmentation of contractility. Of all the available inotropic agents, dobutamine (Dobutrex) is probably tolerated best by patients with heart disease. Other inotropes may be more powerful and should be considered if the patient has profound hypotension and hypoperfusion. However, drugs such as norepinephrine (Levophed) or epinephrine cause vasoconstriction, as well as improved contractility. Vasoconstriction of veins and arteries increases preload and afterload and puts a greater burden on the failing ventricle. Although this strategy may improve the patient's BP, the increased ventricular workload does not improve long-term survival.

Vasodilators can pharmacologically achieve dilation of veins and arteries to unload the failing heart. They are effective in reducing preload and afterload, but require careful titration. In cardiogenic shock, a modest drop in SVR would likely improve CO with little or no change in BP. If needed, inotropes may be added to augment BP, but vasopressors should be avoided in noninflammatory cardiogenic shock.

In addition to pharmacologic support, myocardial ischemia should be corrected, and electrolyte, acid-base, and mechanical imbalances that can depress muscle function should be addressed. Emergency surgical repair may be warranted in the event of structural complications such as tamponade, acute valvular regurgitation, or septal defects.

Thus far in this discussion of cardiogenic shock, the focus has been on failure of the left side of the heart. Acute right-sided failure is common in patients with RV infarction. RV infarction complicates the clinical course in up to 50% of patients with inferior STEMI (and occasionally anterior wall STEMI). The RV is relatively resistant to infarction, and usually recovers even after occlusion. The term *RV infarction* is often regarded as a misnomer, because in most cases, acute RV ischemia dysfunction appears to represent predominantly viable myocardium. It is often due to proximal occlusion of the right coronary artery and is associated with higher risk of mortality. It is characteristic to see a clinical triad consisting of hypotension, clear lung fields, and elevated jugular venous pressure. RA ischemia would further exacerbate hemodynamic compromise. Patients with acute RV infarction are at increased risk for both high-grade AV block and bradycardia hypotension from LV preload deficit. Ventricular tachycardias may also develop either during the occlusion, abruptly after reperfusion, or later.[20]

RV infarction often escapes detection, and early recognition and diagnosis are imperative for preventing hypoperfusion and its complications. Transthoracic echocardiogram can be helpful in patients with initially nondiagnostic findings. The presence of a 1-mm ST elevation in lead V1 and in right precordial lead V4 R is the most sensitive electrocardiogram (ECG) marker of RV injury.[47] Right heart catheterization may reveal a disproportionate elevation of right-sided filling pressures compared to the left side, and include right atrial pressure (RAP) greater than 10 mm Hg, a RAP to PAOP ratio greater than 0.8, or a RAP within 5 mm Hg of the PAOP.[48] Cardiac magnetic resonance has been used recently to detect RV infarction in STEMI patients.[21]

The management of hypoperfusion in RV infarction is drastically different from that of the left ventricular MI. The treatment includes maintenance of RV preload, reduction of RV afterload, and immediate reperfusion. Hypotension may respond to volume resuscitation with caution against excessive volume loading. Restoration of physiologic rhythm and atrioventricular synchrony are also essential to sustain adequate CO. All these therapeutic options improve recovery of RV performance, stabilize the clinical course, and increase survival of patients with RV infarction.[27] Nitrates and diuretics should be avoided. However, when diagnosed and treated early, the RV is relatively resistant to infarction, and usually recovers, even after occlusion.[47]

Mechanical Circulatory Support in Cardiogenic Shock

The short-term goal in managing cardiogenic shock is to decrease the heart's workload to allow for cardiac recovery. In the past decade, advances in mechanical circulatory support (MCS) devices have emerged. Mechanical support from nondurable MCS is indicated as a first step or in conjunction with pharmacologic therapy in patients with refractory cardiogenic shock. Nondurable MCS devices are used as temporary support until more definitive therapies are employed, and they include the intraaortic balloon pump (IABP), extracorporeal membrane oxygenation (ECMO), surgically implanted extracorporeal devices, and percutaneous devices.

The IABP is commonly the first step in the treatment of cardiogenic shock. The IABP provides hemodynamic support by diastolic augmentation of aortic pressure, LV afterload reduction, and coronary perfusion enhancement. However, it may be insufficient in the setting of marked cardiac failure.[49]

ECMO is a nonpulsatile pump used to treat medically refractory cardiogenic shock when there is poor oxygenation, and can be a rapid option for emergency biventricular support. Major limitations are its lack of durability, limited availability, necessary perfusion support, and complications related to vascular access.[49]

Extracorporeal devices are implanted via a traditional sternotomy with an external pumping chamber and drive console. These include the Abiomed, Thoratec Paracorporeal Ventricular Assist Device II, and CentriMag. All of these systems are capable of generating flows up to 10 L/min under normal physiological conditions. The CentriMag may also be used to provide temporary RV support. Various mortality survival rates for each nondurable device are reported in the literature. Some centers use the CentriMag device for ECMO support, allowing rapid initiation of biventricular support.[49]

Percutaneous devices include TandemHeart and Impella. These devices can be placed in the cardiac catheterization laboratory and can generate flow rates of 2.5 to 5.0 L/min. They may also be used to temporarily support patients during high-risk percutaneous interventions, and are appealing in refractory cardiogenic shock because they have the potential to avoid the morbidity and mortality associated with surgical device placement.[49]

An increasing number of centers are using nondurable MCS as a means to achieve clinical stability before transfer to a specialized advanced heart failure center for more definitive therapy. Nondurable MCS are limited to short durations of support because of potential complications and the inability to mobilize patients. Considering the rapid evolution of these devices with concomitant improvements in efficacy and safety, it is recommended that the healthcare team be familiar with these devices to best serve the needs of the patient.[49]

Distributive Shock

Distributive shock has several widely varied etiologies, all of which result in an inappropriate loss of vessel tone, hypotension, and hypoperfusion. Some forms have a dual derangement, with vasodilation along with vessel leakage. Third spacing of vascular volume adds a hypovolemic component to the clinical picture, further complicating therapy. In either case, fluid resuscitation is appropriate, and guidelines are similar to those discussed under hypovolemic shock. In addition to refilling the expanded and potentially depleted vascular space, perfusion pressure is restored by reversing dilation with vasopressive agents. Many distributive shock states are transient and respond to therapies other than hemodynamic medications. Drug overdose, for example, may respond to naloxone (Narcan), and spinal shock may respond to the simple lapse of time and the body's assimilation of the loss of sympathetic innervation.

Sepsis is a common etiology of distributive shock, in which microorganisms in the bloodstream evoke widespread inflammation and trigger a cascade of cardiovascular insults, resulting in hemodynamic instability. In addition to vasodilation (distributive shock) and capillary leakage (hypovolemic shock), the toxins and mediators of sepsis can cause severe myocardial depression (cardiogenic shock). Thus, it is said that septic patients suffer from three forms of shock (Fig. 29.11). In February 2004, the Surviving Sepsis Campaign (SSC) was launched, releasing 45 therapeutic recommendations intended to reduce mortality from sepsis by 25% over a 5-year period.[11] A complete review of sepsis and the updated SSC 2012 can be found in Chapter 31; this section will review only the hemodynamic management of septic shock.[13] The most recent Surviving Sepsis Guidelines 2013 may also be downloaded from http://www.survivingsepsis.org/guidelines/Pages/default.aspx.

Several landmark studies and papers have been written in the past two decades addressing the cardiovascular support of septic patients.[54] In 2001, Rivers et al. published a breakthrough document describing a method termed EGDT.[54] In the past, goal-directed therapy had been tried, but there was little emphasis on intervening "early" and much focus on attaining "supranormal" levels of CO, all with inconclusive results.[31] However, Rivers' EGDT modality was found to decrease mortality by 34%,

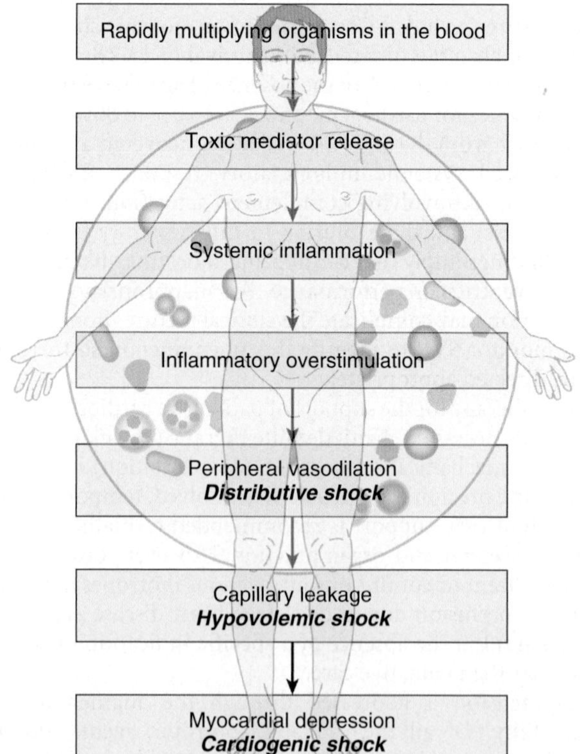

FIG. 29.11 Septic shock has a complicated pathophysiology. This diagram is only a reflection of the changes that lead to hemodynamic imbalance. As noted, the changes to the cardiovascular system give sepsis the characteristics of all three forms of shock.

decrease length of stay by 3.8 days, and decrease cost of care. The premise of the study was early identification (even before hemodynamic findings of shock were apparent) and aggressive intervention to predetermined measures of perfusion. Occult hypoperfusion was uncovered by examining lactate levels. Patients with lactate levels greater than or equal to 4 mmol/L were treated the same as patients with hypotension and overt shock. Once identified, rapid restoration of normal cardiovascular function was sought primarily through fluid resuscitation at volumes approximately 50% higher than standard therapy (i.e., 5 L of crystalloid or more). Dobutamine, packed red blood cells, and vasopressors (dopamine [Intropin], norepinephrine, and vasopressin [Pitressin]) were also used to maintain the following end points:

- UO ≥ 5 mL/kg/min
- MAP ≥ 65 mm Hg
- CVP 8 to 12 mm Hg (12–15 if on a mechanical ventilator)
- $Scvo_2 > 70\%$

Consequent to its success, EGDT was embraced by the SSC and the Institute of Healthcare Improvement and was included in the Sepsis Resuscitation Bundle recommendation (Box 29.6).[13]

As in hypovolemic shock, fluid resuscitation plays a key role in EGDT in septic shock to restore hemodynamic balance and maintain tissue perfusion. One of the challenges in fluid therapy is evaluating hemodynamic response and preload status, a concept currently referred to as *fluid responsiveness*. Fluid responsiveness is defined by a cardiac preload challenge with fluid infusion, resulting in augmented SV and CO.[12,67] When managing septic shock, it is difficult to determine the optimal level of preload. The key is to detect when fluid loading translates to an increase in SV and CO, while avoiding potential harmful effects of fluid infusion such as pulmonary edema. Thus, determining the appropriate volumetric markers of cardiac preload as predictors of fluid responsiveness remains challenging.

Another aspect of cardiovascular support in sepsis relates to the use of steroid therapy. Annanc et al. found that septic patients requiring vasopressive agents frequently suffered from relative adrenal insufficiency.[3] High-dose steroid therapy has been ineffective; however, this 2004 study evaluated 7 days of replacement-dose steroid therapy only, and demonstrated earlier weaning of vasopressors and a significantly lower risk of death.[3]

BOX 29.6 Surviving Sepsis Campaign Bundle

To Be Completed Within 3 Hours:

Measure lactate level
Obtain blood cultures prior to administration of antibiotics
Administer broad spectrum antibiotics
Administer 30 mL/kg crystalloid for hypotension or 4 mmol/L lactate

To Be Completed Within 6 Hours:

Apply vasopressors (for hypotension that does not respond to initial fluid resuscitation) to maintain a mean arterial pressure (MAP) ≥ 65 mm Hg
In the event of persistent arterial hypotension despite volume resuscitation (septic shock) or initial lactate at 4 mmol/L (36 mg/dL):

- Measure central venous pressure (CVP)*
- Measure central venous oxygen saturation ($Scvo_2$)*

Remeasure lactate if initial lactate was elevated*

*Targets for quantitative resuscitation included in the guidelines are CVP of ≥ 8 mm Hg, $Scvo_2$ of 70%, and normalization of lactate.[13]

TITRATABLE MEDICATIONS USED IN MANAGING SHOCK

This section reviews three medication categories used in the treatment of hemodynamic compromise: cardiac inotropes, vasopressors, and vasodilators. Several of these drugs have more than one mechanism of action, and are referred to as *inodilators* (combined inotropic and vasodilatory effects) or *inoconstrictors* (combined inotropic and vasoconstrictor effects). They are discussed under the heading that most describes their primary effect or clinical use. Many of the agents act on the SNS through the alpha- and beta-receptors (Fig. 29.12).

In discussing the uses of titratable drugs for shock, it is a prerequisite to recognize that there are no data definitively supporting the use of one cardiac inotrope or vasoactive agent over another.[66] In addition, because these drugs are generally titrated based on patient response, establishing dosage ranges is difficult. Titration implies infusing small increments until established goals or end points are reached. There is variation in what end points clinicians use. In addition, dosage ranges may vary in the literature and are often reported in mg/min, mcg/min, mcg/kg/min, and units/min. Most of these drugs have very short half-lives, and effects quickly subside when dosages are decreased or when the drug is stopped.

There is no absolute maximum dose for any of the commonly used agents (vasopressin is an exception, and is discussed later). As with most medications, every drug used for shock has positive (therapeutic) and negative (nontherapeutic) effects. These are outlined in Table 29.3. The most critical guides for titration

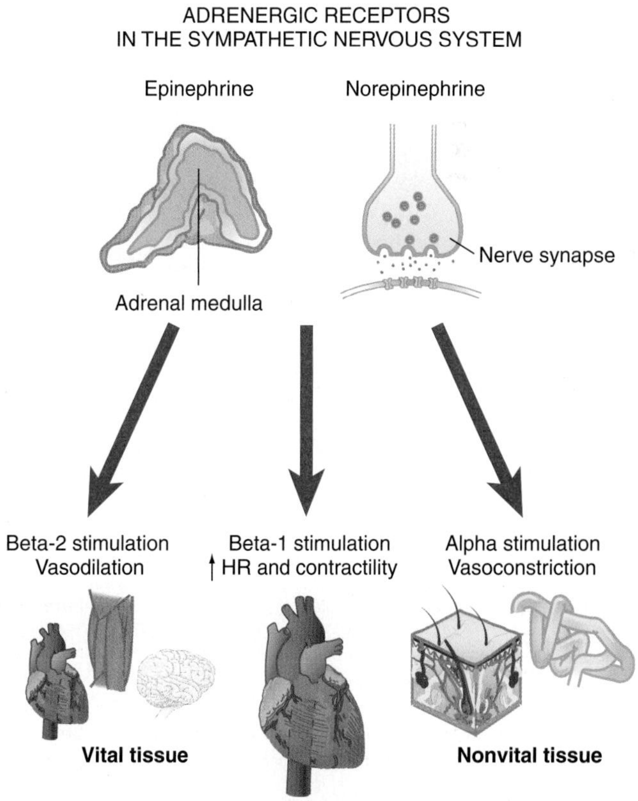

ADRENERGIC RECEPTORS IN THE SYMPATHETIC NERVOUS SYSTEM

Epinephrine — Norepinephrine

Adrenal medulla — Nerve synapse

Beta-2 stimulation Vasodilation | Beta-1 stimulation ↑ HR and contractility | Alpha stimulation Vasoconstriction

Vital tissue — Nonvital tissue

FIG. 29.12 The stress response involves release of chemicals from both the adrenal gland and the sympathetic nervous system. These chemicals act on adrenergic receptors at many body sites, including the heart and vasculature. *HR*, Heart rate.

TABLE 29.3 Action, Dosing, and Special Considerations For Commonly Used Cardiotonic And Vasoactive Drugs

Medication	Action	Dose	Special Considerations
Dobutamine (Dobutrex) *Inotrope*	Adrenergic stimulant. Beta-1 and beta-2 receptor effects. Used to improve contractility in cardiogenic shock. Effects on afterload insignificant due to mild vasodilation limited to vital organ vessels (heart, brain, skeletal muscle).	**Continuous infusion only.** Titrate for desired effect. 2.5–10 mcg/kg/min on average. Occasionally 20–40 mcg/kg/min for desired effect. Dosage at 5 mcg/kg/min has been shown to improve gastrointestinal tract perfusion in shock.	A first-line drug for pump failure, including failure following cardiac surgery. As with any inotrope, should not be used for the treatment of heart failure without signs of hypoperfusion. Increases stroke volume, cardiac index, and coronary artery perfusion. Decreases pulmonary artery occlusion pressure (preload). Generally, increases blood pressure, but may have little effect. May increase myocardial oxygen consumption, heart rate (especially with atrial fibrillation), and dysrhythmias, but less than other inotropes. May decrease blood pressure, especially with incomplete fluid resuscitation.
Dopamine (Intropin) Inotrope *(Vasopressor at higher dosages)*	Adrenergic stimulant. Used as first-line support of blood pressure in hypotension of uncertain etiology. Effects are dose dependent. *Low dose:* *dopaminergic receptor effects;* up to 5 mcg/kg/min, primarily dopaminergic receptors are activated, may increase renal and splanchnic blood flow. It may cause a decrease in vascular resistance and mild increase in cardiac output. *Moderate dose*: *beta-1 receptor effects;* increases stroke volume, cardiac index, and blood pressure; decreases pulmonary artery occlusion pressure; may be best range for cardiogenic shock states. *High dose*: *alpha-receptor effects;* increases systemic vascular resistance and blood pressure; may be best range for vasogenic shock states.	**Continuous infusion only.** Titrate for desired effect. *Low dose:* 2–5 mcg/kg/min *Moderate dose:* 5–10 mcg/kg/min *High dose*: 10–20 mcg/kg/min	Increases myocardial oxygen consumption, heart rate, and dysrhythmias. May decrease stroke volume, cardiac index, and organ perfusion (especially mesenteric perfusion) at high doses. Does not provide protection against renal failure and should be avoided, especially in the septic patient. In cardiogenic shock, vasoconstricting effects are undesirable and may increase preload and afterload and decrease cardiac output, aggravating pump dysfunction. May be administered concomitantly with low-dose vasodilators to support patients with poor pump function. May be difficult to wean due to depletion of norepinephrine stores in synaptic nerve endings with long-term use. Consider switching to norepinephrine at doses greater than 20 mcg/kg/min.
Esmolol (Brevibloc) *Negative inotrope*	Adrenergic blocker. Beta-1 effects. Slows heart rate primarily; decreases contractility and cardiac output. Used to decrease blood pressure. Used to slow supraventricular tachycardias and rapid ventricular rates in atrial fibrillation and atrial flutter.	**Intravenous infusion only.** Titrate for desired effect. Immediate-control dosing: 80 mg bolus (approximately 1 mg/kg) over 30 s followed by 150 mcg/kg/min infusion if needed; may titrate up to 300 mcg/kg/min. Gradual-control dosing: loading dose: 0.25–0.5 mg/kg/min bolus IV over 1–2 min followed by a continuous infusion of 50–200 mcg/kg/min.	Should be avoided in situations of inadequate cardiac output. Hypotension is greatest during the first 30 min of infusion. Rapid, short-term control of ventricular rate. May cause cardiac failure, cardiogenic shock, bradycardic rhythms, heart block greater than first degree, myocardial ischemia, bronchospasm, and glycemic imbalances. Shortest half-life of all beta-blockers.
Epinephrine (Adrenalin) *Inotrope vasopressor*	Adrenergic stimulant. Beta-1 and beta-2 receptor effects predominate at lower doses. Alpha receptor effects predominate at higher doses. Used to improve contractility associated with severe systolic dysfunction in cardiogenic shock. Used to improve vascular tone in vasogenic shock. May be best reserved for bolus therapy in cardiac arrest or anaphylaxis (beyond the scope of this table).	**Intravenous infusion only.** Titrate for desired effect. Beta-1 and beta-2 effects predominate at 0.01–0.05 mcg/kg/min. Beta-1 and alpha effects predominate at 0.05–2 mcg/kg/min. Pure alpha effects at dosages greater than 2 mcg/kg/min.	Powerful and indicated when other inotropes fail. Effects on heart rate may be beneficial with bradycardia. Reverses bronchoconstriction associated with anaphylactic reactions. Increases cardiac index, systemic vascular resistance, and blood pressure. Extreme increases in myocardial oxygen consumption, heart rate, and dysrhythmias possible. May decrease stroke volume, cardiac index, and organ perfusion at excessive doses. May cause cardiac ischemia. Best reserved for patients without coronary artery disease. Has been shown to increase mesenteric ischemia, serum lactate, and blood sugar.

TABLE 29.3 **Action, Dosing, and Special Considerations For Commonly Used Cardiotonic And Vasoactive Drugs—cont'd**

Medication	Action	Dose	Special Considerations
Labetalol (Normodyne) *Negative inotrope* *Vasodilator*	Adrenergic blocker. Alpha, beta-1, and beta-2 blockade; beta effects greater than alpha. Decreases heart rate, contractility, and systemic vascular resistance. Used to decrease blood pressure.	**Intravenous infusion only.** Titrate to effect. Intermittent boluses of 20–40 mg IV administered over 2 min, or as an infusion at 1–4 mg/min.	Longer-acting antihypertensive than esmolol. Helpful in the setting of acute aortic dissection to decrease blood pressure without reflexive increases in cardiac output and heart rate. May cause life-threatening hyperkalemia, especially in patients with renal failure. Use cautiously; may cause profound hypotension. May cause cardiac failure, cardiogenic shock, bradycardic rhythms, heart block greater than first degree, myocardial ischemia, bronchospasm, and glycemic imbalances. Possible myocardial depression when used in conjunction with halothane, isoflurane, and cyclopropane anesthesia.
Milrinone (Primacor) *Inodilator*	Phosphodiesterase inhibitor (nonadrenergic). Increases systolic contractility and diastolic relaxation. Dilates veins and arteries. Long duration of action; dosage changes only every 4–8 h. Optional bolus; maintenance 0.375–0.75 mcg/kg/min.	**Intravenous infusion only.** Relatively weak inotrope; inappropriate monotherapy for shock. Increases stroke volume and cardiac index. Decreases central venous pressure, pulmonary artery occlusion pressure, and systemic vascular resistance. Does not increase myocardial oxygen consumption. Effective with beta blockade and overdose.	May increase heart rate and dysrhythmias. Less arrhythmogenic than catecholamines. May decrease blood pressure, especially with hypovolemia. Not titratable; long half-life. May cause thrombocytopenia.
Nesiritide (Natrecor) *Vasodilator* *Natriuretic*	B-type natriuretic peptide (nonadrenergic). Dilates veins and arteries. Stimulates natriuresis and diuresis. Used to decrease preload and afterload in pump dysfunction.	**Continuous infusion only.** Optional bolus: 2 mcg/kg over 1 min. Maintenance dose: 0.01 mcg/kg/min. Do not exceed recommended dosage.	Neurohormonal modulator. Decreases central venous pressure, pulmonary artery occlusion pressure, and systemic vascular resistance. Increases stroke volume and cardiac index without increasing myocardial oxygen consumption. May decrease blood pressure and increase heart rate, especially with inadequate vascular volume. Discontinue infusion for 2 h before drawing a BNP level. 30-day mortality *may* be higher than in patients managed with other vasodilators and diuretic medications; further research required.
Nicardipine (Cardene) *Vasodilator*	Calcium channel blocker (nonadrenergic). Blocks calcium channels primarily in the vasculature to decrease systemic vascular resistance. May have slight negative inotropic effects. Used to decrease blood pressure.	**Intravenous infusion only.** 2.5 mg IV over 5 min (may repeat × 4), followed by an infusion at 2–4 mg/h.	Provides stable control of blood pressure without the negative inotropic effects of other calcium channel blockers. May be used to treat angina. May also be used at a low dose (0.25 mcg/kg/min) to prevent spasm in radial artery grafts. Reduce dose in hepatic dysfunction.
Nitroglycerin (Tridil) *Vasodilator*	Nitric oxide releaser (nonadrenergic). Dilates primarily veins. Dilates arteries at higher dosages. Used to decrease preload and afterload in pump failure and cardiogenic shock (small amounts). Used to decrease blood pressure in hypertensive states.	**Continuous infusion only.** Titrate for desired effect. Ranges vary greatly; 0.1–100 mcg/kg/min or 5–200 mcg/min (higher doses have been reported). Venous dilation at rates less than 50 mcg/min (1 mcg/kg/min).	Increases stroke volume and cardiac index. Decreases central venous pressure, pulmonary artery occlusion pressure, and systemic vascular resistance. Does not increase myocardial oxygen consumption. Effective coronary dilator. May decrease blood pressure and increase heart rate, especially with inadequate vascular volume or excessive dosage. Must be titrated slowly and in small increments for pump dysfunction, causing hypoperfusion. Less effective for the prevention of postoperative internal mammary artery vasospasm than diltiazem.

Continued

TABLE 29.3 Action, Dosing, and Special Considerations For Commonly Used Cardiotonic And Vasoactive Drugs—cont'd

Medication	Action	Dose	Special Considerations
Nitroprusside (Nipride) *Vasodilator*	Nitric oxide releaser (nonadrenergic). Dilates veins and arteries; balanced effect. Used to decrease blood pressure in hypertensive states. May be used to decrease preload and afterload in pump failure and cardiogenic shock (small amounts).	**Continuous infusion only.** Titrate to desired effects. Initiate slowly, 0.1–8 mcg/kg/min.	Increases stroke volume and cardiac index. Decreases central venous pressure, pulmonary artery occlusion pressure, and systemic vascular resistance. Does not increase myocardial oxygen consumption. Better afterload reducer than nitroglycerin. May cause undesirable decrease in blood pressure and increase in heart rate, especially with inadequate vascular volume or excessive dosage. Must be titrated slowly and in small increments for pump dysfunction, causing hypoperfusion. May cause coronary steal and cardiac ischemia. Inhibits hypoxic vasoconstriction and may reverse pulmonary autoregulation and decrease Pao_2 levels. Can cause methemoglobinemia, thiocyanate production, and cyanide toxicity, especially with high doses and/or prolonged therapy. Must not be used in patients with liver failure or renal failure (unless the patient is being dialyzed).
Norepinephrine *(Levophed)* *Vasopressor* *(Inotrope at lower dosages)*	Adrenergic stimulant. Alpha and beta-1 receptor effects. Used to improve contractility associated with severe systolic dysfunction in cardiogenic shock. Used to improve vascular tone in vasogenic shock, especially sepsis.	**Continuous infusion only.** Titrate to desired effects. Mean dosage range: 0.2–1.3 mcg/kg/min. Maximum dosage: 3.3 mcg/kg/min.	More potent than dopamine. Increases systemic vascular resistance and blood pressure. Increases stroke volume and cardiac index at low doses only. In cardiogenic shock, vasoconstricting effects may increase preload and afterload, decrease cardiac output, and aggravate pump dysfunction. Should be administered concomitantly with vasodilators in patients with poor pump function to counteract the negative effects of vasoconstriction on cardiac output. Increases myocardial oxygen consumption, heart rate, and dysrhythmias. May decrease stroke volume, cardiac index, and organ perfusion at excessive dosages (alpha effect). Associated with improved survival in patients with septic shock.
Phenylephrine (Neo-Synephrine) *Vasopressor*	Adrenergic stimulant. Alpha receptor effects only. Used to increase vascular tone and blood pressure in vasogenic forms of shock.	**Continuous infusion only.** Titrated to desired effect. Optional bolus dosing possible with severe hypotension: 2–5 mg. Infusion doses: average 40–60 mcg/min, and can be as high as 180 mcg/min.	Increases systemic vascular resistance and blood pressure. Ideal in vasogenic shock states involving vasodilation only, such as spinal shock, spinal anesthesia, dilating drug overdose, and neurogenic shock. May decrease stroke volume, cardiac index, and organ perfusion at high doses. Generally, does not increase heart rate. High doses can cause excessive vasoconstriction and a reflexive bradycardia.
Vasopressin (Pitressin) *Vasopressor*	Antidiuretic hormone (nonadrenergic). Stimulates V1 receptors. Used to increase vascular tone and blood pressure in vasogenic forms of shock when other vasopressors have failed. May be best reserved for bolus therapy in cardiac arrest (beyond the scope of this table).	**Intravenous infusion only.** Titrate only within specific parameters. Dosage safest at 0.01–0.04 unit/min. Do not exceed stated dosage ranges.	May decrease stroke volume, cardiac index, and perfusion to nonvital organs, especially the mesentery. Increases systemic vascular resistance and blood pressure. May be helpful in catecholamine-resistant shock, and should be used primarily as salvage therapy. Should never be used as monotherapy for blood pressure control, but instead as a companion drug to catecholamines. May be most efficacious in treating the hypotension seen with sepsis and cardiopulmonary bypass, due to hormone deficiency and a replacement effect. May be helpful in improving blood pressure in patients with massive blood loss until blood can be replaced. Incompletely studied except in cardiac arrest. Important to monitor for hyponatremia (water retention) and correct as needed. Use with caution; do not exceed dosage maximum.

BNP, B-type natriuretic peptide; *IV*, intravenous; *Pao_2*, partial pressure of arterial oxygen.
From Reference 13.

of cardiotonic and vasoactive drugs are an understanding of hemodynamics, an appreciation of cellular oxygenation, and a determination to use them to obtain the best cost-benefit ratio for the patient.

Inotropic Agents

Intravenous inotropes amplify the contractile force of the heart, and are indicated for the support of pump failure that is causing hypoperfusion. All inotropes increase the influx of calcium into cardiac muscle cells to aid in myofibril shortening. One mechanism for augmenting calcium influx is to increase levels of cyclic adenosine monophosphate (cAMP), a molecule often referred to as the *second messenger*, which regulates many cellular processes. Catecholamine drugs mimic SNS effects and increase contractility by increasing the production of cAMP. Pure beta-stimulating drugs include isoproterenol (Isuprel) and dobutamine. Although dopamine, norepinephrine, and epinephrine are beta-stimulating, they also have alpha effects and are generally thought of as *inoconstrictors*. Another mechanism for increasing cAMP to improve calcium influx and contractility is by blocking its enzymatic degradation by phosphodiesterase. Phosphodiesterase inhibitors (PDIs) are noncatecholamine drugs used for inotropic support.

Dobutamine

Dobutamine is a common choice for treating cardiac dysfunction. Because it lacks vasoconstrictive effects, it is thought to cause a smaller increase in the workload of the heart than most other inotropic agents. When compared with isoproterenol, a similar but older drug with pure beta-stimulating effects, it causes less of an increase in mixed venous oxygen saturation (Mvo_2). Dobutamine has balanced beta-1 and beta-2 effects that improve not only contractility, but also coronary artery perfusion. Because it lacks vasopressor effects, some clinicians will consider initiating dobutamine only when systolic BP is greater than 80 mm Hg. Owing to its dromotropic effects (affecting conduction speed), patients with atrial fibrillation may need rate or rhythm control prior to initiating dobutamine to avoid rapid ventricular response. Dosages for dobutamine usually range from 2.5 to 10 mcg/kg/min, but can range up to 20 mcg/kg/min. In rare circumstances, rates up to 40 mcg/kg/min have been required to reach the desired effect. Besides its use in cardiogenic shock, dobutamine is indicated in septic patients when CO measures indicate pump dysfunction.[54] Infusion of dobutamine at a rate of 5 mcg/kg/min has also been reported to improve gastrointestinal perfusion in patients with septic shock.[12]

In chronic heart failure (HF), beta-1 receptors are less prevalent and less sensitive to stimulation (downregulation), causing the myocardium to become beta-2–dependent. Thus, HF patients may respond better to dobutamine than other inotropes because of its beta-2 effect. There is much confusion surrounding the vasodilatory effects of dobutamine, with some considering it an inodilator. However, the vasodilatory effects of dobutamine are mild and primarily limited to vital tissue vessels (beta-2), a relatively small portion of the overall vascular bed. If vasodilation is a prominent effect, as in sepsis, dobutamine is not recommended. Dobutamine may best be considered an inotrope that favors vital organ perfusion. Most of the afterload-lowering effects of dobutamine can be attributed to improvements in CO, leading to a reflexive decline in sympathetic tone, rather than direct vasodilation. Dobutamine's mild vasodilatory effects can decrease BP if volume is not optimized prior to initiation. If dobutamine initiation results in a drop in BP, an evaluation of volume status or fluid challenge should be considered. Like gravitational forces (orthostatic/postural hypotension) and increased intrathoracic pressures (ventilator-induced hypotension), mild vasodilation can have a detrimental effect on BP, even in the presence of borderline hypovolemia.

Dopamine

Dopamine is a beta-1, alpha, and dopaminergic stimulant, depending on dosage being delivered. Low-dose infusions have been used to improve renal and mesenteric perfusion. It was previously believed that dopaminergic levels of dopamine would help prevent renal failure and mesenteric ischemia. A landmark meta-analysis performed by Kellum et al. virtually dispelled this belief.[29] Besides not helping with perfusion of nonvital organs, some studies have indicated that dopamine may even have detrimental effects, especially in septic patients. The SSC does not support the use of dopamine in low doses for septic patients.[13]

Despite these challenges, dopamine is a versatile drug that can be used as an inotrope, an inoconstrictor, or a vasopressor, depending on the clinical situation. Myocardial depression responds best to ranges between 5 and 10 mcg/kg/min, which augments contractility. Sepsis, involving both vasodilation and pump dysfunction, might be treated best at levels from 10 to 20 mcg/kg/min, which augments contractility and afterload. With primary vasodilatory states causing hypotension, levels at 20 mcg/kg/min or higher may be considered, to augment afterload. Dopamine is more dysrhythmogenic than dobutamine. Although it may increase HR as one of its expected effects, tachycardia at low dosages warrants an assessment of fluid status. Hypovolemic states can exaggerate HR responses with virtually any inotropic agent.

Because of its varying and dosage-dependent effects, dopamine should be used cautiously. This is especially true with cardiogenic shock patients. Hypotension resulting from myocardial depression benefits most from inotropic levels of dopamine (5–10 mcg/kg/min). Beyond this range, or even at doses of less than 10 mcg/kg/min in some patients, tachycardia and vasoconstriction (alpha effects) can occur, placing a further burden on the already failing heart. In situations such as this, it is important to consider alternative drugs, such as dobutamine.

Dopamine's effects on the cardiovascular system are both direct and indirect. The indirect effects come from its ability to trigger the release of norepinephrine at nerve endings. Thus, when synaptic stores of norepinephrine are depleted, dopamine's effectiveness is attenuated. The time frame for depletion is variable, but is generally seen after approximately 48 hours of continual use, and should be recognized as a characteristic of the drug and not deterioration of the patient. This same norepinephrine depletion can cause difficulty during weaning off the drug. Some patients become dependent on small amounts to maintain normal cardiovascular function, secondary to the lack of synaptic norepinephrine. Patients on as little as 0.5 mcg/kg/min have been known to decompensate into hypotension with drug termination. In these situations, it can be helpful to switch hemodynamic support to a low-dose norepinephrine infusion. This allows the synaptic granules to rebuild their stores of norepinephrine so that drug therapy can be successfully discontinued.

Epinephrine

Epinephrine is a beta-1, beta-2, and alpha stimulant, and is the most potent inoconstrictor available. Like dopamine, its actions are dose dependent. At 0.01 to 0.05 mcg/kg/min, it is mostly a beta-1 and beta-2 stimulant. At 0.05 to 2 mcg/kg/min, beta-1 and alpha receptors are activated, with more alpha effects as dosages increase. At dosages greater than 2 mcg/kg/min, epinephrine is strictly an alpha adrenergic stimulant. Appropriate uses for epinephrine include the reversal of laryngospasm and vasodilation in anaphylaxis, management of refractory bronchospastic asthma, and treatment of refractory bradycardia, as well as a general cardiovascular stimulant in arrest states.[61] Although it has never been shown to be better than placebo for cardiac arrest, epinephrine continues to be the first choice, despite recommendations for vasopressin.[68] Most of the data available on epinephrine use are from animal studies. It has been shown to elevate serum lactate concentrations, induce myocardial ischemia, lower mesenteric and renal circulation, and induce hyperglycemia and hypokalemia.[14] Epinephrine is highly dysrhythmogenic, but is generally safe for use in children and in heart transplant patients because of normal coronary circulation and the lack of ischemic substrate. Epinephrine administration triggers sensations of anxiety and fear in most patients, requiring frequent reassurance and appropriate sedation. Most experts agree that, because of its potency and potential toxicity, epinephrine should be reserved for situations in which other agents have failed to improve hemodynamics.

Despite abundant precautions regarding epinephrine use, it remains a favorite in cardiovascular surgery settings. Postoperative hypotension is common following cardiac surgery, and its etiologies are varied. A thorough assessment is required to identify the source of hemodynamic compromise so therapy may be properly directed. The most prevalent cause of any postoperative hypotension is hypovolemia, which is particularly common with surgeries requiring cardiopulmonary bypass (CPB). Postoperative vasoconstriction can contribute to poor CO and a fall in BP. Another cause of hypotension following CPB is an inflammatory response compounded by the vasodilatory effects of certain anesthetic agents. This distributive form of shock accounts for less than 10% of postoperative hypotension, and may be the only type requiring the vasopressor support that epinephrine supplies.

A review of the literature conducted by Gillies et al. reported that the best-studied beta agonist with the most favorable cost-benefit ratio is dobutamine.[19] Milrinone was found to enhance the likelihood of successful weaning from CPB support, magnify flow through arterial grafts, reduce mean pulmonary artery pressure, and improve right heart performance in pulmonary hypertension.[19]

Milrinone

Milrinone (Primacor) belongs to a unique class of inotropes known as bipyridines, and has both inotropic and vasodilatory effects. Its ability to reduce preload and afterload allows it to stimulate contractility without increasing myocardial oxygen demands. Its mechanism of action is phosphodiesterase inhibition. Phosphodiesterase induces the breakdown of cAMP, which in turn reduces calcium uptake. By inhibiting this enzyme, cAMP is retained in greater concentrations, and more calcium is available to enhance contractility. The fact that milrinone works outside the realm of the SNS affords certain advantages in the treatment of heart failure. With the widespread use of beta-blocking agents, beta stimulants may not be as effective, secondary to diminished receptor availability. The ability of milrinone to improve contractility without accessing beta receptors is most advantageous in situations of beta-blocker overdose. Milrinone improves systolic function, as well as diastolic relaxation, a plus for patients with lusitropic (myocardial relaxation) disturbances.

Despite the benefits of milrinone, it is a comparatively weak inotrope, and is rarely effective with hypotensive cardiac failure when administered alone. Coupling milrinone with a more powerful beta stimulant, such as dobutamine, can have a synergistic effect by promoting inotropy on two levels. In addition, preload and afterload reduction can profoundly improve CO despite only modest improvements in BP. Milrinone is a far more potent vasodilator than dobutamine, and cannot be expected to increase BP as much as it can improve hemodynamics and perfusion. The combination of inotropic and vasodilatory effects seen with milrinone generated interest in its use to "tune up" the myocardium of chronic heart failure patients in acute decompensation. The Outcomes of a Prospective Trial of Intravenous Milrinone for Exacerbations of Chronic Heart Failure (OPTIME-CHF) study, however, did not support this strategy, showing no decrease in length of stay and an increase in adverse events (mostly dysrhythmias).[17] Thus, the use of chronic IV inotropic therapy, either as a continuous or intermittent infusion in patients with heart failure, remains controversial. There does not appear to be any significant difference in outcome between dobutamine and milrinone in the treatment of these patients, but milrinone does have a significantly higher cost.[69]

The pharmacokinetics of milrinone are different from those of other drugs used for hemodynamic support in hypoperfusion states. It is slower in reaching therapeutic levels, and it has a long half-life, especially in patients with liver and renal insufficiency. Dosing involves an optional bolus of 50 mcg/kg over 10 minutes followed by a maintenance infusion of 0.375 to 0.75 mcg/kg/min. Because of its prolonged effect, dosage adjustments are generally made only every 4 to 8 hours. Therefore, milrinone is best used as a companion drug in the setting of cardiogenic hypotension, with more potent and titratable inotropes used as primary agents. Milrinone can also propagate thrombocytopenia. Therefore, platelet levels should be monitored, and milrinone should be used cautiously with other platelet-lowering medications such as H_2 antagonists and heparin.

Vasopressor Agents

Vasopressor agents constrict vascular beds, increasing both preload and afterload. Vasoconstriction as a treatment for hypotension is best reserved for the reversal of a widespread loss of vascular tone, such as is seen in distributive shock. However, because vasopressors are so reliable in raising BP, they are a common first choice in any hypotensive crisis. Recall that shock is not poor pressure but poor perfusion, and raising BP is not the same as resolving shock. BP is dependent on heart function and vascular tone ($BP = CO \times SVR$). One can either augment CO or increase SVR to improve BP. Increasing SVR is a reliable and relatively easy way to improve BP. Increasing CO is more challenging, more time-consuming, and not as dependable. It is easy to understand why vasopressors are widely used in shock.

Vasopressors have several harmful effects. By increasing SVR, they may create enough afterload to decrease CO and even induce pump failure. In addition, excessive vasoconstriction can intensify hydrostatic pressure and force fluid out of the vessels, creating a relative hypovolemia. Vasopressors can also divert blood flow from enough organ beds to further aggravate cellular hypoxia and perpetuate shock. In short, the misuse of vasopressor drugs can promote cardiogenic shock, hypovolemic shock, and even the multiple organ failure seen in distributive shock (sepsis). At best, vasopressors can dramatically improve perfusion pressure to the body. At worse, they can be as bad as the underlying hypoperfusion they were meant to correct. Vasopressor overuse can mimic the effects of critical illness and organ failure, allowing their negative side effects to be attributed to the underlying disease instead of being recognized as a possible adverse drug event.

Norepinephrine

Norepinephrine is a natural catecholamine with both beta-1 and alpha-stimulating effects. It is a powerful inoconstrictor, and like dopamine, the higher the dose, the greater the vascular effects. Because of the wide variability in vasopressor use, average doses of norepinephrine are difficult to confirm. Mean dosages range from 0.2 to 1.3 mcg/kg/min, with a maximum dosage of 3.3 mcg/kg/min.

Norepinephrine is recommended in the treatment of sepsis-induced hypoperfusion to reverse abnormal vasodilation and maintain perfusion pressure when fluid resuscitation is insufficient. Septic patients with poor CO may require dobutamine along with norepinephrine to treat their cardiovascular collapse. This combination can be advantageous for many reasons. Data support the use of dobutamine for the improvement of mesenteric perfusion, a potential threat in septic patients.[12] In addition, its weak beta-2 vasodilation effects may temper some of the alpha vasoconstriction effects of norepinephrine to better support perfusion.

Norepinephrine also can be used to manage cardiogenic shock. It is a more potent beta stimulant than dobutamine or dopamine, and is possibly safer than epinephrine. However, when administered as monotherapy and titrated to BP in this type of shock, norepinephrine can be harmful, because its vasoconstricting effects can stress the LV. Vasoconstriction increases both preload and afterload, which could be detrimental, unless there is evidence of vasodilation. Vasodilation may be present with severe pump failure due to inflammation, or in late-stage shock due to acidosis. In cardiogenic shock, BP improvement is seen with norepinephrine, but it is generally transient, because vasoconstriction can decrease CO. To use this drug optimally in cardiogenic shock, it is best to couple it with a vasodilator such as nitroglycerin or nitroprusside to isolate the desired beta effects and reduce the undesired alpha response. It also can be used with milrinone. By stimulating inotropy through both beta stimulation and phosphodiesterase inhibition, this combination may be especially beneficial to patients on beta-blockers and those with a diastolic component to their ventricular failure.

Phenylephrine

Phenylephrine (Neo-Synephrine) is a pure alpha stimulant and has no direct effect on the heart. Therefore, it is used in hypotensive situations that do not require cardiac stimulation. Because phenylephrine does not affect beta receptors, less tachycardia and dysrhythmia is seen with its use than with other vasoactive agents. It is used effectively following spinal or epidural blocks, which cause widespread vasodilation. Drug overdose and drug hypersensitivity causing vasodilation and hypotension respond well to phenylephrine. For severe hypotension, a bolus of 2–5 mg can be attempted. Continuous infusion rates average 40–60 mcg/min, but can be as high as 100–180 mcg/min when rapid BP improvement is vital. Bradycardia is a side effect of any vasopressive agent, but most commonly with phenylephrine. Because of its lack of beta effects, phenylephrine's unopposed alpha constriction can stimulate a reflexive slowing of the heart by cardiopulmonary centers in the brain in an attempt to prevent excessive BP. This reflex reaction was employed for the treatment of supraventricular tachycardia before the beta-blocker propranolol (Inderal) became available.

Vasopressin

Vasopressin is an endogenous chemical known more commonly as antidiuretic hormone (ADH). It is produced by the hypothalamus and stored and secreted by the posterior pituitary gland in response to reduced plasma volume or increased serum sodium concentration. Physiologically, the role of vasopressin is to regulate daily fluid balance by promoting the retention of free water. During hypotensive states, however, vasopressin serum levels rise to levels similar to epinephrine, cortisol, and other stress hormones. It is believed to be an influential vasoconstrictor mechanism in shock states. The pressor actions of vasopressin are complex and incompletely understood. It is distinctively different from other vascular constrictors, however, because it does not affect adrenergic receptors. Specialized arterial smooth muscle receptor sites for vasopressin are termed V1 receptors.[41,56] Three situations are associated with inadequate endogenous levels of vasopressin: massive hemorrhage, severe sepsis, and cardiopulmonary bypass.[41,56] The development of this relative vasopressin deficiency is poorly understood, but may be related to exhaustion of secretory stores following prolonged stimulation or impaired autonomic function with depressed baroreceptor-mediated release.[52]

Early research on vasopressin suggested beneficial effects and possible superior efficacy to epinephrine in the treatment of refractory ventricular fibrillation, pulseless ventricular tachycardia, and asystole.[41,68] This led to the addition of vasopressin to standard dose epinephrine in subsequent advanced cardiac life support (ACLS) protocols. However, a 2012 meta-analysis and review of randomized controlled trials on vasopressin in the setting of cardiac arrest showed that efficacy of the two drugs is similar, and that there is no demonstrable benefit from administering both epinephrine and vasopressin as compared with epinephrine alone.[41] This finding is reflected in the changes to the 2015 ACLS algorithms.[46]

Vasopressin's clinical use has expanded to the treatment of hypotension of any etiology in the critical care setting, particularly in postcardiac surgery patients and septic patients. Recall that in the cardiac surgery population, less than 10% of patients are estimated to have vasodilatory hypotension warranting pressor support. Fluid, inotropic, and even vasodilator therapy may be more effective in treating this cohort of patients.[41,52,56]

Several small studies have documented the potential benefits of vasopressin therapy in septic shock.[51,52,56] Vasopressin infusions are associated with decreases in norepinephrine dosing requirements, as well as increases in creatinine clearance and urine output.[52,55] It is not associated with decreased CO or oxygen delivery and consumption, even in higher doses. The Vasopressin and Septic Shock Trial (VASST), a randomized, double-blind trial of 778 patients (vasopressin, $n = 396$; norepinephrine, $n = 382$), compared vasopressin with norepinephrine in the management of septic shock.[55] There was no significant difference between the vasopressin and norepinephrine groups in terms of 28-day mortality (35.4% and 39.3%, respectively; $p = 0.26$) or 90-day mortality (43.9% and 49.6%, respectively; $p = 0.11$). Additionally, there were no significant differences in the overall rates of serious adverse events. Post hoc analyses of VASST showed that in patients who received corticosteroids, use of vasopressin was associated with a significant decrease in mortality compared with norepinephrine plus corticosteroids (35.9% versus 44.7%, $p = 0.03$). This suggests a positive interaction between corticosteroids and vasopressin, requiring further investigation.[70]

Whereas VASST was unable to demonstrate a clear superiority of vasopressin to norepinephrine, emerging data suggest that vasopressin may be a reasonable second-line agent in patients deemed to have an insufficient response to norepinephrine. The SSC guidelines do not recommend vasopressin as a single agent for the management of septic shock, and instead suggest that it could be added to norepinephrine with the intent of either increasing MAP or decreasing the dose of norepinephrine.[10-12]

Adult rates for vasopressin infusion are 0.01 to 0.04 unit/min. When used in patients with sepsis, the SSC guidelines recommend a maximum vasopressin dose of 0.03 unit/min. The patient should be closely monitored and dosed appropriately to avoid deleterious side effects, particularly mesenteric ischemia. Another consideration with the use of vasopressin is the need to monitor serum sodium levels closely for the development of hyponatremia and water retention.

Emerging data on vasopressin suggest that it significantly reduces mortality in general patients, and specifically in patients with septic shock; however, further investigation in large randomized controlled trials is needed.[41,45,51]

Vasodilator Agents

The body's response to hypotension is not helpful in the case of cardiogenic shock. The SNS and RAAS provide support in hypovolemic and vasogenic states, but they are detrimental in pump failure. Vasodilators can reverse the harmful cardiac effects of the stress response in patients with pump failure. Their efficacy is achieved through venous and arterial dilation and the resultant preload and afterload reduction. Reversing vascular constriction conserves cardiac energy and allows the heart to focus on contracting and moving blood, instead of overcoming the burdens placed on it by the body.

Vasodilators have been shown to be associated with significantly lower in-hospital mortality from acute decompensated heart failure than inotropes.[1] The patient with cardiogenic shock should be stabilized with inotropes prior to adding vasodilators. Vasodilators will then assist in lowering PAOP and the ventricular overstretch that compromises contractility beyond the original insult. They will also reduce SVR and the resistance to moving blood out to the body tissues. Preload and afterload reduction can actually improve CO and help reduce the need for inotropic support. In summary, vasodilators allow the heart to move blood more efficiently and with less oxygen consumption.

Nitroglycerin

William Murrell published the first article describing the therapeutic properties of nitroglycerin in the *Lancet* in 1879, and more than a century later it remains a staple in coronary critical care.[44a] Nitroglycerin induces the release of nitric oxide for the dilation of both veins and arteries. It is primarily a venodilator and preload reducer, especially at dosages of less than 50 mcg/min (1 mcg/kg/min). It is used in treating acute coronary syndromes to balance oxygen supply and relieve ischemic pain, and can be titrated up to 200 mcg/min. Because of its short duration of action, and a tendency for patients to become tolerant to it, higher doses have been reported. In cardiogenic shock secondary to myocardial infarction, nitroglycerin is often selected for vasodilation because of its effective dilation of coronary arteries. In the setting of hypotension, nitroglycerin should be started at the lowest possible rate and titrated up according to patient tolerance. As with all vasodilators, it is critical that volume status be optimized before initiating the drug. If RV infarction is present, the preload-reducing characteristics of nitroglycerin may not be tolerated.

Nitroprusside

Although generally thought of as an antihypertensive agent, nitroprusside (Nipride) can be used in minute doses to reduce preload and afterload in pump failure. It rapidly and markedly improves cardiac function in patients with decompensated heart failure secondary to severe LV systolic and aortic valve dysfunction. It may provide a safe and effective bridge to aortic valve replacement or oral vasodilator therapy. However, cyanide toxicity and significant hypotension are concerning in long-term use.

Nitroprusside is a balanced venous and arterial dilator that causes the release of NO, but through a different mechanism than nitroglycerin, and without the problem of tolerance. Nitroprusside is a potent vasodilator and should be started at no more than 0.2 mcg/kg/min. It dilates the coronary arteries, but affects the smaller resistance vessels, and can result in coronary steal in some patients. Chest pain, ST segment depressions, or ischemic ventricular ectopy should warrant a change to nitroglycerin. In pulmonary edema, which is common in cardiogenic states, nitroprusside has been known to reverse normal autoregulation in the lungs, causing arteriovenous shunting and a fall in partial pressure of arterial oxygen tension (Pao_2). For patients with borderline Pao_2, it is prudent to adjust oxygen and ventilator settings before initiating nitroprusside.

Nesiritide

Nesiritide (Natrecor) is not approved for the treatment of shock, but because of its use in the management of cardiac failure, it is reviewed here. Nesiritide is a recombinant form of BNP, an innate secretion of the ventricles that serves to counteract the effects of the SNS and RAAS. It is a vasodilator and a natriuretic that causes the excretion of sodium in the urine to reduce vascular volume. It lowers preload and afterload and indirectly improves CO.[28] It is initiated with an optional bolus of 2 mcg/kg, followed by a maintenance infusion of 0.01 mcg/kg/min. The primary side effect of nesiritide is hypotension, so dosages may need to be reduced in the setting of pump failure with hypoperfusion. Coupled with inotropic support, nesiritide has been shown to be at least as effective as standard vasodilator and diuretic therapy, and to result in a higher rate of survival to discharge than dobutamine or milrinone therapy.[1] There have been questions regarding the safety of nesiritide and its effect on mortality beyond the hospital stay. A pooled analysis of seven nesiritide trials published by Sackner-Bernstein et al. reported a 30-day mortality rate of 5.3% in the nesiritide group, compared with 4.3% in the group treated with other standard medications.[58] Many have been skeptical of this finding, and currently nesiritide remains a questionable pharmacologic modality. One positive outcome from experiences with nesiritide is the revival of interest in vasodilators for the reduction of preload and afterload in the treatment of acutely decompensated heart failure.[64]

Others

Intravenous vasodilators such as nicardipine (Cardene) and enalaprilat (Vasotec) are available, and are effective preload and afterload reducers. However, because of negative inotropic effects and lengthy durations of action, they are better suited for the treatment of hypertension.

NURSING CARE OF THE HYPOPERFUSED PATIENT

The complexities of caring for patients with hemodynamic compromise and oxygenation threats are challenging. Vigilant monitoring of all body organs for cellular dysfunction due to hypoperfusion is crucial, and may stimulate a reevaluation of therapy to improve oxygenation (Box 29.7). Critical care nurses make their greatest contribution by participating in interprofessional care focused on determining the best available therapies. The role of patient advocate includes making research-based recommendations accessible to all clinicians involved and developing protocols and daily goal sheets for improving care for future patients. The nurse needs to ensure that hypovolemic patients are adequately fluid-resuscitated. If patients have cardiogenic shock secondary to MI, implementation of the ACC/AHA guidelines[47] should be encouraged. With sepsis, EGDT should be considered for either hypotension or a lactate level of greater than 4 mmol/L. Bridging the gap from bench to bedside is vital in achieving the best patient outcome.

While caring for hemodynamically unstable patients, it is easy to prioritize the manipulation of cardiovascular status and overlook less life-threatening needs. Skin breakdown is common in the shock patient, and preventive care, including frequent turning and relief of pressure points, is important. Patients in shock require prophylaxis for deep vein thrombosis and pulmonary emboli. Anticoagulants may be contraindicated in certain trauma patients, and pneumatic compression devices are advised. Because most hypotensive patients require mechanical ventilation, peptic ulcer disease prophylaxis and head of bed elevation are also essential. Maintaining the patient with hypotension in a semi-Fowler's position at 30 to 45 degrees is challenging, but this strategy can significantly reduce the chances of ventilator-associated pneumonia (VAP). Oral care, though not definitively proven to reduce the incidence of VAP, is important for good hygiene and patient comfort. Central catheter placement and replacement should be managed with maximum barrier precautions and chlorhexidine site preparation to prevent infection.

The nutritional needs of the hypoperfused patient are important to address. Enteral feeding is recognized as the preferred route. However, the gastrointestinal tract may not be adequately perfused during shock states, and a nutritional load could precipitate an oxygen imbalance and necrosis in addition to poor absorption of nutrients. The parenteral route for nutritional supplementation may be necessary. Intensive insulin therapy for tight glycemic control is becoming a standard of practice for all critically ill patients, and should be considered for this population as well.

Throughout critical illness, it is important to maintain open lines of communication with the patient (when possible) and the family regarding treatment and prognosis. If the patient's chances of survival become unlikely, consideration should be given to limiting support. Critical care has traditionally focused on curative therapy; however, this may not be consistent with the patient's or family's wishes. A realistic assessment of outcome must be made and shared. It is paramount to accept that a less aggressive approach to treatment or the withdrawal of life support may be in the best interest of the patient. Palliative care in critical care is becoming more prevalent, and allowing patients to die with dignity is becoming more acceptable.

BOX 29.7 Signs of Organ Dysfunction

Central Nervous System Dysfunction

Confusion
Psychosis
Deepening level of consciousness

Respiratory Dysfunction

Tachypnea
Pao_2 less than 70 mm Hg
Sao_2 less than 90%
Pao_2/Fio_2 ratio (P/F ratio) ≤ 300

Gastrointestinal Dysfunction

Excessive nasogastric drainage
Abdominal pain (ischemia)
Elevated liver enzymes
Jaundice
Decreased albumin

Renal Dysfunction

Oliguria
Elevated creatinine

Hematologic Dysfunction

Decreased platelets
Decreased activated partial thromboplastin time
Increased D-dimer
Acral cyanosis
Bleeding

Metabolic Dysfunction

Elevated lactate
Metabolic acidosis

Fio_2, Fraction of inspired oxygen; *Pao_2*, partial pressure of arterial oxygen tension; *Sao_2*, arterial oxygen saturation.

CONCLUSION

Managing patients with hemodynamic compromise is a challenging task with inadequate evidence-based guidelines for practice. Despite this, shock patients require our best scientific effort in reversing hypoperfusion and our most compassionate care when treatment becomes futile at the end of life.

CASE STUDY 29.1

J.Q. is a 68-year-old man who was admitted to the cardiovascular surgery critical care unit following abdominal aortic aneurysm repair. He has multiple risk factors for cardiovascular disease, including cigarette smoking, obesity, and hypertension. J.Q.'s history includes coronary artery and peripheral vascular disease, with coronary artery bypass surgery 3 years ago. His current problem started 18 months prior with the identification of an asymptomatic abdominal aortic aneurysm during a routine physical. The aneurysm was monitored for enlargement, and when it reached 5 cm, surgical repair was scheduled.

On arrival to critical care, J.Q. was lethargic but arousable. He was being mechanically ventilated, and a warming blanket had been applied. He was in sinus rhythm with occasional premature ventricular contractions (PVCs), and lower extremity pulses were equal bilaterally. J.Q. had an arterial line, a PAC, and a large abdominal dressing that was dry and intact. His vital signs on admission were: temperature 96°F, HR 116 beats/min, RR 12 breaths/min, BP 158/86 mm Hg.

Approximately 2 hours after his arrival, J.Q. became cool and clammy, hypotensive, and tachycardic. At this time, the following profile was obtained: temperature 98.8°F, HR 122 beats/min, RR 16 breaths/min, BP 92/50 mm Hg, CVP 5 mm Hg, PAOP 9 mm Hg, PAP 24/10 mm Hg, CO 3.6 L/min, CI 2.2 L/min, SVR 1311 dynes.

Decision Point:

To what do you attribute J.Q.'s hypotensive state?

He remained sedated throughout the night and was maintained on dobutamine at 0.5 mcg/kg per min and nitroglycerin at 1.5 mcg/kg per min. Early on postoperative day (POD) 1, he remains sedated and a decision is made to postpone ventilator weaning until the following day. On POD2, J.Q. spikes a temperature of 102.4°F. Urine and blood cultures are drawn, and a chest film is taken. No obvious source of infection is found, and empiric antibiotics are initiated. In the early morning hours of POD3, J.Q. becomes hypotensive once again.

Temp, 101.3°F; HR, 128 beats/min; RR, 30 breaths/min; BP, 80/42 mm Hg; CVP, 8 mm Hg; PAWP, 14 mm Hg; PAP, 30/16 mm Hg; CO, 5.3 L/min; CI, 3.2 L/min; SVR, 709 dynes.

Decision Point:

From this information, what is the source of J.Q.'s hypotension at this juncture, and what treatments are indicated?

J.Q.'s hospital course was long and protracted, but with continued adherence to the principles of EGDT and the Surviving Sepsis Campaign, he began to improve. He was gradually weaned from all vasoactive and inotropic agents (dobutamine and norepinephrine). Respiratory failure proved to be his biggest obstacle, and he required mechanical ventilation for a total of 18 days. After leaving critical care and going through rehabilitation therapy, he was discharged home on the 27th hospital day.

REFERENCES

1. Abraham, W. T. (2005). In-hospital mortality in patients with acute decompensated heart failure requiring intravenous vasoactive medications: an analysis from the Acute Decompensated Heart Failure National Registry (ADHERE). *J Am Coll Cardiol, 46*(1), 65–67.
2. American Association of Critical-Care Nurses (AACN) Practice Alert (2016). Pulmonary artery/central venous presure monitoring in adults. http://www.aacn.org/WD/Practice/Content/practicealerts.content?menu=Practice.
3. Annane, D., et al. (2004). Corticosteroids for severe sepsis and septic shock: a systematic review and meta-analysis. *BMJ, 329*, 480–488.
4. Augusto, J. F., Teboul, J. L., Radermakker, P., & Asfar, P. (2011). Interpretation of blood pressure signal: physiological bases, clinical relevance, and objectives during shock states. *Intensive Care Med, 11*, 411–419.
5. Babaev, A., et al. (2005). Trends in management and outcomes of patients with acute myocardial infarction complicated by cardiogenic shock. *JAMA, 294*(4), 448–454.
6. Benington, S., Ferris, P., & Nirmalan, M. (2009). Emerging trends in minimally invasive haemodynamic monitoring and optimization of fluid therapy. *Eur J Anaesthesiol, 25*(11), 893–905.
7. Buist, M., et al. (2004). Association between clinically abnormal observations and subsequent in-hospital mortality: a prospective study. *Resuscitation, 62*(2), 137–141.
8. Casserly, B., et al. (2011). Hemodynamic monitoring in sepsis. *Crit Care Nurs Clin North Am, 23*, 149–169.
9. Cooper, H. A., Najafi, A. H., Ghafourain, K., et al. (2015). Diagnosis of cardiogenic shock without the use of a pulmonary artery catheter. *Eur Heart J Acute Cardiovasc Care, 1*, 88–95.
10. Cordemans, C., DelLaet, I., Van Regenmortel, N., et al. (2012). Fluid management in critically ill patients: role of extravascular lung fluid, abdominal hypertension, capillary leak and fluid balance. *Ann Intensive Care, 3*(Suppl. 1), 1–12.
11. Dellinger, R. P., et al. (2004). Surviving Sepsis Campaign guidelines for management of severe sepsis and septic shock. *Crit Care Med, 32*(3R), 858–873.
12. Dellinger, R. P., et al. (2008). Sepsis Campaign: international guidelines for management of severe sepsis and septic shock: 2008. *Crit Care Med, 36*, 296–327.
13. Dellinger, R. P., et al. (2012). Surviving Sepsis Campaign: international guidelines for management of severe sepsis and septic shock. *Crit Care Med, 41*(2), 580–637.
14. Di Giantomasso, D., Bellomo, R., & May, C. N. (2005). The hemodynamic and metabolic effects of epinephrine in experimental hyperdynamic septic shock. *Intensive Care Med, 31*(3), 454–462.
15. Dueck, M. H., et al. (2005). Trends but not individual values of central venous oxygen saturation agree with mixed venous oxygen saturation during varying hemodynamic conditions. *Anesthesiology, 103*(2), 249–257.
16. Dzavik, V., et al. (2005). Outcome of patients aged greater than or equal to 75 years in the SHould we emergently revascularize Occluded Coronaries in cardiogenic shocK (SHOCK) trial: do elderly patients with acute myocardial infarction complicated by cardiogenic shock respond differently to emergent revascularization? *Am Heart J, 149*(6), 1128–1134.
17. Felker, G. M., et al. (2003). Heart failure etiology and response to milrinone in decompensated heart failure: results from the OPTIME-CHF study. *J Am Coll Cardiol, 41*(6), 997–1003.
18. Fink, M. P. (2005). Non-invasive and invasive cardiovascular monitoring. In M. P. Fink (Ed.), *Textbook of critical care*. Saunders: Philadelphia.
19. Gillies, M., et al. (2005). Bench-to-bedside review: inotropic drug therapy after adult cardiac surgery, a systematic literature review. *Crit Care, 9*(3), 266–279.
20. Goldstein, J. A. (2012). Acute right ventricular infarction: insights for the interventional era. *Curr Probl Cardiol, 37*, 533–557.
21. Grothoff, M., et al. (2012). Right ventricular injury in STEMI: risk stratification by visualization of wall motion, edema, and delayed-enhancement cardiac magnetic resonance. *Cir Cardiovasc Imaging, 5*, 60–68.
22. Haddad, S. H., & Arabi, Y. M. (2012). Critical care management of severe traumatic brain injury in adults. *Scand J Trauma Resusc Emerg Med, 20*(12), 1–15.
23. Harvy, S., et al. (2005). Assessment of the clinical effectiveness of pulmonary artery catheters in management of patients in intensive care (PAC-Man): a randomized controlled trial. *Lancet, 366*(9484), 472–477.
24. Holcomb, J. B., Tilley, B. C., Baraniuk, S., et al. (2015). Transfusion of plasma, platelets, and red blood cells in a 1:1:1: vs. a 1:1:2 ratio and mortality with severe trauma. The PROPPR randomized clinical trial. *JAMA, 313*(5), 471–482.
25. Holcomb, J. B., Zarazabal, L. A., Michalek, J. E., et al. (2011). Increased platelet:RBC ratios are associated with improved survival after massive transfusions. *J Trauma, 71*, S318–S328.
26. Hollenberg, S. M. (2004). Recognition and treatment of cardiogenic shock. *Semin Respir Crit Care Med, 25*(6), 661–671.
27. Inohara, T., et al. (2013). The Challenges in the management of right ventricular infarction. *Eur Heart J Acute Cardiovasc Care, 2*(3), 226–234.
28. Iyengar, S., et al. (2004). Nesiritide for the treatment of congestive heart failure. *Expert Opin Pharmacother, 5*(4), 901–907.
29. Kellum, J. A., & Decker, J. M. (2001). Use of dopamine in acute renal failure: a meta-analysis. *Crit Care Med, 29*(8), 1526–1531.
30. Kent, A., et al. (2013). Sonographic evaluation of intravascular volume status in the surgical intensive care unit: a prospective comparison of subclavian vein and inferior vena cava collapsibility index. *J Surg Res, 184*(1), 561–566.

31. Kern, J. W., & Shoemaker, W. C. (2002). Early goal-directed therapy in shock. *Crit Care Med, 30*(8), 1686–1692.
32. Khalaf, S., & DeBlieux, P. M. (2001). Managing shock: the role of vasoactive agents, part 1. *J Crit Illn, 16*(6), 281.
33. Klijn, E., et al. (2015). Tissue perfusion and oxygenation to monitor fluid responsiveness in critically ill, septic patients after initial resuscitation: a prospective observational study. *J Clin Monit Comput, 29*(6), 707–712.
34. Kolte, D., Khera, S., Aronow, W. S., et al. (2014 Jan 13). Trends in incidence, management, and outcomes of cardiogenic shock complicating ST-elevation myocardial infarction in the United States. *J Am Heart Assoc, 3*(1), e000590.
35. Lough, M. E. (2016). *Hemodynamic monitoring: evolving technologies and clinical practice*. St. Louis: Elsevier.
36. Madger, S. A. (2014). The highs and lows of blood pressure: toward meaningful clinical targets in patients with shock. *Critical Care Med, 42*(5), 1241–1251.
37. Mahjoub, Y., J, et al. (2010). The passive leg-raising maneuver cannot accurately predict fluid responsiveness in patients with intra-abdominal hypertension. *Crit Care Med, 38*(9), 1824–1829.
38. Marik, P. (2013). Obituary: pulmonary artery catheter 1970-2013. *Ann Intensive Care, 3*(38), 1–6.
39. McKie, P. M., & Burnett, J. C., Jr. (2005). B-type natriuretic peptide as a biomarker beyond heart failure: speculations and opportunities. *Mayo Clin Proc, 80*(8), 1029–1036.
40. Mehta, N., et al. (2014). A review of intraoperative goal-directed therapy using arterial waveform analysis for assessment of cardiac output. *The Sci World J*, 1–8.
41. Mentzelopoulos, S. D. (2012). Vasopressin for cardiac arrest: meta-analysis of randomized controlled trials. *Resuscitation, 83*(1), 32–39.
42. Mohsenin, V. (2015). Assessment of preload and fluid responsiveness in intensive care unit. How good are we? *J Crit Care, 30*, 567–573.
43. Monge Garcia, M. I., et al. (2012). Non-invasive assessment of fluid responsiveness by changes in partial end-tidal CO_2 pressure during a passive leg-raising maneuver. *Ann Intensive Care, 2*(9), 1–10.
44. Monnet, X., & Teboul, J. L. (2013). End-tidal carbon dioxide and arterial pressure for predicting volume responsiveness by the passive leg raising test: reply to Piagnerelli and Biston. *Intensive Care Med, 39*(6), 1165.
44a. Murrell, W. (1879). Nitro-glycerine as a remedy for angina pectoris. *Lancet, 1*, 80–81, 113-115, 151-152, 225–227.
45. Neto, A. S., et al. (2012). Vasopressin and terlipressin in adult vasodilatory shock: a systematic review and meta-analysis of nine randomized controlled trials. *Crit Care, 16*(4), R154.
46. Neumar, R. W., Shuster, M., Callaway, C. W., Gent, L. M., Atkins, D. L., et al. (2015). American Heart Association guidelines update for cardiopulmonary resuscitation and emergency cardiovascular care. *Circulation*. 132-S315-S367.
47. O'Gara, P. T., et al. (2013). Update: ACCF/AHA guideline for the management of ST-elevation myocardial infarction. *J Am Coll Cardiol, 61*(4), e78–e140.
48. Ondrus, T., et al. (2013). Right ventricular myocardial infarction: from pathophysiology to prognosis. *Exp Clin Cardiol, 10*(1), 27–30.
49. Peura, J. L., et al. (2012). Recommendations for the use of mechanical circulatory support: device strategies and patient selection: a scientific statement from the American Heart Association. *Circulation, 126*, 2648–2667.
50. Pinsky, M. R., & Vincent, J. L. (2005). Let us use the pulmonary artery catheter correctly and only when we need it. *Crit Care Med, 33*(5), 1119–1124.
51. Polito, A., et al. (2012). Vasopressin and terlipressin in adult vasodilatory shock. *Crit Care, 16*(6), 470.
52. Pollard, S., et al. (2015). Vasopressor and inotropic management of patients with septic shock. *PT, 40*(7), 438–450.
53. Ramsingh, D., et al. (2013). Clinical review: does it matter which hemodynamic monitoring system is used? *Crit Care, 17*, 208.
54. Rivers, E. P., et al. (2001). Early goal-directed therapy in the treatment of severe sepsis and septic shock. *N Engl J Med, 345*(19), 1368–1377.
55. Russell, J. A., et al., for the VASST Investigators (2008). Vasopressin versus norepinephrine infusion in patients with septic shock. *N Engl J Med, 358*(9), 877–887.
56. Russell, J. A. (2011). Bench-to-bedside review: vasopressin in the management of septic shock. *Crit Care, 15*(4), 226.
57. Sabatine, M. S., et al. (2005). Association of hemoglobin levels with clinical outcomes in acute coronary syndromes. *Circulation, 111*(16), 2042–2049.
58. Sackner-Bernstein, J. D., et al. (2005). Short-term risk of death after treatment with nesiritide for decompensated heart failure: a pooled analysis of randomized controlled trials. *JAMA, 293*(15), 1900–1905.
59. SAFE Study Investigators. (2004). A comparison of albumin and saline for fluid resuscitation in the intensive care unit. *N Engl J Med, 350*, 2247–2256.
60. Shah, M. R., et al. (2005). Impact of the pulmonary artery catheter in critically ill patients: meta-analysis of randomized clinical trials. *JAMA, 294*(13), 1664–1670.
61. Smith, M. A. (2005). Use of vasopressors in the treatment of cardiac arrest. *Crit Care Nurse Clin North Am, 17*(1), 71–75.
62. Strandvik, G. F. (2009). Hypertonic saline in critical care: a review of the literature and guidelines for use in hypotensive states and raised intracranial pressure. *Anaesthesia, 64*(9), 990–1003.
63. Summerhill, E. M., & Baram, M. (2005). Principles of pulmonary artery catheterization in the critically ill. *Lung, 183*(3), 209–219.
64. Tang, W. H., & Hobbs, R. E. (2005). Novel strategies for the management of acute decompensated heart failure. *Curr Cardiol Rev, 1*(1), 1–5.
65. Thiel SW, S. W., Kollef, M. H., & Isakow, W. (2009). Non-invasive stroke volume measurement and passive leg raising predict volume responsiveness in medical ICU patients: an observational cohort study. *Crit Care, 13*(4), R111.
66. Valler-Jones, T., & Wedgbury, K. (2005). Measuring blood pressure using the mercury sphygmomanometer. *Br J Nurs, 14*(3), 145–150.
67. Vincent, J. L., & Weil, M. H. (2006). Fluid challenge revisited. *Crit Care Med, 34*, 1333–1337.
68. Wenzel, V., et al. (2004). A comparison of vasopressin and epinephrine for out-of-hospital cardiopulmonary resuscitation. *N Engl J Med, 350*, 105–113.
69. Yancy, C. W., et al. (2013). ACCF/AHA Heart Failure Guideline. *J Am Coll Cardiol, 15;62*(16), e147–e239.
70. Zhou, F., & Song, Q. (2014). Clinical trials comparing norepinephrine with vasopressin in patients with septic shock: a meta-analysis. *Mil Med Res, 1*, 6.

30

Trauma

Roy Ball

INTRODUCTION

The trauma patient population is one of the most diverse groups of patients seen in critical care, composed of people of all ages, a variety of socioeconomic statuses, and diverse preexisting conditions leading to a variety of complications. Advancements in technology and the proliferation of coordinated trauma care systems have dramatically improved the trauma patient's prospects for recovery and return to a productive life. For those who are critically injured, recovery is dependent on prompt, aggressive, appropriate resuscitation, and ongoing critical care management.

Unique to the trauma patient population is the phenomena of kinetic energy transfer resulting in multisystem injuries. Although some principals of assessment, diagnostic testing, and resuscitative intervention are unique to the trauma population, these patients face similar physiologic challenges to other critically ill patients: acute respiratory distress syndrome (ARDS), shock, neurologic compromise, gastrointestinal (GI) compromise, acute tubular necrosis (ATN), and infection, to name a few. Detailed information about the full spectrum of trauma care is covered in textbooks specific to the topic; this chapter focuses on issues essential for any critical care nurse caring for injured patients.

In modern times, trauma has been viewed as a disease of the young; however, traumatic injury spans the spectrum of age and socioeconomic status. Trauma results from unintentional incidents such as motor vehicle crashes (MVCs), falls, burns, and recreational and occupational mishaps. Intentional injury results from deliberate acts of violence such as assaults, child or elder abuse, shootings, and stabbings (the incidence and prevalence of trauma are described in Box 30.1). Alcohol use has a disturbingly high prevalence in trauma, especially MVCs. Influences of alcohol in trauma are listed in Box 30.2.

Development of the Trauma System

Military experience demonstrates that optimal trauma care is provided when there is a coordinated, systematic approach to patient management utilizing the best available resources. The first attempt at a regional trauma system was the Maryland Institute for Emergency Medical Services System/R. Adams Cowley Shock Trauma Center in Maryland in the late 1960s. This system identified specific facilities for trauma care, categorized those facilities into different tiers based on capability, and triaged injured patients to the most appropriate trauma center based on resources. The success of this first trauma system led to development of similar systems in the United States that now follow national standards developed by the American College of Surgeons Committee on Trauma (ACSCOT). Since then, ACSCOT has facilitated the development of numerous trauma systems in collaboration with National Highway Traffic Safety Administration (NHTSA). Patient morbidity and mortality have significantly improved nationally and internationally with the advent of trauma care systems.[67,91,105] Fundamental components of any trauma care system include coordination of prehospital care, distribution of trauma centers based on population and geography, designation and periodic redesignation of trauma care facilities by a central agency, and the administration of statewide rules and regulations.

A network of trauma centers is the backbone of a successful trauma care system. Trauma centers are categorized from Level I-IV depending on their availability of resources.[4,40] Characteristics of trauma centers are described in Table 30.1.

MECHANISM OF INJURY

The term *mechanism of injury* refers to the underlying causes and physical forces resulting in physical injury. Knowledge of mechanism of injury provides for increased ease in injury identification and prediction of eventual patient outcomes.[148] In addition, it guides initial resuscitation and diagnostic activities and allows the critical care team to discover missed injuries and anticipate complications associated with specific injuries. Injuries are commonly diagnosed because a suspicious healthcare provider compared the physical findings with the patient's history, initiated further diagnostic workup, and identified a previously undiscovered injury.

Trauma occurs when an acute exchange of mechanical, thermal, electrical, or chemical energy results in structural changes or physiologic imbalance.[68] Energy exchange is dependent on three basic principles of physics: an object in rest or motion will remain in that state until acted on by some outside force (Newton's first law of motion); energy is changed from one form to another, not created or destroyed; and the force of energy is a function of size and speed. Doubling the size of an object will result in a doubling of kinetic energy. Doubling the speed of an object results in a quadrupling of kinetic energy (kinetic energy: KE = mass × velocity^1).[68] Force applied slowly and over a large surface area will result in less tissue destruction than force applied quickly over a small surface area.[148] Force puts an object in motion; this motion will not change until a second force equal to or greater than the initiating force stops it. For example, a car will remain at a certain speed until acted on by an outside force, such as the application of brakes, another vehicle, or a tree. Rather than disappear, the kinetic energy of the moving car is absorbed by the other objects and body tissues of any passengers.

Tissue damage occurs as a result of acceleration, deceleration, shearing, or compressive forces. Acceleration is a change in

BOX 30.1 Incidence and Prevalence of Trauma

- Trauma is the fourth leading cause of death for all ages in the United States and the leading cause of death in people between ages 1 and 46.
- People older than the age of 85 have a greater likelihood of dying despite lower injury severity.
- Men are injured more frequently than women until the age of 70, after which time injuries to women are more common.
- Primary causes of unintentional injury are motor vehicle crashes (MVCs), falls, and burns.
- One out of three adults over age 65 will fall each year; the peak incidence occurs after age 80.
- Alcohol is a factor in 40% of all traffic-related fatalities in which at least one driver or nonoccupant had a blood alcohol concentration (BAC) of 0.01 g/dL or higher.
- Alcohol is a major factor in intentional and interpersonal trauma, recreational trauma, and plays a large role in the incidence of traumatic brain injury.

From References 13, 23, 80, 106, and 121.

BOX 30.2 Influences of Alcohol in Trauma

- Habitual drunken drivers have an increased risk of dying in an alcohol-related crash.
- There is no increase in complications in trauma patients who are acutely intoxicated at the time of injury, but there is a twofold-increased risk of complications in patients with a history of chronic alcohol abuse.
- Intoxicated drivers are less likely to use seatbelts and are more likely to drive at high speeds.
- 69% of car occupants between 21 and 44 years of age killed in car crashes had blood alcohol concentration levels at or above 0.08 g/dL.
- More than 36% of all pedestrians older than 16 years of age killed in traffic crashes have elevated BAC.
- 47% of children killed in motor vehicle crashes are in crashes in which the driver had elevated BAC.
- The rate of alcohol involvement in fatal crashes is more than 3 times higher at night than during the day.
- 53% of all fatal crashes involving alcohol occur on the weekend, compared to 30% on weekdays.
- Intoxicated drivers involved in fatal crashes are 9 times more likely to have prior drinking and driving convictions than nonintoxicated drivers.
- Drinking drivers have higher hospitalization costs and longer lengths of stay independent of their age, gender, or injury severity.

From References 76, 86, 104, and 106.

the speed of a moving object (e.g., a person standing by the side of the road is accelerated into motion when hit by an oncoming car).[148] Conversely, deceleration is a decrease in the speed of a moving object (e.g., a person riding a bicycle suddenly stops after hitting a parked car).[148] Many injuries occur from a combination of acceleration and deceleration forces (e.g., a person is thrown into motion after being hit by a car, and suddenly stopped by landing on the ground).[68]

Shearing injuries result when structures move in opposite directions from each other, stretching and disrupting tissue planes and pulling organs away from their attachment points (e.g., when the heart swings forward in the chest cavity while the aortic arch remains fixed to the thoracic spine).[148] Finally, compressive forces overwhelm the ability of tissues to resist squeezing (e.g., a person who falls from a height to land on their feet will sustain vertebral and long bone fractures along the axial

TABLE 30.1 Characteristics of Trauma Centers

Level	Characteristics
Level I	• Typically located in larger cities or population dense areas. • Expected to admit at least 1200 trauma patients per year or at least 20% of admitted patients must be severely injured. • Responsible for teaching, research, and development of the regionalized trauma system. • Usually tertiary academic facilities with dedicated resources to support the personnel, education, equipment, and capacity to provide care for all phases of trauma care.
Level II	• Larger community hospitals that may or may not be academic centers. • Provide definitive trauma care to patients, but when resources are exceeded may need to transfer patient to the highest level of care. • Does not have same expectations for education and research as Level I centers.
Level III	• Community hospital typically in a rural or suburban area. • Has the capability to resuscitate and initially manage the majority of trauma patients. • Provides safe transfer to a higher level of care when the patient's needs exceed facility resources.
Level IV	• Usually smaller hospital in less-populated, rural areas. • Provides timely resuscitation and transfer of injured patients to higher level of care. • Establishes transfer agreements protocols with Level I and II centers.

From Reference 4.

plane, or when inflated lungs are squeezed during a sudden stop against a steering wheel, popping much like a closed paper bag).[148]

Injuries can occur through either blunt or penetrating mechanisms, with the resultant injury dependent on the amount of energy delivered and the area of the body affected.[148] A thorough discussion of these mechanisms is beyond the scope of this chapter; however, an overview is provided here so that the critical care nurse can appreciate the forces responsible for the patient's injuries.

BLUNT TRAUMA

The combination of deceleration, acceleration, shearing, crushing, and compression result in blunt trauma. Blunt trauma is often more life threatening than penetrating trauma because distribution of destructive energy occurs across several body tissues. As a consequence, multiple injuries are common and identification of injuries can be difficult. MVCs, falls, assaults, and contact sports are associated with blunt force injuries.[68,148]

Motor Vehicle Crash

Different types of vehicle crashes produce predictable injury patterns. Types of MVCs include frontal impact collisions (with both "up-and-over" and "down-and-under" patient trajectories), lateral impact collisions, rear impact collisions, rotational collisions, and rollover crashes[41] (Fig. 30.1). Having a high index of suspicion for specific injuries serves as a starting point to look for injuries varying from usual patterns. Four collisions occur with any car crash, all of which have the potential to injure a

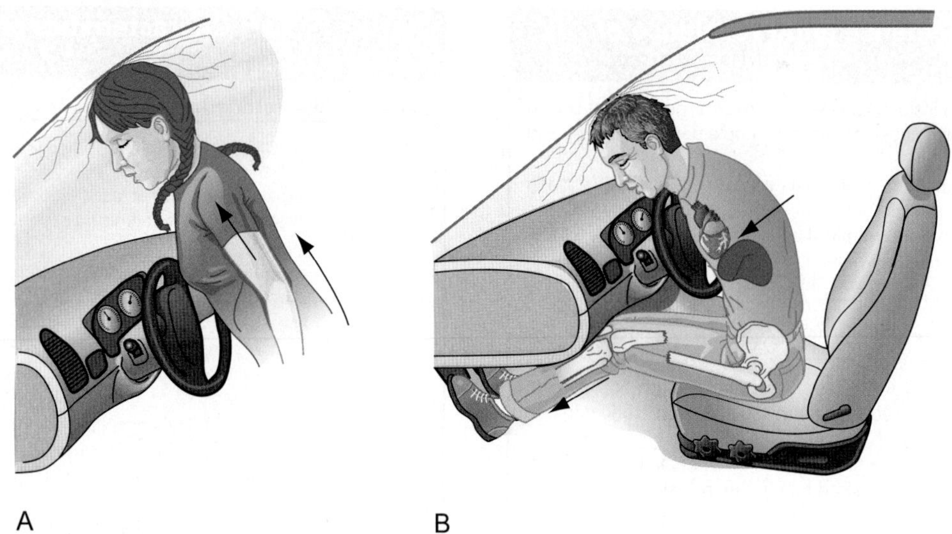

FIG. 30.1 Up-and-over and down-and-under injury patterns. **A,** Up-and-over pathway. **B,** Down-and-under pathway.

TABLE 30.2 Types of Car Collisions ("Alphabet of Collisions")

Type	Description
A: Auto collision	The collision of the vehicle into some object. The force involved depends on the distance required for the vehicle to stop. The extent of damage to the vehicle is a good indicator of the forces transmitted to the occupants.
B: Body collision	The collision of the occupant's body with the inside of the vehicle. Energy is transferred to the vehicle's interior and subsequently transmitted into tissue deformity, compression, stretching, and shearing.
C: Cavity contents collision	The collision of internal body contents against rigid body surfaces. Energy transmission damages tissues and organs as they collide with each other.
D: Debris collision	Loose objects in the car strike occupants as the car accelerates or decelerates. Coffee mugs, purses, briefcases, toolboxes, telephones, and even unrestrained passengers and animals become "debris" as they are thrown about the inside of the vehicle.

From Reference 68.

passenger. They are often referred to as the *alphabet of collisions* and are described in Table 30.2.[122]

Frontal impact collisions occur when a vehicle strikes an object ahead of it. Two injury patterns are seen as a result of the unrestrained occupant's movement. The up-and-over pathway occurs as the head becomes the leading point of the body, striking the windshield or other supporting structures of the car. Once the head stops, the continued momentum of the torso pulls the body upward, forcing the chest and abdomen into the steering column or dashboard. The down-and-under pathway results as the occupant moves forward and down under the dashboard. The knee and femur are forced into the dash; the driver's chest and abdomen collide with the steering wheel. As intrathoracic structures move forward, shearing acceleration forces result in tearing of organs from their vascular pedicles.[68]

Lateral impact collisions occur when the vehicle is struck at a 90-degree angle, changing the direction from a purely forward motion to a forward-lateral motion. Resultant injuries are due to compression and shearing as the occupants are hit on the side of impact or are thrown across the vehicle to hit the opposite side.[68]

Rear impact collisions cause the occupants to move forward at a faster speed than the vehicle's speed. If there is no head restraint, the head will fling backward and serious cervical spine injuries may result.[68]

Rotational collisions occur when an off-center part of the vehicle is struck by an object of lower speed, causing the vehicle to rotate around the point of impact. Occupants will continue movement in the original direction until they strike some object within the car. Shearing and compression injuries occur during rollover crashes as occupants are tossed in multiple directions in subsequent collisions as the car repeatedly rolls.[68] Injury patterns associated with specific collision types are illustrated in Fig. 30.2.

Restraint-System Injuries

The primary protective mechanism of any motor vehicle is the structural design of its frame. Seatbelts, airbags, and infant restraint seats have decreased morbidity and mortality of trauma victims.[148]

When restraints are properly applied, occupants slow at the same pace as their vehicles, rather than being abruptly thrown against vehicle structures or ejected.[149] Even when restraints are worn correctly, injuries may still result, requiring the healthcare team to consider associated injuries. Seatbelts have been shown to prevent deaths by 40%; however, there is an increased incidence of abdominal viscous injury.[149]

A properly applied seatbelt uses a three-point restraint system that crosses over the shoulder and the bony prominences of the pelvis, using these rigid body structures to hold the body securely in the seat. When the shoulder strap and the lap belt are used independently of each other, protective capabilities are significantly diminished and life-threatening injuries may result.[148] The classic Chance fracture occurs when a passenger violently flexes forward against a singular lap belt;

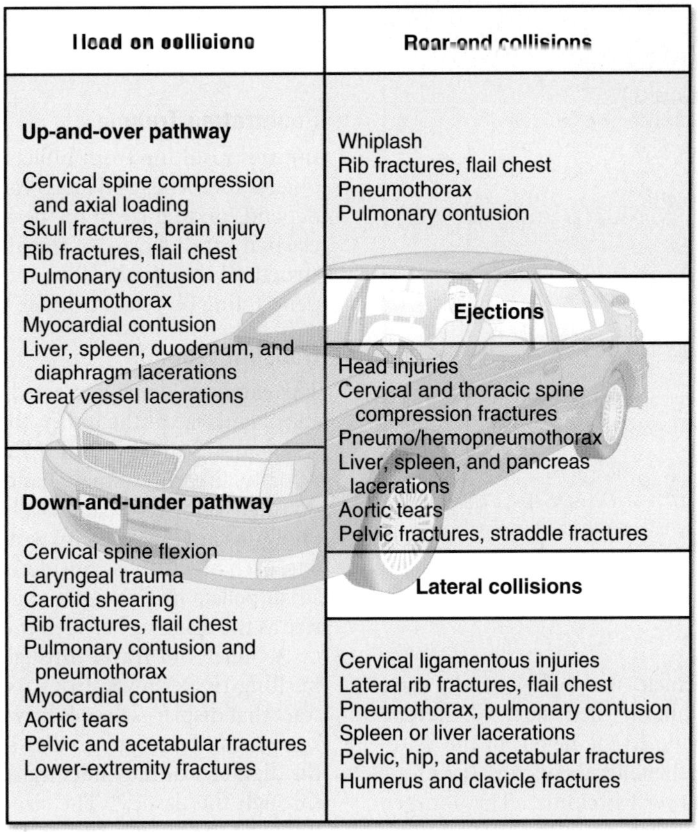

Head-on collisions

Up-and-over pathway

Cervical spine compression and axial loading
Skull fractures, brain injury
Rib fractures, flail chest
Pulmonary contusion and pneumothorax
Myocardial contusion
Liver, spleen, duodenum, and diaphragm lacerations
Great vessel lacerations

Down-and-under pathway

Cervical spine flexion
Laryngeal trauma
Carotid shearing
Rib fractures, flail chest
Pulmonary contusion and pneumothorax
Myocardial contusion
Aortic tears
Pelvic and acetabular fractures
Lower-extremity fractures

Rear-end collisions

Whiplash
Rib fractures, flail chest
Pneumothorax
Pulmonary contusion

Ejections

Head injuries
Cervical and thoracic spine compression fractures
Pneumo/hemopneumothorax
Liver, spleen, and pancreas lacerations
Aortic tears
Pelvic fractures, straddle fractures

Lateral collisions

Cervical ligamentous injuries
Lateral rib fractures, flail chest
Pneumothorax, pulmonary contusion
Spleen or liver lacerations
Pelvic, hip, and acetabular fractures
Humerus and clavicle fractures

FIG. 30.2 Injury patterns resulting from different types of motor vehicle crashes.

the resulting low thoracic and lumbar spine fractures are associated with small bowel injuries. This association between lap belts, lower spine fractures, and small bowel lacerations is so strong that if a Chance fracture is diagnosed, a subsequent exploratory laparotomy is recommended to rule out intestinal injury.[35,68] This and similar injury patterns have led to the current requirements that all seatbelts in a vehicle have a three-point system.

Since 1997, dual airbags have been federally required standard equipment in passenger vehicles in the United States. Recent years have seen the development of side impact, or curtain, airbags in many passenger vehicles. Side impact airbags can be effective at reducing the incidence of traumatic brain injury.[58] Airbag injuries occur when occupants are out of position relative to the airbag compartment at the time of impact (e.g., with a person who is extremely short). They also occur if the occupant was bending over at the time of impact, had a precrash loss of consciousness, was asleep, or if an object was being held close to the face at the time of impact, such as a coffee cup or cellular phone.[68] Airbags inflate and deflate in less than 50 microseconds via a contained explosion of nitrogen, carbon dioxide, and other gases. Airbags inflate only once and therefore offer no protection should there be an immediate second collision[68,107,108] (Box 30.3 lists injuries that occur from inappropriately worn seatbelts and airbag deployment).

BOX 30.3 Injuries From Inappropriately Worn Seatbelts and Airbag Deployment

Seatbelts

Lap Belt Only

- Fractured sternum, ribs, clavicles
- Blunt cardiac injury
- Torn thoracic aorta
- Mesenteric tears, bowel perforations, torn abdominal aorta
- Bladder rupture
- Chance fracture of lower thoracic or lumbar vertebrae

Shoulder Harness Only

- Cervical spine injuries
- Abrasions to neck, chest, abdomen
- Carotid artery, laryngeal injuries

Airbags

- Cervical spine injuries
- Bag slap injuries to face and neck
- Temporary hearing deficits
- Corneal abrasion, retinal detachment
- Upper extremity contusions
- Fracture/dislocations of thumb and wrist

From References 40, 68, 107, and 108.

Key Crash Information

Caregivers of the trauma patient should review the prehospital record to learn about the circumstances of the crash; many emergency medical services (EMS) systems now use digital cameras to photograph an accident scene. The images are downloaded for trauma team review for better appreciation of the amount of energy transfer involved. Important information to know about the crash is listed in Box 30.4.

BOX 30.4 Key Questions Regarding Motor Vehicle Crashes

- What was the size and speed of the car(s)?
- What did the car hit? A guardrail? An oncoming vehicle?
- What was the size and speed of the other vehicle?
- Where was the patient in the car? Driver? Front-seat passenger? Rear-seat passenger on the right or left?
- Were restraint devices used, type of device, and were they used correctly?
- Did airbags deploy?
- What was the amount of damage to the vehicle? How much intrusion was there into the passenger space?
- Where is the damage to the vehicle? Side of the car? Dashboard? Windshield? Steering wheel?
- What was the extrication time? A prolonged extrication time implies a delay of definitive treatment, as well as extensive transfer of energy to the vehicle and its passengers.
- Was there death of an occupant in the car? What is the injury severity of others involved in the accident? The answers to these questions suggest the magnitude of energy transferred during the accident.

From References 40, 68, and 148.

Auto-Pedestrian Accidents

When adults see an oncoming vehicle, they will generally turn and run and are subsequently hit on their side.[68] Different heights of the victim in relationship to the height of the vehicle also influence injury patterns; the taller the victim, the more likely the injuries will be in the lower extremities. The bumper initially strikes adults, resulting in fractures of the tibia and fibula. As they bend, their pelvis and upper femur are struck by the vehicle's hood, resulting in head, abdominal, and thoracic injuries as well as femur, pelvis, and spinal fractures. As they slide off of the hood, a third impact occurs in which the victim's head hits the ground, resulting in brain and cervical spine injuries.[68,107,108]

Falls

Falls from more than three times the victim's height result in severe injury.[68] Circumstances of the fall allow anticipation of the amount of energy involved and likely injuries. Lower extremity fractures, dislocations, and abdominal shearing injuries are common in falls when the victim lands on their feet. In particular, bilateral calcaneal fractures are common if the person fell from a significant height and landed on a hard surface such as asphalt. Compressive forces are transmitted upward from the bottom of the foot to the tibia, femur, and spinal vertebrae, commonly referred to as the "Don Juan" syndrome. Should the victim land on his or her head, as commonly seen in diving injuries, serious head and cervical spine injuries result. In addition to how the victim landed, other influences on injury severity include the surface on which the person landed (a soft bush versus hard concrete), how far the victim fell, and whether anything was hit on the way down.[41,68]

Blast Injuries

Injuries sustained during explosion are the result of heat, chemicals, concussive, and acceleration-deceleration forces because victims are often thrown into the air.[68,148] Victims of an explosion may experience four distinct phases of blast injury: primary, related to over-pressurization; secondary, related to fragmentation of nearby objects and projectiles; tertiary, caused by the victim impacting a nearby object; and quaternary, injures associated with burns, chemicals, etc. Knowledge of the circumstances of the explosion is necessary to discover potential injuries, including thermal and chemical burns, blowout injuries of the lungs, and shearing injuries of abdominal organs.

Penetrating Trauma

Injuries resulting from bullets, knives, and impalements from objects (branches and nails) cause penetrating wounds. Damage depends on the size of the penetrating object, its speed, and the elasticity and density of the affected tissues. In addition to the structural damage, serious infections are highly likely because penetrating objects introduce bacteria.[148]

Gunshot Wounds

The extent of damage created by firearms is influenced by the speed and size of the bullet, the distance of the victim from the weapon, and the amount of air friction on the missile. Low-velocity firearms (small handguns) create less damage than do high-velocity weapons (hunting rifles, large handguns). Shotguns are low-velocity weapons; they fire multiple lead pellets, each of which is considered a separate missile. The 9 to 200 small pellets in a shotgun shell create wounds that increase in size as the distance between the victim and weapon increases.[148]

A bullet will travel through and transfer energy to tissues, pushing tissues away from its path and creating a temporary tract that displaces tissues forward and laterally.[148] This process, known as cavitation, creates a temporary tract 20 to 25 times the diameter of the bullet that disappears once the bullet passes through the tissue.[68] The size of the cavity is directly proportional to the bullet's size and speed and produces injuries outside of the bullet's direct trajectory.[148] Muscle tissue expands to absorb energy with only a moderate amount of tissue damage; in contrast, liver, spleen, and especially bone do not expand to absorb the energy, and burst.[68,148]

Motion of the bullet as it travels through air and tissue contributes to tissue damage as well. Yawing occurs when the nose of the bullet wobbles back and forth as it moves forward after leaving the weapon's muzzle, creating a larger space than the diameter of the bullet. Yawing will cause a bullet to hit the body at an angle, rather than straight-on. Tumbling occurs when momentum carries the tail of the bullet forward in front of the nose, resulting in an end-over-end motion as it continues to move through air and tissue. Fragmentation occurs when bullets break apart on impact to produce several smaller fragments, each causing damage to surrounding tissues.[68,148] Bullets yaw, tumble, and fragment as they pass through tissue, increasing the surface area damaged by the bullet. As a result, exit wounds are often larger than entrance wounds. Yaw and tumble are illustrated in Fig. 30.3, and cavitation is shown in Fig. 30.4.

Stab Wounds and Impalements

Stab wounds are penetrating injuries occurring at lower energy than gunshot wounds. Damage depends on the length and width of the blade, affected tissues and vasculature, and angle at which the device enters the body. Damage is contained within the area of the wound. The concern with stab wounds, however, is that there may be multiple stab wounds, and each wound can extend into several body cavities. For example, any stab wound between the nipple line and the costochondral margin could involve thoracic as well as abdominal organs (Fig. 30.5).[148]

Impalements occur when a victim forcefully collides with an object that penetrates tissue.[148] Impaled objects can be anything in the victim's path: a car door handle during an MVC, fence

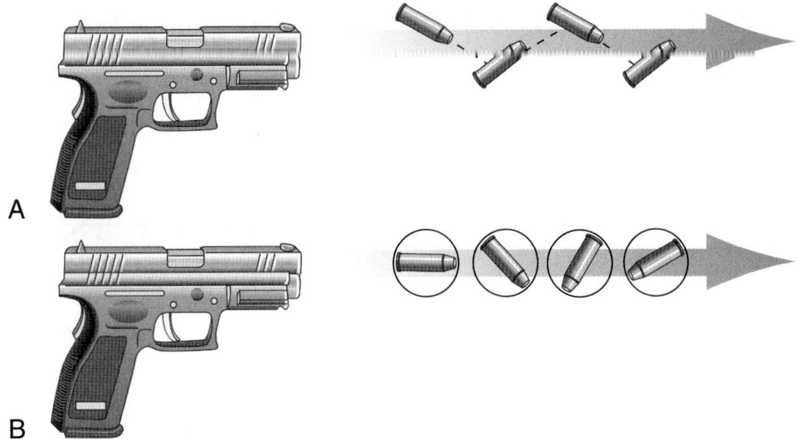

FIG. 30.3 Wounding potential of a bullet. A, Yaw. B, Tumble.

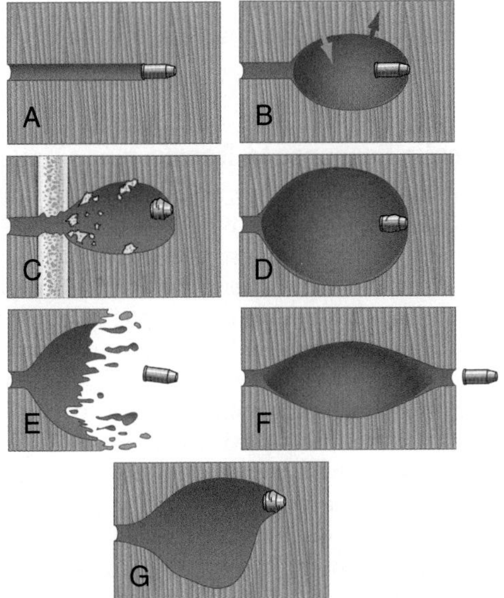

FIG. 30.4 Wounds seen with cavitation and fragmentation. A, Low-velocity missile with small entrance and exit wounds and no cavitation. B, Higher-velocity missile with cavitation; tissue displaced in the direction of the arrows. C, High-velocity missile with cavitation of tissue and penetration of bone; bone fragments become secondary missiles. D, Extremely high-velocity missile with a small entry, resulting in significant cavitation; small exit wound. E, Extremely high-velocity missile with thin target; large exit wound with ragged edges. F, Relationship of missile velocity, size, and tissue thickness creates deep cavitation and small entrance and exit wounds. G, Cavity shape becomes irregular as bullet deforms and tumbles through tissue.

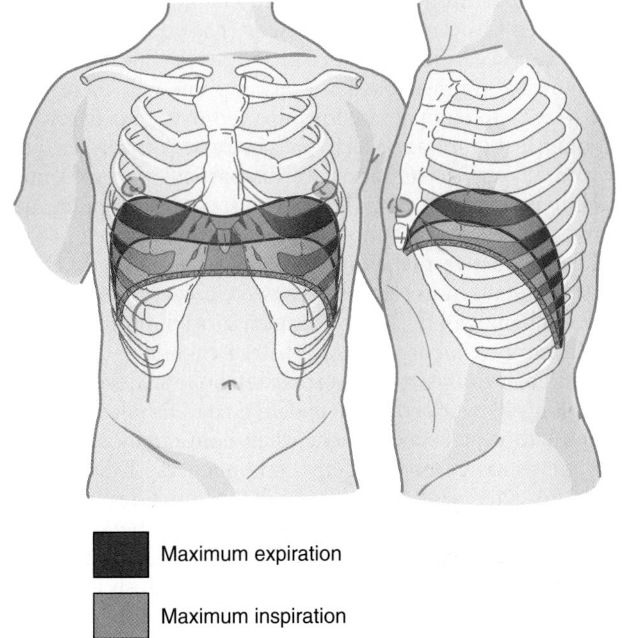

FIG. 30.5 Thoracic and abdominal areas that may be injured with a single stabbing incident.

posts during a fall, arrows during bow hunting, or nails from hydraulic construction nail guns. Clothing fragments, organic materials, and bacteria are often introduced into these wounds, predisposing the patient to significant infection.[148]

APPLIED PATHOPHYSIOLOGY

The body's response to trauma is a global event; multiple processes are initiated at the moment of injury that respond to physiologic insult and promote healing. Compensatory, inflammatory, and hypermetabolic responses occur simultaneously while individual body structures react to injury and the hypoperfusion associated with shock. A comprehensive review of these responses is beyond the scope of this chapter; the reader is referred to Chapter 28 for additional information. This section provides an overview of the role of the physiologic responses to trauma, common physiologic sequelae that occur during the resuscitation phase, and pathophysiology of specific injuries.

Shock

The most common type of shock following trauma is hypovolemic shock from overt hemorrhage; significant third-space fluid losses may also occur from severe burns, large crush injuries, ischemic gut, and GI injuries.[140] Intraperitoneal fluid accumulation can lead to abdominal hypertension and abdominal compartment syndrome, further compromising venous return to the heart and contributing to hypotension.[50] Hyperglycemia and administration of osmotic diuretics also deplete the vascular compartment.[140] Hemorrhagic shock not only results in life-threatening volume depletion, but also leads to inadequate oxygen-carrying capacity associated with red blood cell loss.[140]

Additional types of shock seen in trauma patients are obstructive shock, neurogenic shock, and cardiogenic shock. It is common for hypovolemic shock to occur simultaneously with these other causes of shock. Obstructive shock occurs when blood flow into or out of the heart is obstructed, commonly a result of tension pneumothorax, pericardial tamponade, and abdominal compartment syndrome. Neurogenic shock results when high-level cervical spine injuries transect or compress the sympathetic outflow tracts of the spinal cord, controlling peripheral vascular tone and heart rate (HR). It is not associated with injuries to the brain. Profound hypotension is caused by vasodilation and bradycardia, differentiating neurogenic shock from the other types. Cardiogenic shock occurs after a blunt force bruises the heart. The right ventricle is most often affected because it swings forward in the thoracic cavity and hits the sternum during acceleration injuries. The contused and swollen myocardium is dyskinetic (has poor contractility), and decreased cardiac output results in cardiogenic shock.[16]

Following trauma, oxygen consumption will increase by 15% to 35% to compensate for impaired oxygen delivery.[32,130] Although tachycardia and tachypnea increase both oxygen delivery and oxygen consumption, this is particularly problematic in the hypovolemic trauma patient with cardiac or pulmonary injury. Oxygen consumption is significantly impaired because of failed oxidative metabolism within compromised cells; in late shock, oxygen use drops because cells cannot extract oxygen from hemoglobin (Hgb). Compensatory shunting of blood away from the vital organs exacerbates ischemia in distal tissue beds and contributes to the overall metabolic acidosis.[140]

Prolonged hypoperfusion and hypoxia stimulate multiple inflammatory pathways which, when continually stimulated, have devastating, multisystem consequences. Inflammatory mediators alter vascular and metabolic functions to such a degree that microvascular flow is impaired, metabolic functions become inadequate, and intracellular processes are disrupted. Anaerobic metabolism with profound lactic acidosis is the inevitable result; if they are not reversed, organ failure and death will occur.[78,140]

Systemic Inflammatory Response During Traumatic Shock

Under normal circumstances, a delicate balance exists between proinflammatory and antiinflammatory mediators, or cytokines. Following trauma, a complex inflammatory response is initiated that can overwhelm physiologic reserves. Appropriate and controlled release of inflammatory cytokines contains the insult, prevents bacterial invasion, and promotes healing. However, uncontrolled mediator release (e.g., severe trauma, under resuscitation, or sepsis) results in the systemic inflammatory response syndrome (SIRS). SIRS overwhelms an already compromised host because inflammatory mediators are continuously stimulated, adding to preexisting anaerobic metabolism and perpetuating secondary inflammatory responses. Cytokine release also initiates the immune and coagulation cascades, altering microvascular function, catecholamine release, neutrophil adhesion, chemotaxis, coagulation, and oxygen free radical and protease production.[78,140] Inflammatory mediators contribute to the cardiovascular manifestations of shock as well as end-organ dysfunction,[140] making prompt recognition and treatment of hypovolemia essential for the prevention of severe multisystem complications.

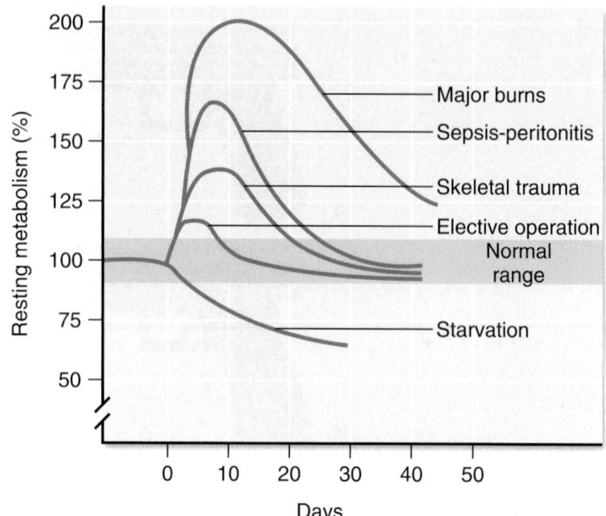

FIG. 30.6 Stress-induced changes in resting metabolic expenditure.

Hypermetabolic Response to Trauma

Following trauma, the body uses endogenous substrates, protein, and fat to support high physiologic demands. Glycogen stores are rapidly depleted because increased demands are coupled with poor intake (e.g., patients unable to ingest or digest food), quickly placing patients into catabolic states. Accelerated catabolic processes (e.g., proteolysis, gluconeogenesis, lipolysis, ketogenesis, and glycogenolysis) occur at a time when the patient needs maximal metabolic support to heal multiple injuries.[82] Basal metabolic rates increase immediately following injury because of increased catecholamine and other hormonal activity, a condition referred to as hypermetabolism. The hypermetabolic response supports survival, minimizes catabolism, and facilitates recovery by providing a constant supply of endogenous carbohydrates, proteins, and fats.[82] During hypermetabolism, the patient's resting energy expenditure may be elevated 120% to 155% above normal during the 10 days following injury (Fig. 30.6).[14,46,69,115] Sustained hypermetabolism results in significant loss of lean body mass and malnutrition, adversely affecting immune function and wound healing, and complicating recovery.[9] However, the ability to establish and maintain a hypermetabolic response to injury positively influences patient outcomes; patients unable to mount or maintain a stress response are likely to die from their injuries.[83,90]

Multiple factors influence the severity and duration of the hypermetabolic response, including the extent of injury, severity of complications, loss of protective barriers to infection, baseline nutritional status, age, and sex.[82] During the first 24 hours following injury, hypoxia, anoxia, and temperature decrease, whereas catecholamines, glucagon, lactate, glucose, and free fatty acids (FFA) increase.[139] The nervous system and inflammatory cytokines (interleukin-1 and tumor necrosis factor) stimulate sustained glucagon, catecholamine, and cortisol release to increase the overall metabolic rate. In addition, catecholamines and cortisol promote lipolysis and the subsequent release of harmful FFAs. (The hypermetabolic response does not occur in patients with spinal cord transection above the level of tissue damage.)[139] The "flow phase" begins when resuscitation is complete and injuries are treated, during which time the previously described responses resolve and physiologic parameters begin to normalize (Fig. 30.7).[139]

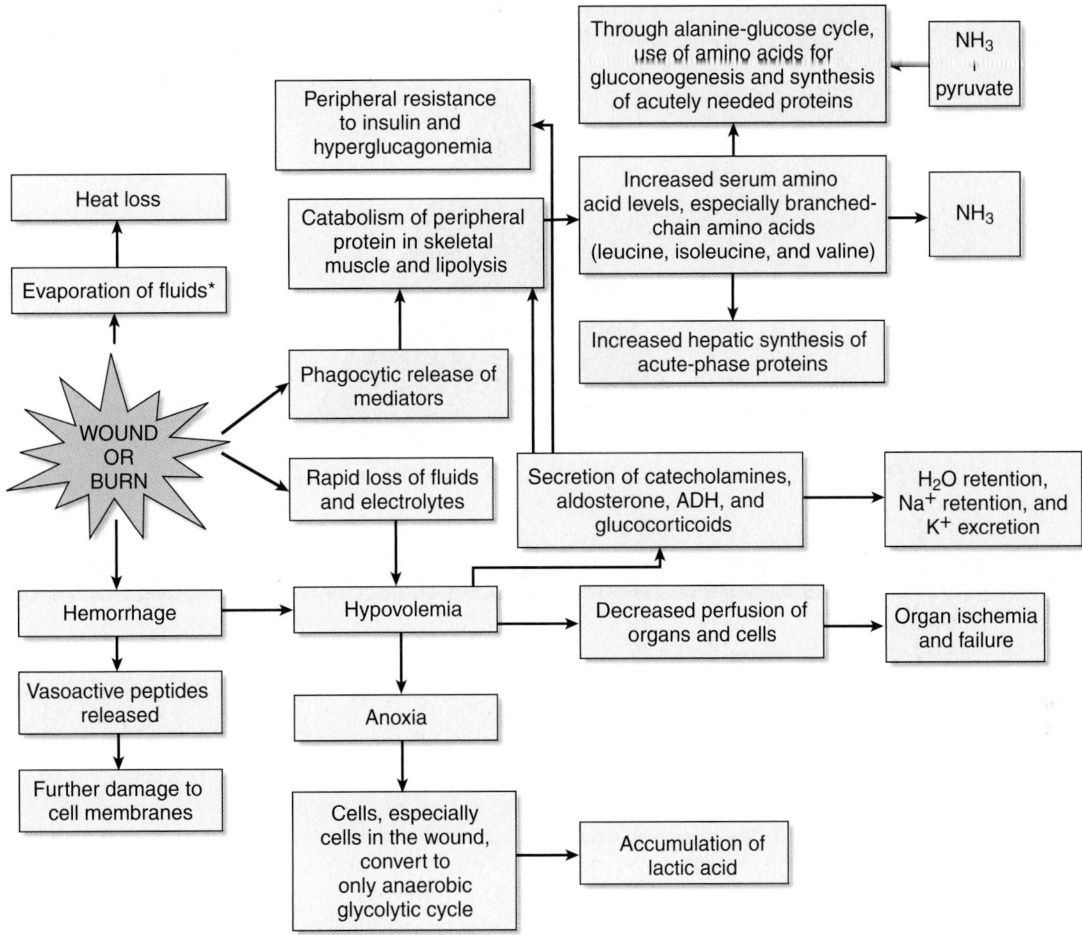

FIG. 30.7 Physiologic and metabolic changes immediately after an injury. *Occurs mainly in patients with extensive burns. *ADH,* Antidiuretic hormone; *NH_3,* ammonia; *Na^+,* sodium; *K^+,* potassium.

Physiologic Sequelae During Trauma Resuscitation

Shock, inflammatory responses, and hypermetabolism following injury contribute to physiologic sequelae common in trauma. These clinical complications add to the physiologic stress in the already compromised patient and can be as difficult to manage as the original injuries themselves. The critical care team must be alert at all times for these complications.

An altogether too common challenge in the critical care phase of trauma care is the lethal triad of hypothermia, acidosis, and coagulopathy. The triad presents early in the patient's course and is not only an indication of the interplay between the inflammatory and coagulation cascades, but is also considered an early sign of physiologic exhaustion.[38] As such, the triad is associated with more complications and high mortality.[29,55,101] Hypothermic trauma patients who are acidotic despite adequate volume resuscitation are prone to coagulopathy.[45] The physiologic consequences associated with each factor have an additive effect, further impairing oxygen delivery and consumption. The physiologic consequence common to each of the three factors is inadequate oxygen delivery to the tissues (Fig. 30.8).

Hypothermia

The causes of hypothermia in trauma are multifactorial and somewhat unique. In normal circumstances, the baseline rate of thermogenesis adequately balances with ongoing heat losses to maintain normal body temperature. The environmental temperature range in which humans can maintain normal body temperature is between 25°C and 30°C. Maintenance of normothermia in a cold environment requires additional oxygen as a substrate for heat production. Impaired oxygen delivery and consumption from hemorrhagic shock in a cool environment overwhelm thermoregulation and result in hypothermia.[62]

Trauma patients become hypothermic simply by being exposed to their environment, as described in Box 30.5. Hypothermia may also be a compensatory response to hemorrhagic shock.[87] During shock it is suggested that poor blood flow to the hypothalamus results in a lowering of the thermoregulatory set point, inhibiting shivering in hypotensive and hypoxic patients.[135]

Another possible explanation for hypothermia is that during refractory hemorrhagic shock, cells have extracted all available oxygen from hemoglobin. This results in inefficient cellular metabolism and lactic acid accumulation, and the stressed, hypoxic cells can neither use oxygen nor do cellular work to produce heat. Lactic acid accumulation in hypothermic and severely injured patients is common and supports this theory.[128]

Several studies show that mortality in trauma patients increases significantly when the core temperature falls below 34°C and that serious hypothermic coagulopathies are present at slightly higher temperatures.[96,124,134,151] Hypothermia in trauma patients has multiple physiologic consequences (see Box 30.5).

Perhaps the most serious consequences of hypothermia in trauma are coagulopathy and cellular hypoxia. These

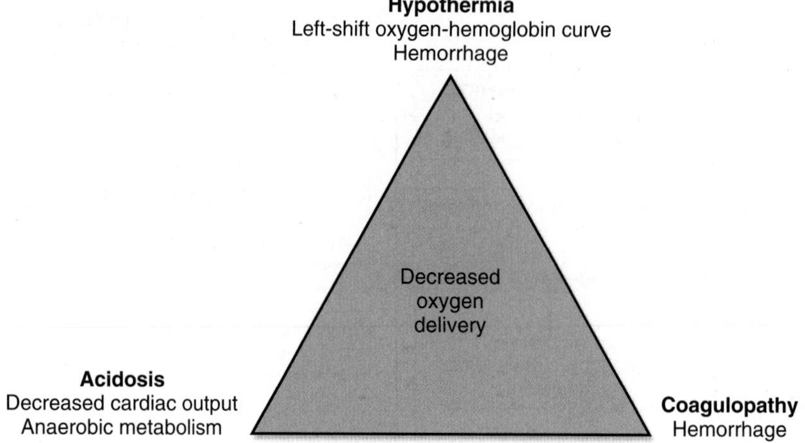

FIG. 30.8 Consequences of hypothermia, acidosis, and coagulopathy.

Box 30.5 Causes and Physiologic Consequences of Hypothermia in Trauma

Causes

Conduction
- Lying on cold examination tables
- Infusion of room temperature or cold resuscitation fluids and blood products
- Application of cold solutions for skin preparation
- Use of room-temperature irrigation solutions
- Cooled ventilator circuit

Convection
- Skin exposure to the environment at the trauma scene
- Ambient air currents moving over the uncovered patient in the emergency department, radiology suite, or operating room
- Ambient air drafts as uncovered patient is moved along hallways

Evaporation
- Exposed internal organs
- Diaphoresis
- Burned patients
- Cooled ventilator circuit

Radiation
- Patient's body temperature higher than room temperature

Medications
- Remove the ability to initiate heat-generating activities such as shivering, pulling on a warm blanket
- Alcohol
- Paralytics
- Sedative agents

Pathophysiologic consequences

Cardiovascular
- Initial increase in blood pressure due to release of catecholamines
- Subsequent decreases in blood pressure and cardiac output
- Increase in heart rate followed by bradycardia when body temperature falls below 32°C
- Increased myocardial workload from increased peripheral vascular resistance
- Increased CVP due to volume shunting from vasoconstriction
- T-wave inversion
- Prolonged PR, QRS, and QT intervals
- Atrial fibrillation
- J wave

Pulmonary
- Increased respiratory rate and drive, followed by a decrease in both when body temperature falls below 32°C
- Decreased hypoxic ventilatory drive
- Increased dead space and worsening $\dot{V}/\dot{Q}$ mismatch
- Increased pulmonary vascular resistance
- Worsening compliance
- Decreased cough and gag reflexes

Box 30.5 Causes and Physiologic Consequences of Hypothermia in Trauma—cont'd

Hematologic

- Decreased leukocyte and platelet counts
- Sequestration of both leukocytes and platelets in liver
- Change in platelet morphology, function, and response time
- Release of thromboplastin
- Increased fibrinolysis
- Increased bleeding due to reduced activity of clotting enzymes
- Hemodilution of coagulation factors due to fluid resuscitation and transfusions of blood products

Metabolic

- Hyperglycemia due to insulin resistance
- Release of catecholamines
- Initial increase in metabolic rate followed by a decrease with profound hypothermia
- Left shift of oxygen-hemoglobin dissociation curve, resulting in decreased oxygen availability at the cellular level
- Combined respiratory and metabolic acidosis

Neurologic

- Confusion, anxiety, poor judgment, psychosis, short-term memory loss, and decreased level of consciousness
- Prolonged neurologic recovery time from anesthesia

Gastrointestinal

- Ileus
- Pancreatitis
- Oliguria
- Delayed hepatic lactate clearance
- Metabolic acidosis from poor renal buffering and excretion of organic acids
- Bacterial translocation from gut, predisposing patient to sepsis

Pharmacologic metabolism

- Increased medication half-life
- Decreased effects of medications on target organs
- Resistance to catecholamines

CVP, Central venous pressure; $\dot{V}/\dot{Q}$, ventilation/perfusion.
From References 48, 60, 61, 122, 123, and 126.

two consequences worsen the situation in the patient who is already hemorrhaging from injuries and has inadequate oxygen delivery. Coagulopathy results in the loss of Hgb and its oxygen-carrying capacity. Cellular hypoxia results in a left shift of the oxygen-hemoglobin dissociation curve, representing an increase in hemoglobin's affinity for oxygen. The Hgb is well saturated, but oxygen is not released to the tissues.[61] The oxygen saturation as measured by pulse oximetry may be excellent, but this does not reflect the fact that the hemoglobin is not releasing oxygen at the cellular level where it is needed the most.[96,124,134,151]

Acidosis

Although respiratory acidosis may occur in trauma (e.g., hypoventilation from brain injury, spinal cord injury, or pulmonary injury), metabolic acidosis is of greater concern because it reflects the patient's degree of oxygen debt and resuscitation status. If the underlying cause of shock is not corrected, acidosis will worsen. Both respiratory and metabolic acidosis can be present in trauma patients with airway compromise or pulmonary injury and hypovolemic shock. Acidosis with a pH of less than 7.20 can cause cardiac irritability, left ventricular failure, poor coronary perfusion, decreased catecholamine responsiveness, altered glucose metabolism, and cerebral swelling.[38,61] If unresolved, acidosis results in cellular death, disruption of cellular membranes, and release of intracellular toxins into the circulation. Cell death leads to organ death, multisystem organ dysfunction, and mortality.[61]

A *washout* phenomenon has been described in which the serum lactic acid (LA) level actually rises despite other resuscitation indicators within normal limits. This is thought to be due to reestablishment of perfusion in previously ischemic tissue beds with mobilization of LA into the general circulation.[38] Metabolic acids, potassium (K^+), polymorphonuclear leukocytes, and other inflammatory mediators enter the circulation and may cause life-threatening hyperkalemia and cardiac dysrhythmias.[131]

Coagulopathy

Hemorrhage is the cause of death in a large percentage of trauma patients.[17,123] The presence of clotting abnormalities is an independent predictor of mortality, even in the presence of other risk factors such as injury severity.[88] Coagulopathic trauma patients who survive are more likely to develop organ dysfunction and have longer critical care stays.[51] A life-threatening coagulopathy is present when the prothrombin time (PT) and activated partial thromboplastin time (aPTT) are more than two times that of laboratory control.[29,33]

Blood loss may be directly due to the injury itself, but several additional factors compound the coagulopathy. Cellular and humoral mediators cause a combination of consumption coagulopathy, excessive fibrinolysis, and activation of inflammatory pathways.[17] Tissue factor, a powerful anticoagulant, is released during massive tissue damage; the brain, mesenteric fat, and long bones are associated with profound clotting abnormalities from tissue factor release.[66,154] Hypothermia, as discussed earlier, causes inactivation of clotting enzymes, platelet sequestration and dysfunction, and increased fibrinolysis. Dilutional coagulopathy is seen when large volumes of crystalloids and red cells are infused without a balanced transfusion of coagulation factors. Consumptive coagulopathy occurs with consumption of clotting factors in excess of supply. Thrombocytopenia is common in patients receiving more than 1.5 times their blood volume in transfusions and exacerbated by consumption of platelets at injury sites.[33,38] Accelerated fibrinolysis destroys clots using plasmin, a proteolytic enzyme that breaks down many coagulation factors and plasma proteins.[85] Coagulopathies via the intrinsic pathways are exacerbated by severe acidosis.[38]

Abdominal Compartment Syndrome

A number of clinical conditions are associated with intraabdominal hypertension and abdominal compartment syndrome (ACS); in trauma patients, ACS can be a clinical consequence of aggressive fluid resuscitation leading to profound tissue edema and accumulation of free fluid within the abdomen. It also can occur from intraabdominal hemorrhage and abdominal packing left in place after surgery.[75,111] ACS is yet another insult in the critically ill trauma patient who often has ongoing blood loss and severe multisystem injuries. In times past, these patients died a dramatic death because they could not be ventilated or perfused due to high abdominal pressure. With today's sophisticated ventilators and rapid infusers, these patients often survive.

Rhabdomyolysis

Rhabdomyolysis is the release of injured skeletal muscle components into the circulation. There are many etiologies for rhabdomyolysis, but those most likely to be associated with trauma involve muscle compression with crush injury, vascular compromise of an extremity, soft-tissue infections, and electrical injuries.

The hallmark of rhabdomyolysis is the release of large amounts of myoglobin into the circulation, threatening kidney function.[89] Acute renal failure (ARF) occurs in 4% to 33% of patients with rhabdomyolysis, with a mortality rate of 3% to 50%.[132,145] ARF occurs from decreased renal perfusion, cast formation with renal tubular obstruction, and myoglobin toxicity. Myoglobin is a pigment protein in skeletal muscle that is filtered by the kidney. Increased levels of circulating myoglobin cause a dark, tea-colored urine from myoglobinuria because the myoglobin molecule is not reabsorbed in the renal tubules.[89]

PATHOPHYSIOLOGY OF SPECIFIC INJURIES

A thorough discussion of the pathophysiology of specific injuries is beyond the scope of this chapter. A brief overview of individual injuries is included here.

Brain and Spinal Cord Injury

Traumatic brain injury (TBI) and spinal cord injury are presented in detail in Chapters 12 and 14.

Facial Trauma

Injuries to the face are often associated with severe brain and cervical spine injuries. The initial concern is for airway patency because profound swelling and significant bleeding are common; hemorrhagic shock can result because facial arteries do not constrict like arteries elsewhere in the body. The extent of injury is directly correlated with the velocity of the face at the time of impact. Penetrating wounds to the face are less common than those from lower-speed, blunt forces.

- Zygoma and orbital floor fractures involve the trigeminal nerve and affect eye movement. Severe comminuted zygomatic fractures cause acute enophthalmos because of severe loss of skeletal support. Entrapment of the facial nerves and muscle within the fracture lines restricts upper eye movement and causes facial paralysis and numbness. Occasionally the zygomatic arch can be displaced downward in such a way that it impedes opening of the mouth.[129]
- Mandibular fractures most frequently involve the body and condylar-subcondylar areas of the mandible. This results in malocclusion of the jaw. Although not directly life threatening, swelling from this and other facial injuries threatens airway patency.[129]
- Le Fort maxillary fractures occur in three consistent patterns after significant blunt injury to the midface. Although not directly life threatening, patients often require tracheostomy for airway control until swelling resolves. LeFort I fractures separate the maxilla from the face; LeFort II fractures are a triangle-shaped separation of the nasomaxillary segment of the midface; and Le Fort III fractures, also known as craniofacial dissociation, are characterized by a complete separation of the midface from the cranium. Fractures of the maxilla, zygomas, and nose are common. Distortion and movement of the midface suggest airway patency is threatened by severe swelling (Fig. 30.9).[129]

Chest Trauma

These injuries may occur as the result of blunt and penetrating trauma and often have extremely high mortality rates. Blunt chest trauma is often associated with severe head and abdominal trauma.

- Pneumothorax, hemothorax, and tension pneumothorax are due to accumulation of air or blood in pleural space, often from a lung laceration, a fractured rib, or a penetrating injury. These injuries may be unilateral or bilateral and, if unresolved, full respiratory and cardiovascular collapse result. Blood loss from hemothorax is not usually from pulmonary tissue but rather from injuries involving thoracic structures, including adhesions between pleura and the chest wall, the main pulmonary vessels, chest wall vessels, internal mammary arteries, and intercostal vessels.[37,47] Hemothorax of 1.5 to 4 L, or at least half of the patient's circulating blood volume, is considered a life-threatening injury because the chest has the capacity to hold most of the patient's circulating volume. It is usually associated with trauma to large systemic blood vessels or mediastinal structures; left-sided hemothorax frequently accompanies injuries to the thoracic aorta.[47]
- Tracheobronchial tears involve injuries at any bronchial level to within an inch of the carina. They are often fatal, with death occurring at the scene. For those who survive to hospital, continuity of the airway may have been maintained by surrounding fascia, or decompensation did not occur until after endotracheal intubation and positive pressure ventilation.[47]
- Rib fractures of the first and second ribs suggest high-energy impact and injury to underlying major vascular structures. Fractures of ribs three through nine are common with blunt trauma and are associated with lung injury; the lower ribs are frequently seen in abdominal trauma. Significant pain associated with these fractures impairs ventilation and secretion clearance, placing the patient at risk for both immediate and

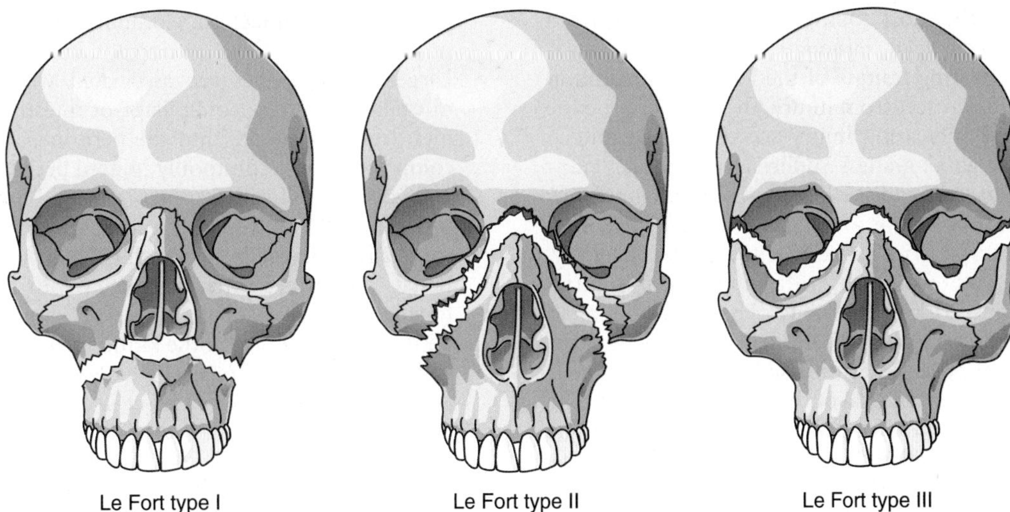

FIG. 30.9 Le Fort fractures. Le Fort type I, transverse fracture of the maxillary process from the base of the maxilla and midface. Le Fort type II, triangular fracture involving the entire maxilla and nasal bones. Le Fort type III, craniofacial-midface disassociation.

prolonged respiratory compromise.[47] A higher mortality is seen in the older adult even with only one or two fractures, when compared with younger patients with the identical injury.[18]

- Flail chest occurs when multiple fractures are present in two or more ribs on one side, resulting in paradoxical movement of the chest wall during respiration. Significant pulmonary contusion usually accompanies this injury. Hypoxia requiring mechanical ventilation is common because of altered dynamics of breathing and increased dead space from severe pain.[47]
- Pulmonary contusion is a direct bruise of the lung followed by alveolar hemorrhage, inflammation, and edema around the injury site. Pulmonary contusions may be unilateral or bilateral and are frequently associated with rib fractures and flail chest. Contusion develops 24 to 48 hours after injury and can cause life-threatening ventilation-perfusion mismatch and shunting. Aggressive fluid resuscitation may exacerbate the contusion because it contributes to pulmonary interstitial edema.[37,47]
- Cardiac tamponade occurs when bleeding into the pericardium or a small pericardial rupture follows high-speed blunt injury or penetrating trauma. The pericardium is a stiff, noncompliant sac; accumulation of more than 100 mL of air or blood into the pericardium produces cardiovascular collapse. The size of the pericardial leak and the opposing intrathoracic pressure determine the speed at which tamponade advances; thus cardiogenic shock may not occur until well after the patient's admission to critical care.[47]
- Thoracic aorta injuries occur when the mobile aorta is torn at points of anatomic fixation with the thoracic spine. The most common sites for tears are at the aortic isthmus, distal to the left subclavian artery, the ascending aorta where it leaves the pericardial sac, and where the aorta enters the diaphragm. Torn vascular intimal and medial layers bleed into the outer adventitial layer, creating a balloon, or pseudoaneurysm. If the expanding pseudoaneurysm is tamponaded by surrounding tissue, the patient may survive long enough to get to definitive repair.[143] Injuries to the thoracic aorta are the leading cause of immediate death from MVC, auto-pedestrian collisions, and falls. Thirty-seven percent of those who survive to hospital die during initial resuscitation or while in surgery, 14% die postoperatively, and 19% of survivors develop paraplegia or sepsis.[103,143]
- Blunt cardiac injuries (BCIs) include small symptomatic contusions, valvular tears, coronary artery dissection, or ventricular rupture. Rarely, BCIs are associated with *blowout* of the ventricular septum or flail injuries to mitral or tricuspid valves. Cardiac contusions are the most common result of BCIs. Dysrhythmias and dyskinesia of the right ventricle cause greatest concern.[143]

Abdominal Trauma

Knowledge of mechanism of injury is essential to determining site of injury. Abdominal injuries occur following both blunt and penetrating mechanisms, with the former being more common. Seldom is only one structure involved; furthermore, abdominal injuries are highly associated with multisystem trauma, particularly TBI and chest injuries. They carry high risk of exsanguination from blunt organ injury as well as transection of major mesenteric vessels. Late mortality from abdominal injuries is frequently caused by infection from spilled abdominal contents into the peritoneum at the time of injury.[75]

- Diaphragmatic injury carries an extremely high morbidity and mortality and is associated with trauma to other chest structures. It is commonly the result of penetrating trauma; blunt injuries occur from sudden rises in intraabdominal pressure (at the time of impact) resulting in a blowout type of injury. It is easier to identify on the left side because the liver *splints* the diaphragm on the right side. Diaphragmatic tears allow intestinal structures to enter the mediastinum impeding respiration, contaminating the mediastinum, and causing severe pain. Late complications are the result of infection and inflammation of the mediastinum and include severe ARDS, pulmonary contusion, and infection.[75]
- Esophageal rupture is most commonly caused by penetrating trauma and usually involves the cervical esophagus; blunt esophageal injuries are extremely rare. Stomach contents escape into the mediastinum, causing severe life-threatening infection, abscess, empyema, fistulas, and ARDS. If definitive treatment is delayed, mortality is very high and is usually related to paraesophageal contamination and infection.[75]

- Splenic injury is the most common injury resulting from blunt trauma mechanism, although it is frequently associated with penetrating trauma of the left upper quadrant. Although the ribs protect from injury, they also may be the source of injury. Increasing injury severity is categorized by grades I through V: grade I implies a subcapsular, nonexpanding hematoma, and grade V describes a completely shattered, hemorrhaging, or avascular spleen. Isolated, low-grade splenic injury carries low mortality risk.[75] Conversely, high-grade injuries associated with multisystem injuries carry much higher risk of mortality. The initial threat to mortality is from uncontrolled hemorrhage.[75,152] Late mortality is a result of postsplenectomy sepsis, which can occur from 1 to 5 years after removal of the spleen. Because of the lifelong threat of infection for patients who have undergone splenectomy, the surgical team will make every effort to salvage, rather than remove, this organ.[75,152]
- Liver injury is a high-risk injury following both blunt and penetrating trauma because of its size and location in the right upper quadrant. Liver injuries carry high mortality rates when associated with other severe injuries. Increasing injury severity is described as grades I through VI: grade I describes a subcapsular, nonexpanding lesion involving a less than 10% surface area that may not require surgery. Grade V describes a large laceration involving at least 50% of a hepatic lobe with injuries to vascular structures around the liver. Grade VI describes complete hepatic avulsion.[75] Life-threatening blood loss is common when major vascular structures (e.g., the portal vein, hepatic artery, or hepatic vein) are involved, and significant coagulopathies develop when the injured liver cannot synthesize coagulation proteins necessary for hemostasis. Hypothermia and refractory acidosis are common challenges in resuscitating patients with high-grade liver injuries.[152] Later complications include ARDS, ATN, infection, hemobilia, hyperpyrexia, biliary fistula, arterial-portal venous fistula, difficulties with nutritional support due to altered liver metabolism, and liver failure.[75,152]
- Pancreatic injuries do not pose early threats to survival unless the splenic artery is involved. Although uncommon, most are caused by penetrating trauma; blunt injuries are the result of direct blows to the epigastric area.[10] Diagnosis of pancreatic injury is difficult and often delayed because of its proximity to other injured organs, particularly the spleen and the C-loop of the duodenum. As a consequence, prolonged spillage of highly caustic pancreatic enzymes contaminates the peritoneum, and subsequent pancreatitis is well established before injury is discovered. Major pancreatic complications such as pseudocyst, abscess, and sepsis are common.[10,75] The profound systemic inflammatory process associated with pancreatitis causes common complications of ARDS and left-sided pleural effusions.[10]
- Small-bowel injuries are common and are caused by penetrating and blunt trauma although they are more common with penetrating mechanisms. There is an especially high incidence of duodenal injures in high-speed MVCs when a patient wearing only a lap belt is thrown violently forward against the restraint and sustains an anterior lumbar spinal fracture (Chance fracture). Blood loss with small-bowel injuries is usually insignificant. However, shearing and penetrating injuries open the intestinal lumen, allowing spillage of intestinal contents into the peritoneum resulting in peritonitis and infection. Complications include hypovolemia secondary to third spacing and infection.[10,75]
- Large-bowel injuries are associated with extremely high mortality as a result of spillage of intestinal contents with high bacterial counts into the peritoneum. The transverse colon is the most commonly injured because of its location, and is associated with lap-belt injuries. Blood loss is usually insignificant. Continued infection from ruptured bowel is surgically managed by a diverting colostomy.[75]
- Renal injuries are often associated with low posterior rib fractures and abdominal injuries. Technically in the retroperitoneum, avulsion of the kidney from its vascular pedicle and ureters is common in high-speed acceleration-deceleration crashes. The kidney is set in motion on its pedicle in relation to the more stable aorta; rotation around the pedicle tears the renal artery or vein and may cause renal artery thrombosis.[133] Renal contusion and fractures are seen with assaults and sports injuries. Penetrating injuries are also common. Ureteral trauma is usually caused by stretching when the kidney is compressed against the lower rib cage and upper lumbar spine.[56] Although not usually a life-threatening injury, mortality increases with injuries that extend deep into the renal cortex and medulla and when ATN and renal failure develop as complications.[133]

Musculoskeletal Injuries

Musculoskeletal injuries involve bone, muscles, tendons, ligaments, cartilage, nerves, blood vessels, and skin. The mechanism of injury is usually blunt trauma associated with MVCs, falls, assaults, and recreational injuries, but penetrating mechanisms seen with gunshot wounds (GSW) can result in significant bone and soft tissue injury. The direction and intensity of energy transferred to bones often influences the injury pattern (e.g., a patient landing on their feet after a fall from a significant height is likely to have fractures in both feet, calcanei, tibias, femurs, pelvis, and spine). Most musculoskeletal injuries are not immediately life threatening, but many require prolonged recovery and result in serious disability. Injuries posing an immediate threat to life include those associated with significant blood loss and shock, such as traumatic amputations and massive pelvic fractures. Late complications and even death can result from infection when bacteria are introduced at the time of injury into open wounds accompanying fractures.[144]

An immediate limb-threatening complication is compartment syndrome, in which severe swelling and bleeding cause increased pressure and ischemic injury within a muscle compartment.[144] Additionally, burns and overly tight external splints can cause compartment syndrome. The immediate inflammation following an extremity injury results in decreased distal blood flow and tissue hypoxia, release of inflammatory mediators, and permeability of capillary walls within the soft tissue. A vicious cycle of edema and ischemia is repeated and threatens limb viability.[114] Muscle ischemia occurs with intracompartmental pressures in excess of 30 to 40 mm Hg; irreversible muscle death occurs with pressures greater than 55 to 65 mm Hg.[114]

Another early complication occurring during resuscitation is fat embolism syndrome (FES). FES occurs in 3% to 4% of patients with long bone fractures related to the release of fat globules and inflammatory free fatty acids into the circulation. It can occur within 1 to 96 hours following injury, causing increased pulmonary capillary permeability, alveolar collapse, and hypoxia (Fig. 30.10).[19,20]

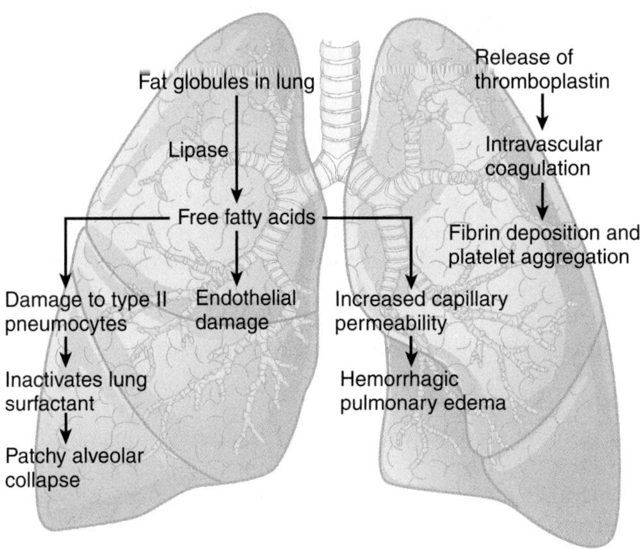

FIG. 30.10 Pathophysiology of fat embolism syndrome.

Extremity Injuries

A fracture in which the skin integrity has not been broken is considered a closed fracture; any fracture associated with a wound is an open fracture. Fractures are classified based on the fracture line, whether the fracture line is oblique or comminuted, the anatomic location of the fracture, the type of displacement, and the position of displacement relative to bony fragments (Fig. 30.11). Open wounds accompanying fractures increase the severity score of the fracture. Bleeding associated with long bone fractures can be significant, with accumulations of blood from 500 mL (humerus fractures) to 3 L (femur fractures) in the surrounding soft tissues.[144]

Dislocation Injuries

Injuries to articulating joints are called dislocations. Joint movement is absent or limited and becomes unstable ("loose") when surrounding ligamentous structures are severely stretched or completely disrupted. Neurovascular structures are often injured, compromising sensation and perfusion of the distal extremity.[144] Subluxation injury occurs when only one portion of the articulating surface of a joint is disrupted. Neurovascular compromise often accompanies subluxation injuries, similar to dislocations.

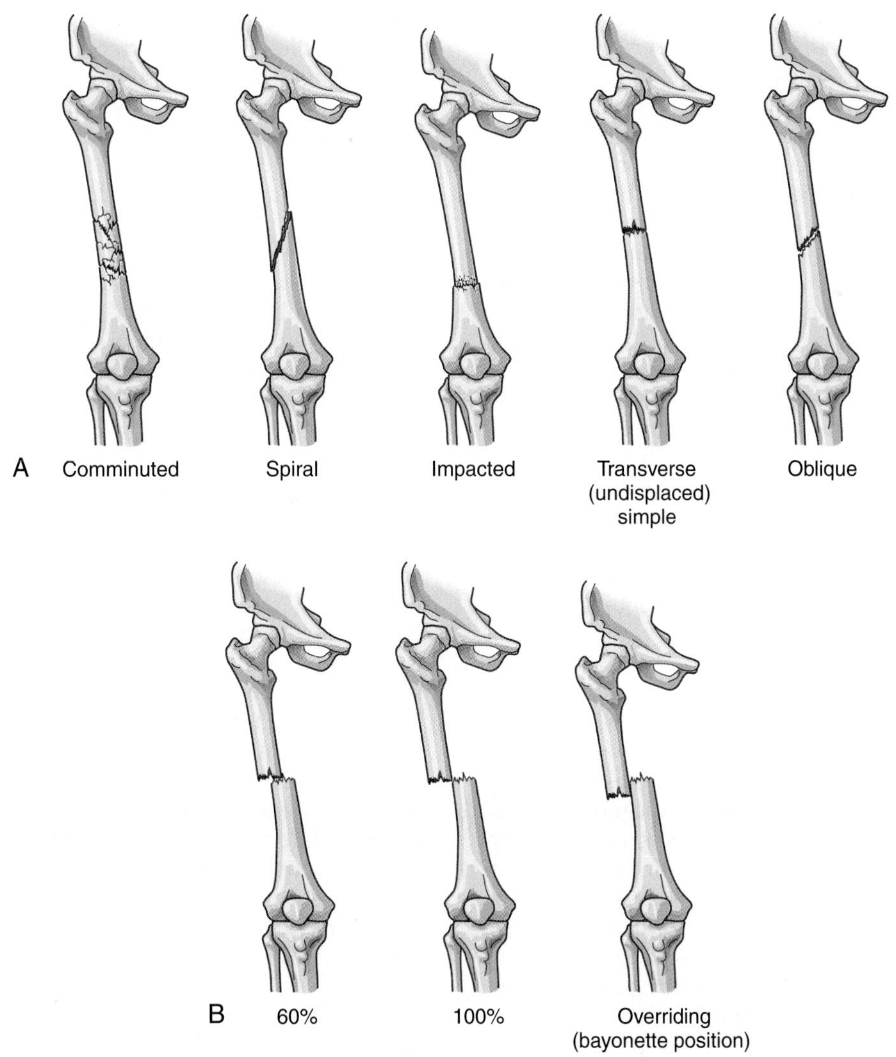

FIG. 30.11 A, Types of fractures. B, Degree of displacement.

Pelvic Ring Fractures

Pelvic ring fractures are the third most common cause of death following MVCs, largely because of associated significant blood loss and injuries to neighboring organs. The pelvis has a large vascular network of collateral arterial and venous structures; disruption of the pelvic ring often involves laceration of multiple vascular structures and subsequent hemorrhage. Up to 6 L of blood can accumulate within the pelvis. The sciatic nerve, which innervates the pelvis and lower extremities, arises from the lumbosacral plexus and passes through the pelvis; injuries result in pelvic pain and decreased sensation in the lower extremities. Both the lower GI tract and genitourinary system have key structures that pass through the floor of the pelvis; fractures often perforate these structures, causing gross contamination and infection. FES (discussed later in this chapter) also contributes to mortality associated with pelvic fractures.[144]

- Whereas they are less common, unstable pelvic ring fractures are accompanied by hemorrhage, genitourinary trauma, sepsis, and chronic pain. Pelvic ring fractures carry the potential for lifelong disability. Mortality from these injuries increases with open wounds and may be as high as 70%, especially if puncture of the rectum or vagina occurs.[153]
- A result of high-energy forces, a common type of pelvic injury occurs when the anterior sacrum is crushed and the anterior pubic rami are displaced. This exerts pressure on the greater trochanter, disrupting the pubic rami into the anterior acetabulum. Even though these injuries are often considered stable, there may be significant soft tissue injury. An open book fracture occurs when a break of the symphysis pubis occurs in conjunction with rupture of the anterior sacroiliac and sacrospinous ligaments causing the anterior components to separate, giving the appearance of an open book.[144] Malgaigne fractures are unstable injuries involving both bone and soft tissue disruption and are the result of significant vertical shearing forces, such as those seen with falls and crush mechanisms. These fractures have the highest morbidity and mortality rates because of the high incidence of associated injuries to GI and genitourinary organs, as well as to vascular and neurologic structures.[144] Immediate complications of these injuries include hemorrhage, pain from muscle spasms and overriding bone ends, decreased venous and lymphatic return, increased swelling, neurovascular injury, and fat embolism. Long-term complications of pelvic fractures include chronic pain, decreased mobility, painful ambulation, and infection.[144]

ASSESSMENT AND INTERVENTION

The primary role of prehospital and emergency department (ED) personnel is to immediately identify life-threatening injuries and intervene accordingly. Multiple diagnostic procedures are performed in the ED to locate and quantify injury, with the goal to transport patient(s) to the operating room or interventional suites within minutes of their arrival. By the time the patient arrives in critical care, major life-threatening injuries have been addressed; their sequelae (e.g., persistent shock, refractory coagulopathy) become the primary focus of care of the critical care team. Although a complete discussion of trauma resuscitation in the ED is not presented here, it is essential that the critical care nurse understand this phase of the patient's care to appreciate the severity of injury, plan for the patient's admission, anticipate complications, and be familiar with diagnostic procedures that may still need to be completed.

Courses in trauma resuscitation such as Advanced Trauma Life Support and Advanced Trauma Care for Nurses teach the use of primary and secondary surveys to guide systematic and organized assessment and treatment of injuries.[5,39] An "ABCDE" mnemonic is used to prioritize care: *a*irway-*b*reathing-*c*irculation-*d*isability-*e*xposure and *e*nvironmental control. In critical care, nurses should perform a primary and secondary survey whenever a patient condition decompensates in order to identify complications and initiate further resuscitation.

Primary Survey

The primary survey identifies life-threatening problems of the ABCDEs, keeping in mind their trauma etiology (Box 30.6). Problems identified during the primary survey are addressed before progressing to the secondary survey.[16,39]

Airway

Airway and breathing are top priorities in trauma resuscitation. Assessment and treatment of the airway are completed while maintaining cervical spine immobilization. Inability to speak suggests a compromised airway. Common causes of airway obstruction include blood, vomitus, loose teeth, other foreign bodies, facial and mandibular fractures, and swelling of the tongue and facial soft tissues. The jaw-thrust–chin-lift maneuver is used to initially open the airway, maintain spinal alignment, and inspect for obstruction. Oral airways may be used in unconscious patients, but in most cases rapid-sequence intubation will be needed to secure a definitive airway. Occasionally, airway problems require surgical management (needle cricothyrotomy or emergent tracheostomy). Surgical airways are performed only for patients in extreme distress with high probability of significant anoxic insult. Performing either of these two procedures in an emergent situation can be challenging because of the presence of severe swelling and blood in the operative field.[16,39]

Breathing

Once the airway is secured, adequate oxygenation and ventilation must be assessed. Breathing is assessed by observing for spontaneous respirations, symmetry, and depth of chest movement, respiratory rate (RR), pattern of breathing, use of accessory muscles, and auscultation of breath sounds. Skin color, thoracic bruises and wounds, chest wall tenderness, and the presence of neck vein distention or tracheal deviation should also be assessed. The patient with effective breathing should receive high-flow oxygen with a nonrebreather mask; the patient with ineffective or absent breathing should be supported with bag-valve-mask ventilation using an attached oxygen reservoir system until endotracheal intubation can be achieved. Life-threatening injuries that compromise breathing (e.g., tension pneumothorax, open pneumothorax, flail chest with pulmonary contusion, and hemothorax) require definitive intervention such as needle thoracostomy and chest tube placement.[16,39]

Circulation

Once the airway and breathing dynamics have been addressed, the circulatory system needs to be assessed. Cardiopulmonary resuscitation is indicated for the trauma patient without a

Box 30.6 Primary Survey for Trauma

Assessments	Interventions
A = Airway With Simultaneous Cervical Spine Stabilization or Immobilization	
While maintaining spinal stabilization:	
• Vocalization	• Position the patient
• Tongue obstruction	• Jaw thrust or chin lift
• Loose teeth or foreign objects	• Suction or remove foreign objects
• Bleeding	• Oro/nasopharyngeal airway
• Vomitus or other secretions	• Cervical spine stabilization
• Edema	• Endotracheal intubation
	• Needle or surgical cricothyrotomy
B = Breathing	
• Spontaneous breathing	• Supplemental oxygen
• Chest rise and fall	• Bag-valve-mask ventilation
• Skin color	• Needle thoracentesis
• General rate and depth of respirations	• Chest tube
• Soft tissue and bony chest wall integrity	• Nonporous dressing taped on 3 sides
• Use of accessory and/or abdominal muscles	
• Bilateral breath sounds	
• Jugular veins and position of trachea	
C = Circulation	
• Pulse rate and quality	• Direct pressure over uncontrolled bleeding sites
• Skin color, temperature, degree of diaphoresis	• Two large-bore intravenous catheters with warmed lactated Ringer's solution or normal saline
• External bleeding	• Infuse fluid rapidly with blood tubing
	• Blood sample for typing
	• Pneumatic antishock garment
	• Pericardiocentesis
	• ED thoracotomy
	• Cardiopulmonary resuscitation and advanced life support measures
	• Blood administration
	• Surgery
D = Disability (neurologic status)	
• Level of consciousness (AVPU)	• Perform further investigation
• Pupils (PERRL)	• Hyperventilation, if indicated

AVPU, Alert, verbal, responsive to painful stimuli, responsive to verbal stimuli; *PERRL*, pupils equal, round, and reactive to light.
From Reference 42.

palpable carotid pulse. Hemorrhage is the most common cause of shock in the trauma patient, although shock can also exist from cardiac tamponade or blunt cardiac injury (cardiogenic shock), tension pneumothorax (obstructive shock), or spinal cord injury (neurogenic shock). The patient is assessed for tachycardia, hypotension, narrowed pulse pressure, poor peripheral pulses, cool and clammy skin, pallor, and any obvious signs of bleeding. An altered mental status, abnormally flattened or distended neck veins, and distant heart sounds are also signs of shock in the trauma patient. Recent military experience has dramatically broadened the approach to management of uncontrolled external bleeding. A variety of hemostatic dressings are available that utilize impregnated gauze to aid hemostasis.[119] Tourniquets have returned to broad use in the civilian setting as a primary means of managing exsanguinating hemorrhage.[70,113,119]

All trauma patients should receive two large-bore peripheral intravenous catheters; patients in shock should also receive at least one large single-lumen central venous catheter for rapid infusion of blood and resuscitation fluids. Fluids should be warmed to prevent hypothermia.[16,39] Uncrossmatched blood (O negative for females, O positive for males) may need to be given for the patient who is exsanguinating and cannot wait for typed and crossmatched blood products.[16,41]

Damage Control Resuscitation

Damage control is a term borrowed from the US Navy and is broadly used in trauma care to indicate any procedure or technique whose aim is to stabilize a patient yet not return them to homeostasis.[7] Damage control resuscitation is utilized in patients with profound and ongoing hemorrhage. Typically damage control resuscitation incorporates three concepts: massive transfusion, permissive hypotension, and immediate hemorrhage control.[7]

Massive transfusion occurs when a patient receives greater than 10 units of red blood cells within 24 hours.[6] Whereas this occurs in a small portion of trauma patients, a massive transfusion frequently involves the coordination of many different providers, ancillary services, and staff. Closely aligned with massive transfusion is the concept of hemostatic resuscitation. Hemostatic resuscitation is resuscitation utilizing blood products in a ratio, approximating whole blood and minimizing the use of crystalloid fluids. Typically, a patient undergoing massive transfusion and hemostatic resuscitation will receive a large volume of blood and blood products in a ratio approaching 1:1:1, red blood cells to plasma to platelets.[74]

Permissive hypotension is the second concept in damage control resuscitation. The principle is straightforward; resuscitate the patient to a systolic blood pressure of 90 mm Hg in order to reduce pressure on a newly formed clot.[63] At a systolic of 90 mm Hg, perfusion is maintained to vital organs while reducing the pressure being exerted upon newly formed platelet plugs or clots. Patients with known or suspected head injury are not candidates for permissive hypotension as the lower blood pressure in combination with elevated intracranial pressure will compromise perfusion to the brain. Permissive hypotension is maintained until the final concept of damage control resuscitation is implemented: immediate hemorrhage control.

Immediate hemorrhage control can be achieved via damage control surgery, which will be discussed further in the chapter, or via interventional radiology. Advances in angiography and transcatheter techniques have led to interventional radiology being an essential partner in the management of traumatic injury.[117,156] Many vascular and solid organ injuries can be successfully managed using angiography alone, sparing patients from an invasive surgical procedure.[117]

Disability

A brief neurologic assessment is performed once the airway, breathing, and circulation have been established and life-threatening injuries have been addressed. It is not practical to perform a thorough exam during aggressive resuscitation, nor is it likely to be accurate. A Glasgow Coma Scale (GCS) score and pupillary size and reaction are all that is needed during initial resuscitation. A head computed tomography (CT) exam is recommended for any patient with a GCS score of 12 or who experiences a decrease in their GCS of more than 2 points.[21] Alcohol and other drugs may affect the pupillary exam as well as the overall neurologic assessment.[16,41] Further neurologic assessment is deferred to the secondary survey.

Secondary Survey

Once life-threatening injuries have been identified and treated, a thorough secondary survey is performed to identify and manage remaining injuries. While a thorough head-to-toe assessment is performed, clothing must be removed, and hypothermia must be prevented by using warmers, warming blankets, and warmed IV fluids.[126] A full set of vital signs are obtained, including BP, HR, RR, and temperature (T); BP should be performed in both arms if the patient sustained trauma to the chest. Electrocardiogram monitoring, pulse oximetry, and end-tidal carbon dioxide (CO_2) monitoring should be initiated.[39]

A gastric tube is placed to prevent aspiration of stomach contents; gastric tubes should not be placed until facial and skull base fractures have been evaluated. Laboratory studies including blood typing, hematocrit (Hct), Hgb, coagulation studies, electrolytes, glucose, blood urea nitrogen (BUN), creatinine (Cr), blood alcohol, toxicology screen; arterial blood gas (ABG), base deficit (BD), or serum LA should be obtained; and blood or urine should be sent for pregnancy tests for female patients of childbearing age.[39]

A full history of the incident is obtained, along with the patient's medical history, if known. Particular attention should be given to the patient's tetanus immunization history, allergies, and preexisting medical conditions. A full head-to-toe assessment, as described in Box 30.7, is performed. Assessment of pain and sedation should also occur, which is often difficult in the confused or unresponsive patient. Of special note, providing analgesia in new trauma patients can be a challenge: although minimizing pain is important, the presence of pain helps identify injuries. During assessment,

BOX 30.7 Secondary Survey for Trauma

E = Expose Patient/Environmental Control (Remove Clothing and Keep Patient Warm)

- Remove clothing
- Provide blankets
- Warming lights

F = Full Set of Vital Signs: Five Interventions: Facilitate Family Presence

- Complete set of vital signs
- Consider the five interventions:
  - Cardiac monitor
  - Pulse oximetry
  - Urinary catheter if not contraindicated
  - Gastric tube
  - Laboratory studies
- Facilitate family presence

G = Give Comfort Measures

- Verbal reassurance
- Touch
- Pain control

H = History

- Mechanism of injury, injuries sustained, vital signs, treatment (MIVT)
- Patient-generated information
- Past medical history

H = Head-to-Toe Assessment

- Head and face
  - Inspect for wounds, ecchymosis, deformities, drainage from nose and ears, assess pupils.
  - Palpate for tenderness; note bony crepitus, deformity.
- Neck
  - Remove the anterior portion of the cervical collar to inspect and palpate the neck. Second team member stabilize the patient's head while the collar is removed and replaced.
  - Inspect for wounds, ecchymosis, deformities, and distended neck veins.
  - Palpate for tenderness; note bony crepitus, deformity, subcutaneous emphysema, and tracheal position.
- Chest
  - Inspect for breathing rate and depth, wounds, deformities, ecchymosis, use of accessory muscles, paradoxical movement.
  - Auscultate breath and heart sounds.
  - Palpate for tenderness; note bony crepitus, subcutaneous emphysema, and deformity.
- Abdomen and flanks
  - Inspect for wounds, distention, ecchymosis, and scars.
  - Auscultate bowel sounds.
  - Palpate all four quadrants for tenderness, rigidity, guarding, masses, and femoral pulses.
- Pelvis and perineum
  - Inspect for wounds, deformities, ecchymosis, priapism, and blood at the urinary meatus or in the perineal area.
  - Palpate the pelvis and anal sphincter tone.
- Extremities
  - Inspect for ecchymosis, movement, wounds, and deformities.
  - Palpate for pulses, skin temperature, sensations, tenderness, and deformities; note bony crepitus.

I = Inspect Posterior Surfaces

- Maintain cervical spine stabilization and support injured extremities while the patient is log-rolled.
- Inspect posterior surfaces for wounds, deformities, and ecchymosis.
- Palpate posterior surfaces for tenderness and deformities.
- Palpate anal sphincter tone (if not performed previously).

From Reference 43.

smaller doses of analgesics and sedatives may be given; full doses of these agents then can be given following identification of all injuries.[15]

Finally, additional diagnostic tests may be performed as part of the secondary survey to gather more information about injury location and severity. The chest radiograph will identify lethal pulmonary injuries and correct placement of chest tubes and central venous catheters. A *f*ast *a*bdominal *s*onography for *t*rauma (FAST) assesses for bleeding in the hemodynamically unstable patient with likely abdominal injuries (Fig. 30.12).[65,97,110] A pelvic radiograph will demonstrate any potentially life-threatening pelvic fractures. CT scans of the head, spine, and thoracoabdominal cavity will be performed to identify or rule out injury. Magnetic resonance imaging (MRI) scans to identify spinal cord injury must be delayed until the patient is completely hemodynamically stable.[21] Extremity and facial films are taken once the patient is stable and considered safe to spend the several hours in radiology to obtain all of the requested radiographs at one time.[79]

Early interventions for non–life-threatening injuries may be initiated during the secondary assessment. These basic interventions may include applications of ice, splinting and elevation of fractures, administration of tetanus toxoid, and provision of emotional support and comfort. Repeated assessments of vital signs are important to determine resuscitation status and the need for additional interventions and diagnostic workup.[39] Following initial stabilization and identification of injuries, the patient may be admitted to critical care for continued resuscitation or taken to surgery or interventional suites.

Definitive surgical repair is frequently not performed on patients during their first operative procedure. *Damage control surgery* is a term applied to any initial surgical procedure performed to control life-threatening hemorrhage and contamination.[125] These abbreviated operations are performed in patients with unresolved metabolic failure characterized by severe hypothermia, persistent acidosis, and coagulopathy refractory to surgical control. Time is of the essence because these patients are more likely to die from prolonged surgery and intraoperative metabolic failure than from the failure to perform definitive organ repairs.[45]

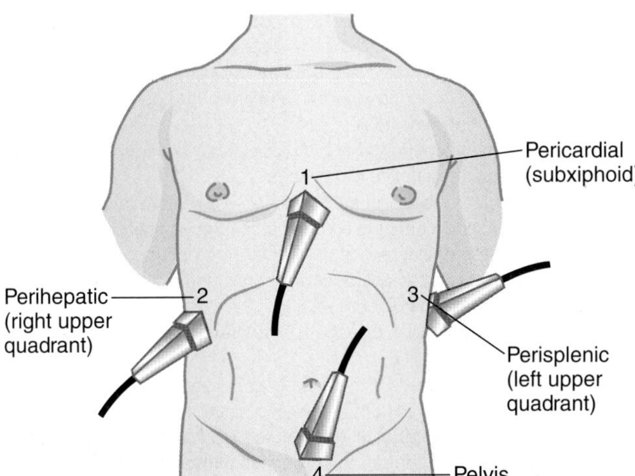

FIG. 30.12 Differentiation of fast abdominal sonography for trauma (FAST) and diagnostic peritoneal lavage (DPL) for abdominal trauma. A bedside FAST scan rapidly assesses the pelvis, pericardium, perisplenic, and perihepatic regions for fluid (blood) accumulation. Easily repeated in the event of sustained hypotension, it identifies location and volume of fluid but does not differentiate type of fluid. FAST is unreliable in patients with morbid obesity, multiple abdominal adhesions, ascites, or subcutaneous emphysema. (From References 75, 90, 97, 131, and 155.)

There are three stages of damage control.[45,125] During the first stage the operation is limited to control of hemorrhage and contamination. Conservative management of solid organ injuries may occur, along with resection without reanastomosis for major GI injuries and control of major vascular injuries in the trunk and extremities. Exploratory laparotomy, exploration of a hemorrhaging extremity, and packing of organs or spaces to control coagulopathy are also performed during the first stage.

The second stage occurs in the critical care unit, where priorities include vigorous rewarming, restoration of normal cardiovascular function, correction of clotting abnormalities, and supportive care for stunned lungs and kidneys. During the third and final stage of damage control, definitive surgical repair, identification of previously missed injuries, and incision closure occur. Trauma patients may return to surgery many times for follow up to their initial operation. Each visit to the OR presents additional physiologic stresses from anesthesia and associated hypotension.[45,125]

Assessment and Intervention of Specific Injuries

Assessment and intervention of specific organ injuries involves multiple components, including the initial physical exam, laboratory results, and diagnostic procedures, followed by surgical and nonsurgical interventions. A detailed discussion of every injury is beyond the scope of this text but is summarized in Table 30.3.

EARLY CRITICAL CARE RESUSCITATION

On arrival in critical care, the patient is settled and priorities for continued resuscitation are established. A quick primary and secondary survey should be done on admission to establish a critical care baseline and allow comparison to the ED assessment. Clinical assessment of the patient's color, skin temperature, vital signs, urine output, wound and drain output, and bleeding should be frequently repeated.

Despite aggressive resuscitation in the ED and OR, during which time multiple liters of fluid and units of blood and blood components may have been given, the patient can still be in shock and require additional fluid resuscitation. Vasopressors may be added if the patient remains hypotensive despite adequate fluid resuscitation. Chapter 28 includes a detailed discussion of the use of crystalloids, colloids, and vasopressors for the resuscitation of hemorrhagic, neurogenic, and obstructive shock. Chapter 26 discusses the use of blood and blood components during the massive transfusion scenarios common in trauma. Frequent monitoring of tests such as lactate and base deficit will help reveal the patient's metabolic state and to what extent that may be due to ongoing hemorrhage. The patient will return to the OR for surgical control of bleeding for persistent hypotension caused by ongoing hemorrhage.

Using Hemodynamic Monitoring to Guide Resuscitation

Identifying optimal volume status and preload is difficult; a comprehensive review of hemodynamic monitoring in shock was addressed in Chapter 28 and will be discussed here only as it pertains to trauma. Traditional filling pressures such as central venous

TABLE 30.3 Assessment and Intervention of Specific Organ Injuries

Assessment	Intervention
Brain Injury	Addressed in Chapter 12
Spinal Cord Injury	Addressed in Chapter 14
Facial Injury Highly associated with brain and cervical spine injuries. Initial concern is for airway patency, requiring intubation and mechanical ventilation until swelling resolves and operative repair complete. Anticipate massive facial swelling; patient may be unrecognizable to family. • Zygoma and orbital floor fractures: ecchymosis, tenderness along lower orbital rim, enophthalmos, and decrease in the height of the zygoma compared with the opposite side. Palpate for irregularities of the supraorbital and infraorbital ridges, depression of the zygomatic arch. Possible restriction in upper eye movement from entrapment of facial muscle in fracture line and associated damage to facial nerve. Assess visual acuity, pupillary response, full range of eye movement, and conjunctiva for hemorrhage or ruptured globe. • Mandibular fractures: assess for pain, sublingual hematoma, offset of the bite, inability to open or close the jaw, pain with chewing. • Le Fort maxillary fractures: assess for facial asymmetry, swelling, and ability to breathe through the nose. Palpate for crepitus, tenderness, and irregularity along bony prominences. Gently manipulate the maxilla to assess for abnormal motion. Epistaxis and/or CSF may be present. Alterations of vision, smell, facial sensation should be assessed. Evaluate range of motion to determine cranial nerve involvement. Diplopia or dysconjugate gaze also may be present.	• Priorities of care are to protect the airway and stop hemorrhage. If injuries are not immediate threats to airway, breathing, and circulation, definitive operative repair is delayed. • Photographs of the patient can help guide the surgeons during facial reconstruction. • Tracheostomy is often required. • Fractures are repaired using fixation devices, plates, and screws. Soft tissues are repaired with muscle, adipose, and vascular grafts. • If the jaws are wired, wire cutters and suction should be kept at the bedside to clear the airway and mouth in the event of vomiting. • Head of the bed should be elevated to help minimize swelling. • Because the face so strongly influences self-image, provision of psychological support is essential to help patients tolerate the emotional sequelae to their injury.
Chest Injuries A general inspection of the chest will help focus detailed assessment for specific injuries. Important to fully expose the chest to adequately assess for injuries. Observe and palpate all surfaces, looking for contusions, steering wheel marks, seatbelt marks, open wounds, bony asymmetry. Palpate for crepitus and unstable bone fragments. Assessment for upper abdominal bruising and wounds is necessary because organs extend to both compartments. • Pneumothorax, hemothorax: respiratory distress or dyspnea, use of accessory respiratory muscles, loss of breath sounds on the affected side, increased tympany on the affected side of pneumothorax, dullness to percussion with hemothorax. Patient may be anxious or confused. Cyanosis is a late sign of impaired oxygenation and ventilation. Subcutaneous emphysema over the chest wall may be palpated. Pain may be present from associated rib fractures. Decrease in oxygen saturation. ABGs reflect a fall in Pao_2 and a rise in $Paco_2$. A CXR is required to definitively determine whether blood or air occupies the pleural space. Signs and symptoms of hypovolemic shock with massive hemothorax (1.5–4 L of intrathoracic blood loss). Both can progress to tension pneumothorax unless treated. • Tension pneumothorax: same as for simple pneumothorax or hemothorax, but has progressed to the point of cardiopulmonary collapse. Early signs may be masked by shock and other injuries until significant tension pneumothorax has developed. Neck veins distended unless the patient is profoundly hypovolemic. Breath sounds decreased bilaterally, tracheal deviation, hypotension, tachycardia. CVP, PA, and PAOP will be elevated with dampened waveforms. If the patient is mechanically ventilated, high inspiratory pressure and low exhaled volume alarms will sound. • Tracheal bronchial tears: dyspnea, hemoptysis, mediastinal subcutaneous emphysema, airway obstruction, difficulty with intubation, pneumothorax unresolved after chest tube insertion, tension pneumothorax. If chest tube present, persistent pleural air leak will be noted in the drainage collection unit; increases in amount of bloody drainage or size of air leak require immediate notification of the provider. CXR demonstrates early and significant atelectasis from blood and secretions obstructing the bronchus. Air embolism is manifested by sudden cardiovascular collapse without signs of bleeding and a change in level of consciousness. • Rib fractures. • Simple, single fractures: pain aggravated by breathing and coughing, tenderness to palpation over fracture site.	• High-flow oxygen via nonrebreathing mask or bag-valve-mask device. Airway support and intubation may be required. • Emergent decompression accomplished with insertion of 14- to 16-gauge needle into pleural space between 2nd and 4th intercostal space. • Additional chest tubes may be required if ventilation does not improve; bilateral chest tubes are quickly placed in severely compromised patients even before the specific side of injury is identified. • Patient may require surgery if bleeding is excessive without signs of stopping. Post insertion CXR identifies placement of the tube and whether the lung(s) have expanded. • Following placement, continually assess respiratory effort (if unintubated) or ventilator inspiratory pressures and exhaled tidal volumes (if intubated) for reaccumulation of pneumothorax, hemothorax, or tension pneumothorax. • Medicate patient for pain during insertion and afterward because chest tubes are extremely uncomfortable. • Chest tube dressing according to hospital policy and procedure. Document amount and characteristics of drainage. • Airway is obtained with endotracheal intubation with a standard ETT or tracheostomy. Double-lumen ETTs allow double lung ventilation: the uninjured lung is ventilated while ventilation to the affected lung is blocked. • Persistent pneumothorax, tension pneumothorax, and mediastinal air may require additional chest tube placements. • Care must be taken to not dislodge the ETT to prevent hypoxia, asphyxia, or reinjury of the bronchus. • Thoracotomy may be indicated if there is no air movement. • Diagnostic bronchoscopy will identify size and location of injury and determine needed repairs. Surgical repair is required for larger tears; small tears can be managed by stenting the bronchus with an ETT so that air movement is distal to the site of the tear. • Tension on postoperative incisions must be avoided; use gentle suctioning and manipulation of the head and neck. • If air embolus suspected, patient should be placed in Trendelenburg position to facilitate collection of air in the left ventricle; the nurse should prepare to assist with cardiocentesis or thoracotomy for control of the air leak. • Ensure that airway is patent and breathing is adequate; support as necessary as previously described. All rib fractures require good pain control, which may include intercostal nerve blocks, intrapleural narcotic administration, patient-controlled analgesia, and epidural analgesia. A TENS unit also may be applied to decrease pain. Adequate analgesia is essential so that the patient tolerates the aggressive pulmonary care needed to prevent atelectasis and pneumonia.

TABLE 30.3 Assessment and Intervention of Specific Organ Injuries—cont'd

Assessment	Intervention
• Complicated fractures with multiple fractures or underlying lung injury: severe chest wall pain, pneumothorax, hemothorax, atelectasis from decreased cough and accumulation of secretions. Associated injuries to liver and spleen with lower rib fractures. Upper rib fractures associated with clavicular fractures and neurovascular neck structures. • Flail chest: common triad of symptoms includes severe pain with respiration, accumulation of secretions, and ineffective ventilation from paradoxical movement (e.g., asymmetrical chest wall movement during respiration). Respiratory distress, tachypnea, decreased oxygen saturation, hypoxia, respiratory acidosis, tachycardia, cyanosis, and crepitus. • Pulmonary contusion: during initial resuscitation, there may be respiratory distress, PAO_2 less than 60 mm Hg on room air, infiltrates on CXR, and bloody sputum. In critical care, CXRs show persistent patchy infiltrates and the sputum may have old blood clots, or fresh blood. Wheezing may be evident, along with increased work of breathing. If the patient is mechanically ventilated, pulmonary compliance worsens, inspiratory and peak airway pressures increase, and Pao_2 falls despite appropriate ventilator changes. • Cardiac tamponade: chest bruising and mechanism of injury suggest potential for immediate or delayed tamponade. Symptoms include distended neck veins, hypotension, narrowed pulse pressure, pulsus paradoxus, flattened hemodynamic waveforms, and rapidly falling cardiac output despite resuscitation. • Thoracic aorta injuries: associated findings suggestive of these injuries include a pulse deficit in extremities, particularly the left arm; hypotension unexplained by other injuries, upper extremity hypertension compared with lower extremities, sternal pain, precordial or interscapular systolic murmur, hoarseness, dyspnea, or respiratory distress, and lower extremity neuromuscular or sensory deficit. CXR demonstrates a widened mediastinum and requires confirmatory angiogram. Some institutions use a dynamic helical CT scan as the confirmatory test because it carries less risk than angiography. Following surgery or stenting, graft failure may present with increased bloody chest tube drainage, sudden hypotension, and high-pressure alarms on the ventilator. Monitor for postoperative complications such as paraplegia, bowel ischemia, and renal failure because these common complications are a result of aortic obstruction from the dissection or cross-clamping of the aorta during surgery. • Blunt cardiac injury: a history of blunt trauma to the chest, presence of chest wall bruising, and fractures of the sternum and ribs raise the index of suspicion for BCI; 12-lead ECG shows abnormalities in only half of patients with BCI. There is no definitive test for BCI; elevations in cardiac enzymes, particularly the CK-MB and troponin, may be present in some patients, although the literature does not strongly support serial monitoring of these enzymes. Continuous ECG monitoring and close clinical observation are necessary for symptomatic ventricular dysrhythmias and conduction defects. Echocardiogram or multigated angiography may detect cardiac wall movement abnormalities with low SV and EF. Chest pain may mimic angina and be difficult to differentiate from chest wall tenderness.	• Mechanical ventilation may be required if underlying pulmonary injuries are present. • Flail chest injuries require definitive airway control, adequate analgesia, and oxygen. • Stabilization of the flail segment can be accomplished by placing the patient on the injured side, but is contraindicated if spinal injuries have not been ruled out. Internal "splinting" of the fractures is achieved using positive pressure ventilation. Internal fixation to stabilize the fracture is rarely required, but if necessary is accomplished by wiring bone fragments together or inserting metal plates. • Sedation and analgesia may be required in order to synchronize respiratory effort with the ventilator cycle and prevent unnecessary movement of the fractures. • Aggressive pulmonary care to include postural drainage, light percussion, and suctioning is necessary to prevent atelectasis and ventilator-associated pneumonia. • Oxygen therapy may be adequate initially, but early mechanical ventilation is required for adequate gas exchange. Severe contusions may require high-frequency ventilation or inverse I:E ventilation to minimize secondary inflammatory injury from barotrauma. • Aggressive fluid resuscitation necessary to achieve hemodynamic stability has been associated with severity of pulmonary contusion. Continued fluid administration should be carefully guided by monitoring of clinical and hemodynamic parameters in patients with persistent shock and pulmonary contusion. • Meticulous pulmonary care is needed to clear the lungs of bloody secretions, clots, and pieces of dead tissue. • Continued monitoring of oxygen saturation, blood gases, capnography, and pulmonary compliance guides subsequent ventilator management. • In the case of sudden or progressive decompensation, emergent needle pericardiocentesis may be required in the critical care unit. Following this, the patient will be taken to surgery for thoracotomy for identification and repair of the source of bleeding. • An emergency pericardiocentesis tray should be kept at the bedside for any patient at high risk for tamponade (e.g., high-force blunt injury to the sternum, penetrating trauma involving the myocardium, patients who had pericardotomy during their initial surgery). • Rupture requires initial resuscitation of the ABCs and treatment of other life-threatening injuries. Massive fluid and blood resuscitation is often required. • Dissecting injuries may require aggressive resuscitation, but if surgery is delayed, strict medical control of the blood pressure to keep MAP under 90 mm Hg is necessary because hypertension extends the dissection. • Surgery or stenting is required to treat the aneurysm, and cardiopulmonary bypass is often used. • Postoperative critical care management includes continued resuscitation and blood pressure control and monitoring for multisystem complications if the patient is in shock for an extended period. Invasive hemodynamic monitoring, frequent ABGs, lactic acid and/or base deficit, hematocrit, and coagulation tests should be drawn frequently to guide resuscitation. • Support of oxygenation and ventilation should be provided as indicated by the patient's condition. • Dysrhythmias are treated according to ACLS standards. • SV and EF may require treatment with dopamine, dobutamine, and digitalis. • Care must be taken to avoid overresuscitation with fluids because this may cause right ventricular dilation, which adversely affects contractility.
Abdominal Injury Knowledge of mechanism of injury is essential for identifying injuries. A common preventable cause of death is unidentified abdominal trauma associated with severe head and chest injuries. Diagnosis of abdominal injury is made by combining physical signs and symptoms with FAST in unstable patients (see Fig. 30.12) and abdominal CT scan in hemodynamically stable patients.	• Support respiratory function and hemodynamics as indicated. Care must be taken for chest tube placement on affected side to avoid perforation of the abdominal organs and contamination of the chest with intestinal contents. Emergent surgical repair is usually required, although repair of right-sided tears may be deferred in patients with stable hemodynamic and respiratory status.

Continued

TABLE 30.3 Assessment and Intervention of Specific Organ Injuries—cont'd

Assessment	Intervention
• Diaphragmatic injury: respiratory distress, decreased breath sounds on the affected side, auscultation of bowel sounds in the chest, hemodynamic instability, difficulty in passing gastric tube, and chest pain. CXR may show stomach or loops of bowel in the chest field. Often complicated by severe ARDS, pulmonary contusion, and infection. Identification of right-sided rupture often delayed as liver covers the diaphragmatic tear. • Esophageal rupture: acute signs include respiratory distress, CXR infiltration, and pain at the site of injury that may radiate to the neck, chest, shoulders, or abdomen, dysphagia, and intraperitoneal fluid or air. CXR changes and signs of sepsis (fever, elevated WBC) may be first indications of a small esophageal rupture; therefore, a high index of suspicion for esophageal rupture is important if the mechanism of injury suggests a possibility of this injury. • Splenic injury: LUQ pain, Kehr's sign (referred shoulder pain), and pain around the injury site. Hemodynamic instability may be present if bleeding is not contained within the subcapsular space. Diagnostic tests include FAST scan for unstable patients and abdominal CT scan for stable patients. • Liver injury: abdominal pain, distention, bruising over RUQ, and hemodynamic instability from hemorrhagic shock. Lower right rib fractures may be present. Frequent hematocrit and coagulation tests are essential if nonoperative management is chosen and postoperatively if surgery was required. • Pancreas injury: not usually an immediately life-threatening issue unless splenic artery is involved. Symptoms may be delayed for 24–72 hours until leakage of pancreatic fluids and bile cause fever, elevated WBC, a continued need for fluid support, and abdominal pain. Continued postoperative assessment for development of pancreatitis is important for early management of sepsis. • Small and large bowel injuries: knowledge of mechanism of injury is an important guide in locating injury. Predominant finding is abdominal pain with signs of peritonitis, but this may be delayed if injury is subtle. FAST scan is not sensitive to bowel injuries, but DPL is very sensitive to the presence of WBC, bacteria, and intestinal contents suggestive of disruption of bowel integrity. Postoperative monitoring includes observation for sepsis, fistula formation, small bowel obstruction, suture line breakdown, bowel ischemia, and short-gut syndrome. • GU injuries: associated with complex or open pelvic fractures. Bleeding at the urinary meatus; genital bruising and swelling; flank, abdominal, and lumbar rib pain; and flank mass. Palpation over the flanks or suprapubic region may indicate extravasation of blood or urine. Inability to void voluntarily or place an indwelling catheter suggests lower urinary tract injuries. Evaluation for vaginal tears should be deferred until bleeding from severe pelvic fractures has stopped because positioning of the legs may result in exsanguinating blood loss. Gross hematuria correlates with lower urologic injury; microscopic hematuria suggests minor injury and may not require further diagnostic workup. • Major renal injuries present with palpable flank mass, gross hematuria, hemorrhagic shock, bruising over lower ribs, abdominal tenderness, or microscopic hematuria. • Radiographic studies include KUB radiograph, intravenous pyelogram, retrograde urethrogram, cystogram, ultrasound, renal angiography, and CT scan. Reabsorption of urine in patients with bladder rupture results in hyperkalemia, hypernatremia, uremia, and acidosis.	• Support of hemodynamic and pulmonary function. Emergent surgical repair is indicated. Continued observation for and management of infection. Mechanical ventilation may be required if mediastinitis has resulted from a tear in the upper esophagus. • Low-grade splenic injuries may not require surgery when close observation in critical care for at least 24 hours is an option. When surgery is needed, efforts to salvage the spleen by packing or resection are made to preserve long-term immunocompetence. In the case of life-threatening hemorrhage from multiple abdominal sources, the spleen will be removed as a quick fix to control a known source of bleeding while other abdominal sources are identified. Vaccinations for postsplenectomy sepsis are required after the patient transfers to acute care and before discharge from the hospital. • Every effort is made to not take the patient to surgery for liver injury alone because mortality risk increases simply by having surgery. A transfusion threshold of 4 to 6 units of PRBCs in 24 hours is often the decision criterion for surgery. Aggressive fluid, blood, and blood component resuscitation with warming measures is indicated pre- and postoperatively for hemodynamically unstable patients. During surgery, packing or resection may be required to control hemorrhage. Multiple trips to the OR may be required before bleeding is stopped and packs are removed. • Surgical debridement, bleeding control, resection, and placement of drains to manage pancreatic fluids are required. Distal pancreatectomy or pancreatic duodenectomy may be needed for major injuries. Postoperative management includes pulmonary and hemodynamic support as indicated by the patient's condition. • Patients are taken to surgery for exploratory laparotomy if bowel injury is suspected for debridement, primary closure, and ligation of bleeding vessels. Resection is warranted if tears are multiple or are in proximity to each other, for massive destruction, and for significant mesenteric vascular injury, causing ischemia to distal bowel. Diverting colostomy or ileostomy may be required. Antibiotics are essential. Enteral feeding may be initiated if feeding tube can be placed well below the injury site. • Medical management varies widely and is dependent on location of injury. Definitive reconstruction of injuries is deferred until after the patient is stable from other life-threatening injuries. • Catheterization should be avoided if blood is present at the urinary meatus. Only one catheterization attempt should be made in patients with suspected GU trauma; if unsuccessful, a urologist should be consulted. Catheters or stents may be placed by a urologist. Suprapubic catheter may be required to divert urine from the injury if a catheter cannot be placed. Infection must be prevented with antibiotic coverage for both gram-positive and gram-negative bacteria.
Orthopedic Injuries	
• Fractures: signs and symptoms of fractures include pain, bruising, swelling, and changes in movement and distal sensation. Angulation, shortening, deformity, crepitus, muscle spasm, open wounds, and abrasions also may be present. Changes in color and decreases in peripheral pulses and capillary refill time indicate involvement of vascular structures. Hemorrhagic shock may accompany femur and pelvic fractures. Diagnostic studies include anterior and posterior plain x-rays. Inlet and outlet views are done for pelvic ring fractures. • Traumatic amputations: signs of hemorrhagic shock are the hallmark presentation of amputations along with pain. Assess for wound infection. Postoperative assessment following reimplantation involves monitoring of color, temperature, swelling, bleeding, and sensation of the affected extremity.	• Long bone fractures require initial immobilization with splints, elevation, and application of ice packs to minimize swelling. Surgery for debridement and placement of external fixation devices is delayed until after the patient is hemodynamically stable. • Pelvic fractures with severe hemorrhage may require PASG, external wrapping of sheets around the pelvis, or external fixation to control bleeding. Definitive control of hemorrhage is most often achieved via angiographic embolization. • Antibiotics are indicated for any open wound or fracture requiring open fixation. • Hemodynamic support, as indicated, for life-threatening hemorrhage associated with orthopedic injury.

TABLE 30.3 Assessment and Intervention of Specific Organ Injuries—cont'd

Assessment	Intervention
• An early complication of orthopedic injuries that occurs even during resuscitation is compartment syndrome. Compartment syndrome presents as pain disproportionate to the injury and unrelieved by narcotics, numbness, and firmness to palpation. Early stages may present with rubor and bounding pulses, compensatory attempts to improve local blood flow. Coolness of the extremity, pallor, and decreased movement also may be noted. Late signs include loss of distal pulses and paralysis. When compartment syndrome is suspected or likely, slit and wick catheters connected to pressure monitoring systems may be placed within the muscle compartments to monitor pressures. • FES presents with sudden pulmonary and cardiovascular collapse. There is a transient appearance of petechiae about the trunk, face, mucous membranes, and conjunctiva. A rapid fever spike up to 40°C is a hallmark sign of FES. Lipuria (fat in the urine) and hematuria may be present. Thrombocytopenia as low as 50,000/mm^3 reflects platelet aggregation around fat globules. The diagnosis of FES cannot be made with laboratory tests or x-rays; it is a clinical diagnosis often made when there is no other explanation for the patient's sudden deterioration.	• Fluid resuscitation as guided by physiologic and laboratory parameters. Efforts at reimplantation are considered in the context of "life-over-limb;" the patient's life should be salvaged even at the cost of sacrificing a limb. Care of the patient with a reimplanted limb includes pain control, elevation of the extremity, and a warm and humid room to promote vasodilation. Occasionally, medicinal leeches may be applied to remove venous congestion that is not drained by veins due to swelling. • Fasciotomy is indicated for intracompartmental pressures between 30–60 mm Hg. When patients are unconscious or unable to reliably describe pain and sensation, fasciotomy is usually recommended at lower compartmental pressures. Mannitol may relieve compartmental pressures by promoting osmotic diuresis. Fluid and blood resuscitation may be indicated following fasciotomy. Pain management and meticulous wound care are also essential. • Management involves hemodynamic and pulmonary support until FES resolves, and early fixation of fractures.

ABC, Airway, breathing, circulation; *ABGs,* arterial blood gases; *ACLS,* advanced cardiac life support; *ARDS,* acute respiratory distress syndrome; *BCI,* blunt cardiac injury; *CK-MB,* creatine kinase-myocardial bands; *CSF,* cerebrospinal fluid; *CT,* computed tomography; *CVP,* central venous pressure; *CXR,* chest X-ray; *DPL,* diagnostic peritoneal lavage; *ECG,* electrocardiogram; *EF,* ejection fraction; *ETT,* endotracheal tube; *FES,* fat embolus syndrome; *GU,* genitourinary; *I:E,* inspiratory:expiratory ratio; *KUB,* kidney, ureter, bladder; *LUQ,* left upper quadrant; *MAP,* mean arterial pressure; *OR,* operating room; *PA,* pulmonary artery; $Paco_2$, partial pressure arterial carbon dioxide; Pao_2, partial pressure arterial oxygen tension; *PASG,* pneumatic antishock garment; *PAOP,* pulmonary artery occlusion pressure; *PRBCs,* packed red blood cells; *RUQ,* right upper quadrant; *SV,* stroke volume; *TENS,* transcutaneous electrical nerve stimulation; *WBC,* white blood cell.
From References 5, 19, 20, 35, 37, 39, 47, 65, 72, 75, 77, 79, 129, 133, 144, and 150.

pressure (CVP) and pulmonary artery occlusion pressure (PAOP) also called pulmonary artery wedge pressure (PAWP) are measurements of volume under pressure, rather than specific volume measurements. Particularly in trauma, they are greatly influenced by many factors such as positive end-expiratory pressure (PEEP), pericardial tamponade, noncompliant myocardium, rigid chest or abdominal wall, ACS, and technical errors in measurement. A patient can be hypovolemic despite seemingly high filling pressures. Several studies suggest that these parameters are unreliable guides to determining volume status in trauma patients; using right ventricular end diastolic volume index (RVEDVI) better reflects preload in trauma patients.[24,34,98,142]

Oxygen delivery index (Do_2I) and consumption index (Vo_2I) can supplement traditional pulmonary artery (PA) measurements and focus trauma resuscitation. Frequently, aberrations in all three components of oxygen delivery (cardiac output, hemoglobin saturation, and pulmonary function) can exist in the trauma patient. Analysis for the source of poor cardiac output, Hgb malfunction, and pulmonary dysfunction will identify the appropriate interventions to improve the Do_2I. Whereas normal Do_2I is 500 mL/min/m^2, one study suggests that a Do_2I of 600 mL/min/m^2 may improve outcomes.[93] Oxygen consumption levels can increase four to five times above normal in a critically injured trauma patient. Tachycardia, pain, agitation, shivering, posturing, and increased respiratory work will elevate oxygen demand beyond oxygen delivery. In late shock, oxygen use drops as cells are compromised and cannot extract oxygen from hemoglobin. Patients with abnormally high or low Vo_2I levels are not using oxygen at the cellular level and are in cellular shock.[3,126,140] Interventions to augment delivery and lower consumption in trauma patients to return the delivery-to-consumption ratio closer to the normal ratio of 4:1 are listed in Table 30.4.

PA catheters are not the mainstay of hemodynamic assessment in critically ill and injured patients that they once were because of concerns over complication rates, measurement error, and variability in treatment.[28] Parameters measured with PA catheters do not measure cellular perfusion, the actual end point of resuscitation. Global and organ-specific parameters help clinicians assess end products of anaerobic metabolism. Global indexes (e.g., mixed venous oxygen saturation [Svo_2], LA, BD, and the difference between the $Paco_2$ and the mixed venous CO_2) reflect a mixing of oxygen debt from multiple vascular beds and quantify the patient's overall degree of hypoperfusion. Global indexes are influenced by a number of extraneous variables and are therefore more valuable as trended values than as isolated values. Organ-specific parameters (e.g., gastric tonometry, sublingual capnometry, and near infrared spectroscopy) measure end-organ metabolic status because some organ beds remain under perfused despite global markers within normal limits.[26,30,57,73,92,99,126,146]

Ideally, the healthcare team should use multiple parameters and their interrelationships to guide resuscitation of the trauma patient. When considered together, traditional vital signs, hemodynamic targets, global end points, and organ-specific end points will identify the appropriate course of action.

Reversing the Lethal Triad of Hypothermia, Acidosis, and Coagulopathy

Hypothermia

Prompt reversal of hypothermia in trauma patients is a top priority because rewarming assists to correct coagulation and return the oxygen-hemoglobin dissociation curve to normal. Patients who are more rapidly rewarmed are more likely to survive resuscitation.[55] Traditional active and passive methods for rewarming have been reserved for mildly hypothermic patients because they may take hours to rewarm a patient (see Box 30.6). Peripheral rewarming techniques warm the extremities and superficial body surfaces first, whereas core body rewarming interventions use invasive techniques to warm the internal organs first.

TABLE 30.4 Causes of and Interventions for Inadequate Oxygen Delivery and Consumption in Trauma Patients

Causes	Interventions
INADEQUATE DELIVERY	
Poor Cardiac Output	
• Hypovolemia • Blunt cardiac injury • Pericardial tamponade • Tension pneumothorax • Cervical spine injury (neurogenic shock) • Septic shock (late response) • Liver shock (release of inflammatory mediators causing vasodilation)	• Fluid resuscitation • Blood product administration • Blood component transfusion • Inotropes for BCIs • Chest decompression • Vasopressors, once volume is adequate • Pericardiocentesis
Hemoglobin Dysfunction	
• Hypothermia • Carbon monoxide poisoning (burns) • Decreased 2,3, DPG (from multiple blood transfusions) • Alkalosis (cerebral hyperventilation)	• Rewarming • Control of mechanical ventilation • Limit blood product transfusions as soon as possible • Give fresh PRBCs, if possible, to optimize 2,3 DPG function • High-flow oxygen
Pulmonary Dysfunction	
• Inadequate airway • Pneumothorax, hemothorax, tension pneumothorax • Pulmonary contusion • Fat embolus syndrome • Pulmonary embolus • Bronchopleural fistula • ARDS • Preexisting COPD • Pneumonia	• Airway control • Oxygen administration • Mechanical ventilation • Chest decompression • Bronchodilator therapy • Antibiotics • Suctioning • Positioning
INADEQUATE CONSUMPTION	
Increased Consumption (Vo_2I >150 mL/min/m²)	
• Tachycardia • Increased respiratory work • Brain injury • Pain • Agitation • Shivering • Posturing • Seizures • Fever	• Support of ventilation • Analgesics • Sedatives • Rewarming • Paralysis • Antipyretics, cultures, antibiotics • Antiepileptic agents • Coordinate nursing care to minimize oxygen needs • Tachycardia will improve if oxygen delivery is adequate
Decreased Oxygen Consumption (Vo_2I <100 mL/min/m²)	
• Paralysis • Hypothermia • Deep sedation • Anesthesia • Sepsis • Profound shock	• Evaluate and treat for refractory shock or sepsis • Reverse induced paralysis if clinically indicated • Rewarm • Reverse anesthesia/deep sedation when clinically indicated

ARDS, Acute respiratory distress syndrome; *BCIs,* blunt cardiac injuries; *COPD,* chronic obstructive pulmonary disease; *DPG,* diphosphoglycerate; *PRBCs,* packed red blood cells; *Vo_2I,* oxygen consumption index.
From References 3, 126, and 140.

Acidosis

Trauma patients should undergo repeated ABG, LA, or BD testing to evaluate for severity and trend metabolic acidosis. A single value of either is not informative, but repeated measurements over time better assess resuscitation progress. Practically speaking, if the LA or BD is worsening, then resuscitation activities need to be evaluated and revised.

Treatment of metabolic acidosis includes reversal of the underlying source of shock; if the etiology of shock is controlled, the acidosis will be corrected. Multiple interventions should be initiated to improve oxygen delivery in trauma patients. The first is augmentation of preload using IV fluids to expand intravascular volume and red blood cell (RBC) transfusions to increase oxygen transport. Fluid resuscitation should be guided by several parameters, all of which are complementary (vital signs, urine output, PA pressures, cardiac index [CI], oxygen delivery and consumption, ABGs, LA and BD, and Hct and Hgb). When the CI, Do_2I, and Vo_2I do not improve with additional fluids, vasoactive medications can be added to support cardiac output. Although vasopressor choice varies among clinicians; epinephrine, dopamine

(Intropin), and phenylephrine (Neo-Synephrine) are commonly used.[140] The patient should be warmed to facilitate oxygen off-loading of Hgb. Buffer therapy, such as sodium bicarbonate, is rarely justified because it does not treat the underlying cause of acidosis. Unfortunately, a paradoxical worsening of intracellular acidosis may occur as the bicarbonate binds with excess CO_2 associated with pulmonary compromise.[3] Shivering, anxiety, pain, and restlessness should be addressed to decrease oxygen demands in the face of impaired oxygen delivery.[126,140]

Coagulation

The mainstay of coagulopathy monitoring is the clinical assessment of ongoing blood loss, either in the form of frank hemorrhage or diffuse oozing from wound punctures, IV sites, surgical drains, or mucous membranes. The most beneficial lab studies with the fastest turnaround times include Hgb, platelet count, PT, aPTT, and fibrinogen.[38] Disseminated intravascular coagulation (DIC) screens, which include D-dimers and fibrinogen split products, provide useful information about the consumptive component of the coagulopathy but have long turnaround times that are often impractical during critical care resuscitation.[33]

Management of coagulopathy includes surgical control of hemorrhage, rewarming, reversal of acidosis, and replacement coagulation factors. The current recommendation is to replace RBCs and coagulation factors based on actual lab values to conserve resources.[3,33,140] At times, providers may order blood products based on the clinical picture rather than wait for lab results and risk coagulopathy. When the laboratory cannot provide results quickly enough to keep up with excessive blood loss, platelets and plasma can be transfused while waiting for lab results. Plasma is indicated when the PT and aPTT are greater than 1.5 times laboratory control values and should not be used as a volume expander alone. Cryoprecipitate is indicated with fibrinogen levels less than 100 mg/dL. Platelets are infused when the platelet count is less than 50,000 in the presence of ongoing hemorrhage.[33,85]

New hemostatic dressings are used by the military to control hemorrhage following trauma. More research is needed before these products can be integrated into routine clinical practice, but preliminary results are very encouraging (Box 30.8).

Managing Abdominal Compartment Syndrome

Often the patient may be too unstable to be transported to the OR, and a decompressive laparotomy to relieve ACS must be done in the critical care unit. The decision to perform a bedside decompression depends on a number of factors including the patient's age and underlying comorbidities; resources to support aggressive fluid resuscitation; confidence that the hypertension is caused by edema and not ongoing hemorrhage; and availability of surgical instruments and bedside cautery. Decompressive laparotomy is recommended only when significant cardiopulmonary compromise is present rather than as a response to a measurement.[49,71]

A high index of suspicion is critical for the early identification of ACS before it reaches a crisis point. Clinical examination alone does not consistently identify whether ACS is present. Intraaortic pressure (IAP) monitoring should be initiated in any patient with an inflammatory response causing capillary leak that requires volume resuscitation or vasopressor support because such patients are at risk for bowel edema, IAP, and ACS.[81,136]

BOX 30.8 Hemostatic Dressings

Dry fibrin sealant dressings	Dry, powdered human thrombin and fibrinogen compressed on a removable backing. Unlike fibrin glue used in the OR, this product requires no preparation, is stable at room temperature, and presents no infectious risk. When pushed into a wound, it coagulates on contact. The only limiting factor is that the product is dependent on adequate blood bank reserves because it is made from human blood.
Rapid deployment hemostat (RDH)	An acetylated poly-*N*-acetyl glucosamine dressing isolated from controlled aseptic, microalgal cultures. It is thought to work outside the coagulation cascade through red cell aggregate adhesion and vasoconstriction. FDA approval for its use in humans is pending.
Chitosan	A product made from shrimp shells, it is a biodegradable, nontoxic, complex carbohydrate derivative of chitin. It is FDA approved and has been successfully used in military conflicts in the Middle East.
QuickClot	A granular zeolite that absorbs water and promotes clot formation. Because it contains no biological or botanical substances, it eliminates the danger of allergic reactions or disease transmission. A major drawback, however, is an exothermic reaction that produces heat when it absorbs fluids. The FDA has approved its use with external wounds.

FDA, US Food and Drug Administration; *OR,* operating room.
From References 2, 64, 118, and 141.

Identifying, Preventing, and Managing Rhabdomyolysis

Early identification of rhabdomyolysis is crucial and facilitated by having a high index of suspicion in patients with significant soft tissue crush or avulsion injuries. Patients with painful, swollen extremities following crush injuries should be monitored for rhabdomyolysis as well as compartment syndrome.[89] Dark, tea-colored urine that is positive for blood despite the absence of RBC on urinalysis suggests rhabdomyolysis is developing.[133] Serum creatinine phosphokinase (CPK) levels are the quickest and least expensive screening test for rhabdomyolysis, but cardiac muscle must be ruled out as a source of the CPK elevation.[89] CPK levels are used instead of myoglobin levels because the results can be quickly obtained, are available in most institutions, and are relatively inexpensive.[132] A trigger for identifying and treating patients at risk for ARF secondary to rhabdomyolysis is a CPK level of equal to or greater than 20,000 units/L.[89]

The primary goal of rhabdomyolysis treatment is prevention of renal failure by early and aggressive resuscitation. This is accomplished by achieving hemodynamic stability without volume overload and maintaining urine output.[132] Large-volume resuscitation treats the hypovolemia and hypokalemia that contribute to rhabdomyolysis. Patients who receive large amounts of fluid before extrication have significantly better outcomes than those whose resuscitation was delayed.[8] Mannitol (Osmitrol) may be used to diurese the patient and wash out tubular myoglobin, but can be used only when the patient is fully volume resuscitated and urine is being produced. It also functions as a free radical scavenger and may therefore offer some renal protective effects.[155] Urine is alkalized with sodium bicarbonate to decrease cast formation and lessen myoglobin toxicity.[8] Large amounts of bicarbonate may be necessary to alkalize the urine to a pH of greater than 6.5.[89]

Early signals of ARF include persistent hyperkalemia and acidosis despite volume resuscitation and bicarbonate administration. ARF from rhabdomyolysis is associated with poor outcomes in patients. Early initiation of continuous venovenous hemofiltration or daily hemodialysis to filter myoglobin and correct fluid overload and electrolyte abnormalities is recommended. These patients stand an excellent chance of full renal recovery if treated early and aggressively.[89]

The source of inflammation and muscle necrosis causing the rhabdomyolysis may need to be removed. Crushed extremities may require early fasciotomy or amputation, forcing the trauma surgeon to sacrifice a limb in order to save the patient's life.[89]

Providing Analgesia and Sedation

Pain and anxiety contribute to morbidity and mortality in the critical care unit as they increase physiologic stress in an already compromised patient. Three general principles guide appropriate pain and sedation management of the trauma patient while in critical care. First, traumatic injuries are typically very painful, requiring aggressive analgesic therapy while avoiding hypotension. Analgesia should not be withheld for the patient in pain with low blood pressure; rather, the blood pressure should be supported with IV fluids and, if necessary, vasopressors. This is frequently a challenge in the initial stages of critical care. Second, high injury severity often leads to lengthy stays in critical care and a prolonged need for sedation. Third, trauma patients often have a history of polysubstance abuse and are therefore at risk for potentially serious problems such as acute withdrawal syndromes and opioid and benzodiazepine tolerance.[27,54] A variety of opioid analgesics, anxiolytics, and antidelirium medications should be administered according to unit protocol. The critical care nurse plays a key role in ensuring that patients receive adequate pain control and sedation without physiologic compromise.

Evaluation for Missed Injuries

The initial evaluation and resuscitation of a trauma patient can be described as controlled chaos. The focus of the primary and secondary surveys is on immediate life threats in the critically ill patient.[16] Upon the completion of resuscitation, all trauma patients should undergo a tertiary survey to evaluate for missed or unidentified injuries. This survey is a methodical and purposeful physical exam.[59] The effectiveness of the tertiary survey can be impacted by the patient's ability to interact and may need to be repeated once the patient is able to answer questions and participate.[59] Identification of missed injuries is vital in the management of the trauma patient; missed injuries often result in prolonged hospital stays, intensive rehab therapy needs, and increased morbidity associated with delayed repair.[116]

CRITICAL CARE MANAGEMENT OF COMPLICATIONS FOLLOWING TRAUMA

Following successful trauma resuscitation, multisystem sequelae and complications must be addressed (many of these considerations are addressed in other chapters in this book; those issues with especially unique considerations related to trauma are briefly discussed here).

Acute Respiratory Distress Syndrome

Originally known as *wet lung, shock lung,* and *Da Nang lung,* ARDS was first recognized as a complication of hypotension associated with trauma. It is a secondary insult following injury, hypoperfusion, and resuscitation. Risk factors for ARDS associated with trauma include any type of shock, significant soft tissue destruction, direct pulmonary contusion, multiple orthopedic fractures, large-volume fluid resuscitation, multiple transfusions, aspiration, pneumonia, and major head injuries.[47,137] Critical care nurses must be alert for signs and symptoms of ARDS during resuscitation, in the days that follow initial resuscitation, and with any episode of sepsis. Clinical presentation and management of ARDS are discussed in detail in Chapter 9.

Nutritional Considerations for the Trauma Patient

Nutritional therapy is a critical component of severely injured patients. Even in trauma patients who are young and well nourished, an unsupported hypermetabolic postinjury response will rapidly result in a starvation state. Immediate access to essential amino acids is required to facilitate healing and prevent infection. Early nutritional support prevents development of sepsis and multiorgan dysfunction syndrome in trauma patients.[82,84] Glycogen stores are rapidly depleted following trauma, forcing the body to use endogenous substrates, protein, and fat to support hypermetabolism following injury. The usual balance between anabolism and catabolism is disrupted, favoring protein catabolism. Profound catabolism, particularly in healthy, muscular patients, occurs when muscles are broken down to supply proteins for metabolic processes. An average loss of 6.4 kg of skeletal muscle can occur in blunt trauma patients within 21 days. Negative nitrogen balance following trauma is an indicator of the magnitude of injury rather than an indicator of how much protein is needed. Sacrifice of lean body mass results in poor wound healing, impaired immunologic function, inadequate pulmonary ventilation, cardiac insufficiency, and sustained elevations in oxygen consumption. The hypermetabolic phase peaks within 10 days following injury, and then gradually decreases.

Providing adequate nutritional support to trauma patients is a challenge for multiple reasons. GI function is impaired in most trauma patients because many have undergone extensive surgical interventions and have subnormal albumin and prealbumin concentrations secondary to the stress response. Direct injury to the GI tract and subsequent surgical repair can be a contraindication for the use of enteral nutrition unless a jejunostomy tube can be used for feeding. The patient with head and facial injuries may be unable to tolerate oral feedings because of altered level of consciousness, poor gag and swallow reflexes, or surgical fixation of the mandible.

A nutritional assessment within 24 hours after admission is indicated for trauma patients. High-risk patients are those who are young (e.g., males with significant muscle mass), sustained brain and facial trauma, multisystem injury, GI injury, or preexisting malnutrition (e.g., older adults). Indirect calorimetry is the best method to calculate energy expenditure and prevent overfeeding in trauma patients. Nutritional status should also be assessed on an ongoing basis; components of this assessment include evaluation of blood chemistries (calcium, magnesium, phosphate, creatine, and BUN), serum triglycerides, albumin, and prealbumin. Enteral nutrition is the preferred method of providing nutrition to the trauma patient and should be initiated as soon as possible.[84] If the initiation of enteral nutrition will be delayed for 5 days, or if the patient does not tolerate enteral nutrition, parental nutrition should be initiated. Use of stool softeners, bulk forming agents, and bowel stimulants should be initiated with enteral feedings. Promobility agents may be of benefit in increasing gastric and GI motility.

Assessing and Treating Infection

Infection is a common complication and a major cause of morbidity and mortality in the trauma patient; this chapter will provide a brief overview of the incidence of infection and of wound management following trauma. Infections can occur with any wound and as a hospital acquired event.[22] To prevent or control infection, the critical care nurse should assess the patient daily for signs of inflammation and infection, practice aseptic technique and impeccable hand hygiene, and perform wound care as ordered.

Traumatic wound infections can occur with any wound and have a variety of presentations. Knife wounds, for example, are relatively clean, whereas wounds from jagged instruments such as chain saws and farm equipment are associated with significant tissue destruction, wound hematomas, bacteria, and foreign bodies. Gangrene is a deep infection often seen with puncture wounds, which may lead to compartment syndrome, deep myonecrosis, and a "dishwater" appearance to wound drainage.[147] Special consideration should be given to abdominal wounds that penetrate the fascia due to the likelihood of gastrointestinal contamination.[102]

Prevention of wound infections involves initial debridement and cleansing of the injury site, with removal of tissue until only viable, bleeding tissue remains. This may be done in the OR, but is frequently performed at the critical care bedside for smaller, less severe wounds. Management of wound infections requires judicious use of antibiotics to minimize the development of *Clostridium difficile (C. diff)* and antibiotic resistance. Aggressive deep fascial debridement and amputation are required to arrest the progression of necrotizing fasciitis and gangrene; hyperbaric oxygen therapy also may be considered.[147]

Open fractures are at risk for infection as they can contain skin fragments, devitalized bone, and foreign bodies such as the patient's clothing. Infection is prevented by thorough irrigation and debridement as soon as possible after the injury; this may be done in the critical care unit if the patient is too hemodynamically unstable to go to the operating room for the procedure. The wound may be closed several days after the injury once it is clear that no infection is present. Repeated debridement and irrigation will be necessary as long as infection persists. The removal of infected internal fixation hardware may be needed for deep infections. Amputation is performed when irreparable vascular injury or osteomyelitis leaves little hope for a functional limb, or systemic compromise from infection threatens mortality.[144]

Intraabdominal infection usually begins with an injury that disrupts the GI tract or biliary tree. Likelihood of infection is based on where the damage occurred; the risk is relatively small for stomach and duodenal injuries; however, there is significant risk if the lower intestinal tract, with high bacterial counts, is injured. Prevention of abdominal infection begins with prompt exploratory laparotomy; if intestinal contamination is found, reoperation and delayed closure may be necessary. Aggressive antibiotic therapy to cover both anaerobic and aerobic bacteria must be started immediately with frequent reevaluation of appropriateness of therapy.[147]

Hospital acquired chest infections secondary to retained hemothorax after chest tube placement can be common.[36] The infections may be a result of contamination from a penetrating injury, but they also may be caused by tube placement under less than ideal conditions. Ideally, strict sterile technique is followed during placement in controlled situations, but chaos during trauma resuscitation frequently allows for breaks in sterility and inadequate skin preparation. Pulmonary infection and empyema create additional respiratory compromise in patients with decreased level of consciousness, disrupted chest wall integrity, thoracic or abdominal incisions, and paralysis.[22]

Empyema presents with fever, leukocytosis, and purulent chest tube drainage, and is more likely in patients who had large amounts of bloody drainage or who have had their tube for more than five days. Empyemas are managed by antibiotics and placement of a second chest tube or catheter directly into the empyema cavity itself; this is occasionally done in CT scan to better guide placement of the tube. Daily chest radiographs monitor the response to therapy. Unresolved empyemas develop a thick "rind," requiring decortication of the pleural space, a surgical procedure that results in significant blood loss and postoperative pain.[147] The critical care nurse plays a key role in preventing empyema by performing daily chest tube care. Anchoring the tube to the chest wall will help prevent to-and-fro movements at the insertion site that drag bacteria into the wound.[47]

Central nervous system (CNS) infections can occur, such as meningitis, brain abscess, and empyema. They may be associated with open skull fractures and with facial fractures that involve the sinuses. CNS infections are a potential complication of intracranial monitoring catheters. Sinusitis is associated with midface fractures and nasotracheal or nasogastric tubes because sinus drainage may be obstructed by edema and injury.[22] Sinus infections may be the underlying source of infection in a trauma patient when other obvious sources of fever have been ruled out.

Postsplenectomy sepsis is a life-threatening, fulminating infection in patients who underwent splenectomy for trauma; although it is more common in children, it is increasingly present in adults and is often fatal. The spleen has essential immunologic functions; when it is removed, patients become at risk for fulminant disseminated bacteremia.[147] The best preventive strategy is to salvage the spleen when possible. In the case of splenectomy, vaccination for *Streptococcus pneumoniae* (pneumococcus), *Neisseria meningitidis* (meningococcus), and *Haemophilus influenzae* must be administered before discharge.[22]

C. diff enterocolitis is a colitis associated with antibiotics. The infection occurs in patients who were colonized by the microbe before injury, which becomes opportunistic when normal gut flora is suppressed by IV antibiotics used to treat other infections. The best way to prevent *C. diff* is with shorter courses of antibiotics. Severe cases, associated with toxic megacolon, may require surgical resection of the colon.[147]

Lastly, hospital-acquired infections are as common in this patient population as in other critically ill patients. Ventilator-associated pneumonia, aspiration-associated pneumonia, urinary tract infection, intravascular device infection, and GI microbial translocation all contribute to the overall morbidity and mortality of trauma patients.

Preventing Deep Venous Thrombosis

After the coagulopathy during initial resuscitation has resolved, the trauma patient develops a hypercoagulable state in the postinjury recovery period; deep venous thrombosis (DVT), pulmonary embolism (PE), and even death can occur. The relationship between trauma and venous thrombosis is well known, with more than half of patients developing lower extremity thrombosis.[52]

The components of Virchow's triad (e.g., venous stasis, endothelial damage, and hypercoagulability) are well described in trauma. Immobility, often seen with head and spinal cord injury and lower extremity fractures, leads to venous stasis from loss of the leg muscle pump.[120] Direct vessel wall damage from penetrating injury, blunt energy forces, or stretch injury may directly damage endothelium and initiate the coagulation cascade. Thrombosis can occur near the sites of traumatic and iatrogenic injury (e.g., central venous catheter insertion sites).[95] Trauma patients have low levels of antithrombin III, protein C, and protein S, leading to a procoagulant state, compounded by increased platelet adhesion and decreased fibrinolysis.[44,100,112] Risk factors for DVT and PE in trauma patients can be separated into three groups, listed in Table 30.5.

Traditional interventions to prevent DVT are early ambulation, graded sequential compression devices, and low-dose anticoagulation. Depending on the patient's injuries, early ambulation may not be an option and anticoagulation is often contraindicated because of bleeding potential from injuries. Therefore, sequential compression devices are recommended for patients with moderate risk of DVT. For high-risk patients who cannot be anticoagulated, a temporary or permanent inferior vena cava (IVC) filter may be indicated. IVC filters have resulted in a decreased incidence of PE, although additional studies regarding efficacy and long-term consequences are needed. Many guidelines exist about how to best prevent DVT and subsequent PE development.[53,109]

Providing Psychosocial Support

Crisis following trauma provides unique challenges to patients and their families as a result of lengthy hospital stays, with many emergencies and complications during that time. Recovery may be prolonged and uncertain, subjecting families to anxiety and emotional stress. During the critical care phase of trauma care, patients may not be alert to manifest stress and require intervention. Families, however, may feel overwhelmed, out of control or angry, have difficulty breathing, be unable to concentrate, and experience mood swings. Early psychosocial intervention by critical care nurses, social workers, and pastoral services is important to support patients and families struggling with an uncertain future.[31,89]

Both the patient and the family are at risk for the development of posttraumatic stress disorder (PTSD) following a traumatic event. Symptoms can begin immediately after the event and persist for months, predisposing the person to long-term mental and emotional health challenges. Those most likely to experience PTSD either experienced or witnessed an incident that resulted in death, spinal cord injuries, or facial injuries.[2,11,12] Patients experience powerful flashbacks of the event, producing feelings of intense fear, helplessness, or horror that are so real they feel as if they are reliving the event. Victims are in a constant state of hyperarousal; extreme fear, grief, and anger cause continuous emotional distress. Relationships with family and friends often suffer, as victims may be distant and unapproachable. Other symptoms include gastric upset, headaches, difficulty concentrating, insomnia, and irritability.[2]

PTSD is not always identified while the patient is in the critical care unit, but nurses should identify those at risk for the disorder and consult with appropriate services to provide early screening and interventions. Social workers, hospital chaplains, psychologists, and psychiatrists are skilled professionals who help patients and families cope with PTSD. Many patients respond well to counseling and other nonpharmacologic interventions, but occasionally benzodiazepines and selective serotonin reuptake inhibitors may be needed. Early interventions that restore a sense of control, reduce hyperarousal, and decrease feelings of guilt will facilitate full recovery.[2]

TABLE 30.5 Risk Factors for Deep Venous Thrombosis and Pulmonary Embolus Specific to Trauma

At risk	Injury severity score > 9 Blood transfusion(s) Surgical procedure ≥ 2 hours Lower-extremity fracture Spinal cord injury Immobilization Excessive soft tissue trauma Shock states
At high risk	Femoral central venous catheter Glasgow Coma Scale score ≤ 8 Spinal cord injury Pelvic fracture Femur/tibia fracture Venous injury
At very high risk	Spinal cord injury with paralysis Severe pelvic fracture Multiple long bone fractures (≥3)

From References 25, 53, 94, 109, and 144.

CONCLUSION

Trauma is a multisystem phenomenon with immediate threat to life and long-term complications for the survivors of critical injury. The first hour after trauma, known as the *golden hour*, sees the highest number of patient deaths;[138] for those who survive, the subsequent hours and days spent in critical care are no less important. An organized, systematic approach to managing these patients provides the best chance for meaningful outcome. The critical care nurse assesses and reassesses, monitors, infuses, assists, transports, applies pressure, educates, and comforts: a seemingly endless myriad of critical thinking and nursing activities. The nurse's attention to the clinical challenges addressed in this chapter, along with a high index of suspicion for decompensation at any time, are the patient's best chance for leaving the critical care unit in optimal condition to begin the long and difficult road of recovery.

CASE STUDY 30.1

D.M., an obese (201 pounds) 17-year-old girl, was found by emergency medical personnel after her open-top jeep rolled several times before its front end hit a tree. She had been traveling at a high rate of speed on an isolated rural highway. Initial vital signs (VS) for EMS: BP: 88/64 mm Hg; HR: 125 beats/min; RR: 28 breaths/min.

After extrication and initiation of prehospital care, DM was transported to the closest Level I trauma center, 30 minutes away.

When D.M. arrived in the emergency department, primary and secondary surveys were performed. Her airway was patent; breathing was rapid, with equal breath sounds bilaterally. Her skin remained cool and slightly diaphoretic. She remained alert and oriented to person and place.

Her vital signs in the ED: T: 34.2°C; BP: 78/50 mm Hg; HR: 135 beats/min; RR: 32 breaths/min.

From the ED, D.M. was quickly taken to surgery for an emergency exploratory laparotomy. In the OR, the following injuries were discovered: a grade V splenic laceration requiring splenectomy, avulsion of the duodenum from the base of her stomach with spillage of intestinal contents into the peritoneum, a pancreatic contusion with laceration of the pancreatic duct, and a right renal thrombosis, assumed to be caused by shearing injury during the multiple rollovers and constriction of the lap belt. Vascular grafts were performed to salvage the injured kidney. On arrival in critical care, the patient was hypotensive, hypothermic, and on a ventilator. After additional volume and PRBC resuscitation, her VS were: T: 34.3°C; BP: 88/60 mm Hg; HR: 122 beats/min; RR: 14 breaths/min on pressure control of 25. Hemodynamics included the following: CVP: 6 mm Hg, Hgb: 7.4 g/100 mL, LA: 4.5 mmol/L, base deficit 4.8 mEq/L, pH: 7.30, Pao_2: 125 mm Hg, $Paco_2$: 42 mm Hg.

Decision Point:

What are the likely explanations for her hemodynamic profile in the critical care unit?

Decision Point:

What are additional resuscitation and assessment priorities in the first hours following admission to critical care?

REFERENCES

1. Aguilera, D. (1998). *Crisis intervention: theory and methodology* (8th ed.). St. Louis: Mosby.
2. Alam, H. G., et al. (2004). Application of a zeolite hemostatic agent achieves 100% survival in a lethal model of complex groin injury. *J Trauma, 56*(5), 974–983.
3. Alarcon, L. H., Puyana, J. C., & Peitzman, A. B. (2013). Management of shock. In K. L. Mattox, D. V. Feliciano, & E. E. Moore (Eds.), *Trauma* (7th ed.) (pp. 189–215). New York: McGraw-Hill.
4. American College of Surgeons Committee on Trauma. (2015). *Resources for optimal care of the injured patient.* Chicago: American College of Surgeons.
5. American College of Surgeons Committee on Trauma. (2012). *Advanced trauma life support course* (9th ed.). Chicago: American College of Surgeons.
6. American College of Surgeons Trauma Quality Improvement Program. (2013). *Massive transfusion in trauma guidelines.* Chicago: American College of Surgeons.
7. Ball, C. (2014). Damage control resuscitation: history, theory and technique. *Can J Surg, 57*(1), 55–60. http://dx.doi.org/10.1503/cjs.020312.
8. Better, O. S., & Stein, J. H. (1990). Early management of shock and prophylaxis of acute renal failure in traumatic rhabdomyolysis (comment). *N Engl J Med, 322*(12), 825–829.
9. Biesel, W. R. (1995). Herman award lecture, 1995: infection induced malnutrition from cholera to cytokines. *Am J Clin Nutr, 62*, 813–819.
10. Biffl, W.L. (2013). Duodenum and pancreas. In K. L. Mattox, D. V. Feliciano, & E. E. Moore (Eds.), *Trauma* (7th ed.) (pp. 603–619). New York: McGraw-Hill.
11. Binks, T. M., et al. (1997). Relationship between level of spinal cord injury and posttraumatic stress disorder symptoms. *Ann N Y Acad Sci, 821*, 430–432.
12. Bisson, J. I., Shepherd, J. P., & Manish, D. (1997). Psychological sequelae of facial trauma. *J Trauma, 43*, 496–500.
13. Bombardier, C. H., & Thurber, C. A. (1998). Blood alcohol level and early cognitive status after traumatic brain injury. *Brain Inj, 12*, 725–734.
14. Boulanger, B. R., Nayman, R., & McLean, R. F. (1994). What are the clinical determinants of early energy expenditure in critically injured adults? *J Trauma, 37*, 969–974.
15. Bower, T. C., & Reuter, J. P. (2009). Analgesia, sedation, and neuromuscular blockade in the trauma patient. In K. A. McQuillan, et al. (Ed.), *Trauma nursing: from resuscitation through rehabilitation* (4th ed.) (pp. 371–413). Philadelphia: Saunders.
16. Brasel, K. J., & Codner, P. A. (2013). Initial assessment and management. In K. L. Mattox, D. V. Feliciano, & E. E. Moore (Eds.), *Trauma* (7th ed.) (pp. 154–166). New York: McGraw-Hill.
17. Brohi, K., et al. (2003). Acute traumatic coagulopathy. *J Trauma, 54*(6), 1127–1130.
18. Bulger, E. (2000). Rib fractures in the elderly. *J Trauma, 48*(6), 1040–1047.
19. Bulger, E. M., et al. (1997). Fat embolism syndrome. *Arch Surg, 132*, 435–439.
20. Bulger, E. M., Smith, D. G., & Maier, R. V. (1997). Fat embolus syndrome: a 10-year review. *Arch Surg, 132*, 435–439.
21. Bullock, M. R., Chesnut, R. M., & Clifton, G. L. (2000). Guidelines for the management of severe traumatic brain injury. In Brain Trauma Foundation and American Association of Neurological Surgeons (Ed.), *Management and prognosis of severe traumatic brain injury.* Brain Trauma Foundation: New York (pp. 7–165).
22. Casper, P. B., Joshi, M., & Algire, M. C. (2009). Infection and infection control. In K. A. McQuillan, et al. (Ed.), *Trauma nursing: from resuscitation through rehabilitation* (4th ed.) (pp. 252–299). Philadelphia: Saunders.
23. CDC/National Center for Health Statistics. (2014). Injuries. http://www.cdc.gov/nchs/fastats/accidental-injury.htm#.
24. Chang, M. C., et al. (1996). Preload assessment in trauma patients during large-volume shock resuscitation. *Arch Surg, 131*, 728–731.
25. Clagett, P. C., et al. (1998). Prevention of thromboembolism. *Chest, 111*, 531S–560S.
26. Cohn, S. M., Crookes, B. A., & Proctor, K. G. (2003). Near-infrared spectroscopy in resuscitation. *J Trauma, 54*(Suppl. 5), S199–S202.
27. Coimbra, R., Doucet, J., & Bansal, V. (2013). Principles of critical care. In K. L. Mattox, E. E. Moore, & D. V. Feliciano (Eds.), *Trauma* (7th ed.) (pp. 1006–1040). New York: McGraw-Hill.
28. Connors, A. F., et al. (1996). The effectiveness of right heart catheterization in the initial care of critically ill patients. *JAMA, 276*, 889–897.
29. Cosgriff, N., et al. (1997). Predicting life-threatening coagulopathy in the massively transfused trauma patient: hypothermia and acidoses revisited. *J Trauma, 42*(5), 857–861.
30. Reference removed in page proofs.
31. Cross, M. L., et al. (1996). Interaction between the trauma team and families: lack of timely communications. *Am J Emerg Med, 14*, 548–550.
32. Cuthbertson, D. P. (1942). Post-shock metabolic response. *Lancet, 1*, 433–436.
33. DeLoughery, T. G. (2004). Coagulation defects in trauma patients: etiology, recognition, and treatment. *Crit Care Clin, 20*(1), 13–24.
34. Diebel, L. N., et al. (1992). End-diastolic volume: a better indicator of pre-load in the critically ill. *Arch Surg, 127*, 817–822.
35. Diebel, L. N. (2013). Stomach and small bowel. In K. L. Mattox, D. V. Feliciano, & E. E. Moore (Eds.), *Trauma* (7th ed.) (pp. 581–602). New York: McGraw-Hill.
36. Dubose, J., et al. (2012). Development of posttraumatic empyema in patients with retained hemothorax: results of a prospective, observational AAST study. *J Trauma Acute Care Surg, 73*(3), 752–757.
37. DuBose, J. A., O'Connor, J. V., & Scalea, T. M. (2013). Lung, trachea and esophagus. In K. L. Mattox, D. V. Feliciano, & E. E. Moore (Eds.), *Trauma* (7th ed.) (pp. 468–484). New York: McGraw-Hill.
38. Eddy, V. A., Morris, J. A., & Cullinane, D. C. (2000). Hypothermia, coagulopathy and acidosis. *Surg Clin North Am, 80*(3), 845–854.
39. Emergency Nurses Association. (2000). Initial assessment. In Emergency Nurses Association (Ed.), *Trauma nursing core course* (5th ed.) (pp. 39–64). Des Plaines, IL: Emergency Nurses Association.
40. Emergency Nurses Association. (2000). Mechanism of injury. In Emergency Nurses Association (Ed.), *Trauma nursing core course* (5th ed.) (pp. 11–38). Des Plaines, IL: Emergency Nurses Association.
41. Emergency Nurses Association. (2000). Stabilization, transfer, and transport. In Emergency Nurses Association (Ed.), *Trauma nursing core course* (5th ed.). Des Plaines, IL: Emergency Nurses Association.
42. Emergency Nurses Association. (2001). *Presenting the option of family presence* (2nd ed.). Des Plaines, IL: Emergency Nurses Association.

43. Emergency Nurses Association. (2000). Primary assessment. In Emergency Nurses Association (Ed.), *Trauma nursing core course* (5th ed.) (p. 313). Des Plaines, IL: Emergency Nurses Association. Table 38.
44. Engelman, D. T., et al. (1996). Hypercoagulability following multiple trauma. *World J Surg, 20*(5).
45. Feliciano, D. V., & Wyrzykowski, A. D. (2013). Trauma damage control. In K. L. Mattox, D. V. Feliciano, & E. E. Moore (Eds.), *Trauma* (7th ed.) (pp. 725–746). New York: McGraw-Hill.
46. Frankenfield, D. C., Omert, L. A., & Badelline, M. M. (1994). Correlation between measured energy expenditure and clinically obtained variables in trauma and sepsis patients. *JPEN, 18*, 398–403.
47. Frawley, P. M. (2009). Thoracic injuries. In K. A. McQuillan, et al. (Ed.), *Trauma nursing: from resuscitation through rehabilitation* (4th ed.) (pp. 614–671). Philadelphia: Saunders.
48. Fritsch, D. E. (1991). Hypothermia in the trauma patient. *AACN Clin Issues, 6*, 196–211.
49. Fritsch, D. E., & Steinmann, R. A. (2000). Managing trauma patients with abdominal compartment syndrome. *Crit Care Nurse, 20*, 48–58.
50. Gallagher, J. J. (2006). Abdominal compression monitoring: ask the experts. *Crit Care Nurse, 26*(1), 67–70.
51. Gando, S., Tedo, L., & Kubota, M. (1992). Post-trauma coagulation and fibrinolysis. *Crit Care Med, 20*, 594–600.
52. Geerts, W. H., et al. (1994). A prospective study of venous thromboembolism after major trauma. *N Engl J Med, 331*, 1601.
53. Geerts, W. H., et al. (2004). Prevention of venous thromboembolism: the seventh ACCP conference on antithrombotic and thrombolytic therapy. *Chest, 126*(3), 338S–400S.
54. Gentilello, L. M. (2013). Alcohol and drugs. In K. L. Mattox, D. V. Feliciano, & E. E. Moore (Eds.), *Trauma* (7th ed.) (pp. 850–858). New York: McGraw-Hill.
55. Gentilello, L. M., Jurkovich, G. J., & Stark, M. S. (1997). Is hypothermia in the victim of major trauma protective or harmful? A randomized prospective study. *Ann Surg, 226*, 642–647.
56. Ghali, A. M. A., El Malik, E. M. A., & Ibrahim, A. I. A. (1999). Ureteric injuries: diagnosis, management, and outcome. *J Thromb Haemost, 46*, 150–158.
57. Gommersall, C. D., et al. (2000). Resuscitation of critically ill patients based on the results of gastric tonometry: a prospective, randomized controlled trial. *Crit Care Med, 28*(3), 607–614.
58. Griffin, R., et al. (2012). Association between side-impact airbag deployment and risk of injury: a matched cohort study using CIREN and the NASS-CDS. *J Trauma Acute Care Surg, 73*(4), 914–918. http://dx.doi.org/10.1097/TA.0b013e31825a7636.
59. Grossman, M. D., & Born, C. (2000). Tertiary survey of the trauma patient in the intensive care unit. *Surg Clin North Am, 80*(3), 805–824.
60. Gubler, K. D., et al. (1994). The effect of hypothermia on dilutional coagulopathy. *J Trauma, 36*, 847–851.
61. Guyton, A. C., & Hall, J. E. (2006). *Textbook of medical physiology* (11th ed.) (pp. 383–401). Philadelphia: Elsevier.
62. Hildebrand, F., et al. (2004). Pathophysiologic changes and effects of hypothermia on outcome in elective surgery and trauma patients. *Am J Surg, 187*, 363–371.
63. Holcomb, J., et al. (2007). Damage control resuscitation: directly addressing the early coagulopathy of trauma. *J Trauma, 62*(2), 307–310. http://dx.doi.org/10.1097/TA.0b013e3180324124.
64. Holcomb, J. B., et al. (1998). Efficacy of a dry fibrin sealant dressing for hemorrhage control after ballistic injury. *Arch Surg, 133*(1), 32–35.
65. Hoyt, D. B., Coimbra, R., & Potenza, M. D. (2004). Management of acute trauma. In C. M. Townsend, et al. (Ed.), *Sabiston textbook of surgery: the biological basis of modern surgical practice* (17th ed.) (pp. 483–532). Philadelphia: Elsevier.
66. Hulka, F., Mullins, R. J., & Frank, E. H. (1996). Blunt brain injury activates the coagulation process. *Arch Surg, 131*, 923–927.
67. Hulka, F., et al. (1997). Influence of a statewide trauma system on pediatric hospitalization and outcome. *J Trauma, 42*(3), 268–276.
68. Hunt, J. P., Marr, A. B., & Stuke, L. E. (2013). Kinematics. In K. L. Mattox, D. V. Feliciano, & E. E. Moore (Eds.), *Trauma* (7th ed.) (pp. 2–17). New York: McGraw-Hill.
69. Hwang, T., Shuang, S., & Chen, M. (1993). The use of indirect calorimetry in critically ill patients: the relationship of measured energy expenditure to injury severity score, septic severity score, and APACHE II score. *J Trauma, 34*, 247–251.
70. Inaba, K., et al. (2015). Tourniquet use for civilian extremity trauma. *J Trauma Acute Care Surg, 79*(2), 232–237. http://dx.doi.org/10.1097/TA.0000000000000747.
71. Ivatury, R. R., Sugerman, H. J., & Peitzman, A. B. (2001). Abdominal compartment syndrome: recognition and management. In J. L. Cameron (Ed.), *Advances in surgery* (vol. 35) (pp. 1–19). St. Louis: Mosby.
72. James, M. D., & Gregis, R. M. (1998). Mannitol treatment for acute compartment syndrome. *Nephron, 79*(4), 492.
73. Jin, S., et al. (1998). Decreases in organ blood flows associated with increases in sublingual $Paco_2$ during hemorrhagic shock. *J Appl Physiol, 85*(6), 1838–1843.
74. Johansson, P. I., & Stensballe, J. (2010). REVIEWS: hemostatic resuscitation for massive bleeding: the paradigm of plasma and platelets—a review of the current literature. *Transfusion, 50*(3), 701–710. http://dx.doi.org/10.1111/j.1537-2995.2009.02458.x.
75. Jones, B., & K. (2009). Abdominal injuries. In K. A. McQuillan, et al. (Ed.), *Trauma nursing: from rehabilitation through resuscitation* (4th ed.) (pp. 678–704). Philadelphia: Saunders.
76. Jurkovich, G. J., Frederick, P., & Rivara, F. J. (1993). The effect of acute alcohol intoxication and chronic alcohol abuse on outcome from trauma. *JAMA, 270*, 51–56.
77. Kalb, R. L. (1999). Preventing the sequelae of compartment syndrome. *Hosp Pract, 34*(1), 105–107.
78. Kearney, M. L. (1996). Imbalance of oxygen supply and demand. In V. H. Secor (Ed.), *Multiple organ dysfunction and failure* (pp. 135–147). St. Louis: Mosby.
79. Kellman, R. M. (2013). Face. In K. L. Mattox, D. V. Feliciano, & E. E. Moore (Eds.), *Trauma* (7th ed.) (pp. 395–413). New York: McGraw-Hill.
80. Kelly, M. P., et al. (1997). Substance abuse, traumatic brain injury, and neuropsychological outcome. *Brain Inj, 11*, 391–402.
81. Kirkpatrick, A. W., et al. (2000). Is clinical examination an accurate indicator of raised intra-abdominal pressure in critically injured patients? *Can J Surg, 43*, 207–211.
82. Klein, C. J., & Stanek, G. S. (2009). Metabolic and nutritional management of the trauma patient. In K. A. McQuillan, et al. (Ed.), *Trauma nursing: from resuscitation through rehabilitation* (4th ed.) (pp. 330–365). Philadelphia: Saunders.
83. Kreymann, G., Grosser, S., & Buggish, P. (1993). Oxygen consumption and resting metabolic rate in sepsis, sepsis syndrome, and septic shock. *Crit Care Med, 21*, 1012–1019.
84. Kudsk, K. A., & Curtis, C. (2013). Nutritional support and electrolyte management. In K. L. Mattox, D. V. Feliciano, & E. E. Moore (Eds.), *Trauma* (7th ed.) (pp. 1100–1127). New York: McGraw-Hill.
85. Lapointe, L. A., & von Rueden, K. T. (2002). Coagulopathies in trauma patients. *AACN Clin Issues, 13*(2), 192–203.
86. Li, G., Keyl, P. M., & Smith, G. S. (1997). Alcohol and injury severity: reappraisal of the continuing controversy. *J Trauma, 42*, 562–569.
87. Little, R. A., & Stoner, H. B. (1981). Body temperature after accidental injury. *Br J Surg, 68*, 221–227.
88. MacLeod, J. B., et al. (2003). Early coagulopathy predicts mortality in trauma. *J Trauma, 55*(1), 39–44.
89. Malinoski, D. J., Slater, M. S., & Mullins, R. J. (2004). Crush injury and rhabdomyolysis. *Crit Care Clin, 20*, 191–192.
90. McClave, S. A., & Snider, H. L. (1994). Understanding the metabolic response to critical illness: factors that cause patients to deviate from the expected pattern of hypermetabolism. *New Horiz, 2*, 139–146.
91. McConnell, K. J., et al. (2005). Mortality benefit of transfer to level I versus level II trauma centers for head-injured patients. *Health Serv Res, 40*(2), 435–457.
92. McKinley, B. A., et al. (2000). Tissue hemoglobin O_2 saturation during resuscitation of traumatic shock monitored using near infrared spectrometry. *J Trauma, 48*(4), 637–642.

93. McKinley, B. A., Valdivia, A., & Moore, F. A. (2003). Goal-oriented shock resuscitation for major torso trauma: what are we learning? *Curr Opin Crit Care*, *9*, 292–299.
94. McMahon, D. J., et al. (1997). Efficacy of inferior vena cava filters in selected patients with very high risk for fatal pulmonary embolism. *Chest*, *110*, 2S.
95. Meredith, J. W., et al. (1993). Femoral catheters and deep venous thrombosis: a prospective evaluation with venous duplex. *J Trauma*, *35*, 187–190.
96. Michelson, A. D., McGregor, H., & Barnard, M. R. (1994). Reversible inhibition of human platelet activation by hypothermia in vivo and in vitro. *J Thromb Haemost*, *71*, 633–640.
97. Miller, M. T., et al. (2003). Not so fast. *J Trauma*, *52*(1), 52–60.
98. Miller, P. R., et al. (1999). Randomized, prospective comparison of increased preload versus inotropes in the resuscitation of trauma patients: effects on cardiopulmonary function and visceral perfusion. *J Trauma*, *44*, 107–113.
99. Miller, P. R., et al. (1998). Threshold values of intramucosal pH and mucosal-arterial CO_2 gap during shock resuscitation. *J Trauma*, *45*(5), 868–872.
100. Miller, R. S., et al. (1994). Antithrombin III and trauma patients: factors that determine low levels. *J Trauma*, *37*, 442–445.
101. Mizushima, Y., Wanag, P., & Cioffi, W. G. (2000). Should normothermia be restored and maintained during resuscitation after trauma and hemorrhage? *J Trauma*, *48*, 58–65.
102. Morales, C. H., et al. (2004). Intra-abdominal infection in patients with abdominal trauma. *Arch Surg*, *139*(12), 1278–1285.
103. Morgan, P. B., & Buetcher, K. J. (2000). Blunt thoracic aortic injuries: initial evaluation and management. *South Med J*, *93*(2), 173–175.
104. Mueller, B. A., Kenaston, T., & Grossman, D. (1998). Hospital charges to injured drinking drivers in Washington state: 1989–1993. *Accid Anal Prev*, *30*, 597–605.
105. Mullins, R. J., et al. (2002). Survival of seriously injured patients first treated in rural hospitals. *J Trauma*, *52*(6), 1019–1029.
106. National Center for Statistics and Analysis. (2003). *Alcohol-related crashes and fatalities*. Washington, DC: National Highway Traffic Safety Administration.
107. National Highway Traffic Safety Administration. (1998). *Questions and answers regarding air gas, new occupant protection technology in 1998 vehicles, and supplemental questions and answers regarding air bags*. http://www.nhtsa.dot.gov.
108. National Highway Traffic Safety Administration. (1999). *Fourth report to congress effectiveness of occupant protection systems and their use*. Washington, DC: National Highway Traffic Safety Administration.
109. National Quality Forum. (2004). September. *National consensus standards for the prevention and care of deep vein thrombosis*. http://www.qualityforum.org/Publications/2006/12/National_Voluntary_Consensus_Standards_for_Prevention_and_Care_of_Venous_Thromboembolism__Policy,_Preferred_Practices,_and_Initial_Performance_Measures.aspx.
110. Ng, A. (2003). *Trauma ultrasonography: the FAST and beyond*. http://www.trauma.org.
111. O'Keefe, G. E. (2003). Abdominal compartment syndrome. *Crit Care Alert*, *11*(3), 29–32.
112. Owings, J. T., et al. (1996). Effect of critical injury on plasma antithrombin activity: low antithrombin levels are associated with thromboembolic complications. *J Trauma*, *41*, 396–405.
113. Passos, E., et al. (2014). Tourniquet use for peripheral vascular injuries in the civilian setting. *Injury*, *45*(3), 573–577. http://dx.doi.org/10.1016/j.injury.2013.11.031.
114. Pellino, T. A., Polacek, L. A., & Preston, M. A. S. (1998). Complications of orthopaedic disorders and orthopaedic surgery. In A. B. Maher, S. W. Salmond, & T. A. Pellino (Eds.), *Orthopaedic nursing* (pp. 646–689). Philadelphia: Saunders.
115. Peterson, S. R., Holday, N. J., & Jeevanandam, M. (1994). Enhancement of protein synthesis efficiency in parenterally fed trauma victims by adjuvant recombinant human growth hormone. *J Trauma*, *36*, 726–733.
116. Pfeifer, R., Pape, H.C., (2008). Missed injuries in trauma patients: a literature review. *Patient Safety in Surgery*, *20*(2). http://dx.doi.org/10.1186/1754-9493-2-20.
117. Pryor, J. P., et al. (2010). The evolving role of interventional radiology in trauma care. *J Trauma*, *59*(1), 102–104.
118. Pusateri, A., et al. (2003). Effect of a chitosan-based hemostatic dressing on blood loss and survival in a model of severe venous hemorrhage and hepatic injury in swine. *J Trauma*, *54*(1), 177–182.
119. Rall, J. M., et al. (2013). Comparison of novel hemostatic dressings with QuikClot combat gauze in a standardized swine model of uncontrolled hemorrhage. *J Trauma Acute Care Surg*, *75*(2 Suppl 2), S150–S156. http://dx.doi.org/10.1097/TA.0b013e318299d909.
120. Rhodes, M., & Cipolle, M. D. (1996). Deep venous thrombosis and pulmonary embolism. In K. Maull, A. Rodriguez, & C. E. Wiles (Eds.), *Complications in trauma and critical care* (p. 81). Philadelphia: Saunders.
121. Rivara, F. J., Jurkovich, G. J., & Gurney, J. G. (1993). The magnitude of acute and chronic alcohol abuse in trauma patients. *Arch Surg*, *128*, 907–912.
122. Rueler, J. B. (1978). Hypothermia: pathophysiology, clinical setting, and management. *Ann Intern Med*, *89*, 519–527.
123. Sauaia, A., Moore, F. A., & Moore, E. E. (1995). Epidemiology of trauma deaths: a reassessment. *J Trauma*, *38*, 185–193.
124. Schmied, H., Kurz, A., & Sessler, D. I. (1996). Mild hypothermia increases blood loss and transfusion requirements during total hip arthroplasty. *Lancet*, *347*, 289–292.
125. Schreiber, M. A. (2004). Damage control surgery. *Crit Care Clin*, *20*(1), 101–118.
126. Schulman, C. S. (2002). End points of resuscitation: choosing the right parameters to monitor. *DCCN*, *21*(1), 2–12.
127. Schulman, C. S., & Pierce, B. (1999). Continuous arteriovenous rewarming: a bedside technique. *Crit Care Nurse*, *19*(6), 54–63.
128. Seekamp, A., et al. (1999). Adenosine-triphosphate in trauma-related and elective hypothermia. *J Trauma*, *47*, 673–683.
129. Sherwood, S. F., McQuillan, K. A., & McQuillan, K. A. (2009). Maxillofacial trauma. In K. A. McQuillan, et al. (Ed.), *Trauma nursing: from resuscitation through rehabilitation* (4th ed.) (pp. 519–539). Philadelphia: Saunders.
130. Siegel, J. H., et al. (1990). Early predictors of injury severity and death in blunt multiple trauma. *Arch Surg*, *125*, 498–508.
131. Sise, M. J., & Shackford, S. R. (2013). Peripheral vascular injury. In K. L. Mattox, D. V. Feliciano, & E. E. Moore (Eds.), *Trauma* (7th ed.) (pp. 816–847). New York: McGraw-Hill.
132. Slater, M. S., & Mullins, R. J. (1998). Rhabdomyolysis and myoglobinuric renal failure in trauma and surgical patients: a review. *J Am Coll Surg*, *186*(6), 693–716.
133. Snyder, K. A., & Veronese, V. R. (2009). Genitourinary injuries and renal management. In K. A. McQuillan, et al. (Ed.), *Trauma nursing: from resuscitation to rehabilitation* (4th ed.) (pp. 706–731). Philadelphia: Saunders.
134. Steinemann, S., Shackford, S. W., & Davis, J. S. (1990). Implications of admission hypothermia in trauma patients. *J Trauma*, *30*, 200–202.
135. Stoner, H. B. (1969). Studies on the mechanisms of shock: the impairment of thermoregulation by trauma. *Br J Exp Pathol*, *52*, 650–656.
136. Sugrue, M., et al. (2002). Clinical examination is an inaccurate predictor of intraabdominal pressure. *World J Surg*, *26*, 1428–1431.
137. Sutchyta, M. R., et al. (1999). Epidemiology in ARDS. *Intensive Care Med*, *25*(5), 538–539.
138. Trunkey, D. D. (1983). Trauma. *Sci Am*, *249*, 28–35.
139. Vitello, J. M. (1999). *Metabolic response to stress*. San Diego, Calif. Paper presented at the 23rd Clinical Congress of the American Society for Parenteral and Enteral Nutrition: Nutrition support in stress and sepsis. Jan 31-Feb 3, 1999.
140. Von Rueden, K. T., Bolton, P., & Vary, T. C. (2009). Shock and multiple organ dysfunction syndrome. In K. A. McQuillan, et al. (Ed.), *Trauma nursing: from resuscitation through rehabilitation* (4th ed.) (pp. 200–223). Philadelphia: Saunders.
141. Vournakis, J. N., et al. (2003). The RDH bandage: hemostasis and survival in a lethal aortotomy hemorrhage mode. *J Surg Res*, *113*(1), 1–5.
142. Wagner, J. G., & Leatherman, J. W. (1998). Right ventricular end-diastolic volume as a predictor of the hemodynamic response to a fluid challenge. *Chest*, *113*(4), 1048–1054.

143. Wall, M. J., Tsai, P., & Mattox, K. L. (2013). Heart and thoracic vascular injuries. In K. L. Mattox, D. V. Feliciano, & E. E. Moore (Eds.), *Trauma* (7th ed.) (pp. 485–511). New York: McGraw-Hill.
144. Walsh, C. R. (2009). Musculoskeletal injuries. In K. A. McQuillan, et al. (Ed.), *Trauma nursing: from resuscitation through rehabilitation* (4th ed.) (pp. 735–774). Philadelphia: Saunders.
145. Ward, M. M. (1988). Factors predictive of acute renal failure in rhabdomyolysis. *Arch Intern Med, 148*(7), 1553–1557.
146. Weil, M. H., et al. (1999). Sublingual capnometry: a new noninvasive measurement for diagnosis and quantitation of severity of circulatory shock. *Crit Care Med, 27*(7), 1225–1229.
147. West, M. A., & Yeh, D. D. (2013). Infections. In K. L. Mattox, D. V. Feliciano, & E. E. Moore (Eds.), *Trauma* (7th ed.) (pp. 330–354). New York: McGraw-Hill.
148. Wiegelt, J. A., Brasel, K. J., & Klein, J. D. (2009). Mechanism of injury. In K. A. McQuillan, et al. (Ed.), *Trauma nursing: from resuscitation through rehabilitation* (4th ed.) (pp. 178–195). Philadelphia: Saunders.
149. Wild, B. R., Kenwright, J., & Rastogi, S. (1985). Effects of seatbelts on injuries to front and rear seat passengers. *BMJ, 290*(6482), 1621–1623.
150. Willy, C., Gerngross, H., & Sterk, J. (1999). Measurement of intracompartmental pressure with use of a new electronic transducer-tipped catheter system. *J Bone Joint Surg, 81*(2), 158–168.
151. Winkler, M., Akca, O., & Birkenberg, B. (2000). Aggressive warming reduces blood loss during hip arthroplasty. *Anesth Analg, 91*, 978–984.
152. Wisner, D. H. (2013). Injury to the spleen. In K. L. Mattox, D. V. Feliciano, & E. E. Moore (Eds.), *Trauma* (7th ed.) (pp. 561–580). New York: McGraw-Hill.
153. Woods, R. K., et al. (1998). Open pelvic fractures and fecal diversion. *Arch Surg, 133*(3), 281–287.
154. Wright, M. M. (1999). Resuscitation of the multitrauma patient with head injury. *AACN Clin Issues, 10*, 32–45.
155. Zager, R. A. (1992). Combined mannitol and deferoxamine therapy for myohemoglobinuric renal injury and oxidant tubular stress: mechanistic and therapeutic implications. *J Clin Invest, 90*(3), 711–719.
156. Zealley, I. A., & Chakraverty, S. (2010). The role of interventional radiology in trauma. *BKJ, 340*, c497. http://dx.doi.org/10.1136/bmj.c497.

31

Sepsis and Multiple Organ Dysfunction Syndrome

Teresa A. Wavra

Sepsis and multiple organ dysfunction syndrome (MODS) continue to be key contributors to disability and death in adult critical care patients. Studies have found that patients do not die from a single complication of their underlying disease, but rather from multiple organ failure.[7,22,40,96] Despite the significant strides made in life support technology, pharmacology, and science as a whole, the mortality rate for patients with two failing organ systems is 20% to 30%.[8,67] Although sepsis and septic shock are the most common causes of organ failure, MODS can also be initiated by any critical illness or traumatic injury that activates a massive systemic inflammatory response in acutely ill patients.[3,12] Other common triggers of MODS include major surgery, burns, shock, acute pancreatitis, acute renal failure, acute respiratory distress syndrome (ARDS), and necrotic tissue.[12]

In order to have a significant impact on this lethal syndrome, healthcare providers must be knowledgeable of the underlying pathophysiology of sepsis and MODS. This chapter focuses on current definitions, developing theories of the underlying pathophysiology, early signs and symptoms, and current guidelines for evidence-based management of patients with sepsis and MODS.

DEFINITIONS AND PATIENT IDENTIFICATION

Since the early 1990s there have been a variety of important improvements in clinical care of patients with sepsis. In 1992, an American College of Chest Physicians (ACCP) and Society of Critical Care Medicine Consensus Conference developed a set of definitions for systemic inflammatory response syndrome (SIRS), sepsis, and MODS.[20] The goal of the conference was to provide standard definitions for researchers and detailed physiologic parameters to assist bedside clinicians in early identification, diagnosis and treatment of patients.[20] In 2003, the European Society of Intensive Care Medicine and the Society of Critical Care Medicine partnered together to develop the *Surviving Sepsis Campaign* (SSC), an international effort to improve diagnosis and treatment of sepsis using the best practice and latest research with the common goal of reducing mortality from sepsis.[100] The goal was to develop evidence-based clinical guidelines to assist clinicians in the care and management of severe sepsis and septic shock to mitigate or eliminate MODS. The SSC has published three editions of guidelines since its inception[39] (Table 31.1).

SIRS is a physiologic response due to an insult or injury from either an infectious or noninfectious source. SIRS is diagnosed when at least two of the following criteria are present: temperature greater than 38°C or less than 36°C; heart rate (HR) greater than 90 beats per minute; respiratory rate (RR) greater than 20 breaths per minute or partial pressure of arterial carbon dioxide ($Paco_2$) less than 32 mm Hg or need for mechanical ventilation secondary to respiratory failure; or white blood cell (WBC) count greater than 12,000 mm^3 or less than 4000 mm^3 or greater than 10% immature neutrophils.[20,21,39] In 2016 the Third Annual International Censuses Definition for Sepsis and Septic Shock task force updated the sepsis definition. Sepsis is now defined as "life-threatening organ dysfunction caused by a dysregulated host response to infection." The task force has also eliminated the definition of severe sepsis.[99a] Septic shock is defined as a subset of sepsis in which underlying circulatory and cellular/metabolic abnormalities are profound enough to substantially increase mortality.[99a] The clinical assessment of sepsis shock includes persistent hypotension requiring vasopressors to maintain mean arterial pressure (MAP) ≥65 mm Hg and having a serum lactate level >2 mmol/L (18 mg/dL) despite adequate volume resuscitation.[99a] Prior to the new definition sepsis was defined as a systemic inflammatory response to probable or documented infection.[39] With the new definition, SIRS criteria has been redefined. SIRS criteria does not necessarily indicate a dysregulated, life-threatening response and has poor validity since it is often present in many hospitalized patients.[26a]

Under normal conditions, the inflammatory response is an essential and tightly regulated protective mechanism of local response to invasion of microorganism or local tissue damage. One of the complications of sepsis is MODS, which is defined as the presence of altered organ function in an acutely ill patient such that homeostasis cannot be maintained without the intervention of healthcare providers.[69] MODS is characterized by the development of progressive and potential reversible physiologic function of two or more organs.[13]

EPIDEMIOLOGY OF SEPSIS AND MULTIPLE ORGAN DYSFUNCTION SYNDROME

Since the consensus definition of sepsis there have been numerous epidemiologic studies to evaluate the impact of sepsis on the healthcare system. One study conducted in the United States between 1979 and 2000 showed an 8.7% increase in patients hospitalized with sepsis-related diagnosis.[78] Sepsis occurs in approximately 2% of all hospitalized patients and is accountable for 17% of in-hospital deaths.[79,83,84] It is estimated that \$14.6 billion is spent in caring for patients with sepsis-related diagnoses.[84] There are a variety of patient-specific factors and

TABLE 31.1 Definitions of Sepsis and Organ Failure

Infection, documented or suspected, and some of the following:
General variables
Fever (core temperature >38.3°C)
Hypothermia (core temperature <36°C)
Heart rate >90/min or >2 SD above the normal value for age
Tachypnea
Altered mental status
Significant edema or positive fluid balance (>20 mL/kg over 24 h)
Hyperglycemia (plasma glucose >110 mg/dL or 7.7 mmol/L) in the absence of diabetes
Inflammatory variables
Leukocytosis (WBC count >12,000 µL)
Leukopenia (WBC count <4000 µL)
Normal WBC count with >10% immature forms (bands)
Plasma C-reactive protein >2 SD above the normal value
Plasma procalcitonin >2 SD above the normal value
Hemodynamic variables
Arterial hypotension (SBP <90 mm Hg, MAP <70, or an SBP decrease >40 mm Hg in adults or <2 SD below normal for age)
Organ dysfunction variables
Arterial hypoxemia (Pao_2/Fio_2<300)
Acute oliguria (urine output <0.5 mL/kg/h or 45 mmol/L for at least 2 h)
Creatinine increase > 0.5 mg/dL or 44.2 mmol/L
Coagulation abnormalities (INR >1.5 or aPTT >60 sec)
Ileus (absent bowel sounds)
Thrombocytopenia (platelet count <100,000 μL^{-1})
Hyperbilirubinemia (plasma total bilirubin >4 mg/dL or 70 mmol/L)
Tissue perfusion variables
Hyperlactatemia (>1 mmol/L)
Decreased capillary refill or mottling

aPTT, Activated partial thromboplastin time; *Fio_2*, fraction of inspired oxygen; *INR*, international normalized ratio; *MAP*, mean arterial pressure; *Pao_2*, partial pressure of arterial oxygen; *SBP*, systolic blood pressure; *SD*, standard deviation; *WBC*, white blood cell. From Reference 40.

comorbidities that increase the potential to develop sepsis. These factors include age, race, ethnicity, and gender, as well as comorbidities that occur in immune compromised patients such as diabetes, HIV, and cancer. The literature identifies other factors that may be responsible for the increase in sepsis mortality, including the rise in invasive procedures, use of catheters, increase in microbial resistance, and the broader use of immunosuppressive and chemotherapeutic agents.[72,84] Respiratory infection is the most common cause of sepsis-related diagnosis. The second most common causes are genitourinary and abdominal sources. Regardless of the source, appropriate antimicrobial therapy is the cornerstone of treatment and improved survival.

Patients with sepsis are at high risk for complications and death related to organ dysfunction. MODS is estimated to develop in approximately 15% of all patients admitted to critical care units.[13] Mortality rates for MODS range from 27% to 100% in medical and surgical critical care units depending on the number of organs involved.[42] The estimated cost of MODS in critical care is $100,000 per patient, with a cost of $500,000 per patient survivor.[30,78] In order to continue tracking the true incidence and mortality of MODS, providers need to document it as a unique diagnosis as opposed to "respiratory failure" or "renal failure."[12,30,78]

PATHOPHYSIOLOGY OF SEPSIS

The immune system has two cooperative defense systems to fight microbial invasion: innate immunity and acquired immunity. Innate immunity is a nonspecific response that does not depend on the host's prior exposure to the pathogen and includes the acute phase response. It is designed to eliminate the infection or keep it in check until the second defense system can respond. Acquired immunity is a specific response tailored to an individual microbe.

Innate immunity consists of cells and proteins that are always present and ready to mobilize to fight pathogens at the site of infection. Cells present in the tissues, such as macrophages, dendritic cells, histiocytes, Kupffer cells, and mastocyte cells, interact with the pathogen.[46] These cells present receptors on the surface or in the cell called pattern-recognition receptors (PRRs). The PRRs recognize and bind to molecules and share a number of different recognizable biochemical features that are broadly utilized by pathogens called pathogen-associated molecular receptors (PAMPs). When the PRR recognizes a PAMP, the macrophage engulfs the pathogen and releases several inflammatory mediators. This local inflammatory response activates endothelial cells near the initial insult, releasing vasodilating mediators, such as histamine, bradykinin, serotonin, leukotrienes, prostaglandin, and nitric oxide (NO). The macrophage releases protein chemokines, which attract cells with chemokine receptors from the blood stream such as neutrophils and monocytes. The chemical mediators released during this acute phase are responsible for vasodilation of blood vessels at the local site of infection and the clinical signs of inflammation. This process can also be activated by damage-associated molecular patterns (DAMPS), which are markers of cell damage.[46,47]

Phagocytes such as neutrophils then trigger other parts of the immune system by releasing factors that summon leukocytes, which include natural killer cells, mast cells, basophils, and the phagocytic cells. Leukocytes produce the cytokines interleukin-1 (IL-1), IL-6, and tumor necrosis factor alpha (TNFα). These cytokines in turn activate the release of several other chemical mediators including IL-8, complement, histamine, kinins, serotonin, selectins, eicosanoids, and neutrophils, which results in local vasodilatation. This provides a physical and chemical barrier around the pathogen.

Interleukins stimulate liver cells to secrete proteins that bind to bacteria and activate complement proteins that destroy the pathogen. Phagocytic cells ingest the pathogen while the macrophage or neutrophil release chemicals that degrade the bacterial cell walls and proteins. Interleukins are also responsible for stimulating the increased number of circulating neutrophils and eosinophils, which help fight infection.

At the same time the endothelial cell lining of the blood vessels expresses adhesion proteins (cytokine and complement fragments) that facilitate the attachment of circulating leukocytes. The adhesion of proteins results in occlusion of the local small blood vessel, which prevents the pathogen from spreading to other parts of the body.[47,99] The attached leukocytes are attracted to the chemokines and migrate (diapedesis) into the tissue to the site of infection.

The inflammatory process manifests clinically as capillary leak, microvascular thrombi, tissue hypoxia, impaired vascular tone, and free radical damage (Fig. 31.1).[33,47,60] The inflammatory process is directed at eliminating the invading pathogen by isolating the damaged area, mobilizing chemical mediators, and promoting healing of any damaged tissue following the clearance of pathogens.[9,27,41,48] To maintain a system balance there is a compensatory antiinflammatory response syndrome (CARS), which produces antiinflammatory cytokine such as

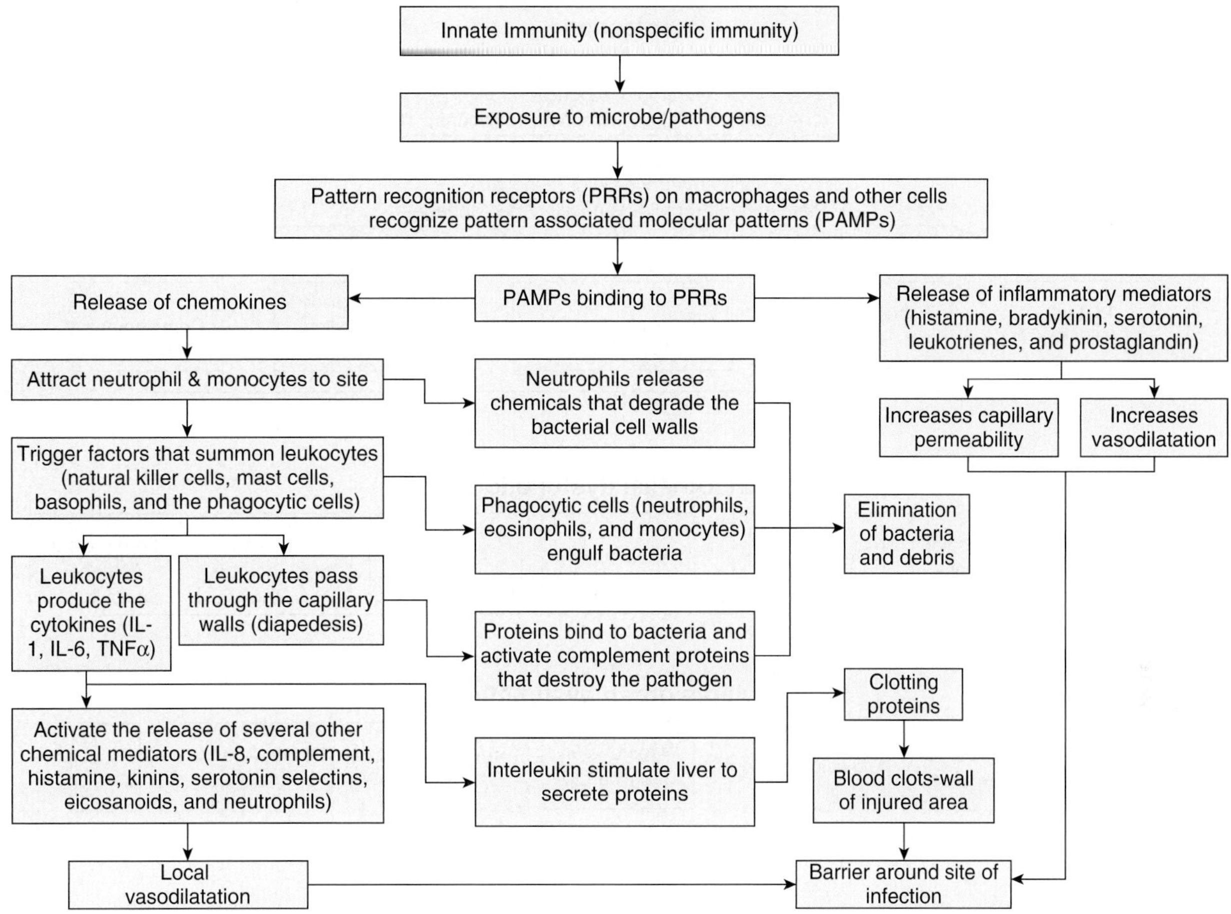

FIG. 31.1 Innate immunity. *IL*, Interleukin; *TNFα,* tumor necrosis factor alpha.

IL-6 and IL-10.[9,99] CARS, focus is to limit the damage caused by the proinflammatory response while not interfering with the pathogen elimination.

An appropriate inflammatory response eliminates the invading microorganisms without causing damage to tissues, organs, or other systems. When there are a limited number of microbes, the local responses are sufficient to clear the pathogen and the body returns to homeostasis.[48,86] If the microbial load is high or the host genetics, medications, preexisting illness, or environment are not conducive to eradicating the microbe, the potential consequence is an exaggerated inflammatory process that causes collateral tissue damage and necrotic cell death.

With necrotic cell death there is a release of DAMPS that acts on the same PRRs that were triggered by initial pathogens.[48,86] This results in a continuation of the inflammatory process. The complex array of intersecting pathways can become dysfunctional, with either excessive activation or depressed function, resulting in a self-destructive process that can be more fatal than the original infection.[9,27]

When patients have a life-threatening organ dysfunction related to a dysregulation of the host response to infection they are considered to have sepsis.[99a] Septic shock is defined as a subset of sepsis in which there is profound circulatory, cellular, and metabolic abnormalities.[99a] Sepsis and its sequelae, septic shock, represent a continuum of clinical and pathophysiologic severity that affects prognosis.

It is the innate immune response that plays a major role in sepsis pathophysiology. Sepsis can develop excessive immune response, leading to an imbalance between proinflammatory and antiinflammatory responses. In SIRS, the inflammatory response becomes systemic, impacting the entire body. The body is overwhelmed by unregulated inflammation, impaired coagulation, fibrinolysis, and endothelial dysfunction. Clinically, this manifests as fever, peripheral edema, hypotension, tachycardia, impaired oxygenation, and elevated white blood cell count.[20,33,69]

PATHOPHYSIOLOGY OF MULTIPLE ORGAN DYSFUNCTION SYNDROME

MODS is a complex and unpredictable clinical syndrome. The pathophysiology of MODS is related to a dysregulation of the immunologic response. It is associated with multiple integrated responses. These major responses include increased inflammation, tissue ischemia or necrosis, altered coagulation, and impaired fibrinolytic activity. There is also involvement of the endothelium, which becomes a central player in the development of SIRS and MODS.

Inflammation

As shown in Fig. 31.2, when the body is exposed to bacteria, bacterial products, necrotic tissue, or other insult, an inflammatory cellular response is initiated. There is an increased production of inflammatory cytokines in the form of IL-1, IL-6, and TNFα.[33] Although the early response of these cytokines plays a major role in the host's defense by attracting neutrophils to

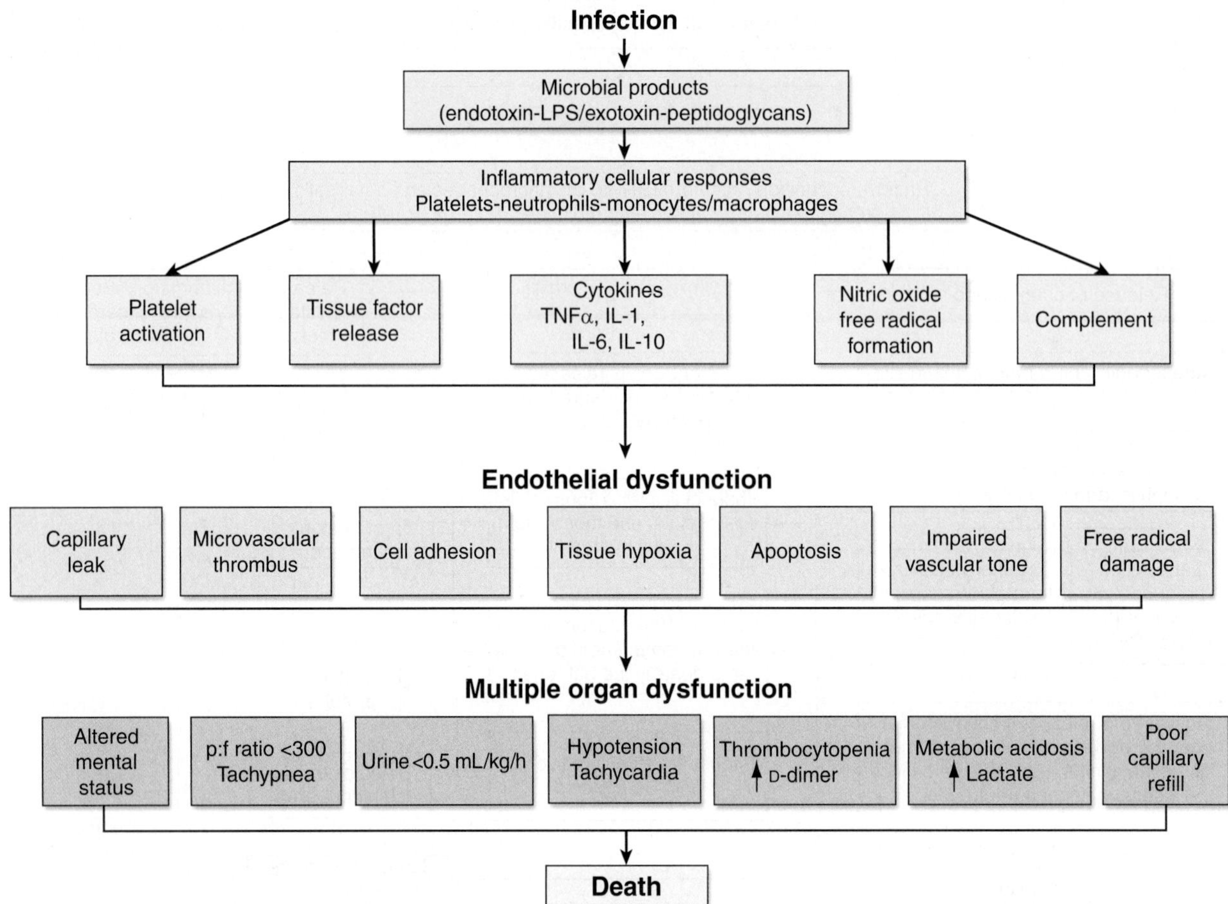

FIG. 31.2 Endothelial dysfunction and multiple organ dysfunction. *IL*, Interleukin; *p:f*, partial pressure of arterial oxygen tension (Pao_2)/fraction of inspired oxygen (Fio_2); *TNF*, tumor necrosis factor.

an infected site, it also contributes to the manifestations of the systemic inflammatory response.[33] The body attempts to maintain homeostasis by releasing antiinflammatory cytokines such as IL-4 and IL-10. Release of both the inflammatory and antiinflammatory mediators may lead to a state of primed inflammatory response (Fig. 31.3).[33]

Mitochondrial Dysfunction

Mitochondria are responsible for energy production, various cell signaling pathways, and regulation of cell death. Mitochondrial dysfunction occurs in sepsis when superoxide from the neutrophils and NO production from the vascular endothelium combine to form peroxynitrite. This inhibits several aspects of mitochondrial respiration and the synthesis of ATP, resulting in cytotoxic hypoxia. When the antioxidant is overwhelmed, the result is oxidative stress, which can cause damage to proteins, lipids, and nucleic acids within the mitochondria and cells. This process promotes cell death by apoptosis, which is the genetically directed process of cell self-destruction.[41]

Activation of Coagulation

Coagulation and inflammation are closely linked. It is believed that tissue factor, a protein, expressed by monocytes and endothelial cells following exposure to bacteria, initiates the extrinsic coagulation cascade.[3,14,33,47] Through cross talk and feedback mechanisms, the intrinsic coagulation pathway also can be initiated.[3,4,14,33,47] Both pathways play an important role in coagulation. The intrinsic pathway is considered the initiator of coagulation and the extrinsic pathway is considered the amplifier. This accelerated coagulation process occurs at the capillary level of the various organs. When clots form at the microcirculatory level, distal cells become anoxic and consequently, if not dissolved, the organ becomes dysfunctional and eventually dies.[3,4,14,26,33,47] As a rule, coagulation reactions occur on activated cell surface membranes. This reaction is believed to be initiated by activated tissue factor. In the case of MODS, the coagulation cascade may be activated by the inflammatory cytokine IL-6 acting on factor VIII.[33,36] Thrombin circulates in the form of prothrombin. The conversion of prothrombin to thrombin is mediated by factor Xa, which is activated by either factor VIIa of the extrinsic pathway or factor IXa of the intrinsic pathway. The result is that thrombin cleaves fibrinogen, forming fibrin, which then produces a clot.[3,4,14,26,33,47]

Impairment of Fibrinolysis

Normally clots are formed when bleeding occurs, but the vascular endothelium also has the ability to dissolve these clots using tissue plasminogen activator (tPA), which is released by endothelial cells. As the severity of sepsis progresses, fibrinolytic activity is impaired due to increased production of plasminogen activator inhibitor-1 (PAI-1) and thrombin-activated fibrinolysis inhibitor (TAFI). These mediators suppress the activity of tPA, resulting in the loss of ability to dissolve clots.

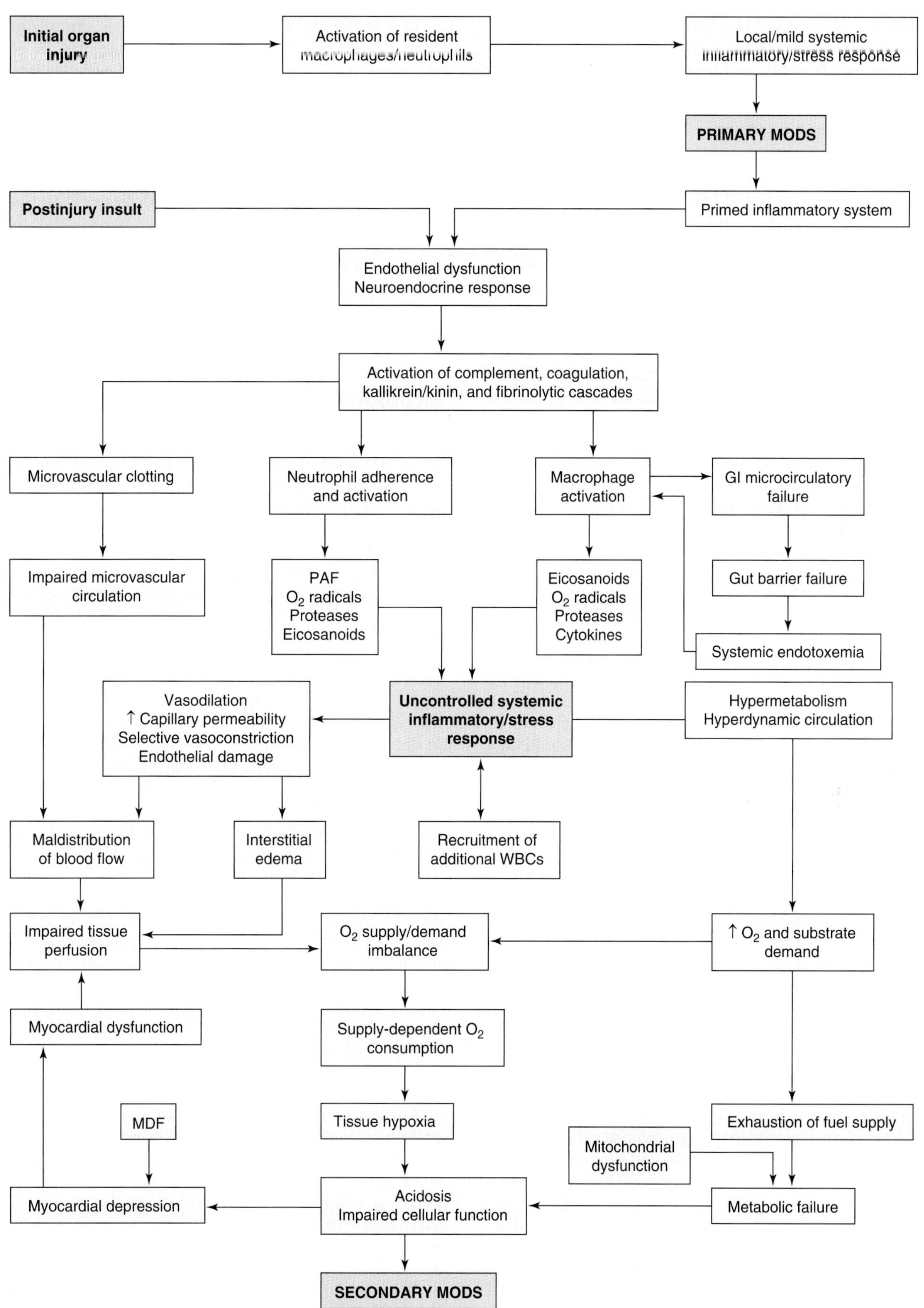

FIG. 31.3 Pathophysiology of multiple organ dysfunction syndrome (MODS). *GI*, Gastrointestinal; *MDF*, myocardial depressant factor; *PAF*, platelet activating factor; *WBC*, white blood cell. (From McCance, K. L., & Huether, S. E. (2014.) *Pathophysiology: the biologic basis for disease in adults and children* (7th ed.). Philadelphia: Mosby.)

Consequently, an increase in the production of clot formation is compounded when the ability to lyse clots is impaired, resulting in diminished blood flow at the microcirculatory level and organ damage.[3,4,14,33,47]

Alteration in Microcirculation

Microcirculation alterations play a major role in organ dysfunction. Trials have shown an association between the severity of microvascular dysfunction and organ dysfunction. There are various mechanisms that are potentially responsible for the impaired microcirculation, which include endothelial dysfunction, impaired inter-cell communication, altered glycocalyx, adhesion and rolling of white blood cells and platelets, and altered red blood cell deformability.[36,75]

In septic shock and MODS, there is a decrease in capillary density, which results in an increase in diffusion distance for oxygen. There is also heterogeneity of perfusion, which translates to perfused capillaries in close proximity to intermittent or nonperfused capillaries. Heterogeneity in perfusion results in altered oxygen extraction as compared to homogenously decreased perfusion. Changes also occur in the membrane properties of red blood cells, which have been postulated to be related to membrane damage from reactive oxygen species. Red blood cell deformity results in reduced flow in the microcirculation and contributes to impaired oxygen delivery and organ dysfunction.[5]

For many years the endothelium was considered an inert layer, separating blood from underlying tissue. Over time we have learned that the endothelium is a highly active cell layer that has several functions including controlling vasomotor tone, trafficking nutrients, and maintaining blood fluidity.[26] The largest organ in the body, the endothelium plays a key role in the inflammatory, prothrombotic, and impaired fibrinolytic components of SIRS and MODS.[3,4,26,27,33,47,48,102] Progression of endothelial dysfunction results in maldistribution of blood flow secondary to increased microvascular permeability and formation of microthrombi (see Fig. 31.2).[33,102] This is believed to be caused by either the production of inflammatory mediators and/or by the infecting organism or endotoxin.[34,102]

Normal endothelium has anticoagulant properties. A thin outer layer called the glycocalyx covers the endothelial surface. The glycocalyx is embedded with substances (superoxide dismutase and antithrombin) that facilitate the flow of red blood cells and limit adhesion of white bloods cells and platelets. Its outer membrane normally expresses various membrane-associated components with anticoagulant properties; among these is a cell surface heparin-like molecule. In SIRS and MODS, proinflammatory mediators are released from monocytes and macrophages, which cause injury to the endothelium.[33] These mediators promote recruitment of neutrophils and accumulation of platelets to wall off infection but they can also continue to damage the endothelial layer. After injury, the endothelial cells may down-regulate the synthesis and expression of antithrombin molecules, such as thrombomodulin, endothelial cell receptors for protein C, and tissue factor pathway inhibitor.[4,33,48]

Normally the endothelium produces a low level of adhesion molecules such as selectin. However, in septic shock and MODS, up-regulation of the adhesion molecules promotes interaction among the endothelium, white blood cells, and platelets. This interaction promotes accumulation of neutrophils and platelets that adhere to the endothelial wall and form further thrombi.[4,47]

In addition to the formation of clots, proinflammatory cytokines increase vascular permeability within 6 to 24 hours of the insult.[34] Physical disruption of the endothelium allows fluid and cells to move from the vascular compartment into the interstitial compartment, further adding to endothelial cell dysfunction, inflammation, and formation of edema. This is the mechanism responsible for the anasarca that critically ill patients may develop.[4,20,33,47]

Vasomotor tone can also be affected. Normally the endothelium secretes substances such as NO and epoprostenol that promote a steady level of vasodilation. This becomes impaired when increased production of NO leads to abnormal and persistent vascular relaxation.[93,98,106] As MODS progresses, alterations in vasoregulation result in vasodilation, refractory hypotension, and impaired microcirculatory blood flow, which eventually lead to system-wide organ dysfunction (see Fig. 31.2).[93,98]

MECHANISMS OF ORGAN DYSFUNCTION IN MODS

Cardiovascular System

In MODS there is an alteration in both cardiac and vascular tone. The direct cardiac abnormalities include reduction of both right and left ventricular ejection fraction and ventricular dilation related to the decrease in pulmonary compliance and injury. Cardiovascular dysfunction is both the result and cause of hypoperfusion through several mechanisms. The high levels of circulating inflammatory cytokines and DAMPS result in decreased vascular resistance and an increase in microvascular permeability. Initially, ventricular function increases cardiac output (CO) to maintain adequate BP in the presence of vasodilation because of the Frank-Starling mechanism.[36] The initial hyperdynamic response result is tachycardia and unstable systolic and mean arterial pressures. These changes result in decreased CO. However, older adult patients and those with profound SIRS and preexisting heart disease have an impaired ability to increase CO using contractility, resulting in hypoperfusion.[44] Myocardial contractility also may be depressed by the effects of hypoxia and acidosis of the myocardium or proinflammatory cytokines such as TNFα, IL-1, or the myocardial depressant factor.[44]

In the regional circulation, vascular hyporesponsiveness induced by SIRS or MODS leads to considerable maldistribution of systemic blood flow among organ systems as well as hypotension. For example, organ dysfunction interferes with the normal ability to redistribute blood away from splanchnic organs (e.g., liver, gastrointestinal system) to essential organs (e.g., heart, brain) when oxygen delivery is depressed.[33,49] Blood volume pools in the distal organ beds rather than actively circulating to essential organs, creating a relative hypovolemia further contributing to poor CO and cardiovascular dysfunction.[33]

Microcirculatory blood flow may present as either *no flow* or *intermittent flow*.[34] Techniques including reflectance spectrophotometry and orthogonal polarization spectral imaging allow for in vivo visualization of the sublingual and gastric microvasculature. Compared with normal controls and critically ill patients without organ dysfunction, patients with severe organ dysfunction have an overall decrease in vessel density.[34] These changes may be due to extrinsic compression of the capillary by tissue edema and endothelial swelling, or plugging of the capillary lumen by leukocytes or red blood cells.[89] This capillary obstruction prevents blood flow to distal tissues, creating a significant derangement in metabolic autoregulation. The increased microvascular permeability, depletion of intravascular volume, and peripheral edema result in worsening circulatory shock.

Metabolic autoregulation matches oxygen availability to changing tissue oxygen needs at the microvascular level. The initial release of inflammatory mediators causes appropriate vasodilation and increases microvascular permeability at the site of infection, a response intended to facilitate WBC movement through narrowed capillaries and into the interstitium to destroy bacteria. Among these mediators are the vasodilators epoprostenol and NO.[1,33,98,106] During septic shock, however, normal compensatory mechanisms become overwhelmed, and profound vasodilation and capillary permeability cause refractory hypoperfusion.[33] Subsequent blood flow stasis fails to deliver oxygen to the capillaries and cells, resulting in additional tissue ischemia and hypoperfusion (see Fig. 31.2).[1,34]

In particular, NO has additional influences on cardiovascular failure accompanying septic shock.[98] NO depresses the control mechanisms that match oxygen delivery to oxygen needs at all the central, regional, and microregional levels of the circulation. In addition, NO may trigger injury in the central nervous system in areas that regulate autonomic control such as HR and BP via apoptosis or programmed cell death of the neurons located in the critical area of the central nervous system.[98] NO can react with superoxide radical anions to form peroxynitrite. This potent oxidizing agent not only induces lipid peroxidation, thus compromising cell wall integrity, but also damages deoxyribonucleic acid (DNA). When DNA is damaged, the enzyme poly-ADP-ribosyl polymerase-1 is activated and uses nicotinamide adenine dinucleotide (NAD), an essential cofactor in a number of cellular reactions, including the consumption of oxygen by the mitochondria, to repair DNA. During the repair process, NAD is consumed; without the availability of NAD, the cell's mitochondria cannot use oxygen.[14,22,32,43]

Another factor contributing to persistent cardiovascular dysfunction is impaired compensatory secretion of antidiuretic hormone (vasopressin). Vasopressin is a nonapeptide synthesized in the hypothalamus.[54,55,74,101] Vasopressin release is stimulated by hyperosmolality, hypotension, and hypovolemia, as well as acidosis, pain, hypoxia, and hypercapnia.[54,55,74,101] Vasopressin acts on several different vasopressin receptors. Vasopressin-1 (V1) receptors stimulate vasoconstriction, V2 receptors regulate water balance, and V3 receptors stimulate adrenocorticotropin hormone (ACTH) release.[54,55,74,101] Normal vasopressin levels are 0.5 to 5.0 pg/mL in humans. In one report, plasma vasopressin levels were much lower in 19 patients with septic shock (3.1 pg/mL) than in 12 patients with cardiogenic shock who had similar systemic blood pressures (22.7 pg/mL).[50]

Yet another probable etiology of cardiovascular dysfunction in SIRS and MODS is relative adrenal insufficiency. In a double-blind, randomized study, 300 patients underwent corticotropin stimulation testing; they were randomly assigned to receive either hydrocortisone, fludrocortisone, or a matching placebo.[10] In this trial, those who met the criteria of relative adrenal insufficiency and received steroids had a lower incidence of death than those who received the placebo. Vasopressors were also withdrawn earlier in the steroid group.[10]

Respiratory System

Pulmonary dysfunction both results from and causes MODS. Acute lung injury (ALI) and ARDS can occur from either direct or indirect insult. Sepsis and pneumonia are the most common sources for initiating the inflammatory process leading to pulmonary endothelial dysfunction and ARDS.[12,15,96]

ARDS is defined by a partial pressure of arterial oxygen tension (Pao_2)/fraction of inspired oxygen (Fio_2) (P/F) ratio lower than 200 mm Hg, in association with bilateral fluffy pulmonary infiltrates and pulmonary artery occlusion pressure (PAOP) also called pulmonary capillary wedge pressure (PAWP) lower than 18mm Hg, or no evidence of left atrial hypertension.[15] In ARDS, endothelial dysfunction in the pulmonary vasculature leads to disturbed capillary blood flow and increased microvascular permeability over a large surface area, resulting in interstitial and alveolar edema.[9,15,60] Neutrophil entrapment within the lungs' microcirculation initiates and/or amplifies this injury to the alveolar-capillary membrane.[32,34] Pulmonary edema is the clinical result, and is accompanied by ventilation-perfusion mismatch and arterial hypoxemia. As the acute inflammatory process resolves there is further lung injury as a result of fibrosis and hyaline material disposition. Approximately 25% to 40% of ARDS cases originate from sepsis.[8,14,60]

Gastrointestinal System

The gastrointestinal (GI) tract is a particularly important target organ system for injury in organ dysfunction because it has the potential to provide a positive feedback loop in propagation of the injury.[33,34] This is even truer when the patient is intubated and unable to eat because bacteria may overgrow the upper GI tract and be aspirated into the lung, causing nosocomial pneumonia. Furthermore, the circulatory abnormalities seen during hypoperfusion may depress the gut's normal barrier function, allowing translocation of bacteria and endotoxin to enter the systemic circulation (possibly via the lymphatics), extending the inflammatory process.[33,36,60,64] Bacteria can be found in mesenteric lymph nodes as well as in the spleen and liver. Whether these findings are clinically important is not clear, although late infectious complications in SIRS/MODS are commonly caused by *Pseudomonas*, coagulase-negative staphylococcus, *Candida*, and *Eenterococcus*, all common organisms found in the GI tract of critically ill patients.[49,64]

Hepatic System

By virtue of the liver's role in host defense and synthetic functions, liver dysfunction contributes to both the initiation and progression of SIRS and MODS. The reticuloendothelial system of the liver normally acts as the first line of defense in clearing bacteria and bacteria-derived products that entered the portal system from the gut. Liver dysfunction prevents the elimination of enteric-derived endotoxin and bacteria-derived products, precluding appropriate local cytokine response and permitting direct entry of these potentially injurious products into the systemic circulation.[33,36,49,60,85] The liver may also serve as a site for the release of acute-phase reactants (e.g., proinflammatory and antiinflammatory cytokines) during a hypoperfused state, leading to the development of centrilobular necrosis. If the liver is already at risk from other causes such as cirrhosis, hepatic failure will significantly affect formation and release of coagulation factors, also affecting any ongoing blood loss. Lastly, liver failure decreases albumin production. Hypoalbuminemia causes movement of intravascular fluids into interstitial compartments and peripheral and organ edema, further contributing to MODS.[33,49]

Renal System

The mechanisms by which endotoxemia and MODS might lead to acute kidney injury (AKI) are attributed to systemic hypotension and decreased renal blood flow. It may also be the result of direct renal vasoconstriction from the release of cytokines such as TNF, and activation of neutrophils by endotoxin.

AKI may also be a cause in the development of SIRS or MODS via the activation of endothelium located in the renal system, which induces the release of the vasoconstrictor, endothelin, and decreases production of the vasodilators NO and prostacyclin.[36,60] The intrarenal vasoconstriction reduces the glomerular filtration rate and the hypoxic injury to tubular epithelial cells results in desquamation of injured cells into the tubules. This damage causes leakage of filtrate back into the renal interstitium, evoking neutrophil-mediated inflammation that causes further local tissue injury.

Neurologic System

Altered level of consciousness is the most recognized result of neurologic dysfunction in MODS, but the pathogenesis is poorly defined. It is postulated that the encephalopathy is the result of the metabolic alteration related to the direct effects of the proinflammatory mediators on cerebral function; dysfunction of neuronal communication; vasogenic cerebral edema, and reduced cerebral perfusion pressure; hepatic encephalopathy and hypotension that causes cerebral hypoxia and infarcts; and the iatrogenic effects of sedatives and analgesics.[13]

It is also possible that with growing endothelial dysfunction, microvascular hypoperfusion will have an impact on the development of encephalopathy.[2,12,33,57] Continued hypoperfusion, seen with shock and cardiac arrest, leads to neurologic dysfunction and cerebral microvascular changes, causing cerebral edema, increased intracranial pressure, and herniation. Loss of cerebral autoregulation function causes continued cerebral and systemic hypotension, potentiating ischemic and inflammatory processes in the brain and throughout the body; that is, central nervous system infection and stroke can cause global hypoperfusion, leading to inflammatory processes and MODS.[33]

Epidemiologic studies suggest that at least 25% of patients admitted to medical or surgical intensive care units have some degree of acquired paresis.[30,40,61,78] Most episodes present 7 or more days after the onset of critical illness. Affected patients manifest a sensorimotor polyneuropathy characterized clinically by limb muscle weakness and atrophy, reduced or absent deep tendon reflexes, loss of peripheral sensation to light touch and pinprick, and relative preservation of the cranial nerve function. Critical illness polyneuropathy is strongly associated with organ dysfunction and probably represents neurologic manifestations of the systemic inflammatory response.[33]

Hematologic System

Anemia is the most common hematologic abnormality noted in MODS. The etiology of anemia is unclear but could be related to crystalloid dilution, iatrogenic phlebotomy or the ongoing red cell destruction.[13] It could also be related to erythropoietin and hormonal deficiencies and global hyper-inflammation resulting in bone marrow suppression.[13]

Although disseminated intravascular coagulation (DIC) can occur in patients with organ dysfunction, the activation of the hemostatic system in patients with SIRS or MODS is not DIC. Increased D-dimers and decreased protein C levels are consistently seen in patients with organ dysfunction, but thrombocytopenia, prolonged activated partial thromboplastin time (aPTT), prothrombin time (PT), or any combination is distinctly uncommon.[36,40] DIC can occur because of increased activation of coagulation and inhibition of fibrinolysis. There are two phenotypes in DIC. One is the fibrinolytic (hemorrhagic) and the other is antifibrinolytic (thrombotic) phenotypes. DIC in sepsis is related to the PAI-1 mediated inhibition, which is the thrombotic phenotype.[46] The diagnosis of DIC is a clinicopathologic one; laboratory data suggest that the inflammatory and hemostatic changes of organ dysfunction are similar.[36,40] However, it is uncommon for the abnormal laboratory criteria seen with DIC, SIRS, or MODS to produce clinical bleeding.[3,8]

Decreases in protein C levels play an active role in the development of the hypercoagulable state in patients with septic shock, and are linked to the development of organ dysfunction and increased mortality.[14,36] A study of patients with cancer, chemotherapy-induced neutropenia (absolute neutrophil count [ANC] less than 1000/μL), and septic shock demonstrated that protein C concentrations fall before the onset of fever or alterations in the leukocyte count. In fact, protein C levels decline 16 hours before septic shock is clinically diagnosed.[14] Protein C is a glycoprotein that is synthesized in the liver and circulates in the bloodstream. Activated protein C (APC) binds to the cell-surface-bound anticoagulant cofactor, protein S. The APC/protein S complex then lyses activated procoagulant cofactors such as factor VIII and factor V, reducing fibrin formation by preventing activation of procoagulant proteins such as factor X and prothrombin. Protein C deficiency is associated with an increased risk of thrombus formation. In addition to having anticoagulant properties, APC also appears to have profibrinolytic and antiinflammatory properties and preserves endothelial function.[14,60]

In one study, both tissue plasminogen activator and PAI-1 were high in survivors and nonsurvivors of sepsis, but survivors showed a progressive normalization of fibrinolytic parameters during the study period.[14] Low plasminogen levels and plasminogen/alpha 2-antiplasmin ratios were found in both groups, with a trend toward normalization noted only in survivors. The differences reported were not apparent at the time of hospital admission. The investigators concluded that in the presence of fibrin formation, nonsurvivors maintained an imbalance in the fibrinolytic response determined by a higher PAI-1 plasma concentration.[14]

ASSESSMENT OF MULTIPLE ORGAN DYSFUNCTION SYNDROME

Much of our understanding of the progression of MODS comes from the work of Knaus et al., using the Acute Physiology and Chronic Health Evaluation (APACHE) scoring systems at George Washington University.[61] Their work gave rise to a more consistent method for quantifying organ dysfunction and patient outcomes associated with MODS.[61] Organ dysfunction has been described using physiologic criteria that are based on clinical presentation and laboratory markers for the neurologic, pulmonary, hepatic, cardiovascular, renal, and hematologic systems.[60] The degree of physiologic derangement present on admission is a determining factor of morbidity and critical illness survival. These criteria, along with general clinical presentation of patients with MODS, are described hereafter; a complete review of the pathophysiology and clinical presentation of individual organ dysfunction or failure is presented in organ-specific chapters elsewhere in this book.

A change in the level of consciousness is one of the most sensitive indicators of a failing neurologic system (Box 31.1). This change in mental status can be as subtle as an alteration in mental status to confusion or even deep coma. Most often, the critical care nurse will assess neurologic status using a specific scale such as the Glasgow Coma Scale (GCS).[61] The GCS is based on eye opening, verbal response, and motor response. The total possible score is 15; the lowest is a 3, indicating a patient in a total coma state. A patient with MODS will often have a GCS score of less than 6 in the absence of sedation.[61]

Manifestations of respiratory failure in MODS include a $Paco_2$ of greater than 50 mm Hg, ventilator or continuous positive airway pressure dependence on the second day of organ dysfunction, and a P/F ratio equal to, or less than, 300. The ACCP defines a P/F ratio of less than 200 as ARDS, and P/F ratio of less than 300 as ALI.[1,30] Clinical presentation also may include tachypnea, severe dyspnea, decreased oxygen saturation, cyanosis, respiratory acidosis, and refractory hypoxemia.[16,60]

Manifestations of hepatic failure include jaundice with bilirubin levels of greater than 4 mg/dL or 70 mmol/L. Liver enzymes are also elevated, including aspartate aminotransferase (AST), alanine aminotransferase (ALT), lactic dehydrogenase (LDH), and alkaline phosphatase. An increase in serum ammonia and decreases in serum albumin, prealbumin, and transferrin levels also may be present. A dysfunction in the regulation of the coagulation cascade is demonstrated by INR greater than 1.5 or aPTT greater than 60 seconds. Any time a coagulopathy is noted in the absence of anticoagulant therapy, a full workup of liver function should be performed.[2,33,39,60] The clinical manifestation of hepatic dysfunction in MODS is hepatomegaly, jaundice, bleeding, and hepatic encephalopathy.[60]

Cardiovascular dysfunction associated with MODS presents in a number of ways. Early signs and symptoms of cardiovascular challenges include tachycardia, hypotension, pale mottled skin that is cool to the touch, and weak peripheral pulses.[60] Fulminant cardiac dysfunction in MODS is an ominous indication that compensatory requirements of hypoperfusion and shock are overwhelming.[2,33,60] As systemic hypoperfusion continues, the microcirculation continues to deteriorate; decreased oxygen delivery, as well as decreased consumption, are evidenced by a serum pH less than 7.24 and a $Paco_2$ greater than 49 mm Hg.[33,60]

Criteria for renal dysfunction in MODS include urine output less than 479 mL/24 hours or less than 159 mL/8 hours, serum blood urea nitrogen (BUN) greater than 100 mg/dL, and/or serum creatinine greater than 3.5 mg/dL.[2,33,60] The cause of renal dysfunction in MODS may be due to renal hypoperfusion or possibly acute tubular necrosis. The clinical manifestation may be oliguria or anuria along with elevated BUN and serum creatinine.[60]

The last markers of organ dysfunction in MODS are abnormalities in hematologic function. Manifestations of hematologic failure include thrombocytopenia (platelet count < 100,000 μL^{-1}), prolonged international normalized ratio (INR) greater than 1.5 or aPTT greater than 60 seconds, decreased protein C (normal level is 4 mcg/mL), leukopenia (< 4000 cells/mm^3), and an elevated D-dimer level (normal range is 0 to 0.4 mcg/mL).[4,14,60]

Quantification of organ function may be measured with one of several outcome prediction scores. The Logistic Organ Dysfunction Score (LODS) (Table 31.2), MODS score (Table 31.3), or the Sequential (formerly Sepsis-Related) Organ Failure Assessment (SOFA) (Table 31.4) are based on dysfunction of the respiratory, renal, hepatic, cardiovascular, hematologic, and neurologic systems and combine the severity of organ dysfunction from MODS into a single score. In 2002, Pettila et al. compared the predictive power for hospital mortality using the LODS, MODS, and SOFA tools along with the APACHE III and found that the discriminative power was strong among all the tools tested.[88] The study demonstrated that the greater the score and duration of organ dysfunction, the higher the mortality from MODS.[30,40,61,88] The APACHE is more predictive of mortality at admission and the MODS and SOFA score are more useful in monitoring disease progression.[81] The European Society of Intensive Care Medicine has proposed the use of the SOFA tool in sepsis-related diagnosis.[105] The International Consensus Definitions for Sepsis and Septic shock task force recommended a simplified SOFA score called a quick SOFA (qSOFA). The qSOFA score incorporates the following three clinical criteria: altered mentation, systolic blood pressure of 100 mm Hg or less, and respiratory rate of 22 per minute or greater. The presence of two or more of the criteria in adult patients with suspected infections should prompt the clinician to escalate therapy since these patients are more likely to have poor outcomes.[99a]

The scoring systems were designed to describe the evolving morbidity and mortality and are employed primarily in clinical evaluation of interventions to treat MODS and sepsis.[30,40,61,88] In most of the scoring tools, the disease severity is evaluated using clinical presentation and laboratory data on the six specific organ systems.[30,40,61,88] In clinical practice, treatment is initiated as the scores increase, although there is no research defining at exactly what point on each scale interventions should start. The

BOX 31.1 Commonly Used Markers of Acute Organ System Dysfunction

Cardiovascular

Tachycardia
Dysrhythmias
Hypotension
Elevated central venous and pulmonary artery pressures

Respiratory

Tachypnea
Hypoxemia
Renal
Oliguria
Anuria
Elevated creatinine levels

Hematologic

Jaundice
Elevated levels of liver enzymes
Decreased concentration of albumin
Coagulopathy

Hepatic

Thrombocytopenia
Coagulopathy
Decreased levels of protein C
Increased levels of D-dimers

Neurologic

Altered consciousness
Confusion
Psychosis

From Reference 60.

TABLE 31.2 Logistic Organ Dysfunction Score System

Variables	0	1	2	3	4
Glasgow Coma Scale	14–15	9–13	6–8	4–5	3
Pao_2/Fio_2	No ventilator	>250	150–249	50–149	<50
Heart rate	130–139	140–159	160	<30	
Blood urea nitrogen	<6	6–9.9	10–19.9	>20	
Creatinine	<1.2	1.2–1.6	>1.6		
Urine output (L/day)	0.75–9.99	0.5–0.74	<0.5		
White blood cell count	2.5–49.9	1.0–2.4 or >50	<1.0		
Bilirubin	<34.2	34.2–68.3	>68.3		
Platelets	≥ 50	<50			
Prothrombin time	≥ 25%	<25%			

Fio_2, Fraction of inspired oxygen; *Pao_2*, partial pressure of arterial oxygen.
From Reference 68.

TABLE 31.3 Multiple Organ Dysfunction Syndrome Scoring System

Organ System	0	1	2	3	4
Cardiovascular (heart rate, inotropes, lactate)	≤ 120	120–140	>140	Inotropes	Lactate >5
Respiratory, Pao_2/Fio_2	>300	226–300	151–225	76–150	≤ 75
Renal (creatinine, mmol/L)	≤100	101–200	201–350	351–500	>500
Central nervous system (Glasgow Coma Scale score)	15	13–14	10–12	7–9	≤ 6
Hepatic (total bilirubin, mmol/L)	≤20	21–60	61–120	121–240	>240
Hematologic (platelet count × 10^3)	>120	81–120	51–80	21–50	≤ 20

Six domains of multiple organ dysfunction syndrome (MODS). The original cardiovascular component was defined by the heart rate times right atrial pressure. The modified cardiovascular component of MODS is defined as follows: 0, heart rate <120 beats per minute (bpm); 1, heart rate 120–140 bpm; 2, heart rate >140 bpm; 3, need for inotropes more than dopamine >3 mcg/kg/min; 4, serum lactate >5 mmol/L.
Fio_2, Fraction of inspired oxygen; *Pao_2*, partial pressure of arterial oxygen.
From Reference 77.

TABLE 31.4 Sequential Organ Failure Assessment Scoring System

	SCORE				
Organ System	0	1	2	3	4
Respiratory Pao_2/Fio_2	>400	≤ 400	≤ 300	≤ 200	≤ 100
Renal creatinine, mmol/L	≤ 110	110–170	171–299	300–440	>440
Hepatic bilirubin, mmol/L	≤ 20	20–32	33–101	102–204	>204
Cardiovascular hypotension	No hypotension	Mean arterial pressure <70 mm Hg	Dopamine ≤ 5	Dopamine >5 or epinephrine ≤ 0.1 or norepinephrine ≤ 0.1	Dopamine >15 or epinephrine > 0.1 or norepinephrine >0.1
Hematologic platelet count (× 10^{12}/L)	>150	≤ 150	≤ 100	≤ 50	≤ 20
Neurologic Glasgow Coma Scale score	15	13–14	10–12	6–9	<6

Fio_2, Fraction of inspired oxygen; *Pao_2*, partial pressure of arterial oxygen.
From Reference 105.

key for the critical care nurse is the early detection and treatment of dysfunctional organ systems to avoid subsequent organ failure. Mortality from MODS with failure of just two organ systems is 20% to 30%, and increases significantly to 100% when five or more systems have failed.[12]

INTERVENTIONS

Early detection or prevention of organ dysfunction is extremely important because there is no specific therapy for MODS once it occurs. In October 2003, 11 international critical care and infectious disease organizations collaborated to develop and publish management guidelines for the care of patients with sepsis and severe sepsis, known as the SSC.[38] This international effort focused on increasing the awareness and improving the outcomes of severe sepsis. The third edition of the guidelines was published in 2012 and another revision in the bundles was published in 2015.[39,100] Because sepsis is the most common etiology for MODS, many of the recommendations from the SSC may be applicable for any patient with multiple organ dysfunction. The majority of their recommendations are grouped by category and not supported by evidence but only by expert opinion.[38,45] A interprofessional plan of care should be developed when caring for patients with sepsis and/or MODS. The overall goal of the SSC is to prevent and respond to organ dysfunction before it becomes irreversible. A full review of individual organ system support is beyond the scope of this chapter, but is found elsewhere in this text. The following discussion focuses on the specific interventions prioritized by the SSC to avert MODS resulting from increased severity of sepsis and septic shock.

Initial Resuscitation

Reducing the time to diagnosis and treatment of sepsis is paramount in decreasing mortality. Early recognition requires routine screening for sepsis not only in emergency departments but also throughout the hospital. The primary goal in initial resuscitation is to achieve adequate tissue perfusion.

The third update of the SSC guidelines in 2012 recommends two treatment bundles to be completed within 6 hours.[39] The first bundle, to be completed within 3 hours, includes measuring initial lactic acid level, obtaining blood cultures before administering antibiotics, administering broad spectrum antibiotics, and administering 30 mL/kg crystalloid for hypotension or lactate acid level of 4 mmol/L or greater. In patients who exhibit signs of decreased tissue perfusion, it is important not to delay administering antibiotics if it is going to take longer than 45 minutes to obtain blood cultures.[12] The second bundle, to be completed within 6 hours, includes intravenous vasopressors and monitoring central venous pressure (CVP) and/or mixed venous oxygen saturation (Svo_2) when there is persistent arterial hypotension after initial volume resuscitation, or the patient's initial lactate is 4 mmol/L or greater, and finally to remeasure lactic acid levels to determine if the treatment has improved the patient's tissue perfusion.

During the first 6 hours of treatment, resuscitation goals should include all of the following: CVP, 8 to 12 mm Hg (12 to 15 mm Hg if mechanically ventilated); MAP equal to or greater than 65 mm Hg, or systolic BP greater than 90 mm Hg; urinary output equal to or greater than 0.5 mL/kg/hour; and central venous oxygen saturation ($Scvo_2$) equal to or greater than 70%, or Svo_2 equal to or greater than 65%, as well as normalizing lactate levels if initially markers were elevated.[39,58]

The Australasian Resuscitation in Sepsis Evaluation (ARISE) trial in 2009 did not use protocols or $Scvo_2$ to direct resuscitation and the mortality was similar to other international sepsis trials.[37] The Protocol-Based Care for Early Septic Shock (ProCESS) multicenter randomized trial in 2014 concluded that protocol-based resuscitation in septic shock patients did not improve outcomes.[93] ProCESS enrolled 1341 patients with recognized septic shock in the emergency department. Patients were randomly assigned to protocol-based, early goal directed therapy (EGDT), protocol-based standard therapy, and usual care. There were different resuscitation strategies with respect to the monitoring of CVP, oxygenation, use of intravenous fluids, vasopressors, inotropes, and blood transfusions.[93] The investigators found no significant benefit with the use of central venous catheterization or hemodynamic monitoring.

The Protocolised Management in Sepsis (ProMISe) trial, in 2015, compared EGDT versus *usual* care.[82] The study enrolled 1260 patients, with 630 assigned to EGDT and 630 to usual care. The results of that trial did not show any statistical difference in 90-day mortality between the two groups. The three studies confirm that early identification and intravenous fluid resuscitation are the hallmarks to improve patient outcomes. The studies invalidated the need for CVP and $Scvo_2$ monitoring to dictate care.[82]

Traditionally, static indicators such as CVP have guided fluid resuscitation. In sepsis it is important to identify patients who are preload (fluid) responsive. Recent and historic literature indicates CVP is a poor predictor of volume status or preload responsiveness.[76] The SSC continues to have CVP guided fluid responsiveness in the guidelines because many centers do not have access to other dynamic variable technology and removal may result in inadequate volume resuscitation.[73] There is evidence that dynamic variables are accurate predictors of fluid responsiveness in patients who are in sinus rhythm and mechanically ventilated with sufficient tidal volumes.

With the publication of these three trials, the SSC revised the 6-hour bundle to include a repeat focused exam after initial fluid resuscitation by a licensed independent practitioner. The recommendations for reassessment include documentation of vital signs, cardiopulmonary assessment, capillary refill, pulse, and skin findings or two of the following: CVP, $Scvo_2$, bedside cardiovascular ultrasound, and dynamic assessment fluid responsiveness with passive leg raise or fluid challenge.[100]

To achieve the resuscitation goals in patients with sepsis-induced tissue hypoperfusion, initial fluid resuscitation should be 30 mL/kg.[29,40,44,97] Additional boluses of crystalloids (e.g., 0.9% saline or lactated Ringer's [LR] 500 to 100 mL) and colloids (e.g., albumin 300 to 500 mL) may be given and repeated as long as there is hemodynamic improvement either based on dynamic (e.g., change in pulse pressure, stroke volume variation) or static (e.g., arterial pressure, heart rate) variables.[24,29,75,76] The choice of using colloids or crystalloids remains controversial.[90] One issue that is not controversial is that crystalloid use requires approximately three times as much fluid as colloids to reach the same end point. Crystalloids have a larger distribution space and do not remain in the intravascular space, putting the patient at risk for significant edema.[11,87]

There are few studies that compare balanced crystalloid solutions such as LR with 0.9% saline in sepsis patients. Literature shows that 0.9% saline is high in chloride content and can lead to pathophysiologic changes that are not seen when using balanced crystalloid solutions. Research in animal models shows an increase in inflammatory cytokines, worsened hypotension, and hyperlactatemia with the administration of 0.9% saline.[70] Animal sepsis models have shown 0.9% saline may cause or worsen hyperchloremic acidosis and has been associated with increased risk of renal injury.[70] Hyperchloremia is associated with progressive renal vasoconstriction and a fall in glomerular filtration rate.[70] Raghunathan et al. examined 53,448 patients with sepsis who were treated with vasopressors and crystalloid. The study found a lower risk of in-hospital mortality with balanced fluids such as LR.[20,94]

Balanced solutions should not be used in patients with alkalosis and hypochloremia. LR, which is hypoosmolar, may not be suitable to use in patients with head injuries. It is obvious that one size does not fit all and fluid resuscitation should be individualized to the patient's condition. These findings could have significant implications for the choice of fluids used for resuscitation in the future.

Management of Infection

Source Identification

Early diagnosis along with source identification and control are essential interventions for sepsis before it develops into septic shock. These activities should occur simultaneously with ongoing resuscitation, as indicated by the patient's clinical condition. Whenever possible, cultures of all potential infection sites should be obtained before antibiotics are given. To optimize identification of the causative organisms, at least two blood cultures should be obtained, with one drawn from a vascular access and the other from venipuncture.[18] If both cultures are positive, it suggests that the same organism is causing the sepsis. Moreover, if the culture from the vascular access is positive at a time earlier than the peripheral sample was drawn, it may offer support that the access is the source of the infection.[6] Other diagnostic studies (chest x-ray, ultrasound, computed tomography [CT] scan, lumbar puncture) should be performed promptly to determine the source of infection and the causative organism. However, the patient's safety and ongoing resuscitation should never be jeopardized for the sake of obtaining the cultures.[6]

Antibiotic Therapy

After appropriate cultures are obtained, broad-spectrum antibiotics should be started within the first hour of recognizing severe sepsis. Once the pathogen is identified, the drugs should be changed to organism-specific antibiotics to prevent superinfection and minimize development of resistant pathogens.[9,12,36] Forty-eight to seventy-two hours after starting antibiotics, the response to treatment should be reevaluated and changed as indicated.[66] Antibiotics should be administered for 7 to 10 days and be guided by clinical response.[50,65] Antibiotics should be discontinued if the clinical syndrome is due to a noninfectious source.[17,18]

Source Control

Patients should be examined for the source of infection and evaluated by an appropriate service for source control (e.g., interventionalist for abscess drainage or surgeon consult for surgery). When a source of infection is identified, source control should be initiated as soon as possible after resuscitation. If an intravenous catheter is the likely source of infection, the device should be promptly removed after another access can be established. Benefit of the method of source control must outweigh the risk and the treatment used should be the one with the least physiologic upset.[12,38]

Additional Hemodynamic Support

Vasopressors

Vasopressors can be used if adequate fluid volume fails to restore blood pressure and organ perfusion. (The medication table in Chapter 29 provides comprehensive information about vasopressor agents.) Norepinephrine (Levophed) is the first choice vasopressor. The goal is to target vasopressor therapy to a MAP of 65 mm Hg. Norepinephrine at 0.5 mcg to 30 mcg/min has been shown to be an excellent first choice for septic shock because it has less chronotropic effect, especially for patients who are already tachycardic.[35] Either epinephrine or vasopressin can be added if an additional agent is needed to maintain target MAP.[39] Dopamine is only recommended in patients with low risk of tachyarrhythmias and absolute or relative bradycardia.[39] Phenylephrine (Neo-Synephrine) is only recommended if norepinephrine is associated with serious arrhythmias or CO is known to be high and BP persistently low. It can also be used as a salvage therapy when combined inotrope/vasopressor drugs and low dose vasopressin have failed to achieve target MAP.

Several studies show that during early septic shock, vasopressin levels are elevated.[54,55,74] However, with continued shock, vasopressin concentration decreases to within a normal range in the majority of the patients within 24 to 48 hours. This is referred to as *relative vasopressin deficiency* because in the presence of hypotension, vasopressin should be elevated. Vasopressin is a direct vasoconstrictor without inotropic or chronotropic effects and may result in decreased CO and hepatosplanchnic flow. There are unique vasopressin receptor sites in the peripheral vasculature, explaining why this agent may be used when adrenergic agents have been ineffective. The guidelines recommend vasopressin should be added to norepinephrine at a rate of 0.03 unit/min to maintain MAP greater than 65 mm Hg. The use of higher doses of 0.03 to 0.04 unit/min should only be used if salvage therapy is required. Doses of greater than 0.04 unit/min have been associated with myocardial ischemia, significant decreases in CO, and cardiac arrest.[47-49,55]

Inotropic Therapy

Dobutamine to augment myocardial contractility may be used in patients with low CO despite adequate fluid resuscitation. Combined with vasopressor therapy, it can be used to increase BP and CO.[38] Infusion doses range from 2.5 to 20 mcg/minute. Increasing cardiac index to supranormal levels in order to achieve arbitrarily predefined targets is not recommended. Two large prospective clinical trials in critically ill patients failed to demonstrate benefit by increasing oxygen delivery to supranormal levels by using dobutamine.[35,51]

Steroids

For patients with persistent septic shock despite adequate fluid resuscitation and vasopressors, intravenous corticosteroids are indicated.[38] One multicenter, randomized, controlled trial with patients in septic shock showed a high incidence of *relative* adrenal insufficiency as determined by a cortisol stimulation test.[104] To perform this test, three cortisol levels were drawn: a preadministration dose, immediately following the administration of 250 mcg of ACTH, and 30 to 60 minutes after administration. Those patients whose serum cortisol levels were less than or equal to 9 mcg/dL were classified as nonresponders and found to have a reduced mortality with the full course of steroid administration. With hypotensive patients, clinicians should not wait for ACTH results to administer corticosteroids.[10,19,31,38,104]

Hydrocortisone 200 mg/day is recommended for 7 days by continuous infusion.[19,31,38] Doses of corticosteroids greater than 300 mg daily should not be used in septic shock for the purpose of treating septic shock because high doses have been shown to be ineffective and even harmful.[19,31,38,104] In the absence of shock, corticosteroids should not be administered for the treatment of sepsis.

Blood Product Administration

Red blood cell transfusion should be continued if hemoglobin (Hgb) remains below 7 g/dL. A level of 7 to 9 g/dL should be targeted as more conservative transfusion thresholds are associated with improved mortality in critically ill patients.[52] Red blood cell transfusion in septic patients improves oxygen delivery but not consumption.[71] Erythropoietin is not recommended as a specific treatment of anemia associated with sepsis but may be used for septic patients who may have other reasons for its administration, such as renal failure.[38]

Coagulopathy accompanying sepsis often requires administration of several blood products. Professional organizations have recommended fresh frozen plasma to treat coagulopathy associated with a documented deficiency of coagulation factors.[91,92] Routine use of fresh frozen plasma for volume resuscitation alone or to correct laboratory clotting abnormalities in the absence of bleeding or planned invasive procedure is not recommended.[91,92] Antithrombin administration is not recommended for the treatment of severe sepsis or septic shock.[107] In particular, high-dose antithrombin is associated with an increased risk of bleeding, especially when given with heparin.[107] Platelets should be administered to patients with sepsis when counts are less than 10,000/mm^3, regardless of apparent bleeding. Platelet transfusion may be considered when counts are less than 20,000/mm^3 and there is significant risk of bleeding. Platelet counts greater than 50,000/mm^3 are typically required for surgery or invasive procedures.[39,91,92]

Mechanical Ventilation

High tidal volumes coupled with high plateau pressures should be avoided in ALI/ARDS because overventilation of affected alveoli potentiates the pulmonary inflammatory response.[1,53] Tidal volume should be targeted to 6 mL/kg of predicted body weight in conjunction with inspiratory plateau pressures of less than 30 cm H_2O.[23,38,53] Hypercapnia (allowing $Paco_2$ to increase above normal, called *permissive hypercapnia*) can be tolerated in patients with ALI/ARDS who require minimized plateau pressures and tidal volumes for oxygenation without barotrauma.[16,53] The use of permissive hypercapnia is limited in patients with preexisting metabolic acidosis and is contraindicated in patients with increased intracranial pressure. In patients with preexisting metabolic acidosis, sodium bicarbonate infusion may be considered.[2,80]

Sedation, Analgesia, and Neuromuscular Blockade

Protocols should be used when sedation of critically ill mechanically ventilated patients is required. The protocol should include the use of a sedation goal as measured by a standardized subjective sedation scale.[38] Although either intermittent bolus or continuous drips may be used, the protocol should include a daily interruption or lightening of a continuous sedative infusion to determine whether sedative agents may be decreased.[62] This practice has been shown to decrease ventilator and critical care days and ventilator-associated pneumonia, thereby decreasing the risk of sepsis and MODS.[63]

Neuromuscular blockade agents should be discontinued as soon as possible. Train-of-four monitoring should be used to monitor the depth of block.[63] Chapter 39 discusses specific management strategies for sedation and neuromuscular blockade.

Glucose Monitoring

In a large, single center trial of postoperative surgical patients, a significant improvement in survival was demonstrated when continuous insulin infusion was used to maintain glucose levels between 80 and 110 mg/dL.[103] Following initial stabilization of patients with sepsis or septic shock, blood glucose should be maintained at a level of less than or equal to 180 mg/dL. With any protocol, glucose should be monitored frequently after initiation of insulin (every 1 to 2 hours) and on a regular basis (every 4 hours) once the blood glucose concentration has been stabilized.[38,103] Glycemic control should also include a nutrition protocol with preferential use of the enteral route.[33,88]

Considerations for Nutrition

Patients with sepsis and MODS have increased energy requirements, numerous metabolic derangements, and are extremely hypermetabolic. Total energy expenditure may be increased 15% to 100% above normal. Even though they appear quiet and sedated in a critical care bed, these patients are running a physiologic marathon. Typical findings of the septic patients include hyperglycemia, elevated free fatty acids, accelerated protein catabolism, and negative nitrogen balance.[25] The goal of nutrition support for septic patients is to provide enough calories, protein, and water to meet patients' metabolic demand and prevent catabolism.[25,38] Ultimately, adequate nutritional support improves resistance to the development of MODS.[25]

Calories. Indirect calorimetry is generally considered the standard for measuring energy expenditure through the measures of oxygen consumption, carbon dioxide production, and the ratio of carbon dioxide produced to oxygen consumed employing a metabolic cart. This method is relatively accurate in measuring calorie need of the mechanically ventilated critically ill patient, except for the patient with severe ARDS. Another reliable way to estimate calories needed for a patient with MODS is employing the Harris-Benedict equation, which is an estimation of the patient's basal energy expenditure (BEE). Multiply the BEE by the patient's activity factor and stress factor.

$$\textit{Men: } \text{BEE (kcal/24 h)} = 66 + (13.7 \times \text{weight}) + (5 \times \text{height in cm}) - (6.7 \times \text{age in years})$$

$$\textit{Women: } \text{BEE (kcal/24 h)} = 655 + (9.6 \times \text{weight}) + (5 \times \text{height in cm}) - (4.7 \times \text{age in years})$$

Activity factor: confined to bed = 1.2; out of bed = 1.3

Stress factor for sepsis = 1.8

Protein. In septic shock, the recommendation is to provide oral or enteral feedings as tolerated. Even though septic shock create a hypermetabolic physiologic state, it is recommended to start with low-dose feedings of up to 500 kcal per day for the first 7 days after diagnosis. There is evidence that early enteral feeding has an impact on outcomes by reducing the incidence of infectious complications, ventilator, and critical care days.[39,64]

Fluid, electrolytes, vitamins, and minerals. MODS generates increased fluid requirements. To provide adequate fluids use the following formula: 30 cm^3/kg body weight per day. Glucose-containing intravenous solutions should be employed with caution because they can contribute to the hyperglycemia state. Electrolytes within normal limits are to be achieved and maintained. Provide supplementation as needed.

Renal Replacement

Intermittent hemodialysis and continuous renal replacement therapy (CRRT) result in equivalent outcomes in septic patients.[59] CRRT offers easier management in hemodynamically unstable patients. There is no current evidence to support the use of CRRT for the treatment of sepsis independent of renal replacement needs.[38,59]

Bicarbonate Therapy

Bicarbonate therapy for the purpose of improving hemodynamics or reducing vasopressor requirements is not recommended for treatment of hypoperfusion-induced lactic acidemia with pH greater than or equal to 7.15.[38,80] Administration of bicarbonate solely for metabolic acidosis masks the underlying cause: persistent hypoperfusion. Therefore, effectiveness of resuscitation strategies should be evaluated and changed, if necessary, before the addition of a bicarbonate infusion.[80] The effect of bicarbonate administration on hemodynamics and vasopressor requirement at lower pH has not been studied.[80]

Deep Vein Thrombosis Prophylaxis

Septic shock patients should receive deep vein thrombosis (DVT) prophylaxis with low doses of either low-molecular-weight or unfractionated heparin. For septic patients with contraindications to heparin use, mechanical prophylactic devices or intermittent compression devices are recommended. For very high-risk patients such as those with severe sepsis or previous history of DVT, a combination of pharmacologic and mechanical therapy is recommended.[38,95]

Stress Ulcer Prophylaxis

Stress ulcer prophylaxis should be given to all patients with septic shock.[38] H_2 blockers are more effective than sucralfate (Carafate) and are the preferred agent.[28] Proton pump inhibitors have not been assessed in a direct comparison and therefore their relative efficacy is unknown.

Consideration for Limitation of Support

A final consideration must be given to limitation of support due to futility.[38] Advance care planning, including the communication of likely outcomes and realistic goals, should be discussed with patients and families. Decisions for less aggressive support or withdrawal of support may be in the patient's best interest.

CONCLUSION

Patients with MODS do not die from their present disease or even a single complication, but rather from progressive and sequential organ dysfunction.[12] Goals for the bedside critical care nurse are the early identification and treatment of those patients whose organs are at risk for failure. The initial insult leads to microvascular hypoperfusion within each organ system. It is difficult to monitor, let alone identify, impending MODS. If unrecognized and untreated, hypoperfusion initiates systemic inflammatory responses, activates the coagulation cascade, impairs the fibrinolytic system, and causes endothelial dysfunction. This exacerbates hypoperfusion and results in further maldistribution of blood flow within individual organs, eventually leading to single organ failure and MODS. Despite the significant strides made in life-support technology, pharmacology, and science as a whole, the key to positive outcomes is early detection and treatment of every organ system at risk. The critical care nurse is in a strategic position to detect, identify, and facilitate treatment of those patients at risk for developing MODS.

CASE STUDY 31.1

Evidence-Based Care of the MODS/SIRS Patient

L.M. is a 50-year-old Caucasian male who was brought to the emergency center by his wife with a 2-day history of hematemesis and melena. Three days earlier he was seen by his primary care provider with symptoms of anorexia, weakness, dizziness, and pain in bilateral lower extremities. He was given an acetaminophen 325 mg/oxycodone 5 mg (Percocet) prescription for presumptive peripheral neuropathy and sent home. His medical history was significant for alcohol abuse and hepatitis C diagnosed by liver biopsy. The patient stated he had abused alcohol in the past, but recently restarted because of being laid off from his job and admitted to drinking a bottle of wine and several beers daily. On initial assessment, his physical examination was as follows: temperature 36°C, HR 104 beats/min, RR 22 breaths/min, BP 88/57 mm Hg, weight 71 kg, moderate distress, awake and oriented × 3, positive asterixis, scleral icterus, 2 + edema bilateral lower extremities, erythematous, warm and tender to palpation, especially both feet, palpable pulses, spider angiomata, jaundice, abdomen mildly distended, nontender, with normal active bowel sounds. Laboratory Values: sodium: 132 mEq/L; potassium: 3.9 mEq/L; chloride: 97 mEq/L; CO_2: 17 mEq/L; BUN: 54 mg/dL; creatinine: 1.8 mg/dL; glucose: 114 mg/dL; WBC: 12.9 cells/mm^3; Hgb: 9.9 g/dL; Hct: 29.7%; Platelets: 112,000/µL; neutrophils: 83%. Amylase, lipase, and liver function tests were normal except for a slight hyperbilirubinemia of 1.8. Ethanol (ETOH) was negative. His magnesium (Mg^{2+}) was 1 mEq/L. He was admitted and transferred to the critical care unit with an initial diagnosis of a GI bleed. Cultures were sent and empiric antibiotics started pending culture results. Four hours later, more laboratory tests were obtained.

Laboratory Values: pH: 7.33; $Paco_2$: 19.3 mm Hg; Pao_2: 79.2 mm Hg; HCO_3^-: 9.8 mEq/L; base excess: 14.6 on O_2 3 L/nasal cannula; WBC: 2.9 cells/mm^3; Hct: 26.2%; platelets: 93,000/µL; neutrophils: 33%; bands: 34%. Admitting orders included normal saline infusion at 125 mL/h; pantoprazole (Protonix) infusion at 40 mg/h; ETOH withdrawal prophylaxis including lorazepam (Ativan), thiamine, folate, and multiple vitamins; Mg^{2+} replacement, ultrasound of abdomen, and repeat Hgb, Hct, and electrolytes every 4 hours. A GI consult was obtained and the gastroenterologist concluded that the bleeding may be secondary to gastritis, varices, or ulceration.

L.M. developed acute respiratory failure and was emergently intubated by the intensivist. His pulmonary status continued to worsen, requiring maximal ventilatory support: Fio_2 100%, assist control rate of 34, inverse inspiratory/expiratory ratio (I:E) of 2:1, positive end-expiratory pressure (PEEP) of 14, with tidal volumes of 350 mL. He was sedated with fentanyl (Sublimaze) and propofol (Diprivan) infusions to tolerate the ventilator and for comfort; protocols for daily sedation holidays were initiated. A right subclavian $Scvo_2$ catheter and an arterial catheter were inserted with an $Scvo_2$ value of 55%. Because the patient remained hypotensive despite a CVP of 15, norepinephrine (Levophed) was started for worsening hypotension. Piperacillin sodium/tazobactam sodium (Zosyn) and gentamicin sulfate were empirically started. Delirium tremens (DTs) prophylaxis was continued (multivitamins, thiamine, folate, and magnesium 4 g).

Although some of his laboratory values appeared better at 6:00 a.m. the next day, he was still critically ill. He was in septic shock and was developing MODS. Assessment: BP 88/50 on norepinephrine, HR 132, sinus tachycardia with a few unifocal premature ventricular contractions (PVCs), Doppler-detected peripheral pulses, capillary refill >5 seconds, and cyanotic, mottled extremities. CVP of 16, $Scvo_2$ 55%; bilateral interstitial infiltrates on the same ventilator settings. pH: 7.28, Pao_2: 66, $Paco_2$: 56, HCO_3^-: 16, oxygen saturation 94%; urinary output 10 to 15 mL/h of dark amber/brown, cloudy urine; extremities pitting edema, mottled, cold below the knees, hot around the thighs, Doppler-detected pulses, and small bilateral bullous skin lesions. Laboratory Values: sodium: 130mEq /L; potassium: 3.6 mEq /L; chloride: 95 mEq /L; CO_2: 20 mEq /L; BUN: 52 mg/dL; creatinine: 2 mg/dL; glucose: 358 mg/dL; WBC count: 1.2 cells/mm^3; Hgb: 6.7 g/dL; Hct: 18.8%; platelets: 45/µL; neutrophils: 11%; bands: 13%; PT/INR: 22.5/3.8%; AST: 132 mc/L; ALT: 63 mc/L; lactate: 12.4 mg/dL.

Decision Point:

Does L.M. show any signs of SIRS?

Decision Point:

What are appropriate interventions and further diagnostic tests for the patient at this time?

Decision Point:

What interventions should the critical care nurse anticipate in the event that the patient decompensates further?

Decision Point:

What other interventions are needed to provide multisystem support of this critically ill patient with MODS?

REFERENCES

1. The Acute Respiratory Distress Syndrome Network. (2000). Ventilation with lower tidal volumes as compared with traditional tidal volumes for acute lung injury and the acute respiratory distress syndrome. *N Engl J Med, 342,* 1301–1308.
2. Ahrens, T., & Tuggle, D. (2004). Surviving severe sepsis: early recognition and treatment. *Crit Care Nurse,* (supplement to October 2004) 2–15.
3. Aird, W. C. (2001). Vascular bed specific homeostasis and role of endothelium in sepsis pathogenesis. *Crit Care Med, 29*(Suppl. 7), 528–535.
4. Aird, W. C. (2003). The role of the endothelium in severe sepsis & MODS. *Blood, 101,* 3756–3777.
5. Aird, W. C. (2003). The hematologic system as a marker of organ dysfunction in Sepsis. *Mayo Clin Proc, 78,* 869–881.
6. Amsden, G. W., Ballow, C. H., & Bertino, J. S. (2000). Pharmacokinetics and pharmacodynamics of anti-infective agents. In G. L. Mandell, J. E. Bennett, & R. Dolin (Eds.), *Principles and practice of infectious diseases* (5th ed.). Philadelphia: Churchill Livingstone.
7. Angus, D. C., et al. (2000). Caring for the critically ill patients: current & projected work force requirement for care of the critically ill and patients with pulmonary disease: can we meet the requirement of an aging population? *JAMA, 284,* 2762–2770.
8. Angus, D. C., et al. (2001). Epidemiology of severe sepsis in the United States: analysis of incidence outcome, and associated costs of care. *Crit Care Med, 29,* 1301–1310.
9. Angus, D. C., & van der Poll, T. (2013). Severe sepsis and septic shock. *N Engl J Med, 369,* 840–851.
10. Annane, D., et al. (2002). Effects of treatment with low doses hydrocortisone and fludrocortisone on mortality in patients with septic shock. *JAMA, 288,* 862–887.
11. Annane, D., et al. (2013). Effects of fluid resuscitation with colloids vs crystalloids on mortality in critically ill patients presenting with hypovolemic shock: the CRISTAL randomized trial. *JAMA, 6,* 1809–1817.
12. Awad, S. S. (2003). State-of-the-art therapy for severe sepsis and multisystem organ dysfunction. *Am J Surg, 186*(Suppl), 23S–30S.
13. Bansal, V., & Doucet, J. (2015). Multiple organ dysfunction syndrome. *Scientific American Surgery,* 1–20.
14. Bernard, G. R., et al. (2001). Efficacy and safety of recombinant human activated protein C for severe sepsis. *N Engl J Med, 344,* 699–709.
15. Bernard, G. R. (2005). Acute respiratory distress syndrome: a historical perspective. *Am J Respir Crit Care Med, 172*(7), 798–806.
16. Bidani, A., et al. (1992). Permissive hypercapnia in acute respiratory failure. *JAMA, 272,* 957–962.
17. Bisharat, N., et al. (1999). Clinical, epidemiological, and microbiological features of *Vibrio vulnificus* biogroup 3 causing outbreaks of wound infection and bacteremia in Israel. *Lancet, 354,* 1421–1424.
18. Blot, F., et al. (1998). Earlier positivity of central venous versus peripheral blood cultures is highly predictive of catheter-related sepsis. *J Clin Microbiol, 36,* 105–109.
19. Bone, R. C., Fisher, C. J., & Clemmer, T. P. (1987). A controlled clinical trial of high-dose methylprednisolone in the treatment of severe sepsis and septic shock. *N Engl J Med, 317,* 653–658.
20. Bone, R. C., et al. (1992). Definitions for sepsis and organ failure and guidelines for the use of innovative therapies in sepsis. The ACCP/SCCM Consensus Conference Committee. *Chest, 101*(6), 1644–1655.
21. Bota, D. P., et al. (2004). Body temperature alterations in the critically ill. *Intensive Care Med, 30,* 811–816.
22. Brealey, D., et al. (2002). Association between mitochondrial dysfunction and severity and outcome of septic shock. *Lancet, 360,* 219–223.
23. Burns, K., et al. (2011). Pressure and volume limited ventilation for ventilator management of patient with acute lung injury: a systematic review and meta-analysis. PLoS One 6;e14623. http://journals.plos.org/plosone/article/asset?id=10.1371/journal.pone.0014623.PDF
24. Caironi, P., Tognoni, G., Masson, S., et al. (2014). Albumin replacement in patients with severe sepsis or septic shock. *N Engl J Med, 370,* 1412–1421.
25. Cartwright, C. M. (2004). The metabolic response to stress: a case of complex nutrition support management. *Crit Care Nurs Clin North Am, 16,* 467–487.
26. Cheek, D. J., Smith, H., & Good, J. (2006). New respect for the humble endothelium. *Nursing,* 2006, *36*(3), 44–47.

26a. Churpek, M.M., Zadravecz, F.J., Winslow, C., Howell, M.D., Edelson, D.P. (2015). Incidence and prognostic value of the systemic inflammatory response syndrome and organ dysfunctions in ward patients. *Am J Respir Crit Care Med, 192*(8): 958–964.

27. Coletta, C., et al. (2014). Endothelial dysfunction is a potential contributor to multiple organ failure and mortality in aged mice subjected to septic shock: preclinical studies in a murine model of cecal ligation and puncture. *Crit Care, 18*(5), 511.
28. Cook, D., et al. (1998). A comparison of sucralfate and ranitidine for the prevention of upper gastrointestinal bleeding in patients requiring mechanical ventilation. Canadian Critical Care Trials Group. *N Engl J Med, 338,* 791–797.
29. Cook, D., & Guyatt, G. (2001). Colloid use for fluid resuscitation: evidence and spin. *Ann Intern Med, 135,* 205–208.
30. Cook, R., et al. (2001). Multiple organ dysfunction: baseline and serial component scores. *Crit Care Med, 29*(11), 2046–2050.
31. Cronin, L., et al. (1995). Corticosteroid treatment for sepsis: a critical appraisal and meta-analysis of the literature. *Crit Care Med, 23,* 1430–1439.
32. Crouser, E. D., et al. (2002). Endotoxin induced mitochondrial damage correlates with impaired respiratory activity. *Crit Care Med, 30,* 276–284.
33. Cunneen, J., & Cartwright, M. (2004). The puzzle of sepsis: fitting the pieces of the inflammation response with treatment. *AACN Clin Issue, 15*(1), 18–44.
34. De Backer, D., et al. (2002). Microvascular blood flow is altered in patients with sepsis. *Am J Respir Crit Care Med, 166,* 98–104.
35. De Backer, D., et al. (2003). Effects of dopamine, norepinephrine, and epinephrine on the splanchnic circulation in septic shock: which is best? *Crit Care Med, 31,* 1659–1667.
36. De Backer, D., et al. (2014). Pathophysiology of microcirculation dysfunction and the pathogenesis of septic shock. *Virulence, 5,* 73–79.
37. Delaney, A. P., et al. (2013). ARISE investigators. The Australasian Resuscitation in Sepsis Evaluation (ARISE) trial statistical analysis plan. *Crit Care Resusc, 15*(3), 162–171.
38. Dellinger, R., et al. (2004). Surviving sepsis campaign guidelines for management of severe sepsis and septic shock. *Crit Care Med, 32,* 855–873.
39. Dellinger, R. P., Levy, M., Andrew Rhodes, A., et al. (2013). Surviving sepsis campaign: international guidelines for management of severe sepsis and septic shock 2012. *Crit Care Med, 41*(2), 581–637.
40. Doig, C. J., et al. (2004). Study of clinical course of organ dysfunction in intensive care. *Crit Care Med, 32*(2), 384–390.
41. Duran-Bedolla, J., et al. (2014). Sepsis, mitochondrial failure and multiple organ dysfunction. *Clin Invest Med, 37,* E58–E69.
42. El-Menyar, A., et al. (2012). Multiple organ dysfunction syndrome (MODS): is it preventable or inevitable? *Int J Clin Med, 3,* 722–730.
43. Futterman, L. G., & Lemberg, L. (2006). Coronary endothelium: a key to life expectancy. *Am J Crit Care, 15*(3), 315–320.
44. Gattinoni, L., et al. (1995). A trial of goal-oriented hemodynamic therapy in critically ill patients. *N Engl J Med, 333,* 1025–1032.
45. Girard, T. D., Opal, S. M., & Ely, E. W. (2005). Insights of severe sepsis in older patients: the epidemiology to evidence based management. *Clin Infect Dis, 40,* 719–727.
46. Gando, S., & Ottoomo, Y. (2015). Local hemostasis, immunothrombosis, and system disseminated intravascular coagulation in trauma and traumatic shock. *Crit Care, 19,* 72. http://link.springer.com/article/10.1186%2Fs13054-015-0735-x#.
47. Gross, P. L., & Aird, W. C. (2000). The endothelium and thrombosis. *Semin Throm Hemost, 26,* 463–478.
48. Hack, C. E., & Zeerleder, S. (2001). The endothelium in sepsis: source of and a target for inflammation. *Crit Care Med, 29*(Suppl. 7), 521–527.
49. Hassoun, H. T., et al. (2001). Post injury multiple organ failure. The role of the gut. *Shock, 15,* 1–10.

50. Hatala, R., Dinh, R., & Cook, D. J. (1996). Once-daily aminoglycoside dosing in immunocompetent adults: a meta-analysis. *Ann Intern Med, 124*, 717–725.
51. Hayes, M. A., et al. (1994). Elevation of systemic oxygen delivery in the treatment of critically ill patients. *N Engl J Med, 330*, 1717–1722.
52. Hébert, P. C., et al. (1999). A multicenter, randomized, controlled clinical trial of transfusion in critical care. *N Engl J Med, 340*, 409–417.
53. Hickling, K. G., et al. (1994). Low mortality rate in adult respiratory distress syndrome using low-volume, pressure-limited ventilation with permissive hypercapnia: a prospective study. *Crit Care Med, 22*, 1568–1578.
54. Holmes, C. L., et al. (2001). Physiology of vasopressin relevant to management of septic shock. *Chest, 120*, 989–1002.
55. Holmes, C. L., et al. (2001). The effects of vasopressin on hemodynamics and renal function in severe septic shock: a case series. *Intensive Care Med, 27*, 1416–1421.
56. Reference deleted in page proof.
57. Iwashyna, T. J., Ely, E. W., Smith, D. M., & Langa, K. M. (2010). Long-term cognitive impairment and functional disability among survivors of severe sepsis. *JAMA, 304*(16), 1787–1794.
58. Jones, A. E., et al. (2010). Emergency Medicine Shock Research Network (EMShockNet) Investigators: lactate clearance vs central venous oxygen saturation as goals of early sepsis therapy: a randomized clinical trial. *JAMA, 303*, 739–746.
59. Kellum, J., et al. (2002). Continuous versus intermittent renal replacement therapy: a meta analysis. *Intensive Care Med, 28*, 29–37.
60. Kleinpell, R. (2002). Advances in treating patients with severe sepsis. *Crit Care Nurse, 23*(3), 16–28.
61. Knaus, W. A., et al. (1991). The APACHE III prognostic system prediction of hospital mortality for critically ill hospitalized adults. *Chest, 100*, 1616–1640.
62. Kolleff, M. H., et al. (1998). The use of continuous IV sedation is associated with prolongation of mechanical ventilation. *Chest, 114*, 541–548.
63. Kress, J. P. (2000). Daily interruptions of sedative infusions in critically ill patients undergoing mechanical ventilation. *N Engl J Med, 342*, 1471–1477.
64. Kudsk, K. A. (2001). Importance of enteral feeding in maintaining gut integrity. *Tech GI Endo, 3*, 2–8.
65. Kumar, A., et al. (2006). Duration of hypotension prior to initiation of effective antimicrobial therapy is the critical determinant of survival in human septic shock. *Crit Care Med, 34*, 1589–1596.
66. Kumur, A., Safdar, N., Kethireddy, S., & Chateau, D. A. (2010). Survival benefit of combination antibiotic therapy for serious infections associated with sepsis and septic shock is contingent only on the risk of death: a meta-analytic/meta-regression study. *Crit Care Med, 38*, 1651–1664.
67. Kumar, G., et al. (2011). Milwaukee Initiative in Critical Care Outcomes Research Group of Investigators. Nationwide trends of severe sepsis in the 21st century (2000-2007). *Chest, 140*(5), 1223–1231.
68. Le Gall, R., et al. (1996). The logistic organ dysfunction system. A new way to assess organ dysfunction in the intensive care unit. *JAMA, 276*, 802–810.
69. Levy, M. M., et al. (2003). 2001 SCCM/ESICM/ACCP/ATS/SIS international sepsis definition conference. *Crit Care Med, 31*(4), 1250–1256.
70. Lobo, D. N., & Awad, S. (2014). Should chloride-rich crystalloids remain the mainstay of fluid resuscitation to prevent 'pre-renal' acute kidney injury? con. *Kidney International, 86*, 1096–1105.
71. Lorente, J. A., et al. (1993). Effects of blood transfusion on oxygen transport variables in severe sepsis. *Crit Care Med, 21*, 1312–1318.
72. Liu, V., Escobar, G. J., Greene, J. D., Soule, J., Whippy, A., Angus, D. C., et al. (2014). Hospital deaths in patient with sepsis from 2 independent cohorts. *JAMA, 312*(1), 90–92. http://dx.doi.org/10.1001/jama.2014.5804.
73. Madhusudan, P., Vijayaraghavan, B. K. T., & Covel, M. E. (2014). Fluid resuscitation in sepsis: reexamining the paradigm. *BioMed Res In, 2014*, 1–9.
74. Malay, M. B., et al. (1999). Low-dose vasopressin in the treatment of vasodilatory septic shock. *J Trauma, 47*, 699–705.
75. Marik, P. E. (2014). Early management of severe sepsis: concepts and controversies. *Chest, 145*, 1407–1418.
76. Marik, P. E., Cavallazzi, R., Vasu, T., & Hirani, A. (2009). Dynamic changes in arterial waveform derived variables and fluid responsiveness in mechanically ventilated patients: a systematic review of the literature. *Crit Care Med, 37*(9), 2642–2647.
77. Marshall, J. C., et al. (1995). Multiple organ dysfunction score: a reliable descriptor of a complex clinical outcome. *Crit Care Med, 23*(10), 1638–1652.
78. Martin, G. S., et al. (2003). The epidemiology of sepsis in the United States from 1979 through 2000. *N Engl J Med, 348*, 1540–1546.
79. Martin, G. (2012). Sepsis, severe sepsis and septic shock: changes in incidence, pathogens and outcomes. *Expert Rev Anti Infect Ther, 10*(6), 701–706.
80. Mathieu, D., et al. (1991). Effects of bicarbonate therapy on hemodynamic and tissue oxygenation in patients with lactic acidosis: a prospective, controlled clinical study. *Crit Care Med, 19*, 1352–1356.
81. Minne, L., Abu-Hanna, A., & de Jonge, E. (2008). Evaluation of SOFA-based models for predicating mortality in the ICU: a systematic review. *Crit Care, 12*, R161.
82. Mouncey, P. R., et al. (2015). Trial of early, goal-directed resuscitation for septic shock. *N Engl J Med, 372*, 1301–1311.
83. National Institute of General Medical Sciences. (2009). National Institutes of Health. *Sepsis fact sheet*. Available from: http://www.nigms.nih.gov/Publications/factsheet_sepsis.htm.
84. National Center for Health Statistics Data Brief No. 62. (June 2011). *Inpatient care for septicemia or sepsis: a challenge for patients and hospitals.*
85. Nesseler, N., et al. (2012). Clinical review: the liver in sepsis. *Crit Care, 16*, 235. http://www.ncbi.nlm.nih.gov/pmc/articles/PMC3682239/.
86. Okazaki, Y., & Matsukawa, A. (2009). Pathophysiology of sepsis and recent patents on the diagnosis, treatment and prophylaxis for sepsis. *Recent Pat Inflamm Allergy Drug Discov, 3*, 26–32.
87. Perel, P., Roberts, I., & Ker, K. (2013). Effects of fluid resuscitation with colloids vs crystalloids on mortality in critically ill patients presenting with hypovolemic shock: the CRISTAL randomized trial. *JAMA, 310*, 1809–1817. http://dx.doi.org/10.1001/jama.2013.280502.
88. Pettila, V., et al. (2002). Comparison of multiple organ dysfunction scores in the prediction of hospital mortality in the critically ill. *Crit Care Med, 30*(8), 1705–1711.
89. Piagnerelli, M., et al. (2003). Modification of red blood cell shape & glycoproteins membrane content in septic patients. *Adv Exp Med Biol, 510*, 109–114.
90. Phillips, D. P., Kaynar, A. M., Kellum, J. A., & Gomez, H. (2013). Crystalloids vs. colloids: KO at the twelfth round? *Critical Care, 17*, 319. http://dx.doi.org/10.1186/cc12708.
91. Practice guidelines for blood component therapy. A report by the American Society of Anesthesiologists Task Force on Blood Component Therapy. (1996). *Anesthesiology, 84*, 732–747.
92. Practice parameter for the use of fresh frozen plasma, cryoprecipitate, and platelets. Fresh-Frozen Plasma, Cryoprecipitate, and Platelets Administration Practice Guidelines Development Task Force of the College of American Pathologists. (1994). *JAMA, 271*, 777–781.
93. The ProcCESS investigators. (2014). A randomized trial of protocol-based care for early septic shock. *N Engl J Med, 370*, 1683–1693.
94. Raghunathan, K., et al. (2013). Association between the choice of IV crystalloid and in-hospital mortality among critically ill adults with sepsis. *Crit Care Resusc, 15*, 311–317.
95. Samama, M. M., et al. (1999). A comparison of enoxaparin with placebo for the prevention of venous thromboembolism in acutely ill medical patients. Prophylaxis in medical patients with enoxaparin study group. *N Engl J Med, 341*, 793–800.
96. Sands, K., et al. (1997). Epidemiology of sepsis syndrome in 8 academic medical centers. *JAMA, 278*, 234–240.
97. Schierhout, G., & Roberts, I. (1998). Fluid resuscitation with colloid or crystalloid solutions in critically ill patients: a systematic review of randomized trials. *BMJ, 31*, 961–964.
98. Sharshar, T., et al. (2003). Apoptosis of neurons in cardiovascular autonomic centers triggered by inducible nitric oxide synthase after death from septic shock. *Lancet, 362*, 1799–1805.
99. Schulte, W., Bernhagen, J., & Bucala, R. (2013). Cytokines in sepsis: Potent immunoregulators and potential therapeutic targets – an updated view. Available from: http://www.ncbi.nlm.nih.gov/pmc/articles/PMC3703895/pdf/MI2013-165974.pdf.

99a. Singer, M., et al. (2016). The third international consensus definitions for sepsis and septic shock (Sepsis-3). *JAMA, 315*(8): 801–810.

100. Surviving sepsis campaign. Updated bundles in response to new evidence. Available from: http://www.survivingsepsis.org/sitecollectiondocuments/ssc_bundle.pdf.
101. Tsuneyoski, I., et al. (2002). Hemodynamic and metabolic effects of low dose vasopressin infusions in vasodilatory septic shock. *Crit Care Med, 29*, 487–493.
102. Vallet, B., & Weil, E. (2001). Endothelial cell dysfunction and coagulation. *Crit Care Med, 29*(Suppl. 7), 536–541.
103. Van den Berghe, G., et al. (2001). Intensive insulin therapy in the critically ill patients. *N Engl J Med, 345*, 1359–1367.
104. The Veterans Administration Systemic Sepsis Cooperative Study Group. (1987). Effect on high-dose glucocorticoid therapy on mortality in patients with clinical signs of sepsis. *N Engl J Med, 317*, 659–665.
105. Vincent, J. L., et al. (1996). The sepsis-related organ failure assessment (SOFA) scores to describe organ dysfunction/failure. *Intensive Care Med, 22*, 707–710.
106. Vincent, J. L., et al. (2000). Effects of nitric oxide in septic shock. *Am J Respir Crit Care Med, 161*, 1781–1785.
107. Warren, B. L., et al. (2001). High dose antithrombin III in severe sepsis: a randomized controlled trial. *JAMA, 286*, 1869–1878.

32

Caring for the Immunocompromised Patient

Anna Dermenchyan

INTRODUCTION

The function of the immune system is to protect the human body against disease. Complications may arise when the immune system does not function properly. Immune deficiencies, which compromise and affect different components of the immune system, may occur temporarily or permanently. Disorders may be genetically linked and present at birth, acquired through exposure to specific clinical toxins, or the secondary effect of another disease process. In the past few decades, increasing numbers of patients have been admitted to critical care with significant preexisting immune compromise.[40] Medications, nutritional deficits, invasive procedures, chronic illness, and exposure to resistant microbes contribute to immune compromise for most critically ill patients, although intrinsic hematopoietic failure also may occur.

The assessment and management of patients with different immune defects may vary in some aspects, but general clinical care is universal. The admission of immune-incompetent patients to critical care creates unique challenges for critical care practitioners. The experienced critical care nurse serves as a critical link in providing specialized care for these patients. The greatest risk for morbidity in all immunocompromised patients is development of life-threatening infections; however, immunologic deficits and subtle clinical presentation may make it difficult to diagnose potentially life-threatening infections. All patients who enter critical care should be assessed for factors that interfere with their normal immune capacity so recognition and appropriate management of their immunocompromised state and infection risk can be instituted. Diagnostic tests and interventions are directed at specific immune defects and the anticipated complications unique to that defect. For example, patients with T-lymphocytic suppression to prevent organ transplant rejection are more prone to viral and opportunistic infections that correlate with the usual functions of the T-lymphocyte. These patients are routinely prescribed acyclovir (Zovirax) to prevent herpes simplex and trimethoprim-sulfamethoxazole (Bactrim) for prevention of *Pneumocystis jiroveci*. If immune-supportive interventions are not implemented in time to prevent infection, knowledge of immune deficit and infection history is used to treat the most probable microbe based upon the patient's defined risk factors and probable site of infection. The patient with prolonged granulocytopenia who continues to be febrile despite extensive antibacterial antibiotic coverage is usually treated with antifungal medications with the realization that fungal infection often occurs after granulocytes are suppressed for more than 7 to 10 days.[39]

DEFINITIONS

Immunocompromise is a broad term indicating inadequate white blood cell (WBC) response.[38] It may involve the nonspecific immune system or specific immunity. A comparison of the key features of immunologic impairment based on type of physiologic defect is described in Fig. 32.1. Nonspecific immune functions include barrier defenses and the actions of complement proteins or granulocytes. The nonspecific immune response is most important in mounting a defense against bacteria and is active in the inflammatory response. B and T lymphocytes, and their activated immune chemicals essential for recognition and destruction of viral or opportunistic pathogens, coordinate the specific immune response. Monocytes have combined specific and nonspecific actions, usually at a tissue level, because monocytes differentiate into tissue macrophages early in their development. Within the term immunocompromise there are several different types of immune dysfunction.

Primary immunodeficiency disorders are immune disorders caused by inherited genetic mutations. Primary disorders include: X-linked agammaglobulinemia (XLA), common variable immunodeficiency (CVID), severe combined immunodeficiency (SCID), and alymphocytosis. Secondary disorders occur when an outside source, such as a toxic chemical or infection, attacks the body. Secondary disorders include: AIDS, cancers of the immune system (e.g., leukemia), immune-complex diseases (e.g., viral hepatitis), and multiple myeloma.[34,37]

Leukopenia is defined as an abnormal reduction of disease-fighting WBCs circulating in the blood. This may be due to reduced production of WBCs or increased utilization and destruction, or both. Infection, medications, malignancy, megaloblastosis, hypersplenism, and immunoneutropenia are responsible for most cases of leukopenia. The threshold for a low WBC count varies from one medical practice to another. A count lower than 4000 WBCs per microliter of blood is generally considered a low WBC count. The term leukopenia is often used interchangeably with neutropenia.[34,37]

Granulocytopenia (used interchangeably with neutropenia) is defined as inadequate circulating cells to combat bacterial microbes. The most common granulocytes are the neutrophils.

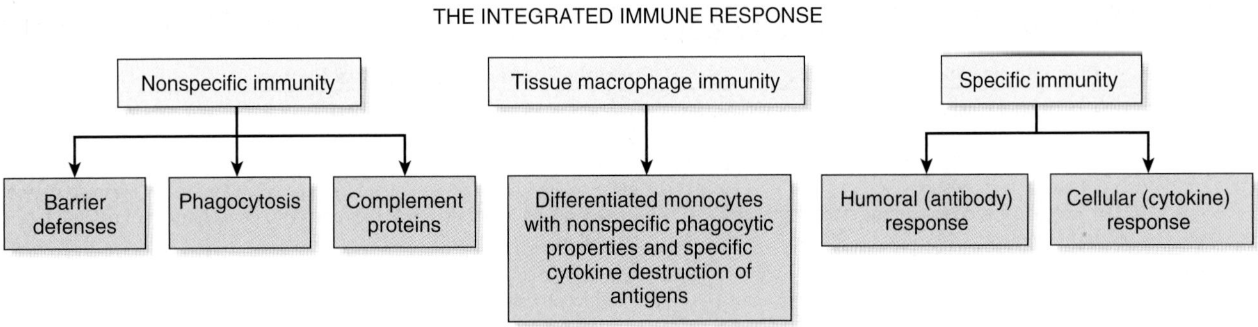

THE INTEGRATED IMMUNE RESPONSE

FIG. 32.1 Comparison of nonspecific and specific immune function.

They are the only WBC that can be released immaturely (referred to as a *band*) in response to infection. The presence of a high percentage of bands (> 20%) when the total WBC count is elevated is indicative of a bacterial infection.[38,39]

Lymphopenia is defined as a low absolute lymphocyte count (manual count rather than machine averaged). Cellular dysfunction rather than number of cells may also measure immune compromise. Individuals who inject unpurified recreational drugs develop impaired T-lymphocytic function even without acquiring an infectious disease, such as hepatitis or human immunodeficiency virus.[21,38]

PATIENTS AT RISK

Immune compromise can occur as a result of a wide variety of health maintenance disorders, comorbid diseases (e.g., diabetes, heart disease), medications, and environmental influences. The degree of compromise and clinical consequences vary according to the specific cells involved and number or severity of dysfunction. In general, patients with granulocytic defects are at greatest risk for bacterial infections; monocyte defects increase the risk for deep-seated organ infections and lymphocyte abnormalities result in viral illness, infection with atypical bacteria, or development of malignancy.[38] A detailed listing of patients at risk for common immune defects and the clinical characteristics of such disorders is given in Table 32.1.[39] Obtaining a comprehensive clinical history can aid the critical care nurse in identifying patients with risk factors for immune compromise. The level of vigilance and specialized therapies to compensate for immune incompetence and propensity for infection is determined by patient risk. For example, patients receiving chemotherapy for any diagnosis are at risk for the development of immune compromise, as the WBC count is suppressed for 3 to 10 days.[33,34] The depth and length of the neutropenia are a reflection of the fact that the bone marrow is recovering and new blood cells are beginning to grow and mature. A patient is less likely to have prolonged neutropenia early in the treatment plan unless other risk factors are present. Contributing factors that may prolong the length of neutropenia include older age, viral illness, malnutrition, intravenous drug use, previous chemotherapy, antimicrobials, and antiretrovirals.[9,25] The experienced critical care nurse should recognize the reversibility of this current medical crisis and consider the patient's health and medication profile to predict the course of neutropenia.

Both the presence of tumor and radiation treatment will result in damaged ciliary action, disrupted lymphatic drainage, and altered cough or ability to mobilize secretions. The tumor may also obstruct natural drainage of secretions, causing a postobstructive pneumonia.[42] These risks will not be alleviated after treatment of this specific infectious episode, and should be acknowledged in future treatment plans to reduce the risk of recurrent infectious episodes. This may include the prescription of prophylactic antimicrobial agents or hematopoietic growth factors immediately following administration of the chemotherapy regimen.[16]

Many oncology patients receiving chemotherapy have a semipermanent or permanent central venous catheter. Even if there are no current signs of a line-related infection, careful and frequent assessment of the insertion site, exit site, and tunnel should be performed.[13,33,34] Although many central lines are treated with clean technique in the home setting, strict sterile technique should be used for all in-hospital manipulations.[4,13] The microbes that produce hospital-acquired infections are usually more virulent and resistant to antimicrobial therapy.[13,20] Many specific organisms do not easily resolve after they have infected a central line (e.g., *Candida, Giardia, Pseudomonas,* and *Staphylococcus*), necessitating removal of the central intravenous line when a single episode of infection occurs.[3,13] Research has been inconclusive identifying specific practices in managing venous access devices that reduce the risk of infection for these patients.[13] More frequent fluid and tubing changes, accessing the line with sterile technique, or antimicrobial lock solutions may be part of an institutional standard of care, although the benefit of these practices has not been fully supported.[8,13,15]

Patients who are receiving broad-spectrum antimicrobials have concomitant destruction of the normal flora that resides in the mouth, gastrointestinal (GI), and genitourinary systems. The overgrowth of nonbacteria, such as the fungus *Candida albicans,* may result in superinfections manifesting as oral thrush, an erosive rash in skin folds, diarrhea from *Candida,* or fungal urinary tract infections.[20] It is often the bedside nurse who detects these subtle, but potentially fatal infections. Oral care in the immunocompromised patient to avoid ventilator-associated pneumonia is an example of critical care nurse led intervention that can prevent and decrease mortality in immunocompromised patients. Oral care provided to intensive care patients can be best improved by providing staff education on the importance and potential benefits of this practice, having a staffing pattern that supports this practice, and helping all staff perceive this activity as a top priority of patient care.[17,26]

ASSESSMENT

Physical Findings

When assessing patients who have compromised immune systems, it is essential to be attentive to subtle changes in the patient's baseline assessment. Immune dysfunction blunts normal inflammatory responses, leading to diminished signs and symptoms of infection. The usual WBC responses create infectious exudates, such as wound drainage or sputum, but these are

TABLE 32.1 Characteristics and Risks for Immunocompromised Patient Populations

Characteristics	Physiologic Mechanism of Risk	Possible Consequences of Risk Factor
Frequent hospitalizations	• Frequent exposure to environmental organisms other than one's own normal environment • Exposure to other people's organisms via staff, equipment, or supplies • Potential exposure to resistant organisms	Hospitalizations are avoided whenever possible to reduce exposure of patient to foreign microbes that are more pathogenic than those in normal living environment. When hospitalizations cannot be avoided, careful separation of patient care items, single patient use items, and thorough cleaning between uses reduces transference of microbes and development of resistant microbes.
Gastrointestinal disease	• Decreased bowel motility allows normal flora to translocate across GI wall to bloodstream • Breaks in mucosal integrity of GI tract predispose patients to microbial transference into bloodstream • Poor circulation to GI tract causes decreased peristalsis and mucosal atrophy; normal flora and intestinal gram-negative organisms can become pathogenic	Maintaining minimal normal GI motility and mucosal integrity reduces amount of infection via GI tract. Using the gut consistently for food and fluid consumption helps maintain normal function. Enteral feeding is always attempted, if at all possible, to enhance GI integrity and function.
HIV disease	• Viral incorporation into the RNA, then the DNA of immune cells having the $CD8^+$ molecule disrupts normal WBC function and replication, leading to lymphopenia, lymphocyte dysfunction, and macrophage dysfunction • Disruption of these cells leads to many different infections (e.g., unusual bacteria, fungi, opportunistic bacteria, and viruses) and lymphoproliferative disorders/malignancies (e.g., Kaposi's sarcoma, lymphoma)	HIV disease is directly treated with antiretrovirals and immune-reconstituting agents, such as interleukin-2. Stabilization of lymphocyte counts reduces risk and incidence of opportunistic infections. When lymphocyte count does drop, prophylactic antimicrobial agents specific to organisms likely to infect these patients are prescribed in a well-defined and protocol-determined manner. Avoidance of activities likely to expose patients to infection and attempts to maintain care in the ambulatory environment may also reduce risk of serious or resistant infections.
Immunosuppressive agents and corticosteroids	• Decreased phagocytic activity • Altered T-cell recognition of pathogens, especially viral • Lack of immune memory to recall antibodies to previously encountered pathogens	Immune-suppressing agents have multiple immune-depressing functions, putting patients at risk for all kinds of infections. Special precautions are implemented and prophylactic antimicrobial agents against common opportunistic organisms may be indicated. These patients also lose immune memory and are candidates for vaccinations, provided that the vaccine does not contain live agents. Patients are taught that they will have blunted inflammatory responses and that subtle symptoms may indicate infections
Indwelling intravenous catheters	• Indwelling venous or arterial access devices break barrier defenses, with subsequent risk of microbial invasion • Presence of an intravenous device may irritate venous wall and induce inflammatory damage, resulting in a higher risk for microbial invasion	Intravenous catheters breach barrier defenses and increase risk of microbial invasion into the body. Some companies have developed catheters that have been coated or treated with active antimicrobial agents, such as silver ions, chlorhexidine, or heparin. Catheters have also been designed with structural variations in an attempt to reduce irritation of veins, thereby minimizing phlebitis and infection (e.g., angled catheter tips, modified catheter anchoring devices). Clinicians must choose the smallest lumen size, least number of lumens, and most appropriate permanence of a device to reduce infection rates. Heightened sterile technique when accessing these devices may also reduce rate of associated infection.
Infants/older adults	• Immature thymus gland in infants increases viral and opportunistic infections • Atrophy of thymus gland in older adults increases viral infection • Decreased antigen-specific immunoglobulins in older adults diminishes immune memory, and delayed hypersensitivity reactions	Immature and atrophied immune systems can lead to infection with a variety of organisms from any additional breach in the body's defenses. Frequent, complex, or polymicrobial infections are expected and are guarded against by careful infection prevention techniques and strategies. Recognition of the variety of infectious complications and the potential for their rapid dissemination causes increased vigilance in monitoring and early aggressive interventions for infection. Prophylactic strategies are not usually recommended in these populations, but a low threshold for treatment is implemented.
Invasive devices (e.g., Foley catheter, nasogastric tube)	• Altered barrier defenses allow pathogen entry, especially skin organisms	Invasive devices breach barrier defenses and increase risk of microbial invasion into body. Catheters and other invasive devices have been coated with active antimicrobial agents such as silver ions, chlorhexidine, or heparin in an attempt to reduce related infection. Some devices also have structural variations (e.g., altered bluntness of the tip of tracheal suction catheter) that reduce irritation or mucosal injury, with the hope of reducing infection rate. Infection monitoring for microbial colonization may also help detect early presence of potential pathogens in high-risk patients.
Malnutrition	• Inadequate WBC count • Reduced neutrophil activity	Altered nutrition increases risk of all infections. Efforts to boost immune-related nutrition deficits may focus on inclusion of glutamine, arginine, and other essential amino acids in nutrient supplements as well as other measures aimed at enhancing nutritional well-being.
Hepatic disease	• Decreased neutrophil count • Decreased phagocytic activity • Lost immunoglobulin production	Hepatic disease increases risk of bacterial infection and rapid dissemination of that infection. Loss of immunoglobulins leads to failed immune memory. Special infection precautions for immunocompromised patients are implemented.

TABLE 32.1 **Characteristics and Risks for Immunocompromised Patient Populations—cont'd**

Characteristics	Physiologic Mechanism of Risk	Possible Consequences of Risk Factor
Neutropenia	• Inadequate neutrophils to combat infection	Lack of neutrophils places patient at high risk for bacterial infections that will rapidly disseminate and potentially cause septic shock. Hematopoietic growth factors may be administered as primary or secondary prophylaxis to abrogate the severity (depth of nadir) or longevity of the period of neutropenia.
Pulmonary disease	• Inadequate oxygenation decreases neutrophil activity	Infection risk is increased and can be abrogated by implementing immunocompromised precautions.
Radiation therapy	• Radiation to long bones will interfere with WBC production • Radiation in area of certain endocrine organs can lead to endocrine failure (hypoadrenalism, hypothyroidism) and infection risk • Radiation damage to barrier defenses will predispose patient to invasion by microbes	Destruction of stem cells and existing bone marrow reserve of hematopoietic cells is a common dose-limiting toxicity of radiation therapy involving the long bones, where cells are produced. Destruction of the normal skin and soft tissue barriers is treated with specialized skin care to reduce incidence of infection.
Renal disease	• Decreased neutrophil activity • Decreased immunoglobulin activity	Patients with renal dysfunction are provided extra precautions against bacterial infection, recognizing that they may also show blunted or reduced symptoms of infection. These patients are appropriate candidates for vaccinations against many microorganisms.
Splenectomy	• Inability to recognize and remove encapsulated bacteria (e.g., streptococci, mycobacteria)	Postsplenectomy, either functional or anatomical, the patient is at risk for specific infections. Vaccination against pneumococci is recommended for these patients. A low threshold of suspicion for streptococci with oropharyngeal or urinary tract symptoms may allow for early antimicrobial therapy.
Surgical procedure/ wounds	• Normal flora may be translocated by surgical procedure • Altered barrier defenses because of surgical entry • Stress of surgery or anesthetic agents may reduce neutrophil activity	Careful surgical preparation of planned surgical site with chlorhexidine scrub is recommended before many surgical procedures. Shaving involved area remains a debatable practice, with some believing that hair removal reduces risk, and others believing that skin nicks from razor may increase risk of infection. Operating room staff may perform a surgical scrub of site followed by placement of a clear sterile barrier film, which is subsequently cut through for actual procedure. Conscientious postoperative care with fluids, coughing, deep breathing, and early mobilization may decrease risk of infection. Being aware of previous colonization or infection before surgery may assist in defining source of fever postoperatively.
Traumatic injuries	• Altered barrier defenses allow pathogen entry • Type of infection dependent upon source and severity of injury (e.g., soil contamination, water contamination, skin flora)	Altered barrier defenses are treated with frequent cleansing, antimicrobial cleansing, covering with sterile dressings to prevent infectious organisms from entering the bloodstream via the open wound. Antimicrobial ointments have not been proven effective. If a wound is thought to be clean and sterile, a clear protective barrier dressing may provide better occlusiveness and guard against microorganism entry.

GI, Gastrointestinal; *WBC*, white blood cell count.
From Reference 39.

often not present in immunocompromised patients. Organism-specific lesions may also appear differently in immunocompromised patients. For example, herpes simplex oral lesions usually manifest as a shallow ulcer with a raised red border. This may appear as a flat ulceration without inflammation or border in an immunocompromised patient.[12] A complete physical examination to detect infection includes careful examination of all skin surfaces and orifices where infections are most likely to arise. All suspicious changes in skin integrity should be cultured for both common and uncommon pathogens.[16]

For immunocompromised patients, the only symptoms of infection may be fever or pain.[18] If patients are lymphocyte suppressed or receiving corticosteroids, a fever may not be present.[16] In fact, subnormal temperatures may be equally indicative of infection in the immunocompromised patient, a finding more common in these patients than those with normal immune responses.[8,15]

Immunocompromised patients have such limited protective function that infections rarely remain localized.[8,15] Because microbial invasion extends systemically, sepsis is often evident. Again, these individuals have reduced symptoms of the severity of infection. Common symptoms such as myalgias or arthralgias occur, but are not accompanied by inflammation.[8,15] Compensatory tachycardia and a low diastolic blood pressure are common and reflect the degree of vasodilation that accompanies severe sepsis. Surprisingly, these patients do not progress to organ failure as rapidly as individuals with normal inflammatory responses, which is thought to be related to the lack of WBC cytokines that are the etiology of organ failure during sepsis.[36]

An important aspect of assessment in patients with short-term granulocytopenia is the recognition that the absence of symptoms during neutropenia is followed by exacerbated symptoms at the site of infection when the cells begin to repopulate. Patients presenting with infection while neutropenic may develop more severe symptoms and WBC infiltration at the site of infection as the bone marrow recovers.[27,38,39]

Diagnostic Test Results

Physical findings are complemented with diagnostic test results to identify clinical immune suppression disorders. Immune compromise has been referred to as the silent complication because the actual absence of cells or cell function is the defined disorder, but it is asymptomatic unless the individual is infected. There are several tests of immunologic function that are important to evaluate the level of immune competence in at-risk individuals. A summary of diagnostic tests of immune function and the significance of their abnormal results is given in Table 32.2.[2,5,6,33,34,38,39]

TABLE 32.2 Diagnostic Tests of Immune Function

Study	Description and Purpose	Normal Values
WBC count	Measurement of total number of leukocytes. When WBC count is very low, machine counting may be inaccurate and laboratory personnel may hand-count WBCs on slide.	5000–10,000/mm^3
WBC differential	Determination of whether each kind of WBC is present in proper proportion; determination of absolute value by multiplying percentage of cell type by total WBC count and dividing by 100. When calculating absolute neutrophil count, both mature neutrophils (segmented neutrophils) and bands are included in calculation. In addition to common WBCs, immature neutrophils, called bands, may be noted as a percentage of total WBC count.	Neutrophils: 55%–70% (2500–8000/mm^3) Neutrophil bands: 26% of total WBC count Eosinophils: 1%–4% (50–500/mm^3) Basophils: 0.5% –1% (25–100/mm^3) Lymphocytes: 20%–40% (1000–4000/mm^3)
Absolute neutrophil count (ANC)	Calculates number of neutrophils available for combating bacterial infection. Lower than normal values increase risk of infection with typical and atypical bacteria. Severity scoring system for abnormal values is as follows:[9] ANC = WBC × (% neutrophils + % bands) Grade 1: >1500/mm^3, but <2500/mm^3 Grade 2: >1000/mm^3, but <1500/mm^3 Grade 3: >500/mm^3, but <1000/mm^3 Grade 4: <500/mm^3	> 2500/mm^3
Absolute lymphocyte count (ALC)	Calculates number of lymphocytes available to combat viral and opportunistic infections. Severity scoring system for abnormal values is as follows:[9] Grade 1: >800/mm^3 Grade 2: >500/mm^3, but <800/mm^3 Grade 3: >200/mm^3, but <500/mm^3 Grade 4: <200/mm^3	800–1500 cells/mm^3
Erythrocyte sedimentation rate (ESR)	Screening tool for serum evidence of the presence of an inflammatory process.	Age and gender related normal values may apply; Male: up to 15 mm/h Female: up to 20 mm/h
Immunoglobulin G levels (IgG)	Of all immunoglobulins, the largest percentage and most universally important is IgG; therefore other specific immunoglobulin levels are not measured.	150–300 mcg/dL
C-reactive protein	Whereas not usually present, it will be detectable in the presence of inflammation or tissue destruction.	Not present
Complement CH_{50} (total complement)	Total amount of complement components in serum. Can be affected by secondary immune deficiency and autoimmune disorders.	30–75 units/mL
Complement C3 level	Amount of C3 in serum. When reduced, can increase risk of sino-pulmonary infections.	75–175 mg/dL
Complement C4 level	Amount of C4 in serum. When reduced, can indicate immune-complex disease.	22–45 mg/dL
C1 inhibitor functional assay	Function of C1 esterase inhibitor that is abnormal may indicate hereditary angioedema.	13.2–24 mg/dL
Complement fixation ratio	Immunofluorescence detection of complement complexes indicative of nonspecific immunologic antigen-antibody reactions.	None
HIV antibody test	ELISA test for presence of antibodies to HIV virus can detect reactive antibodies indicative of recent HIV disease.	None
HIV core protein antigen P24	Immunofluorescence detection of core antigen protein of HIV: P24 antigen.	None
HIV envelope glycoprotein GP41	Immunofluorescence detection of envelope protein GP41.	None
HIV cultures	Polymerase chain reaction amplification of viral proteins can be detected early in disease.	Absent
CD4 count (detection of surface marker of some macrophages and some lymphocytes)	CD4 counts are used to monitor progression or response to therapy of anti-HIV therapies. CD4 level is predictive of risk for opportunistic infections, and used as a guide for prescription of prophylactic antimicrobial therapy. Severity scoring system for abnormal values is as follows:[9] Grade 1: >500/mm^3, but less than the lower limit of normal Grade 2: >200/mm^3, but <500/mm^3 Grade 3: >50/mm^3, but <200/mm^3 Grade 4: <50/mm^3	60%–75% 600–1500/mL
Antibody panels: Hepatitis A, Hepatitis B, CMV, RSV	Immunofluorescence detection of antibodies or core antigens to specific viruses.	Absent
Tissue anergy panel	Antigens are injected intradermally, and individuals with normal immune function will activate immunoglobulins, producing a localized *wheal response*. Absence of response is indicative of lymphocyte suppression.	Positive wheal reaction to intradermal: tuberculosis, *Candida*, and *Clostridium difficile*
Bone marrow aspirate and biopsy	Technique involves removal of bone marrow through a locally anesthetized site to evaluate status of blood-forming tissue. It is used to diagnose or assess status of hematologic malignancies, to stage solid tumors (e.g., breast cancer), and for diagnosis of primary bone marrow cell development disorders (e.g., aplastic anemia).	Normal mature cells in adequate numbers, absence of clonal immature cell lines

CMV, Cytomegalovirus; *ELISA*, enzyme-linked immunosorbent assay; *IgG*, immunoglobulin G; *RSV*, respiratory syncytial virus; *WBC*, white blood cell.
From Reference 35.

BOX 32.1 Calculation of Absolute Neutrophil and Lymphocyte Counts

Percentage of cells multiplied by total WBC = absolute count subtype

Absolute neutrophil count (ANC) 0.40 (% neutrophils) × 800 = 320

Absolute lymphocyte count (ALC) 0.40 (% lymphocytes) × 800 = 320

The absolute neutrophil count, lymphocyte counts, and cluster of differentiation 4 (CD4) counts are important diagnostic laboratory tests that demonstrate the severity of immune deficiency. The neutrophils are key components in the system of defense against infection. An absence or shortage of neutrophils (e.g., neutropenia) makes a person vulnerable to infection. The absolute neutrophil count (ANC) is the actual number of WBCs that are neutrophils. The ANC is not measured directly: it is derived by multiplying the WBC count times the percentage of neutrophils in the differential WBC count. Many laboratories report these values as percentages of the total count, and individual practitioners must mathematically calculate the absolute count. The experienced critical care nurse routinely performs this mathematical calculation, shown in Box 32.1, for patients at risk for neutropenia or lymphopenia, interprets the results, and modifies the patient's plan of care as the risk for infection increases.

Grading blood cell deficiency in terms of its severity and risk for infection is a common practice. The National Cancer Therapy Evaluation Program has defined toxicity levels: mild (grade 1), moderate (grade 2), severe (grade 3), life-threatening (grade 4), and death (grade 5).[5] Specific toxicity scales are included within Table 32.2. Lower lymphocyte counts increase the risk of certain common infections, malignancies (e.g., Kaposi's sarcoma, metastatic cervical cancer, malignant lymphoma), and unusual infections (e.g., *Pneumocystis jiroveci*).[2,7,28,37]

INFECTION PREVENTION

The general care of patients with immune compromise is supportive and heavily focused on protection from infection. Immunocompromised patient infection precautions are based upon multiple documents published by the Centers for Disease Control,[13,22] the Society of Hospital Infectious Disease,[14] and the National Comprehensive Cancer Network.[16] Precautions involve environmental control, personal care routines, and active immune supportive measures. The precautions may vary slightly from one institution to another and between different patient populations (granulocyte dysfunction versus lymphocyte dysfunction).

Immunocompromised patients differ in their susceptibility to nosocomial infections, depending on the severity and duration of immunosuppression. They are at increased risk for bacterial, fungal, parasitic, and viral infections from both endogenous and exogenous sources. The Centers for Disease Control and Prevention no longer advocates a category of isolation, termed protective isolation, for patients with immune compromise because research has demonstrated that simple protective isolation offers no advantage over routine care for most immunocompromised patients.[14,22] The prevention of infection in immunocompromised patients relies heavily on implementation of rigorous infection control precautions. In critical care settings, this may include using private rooms normally reserved for patients with resistant infections or wearing protective attire such as gloves and masks because of the highly infectious environment of critical care. When the patient leaves the room for a diagnostic test, the application of a mask on the patient may reduce exposure to environmental molds (e.g., *Aspergillus*) or infectious diseases existing in other people the patient encounters, but is not advocated by all institutions.[30,31]

Critical care nurses can prevent infections by performing, monitoring, and assuring compliance with aseptic work practices. The experienced critical care nurse routinely performs mathematical calculations of absolute counts for patients at risk for neutropenia or lymphopenia, interprets the results, and modifies the patient's care as the risk for infection increases.[5,11,33,34] Invasive procedures are limited when possible, and some critical care routines may be modified to reduce infections in these high-risk patients. For example, rectal temperature probes and drainage tubes are discouraged because of the chance for perirectal infection if the anal mucosa is damaged.[13] Specific precautions are defined by individual institutions based upon their level of experience and comfort in management of these patients.

Active measures to prevent infection are particularly important for these patients. Healthy living and nonspecific immune support (such as adequate sleep and nutritional support), as well as avoidance of infection risks (such as invasive procedures), are implemented to avoid infection until immune function is restored. *Immune nutrition* is a new term used to imply a base nutrition aimed at supporting the growth and activity of WBCs. Diets high in protein and vitamins and low in complex carbohydrates and sugar are generally recommended. The addition of nutritional supplements such as arginine and glutamine is thought to target immune function, but is not yet supported by a large body of evidence.[41] New information is available that demonstrates the importance of using the GI tract, even for small amounts of feeding, as a means to maintain GI mucosal integrity to reduce translocation of bacteria from the GI tract into the bloodstream.[19]

For the immunocompromised patient, balanced calories from a variety of healthy food choices are encouraged. At this time no specific calorie limitations exist, but protein intake is encouraged to enhance tissue maintenance and repair. In addition, fluids are generally encouraged and improved hydration can enhance natural clearance of microbes via excretions, such as sputum or urine. Supplemental vitamins and minerals are encouraged to enhance tissue maintenance and repair. Special considerations include avoidance of fermented and unpasteurized drinks and foods, and discouraging ingestion of raw or partially cooked eggs and meat. Food substances that can be consumed after careful cleaning and evaluation of contamination include: salads, uncooked fresh fruit or vegetables, fresh shell nuts, and cheeses.

Vaccinations to prevent common infections, such as meningitis and pneumococcus, are recommended for patients with special risk factors, provided that the vaccine does not contain live organisms.[13,23,24,29] Organ transplant recipients should receive vaccinations against influenza, pneumococcus, and meningitis at a minimum.[23,24] Patients with surgical (e.g., treatment for traumatic injury or chronic leukemia) or functional splenectomy (e.g., infarcted spleen with sickle cell crisis) should receive a pneumococcal vaccine as this is an important organism normally removed by splenic macrophages.[10] Other immunocompromised patients who may be candidates for specific vaccinations include the following: older adults, organ transplant recipients, intravenous drug users, HIV-infected individuals, and those with renal or hepatic impairment.[2,14,16] In situations in which the immune compromise is related to a reversible etiology, the priority is to eliminate the causative agent and provide symptomatic support until the disorder is reversed.[16] This may be the objective when immune compromise is due to medications that can be discontinued, or diseases that can be stabilized. For example, if immune compromise is related to infection with HIV, antiretroviral therapy may restore lymphocyte counts and reduce the severity of immune compromise.[2,7,28]

In patients who are at particular risk for defined microorganisms, prophylactic antimicrobial therapy may be employed. Prophylactic antimicrobial agents are approved for routine use in patients with prolonged neutropenia or HIV infection, or in recipients of immunosuppressant agents for autoimmune disease, or to prevent rejection after organ transplant.[2,7,13,14,16,28,37] The regimen prescribed will be based on host variables, the type of immune defect, and anticipated infectious organisms. For example, the prophylactic regimen for HIV-infected individuals is well defined. Once the CD4 count is below 200/mm^3, pneumocystis prophylaxis with trimethoprim-sulfamethoxazole is started. When the CD4 count further decreases below 200/mm^3, antimycobacterial therapy is initiated, and as the count drops below 50/mm^3, agents against cytomegalovirus are prescribed.[2,7,28,37]

ENHANCEMENT OF IMMUNE FUNCTION

As outlined in Table 32.3, specific interventions to enhance immunologic function may be indicated for patients who are

TABLE 32.3 Immune Support Therapies

Growth Factor	Indications	Dose	Nursing Considerations
Hematopoietic Factors/Growth Colony-Stimulating Factors			

Granulocyte colony-stimulating factor (GCSF, filgrastim, pegfilgrastim)	• Chemotherapy-induced neutropenia
	• Antiretroviral-induced neutropenia
	• Under investigation:
	  • Sepsis in children
	  • Autoimmune neutropenia
	  • Neutropenia of chronic illness
		Filgrastim: single daily dose of 5–20 mcg/kg IV or subcutaneously every day for up to 2 weeks based upon post-chemotherapy nadir; administer slowly subcutaneously over 1 min; administer over 30 min IV pegfilgrastim: single one-time dose of 6 mg IV or subcutaneous dose once per chemotherapy cycle, and no more frequently than every 21 days	• For patients receiving pegfilgrastim with chemotherapy, pegfilgrastim administered 24 hours after chemotherapy completion is recommended.
			• In daily dosing agent, therapy should be continued within this two-week time frame until WBC count reaches 10,000 cells/mm.
			• Hypersensitivity reactions may occur. Administer slowly, observing for rash, hives, or respiratory distress.
			• Monitor total WBC count and differential.
			• Prepare patient for possible adverse effects: fever, bone pain, and redness at injection site.
			• Advise patients how to manage adverse effects with over-the-counter medications, such as acetaminophen.

Granulocyte macrophage colony-stimulating factor (sargramostim, IL-3)	• Post–hematopoietic stem cell transplant • Chemotherapy-induced neutropenia	• Single daily dose of 250 mcg/m^2; administer IV over 2 hours	• Should not be used 24 hours before to 24 hours after administration of antineoplastic chemotherapy. • Caution if pleural effusion, pericardial effusion, HF, or arrhythmias. • CBC w/diff 2×/week. • BUN/Cr or LFTs at least every 2 weeks if renal/liver impairment. • Avoid use of bacteriostatic water for injection in neonates, which can cause potentially fatal syndrome called *gasping syndrome.*
Immune Globulin Replacement			

Intravenous immune globulin (Gammagard, Gammar-IV, Iveegam, Sandoglobulin, Venoglobulin-S)	• Primary immunodeficiency syndromes
	• Immune thrombocytopenia
	• Chronic lymphocytic leukemia
	• Immune reconstitution after hematopoietic stem cell transplantation
	• Specific products indicated for defined viral infections (e.g., cytomegalovirus, respiratory syncytial virus)
	• Under investigation for:
	  • Chronic disease-related IgG deficiency
	  • Sino-pulmonary infections
		Single dose of 200–800 mg/kg IV may be given for 3 to 4 weeks. IV dosing and duration of therapy are variable according to clinical situation. Also available in a subcutaneous formulation for primary immunodeficiency syndromes.	• Retest IgG levels after administration (should be > 300 mg/dL).
			• Reconstitution or dilution is required for all products.
			• Determine special requirements for each specific product: may require a 15-micrometer filter; some may only be administered centrally; some are contraindicated in patients with renal dysfunction.
			• Hypersensitivity may occur. Administer by slow titration (increasing rate every 15–30 min over a 1–2 h period) with frequent observation and assessment of vital signs and respiratory function.
			• Black box warning: thrombosis may occur with any route of administration.

Colony stimulating factors (epoetin alfa)	• Anemia, chronic kidney disease associated, chemotherapy, transfusion or HIV associated anemia		• Increase risk for mortality and tumor progression in cancer patients. • Increase risk for cardiovascular events in chronic kidney disease patients especially when administered to reach target levels of Hgb greater than 11 g/dL. • Contraindicated in neonates or infants.

HF, Heart failure; *Hgb,* hemoglobin; *IgG,* immunoglobulin G; *WBC,* white blood cell.
Data from References 3 and 4.

at high risk for life-threatening infections. The specific type of immune support will depend upon the identified deficit. Bone marrow growth factors, also called colony-stimulating factors, support bone marrow regrowth after chemotherapy so that the depth and length of neutropenia are diminished, reducing the risk of infection.[1,9,16,25] These are usually administered approximately 24 hours after the last dose of chemotherapy. These agents are available as a single injection , or every three- to four-week injection, or daily injections that start the day after chemotherapy and continue for approximately 10 days, or until the blood count begins to return to normal.[33,34] If immunoglobulin (Ig) deficiency (IgG levels < 300 mg/dL) is present, intravenous immunoglobulin is available as replacement therapy.[14,16] Intravenous immunoglobulin infusions are administered slowly, with careful monitoring for hypersensitivity reactions. When lymphocyte activity is altered, there are no clear treatments. The experienced critical care nurse can recognize patients who are candidates for immune replacement therapies and the specific nursing care required during administration of these agents.

TREATMENT OF INFECTION

When infections occur in patients with immune compromise, the list of possible pathogens is extensive and challenging to anticipate. When symptoms of infection are present, broad-spectrum bactericidal antibiotics aimed to target both gram-positive and gram-negative organisms are prescribed.[16] Unlike other patients with infections, antimicrobials are initiated at the first sign of infection rather than after the return of positive cultures.[16] These patients have been reported to progress from infection to septic shock in mere hours without comprehensive antimicrobial therapy. This often dictates administration of agents normally requiring approval from the appropriate infectious disease authority.[18] Efficient standing order sets or automated approval processes for management of these patients exist in many institutions.[31] An experienced critical care nurse should be familiar with these policies and facilitate administration of appropriate antimicrobial therapy within two hours of the onset of symptoms.[33,34] Antimicrobials administered in the setting of immune compromise may require higher doses for a longer time.[16] Sometimes multiple antibiotics are administered simultaneously to cover the same microorganism.[18]

Patients who develop severe, refractory infections and remain immune compromised have little chance of full recovery. Granulocyte transfusions can temporarily combat severe microbial infections, but their infusion is associated with a high incidence of hypersensitivity reactions.[16,32] Guidelines for administration of granulocyte transfusions are included in Box 32.2.[32-34]

Oral infection is a common occurrence among immunocompromised patients. Before administration of antimicrobial therapy, a culture of one of the oral ulcerations is performed and sent for bacteria, mycology, and virology evaluation. Although the lesions do not appear infected, immunocompromised patients often do not display traditional symptoms of infection. Additionally, lesion appearance may be atypical for well-known organisms, and the open lesions may actually be herpes simplex virus, not simply a result of chemotherapy. Oral ulcerations in granulocytopenic patients may appear to be nonspecifically erythematous, yet culture positive for fungus or virus. This is particularly concerning in patients who have had previous immunosuppression therapy (such as renal and heart transplant patients) and then are administered long-term lymphocyte suppression after the transplant, predisposing them to herpes simplex infection.

CONCLUSION

Patients with compromised immune systems are cared for in critical care far more frequently than credited in the literature. Although hematologic and immunologic disorders comprise some of these patients, it is often a more subtle state of

BOX 32.2 Administration of Granulocyte Transfusions

Candidate Selection

- Refractory infection
- Presumed fungal infection
- Persistent and refractory granulocytopenia

Administration Guidelines

- Cell preparation
  - Granulocytes must be gamma irradiated before administration.
  - Blood bank requires several hours to prepare granulocytes.
- Before starting the infusion
  - Obtain baseline vital signs, oxygen saturation, and breath sounds. Notify the provider of any abnormalities.
  - Premedicate routinely with diphenhydramine (Benadryl) 25–50 mg IV/PO and acetaminophen (Tylenol) 650 mg IV/PO.
  - Some patients may also require hydrocortisone (Solu-Cortef) 100 mg before transfusion.
  - Administer premedications 15 to 30 minutes before beginning transfusion.
  - Prime standard blood tubing without additional filters with normal saline.
- During infusion
  - Administer granulocytes by gravity only. Infusion pumps may damage the cells.
  - Transfusion must begin within 30 minutes of arrival on unit, and infused at a rate of 1×10^{10} cells per 30 minutes, not to exceed 500 mL/h.
  - Gently agitate bottom of bag every 15 minutes to ensure mixing of cells suspended in plasma. Cells settling in the bottom of bag may infuse too quickly, resulting in bolus effect.
  - Ongoing assessments of vital signs and breath sounds are performed frequently during the infusion.

Nursing Implications

- Reactions are common and may range from a mild to moderate rash and hives to severe hypersensitivity reaction with severe respiratory distress.
- WBCs should migrate to the site of infection, and the patient may demonstrate symptoms reflecting WBC infiltration (e.g., dyspnea, crackles in the presence of pneumonia).
- Have emergency equipment, oxygen delivery system, and suction available.
- For rigors during transfusion, administer meperidine (Demerol) 10 mg IV every 5 minutes up to a total dose of 50 mg. Alternative medications for rigors may be morphine in 0.5 mg increments or small doses of benzodiazepines.
- Avoid infusion of amphotericin or other blood products within 6 hours of WBC transfusion if at all possible.

WBC, White blood cell.
Adapted from References 33 and 34.

compromise from medical-surgical disorders or therapies that affects patients. The role of the critical care nurse in recognizing high-risk patients and implementing heightened surveillance cannot be underestimated. Preventive and proactive management of the immune system dysfunction before the onset of infection is key for successful recovery. Extra infection prevention strategies can be taken for granted, but unless conscientious attention is paid to everyday elements of care, serious infection threatens the lives of these patients. A number of strategies aimed at this specialized care can be incorporated into routine critical care nursing orientations. Key pearls of care for immunocompromised patients in the critical care unit are included in Box 32.3.

BOX 32.3 Nursing Practice Pearls for Immunocompromised Patients

1. Have a high index of suspicion.
   Immunocompromise is NOT just found in patients with hematologic or immune disorders.
2. Be a detective.
   Immunocompromised patients do NOT exhibit the usual common signs and symptoms of infection, and subtle symptoms should not be overlooked.
3. Beware—the patient may get worse before getting better.
   Return of immune function often heralds symptom exacerbation. As WBC and other supportive immune function returns to normal in patients with temporary deficits, the WBC response causes white out on the chest radiograph that leads to symptom exacerbation.
4. Assess and culture every opening or potential opening.
   Immune-compromised patients can be colonized with large quantities of normal nonpathogenic flora or resistant microbes. These can become the source of infection. Keep a broad view of possible infectious organisms, uncommon and resistant microbes may be the culprits.
5. Proactively prevent infection in every aspect of care.
   Realize that the smallest infractions in infection control technique can cause life-threatening infection, and take special care to protect the patient.
6. Learn which antimicrobial agents target specific microbes and understand unique infection risks.
   Understanding the risk factors for infection dictate which antimicrobial agent choices during early signs of infection can help the interprofessional team be comprehensive in consideration of therapy choices.
7. Think of creative options.
   Advocate exploring additional risks for infection or avenues for treatment such as IgG replenishment or granulocyte transfusions.

IgG, Immunoglobin G; *WBC,* white blood cell.

CASE STUDY 32.1

Evidence-Based Management of the Immunocompromised Patient

S.E. is a 49-year-old diabetic male patient who had a live donor kidney transplant 8 years ago. Immunosuppressive medications were discontinued 5 years ago, and he has not demonstrated rejection. He most recently presented 3 months ago to the oncology clinic with right axillary lymphadenopathy and dyspnea. Axillary lymph nodes and a 2 cm by 2 cm mass in the right hilar region of the lung were biopsy-positive for follicular lymphoma, a malignancy that affects the antibody-producing B-lymphocytes. He received radiation therapy delivered in 7 fractions over 9 days for immediate reduction of the hilar mass obstructing the airway, followed by a multimedication chemotherapy regimen. He has received two cycles of chemotherapy, the last doses given 9 days ago. Today, he was admitted from the emergency department for high spiking fevers and hypoxemia. His admission data are as follows:

S.E.'s Admission Findings Subjective Symptoms

- Headache
- Dyspnea
- Nonproductive cough

Physical Examination

- Vital signs: T 39.5°C, Pulse 134 beats/min with occasional premature atrial contractions (PACs), Respiration rate (RR) 32 breaths/min, Blood pressure (BP) 108/42 mm Hg (normally 120–130/76–84 mm Hg)
- Breath sounds: faint crackles in bases and diminished in right mid-anterior chest extending into the axilla
- Soft, nontender abdomen with hypoactive bowel sounds
- Oral mucosa is erythematous with ulceration of the buccal mucosa and a white coated tongue
- Semipermanent double-lumen soft silastic tunneled catheter is noted on the right chest with the tunnel up into the right neck; line is not reddened, swollen, tender, or presenting with exudates

Diagnostic Tests

- Pulse oximetry 86% on room air
- Arterial blood gases: pH: 7.30, partial pressure of carbon dioxide ($Paco_2$): 45 mm Hg, partial pressure of arterial oxygen (Pao_2): 58 mm Hg, HCO_3^-: 19 mEq/L
- Chest radiograph: slight haziness in right lateral lung, blunted costophrenic angles bilaterally
- Complete blood cell count with WBC differential pending

Decision Point:
What does his admission lab work indicate?

Decision Point:
Given his symptoms, what diagnosis would be made?

Decision Point:
What are S.E.'s infection risks?

REFERENCES

1. Aapro, M. S., Bohlius, J., Cameron, D. A., et al. (2011). 2010 update of EORTC guidelines for the use of granulocyte-colony stimulating factor to reduce the incidence of chemotherapy-induced febrile neutropenia in adult patients with lymphoproliferative disorders and solid tumours. *Eur J Cancer, 47*(1), 8–32.
2. Bartlett, J. G. (2005). *The Johns Hopkins Hospital 2004–2005 guide to care of patients with HIV infection*. Philadelphia: Lippincott Williams & Wilkins.
3. Bouza, E., Burillo, A., & Guembe, M. (2011). Managing intravascular catheter-related infections in heart transplant patients: how far can we apply IDSA guidelines for immunocompromised patients? *Curr Opin Infect Dis, 24*(4), 302–308.
4. Burris, H. A., Belani, C. P., Kaufman, P. A., et al. (2010). Pegfilgrastim on the same day versus next day of chemotherapy in patients with breast cancer, non-small-cell lung cancer, ovarian cancer, and non-Hodgkin's lymphoma: results of four multicenter, double-blind, randomized phase II studies. *J Oncol Pract, 6*(3), 133–140.
5. Cagen, D., Franco, M., & Vasquez, D. (2002). The ABCs of low blood cell count. *Clin J Oncol Nurs, 6*(1), 34–35.
6. Cancer Therapy Evaluation Program. (2015). *Common terminology criteria for adverse events*. Bethesda, MD: v. 5.0 (CTCAE) DCTD, NCI, NIH, DHHS. http://ctep.cancer.gov.
7. Center for Disease Control & U.S. Department of Health. (2012). Integrated prevention services for HIV infection, viral hepatitis, sexually transmitted diseases, and tuberculosis for persons who use drugs illicitly: summary guidance from CDC and the U.S. Department of Health and Human Services. *MMWR Recomm Rep, 61*(RR-5), 1–40.
8. Ching, L. C. (2013). Cochrane review summary for cancer nursing: low-bacterial diet versus control diet to prevent infection in cancer patients treated with chemotherapy causing episodes of neutropenia. *Cancer Nurs, 36*(6), 493.

9. Crawford, J., et al. (2014). *NCCN Clinical practice guidelines in oncology. Myeloid growth factors.* Jenkintown, PA: v.2.2014 National Comprehensive Cancer Network. https://www.nccn.org/professionalsphysician_gls_guidelines.asp.
10. Dahyot Fizelier, C., Debaene, B., & Mimoz, O. (2013). Management of infection risk in asplenic patients. *Ann Fr Anesth Reanim, 32*(4), 251–256.
11. Ehrenkranz, N. J., MacIntyre, A. T., Hebert, P. R., et al. (2011). Control of health care-associated infections (HAI): winning both the battles and the war. *J Gen Intern Med, 26*(3), 340–342.
12. Fernández González, F., Betancourt, J., Malpica, J. C., et al. (2013). An unusual presentation of herpes simplex in an immunocompromised patient. *Bol Asoc Med P R, 105*(1), 48–50.
13. Feider, L., Mitchell, P., & Bridges, E. (2010). Oral care practices for orally intubated critically ill adults. *Am J Crit Care, 19*(2), 175–183.
14. Foster, M. (2014). Reevaluating the neutropenic diet: time to change. *Clin J Oncol Nurs, 18*(2), 239–241.
15. Fox, N., & Freifeld, A. G. (2012). The neutropenic diet reviewed: moving toward a safe food handling approach. *Oncology, 26*(6), 572–575, 580, 582 passim.
16. Freifeld, A. G., et al. (2012). *NCCN practice guidelines for fever and neutropenia.* Jenkintown, PA: v.1.2012 National Comprehensive Cancer Network. 2012. http://www.nccn.org.
17. Goss, L. K., Coty, M., & Myers, J. A. (2011). A review of documented oral care practices in an intensive care unit. *Clin Nurs Res, 20*(2), 181–196.
18. Gille Johnson, P., Hansson, K. E., & Gårdlund, B. (2013). Severe sepsis and systemic inflammatory response syndrome in emergency department patients with suspected severe infection. *Scand J Infect Dis, 45*(3), 186–193.
19. Huynh, D., Chapman, M. J., & Nguyen, N. Q. (2013). Nutrition support in the critically ill. *Curr Opin Gastroenterol, 29*(2), 208–215.
20. Jubelirer, S. J. (2011). The benefit of the neutropenic diet: fact or fiction? *Oncologist, 16*(5), 704–707.
21. Katz, M. H. (2015). Mitigating the dangers of opioids. *JAMA Intern Med, 175*(4), 616.
22. Kaufman, C. (2011). The secret life of lymphocytes. *Nursing, 41*(6), 50–54.
23. Kumar, D. (2014). Immunizations following solid-organ transplantation. *Curr Opin Infect Dis, 27*(4), 329–335.
24. Kumar, D., Blumberg, E. A., Danziger Isakov, L., et al. (2011). Influenza vaccination in the organ transplant recipient: review and summary recommendations. *Am J Transplant, 11*(10), 2020–2030.
25. Lyman, G. H., & Kleiner, J. M. (2011). Summary and comparison of myeloid growth factor guidelines in patients receiving cancer chemotherapy. *Cancer Treat Res, 157*, 145–165.
26. Lin, Y., Chang, J., Chang, T., et al. (2011). Critical care nurses' knowledge, attitudes and practices of oral care for patients with oral endotracheal intubation: a questionnaire survey. *J Clin Nurs, 20*(21-22), 3204–3214.
27. Marrs, J. A. (2006). Care of patients with neutropenia. *Clin J Oncol Nurs, 10*(2), 164–166.
28. Masur, H., Brooks, J. T., Benson, C. A., et al. (2014). Prevention and treatment of opportunistic infections in HIV-infected adults and adolescents: Updated Guidelines from the Centers for Disease Control and Prevention, National Institutes of Health, and HIV Medicine Association of the Infectious Diseases Society of America. *Clin Infect Dis, 58*(9), 1308–1311.
29. Mayhill, C. G. (2011). *Hospital epidemiology and infection control* (4th ed.). Philadelphia: Lippincott Williams & Wilkins.
30. Menegueti, M. G., Ferreira, L. R., Silva, M. F., et al. (2013). Assessment of microbiological air quality in hemato-oncology units and its relationship with the occurrence of invasive fungal infections: an integrative review. *Rev Soc Bras Med Trop, 46*(4), 391–396.
31. Nash, A., Dalziel, R. G., & Fitzgerald, J. R. (2015). *Mims' pathogenesis of infectious disease* (6th ed.). San Diego: Academic Press.
32. Netelenbos, T. (2013). Therapeutic granulocyte transfusions in adults: more evidence needed. *Transfus Apher Sci, 48*(2), 139–140.
33. Nirenberg, A., Reame, N. K., Cato, K. D., et al. (2010). Oncology nurses' use of National Comprehensive Cancer Network clinical practice guidelines for chemotherapy-induced and febrile neutropenia. *Oncol Nurs Forum, 37*(6), 765–773.
34. Olsen, J. P., Baldwin, S., & Houts, A. C. (2011). The Patient Care Monitor-Neutropenia Index: development, reliability, and validity of a measure for chemotherapy-induced neutropenia. *Oncol Nurs Forum, 38*(3), 360–367.
35. Pagana, K. D., Pagana, T. J., & Pagana, T. N. (2015). *Mosby's diagnostic and laboratory test reference* (12 ed.). St. Louis: Elsevier.
36. Sehulster, L., & Chinn, R. Y. (2003). Guidelines for environmental infection control in health-care facilities. Recommendations of CDC and the Healthcare Infection Control Practices Advisory Committee (HICPAC). *MMWR Recommen Rep, 52*(RR-10), 1–42.
37. Shelton, B. K. (2001). Hematological and immune disorders. In M. L. Sole, M. L. Lamborn, & J. C. Hartshorn (Eds.), *Introduction to critical care nursing* (3rd ed.). Philadelphia: Saunders.
38. Shelton, B. K. (2005). Infections. In C. H. Yarbro, M. H. Frogge, & M. Goodman (Eds.), *Cancer nursing principles and practice* (6th ed.) (pp. 698–722). Boston: Jones & Bartlett Publishers.
39. Sullivan, K. M., et al. (2001). Preventing opportunistic infections after hematopoietic stem cell transplantation: the Centers for Disease Control and Prevention, Infectious Diseases Society of America, and American Society for Blood and Marrow Transplantation Practice guidelines and beyond. *Hematology Am Soc Hematol Educ Program*, 392–421.
40. Sydnor, E. R. M., & Perl, T. M. (2011). Hospital epidemiology and infection control in acute-care settings. *Clin Microbiol Rev, 24*(1), 141–173.
41. Tsang, V. (2012). Vaccination recommendations for the hematology and oncology and post-stem cell transplant populations. *J Adv Pract Oncol, 3*(2), 71–83.
42. Tsoutsou, P. G. (2014). The interplay between radiation and the immune system in the field of post-radical pneumonitis and fibrosis and why it is important to understand it. *Expert Opin Pharmacother, 15*(13), 1781–1783.

Additional Reading

Centers for Disease Control and Prevention. (2002). Guidelines for the hand hygiene in healthcare settings. *MMWR, 51*(No, RR-16), 1–44.
Heitkamp, D. E., Albin, M., Chung, J. H., et al. (2015). ACR appropriateness criteria acute respiratory illness in immunocompromised patients. *J Thorac Imaging, 30*(3), W2–W5.
Rubin, L. G., Levin, M. J., Ljungman, P., et al. (2014). 2013 IDSA clinical practice guideline for vaccination of the immunocompromised host. *Clin Infect Dis, 58*(3), 309–318.

Additional Resources

Centers for Disease Control and Prevention (CDC). http://www.cdc.gov/.
National Comprehensive Cancer Network (NCCN). http://www.nccn.org/.
Oncology Nursing Society (ONS). https://www.ons.org/.
Society of Healthcare Epidemiology of America (SHEA). http://www.shea-online.org/.

33

Caring for the Patient in the Immediate Postoperative Period

Denise O'Brien and Sharon Dickinson

The immediate postanesthesia period is a time when patients are vulnerable and dependent secondary to the residual physiologic effects of anesthesia on the respiratory and cardiovascular systems, as well as the specific surgical procedure. Nursing care during this time should focus on assessment, anticipation, and prevention of adverse outcomes and complications, especially those related to the respiratory and cardiovascular systems. From the arrival of the patient into the postanesthesia care unit (PACU) or critical care unit until the patient is ready for discharge or transfer to the next level of care, the patient requires intensive and observant monitoring by nurses who are prepared to address the special needs of this population.

Patients with comorbidities who have undergone major surgical procedures, or those who have suffered perioperative complications, may require recovery, observation, and monitoring in the critical care setting. Practices vary among institutions regarding the disposition of the immediate postanesthesia patient; some institutions initiate direct operating room (OR) to critical care transfers; others require an initial transfer from the operating room to the PACU and then to critical care when the patient stabilizes and can be safely transferred. Wherever recovery from anesthesia occurs, the patient should receive the same standard of nursing care. Understanding anesthesia agents and techniques, anticipating common postanesthesia complications and emergencies, and knowledge of and adherence to the American Society of PeriAnesthesia Nurses (ASPAN) *Perianesthesia Nursing Standards, Practice Recommendations and Interpretive Statements* will assist the critical care nurse to provide quality patient care regardless of the practice setting.[5]

PATIENTS AT RISK FOR POSTOPERATIVE COMPLICATIONS

Patients undergoing operative procedures with anesthesia may be at increased risk for intraoperative and postoperative complications because of preexisting medical conditions or medications. For elective surgical procedures, these comorbidities require preoperative evaluation and potential intervention to optimize the patient's physical condition for surgery.

First introduced by Saklad in 1941, the American Society of Anesthesiologists (ASA) physical status classification scale identifies patient risk for anesthetic morbidity and mortality based on history and physical examination.[59] The classification system concisely and simply offers the anesthesia provider information regarding the patient's status. The ASA physical status classification predicts risk for anesthesia based on the patient's coexisting medical conditions and not based on the surgical procedure (Table 33.1).

Factors known to increase the patient's risk for intraoperative and postoperative complications include history of pulmonary disease (e.g., chronic obstructive pulmonary disease [COPD], smoking, asthma), extremes of body mass index (BMI), obstructive sleep apnea, cardiovascular disease (e.g., coronary artery disease, hypertension, peripheral vascular disease), diabetes, extremes of age, poor nutritional status, operative procedures over 3 hours long, significant blood loss, renal or hepatic disease, and use of herbal and vitamin supplements.[6,15,51,53,55,62,63,66,68,70]

These preexisting conditions can lead to increased length of hospitalization, impaired wound healing, surgical site infection, prolonged postoperative mechanical ventilation, and an overall increase in morbidity and mortality.[12,23,34]

OVERVIEW OF ANESTHESIA AND THE ANESTHETIC AGENTS

Prior to administering any anesthesia, the anesthesia care provider evaluates the patient and develops a plan based on the patient's physical status, operative procedure, and surgeon preference. Anesthesia can consist of general or regional techniques or a combination of both techniques. Knowledge of anesthetics and anesthesia techniques helps the nurse anticipate recovery and emergence of the patient, potential side effects, and plan care based on the anesthesia given to the patient.

GENERAL ANESTHESIA

General anesthesia is defined as "a reversible state of unconsciousness, produced by anesthetic agents, with absence of pain sensation over the entire body and a greater or lesser degree of muscular relaxation. The drugs producing this state can be administered by inhalation, intravenously, intramuscularly, or rectally."[20] Therefore general anesthesia produces unconsciousness, amnesia, analgesia, blunting of autonomic nervous system reflexes, and some degree of muscle relaxation.[13]

Inhalation agents, introduced in the mid-1800s, are administered as vapors or gases that diffuse across air spaces and are carried by the blood to the brain to produce anesthesia. The inhalation agents first introduced included ether and nitrous oxide.[41] Ether was used until the 1960s and was replaced by halothane, the first halogenated inhalation agent.[65] Halothane was nonflammable and sweet smelling. Today, newer inhalation agents that are less toxic and less soluble have replaced halothane. Nitrous oxide, although still in use after 170 years, is not a complete anesthetic agent. It is used primarily as a carrier agent for the other gases and to diminish awareness under anesthesia.

Although inhalation agents are defined as gases, nitrous oxide is technically the only gas; the other agents are vapors of volatile (i.e., evaporate) liquids.[65] Speed of action and administration via the lungs are unique features of the inhalation agents. Establishing a partial pressure gradient in the lung helps propel the agent across tissues to sites of action in the central nervous system to produce the anesthetic state. Recovery, like induction, depends on the agent's solubility as well as the patient's ventilation and cardiac output (CO). The inhalation agents all produce respiratory depression, vasodilation, and some degree of myocardial depression. In general, minimal metabolism of the agents occurs in the body, and elimination is primarily through the lungs. Table 33.2 lists medications used as inhalation agents for general anesthesia.

Postoperatively, patients who have received the inhalation anesthetic agents require monitoring of respiratory rate and rhythm, oxygen saturation monitoring, supplemental oxygen if desaturation occurs, and stimulation and encouragement to ventilate (deep breathe). Depending on the surgical procedure and hemodynamic status, elevation of the head of bed may help the patient's oxygenation and ventilation. The newer volatile agents are rapidly eliminated from the lungs in the spontaneously breathing patient. Patients with airway obstructions or inadequate ventilatory efforts may require additional supportive care.

TABLE 33.1 ASA Physical Status Classification

ASA Physical Status	Classification
ASA or PS 1	A normal healthy patient
ASA or PS 2	Patient with mild systemic disease
ASA or PS 3	Patient with severe systemic disease
ASA or PS 4	Patient with severe systemic disease that is a constant threat to life
ASA or PS 5	Patient critically ill who will die within 24 hours with or without operative procedure
ASA or PS 6	Declared brain dead patient whose organs are being removed for donor purposes
E	Emergency, added to any of the above

ASA, American Society of Anesthesiologists; *E, emergency*; *PS*, physical status.

INTRAVENOUS AGENTS

Intravenous agents used to provide anesthesia include hypnotics/nonhypnotics, barbiturates, benzodiazepines, and analgesics. Combining intravenous agents to produce analgesia, amnesia, and muscle relaxation is called *balanced anesthesia*, or "anesthesia that uses a combination of drugs, each in an amount sufficient to produce its major or desired effect to the optimum degree and keep its undesirable or unnecessary effects to a minimum."[20]

Barbiturates, such as sodium thiopental (Pentothal) and methohexital (Brevital), are mostly unavailable and have been replaced by newer agents. Nonhypnotic agents used for induction are propofol (Diprivan) and etomidate (Amidate). The benzodiazepines (diazepam [Valium], midazolam [Versed], and lorazepam [Ativan]) are agents used for anxiolysis and to produce amnesia before induction and intraoperatively. Dexmedetomidine (Precedex) is used for preoperative and maintenance sedation. Ketamine is an older agent that may be used as an induction agent or for anesthesia maintenance to help reduce opioid requirements. Analgesics are used to blunt cardiovascular stimulation during induction and intraoperatively, and for pain relief. Table 33.3 lists medications commonly used for intravenous anesthesia techniques and in combination with inhalation anesthetic agents to produce general anesthesia.

In addition, other agents such as antacids, gastrokinetic agents, and histamine blockers are routinely administered as part of the anesthesia plan. Antacid prophylaxis may be administered to patients at increased risk for aspiration because of a history of hiatal hernia, gastroesophageal reflux disease, and gastroparesis.[56]

NEUROMUSCULAR BLOCKING AGENTS

Neuromuscular blocking agents (NMBAs) are used to facilitate intubation and for paralysis of skeletal muscles to improve operative access. NMBAs include depolarizing agents (agents

TABLE 33.2 Medications Used as Inhalation Agents for General Anesthesia

Agent	Metabolism/Elimination	Advantages	Disadvantages
Nitrous oxide (N_2O) "gas" (1844)	Elimination via exhalation	Carrier agent Amnesia Analgesia	Fills air-containing spaces (avoid in ear, brain, bowel procedures) May increase risk of postoperative nausea and vomiting
Isoflurane (Forane) (1970)	Primary: exhalation	Inexpensive Nontoxic Coronary artery vasodilator	Malignant hyperthermia triggering agent
Sevoflurane (Ultane) (1984)	Primary: exhalation	Minimal odor, pungency; potent bronchodilator	Expensive May precipitate emergence agitation/delirium, pediatrics more than adults (up to 15% of patients) Malignant hyperthermia-triggering agent
Desflurane (Suprane) (1990)	Least soluble, rapid elimination-exhalation	Very rapid emergence	Airway irritant Requires specialized vaporizer Expensive Malignant hyperthermia-triggering agent

Data from References 19 and 46.

TABLE 33.3 Medications Used for Intravenous Anesthesia

Medication	Action	Dose Range	Special Considerations
Induction Agents(Promote Unconsciousness)			
Propofol (Diprivan)	Nonbarbiturate hypnotic agent for induction/general anesthesia	2–2.5 mg/kg elderly, debilitated: 1–1.5 mg/kg Maintenance: 0.1–0.2 mg/kg/min	Antiemetic properties; pain at injection site; systemic vasodilator
Etomidate (Amidate)	Nonbarbiturate hypnotic agent; induction/maintenance of general anesthesia; useful for hemodynamically unstable patients	0.2–0.6 mg/kg over 30–60 sec Maintenance: 5–20 mcg/kg/min	Pain at injection site; blocks normal stress-induced increase in adrenal cortisol production for 4–8 h; myoclonus
Ketamine (Ketalar)	Nonbarbiturate anesthetic/analgesic	1–4.5 mg/kg single dose; 1–2 mg/kg infusion for induction; 0.01–0.03 mg/kg/min continuous infusion for maintenance	Produces analgesia, normal pharyngeal-laryngeal reflexes, cardiovascular/respiratory stimulant; may cause emergence agitation/delirium
Methohexital (Brevital)	Barbiturate; induction of general anesthesia, cardioversion, electroconvulsive shock therapy	50–120 mg initially, 20–40 mg every 4–7 min IV	Myoclonus, hiccups, seizures; rare use
Sedatives/Amnesic Agents (Provide Amnesia and Anxiolysis)			
Midazolam (Versed)	Benzodiazepine; anxiolysis, sedation	Preoperative sedation: 0.02–0.04 mg/kg, repeat every 5 min; titrate to effect Sedation for procedures: 0.05–0.2 mg/kg	Dose needs to be individualized: reduce dose in hepatic dysfunction, elderly, COPD, CHF, concomitant CNS depressants
Dexmedetomidine (Precedex)	Selective alpha-2 adrenergic agonist	0.5–1.0 mcg/kg for premedication; 0.2–0.7 mcg/kg/h for maintenance	Bradycardia; hypotension; respiratory depression
Diazepam (Valium)	Benzodiazepine; anxiolysis, sedation	2–10 mg	Paradoxical excitement/rage may be seen; phlebitis, pain with injection; available but not widely used
Lorazepam (Ativan)	Benzodiazepine; anxiolysis, sedation	Preoperative sedation: 0.04–0.05 mg/kg IV, maximum 2 mg; induction agent 0.1–0.25 mg/kg IV	Given slowly and diluted
Analgesics (Blunt Response to Surgical Stimulus and for Pain Intraoperatively)			
Morphine	Opioid analgesic; preanesthetic medication, adjunct to general or regional anesthesia	2.5–20 mg	Hypotension, nausea, vomiting, respiratory depression
Fentanyl (Sublimaze)	Synthetic opioid analgesic; preoperative medication, adjunct to general or regional anesthesia	Preoperative sedation: 25–100 mcg Adjunct to general anesthesia (GA): 2–50 mcg/kg IV	Rapid infusion may lead to chest wall rigidity: hypotension, nausea/vomiting, respiratory depression
Remifentanil (Ultiva)	Synthetic opioid analgesic; induction (in combination with other agents)/maintenance of general anesthesia	Induction or sedation: 1 mcg/kg IV; continuous infusion: 0.5–1 mcg/kg/min	Risk of respiratory depression/muscle rigidity; ultra-short-acting; potent
Hydromorphone (Dilaudid)	Opioid analgesic; blunt surgical stimulus	1–4 mg IV titrated doses	Respiratory depression; less nausea/vomiting than morphine/fentanyl
Meperidine (Demerol)	Synthetic opioid analgesic; postoperative shivering	12.5–25 mg	Not recommended for analgesia; may precipitate serotonin syndrome*; active metabolite: normeperidine; not reversible with naloxone

*Serotonin syndrome can be triggered by a drug or combination of drugs (e.g., selective serotonin reuptake inhibitors [SSRIs], tricyclic antidepressants [TCAs], monoamine oxidase inhibitors [MAOIs], and other serotonergic drugs) that increase CNS serotonin receptor stimulation. Signs and symptoms include cognitive changes (disorientation, confusion), altered behavioral status (agitation, restlessness), autonomic nervous system instability (fever, shivering, diaphoresis, tachycardia, diarrhea), and neuromuscular changes (tremors, hyperreflexia, myoclonus, ataxia). The addition of a second serotonergic drug may trigger these symptoms.[26,52]

CHF, Congestive heart failure; *CNS,* central nervous system; *COPD,* chronic obstructive pulmonary disease; IV, intravenous.

Data from References 19 and 46.

that mimic acetylcholine) and nondepolarizing agents (agents that interfere or block the action of acetylcholine).[65] The only depolarizing agent used in the United States is succinylcholine (Anectine), a rapid-acting skeletal muscle relaxant used for intubation and rapid-sequence induction of anesthesia. It has an onset of approximately 30 to 60 seconds and duration of 3 to 5 minutes. Adverse effects of succinylcholine include myalgias, hyperkalemia, increased intracranial pressure, and increased intraocular pressure. It is also known to be a triggering agent for malignant hyperthermia. Patients with histories of pseudocholinesterase deficiency, either hereditary or from disease processes (e.g., febrile disorders, hepatic disease, use of echothiophate eye drops), will have prolonged neuromuscular blocks, often requiring endotracheal intubation and mechanical ventilation.[65] Drugs such as the anticholinesterases do not antagonize succinylcholine.[24]

Nondepolarizing agents are either spontaneously reversible or reversible with pharmacologic intervention. Pharmacologic reversal includes an anticholinesterase (e.g., neostigmine [Prostigmin]) and anticholinergic (e.g., glycopyrrolate to

TABLE 33.4 **Medications Commonly Used as Local Anesthetics**

Agent	Use	Special Considerations
Amides		
Lidocaine	Topical, infiltration, field block, spinal, epidural, caudal (also used as an antidysrhythmic)	Most versatile; rapid onset, intense analgesia Class Ib antidysrhythmic agent
Bupivacaine	Infiltration, nerve block, spinal, epidural	Most widely used
Ropivacaine	Spinal, epidural (labor), nerve block	Less cardiotoxic, less potent than bupivacaine
Mepivacaine	Infiltration, nerve block	Derivative of lidocaine, slower metabolism, ineffective topically
Esters		
Cocaine	Topical	CNS depression/stimulation; tachydysrhythmias
Chloroprocaine	Nerve block, epidural	

CNS, Central nervous system.
Data from References 11, 38, 46, and 47.

counteract the muscarinic effects of the anticholinesterase agent). Muscarinic effects include bradycardia, salivation, miosis, and hyperperistalsis.[21] The nondepolarizing agents are not known to trigger malignant hyperthermia crisis.

Metabolism and elimination of the NMBAs vary with the agents. Atracurium (Tracrium) and cisatracurium (Nimbex) are unique nondepolarizing agents that are eliminated through Hofmann degradation; warming may speed reversal of these agents. Hofmann degradation, or elimination, is a spontaneous, nonbiologic process in plasma at normal pH and temperature and does not depend on circulating esterases.[21,36] Pancuronium (Pavulon) is primarily excreted by the kidneys; vecuronium (Vecuron) undergoes both renal and hepatic elimination. Rocuronium (Zemuron) is primarily excreted by the liver with some renal excretion.

REGIONAL ANESTHESIA

Regional anesthesia is "the production of insensibility of a part by interrupting the sensory nerve conductivity from that region of the body. It may be produced by field block, the creation of walls of anesthesia encircling the operative field by means of injections of a local anesthetic; or nerve block, injection of the anesthetic agent close to the nerves whose conductivity is to be cut off. These are also called blocks, blockages, block a., and conduction a."[20]

Local Anesthetics

Local anesthetics are used to produce the anesthesia or analgesia when using regional techniques, as indicated in Table 33.4. The agents are either esters or amides. Ester local anesthetics include cocaine (used topically) and chloroprocaine (Nesacaine) (low risk of systemic toxicity). These agents are not as widely used as the amide local anesthetics. Esters are less stable than amides and may cause rare allergic reactions.[11,39]

Amide local anesthetics include lidocaine (Xylocaine), bupivacaine (Marcaine), mepivacaine (Carbocaine), and ropivacaine (Naropin). Allergic reactions are extremely rare with amide local anesthetic agents.

Systemic toxicity may occur following an inappropriately high dose or accidental intravascular injection of any type of local anesthetic.[39] Early signs involve the central nervous system and include circumoral numbness, dizziness, slurred speech, tinnitus, confusion, and restlessness. Cardiovascular signs may include bradycardia, with subsequent conduction block, multifocal ectopic beats, reentrant dysrhythmias, tachycardia, and ventricular fibrillation. Treatment is supportive and may include oxygen supplementation, fluids, anticonvulsants, and vasoconstrictor and inotropic medications. Dysrhythmias may be treated with amiodarone (Cordarone). Recent evidence suggests lipid emulsion infusions may be useful in these toxic reactions.[48]

The following blocks are rarely used; however, it is important for the critical care nurse to be aware of them. Further information regarding assessment and management of patients receiving these blocks is beyond the scope of this chapter and can be found in other references.

Central Neuraxial Blocks

Spinal anesthesia, also referred to as intrathecal, subarachnoid, or SA block, produces sensory, motor, and sympathetic blocks of the nerve roots. Injection of the local anesthesia agents into the cerebrospinal fluid at the level of L3-4 or L4-5 provides variable duration of lower abdominal and lower extremity anesthesia. Loss of sympathetic tone can result in significant hypotension, usually responsive to ephedrine intravenously. Other complications include bladder atony, high spinal block, hematoma formation, postdural puncture headache, and lower back pain.[47,48] Infrequently, neurologic injury can occur from local anesthetic toxicity or inadvertent intravascular injection.

Epidural anesthesia (injection of local anesthesia into the epidural space) provides sensory and motor blockade, and less sympathetic block than spinal anesthesia. Epidural approaches may be used as the sole anesthetic or in combination with spinal anesthesia or general anesthesia techniques. Lumbar and thoracic approaches are used depending on the level of anesthesia or analgesia required for the operative procedure (Fig. 33.1). The epidural catheter may remain in place after the surgery for postoperative pain management or removed following the operative procedure. An epidural catheter may also be placed preoperatively for postoperative analgesia and attached to a pump after surgery for continued postoperative pain management. Potential complications include epidural hematoma formation, catheter migration or break, intravascular injection, postdural puncture headache, and local anesthetic systemic toxicity.[14,47]

Local anesthesia that is injected through the lower back into the caudal space leading to sacral and perineal sensory block is called *caudal anesthesia*. Although useful in pediatric patients, it is rarely used in adults and has a failure rate of 3% to 5%.[14]

Peripheral Nerve Blocks

Peripheral nerve blocks are used for anesthesia and postoperative analgesia. Blocks may be appropriate as adjuncts

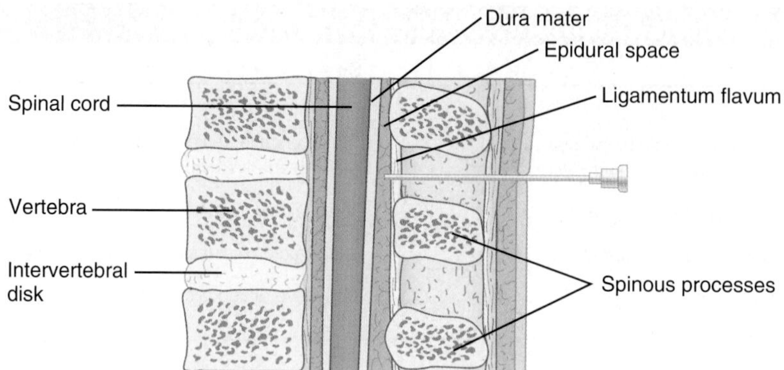

FIG. 33.1 Anatomy for epidural placement.

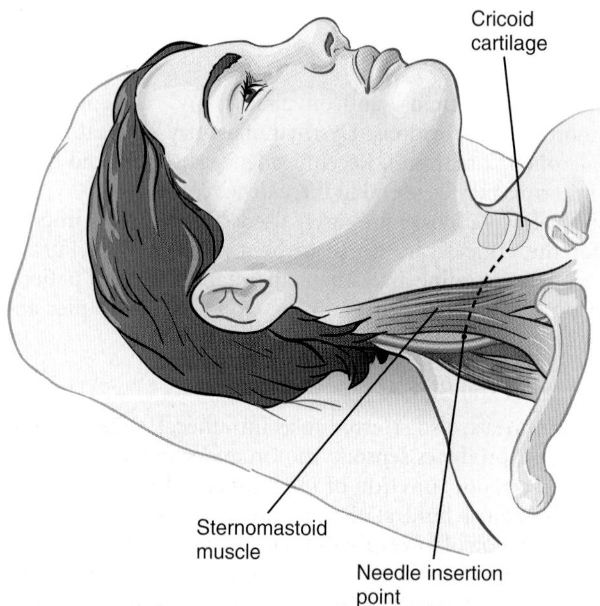

FIG. 33.2 Superficial cervical plexus block.

to general anesthesia or used as the sole anesthetic. Benefits include decreased pain and use of postoperative opioids, and subsequently less nausea, vomiting, and sedation.[22] Patients who have had these blocks may be seen in critical care either postoperatively after procedures during which the blocks were used, or as the result of complications resulting from block placement or local anesthetic side effects.

Cervical Plexus

Cervical plexus blocks provide anesthesia for surgical procedures in the distribution of C2 to C4, including lymph node dissections, plastic repairs, and carotid endarterectomy (Fig. 33.2).[32] Patients remain awake; neurologic status should be monitored continuously. Tracheostomy and thyroidectomy can be performed using a bilateral cervical plexus block. Complications include intravascular injection producing blockade of the phrenic and superior laryngeal nerves, and spread of local anesthetic solution into the epidural and subarachnoid spaces.

Brachial Plexus

An interscalene brachial plexus block is commonly used to provide anesthesia and analgesia for shoulder and upper arm surgery (Fig. 33.3).[32] Complications include ipsilateral phrenic nerve block with diaphragmatic paralysis and, rarely, severe hypotension and bradycardia (i.e., Bezold-Jarisch reflex).[32]

Supraclavicular blocks are indicated for operations on the elbow, forearm, and hand (Fig. 33.4). Pneumothorax is a potential complication of this block, and onset of symptoms is usually delayed for up to 24 hours. Other complications include frequent phrenic nerve block (40% to 60%), Horner syndrome, and neuropathy.[31] Horner syndrome, caused by paralysis of the cervical sympathetic nerve trunk, is characterized by contraction of the pupil, partial ptosis of the eyelid, enophthalmos, and sometimes loss of sweating on the ipsilateral side of the block.[69] The phrenic block, or cervical sympathetic block, is self-limited. The patient needs reassurance that the effects are temporary and will resolve in time.

The infraclavicular block provides anesthesia to the arm and hand. The approach to the plexus is blind, thus increasing the risk of intravascular injection.[32] Other complications include pneumothorax, infection, and hematoma.[32]

Forearm, hand, and elbow surgery may be performed with an axillary block (Fig. 33.5).[32] This technique may be used for vascular access procedures. Significant complications include nerve injury and systemic toxicity from intravascular injection. Hematoma and infection are rare complications. Unlike the risk with the other brachial plexus approaches, central neural blockade and pneumothorax are not complications of the axillary approach.[32]

Intercostal Nerve Block and Interpleural Catheter Placement

Patients with contraindications to neuraxial blockade may have intercostal nerve blocks or interpleural catheters placed (Figs. 33.6 and 33.7). When combined with celiac plexus blocks and light general anesthesia, they may also be used for intraabdominal procedures.[32] Pneumothorax is the most common complication of the intercostal nerve block.[32]

Celiac Plexus Block

The celiac plexus block can be combined with intercostal block to provide anesthesia for intraabdominal surgery (Fig. 33.8).[32] Reduction of stress and endocrine responses to operative procedures is possible with this block because of autonomic nervous system blockade. Complications that may occur include hypotension; spinal, epidural, or intravascular injection; pneumothorax; puncture of the kidney, ureter, or intestine; and retroperitoneal hematoma.[32] The paravertebral block may be used to provide anesthesia and analgesia for thoracic, abdominal, pelvic, and upper leg surgery (Fig. 33.9). Local anesthetic injection in the epidural or subarachnoid space is possible because of

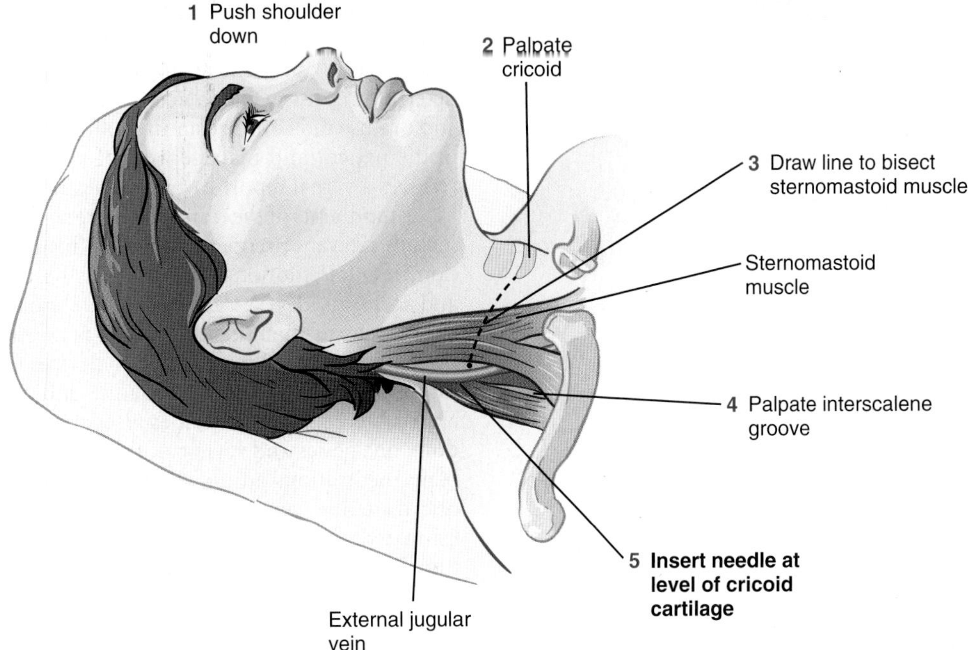

FIG. 33.3 Interscalene approach to brachial plexus block.

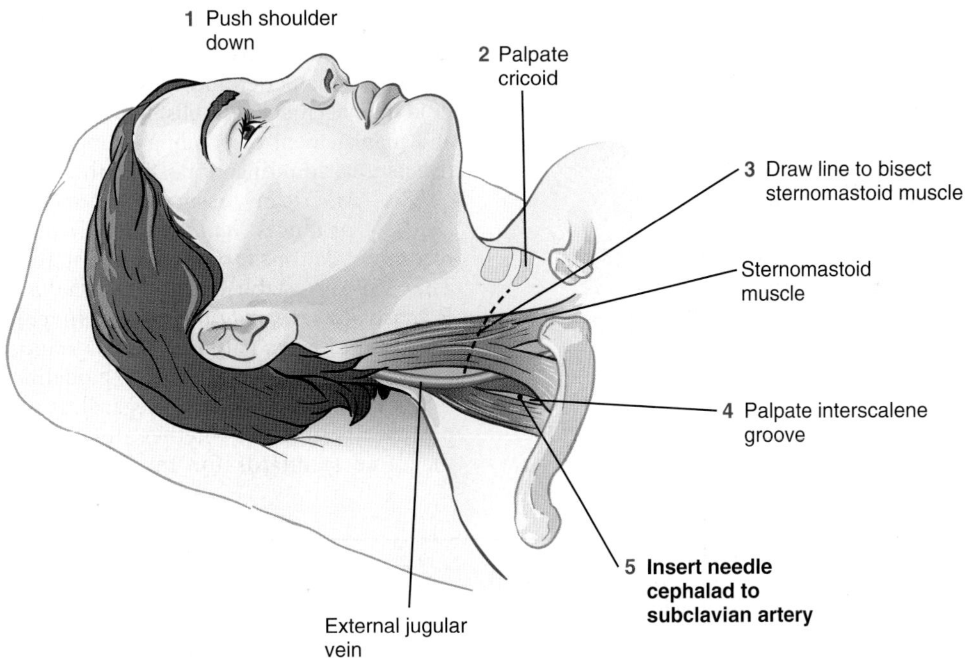

FIG. 33.4 Supraclavicular approach to brachial plexus block.

the proximity of the central neuraxis during placement.[32] There is a risk of intravascular injection through the lumbar vessels, vena cava, or aorta. Although this block has multiple uses and advantages over thoracic epidural anesthesia and is less difficult to place, it is not widely used at this time.[22]

Lumbar Plexus

Three main terminal nerves (femoral, lateral femoral cutaneous, and obturator) can be reliably anesthetized for knee and hip procedures with a block of the lumbar plexus (Fig. 33.10). Prolonged postoperative analgesia can be achieved using continuous catheter techniques.[22] Single-injection blocks may regress over 10 to 18 hours after the local anesthetic injection, reducing the benefits of blocks for postoperative pain management. Potential risks include epidural, subarachnoid, or intravascular injection and peripheral nerve damage.[32]

PATIENT TRANSFER TO THE PERIANESTHESIA CARE UNIT OR CRITICAL CARE UNIT FROM THE OPERATING ROOM

Upon arrival to the receiving unit, PACU or critical care, the nurse assesses the patient, focusing on airway, breathing (i.e., ventilation and oxygenation), and circulation (i.e., heart rate/

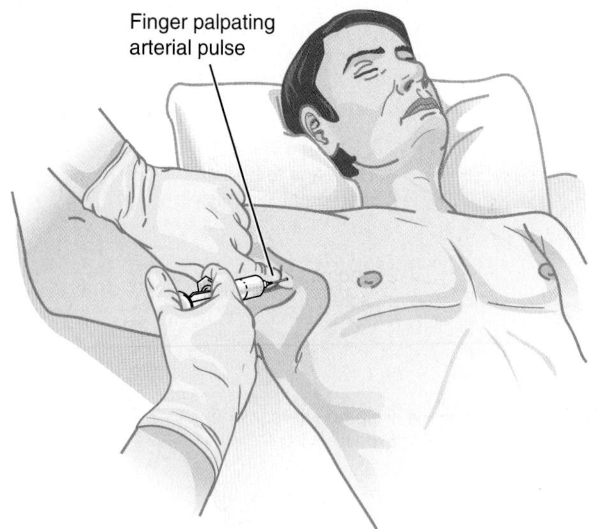

FIG. 33.5 Approach and needle insertion position for axillary block.

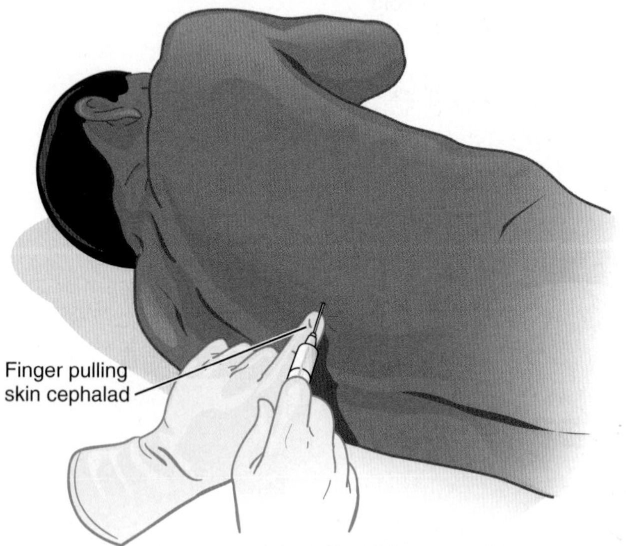

FIG. 33.6 Approach and needle insertion position for intercostal nerve block.

rhythm, blood pressure [BP]) including temperature assessment. After the initial evaluation of these parameters, the nurse completes a quick "head-to-toe" assessment of the patient, determining intravenous access; condition of skin, dressings, and drains; and comfort status. Following the initial assessment of the patient and management of any acute issues, the nurse receives a verbal report from the anesthesia care provider.

Components of the transfer of care summary from anesthesia include relevant preoperative status (history, physical examination, mental/emotional status); anesthesia/sedation technique and agents used; reversal agents given; procedure(s) performed; airway management including airway assessment (i.e., status of upper airway, need for adjunctive devices for intubation), tube location (depth at lips/teeth/nares) and time of extubation if applicable; length of anesthesia/sedation and operative procedure; analgesics and review of postoperative pain management plan; medications administered including time of next antibiotic dose and venous thromboembolism (VTE) prophylaxis; estimated fluid/blood loss and replacement; and complications during anesthesia and operative course, treatment, and response (Table 33.5).[5]

Following report, the nurse indicates verbal acceptance of transfer of care and responsibility for the patient from the anesthesia care provider. If questions remain related to the patient's safety or physical status, the nurse should not accept the transfer until the questions are answered and the nurse can safely assume care of the patient. The plan of care for the immediate postanesthesia period includes pain and comfort management, fluid management, establishment of hemodynamic stability, and management of potential complications (e.g., postoperative nausea, vomiting, or postanesthetic shivering).

The American Association of Critical-Care Nurses (AACN) produces *Standards for Critical Care Nursing* with recommendations for monitoring, staffing, and patient care.[4] The ASPAN establishes *Perianesthesia Nursing Standards, Practice Recommendations and Interpretive Statements* for all postanesthesia patients.[5] These standards include assessment, monitoring, and staffing guidelines for this postanesthesia patient population. Regardless of the location of the postanesthesia care, whether in critical care or the PACU, the same standards for recovery and stabilization apply.

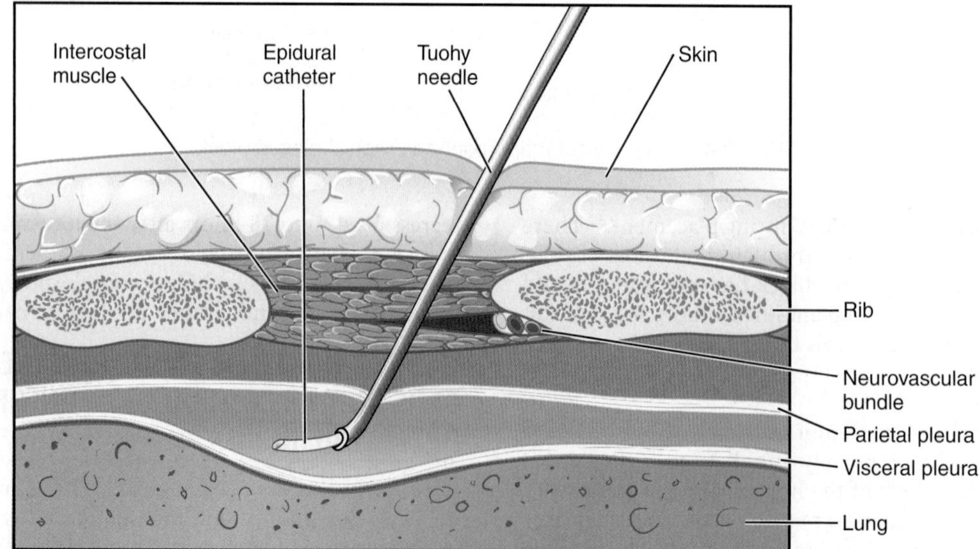

FIG. 33.7 Placement of epidural catheter for interpleural block.

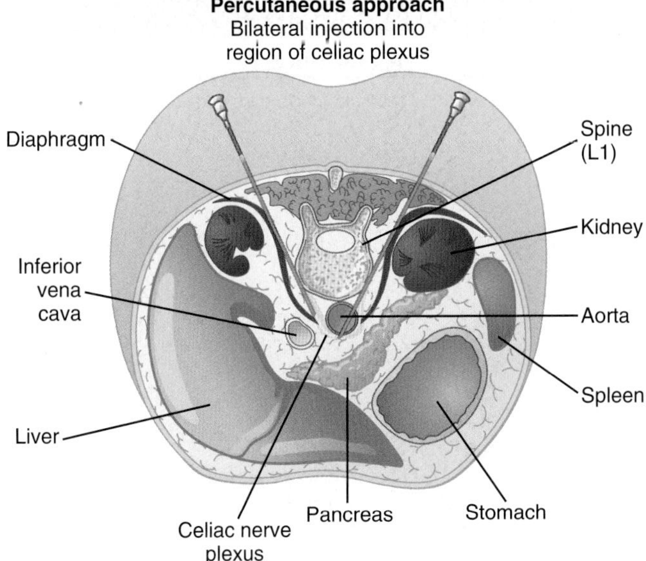

FIG. 33.8 Celiac plexus block.

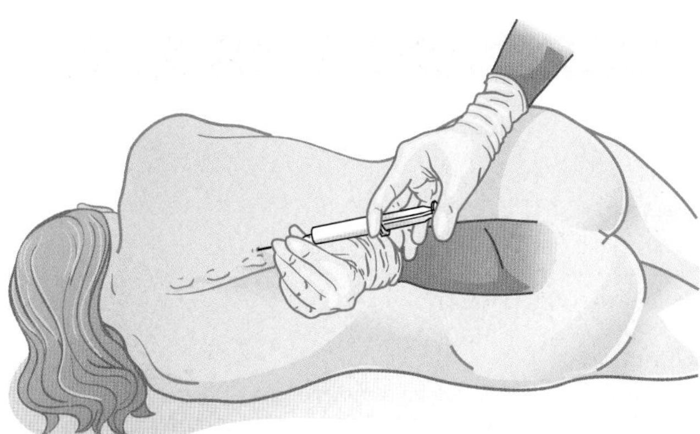

FIG. 33.9 Approach and needle insertion position for thoracic paravertebral block.

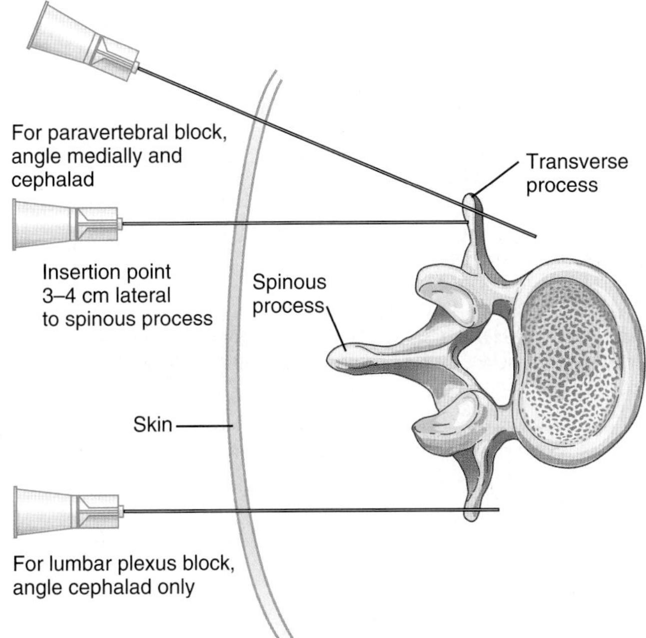

FIG. 33.10 Needle insertion points for lumbar plexus blocks.

Full details can be found in the AACN/ASPAN/ASA Joint Statement on ICU Overflow.[1]

Although one normally thinks of operative complications occurring in the OR, they often occur wherever the patient is during the postoperative period. For example, decreased stimulation, delayed drug absorption, or slow drug elimination may contribute to residual sedation or cardiopulmonary depression. Currently, there are insufficient data to examine the effects of postprocedural monitoring on patient outcomes in the postoperative period. However, it is widely accepted that continuous observation and monitoring of the patient during this critical period can decrease the likelihood of adverse events. Therefore patients should be observed in an appropriately staffed and equipped area (i.e., PACU or critical care) until they are near their baseline level of consciousness and are no longer at risk for cardiopulmonary compromise. See Table 33.6 for an example of the elements included in postanesthesia Phase 1 discharge criteria based on the American Society of PeriAnesthesia Nurses Practice Recommendation 1.[5]

Initial postanesthesia care should be managed in terms of the ABCs: airway (patency), breathing (respiratory status, breath sounds, oxygen therapy, and oxygen saturation), and circulation (BP, pulse, cardiac rhythm, fluid and electrolyte balance, including urine output, temperature, and hemodynamic readings from central venous catheters and pulmonary artery catheters [PACs]). After the ABCs are stabilized, ongoing assessment and management should include, but not be limited to, monitoring neurologic status, including level of consciousness, mentation, and sensorimotor functioning; thermoregulation, promoting normothermia; pain management; emotional comfort; promoting skin integrity and mobility, as well as procedural/surgical specific care.[64] Institutional practice standards and specific provider orders define monitoring parameters to guide the nurse caring for the postanesthesia patient.

Respiratory Care and Complications

Respiratory complications are perhaps the most common and dangerous in the immediate postoperative patient. PACU and critical care staff should anticipate and closely monitor the development of respiratory compromise. The signs and symptoms of respiratory compromise include altered level of consciousness, agitation, tachypnea, dyspnea, increased work of breathing, shallow respirations, and decreased oxygen saturation.

Respiratory complications can be divided into upper airway dysfunction and alterations in lower airway function or breathing.[43,60] Upper airway dysfunction can be subtle in the postoperative patient. Initially, there may only be some dyspnea that can be easily overlooked. However, even though the work of breathing has increased, observant staff will notice a decrease in breath sounds and air movement. This is followed by a decrease in oxygen saturation. The most common cause of upper airway obstruction is a loss of muscle tone, often with the tongue falling posteriorly. This can be treated with a jaw thrust that pulls the tongue anteriorly (Fig. 33.11) or with placement of an oral airway. Occasionally the loss of muscle tone can result from oversedation. In this instance, it can be effectively treated with pharmacologic reversal agents. Laryngospasm, either partial or complete closure of the vocal cords with wheezing, stridor (partial), or absence of ventilation (complete), is another cause of upper airway obstruction that generally requires intubation. Lastly, upper airway obstruction can occur as the result of external trauma or by airway damage, or edema as the result of the

TABLE 33.5 Transfer of Care Summary

Preoperative	Operative	Postoperative
History: including chronic medical conditions	Procedure performed and complications	Procedure performed and complications
Allergies	Allergies Pertinent history and medications	Level of consciousness
Physical exam (focus on cardiovascular, respiratory, endocrine, skin assessment)	Airway management (e.g., ease of intubation or difficult airway management) Hemodynamic status	Vital signs
Mental/emotional status	Anesthetics given Length of anesthesia	Airway and ventilation status
Medications: pertinent (status of medications: taken, held)	Reversal agents used	IV access points, fluid rates, blood products, intake/output
Fasting status	Other medications given (including antiemetics, anxiolytics/sedatives, analgesics)	Analgesics given
Pain assessment and management plan	Estimated blood loss, urinary output, other losses/output Fluids and blood products given Pain management plan	Pain management plan Other medications given Medications/allergies

TABLE 33.6 Example of Postanesthesia Phase 1 Discharge Criteria

Example of Elements Included in Phase 1 Discharge Criteria
Basic Systemic Criteria
(Tolerance of criteria outside of these is at the discretion of the anesthesia faculty)

Respiratory

- Oxygen saturation ≥ 92% or preoperative baseline

Temperature

- 36–38 degrees Celsius (core temperature)

Cardiovascular

- Intravenous access patent/without redness (signs/symptoms of infiltration)
- Heart rate (HR) and rhythm regular without arrhythmia or with preoperative baseline
- Blood pressure (BP) within 20% of baseline

Neurologic

- Pupils equal, round, reactive, to light accommodation (PERRLA)
- Speech clear
- No facial asymmetry (droop)
- Opens eyes spontaneously
- Conversant
- Follows verbal commands
- Movement of extremities (MOE)/strength/sensation function normal or at preoperative baseline
- Exception: patient will return to baseline neurologic function if there are preexisting deficits

Surgical Site

- Drains patent/intact
- Dressings: minimal drainage
- Suture line(s) intact (if visible)

Rest/Comfort

- Pain score "4" or less (or return to baseline) and acceptable to patient
- Postoperative Nausea/Vomiting (PONV): tolerable level, minimal side effects associated with treatment of PONV

Considerations for Blocks/Monitored Anesthesia Care

Spinal Anesthesia

- Sensory dermatome level of T-12 or below
- Absence of orthostatic hypotension (with head of bed elevated)

Epidural

- If used only for intra-operative anesthetic technique (assess for dense epidural block) see Spinal Anesthesia above
- Epidural catheter can only be removed by an anesthesia provider

MAC

- Must be observed and have 2 sets of vital signs (BP, HR, RR, Spo_2) recorded before discharge eligible

IV Regional/Peripheral Nerve Blocks

- Must be observed and have vital signs recorded every 15 minutes × 2 Observe for signs and symptoms of systemic infiltration/toxicity of local anesthesia

NOTE: Discharge criteria will be developed with nursing and anesthesiology; discharge criteria are medically approved by anesthesiology and medical staff in each facility.
MAC, Monitored anesthesia care; *RR*, respiratory rate; Spo_2, blood oxygen saturation level.

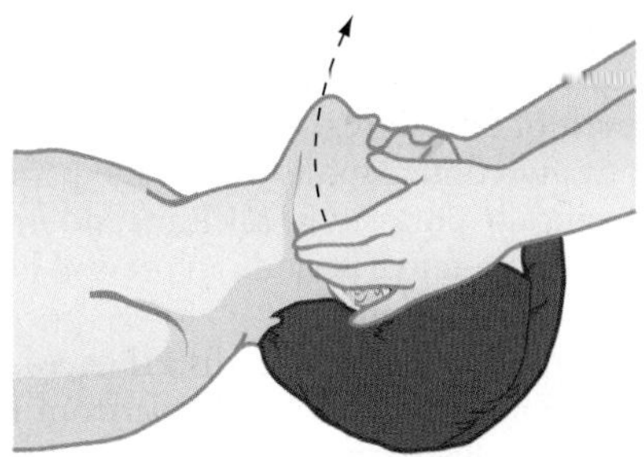

FIG. 33.11 Jaw-thrust airway maneuver.

operative procedure itself. In this situation, intubation or tracheostomy may be necessary.

Postoperative patients are also at risk for developing alterations in breathing or lower respiratory tract dysfunction. This most commonly results from atelectasis. Effects of pain (especially from chest or abdominal incisions) and sedation can increase the incidence of atelectasis. Diminished breath sounds, rales, or crackles can often be auscultated in dependent portions of the lungs of patients with atelectasis. Atelectasis can be treated with adequate pain control to encourage coughing and deep breathing and use of incentive spirometry.[71] Although limited evidence supports the use of incentive spirometry, it remains an intervention commonly prescribed for postoperative patients.[12] Pneumothorax can develop, compressing the lung, and may be a complication of chest or neck surgery or central line placement. Occasionally patients with preexisting significant COPD can rupture a bleb (a small subpleural thin walled air containing space 1–2 cm in diameter) while being ventilated, causing a pneumothorax. With a pneumothorax, reduced breath sounds will be auscultated on the affected side. Accumulation of more air in the pleural space may lead to further collapse of the affected lung and displacement of the trachea and mediastinal structures to the opposite side. In general, a pneumothorax of less than 20% is asymptomatic and will not require chest tube placement. In patients who are symptomatic, a chest tube may be needed.

Pulmonary edema may cause lower respiratory tract dysfunction in postoperative patients. Operative patients often accumulate interstitial fluid, requiring additional fluids throughout the procedure to maintain preload and CO. These additional fluids may lead to hypervolemia; occasionally this fluid accumulates in the lungs, resulting in pulmonary edema. The stress of surgery can also lead to cardiac dysfunction, further exacerbating pulmonary edema. Treatment of pulmonary edema involves fluid restriction or diuretics. An additional sign of fluid overload may be a falling hematocrit (Hct) as the excess intravascular fluid dilutes the red blood cells. However, extreme caution should be used in assuming that a falling Hct is a sign of fluid overload. It may be a sign of blood loss and the need for additional fluids.

Cardiovascular Care and Complications

Postoperative patients frequently develop cardiovascular complications. The primary manifestation of cardiovascular dysfunction is poor perfusion. Signs and symptoms of this include tachycardia, hypotension, and poor peripheral perfusion as demonstrated by cool, pale extremities and poor capillary refill (>3 seconds). However, poor peripheral perfusion can be misleading in patients with preexisting peripheral vascular disease.

Diminished CO could be due either to primary cardiac dysfunction or to insufficient preload causing secondary cardiac dysfunction. Differentiation between these two states can best be made by examining the central venous pressure (CVP), the pulmonary artery occlusion pressure (PAOP) also known as pulmonary artery wedge pressure (PAWP), or esophageal Doppler monitoring (EDM).[8,30] In cardiac disease, these pressures are often elevated, whereas if insufficient preload is the problem, CVP, PAOP, and flow times will be low. Insufficient preload is common in the postoperative patient.

Insufficient preload in the postoperative patient can result from bleeding at the operative site, occult bleeding in the gastrointestinal tract (e.g., stress gastritis or peptic ulcer disease), or bleeding from other organs. If bleeding is suspected, the Hct should be checked and vital signs monitored closely. Large amounts of blood can escape the vascular space without obvious outward signs. The abdominal cavity, pleural space, or thighs may sequester large blood volumes following injury or operative procedures with inadequate hemostasis. When bleeding is present, red blood cells should be replaced, along with attempts made to correct low platelet counts and abnormal blood coagulation as measured by the prothrombin time (PT) and partial thromboplastin time (PTT), if necessary. A more common cause of insufficient cardiac preload is the movement of fluid into the interstitial space due to a systemic inflammatory response that often occurs during surgery. Frequently, patients just out of the OR will continue to require large amounts of crystalloid solution to maintain their CVP and CO. Lastly, some surgeries include treatment of infectious sites, such as abscesses. This can lead to endotoxemia, sepsis, and interstitial fluid movement in the immediate postoperative period. Additional fluids may be required.

Cardiac causes of poor CO are also quite common in the postoperative patient. The stress of a major surgery, stimulating a neuroendocrine response, especially in patients with preexisting coronary artery disease, may lead to myocardial infarction (MI). Unlike a nonoperative patient, postoperative patients are often sedated or given analgesics. Therefore patients may not complain of chest pain even in the presence of a significant MI. As the result of the interstitial fluid shifts, another cause of cardiac dysfunction is pulmonary edema.

Stressful stimuli (e.g., surgical incisions, organ manipulation) can elicit an adrenergic response precipitating transient increases in heart rate and BP.[58] This stress of surgery can lead to cardiac dysfunction and exacerbate pulmonary edema. Patients with histories of coronary artery disease are frequently taking beta-blocker medications. According to Zaugg et al., the neuroendocrine response is not enhanced by the use of beta blockade.[73] However, advantages can be obtained from use of beta blockers, including decreased analgesic requirements, faster recovery from anesthesia, and improved hemodynamic stability.[72,73]

Hypertension in postoperative patients is usually the result of a preexisting condition, aggravated by withholding the patient's medications before or during surgery.[28,49] Although postoperative patients often require large amounts of crystalloid, too much fluid may also lead to hypertension, especially in patients with a history of renal disease or after operations that involve the urinary tract. Hypertension can also be an early sign of pain or fluid overload.

Postoperative patients are often immobilized for prolonged periods of time both in the OR and in critical care, leading to deep vein thrombosis (DVT). There are several therapeutic maneuvers to prevent this often life-threatening complication, starting with evaluating a patient's risk and then providing low molecular weight heparin (LMWH) and/or mechanical prophylaxis based on their risk.[27] Previously, restrictive stockings were thought to be sufficient to prevent DVTs. However, intermittent pneumatic compression (IPC) devices and foot-pump devices have been found more effective.[35] IPC devices encircle the lower extremities and are sequentially inflated and deflated to compress the legs and move venous blood to the heart. Although IPC devices are somewhat effective for the legs, DVTs can form in other large veins. Thus anticoagulation with subcutaneous heparin, including LMWH, is more effective. Warfarin (Coumadin) can take several days to fully anticoagulate a patient and is not used in the immediate postoperative period. Although anticoagulation is often the preferred method of DVT prophylaxis for hospitalized patients, great care should be used because of the risk of bleeding at the operative site. Thus many postoperative patients receive IPC devices.

Central Nervous System Care and Complications

Unless patients are intentionally sedated postoperatively, emergence from anesthesia should occur rapidly and predictably. The Glasgow Coma Scale is commonly used to quickly and consistently monitor neurologic status. Return to baseline neurologic status is expected in the immediate postanesthesia period. Level of consciousness, response to commands, pupillary response and purposeful extremity movement are assessed and documented. Orientation to person, place, and time begins as the patient awakens. Facial symmetry, speech and muscle strength (hand grasps, ability to raise head, and plantar extension) are evaluated to identify possible stroke.[44] Any deviation from baseline status is noted and reported in the event the patient requires further evaluation of the neurologic changes.

Infrequently, either patients will awaken abruptly, agitated and unresponsive to commands, or emergence will be delayed. Emergence delirium or excitement is characterized by restlessness, disorientation, crying, moaning, and inappropriate behavior.[50] Oxygenation and ventilation status is assessed to rule out hypoxemia or pain as a cause of the excitement. Other causes include preexisting agitation or anxiety, medications, incomplete reversal of neuromuscular blocking agents, withdrawal from alcohol or drugs, full bladder or bowel, acid-base disturbances, and electrolyte abnormalities. Allowing the agitated patient to return to a full consciousness before analgesic administration may result in unnecessary pain. However, premature analgesic or sedative administration may delay the treatment of other causes of agitation.

Delayed emergence from anesthesia may be due to prolonged drug effects, metabolic problems, or neurologic injury.[50] Drug effects may include overdosage, inadequate reversal, or altered metabolism or elimination of drugs. Electrolyte imbalances may result in decreased awareness or an altered level of consciousness. Neurologic injury may be the result of tissue damage or an anoxic event. The response is that the patient fails to respond as expected during emergence from anesthesia. Maintenance of adequate ventilation, oxygen saturation, and CO is essential while potential causes are evaluated. A thorough review of the anesthesia course is initiated, metabolic disturbances are corrected, and, if no other cause is identified, a complete neurologic examination is performed.

Electrolytes

Assessment of the serum electrolyte values and potential interventions are a vital component in caring for a critically ill patient in the postoperative period. Electrolyte concentrations influence metabolic activities as well as fluid movement within and between body compartments. Abnormal electrolyte values may be the result of fluid shifts, acid-base imbalances, or renal or endocrine dysfunction. Monitoring of the patient's electrolyte status, specifically potassium, calcium, and magnesium, in the immediate postoperative period can prevent hemodynamic instability and cardiac dysfunction.

The most common electrolyte disturbances seen in the postoperative period include hypokalemia from fluid resuscitation or nasogastric losses; hyperkalemia from tissue catabolism or acidosis; hypocalcemia from alkalosis, administration of citrated blood, or hemodilution; and hypomagnesemia from gastrointestinal or urinary losses. Hypomagnesemia has been associated with a higher mortality and worse clinical outcomes in the critical care setting.[67]

Nutrition

Nutrition is important for the rapid and complete recovery of the postoperative patient. Good nutrition improves wound healing, decreases the time patients require mechanical ventilation, results in fewer infectious complications, and reduces length of stay.[45] A nutritional assessment should be made soon after the patient is admitted to critical care.

The first consideration is to determine if the patient is already malnourished. Many critically ill postoperative patients have had prolonged illnesses before surgery that can result in malnutrition. The nutritional assessment should include pertinent historical data such as weight loss or decreased caloric intake. On physical exam, malnourished patients may have a decrease in weight and a loss of subcutaneous fat in the triceps or buttocks. If a patient is malnourished, nutritional management should be considered as soon as the patient is stabilized.[45] Current recommendations suggest starting gastric feeding, while also providing micronutrients, once the patient has stabilized to allow macronutrient intake during the first week of critical illness.[16] The gastrointestinal tract is the preferred choice because it has far fewer complications (e.g., infection) than intravenous or parenteral nutrition. Most critically ill patients cannot take sufficient calories orally, and a feeding tube must be used.[16] Tube feedings are usually begun continuously at small volumes and then increased as tolerated by the patient. It should be remembered that even very small amounts of tube feedings (5 to 10 mL/h) have beneficial effects on the gut.[45] Patients usually cannot tolerate the large glucose loads initially, because they may precipitate hyperglycemia. Hyperglycemia is associated with increased mortality and morbidity in critically ill patients. Surgical patients develop hyperglycemia related to the hypermetabolic stress response, which increases glucose production and causes insulin resistance. Hyperglycemia is associated with worse outcomes, but the treatment of hyperglycemia with insulin infusions has not provided consistent benefits. Early results suggested decreased mortality but later investigations found no benefit or increased mortality when hyperglycemia was aggressively treated with insulin. The optimal blood glucose range to target in hospitalized patients remains uncertain, but a recent systematic review from the American College of Physicians (ACP) suggests targeting blood glucose levels between 80–180 mg/dL.[57] In the immediate postoperative period, blood sugar levels should be checked routinely on admission and at 1 to 2 hour intervals. If the nurse obtains two blood sugars greater than 180 mg/dL or one blood sugar greater than 200 mg/dL, an insulin drip should be started.[57]

Thermoregulation

Thermoregulation during the perioperative period ranges from the hypothermic to the hyperthermic state. Normothermia is defined as a core temperature between 36°C and 38°C. Temperature is assessed when the patient arrives in the PACU or critical care unit and periodically throughout the patient's recovery and postoperative care.

Hypothermia is defined as a core temperature below 36°C. Patients who are hypothermic should have temperatures assessed every 30 minutes until normothermia is achieved.[31] Hypothermia normally results in an increased catecholamine level, causing tachycardia, peripheral vasoconstriction, and hypertension. However, anesthetic agents blunt the peripheral vasoconstriction, resulting in little change in BP in the postoperative patient. Hypothermia can produce patient discomfort, untoward cardiac events, adrenergic stimulation, impaired platelet function, altered drug metabolism, and impaired wound healing with increased risk of infection.[31] Active warming measures include application of a forced-air warming system, passive insulation (with warm blankets, socks, head coverings, circulating water mattress/pads), increased room temperature, warmed intravenous solutions, and humidified and warmed supplemental oxygen.[31]

Hyperthermia, at the other end of the temperature spectrum, is rare in the postanesthesia population. Core temperatures above 38°C may be due to sepsis, preexisting infectious processes, drug fever, trauma, blood transfusions, or, rarely, malignant hyperthermia. Hyperthermic patients may also have tachycardia with increased CO, increased respiratory rates, and peripheral vasodilation with a widening of the pulse pressure; all are designed to remove heat from the body. Five syndromes of drug-induced hyperthermia have been described. The syndromes include malignant hyperthermia (MH), neuroleptic malignant syndrome, anticholinergic poisoning, sympathomimetic poisoning, and serotonin syndrome.[29,52] Treatment includes medications (antiinfectives, antipyretics) and cooling measures (cool cloths, cooling blankets).

MH, known as the disease of anesthesia, is a rare, life-threatening pharmacogenetic disorder triggered by volatile anesthetic agents (halothane, isoflurane, sevoflurane, desflurane) and succinylcholine in genetically susceptible patients. It is a state of hypermetabolism and skeletal muscle rigidity. The incidence ranges from 1:10,000 to 1:50,000 patients.[42,61] It occurs more frequently in children, but has been reported in older adults. Development of MH during the perioperative period frequently led to death (over 70%) before the introduction of dantrolene (Dantrium) in 1975.[61] When triggering agents are given to susceptible individuals, the initial response may be doubling or tripling of the end-tidal carbon dioxide concentration and unexplained tachycardia (Box 33.1). This can occur within 30 minutes of induction of anesthesia or up to 24 hours after the triggering agent is administered. Temperature elevation is a late indicator and is sometimes absent. Prompt recognition and treatment with dantrolene can reduce morbidity and mortality to less than 5% to 10%.[42,61]

Treatment begins with recognition. Once recognized, triggering agents are stopped, 100% oxygen is administered, and dantrolene is administered. Additional treatment includes monitoring of cardiac rhythm, urine output, and temperature (Box 33.2). Every anesthetizing location needs to be prepared for the potential development of MH. An MH kit or cart stocked with recommended supplies and resource materials (posters, pocket cards, reference guides) should be readily available to the nursing and medical staff. The Malignant Hyperthermia Association of the United States (MHAUS) offers telephone support (1-800-MHHYPER) 24 hours daily to assist providers managing an MH crisis.

BOX 33.1 Signs of Malignant Hyperthermia

Early
- Doubling or tripling of end-tidal CO_2
- Hypoxemia
- Metabolic acidosis
- Muscle rigidity
- Masseter spasm
- Skin flushing
- Tachycardia
- Tachypnea
- Ventricular dysrhythmias

Late*
- Elevated creatinine phosphokinase
- Hyperkalemia
- Hyperthermia†
- Mixed metabolic and respiratory acidosis
- Hypotension
- Rhabdomyolysis
- Myoglobinuria
- Skin mottling
- Sweating

*These signs may not be present with early recognition and treatment.
†Correlates with severity of malignant hyperthermia.
Data from References 42 and 61.

BOX 33.2 Treatment of a Malignant Hyperthermia Crisis

- Call for help.
- Stop triggering agents.
- Evaluate need for invasive monitoring, mechanical ventilation.
- Hyperventilate with 100% oxygen (increase minute ventilation to decrease end-tidal carbon dioxide concentration).
- Prepare and administer dantrolene (2.5 mg/kg initial dose, up to 10 mg/kg recommended but may be exceeded).
- Monitor temperature continuously.
- Begin cooling measures for hyperthermia: iced solutions; ice packs to axilla/groin, neck; iced nasogastric lavage; cool water mist and fans. Stop cooling at 38.5°C.
- Treat dysrhythmias: do not use calcium channel blockers; may use lidocaine.
- Obtain blood gases, electrolytes, creatine kinase (CK) level, coagulation studies, blood and urine for myoglobin level.
- Treat hyperkalemia with bicarbonate, IV glucose, and insulin.
- Maintain urine output at 1 mL/kg/h with mannitol, furosemide, fluids.
- Observe in intensive care unit for 24 hours minimum.
- Postacute episode: continue dantrolene at 1 mg/kg IV every 4–6 hours for 24 hours.
- Report episode to MHAUS.
- Counsel patient and family; refer patient and family to Malignant Hyperthermia Association of the United States.

MHAUS, Malignant Hyperthermia Association of the United States.
Data from References 40, 42, 52, and 61.

Postanesthesia Shivering

Postanesthesia patients frequently experience shivering.[3] Shivering is more common in young adults, with longer anesthesia or surgery times, and if no active perioperative rewarming was used.[3] There is no definitive explanation for why postanesthesia shivering occurs. Most common causes are thought to include perioperative hypothermia and postoperative pain, although hypotheses suggest perioperative heat loss, the direct effect of certain anesthetics, hypercapnia or respiratory alkalosis, pyrogens, hypoxia, early recovery of spinal reflex activity, and sympathetic overactivity may contribute. Consequences of shivering include discomfort, increased pain at the operative site because of muscle contractions, increased intraocular pressure after ophthalmologic surgery, and an increase in oxygen consumption by 200% to 500%.[3,7,10] Hypothermia may cause vasoconstriction, with increased vascular resistance further compromising myocardial function in the patient with preexisting decreased myocardial oxygen supply secondary to arteriosclerosis.[37]

Postanesthetic shivering caused by perioperative hypothermia may be prevented by skin surface rewarming before induction, raising the temperature in the OR, or using rewarming intravenous solutions and active warming during the surgical procedure. Shivering may also exist in the absence of hypothermia (cutaneous vasodilation or nonthermoregulatory shivering); its cause is not known. Treatment may include low doses of meperidine (Demerol).[7]

Acute Postoperative Pain and Comfort Management

Evidence exists that postoperative pain remains suboptimally treated.[9] Pain may cause changes in immune system function, decreased healing, catabolic hypermetabolism resulting in hyperglycemia and breakdown of muscle, diminished ability to function, needless suffering, and chronic pain. Acute postoperative pain needs to be assessed and reassessed frequently and managed aggressively. Treatment of pain, in the critically ill patient, can include opioids (morphine, fentanyl, hydromorphone, remifentanil and methadone), pain modulating medications such as local and regional anesthetics delivered through continuous catheter techniques (epidural, other peripheral nerve blocks), such as bupivacaine, nonsteroidal antiinflammatories (ibuprofen, ketorolac). Intravenous (IV) acetaminophen and anticonvulsants have been used as adjunctive to help reduce opioid doses. If there is adequate gastrointestinal absorption, neuropathic pain can be treated with enteral gabapentin and carbamazepine.

There are also a variety of nonpharmacologic, complementary pain management strategies that should be considered, such as diversional, music, and massage therapy.[33]

Pain and comfort guidelines have been published for the assessment and management of acute postoperative pain.[9,54] The reader is directed to the Society of Critical Care Medicine (SCCM), *Clinical Practice Guidelines for the Management of Pain, Agitation and Delirium in Adult Patients in the Intensive Care Unit*, and the *Practice Guidelines for Acute Pain Management in the Perioperative Setting: An Updated Report by the American Society of Anesthesiologists Task Force on Acute Pain Management* for an in-depth discussion of pain assessment and management in the critical care setting.

Postoperative Nausea and Vomiting

Nausea and vomiting occur in 25% to 30% of postoperative patients; an incidence that has remained unchanged over the past 40 years.[25] Risk factors for postoperative nausea and vomiting (PONV) are female gender, nonsmoker, history of motion sickness, history of previous PONV, and an operative procedure longer than 180 minutes. Certain anesthetic agents (nitrous oxide) and commonly used drugs (opioids, anticholinesterases) are known to increase the risk of PONV, while other agents (propofol) may help minimize the incidence. Adequate hydration, pain management, antiemetic prophylaxis, and avoidance of triggering agents and other stimuli may minimize PONV.[25]

Treatment includes medications that are antagonists of serotonin (e.g., ondansetron), dopamine (e.g., haloperidol), and histamine (e.g., diphenhydramine). Nonpharmacologic treatment may also be recommended (e.g., ginger gum, acupressure [P-6] bands). Studies have shown that the effectiveness of these nonpharmacologic therapies varies, and further research is necessary.[25]

Skin Integrity and Mobility

Preoperative skin assessment and evaluation of preoperative risk factors are important first steps in preventing postoperative pressure ulcer development. Attention must be paid to all patients undergoing operative procedures and especially those patients with known risk factors. These include advanced age, hypotension, diabetes, renal insufficiency, low BMI, sepsis, vascular disease, prolonged operative times (> 180 minutes) and use of vasopressors and steroids.[2,17,18]

Upon arrival in the PACU or critical care unit, skin is assessed, focusing on pressure points associated with the patient's position during the procedure. Any areas of concern are noted and monitored on a continuing basis. Early initiation of mobility activities, including repositioning, head of bed elevation, active or passive range of motion, and use of pressure reduction surfaces, promotes skin integrity and enhances patient comfort and recovery.[18]

CONCLUSION

The immediate postoperative period is challenging for the patient and the nurse. The patient is vulnerable to pain and discomfort, hemodynamic alterations, respiratory compromise, and other complications. Nurses must remain vigilant and aware of the risks associated with anesthesia and surgical intervention. Critical and comprehensive monitoring along with an understanding of anesthesia agents and adjuncts, postoperative care, and complications will provide a sound basis for caring for patients in the immediate postoperative period.

CASE STUDY 33.1

Assessing Risk Factors of a Patient

M.F. is a 68-year-old female, ASA physical status classification 3, recently diagnosed with colon cancer and subsequent bowel obstruction after a 3-month history of abdominal pain and passage of pencil shaped stools and unintentional 20-pound weight loss. Her medical history is significant for hypertension, 75 pack/year smoking history, obesity, gastroesophageal reflex, and anxiety disorder. She is married with one child and works as a secretary. Medications include simvastatin 20 mg daily, enalapril 10 mg daily, Atrovent two puffs twice a day, omeprazole 20 mg daily, and vitamin C 500 mg daily. No previous hospitalizations or surgery. One hour before the surgical procedure M.F received metronidazole 500 mg and gentamycin 80 mg. General anesthesia was planned and she was induced with propofol, intubated, and anesthesia maintained using isoflurane, nitrous oxide, morphine, and neuromuscular blockade with rocuronium.

M.F had a left hemicolectomy with no ostomy, which took 6 and 1/2 hours. She was moved to the critical care unit due to an inability to extubate. On admission the patient was sedated, vital signs were blood pressure of 140/70 mm Hg, heart rate 110 BPM, respiratory rate 14. The ventilator parameters were a fraction of inspired oxygen (FiO_2) 100% on

CASE STUDY 33.1

a synchronized intermittent mandatory ventilation with a tidal volume of 500 mL. The pulse oximeter was reading 94%, temperature 36°C. She had an estimated blood loss of 500 mL and was replaced with 6 liters of crystalloid. Urine output during the case was 250 mL. She was not responsive to verbal cues, extremities were warm and well perfused, capillary refill was less than 2 seconds, color was pale pink, lungs were clear to auscultation, anteriorly, heart sounds S1, S2, and an S4. She had a nasogastic tube draining pale green fluid, a urine catheter draining pale yellow urine. Laboratory values reported by anesthesia were hemoglobin of 10 g/dL, white count 17.3, platelets 143,000, sodium of 138, potassium of 3.4, chloride 103, bicarbonate 22, blood urea nitrogen 23, and creatinine 1.4.

Decision Point:
What comorbid conditions influence her risk for anesthesia and surgery?

Decision Point:
What information does the receiving nurse need to obtain during report?

Decision Point:
What complications are likely to arise in the immediate postoperative period?

Decision Point:
How should pain and sedation be managed postoperatively?

Decision Point:
When can she start to receive mobility?

REFERENCES

1. AACN/ASPAN/ASDA Joint Statement on ICU Overflow. http://www.aspan.org/Portals/6/docs/ClinicalPractice/PositionStatement/Current/PS4_2015.pdf.
2. Alderden, J., Whitney, J. D., Taylor, S. M., & Zaratkiewicz, S. (2011). Risk profile characteristics associated with outcomes of hospital-acquired pressure ulcers: a retrospective review. *Crit Care Nurse, 31*(4), 30–43. http://dx.doi.org/ 31/4/30 [pii]10.4037/ccn2011806.
3. Alfonsi, P. (2001). Postanaesthetic shivering. *Drugs, 61*(15), 2193–2205. http://dx.doi.org/10.2165/00003495–200161150–00004.
4. American Association of Critical-Care Nurses. (2015). *AACN scope and standards for acute and critical care nursing practice.* Aliso Viejo, CA: American Association of Critical-Care Nurses.
5. American Society of PeriAnesthesia Nurses. (2015). *2015–2017 Perianesthesia nursing standards, practice recommendations and interpretive statements.* Cherry Hill, NJ: American Society of PeriAnesthesia Nurses.
6. Ang-Lee, M. K., Moss, J., & Yuan, C. (2001). Herbal medicines and perioperative care. *JAMA, 286*(2), 208–216. http://dx.doi.org/10.1001/jama.286.2.208.
7. Apfelbaum, J. L., Silverstein, J. H., Chung, F. F., Connis, R. T., Fillmore, R. B., Hunt, S. E., et al. (2013). Practice guidelines for postanesthetic care: an updated report by the American Society of Anesthesiologists Task Force on Postanesthetic Care. *Anesthesiology, 118*(2), 291–307. http://dx.doi.org/10.1097/ALN.0b013e31827773e9.
8. Barone, C. P., Pablo, C. S., & Barone, G. W. (2004). Postanesthetic care in the critical care unit. *Crit Care Nurse, 24*(1), 38–45.
9. Barr, J., Fraser, G. L., Puntillo, K., Ely, E. W., Gélinas, C., Dasta, J. F., et al. (2013). Clinical practice guidelines for the management of pain, agitation, and delirium in adult patients in the intensive care unit. *Crit Care Med, 41*(1), 263–306. http://dx.doi.org/10.1097/CCM.0b013e3182783b72.
10. Bay, J., Nunn, J. F., & Prys-Roberts, C. (1968). Factors influencing arterial PO_2 during recovery from anaesthesia. *Br J Anaesth, 40*(6), 398–407. http://dx.doi.org/10.1093/bja/40.6.398.
11. Berde, C. B., & Strichartz, G. R. (2015). Local anesthetics. In R. D. Miller (Ed.), *Miller's anesthesia* (8th ed.) (pp. 1028–1054). Philadelphia, PA: Elsevier/Saunders.
12. Branson, R. D. (2013). The scientific basis for postoperative respiratory care. *Respir Care, 58*(11), 1974–1984. http://dx.doi.org/10.4187/respcare.02832.
13. Brown, E. N., Solt, K., Purdon, P. L., & Johnson-Akeju, O. (2015). Monitoring brain state during general anesthesia and sedation. In R. D. Miller (Ed.), *Miller's anesthesia* (8th ed.) (pp. 1524–1540). Philadelphia, PA: Elsevier/Saunders.
14. Brull, R., MacFarlane, A. J. R., & Chan, V. W. S. (2015). Spinal, epidural, and caudal anesthesia. In R. D. Miller (Ed.), *Miller's anesthesia* (8th ed., vol. 1, pp. 1684–1720). Philadelphia, PA: Elsevier/Saunders.
15. Canet, J., & Gallart, L. (2014). Postoperative respiratory failure: pathogenesis, prediction, and prevention. *Curr Opin Crit Care, 20*(1), 56–62. http://dx.doi.org/10.1097/MCC.0000000000000045.
16. Casaer, M. P., & Van den Berghe, G. (2014). Nutrition in the acute phase of critical illness. *N Engl J Med, 370*(13), 1227–1236. http://dx.doi.org/10.1056/NEJMra1304623.
17. Cox, J. (2011). Predictors of pressure ulcers in adult critical care patients. *Am J Crit Care, 20*(5), 364–375. http://dx.doi.org/10.4037/ajcc2011934.
18. Dickinson, S., Tschannen, D., & Shever, L. L. (2013). Can the use of an early mobility program reduce the incidence of pressure ulcers in a surgical critical care unit? *Crit Care Nurs Q, 36*(1), 127–140. http://dx.doi.org/10.1097/CNQ.0b013e31827538a1.
19. Donnelly, A. J., et al. (2008). *Anesthesiology & critical care drug handbook* (8th ed.). Hudson, Ohio: Lexi-Comp.
20. Dorland, W. A. N. (2007). *Dorland's illustrated medical dictionary* (29th ed.). Philadelphia: Saunders.
21. Drain, C. B. (2012). Neuromuscular blocking agents. In J. L. Forren (Ed.), *Perianesthesia nursing: a critical care approach* (6th ed.) (pp. 291–310). Philadelphia: Elsevier/Saunders.
22. Evans, H., Steele, S. M., Nielsen, K. C., Tucker, M. S., & Klein, S. M. (2005). Peripheral nerve blocks and continuous catheter techniques. *Anesthesiol Clin North America, 23*(1), 141–162. http://dx.doi.org/10.1016/j.atc.2004.11.003.
23. Evans, C. H., Lee, J., & Ruhlman, M. K. (2015). Optimal glucose management in the perioperative period. *Surg Clin North Am, 95*(2), 337–354. http://dx.doi.org/10.1016/j.suc.2014.11.003.
24. Fisher, D. M. (1997). Muscle relaxants. In D. E. Longnecker, & F. L. Murphy (Eds.), *Dripps/Eckenhoff/VanDam introduction to anesthesia* (9th ed.). Philadelphia: Saunders.
25. Gan, T. J., Diemunsch, P., Habib, A. S., Kovac, A., Kranke, P., Meyer, T. A., et al. (2014). Consensus guidelines for the management of postoperative nausea and vomiting. *Anesth Analg, 118*(1), 85–113. http://dx.doi.org/10.1213/ane.0000000000000002.
26. Golembiewski, J. (2002). Safety concerns with meperidine. *J Perianesth Nurs, 17*(2), 123–125.
27. Gould, M. K., Garcia, D. A., Wren, S. M., Karanicolas, P. J., Arcelus, J. I., Heit, J. A., et al. (2012). Prevention of VTE in nonorthopedic surgical patients: Antithrombotic therapy and prevention of thrombosis, 9th ed: American College of Chest Physicians evidence-based clinical practice guidelines. *Chest, 141*(Suppl. 2), e227S–e277S. http://dx.doi.org/10.1378/chest.11–2297.
28. Halaszynski, T. M., et al. (2004). Optimizing postoperative outcomes with efficient preoperative assessment and management. *Crit Care Med, 32*(Suppl. 4), S76–S86.
29. Halloran, L. L., & Bernard, D. W. (2004). Management of drug-induced hyperthermia. *Curr Opin Pediatr, 16*(2), 211–215.
30. Hamilton, M. A., Cecconi, M., & Rhodes, A. (2011). A systematic review and meta-analysis on the use of preemptive hemodynamic intervention to improve postoperative outcomes in moderate and high-risk surgical patients. *Anesth Analg, 112*, 1392–1402.
31. Hooper, V. D., Chard, R., Clifford, T., Fetzer, S., Fossum, S., Godden, B., et al. (2010). ASPAN's Evidence-based clinical practice guideline for the promotion of perioperative normothermia: second edition. *J Perianesth Nurs, 25*(6), 346–365. http://dx.doi.org/10.1016/j.jopan.2010.10.006.
32. Horlocker, T. T., Kopp, S. L. W., & Denise, J. (2015). Peripheral nerve blocks. In R. D. Miller (Ed.), *Miller's anesthesia* (8th ed.) (pp. 1721–1751). Philadelphia, PA: Elsevier/Saunders.

33. Hshieh, T. T., Yue, J., Oh, E., et al. (2015). Effectiveness of multicomponent nonpharmacological delirium interventions: a meta-analysis. *JAMA Intern Med*, *175*(4), 512–520. http://dx.doi.org/10.1001/jamainternmed.2014.7779.
34. Kaafarani, H. M., Itani, K. M., Thornby, J., & Berger, D. H. (2004). Thirty-day and one-year predictors of death in noncardiac major surgical procedures. *Am J Surg*, *188*(5), 495–499. http://dx.doi.org/10.1016/j.amjsurg.2004.07.018.
35. Kaboli, P., Henderson, M. C., & White, R. H. (2003). DVT prophylaxis and anticoagulation in the surgical patient. *Med Clin North Am*, *87*(1), 77–110. http://dx.doi.org/10.1016/S0025–7125(02)00144-X.
36. Kim, T. K., Obara, S., & Johnson, K. B. (2015). Basic principles of pharmacology. In R. D. Miller (Ed.), *Miller's anesthesia* (8th ed., pp. 590–613). Philadelphia, PA: Elsevier/Saunders.
37. Kranke, P. P. (2002). Pharmacological treatment of postoperative shivering: a quantitative systematic review of randomized controlled trials. *Anesth Analg*, *94*(2), 453–460.
38. Lagan, G., & McLure, H. A. (2004). Review of local anaesthetic agents. *Curr Anaesth Crit Care*, *15*(4–5), 247–254. http://dx.doi.org/10.1016/j.cacc.2004.08.007.
39. Lane, J. L. (2007). Postoperative respiratory insufficiency. In J. L. Atlee (Ed.), *Complications in anesthesia* (2nd ed., pp. 877–880). Philadelphia, PA: Elsevier/Saunders.
40. Larach, M. G., Gronert, G. A., Allen, G. C., Brandom, B. W., & Lehman, E. B. (2010). Clinical presentation, treatment, and complications of malignant hyperthermia in North America from 1987 to 2006. *Anesth Analg*, *110*(2), 498–507. http://dx.doi.org/10.1213/ANE.0b013e3181c6b9b2.
41. Larson, M. D. (2011). History of anesthesia. In R. D. Miller, & M. C. Pardo (Eds.), *Basics of anesthesia* (6th ed., pp. 3–10). Philadelphia, PA: Elsevier/Saunders.
42. Malignant Hyperthermia Associate of the United States. (2015). Retrieved from: http://www.mhaus.org/healthcare-professionals/managing-a-crisis.
43. Mandel, M. B. (2005). *Respiratory complications*. Retrieved from: http://www.pitt.edu/~mandel/resp.htm.
44. Mashour, G. A., Woodrum, D. T., & Avidan, M. S. (2015). Neurological complications of surgery and anaesthesia. *Br J Anesth*, *114*(2), 194–203. http://dx.doi.org/10.1093/bja/aeu296.
45. McClave, S. A., Martindale, R. G., Vanek, V. W., McCarthy, M., Roberts, P., Taylor, B., et al. (2009). Guidelines for the provision and assessment of nutrition support therapy in the adult critically ill patient: Society of Critical Care Medicine (SCCM) and American Society for Parenteral and Enteral Nutrition (A.S.P.E.N). *JPEN J Parenter Enteral Nutr*, *33*(3), 277–316. http://dx.doi.org/10.1177/0148607109335234.
46. Micromedex 2.0, (electronic version). Truven Health Analytics, Greenwood Village, CO. http://www.micromedexsolutions.com.proxy.lib.umich.edu/ (cited: *8/16/2015*).
47. Moos, D. D. (2012). Local anesthetics. In J. L. Forren (Ed.), *Perianesthesia nursing: a critical care approach* (6th ed., pp. 311–324). Philadelphia: Elsevier/Saunders.
48. Moos, D. D. (2012). Regional anesthesia. In J. L. Forren (Ed.), *Perianesthesia nursing: a critical care approach* (6th ed., pp. 325–341). Philadelphia: Elsevier/Saunders.
49. Nicholau, T. K. (2015). The postanesthesia care unit. In R. D. Miller (Ed.), *Miller's anesthesia* (8th ed., pp. 2924–2946). Philadelphia, PA: Elsevier/Saunders.
50. O'Brien, D. (2012). Patient education and care of the perianesthesia patient. In J. L. Forren (Ed.), *Perianesthesia nursing: a critical care approach* (6th ed., pp. 381–393). Philadelphia: Elsevier/Saunders.
51. Ortiz, V. E., & Kwo, J. (2015). Obesity: physiologic changes and implications for preoperative management. *BMC Anesthesiol*, *15*, 97. http://dx.doi.org/10.1186/s12871–015–0079–8.
52. Paden, M. S., Franjic, L., & Halcomb, S. E. (2013). Hyperthermia caused by drug interactions and adverse reactions. *Emerg Med Clin North Am*, *31*(4), 1035–1044. http://dx.doi.org/10.1016/j.emc.2013.07.003.
53. Posadzki, P., Watson, L., & Ernst, E. (2013). Herb–drug interactions: an overview of systematic reviews. *Br J Clin Pharmacol*, *75*(3), 603–618. http://dx.doi.org/10.1111/j.1365–2125.2012.04350.x.
54. American Society of Anesthesiologists Committee. (2012). Practice guidelines for acute pain management in the perioperative setting: an updated report by the American Society of Anesthesiologists Task Force on Acute Pain Management. *Anesthesiology*, *116*(2), 248–273. http://dx.doi.org/10.1097/ALN.0b013e31823c1030.
55. American Society of Anesthesiologists Committee. (2015). Practice guidelines for perioperative blood management: an updated report by the American Society of Anesthesiologists Task Force on Perioperative Blood Management. *Anesthesiology*, *122*(2), 241–275. http://dx.doi.org/10.1097/ALN.0000000000000463.
56. American Society of Anesthesiologists Committee. (2011). Practice guidelines for preoperative fasting and the use of pharmacologic agents to reduce the risk of pulmonary aspiration: application to healthy patients undergoing elective procedures: an updated report by the American Society of Anesthesiologists Committee on Standards and Practice Parameters. *Anesthesiology*, *114*(3), 495–511. http://dx.doi.org/10.1097/ALN.0b013e3181fcbfd9.
57. Qaseem, A. A. (2011). Use of intensive insulin therapy for the management of glycemic control in hospitalized patients: a clinical practice guideline from the American College of Physicians. *Ann Intern Med*, *154*(4), 260–267. http://dx.doi.org/10.7326/0003-4819-154-4-201102150-00007.
58. Reves, J. G., & Flezzani, P. (1985). Perioperative use of esmolol. *Am J Cardiol*, *56*(11), F57–F62. http://dx.doi.org/10.1016/0002-9149(85)90917-8.
59. Saklad, M. D. M. (1941). Grading of patients for surgical procedures. *Anesthesiology*, *2*(3), 281–284.
60. Sasaki, N., Meyer, M. J., & Eikermann, M. (2013). Postoperative respiratory muscle dysfunction: pathophysiology and preventive strategies. *Anesthesiology*, *118*(4), 961–978. http://dx.doi.org/10.1097/ALN.0b013e318288834f.
61. Schneiderbanger, D., Johannsen, S., Roewer, N., & Schuster, F. (2014). Management of malignant hyperthermia: diagnosis and treatment. *Ther Clin Risk Manag*, *10*, 355–362. http://dx.doi.org/10.2147/TCRM.S47632.
62. Shah, T. R., Veith, F. J., & Bauer, S. M. (2014). Cardiac evaluation and management before vascular surgery. *Curr Opin Cardiol*, *29*(6), 499–505. http://dx.doi.org/10.1097/HCO.0000000000000117.
63. Shander, A., Fleisher, L. A., Barie, P. S., Bigatello, L. M., Sladen, R. N., & Watson, C. B. (2011). Clinical and economic burden of postoperative pulmonary complications: patient safety summit on definition, risk-reducing interventions, and preventive strategies. *Crit Care Med*, *39*(9), 2163–2172. http://dx.doi.org/10.1097/CCM.0b013e31821f0522.
64. Society of Critical Care Medicine. (2015). ABCDEF liberation. http://www.iculiberation.org/Bundles/Pages/default.aspx.
65. Stoelting, R. K., & Hillier, S. C. (2006). Inhaled anesthetics. In *Handbook of pharmacology & physiology in anesthetic practice* (2nd ed., pp. 45–79). Philadelphia: Lippincott Williams & Wilkins.
66. Taylor, A., DeBoard, Z., & Gauvin, J. M. (2015). Prevention of postoperative pulmonary complications. *Surg Clin North Am*, *95*(2), 237–254. http://dx.doi.org/10.1016/j.suc.2014.11.002.
67. Tong, G. M., & Rude, R. K. (2005). Magnesium deficiency in critical illness. *J Intensive Care Med*, *20*(1), 3–17. http://dx.doi.org/10.1177/0885066604271539.
68. Vasu, T. S., Grewal, R., & Doghramji, K. (2012). Obstructive sleep apnea syndrome and perioperative complications: a systematic review of the literature. *J Clin Sleep Med*, *8*(2), 199–207. http://dx.doi.org/10.5664/jcsm.1784.
69. Venes, D. (2013). *Taber's cyclopedic medical dictionary* (22nd ed.). Philadelphia: F.A. Davis.
70. Visser, A., Geboers, B., Gouma, D. J., Goslings, J. C., & Ubbink, D. T. (2015). Predictors of surgical complications: a systematic review. *Surgery*, *158*(1), 58–65. http://dx.doi.org/10.1016/j.surg.2015.01.012.
71. Westerdahl, E. E. (2005). Deep-breathing exercises reduce atelectasis and improve pulmonary function after coronary artery bypass surgery. *Chest*, *128*(5), 3482–3488. http://dx.doi.org/10.1378/chest.128.5.3482.
72. Wijeysundera, D. N., Duncan, D., Nkonde-Price, C., Virani, S. S., Washam, J. B., Fleischmann, K. E., et al. (2014). Perioperative beta blockade in noncardiac surgery: a systematic review for the 2014 ACC/AHA Guideline on Perioperative Cardiovascular Evaluation and Management of Patients Undergoing Noncardiac Surgery: a report of the American College of Cardiology/American Heart Association Task Force on Practice Guidelines. *Circulation*, *130*(24), 2246–2264. http://dx.doi.org/10.1161/CIR.0000000000000104.
73. Zaugg, M., Tagliente, T., Lucchinetti, E., Jacobs, E., Krol, M., Bodian, C., et al. (1999). Beneficial effects from β-adrenergic blockade in elderly patients undergoing noncardiac surgery. *Anesthesiology*, *91*(6) 1674–1674.

Caring for the Critically Ill Pregnant Patient

Julene (Julie) B. Kruithof

INTRODUCTION

Caring for the critically ill obstetric patient presents the critical care team with unique management challenges. It is estimated that 1% to 3% of pregnant women require critical care each year.[5,38] In the past, the specialties of obstetrics and critical care have been widely separated; the usual normalcy of pregnancy and the severe illness-orientation of critical care seem diametrically opposed. However, current trends, including higher maternal age and pregnancy in women with preexisting diseases, have led to an increase in the number of pregnant women cared for in critical care. Global health priorities included the goal of reducing maternal mortality by 75% between 1990 and 2015.[21,30] However, instead of a persistent decrease, the United States has seen an increase in maternal mortality, with a current rate approximated between 14.5 and 21 maternal deaths per 100,000 live births.[18,27,29] Race-specific pregnancy-related mortality trends demonstrate that African-American women are three to four times as likely to die from pregnancy-related causes as are Caucasian women.[27,30] Many efforts are focused on improving maternal mortality. Examples include, but are not limited to, global advocacy agencies and programs, professional association programs, and promotion of state Maternal Mortality Review Boards.[30] Experts have advocated for clinical emergency preparedness efforts, and work has been initiated to enhance early recognition and management of maternal compromise.[11,16,18,22] The concerning mortality trends underscore the need for critical care nurses who, in addition to their critical care knowledge and skills, also understand the unique needs of the critically ill obstetric patient.

There are three management priorities for the critically ill pregnant patient: optimizing maternal physiologic functioning, enhancing fetal growth and development, and supporting the maternal and family experience. Understanding the unique body of knowledge surrounding critical care obstetrics will help to achieve positive outcomes for both the mother and the child. Common obstetric terms are highlighted in Box 34.1, and a broad overview of fetal development is provided in Fig. 34.1.

PREGNANCY AND CRITICAL ILLNESS

Obstetric patients requiring critical care fall into two groups. The first group includes women with preexisting disease who become pregnant and require advanced care and management. Examples of preexisting diseases that might compromise a woman's condition and necessitate admission to critical care include diabetes, heart valve disease, corrected or uncorrected congenital heart disease, asthma, spinal cord injury, and neuromuscular disease (e.g., multiple sclerosis). The second group includes women who experience critical illness or injury during an otherwise normal pregnancy. Examples of critical illnesses or injury that may arise during or as a result of pregnancy include thromboembolic disease, myocardial infarction, peripartum cardiomyopathy, anaphylactoid syndrome, pneumonia, sepsis, or trauma. The most common causes of intensive care unit (ICU) admission are hemorrhage and hypertension.[5] Critical care nurses must be prepared to handle the unique management concerns during pregnancy or in the immediate postpartum period.

NORMAL PHYSIOLOGIC CHANGES IN PREGNANCY

Physiologic changes occur during pregnancy impacting nearly every organ system. These changes alter baseline assessment and laboratory data findings, potentially confounding diagnosis and management. These physiologic changes occur to maintain the pregnancy and allow for fetal growth and development. Hormonal increases in progesterone, estrogen, and human placental lactogen account for many of these changes. Nearly every body system is affected. Some adaptations are so profound that they would be considered pathologic if they occurred outside of pregnancy. The physiologic changes begin as early as the first week of gestation and continue up to 6 weeks or more following delivery. Changes associated with critical illness or injury are highlighted within this chapter.

Reproductive System

Reproductive organs undergo dramatic changes during pregnancy. The capacity of the uterus grows from 10 mL to between 4.5 and 5.0 L. As the uterus grows out of the pelvis, abdominal contents are displaced, and diaphragmatic elevation occurs. The uterine vascular bed expands dramatically, and uterine blood flow increases from 50 mL/min at 10 weeks to 500 mL/min at 40 weeks.[47]

Cardiovascular System

During pregnancy, the cardiovascular system undergoes dramatic changes in blood volume and cardiac output (CO). The total blood volume increases approximately 45% to 50%, which is approximately 1.0 to 1.5 L greater than the normal volume.[35,38] This increase in volume peaks between weeks 26 and 34 of gestation. The red blood cell volume increases approximately 20% to 30%, the plasma volume increases 45% to 50%, and the total

BOX 34.1 Common Obstetric Terms

- Acceleration: visually apparent abrupt increase in fetal heart rate above the baseline
- Deceleration: visually apparent decrease in fetal heart rate
- Effacement: shortening and thinning of the cervix during the first stage of labor
- First trimester: weeks 1 through 13 of pregnancy
- *Gravida:* woman who is pregnant
- *Multipara:* woman who has completed two or more pregnancies to the stage of fetal viability
- *Nullipara:* woman who has not completed a pregnancy with a fetus who has reached the stage of viability
- Preterm: pregnancy that has reached 20 weeks of gestation, but before completion of 37 weeks of gestation
- *Primigravida:* woman who is pregnant for the first time
- Second trimester: weeks 14 through 26 of pregnancy
- Term: describes a pregnancy from the beginning of the 38th week of gestation to the end of the 42nd week of gestation
- Third trimester: weeks 27 through 40 of pregnancy
- Viability: capacity to live outside the uterus; currently approximately 22 to 24 weeks of gestation, or fetal weight greater than 500 g

From References 6, 39, 40, 41, and 42.

body water increases by approximately 6 to 8 L.[19,35,38] Together, these changes produce a dilutional anemia and a decrease in colloid oncotic pressure. Expected hemoglobin (Hgb) and hematocrit levels (Hct) in pregnancy are approximately 10 to 11 g/dL and 30% to 35%, respectively.[35] Pregnancy is considered a hypercoagulable state, with increases in the levels of factors VII, VIII, IX, and X.[5,35] In addition to the increased levels of clotting factors, fibrinolytic activity is decreased, further promoting coagulability.[38]

Along with the volume changes, structural changes in the cardiovascular system occur. The heart is displaced upward and to the left because of the elevation of the diaphragm. Left axis deviation can occur as a result of the mechanical displacement, but there are no other characteristic electrocardiographic changes. Hypertrophy of the cardiac muscle can occur to meet the volume demands. During physical assessment, changes in heart sounds may be noted, such as S_1 split, development of an S_3, or systolic murmur.[47] These are typically considered normal physiologic changes in pregnancy.

Pregnancy also brings many blood pressure (BP) variations. Typically, BP decreases slightly during the first trimester, reaches a low point during the second trimester, and then returns to normal. Supine positioning can cause vena cava compression by the gravid uterus, decreasing venous return and CO, potentially causing postural hypotension. To meet the physiologic demands of pregnancy, CO undergoes dramatic changes. Normal CO during pregnancy is considered to be 6 to 7 L/min, generally a 30% to 50% increase from prepregnancy values.[29,34] Changes in CO begin in the first trimester and peak during early- to mid-third trimester. One study concluded that the initial increase in CO can be attributed to an increase in heart rate, and the progressive increase is due to an increase in stroke volume.[29] Unique to pregnancy are the positional CO changes that occur (Table 34.1). Normal hemodynamic values in pregnancy are referenced in Table 34.2. Cardiac index is not accurately calculated during pregnancy.[34]

Pulmonary System

As pregnancy progresses, diaphragmatic elevation occurs, shortening lung length by approximately 4 cm. However, hormonal changes allow anteroposterior and circumferential enlargement, compensating for the shorter thoracic cavity.[51] Tidal volume increases approximately 40%, to a normal range of 500 to 600 mL, and the respiratory rate increases slightly. Respiratory reserve volume and functional residual capacity both decrease. Together, these changes enhance minute ventilation to 9 to 13 L/min. Altogether pulmonary physiologic changes allow the mother to have increased minute ventilation by approximately 50% at term. This normal hyperventilation causes changes in arterial blood gas values during pregnancy. Hyperventilation causes the maternal partial pressure of arterial carbon dioxide ($Paco_2$) level to drop between 26 and 32 mm Hg, with a resultant mild respiratory alkalosis.[38,51]

Maternal oxygen demands increase 15% to 25% during pregnancy, primarily to meet fetal oxygen demands. To meet these requirements, normal maternal partial pressure of arterial oxygen tension (Pao_2) is 101 to 108 mm Hg, and arterial oxygen saturation should be maintained at greater than 95%.[20] To facilitate oxygen exchange from the mother to the fetus, the maternal oxyhemoglobin dissociation curve shifts slightly to the right.

Gastrointestinal System

The maternal gastrointestinal (GI) system undergoes changes in both structure and function, attributable to hormonal changes, as well as interference from the growing uterus. GI motility decreases, intestinal secretion slows, and water absorption increases, placing the woman at risk for constipation and aspiration. In addition, the gravid uterus causes displacement and potential incompetence of the gastroesophageal junction, further enhancing aspiration risk. Due to the influence of estrogen, vascular congestion (hyperemia) occurs in many mucosal tissues, including the gums, nose, pharynx, larynx, trachea, bronchi, urethra, and bladder.[42] Hyperemia can lead to bleeding gums and impaired gallbladder emptying, as well as decreased gallbladder activity, leading to gallstones and cholecystitis.

Renal System

Functional renal changes are primarily caused by changes in renal blood flow. Renal blood flow increases 30% to 50%, and glomerular filtration increases approximately 50%.[13,35] Because glomerular filtration increases more than blood flow, renal clearance is enhanced, lowering the plasma concentration of many substances, including maternal creatinine and blood urea nitrogen (BUN). As these waste products are excreted more effectively, serum levels in pregnant women are reduced. The normal values for serum creatinine level in pregnancy are 0.5–1.1 mg/dL, and normal BUN levels are 10 to 20 mg/dL.[35,41] Although glomerular filtration is enhanced, the maternal tubular capacity to reabsorb glucose and protein does not change; therefore, both glycosuria and proteinuria are common in pregnancy. These findings may be normal, but require further investigation, as they may be indicators of serious pathology.

MONITORING OF THE CRITICALLY ILL OBSTETRIC PATIENT

Monitoring of both mother and fetus is essential to provide the healthcare team with information regarding the status and tolerance of therapies and activities. Gestational age plays a significant role in the decision-making process for determining appropriate monitoring strategies. The current range for

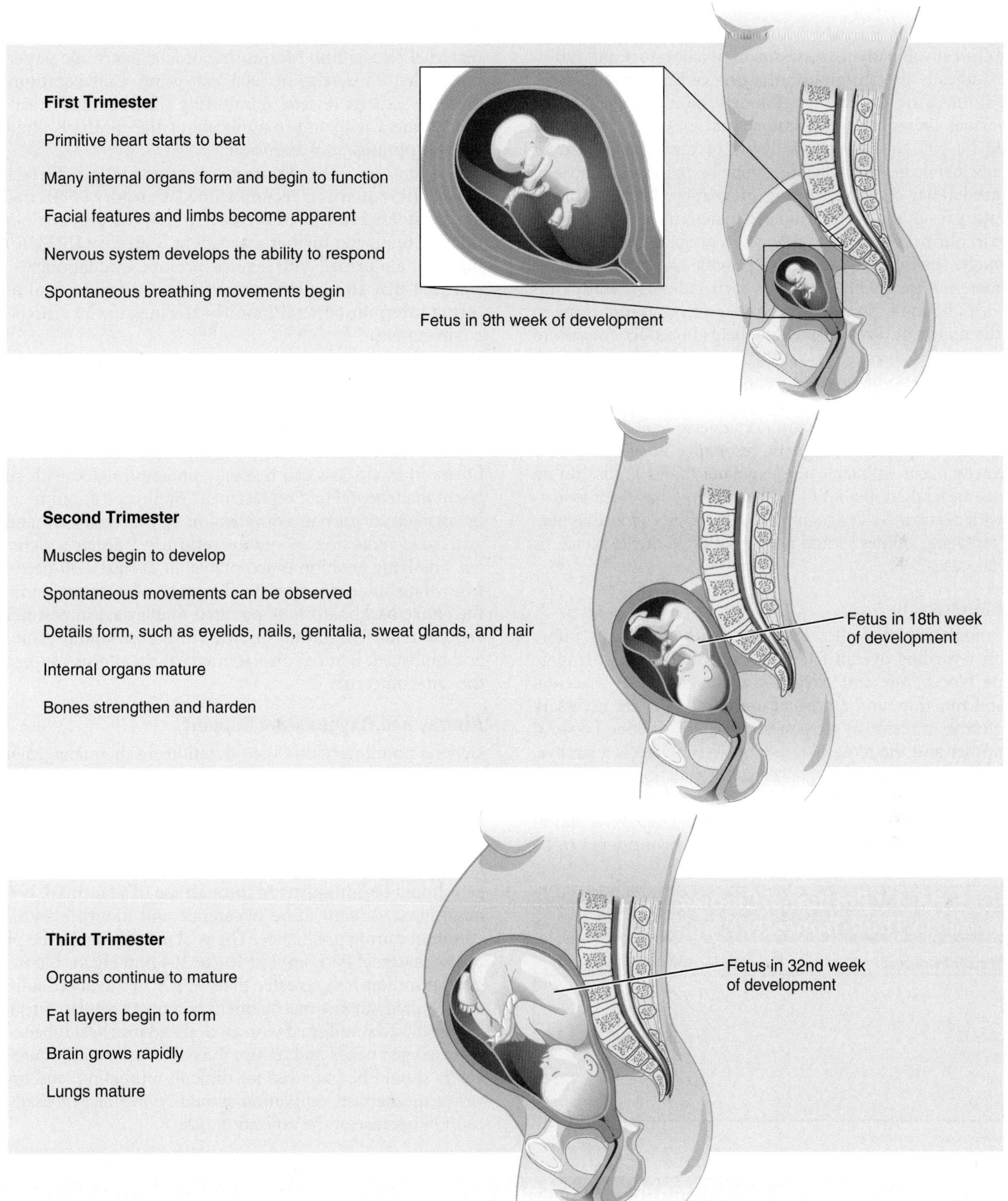

First Trimester
Primitive heart starts to beat
Many internal organs form and begin to function
Facial features and limbs become apparent
Nervous system develops the ability to respond
Spontaneous breathing movements begin
Fetus in 9th week of development
Second Trimester
Muscles begin to develop
Spontaneous movements can be observed
Details form, such as eyelids, nails, genitalia, sweat glands, and hair
Internal organs mature
Bones strengthen and harden
Fetus in 18th week of development
Third Trimester
Organs continue to mature
Fat layers begin to form
Brain grows rapidly
Lungs mature
Fetus in 32nd week of development

FIG. 34.1 Stages of fetal development.

fetal viability is between 22 and 24 weeks of gestation, with fetal weight greater than 500 grams (0.5 kg).[41] In light of these parameters, management efforts should be focused primarily on maternal outcomes before 26 weeks of gestation. Once fetal viability has been reached, however, it is critical to evaluate both maternal and fetal response to interventions and physiologic status. Many authorities concur that until approximately 32 to 34 weeks of gestation, the fetus is generally supported better *in utero* rather than outside of the uterus. Situations may be encountered where fetal viability, fetal outcome, and maternal stability are uncertain. Each clinical decision must be weighed while considering maternal and fetal risk and benefit.

Maternal Monitoring

Monitoring of the pregnant woman is similar to monitoring other critically ill patients. Assessment of laboratory and radiologic studies is also an important aspect of caring for the critically ill obstetric patient. Practitioners should keep in mind the normal alterations in laboratory studies. Careful attention should be paid to therapeutic levels of medications. Larger than normal doses of medications may be required because of enhanced renal clearance during pregnancy. Each abnormal laboratory result should be evaluated to determine if the change is due to normal physiologic changes in pregnancy or potential pathology. Radiologic studies also provide important insights into maternal treatment. However, each radiologic study may provide radiation exposure to the growing fetus, posing a risk to fetal development. Proper shielding helps to reduce the risk to the fetus, and each radiologic study should be considered with a risk/benefit ratio before performing it. If possible, consideration should be given to use of imaging procedures that are not associated with ionizing radiation or adverse fetal effects, such as ultrasonography and magnetic resonance imaging.[1] Severe defects can occur with exposure to greater than 10 rads, but no increase in fetal anomalies or pregnancy loss has been associated with exposure to less than 5 rads.[1,36] Experts agree that necessary imaging studies should not be withheld due to concerns for fetal status.[5,34]

Fetal Monitoring

Fetal monitoring provides caregivers with important information regarding overall fetal and maternal status. Adequate uterine blood flow and oxygen content, sufficient placental size and function, and a normal umbilical cord are necessary for effective transfer of oxygen and carbon dioxide between the mother and the fetus. The uteroplacental bed is a passive, low-resistance system that has no autoregulation and few, if any, compensatory mechanisms. Therefore, changes in uteroplacental perfusion can significantly affect fetal oxygenation and well-being. The uteroplacental system is considered to be a peripheral, nonessential organ during physiologic stress, preferentially shunting perfusion away from the fetus and back into maternal circulation. Monitoring of fetal heart rate patterns is undertaken to determine fetal well-being. Collaboration with obstetric experts in fetal monitoring will provide critical care practitioners with information about the mother's ability to provide optimal fetal perfusion.

Currently, a 3-tiered system for categorization of fetal heart rate (FHR) patterns is recommended. Category I FHR tracings are considered normal. Category II FHR tracings are indeterminate, requiring further assessment. Category III FHR tracings are abnormal and require prompt evaluation.[6,44] It is essential that an obstetric practitioner trained in fetal monitoring interpret all fetal monitor tracings in the critical care environment.

TABLE 34.1 Positional Cardiac Output Changes in Third-Trimester Pregnancy

Maternal Position	Cardiac Output (L/min)
Knee-chest	6.9 ± 2.1
Right lateral	6.8 ± 1.3
Left lateral	6.6 ± 1.4
Sitting	6.2 ± 2.0
Supine	6.0 ± 1.4
Standing	5.4 ± 2.0

From References 23, 24, and 25.

Maintenance of Cardiac Output

Ensuring adequate blood volume and correct positioning of the critically ill obstetric patient is essential to optimize CO. The normal hypervolemic state of pregnancy should be maintained; however, blood loss can be easily underestimated with subsequent inadequate fluid replacement. Supine positioning should be avoided to prevent compression of the vena cava and the associated reduction in venous return.[35,39] Either a right or a left side-lying position is acceptable, or at least a 30-degree tilt from the supine position. In the event of a traumatic injury, the entire backboard may be tilted to alleviate impairment of venous return. If tilting or side-lying positioning cannot be accomplished, manual displacement of the uterus can provide the same outcome.

Airway and Oxygenation Support

General pulmonary care considerations in the management of critically ill obstetric patients include continuous assessment, as well as maintenance of maternal oxygenation, protection of the airway, and provision of ventilatory support. Assessment of maternal status may be confounded by the normal hyperventilation and dyspnea associated with pregnancy. High-flow oxygen should be administered through use of a facemask because nasal passages tend to be hyperemic and mouth breathing is common during pregnancy. The goal is to maintain the physiologic maternal Pa_{O_2} level of 101 to 104 mm Hg, or blood oxygen saturation Sp_{O_2} greater than 95%.[20] If advanced adjuncts are required, airway management in a pregnant patient should be rapidly accomplished with an oral endotracheal tube to help meet oxygen needs and reduce the risk of aspiration. Care providers should be prepared for difficult intubation, and noninvasive mechanical ventilation should be avoided or used with caution because of the aspiration risk.[34]

TABLE 34.2 Hemodynamic Changes Associated with Term Pregnancy

Parameter	Normal Value	Change
Central venous pressure	4–8 ± 2 mm Hg	No significant change
Pulmonary artery occlusion pressure	4–7 ± 2–3 mm Hg	No significant change
Heart rate	75–95 beats/min	Increase 10–20 beats/min
Cardiac output	6.2 ± 1 L/min	Increase 30%–50%
Systemic vascular resistance	1210 ± 266 dynes/sec/cm^{-5}	Decrease 20%
Pulmonary vascular resistance	78 ± 22 dynes/sec/cm^{-5}	Decrease 34%
Left ventricular stroke work index	43–48 ± 6–9 g/m^2	No significant change

From References 23, 24, and 25.

Ventilatory support should target lung-protective ventilation; target a tidal volume less than or equal to 6 mL/kg of ideal body weight and airway pressures of less than 30 cm H_2O, whenever able.[34,39] Gastric decompression with an orogastric or small nasogastric tube should be accomplished to prevent gastric reflux and aspiration. If emergency cricothyrotomy or tracheotomy is needed, it should be performed above the usual site because of the upward displacement of thoracic structures. In addition, the entry point for chest tube insertion may need to be reassessed because of the increase in the anteroposterior diameter of the chest and decrease in length.

Pharmacologic Concerns

Use of medications in critically ill obstetric patients requires thoughtful consideration of the likelihood of obtaining therapeutic results and the risk/benefit ratio for both mother and fetus.

Historically, the US Food and Drug Administration (FDA) developed pregnancy categories of A, B, C, D, and X for drug use in pregnancy that were useful in guiding decision making. The FDA has updated the guidelines, and as of June 30, 2015, pregnancy categories are required to be removed from drug product labeling, with new requirements for three subsections: "Pregnancy," "Lactation," and "Females and Males of Reproductive Potential."[28,55] The new guidelines provide more robust information and guidance regarding safe medication use during pregnancy and lactation.

Other considerations include careful attention to therapeutic levels of medications due to enhanced physiologic clearance of some substances. In addition, certain medications may have teratogenic effects on the developing fetus. Many vasoactive medications commonly used in the critical care setting (e.g., epinephrine, dopamine) may have negative effects on uteroplacental perfusion. Use requires consideration of the risk/benefit ratio, keeping in mind that adequate maternal perfusion is required, in spite of vasoconstriction, for fetal perfusion to occur. Experts agree that necessary medications should not be withheld because of fetal concerns.[5] All pharmacologics used in the management of a critically ill obstetric patient should be individualized with consideration given to the risk/benefit ratio.

Nutritional Considerations/Glycemic Control

The maternal metabolic rate increases during pregnancy.[41] Nutritional support provided during critical illness or injury must meet these increased demands. Total daily caloric intake should be based on ideal body weight. Glucose maintenance during pregnancy can present significant challenges during critical illness or injury. Maternal hypoglycemia is anticipated due to increased insulin levels.[5] Diabetes during pregnancy, either preexisting or gestational, causes both maternal and fetal complications and increases morbidity. Major tenets of diabetic care in pregnancy are similar to conventional diabetic therapy: blood glucose level monitoring, diet, exercise, and patient education. Glycemic control should be reassessed frequently throughout pregnancy and in the postpartum period.

Prevention of Thromboembolism

The risk of thromboembolism is four to five times higher in pregnant women as compared with nonpregnant women, and risk continues into the postpartum period.[7] Major underlying factors in venous thromboembolism—hypercoagulability, venous stasis, vena caval compression, and decreased mobility—all occur in pregnancy. Diagnosis of thromboembolism in the pregnant patient is as difficult as in the nonpregnant patient because some do not exhibit classic signs and symptoms. Thromboembolism in pregnancy can be associated with lower abdominal pain that can confound the diagnosis. Whereas most diagnostic tests are identical to those for nonpregnant patients, D-dimer testing is not reliable in pregnancy.[7,13]

Management of thromboembolism is generally completed with heparin compounds. Patients who are anticoagulated require a carefully planned delivery and anticoagulation resumption plan to avoid potentially negative outcomes. Pneumatic compression devices should be placed prior to cesarean delivery and left in place until the patient is ambulatory and anticoagulation is resumed.[7,24] Postpartum patients should continue treatment for between 6 weeks and 6 months after delivery to reduce the risk of pulmonary embolism.

Labor and Delivery Considerations

Additional stress is incurred during labor and delivery. Critical care nurses caring for antepartum patients should monitor for signs of labor. These may include increased urinary frequency because of lightening (descending of the fetal presenting part into the pelvis), an increase in vaginal mucus *(bloody show)*, backaches, contractions, nausea, or rupture of membranes. Normal labor includes a regular progression of uterine contractions, effacement (thinning), dilation of the cervix, and progress in the descent of the presenting part of the fetus through the birth canal.[43] Collaboration with obstetric resources is essential once any indication or suspicion of labor is evident.

The normal labor and delivery process occurs in four stages (Table 34.3 and Fig. 34.2). Throughout each of these stages, dramatic physiologic changes occur. These changes are due in part to the pain and anxiety associated with labor, but are also due to physiologic alterations. The most dramatic changes are seen in the cardiovascular system. Each contraction produces an autotransfusion of approximately 300 to 500 mL, and therefore CO changes during each phase of labor, with the most dramatic changes during the immediate postpartum period.[37] Blood loss also occurs during delivery, and is generally estimated to be approximately 500 mL from a vaginal birth and 1,000 mL from a cesarean birth.[23] Because these dramatic changes typically occur over a short length of time, mothers must be monitored carefully to assess tolerance and to watch for potential decompensation. Obstetric emergencies during the labor process include the development of fetal stress, inadequate uterine relaxation, vaginal bleeding, or umbilical cord prolapse.[43]

TABLE 34.3 Stages of Labor

Labor Stage	Definition/Characteristics
First stage	Onset of regular uterine contractions through full dilation of cervix. Typically lasts between 1 and 20 hours.
Second stage	From full cervical dilation through fetal delivery. Typically lasts 20 to 50 minutes.
Third stage	Birth of fetus through placental delivery. Typically lasts between 3 and 30 minutes.
Fourth stage	First 2 hours after placental delivery. Immediate recovery phase and until initial homeostasis is achieved.

From Reference 41.

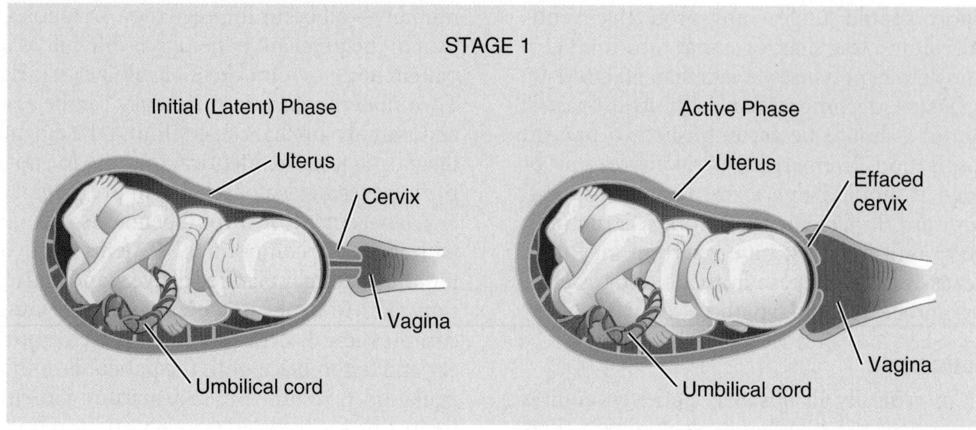

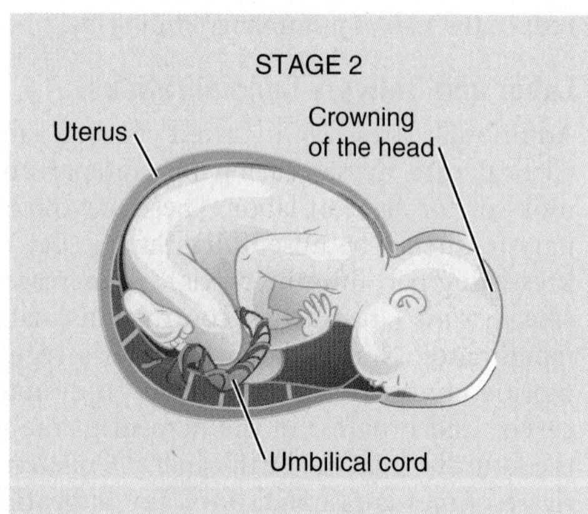

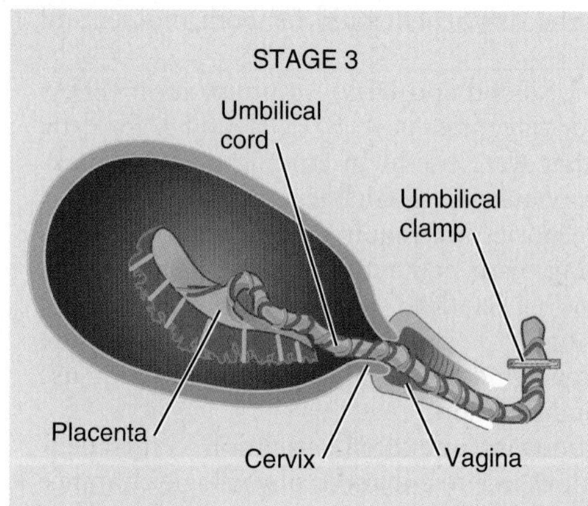

FIG. 34.2 Stages of labor.

Preterm labor is defined as cervical change and uterine contractions occurring between 20 weeks and 37 weeks of pregnancy. Preterm labor is multifactorial in nature and can lead to preterm birth, which is defined as any birth occurring before the end of 37 weeks of pregnancy.[50] Management of preterm labor includes prevention with prenatal care, lifestyle modifications to avoid activities presumed to initiate preterm labor, and restriction of physical activity. Tocolytic therapy (the administration of pharmaceutical agents that suppress uterine activity) is a mainstay of therapy. Tocolytic therapy can provide a window of opportunity for administration of glucocorticoids that can stimulate fetal lung maturity and reduce infant complications if labor cannot be stopped.

Labor induction is the chemical or mechanical initiation of uterine contractions before the natural onset of spontaneous labor. Labor induction is usually performed when the maternal and fetal risks of labor and birth are less than the risk of continuing the pregnancy. The most common methods for labor induction include cervical ripening with prostaglandin agents or mechanical induction through artificial rupture of the membranes, along with administration of oxytocin (Pitocin) to stimulate uterine contractions.

Environment of Safety

Central to the care of the critically ill obstetric patient is ensuring an optimal environment for safe care of the mother and fetus. Collaborative decision making should occur during the admission process, beginning with placement decisions addressing whether the mother is best cared for in critical care, labor and delivery, or an antepartal unit. Decisions should be based upon optimal care for the mother, and resources should then be mobilized to meet those needs. If care will be provided in critical care, rapid access to and availability of essential obstetric and neonatal resources should be ensured. Regardless of patient location, collaboration, teamwork, and open communication among practitioners provide the optimal benefit to the patient (Box 34.2).

BOX 34.2 Infection Prevention

Pregnancy poses several infection risks to maternal well-being. Several pulmonary-related considerations are essential. Seasonal influenza vaccination is encouraged because pregnant women are at an increased risk of serious illness secondary to influenza. In addition, current recommendations advocate for administration of the tetanus toxoid, reduced diphtheria toxoid, and acellular pertussis vaccine (Tdap) between 27 and 36 weeks of gestation Incompetence of the gastroesophageal mechanism and delays in gastric emptying enhance the aspiration risk. Obstetric patients are generally treated as *full stomach* patients. If mechanical ventilator support is required, careful attention should be paid to ventilator-associated event prevention techniques, including oral care and elevation of the head of the bed. The potential for urinary stasis also increases the risk for urinary tract infections during pregnancy. Over 5 million new cases of maternal sepsis occur annually, accounting for between 2% and 11.6% of maternal deaths. Causes of maternal sepsis vary related to the stage of pregnancy. Early pregnancy-specific causes include miscarriage or termination of pregnancy; whereas chorioamnionitis associated with premature rupture of membranes can occur in the second or third trimester. Postdelivery sepsis can be caused by perineal infections, endometritis, wound infections, or mastitis. As in the general population, early resuscitation and antibiotic administration are essential, along with aggressive supportive therapies. Careful consideration of the physiologic changes that occur during pregnancy must be undertaken, to avoid missing early warning signs and to ensure maximal therapy.

From References 9, 10, and 15.

Psychosocial Care

Pregnancy has an inherent set of maternal psychosocial tasks, and fathers have specific psychological tasks to accomplish as well. One of the confounding factors of critical care obstetrics is that the normalcy and joyful expectation typically associated with pregnancy and delivery is marred. Encountering critical illness or injury during pregnancy challenges the coping mechanisms of the individual and the family unit. In addition, stress may occur because of a real or perceived threat to the life or functional outcome of both mother and baby. In the event of fetal demise, collaboration with individuals who have received advanced training in fetal demise can provide essential support to the maternal family unit through that experience. Critical situations may bring a variety of personal, cultural, social, spiritual, or ethical values into conflict. All members of the healthcare team should discuss management options and proceed with collaborative decision making with patient or family members.

Pain Management

Pain management in critically ill obstetric patients, outside of labor pain management, is essentially similar to that for other critically ill patients. Consideration must be given to maternal and fetal tolerance of medications administered. Many narcotics decrease maternal BP, which can, in turn, reduce uteroplacental perfusion and cause fetal stress. Unique to the critically ill obstetric patient's pain management plan is pain management during labor. The Committee on Obstetric Practice of the American College of Obstetricians and Gynecologists (ACOG) states that pain management should be provided whenever medically indicated, and that maternal request is a sufficient medical indication for pain relief during labor.[2] Labor pain management is best managed with collaborative expertise from obstetric and anesthesia colleagues. This is frequently accomplished with epidural analgesia, allowing the woman to maintain alertness and participation in the labor process with the fewest negative effects for the fetus. Epidural placement can cause vasodilation, and is commonly managed with a preplacement fluid bolus. Careful consideration of the mother's ability to tolerate the fluid bolus must be undertaken before administration.

POSTDELIVERY CARE

Management of the postdelivery patient requires expert teamwork between critical care and obstetric practitioners. Highlights of postpartum care are presented here in three broad categories: prevention of hemorrhage, support of breastfeeding, and support of maternal-infant bonding.

Prevention of Hemorrhage

Hemorrhage is the leading cause of maternal death; therefore, careful attention to monitoring of lochial flow is essential.[51] Immediate postdelivery lochial flow is generally considered to be normal if it is less than or equal to one pad per hour. Clots, the size of a quarter or smaller, can be expected, but greater flow or larger clots warrants further investigation. Lochial flow is generally bright red for the first day (ruborous) and progresses to a more normal serosanguineous color after 2 to 3 days. Patients experiencing more than normal bleeding postdelivery should be assessed to determine the source of bleeding and to identify potential signs of shock. Appropriate lab studies (e.g., complete blood cell count, type and crossmatch, coagulation studies) should be obtained and venous access ensured for volume resuscitation.

Primary postpartum hemorrhage occurs with 24 hours postdelivery, whereas secondary postpartum hemorrhage occurs between 24 hours and 6 to 12 weeks postpartum.[3] Uterine atony is the most common cause of primary postpartum hemorrhage. Careful assessment of fundal height and character is essential to ensure uterine firmness and regression. The top of the fundus is described as the number of fingerbreadths below the umbilicus, and the fundus should be firm, not boggy or mushy. If the fundus is not firm, uterine massage may be performed to stimulate uterine contractions and regression. Concerns about fundal height and character or the presence of continued bleeding require immediate consultation with obstetric colleagues. Other causes of primary postpartum hemorrhage include retained placenta, coagulopathy, lacerations, and uterine inversion.[3] Management of primary postpartum hemorrhage includes appropriate fluid and blood replacement therapy; pharmacologic support with uterotonic agents, vasopressors, or coagulation factors; and cause-specific interventions or surgical intervention. New trends include hemostatic resuscitation with use of mass transfusion protocols, which require further study in the obstetric population.[48]

Support of Breastfeeding

Many mothers wish to breastfeed their newborn infants; this request should be honored and supported unless absolutely impossible. Consideration must be given to maternal medications and their safety for the infant. Consultation with obstetric and pharmacy colleagues is recommended to determine whether the mother's milk can be stored for later infant consumption or whether it should be discarded. If it is to be stored for later consumption, strict attention should be paid to institution policies for handling and storage of breast milk. Pumping with a hospital-grade electric pump should be initiated as soon as possible. General guidelines for pumping are to pump simultaneously for a minimum of 15 minutes on each breast every 2 to 4 hours. Assisting the mother with donning a nursing support bra should be accomplished as soon as is feasible. Consultation with lactation or obstetric colleagues can enhance success for all involved.

Support of Maternal-Infant Bonding

Maternal-infant bonding is essential during the immediate postpartum period, and of special significance is the ability of the mother to have skin contact with and hold her newborn infant. Although severe physiologic instability of either the infant or the mother may prohibit visitation, great strides should be taken to facilitate visitation if at all possible. Other mechanisms, such as pictures and recordings of infant or maternal voices, should be employed to enhance bonding as much as possible. Infant visitation in critical care should be accomplished whenever possible, and collaboration with neonatal or nursery staff can facilitate this experience. There is no increased risk of infection to either the mother or the infant during visitation.

CARDIAC DISEASE IN PREGNANCY

General Considerations

Cardiac disease occurs in 4% of pregnancies; it may be the result of preexisting conditions, or may develop during pregnancy.[38] Prepregnancy counseling is highly recommended for women with known cardiac disease to provide insight into the maternal and fetal risks associated with pregnancy, as well as open the discussion into appropriate timing of pregnancy. Some preexisting or congenital cardiac diseases may require intervention before conception to maximize maternal and fetal outcomes. The four strongest predictors of maternal outcomes in cardiac disease during pregnancy have been documented as: (1) history of heart failure, transient ischemic attack, stroke or arrhythmia; (2) prepregnancy New York Heart Association (NYHA) class (> II equals better maternal outcomes); (3) left heart outflow obstruction; and (4) an ejection fraction that is compromised by less than 40%.[33]

General principles of antenatal management address four areas: coagulation, heart rate, volume status, and antibiotic prophylaxis. Anticoagulation is frequently recommended because of the normal hypercoagulable state of pregnancy. As mentioned previously, anticoagulation with heparin is recommended because of the teratogenic effects of oral agents.[33] Heart rate must be carefully monitored, and although mild tachycardia is expected, caution must be taken to avoid significant tachycardia, which could compromise CO. Management is generally accomplished with beta blockade. Careful attention must be paid to maternal volume status to maintain optimal euvolemia as far as possible. Pulmonary edema may be easily induced because of the natural decrease in colloid osmotic pressure. Antibiotic prophylaxis may be used to prevent endocarditis.

Physiologic changes that occur during pregnancy (e.g., murmur development, shortness of breath) and may be problematic may sometimes be accepted as routine when they are actually due to pathology. Cardiac monitoring is recommended through all stages of labor. Management of the pregnant woman with cardiac disease mandates collaboration between obstetric and cardiology colleagues to carefully monitor progress throughout pregnancy, as well as plan for delivery. The method and timing of delivery are decided primarily by obstetric needs, but must consider the woman's ability to tolerate the stress and cardiac demands of labor. Induction or shortening the second, or pushing, stage of labor may be advised to alleviate prolonged cardiac stress. Patients who have received antenatal anticoagulation are generally changed to intravenous anticoagulation in the inpatient setting to allow careful titration of therapy. Pain management is crucial, as pain and anxiety can lead to tachycardia, and may have a negative impact on cardiac function. As a general rule, most patients tolerate epidural anesthesia better than general anesthesia, although attention must be paid to the risk of vasodilation and subsequent hypotension. Intravenous fluid resuscitation should be immediately available. Aggressive control of bleeding should be accomplished in order to lessen fluid volume shifts in the immediate postpartum period.

Women with Preexisting Valvular Heart Disease

The significant physiologic changes that occur during pregnancy can pose problems for patients with preexisting valvular heart disease, whether congenital or rheumatic in origin. Mild aortic or mitral stenosis is generally well tolerated during pregnancy, in spite of the relatively fixed CO that occurs due to the disease processes.[38] However, changes in preload, heart rate, or vascular resistance can lead to decompensation and maternal instability. Special attention should be paid to vasodilation-associated preload changes that could occur with epidural anesthesia, autotransfusions that occur with labor and delivery, and preload reduction that could occur with postpartum hemorrhage. Careful monitoring of patient status is warranted. Regurgitant valve disease is typically rheumatic in origin, and is usually well tolerated in pregnancy.[38,52]

Women with Congenital Heart Disease

Women with congenital heart disease must face two realities during pregnancy: the risk of cardiac decompensation, and the potential for transmission of the congenital defect to the fetus. Proactive correction of maternal congenital defects may be advised. In general, women with corrected lesions tolerate pregnancy and the associated cardiac demands well. In addition to the general considerations and management during pregnancy, patients with congenital disease should be monitored with serial echocardiography and evaluated for the development of pulmonary hypertension. The development of pulmonary hypertension has a negative and rather dramatic impact on both maternal and fetal prognosis.[51,52] Several congenital defects are highlighted here.

Left to Right Shunts

Defects causing a left to right shunt (e.g., atrial septal defects, ventricular septal defects) are commonly well tolerated during pregnancy because of the natural hypervolemia. Logically, the size of the defect impacts the woman's ability to meet the increased cardiac demands. The most typical complications are dysrhythmias, heart failure, and thromboembolism; proactive management should be employed to maximize outcome.

Marfan Syndrome

The prognosis of a pregnant woman with Marfan syndrome is primarily based upon aortic root diameter, with a significant increase in aortic dissection and mortality when the aortic root diameter exceeds 4.0 to 4.5 cm.[33,52] Hypertension and aortic wall stress should be avoided, which is typically managed with beta blockade.

Cyanotic Lesions

Cyanotic congenital heart diseases, such as tetralogy of Fallot, transposition of the great arteries, tricuspid atresia, and others, are frequently significant enough to require repair during the childhood years. Women with corrected cyanotic lesions often tolerate pregnancy well, although careful observation for and management of dysrhythmias, heart failure, thromboembolism, and pulmonary hypertension are essential.

Cardiac Disease Arising During Pregnancy

Peripartum Cardiomyopathy

Peripartum cardiomyopathy (PPCM) is defined as the onset of cardiac failure in the last month of pregnancy or within 5 months postpartum in patients with no identifiable cause and no known heart disease.[33,52,53] The etiology is unknown, although multiple hypotheses have been proposed, including viral myocarditis, immune-mediated injury, selenium deficiency, the cardiac stress of pregnancy, and myocarditis. PPCM has been associated with older maternal age, obesity, African descent, multiparity, infectious diseases, autoimmune diseases, cesarean section, use of tocolytic therapy, and hypertensive disease.[33,38,53] Symptoms and management of peripartum cardiomyopathy are similar to those seen with classic heart failure. Management is typically accomplished with preload optimization, afterload reduction, and inotropic support. Unique to pregnancy is the inability to provide afterload reduction with angiotensin-converting enzyme (ACE) inhibitors. Administration of ACE inhibitors during the second and third trimesters of the antenatal period is associated with fetal renal dysfunction.[46] Indicators of overall prognosis are the severity of cardiac dysfunction at time of diagnosis and the length of time to recover baseline cardiac function.[53]

Ischemic Heart Disease

The incidence of myocardial infarction during pregnancy is increasing. Risk factors include hypertension, diabetes, advanced maternal age, thrombophilia, African-American race, hypertensive disease, postpartum hemorrhage, and blood transfusion.[38] Diagnosis and management of acute ischemic heart disease during pregnancy are similar to conventional management, with general and pharmacologic considerations for pregnancy taken into consideration.

Shock

Shock requires aggressive management of both the underlying cause and the current clinical status. Management must consider the enhanced physiologic cellular oxygen requirements during pregnancy. Therapies used are similar to conventional therapy, and practitioners must focus on maternal stabilization in order to provide an optimal uterine environment for the fetus. Special consideration should be given to fetal well-being when vasoconstrictors are employed, because uteroplacental insufficiency may result. *Abruptio placentae,* uterine rupture, *placenta previa,* and postpartum hemorrhage are examples of causes of hemorrhagic shock that are unique to pregnancy. Unique causes of septic shock in the pregnant patient include chorioamnionitis, septic abortion, and postpartum pyelonephritis.[15] Physiologic changes in pregnancy may obscure initial recognition of early sepsis; therefore, a high index of suspicion should be maintained, along with astute assessment and rapid initiation of established sepsis resuscitation guidelines.[15,38]

Cardiac Arrest

Should cardiac arrest occur during pregnancy, the primary goal is to resuscitate the mother rapidly, thereby minimizing negative fetal effects. With a viable fetus, survival and outcome of the infant are directly proportional to the interval of time between maternal death and delivery. Fetal outcomes are usually enhanced if delivery is accomplished as soon as possible, and preferably within 5 minutes of cardiac arrest.[39] Perimortem cesarean section may improve CO and actually play a role in maternal survival as well. If the fetus has not yet reached the age of viability, there is little evidence as to whether perimortem cesarean section is beneficial.

American Heart Association recommendations for basic life support for the pregnant patient include minor changes from standard procedures.[12] Ensuring venous return is essential, and can easily be accomplished through lateral displacement of the uterus. Manual uterine displacement or placement of a wedge under the woman's hip will reduce vena caval compression and facilitate venous return. The risk of complications from cardiopulmonary resuscitation, including fractured ribs or sternum, hemothorax, hemopericardium, and internal organ damage, is greater during pregnancy. There are no specific alterations of advanced life support guidelines for resuscitation during pregnancy.

Hypertensive Disease

In the obstetric population, hypertensive disease accounts for 12% to 75% of ICU admissions.[38] Whereas multifactorial in nature, the main pathophysiologic characteristic is vasospasm and vasoconstriction related to endothelial dysfunction.[14,38] Whereas historically associated with antepartum states, hypertensive disease can affect the postpartum mother as well.[54] Maternal compromise can be seen in the cardiovascular, pulmonary, renal, neurologic, and hepatic systems.[14,54] Fetal consequences include uteroplacental insufficiency, fetal growth restriction, placental abruption, or intrauterine fetal death.[14,39,49]

Classification

There are four classifications of hypertension during pregnancy. Common to the definitions are systolic BP greater than or equal to 140 mm Hg and a diastolic pressure greater than 90 mm Hg. Preeclampsia is defined as elevated BP after 20 weeks gestation with either proteinuria or any other new onset systemic finding. Severe disease criteria include BP elevations to 160 mm Hg or greater systolic and 110 mm Hg or greater diastolic, along with additional symptomatology.[8,49] The presence of seizures advances the diagnosis from preeclampsia to eclampsia. Chronic hypertension is defined as hypertension that is present prior to pregnancy, occurs before 20 weeks gestation, or persists for more than 12 weeks following delivery.[8] Gestational hypertension occurs after 20 weeks of pregnancy, but lacks the proteinuria or other systemic systems of preeclampsia. Either preeclampsia or eclampsia can be superimposed upon chronic hypertension.

Management

Hypertensive disease in pregnancy should be managed to maximize maternal and fetal outcomes. Accurate assessment of BP is paramount. Commonly used agents include beta blockers (labetalol) and/or calcium channel blockers (nifedipine), alpha-adrenergic agonists (methyldopa), and peripheral vasodilators (hydralazine).[14,39] Oral therapy is preferred, with intravenous agents being employed when required. The goal of therapy is to target a systolic pressure of less than 140 to 150 mm Hg and a diastolic pressure of less than 80 to 90 mm Hg, to reduce the risk of intracranial hemorrhage and other adverse events.[14,39] Concurrent optimization of maternal fluid status is essential, taking caution to avoid volume overload, which could lead to pulmonary edema.

In addition to BP control, continuous assessment and management of both mother and fetus should be a collaborative effort between obstetric and critical care practitioners. Ongoing assessment of cardiovascular, pulmonary, renal, and neurologic systems provides early indications of potential maternal complications secondary to hypertension. Ongoing monitoring of fetal well-being is required, and is accomplished through fetal monitoring, biophysical profile assessment, and fetal lung maturity testing through amniocentesis. Management strategies include bedrest, seizure prevention, and delivery. Bedrest reduces the mother's oxygen demand, allowing for fetal oxygenation. Seizure prevention and management are essential therapy components.

Magnesium sulfate is the mainline therapy in the obstetric population, rather than anticonvulsant therapies, because of the vasospastic nature of the disease. Magnesium decreases neuromuscular irritability, decreases cardiac conduction, and decreases central nervous system irritability. Magnesium infusions of 1 to 2 g/hour are given following a loading bolus dose of 4 to 6 g, in order to achieve serum magnesium levels of 4 to 7 mEq/L. Ongoing assessment during magnesium therapy includes monitoring of BP, heart rate, respiratory rate, urine output, and deep tendon reflexes. Anticonvulsants such as phenytoin (Dilantin) may be indicated if magnesium is ineffective or cannot be tolerated. The ultimate management strategy is delivery of the fetus.

Complications

Complications of hypertensive disease include stoke; *h*emolysis, *e*levated *l*iver enzymes, and *l*ow *p*latelet count (HELLP) syndrome; and disseminated intravascular coagulation (DIC). The presence of hypertensive disease increases stroke risk 5.2 times; women with other traditional stroke risk factors are at even higher risk.[40] HELLP syndrome is a cluster of symptoms reflecting the negative impact of arteriolar vasospasms. Vasospasm causes red blood cell hemolysis. Liver dysfunction causes elevated liver enzymes and platelet consumption, evidenced as thrombocytopenia. Management of HELLP syndrome is supportive, with delivery of the fetus being definitive therapy. There is ongoing controversy regarding the role of corticosteroids in the management of HELLP syndrome.[17] Although it is associated with hypertensive disease, not all pregnant patients with HELLP syndrome will have elevated BP.[26,52] Preeclampsia, HELLP syndrome, obstetric hemorrhage, acute fatty liver of pregnancy, chorioamnionitis, septic shock, intrauterine fetal demise, and amniotic fluid embolism are all obstetric-related causes of DIC.[39] Management is similar to conventional management, with the additional caveats of treating the obstetric-specific cause, if applicable.

PULMONARY DYSFUNCTION IN PREGNANCY

Oxygen requirements are elevated during pregnancy, and, because fetal oxygenation is directly dependent on maternal oxygen supply, compromise of maternal respiratory function places both mother and fetus at risk for harm. Maternal hypoxia can be caused by various conditions, including, but not limited to, pneumonia, asthma, trauma, acute respiratory distress syndrome (ARDS), and pulmonary embolism (PE).

Mechanical Ventilation

Mechanical ventilation settings should mimic physiologic tachypnea, increased tidal volume, enhanced minute ventilation, and decreased functional residual volumes of pregnancy. $Paco_2$ less than 45 mm Hg should be maintained to both mimic physiologic changes and lower the risk of fetal acidosis.[39] Sedation and analgesia to enhance tolerance of therapy are similar to conventional therapy. The fetal impact of the sedative and analgesic agents administered must be considered; obstetric colleagues should be aware of the medications used when analyzing fetal well-being. Neuromuscular blocking agents may be required during pregnancy for facilitation of mechanical ventilation. Care providers must recognize that only skeletal muscle is affected; therefore, the uterine smooth muscle can still contract. In addition, neuromuscular blocking agents cross the placental barrier and paralyze the fetus as well. If delivery occurs, neonatal resuscitation will be required for fetal support.

Asthma

Adverse outcomes associated with asthma include preterm labor and low birth weight infants.[4,38] Approximately one-third of women will see their symptoms worsen during pregnancy. Management recommendations are similar to conventional therapies, including avoidance of triggers, monitoring of pulmonary function through peak flow or spirometry, and routine use of medications. Pharmacologic therapies such as inhaled corticosteroids, cromolyn sodium, or beta-2 agonists are considered safe during pregnancy and while breastfeeding. The ACOG recommends that pregnant women be treated with asthma medications rather than experience symptoms and exacerbations, in order to preserve adequate fetal oxygenation.[4]

Acute Respiratory Distress Syndrome

ARDS can result from a variety of conditions. Pregnancy-specific risks for acute lung injury include sepsis, hemorrhage, amniotic fluid embolism, ovarian hyperstimulation syndrome, tocolytic use, air embolism, preeclampsia, and aspiration.[38] However, regardless of whether the cause of ARDS is unique to pregnancy or is seen in the general population, management is similar to conventional therapy, with the addition of the pregnancy-specific pulmonary management considerations mentioned previously.[51] Caution must be used to avoid significant hypercarbia, because of the normal respiratory alkalosis of pregnancy. Prone therapy can be accomplished during the antenatal period, if indicated.

Pulmonary Embolism

Pulmonary embolism (PE) is one of the leading causes of maternal death, and is linked to the incidence of venous thromboembolism.[39] Obstetric patients are at risk for PE during pregnancy and in the immediate postpartum period from emboli in the legs or pelvis due to the hypercoagulable state and impaired venous return. Presentation and diagnosis of PE are similar to those in nonpregnant patients, although practitioners must have a high index of suspicion. Management is accomplished with standard supportive care, anticoagulation, or temporary vena caval filters.

Amniotic Fluid Embolism/Anaphylactoid Syndrome of Pregnancy

Amniotic fluid embolism (AFE), also known as anaphylactoid syndrome of pregnancy, is a highly catastrophic condition that typically occurs within 24 hours of delivery.[38] Whereas the mechanisms are not clearly understood, and range from amniotic fluid/vasoactive substances being released into the maternal circulation to an anaphylactoid reaction, acute ventilatory and cardiac failure are the hallmark features.[32,51] Total cardiovascular collapse, seizures, and DIC may rapidly follow. Diagnosis is essentially clinical, made on the basis of the clinical presentation of a woman presenting with profound shock, cardiovascular collapse, and severe respiratory distress while in labor or shortly after delivery. Management requires aggressive airway management, oxygenation, cardiovascular support with fluids and inotropic therapy, rapid delivery, and correction of coagulopathies. Fortunately, the incidence is low, with a range of 1 in 8000 to 1 in 80,000 deliveries, and mortality rates between 26% and 80%.[13,32,38]

ACUTE FATTY LIVER OF PREGNANCY

Acute fatty liver of pregnancy (AFLP) occurs rarely, with an incidence of approximately 1 in 12,000 births.[13] AFLP most likely occurs because of an enzyme deficiency that increases levels of long chain fatty acids, causing hepatic overload and hepatotoxicity. Women may present with the following signs and symptoms: abdominal pain, fatigue, nausea, or vomiting. Unfortunately, these symptoms can be easily overlooked; therefore, jaundice, altered mentation, hepatic encephalopathy, or hypoglycemia are sometimes the initial presenting symptoms. As the disease progresses, renal failure, acidosis, and coagulopathies ensue. Frequently, AFLP is associated with hypertensive diseases or HELLP syndrome. Diagnosis is confirmed by liver biopsy. Management includes delivery, which stops the overload of long chain fatty acids, and appropriate supportive therapies.[13]

TRAUMA IN PREGNANCY

Trauma in pregnancy requires systematic evaluation and collaborative management from the interprofessional team in an effort to optimize maternal and fetal outcomes. Traumatic injury is estimated to complicate 1 in 12 pregnancies, and is the leading nonobstetrical cause of maternal death.[31,45,51] Trauma places the mother and fetus at risk for maternal or fetal injury or death, premature rupture of membranes, preterm birth, spontaneous abortion, and uterine rupture. Management of pregnant trauma patients is essentially identical to management of nonpregnant patients, with some specific considerations. This section will briefly review types of trauma in pregnancy and highlight gestational considerations and management strategies.

Causes/Types/Incidence

Motor vehicle crashes are the leading cause of trauma in pregnancy.[35] Strain placed on the uterus from either initial direct force or a *coup-contrecoup* injury significantly increases the risk of placental abruption.[31,45] Falls and slips occur easily during pregnancy, especially in the third trimester, and are attributed primarily to weight gain and the physiologic changes in joint stability. Assaults or intentional trauma account for approximately 18% of trauma during pregnancy, and are most typically related to domestic or intimate partner violence.[31,51] Burns are rare during pregnancy; however, significant maternal and fetal mortality are associated with body surface area injury greater than 40% to 50%.[31,45] Other assorted causes such as electrocution, poisoning, suicide, and penetrating trauma have been reported. Of special interest to the interprofessional team is the finding that splenic and retroperitoneal injury and hematomas occur more frequently in pregnant women with any type of blunt trauma, due to the normal increased vascularity of pregnancy.[31]

Gestational Considerations

Prior to fetal viability, efforts should be focused on maternal stabilization. The impact of blunt trauma on the fetus is directly related to gestational age and the location of the uterus in the abdomen. Before 13 weeks, the uterus (and therefore the fetus) is fairly well protected by pelvis, so injury is less common.[31] Once the uterus begins to ascend into the abdominal cavity, the fetus may be afforded some protection from the uterine wall and the amniotic fluid, but becomes more vulnerable. Once past 10 to 20 weeks of gestation, the gravid uterus can induce significant vena caval compression, so uterine displacement is recommended.[31,45] Alleviation of vena caval compression can be accomplished through either a maternal lateral tilt or manual uterine displacement.

Management

Fetal outcomes are correlated with early and aggressive maternal resuscitation; the primary management goal of trauma during pregnancy is to stabilize the mother. If delivery is clinically warranted, it should not be delayed with the hopes of improving outcomes.[45] Initial management of the pregnant trauma patient includes the primary survey, which should include uterine displacement and initiation of electronic fetal monitoring as soon as possible, because it can serve as an early warning sign of decreased maternal circulation.[31,51] Secondary assessment should include appropriate diagnostic studies with fetal shielding if able, and ultrasound examination to assess abdominal injury and fetal viability. The Focused Assessment with Sonography for Trauma (FAST) examination is as useful during pregnancy as it is in nonpregnant patients.[45,51] Secondary survey should include comprehensive obstetric assessment.

There are also some unique management considerations during pregnancy. Assessment findings may be altered, and signs and symptoms may be in alternate locations or masked due to the normal physiologic changes of pregnancy. Airway management may be more difficult, due to the higher risk of aspiration. Placement of chest tubes may require insertion one or two intercostal spaces above the usual landmarks.[45] Volume resuscitation should take into consideration the normal hypervolemic state of pregnancy. Displacement of the gravid uterus is essential to avoid vena caval compression. In situations of major trauma in Rh-negative mothers, the Kleihauer-Betke (KB) test can be used to calculate the total required dose of Rh immune globulin to protect the mother from fetal blood. A 300 mcg dose of Rh immune globulin will protect the mother against 30 mL of fetal blood exposure.[35,45,51] Vaginal birth can be safely accomplished following pelvic fracture.[45]

Placental abruption is the major complication that is feared following abdominal trauma. Because ultrasound cannot necessarily exclude the presence of abruption, electronic fetal monitoring is a mainstay of maternal and fetal assessment following trauma. Continuous fetal monitoring is recommended for women at 23 weeks or more of gestation. There is a lack of consensus regarding the recommended time frame for electronic fetal monitoring; 4 to 48 hours has been documented, but authorities recommend a minimum of 4 to 6 hours posttrauma, discontinuing after 4 hours if contractions are occurring less than every 10 minutes, the fetal tracing is reassuring, and the mother reports no abdominal pain or bleeding.[31,35,51] In situations of maternal arrest, perimortem cesarean section may be required. As previously discussed, delivery should be initiated within 4 minutes of maternal cardiac arrest, with delivery of fetus occurring within 5 minutes.

CONCLUSION

Caring for the critically ill obstetric patient presents unique challenges to critical care practitioners. Optimizing care for the mother and the fetus requires interprofessional collaboration between the critical care and obstetrics teams and a conscious assessment of the risk/benefit ratio of the impact of all interventions or medications on both mother and fetus. Maternal assessment and management must be undertaken with constant consideration of the physiologic alterations that occur during pregnancy. Immediate access to obstetric colleagues is essential. The interprofessional team should continually focus on the maternal-fetal relationship, with the goal of optimizing maternal status so as to provide an optimal *in utero* environment for the fetus. Obstetric patients may require critical care services during pregnancy because of preexisting disease, critical illness, or injury that arises during pregnancy. Each interaction brings unique challenges, but is also an opportunity for expert collaboration to optimize outcomes for the maternal-family experience.

CASE STUDY 34.1

M.P. is a 36-year-old *primigravida* at 32 weeks gestation. M.P.'s husband brought her to the hospital due to a severe headache and epigastric discomfort. He relates that M.P. threw up a couple of times and has been acting "weird." Admission vital signs included a temperature of 36.8°C, pulse rate of 96, respiratory rate of 22, and BP of 184/112 mm Hg. An indwelling urinary catheter was placed, and returned 40 mL of dark urine. An intravenous infusion of normal saline was initiated. M.P. was given a 500 mL bolus, and that was followed by an infusion of 150 mL/h. M.P. was not experiencing any contractions, and the electronic fetal heart rate (FHR) tracing revealed a rate of 170 with minimal variability.

Within the next hour, M.P. experienced a full-blown *grand mal* seizure lasting 90 seconds. During the seizure, the FHR dropped to 70. Following the seizure, M.P. was unresponsive and pulseless.

Decision Point:

Prior to the seizure, what initial stabilization measures should be taken?

Decision Point:

What is the significance of the FHR tracing?

Decision Point:

After the seizure, what are the current management priorities?

REFERENCES

1. American College of Obstetricians and Gynecologists. (2004). Guidelines for Diagnostic Imaging During Pregnancy: ACOG Committee Opinion No. 299. *Obstet Gynecol, 104,* 647–651.
2. American College of Obstetricians and Gynecologists. (2004). Pain Relief During Labor: ACOG Committee Opinion No. 295. *Obstet Gynecol, 104,* 213.
3. American College of Obstetricians and Gynecologists. (2006). *ACOG Practice Bulletin #76: postpartum hemorrhage.* Volume 108, No 4. Washington, DC: ACOG.
4. American College of Obstetricians and Gynecologists. (2008). *ACOG Practice Bulletin #90: asthma in pregnancy.* Volume 111, No 2, Part 1. Washington, DC: ACOG.
5. American College of Obstetricians and Gynecologists. (2009). *ACOG Practice Bulletin #100: critical Care in pregnancy.* Volume 113, No 2, Part 1. Washington, DC: ACOG.
6. American College of Obstetricians and Gynecologists. (2009). *ACOG Practice Bulletin #106: intrapartum fetal heart rate monitoring: nomenclature, interpretation, and general management principles.* Volume 114, No 1. Washington, DC: ACOG.
7. American College of Obstetricians and Gynecologists. (2011). *ACOG Practice Bulletin #123: thromboembolism in pregnancy.* Volume 118, No 3. Washington, DC: ACOG.
8. American College of Obstetricians and Gynecologists. (2013). Hypertension in pregnancy. Report of the American College of Obstetricians and Gynecologists Task Force on hypertension in pregnancy. *Obstet Gynecol, 122*(5), 1122–1131.
9. American College of Obstetricians and Gynecologists. (2013). Update on immunization and pregnancy: tetanus, diphtheria and pertussis vaccination: ACOG Committee Opinion No. 566. *Obstet Gynecol, 121,* 1411–1414.
10. American College of Obstetricians and Gynecologists. (2014). Influenza vaccination during pregnancy: ACOG Committee Opinion No. 608. *Obstet Gynecol, 124,* 648–651.
11. American College of Obstetricians and Gynecologists. (2014). Preparing for clinical emergencies in obstetrics and gynecology. ACOG Committee Opinion No. 590. *Obstet Gynecol, 123,* 722–725.
12. American Heart Association. (2011). *Advanced cardiovascular life support provider manual.* Dallas, TX: American Heart Association.
13. Anthony, J. (2011). Critical care of the obstetric patient. In D. James, P. Steer, P. Weiner, & B. Gonik (Eds.), *High Risk Pregnancy.* (Chapter 78). Philadelphia: Saunders.
14. Arulkumaran, N., & Lightstone, L. (2013). Severe pre-eclampsia and hypertensive crises. *Best Pract Res Clin Obstet Gynaecol, 27,* 877–884.
15. Arulkumaran, N., & Singer, M. (2013). Puerperal sepsis. *Best Pract Res Clin Obstet Gynaecol, 27,* 893–902. http://dx.doi.org/10.1016/j.bpobgyn.2013.07.004.
16. Baird, S., & Graves, C. (2015). REACT: an interprofessional education and safety program to recognize and manage the compromised obstetric patient. *J Perinat Neonatal Nurs, 29*(2), 138–148.
17. Basaran, A., Basaran, M., Basaran, B., Sen, C., & Martin, J. (2015). Controversial clinical practices for patients with preeclampsia or HELLP syndrome: a survey. *J Perinat Med, 43*(1), 61–66.
18. Behling, D., & Renaud, M. (2015). Development of an obstetric vital sign alert to improve outcomes in acute care obstetrics. *Nurs Womens Health, 19*(2), 128–141.
19. Blackburn, S. (2012). *Maternal, fetal and neonatal physiology: a clinical perspective* (4th ed.). Philadelphia: Saunders Elsevier.
20. Blackburn, S. (2014). Physiologic changes of pregnancy. In K. Simpson, & P. Creehan (Eds.), *Perinatal nursing* (4th ed.). Philadelphia: Wolters Kluwer/Lippincott Williams & Wilkins.
21. Cabero, L., & Chervenak, F. (2015). Maternal mortality: an ongoing challenge to perinatal medicine. *J Perinat Med, 43*(1), 1–3. http://dx.doi.org/10.1515/jpm-2014-0367.
22. Carle, C., Alexander, P., Columb, M., & Johal, J. (2013). Design and internal validation of an obstetric early warning score: secondary analysis of the intensive care national audit and research centre case mix programme database. *Anaesthesia, 68,* 354–367. http://dx.doi.org/10.1111/anae.12180.
23. Cashion, K. (2010). Maternal physiologic changes. In D. Lowdermilk, S. Perry, & K. Cashion (Eds.), *Maternity nursing* (8th ed.). St. Louis, MO: Mosby Elsevier.
24. Clark, S. (2015). Peripartum venous thromboembolism prophylaxis: where do we go from here? *Obstet Gynecol, 125*(1), 16–17.
25. Clark, S., Cotton, D., Lee, W., Bishop, C., Hill, T., & Southwick, J. (1989). Central hemodynamic assessment of normal term pregnancy. *Am J Obstet Gynecol, 161*(6), 1439–1442.
26. Clark, S., Cotton, D., Pivarnik, J., Lee, W., Hankins, G., & Benedetti, T. (1991). Position change and central hemodynamic profile during normal third-trimester pregnancy and postpartum. *Am J Obstet Gynecol, 164*(3), 883–887.
27. Creanga, A., Berg, C., Syverson, C., Seed, K., Bruce, F., & Callaghan, W. (2015). Pregnancy-related mortality in the United States, 2006–2010. *Obstet Gynecol, 125*(1), 5–12.
28. Department of Health and Human Services Food and Drug Administration. (2014). Content and format of labeling for human prescription drug and biological products; requirements for pregnancy and lactation labeling; pregnancy, lactation and reproductive potential: labeling for human prescription drug and biological products – content and format; draft guidance for industry; availability; final rule and notice. *Fed Regist*

79(233). http://www.gpo.gov/fdsys/pkg/FR-2014-12-04/pdf/2014-28241.pdf.
29. Desai, D., Moodley, J., & Naidoo, D. (2004). Echocardiographic assessment of cardiovascular hemodynamics in normal pregnancy. *Obstet Gynecol, 104*(1), 20–29.
30. Edwards, J., & Hanke, J. (2013). An update on maternal mortality and morbidity in the United States. *Nurs Womens Health, 17*(5), 376–388.
31. Foroutan, J., & Ashmead, G. (2014). Trauma in pregnancy. *Postgraduate Obstet Gynecol, 34*(14), 1–6.
32. Fox, N., Goldberg, J., & Smith, R. (2013). Critical care obstetrics. In A. DeCherney, L. Nathan, N. Laufer, & A. Roman (Eds.), *CURRENT diagnosis and treatment: obstetrics & gynecology* (11th ed.). New York: McGraw-Hill. http://accessmedicine.mhmedical.com/content.aspx?bookid:498§ionid=41008613.
33. Gaddipati, S., & Troiano, N. (2013). Cardiac disorders in pregnancy. In N. Troiano, C. Harvey, & B. Chez (Eds.), *High-risk & critical care obstetrics* (3rd ed.). Philadelphia: Wolters Kluwer/Lippincott Williams & Wilkins.
34. Gaffney, A. (2014). Critical care in pregnancy – is it different? *Semin Perinatol, 38*(6), 329–340.
35. Gianopoulos, J., & Critchlow, J. (2011). Management of the obstetrical patient in the intensive care setting. In R. Irwin, & J. Rippe (Eds.), *Irwin & Rippe's intensive care medicine* (7th ed.). Philadelphia: Lippincott Williams & Wilkins.
36. Groen, R., Bae, J., & Lim, K. (2012). Fear of the unknown: ionizing radiation exposure during pregnancy. *Am J Obstet Gynecol, 206*(6), 456–462.
37. Hill, W., & Harvey, C. (2013). Induction of labor. In N. Troiano, C. Harvey, & B. Chez (Eds.), *High-risk & critical care obstetrics* (3rd ed.). Philadelphia: Wolters Kluwer/Lippincott Williams & Wilkins.
38. Kamel, I., & Mastrogiannis, D. (2015). The critically ill obstetric patient part 1: epidemiology and pathophysiology. *Postgraduate Obstet Gynecol*, (35), 11.
39. Kamel, I., & Mastrogiannis, D. (2015). The critically ill obstetric patient part 2: management. *Postgraduate Obstet Gynecol*, (35), 12.
40. Leffert, L., Clancy, C., Bateman, B., Bryant, A., & Kuklina, E. (2015). Hypertensive disorders and pregnancy-related stroke: frequency, trends, risk factors, and outcomes. *Obstet Gynecol, 125*(1), 124–131.
41. Lowdermilk, D. (2010). Anatomy and physiology of pregnancy. In D. Lowdermilk, S. Perry, & K. Cashion (Eds.), *Maternity nursing* (8th ed.). St. Louis: Mosby Elsevier.
42. Lowdermilk, D. (2010). Nursing care of the family during pregnancy. In D. Lowdermilk, S. Perry, & K. Cashion (Eds.), *Maternity nursing* (8th ed.). St. Louis: Mosby Elsevier.
43. Lowdermilk, D. (2010). Labor and birth processes. In D. Lowdermilk, S. Perry, & K. Cashion (Eds.), *Maternity nursing* (8th ed.). St. Louis: Mosby Elsevier.
44. Lyndon, A., O'Brien-Abel, N., & Simpson, K. (2014). Fetal assessment during labor. In K. Simpson, & P. Creehan (Eds.), *Perinatal nursing* (4th ed.). Philadelphia: Wolters Kluwer/Lippincott Williams & Wilkins.
45. Mendez-Figueroa, H., Dahlke, J., Vrees, R., & Rouse, D. (2013). Trauma in pregnancy: an updated systematic review. *Am J Obstet Gynecol, 2009*(1), 1–10.
46. Merlob, P., & Weber-Schondorfer, C. (2015). Cardiovascular drugs and diuretics. In C. Schaefer (Ed.), *Drugs during pregnancy and lactation* (3rd ed.). St. Louis: Elsevier.
47. Monga, M. (2009). Maternal cardiovascular, respiratory and renal adaptation to pregnancy. In R. Creasy, R. Resnik, J. Iams, C. Lockwood, & T. Moore (Eds.), *Creasy & Resnik's maternal-fetal medicine: principles and practice* (6th ed.). Philadelphia: Saunders Elsevier.
48. Pacheco, L., Saade, G., Constantine, M., Clark, S., & Hankins, G. (2012). The role of massive transfusion protocols in obstetrics. *Am J Perinatol, 2013*(30), 1–4. http://dx.doi.org/10.1055/s-0032-1322511.
49. Pfaff, N. (2014). The new hypertensive guidelines for pregnancy: what every nurse should know. *J Perinat Neonatal Nurs, 28*(2), 91–93.
50. Reedy, N. (2014). Preterm labor and birth. In K. Simpson, & P. Creehan (Eds.), *Perinatal nursing* (4th ed.). Philadelphia: Wolters Kluwer/Lippincott Williams & Wilkins.
51. Robbins, K., Martin, S., & Wilson, W. (2014). Intensive care considerations for the critically ill parturient. In R. Creasy, R. Resnik, J. Iams, C. Lockwood, & T. Moore (Eds.), *Creasy & Resnik's maternal-fetal medicine: principles and practice* (6th ed.). Philadelphia: Saunders Elsevier.
52. Shah, S., & Rubin, S. (2012). Cardiac disease. In V. Berghella (Ed.), *Maternal-fetal evidence-based guidelines* (2nd ed.). New York: Informa Healthcare.
53. Shani, H., Kuperstein, R., Berlin, A., Arad, M., Goldenberg, I., & Simchen, M. (2015). Peripartum cardiomyopathy – risk factors, characteristics and long-term follow up. *J Perinat Med, 43*(1), 95–101.
54. Sibai, B. (2012). Etiology and management of postpartum hypertension-preeclampsia. *Am J Obstet Gynecol, 102*(1), 181–192. http://dx.doi.org/10.1016/j.ajog.2011.09.002.
55. Tillett, J. (2015). Medication use during pregnancy and lactation: the new FDA drug labeling. *J Perinat Neonatal Nurs, 29*(2), 97–99.

SUGGESTED READINGS

Anthony, J. (2011). Chapter 78. Critical care of the obstetric patient. In D. James, P. Steer, P. Weiner, & B. Gonik (Eds.), *High risk pregnancy*. Philadelphia: Saunders.

Engstrom, A., & Lindberg, I. (2013). *Critical care nurses' experiences of nursing mothers in an ICU after complicated childbirth.*

Gaffney, A. (2014). Critical care in pregnancy – is it different? *Semin Perinatol* (38), 329–340.

Robbins, K., Martin, S., & Wilson, W. (2014). Chapter 77. Intensive care considerations for the critically ill parturient. In R. Creasy, R. Resnik, J. Iams, C. Lockwood, & T. Moore (Eds.), *Creasy & Resnik's maternal-fetal medicine: principles and practice* (6th ed.). Philadelphia: Saunders Elsevier.

Troiano, N., Harvey, C., & Chez, B. (2013). *High-risk & critical care obstetrics* (3rd ed.). Philadelphia: Wolters Kluwer Health.

35

Caring for the Pediatric Patient in an Adult Critical Care Unit

Mary Frances Pate and Serena Phromsivarak Kelly

INTRODUCTION

This chapter is designed to be a resource for those nurses who care predominantly for critically ill adults. There is a saying that "children are not little adults." Skilled adult critical care nurses are acutely aware of this fact; especially when faced with pediatric patients admitted to the adult critical care unit. Maintaining pediatric skills and competencies becomes an ongoing challenge for adult critical care nurses when they rarely care for pediatric patients.

Critically ill children should primarily be admitted to designated pediatric critical care beds.[6,96] This goal may be difficult to achieve when there are 67,357 adult intensive care beds in the United States compared to approximately 4044 Pediatric Intensive Care Unit (PICU) beds, with the majority located in urban areas.[57,90] Whereas the reasons for admission to a PICU vary, guidelines for the development of admission and discharge criteria have been published by the American Academy of Pediatrics (AAP) in collaboration with the Society of Critical Care Medicine (SCCM), so that available beds can be optimized and care appropriate to a child's condition can be provided[96] (Box 35.1).

LEVELS OF PICU CARE

Guidelines and levels of care for PICUs were developed and represent the elements necessary to provide the highest quality of care possible.[92] Level 1 PICUs provide interprofessional care for a wide range of complex, progressive, rapidly changing medical, surgical, and traumatic disorders for pediatrics (excluding premature newborns). Level 2 PICUs care for patients who are less complex, with some units providing care for children with moderate illness severity. Level 2 PICUs may also provide stabilization to children requiring transfer a higher level of care.[92] Regardless of the level of PICU, the same standards of care must be maintained.

MODELS OF CO-RESIDENCE

In the United States, some hospitals without PICUs provide co-residence of adult and pediatric patients. These co-residential units can provide mechanical ventilation, cardiovascular monitoring, and intracranial pressure monitoring. Fewer of these types of patient care settings offer nitric oxide, hemodialysis, or hemofiltration for children. Two models regarding the co-residence of children and adults have been described in the literature: service line model and geographic model.[29]

Service Line Model

The service line model places children and adults in the same critical care unit along service lines. An example is a cardiac or trauma critical care unit where the staff cares for patients along the age continuum; or in the reverse where adults are placed in pediatric units for issues such as congenital heart disease.[29]

Geographic Model

The geographic model of co-residence intermingles adult and pediatric patients in the same general medical-surgical units.[29] Some primarily adult critical care units where children are cared for have designated pediatric areas within the unit. These areas may be decorated for the pediatric population and stocked with pediatric equipment and supplies. Other co-residential units may instead intermingle pediatric patients with adult patients while having pediatric-focused carts that can be rolled to the bedside of children who are admitted to critical care. These carts can be stocked with pediatric supplies, equipment, and pediatric reference materials.[81]

REGIONALIZATION OF CARE

In 2000, the AAP and SCCM supported the strong evidence recommending regionalized care for critically ill children. Additional studies support the view that regionalization of PICU services in large tertiary centers leads to improved health outcomes when compared to small units with limited tertiary pediatric services.[68,86]

Pediatric Intensivist Coverage

An association has been shown between improved patient outcomes and 24-hour coverage by intensivists in the PICU.[31,86] For units without pediatric intensivists, telemedicine has been implemented and allows for remote PICU management in rural or other locations that lack staffing depth.[44] The use of telemedicine to provide pediatric critical care consultation has yielded decreased mortality rates and length-of-stays comparable to admissions in tertiary PICUs with an intensivist.[69]

Tiered Care

Another solution for providing optimal pediatric critical care is organizing critical care resources in a tiered manner, following the example of trauma centers. Utilizing such a model would channel children in need of more intensive or complex services to the needed resources.[46,90]

BOX 35.1 Common Reasons for Pediatric Intensive Care Unit Admissions

- Respiratory disease processes
- Injuries (leading cause of death in children and young adults)
  - Motor vehicle injuries
  - Pedestrian injuries
  - Bicycle injuries
  - Firearms injuries
  - Nonaccidental trauma
  - Burns
- Submersion accidents
- Congenital heart defect repair
- Infectious processes/sepsis
- Diabetic ketoacidosis
- Ingestions
- Shock

Localized Community Care

Despite clinical evidence for regionalization of pediatric services and insurance plan mandates, the importance of pediatric patients remaining in local communities has been shown to be important to healthcare providers and families.[81] It is also possible that some lengthy, risky, and expensive patient and family transports can be avoided when care is provided locally. Some nontertiary hospitals are set up with the intent of transferring the more critically ill children to the regional PICUs and caring for the less acutely ill patients in their own facility. However, some of the more ill children may remain in the community hospital because of family preferences, whereas children not acutely ill may be transferred to regional tertiary center PICUs, again because of family preference.[69] The development of clear transfer guidelines can assist healthcare providers in the decision-making process of whether or not to transfer pediatric patients to tertiary care centers; patients transferred to PICUs from referring hospitals are often more acutely ill than those transferred from within the same institution to the PICU.[54] Tools such as the Pediatric Early Warning System (PEWS)[101] or Pediatric Advanced Warning Score (PAWS)[17] may be useful in evaluating patients who may be deteriorating.

STANDARDIZING CARE FOR CHILDREN

It is essential that institutions caring for children require pediatric-specific competency validation for all disciplines involved. Pediatric-specific policies, procedures, standards, and protocols can be developed or pediatric-specific information can be integrated into existing adult documents (Box 35.2). Pediatric procedure books and pediatric-specific standards have been developed by the American Association of Critical-Care Nurses (AACN) and the SCCM, and can be used to guide practice.

Ensuring that the entire health system is child-ready can be challenging to implement. In 1993, the AAP and SCCM codeveloped the original *Guidelines and Levels of Care for Pediatric Intensive Care Units*[10] and updated them in 2004.[92] The guidelines are helpful to PICUs in determining the scope of care to pediatric patients, organizational and administrative structures, hospital facilities and services, personnel needs, medications and equipment needs, quality monitoring, and educational needs. Although these guidelines were not written for units without distinct, separate PICUs, they may be helpful for those facilities with small inpatient pediatric populations.[24] Pediatric care considerations are provided in Table 35.1.

BOX 35.2 Admission of the Child to the Adult Critical Care Unit

- Obtain report from emergency department/transport team/acute care floor/other
- Notify interprofessional team
  1. Pediatric respiratory therapist for supplemental oxygen/ventilatory support
  2. Pediatric pharmacist so that medications, maintenance intravenous fluids, vasoactive, analgesic, and anxiolytic drips will be set up and ready to start upon arrival to unit
  3. Child life therapy/pediatric-specific social worker/chaplain to assist with family support
  4. Provider upon patient admission
- Bedside setup
  1. Infusion pumps including syringe pumps with the ability to administer small fluid volumes down to 0.5 mL/h
  2. Pressure tubing for transduced lines
  3. Isolation room/equipment if appropriate
  4. Pediatric-focused documentation
  5. Weight-specific resuscitation medication resources
  6. Cardiorespiratory monitor with pediatric mode activated (i.e., adult/pediatric/neonatal)
- Age/size-specific equipment (as needed)
  1. Resuscitation equipment (defibrillator, code cart, bag and mask)
  2. Electrocardiogram leads
  3. Gown
  4. Diapers
  5. Crib/bed (if scale in bed, zero with linens)
  6. Chest tubes
  7. Foley catheter
  8. Blood pressure cuff
  9. Intravenous catheters
  10. Pulse oximetry probes
  11. Central venous line tray
  12. Pediatric laboratory tubes
  13. Suction catheters/bulb syringes/oral suction
  14. Cervical spine collar (if prehospital collar improperly fitted)

Standardizing Documentation Across the Institution

Pediatric-specific documentation in areas caring for children will also be needed and may be able to be integrated into preexisting adult-focused documentation. An admission database that addresses the pediatric patient's development is essential. This document should include the child's regular routine, food preferences, and comfort items. When normal routines are altered, the child can feel a loss of control and have decreased coping skills. Children may also regress from previously achieved milestones during times of acute/chronic illness.

Standardized Equipment

It is important that all areas of the hospital where children will receive treatment have child-appropriate equipment, resuscitation resources, and clinical services available (e.g., surgery, post anesthesia care unit, radiology, emergency department). Pediatric equipment should be standardized across the institution for safety to include resuscitation equipment and intravenous pumps that can deliver volumes less than 1 mL/hour. Having child-safe hospital beds available to accommodate infants, toddlers, and preschoolers is imperative (Fig. 35.1). Dietary and nutrition services will need to be competent in pediatric diets and nutrition. Blood banks should have the ability to have blood products available in aliquots for the

TABLE 35.1 Pediatric Care Considerations

Focus	Intervention	Rationale
Respiratory Considerations		
Smaller upper and lower airways	In the trauma patient, open the airway using the jaw-thrust maneuver. Repositioning often may be the only intervention needed to maintain a patent airway.	Foreign matter such as blood, mucus, vomit, and teeth easily obstruct small airways. Small amounts of edema can obstruct the airway, markedly increasing airway resistance.
Tongue is larger relative to oropharynx	Oropharyngeal airways can be used in the unresponsive child.	In the trauma patient, open the airway using the jaw-thrust maneuver. Repositioning often may be the only intervention needed to maintain a patent airway.
Cartilage of the larynx is softer	Place child in *sniffing* position with chin-lift maneuver. Use jaw-thrust in the trauma patient.	Hyperextension or hyperflexion of the neck can compress and obstruct the airway.
Larger head/body ratio	Place a small towel roll under the child's shoulders to maintain the sniffing position.	Neck may be in flexion when the child is immobilized on a backboard.
Infants are obligate nose breathers for the first several months of life	Suction nares frequently. Nasopharyngeal airway may be placed.	Obstructed nasal passages can produce significant respiratory distress in the infant.
Larynx is positioned more anteriorly and cephalad	The once recommended use of cricoid pressure to compress the esophagus against the spine during bag-mask ventilation to help prevent gastric insufflation and aspiration is no longer used in the pediatric patient.	There is an increased risk of aspiration. Direct visualization of the vocal cords is more difficult during intubation.
Shorter tracheal length	Pay meticulous attention to initial endotracheal tube position (centimeter mark at the gum). Perform recurrent reassessment of tube placement with post intubation chest x-ray films. Maintain head in midline position and prevent extension or flexion of the neck.	There is an increased chance of mainstem intubation. Changes in head position will cause movement in the endotracheal tube. Flexion of the neck displaces the tube farther into the trachea, and extension of the neck moves the tube farther out of the trachea.
Cricoid cartilage is the narrowest portion of the airway	In the in-hospital setting a cuffed endotracheal tube is as safe as an uncuffed tube for children beyond the newborn period. Cuff pressures should be less than 20 cm H_2O.	Cricoid ring provides a natural seal for the endotracheal tube. Cuffed tubes with high pressure may cause airway damage in younger children.
Cartilaginous ribs of the infant and small child are twice as compliant as those of an adult	Closely observe the child with continuous monitoring of heart rate, respiratory rate and effort, and pulse oximetry. Deliver highest possible concentration of oxygen to infants and children in respiratory distress. Provide nonthreatening environment and avoid noxious stimuli. Allow alert child to maintain own position of comfort to optimize respiratory effort. Allow parents to remain with child if their presence is comforting to the child.	Retractions are more common and reduce the infant's or small child's ability to maintain functional residual capacity or generate adequate tidal volume.
Intercostal muscles are poorly developed	If possible, maintain patient in upright position to support diaphragmatic function. Avoid abdominal distention by inserting a nasogastric or orogastric tube to decompress the stomach.	Generation of tidal volume depends on diaphragmatic function. Anything impeding diaphragm movement can lead to respiratory failure.
The child's respiratory system has less compensatory reserve than the adult's respiratory system	Closely observe the child with continuous monitoring of heart rate, respiratory rate and effort, and pulse oximetry. Deliver highest possible concentration of oxygen in a nonthreatening manner. Consider blood gas analysis.	The younger child may develop respiratory distress and failure more rapidly than an adult.
Infants with respiratory distress often grunt during exhalation	Provide high concentration of supplemental oxygen and consider ventilatory support.	Grunting is a result of premature glottic closure during exhalation. Infants grunt to increase airway pressure, lung volume, and functional residual capacity.
Infants and small children have less elastic and collagen tissue in their lungs	Maintain high index of suspicion for pneumothorax, pneumomediastinum, and pulmonary edema. Obtain chest radiograph as necessary.	Liquid or air can enter an infant's pulmonary interstitium more easily than in the older child or adult, making the infant more susceptible to air leaks and edema.
Infants and small children have thin chest walls	Frequently reassess bilateral breath sounds with side-by-side comparison of difference in pitch and intensity. Breath sounds should be auscultated over the anterior and posterior chest wall and in the axillary areas using a pediatric stethoscope. Obtain chest x-ray films as necessary.	Breath sounds are easily transmitted across the chest wall and over the abdomen.
The ventilated child	Noninvasive ventilation may be an option for some pediatric patients (e.g., cystic fibrosis, musculoskeletal disease) and should be considered first. When conventional ventilation is used, tidal volume may escape around an uncuffed ETT, so the lowest effective tidal volume should be used. Suction catheters should not touch mucosa or the carina, so the end of the catheter should not extend more than 0.5 cm past the end of the ETT. Suctioning and instillation of normal saline should not be performed on a routine basis, but individualized according to patient assessment. Suction settings should be set between 80 and 120 cm H_2O.[83]	Lower tidal volumes, low suction settings, individualized suctioning, and premeasured suction depths prevent barotrauma.

TABLE 35.1 Pediatric Care Considerations—cont'd

Focus	Intervention	Rationale
Circulatory Considerations		
Myocardium is less compliant and has less contractile tissue compared with that of an adult	Provide continuous ECG monitoring with attention to trends in heart rate. Tachycardia is the earliest clinical manifestation in compensated shock, but it also may be a result of anxiety, pain, fever, or increased activity. If other signs of compensated shock are present (delayed capillary refill time, cool extremities, duskiness or mottling of the skin, diminished peripheral pulses, narrowing pulse pressure, tachypnea), rapid intravenous access is established and fluid resuscitation is initiated.	Stroke volume is not easily adjusted; therefore children increase their heart rate in response to falling cardiac output.
Infants and children have a smaller overall blood volume	Carefully estimate blood loss, including blood drawn for laboratory analysis. Serial hemoglobin and hematocrit analysis should be obtained as necessary.	Although the child's circulating blood volume is greater per kilogram of body weight compared with an adult (child 80 mL/kg versus adult 70 mL/kg), the circulating volume is significantly less. Smaller amounts of blood loss can cause volume depletion.
Most dysrhythmias are clinically insignificant in the pediatric patient and do not require treatment	Provide continuous ECG monitoring. Establish and maintain patent airway	Bradycardia and SVT are the two most common significant dysrhythmias in children.
Bradycardia is the most common terminal cardiac rhythm in children, whereas ventricular tachycardia or ventricular fibrillation is the usual terminal rhythm in the adult	Provide adequate oxygenation and ventilation. Establish intravenous access. If severe cardiorespiratory compromise (as evidenced by poor perfusion, respiratory distress, or hypotension) is present, follow the PALS guidelines for bradycardia or tachycardia with poor perfusion.	Bradycardia is often a result of hypoxia and is not well tolerated in children because it significantly reduces cardiac output. SVT usually is well tolerated in infants and children, but can lead to cardiovascular collapse.
A greater percentage of total body weight is water in infants and children	Calculate maintenance fluids based on each child's weight in kilograms and clinical condition.	Infants and young children will lose larger amounts of water through evaporation than will the adult.
There is a larger surface area/volume ratio	Record all sources of fluid intake and fluid loss to calculate fluid balance and adjust fluid therapy accordingly.	Children have greater potential for dehydration. Maintenance fluid requirements per kilogram of body weight are higher in children.
Infants and children have smaller, more difficult to cannulate veins	Establish a protocol that addresses obtaining intravenous and intraosseous access in critically ill or injured children utilizing PALS guidelines.	Rapid establishment of intravenous access is more difficult in infants and children.
Neurologic Considerations		
The head of the infant and young child is larger and heavier in proportion to the rest of the body	Anticipate head injury in the traumatically injured child. Suggest use of stress preventive measures, such as seat belts, car seats, and helmets, to patients and family members.	If an infant or child falls or is thrown a significant distance, the initial impact more often will be to the head, which predisposes the child to head injury.
The skull is thinner during infancy and childhood	Anticipate head injury in the traumatically injured child. Suggest use of stress preventive measures, such as seat belts, car seats, and helmets, to patients and family members.	The thin skull provides less protection for the brain. Head trauma can result in severe brain injury in children.
Cranial sutures do not fuse until approximately age 16 to 18 months	Measure occipital frontal circumference with neurologic examinations in the child up to age 16 to 18 months at risk for increasing intracranial pressure.	If intracranial volume increases during this time, head circumference may increase. The ability to expand may better accommodate gradual increases in intracranial volume than in an adult. Increased intracranial pressure may still develop, especially with acute increase in intracranial volume.
Anterior and posterior fontanelles are open in infants	Assess fontanelles for size and tension in the infant age 16 to 18 months or younger.	The anterior fontanelle is the junction of the coronal-sagittal and frontal bones and does not close until age 16 to 18 months. The posterior fontanelle is the junction of the parietal and occipital bones and closes at approximately age 2 months. The fontanelles will be tense or bulging in the event of increased intracranial pressure and will be sunken if the infant is dehydrated.
Spinal cord injuries are less common in the pediatric trauma patient than in the adult trauma patient	Children with head and/or neck injuries should be presumed to have a spinal cord injury until proven otherwise. Stabilize and immobilize the cervical spine with a hard cervical collar, long spine board, and a commercial immobilization device or foam blocks, rolled towel, and tape. Remember, the child's prominent occiput places the neck in flexion when lying flat on a spine board. Place padding under the child's torso to elevate it approximately 2 cm, bringing the head into neutral position.	The child's spine, especially the cervical spine, is more elastic and mobile. When a child sustains a spinal cord injury, it is often present without radiographic abnormality; described as spinal cord injury without radiographic abnormality.

Continued

TABLE 35.1 Pediatric Care Considerations—cont'd

Focus	Intervention	Rationale
Musculoskeletal Considerations		
Children's bones are more flexible because of incomplete bone calcification	Suspect injury to internal structures underlying fractures and areas subjected to significant forces as evidenced by contusions, swelling, and tenderness. Obtain surgical consultation as necessary. Monitor for signs of internal hemorrhage: decreasing level of consciousness, poor peripheral perfusion, decreased urinary output, tachycardia, tachypnea, and narrowing pulse pressure. Obtain hemoglobin and hematocrit analysis as necessary.	Significant force generally is necessary to break children's bones. Underlying injury may be present without fracture.
There is increased elasticity and compliance of the chest wall because the ribs and sternum are more cartilaginous in infants and young children	Suspect pneumothoraces and/or hemothoraces in the child who has significant chest trauma with or without rib fractures. Monitor respiratory effort and oxygen saturation. Obtain chest radiograph as necessary. Be prepared for needle thoracostomy or chest tube insertion in the event of a tension pneumothorax.	There is a low incidence of rib or sternal fractures in children. Increased chest wall compliance allows traumatic forces to be transmitted to underlying thoracic structures. Pneumothorax is the most common result of thoracic trauma in children and may be more likely to progress to a tension pneumothorax because of the increased mobility of the mediastinal structures.
Abdominal muscles are less developed in children	Obtain surgical consultation as necessary. Monitor for signs of shock secondary to internal hemorrhage. Obtain serial abdominal girth measurements. Follow serial hemoglobin and hematocrit analysis.	Children are at an increased risk of sustaining abdominal injuries. The spleen and the liver are the most commonly injured abdominal organs in children.
Pseudosubluxation of C2 on C3	Maintain cervical spine immobilization and suspect spinal cord injury in any child with head and neck injuries. Perform thorough serial neurologic examination. Do not rule out cervical spine injury on the basis of negative radiographic studies only. Obtain neurosurgical consultation.	Seen in up to 40% of children age less than 7 years and in less than or equal to 20% of children age less than 16 years. This is a normal variation caused by increased ligamentous laxity.
Metabolic and Thermoregulatory Considerations		
Infants and young children have a larger body surface area/body mass ratio, and less insulating subcutaneous tissue and fat stores	Monitor temperature frequently. Cover children with warm blankets or place them under warming lights if they cannot be covered. Use warmed intravenous fluids or blood for volume resuscitation. Warm and humidify supplemental oxygen if possible. Place warming pads (such as K pads) or chemically activated warming devices (such as portable warmers) under children. Follow manufacturer's directions for the use of these devices.	A large amount of heat is lost to the environment through radiation and evaporation, especially from the child's proportionally large head. Infants and children can easily become hypothermic. Hypothermia can cause metabolic acidosis, hypoglycemia, coagulopathies, central nervous system depression, respiratory depression, and myocardial irritability, making resuscitation more difficult.
Infants younger than 3 months old cannot produce heat by shivering and must burn their limited fat stores for thermogenesis	Same as above. Consider placing small infants in isolettes with overbed warmers. Attach skin probe for continuous skin temperature monitoring to avoid overheating and thermal injury.	There is an increased risk of hypothermia in the small infant. The burning of fat increases oxygen consumption, which can lead to hypoxia.
Infants and young children have less glycogen stores than adults	Monitor glucose level frequently during and after resuscitation. Administer glucose as ordered.	The ill or injured child is at increased risk for developing hypoglycemia.
Children have higher metabolic rates than adults	Provide supplemental oxygen to all seriously ill or injured children. Consult with provider and dietitian to provide early nutritional support to the compromised child.	Higher metabolic rates increase oxygen consumption. The child's nutritional needs are higher per kilogram of body weight than an adult.
Pain Management Considerations		
Children may receive too little pain medication or none at all	Maintain awareness of misconceptions regarding pain in children and advocate, assess, and provide for evidence-based pain management.	Children express pain in a variety of ways. Younger children may not say that they are in pain because they feel the pain is punishment for misbehavior, or they may fear an injection. Older children may not admit pain in front of peers. Just because children are asleep does not mean that they are not experiencing pain.

ECG, Electrocardiogram; *ETT*, endotracheal tube; *PALS*, pediatric advanced life support, *SVT*, supraventricular tachycardia.
From References 5, 12, 33, 56, 71, and 78.

small amounts required by pediatric patients. Hospital laboratories will need equipment for testing the small volumes of blood required for pediatric laboratory samples. Pediatric-sized tubes for blood draws should be available in all areas where children are served, because minor blood losses can have a significant impact on a child. Pharmacies must ensure that medications can be delivered in the small doses needed for the pediatric population and that the pharmacists and technicians are educated to prepare and dispense medications for children.[8]

Standardizing Emergency Equipment

Infant and child resuscitation requires medication dosages that are based on the child's weight and the initiation of resuscitation is different than in an adult. In addition, cardiac compression rate and depth as well as the number of resuscitation breaths differ from an adult. Administering weight-based resuscitation medications may be made easier through the use of precalculated emergency medication resources. Software programs are available that allow emergency resources to be prepared upon the child's admission to critical care and placed at the bedside or in the electronic health record (EHR) for quick retrieval in case of deterioration in patient status. If the precalculated resources are not available, a Broselow/Luten pediatric resuscitation tape can be used as a guide (Fig. 35.2). The child is measured with the tape, and at each increment on the tape, the endotracheal tube size, precalculated medication for weight, and joules for defibrillation are noted. Products such as a Broselow/Hinkle resuscitation cart can be used in conjunction with the tape measurement (Fig. 35.3). The drawers on the resuscitation cart are color-coded to match the resuscitation tape and are stocked with equipment accordingly. Some units use the Broselow/Hinkle carts and precalculated medication sheets together. Staff members place colored dots that correspond with the color on the corresponding cart drawer on the precalculated medication resources, so the proper drawer can be retrieved in a rapid manner. Other units print precalculated emergency medication sheets on colored paper that corresponds with the correct code cart drawer so that time will not be lost in crisis situations. Table 35.2 summarizes medications for treatment of pediatric dysrhythmias and Table 35.3 summarizes medications used in nondysrhythmia emergencies.

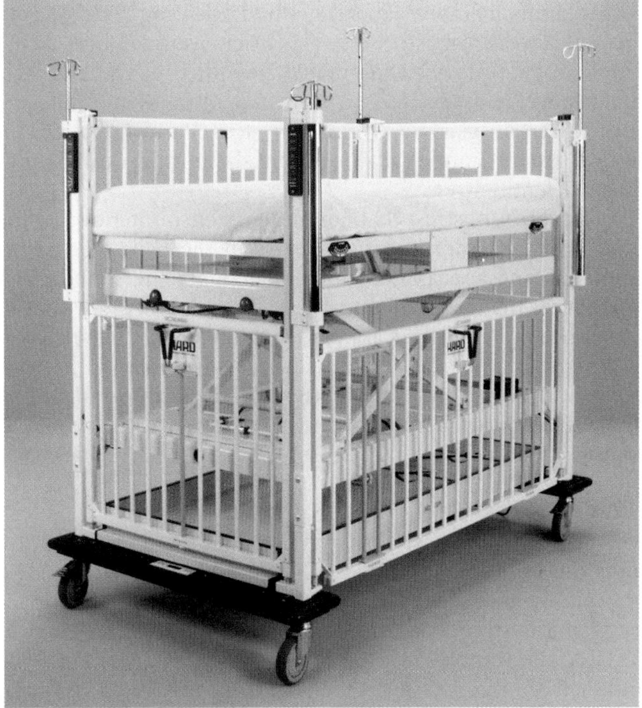

FIG. 35.1 Doernbecher critical care crib. (Courtesy Hard Manufacturing Company, Inc.)

PEDIATRIC RESUSCITATION PRIORITIES

Unlike adults, children exhibit subtle changes that must be identified early to prevent decompensation (Table 35.4). Cardiac arrest is often caused by progressive respiratory failure or shock. Basic life support sequences are dependent on the age of the victim. When children do have cardiac arrest, the American Heart Association algorithms should be followed. Continuous monitoring of a child's end-tidal carbon dioxide ($ETco_2$) can provide information about the quality of chest compressions. If $ETco_2$ is less than 10 to 15 mm Hg, this is suggestive of low cardiac output during cardiopulmonary resuscitation (CPR). Goal $ETco_2$ is greater than 10 to 15 mm Hg. A sudden increase in $ETco_2$ is suggestive of return of spontaneous circulation.

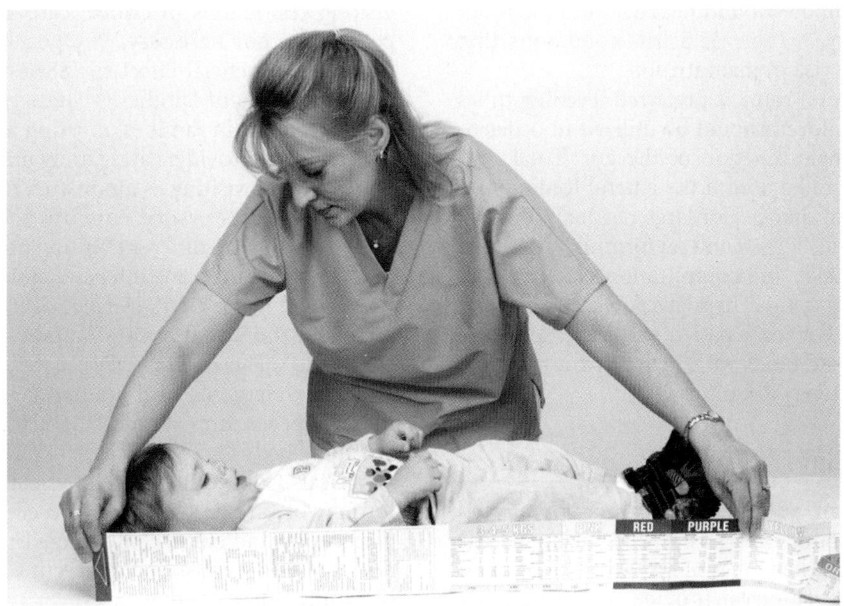

FIG. 35.2 Broselow/Luten tape. (Courtesy Armstrong Medical Industries, Inc.)

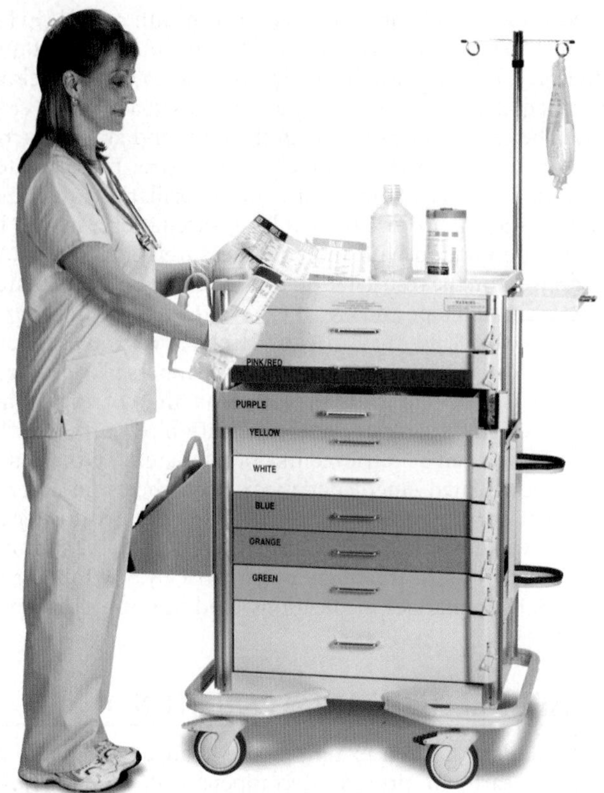

FIG. 35.3 Broselow/Hinkle cart. (Courtesy Armstrong Medical Industries, Inc.)

NUTRITION

Compared to adults, children are more vulnerable to malnutrition in the critical care unit because of increased basal energy requirements and limited nutritional reserves. Unfortunately, children may be admitted to the unit already undernourished. Without adequate nutritional support, children develop protein-calorie malnutrition within 5 to 7 days. Once the resuscitation phase of critical care has resolved, nutritional support should be initiated to promote wound healing, immune function, and overall recovery.[73] Table 35.5 lists conditions that increase pediatric patients risk of malnutrition.

As with adults, the enteral route is preferred. Feeding tubes appropriately sized for children should be utilized in order to promote normal physiologic function of the gut. Total parenteral nutrition (TPN) can be used if the enteral feedings are poorly tolerated because of diarrhea or large residuals. Careful selection of the appropriate TPN or enteral formula is essential to avoid excess protein intake and complications such as electrolyte imbalance, hyperglycemia, hypoglycemia, and fat and carbohydrate imbalances. For those patients able to take in oral nutrition, providing favorite foods with high nutritional value will increase the child's interest in eating.

CHILD AND FAMILY-CENTERED CARE

Highlighting the child's daily routine can also be accomplished by completing an "All About Me" poster that highlights the child's preferences and lists the names of his or her loved ones. Participating in poster completion can provide a needed distraction for families, especially at the time of admission to critical care. Pictures of the child and family are sometimes added to the posters, to allow healthcare providers to see "what the child was like" before the illness/injury.

It has been said that no one knows the child better than loved ones. Members of the family can serve as interpreters of the child's behaviors and symptoms. The Nursing Mutual Participation Model of Care emphasizes the family's role in caring for the child and stresses the importance of a strong partnership with the healthcare team[37,38] (Box 35.3).

Decreasing Family Stressors

The experience of having a child admitted to critical care is stressful for family members. Spending time orienting loved ones to the unit can decrease stressors. This orientation can include the purpose of monitoring equipment, the types of alarms and their significance, and reasons why staff may respond at a different pace to certain alarms.[23,24] Ensuring that alarm limits are set so they are not continually or needlessly sounding can help to decrease family stress.

Other areas of stress that families may encounter during the time in critical care include changes in the child's behavior, emotions, and appearance; unfamiliar sights and sounds; and procedures that are frightening to the child, especially ones in which needles and tubes are placed in the child. The behavior of the critical care staff and "too many people talking" has also been shown to increase family stress. Of the stressors identified by families, parental role change is the hardest with which to cope.[23,24]

Family Presence

A sound scientific basis for restricting visitors in critical care units does not exist. Families who have children admitted to critical care have identified being with their child as their priority need. In carrying out the family-centered care philosophy of AACN that promotes care that is driven by the needs of patients and their families, this need can be met through open visitation policies for all critical care patients, not only for the children. Parents should be given the option of staying to support their child even when procedures are performed, because the majority of parents desire to stay.[50] Berwick and Kotagal write that visiting restrictions in critical care are "neither caring, compassionate, nor necessary."[20] Open visitation has been found to have a beneficial effect for 88% of families and decreased anxiety in 65% of families.[20] These types of open policies also engender trust in families, creating a better working relationship between providers and family members. Adult critical care patients rated visiting as a nonstressful experience because visitors offered reassurance, comfort, and calming effects.[50] There is no need to have different visiting policies for the children and adults sharing the same intensive care unit. The AACN *Practice Alert: Family Presence During CPR and Invasive Procedures* addresses the importance of families in the critical care environment.[11] The practice alert states, "Family members of all patients undergoing cardiopulmonary resuscitation (CPR) and invasive procedures should be given the option of being present at the bedside." The Emergency Nurses Association and the American College of Chest Physicians also support this philosophy of care.[45,58] Family-centered care is an evidence-based philosophy and culture of caring. The philosophy and culture does not involve just one intervention, such as open visitation or family presence, but many.[5,39,72] A lack of family-centered care is when family and friends are referred to as "visitors,"

TABLE 35.2 Medications for Pediatric Dysrhythmias

Medication	Actions	Dosage	Special Considerations
Adenosine (Adenocard, Adenoscan)	Temporarily interrupts conduction through the AV node; Slows impulse formation in the SA node Used for treatment of supraventricular tachycardias	Initial dose: 0.1 mg/kg IV/IO (maximum dose 6 mg); if ineffective, may repeat in 1–2 minutes at 0.2 mg/kg IV/IO (maximum dose 12 mg)	RAPID IV push, followed by 5–10 mL normal saline flush via the most proximal injection site May cause temporary heart block or asystole If possible, record administration with 12-lead ECG
Amiodarone (Cordarone)	Decreases SA node function; slows conduction in the AV node Used for treatment of ventricular dysrhythmias	For pulseless rhythms: 5 mg/kg IV/IO rapid bolus (maximum bolus dose 300 mg); repeat as needed up to maximum daily dose 15 mg/kg IV/IO (2.2 g in adolescent) For SVT, VT (with pulses): 5 mg/kg load over 20–60 minutes (maximum bolus dose 300 mg); may give up to 3 doses to maximum daily dose 15 mg/kg IV/IO (2.2 g in adolescents)	Monitor QT interval Long half-life and multiple potential drug interactions, consult cardiology Give over 20–60 minutes for SVT or VT with pulses. Give rapid bolus in pulseless arrest (VF/pulseless VT)
Atropine	Competes with acetylcholine for binding sites; blocks muscarinic receptors Used for treatment of symptomatic bradycardic arrhythmias	0.02 mg/kg IV/IO; may repeat once after 5 minutes (minimum dose 0.1 mg in children with maximum single dose of 0.5 mg; maximum total child dose 1 mg; maximum adolescent dose 2 mg) 0.04 to 0.06 mg/kg ETT	
Epinephrine (1:10,000 preparation; 0.1 mg/mL or 1:1000 preparation; 1 mg/mL)	Stimulates alpha receptors to cause vasoconstriction and beta receptors to cause increased heart rate and contractility Used in the treatment of pulseless dysrhythmias and symptomatic bradycardia Repeat every 3–5 minutes as needed	0.01 mg/kg IV/IO 1:10,000 (maximum dose 1 mg) 0.1 mg/kg ETT 1:1000 preparation	Monitor blood pressure and ECG continuously
Lidocaine	Decreases automaticity in the myocardium during diastole Used for treatment of ventricular dysrhythmias	1 mg/kg IV/IO; 2–3 mg via ETT Infusion: 20–50 mcg/kg/min	Follow bolus with continuous infusion
Magnesium sulfate	Used for treatment of ventricular dysrhythmias Used in treatment of cardiac arrest when hypomagnesemia is suspected or if the dysrhythmia is torsades de pointes	25–50 mg/kg IV/IO (maximum dose: 2 g)	Usually administered over 10–20 minutes; may be given as a bolus for pulseless VT with torsades de pointes Monitor BP and ECG continuously
Procainamide	Decreases myocardial excitability, conduction velocity, and depresses contractility Used to treat atrial flutter, SVT, VT with pulses	15 mg/kg IV/IO	Give initial bolus slowly over 30–60 minutes; Monitor QT interval

AV node, Atrioventricular node; *BP*, blood pressure; *ECG*, electrocardiogram; *ETT*, endotracheal tube; *IO*, intraosseous; *SA node*, sinoatrial note; *SVT*, supraventricular tachycardia; *VF*, ventricular fibrillation; *VT*, ventricular tachycardia;.
From References 5, 12, 33, and 67.

giving them a perception of decreased significance;[94] however, it is the healthcare providers who are the visitors to the patient and family situation.

Siblings and Childhood Friends

Siblings and friends should also be allowed to visit with the pediatric patient. Before visiting, these special visitors should be screened for exposure to contagious illnesses such as chickenpox, measles, or mumps so that these illnesses are not spread to any patients or families.

Allowing siblings and young friends to visit decreases the chance that their imaginations will have them envision a reality of the hospitalized child's illness or injury that is far worse. Child life therapists (CLTs) can be an important support to siblings and friends, especially if they feel, in a real or imagined way, responsible for the illness/injury. These special visitors will need preparation before visiting the bedside to have their questions addressed.[94] After visiting the critically ill child, a debriefing may be needed by younger loved ones to address any remaining questions or concerns. CLTs are specifically educated to assist with this process.

QUALITY MONITORING

A program of performance improvement must be in place at the outset of the initiation of pediatric care to assess and improve the critical care systems and processes.[86] Taking time to assess indicators such as pain management, unplanned extubations,

TABLE 35.3 Medications Used in Nondysrhythmia Emergencies

Medication	Actions	Dosage	Special Considerations
Calcium chloride 10%	Used in the management of hyperkalemia, hypocalcemia, or calcium channel blocker toxicity	20 mg/kg IV/IO; may be repeated in 10 minutes if needed	IV/IO bolus during cardiac arrest if hypocalcemia known or suspected. Otherwise, infuse over 30–60 minutes. Monitor BP and ECG continuously Central venous administration is preferred Flush between infusing calcium and sodium bicarbonate to avoid formation of precipitate
Dextrose (Glucose)	Used in the treatment of hypoglycemic emergencies	0.5–1 g/kg IV/IO Different glucose preparations are available $D_{50}W$: usual dose 1–2 mL/kg $D_{25}W$: usual dose is 2–4 mL/kg $D_{10}W$: usual dose is 5–10 mL/kg	Maximum recommended concentration for bolus administration is $D_{25}W$ Monitor with point-of-care glucose and continuous infusion if indicated
Naloxone (Narcan)	Displaces opiates on opiate receptors in the central nervous system Used to treat narcotic toxicity, opiate-induced sedation, and respiratory depression	Total reversal: 0.1 mg/kg IV/IO/IM/subcutaneously every 2 minutes as needed up to 2 mg Reversal titrated to effect: 1 to 5 mcg/kg IV/IO/IM/subcutaneously Continuous infusion IV/IO 0.002 to 0.16 mg/kg/h (2–160 mcg/kg/h)	Dose may need to be repeated as half-life of opioid being reversed may be longer than that of naloxone
Sodium bicarbonate (8.4% injection; 1 mEq/mL 4.2% injection; 0.5 mEq/mL	Provides bicarbonate ions used to treat metabolic acidosis, severe hyperkalemia, and sodium channel blocker overdose	1 mEq/kg IV/IO (Maximum dose 50 mEq)	Give SLOWLY. 4.2% concentration recommended for infants less than 1 month of age Monitor pH and ECG

$D_{(50/25/10)}W$, Dextrose $_{(50/25/10)}$ in water; *ECG*, electrocardiogram; *ET*, endotracheal tube; *IM*, intramuscular; *IO*, intraosseous.
From References 5, 12, 33, and 67.

TABLE 35.4 Warning Signs of Potential Decompensation

System	Assessment Findings
Respiratory	Child self-positions Requires interventions (head positioning, suctioning, adjunct airways) Tachypnea* Bradycardia* Hypoxemia Hypercarbia Change in responsiveness Decreased chest movement with respiration Labored breathing, retractions, nasal flaring, grunting, head bobbing, wheezing, or stridor Decreased or absent air exchange upon auscultation
Cardiovascular	Heart rate is absent, irregular, bradycardic, or tachycardic* Blood pressure decreases (sign of late decompensation: 10 mm Hg decrease is significant) Pallor, cyanosis, mottled skin Cool extremities Diminished or absent peripheral pulses Capillary refill greater than 2 seconds despite warm ambient temperature Worried appearance Decreased urine output
Neurologic	Irritable Lethargic Obtunded or comatose Decreased or absent reaction to pain Decreased muscle tone Decreased or absent pupillary response Unequal pupils

*All vital signs must be evaluated according to individual patient's age, baseline values, and clinical condition.
From References 35, 56, 77, and 78.

and evidence-based bundles is important for maintaining quality care. Participation in national PICU databases allows caregivers to compare their outcomes to similar institutions. Regular interprofessional pediatric mortality and morbidity conferences can also provide a time for the interprofessional team to review pediatric cases and make improvements when necessary.

INFECTION PREVENTION

Healthcare-associated infections (HAI) increase mortality and morbidity and occur most in the intensive care unit setting. Patients in the ICU have increased susceptibility to infection due to multiple factors including underlying diseases and conditions, invasive catheters and drains, technology such as ventilators, frequent contact with hospital personnel, and exposure to antibiotics and drug resistant organisms. Children are at particular risk of acquired infections given the potential difficulty of obtaining access and an immature immune system from either vaccinations or natural infections. The younger the child, the more concerning fever or rashes are to the healthcare provider. Newborn infants are more susceptible to serious infections of various organisms than older children due to immaturity of the immune system.[34]

Children with community-acquired infections should be in transmission-based isolation precautions to protect other patients and healthcare professionals. However, the most effective measure to prevent infection is hand hygiene. Hand hygiene reduces the risk of transmission of microorganisms to patients as well as the risks to healthcare workers. The Centers for Disease Control and Prevention (CDC) recommends hand hygiene prior to contact with a patient's intact skin, contact with surfaces close to patients, and after removing gloves. According to its recommendation, a 15-second wash with soap and water

TABLE 35.5 Conditions That May Predispose Patients to Malnutrition

Medical Condition	Associated Clinical Manifestations
Cardiac disease Congenital heart disease Congestive heart failure	Fatigue, dyspnea, diaphoresis, cyanosis, decreased oral intake, vomiting, gastric distention, anorexia, early satiety, and inability to coordinate suck, and swallow
Pulmonary disease Respiratory syncytial virus Bronchopulmonary dysplasia Pneumonia Cystic fibrosis	Fatigue, dyspnea, diaphoresis, cyanosis, decreased oral intake, vomiting, and gastric distention
Liver disease	Anorexia, vomiting, gastric distention, and malabsorption
Renal disease	Vomiting, loss of appetite, anorexia, poor growth, reflux, and uremia
Inborn errors of metabolism	Inability to metabolize various substrates, severe dietary restrictions, and anorexia
Oncology	Anorexia, nausea, vomiting, increased energy demands, and poor growth
HIV/AIDS	Anorexia, nausea, vomiting, diarrhea, malabsorption, failure to thrive, increased energy demands, and medication side effects
Trauma Multiple fractures Burns	Increased energy demands, inability to take oral diet, and nutrient losses from wounds
Gastrointestinal disorders Short-bowel syndrome Inflammatory bowel syndrome Gastroesophageal reflux Gastric surgery	Impaired absorption of nutrients, altered gastric motility, delayed gastric emptying
Developmental disabilities	Poor suck and swallow and impaired motor and oral skills

From Reference 19.

before patient care when hands have visible contaminate and use of an alcohol-based hand rub immediately prior to and after all direct patient contact is paramount to infection prevention.

Shared areas such as playrooms and developmentally appropriate equipment including toys need to be given special attention for cleaning and containment. Family members should room in with their child to prevent transmission of infection to other individuals. Visitor screening of family members, friends, and siblings is essential to prevent transmitting infection to the patient and vice versa. Anyone with a fever or contagious illness, under most circumstances, should not visit.[66] Siblings are encouraged to visit but guidelines should be established to minimize the risk of transmission of pathogens to the hospital, and screening should be completed before visitation.

The average cost per central line associated–bloodstream infection (CLABSI) is estimated at $70,696 with a range of $40,412 to $100,980. The mean cost of CLABSI in pediatric patients is $55,646 with an additional 19-day length of stay.[51] The same recommendations to prevent CLABSI in adults also apply to children. Emphasis on education of personnel who insert and maintain catheters, utilizing sterile barrier precautions, using chlorhexidine skin preparation, and giving careful thought to the risks versus benefits of placing central catheters should be a priority.[1,80]

BOX 35.3 Nursing Mutual Participation Model of Care

Admission

- Extend care to include parents
- Acknowledge importance of entire family

Daily Bedside Contact

- Offer strategies to provide parents with healthcare information: teach and clarify
- Anticipate guidance needed regarding illness trajectory
- Provide instrumental resources
- Facilitate transition to *parent-to-a-critically ill child.* Enhance parent-child unique connectedness
- Role model interactions
- Invite participation in nurturing activity
- Provide options during procedures for family involvement

Establish a Caring Relationship with the Parent Through Communication

- How are you doing today?
  - Assist parental perception of the child's illness
- How does she/he look to you today?
  - Determine parental goals, objectives, and expectations
- What troubles you most?
  - Seek informed suggestions and preferences, and invite participation in care
- How can I help you today?

From References 37 and 38.

Ventilator-associated pneumonia (VAP) is the second most common hospital acquired infection and the most common reason for antibiotic use. Studies show that diagnosis is challenging because clinical, radiologic, and microbiologic criteria lack sensitivity and specificity.[105] Early and appropriate antibiotic treatment is essential in children. VAP in children has not been found to increase mortality rates, but it is associated with increased morbidity, increased duration of ventilation, and overall hospital costs. Implementation of a prevention bundle designed to reduce bacterial colonization, and reduce aspiration, can serve to decrease VAP rates in the ICU.[21]

Catheter-associated urinary tract infection (CAUTI) in children is one of the most common healthcare-associated infections. Indications for catheter placement are the same as in adults: urinary retention, bladder outlet obstruction, need for accurate output measurements in critically ill children, and with select surgical procedures to assist in wound healing.[52] Intermittent catheterization should be considered in children with myelomeningocele and neurogenic bladder. Otherwise, diapers, commodes, and urinals should be used. The initiation of a CAUTI bundle can decrease the incidence of infections. Institution-wide practice standardization and education focused on urinary catheter insertions and maintenance practices, coupled with daily reviews of catheter necessity, and rapid reviews of all CAUTIs has been associated with decreased rates.[40]

The American Academy of Pediatrics (AAP) released a policy statement regarding *Clostridium difficile* infections (CDI) in children in 2013.[4] This bacterium is the most common cause of antimicrobial-associated diarrhea and is typically a healthcare-associated infection. The organism may be found on hospital personnel, baby baths, and hospital equipment.[6] The incidence of CDI in children has increased since 1997.[79] Although children have intestinal flora similar to that of an adult by 1 year of age, risk factors for CDI include antimicrobial therapy, use of proton

BOX 35.4 Age-Specific Variations for Working with Hospitalized Children

Infant
- Give family choices on how to be involved in procedures
- Use analgesics as needed
- Keep family in infant's line of vision
- If family members cannot remain with infant, place familiar object near infant
- Have consistent caregivers and limit stranger contact
- Comfort child during and after procedures
- Keep harmful objects out of reach
- Keep frightening objects out of view
- Use nonintrusive procedures when possible (e.g., oral medications, axillary temperatures)

Toddler
Use same approaches as for infant with these additions:
- Explain what child will see, hear, taste, smell, and feel
- Emphasize when cooperation is needed (e.g., lie still)
- Let child know that it is okay to cry, scream, or yell to express discomfort/fear
- Ignore temper tantrums
- Use distraction techniques
- Use simple terms familiar to child, using one direction at a time
- Show small replicas of equipment and allow child to hold
- Use play to demonstrate procedures, but not child's favorite toy; child's imagination may believe that the toy can feel procedure
- Prepare child immediately before procedures
- Tell child when procedures are complete
- Allow choices and child's participation whenever possible

Preschool-Age Child
- Encourage family presence as a comforter, to avoid restraining child
- Provide analgesia as needed
- Use simple terms to explain procedures
- Demonstrate equipment and allow child to play with equipment or simulated equipment models
- Allow child to use play to demonstrate procedures to clarify misconceptions
- Allow child to point out on doll exact location of procedure to decrease fantasy of multiple body parts being involved
- Allow child to wear underpants and realize that procedures involving genitals are anxiety producing
- Explain all unfamiliar procedures/activities
- Involve child in care, but avoid delays in procedures
- Praise child continually
- Use concrete words (e.g., rolling bed versus stretcher; child may believe bed can *stretch* child)
- Allow child to verbalize
- Provide information regarding procedures shortly before actual procedure
- Explain the reason procedure is being performed and allow child to say why a procedure is done (e.g., children may imagine they are being punished)
- Keep equipment out of sight
- Use nonintrusive procedures when possible (e.g., oral medications, axillary temperatures)
- Apply a bandage; children may fantasize *leakage* of *insides*
- Involve child in care whenever possible, avoiding excessive delays

School-Age Child
- Explain procedures using correct terminology
- Explain procedures by using simple diagrams
- Explain function of equipment in concrete terms and allow to hold and model use
- Allow time before and after procedure for questions and discussion
- Prepare in advance of procedure
- Gain child's cooperation, explaining what is expected of child
- Suggest ways of maintaining control (e.g., taking a deep breath, counting)
- Allow child to assist with simple tasks and include in decision-making when feasible (e.g., time of day to perform, preferred site)
- Encourage active participation (e.g., opening packages)
- Provide privacy during procedures

Adolescent
- Explain procedure including why it is beneficial/necessary, and long-term consequences
- Encourage questioning regarding fears, risks, options, and alternatives
- Provide privacy
- Discuss how procedure may affect appearance and how to minimize
- Realize that immediate effects are more significant than long-term benefits
- Involve in decision making and planning (e.g., clothing to wear)
- Impose as few restrictions as possible, allowing patient to maintain control
- Suggest ways of maintaining control and accept aggression as method of coping
- Realize adolescents may have difficulty accepting new authority figures and may resist complying with procedures
- Allow adolescents to talk with other adolescents who have had same experience

From Reference 26.

pump inhibitors, use of enemas, diapers, presence of gastrostomy and jejunostomy tubes, bowel disease, gastrointestinal track surgery, renal insufficiency, and impaired immunity. Transmission is via the fecal-oral route, and children with suspected CDIs should be placed in standard and contact precautions. Healthcare providers should be aware that hand washing with soap and water is more effective at eliminating *Clostridium difficile* spores than alcohol-based hand sanitizers.[6,32]

THE CHILD'S RESPONSE TO CRITICAL CARE

A child's response to surgery and hospitalization will reflect experience, age, and family support. Children tend to regress to a previous developmental level when stressed. In general, care should be directed toward developmental age rather than chronologic age (Box 35.4). Children who are admitted to critical care are exposed to a multitude of environmental stimuli that can be overwhelming. With the addition of severe illness and invasive procedures endured, the child has the potential to have lasting emotional and physical effects. Some children have been able to recall their intensive care experience in great detail, whereas others have been amnesic of the event. One study found that, for the youngest pediatric patients, the number of invasive procedures endured and the severity of the illness had the longest effects postdischarge. These findings underscore the potential need for long-term support that can be provided by advanced practice nurses, clinical psychologists, child life and music therapists, social workers, discharge planners, and case managers specializing in pediatric care.[3]

CONSIDERATIONS IN PEDIATRIC CARE

Pediatric Assessment

Blood Pressure

The age and size of the child should be considered when obtaining vital signs (Table 35.6). Blood pressure measurement is

TABLE 35.6 Pediatric Vital Signs

Age	Heart Rate (beats/min)	Respirations (breaths/min)	Systolic Blood Pressure (mm Hg)
Infant	100–160	30–60	87–105
Toddler	80–110	24–40	95–105
Preschooler	70–110	22–34	80–110
School-age	65–110	18–30	97–112
Adolescent	60–90	12–16	112–128

Normal Hemodynamic Values in Children

Central venous pressure	4–8 mm Hg
Systolic pulmonary artery pressure	20–30 mm Hg
Diastolic pulmonary artery pressure	<10 mm Hg
Mean pulmonary artery pressure	<20 mm Hg
Pulmonary artery occlusion pressure	4–12 mm Hg

From References 56, 77, and 78.

most accurate when the cuff's bladder encompasses 80% to 100% of the arm's circumference and has a bladder width of approximately 40% of the circumference of the child's upper arm.[14] When attempting to obtain a diastolic blood pressure in children, the disappearance of sound may not occur until zero. Some institutions and healthcare providers may choose to only document a systolic value. If a change occurs in the sounds at a point during auscultation of the blood pressure, this value can also be noted, such as 90/50/0.

Pulse

During auscultation of an apical pulse, the healthcare provider should listen at the fourth intercostal space medial to the left midclavicular line in children under 7 years of age. After age 7, the apical impulse is located at the fifth intercostal space at the left midclavicular line. The healthcare provider should make sure that the stethoscope used during the assessment is the appropriate size for infants and children.

Temperature

Historically, healthcare providers have assumed that rectal temperatures are 1°C higher and that axillary temperatures are 1°C lower than oral temperatures. Studies have demonstrated that the difference is much smaller.[60,61] The temperature measurement site and instrument should be based on the child's physiologic stability and age, not "one size fits all." For consistency, the same method and instrument should be used to trend the individual patient's temperature over time. The axillary route for temperature assessment may be the safest for neonates and small infants, whereas the tympanic and rectal routes may be best for children with poor perfusion.[70] Studies have shown that temporal artery temperature measurement cannot be relied upon in critically ill children, but is useful as a baseline temperature during a general pediatric assessment.[89] It must be noted that the rectal route should not be "the norm," but that the temperature route and instrument should be individualized according to the child's needs.

Respiratory Rate

The respiratory rate should be assessed when the child is at rest. Any condition that increases oxygen needs can cause increased respiration (e.g., fever, fear, respiratory distress). Children with a sustained respiratory rate greater than 60 breaths per minute should be assessed for hypoxemia.[14]

Fluid Balance in Children

Placing an intravenous (IV) catheter into the small vein of a child can be a daunting task. No nurse wants a child to endure repeated attempts at locating a vessel, but pediatric IV placement skills are difficult to maintain without consistent opportunities for practice. Repeated attempts may be a catalyst for negative physiologic consequences in the child (e.g., oxygen desaturations, bradycardia). Many hospitals limit the number of times an individual healthcare provider may attempt IV placement to 2 to 3 times. IV catheter gauge and length selection is individualized for each child. Following catheter insertion, an infusion pump that can deliver low volumes in increments of 0.1 mL is used for fluid and IV medication administration.

In the event an IV line cannot be inserted, intraosseous infusions may be used to gain vascular access in children. This is an effective, safe, and accessible route for fluid resuscitation, blood sampling, blood product transfusion, and vasoactive infusions. Although rare, complications include subcutaneous infiltration and leakage from the puncture site after needle removal. Extended intraosseous infusions and infusion of hypertonic fluids have been associated with infections; therefore, they should be limited.[77]

Small changes in fluid and electrolyte balance may cause complications in a child. Rapid changes in weight are most likely due to accumulation or loss of fluid. Those under the age of 2 years are more dependent on adequate intake than adults, because of the greater proportion of daily fluid losses. Conditions such as fever, increases in metabolic rate, vomiting, and diarrhea may increase fluid losses. Conversely, children may experience fluid excesses from chronic renal disease and rapidly flowing IVs. Maintenance fluids for a child should be calculated based on kilograms of body weight (Table 35.7).

To monitor fluid balance, strict fluid intake and output as well as daily weights (taken at the same time of day with the same scale) are documented so that trends can be assessed. Weighing diapers using a gram scale can measure urinary output for infants and incontinent children; 1 g of weight equals 1 mL of urine volume.[14]

TABLE 35.7 Calculation of Maintenance Fluids (Per 24 Hours) in Children

Weight (kg)	Kilogram Body Weight Formula
0–10	100–120 mL/kg
11–20	1000 mL for first 10 kg and 50 mL/kg for each kilogram over 10 kg
21–30	1500 mL for first 20 kg and 25 mL/kg for each kilogram over 20 kg

From Reference 56.

Additional volume losses can occur when blood is drawn for laboratory specimens. Pediatric tubes should be used, obtaining the smallest sample necessary. Closed blood drawing systems can be used so the blood loss is minimized, and there are no "discards" or wasted blood. The amount of blood drawn should be documented so that cumulative totals of blood loss are easily retrievable.

Medication Administration in Children

The administration of medication in the pediatric population may be challenging to those not accustomed to the small doses and weight-based calculations. Because of the weight variability for each age of child, having standard doses for pediatrics is not possible. Because of variations in child weight, body surface area, and organ maturity, the ability to metabolize and excrete medications may be affected.[8] Pediatric medications are weight-based, so it is critical that an accurate weight in kilograms is obtained upon patient admission and that the weight is documented in a standard area of the patient's chart. According to the United States Pharmacopoeia Medication Reporting Program, incorrect administration of intravenous fluids was the most common pediatric medication error noted.[36] The number of pediatric medication errors has been reported to be as high as 1 in 6.4 orders, and The Joint Commission has reported a higher medication error rate than that of adults (Box 35.5). In response to the high numbers of errors, the AAP developed a policy statement related to the prevention of medication errors in the pediatric inpatient setting as a commitment to preventing such errors.[9]

The presence of critical care pharmacists, as part of the critical care interprofessional team, can enhance patient outcomes related to fluid management, adverse drug events, medication administration errors, and ventilator-associated pneumonias.[64] Institutions caring for children should ensure that they have a pharmacist who specializes in the administration of fluids and medications in the pediatric population to improve quality and safety.

Frequently, medication package inserts are found with the following statement: "Safety and effectiveness has not been established for children." Only one third of the medications used in pediatrics have been studied in this population and have adequate information regarding pediatric utilization. The remaining medications have insufficient information regarding safety and efficacy in children, and the younger the child the less information available.[102] Because the US Food and Drug Administration does not license many medications for use in children and lacks dosing guidelines, an increase in the frequency of medication errors in children versus adults has been reported. It has been suggested that patient and family involvement in the administration of medications may be of value in the reduction of errors.

BOX 35.5 Prevention of Pediatric Medication Errors

1. Provide adequate numbers of nurses and pharmacists that are educated to prepare, dispense, and administer medications to children
2. Establish and maintain a functional pediatric formulary
3. Standardize the following throughout the institution:
   - Pediatric infusion pumps
   - Weight scales
   - Measurement systems, (e.g., all kilograms)
   - Pediatric medication order sets
4. Confirm that child's weight is correct, and dose does not exceed adult dose
5. Avoid use of a terminal zero to minimize 10-fold dosing errors (e.g., use 4 rather than 4.0)
6. Use a zero to the left of a dose less than 1 to avoid dosing errors (e.g., use 0.25 rather than .25)
7. Double-check calculations
8. Verify unusually large or small volumes or dosages
9. Listen when the patient or caregiver questions whether a medication should be administered

From References 63, 87, and 91.

Having so many unstudied medications in the pediatric population limits the number of "known" medications for children and places healthcare practitioners in a difficult situation when prescribing. For example, one major drug company, AstraZeneca, the manufacturer of propofol (Diprivan), distributed a letter in 2001 reminding healthcare providers that this specific medication was "not approved for sedation in pediatric critical care patients in the United States and should not be used for this purpose."[13] Having pediatric-focused medication text can make administration less challenging. A resource that focuses on injectable medications for children is useful in the critical care environment. The American Society of Health-System Pharmacists developed the *Teddy Bear Book: Pediatric Injectable Drugs* for hospitalized children.[84]

PAIN IN CHILDREN

Children who are admitted to critical care have pain and anxiety associated with the illness or injury, from medical and nursing procedures, and anxiety from the experience of the critical care hospitalization, as well as separation from friends and family. Children may deny that they are hurting for fear of "a shot" as the remedy. Intramuscular injections are inappropriate if the child has a functioning intravenous line.[53] During IV placement and needle sticks for blood drawing, the use of local anesthetic creams is desirable. Consultation with an interprofessional Pediatric Pain Service can assist the pediatric healthcare provider with pain management in children with complex pain issues; however, there are estimated to be very few such teams in the United States. The AAP has developed guidelines that can be used to ensure the safe administration and monitoring of patients receiving sedation and analgesia in the pediatric population[7,9] (Box 35.6).

A pain assessment should occur upon admission to the hospital, and on an ongoing basis according to institution policies. It is difficult to assess and measure the pain of another person. Assessment of the child in pain can be a challenging task especially if the child is preverbal or has developmental delays.[59]

BOX 35.6 Overview of Pediatric Sedation Guidelines

1. The child must undergo a documented presedation medical evaluation, including a focused airway examination.
2. There should be an appropriate interval of fasting before sedation.
3. Children should not receive sedative or anxiolytic medications without supervision by skilled medical personnel (i.e., medication should not be administered at home or by a technician without medical supervision from a practitioner who, by virtue of training, education, certification, or applicable licensure, law, or regulation, is qualified to supervise the delivery of medical care). The individual may be a provider, nurse, dentist, or other appropriately educated health professional.
4. Sedative and anxiolytic medications should be administered only by or in the presence of individuals skilled in airway management and cardiopulmonary resuscitation.
5. Age- and size-appropriate equipment and appropriate medications to sustain life should be checked before sedation and be immediately available.
6. All patients sedated for a procedure must be continuously monitored with pulse oximetry and capnography.
7. An individual must be specifically assigned to monitor the patient's cardiorespiratory status during and after the procedure; for deeply sedated patients, that individual should have no other responsibilities and should record vital signs at least every 5 minutes.
8. Specific discharge criteria must be established and consistently utilized.
9. The *Guidelines for Monitoring and Management of Pediatric Patients During and After Sedation for Diagnostic and Therapeutic Procedures* apply regardless of the settings in which sedatives are administered or the specific training or profession of the practitioners involved.
10. At least one individual must be present who is trained in, and capable of, providing pediatric basic life support, and who is skilled in airway management and cardiopulmonary resuscitation; training in pediatric advanced life support is strongly encouraged.
11. Children who receive sedative medication with a long half-life may require extended observation.

From Reference 8.

Nurses have consistently rated children's pain levels lower than the children themselves have rated their pain, and children report undertreatment of preventable pain.[22] Children respond to pain behaviorally and physiologically, and there are pain assessment tools that can be helpful in measuring both types of responses (Boxes 35.7 through 35.9 and Table 35.8). Numerical rating scales (0 – 10) are recommended for children older than 7 years of age. Sedation scales can be used in conjunction with pain assessment scales. One such scale is the Modified Motor Activity Assessment scale (Table 35.9). As with adults, nonpharmacologic strategies for pain relief (e.g., distraction, touch, sucking) can be utilized, but the comfort that they provide may cease when the intervention stops, so adequate pharmacologic sedation/analgesia must still be utilized. Infusion rates listed in Table 35.10 represent suggestions for starting doses. The infusion should be supplemented with as-needed bolus doses to provide the desired level of baseline sedation/analgesia. In patients requiring frequent bolus doses, the infusion rate should be increased by 10% to 20%. If patients require no bolus doses and are excessively sedated, the infusion rate should be decreased by 10% to 20%.

When it is time to wean the patient from sedation/analgesia, weaning protocols that allow these medications to be reduced slowly can decrease the physical signs and symptoms of withdrawal (Box 35.10). These symptoms may be affected by the child's age, underlying illness, and cognitive state.[98,99] Diarrhea, vomiting, problems with feeding, sucking, and swallowing, high-pitched crying, and irritability may be signs of withdrawal in neonates and infants, but may be attributed to reasons other than withdrawal.[15] It is essential to use objective screening tools such as the Withdrawal Assessment Tool 1 (WAT-1) for patient assessment[47,48] (Fig. 35.4).

Delirium in Children

Delirium is defined as acute cerebral dysfunction caused by illness or the effects of treatment. Delirium in children is difficult to diagnose because it is understudied.[100] The ideal screening tool must take into account children of all ages and developmental levels, as well as the various types of delirium whether hyper- or hypoactive.[100] Delirium is associated with increased PICU length of stay, post-traumatic stress symptoms, neurocognitive dysfunction, and can be associated with a decrease in spatial and verbal memory and the ability to sustain attention.[95,100] The Cornell Assessment of Pediatric Delirium has been found to be a rapid, validated, observational nurse-screening tool that may detect delirium in children. This tool takes into account developmental anchor points in determining a delirium score.[100] The ICU environment, pain, and use of sedatives can worsen delirium.[95] Adequate pain control, minimizing unnecessary sedative administration, and optimizing the ICU environment to allow sleep and a day/night schedule, providing familiar and comforting objects all may prevent and treat pediatric delirium.[95]

Neuromuscular Blockade

Chemical relaxation with neuromuscular blocking agents is used in the pediatric population for reasons such as rapid-sequence intubation, ventilatory control, and the prevention of increased arterial blood pressure from isometric muscle contraction. Some care providers continue to mistakenly believe that these agents have analgesic and anxiolytic properties and fail to provide adequate pain relief and sedation for the children receiving them. Train-of-four testing with a peripheral nerve stimulator and medication holidays can be used to assess the appropriate level of chemical relaxation for the patient's condition and to prevent the complication of prolonged weakness following neuromuscular blockade. In children who are chemically paralyzed or who have no blink response, eyes should be kept protected and moist by creating a moisture chamber. This can be achieved by instilling normal saline drops every 2 hours, covering the eyes with plastic wrap, and changing the wrap daily or more frequently to prevent infection. Earplugs can be used to eliminate the noise in critical care. These should be removed any time patients will be touched so they can be apprised of what will be occurring. The nurse should reassure the patient that the inability to move is only temporary. To reduce stress, using the word *relaxation* versus *paralyzed* may be helpful when discussing neuromuscular blockade with the child and family.

INTENTIONAL INJURIES IN THE PEDIATRIC PATIENT

Reports of child abuse in the United States are increasing, and those children who are admitted to PICUs have the highest rates of mortality. These children most often present with severe head injury, and the victims tend to be younger in age.[108] Clinicians

BOX 35.7 Behavioral Indicators of Pain

Infant

- Facial expression: brows lowered and drawn together, broadened nasal root, eyes tightly closed and angular, squarish mouth with a taut tongue
- Irritability
- Restlessness
- Continuous crying/whimpering
- Crying when stimulus applied
- Intense crying
- Knees drawn to chest
- Clenched fists
- Refusal to eat
- Hyperalertness
- Restless sleep, inability to sleep
- Hypersensitivity to touch
- Muscle tension

Toddler

- Says he or she *hurts* or has an *owie*
- Intense or continuous crying
- Aggressive behavior
- Rubbing, pulling, guarding, and touching affected body part
- Inability to be comforted
- Regressive behavior
- Resistance to being helped
- Irritability or restlessness
- Nightmares, inability to sleep
- Decreased activity tolerance
- Lowered frustration tolerance
- Change from usual play behavior
- Seeking of comfort objects (e.g., blanket)
- Seeking of comfort from family

Preschool-Age Child

Similar to toddler with the following additions:

- Denies pain in the presence of other behavioral cues and physical injury
- Repetitive verbalizations such as "it hurts, it hurts, it hurts"
- Refusal to allow touching of affected body part by others

School-Age Child

- Denial of pain in the presence of behavioral cues
- Resistance of movement
- Grimacing
- Nightmares
- Low frustration tolerance
- Guarding
- Emotional withdrawal
- Irritability, restlessness, or thrashing

Teenager

- Muscle tension
- Guarding
- Change in activity level
- Nightmares
- Change in eating pattern
- Irritability, restlessness, or thrashing
- Increased sleeping in the absence of pain control measures
- Low frustration tolerance
- Grimacing
- Nonverbal/neurologic damage
- Facial grimacing or flushing
- Increased muscle tension
- Hypersensitivity to the environment/touch
- Grinding of teeth
- Seizure activity
- Clenched fists
- Inability to be comforted
- Continuous crying
- Extremity spasms
- Vomiting
- Inability to tolerate lying in the same position

From Reference 76.

BOX 35.8 Physiologic Responses to Pain in Children

- Increased pulse rate, blood pressure, respiratory rate
- Increased depth of respirations
- Flushing or pallor
- Diaphoresis
- Dilated pupils
- Decreased oxygen consumption/saturation
- Muscle tension
- Nausea and/or decreased gastric motility

Additionally, infants may have the following:

- Apnea
- Color changes
- Seizures
- Stooping
- Hiccupping

From Reference 25.

BOX 35.9 FACES Pain Rating Scale

Original Instructions

Explain to the person that each face is for a person who feels happy because he has no pain (hurt) or sad because he has some or a lot of pain (hurt).

- **Face 0** is very happy because he doesn't hurt at all
- **Face 1** hurts just a little bit
- **Face 2** hurts a little more
- **Face 3** hurts even more
- **Face 4** hurts a whole lot
- **Face 5** hurts as much as you can imagine, although you don't have to be crying to feel this bad

Ask the child to choose the face that best describes how he/she is feeling. This rating scale is recommended for persons age 3 years and older.

From References 76 and 106.

should also be aware that inconsistencies in the child's patient history might also be indicative of Munchausen syndrome by proxy, the fabrication of a child's illness. A summary of factors to assess in children with suspected intentional injuries is given in Box 35.11.

All healthcare providers are required by law to report any suspected case of abuse to child protective services and law enforcement personnel as soon as possible. The focus should be on care of the patient and family in a professional, nonjudgmental manner, and not on identification of child abusers or perpetrators. Unit visitation policies should be followed in the usual manner unless the child is taken into protective custody or there is a reason to believe the child is in danger. Documentation should be focused on detailed objective data that include history of the injury with timelines, actual behaviors of child and family, and physical

TABLE 35.8 FLACC Scale for Assessing Postoperative Pain in Children Ages 2 to 7

	SCORING*		
Categories	**0**	**1**	**2**
Face	No particular expression or smile	Occasional grimace or frown, withdrawn, uninterested	Frequent to constant quivering chin, clenched jaw
Legs	Normal position or relaxed	Uneasy, restless, tense	Kicking, or legs drawn up
Activity	Lying quietly, normal position, moves easily	Squirming, shifting back and forth, tense	Arched, rigid, or jerking
Cry	No cry (awake or asleep)	Moans or whimpers; occasional complaint	Crying steadily, screams or sobs, frequent complaints
Consolability	Content, relaxed	Reassured by occasional touching, hugging, or being talked to, distractible	Difficult to console or comfort

*Each of the 5 categories—(F) Face; (L) Legs; (A) Activity; (C) Cry; (C) Consolability—is scored from 0 to 2, which results in a total score between 0 and 10.
From References 74 and 75.

TABLE 35.9 Modified Motor Activity Assessment Scale

Score	Description	Definition
-3	Unresponsive	Minimal or no response to noxious* stimulus; does not communicate or follow commands
-2	Responsive only to noxious stimuli	Opens eyes or raises eyebrows or turns head toward stimulus or moves limbs with noxious stimulus
-1	Responsive to touch or name	Opens eyes or raises eyebrows or turns head toward stimulus or moves limbs with touch or when name is spoken; drifts off after stimulation; follows simple commands
0	Calm and cooperative	No external stimulus is required to elicit movement; calm, awakens easily, and follows commands
+1	Restless and cooperative	No external stimulus is required to elicit movement; picking at tubes but consolable
+2	Agitated	No external stimulus is required to elicit movement; attempting to sit or move limbs to get up and inconsolable despite frequent attempts; requires physical restraint, biting ETT
+3	Dangerously agitated, uncooperative	No external stimulus is required to elicit movement; patient unsafe; attempting to pull at ETT/catheters; desaturating; thrashing side-to-side; climbing over rail; striking at staff

*Suctioning or 5 seconds of nail bed pressure.
ETT, Endotracheal tube.
From Reference 41.

findings that may include radiographs, photographs, and body diagrams.

In the event of death from an intentional injury, the child may still be considered for organ donation. It is imperative that there is collaboration between law enforcement, medical examiners, coroners, the critical care team, and the transplant surgeon to ensure that evidence is preserved and there is meticulous documentation of the transplant procedure.[108] Flawed criminal investigations or prosecutions related to organ donation have not been reported and organ donation in suspected child abuse cases is not a contraindication to organ donation.

TABLE 35.10 Suggested Guidelines for Dosing of Sedative and Analgesic Agents

Agent	Dose	Comments
Fentanyl (Duragesic)	1–4 mcg/kg/h	Neonates may be more sensitive to chest wall rigidity and respiratory depression than adults.
Morphine	10–30 mcg/kg/h	Chest wall rigidity and hypotension may occur with rapid administration.
Midazolam (Versed)	0.05–0.15 mg/kg/h	Contains benzyl alcohol 1%, which may cause fatal gasping syndrome in neonates.
Lorazepam (Ativan)	0.025–0.05 mg/kg/h	Contains benzyl alcohol 2% and propylene glycol, which may cause adverse effects in neonates.
Ketamine (Ketalar)	1–2 mg/kg/h	Use with caution in those at risk for increased intracranial pressure. Laryngospasm and apnea may occur.
Pentobarbital (Nembutal)	1–2 mg/kg/h	Is an alkaline solution so may cause tissue necrosis with extravasation.

From References 62 and 99.

BOX 35.10 Sedative/Analgesic Weaning for Administration Longer Than Approximately 5 Days

1. A weaning schedule should be developed for children who have received sedative/analgesic infusions or frequent dosing for greater than approximately 5 days.
2. Medication dosing should be changed from continuous infusions to around-the-clock intermittent IV/oral administration.
3. Intravenous medications the patient is receiving should be converted to equianalgesic oral dosing as soon as possible before discharge.
4. During medication weaning, the baseline original daily dose should be reduced 10% to 20% every 1 to 2 days. For example, a dose of 60 mg would be reduced by 6 to 12 mg every 1 to 2 days. In patients receiving high doses of medication, it may be necessary to decrease the rate by smaller increments every 12 hours to reduce withdrawal symptoms.
5. Use of a withdrawal screening tool during the weaning process is essential for patient assessment.

From References 15, 47, and 99.

WITHDRAWAL ASSESSMENT TOOL VERSION 1 (WAT – 1)

Patient Identifier														
	Date:													
	Time:													
Information from patient record, previous 12 hours														
Any loose /watery stools	No = 0 Yes = 1													
Any vomiting/retching/gagging	No = 0 Yes = 1													
Temperature > 37.8°C	No = 0 Yes = 1													
2 minute pre-stimulus observation														
State	SBS[1] ≤ 0 or asleep/awake/calm = 0 SBS[1] ≥ +1 or awake/distressed = 1													
Tremor	None/mild = 0 Moderate/severe = 1													
Any sweating	No = 0 Yes = 1													
Uncoordinated/repetitive movement	None/mild = 0 Moderate/severe = 1													
Yawning or sneezing	None or 1 = 0 ≥2 = 1													
1 minute stimulus observation														
Startle to touch	None/mild = 0 Moderate/severe = 1													
Muscle tone	Normal = 0 Increased = 1													
Post-stimulus recovery														
Time to gain calm state (SBS[1] ≤ 0)	< 2 min = 0 2 - 5 min = 1 > 5 min = 2													
Total Score (0-12)														

WITHDRAWAL ASSESSMENT TOOL (WAT – 1) INSTRUCTIONS

- Start WAT-1 scoring from the **first day of weaning** in patients who have received opioids +/or benzodiazepines by infusion or regular dosing for prolonged periods (e.g., > 5 days). Continue twice daily scoring until 72 hours after the last dose.
- The Withdrawal Assessment Tool (WAT-1) should be completed along with the SBS[1] at least once per 12 hour shift (e.g., at 08:00 and 20:00 ± 2 hours). The progressive stimulus used in the SBS[1] assessment provides a standard stimulus for observing signs of withdrawal.

Obtain information from patient record (this can be done before or after the stimulus):

- ✓ **Loose/watery stools**: Score 1 if any loose or watery stools were documented in the past 12 hours; score 0 if none were noted.
- ✓ **Vomiting/retching/gagging**: Score 1 if any vomiting or spontaneous retching or gagging were documented in the past 12 hours; score 0 if none were noted
- ✓ **Temperature > 37.8°C**: Score 1 if the modal (most frequently occurring) temperature documented was greater than 37.8 °C in the past 12 hours; score 0 if this was not the case.

2 minute pre-stimulus observation:

- ✓ **State**: Score 1 if awake and distress (SBS[1]: ≥ +1) observed during the 2 minutes prior to the stimulus; score 0 if asleep or awake and calm/cooperative (SBS[1] ≤ 0).
- ✓ **Tremor**: Score 1 if moderate to severe tremor observed during the 2 minutes prior to the stimulus; score 0 if no tremor (or only minor, intermittent tremor).
- ✓ **Sweating**: Score 1 if any sweating during the 2 minutes prior to the stimulus; score 0 if no sweating noted.
- ✓ **Uncoordinated/repetitive movements**: Score 1 if moderate to severe uncoordinated or repetitive movements such as head turning, leg or arm flailing, or torso arching observed during the 2 minutes prior to the stimulus; score 0 if no (or only mild) uncoordinated or repetitive movements.
- ✓ **Yawning or sneezing** > 1: Score 1 if more than 1 yawn or sneeze observed during the 2 minutes prior to the stimulus; score 0 if 0 to 1 yawn or sneeze.

1 minute stimulus observation:

- ✓ **Startle to touch**: Score 1 if moderate to severe startle occurs when touched during the stimulus; score 0 if none (or mild).
- ✓ **Muscle tone**: Score 1 if tone increased during the stimulus; score 0 if normal.

Post-stimulus recovery:

- ✓ **Time to gain calm state** (SBS[1] ≤ 0): Score 2 if it takes greater than 5 minutes following stimulus; score 1 if achieved within 2 to 5 minutes; score 0 if achieved in less than 2 minutes.

Sum the 11 numbers in the column for the total WAT-1 score (0-12).

[1]Curley et al. State behavioral scale: A sedation assessment instrument for infants and young children supported on mechanical ventilation. Pediatr Crit Care Med 2006;7(2):107-114.

FIG. 35.4 Withdrawal assessment tool. (Reprinted with permission from Franck, L. S., Harris, S. K., Soetenga, D. J., Amling, J. K., & Curley, M. A. Q. (2008). The Withdrawal Assessment Tool–1 (WAT–1): an assessment instrument for monitoring opioid and benzodiazepine withdrawal symptoms in pediatric patients. *Pediatr Crit Care Med*, 9(6), 573–580.).

BOX 35.11 Assessment of Intentional Injuries

- Unbelievable or inconsistent patient history
- Delay in seeking medical assistance
- New adult partner in household
- Prior history of abuse or suspected abuse
- Multiple injuries in various stages of healing
- Absence of primary caretaker at onset of illness
- Unexplained neurologic deterioration, shock, or cardiac arrest

From References 30 and 108.

Regardless of the patient's outcome, handling intentional injuries to a child can be difficult. Participation in unit-level debriefing sessions, increased peer-to-peer support, and individual self-care measures can be helpful in coping with this patient situation.

PARENTAL PERMISSION AND CHILD ASSENT

In the United States, parents have legal authority in matters of concern for their minor children, and limits to parental authority occur only when the child's interests are clearly severely threatened by parental action. Some states recognize *mature minors* as those who can understand proposed treatments and the potential consequences. Whereas state statutes vary, emancipated minors are generally recognized as adolescents younger than 18 years of age who are one of the following: in the military, married, an unmarried mother, or not living at home and self-supporting. Those living in states with mature minor statutes, or who are emancipated, are generally allowed to make personal healthcare decisions. The traditional view is that children are not competent to make medical decisions; whereas competent adults are allowed to make medical decisions including refusal of care, children are not afforded the same rights in the United States.[82,107] One may argue that children are not always rational; however, "rationality might not be a necessary criterion for a minor to make his or her own medical decision, given that medical decisions by adults need not be rational."[7,107] Children may only be deemed competent when they make the decision that the doctor wants them to make.[42]

Children may be more capable of making health-related decisions than first thought, and it is reasonable to ask for a child's consent to treatment while giving parents the opportunity to give informed permission. The AAP concluded that, "patients should participate in decision-making commensurate with their development…parents and physicians should not exclude children and adolescents…without persuasive reasons."[7]

The wishes of those children who refuse consent in order to gain a better understanding or refuse because of fear should be respected, and coercion to treat should be avoided. When there is persistent objection, medical interventions performed for the child's "own good" are disrespectful to the child. Any time this occurs, an apology to the child should occur.[16] For healthcare providers who were not treated with this type of decision-making respect as children, it may not be easy for them to respect children in this manner. It may also be hard for parents to view the child as a decision maker when that role may not be supported in the child's home environment. A collaborative model of decision making that involves the child, family, and healthcare providers is optimal.

The best interest of the child must take priority over any controversies and medical tensions. The pediatric critical care nurse is in a prime position to ensure that the child is the focus of all decisions and not the individual personalities involved.

TRANSITIONS FOR THE CHILD AND FAMILY IN CRITICAL CARE

Out of the PICU

As the child's health improves, the child and family must be prepared for transfer out of the critical care unit or for discharge home. Transitioning to a general care unit after a critical care admission may be a source of anxiety for the child and family.[103] Utilization of a transfer protocol for pediatric patients from the critical care unit has been shown to decrease family stress while increasing family satisfaction with the transfer process. Parents often feel unprepared to care for their child after discharge home from a critical care admission.[18] The time following discharge from the PICU is extremely stressful and uncertain. The nurse provides key support throughout the transition from the PICU to another level of care.[18]

Palliative Care

Forty to sixty percent of all deaths in the PICU occur following a decision to limit life-sustaining therapies.[27] Therefore, a commitment and a plan to provide palliative care to children and families is needed in institutions that have made the decision to provide care at the end-of-life for this population.[85] Involvement of a palliative care team can facilitate this transition of care and provide additional support to the family. It is also important to provide interprofessional healthcare provider debriefing sessions and bereavement rounds. These allow for the open discussion of end-of-life issues and opportunity for the healthcare provider team to verbalize stress and emotions.

COMPETENT PEDIATRIC INTENSIVE CARE NURSING

Studies have shown improved patient outcomes related to higher volumes of pediatric critical care admissions.[93,97] Remaining competent in an area with little chance to utilize skills is challenging, and orienting an entire adult critical care unit's staff to pediatric patients and maintaining ongoing competencies may be time and cost prohibitive. Unit leaders should identify an interprofessional team of healthcare providers who have an interest in caring for the pediatric population. This team must receive ongoing education and skills training specific to the pediatric patient. Children and families, especially those who are hospital savvy, are highly skilled at recognizing those who truly enjoy the care of pediatric patients.

Initial Pediatric Orientation

For the identified team of nurses, competency of pediatric advanced life support (PALS) skills is essential. PALS focuses on pediatric emergency care; PALS does not include routine care considerations of a pediatric patient. Preparing to care for children in the adult critical care unit takes initial educational preparation that may include the following: a pediatric-focused internship, didactic lectures by experts/consultants, PALS classes, simulated admissions and emergencies, and bedside pediatric clinical competency validation by an experienced preceptor.[81]

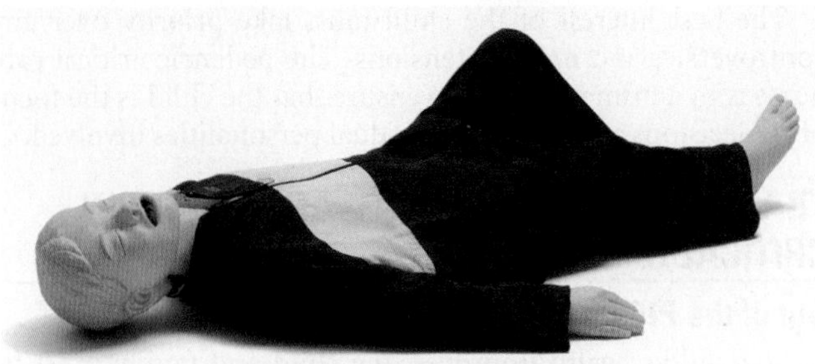

FIG. 35.5 SimJunior. (Courtesy Laerdal Medical Corporation.)

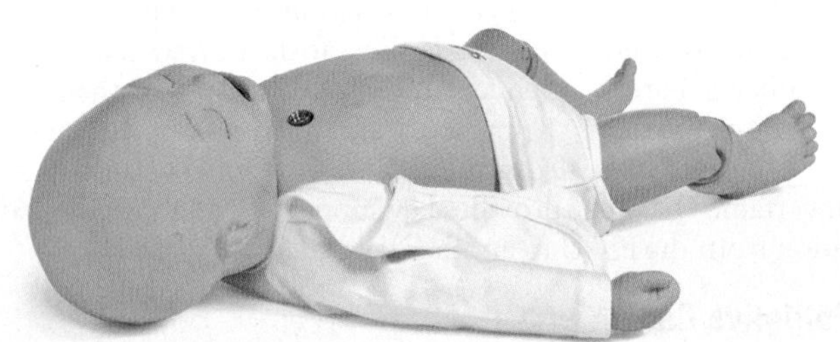

FIG. 35.6 SimBaby. (Courtesy Laerdal Medical Corporation.)

Ongoing Competencies

To provide ongoing pediatric clinical focus after the initial orientation, the following are recommended: reassessment of pediatric skills and bedside competencies, attendance at pediatric educational sessions, and the opportunity to provide care for pediatric patients on a regular basis. If there are not ample pediatric admissions, a repeat precepted bedside experience at a tertiary PICU should be considered. For units with low pediatric admissions, skill labs and simulation labs with products such as SimJunior, MegaCode Baby, and mock resuscitations can provide pediatric content reinforcement. However, simulation can never take the place of actual, hands-on pediatric patient care (Figs. 35.5 and 35.6).

Daily bedside interprofessional pediatric team rounds can also provide an opportunity for learning and have been shown to improve communication and collaboration among the participants and decrease patient length of stay.[43,104] Family members should be given a chance to participate in bedside rounds. With families present at rounds, the importance of family involvement in the care process is reinforced. Pediatric reference guides that can be utilized quickly, such as the *AACN Pediatric Reference Card*, the *PALS Pocket Reference* by the American Heart Association, and the *Harriet Lane Handbook*, are all fingertip resources.

Pediatric advanced practice nurses (APRNs) have specialized population knowledge related to physical assessment, pharmacology, pathophysiology, and can promote evidence-based practice in the critical care environment. These clinical experts can provide mentoring and reinforce pediatric best practices with the bedside nurse.

Nurses working with children, meeting the designated requirements, should strongly consider taking the certification exam to become a pediatric critical care registered nurse. Certification offers employers and patients validation that the nurse possesses the specialty knowledge, skills, and experience to effectively and safely deliver care. Additionally, increased job satisfaction and increased self-confidence have been linked to certification, increasing the job enjoyment of the PICU nurse.[65]

To remain current in the care of pediatric patients, AACN and the SCCM provide pediatric-focused resources in the form of current books, journal articles, web pages, and live educational sessions. Additionally, PICU Listservs provide opportunities for networking with others in the specialty to enhance knowledge of the pediatric patient.

CONCLUSION

Caring for children in an adult critical care unit can be an exciting challenge. With appropriate orientation, competency maintenance, and performance improvement monitoring, the interprofessional team can provide quality care to children and their families. Providers caring for the youngest patients outside of a pediatric setting should remain ever vigilant, continuously assessing the need for transfer to a pediatric-specific center.

CASE STUDY 35.1

Respiratory Syncytial Virus Bronchiolitis

A 3-month-old male presents to the emergency department (ED) with two days of rhinorrhea and decreased oral intake. The patient history reveals a low-grade fever and rapid, noisy breathing, prompting his parents to seek care. The baby was born at 36 weeks gestation, received his 2-month immunizations on time, and usually breast feeds, but has not been feeding well since the illness started. His mother reports a decreased number of wet diapers and denies observing any cough, vomiting, diarrhea, or rashes. The infant lives with his parents and a 3-year-old sibling, and started attending daycare when his mother returned to work two weeks ago. The sibling has also been ill with rhinorrhea and a cough for the last week.

Physical exam reveals a tachypneic infant with grunting, nasal flaring, intercostal and subcostal retractions, intermittent wheezing, and coarse breath sounds throughout. Oxygen saturations were found to be 88% on room air. Oxygen therapy via high flow nasal cannula was started with an improvement in oxygen saturation to 92%. A nasal aspirator was used to suction copious secretions, which further improved the infant's oxygen saturation to 95%. The infant was given an albuterol treatment with minimal improvement in his symptoms. A peripheral intravenous (IV) catheter was placed and IV fluids started. While awaiting an inpatient bed, he became more tachypneic with increased work of breathing and a drop in his oxygen saturations, prompting admission to the intensive care unit (ICU).

Upon arrival, a viral respiratory panel was returned from the lab, revealing a positive identification of respiratory syncytial virus (RSV). Admission vital signs were: temperature 38.2°C, heart rate 160 bpm, blood pressure 72/52 mm Hg, respiratory rate of 60 breaths per minute and a blood oxygen saturation level (Spo^2) of 86%. His nasopharynx was suctioned and respiratory support was provided by high flow nasal cannula. The use of hypertonic saline, albuterol, corticosteroids, helium-oxygen (Heliox), and intubation were discussed but not initiated or required. A nasogastric feeding tube was placed and enteral nutrition of mother's breast milk was initiated.

Decision Point:

Why is the treatment plan in this case study appropriate to the patient situation?

REFERENCES

1. Agency for Healthcare Research and Quality. (2014). *Eliminating CLABSI: a national patient safety imperative: a progress report on the national on the CUSP: stop BSI project*. Rockville, MD. http://www.ahrq.gov/professionals/quality-patient-safety/cusp/onthecusprpt/index.html.
2. Reference deleted in page proofs.
3. Als, L. C., et al. (2015). Mental and physical well-being following admission to pediatric critical care. *Pediatr Crit Care Med*, *16*(5), 141–149.
4. American Academy of Pediatrics. (2013). AAP publications reaffirmed or retired (admission and discharge criteria). *Pediatrics*, *131*(5), e1707.
5. American Academy of Pediatrics. (2012). Committee on Hospital Care and Institute for Patient- and Family-Centered Care: patient- and family-centered care and the pediatrician's role. *Pediatrics*, *129*, 394–404.
6. American Academy of Pediatrics. (2013). Policy statement: *Clostridium difficile* infection in infants and children. *Pediatrics*, *131*(1), 196–200.
7. American Academy of Pediatrics, Committee on Bioethics. (1995). Informed consent, parental permission, and assent in pediatric practice. *Pediatrics*, *95*(2), 314–317.
8. American Academy of Pediatrics, Committee on Drugs. (2006). Guidelines for monitoring and management of pediatric patient during and after sedation for diagnostic and therapeutic procedures: an update. *Pediatrics*, *118*(6), 2587–2602.
9. American Academy of Pediatric Committee on Drugs and Committee on Hospital Care. (2003). Prevention of medication errors in the pediatric inpatient setting. *Pediatrics*, *112*(2), 431–435.
10. American Academy of Pediatrics Committee on Hospitals. (1993). Guidelines and levels of care for pediatric intensive care units. *Pediatrics*, *92*(1), 166–175.
11. American Association of Critical-Care Nurses. (2010). *Practice alert: family presence during CPR and invasive procedures*. Aliso Viejo: AACN.
12. American Heart Association and American Academy of Pediatrics. (2012). *Pediatric advanced life support provider manual*. Dallas: American Heart Association.
13. AstraZeneca. March 26. (2001). *Letter*. Wilmington, DE.
14. Ball, J. W., Bindler, R. C., & Cowen, K. (2014). *Pediatric assessment. principles of pediatric nursing: caring for children* (6th ed.). Upper Saddle River: Pearson.
15. Barnes, S. (2015). Analgesia and procedural sedation. In Johns Hopkins Hospital, B. Engorn, & J. Flerage (Eds.), *The Harriet Lane handbook: mobile medicine series* (20th ed.). Philadelphia: Elsevier Saunders.
16. Bartholome, W. G. (1995). Informed consent, parental permission, and assent in pediatric practice (Letter to the editor). *Pediatrics*, *95*(5), 981–982.
17. Bell, D., et al. (2013). The Texas Children's Hospital pediatric advanced warning score as a predictor of clinical deterioration in hospitalized infants and children: a modification of the PEWS tool. *J Pediatr Nurs*, *28*(6), 2–9.
18. Bent, K. N., Keeling, A., & Rouston, J. (1996). Home from the PICU: are parents ready? *Matern Child Nurs*, *21*, 80–84.
19. Bettler, J., & Roberts, K. A. (2000). Nutrition assessment of the critically ill child. *AACN Clin Issues*, *11*(4), 498–506.
20. Berwick, D. M., & Kotagal, M. (2004). Restricted visiting hours in the ICU: time to change. *JAMA*, *292*(6), 736–737.
21. Bigham, M. T., Amato, R., Bondurrant, P., et al. (2009). Ventilator-associated pneumonia in the pediatric intensive care unit: characterizing the problem and implementing a sustainable solution. *J Pediatr*, *154*, 582–587.
22. Birnie, K. A., et al. (2014). Hospitalized children continue to report undertreated and preventable pain. *Pain Res Manag*, *14*(4), 198–204.
23. Board, R. (2004). Father stress during a child's critical care hospitalization. *J Pediatr Health Care*, *18*, 244–249.
24. Board, R., & Ryan-Wenger, N. (2000). State of the science on parental stress and family functioning in pediatric intensive care units. *Am J Crit Care*, *9*(2), 106–122.
25. Brinker, D. (2003). Pain management in children. In P. A. Moloney-Harmon, & S. J. Czerwinski (Eds.), *Nursing care of the pediatric trauma patient*. St. Louis: Saunders.
26. Brown, T. L. (2012). Pediatric variations of nursing interventions. In M. J. Hockenberry, & D. Wilson (Eds.), *Wong's nursing care of infants and children* (10th ed.). St. Louis: Elsevier.
27. Burns, J. P., & Rushton, C. H. (2004). End-of-life care in the pediatric intensive care unit: research review and recommendations. *Crit Care Clin*, *20*, 467–485.
28. Reference deleted in page proofs.
29. Campbell, J. (2001). Unique solutions in pediatric critical care. *Pediatr Nurs*, *27*(5), 483–491.
30. Campbell, K. A., Olson, L. M., & Keenan, H. T. (2015). Critical elements in the medical evaluation of suspected child physical abuse. *Pediatrics*, *136*(1), 35–43.
31. Carroll, F. A., Sala, K., Fisher, D., & Zucker, A. (2014). Pediatric code events: does in-house intensivist coverage improve outcomes? *Pediatric Crit Care Med*, *15*(3), 250–257.
32. Centers for Disease Control and Prevention. (2002). Guideline for hand hygiene in healthcare settings: recommendations of the healthcare infection control practices advisory committee and the HICPA/SHEA/APIC/IDSA hand hygiene task force. *MMWR*, 51.
33. Chameides, L., & Ralston, M. (Eds.). (2011). American Academy of Pediatrics & American Heart Association. *Pediatric advanced life support*. Dallas: American Heart Association.
34. Cherry, J. D., et al. (Eds.). (2014). *Feigin and Cherry's textbook of pediatric infectious diseases* (7th ed.). St. Louis: Saunders.
35. Conlon, P., & Wilson, D. (2012). The child with respiratory dysfunction. In M. J. Hockenberry, & D. Wilson (Eds.), *Wong's nursing care of infants and children* (10th ed.). St. Louis: Elsevier.
36. Crowley, E., Williams, R., & Cousins, D. (2001). Medication errors in children: a descriptive summary of medication error reports submitted to the United States Pharmacopeia. *Curr Ther Res*, *26*, 627–640.
37. Curley, M. A. Q. (1998). Effects of the nursing mutual participation model of care and parental stress in the pediatric intensive care unit. *Heart Lung*, *17*, 682–688.
38. Curley, M. A. Q., & Wallace, J. (1992). Effects of the nursing mutual participation model of care on parental stress in the pediatric intensive care unit—a replication. *J Pediatr Nurs*, *7*, 377–385.
39. Davidson, J. E., Powers, K., Hedayat, K. M., et al. (2007). Clinical practice guidelines for support of the family in the patient-centered intensive care unit: American College of Critical Care Medicine task force 2004–2005. *Crit Care Med*, *35*, 605–622.
40. Davis, K. F., Colebaugh, A. M., Eithun, B. L., et al. (2014). Reducing catheter-associated urinary tract infections: a quality improvement initiative. *Pediatrics*, *134*(3), e857–e864.
41. Devlin, J. W., et al. (1999). Motor activity assessment scale: a valid and reliable sedation scale for use with mechanically ventilated patients in an adult surgical intensive care unit. *Crit Care Med*, *27*, 1271–1275.
42. Dixon-Woods, M., Young, B., & Henry, D. (1999). Partnerships with children. *BMJ*, *319*, 778–780.
43. Dutton, R. P., et al. (2003). Daily multidisciplinary rounds shorten length of stay for trauma patients. *J Trauma*, *55*(5), 913–919.
44. Ellenby, M. S., & Marcin, J. P. (2015). The role of telemedicine in pediatric critical care. *Crit Care Clin*, *31*(2), 275–290.
45. Emergency Nurses Association. (2012). *Clinical practice guideline: family presence during invasive procedures and resuscitation*. Park Ridge: Emergency Nurses Association.
46. Ewart, G. W., et al. (2004). The critical care medicine crisis: a call for federal action. *Chest*, *125*, 1518–1521.
47. Franck, L. S., Scoppettuolo, L. A., Wypij, D., Curley, M. A. Q., & The RESTORE Investigative Team. (2012). Validity and generalizability of the Withdrawal Assessment Tool-1 (WAT-1) for monitoring iatrogenic withdrawal syndrome in pediatric patients. *Pain*, *153*(1), 142–148.
48. Franck, L. S., Harris, S. K., Soetenga, D. J., Amling, J. K., & Curley, M. A. Q. (2008). The Withdrawal Assessment Tool–1 (WAT–1): an assessment instrument for monitoring opioid and benzodiazepine withdrawal symptoms in pediatric patients. *Pediatr Crit Care Med*, *9*(6), 573–580.
49. Reference deleted in page proofs.

50. Gonzalea, C. E., et al. (2004). Visiting preferences of patients in the intensive care unit and in a complex medical care unit. *Am J Crit Care, 13*(13), 194–197.
51. Goudie, A., Dynan, L., Brady, P. W., et al. (2014). Attributable cost and length of stay for central line-associated bloodstream infections. *Pediatrics, 133*(6), 1–8.
52. Gould, C. V., Umscheid, C. A., Agarwal, R. K., et al. (2010). Health-care infection control practice advisory: guideline for prevention of catheter-associated urinary tract infections 2009. *Infect Control Hosp Epidemiol, 31*(4), 319–326.
53. Gregg, T. L. (1998). Pediatric pain management in an adult critical care unit. *Crit Care Nurs Q, 21*(2), 42–58.
54. Gregory, C. J., et al. (2008). Comparison of critically ill and injured children transferred from referring hospitals versus in-house admissions. *Pediatrics, 121*(4), 906–911.
55. Reference deleted in page proofs.
56. Hazinski, M. F. (2013). Children are different. *In Nursing care of the critically ill child* (3rd ed.). St. Louis: Mosby.
57. Health Forum, L. L. C. (2011). *American Hospital Association Hospital Statistics, 2011 (2009 survey data)*. Chicago: American Hospital Association.
58. Henderson, D. P., & Knapp, J. F. (2006). Report of the national consensus conference on family presence during pediatric cardiopulmonary resuscitation and procedures. *J Emerg Nurs, 32*, 23–29.
59. Herr, K., Coyne, P. J., McCaffery, M., Manworren, R., & Merkel, S. (2011). Pain assessment in the patient unable to self-report: position statement with clinical practice recommendations. *Pain Manag Nurs, 12*(4), 230–250.
60. Holtzclaw, B. J. (1993). Monitoring body temperature. *AACN Clin Issues Crit Care Nurs, 4*(1), 44–55.
61. Holtzclaw, B. J. (1998). New trends in thermometry for the patient in the ICU. *Crit Care Nurs Q, 21*(3), 12–25.
62. Johnson, P. N., Miller, J. L., & Hagemann, T. M. (2012). Sedation and analgesia in critically ill children. *AACN Clin Issues Crit Care Nurs, 23*(4), 415–434.
63. Joint Commission. (2008). Preventing pediatric medication errors. *Sentinel event alert, 11*(39), 1–4.
64. Kane, S. L., Weber, R. J., & Dasta, J. F. (2003). The impact of critical care pharmacists on enhancing patient outcomes. *Intensive Care Med, 29*, 691–698.
65. Kaplow, R. (2011). The value of certification. *AACN Adv Crit Care, 22*(1), 25–32.
66. Kimberlin, D. W., Brady, M. T., Jackson, M., et al. (2015). Report of the committee on infectious diseases. *2015 Red Book* (30th ed.).
67. Kleinman, M. E., Chameides, L., Schexnayder, S. M., et al. (2010). Pediatric advanced life support: American Heart Association guidelines for cardiopulmonary resuscitation and emergency cardiovascular care. *Circulation, 122*(suppl 3), S876–S908.
68. Lorch, S. A., Meyers, S., & Carr, B. (2010). The regionalization of pediatric health care. *Pediatrics, 126*, 1182–1190.
69. Marcin, J. P., et al. (2004). Use of telemedicine to provide pediatric inpatient consultation to underserved rural Northern California. *J Pediatr, 144*, 375–380.
70. Martin, S. A., & Kline, A. M. (2004). Can there be a standard for temperature measurement in the pediatric intensive care unit? *AACN Clin Issues, 15*(2), 254–266.
71. McIntosh, A., & Pollock, A. N. (2010). Psuedosubluxation. *Pediatr Emerg Care, 26*(9), 691–692.
72. Meert, K. L., Clark, J., & Eggly, S. (2013). Family-centered care in the pediatric intensive care unit. *Pediatr Clin North Am, 60*, 761–772.
73. Mehta, N. M., & Duggan, C. P. (2009). Nutritional deficiencies during critical illness. *Pediatr Clin North Am, 56*(5), 1143–1160.
74. Merkel, S. I., et al. (2003). FLACC behavioral pain assessment scale: a comparison with the child's self-report. *Pediatr Nurs, 29*(13), 195–199.
75. Merkel, S. I., et al. (1997). The FLACC: a behavioral scale for scoring postoperative pain in young children. *Pediatr Nurs, 23*(3), 293–298.
76. Merck, T., & McElfresh, P. (2012). Family-centered care of the child during illness and hospitalization. In M. J. Hockenberry, & D. Wilson (Eds.), *Wong's nursing care of infants and children* (10th ed.). St. Louis: Elsevier.
77. Moloney-Harmon, P. A. (2009). Pediatric trauma. In K. McQuillan, M. B. Flynn Makic, & E. Whalen (Eds.), *Trauma nursing: from resuscitation to rehabilitation* (4th ed.). Philadelphia: Saunders.
78. Moloney-Harmon, P. A. (2013). The critically ill pediatric patient. In P. Gonce Morton, & D. K. Fontaine (Eds.), *Critical care nursing: a holistic approach* (10th ed.). Philadelphia: Lippincott Williams & Wilkins.
79. Nylund, C. M., Goudie, A., & Garza, J. M. (2011). *Clostridium difficile* infection in hospitalized children in the United States. *Arch Pediatr Adolesc Med, 165*(5), 451–457.
80. O'Grady, N. P., et al. (2011). *Healthcare Infection Control Practices Advisory Committee (HICPAC). Guidelines for the prevention of intravascular catheter-related infections.* Atlanta: Centers for Disease Control and Prevention.
81. Paladichuk, A. (1998). Children in the adult ICU: interview with Mary Fran Hazinski. *Crit Care Nurse, 18*(6), 82–87.
82. Pate, M. F. (2013). Assent and dissent in pediatric progressive and critical care. *AACN Adv Crit Care, 24*(4), 356–359.
83. Pate, M. F., & Zapata, T. (2002). How deeply should I go when I suction an endotracheal (ETT) or tracheostomy tube (TT)? *Crit Care Nurse, 22*, 130–131.
84. Phelps, S. J., Hagemann, T. M., Lee, K. R., & Thompson, A. J. (Eds.). (2013). *Pediatric injectable drugs: teddy bear book* (10th ed.) Bethesda, MD: American Society of Health-System Pharmacists.
85. Polikoff, L. A., & McCabe, M. E. (2013). End of life care in the pediatric ICU. *Curr Opin Pediatr, 25*(3), 285–289.
86. Pollack, M. M. (2007). Pediatric quality factors. *J Trauma, 63*, S143–S145.
87. Poole, R. L., & Carleton, B. C. (2008). Medication errors: neonates and children are the most vulnerable. *J Pediatr Pharmacol Ther, 13*(2), 65–67.
88. Ralston, S., et al. (2014). Clinical practice guideline: the diagnosis, management, and prevention of bronchiolitis. *Pediatrics, 134*(5), e1474–e1502.
89. Reynolds, M., et al. (2014). Are temporal artery temperatures accurate enough to replace rectal temperature measurement in pediatric ED patients? *J Emerg Nurs, 40*, 46–50.
90. Riley, C., Poss, W. B., & Wheeler, D. S. (2013). The evolving model of pediatric critical care delivery in North America. *Pediatr Clin North Am, 60*, 545–562.
91. Rinke, M. L., et al. (2014). Interventions to reduce pediatric medication errors: a systematic review. *Pediatrics, 134*(2), 338–360.
92. Rosenberg, D. I., & Moss, M. M. (2004). American College of Critical Care Medicine of the Society of Critical Care Medicine: guidelines and levels of care for pediatric intensive care units. *Crit Care Med, 32*(10), 2117–2127.
93. Ruttimann, U. E., Patel, K. M., & Pollack, M. M. (2002). Relevance of diagnostic diversity and patient volumes for quality and length of stay in pediatric intensive care units. *Pediatr Crit Care Med, 1*, 133–139.
94. Slota, M., et al. (2003). Perspectives on family-centered, flexible visitation in the intensive care setting. *Crit Care Med, 31*(5), S362–S366.
95. Smith, H. A. B. (2013). Pediatric delirium monitoring and management in the pediatric intensive care unit. *Pediatr Clin North Am, 60*, 741–760.
96. Society of Critical Care Medicine, Pediatric Section Task Force on Admission and Discharge Criteria in Conjunction with the American College of Critical Care Medicine and the Committee on Hospital Care of the American Academy of Pediatrics. (1999). Guidelines for developing admission and discharge policies for the pediatric intensive care unit. *Crit Care Med, 27*(4), 843–845.
97. Tilford, J. M., et al. (2000). Volume-outcome relationships in pediatric intensive care units. *Pediatrics, 106*, 289–294.
98. Tobias, J. D. (2014). Acute pain management in infants and children part 1. *Pediatr Ann, 43*(7), 163–168.
99. Tobias, J. D. (2014). Acute pain management in infants and children part 2. *Pediatr Ann, 43*(7), 169–175.
100. Traube, C., et al. (2014). Cornell assessment of pediatric delirium: a valid, rapid, observational tool for screening delirium in the PICU. *Crit Care Med, 42*(2), 1–8.
101. Tucker., et al. (2009). Prospective evaluation of a pediatric inpatient early warning scoring system. *J Spec Pediatr Nurs, 14*, 79–85.

102. US Food and Drug Administration. (2001). *Pediatric exclusivity provision: status report to Congress.* Rockville, MD: Food and Drug Administration.
103. Van Waning, N. R., Kleiber, C1, & Freyenberger, B. (2005). Development and implementation of a protocol for transfers out of the pediatric intensive care unit. *Crit Care Nurse, 25*(3), 50–55.
104. Vazirani, S., Hays, R. D., Shapiro, M. F., et al. (2005). Effect of a multidisciplinary intervention on communication and collaboration among physicians and nurses. *Am J Crit Care, 14*(1), 71–77.
105. Venkatachalam, V., Hendley, J. O., & Wilson, D. F. (2011). The diagnostic dilemma of ventilator associated pneumonia in critically ill children. *Pediatr Crit Care Med, 12*(3), 286–296.
106. Wong, D., & Baker, C. (1988). Pain in children: comparison of assessment scales. *Pediatr Nurs, 14*(1), 9–17.
107. Zawistowski, C. A., & Frader, J. E. (2003). Ethical problems in pediatric critical care: consent. *Crit Care Med, 31*(5), 407–410.
108. Zenel, J., & Goldstein, B. (2002). Child abuse in the pediatric intensive care unit. *Crit Care Med, 30*(11), S515–S523.

36

Caring for the Critically Ill Elderly Patient

Rosemarie Hirsch

THE AGING POPULATION

Demographics

Americans are living longer than ever before. Older adults constitute the fastest-growing segment of the US population. The number of Americans aged 65 and over is projected to increase from a current level of 43.1 million to 83.7 million by the year 2050, which will be approximately 20% of the total population. This represents a doubling of the age-group numbers since 2012. In the United States, the definition of older adult or elderly is commonly considered to be 65 years of age and older, the age of Medicare eligibility. This large, heterogeneous population is subdivided into three main subgroups to address the unique and specific physiological, social, and healthcare needs:[19,40,45]

- Young-old: ages 65–74
- Middle-old: ages 75–84
- Old-old: ages 85+

The old-old group is the fastest growing segment of the population, growing at twice the rate of the 65 and over age group and four times faster than the total US population.[43] Females continue to live longer than males but this gap is narrowing.[42] The current cohort of older Americans is more highly educated than previous generations. In 2010, 80% of the elderly population had a high school education and 23% had a Bachelor's degree.[44]

Mortality has declined due to reductions in infections, childhood diseases, and advances in adult healthcare. Thus life expectancy has increased. The increase in life expectancy during the twentieth century has been due in large part to remarkable achievements in treating infectious diseases and chronic diseases in the older population. Although older Americans generally enjoy good heath, a significant proportion of the elderly suffer from chronic health conditions.

FACTORS THAT INFLUENCE AGING

Age-Related Changes

Regardless of chronologic age, the physiologic process of aging is a highly individualized process; no two people age at the same rate or in the same way. Some aging processes are universal. Over time, the number of normally functioning cells in the body is reduced, oxygen consumption is decreased, and response to physiologic stressors is blunted.[19,40] However, a significant interaction between genetic, environmental, physiologic, psychological, and social aspects of life exists. There are major differences between individuals' physiologic reserves and their disease exposure, severity, and its functional impact. As age advances, the incidence of disease increases and cardiovascular and neoplastic diseases become the most common causes of death.[19,29] Although physiologic decline and disease processes influence each other, the body's normal aging process does not produce significant dysfunction or impairment in the absence of disease.[19,29] Therefore it is important to distinguish age-related changes from those associated with chronic conditions or acute illness in order to avoid prematurely attributing findings to advanced age, when they are actually caused by a disease state.[19,29]

Social and Environmental Factors

Some changes commonly associated with aging are a result of long-term exposure to a variety of environmental and social conditions (Box 36.1). Over the course of a lifetime, socioeconomic status, lifestyle, and personal health habits leave their mark on everyone.

Cumulative Health History

Long life span is associated with an increased prevalence of chronic and acute illnesses. Many conditions take years or even decades to manifest, and their number accumulates over time. The cumulative effects of life are borne by all; no one reaches old age without a medical history, often a very extensive one.

Comorbidities

A comorbid condition is defined as any additional disease state that will significantly affect the patient's response to the present illness or injury. Box 36.2 lists comorbidities common among geriatric patients. Each of the environmental, social, and comorbidity factors previously described is strongly influenced by genetics, particularly a family history of certain disorders (e.g., coronary artery disease, stroke, dementia, and cancer).

THE GERIATRIC CRITICAL CARE PATIENT

Demographics

The characteristic processes of tissue and organ changes associated with aging—in conjunction with the prevalence of chronic conditions—contribute to the high number of geriatric patients treated in critical care.[1,23] Driven by demographics and increased life expectancy, the total number of older patients treated in critical care can be expected to rise dramatically over the next quarter century.[23] As of 2014, half of all patients admitted to critical care in the United States were older than 65 years and accounted for 60% of all intensive care days.[41] It is estimated that one in four admissions to critical care are in the 85 and older age group.[37]

BOX 36.1 Environmental and Social Factors Associated with Aging

Environmental Exposures
- Inhalants: tobacco smoke, wood fires, asbestos, coal dust
- Toxins: heavy metals, radon
- Ultraviolet light

Poverty
- Lack of adequate primary care, including immunizations
- Reduced access to care
- Self-care knowledge and skills deficits
- Undertreatment of acute and chronic conditions

Lifestyle
- Absence of an effective social support system
- Chronic stress
- Deficient personal hygiene practices
- Inadequate sleep
- Poor nutritional status, including obesity
- Repetitive-use injuries
- Sedentary behaviors
- Substance abuse: alcohol, tobacco, prescription and recreational drugs

Data from References 1, 6, 19, 21, 22, 25, 26, 29, 36, 37, and 40.

BOX 36.2 Comorbidities Common to the Geriatric Patient

- Arthritis
- Hypertension
- Cardiovascular disease
- Neoplasms
- Chronic pulmonary disease
- Obesity
- Dementia
- Renal insufficiency
- Hepatic disease
- Stroke
- Hyperlipidemia
- Type 2 diabetes

Data from References 6, 19, 24-26, 40, 42, and 45.

The critical care admitting diagnoses for patients over 65 years vary based on the age subgroup. Those 85 and older (old-old) are admitted more often after a surgical procedure, whereas the 75–84 (middle-old) age-group is more likely to be admitted with decompensated heart failure.[6] However, with advancing age, the need for critical care management of chronic disease exacerbations also results in frequent critical care admissions.[6,37] Practitioners caring for critically ill elderly patients are routinely faced with difficult decisions regarding aggressive treatment, outcome optimization, and rationing of resources. In order to understand the basis for such decisions, healthcare providers must appreciate the normal changes associated with aging and their implications for care.[13]

Critical care nurses need to be cognizant of the differences in outcomes and complications experienced by critically ill elders.[24] Aging has a profound impact on individual physiologic performance. In every body system, the elderly patient's physiologic reserves are limited and function can deteriorate rapidly, even with expert medical and nursing attention. Their declining physiologic status can force seniors to use their limited reserves just to maintain homeostasis. Therefore, when reserves are required to meet the increased demands of acute illness or surgical stress, but are no longer present, organ system failure ensues.[24]

Traumatic Injury

In addition to experiencing frequent acute illnesses and exacerbations of chronic conditions, the elderly are overrepresented in the number of trauma patients admitted to surgical critical care units. Trauma, once considered predominantly a disease of the young, has long been the leading cause of death in the United States for individuals between the ages of 1 and 44 years.

Although the incidence of major traumatic injury remains lower in the geriatric population than in any other age group, both longevity gains and increasingly active lifestyles have contributed to rising injury rates.[36] The risk of death after traumatic injury increases over the age of 55. Following major injury, older adults experience in-hospital mortality two to six times greater than younger adults with equivalent injuries. Although older persons comprise only 12.5% of the population, almost one-third of the deaths from injury occur in the 65-plus age group.

In the elderly patient, poor outcomes following traumatic injury are related to both the normal changes of aging and the prevalence of preexisting comorbid conditions. As a result of reduced physiologic reserves and chronic disease, injured older adults are hospitalized for trauma at a rate twice that of the general population.[36] There are significant differences between older and younger patients related both to injury patterns and to the frequency and type of complications experienced following trauma. Despite a typically less severe mechanism of injury, older adults experience a greater number of postinjury complications than do their younger counterparts. Preexisting medical conditions, particularly cardiovascular disease, have a profound effect on patients' abilities to manage the stresses of injury.

Mechanisms of Injury

Falls are the leading trauma mechanism among persons over the age of 65.[36] Many factors associated with aging contribute to the high incidence of falls in this population. In the over-75 age group, falls are also the leading cause of death from trauma.[36] Dementia, decreased visual acuity, obesity, neurologic and musculoskeletal impairments, gait and balance disturbances, and medication use can all be contributory factors. The majority of falls (84%) occur at home, and approximately 13% are attributed to some acute medical condition.[36]

The second cause of accidental death in older adults is motor vehicle accidents. Although the number of miles driven annually decreases in individuals over the age of 55, the elderly have a total motor vehicle crash rate second only to that of 16- to 25-year-olds. However, the elderly (particularly those 75 years or older) suffer a post collision fatality rate greater than any other age group. In contrast to younger individuals, the elderly are more likely to crash during daylight hours, in good weather, and close to home. Older adults are also more prone to collisions involving intersections, traffic sign violations, right-of-way decisions, and another vehicle. However, compared with younger cohorts, the older adult is less likely to have ingested alcohol. Age-related declines in cognitive function, decreased auditory acuity, changes in direct and peripheral vision, impaired coordination, and increased reaction time all contribute to crashes in elderly motorists.[40]

Critical Care Outcomes Following Injury

The elderly are predisposed to serious posttrauma sequelae and suffer an increased incidence of multiple organ system dysfunction, wound healing problems, sepsis, and other infections.[36] The differences between geriatric and younger patients suggest the need for prompt diagnosis and aggressive treatment of the older population. However, there is still considerable debate regarding whether routine critical care admission, invasive hemodynamic monitoring, and hemodynamic optimization really lead to improved survival following trauma in the geriatric patient. Outcomes in the critically injured elderly are often affected by the presence of complications, some of which have significant effects on an individual's long-term status.

Even minor trauma may result in a substantial loss of preinjury function.[36] Nevertheless, most injured older adults without significant neurologic insults will return home and as many as 85% eventually resume independent function.[36] This suggests that an initial aggressive approach to geriatric trauma patient management should be pursued.

However, more attention must be paid to long-term outcomes (e.g., quality of life and functional ability), and not just survival to hospital discharge. Without these long-term predictors, we may fail to treat those older adults who would survive, and instead pursue futile interventions in other critically injured older adults.[36]

Minimizing Potential Critical Care Problems

The goals of patient management in critical care are to maintain optimum cellular oxygen delivery, provide adequate substrate for tissue healing, and control pain. As a result of the physiologic changes and coexisting organ dysfunction common to the elderly population, some of our usual patient care strategies may need to be adjusted.

CARDIOVASCULAR SYSTEM

Cardiovascular decline has been one of the most studied aspects of aging, yet the functional implications of these changes are difficult to separate from normal age-related alterations in body composition, metabolic rate, and general state of fitness, all of which affect cardiac performance.[15] In the healthy elderly, exercise capacity is commonly restricted by noncardiac functions that limit exercise ability (e.g., neurologic, pulmonary, or musculoskeletal disorders).[23]

Age-Related Changes

Decreased Beta-Adrenergic Receptors

Aging is associated with changes in the sympathetic and parasympathetic nervous systems. Receptors present on the senescent myocardium become less sensitive, producing an impaired response to beta-adrenergic stimulation that attenuates maximal heart rate (HR). This is particularly important during exercise or other physiologic stressors such as major injury or critical illness. From a pharmacologic standpoint, HR responses to drugs (e.g., beta blockers, digoxin, and parasympatholytic agents) are less in the elderly population.[29]

Decreased Exercise Tolerance and Cardiac Reserve

In the older patient at rest, cardiac output (CO), stroke volume (SV), and ejection fraction are not substantially changed.[29] These functions are maintained despite the increase in afterload imposed by stiffening of the outflow tract. However, aging is associated with a decline in exercise performance.[29] Patients 65 years and older have decreased pump function as a result of progressive fibrosis of the myocardium. Thickening of the left ventricular wall, along with stiffening of the aortic and mitral valves, makes it more difficult for the aging heart to maintain adequate contractile strength.[29]

Healthy older persons have no major age-associated decline in CO during exercise, but maximal HR, maximal aerobic capacity, peak exercise CO, and peak ejection fraction slowly decline with advancing years. Notably, the mechanism by which CO is maintained during exercise differs between elderly and younger persons. In young adults, output is sustained by increasing HR. In contrast, the aging heart becomes less responsive to beta-adrenergic stimulation and instead maintains CO by recruitment of reserves to increase ventricular filling and SV.[29]

Increased Dysrhythmias

With aging, much of the heart's autonomic tissue is replaced by connective tissue and fat. These progressive changes cause conduction abnormalities throughout the intranodal tracts and bundle of His, contributing to a high incidence of sick sinus syndrome, atrial dysrhythmias, and bundle branch blocks. Approximately 50% of the elderly population have abnormalities on their resting electrocardiograms (ECGs), most commonly PR or QT interval prolongation, intraventricular conduction abnormalities, reduced QRS voltage, and a leftward shift of the QRS axis. Elderly men have ECG abnormalities more frequently than do equivalent-age women.[29]

The most prominent dysrhythmia in older adults is premature ventricular contractions. Other symptoms of increasing myocardial irritability include sinus node and atrioventricular conduction defects, of which atrial fibrillation is the most common sustained arrhythmia in older adults.[12,29] Because the majority of dysrhythmic patients are asymptomatic, the routine use of antidysrhythmics is not recommended. The side effects and toxicities related to antidysrhythmic use frequently pose a greater risk to the elderly than do the dysrhythmia itself. On the other hand, pharmacologic therapy is warranted in symptomatic patients.

Orthostatic Hypotension

Abrupt reductions in blood pressure (BP), caused by alterations in peripheral resistance, CO, or blood volume, are sensed by the baroreceptors. Baroreceptor stimulation results in increased impulse frequency in the medullary vasomotor center. This produces a rise in HR, as well as vasoconstriction of the peripheral vasculature. Both of these effects are designed to restore BP. However, baroreceptor function is blunted with aging, predisposing elderly patients to episodes of orthostatic hypotension that can be further exacerbated by certain common medications. In addition, many geriatric patients can readily become hypotensive as a result of vagal stimulation. In this population, a Valsalva maneuver can easily cause a drop in BP and even produce syncope.

Heart Rate Changes

With advancing age, the heart maintains a rate not substantially changed from that of younger adults. However, the maximal HR achieved during exercise is attenuated. Fortunately, this decreased HR response is accompanied by an increase in both left ventricular end-diastolic volume and SV, which serve to maintain CO during exercise. If the HR response becomes restricted, from diseased myocardium or beta-blockade, an elderly person's capacity to respond to exercise or stress will be severely limited.[29] Conversely, tachycardias are also poorly tolerated in the elderly. When left ventricular filling time is shortened by a tachydysrhythmia, cardiac performance is significantly decreased.[29]

Decreased Diastolic Filling

Despite an age-related reduction in early diastolic filling, preload is maintained because left atrial contraction becomes more vigorous, thereby increasing late diastolic filling of the left ventricle (LV). In a poorly compliant LV, left atrial contraction can contribute up to 50% of LV filling. As a result of this vigorous atrial contraction, it is not uncommon to note a compensatory S_4 heart sound. Loss of atrial kick, the atrial contribution to preload, will substantially impair cardiac function. Consequently, in older adults, the onset of atrial fibrillation can cause a marked reduction in CO.[12] Because ventricular filling and relaxation are energy-dependent processes, even mild hypoxemia can prolong relaxation, increase diastolic pressures, and aggravate pulmonary congestion, subsequently leading to diastolic dysfunction. In patients over the age of 80 years, diastolic dysfunction is responsible for up to 50% of heart failure cases.[29]

Vascular Changes

Aging induces gradual thickening of the intimal vascular layer, primarily the result of an increase in the number of smooth muscle cells and the amount of connective tissue.[29] Arteriosclerosis (thickening and loss of elasticity in the arterial walls) and atherosclerosis (lipid deposition and thickening of the intimal cell layers within the arteries) cause the arteries to become progressively less distensible. The narrowing vascular diameter then alters the vessels' pressure-volume relationship. These changes are clinically significant because even small alterations in intravascular diameter are accompanied by a disproportionate increase in systolic BP.[29] Atherosclerotic disease not only elevates BP but also is associated with a concomitant reduction in blood flow to vital organs, and a decrease in physiologic reserve.

The vascular changes of aging are not limited to the small vessels. Calcification and fibrosis cause progressive stiffening of the cardiac valves, the great vessels, and the heart's outflow tract, resulting in increased resistance to ventricular emptying, a modest increase in pulmonary artery pressure, and compensatory ventricular hypertrophy.[29] Because of these vascular changes, peripheral pulses, particularly in the feet, may be diminished or absent in the elderly.

Blood Pressure Changes

The vascular changes of aging produce a gradual but linear rise in systolic BP. Diastolic pressure is less affected by time and generally remains the same or may even drop as the patient ages.[10,29] Because of the cardiovascular changes with aging, over two thirds of older adults are diagnosed with hypertension and over 80% are 75 years or older. Practitioners must be alert to how a blood pressure measurement is obtained (i.e., correct size blood pressure cuff). The use of a mean arterial pressure (MAP) measurement can provide a more meaningful indication of organ perfusion in the elderly.[15]

Decreased Left Ventricular Compliance

With advancing years, there is progressive loss of myocytes, in both the left and right ventricles, and an increase in myocardial collagen content (type I). Although the muscle fibers that line the endocardium atrophy with age, the LV wall thickens, producing left ventricular hypertrophy (LVH). This LVH is primarily the result of myocyte hypertrophy related to an increase in myocyte cell volume. LVH causes a moderate reduction in left ventricular cavity size and a compensatory rise in systolic BP. These changes all combine to increase myocardial stiffness, limit diastolic filling, and produce an overall decline in ventricular compliance. Therefore, the LV must develop a higher filling pressure for a given increase in ventricular volume. The functional consequence of this is heightened myocardial oxygen consumption, which puts patients at risk for the development of myocardial ischemia.[29]

Decreased Number of Pacemaker Cells

Another change associated with cardiac aging is a progressive reduction in the number of pacemaker cells in the sinus node. This explains the frequency of sinus dysrhythmias in the elderly and partially accounts for elders' reduced compensatory response to stressors.

Common Problems and Management Strategies

Acute Coronary Syndrome

The incidence of acute coronary syndromes (ACSs), coronary artery disease (CAD) and myocardial infarction (MI), all increase markedly with age. Cardiac disease is also the most common comorbid condition in the elderly, with 83% of all cardiovascular deaths occurring in patients over the age of 65. Although the functional impact of this disease significantly affects geriatric morbidity and mortality, its presentation is frequently atypical and nonspecific.[15,29]

Chest pain is still the leading symptom of MI in all age groups, yet the elderly often present a very different clinical picture than younger persons with acute MI. Individuals with altered cardiac pain perception (e.g., the elderly and persons with long-standing diabetes mellitus) regularly present with anginal-equivalent syndromes rather than classic ischemic chest pain. In older patients, typical anginal-equivalent symptoms include unusual fatigue, shortness of breath, syncope, acute confusion, and vomiting. The most frequently encountered anginal-equivalent chief complaint is dyspnea, usually resulting from pulmonary edema. Unexplained sinus tachycardia, cardiogenic asthma, and new-onset lower extremity edema have also been reported as anginal-equivalents in the elderly.[15] Among the old-old, an acute MI may present with neurologic symptoms (e.g., acute mental status changes, new-onset weakness, and stroke).[15] In the Framingham Heart Study, persons aged 75 to 84 years were found to have an asymptomatic MI incidence of greater than 40%.[29]

Myocardial ischemia treatment strategies for patients between the ages of 65 and 75 years are similar to those used in the younger population. Limited data are available regarding the treatment of patients 75 to 84 years of age. In the old-old, diagnosis and therapy must be highly individualized.[15] The high incidence of atypical MI symptoms means that older patients often arrive at the hospital later than their younger counterparts. Unfortunately, this eliminates the possibility of fibrinolytic therapy if the 6-hour window of opportunity has expired. In addition, comorbid conditions (e.g., hypertension, dysrhythmias, or previous stroke) frequently contraindicate fibrinolysis in the elderly.[15]

In older patients undergoing surgery who are at increased cardiac risk, the use of preoperative beta-adrenergic blockade has been shown to reduce the incidence of postoperative cardiac morbidity and mortality. In fact, published guidelines on perioperative cardiac risk management now include the use of beta blockers.[35]

Shock

Normal cardiovascular changes in the elderly affect how the body responds to shock states. LV wall thickening, myocardial irritability, calcification and fibrosis of the heart valves, loss of myocardial compliance, and decreased SV combine to limit the body's response to stress and increased oxygen demands. These age-related cardiac changes make it considerably more difficult for the geriatric patient to respond to hypovolemic, distributive, or cardiogenic shock states.

Because of the prevalence of hypertension in the elderly, BP may appear normal despite significant reduction from baseline. This loss of elasticity and vasomotor tone decreases the body's ability to adapt to changing oxygen needs. In individuals with a history of hypertension, hypotensive episodes may be difficult to detect. Common medications (e.g., digoxin [Lanoxin] and beta blockers) will blunt compensatory reactions to shock by inhibiting the normal tachycardic response.[15] As a result of the elderly patient's dependence on preload, even minor hypovolemia can produce significant compromises in cardiac function.[45] The aging myocardium is less sensitive to both endogenous and exogenous catecholamines, restricting its ability to mount a normal, compensatory tachycardic response to hypovolemia.[45]

Fluid administration in hypovolemic and distributive shock states must be judiciously monitored to provide adequate volume replacement while preventing overload. Nonetheless, underresuscitation must be strictly avoided because CO in the aging heart is highly dependent on adequate preload. Hypovolemia will worsen diastolic dysfunction, decrease renal and coronary perfusion, and impair tissue oxygen delivery, leading to myocardial ischemia and wound-healing failures.[45] Once the geriatric patient has been fluid resuscitated, the need for high doses of vasopressors to achieve adequate BP must be weighed against the increased myocardial workload these agents produce.

Because the elderly are barely able to raise CO to meet oxygen demands, in patients with hypovolemic shock consider early transfusion rather than the infusion of large volumes of crystalloids or colloids. Many elders are at increased risk for bleeding because of the use of warfarin (Coumadin), aspirin, ibuprofen (Advil), and other anticlotting agents. Administration of packed red blood cells promotes oxygen-carrying capacity without fluid overload. Whenever possible, all blood products should be warmed before transfusion. Vasopressors should be used cautiously and only after adequate volume has been restored. When large-volume resuscitation is necessary (e.g., sepsis, hemorrhage), subsequent fluid mobilization may take up to four times as long as it does in younger patients.[45]

Cardiac Arrest

Complications resulting from cardiopulmonary resuscitation increase with age. Even when chest compressions are performed correctly, rib fractures can result. Less frequent complications include sternal fractures, pneumothorax, hemothorax, pulmonary contusions, lacerations of the liver and spleen, and separation of the ribs from the sternum. Each of these conditions is poorly tolerated in the geriatric patient.

RESPIRATORY SYSTEM

As the result of both chest wall and lung changes, a gradual decline in respiratory function accompanies aging. The normal respiratory rate in older adults is 20 to 22 breaths per minute. Typically, these modifications occur progressively as age advances and they should not alter an elderly person's ability to breathe effortlessly.[19] Nonetheless, factors such as frequent exposure to environmental pollutants (particularly cigarette smoke) and recurrent pulmonary infections will accelerate age-related changes, making it difficult to distinguish expected alterations in pulmonary function from disease states.[19] Careful assessment and management of respiratory status are essential even when the patient presents with a nonrespiratory condition.

Age-Related Changes

Decreased Lung Compliance

Physiologic changes in the aging lungs lead to diminished elastic recoil as a result of an increase in the ratio of elastin to collagen in the interlobular septa and pleura.[40] This loss of lung elasticity reduces pulmonary compliance, which leads to small airway collapse, uneven alveolar ventilation, and air trapping. Collapse of the small airways during forced expiration affects dynamic lung volumes and limits flow rates. These anatomic changes are reflected by an increase in residual volume and a decline in forced expiratory volume.[20]

Ventilation/Perfusion Imbalance

Age-associated changes in the morphology of the alveolar parenchyma are related to a reduction in the alveolar surface area available for gas exchange.[40] This produces an increase in the amount of physiologic dead space and leads to a ventilation/perfusion mismatch, which in turn causes a decline in the partial pressure of arterial oxygen tension (Pao_2).[20,40]

Age alone does not affect ventilation. The partial pressure of carbon dioxide ($Paco_2$) in healthy elders remains unchanged despite the increase in dead space.[20] However, because many older patients suffer from pulmonary disorders that reduce carbon dioxide elimination (e.g., chronic obstructive pulmonary disease), elevated $Paco_2$ levels are not an uncommon finding in the elderly population.[40]

Thoracic Changes

With advancing age, the chest wall and vertebrae (thoracic skeleton) undergo progressive osteoporotic changes and vertebral collapse, producing kyphosis. Contractures of the intercostal muscles and calcification of the costal cartilage result in a decline in rib mobility and reduced chest wall compliance. The functional effect of these transformations is a decrease in thoracic wall excursion.[20] Progressive loss of strength in the respiratory muscles is accompanied by a decline in maximum inspiratory and expiratory force by as much as 50%.[40]

Decreased Efficacy of Ventilatory Exchange

Starting at approximately 40 years of age, there is a gradual and linear decrease in the efficacy of ventilatory exchange. Changes include a reduction in the number of functional alveoli and pulmonary capillaries, an increase in atelectasis and fibrosis, and enlargement of the alveolar ducts.[40] Capillary blood volume and surface area also decline with advancing age. In addition to remodeling of the small airways, anatomic alterations occur in the large airways as well. The cartilage of the trachea and bronchi becomes stiffer and less compliant. Bronchial enlargement then displaces inhaled air away from the alveoli that line the alveolar ducts, limiting the area available for gas exchange.[40] These modifications combine to diminish diffusion capacity, which is a function of both surface area and capillary blood volume.[40] A summary of age-associated changes in respiratory parameters is given in Table 36.1.

Decreased Ventilatory Response to Hypoxia and Hypercarbia

The control of ventilation is also affected by aging. Geriatric patients have a diminished response to hypoxia and hypercarbia because chemoreceptor sensitivity is decreased.[40] Therefore ventilatory responses to hypoxemia and hypercapnia fall by 50% and 40%, respectively. The exact mechanism of this decline has not been well defined, but it may be the result of reduced chemoreceptor function either at the peripheral or at the central nervous system level.[40] It is important to remember that respiratory center sensitivity to narcotics increases with advancing age.[40]

Increased Susceptibility to Atelectasis and Infection

A number of age-related changes diminish the elderly patient's respiratory defense mechanisms and increase susceptibility to atelectasis and pulmonary infections. Because of atrophy of the epithelial lining, mucociliary clearance is reduced and it becomes progressively more difficult to clear bacteria from the bronchi. Even the mucus itself changes. The submucosal glands decrease mucus production, causing dryness and thickening of secretions.[20] Impaired mucociliary clearance and thickened secretions promote chronic gram-negative colonization of the upper airways, predisposing patients to pneumonia. Elderly individuals with impaired cough and swallowing mechanisms are at heightened risk for pneumonia secondary to aspiration.[20] In addition, older adults experience alterations in the ability of the respiratory system to protect against pathogens. As an accompaniment of normal aging, cough strength decreases and there is a progressive reduction in T-cell function and decreased IgA production, which unite to increase susceptibility to viral and bacterial infections.[40]

TABLE 36.1 Age-Associated Changes in Respiratory Parameters for the Critically Ill Elderly Patient

Parameter	Change
Chest wall compliance	Decreased
Forced vital capacity	Decreased
Forced expiratory volume	Decreased
Functional residual capacity	Mildly increased
Maximum expiratory force	Decreased
Maximum inspiratory force	Decreased
Pa_{O_2}	No change
Pa_{O_2}	Decreased
P_{CO_2}	No change
Residual volume	Increased
Total lung capacity	No change
Vital capacity	Decreased

From References 15, 19, 20, 29, 40, and 45.

Common Problems and Management Strategies

Pneumonia

Respiratory infections are the fourth leading cause of death of those over 65 years of age. Elderly nursing home patients in particular have a substantially higher mortality rate than other individuals with community-acquired pneumonia.[40] A diminished cough reflex, fewer cilia, a decline in surfactant production, a decrease in immune system effectiveness, and an increased frequency of oropharyngeal colonization with gram-negative organisms all place the elderly patient at risk for the development of pneumonia.[20]

Most pneumonias in older adults result from micro-aspiration. The elderly, particularly those with impaired airway protection or a gastrointestinal condition that predisposes them to reflux, can aspirate large volumes of bacteria.[12] The high incidence of pneumonia among elderly inhabitants of long-term care facilities is largely related to the prevalence of dysphagia.[40]

Pneumonia is also strongly associated with nutritional status because of the relationship between protein adequacy and immune system function. In general, pneumonia symptoms in the elderly are less prominent than in adults under 65 years old. The elderly are prone to atypical pneumonia presentations characterized by subacute illness and nonrespiratory symptoms (e.g., headache and diarrhea). Although cough is the most common finding in approximately 80% of all pneumonia patients,[40] it is less prominent in the elderly, especially nursing home residents and those with serious comorbidities. Other atypical pneumonia symptoms include falling, failure to thrive, altered functional capacity, and deterioration of existing illnesses. Delirium and acute confusion frequently signal pneumonia in older adults.[20,40] Individuals over the age of 80 years are less likely to present with pleuritic chest pain, headache, or myalgias than are younger patients, but are more likely to exhibit altered mental status. The absence of clear-cut respiratory symptoms, the lack of fever, and the presence of pleuritic chest pain are all related to an increased risk of death from pneumonia.[40]

Chest Trauma

As a result of progressive osteoporosis and reduced chest wall compliance, older trauma patients are more likely to have rib fractures, or even a flail segment, than are young adults. Rib fractures and chest wall contusions are intensely painful and lead to splinting and hypoventilation. This is especially detrimental to the patient with little respiratory reserve. Incentive spirometry, early mobilization, and keeping the head of the bed elevated at least 30 degrees are all well-established methods of reducing post chest trauma respiratory complications.[36]

Prompt and adequate pain relief is essential for promoting pulmonary health in the elderly patient with thoracic compromise. Inadequate pain control increases the work of breathing, elevates oxygen demand, and can easily progress to respiratory failure. Epidural catheters are particularly effective for controlling rib fracture and thoracotomy pain without heavy sedation, while simultaneously decreasing the incidence of pulmonary complications. For elderly patients, an epidural infusion of opioids combined with a local anesthetic agent is an excellent method of pain control, providing excellent analgesia with minimum sedation.[36] For epidural analgesia to be most effective, it should be initiated early in the course of care. Unfortunately, because of degenerative changes, the elderly spinal canal may not be easy to cannulate.

Mechanical Ventilation

Obtaining and maintaining a definitive airway is essential in the older patient with respiratory failure. Because even mild hypoxia can initiate a downward spiral in the elderly, it is best to err on the side of early ventilatory support. Evaluation of the need for preintubation removal of dental appliances in the mechanically ventilated older adult patient is essential. Evidence-based studies on the efficacy of ventilator use in the elderly population have not provided definitive guidelines for deciding to "intubate and ventilate." Mechanically ventilated elderly in the critical care areas account for 70% to 80% of patients with delirium.[41] However, these outcomes appear to be more related to the disease process itself than to the patient's age.[45]

Successful weaning from mechanical ventilation does not appear to be directly correlated with age, but age-related changes clearly impact the respiratory fitness of a particular patient and contribute to weaning failure. Few studies have specifically addressed the role of monitoring weaning parameters or other common ventilatory issues (e.g., timing of tracheostomy) in the elderly population. The benefits of several new and heavily promoted devices for the prevention of ventilator-associated pneumonias (e.g., subglottic suction or silver-coated endotracheal tubes) have not been well established in the elderly population.

NEUROLOGIC SYSTEM

The nervous system regulates cognitive, behavioral, motor, sensory, and homeostatic functions throughout the body. Age-related physiologic changes to the nervous system are complex and far-reaching. Sensory perception declines steadily with normal aging; the incidence of neurologic disorders increases with every decade of life.[30,40]

Age-Related Changes

Brain Atrophy

Between the ages of 40 and 70 years, a 10% reduction in brain size occurs as a result of the progressive, scattered loss of approximately 20% of cerebral cortex neurons.[40] As brain weight decreases, cerebral blood flow is concomitantly reduced. The number of neuroglial cells increases as the brain loses neurons. Neuronal loss is associated with slowed impulse conduction through nerves, along nerve fibers, and across synapses.[40] Neuronal loss is accelerated by Alzheimer's disease and alcoholism.[40] Loss of neurons diminishes the body's ability to deal with multiple stimuli, respond to information, and recover from stressors.

Cognitive Decline

Intellectual functioning normally peaks at age 20 to 30 years and then plateaus until the mid-80s, at which time function starts to decline.[40] Cognitive decline is accompanied by a modest loss of short-term memory and reduced sensory and perceptual acuity.[29] Sleep disturbances include taking a longer time to fall asleep, less time spent in rapid eye movement sleep, and alterations in sleep patterns, such as daytime sleeping.[19] Additional neurologic changes include impaired judgment, poor memory, and a reduced ability to process new information.[19,40]

Vascular Disease

The development of age-associated atherosclerotic disease is not limited to the heart. Vessels in the brain are similarly affected, and the incidence of stroke jumps markedly with age. In addition to ischemic strokes, older adults are also at increased risk for hemorrhagic stroke. There is a rising incidence of intracranial aneurysms associated with advancing age and the female gender. Although not as strongly suggestive as genetics and heredity, risk factors acquired over a lifetime are the most important etiologies of intracranial aneurysms and subarachnoid hemorrhage (SAH). Hypertension, smoking, traumatic brain injury, and sepsis are among the acquired factors that contribute to the intracranial aneurysm formation and subsequent SAH in elderly individuals.

Peripheral Nerve and Metabolic Changes

An age-related decline in peripheral nerve function, associated with thickening of the leptomeninges in the spinal cord, reduces the body's ability to maintain homeostasis efficiently.[40] In addition, the elderly blood-brain barrier becomes more permeable, leading to increased sensitivity to many medications.[40]

Sensory Decline

Hearing. Elderly persons lose auditory acuity for a variety of reasons. Normal aging is accompanied by anatomic and functional changes in the auditory and vestibular apparatus, causing decreased sensitivity to sound and altered frequency discrimination. Changes include loss of auditory neurons, angiosclerosis of the ear, and degeneration of neural receptors in the cochlea, eighth cranial nerve, and the central nervous system. These alterations produce both loss of hearing (from high to low frequencies) and difficulty hearing, especially in the presence of background noise or when speech is rapid or involves consonants. Presbycusis, a sensorineural hearing loss, is the most common cause of hearing loss in older adults. This condition is characterized by a gradual, progressive, bilateral, symmetrical high-frequency, perceptive hearing loss associated with poor speech discrimination.[27] In addition, cerumen production increases with age, and impaction may cause conductive hearing loss. Older patients should be evaluated for cerumen impaction and have it removed as necessary. Hearing loss leads to social isolation, but elderly patients may not have adequate resources to obtain auditory aids.[19,27,40]

Vision. With aging, many transformations occur in the eye and the central visual pathways. Anatomic changes include decreased rod and cone function and pigment accumulation. The ciliary muscles atrophy and the iris loses its ability to accommodate rapidly to light and dark.[19,40] The elderly lens yellows, increases in size, and becomes less flexible. Pupils decrease in size and become less responsive to light as a result of pupil sphincter hardening. Intraocular pressure in the aging eye rises, and there is a drop in tear production which causes eye dryness and irritation.[19,40]

These anatomic changes limit visual acuity, depth perception, peripheral vision, tolerance to glare, and speed of eye movements. Impaired light/dark adaptation and other age-related effects heighten an older person's need for ambient light and reduce the elderly patient's ability to differentiate blues, greens, and violets.[19,40] Elevated intraocular pressure and lens inflexibility combine to increase the prevalence of glaucoma in the elderly. In addition, the high incidence of macular degeneration, retinal tears, cataracts, and diabetic retinopathy in the elderly all contribute to visual impairment.[19,40]

Strategies for working with older adults with visual impairment include use of materials with large print, selection of contrasting colors for printed material, assurance of adequate glare-free lighting, and facing the patient directly when speaking. Touch and visual cues can also be used to facilitate communication.[19,40]

Smell and taste. There is a reduction in the number of olfactory and gustatory nerve fibers accompanying normal aging, which limits the ability to perceive and discriminate both pleasant and noxious odors and flavors. Decreased taste perception is associated with a declining food intake in the elderly. In addition to smell and taste, hunger and thirst are affected by age, both at the end-organ level and in the hypothalamus. Older adults develop an increased threshold for certain flavors such as salt. The satiety center in the hypothalamus can become hypersensitive, leading to anorexia, while the hypothalamically mediated thirst response to hyperosmolarity is reduced, making the elderly less sensitive to their need for water.[9,40]

Touch and balance. Two-point discrimination and both tactile and vibratory sensation all diminish with aging. Proprioception, balance, and postural control likewise decline. Elderly persons experience changes in coordination, an altered *righting* reflex, and difficulty with balance. Together, these transformations, in conjunction with distorted depth perception and musculoskeletal deterioration, make the older individual less able to respond to environmental changes and more susceptible to falls, particularly in unfamiliar surroundings (e.g., critical care).[19,40]

Pain. The sensory changes of aging can reduce an elder's ability to perceive, respond to, or express pain, yet pain is one of the most pervasive and undertreated problems of aging.[19] Pain in the elderly, both acute and chronic, is associated with depression, decreased socialization, poor nutrition, sleep disturbances, impaired mobility, and increased healthcare costs.[19] Pain assessment in seniors can be challenging, particularly in those who are cognitively impaired. Pain is frequently expressed nonverbally as facial grimacing, guarding, or restlessness. Other common pain manifestations are psychobehavioral and include withdrawal, irritability, anxiety, crying, or fearfulness.[19]

Age-associated respiratory, neurologic, and gastrointestinal changes complicate pain management in the elderly. Older adults, who are opiate naïve, and those with neuromuscular or pulmonary disease, are very sensitive to the side effects of narcotic analgesics[40] (i.e., respiratory depression, altered mental status, weakness, and constipation).

Common Problems and Management Strategies

Stroke and Transient Ischemic Attack

Stroke is one of the leading health problems in the United States today, with 795,000 new or recurrent cerebral ischemic events occurring annually.[29] Three important factors characterize stroke in the elderly. First, the incidence of stroke is highest in this age group. Seventy-five percent of all cerebrovascular accidents occur in persons age 65 years and older.[29] In fact, age is the single most important risk factor for stroke and reversible ischemic neurologic deficits.[29] Second, the risk factors contributing to stroke continue to increase with age; stroke is now the third most common cause of death among Americans.[40] As a consequence of population aging, the stroke death rate in the United States has been increasing despite advances in care.[40] African Americans have a 38% higher adjusted incidence of ischemic stroke than do Caucasians and therefore suffer greater stroke mortality.[29]

The third reason stroke is a major public health problem in older individuals is that the ongoing burden of this disease is huge. In the United States, stroke has become the principal cause of long-term disability, primarily in the elderly population.[40] There are approximately 4.5 million stroke survivors alive today, most of them over the age of 65. The economic toll of stroke is estimated at $43 billion each year in the United States.[29]

Stroke is a broad category of neurologic deficits with many etiologies. There are several vascular mechanisms that lead to stroke, including large-artery atherosclerosis with occlusion, distal embolization, aneurysm rupture, and small penetrating arterial disease with lacunar infarction. The incidence of each of these conditions increases with advancing age. Approximately 85% of all strokes are ischemic, and almost 60% are attributable to atherothrombotic disease. The location of this disease can be anywhere in the vasculature from the carotid arteries to the small vessels of the brain. Although the smaller vessels are the most common site, extracranial arterial occlusion from carotid atherosclerosis accounts for approximately 20% of all strokes in geriatric patients.[40] Cardiac dysrhythmias, primarily atrial fibrillation, may be either the cause or the consequence of a stroke.[12]

Dysphagia

Dysphagia occurs in a large proportion of adults; it occurs in 20% of adults over 55 years of age and increases to between 60% and 80% in the institutionalized elderly.[29] Many elderly individuals with ischemic or degenerative diseases of the central nervous system, such as Alzheimer's disease, amyotrophic lateral sclerosis, Parkinson's disease, multiple sclerosis, and stroke, will develop dysphagia. Dysphagia generally occurs early in the course of the disease; its severity does not necessarily correlate with the overall severity of the neurologic condition. Aspiration pneumonia is a major cause of death in these patients.[40] This explains the extremely high incidence of pneumonia among residents of long-term care facilities.

Head Trauma

Atrophic changes in the aging brain increase the amount of intracranial dead space. As a result, the distance between the skull and the brain surface increases and the bridging veins between the brain and dura mater are stretched, making them prone to tear and bleed. These anatomic transformations place older patients at a significantly increased risk for acute, chronic, and subacute subdural hematoma formation following even minor traumatic injury.[29] Unfortunately, significant cerebral atrophy can mask signs of an expanding hematoma in the elderly and there may be substantial intracranial hemorrhage before definitive neurologic symptoms are present.[29] Subtle changes in level of consciousness, an early indicator of intracranial hemorrhage, may be difficult to detect, particularly in persons with dementia.[19] In the geriatric trauma patient, computed tomographic brain scans should be used liberally to assess any patient with a potential head injury.[40]

Spinal Cord Injury

Although seniors may sustain a variety of spinal cord injuries, one type of cord trauma is more prevalent in the geriatric age group than in other populations. Central cord syndrome, an incomplete injury, is uncommon in younger individuals and usually occurs in older trauma patients with preexisting cervical spinal stenosis or spondylosis. The elderly most often develop central cord syndrome following a forward fall. This mechanism causes cervical hyperextension. Neurologic dysfunction is secondary to ischemia in the central portion of the spinal cord, particularly near the distribution of the anterior spinal artery. Patients with central cord syndrome generally retain lower extremity motor and sensory function with deficits noted in the upper extremities.

As is true in younger persons, the spine of the geriatric trauma patient must be stabilized with a rigid cervical collar, rigid backboard, and a head immobilization device until the patient is clinically or radiographically cleared. However, because of kyphosis, elderly individuals are frequently difficult to stabilize effectively. Adequate padding to reduce discomfort and removal of all immobilization devices as soon as possible to minimize skin breakdown and other complications of immobility should be encouraged. Magnetic resonance imaging scans may be required to evaluate compression of the spinal cord and detect injury to the stabilizing ligaments.

Dementia and Delirium

The person with dementia has a preexisting or baseline cognitive impairment (e.g., Alzheimer's disease). Although rarely the admitting diagnosis for a critically ill patient, dementia is a common comorbidity in the hospitalized elderly. In fact, the dementia rate in older Americans doubles with every 5-year increase in age, from 1.5% in those ages 65 to 70, to nearly 25% in people over the age of 85.[19] Because dementia is part of a patient's baseline status, interventions focus on symptom management and not on cure.

In contrast, the patient with delirium has a transient organic mental syndrome characterized by a cognition disorder, global attention deficits, a reduced level of consciousness, abnormal psychomotor activity patterns, and disturbed sleep-wake cycles. Delirium adversely affects mental processing, perception, thinking, short-term memory, and, frequently, behavior.[19] Despite its behavioral manifestations, the root cause of delirium is not psychiatric. Any condition that affects brain function can potentially lead to delirium.[19]

Up to one half of persons over the age of 65 admitted to critical care will develop some kind of delirium during their hospitalization.[41] Risk factors for delirium are multifactorial but include advanced age, preexisting cognitive impairment, poor functional status, hemodynamic or respiratory instability, ethanol abuse, sensory overload, hypoxemia, infections, metabolic imbalances, pain, anxiety, alterations in the sleep-wake cycle, malnutrition, bladder catheterization, sleep deprivation, polypharmacy, acute stress, and the use of physical restraints.[2,3,5,14,34,35] Delirium may also be the first manifestation of a previously unrecognized disease. Regrettably, in the critically ill older adult, the behavioral disturbances of delirium are all too often dismissed as critical care psychosis and the patient is treated with sedatives and antipsychotic medications. In older individuals, the likelihood of medication-induced delirium is high. Analgesics can alter cognitive function, especially when used in combination with many other substances. Nevertheless, withholding medications, particularly undertreating pain, can also cause delirium.[41]

Appropriate assessment and intervention are essential for a positive outcome in the patient with delirium. The Confusion Assessment Method for the ICU (CAM-ICU) is one valid and reliable tool used to assess delirium.[3,5,34,41] In studies conducted in 2012 and 2015, findings indicated administration of benzodiazepines, opioids, or haloperidol (Haldol), in conjunction with an acute illness, and preexisting dementia were associated with the duration of delirium experienced in the elderly.[5,35] Pain should be controlled prior to adding medications related to the delirium.[5] Many of the medications administered to critical care patients increase the risk for delirium.[5,9] The primary treatment goal, however, involves identifying and removing the underlying causes of delirium. Nonpharmacological treatments are preferred and patient safety is the highest priority.[41] Mild agitation interventions include decreasing environmental stimuli (lights and noise) and clustering care. Friends or volunteers can help reorient, mobilize, and feed the patient.[28] Clocks, calendars, family photos, glasses, and hearing aids are also means of assisting orientation.[41] The evidence-based Awakening and Breathing Coordination, Delirium Monitoring and Management with early mobility (ABCDE) bundle provides interventions to consider in managing patients with delirium.[3,5,14,41] The strategies are related to awakening from sedation/analgesia, careful sedation selection and titration, coordination of sedation with weaning from the ventilator, delirium monitoring, and progressive early mobility.[41]

The hypoactive form of delirium is the most common type of delirium in the elderly; it is difficult to recognize and is associated with poor outcomes. This condition is manifested by a quiet state of withdrawal, apathy, and decreased arousal.[5]

MUSCULOSKELETAL SYSTEM

Normal aging is accompanied by a number of important changes to the musculoskeletal system. An overall decrease in muscle mass, strength, and agility leads to alterations in gait (wide-based, shorter steps) and posture (flexed forward).[19] These alterations, in combination with loss of bone mass, put older persons at risk for musculoskeletal injury.

Age-Related Changes

Muscular Changes

As the body ages, there is a concomitant decline in the total amount of body water and an increase in the percentage of body fat.[40] Sarcopenia is the age-related loss of muscle mass, strength, and/or function related to a reduction in protein synthesis and an increase in muscle protein degradation.[19,40] Not only is muscle mass diminished, but the remaining myocytes lose functional capacity because of a reduction in myosin adenosine triphosphate (ATP) activity in the cells.[40] This diminishes the muscle cells' ability to extract and utilize oxygen, which increases fatigue. These changes serve to reduce overall muscle strength.[40] This functional loss of muscle strength gradually reduces the independence of the elderly, especially in activities of daily living (ADLs) and promote a more sedentary lifestyle. Studies have shown how detrimental complete bed rest is on deconditioning and functional decline in the elderly. Bed rest can decrease the amount of muscle mass and strength by 1.5% per day and that functional decline can be experienced by the second day of an acute care admission.[19,40]

Skeletal Changes

Osteoporosis. The high incidence of osteoporosis in the elderly population leads to a rate of fractures greater than in any other age group. Osteoporosis occurs as a result of three factors: (1) peak bone mass not reached in early adulthood, (2) increased bone resorption, and (3) decreased bone formation (decreased osteoblastic activity, which reduces production of new bone cells).[40] The resultant loss of bone mass is associated with bone fragility and predisposes the older adult to bony fractures following even minor trauma. Much attention has been given to osteoporosis in women, but both elderly men and women have brittle skeletons and decreased bone density.[40] There is a loss of total body height, attributable in large part to a decrease in the height of the vertebral bodies. Other degenerative changes to the cervical spine include narrowing of the cervical canal secondary to osteophytes (bony spurs).[19,40]

Osteoarthritis. Osteoarthritis, previously known as *degenerative joint disease*, is the most common form of arthritis in the United States. This condition is diagnosed in 50% of those individuals over 65 years of age and is the leading cause of disability. Elderly women are disproportionately affected by osteoarthritis, but this condition also affects many older men.[40]

Osteoarthritis is a disease of both weight-bearing and non–weight-bearing joints. Damage is caused by mechanical stresses that injure areas of articular cartilage and subchondral bone. Biochemical changes in the joint surface, the synovium, and synovial fluid play a role in osteoarthritis etiology as well. Symptoms include joint pain, morning stiffness lasting less than 30 minutes, and loss of function. Pain is related to activity and is initially relieved by rest but progresses to pain at rest over time.[40]

Connective Tissue Changes

The amount of connective tissue and collagen continues to increase with age. This is most prominently manifested by growth of the nose and ears. These transformations are largely cosmetic and have few functional implications. Other changes, such as deterioration and drying of the joints and cartilage, have clinical ramifications, producing joint pain and stiffness.[40]

Common Problems and Management Strategies

Fractures

The incidence of fractures in the elderly is extremely high. Most of the fractures are related to falls in the home environment during the daytime hours. A large number of these fractures are preventable and prevention strategies are tantamount to reducing the incidence and the concomitant sequelae in functional status changes.

The rate of hip fractures increases with advancing years and more than 95% are a result of falls. However, evidence suggests that some individuals have such osteoporotic hips that a spontaneous fracture actually precedes the fall.[40] Cervical spine fractures in older adults tend to involve more than one level, commonly occur at C1-C2, and are frequently unstable.[19] As with hip fractures, the leading cause of pelvic fractures in the elderly is falls. Bone healing time is prolonged in the elderly patient. Patient interventions (e.g., physical therapy, range-of-motion exercises, occupational therapy) focus on facilitating mobility and restoring function, while simultaneously preventing complications of immobility (e.g., thromboembolic disease, pneumonia, renal calculi, contractions, and pressure ulcers).[19,40] Nursing interventions related to early mobilization,[8,16,38] proper nutrition, and the use of incentive spirometry will also decrease the risk of these potential complications.

INTEGUMENTARY SYSTEM

Assessment of the elderly person's skin (i.e., presence of peripheral vascular disease, edema, deformities, lesions, discoloration, wounds, scars, medical devices) can provide a large amount of information about the patient's medical history, surgical history, and current health status. Because of decreased skin elasticity, the common practice of using skin turgor as a measure of hydration status may be inaccurate in the elderly.[19,40]

Age-Related Changes

Decreased Protective Functions

Aging is associated with decreased effectiveness of several of the skin's protective functions. Subcutaneous fat is lost, particularly the fatty pads that protect bony prominences. Both the dermis and the epidermis thin, making delicate, aging skin susceptible to tears.[19] Changes also occur in the structure of interstitial tissues, which predispose to soft tissue injury.[40] Loss of skin moisture, decreased elasticity, diminished tensile strength, and reduced turgor all lead to wrinkling and skin laxity. Both dryness and pruritus are common dermal complaints in older individuals and may lead to scratching.[19,40] The number of nerve cells in the skin also declines with advancing age, making the elderly less aware of dermal injury or ischemia. These age-related changes are accompanied by a reduction in the number of melanocytes, which heightens older adults' need for sun protection.[19]

Delayed Wound Healing

All aspects of wound healing appear to be influenced by aging. Responses in both the inflammatory and the proliferative wound healing phases are decreased. Angiogenesis, epithelialization, and wound remodeling are all delayed. Fibroblast proliferation and collagen synthesis also diminish with aging.[29] Furthermore, the high frequency of routine aspirin or ibuprofen use in the older population, combined with capillary fragility, contributes to wound bleeding tendencies and ecchymosis. Once the body's protective layers are breached, external barriers to bacterial invasion are removed, promoting wound infection. This is aggravated by the immune system alterations that accompany aging, which limit the older adult's ability to mount an adequate response to infection.[19,40] Nutritional deficits, particularly vitamins A and C and trace minerals (e.g., zinc), adversely affect the enzyme systems necessary for wound healing.[29] All of these factors must be considered when implementing wound care protocols.

Common Problems and Management Strategies

Pressure Ulcers

In the elderly patient, atrophic changes in the skin and a limited capacity to heal contribute to the high incidence of pressure ulcer formation. The prevalence of pressure ulcers in hospitalized patients is highest in the critical care units.[11] Skin breakdown in the elderly can be initiated by a variety of factors including sensory or motor loss, bed rest, reduced vasomotor tone, hypovolemia, poor nutrition, and age-related changes in skin composition.[19,40] Wound healing is prolonged and may take twice as long for reepithelialization to occur in the elderly as compared to younger adults.[45] Pressure ulcers may develop virtually anywhere on a patient's body, but are most common over the bony prominences of the sacrum, heels, ischium, elbows, occiput, and pinna.[40] Pressure ulcers can form rapidly in immobilized older adults.

The elderly require exceptional skin care, and skin integrity must be monitored frequently for signs of impairment. Strategies to prevent skin damage in the critically ill older adult include gentle handling of the patient, avoidance of shearing forces, padding of bony prominences with additional layers, and frequent repositioning.[19,40] Use of a nonalcoholic, nondrying cleanser to keep the skin clean may be helpful. Skin moisturizers and protective lotions should be applied liberally, and bony prominence contact with beds and chairs should be minimized. For older adult patients at high risk, and those with signs of skin disruption, the use of special air or rotating beds might be considered. The number of products and treatment options currently available for pressure ulcer care is staggering. Consultation with a wound and ostomy nurse for help with selecting the most appropriate interventions is often beneficial.

Burns

Elderly individuals are at increased risk for thermal injuries because many of the physical and cognitive changes of normal aging render some elderly poorly equipped to respond to fires and smoke. Impaired thermal perception, diminished manual dexterity, slowed reaction time, limited vision, hearing loss, an attenuated sense of smell, and possible cognitive impairment all render the older person vulnerable to burns. Alcohol abuse, cigarette smoking, poverty, sedating medications, and altered sleep patterns also contribute to injury.[29]

Once burned, elderly patients are more adversely affected than are younger individuals with similar injuries.[29] Despite advances in burn care, postburn mortality in the geriatric population remains extremely high. The elderly between the ages of 75 and 85 have a burn-related mortality rate two times higher than the national average.[29] All together, burns claim the lives of approximately 1200 to 1500 persons over the age of 65 each year in the United States.[29]

Variables influencing outcome following thermal injuries in the elderly include previous health status, burn severity (i.e., location, depth, and extent), adequacy of resuscitation, and any postinjury complications. Providing appropriate fluid resuscitation to the geriatric burn patient is especially challenging. Preexisting comorbid conditions, particularly cardiovascular or pulmonary disease, make fluid resuscitation problematic. Postresuscitation, older burn patients are prone to pneumonia and sepsis, particularly those with inhalation injuries.[40] Burn wound care presents special challenges in the elderly, and complications of healing occur frequently in this population. Following even minor burns, wounds generally exhibit poor or delayed healing. Delayed healing, or failure to heal, affects not only partial-thickness wounds but also skin graft beds and split-thickness donor sites as well.[40]

URINARY SYSTEM

With increasing age, a substantial number of anatomic and physiologic changes occur that directly impact the urinary system. The number of comorbidities, such as diabetes, hypertension, and urinary obstruction can decrease renal function.[7] In addition, alterations to other systems (e.g., a decreased sense of thirst and changes in cardiovascular status) have an indirect effect on renal function.

Age-Related Changes

Voiding Pattern Changes

Several normal transformations of aging impact voiding in the elderly, including reduced bladder muscle tone, diminished bladder capacity, and a heightened sense of urgency.[19,40] In the aging bladder, increased collagen content limits distensibility and impairs emptying. In females, decreased circulating levels of estrogen and decreased tissue estrogen responsiveness causes urethral sphincter changes that predispose to urinary incontinence. In older males, prostate enlargement may impede urinary flow, impairing bladder emptying.[19,40] Together, these factors lead to urinary incontinence in approximately 8% to 46% of seniors living in the community and 30% of hospitalized elders.[19]

Nephron Loss

The total number of glomeruli decreases by 30% to 50% by the seventh decade of life.[7] Nephron loss is accompanied by a drop in the number of renal tubular cells. Glomerular sclerosis produces a gradual reduction in blood flow to the glomerular capillary tufts and the small vessel walls, resulting in atrophy of the afferent and efferent arterioles.[29] Sclerotic changes begin in the cortical regions of the kidneys and then progress toward the medullary portion. These processes eventually cause renal blood flow to decline by approximately 50%.[7] To compensate, the remaining functional nephrons hypertrophy. Over time, this nephron loss causes the elderly patient's renal reserve to dwindle.[7]

Decreased Glomerular Filtration Rate

Glomerular filtration rate (GFR) declines with advancing age as a result of both nephron loss and reduced renal blood flow.[7] Total renal blood flow begins to drop after the fourth decade of life because of hyaline arteriosclerosis.

Altered Renal Clearance

Serum creatinine levels do not undergo significant changes in older patients because of the normal decrease in lean body mass, which reduces overall creatinine production. Therefore, a normal serum creatinine level does not necessarily mean normal kidneys; creatinine levels tend to overestimate renal function in the geriatric population. In the aging kidney, the declining GFR is reflected by a slight drop in creatinine clearance (approximately 0.75 mL/min/year in healthy older males). However, creatinine clearance remains a better indicator of renal function than does serum creatinine level.[19,40] The following formula can be used to estimate creatinine clearance in healthy older persons, although it may be influenced by critical illness or medications that affect renal function.[40]

$$\text{Creatinine clearance} = \frac{(140 - \text{Age in years}) \times (\text{Lean weight in kilograms})}{72 \times (\text{Serum creatinine in mg/dL}) \times (0.85 \text{ only if female})}$$

Decreased Ability to Concentrate or Dilute Urine

As renal tubular function declines with age, the kidneys' ability to conserve sodium and excrete hydrogen ions is diminished. This reduces the older adult's capacity to maintain fluid and acid-base balance. Seniors are prone to develop volume depletion (prerenal conditions) because the aging kidney does not compensate for nonrenal sodium and water losses with the typical mechanisms of enhanced renal sodium retention, increased urinary concentration, and heightened thirst.[7] These changes occur secondary to renin-angiotensin system attenuation and decreased end-organ responsiveness to antidiuretic hormone (ADH).[40]

Dehydration in older individuals can be missed because of their limited ability to concentrate urine. In the aged, urine specific gravity will remain relatively low despite significant volume loss.[40] This finding makes urine specific gravity an unreliable indicator of volume status in elderly persons. As age increases, urine production over a 24-hour period becomes more constant (loss of diurnal variation). This reduces the kidneys' ability to conserve fluid volume on demand.[7] Conversely, volume overload can occur because of both a drop in GFR and functional impairment of the diluting segment of the nephron. This phenomenon is exacerbated in critically ill patients by the elevation in levels of ADH seen postoperatively and during other periods of physiologic stress.[24]

Common Problems and Management Strategies

Altered Drug Excretion

Changes in renal status have important implications for the type and dosage of drugs used in the elderly. Although drugs are managed by the kidneys in a variety of ways, most alterations in renal drug processing correspond with the decline in GFR. Therefore, creatinine clearance is a good marker of clearance for most agents processed by the kidneys; dosages can be adjusted accordingly.[40] Two classes of drugs commonly consumed by older individuals are nonsteroidal antiinflammatory agents and angiotensin-converting enzyme inhibitors. Both of these drugs have adverse effects on renal regulatory mechanisms.[7] Other nephrotoxic substances frequently prescribed to critically ill patients include iodinated contrast media and diuretics. Aminoglycosides (e.g., vancomycin and gentamicin) require careful monitoring of serum levels to avoid toxicity in the geriatric patient.[7,9,40]

Acute Kidney Injury

The incidence of chronic kidney disease increases with age because of anatomic and physiologic changes to the kidneys associated with age and comorbidities. In the critically ill older adult, diminished baseline renal function, polypharmacy, and an elevated risk for nephrotoxicity combine to increase the incidence of acute kidney injury (AKI) as well. However, elderly patients may also exhibit atypical signs of uremia. Unexplained exacerbations of well-controlled heart failure and unexplained mental status or personality changes may be evidence of failing renal function.[7,19,40]

AKI in critically ill elders is often found in conjunction with sepsis. This disease combination carries a mortality rate of 65% to 80%.[7] Overall, outcomes for persons with AKI are not improving.[7] The likely explanation for this finding is that we are now treating older and more difficult AKI cases.

Urinary Tract Infections

Urinary tract infections (UTIs) are among the most common infections in older adults in the community, in long-term care facilities, and in critical care. With age, there is an increasing incidence of asymptomatic bacteriuria (significant bacterial counts in the urine, without other symptoms).[40] The prevalence of urinary tract infections increases with age and approximately one out of eight older adults has a UTI annually.[19] Women in the old-old age group may have almost three times the incidence of UTIs.[40]

UTIs are a major source of bacteremia and sepsis in the older adult, causing significant morbidity and mortality.[7] The presence of an indwelling urinary catheter dramatically increases the incidence of bacteriuria, pyuria, and symptomatic UTIs. Early discontinuation of indwelling catheters is recommended.[19,32,40]

GASTROINTESTINAL SYSTEM

Although gastrointestinal (GI) complaints are common in old age, in general, GI function is well preserved in the healthy older adult. Importantly, some of the age-associated changes that affect GI function, such as loss of abdominal muscle strength, reduced appetite, and decreased fluid intake, actually take place in other body systems.[31]

Age-Related Changes

Supragastric Changes

With aging, fibrosis and atrophy of the salivary glands decrease salivation, resulting in dry mouth.[40] There is a concomitant atrophy and loss of taste buds, dulling the sense of taste, particularly altering the ability to distinguish sweet and salty foods. Bitter and sour tastes remain largely unchanged. In addition, esophageal emptying slows, increasing risk for esophageal spasm.[40]

Gastric Changes

Gastric acid secretion does not decrease as a result of normal aging, but there is a rising incidence of gastritis and GI bleeding, commonly caused by *Helicobacter pylori.* Delayed gastric emptying has been demonstrated in some studies of elderly subjects. Aspiration, secondary to unrecognized gastric atony, is not uncommon.[40]

Bowel Changes

Small-bowel motility and the absorption of most nutrients are unchanged with age. Only calcium absorption falls significantly; this is primarily attributed to a decrease in renal production of 1,25-hydroxycholecalciferol and reduced intestinal calcium binding.[19] Iron and many drugs are absorbed more slowly or less effectively in older adults as a result of atrophy of the mucosal lining. In addition, the aging gut stabilizes and absorbs cholesterol less efficiently. Decreased muscle tone in the bowel delays bowel emptying, putting the elderly at risk for constipation, diverticular disease, and bacterial translocation. The etiology of constipation in the elderly is multifactorial; sedentary lifestyle, poor diet, dehydration, anorectal and colonic pathology, systemic illness, and medications can all contribute to abnormal bowel function.[19] A history of multiple abdominal surgeries, tumors, or adhesions increases the incidence of bowel obstruction in geriatric patients.

Hepatobiliary Changes

In association with advancing age, there is a reduction in the number of hepatocytes and overall liver size. Aging causes a decreased hepatic blood flow and may be reduced by 50% in those over 65 years, which could lead to increased drug toxicity.[40] Although standard liver function tests remain unchanged in healthy older adults, metabolism of, and sensitivity to, certain substances is altered.[40] Metabolism of drugs requiring microsomal oxidation (phase I reactions) before conjugation (phase II reactions) slows, whereas substances requiring only conjugation will continue to be cleared at a normal rate. Drugs such as warfarin, which acts directly on the liver cells, will produce therapeutic effects at lower doses in the elderly because of increased hepatocyte sensitivity.[40] There is also a drop in the liver's first-pass extraction of some pharmacologic agents, including propranolol (Inderal) and verapamil (Calan), which reduces hepatic clearance of these substances.[19,29,40]

Common Problems and Management Strategies

Malnutrition

There are countless reasons for malnutrition in the elderly, only some of which involve the GI system. A variety of social, cognitive, functional, and physiologic factors contribute to poor nutritional status in the elderly population. These include limited financial or physical ability to obtain and prepare food, poor dentition, depression, alcohol abuse, anorexia, drug-nutrient interactions, and the loss of a spouse. Additionally, chronic medical conditions, such as congestive heart failure, diabetes, lung disease, and renal failure, make it difficult to keep ill older adults adequately fed and hydrated.[18] Gastroesophageal reflux disease, chronic diarrhea, and many medications also interfere with appetite or nutrient metabolism among this population.[19,40] Moreover, malabsorption secondary to bacterial overgrowth is found in a large percentage of older adults with nutritional deficits unexplained by dietary factors.[29] Measuring nutritional status in older adults can be difficult; criteria for the interpretation of biochemical markers in this age-group have not been well established. Unfortunately, standard anthropomorphic measurements do not take into account the body composition and structural alterations that accompany aging. The caloric needs of the elderly critical care patient must meet the body's needs for increased energy to decrease catabolic response to critical illnesses.[18]

Several simple measurements have been used to predict outcome related to nutritional deficits in critically ill elders, but they should be applied with caution. The simplest of these measures is body mass index (weight in kilograms divided by the height in meters, squared). A body mass index (BMI) less than 22 kg/m^2 signals undernutrition and is associated with an increased mortality risk. The BMI is not a sensitive predictor of overnutrition especially in the middle-old age group and older.[40] Albumin levels, alone, are not strong predictors of malnutrition in critically ill elderly patients. Dehydration and overhydration may cause false albumin levels.[40] Low serum albumin levels (less than 3.3 mg/dL) in the elderly correlate with increased length of stay and an increased rate of all-cause mortality. However, because the half-life of albumin is 20 days, it does not detect early protein malnutrition. Prealbumin has a half-life of only 1 to 2 days. This makes it an excellent marker for recent-onset malnutrition and is more appropriate for assessment of the elderly in a critical care setting.[40] Albumin and prealbumin are acute-phase proteins and levels may decrease during inflammation. In order to verify if the decrease in albumin levels is due to malnutrition or inflammation, it is suggested that inflammatory markers such as C-reactive proteins be monitored.[18] Malnutrition places the elderly at heightened risk for morbidity and mortality.

The incidence of poor wound healing, pneumonia, prolonged ventilatory support, and postoperative complications is increased in patients with nutritional deficits.[18] In fact, impaired nutritional status, present at the time of admission to critical care, has been shown to predict 6-month mortality in older individuals who require ventilatory support.[20] Despite reduced metabolic demands, normal GI changes associated with aging predispose the elderly to nutritional deficits by reducing the absorption of lipids, proteins, and carbohydrates.

An elderly patient's protein needs must be individualized on the basis of preexisting nutritional status and current medical condition. Protein-energy malnutrition, together with immobility, leads to deconditioning, and deconditioning involves changes to all major organ systems. A diet that does not meet the daily recommendations for protein has been associated with a loss of skeletal muscle mass and may affect mobility. Protein supplementation has been shown to increase strength and muscle mass in the elderly.[40] Critically ill older adults with declining renal function may require adjustment in protein needs. However, basal protein requirements may be slightly higher rather than lower.

A decrease in the hypothalamically mediated thirst response to hyperosmolarity makes the elderly less sensitive to their need for water.[19,40] Elderly patients with limited cardiac or renal function poorly tolerate high sodium loads, and individuals taking diuretics frequently require potassium supplementation. Enhanced intake of calcium and vitamin D is instrumental in both the prevention and treatment of osteoporosis in the at-risk elderly population.[17] Routine micronutrient supplementation should be provided because deficiencies are common among the elderly. Enteral vitamins and trace mineral supplementation have been shown to improve immunologic responses and to decrease infections.[24] Steps should be taken to avoid long periods of nothing by mouth in the geriatric patient.

When feasible, enteral nutrition is the preferred route.[4,31] Enteral nutrition (either oral or through a feeding tube) is considerably safer and less expensive than parenteral nutrition.

Moreover, enteral nutrition helps the GI tract maintain its physiologic processes and may protect against bacterial translocation from the gut to the bloodstream via the mesenteric lymph nodes.[39] In elderly patients who are adequately nourished, postoperative parenteral nutrition has actually been associated with increased complications and, therefore, should be used only in older adults with severe nutritional deficits in whom the enteral route is unavailable.[18]

It is important to start early enteral supplementation in the undernourished or malnourished patient. Limited data suggest that enteral protein supplementation preoperatively can reduce negative outcomes in malnourished patients.[7] Studies have reported that enteral feedings were withheld for an average of 6 hours per day. Reasons for withholding feedings related to routine nursing care, interruptions related to procedures, large gastric residual volumes, and unstable hemodynamic status.[11] Underfeeding may be an outcome of this practice. Other interventions to prevent or reverse malnutrition or feeding problems in the critically ill elderly patient include the following: provide small, frequent meals to avoid discomfort and increase intake; encourage fluids and fiber to improve bowel function; and obtain early nutritional consultation.[19,40]

ENDOCRINE/METABOLIC SYSTEM

The metabolic and endocrine changes associated with aging are wide ranging, affecting every system in the body. Metabolic responses, in particular, influence the older adult patient's ability to cope with the stresses of critical illness.

Age-Related Changes

Metabolic Needs

Caloric requirements are lower in older adults. Both basal metabolic rate and daily energy expenditure decrease over time. At age 80, resting energy expenditure is approximately 15% lower than at age 40.[29] Maximum oxygen consumption and maximum energy expenditure are also reduced. These decreases are primarily the result of a decline in physical activity and a loss of lean muscle mass. In the presence of acute illness or injury, resting energy expenditure and oxygen consumption normally rise to support the additional cardiopulmonary work, tissue repair, and immunologic responses that accompany healing. In the elderly, however, the magnitude of this increase is smaller and the hypermetabolic state is less pronounced.[29]

In the face of stress, the older patient's metabolic response is characterized by increased requirements for energy and protein. However, the increase in catabolism, from illness, injury, infection, or surgery, is frequently not matched by an equal rise in energy intake. This condition is further exacerbated in patients with a preexisting poor nutritional status. Endogenous protein stores are depleted just to meet basic metabolic demands. Serum albumin is consumed and hepatic function declines, further impairing protein synthesis. Decreased muscle mass causes a reduction in muscle strength, particularly detrimental in the respiratory muscles. Cells with high turnover (e.g., skin, red and white blood cells, GI organs) fail first, leading to loss of barrier function, delayed wound healing, increased susceptibility to infection, and further impairment of nutrient absorption.[32]

Changes in Insulin Sensitivity

Aging is associated with a decline in glucose tolerance because of decreased peripheral receptor insulin sensitivity. Elderly individuals have a fasting blood glucose level that is normal to slightly elevated under optimal circumstances. An increase in blood glucose level to 200 mg/dL occurs in approximately half of all people over the age of 70 years. In times of acute illness, insulin responsiveness declines even further.[40]

Other Hormonal Changes

Secretion of many hormones decreases with aging. Elderly individuals experience a drop in the production of growth hormone, thyroid hormone, aldosterone, adrenal androgens, testosterone, and estrogen.[40]

Older adults have an increased incidence of thyroid nodularity, thyroid fibrosis, and other thyroid disorders, particularly hypothyroidism. A reduction in thyroid function is manifested by a decrease in triiodothyronine (T_3) levels with a concomitant elevation in levels of thyroid-stimulating hormone. Adrenal androgen levels also decline, limiting patients' immune system responsiveness to stress.[40] Significant changes in sex hormone levels occur with aging but seldom play an important role in critical illness.[40]

Common Problems and Management Strategies

Hyperglycemia

Glycemic control becomes difficult in the geriatric patient because the usual insulin resistance to stress is exacerbated by the declining glucose tolerance associated with normal aging. Careful glucose regulation is particularly important in the elderly patient. Optimal glucose management guidelines in the older population have not been well defined. Lipska et al.[33] discussed the overtreatment of elders when tight glycemic controls were the ideal management strategy. Many elderly patients were overtreated with ensuing hypoglycemia. The consequences of hypoglycemia in the elderly had many poor outcomes. Current recommendations endorse a higher glucose target for this population.[33]

THERMOREGULATION

Thermoregulatory responses are decreased in older persons. Cognitive and functional decline, certain medications, social factors, loss of muscle mass, skin thinning, and systemic conditions (e.g., thyroid disease, diabetes, and malnutrition) all reduce tolerance to temperature extremes. Therefore, abnormalities of body temperature are both more common and more prolonged in older adults.[19] Not surprisingly, the majority of both cold-related and heat-related deaths occur in elderly people.[19]

Age-Related Changes

Hypothalamic Decline

The hypothalamus is the body's thermoregulatory control center. With advancing age, declining hypothalamic function and a decreased basal metabolic rate combine to produce an overall reduction in the older patient's capacity to maintain thermal balance.[40]

Aging is also associated with a normal reduction in the threshold for peripheral vasoconstriction and shivering, reducing the body's ability to generate and conserve heat.[19] Because of sweat gland atrophy, the ability to sweat decreases with normal aging, thus reducing the body's ability to regulate heat when exposed to high ambient temperatures or exertion.[40]

Lower Baseline Temperature

Hypothalamic, metabolic, and body fat changes combine to cause older adults to experience a reduction in baseline body temperature. Normal temperature drops from 35.5°C to 36.1°C.[40] Axillary temperature measurements tend to be poor indicators of core temperature in the elderly population because skin temperature may be several degrees cooler than core temperature as a result of decreased peripheral circulation. Tympanic or oral temperature measurements are generally considered acceptable in the critically ill elderly, but bladder or pulmonary artery thermometers provide a more accurate assessment of core thermal status.[19,40]

Attenuated Febrile Response and Immunosenescence

In addition to a reduced ability to self-warm, geriatric patients have a blunted febrile reaction to infection as a result of immunosenescence. A significantly smaller percentage of older individuals generate a febrile response to stress than do their younger counterparts, and this febrile response is often attenuated.[19,40] With aging, there is a progressive decrease in T-cell function, defects in B-cell function, an increase in the number of autoantibodies and monoclonal immunoglobulins, and increased tumorigenesis.[32] Neutrophil counts do not drop, but the ability of the bone marrow to increase white blood cell production in response to infection is impaired. When combined with the stresses of critical illness, injury, or surgery, these cellular changes make it more likely that the geriatric patient will contract an infectious disease and will then be less able to eradicate it.[32]

Almost 60% of sepsis cases admitted to critical care units were 65 years old and older.[32] The elderly have a greater incidence of sepsis related to many factors: immunosenescence, diminished physiological reserves, presence of comorbidities and atypical presentation of signs and symptoms leading to delayed diagnosis.[31,32] Those who survive have poor outcomes related to functional decline, institutionalization, cognitive impairments, and irreversible organ damage.[32]

Common Problems and Management Strategies

Hypothermia

There are far more cold-related deaths than heat-related deaths in the United States, Europe, and almost all countries outside of the tropics. The majority of deaths are due to common illnesses that are exacerbated by cold rather than the direct result of severe hypothermia. Coronary and cerebral thrombosis constitute approximately 50% of cold-related deaths; respiratory diseases account for almost half of the rest.[40]

Hypothermia has profound effects on all components of the coagulation system. When exposed to cold stress, the body's first adjustment is to limit blood flow to the skin in order to conserve body heat. This vasoconstriction shifts blood from the skin to the core, which increases central blood volume and results in hypertension.[29] To compensate, sodium and water are shunted from the vessels into the interstitial space and are eventually excreted (cold diuresis). Left behind as the plasma volume drops are red cells, white cells, platelets, and fibrinogen. This increase in blood viscosity and concentration of thrombogenic factors promotes clotting.[32] Besides increased clotting, the high incidence of morbid cardiac events among hypothermic elderly is likely attributable to the increased level of circulating norepinephrine required to produce vasoconstriction and maintain shivering. With more severe degrees of hypothermia, conduction abnormalities and myocardial irritability are common. Dysrhythmias in the hypothermic older adult are usually resistant to medications, countershock, and electrical pacing.[29]

The elderly individual may arrive at the hospital in a hypothermic state. However, iatrogenically induced hypothermia also puts elders at risk. Intraoperative hypothermia in the elderly with cardiac risk factors is an independent predictor of postoperative cardiac events. In the postoperative period, ventricular tachycardia, hypertension, angina, and hypoxemia have been demonstrated to occur more frequently in mildly hypothermic elderly patients than in normothermic individuals. Because the elderly are at an increased risk for hypothermia, every effort should be made to prevent heat losses. Use of forced-air heating blankets, warmed intravenous solutions, heated ventilator circuits, and higher room temperatures when patients are uncovered are all appropriate interventions.

Hyperthermia

Like cold-related deaths, most heat-related deaths in the elderly are due to the indirect effects of temperature rather than to high temperature per se. However, when persons are exposed to air close to or above body temperature for long periods, a substantial number of heat-related deaths will be due to simple hyperthermia. Hyperthermia elevates temperature to a point where body proteins denature. In addition to reduced sweating mechanisms, many cognitive, social, and functional changes predispose older adults to heat-related illnesses. A wide range of drugs, particularly psychiatric medications and those with anticholinergic or narcotic actions, further impair sweating and other responses to heat.[19,40]

Coronary and cerebral thromboses account for many heat-related deaths because the salt and water losses from sweating produce hemoconcentration. Other heat-related deaths result from a range of factors that are poorly understood, but which probably include cardiac strain from trying to provide additional blood flow to the skin to increase heat loss. In the frankly hyperthermic patient (above 40°C), immediate and aggressive cooling can be life-saving. However, measures that induce shivering, which causes vasoconstriction and adds excess stress to the elderly heart, should be avoided.

DRUG METABOLISM

Compared to younger adults, the elderly typically take more drugs, have more underlying organ dysfunction, are more susceptible to malnutrition, are more likely to have diminished or exaggerated responses to medications, and experience more interindividual variations in drug disposition.[19,40] The majority of older patients admitted to critical care are already taking a number of medications. Each drug is associated with an adverse risk profile that only worsens when combined with systemic disease and additional medications. This fact underscores the importance of obtaining a thorough medication and health history from the patient, family, or caregiver.[6]

Age-Related Changes

Altered Body Habitus

Several age-associated changes alter drug distribution in the elderly. With aging, the portion of lean body mass decreases, the percent of body water drops, and the relative amount of adipose tissue increases. These alterations result in greater distribution of lipophilic drugs into the fat, producing a longer half-life for agents such as anesthetics, barbiturates, and benzodiazepines.[19,40]

Changes in Drug Processing, Absorption, Metabolism, and Excretion

Although the total amount of drug absorbed is basically unchanged, elderly patients experience a decline in the rate of drug absorption. Decreased serum albumin levels alter drug availability in substances that are protein-bound, enhancing the amount of bioactive agents. Both liver and kidney function decline with advancing age, which reduces clearance of many substances. The net effect of these age-related changes is an increase in the incidence of drug toxicity related to accumulation of metabolites.[19,40]

Common Problems and Management Strategies

Adverse Drug Reactions

Age-related changes in pharmacologic responses place the elderly at increased risk for adverse drug reactions. The number of medications consumed by the elderly range from an estimated 8-13, and more than 40% take more than 5 or more medications per day. The hepatic and renal impairment that occurs with aging can quickly lead to elevated drug concentrations, even in fully compliant patients on standard therapeutic dosing regimens. Also, the risk of drug-drug and drug-food interactions increases dramatically. Agents with a high potential for adverse reactions in older adults include anticoagulants, antidysrhythmics, calcium-channel blockers, digoxin, diuretics, narcotics, and theophylline.[19] Cardioactive substances in particular are problematic for the elderly. These agents have an inherently narrow therapeutic range, which is further reduced in the elderly by an age-related decline in intrinsic HR and slowing of conduction through the atrioventricular node.[19]

The first step in reducing adverse medication reactions in the elderly involves obtaining a complete medication history (drug reconciliation) on each patient at the time of admission. This history must include prescription medications, over-the-counter agents, recreational drugs, and nutritional supplements, as well as herbal, homeopathic, naturopathic, and folk medications.[19,40] Other strategies for reducing adverse medication reactions in the elderly include weaning drugs as appropriate, increasing doses cautiously, monitoring closely for untoward effects, dosing according to renal function, and consulting with a pharmacist regarding age-appropriate dosages.[19,40]

PSYCHOSOCIAL AND FUNCTIONAL FACTORS

Regardless of initial circumstances, when a potentially life-threatening medical condition, injury, or complex surgical procedure has occurred, older persons suddenly find themselves in a strange and scary environment where they experience pain, anxiety, loss of familiar surroundings, loss of independence, and sleep deprivation.[19,40]

Age-Related Changes

As part of the normal aging process, the elderly experience a number of changes in social interaction. Friends, siblings, spouses, and other family members are often dead or dying. Many geriatric patients have lost their life partner as the result of either death or severe cognitive impairment. Even while managing their own healthcare needs, older adults frequently serve as caregivers for a spouse, parent, sibling, neighbor, child, or even great-grandchild. A huge number of elderly persons are cared for by those who are senior citizens themselves. The individual caring for a 94-year-old patient is likely to be the 92-year-old spouse or a 70-year-old child.[28] Despite the decremental losses associated with aging, most elders perceive their lives as satisfying. Older adults exhibit a strong need to remain independent, maintain and develop meaningful relationships, and have a purpose in life.

Common Problems and Management Strategies

Functional Decline

Up to half of all geriatric patients admitted to hospitals experience a significant decline in function, or loss of the ability to perform activities of daily living. Specific factors associated with loss of function in the elderly include preexisting chronic illness, delirium, immobility, malnutrition, depression, and uncontrolled pain.[19,40] Sleep disturbances also accelerate functional decline. Approximately 5 million older Americans have serious sleep disorders.[40] Sleep problems are only exaggerated by the stresses of critical care.

Another condition that can cause severe functional decline in elderly persons is alcoholism. When the older adult patient experiences hallucinations, tremors, or seizures, the possibility of alcohol withdrawal must be considered. The onset of alcohol withdrawal usually occurs in the first 48 to 72 hours of admission. Patients with a known history of alcohol abuse can be treated to prevent or attenuate the effects of delirium tremens. However, unrecognized abuse can lead to life-threatening alcohol withdrawal with consequences that can negatively affect the patient's critical care course and create long-term morbidity.[40]

End-of-Life Concerns

A tremendous amount of healthcare resources, and a large percentage of Medicare expenditures, are being consumed by geriatric patients in the last weeks of life.[13] In general, age alone does not predict a poor outcome for the critically ill.[13] However, a central problem complicating end-of-life decision making is the difficulty predicting outcomes in critically ill older adults. Yet the combination of multiple coinciding medical problems and rapidly changing clinical status makes predicting remaining life span a very difficult task.[21] Attempts have been made to generate models of projected mortality in critically ill seniors. Factors entered into these formulas include such variables as age, gender, HR, independent activities of daily living, dependent activities of daily living, number of critical care interventions, and the number of organ system failures.[21] Despite some predictive success in certain facilities, no system of geriatric critical care mortality determination has yet been widely validated or adopted.[21]

One of the greatest potential critical care problems in the elderly is the decision to withhold or withdraw support. This decision is a complex one that may reflect the personal biases of healthcare providers, patients, and family members.[13] Aggressive treatment of the critically ill geriatric patient may be contrary to the individual's own expressed wishes. Unfortunately, only approximately 15% to 20% of patients have an advance directive at the time of hospital admission. When they exist, advance directives are often inadequate, except in cases of the most obvious treatment decisions, because they are too vague, using phrases such as terminal illness and little chance of recovery. Even when a patient's wishes are clear, many providers are wary of ignoring the requests of a living surrogate, especially if it is a spouse or other close family member.

Research regarding older adults' end-of-life preferences often seems confusing or contradictory. Despite the fact that 90% of Americans polled said that they would prefer to die at home, approximately 80% continue to go to some sort of healthcare facility to die. Sixty percent will die in an acute care hospital, and 20% will die in critical care.[12]

INTERPROFESSIONAL PLAN OF CARE

Meeting the needs of the critically ill geriatric patient requires careful assessment, individualized planning, teamwork, and frequent reevaluation. As mentioned throughout this chapter, areas of special concern in this population include: comorbidities, delirium, diminished physiologic reserves, hypothermia, pain, polypharmacy, potential for skin breakdown, and sensory deficits.

CONCLUSION

Demographic shifts, longevity gains, and advances in healthcare in the last 50 years have dramatically increased the number of older persons in the United States critical care units. The proportion of critically ill patients who are elderly is projected to continue to increase well into the middle of the twenty-first century. Age-related change affects every system in the body, but in the older adult patient, normal age-related transformations can be difficult to distinguish from alterations caused by illness, environmental, social, functional, and comorbid conditions. These changes interact to threaten the older adults' ability to survive and recover from critical illness or injury.

CASE STUDY 36.1

Evidence-Based Care of the Critically Ill Elderly Patient

R.S., a 92-year-old retired accountant, cannot recall what happened, but his neighbor found him lying unconscious on the kitchen floor. On hospital arrival, R.S.'s respirations are regular and unlabored, his oxygen saturation is normal, he denies chest pain, and there are no obvious signs of a head injury. R.S.'s chief complaint is severe pain in his obviously deformed right upper arm. R.S. states that he has had mild diarrhea for the past 2 days. A brief neurologic exam reveals no gross focal or cognitive deficits. R.S. is in sinus rhythm at a rate of 47 beats/min, with frequent premature ventricular beats and a BP of 96/45 mm Hg.

When R.S. reaches critical care, he is alert and cooperative but in a lot of pain from his upper arm injury. R.S. has a history of atrial fibrillation, treated with digoxin and warfarin. R.S. has also been taking metoprolol since his myocardial infarction 3 years ago. In addition, R.S. suffers from gout and osteoarthritis of the knees. A 12-lead ECG indicates an old anterolateral wall infarction, but no acute changes are noted. Basic laboratory studies, including a troponin level, are all within normal limits.

A 2-L infusion of normal saline brings R.S.'s BP up to 127/52 mm Hg and his HR is now 86 beats per minute. The provider orders a computed tomographic scan of R.S.'s head and plain radiographs of his right arm and cervical spine. During the imaging procedure, while still strapped to a long backboard, R.S. begins to vomit. He is turned onto his left side and his secretions are suctioned. However, since the vomiting event, R.S. has had a persistent cough. R.S. receives 5 mg of IV morphine sulfate and obtains some relief from his humeral fracture pain. Thirty minutes later, his nurse notes that R.S.'s room air saturation level has dropped to 87%. He is started on 3 L of oxygen by nasal prongs.

After receiving a third liter of normal saline R.S. states he needs to urinate. R.S. is unable to sit up and cannot void in a supine position, so an indwelling catheter is placed. Because of benign prostatic hypertrophy, catheter insertion is very difficult and results in urethral bleeding. The urine retrieved is cloudy and foul-smelling. The operating room notifies R.S.'s nurse that they are ready to perform R.S.'s humeral repair. As his nurse prepares him for surgery, she notes that R.S. is moderately agitated, cannot remember why he is in the hospital, and is trying to climb out of bed to look for his wife. R.S.'s skin is dry and flushed; his temperature is 37.9°C.

Just 3 hours after hospital arrival, and only 4 hours after waking up in his own home feeling fine, R.S. is on his way to surgery. He leaves critical care still in pain, with a serious orthopedic injury, occasional-to-frequent premature ventricular beats, a large skin tear, a small urethral tear, and early symptoms of fluid overload, aspiration pneumonia, delirium, and a sacral pressure ulcer.

Decision Point:

What are likely etiologies of R.S.'s initial episode of loss of consciousness?

Decision Point:

What impact will routine beta blocker use have on R.S.'s physiologic response to his injury and hospitalization?

Decision Point:

What factors might be responsible for R.S.'s dwindling oxygen saturation?

Decision Point:

What musculoskeletal changes of aging predispose this patient to fractures?

Decision Point:

What additional possible reason for R.S.'s hypotension, flushed skin, and altered level of consciousness is suggested by his cloudy, foul-smelling urine; and moderate temperature elevation?

REFERENCES

1. Adhikari, N., et al. (2010). Critical care and the global burden of critical illness in adults, Lancet. published online, October 9, 2010, *376*, 1–8.
2. Alspach, J. (2012). Acute myocardial infarction without chest pain: a life-threatening variant? [Editorial]. *Crit Care Nurse, 32*(4), 10–13.
3. Andrews, L., Siva, S., Kaplan, S., & Zimbro, K. (2015). Delirium monitoring and patient outcomes in a general intensive care unit. *Am J Crit Care, 24*(1), 48–56.
4. Arabi, Y., et al. (2015). Permissive underfeeding or standard enteral feeding in critically ill adults. *N Engl J Med, 372*, 2398–2408.
5. Balas, M., et al. (2012). Management of delirium in critically ill older adults. *Crit Care Nurse, 32*(4), 15–25.
6. Bell, L. (2014). The epidemiology of acute and critical illness in older adults. *Crit Care Nurs Clin North Am, 26*(1), 1–5.
7. Boling, B. (2014). Renal issues in older adults in critical care. *Crit Care Nurs Clin North Am, 26*(1), 99–104.
8. Campbell, M., Fisher, J., Anderson, L., & Kreppel, E. (2015). Implementation of early exercise and progressive mobility: steps to success. *Crit Care Nurse, 35*(1), 82–88.
9. Campanelli, C. M. (2012). American Geriatrics Society updated Beers Criteria for potentially inappropriate medication use in older adults. *J Am Geriatr Soc, 60*(4), 616–631.
10. Churpek, M. M., et al. (2015). Differences in vital signs between elderly and nonelderly patient prior to ward cardiac arrest. *Crit Care Med, 43*(4), 816–822.
11. Cox, J., & Rasmussen, L. (2014). Enteral nutrition in the prevention and treatment of pressure ulcers in adult critical care patients. *Crit Care Nurse, 34*(6), 15–27.
12. Cutugno, C. L. (2015). Atrial fibrillation: updated management guidelines and nursing implications. *Am J Nurs, 115*(5), 26–38.
13. Dacher, J. (2014). Nursing practice of palliative care with critically ill older adults. *Crit Care Nurs Clin North Am, 26*(1), 155–170.
14. Davidson, J., Winkelman, C., Gelinas, C., & Dermenchyan, A. (2015). Pain, agitation, and delirium guidelines: nurses' involvement in development and implementation. *Crit Care Nurs, 35*(3), 17–31.
15. Davis, L. (2014). Cardiovascular issues in older adults. *Crit Care Nurs Clin North Am, 26*(1), 61–89.
16. Ecklund, M., & Bloss, J. (2015). Progressive mobility as a team effort in transitional care. *Crit Care Nurse, 35*(3), 62–68.
17. Ehlenbach, W., et al. (2010). Association between acute care and critical illness hospitalization and cognitive function in older adults. *JAMA, 303*(8), 763–770.
18. DiMaria-Ghalili, R. A., & Nicolo, M. (2014). Nutrition and hydration in older adults in critical care. *Crit Care Nurs Clin North Am, 26*(1), 31–45.
19. Eliopoulos, C. (2014). *Gerontological nursing* (8th ed.). Philadelphia: Wolters Kluwer Health/Lippincott Williams & Wilkins.
20. Frederick, D. (2014). Pulmonary issues in the older adult. In S. Hardin (Ed.), *Aging and Critical Care, Critical Care Nursing Clinics of North America, 26*(1), 91–97.
21. Fuchs, L., et al. (2012). ICU admission characteristics and mortality rates among elderly and very elderly patients. *Intensive Care Med, 38*, 1654–1661. http://dx.doi.org/10.1007/s00134-012-2629-6.
22. Gehlbach, B., et al. (2011). Patient-related factors associated with hospital discharge to a care facility after critical illness. *Am J Crit Care, 20*(5), 378–386.
23. Gentleman, B. (2014). Focused assessment in the care of the older adult. *Crit Care Nurs Clin North Am, 26*(1), 15–20.
24. Gunn, S., & Fowler, R. (2014). Back to basics: importance of nursing interventions in the elderly critical care patient. *Crit Care Nurs Clin North Am, 26*(4), 433–446.
25. Hardin, S. (2015). Vulnerability of older patients in critical care. *Crit Care Nurse, 35*(3), 55–61.
26. Hardin, S. (2014). Ethnogeriatrics in critical care. *Crit Care Nurs Clin North Am, 26*(1), 21–30.
27. Hardin, S. (2012). Hearing loss in older critical care patients: participation in decision making. *Crit Care Nurs, 32*(6), 43–50.

28. Hardin, S. (2012). Engaging families to participate in care of older critical care patients. *Crit Care Nurs, 32*(3), 35–40.
29. Kennedy-Malone, L., Fletcher, K., & Martin-Plank, L. (2014). *Advance practice nursing in the care of the older adults.* Philadelphia: F.A. Davis.
30. Klein, K., Mulkey, M., Bena, J., & Albert, N. (2015). Clinical and psychological effects of early mobilization in patients treated in a neurologic ICU: a comparative study. *Crit Care Med, 43*(4), 865–873.
31. Kleinpell, R., Aitken, L., & Schorr, C. A. (2013). Implications of the new international sepsis guidelines for nursing care. *Am J Crit Care, 22*(3), 212–222.
32. Lineberry, C., & Stein, D. E. (2014). Infection, sepsis, and immune function in the older adult receiving critical care. *Crit Care Nurs Clin North Am, 26*(1), 47–60.
33. Lipska, K., et al. (2015). Potential overtreatment of diabetes mellitus in older adults with tight glycemic control. *JAMA Intern Med, 175*(3), 356–362.
34. Mangnall, L., Gallagher, R., & Stein-Parbury, J. (2011). Postoperative delirium after colorectal surgery in older patients. *Am J Crit Care, 20*(1), 45–55.
35. Mangusan, R., Hooper, V., Denslow, S., & Travis, L. (2015). Outcomes associated with postoperative delirium after cardiac surgery. *Am J Crit Care, 24*(2), 156–162.
36. Maxwell, C. A. (2015). Trauma in the geriatric population. *Crit Care Nurs Clin North Am, 27*(2), 183–197.
37. Nguyen, Y., Angus, D., Boumendil, A., & Guidet, B. (2011). The challenge of admitting the very elderly to intensive care. *Ann Intensive Care, 1*(29), 1–7.
38. Roberts, M., Johnson, L., & Lalonde, T. (2014). Early mobility in the intensive care unit: standard equipment vs a mobility platform. *Am J Crit Care, 23*(6), 451–459.
39. Stewart, M. L. (2014). Interruptions in enteral nutrition delivery in critically ill patients and recommendations for clinical practice. *Crit Care Nurs, 34*(4), 14–21.
40. Tabloski, P. (2014). *Gerontological nursing* (3rd ed.). Boston: Pearson.
41. Tifuh Amba, K. (2014). Delirium in the elderly adult in critical care. *Crit Care Nurs Clin North Am, 26*(1), 139–145.
42. United States Census Bureau. (June, 2014). *65+ in the United States: 2010.* Available at http://factfinder2.census.gov/.
43. United States Census Bureau. (May, 2014). *An aging nation: the older population in the United States.* Available at http://factfinder2.census.gov/.
44. United States Census Bureau. (November, 2011). *The older population: 2010.* Available at http://factfinder2.census.gov/.
45. Walker, M., Spivak, M., & Sebastian, M. (2014). The impact of aging physiology in critical care. *Crit Care Nurs Clin North Am, 26*(1), 7–14.

37

Caring for the Critically Ill Patient With a Neuropsychiatric Disorder

Charles Walker

INTRODUCTION

The prevalence of patients with neuropsychiatric disorders in acute care settings ranges between 20% to 35%.[50] Deinstitutionalization, a laudable human rights movement that began in the early 1960s, has placed an increasing number of patients with severe and chronic neuropsychiatric disorders into the community and onto the streets.[57] Nurses working in critical care can expect to encounter these patients in their practice. Attitudes of nurses toward patients with neuropsychiatric disorders in a critical care setting are mixed.[43] Perceptions about the purposes of critical care and the appropriateness of caring for patients with neuropsychiatric disorders may be based on unquestioned assumptions, prejudice, and social stigma.

Most neuropsychiatric disorders seen in critical care are co-occurring conditions. These disorders may be preexisting and play a major role in the development of an acute illness or injury, but are usually not responsible for the critical care admission. Neuropsychiatric disorders may develop following the critical care admission and complicate recovery. Dealing with a critically ill patient is challenging enough; neuropsychiatric symptoms and their treatment can further complicate the management of multisystem conditions and may lead to emergency situations. Additionally, the symptoms and treatment of medical conditions may exacerbate neuropsychiatric disorders.

This chapter differs from others in many respects. Whereas other chapters in this book are devoted to single disorders (e.g., acute renal failure), this chapter encompasses many and varied disorders. In the first half of this chapter, six common disorders are classified and described. In the second half, an interprofessional plan of care is provided for treatment of patients who are anxious, confused, elated, hostile, manipulative, suicidal, suspicious, or withdrawn.

DEFINITIONS

Neuropsychiatric illnesses are disorders of the brain. Although these disorders may be associated with gross structural changes (cortical atrophy, enlarged ventricular spaces) of that complex and highly plastic organ, most of the structural changes in neuroanatomy are at cellular and molecular levels. For example, widespread loss of cholinergic neurons is characteristic of Alzheimer's-type dementia, whereas schizophrenia and delusional disorders are caused by an increase in the number and sensitivity of dopaminergic and serotonergic receptors. In short, neuropsychiatric disorders represent flaws in brain chemistry.

Neurochemicals (acetylcholine, dopamine, gamma-aminobutyric acid [GABA], noradrenaline, and serotonin) increase or decrease communication between and among nerve cells. Because the brain's purpose is to transmit electrochemical impulses, these chemicals (known as neurotransmitters) must be present in the right amount. For convenience, neuropsychiatric disorders may be classified as excesses or deficiencies of specific chemicals. Similar to hormone modulation for hyperadrenalism, hypothyroidism, or diabetes, treatment is frequently lifelong and focuses on eliminating surplus chemicals or replacing those chemicals that are in short supply (Table 37.1).

Genetic predisposition for a particular mix of brain chemicals does not necessarily cause a neuropsychiatric disorder. Although brain chemistry is an important factor in the development of neuropsychiatric disorders, environmental triggers usually prompt the onset of symptoms. These triggers may include psychosocial stressors (e.g., surviving physical, emotional, or sexual trauma; living in relentless poverty; or experiencing profound loss, such as the death of a loved one or a disabling disease). Other triggers include autoimmune responses, biological or industrial toxins, viral infections, chronic illnesses, medical emergencies, malnutrition, and crisis events (e.g., the 9/11 terrorist attacks or Hurricane Katrina). Genetics plus environment yield changes in brain chemistry that cause neuropsychiatric disorders.

Neuropsychiatric disorders are defined by behavior. The *Diagnostic and Statistical Manual of Mental Disorders (DSM-5)*[4] is the primary diagnostic compendium used by all mental health professionals. The *DSM-5* lists defining criteria for hundreds of neuropsychiatric, personality, and substance abuse disorders. These defining criteria include specific symptom manifestations such as apathy, irritability, delusions, hallucinations, euphoria, loosely associated thoughts, strange or extreme emotional reactions, impoverished or garrulous speech, poor interpersonal relationships, disturbed sleep, short attention span, impulsivity, and low self-esteem. For a definitive diagnosis, symptoms must be present for a length of time (usually 2 weeks to 3 months). Exhibited behavior is the clinician's clue to chemical substrates causing a neuropsychiatric disorder; therefore, behavior becomes a target for determining treatment effectiveness. Selection and adjustment of pharmacologic and nonpharmacologic interventions is determined by the effect on patient behavior (Table 37.2).

AT-RISK PATIENTS

Patients with a history of psychiatric hospitalization, diagnosis, and treatment are at risk; however, many high-risk

TABLE 37.1 Neuropsychiatric Disorders as Excesses or Deficiencies of Specific Neurochemicals

Neuropsychiatric Disorders	Levels	Neurochemicals
Schizophrenia and other psychoses	Excess Deficiency	Dopamine (D2), norepinephrine (NE), glutamate GABA
Bipolar disorder—mania	Excess Deficiency	D2, NE, serotonin (5-HTP) GABA
Anxiety and related disorders	Excess Deficiency	D2, NE, GABA, serotonin (CSF 5 AA)
Dementia—Alzheimer's type	Deficiency	Acetylcholine, serotonin (5-HTP 2), glutamate*
Depression	Deficiency	D2, NE, serotonin (5-HTP 2)
Delirium	Variable	Synergistic effects

D2, Dopamine; *GABA*, gamma-aminobutyric acid; *NE*, norepinephrine.
*Glutamate controversy, glutamate stimulates the brain, but too much can cause neuronal destruction.

individuals do not have a previous history. Patients who have known genetic susceptibility, a generational trend, recent loss, or other environment triggers are also at risk. Risk factors associated with specific neuropsychiatric disorders are detailed later in this chapter.

Although the official classification system for neuropsychiatric disorders is the *DSM-5*, neuropsychiatric disorders may be classified in various ways. This chapter divides disorders into two general groups with respect to specific neurochemical concentrations and their effects. Delirium, dementia, and depression represent neurochemical deficiencies or synergistic effects, whereas schizophrenia, mania, and anxiety represent excesses of central nervous system (CNS) activity.

NEUROCHEMICAL DEFICIENCIES

This section addresses three conditions that are often confused with one another and are frequently misdiagnosed (e.g., delirium diagnosed as dementia) or underdiagnosed (e.g.,

TABLE 37.2 Common Medications Used for Neuropsychiatric Conditions

Medication	Actions	Dosage	Special Considerations
Antianxiety			
Buspirone hydrochloride (BuSpar)	Binds to serotonin, dopamine at presynaptic neurotransmitter receptors in the CNS.	5 mg 2–3 × daily PO or 7.5 mg 2 times/d PO. May increase in 5-mg increments/d at intervals of 2–4 d. Maintenance: 15–30 mg/d in 2–3 divided doses. Maximum dose 60 mg/d.	Can cause hypotension, sedation, nausea, and dry mouth. Interacts with CNS depressants, alcohol, and other antidepressants. Can cause moderate to severe renal or hepatic impairment. May increase serum transaminase levels. May displace digoxin from serum binding increasing risk for dig toxicity.
Benzodiazepines	Enhances action of gamma-aminobutyric acid (GABA, an inhibitory neurotransmitter) in the brain.	Alprazolam (Xanax): 0.25–0.5 mg PO TID, may titrate to a max dose of 4 mg/d in divided doses. Clonazepam (Klonopin): 1.5 mg PO daily, may titrate. Do not exceed maintenance dosage of 0.2 mg/kg daily. Long-acting. Lorazepam (Ativan): PO: 1–10 mg/d in 2–3 divided doses. IV infusion: 0.01–0.1 mg/kg/h.	Observe for paradoxical reaction. Can cause respiratory depression. Can transiently elevate serum transaminases and alkaline phosphatase. Can reach toxic levels if there is renal impairment. Abrupt withdrawal may result in pronounced restlessness, irritability, and insomnia.
Antidepressants			
1. SSRIs	Inhibit reuptake of serotonin by CNS.	Paroxetine hydrochloride (Paxil): 10–60 mg PO daily. Sertraline hydrochloride: 50–200 mg PO daily. Fluoxetine hydrochloride (Prozac): 10–80 mg PO daily. Escitalopram (Lexapro): 10–20 mg PO daily.	Can cause hypotension, sedation, nausea, and dry mouth. Interacts with CNS depressants, alcohol, and other antidepressants. Patients with hepatic or renal impairment need a lower dose. May cause hyponatremia and abrupt swings in blood glucose levels.
2. SNRIs	Inhibit reuptake of norepinephrine and serotonin from the synaptic gap.	Duloxetine: 40–60 mg PO daily. Venlafaxine: 37.5–75 mg PO daily. Desvenlafaxine: 25–100 mg PO daily.	Can cause sedation, hypertension, dry mouth, somnolence, and sweating. Can interact with alcohol and other CNS depressants. Use cautiously in patients with renal and liver impairment. Can increase suicidal ideation.
3. Atypical	Interfere with dopamine and norepinephrine catabolism.	Bupropion: 75–300 mg PO daily.	Can cause seizure, but more likely to produce transient headache, numbness or tingling of scalp, and residual tremor.
Antipsychotics			
Haloperidol (Haldol)	Blocks postsynaptic dopamine receptors, interrupts nerve impulse movement, increases turnover of dopamine in the brain.	Psychotic disorder: initially, 0.5–5 mg 2–3 times daily. Dosage gradually adjusted as needed. Elderly 0.5–2 mg 2–3 times/d. Maximum dosage 0.15 mg/kg/d in divided doses.	Observe patient for Parkinson's-like extrapyramidal reaction tremors, slurred speech, restlessness, and muscle rigidity. Can cause neuroleptic malignant syndrome, agranulocytosis, laryngospasm, and respiratory depression.

Continued

TABLE 37.2 Common Medications Used for Neuropsychiatric Conditions—cont'd

Medication	Actions	Dosage	Special Considerations
Chlorpromazine (Thorazine)	Blocks dopamine neurotransmission at postsynaptic dopamine receptor sites. Possesses strong anticholinergic, sedative, antiemetic effects.	IM/IV: initially 25 mg; may repeat in 1–4 h. May gradually increase to 400 mg q 4–6 h, maximum 300–800 mg/d. PO: 30–800 mg/d in 1–4 divided doses.	Extrapyramidal symptoms appear to be dose related and are divided into 3 categories: • akathisia • Parkinsonian symptoms • acute dystonias Can cause sudden, unexplained death.
Fluphenazine hydrochloride (Prolixin)	Antagonizes dopamine neurotransmission at synapses by blocking postsynaptic dopaminergic receptors in the brain.	IM: 2.5–10 mg/d in divided doses at 6–8 h intervals. PO: 0.5–10 mg/d in divided doses at 6–8 h intervals.	Extrapyramidal symptoms appear to be dose related and are divided into 3 categories: • akathisia • Parkinsonian symptoms • acute dystonias May cause impaired thermoregulation.
Second Generation Antipsychotics			
Aripiprazole (Abilify)	Provides partial agonist activity at dopamine and serotonin receptors and antagonist activity at serotonin receptors.	10–15 mg/daily. May increase up to 30 mg/d.	Extrapyramidal symptoms, neuroleptic malignant syndrome (NMS) rarely occurs. Monitor diabetics for loss of glucose control. May cause orthostasis.
Olanzapine (Zyprexa)	Antagonizes dopamine, serotonin, muscarinic, histamine, alpha$_1$-adrenergic receptors. Produces anticholinergic, histaminic, CNS depressant effects.	PO: 5–15 mg/d, may titrate to desired effect. Maximum: 20 mg/d. IM: 2.5–10 mg, may repeat in 2 h after 1st dose and 4 h after 2nd dose. Maximum: 30 mg/d.	Neuroleptic malignant syndrome (NMS), extrapyramidal symptoms can occur. May enhance hypotensive effects of antihypertensive medications. Monitor diabetics for glucose control. Monitor liver functions particularly in patients with hepatic disease.
Quetiapine (Seroquel)	Interacts with neurotransmitter receptors, including dopamine, serotonin, histamine, alpha$_1$-adrenergic receptors.	Maintenance dose: 300–800 mg/d PO.	Overdose produces heart block, decreased BP, hypokalemia, and tachycardia. Monitor diabetics for loss of glucose control. Can lower seizure threshold.
Risperidone (Risperdal)	Dopamine, serotonin receptor antagonism.	Psychotic disorder: initially, 0.5–1 mg BID PO, reduce in elderly to 0.25–2 mg/d PO in 1–2 divided doses. Range 2–6 mg/d. Mania: initially, 2–3 mg PO as a single daily dose. May increase at 24-h intervals of 1 mg/d. Range 2–6 mg/d.	Observe patient for signs of NMS and tardive dyskinesia. Can elevate liver functions tests. Monitor diabetics for loss of glucose control. Can prolong QT/QTc interval and cause tachycardia.
Ziprasidone (Geodon)	Antagonizes dopamine, serotonin, histamine, alpha$_1$-adrenergic receptors; inhibits reuptake of serotonin, norepinephrine	Initially 20 mg 2 × d PO with food, titrate at intervals of no less than 2 d. Maximum dose: 80 mg PO BID.	Prolongation of QT/QTc interval as seen on EKG may produce torsades de pointes. Do not administer to patients with known cardiac disease. Monitor diabetics for loss of glucose control.
Iloperidone (Fanapt)	Antagozines dopamine, serotonin, histamine, alpha1-adrenergic receptors; inhibits reuptake of serotonin, norepinephrine	12–24 mg PO daily. Divided doses.	Can cause NMS. Changes in heart rate and blood pressure can cause orthostasis. Risk for tardive dyskinesia. Monitor cholesterol and triglycerides. Monitor diabetics for increased blood glucose. Black box warning: increased risk of stroke or sudden death in elderly patients with dementia-related psychosis.
Lurasidone (Latuda)	Antagozines dopamine, serotonin, histamine, alpha1-adrenergic receptors; inhibits reuptake of serotonin, norepinephrine	20–120 mg PO daily. Divided doses.	Rarely causes NMS; tardive dyskinesia can be permanent. Dyslipidemia increases risk for stroke and coronary artery disease. May raise prolactin levels. Avoid alcohol and CY3A4 inhibitors or inducers. Caution in elderly.
Paliperidone (Invega)	Antagozines dopamine, serotonin, histamine, alpha1-adrenergic receptors; inhibits reuptake of serotonin, norepinephrine	39–234 mg IM/month. Depot dose.	Risk for NMS, tardive dyskinesia, dizziness, weight gain, hyperglycemia, diabetes, and hyperlipidemia. Monitor CBC. Stroke leading to death in elderly patients.
Cholinesterase Inhibitors—Anti-Alzheimer's Dementia Agents			
Donepezil hydrochloride (Aricept)	Enhances cholinergic function by increasing the concentration of acetylcholine through inhibition of the hydrolysis of acetylcholine by the enzyme acetylcholinesterase.	Alzheimer's disease: 5–10 mg/d as a single dose.	Overdosing may result in cholinergic crisis. Use cautiously in patients with cardiac disease, GI bleeding, and pulmonary disease. Monitor for GI bleeding especially if the patient is taking an NSAID.

TABLE 37.2 **Common Medications Used for Neuropsychiatric Conditions—cont'd**

Medication	Actions	Dosage	Special Considerations
Rivastigmine tartrate (Exelon)	Increases the concentration of acetylcholine through reversible inhibition of its hydrolysis by cholinesterase.	Alzheimer's disease: initially, 1.5 mg 2 × day. Increase dosage after a minimum of 1–2 wks. Maximum 6 mg 2 × day.	Overdosing may result in cholinergic crisis. May exacerbate muscle reactions to paralytics. Monitor diabetics for loss of glucose control.
Galantamine (Reminyl)	Elevates acetylcholine concentrations in cerebral cortex by slowing degeneration of acetylcholine released by still intact cholinergic neurons.	Alzheimer's disease: initially, 4 mg 2 × day (8 mg/d). If tolerated after a minimum of 4 wks, may increase dosage. Range is 16–24 mg/d in two divided doses.	Overdosing may result in cholinergic crisis. Not recommended in patients with severe renal or hepatic dysfunction. May cause orthostasis.
Memantine hydrochloride (Namenda)	Decreases the effects of glutamate, the principal excitatory neurotransmitter in the brain.	Alzheimer's disease: initially, 5 mg once/d, with target dose of 20 mg/d. Increase in 5 mg increments to 10 mg/d, 15 mg/d, 20 mg/d. Total dosage should be given in two doses. Recommended dose increases are in 1-wk increments.	Use cautiously in moderate to severe renal impairment. Can cause hypertension, and cardiac failure. Can cause hallucinations, ataxia, aggression, and agitation. Glutamate controversy: although glutamate's excitatory potential may improve cognitive function for a time, excess glutamate can destroy healthy neuronal cells.
Mood Stabilizers			
Lithium (Lithobid)	Accelerates catecholamine destruction, inhibits neurotransmitter release, and decreases the sensitivity of postsynaptic receptors. Displaces Na^+.	Loading dose: total of 1800 mg PO over 24 h in either 600 mg tablets TID or 900 mg sustained-release tablets BID. Maintenance dose: 300 mg tablets PO TID or QID.	NSAIDs, diuretics, and ACE inhibitors increase lithium levels. Theophylline, caffeine, sodium, and acetazolamide decrease lithium levels. Methyldopa, carbamazepine, calcium channel antagonists, antipsychotics, and SSRIs increase the chance for lithium toxicity. Monitor serum L^+ levels which should be below 1.6 mEq/L.
Carbamazepine (Tegretol)	Decreases sodium, calcium ion influx into neuronal membranes, reducing post-tetanic potentiation at synapse.	Initially 100 mg 2 × d. May increase by 100 mg 2 × d up to 400–800 mg/d, maximum dose 1200 mg/d.	Toxic reactions appear as blood dyscrasias. Can cause respiratory depression and heart block. Do not abruptly withdraw medication after long-term use.
Valproic acid (Depakene)	Directly increases concentration of the inhibitory neurotransmitter GABA.	Manic episodes: initially 750 mg/d in divided doses. Maximum dose 60 mg/kg/d.	Observe for hepatotoxicity especially in 1st 6 months of therapy. Can cause liver failure, pancreatitis, and bone marrow suppression. Therapeutic serum level is 50–100 mcg/mL. Toxic reactions appear as blood dyscrasias. Do not discontinue abruptly.

ACE, Angiotensin-converting enzyme; *BID*, twice per day; *BP*, blood pressure; *CNS*, central nervous system; *GI*, gastrointestinal; *IM*, intramuscular; *IV*, intravenous; *NSAID*, nonsteroidal antiinflammatory drug; *PO*, orally; *QID*, four times per day; *SNRI*, serotonin-norepinephrine reuptake inhibitor; *SSRI*, selective serotonin reuptake inhibitor; *TID*, three times per day.

depression). From a neurochemical standpoint, deficiencies or synergistic effects of acetylcholine, dopamine, norepinephrine, and serotonin characterize these disorders. Patients with delirium, dementia, and depression may exhibit highly variable and unpredictable behaviors[43] (Table 37.3).

Delirium

Delirium is an acute confusional syndrome resulting in dramatic yet reversible behavioral and consciousness changes. It is a potentially life-threatening medical emergency but is temporary and reversible with early recognition and intervention.[21,31] Delirium is often misdiagnosed and inappropriately treated as Alzheimer's-type dementia despite its sudden onset and transient course. To complicate matters further, manifestations of delirium are under-recognized, particularly in patients with concomitant dementia.[45]

Delirium increases morbidity and mortality, complicates and prolongs patient hospitalizations, and increases the cost of care.[59] The 3-month mortality rate from a diagnosis of delirium in the acutely delirious patient is 34%.[21] Delirium can occur at any age but is more common in older adults. Delirium is estimated to occur in 5% to 80% of hospitalized patients ages 65 and older, 6% to 30% of the general hospital population,[21] and 7% to 52% of patients following surgery.[3,46]

Risk factors of delirium vary and may include disease exacerbations, preexisting dementia, metabolic disorders, fluid and electrolyte imbalances, and alcohol or medication intoxication or withdrawal. Infections, sepsis, hypoxia, fractures, pain, nutritional deficiencies, sleep deprivation, immobility, sensory deficits, intracranial insults, urinary retention, and fecal impaction may also cause delirium.[3,21,51,68] Underlying medical conditions predisposing patients to delirium include hypertensive encephalopathy, hypertension, seizure, sequelae of head trauma, and focal lesions of the right parietal lobe.[3,60]

Among older adults, delirium commonly results from polypharmacy, medication interactions, and medication toxicity, particularly from sedative hypnotics, diuretics, and anticholinergics (Box 37.1). Many medications have anticholinergic properties that severely alter mental status. Sedatives have consistently been implicated in iatrogenic delirium of the critical

TABLE 37.3 Delirium, Dementia, and Depression Differentiation

Parameter	Delirium	Dementia	Depression
Onset	Rapid, acute, often occurs at night	Slow, insidious	Rapid, related to specific events
Distinguishing feature	Fluctuating levels of consciousness with decreased attention	Memory impairment	Sadness, loss of interest
Duration	Hours or days, less than 1 month	Years	Variable, can be persistent or episodic
Course	Short, fluctuation worse at night	Long-term, progressive course	Variable, related to causative factors
Prognosis	Potentially reversible	Irreversible, progressive	Potentially reversible
Triggers	Multiple physical and psychological factors	Vary with the cause of dementia	Personal loss, stress, medication toxicity
Acuity	Medical emergency	Chronic, progressive disease	Episodic disease
Awareness	Reduced	Clear	Clear, but selective
Alertness	Fluctuates, can be abnormally high or low	Usually normal	Normal
Attention	Impaired, fluctuating	Generally normal	Minimal impairment, but distracted
Activity	Increased or decreased	Decreased in later stages	Lethargic or agitated
Memory	Impaired recent and immediate memory	Impaired recent and remote memory	Forgetfulness
Thinking	Disorganized, distorted, fragmented, can be slow or accelerated	Impaired abstract thinking, word finding, and judgment	Inability to concentrate
Speech	Incoherent and rambling	Inappropriate or incorrect, but may be close to correct	Apathetic. Often responds "Don't know"
Mood/affect	Labile, with rapid swings	Fluctuating, depressed, apathetic, uninterested	Consistent, from extreme sadness to anxiety or irritability
Sleep-wake cycle	Disturbed, cycles reversed	Fragmented, awakens often at night	Insomnia or hypersomnia
Delusions	Yes	Yes	Yes
Hallucinations	Yes	Yes	Not usually
Disabilities	Acute, new deficits	Slow onset and may conceal them	Recognizes deficits

BOX 37.1 Drugs That Can Cause Acute Confusion (Delirium)

Amantadine (Symmetrel)
Amitriptyline (Elavil)
Atenolol (Tenormin)
Atropine (Atropine)
Benztropine (Cogentin)
Chlorpheniramine maleate (Chlor-Trimeton)
Chlorpromazine (Thorazine)
Cimetidine (Tagamet)
Digoxin (Lanoxin)
Diphenhydramine (Benadryl)
Disopyramide (Norpace)
Doxepine (Doxepin)
Furosemide (Lasix)
Homatropine (Isopto)
Hydroxyzine (Vistaril)
Imipramine pamoate (Tofranil)
Lithium (Eskalith, Lithobid)
Meperidine (Demerol)
Methyldopa (Aldomet)
Metoprolol (Lopressor, Toprol)
Nifedipine (Adalat, Procardia)
Quinidine (Quinate)
Prazosin (Minipres)
Prednisolone (Prednisone)
Procainamide (Procanbid)
Prochloroperazine maleate (Compazine)
Promethazine (Phenergan)
Propranolol (Inderal)
Ranitidine (Zantac)
Scopolamine (Scopolamine)
Theophylline (Theodur)
Thioridazine (Mellaril)
Trihexyphenidyl (Artane)
Verapamil (Calan)

care patient. The effects of anticholinergic medications are additive if a patient is taking more than one. Correctly diagnosing and treating the underlying cause is the most important caveat for managing delirium.[21] The Society of Critical Care Medicine suggests using the THINK mnemonic to assist in identifying the cause of intensive care unit (ICU) delirium (Box 37.2).

There are three categories of delirium: hyperactive (the most common), hypoactive, and mixed.[51] Patients with hyperactive delirium are restless and agitated, patients with hypoactive

BOX 37.2 THINK—Potential Causes of Delirium

Toxic situations
- CHF, shock, dehydration
- Deliriogenic medications (tight titration of sedatives)
- New organ failure (e.g., liver, kidney)

Hypoxemia
Infection/sepsis (nosocomial)
Nonpharmacologic interventions (are the following areas being neglected: hearing aids, glasses, sleep protocols, music, noise control, ambulation?)
K^+ or electrolyte problems

delirium may present in stupor and be barely responsive, and those with mixed delirium exhibit hyperactive as well as hypoactive symptoms. Because symptoms vary depending on type, the diagnosis and treatment of delirium become more challenging. Any acute change in cognition, consciousness, or both should be considered delirium until proven otherwise. Delirium is distinguished by a disturbance of consciousness that develops quickly and fluctuates over the course of the day.[4]

Prevention of delirium should be the major goal of care although there is no established, effective protocol. Interventions to prevent or treat delirium can be subdivided into four areas: physiologic, environmental, patient safety, and pharmacologic.[7] Physiologic intervention begins with identification of patients at risk for delirium and proceeds to early diagnosis and treatment of underlying causes. Delirium assessment is key to early identification and should be performed a minimum of once per shift. Early identification and correction of dehydration and electrolyte imbalance, recognition of concomitant dementia, adequate oxygenation, and correction of nutritional deficits are key aspects of physiologic intervention.

Environmental interventions to prevent delirium include early mobilization, adequate and uninterrupted sleep, and noise control, all of which are difficult to regulate in critical care. Using glasses and hearing aids to compensate for sensory deficits, keeping familiar objects in the patient's room, varying light intensity to distinguish night and day, and providing a television or radio for stimulation may delay or prevent delirium. Patient safety interventions include integrating reality orientation into casual conversations with the patient, preventing hospital-acquired infections, allowing the patient to participate in care, using bed alarms and wander guards, placing the patient in a room close to the nurses' station, providing clocks and calendars in the patient's room, and minimizing the number of room changes and transfers.

Pharmacologic interventions for delirium prevention include using neuroleptics or benzodiazepines to manage symptoms, completing a medication evaluation to determine if the additive effects of medicines are the cause of the delirium, managing the patient's pain, and minimizing sedation.[3,14,31] Risperidone (Risperdal) is rapidly replacing haloperidol (Haldol) as the medication of choice for patients with delirium.[24] Haloperidol is notorious for producing brutal Parkinson-like extrapyramidal reactions; however, at only slightly higher than normal doses, risperidone yields similar neuromotor effects, which include tremors, slurred speech, restlessness, and muscle rigidity.

Dementia

Dementia is the eighth leading cause of death in the United States.[6] It has an insidiously gradual onset with progressive cognitive decline. Unlike other chronic illnesses, dementia does not remit, and brain insult results in global loss of intellectual functioning.[49] Alzheimer's disease is the most common type of dementia, and it accounts for 53% to 65% of all dementias.[56] It is followed by vascular dementia, accounting for 15% to 23% of dementias.[56] The remaining 14% to 20% of dementias are caused by other pathologic processes, including diffuse Lewy body disease, Pick's disease, Huntington's disease, Creutzfeldt-Jakob disease, Parkinson's disease, substance-induced dementia, HIV dementia, normal-pressure hydrocephalus, vitamin deficiencies, and endocrine abnormalities.[16,51]

Dementia occurs most commonly in older adults; incidence increases with age. Approximately 1% of individuals younger than age 65 have dementia, in contrast to 10% to 22% of individuals ages 65 to 85, and 40% to 50% of individuals older than age 85.[56] The incidence of Alzheimer's disease and vascular dementia increases with age, so the number of people affected by both processes will rise as the population of older adults mushrooms in the decades ahead.

Alzheimer's disease results in a slow, unrelenting deterioration of mental and self-care capacities that change a patient's personality. The disease usually lasts 8 to 10 years, always culminating in death. Because of its slow course, early identification of Alzheimer's disease may be missed. Memory impairment can be masked in the early stages by social skills and memory aids.[49] Senile plaques and neurofibrillary tangles develop throughout the brain. As these plaques and tangles increase, patients experience difficulty with memory, decision making, communication, and ability to care for themselves.[51] Although the precise cause of Alzheimer's disease is unknown, current theories include loss of neurotransmitter stimulation, genetic mutations, loss of the protein that binds with beta amyloid, and influx of excess calcium into the brain.

Diagnosis of dementia is made by identifying an impairment in two or more of the following brain functions: language, memory, personality, cognition, and visuospatial perception.[51] Several evidence-based assessment tools are used to confirm a diagnosis of dementia. The Confusion Assessment Method; Folstein Mini-Mental State Exam; and the Geriatric Depression Scale all may be used in the critically ill patient because they take little time to complete and do not deplete the patient's reserves.[10,29,55]

Treatment of dementia depends on the cause. If the cause can be corrected, appropriate measures should be taken. Otherwise, the treatment is supportive and includes pharmacologic and nonpharmacologic approaches. Significant dementia research has yielded memory-enhancing medications that can slow the decline of intellectual function, but rarely raise cognitive ability. Known as cholinesterase inhibitors, these medications increase acetylcholine levels and include donepezil (Aricept), rivastigmine (Exelon), and galantamine (Reminyl). Memantine (Namenda) is a medication approved by the US Food and Drug Administration (FDA) for treatment of moderate to severe Alzheimer's disease. When used in conjunction with donepezil or other cholinesterase inhibitors, memantine appears to work by regulating the activity of glutamate, a brain chemical that plays a specialized role in learning and memory functions.[13]

Atypical second-generation antipsychotic medications, such as olanzapine (Zyprexa), aripiprazole (Abilify), risperidone (Risperdal), and quetiapine (Seroquel), have been used to treat behavioral symptoms in dementia; however, the FDA issued a black box warning that they are associated with increased mortality, especially among the elderly. Other medications used for the treatment of dementia include vitamins, ginkgo biloba, antiinflammatory agents, statins, estrogen, antidepressants, and mood stabilizers.[66]

The goals of nonpharmacologic treatment are to maintain functional capacity, independence, and quality of life. Nonpharmacologic treatment measures include reducing stress, providing cues to prompt memory, using sensory enhancements, adjusting daily routines to focus on the person, encouraging socialization to prevent sensory deprivation and isolation, and offering structured activities to alleviate agitation and boredom.[49] Most patients require continual care and institutionalization in the latter stages of dementia. The burden to caregivers who keep patients with dementia at home is significant; therefore, decisions about when and where to discharge the patient should be started early.

Depression

Depression is a common psychiatric disorder. According to an Institute of Medicine report, unipolar depression is the leading cause of global disability.[26] An estimated 8.3% of adolescents, 5.3% of adults, and 6% of elders have been diagnosed with major depression in the United States.[63] Depression is underdiagnosed and undertreated, particularly among older adults, and is seen in 20% to 30% of patients with dementia.[11]

Although the incidence of depression is similar across all races and ethnic groups, there are gender differences; more women than men are affected worldwide.[48] Depression frequently accompanies acute and chronic illness with prevalence rates as high as 70%.[6] Treatment and lost productivity due to depression costs billions of dollars annually. The cause of depression is thought to be dysregulation of the neurotransmitters serotonin, norepinephrine, epinephrine, and dopamine.[48] The underlying medical conditions predisposing people to depression (and carrying the greatest risk for suicide) include chronic, incurable, and painful conditions (e.g., malignancy, spinal cord injury, peptic ulcer disease, Huntington's disease, AIDS, and end-stage renal disease).[4]

Depression slows all bodily processes, including elimination; therefore, clinically depressed patients must be observed for signs of constipation and urinary retention. Depression also slows cognition, leading mental health professionals to use the term *pseudodementia*[6] when referring to depressive symptoms (e.g., poor attention span and memory loss). Diagnosis of depression begins with a comprehensive assessment. Presenting symptoms include insomnia or hypersomnia; tiredness; lack of energy; overeating or undereating; difficulty concentrating and making decisions; lack of interest in personal appearance; sexual dysfunction; avoidance of interpersonal interactions; delusions; hallucinations; vague somatic complaints; feelings of sadness, despair, misery, self-loathing, and guilt; and suicidal ideation. Physiologic processes that mimic depression (e.g., vitamin deficiencies, hypothyroidism) must be ruled out as potential causes.[1]

Treatment of depression is aimed at eliminating symptoms, reducing recurrence, and increasing quality of life.[6] Both pharmacologic and nonpharmacologic therapies are used to treat depression. Major nonpharmacologic therapies for depression are psychotherapy and electroconvulsive therapy. Other therapies include phototherapy, increased physical exercise to raise serotonin levels, transcranial magnetic stimulation, vagus nerve stimulation, and herbal remedies (St. John's wort).[35] The four classes of antidepressant medications are selective serotonin reuptake inhibitors (SSRIs), serotonin-norepinephrine reuptake inhibitors (SNRIs), monoamine oxidase inhibitors (MAOIs), and atypical antidepressants. All antidepressants interact with other medications. The most frequently used and safest medications are the SSRIs, including escitalopram (Lexapro), paroxetine (Paxil), and sertraline (Zoloft); the SNRIs including venlafaxine (Effexor XR) and duloxetine (Cymbalta); and the atypical agent, bupropion (Wellbutrin).[1]

Serotonin syndrome, a rare but potentially lethal condition, occurs when introducing or incrementally increasing the dosage of any serotomimetic agent. Symptoms include autonomic instability, hyperreflexia, shivering, diaphoresis, hypertension, tremors, mental status changes, and ataxia.[20] Immediate recognition and intervention are needed to prevent the potentially fatal complications of rhabdomyolysis, multiple organ dysfunction syndrome, and disseminated intravascular coagulation. The offending medication should be discontinued and the provider notified.

CENTRAL NERVOUS SYSTEM EXCESSES

This section discusses commonalities and differences among psychotic, mood, and anxiety-related disorders. Excesses of dopamine, norepinephrine, serotonin or a deficiency in a CNS inhibitor GABA characterize these disorders. Patients with schizophrenia, mania, or acute anxiety disorders exhibit excitation and hypersensitivity to internal and external stimuli due to the fact that their CNS is supercharged.[37]

Schizophrenia

The schizophrenic spectrum includes a group of psychotic disorders characterized by disturbed or loosely associated thoughts, misperceived or falsified interpretations of reality, altered sense perceptions, apathy, ambivalence, lack of emotional responsiveness, and impaired interpersonal and vocational functioning. To think of schizophrenia as a single disorder is akin to thinking of heart disease as one malady, rather than several clearly distinguishable conditions (myocardial infarction, heart failure, or cardiomyopathy). Despite some common symptom presentations, schizophrenia manifests differently in different people; many are paranoid, others are childlike and silly.

Schizophrenia exists in all cultures and socioeconomic groups. Approximately 1% of the population worldwide will develop this severe and disabling condition over the course of a lifetime.[58] Schizophrenia is responsible for longer hospitalizations, higher costs to individuals and governments, more chaos in families, and more public fear (usually unfounded) than any other neuropsychiatric disorder. Schizophrenia is a condition in which thoughts are fragmented and emotions are compartmentalized. Causes of schizophrenia are complex. Schizophrenia most likely results from a combination of biological, psychological, and environmental influences on a person vulnerable to the illness.[34,65] Abnormal levels of dopamine, norepinephrine, serotonin, and GABA have been implicated.

Schizophrenia usually develops in stages. Premorbid behavior includes aloof indifference to others. People who will later become schizophrenic have difficulty forming and maintaining relationships. As they become more socially withdrawn, their lifestyle grows more eccentric. They begin to neglect personal hygiene, communicate in peculiar ways, and fail to perform in mature adult roles. Tasks that constitute the normal transition from adolescence to adulthood, such as establishing occupational capacities, are the very things that tend to pose the greatest difficulties for schizophrenic patients. Poor prognosis is associated with an earlier onset of symptoms, failure to complete college or high school, inability to hold a job, and lack of familial support. Even when prognostic indicators are in the person's favor, a severely distorted, internal representation of the illness makes sustained compliance with treatment unlikely. People with schizophrenia may not agree that they are ill (or ill enough) to warrant costly treatment.[15]

Schizophrenia is a chronic illness that follows predictable patterns with respect to chronicity. In acute exacerbations or relapses, positive symptoms predominate. Far from positive in the sense of being desired or desirable, positive symptoms of schizophrenia include intense reactions, such as full-blown delusions and hallucinations. Delusions are false ideas unmediated by logic; hallucinations are sensory experiences, usually auditory, without basis in reality. Delusions and hallucinations are stress-related reactions that respond favorably to hospitalization and medication.[40] After stabilization, the person with schizophrenia experiences remission of positive symptoms; however, negative symptoms of schizophrenia remain. Negative symptoms refer to lack of motivation, apathy, thought blocking, and dulled emotions; these are the insidious, often unrecognized silent suffering of schizophrenic patients. If antipsychotic medications are withheld during a critical care stay, some breakthrough of psychotic symptoms, including anxiety, confusion, suspicion, and withdrawal may be expected.

Treatment modalities for schizophrenia and other psychotic disorders may include psychotherapy and social skills training. These therapies are successful, however, only when used in conjunction with antipsychotic medications (neuroleptics). Older medications, including chlorpromazine (Thorazine), fluphenazine (Prolixin), and haloperidol, were effective for curbing positive symptoms, but they possessed troublesome anticholinergic properties and neuromotor side effects. The newer medications, including olanzapine (Zyprexa), ziprasidone (Geodon), and aripiprazole (Abilify), treat positive and negative symptoms and produce fewer neuromotor effects; however, they are known to cause obesity, glucose metabolism errors, and EKG changes, specifically prolongation of the QT interval.[54] Close and careful monitoring of neuroleptic therapy prevents the most serious adverse reactions (e.g., neuroleptic malignant syndrome, tardive dyskinesia, and seizure). Antipsychotic medications achieve their therapeutic benefit by exerting an alpha-adrenergic blockade on the CNS. Sedation and orthostatic hypotension are common side effects. Because these medications are also beta-agonists, tachycardia, leading to fatal dysrhythmias, may occur with moderate to high doses.[18]

Psychosis is a generic term referring to schizophrenia and the schizophrenic-like behaviors of people with other medical conditions, including neoplasms, stroke, meningitis, Huntington's disease, hypoadrenalism, hypoxia, and hypoglycemia.[4] Fluid and electrolyte imbalances and adverse medication reactions may produce similar symptoms. For instance, a rarely reported sequela of procainamide (Pronestyl) use is medication-induced psychosis. Procainamide is used to treat atrial and ventricular dysrhythmias in physiologically compromised patients. If a patient reports experiencing an adverse reaction to procaine in the dentist's office, critical care nurses should be alert to the possibility of procainamide-induced psychosis. To avoid mistaking the schizophrenic-like symptoms for critical care psychosis, listening to family and client cues is helpful. Critical care psychosis is a type of delirium caused by sensory overload, sleep deprivation, or pain; it reportedly occurs after 48 hours. Medication-induced psychosis usually occurs sooner.[25]

Mania

Mania is associated with bipolar illness. The person with bipolar illness experiences a range of moods from incapacitating depression to acute mania. During mania, patients describe their experience as an intense feeling of well-being, extreme cheerfulness, or oneness with the universe. The median age of onset is 19 years.[39] Bipolar illness occurs equally between genders, although depression is more prevalent in women than men.

As the height of the bipolar mood swing, mania begins with euphoria, progresses through expansive exultation, and sometimes ends in frenzy. Symptoms of mania are categorized by severity. Hypomanic symptoms are not sufficiently severe to impair social or occupational functioning, and they do not warrant hospitalization. In acute mania, the person's over joyous mood seems out of proportion to the circumstances. With boundless enthusiasm, energy, and self-confidence, the person with acute mania knows no strangers. Friendly and talkative, manic patients often claim to be on a quixotic quest and frequently grow irritable when others fail to appreciate the great quest they are undertaking. Manic patients can be belligerent, intrusive, and quick to anger. With the belief that they possess great wealth, power, and prestige, they may squander their life savings or accumulate excessive credit card debt. Hospitalization is required for acute mania. Delirious mania is the gravest form of mania, characterized by intense manic symptoms, self-neglect, clouding of consciousness, and psychotic features. According to the kindling theory,[36] one severely manic episode tends to yield another. Increased neuroreceptor sensitivity is responsible for this kindling effect.

Like schizophrenia, the causes of mania are complex; strong hereditary influence has been reinforced by study of the human genome.[39] Physiologic reasons for mania include brain lesions, medication side effects, and electrolyte imbalances, particularly increases in intracellular sodium and calcium. Biochemical abnormalities of dopamine, norepinephrine, serotonin, and GABA have been implicated.[27]

Treatment for mania is primarily pharmacologic. In the high pitch of acute mania, patients require antipsychotic medications to rein in their expansive mood. Mood stabilizers are used to keep the mood on an even keel. Lithium is an effective medication for stabilizing mood; it is a mineral salt with a therapeutic blood level of 0.8–1.3 mEq/L. As a salt, lithium binds freely with sodium receptors. This competition for receptor sites can deplete sodium and cause lithium toxicity (levels ≥ 2 mEq/L). The physiologic signs and symptoms of lithium toxicity are the signs and symptoms of hyponatremia, familiar to critical care nurses. Consequently, other medications that increase the elimination of sodium, including diuretics and angiotensin-converting enzyme inhibitors, should be avoided or used with extreme caution when the patient is taking lithium.[17] Selected anticonvulsants, such as carbamazepine (Tegretol) and valproic acid (Depakene), are also useful as mood stabilizers; each has its own side effect profile, including blood disorders and hepatotoxicity, respectively.

Anxiety

Anxiety is both a symptom and a class of neuropsychiatric disorders. Levels of anxiety range from mild to moderate to severe. Panic is the most extreme form of anxiety. A person with mild to moderate anxiety usually feels energized or tense, exhibits discriminating attention, and solves problems with speed. Conversely, a person with severe to panic-level anxiety often feels threatened, distorts reality, and experiences excessive autonomic stimulation, poor motor coordination, diminished hearing and pain sensation, scattered perception, and inattentiveness.

Anxiety is pathologic if the response is greatly disproportional to the threat, continues after the danger abates, impairs everyday functioning, or leads to somatic consequences (e.g., colitis or dermatitis).[9] Specific types of anxiety disorders include phobias, panic, selective mutism, and social anxiety disorder. As their name suggests, panic attacks are episodic. Their onset is sudden, and patients frequently present in the hospital emergency department with a pervasive feeling of terror, fear of impending doom, and intense physical discomfort. Previous traumas experienced by posttraumatic stress disorder (PTSD) patients may predispose them to flashbacks, nightmares, and confusion in critical care.

Treatment modalities for anxiety disorders include cognitive and behavioral therapies, as well as medications. The medications used depend on the cause or source of the anxiety. Sometimes antidepressants are recommended;[5] because antidepressants are psychostimulants, their use seems paradoxical;

however, their use is justified if the anxiety is symptomatic of an underlying, chronic depression. Anxiolytic (or antianxiety) medications are most often used to treat acute anxiety and incorporate use of the benzodiazepines, including alprazolam (Xanax), clonazepam (Klonopin), and lorazepam (Ativan), along with buspirone (BuSpar) and beta blockers.[38] Buspirone is less potentially addictive than the benzodiazepines and achieves similar CNS depression without compromising patient alertness or arousal. By slowing heart rate, beta blockers relieve the autonomic manifestations that patients associate with anxiety. Any of these medications must be monitored judiciously, particularly in a critical care setting. Interactions with alcohol and other medications are common and can prove catastrophic.

INTERPROFESSIONAL PLAN OF CARE

In this section, behavior-specific strategies for dealing with diverse patients are covered. Eight behaviors frequently seen among patients with neuropsychiatric disorders include anxiety, confusion, elation, hostility, manipulation, suicidal, suspicion, and withdrawal. These behaviors are identifiable and distinguishable through patient actions and statements. Verbal and nonverbal indicators of these behaviors are fairly easy to detect even in complicated clinical situations such as critical care. To respond appropriately, critical care nurses do not need to know the nuances of every *DSM-5* diagnosis,[4] but the nurse must master the ability to identify and distinguish these eight behaviors when patients, family, and visitors manifest the behaviors.

Patients with neuropsychiatric disorders have overt behaviors. The acute and critical care nurse should recognize each behavior and know how to respond quickly, safely, and accurately. Symptom recognition is familiar to critical care nurses. Critical care nurses "know" cardiogenic shock, acute renal failure, and increased intracranial pressure by their symptom presentations. Becoming familiar with behaviors associated with neuropsychiatric disorders will facilitate prompt recognition and, therefore, appropriate intervention for these disorders, too.

The Anxious Patient

In *The Meaning of Anxiety,* Rollo May distinguishes between fear and anxiety.[33] According to May, fear is a threat to the periphery of an individual's experience, but anxiety is a threat to the foundation and center of human existence. The anxious patient exhibits a number of autonomic symptoms that include pupillary dilation, palpitations, sweating, trembling, shortness of breath, dry mouth, throat constriction, choking, chest pain, nausea, dizziness, crying, fear of losing control, numbness, tingling, and chills.

Even under the best of circumstances, critically ill patients can feel afraid and anxious. Gently approaching the anxious patient and demonstrating acceptance of nervously heightened activity or increasingly bizarre behavior are important. Patients who are intubated or delusional cannot express their feelings easily. Giving voice to anxious feelings, particularly if the patient cannot, may be helpful. If a delusional patient becomes more delusional and irrational, the nurse should not appeal to reason, defend her actions, or request detailed explanations. Instead, responding to the patient, it would be appropriate to stop and say, "I think you are getting more anxious," and then sit quietly with the patient. If possible, the nurse should not leave the patient's bedside; leaving or walking to another part of the room may increase the patient's anxiety. Anxious patients may use rituals or avoidance behaviors to manage their anxiety. The nurse should not interfere with ritualistic behaviors unless they pose a legitimate and imminent threat, such as compulsively drinking fluids or repeatedly dialing 911.[2] Patients with PTSD (e.g., combat or rape trauma) may startle easily, so they should be warned about sudden, loud noises or unexpected activity.

Because anxiety can be contagious, the nurse should create as calm an emotional climate as possible. A patient who is anxious may fear losing control. For the patient to whom losing control is a major concern, the nurse should gently explain that a response team and other resources are in place to assist in managing out-of-control behavior. Explaining a plan in matter-of-fact terms may reassure the anxious patient. To avoid sounding like a threat, which heightens rather than allays anxiety, this verbal intervention requires the finesse that comes with experience. The nurse can enlist the help of a psychiatric liaison nurse or clinical nurse specialist as needed.

The Confused Patient

The unfamiliar setting of critical care may be disorienting to a patient, especially if that patient is hypoxemic, ketoacidotic, or otherwise at risk for delirium.[8] A confused patient may be mute or mumble incoherently, appear clueless when asked simple questions, fail to respond or respond slowly when given a command, reply to unseen voices, see people who are not present, or behave in odd and eccentric ways.

When dealing with a critically ill patient who is visibly confused, the nurse should offer explanations that are short and simple. The patient's environment should be structured and the schedule kept as predictable as possible. If a change is necessary, prepare the patient for it as early and as consistently as possible. No more than one caregiver should be assigned per shift. The nurse should set few limits, offer frequent reminders, and be lenient.[43] Tangible and familiar objects should be used to orient and reorient the patient. The nurse should introduce him/herself, casually integrating the date, time, and location into the conversation, but cease reality orientation if the patient reaches a tolerance threshold or becomes agitated. A list can be posted to remind the patient's family and other nurses of the patient's routine activities and care. The nurse should accept regressive or infantile behavior from such patients. If a confused patient exposes himself or openly masturbates, the nurse should realize that he is expressing primitive impulses, much as a young child does; cover the patient and offer privacy.

The nurse should acknowledge hallucinations as "real" for the patient and convey understanding for how the patient is affected by them. For instance, once the nurse has determined that a patient is hearing voices (about which it is okay, even prudent, to ask), the nurse might say, "I don't hear the voices, but I can see how upset you are by them." With a patient who is actively hallucinating, the nurse should avoid abrupt handling, accidental touching, hugging, or other gestures that could be misinterpreted.[58] Confused patients should be reassured that they will not be harmed by frighteningly unfamiliar objects, such as an oxygen compressor, nasal cannula, or rebreather mask. Even common objects such as a hairbrush, cup of lukewarm tea, or "razor-sharp" apple slice may appear strange and scary. The nurse should not assume that a confused patient is in full control of their language and behavior. Exhorting the confused patient to exercise whatever degree of control he can muster at the moment is a reasonable expectation.

The Elated Patient

Although elation is most frequently associated with major mood disorders, other causes include primary endocrine dysfunction (e.g., thyrotoxicosis),[62] steroid use, and psychostimulant intoxication, such as amphetamine or cocaine abuse.[12] Medical treatment is the paramount concern, but managing an elated patient means staying alert to behavioral cues. An elated patient will display a persistently elevated and expansive mood, inflated self-esteem, incessant talkativeness, insomnia, hypersexual impulses, excessive movement, and racing thoughts. Intrusiveness, distractibility, irritability, and agitation are commonly observed.

When addressing the critically ill patient who is elated, the nurse may use mild persuasion and distraction. Despite the patient's constant motion and flightiness, an elated patient does not respond positively to being hurried.[19,37] Too many people and too much activity can easily agitate an elated patient. It is important to limit choices and reduce environmental stimuli, which are ubiquitous in critical care. As the main source of stimulation in the patient's environment, the nurse should speak and move slowly. The nurse should avoid calling the elated patient by his nickname or speaking sharply. If elation reaches a feverish and frenzied pitch, the nurse can encourage hygiene, nutrition, and rest. Fluid and electrolyte imbalances should be monitored closely and provide replacement therapy, especially if the client is taking lithium.

The Hostile Patient

Aggression and hostility are more common in nonpsychiatric settings than they once were. Because patients are sicker and healthcare resources are limited, patients, as well as their families, experience frustration without an appropriate outlet for expression. Contrary to the popular stereotype, people with schizophrenia are no more likely than members of the general population to exhibit violent behavior.[52] Other risk factors for aggressive or hostile behavior include a diagnosis of delirium or dementia, alcohol intoxication, misuse of medications, youthfulness, overt threats against others, angry outbursts, and direct provocation within the treatment milieu. The number one risk factor for hostile behavior is a history of violence.[23,30] Shouting, shoving, and brandishing a weapon are the most salient clues.

When dealing with a hostile and potentially violent patient, the nurse must be alert, evaluate the situation, and solicit help. The nurse should listen to the aggressive patient, let him/her vent frustration or anger, and not argue or demand better behavior. While striving to communicate an expectation of self-control, the nurse should psychologically disarm a hostile person. For example, the nurse might calmly say, "I can see that you're worried. Tell me what's bothering you in a way that doesn't hurt you or anyone else." Saying no too quickly and insisting that patients do things the hospital's way are the biggest mistakes nurses make.[23] The nurse should avoid taking verbal or physical attacks personally, lower her voice, and adopt a nonconfrontational posture. Standing at a right angle to the hostile person and keeping hands visible are ways to minimize the patient's perception of a threat. Demonstrating the universal "no weapons" gesture and avoiding a locked stare with the patient send the same message.

The nurse can ensure safety of other patients and staff by assisting the hostile person to a safe place. Seclusion or restraint should only be used as a last resort and always in the least restrictive way possible. A nurse should never approach a hostile person from behind, never block access to an exit, and never attempt to subdue a patient or visitor who has a weapon. For example, suppose an agitated critical care visitor grabs a large pair of scissors from the nurses' station and displays them menacingly. The nurse would move a safe distance away, motion others to do the same, and firmly instruct, "Put the scissors down."

The Manipulative Patient

When critically ill patients cannot express their wishes clearly or are unable to read cues about acceptable behavior, they may try to manipulate nurses and other healthcare professionals. Manipulative behavior may be difficult to detect. People who frequently resort to manipulation may appear sincere and quite charming initially. They present themselves as victims; their stories are convincing. The target of manipulative behavior feels used and angry. Nurses may experience tremendous guilt for being angry at a patient, and they may need to debrief with a colleague or supervisor about the incident.

To deal effectively with manipulative patients, critical care nurses should establish and enforce limits firmly, consistently, and without exception. (NOTE: This approach to enforcing limits departs dramatically from the tactic taken with a confused patient.) Avoid giving ultimatums and making deals; limit responses to the present situation. The nurse should not offer choices when there are none, and should not argue facts. The nurse should identify his/her feelings in order to avoid being drawn into defending his/her position.[41,67] Respond to suggestive talk and sexually inappropriate behavior in a no-nonsense manner. The manipulative patient will be disappointed when he/she does not get their way, so the nurse must be prepared for sweet seduction to morph into rage when the patient is thwarted. Acknowledgment by the nurse that the manipulative patient has been deprived of something is important. Explain that the patient's manipulative behavior may cause others to reject him/her. The patient should be held to standards; his/her self-esteem can be built with praise for socially appropriate accomplishments.

The Suicidal Patient

Although Thomas Szasz, professor emeritus of psychiatry at Syracuse University, asserts that suicide is the most autonomous human act, the majority of healthcare providers and bioethicists argue against the right of a suicidal person to kill himself.[53] Suicide intervention is mandated in order to preserve the person's autonomy for the future. Despite the link to major depression, a suicidal impulse, plan, or attempt is not a neuropsychiatric diagnosis.

Suicidal patients are not merely acting out or staking a dramatic bid for attention. A suicidal gesture is an intentional act of self-harm, which seems to contradict the value of human life that nurses hold sacrosanct. Suicidal patients present a great challenge to nurses, particularly those who work in intensive care. Critical care nurses experience mixed emotions about treating patients who have attempted suicide and wish to die. Critical care nurses may question the appropriateness of caring for suicidal patients in critical care, and they often feel inadequately prepared to manage suicidal patients.[22,43] Nurses without a background in psychiatric care often fear that if patients are suicidal, then talking about suicide will precipitate suicidal behavior. On the contrary, patients may experience relief that someone is willing to listen to their concerns, rather than leaving them to feel alone and isolated in a conspiracy of silence. If a nurse does not have the time or feels uncertain of how to handle a suicidal patient, he/she can solicit help from the psychiatric consultation team or from a clinical nurse specialist.

Suicidal patients may have a history of physical, verbal, or sexual abuse. They may have survived the suicide or sudden death of a close friend or family member. Besides bereavement, other risk factors include loss of job, onset or progression of a chronic, disabling, or terminal illness, threat of incarceration, and social isolation. Suicidal patients may voice veiled intent or speak openly about suicide; they may give away personal belongings, make funeral arrangements, write a will, and withdraw from loved ones. Suicidal patients typically exhibit a deadly triad of depression, hostility, and impulsivity.[32]

When caring for a critically ill patient who is suicidal, the critical care nurse must maintain close surveillance and activate suicide precautions. Recognition by the nurse of a sudden burst of energy, improved appetite and sleep, or an unexpected lift in mood as a cue that the depressed patient has mobilized the wherewithal to devise a plan and act on it. All suicide threats should be taken seriously and the lethality of the threat should be determined. Even indirect statements such as, "I don't see much hope for the future," should alert the nurse to inquire directly about suicide plans. Although most suicidal patients are not psychotic, the nurse should ask the actively hallucinating patient to describe auditory imperative or command hallucinations (e.g., "What are the voices telling you to do?"). Potentially harmful devices and instruments of mutilation should be removed from the patient's room. The patient should be observed for opportunities to hoard and overdose on antidepressants or other medications.

A suicidal patient may speak in ironic terms (e.g., "I don't like it here"), which nurses tend to interpret literally. Rather than clarify lived ironies or delve deeply into their meaning, the nurse should encourage the patient to talk (e.g., "Tell me more"). Evidence of the patient's ambivalence should be observed. Glimmers of hopefulness, happy memories, or expressions of moral uncertainty (e.g., "I can't leave my kids alone") provide occasions for the nurse to intervene by providing genuine reassurance and life support if an attempt is made. Sensitivity should be maintained to the fact that a failed suicide is construed by the suicidal patient as an example of their ineptitude, another failure in a life characterized by a long succession of perceived failures.[32,64]

The Suspicious Patient

Even mentally healthy patients who voluntarily enter the hospital acknowledge that events and activities done on their behalf seem to be done to them rather than for them. If the patient is psychotically suspicious, this perception is multiplied exponentially. Although the structured environment and treatment patterns of critical care may mitigate external and internal stimuli that fuel perceptual distortions of a suspicious patient, critical care nurses must proceed with caution.[28] A suspicious patient generally is not reassured by touch. It may be misinterpreted as an assault or a sexual advance. If the nurse must touch the patient to administer care, explain why and limit contact to only what is necessary.

Most suspicious patients are uncomfortable in open spaces. They may think that someone is coming up behind them. They should not be positioned in bed with their backs toward the door. If a suspicious patient must sit out of bed, the chair should be arranged so that the patient's back is against the wall. Extremes of light or darkness may be another source of stress. Suspicious patients exhibit hypervigilance; they frequently dart their eyes around the room, turn their heads from side to side, and hide their personal belongings. They have a low tolerance for ambiguity, become impatient with routine questions, and may make insulting or derogatory remarks meant to offend or repel others.[61]

The critical care nurse should try to maintain a physical and emotional distance from the suspicious patient. Communication should be honest and direct; make promises clear and abide by them, speak in brief declarative sentences, and avoid making critical statements. Communication should avoid secretive gestures, whispering, or figures of speech. Even common medical abbreviations may be ominously misconstrued with an unintended message (e.g., "PRN" may be interpreted as "Persecute Robert Now!").

Gaining and preserving trust are goals with a suspicious patient. The patient's delusion should never be challenged or denied. The nurse who either validates or denies a patient's delusion will become part of the perceived conspiracy against the suspicious patient. Instead, the nurse should look for and respond to the underlying concern. For example, if the suspicious patient says, "You're out to kill me; I have to leave," the nurse should not argue, defend, or openly disagree with the delusion. Empathy should be conveyed by saying, "Being in a strange hospital and not knowing what's going on must be very frightening." Focus on what is real in the patient's immediate situation and anticipate the patient's refusal to accept food or prescribed treatment.[42] To decrease suspicion, foods and medicine may be offered whole or in "tamper-proof" containers. For instance, a whole pear, rather than fruit cocktail, can be requested for the patient's dinner tray, and the patient can be allowed to tear open individually wrapped, unit-dose oral medications.

The Withdrawn Patient

Admission to critical care is an overwhelming experience for patients and their families. It may be so overwhelming that critically ill patients may shut down emotionally to preserve their sanity over the short term. For clinically depressed or catatonic patients, the social and emotional withdrawal will be more pronounced and can interfere with medical treatment. Symptoms of withdrawal include little or no eye contact, a blank facial expression, slowed responses, barely discernible speech, blunted or dulled affect, sluggish or no movement, urinary retention, constipation, and poor personal hygiene. Grooming may underscore separation from others. For example, a bushy mustache or unkempt beard covers the patient's mouth, and oily hair worn in long bangs conceals the patient's eyes.

When caring for a severely withdrawn patient, the critical care nurse must urge the patient to express feelings of anger, fear, or guilt. Clinical depression is not the same as sadness; in fact, the critically ill patient who presents tearfully and feels sad is exhibiting a normal response to a stressful situation. A clinically depressed or catatonic patient experiences an emotional vacuum or void. The nurse should provide simple diversion and distracting conversation without obligating the withdrawn patient to participate and can enlist the patient's help with basic care.

Malignant catatonia and clinical depression often look alike. Both conditions exacerbate the critically ill patient's medical compromise and hamper recuperation.[13,44,47] The stuporously withdrawn patient must be protected from the effects of self-neglect. The nurse should assist with feeding, perform passive range-of-motion exercises, and administer medications that prevent thrombus formation, aid with elimination, and promote restful sleep. The severely withdrawn patient should be approached slowly and cautiously. Although the withdrawn patient seems totally unresponsive and motionless, he/she may react suddenly and forcefully when startled.

CONCLUSION

Underlying unrecognized baseline neuropsychiatric disorders complicate the care of critically ill patients with serious medical illnesses or traumatic injuries. This chapter provided an overview of selected neuropsychiatric disorders and eight behaviors frequently seen in patients experiencing such disorders. Nursing interventions to treat patients exhibiting these eight behaviors are provided with the primary goal of maintaining the psychological and physical safety of the patient. The nursing care goal should be early recognition of neuropsychiatric disorders and rapidly instituted, appropriate treatment interventions to decrease or prevent morbidity and mortality. Collaboration with a mental health professional for diagnosis and treatment recommendations will facilitate patient-centered care for the critically ill patient with a neuropsychiatric disorder.

REFERENCES

1. Adams, M. P., Josephson, D. L., & Holland, L. N. (2013). *Pharmacology for nurses: a pathophysiologic approach*. Upper Saddle River, NJ: Pearson Prentice Hall.
2. Adetoki, A., Evans, R., & Cassidy, G. (2013). Polydipsia with water intoxication in treatment-resistant schizophrenia. *Prog Neurol Psychiatry, 17*, 20–23.
3. American Association of Critical Care Nurses. (2011). AACN Practice Alert: delirium assessment and management. Accessed from: http://www.aacn.org.
4. American Psychiatric Association. (2013). *Diagnostic and statistical manual of mental disorders—DSM 5*. Washington, DC: American Psychiatric Association.
5. Antidepressants are the main option for the long-term pharmacological treatment of generalized anxiety disorder. (2010). *Drugs Ther Perspect, 26*, 12–15.
6. Arnold, E. (2005). Sorting out the 3 D's: delirium, dementia, depression: learn how to sift through overlapping signs and symptoms so you can improve an older patient's quality of life. *Holistic Nurs Pract, 19*, 99–105.
7. Barr, J., Fraser, G. L., Puntillo, K., et al. (2013). Clinical practice guidelines for the management of pain, agitation, and delirium in adult patients in the intensive care unit. *Crit Care Med, 41*(1), 263–306.
8. Bone, Y., & Smith, G. B. (2012). Critical care nurses and delirium management in the mentally ill client. *Crit Care Nurs Clin North Am, 24*, 101–104.
9. Ceide, M., & Kennedy, G. (2014). Addressing psychosomatic illness in the elderly: integrated care. *Psychiatr Times*, 1–4.
10. Choe, J. Y., et al. (2014). A new scoring method of the Mini-Mental Status Examination to screen for dementia. *Dement Geriatr Cognit Disord, 37*, 347–356.
11. Choi, S., Morrow-Howell, N., & Proctor, E. (2006). Configuration of services used by depressed older adults. *Aging Ment Health, 10*, 240–249.
12. Ciraulo, D. A., et al. (2005). Nefazodone treatment of cocaine dependence with comorbid depressive symptoms. *Addiction, 100*(Suppl. 1), 23–31.
13. Collins, T. R. (2013). New analysis finds benefit of combination memantine-donepezil. *Neuro Today, 13*, 45–49.
14. Davidson, J. E., Winkelman, C., Gelinas, C., & Dermenchyan, A. (2015). Pain, agitation, and delirium guidelines: nurses' involvement in development and implementation. *Crit Care Nurse, 35*(3), 17–31.
15. Dearing, K. S. (2004). Getting it together: how nurse patient relationships influence treatment compliance for patients with schizophrenia. *Arch Psychiatr Nurs, 18*, 155–163.
16. de la Torre, J. C. (2009). Carotid artery ultrasound and echocardiography testing to lower the prevalence of Alzheimer's disease. *J Stroke Cerebrovasc Dis, 18*, 319–328.
17. Fasanello, R. A. (2012). Paradoxical hyponatremia and polyurodipsia in a patient with lithium-induced nephrogenic diabetes insipidus. *J Am Osteopath Assoc, 112*, 588.
18. Glassman, A. H. (2005). Schizophrenia, antipsychotic drugs, and cardiovascular disease. *J Clin Psychiatry, 66*(Suppl. 6), 5–10.
19. Goossens, P. J., van Achterburg, T., & Knoppert-van der Klein, E. (2007). Nursing processes used in the treatment of patients with bipolar disorder. *Int J Ment Health Nurs, 16*, 168–177.
20. Greenier, E., Lukyanova, V., & Reede, L. (2014). Serotonin syndrome: fentanyl and selective serotonin reuptake inhibitor interactions. *AANA J, 82*, 340–345.
21. Grover, S., et al. (2013). Risk factors for delirium and inpatient mortality with delirium. *J Postgrad Med, 59*, 263–270.
22. Guptill, J. (2011). After an attempt: caring for the suicidal patient on the medical-surgical unit. *Medsurg Nurs, 20*, 163–168.
23. Haddad, A. (2005). Ethics in action: where do you draw the line between protecting yourself and caring for a potentially violent patient? *RN, 68*, 30.
24. Hakim, S. M., Othman, A., & Naoum, D. O. (2012). Treatment with risperidone for subsyndromal delirium after on-pump cardiac surgery in the elderly: a randomized controlled trial. *Anesthesiology, 116*, 987–997.
25. Harrington, L. (1993). Procainamide-induced psychosis. *Crit Care Nurs, 13*, 70–72.
26. Institute of Medicine. (2014). *Improving access to essential medicines for mental, neurological, and substance abuse disorders in Sub-Saharan Africa—Workshop Summary*. Washington, DC: IOM Board on Global Health.
27. Johnson, S. L., Edge, M. D., Holmes, M. K., & Carver, C. S. (2012). The behavioral activation system and mania. *Annu Rev Clin Psychol, 8*, 243–267.
28. Kotowski, A. (2012). Case study: a young male with auditory hallucinations in paranoid schizophrenia. *Int J Nurs Know, 23*, 41–44.
29. Lach, H. W., Chang, Y., & Edwards, D. (2010). Can older adults with dementia accurately report depression using brief forms? Reliability and validity of the Geriatric Depression Scale. *J Gerontol Nurs, 36*, 30–37.
30. MacKay, I., Paterson, B., & Cassells, C. (2005). Constant or special observations of inpatients presenting risk of aggression or violence: nurses' perceptions of the rules of engagement. *J Psychiatr Ment Health Nurs, 12*, 464–471.
31. Marino, J., Bucher, D., Beach, M., Yegneswaran, B., & Cooper, B. (2015). Implementation of an intensive care unit delirium protocol. *Dimens Crit Care Nurs, 34*(5), 273–284. http://dx.doi.org/10.1097/DCC.0000000000000130.
32. Matarazzo, B. B., Homaifar, B. Y., & Hal, S. (2014). Therapeutic risk management of the suicidal patient: safety planning. *J Psychiatr Pract, 20*, 220–224.
33. May, R. (1979). *The meaning of anxiety*. New York: Pocket Books (classic).
34. McCarthy, S. E., McCombie, W. R., & Corvin, A. (2014). Unlocking the treasure trove: from genes to schizophrenia biology. *Schizophr Bull, 40*, 492–496.
35. Mintz, D. L., & Flynn, D. F. (2012). How (not what) to prescribe: nonpharmacologic aspects of psychopharmacology. *Psychiatr Clin North Am, 35*, 143–163.
36. Mula, M. (2010). The clinical spectrum of bipolar symptoms in epilepsy: a critical reappraisal. *Postgrad Med, 122*, 17–23.
37. Murphy, K. (2005). The separate reality of bipolar disorder and schizophrenia. *Nursing Made Incredibly Easy, 3*, 6–19.
38. Nutt, D. J. (2005). Overview of diagnosis and drug treatments of anxiety disorders. *CNS Spectrums, 10*, 49–56.
39. Oostervink, F., Nolen, W. A., & Kok, R. M. (2015). Two years' outcomes of acute mania in bipolar disorder: different effects of age and age of onset. *J Geriatr Psychiatry, 30*, 201–209.
40. Pandya, S. (2012). Risks associated with antipsychotic drugs. *Nursing and Residential Care, 14*, 400–404.
41. Porter, K. (2009). Managing manipulative patients. *Independent Nurse*, 5, 43.

42. Pullen, J., & Teller, J. (2012). Delusional disorder leading to precipitous weight loss. *Ann Long Term Care, 20,* 32–36.
43. Reed, F., & Fitzgerald, L. (2005). The mixed attitudes of nurses to caring for people with mental illness. *Int J Ment Health Nurs, 14,* 249–257.
44. Rizos, D. V., & Peritogiannis, V. (2015). Catatonia in the ICU. *Crit Care Med, 43,* e48.
45. Roden, M., & Simmons, B. B. (2014). Delirium superimposed on dementia and mild cognitive impairment. *Postgrad Med, 126,* 129–137.
46. Russell-Babin, K. A., & Miley, H. (2013). Implementing the best available evidence in early delirium identification in elderly hip surgery patients. *Int J Evid Based Healthc, 11,* 39–45.
47. Saddawi-Konefka, D., Berg, S. M., Nejad, S. H., & Bittner, E. A. (2014). Catatonia in the ICU: an important and underdiagnosed cause of altered mental status. *Crit Care Med, 42,* e234–e241.
48. Saveanu, R. V., & Nemeroff, C. B. (2012). Etiology of depression: genetic and environmental factors. *Psychiatr Clin North Am, 35,* 51–71.
49. Smith, M., & Bockwalter, K. (2005). Behaviors associated with dementia. *Am J Nurs, 105,* 40–52.
50. Solomon, P., Hanrahan, N. P., Hurford, M., DeCesaris, M., & LaKeetra, J. (2014). Lessons learned from implementing a pilot RCT of transitional care model for individuals with serious mental illness. *Arch Psychiatr Nurs, 28,* 250–255.
51. Somes, J., Donatelli, N. S., & Barrett, J. (2010). Sudden confusion and agitation: Causes to investigate! Delirium, dementia, depression. *J Emerg Nurs, 36,* 486–488.
52. Struble, L. M., Sullivan, B. J., & Hartman, L. S. (2014). Psychiatric disorders impacting critical illness. *Crit Care Nurs Clin North Am, 26,* 115–138.
53. Szasz, T. (2002). *Fatal freedom: the ethics and politics of suicide.* Syracuse, NY: Syracuse University Press.
54. Taylor, D. M. (2002). Prolongation of QTc interval and antipsychotics. *Am J Psychiatry, 159,* 1062–1064.
55. Thomas, C., et al. (2012). Diagnosing delirium in older adults with dementia: adapting the Confusion Assessment Method to International Classification of Diseases. *J Am Geriatr Soc, 60,* 1471–1477.
56. Tom, S. E., et al. (2015). Characterization of dementia and Alzheimer's disease in an older population: updated incidence and life expectancy with and without dementia. *Am J Public Health, 105,* 408–413.
57. Walker, C. (1998). Homeless people and mental health: a nursing concern. *Am J Nurs, 98,* 26–32.
58. Walker, C. A. (2015). Care of the acutely psychotic patient. *Nursing Made Incredibly Easy, 13*(3), 40–47.
59. Wand, A. P. F., Thoo, W., Sciuriaga, H., Ting, V., Baker, J., & Hunt, G. E. (2014). A multifaceted educational intervention to prevent delirium in older inpatients. *Int J Nurs Stud, 51,* 974–982.
60. Webb, J. M., Carlton, E. F., & Geehan, D. M. (2000). Delirium in the intensive care unit: are we helping the patient? *Crit Care Nurs Q, 22,* 47–60.
61. White, R. G., & Gumley, A. I. (2009). Postpsychotic posttraumatic stress disorder: associations with fear of recurrence and intolerance of uncertainty. *J Nerv Ment Dis, 197,* 841–849.
62. Woodhouse, K. N. (2012). Thyrotoxicosis: evaluation and treatment of a multinodular goiter. *Nurse Pract, 37,* 6–10.
63. Wong, E., & Miles, J. (2014). Prevalence and correlates of depression among US immigrants. *J Immigr Minor Health, 16,* 422–428.
64. Wortzel, H. S., Homaifar, B., Matarazzo, B., & Brenner, L. A. (2014). Therapeutic risk management of the suicidal patient: stratifying risk in terms of severity and temporality. *J Psychiatr Pract, 20,* 63–67.
65. Wright, B., Peters, E., Elrich, U., Kuipers, E., & Kumari, V. (2014). Understanding noise stress-induced cognitive impairment in healthy adults and its implications for schizophrenia. *Noise Health, 16,* 166–176.
66. Xiong, G., & Doraiswamy, M. (2005). Combination therapy for Alzheimer's disease: what is evidence-based and what is not? *Geriatrics, 60,* 22–26.
67. Yeandle, J., Fawkes, L., Beeby, R., Gordon, C., & Challis, E. (2015). A collaborative formulation framework for service users with personality disorders. *Ment Health Pract, 18,* 25–28.
68. Zaal, I. J., Devlin, J. W., Peelen, L. M., & Slooter, A. J. C. (2015). A systematic review of risk factors for delirium in the ICU. *Crit Care Med, 43*(1), 40–47. http://dx.doi.org/10.1097/CCM.0000000000000625.

38

Caring for the Bariatric Patient

Carmela M. Pontillo

Bariatrics represents a branch of medicine focusing on the etiology, prevention, and treatment of obesity. The term *bariatric* is derived from the Greek words *baro*, meaning "weight," and *iatric*, meaning "treatment." Worldwide, obesity has become a serious public health challenge. According to the World Health Organization (WHO), in 2014 more than 1.9 billion adults were overweight, and of these, over 600 million were obese.[134] Between 1980 and 2014, the prevalence of obesity more than doubled worldwide. In 2013, the Centers for Disease Control and Prevention (CDC) reported that 35% of the US adult population was obese, with 20 states reporting rates of obesity in excess of 30%. The CDC projects that by 2030, 42% of the US population will be obese.[27] It is estimated that 300,000 deaths per year in the United States are attributable to obesity, making it the second leading cause of preventable death today. Compared with individuals of normal weight, individuals who are obese have a 50% to 100% increased risk of premature death from all causes.[102] In addition to the risk of premature death, being overweight and obese results in many debilitating conditions that negatively impact physical, behavioral, and emotional health. The most common obesity-associated conditions include type 2 diabetes, coronary artery disease (CAD), hypertension, dyslipidemia, stroke, sleep apnea, osteoarthritis, and certain cancers. The cost of obesity-related illnesses is staggering. In 2008, the estimated annual medical cost of obesity for the United States was $147 billion. By 2018, the projected cost will be $344 billion per year.[125] When compared to the normal weight individual, the obese incur 46% greater inpatient costs, have 27% more provider visits, and spend 80% more on prescription medications.[42]

DEFINING AND CLASSIFYING OBESITY

Obesity has been defined as a complex, multivariate, chronic disease. In 1991, the WHO and the National Institutes of Health (NIH) defined being overweight or obese according to body mass index (BMI).[96] BMI is determined by dividing the weight in kilograms by the height in meters squared, using the following equation:

$$\text{BMI} = \text{weight (kg)}/\text{height(m)}^2$$

A healthy BMI falls between 18.5 and 24.9 kg/m^2. Overweight is defined as a BMI from 25 to 29.9 kg/m^2, and obesity is defined as a BMI of greater than 30 kg/m^2. Obesity is further classified into three classes or subsets: Class I obesity is a BMI of 30 to 34.9 kg/m^2; Class II obesity is defined as a BMI of 35 to 39.9 kg/m^2; and a BMI of 40 kg/m^2 or more defines Class III and is considered extreme obesity (Table 38.1).

It is important to note that BMI represents an estimate rather than an accurate measurement of obesity. The limitation of this measurement is that it fails to accurately quantify body composition with regards to adiposity versus muscle mass. The waist to hip ratio has also been used as a measurement for obesity, but BMI is the more common standard used in clinical guidelines.

CAUSES OF OBESITY

Obesity is a chronic, complex, multifactorial metabolic disease in which there is an imbalance of energy ingested (in calories) over the energy expended. It represents a condition of excess body fat relative to lean body mass. The exact etiology of obesity is unknown, but is believed to involve a complex interaction of genetic, environmental, behavioral, psychological, physiologic, and metabolic factors.[135] Prentice described the obesity epidemic as partly caused by a "genetic heritage" that protected against famine and ensured human survival through evolution.[108] However, this genetic heritage, which once protected us against starvation, is now nonbeneficial and detrimental in the modern obesogenic environment.

Environmental influences on obesity include lifestyle behaviors such as dietary choices and physical activity. Modern society provides readily available, oversized portions and highly processed, high-calorie, and high-fat foods. These products are heavily marketed and very affordable, making them an easy choice for today's fast-paced consumers. Physical activity has changed dramatically in the past several decades. Advances in technology, including the development of many energy-sparing devices, have given rise to a much more sedentary lifestyle and a consequent reduction in the number of calories being used on a daily basis. The National Health and Nutrition Examination Survey found that the rate of Americans who exercise has decreased significantly from 1994 to 2010: the number of women who claimed they never exercised increased from 19.1% to 51.7%, and for men from 11.4% to 43.5%. It is believed that environmental changes affecting both energy intake and expenditure have played a large role in the development of our current obesity epidemic.[28]

Other factors that have been identified as contributing to the obesity epidemic include commonly used medications such as antipsychotics, antidepressants, antiepileptics, and diabetic medications; sleep deprivation; smoking cessation; exposure to adenovirus 36; increasing maternal age; and improved reproductive outcomes for childbearing woman with higher BMIs.[135] Socioeconomic factors may also play a role, as obesity appears to be more prevalent in lower socioeconomic groups. This may be related to lower education levels, poor food choices, and physical environments that are less conducive to physical activity.[37,38]

TABLE 38.1 Obesity Classification by Body Mass Index

Classification	Body Mass Index	Obesity Class
Underweight	<18.5	N/A
Normal	18.5–24.9	N/A
Overweight	25–29.9	NA
Obese	30–34.9	I
Moderately obese	35–39.9	II
Morbidly obese	40–49.9	III
Super morbidly obese	≥50	IV

The role of genetics in the development of obesity is complex. Twin and adoption studies from the 1980s provided evidence that genetic factors play an important role in the development of obesity. The discovery of leptin in the 1990s marked the beginning of extensive biomedical research into genetics and obesity. A more recent hypothesis states that obesity is a neuroendocrine disorder marked by the interplay between environment and genetic predisposition.[61]

Increased efforts in gene identification are beginning to provide a more comprehensive picture of the complex biological mechanisms involved in the development of obesity. Research into human monogenic obesities has focused on mutations in molecular elements involved in mechanisms that control energy balance. Genes have been identified that regulate food/energy intake, energy expenditure, and adipogenesis. Currently, over a dozen genetic mutations have been studied, including mutations in the genes coding for leptin *(LEP)*, leptin receptor *(LEPR)*, proopiomelanocortin *(POMC)*, melanocortin 4 receptor *(MC4R)*, neuropeptide Y *(NPY)*, and ghrelin receptor, as well as mutations in genes related to food preferences. The most commonly exhibited feature of these mutations is hyperphagia. Monogenic obesity is believed to be involved in approximately 5% of all extreme obesity cases.[30,116]

Syndromic forms of obesity include pleiotropic syndromes that produce multiple phenotypic expressions of the same gene mutation and syndromes caused by chromosomal rearrangement. The most frequently occurring syndrome is Prader-Willi syndrome, with a population prevalence of 1 in 50,000. It is characterized by obesity, hyperphagia, hypotonia, mental retardation, short stature, and central hypogonadism. Bardet-Biedl syndrome, with a prevalence of 1 in 100,000, is characterized by central obesity, polydactyly, learning disabilities, rod-cone dystrophy, hypogonadism, and renal abnormalities. Continued research on the interaction of genetics with the modern environment will further our understanding of the obesity epidemic and contribute to discoveries of novel treatment options.

THE PATHOPHYSIOLOGY OF OBESITY

Obesity is the result of a complex interaction involving the brain and gastrointestinal system. Central to the control of eating behavior is the ventral hypothalamus. Within the arcuate nucleus of the hypothalamus exist two opposing sets of neurons that stimulate and repress the appetite (orexigenic and anorexigenic neurons, respectively). NPY and agouti-related protein (AGRP) both stimulate feeding and inhibit satiety. POMC and cocaine amphetamine-regulated transcript (CART) neurons have the opposite effect and stimulate satiety. The discovery of leptin led to further investigation into a collection of proteins that regulate food intake. These include adipokines, gut hormones, and cytokines. Leptin plays an important role in long-term satiety. It directly inhibits NPY receptors and stimulates POMC receptors. It is secreted by white adipose tissue in direct relation to the total amount of body fat. Central resistance to leptin has been implicated as a prominent feature of obesity. The obese patient appears to be resistant to the hypothalamic effects of leptin, and maintains excess body weight due to the interruption or inactivation of the neural triggers designed to reduce appetite and increase energy expenditure. Leptin has also been linked to the increased sympathetic activity and the increased inflammatory state found in obesity. Leptin and its receptors share structural and functional similarities to the proinflammatory interleukin-6 (IL-6) cytokine family. IL-6 cytokines stimulate the release of tumor necrosis factor-alpha (TNFα), which increases inflammation. Additionally, insulin acts as an anorexigenic resulting in suppression of NPY and stimulation of POMC.[110]

Adiponectin, which is also an adipokine, is secreted by adipocytes and appears to have a more modest effect on food intake. Adiponectin stimulates insulin secretion, inhibits beta cell destruction, and minimizes the inflammatory response. Adiponectin levels are inversely related to obesity.

Gut hormones from the gastrointestinal tract play an important role in regulating appetite. Incretins are a class of gut hormones that stimulate a reduction in blood glucose levels. Two commonly studied hormones are glucose-dependent insulinotropic polypeptide (GIP) and glucagon-like peptide 1 (GLP-1). Both of these mediators are anorexigenic. GIP is secreted by K-cells in the duodenum and jejunum in response to a glucose load. It induces insulin secretion and stimulates fatty acid synthesis in adipocytes. GLP-1 is secreted by L-cells in the ileum in response to food. It reduces gastric mobility and emptying. GLP-1 augments postprandial insulin secretion and increases insulin sensitivity. It has also been shown to have antiinflammatory properties. GIP and GLP-1 are believed to be responsible for approximately 50% of all postprandial insulin secretion. A gut hormone with the opposite effect is the orexigenic hormone ghrelin. Ghrelin has been commonly referred to as the appetite hormone. It stimulates appetite and promotes food intake. Ghrelin is secreted in the gastric fundus cells in response to fasting. This hormone has antiinflammatory properties but results in insulin resistance. In the obese individual, there is no apparent postprandial decline in ghrelin levels, which may lead to increased appetite and eating.[98,110]

Cytokines are yet another group of mediators that regulate food intake, satiety, and hunger. In this class of mediators, TNFα and IL-6 are considered proinflammatory and diabetogenic, whereas IL-8 and IL-1 exert the opposite effect, as they are antiinflammatory and insulinomimetic. TNFα is produced by adipocytes throughout the body, but especially by those found in the waist-hip region. Studies have shown a strong correlation between waist-hip ratio and TNFα. IL-6 levels have been shown to be elevated in obese individuals, and correlate with TNFα levels, BMI, and waist to hip ratio.[98,110]

Multiple other mediators are involved in regulating eating behavior. This speaks to the overall complexity of just one aspect of the regulatory systems involved in weight and energy balance.

An area of increased research is the role of the gut microbiome in obesity and metabolic disorders. Studies have found profound changes in the composition and metabolic function

TABLE 38.2 Obesity-Related Medical Complications and Comorbidities

Pulmonary	Poor quality of life
Obstructive sleep apnea	Body image disturbance
Obesity hypoventilation syndrome/Pickwickian syndrome	
Gastroesophageal reflux–induced asthma or aspiration	**Gastrointestinal/Abdominal**
Pulmonary hypertension	Gallbladder disease (usually associated with cyclic weight loss and gain)
	Gastroesophageal reflux disease
Cardiovascular	Recurrent ventral hernias
Hypertension	Nonalcoholic fatty liver disease
Atherosclerotic coronary artery disease	
Cardiomyopathy	**Endocrine**
Congestive heart failure	Type 2 diabetes
Dyslipidemia	Metabolic syndrome
Stroke	Gout
Pulmonary embolism	Impaired glucose tolerance
Varicose veins	Insulin resistance
Venous thromboembolic disease	Hyperlipidemia
Cor pulmonale	Hypercholesterolemia
Neurovascular	**Genitourinary/Reproductive**
Intracranial hypertension	Recurrent urinary tract infections
Pseudotumor cerebri	Stress urinary incontinence
	Irregular menstruation
Hematologic	Infertility
Hypercoagulability	Polycystic ovarian syndrome
	Obstetric complications
Dermatologic	Fetal abnormalities
Hirsutism	
Cellulitis	**Musculoskeletal**
Venous and stasis ulcers	Degenerative osteoarthritis of the knees, hips, and feet
Acne	Intervertebral disk herniation
Intertrigo	Restrictive mobility
Striae distensae (stretch marks)	Chronic low back pain
Acanthosis nigricans/skin tags	
Lymphedema	**Other**
Stasis pigmentation of the legs	Cancer (breast, endometrium, colon, and prostate)
	Increased susceptibility to accidents
Psychological	Social stigmatization
Depression	
Poor self image	

of the gut microbiome in the obese. It appears that in obese individuals, the gut microbiome is capable of extracting more energy from the diet. Other studies have shown how the gut microbiota interacts with epithelial cells to indirectly affect energy expenditure and storage.[126,127] Diet and antibiotics have also been shown to strongly affect the composition of the gut microbiota, with changes in microbiota composition occurring as rapidly as 24 hours after a dietary change or after ingesting an oral medication.[56]

This section served to illustrate a sampling of the vast variety of research on the causes and development of obesity. It is clear that the current understanding of this disease is in its infancy. It is imperative that we as healthcare providers realize that obesity is not a character flaw, but rather a complex interplay between genetic makeup, the modern obesogenic environment, and powerful, poorly understood physiologic mechanisms.

PHYSIOLOGIC CONSEQUENCES OF OBESITY

Inflammation, hypercoagulability, and insulin resistance characterize obesity. These derangements lead to numerous medical complications, including increased mortality and comorbid conditions (Table 38.2).[132] The physiologic consequences of obesity affect virtually every organ and body system (Table 38.3).

In a survey of the US population, the overweight and obese had a higher relative risk of hypertension, hypercholesterolemia, and type 2 diabetes when compared to normal weight individuals.[100] Of significance is the increased distribution of intra-abdominal fat and its link to the previously mentioned conditions. Abdominal fat is predictive of insulin resistance and the abnormalities characteristic of metabolic syndrome.[124] The mechanisms by which visceral obesity affects metabolic syndrome remain unclear. It has been proposed that the hyperlipolytic visceral adipose tissue is resistant to the action of insulin, and thereby exposes the liver to free fatty acids, resulting in impaired hepatic metabolic processes. This disruption leads to hyperinsulinemia, glucose intolerance, and hypertriglyceridemia. An alternate mechanism proposes that adipose tissue represents a powerful endocrine organ that contributes to insulin resistance and proinflammatory, thrombotic, and hypertensive states. Adiponectin and the inflammatory cytokines IL-6

TABLE 38.3 Physiologic Consequences of Obesity

System	Pathophysiology	Clinical Manifestations
Pulmonary	Decreased residual lung volume from abdominal pressure on the diaphragm Pulmonary shunting following alveolar collapse Decreased compliance Increased carbon dioxide production Increased chest wall thickness Increased intrathoracic pressure	Decreased functional residual capacity Atelectasis Hypercarbia Hypoxemia Sleep apnea
Cardiovascular	Hypertension Increased blood volume (increased preload and afterload) Hyperkinetic circulation	Hypertension Elevated central venous pressure, pulmonary artery pressure, pulmonary artery occulsion pressure, systemic vascular resistance, cardiac output Tachycardia
Renal	Increased renal blood flow Increased renin and aldosterone levels	Increased clearance of renally excreted medications Fluid and electrolyte abnormalities
Hematologic	Increased blood viscosity Decreased fibrinolysis Increased plasminogen activator inhibitor Antithrombin III deficiency	Elevated fibrinogen levels Venous stasis leading to venous thrombosis Pulmonary embolism
Gastrointestinal	Increased intra-abdominal pressure	Increased incidence of hiatal hernia
Metabolic/endocrine	Increased production of insulin and pancreatic polypeptides Insulin resistance	Hyperglycemia
Immunologic	Endothelial inflammation Changes in cellular immunity Impaired neutrophil function	Increased tumor necrosis factor-alpha Increased interleukin-6 Increased risk for infection

BOX 38.1 Cardiovascular Risk Factors Associated with Visceral Obesity

- Blood pressure greater than 135/85 mm Hg
- Insulin resistance or hyperinsulinemia
- Low high-density lipoprotein cholesterol concentrations
- High triglyceride concentrations
- Increased apolipoprotein B concentrations
- Small, dense low-density lipoprotein cholesterol particles
- Increased fibrinogen concentrations
- Increased plasminogen activator inhibitor levels
- Increased C-reactive protein levels
- Increased tumor necrosis factor-alpha levels
- Increased interleukin-6 levels
- Microalbuminuria
- Increased blood viscosity
- Increased systolic and pulse pressures
- Increased left ventricular hypertrophy
- Premature atherosclerosis (coronary heart disease and stroke)
- Nonalcoholic fatty liver disease

and TNFα have all been identified as playing a role in altering the metabolic profile of the obese individual.[33] The rates of insulin resistance, hypertension, diabetes, unfavorable lipid profiles, stroke, and CAD are all higher in persons with upper body fat patterns when compared to those with lower body fat distributions. Box 38.1 lists cardiovascular risk factors associated with visceral obesity.

Cardiovascular Complications

Changes to the cardiovascular system can be categorized as those related to changes in cardiac performance and cardiac structure. A linear relationship exists between increases in body weight and increases in total circulating blood volume, which leads to an increased stroke volume and cardiac output. Increased cardiac output may occur as a compensatory response to the increased need to perfuse excess mass and the increased oxygen consumption needs.[64] Increased wall tension from a higher preload may lead to eccentric left ventricle hypertrophy. Systolic and diastolic left ventricular dysfunction may occur, and ultimately result in left ventricular (LV) failure. Systolic and diastolic LV dysfunction, left atrial enlargement, and atrial fibrillation are common in the obese patient population. The increased cardiac work associated with obesity may produce cardiomyopathy and heart failure in the absence of diabetes, hypertension, or atherosclerosis. Patients with longstanding obesity greater than or equal to 40 kg/m^2 may be at increased risk of obesity cardiomyopathy.[64,115]

Visceral obesity is linked to a number of metabolic alterations that directly impact cardiovascular disease, hypertension, and dyslipidemia. It is estimated that approximately 75% of the overall incidence of hypertension is directly related to obesity.[9] The physiologic mechanisms responsible for obesity-related hypertension are not completely understood. Our current understanding seems to point toward an interaction between dietary, genetic, environmental, and behavioral factors. Potential mechanisms explaining the association between obesity and hypertension include insulin- and leptin-mediated stimulation of the sympathetic nervous system; renin-angiotensin-aldosterone activation; sodium retention and glomerular hyperfiltration; proteinuria; decreased adiponectin; and altered immune and inflammatory responses.[77] Growing evidence suggests that the gut microbiota may also represent a potentially important factor in the development of hypertension in the obese.[126] Fig. 38.1 illustrates the role of increased body fat mass in the pathophysiology of hypertension and congestive heart failure.

Excess central adiposity is linked with dyslipidemia. Changes in the lipoprotein profile of the obese include high triglycerides, with an increased proportion of large very low density

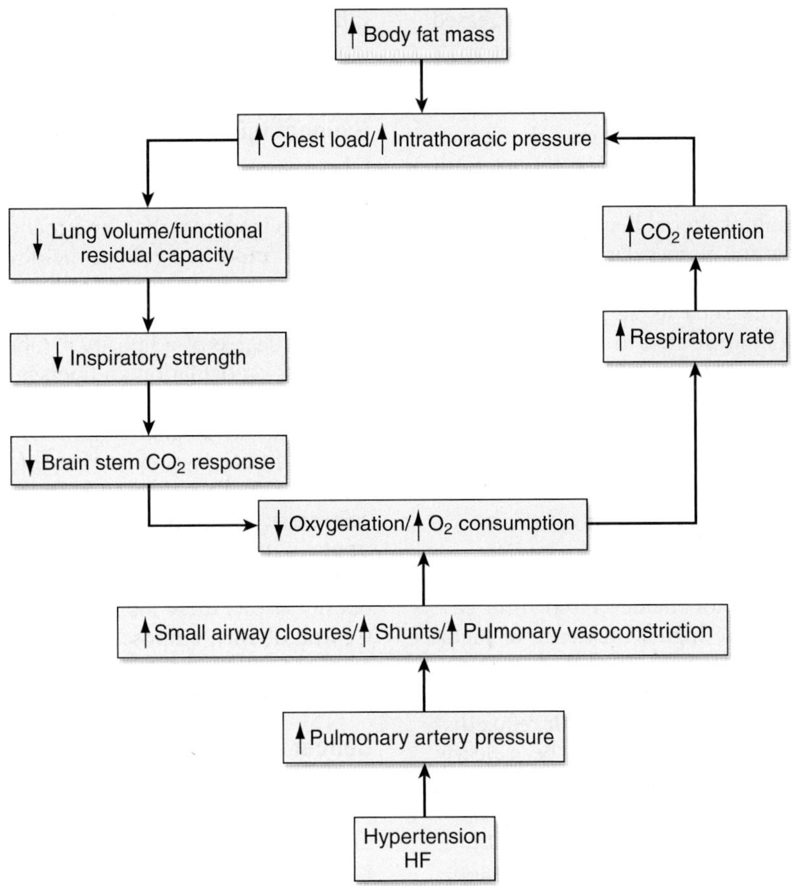

FIG. 38.1 Role of increased body fat mass in the pathophysiology of hypertension and heart failure. *CO_2,* Carbon dioxide; *O_2,* oxygen; *HF,* heart failure.

lipoproteins (VLDLs). Low density lipoprotein (LDL) cholesterol levels may be normal or slightly elevated, with an increased proportion of small LDLs. And finally, high density lipoprotein (HDL) cholesterol levels may be lower, with a decreased level of large HDL particles (HDL_2s).[124]

Pulmonary Complications

Obesity greatly decreases total respiratory compliance in the obese individual. Reduced lung compliance in the obese is exponentially related to BMI. Increased pulmonary blood volume, closure of dependent airways, and increased alveolar surface tension due to reduced functional residual capacity (FRC) are all involved in altering lung compliance in the obese. The most characteristic change in lung function in the obese is a reduction in FRC. This alteration is due to the presence of excess adipose tissue around the rib cage and abdomen. The expiratory reserve volume (ERV) decreases due to the displacement of the diaphragm into the chest cavity and the increased chest wall mass. Total lung capacity and vital capacity both decrease with rising BMI. Abdominal obesity is strongly correlated with a reduction in forced expiratory volume in one second (FEV1) and forced vital capacity (FVC). Tidal volumes are reduced in the obese, resulting in rapid shallow breathing and increased work of breathing. Loss of volume leads to airway closure and alveolar collapse. This results in decreased ventilation to the base of the lungs, with ventilation-perfusion mismatch and hypoxemia.[109]

Obese individuals are also at high risk of sleep apnea from recurrent upper airway obstruction. It is believed that approximately 65% of the US adult population suffers from varying degrees of sleep apnea.[34] The incidence of obstructive sleep apnea (OSA) is twice as high in men as it is in women.[70] With the obesity epidemic, we have seen an eightfold increase in the occurrence of OSA.[5] One study found that 70% of all patients presenting for bariatric surgery suffered from sleep apnea.[41] During sleep apnea, the upper airway and pharynx relax and obstruct the airway. This results in periods of apnea with hypoxia and hypercarbia, which eventually arouse the individual from sleep. This pattern can repeat itself hundreds of times per night, preventing deep sleep. These individuals often present with daytime somnolence and morning headaches.[34] Ultimately, this may lead to systemic hypertension, a worsening of current hypertension, and eventually, pulmonary hypertension.

It is estimated that approximately 30% of patients suffering from morbid obesity have obesity hypoventilation syndrome (OHS), also known as *Pickwickian syndrome*.[80] OHS is defined as having a BMI greater than or equal to 30 kg/m^2 and chronic hypercapnia during wakefulness in the absence of other cardiorespiratory diseases. This syndrome is often underdiagnosed in this patient population. Several mechanisms have been suggested to explain this syndrome. These include excess loading of respiratory muscles by centrally located adipose tissue, increased work of breathing, impaired gas exchange, obesity-related upper airway narrowing, and disordered ventilatory drive.[20]

Renal Complications

Many of the comorbid conditions associated with obesity, including hypertension, diabetes, and metabolic syndrome, are all known to compromise renal function. However, obesity has been shown to be independently associated with an increased risk of developing chronic kidney disease (CKD) and end-stage renal disease (ESRD). In the obese patient, CKD and ESRD are directly proportional to increments in BMI, independent of diabetes and hypertension. Focal segmental glomerulosclerosis (FSGS) and obesity-related glomerulopathy (ORG) are both associated with proteinuria in the obese. Traditionally, ORG was thought to occur as a result of altered hemodynamics (i.e., elevations in renal plasma flow and glomerular filtration rate).[88] The focus has now shifted to the effect of adipose tissue on kidney disease. Circulating factors such as adiponectin, leptin, TNFα, and IL-6 have been demonstrated to play roles in the development of kidney disease. Obesity-related nephropathy covers a wide spectrum of diseases, including hyperfiltration, glomerulomegaly, mild proteinuria, and tubulointerstitial disease. Progression of disease may result in impaired clearance, glomerulosclerosis, nephrotic range proteinuria, and interstitial fibrosis, possibly leading to end-stage renal failure.[95]

Gastrointestinal Complications

Obesity is a significant risk factor for the development of gastroesophageal reflux disease.[44] The higher incidence of hiatal hernias, weakened esophageal sphincters, increased intra-abdominal pressure (IAP), and slowed gastric emptying all affect the obese patient and place them at increased risk for reflux disease. Abnormal elevations in IAP in the obese have been clearly documented. In one study, normal weight patients undergoing abdominal surgery had a mean IAP of 0 mm Hg, in comparison to a mean IAP of 12 mm Hg in the morbidly obese patient presenting for bariatric surgery.[76] This baseline elevated intra-abdominal pressure may place the obese patient at increased risk for compartment syndrome during critical illness.

Obese individuals are at increased risk for the development of gallstones. This is due in part to the increased production of cholesterol and increased biliary excretion. Cholesterol production is directly related to increased body fat.[85]

Obesity is also a risk factor for the development and progression of nonalcoholic fatty liver disease (NAFLD). Free fatty acids from visceral adipose tissue are released directly into the portal circulation, resulting in hepatic injury. NAFLD may progress to become nonalcoholic steatohepatitis (NASH), in which steatosis is combined with inflammation and fibrosis. This may further progress into frank cirrhosis of the liver. NASH is often underdiagnosed in the obese. In one study, 91% of patients presenting for bariatric surgery had histologic evidence of steatosis, and 1.7% had unexpected cirrhosis. Symptoms of the progression of this disease include hepatomegaly, abnormal liver function tests, and abnormal liver histology.[85]

Degenerative Joint Disease

Obesity significantly impacts the musculoskeletal system, due to excess joint loading. Obesity is also associated with the development and progression of osteoarthritis (OA). This degenerative joint disorder negatively impacts quality of life, due to decreased mobility and pain. There appears to be a dose-dependent relationship between BMI and the risk of OA in the knees and hips. A five unit increase in BMI is associated with a 35% increased risk of knee OA and an 11% increased risk of hip OA. Obesity also increases the risk of osteoarthritis in non–weight-bearing joints such as the hands. The cause of these structural joint changes is believed to be multifactorial, including a variety of both mechanical and metabolic factors. Increased joint load, decreased muscle strength, altered biomechanics, a chronic inflammatory state, and increased levels of adipokines and leptin have all been identified as potential factors in the development and progression of this degenerative joint disease.[49,73]

Gynecologic Complications

Obese women are at risk for many gynecologic and reproductive disorders. Problems with menstruation may include amenorrhea, oligomenorrhea, and menorrhagia. Increased adiposity plays an important role in the development and maintenance of polycystic ovarian syndrome (PCOS). Studies have shown a close correlation between the severity of PCOS symptoms and the degree of adiposity.[16] Obesity impairs fertility due to its effects on ovulation and oocyte, embryo, and endometrium development. Infertility is also associated with implantation problems and pregnancy loss. Obese women are at increased risk for miscarriage, even after infertility treatment. Pregnancy may be complicated by an increased risk of hypertension, preeclampsia, gestational diabetes, and cesarean section. The fetuses of obese pregnant women are at increased risk of prematurity, stillbirth, and congenital anomalies.[7] The mechanisms by which obesity affects these disorders have yet to be fully understood. Central obesity, adipose tissue, insulin, adipokines, and leptin all play a role in the disruption of the complex hormonal environment needed for reproductive health.[22]

Cancer Risk

Certain types of cancers are more prevalent in the obese patient population. Among women, there appears to be a strong relationship between higher BMIs and endometrial, gallbladder, kidney, and esophageal cancer. Weaker associations have been noted between obesity and leukemia, thyroid cancer, postmenopausal breast cancer, pancreatic cancer, colon cancer, and non-Hodgkin's lymphoma. In men, strong relationships have been noted with esophageal adenocarcinoma, thyroid cancer, kidney cancer, and colon cancer. Weaker associations have been found between obesity and malignant melanoma, rectal cancer, leukemia, and non-Hodgkin's lymphoma in men.[17] Several possible mechanisms have been suggested to explain the association between obesity and cancer. Factors identified as part of these mechanisms include: high estrogen levels in obese women, increased insulin and insulin-like factor-1, the effects of adipokines on cell growth, tumor growth regulators, and chronic inflammatory processes.

Genitourinary Complications

Obesity is a risk factor for all forms of female urinary incontinence. The mechanism is unknown, but it is believed that the excess body weight increases abdominal pressure, which in turn increases bladder pressure and urethral mobility, leading to incontinence. It has been suggested that the degree of obesity also influences the severity of urinary incontinence, with each five unit increase in BMI being associated with a 20% to 70% increase in the risk of urinary incontinence.[122] In males, obesity is associated with lower urinary tract symptoms (LUTS) and benign prostatic hyperplasia (BPH). Mechanisms linking obesity to LUTS/BPH remain unclear.[93]

Dermatologic Complications

The skin, the largest human organ, is affected by obesity, which can cause an array of dermatologic conditions. Stretch marks, or *striae distensae*, are smooth linear bands of skin. The color progresses from red to purple to white. These lesions tend to present in a perpendicular direction to that of the greatest tension on the skin. *Acanthosis nigricans* is characterized by leathery, hyperpigmented, irregularly-shaped plaques. This condition is most often a manifestation of endocrine disease. It may also be associated with cancer, especially gastric cancer. Lesions typically occur in the axilla or on the back of the neck. Less common presentations may also be seen on the scalp, elbows, umbilical area, knees, and knuckles. Friction and excessive moisture between skin folds may result in intertrigo, yeast dermatitis, and fissures. The skinfolds are also at risk of breakdown and maceration. Lower extremity edema, lymphedema, stasis dermatitis, and leg ulcers are common. Lymphedema, in turn, may lead to or exacerbate lower extremity cellulitis. Cellulitis presents with edema, erythema, pain, and warmth. Wound healing may be compromised in the obese postoperative patient. Surgical wounds are more prone to dehiscence, given the increased tension on the wound edges. Poor nutrition, reduced tissue perfusion, and reduced oxygen delivery may result in slower wound healing and increase the risk of infection.[52]

Cerebrovascular Effects

Obese individuals have an increased risk of developing pseudotumor cerebri (PTC), also known as *idiopathic intracranial hypertension*. The clinical syndrome consists of elevated cerebrospinal fluid pressure in the absence of a space-occupying lesion, vascular lesions, or enlargement of cerebral ventricles with no identifiable causative factor. Symptoms include headaches, nausea, vomiting, tinnitus, blurred vision, diplopia, and eye pain. The etiology remains unknown; however, it has been hypothesized to be the result of increased intra-abdominal pressure in the obese. This, in turn, leads to increased intrathoracic pressure, which leads to elevations in intracranial pressure.[53] It also remains unclear whether the degree of obesity affects the severity of symptoms and outcomes. Individuals with a BMI of greater than or equal to 40 kg/m^2 seem to be at higher risk of developing more severe visual field defects.[11]

Hematologic Effects

The body size of obese individuals places them at increased risk of venous thromboembolism (VTE). Increased adiposity, elevated intra-abdominal pressure, increased plasma viscosity, and immobility may all contribute to thrombogenesis. A variety of abnormalities have been described in the obese, such as increased levels of platelet activator inhibitor-1 (PAI-1), increased platelet activation, and increased levels of factor VII, factor VIII, von Willebrand factor, and fibrinogen.[6,112]

Immunologic Effects

The state of excess adiposity in the obese greatly increases susceptibility to infection. Much remains to be learned about the association between obesity and immune function. However, the link between obesity and the immune system appears to involve adipose tissue. It has been proposed that adipose tissue is the site for formation and maturation of precursors to the immune cells. Excess body fat is associated with elevated counts of leukocytes, neutrophils, monocytes, and lymphocytes, but reduced mitogen-induced proliferation of T-cells and B-cells.[58] Immune dysfunction places the obese at increased risk for surgical site infections, periodontitis, influenza, and respiratory, skin, and urinary tract infections.[15]

Psychosocial Impacts

There is significant prejudice towards and discrimination against the obese individual. These biases continue to persist with the increased population of obese individuals. There is a strong anti fat bias in the media, schools, businesses, and every day life. Healthcare providers are also among those who misunderstand, ridicule, and reject the obese.[23] The view is that obese individuals are responsible for their excess weight. They are often viewed as lazy, unmotivated, and lacking in discipline. Consequently, the obese individual is often told by healthcare providers to simply try harder at diet and exercise. Negative societal views and biases may place the obese individual at greater risk for mood and anxiety disorders and low self-esteem.

The relationship between extreme obesity and mental health is not well understood. Studies have demonstrated conflicting data. For example, a systematic review of over 4500 studies revealed a weak relationship between obesity and increased risk of depression.[21] Another study, however, demonstrated a positive correlation between BMI and depression, but no association between BMI and anxiety.[14] Research in this area is confounded by the great variety in psychopathology measures and the failure to account for demographic and socioeconomic variables. In a multinational study involving over 62,000 individuals, researchers utilized standardized diagnostics to investigate the relationship between obesity and mental health disorders, while considering demographic data. Their results showed a statistically significant association between obesity and depressive and anxiety disorders among female subjects. Age and education had variable effects across disorders.[24]

In addition to depression and anxiety disorders, the obese individual may also be at increased risk for problematic eating behaviors such as mindless eating, using food as a coping mechanism, night eating, and binge eating. Most obese individuals have repeatedly lost and then regained weight. This "yo-yo dieting" with no long-term success results in discouragement, frustration, hopelessness, and helplessness.[31]

TREATMENT OF OBESITY

The goals of any weight loss therapy are to produce a negative energy balance, prevent or reduce disability/morbidity, and improve the quality of life of the individual. There are multiple strategies designed to promote weight loss, including dietary therapy, physical activity, behavioral modification therapy, pharmacotherapy, combination therapy, and metabolic and bariatric surgery. When evaluating strategies for a weight loss program, it is important to assess patient expectations and set realistic patient goals.

Recommendations for the treatment of obesity are determined by the patient's BMI and comorbid conditions. At a BMI of greater than or equal to 25, lifestyle modification, which combines dietary changes, physical activity, and behavior modification, is the recommended treatment. A meta-analysis of lifestyle modification showed an average weight loss of approximately 4% within six months of initiation of treatment.[79] For most individuals, behavior modification is ineffective at producing sustained long-term weight loss.[133] However, even a modest weight loss of 5% to 10% decreases the risk of developing conditions such heart disease and diabetes.[129] Dietary strategies for weight loss may include:[101]

- A 1200–1500 kcal/day diet for women or a 1500–1800 kcal/day diet for men;
- A diet producing a 500–750 kcal/day energy deficit; or
- A diet restricting certain food types such as high carbohydrate foods or high fat foods, in order to create energy deficit.

It is important to consider patient preferences and health status when prescribing a calorie-restricted diet. Whenever possible, it is recommended to refer patients to nutritional counseling. Comprehensive lifestyle intervention programs should include a reduced calorie diet, a program designed to increase physical activity, and the use of behavioral therapy to facilitate the necessary changes in lifestyle. Comprehensive lifestyle programs can produce a weight loss of approximately 5% to 10% within the first six months.[101]

However, even with the support of a comprehensive program, less than 20% of individuals are capable of achieving and sustaining a 10% weight loss after one year.[75] It has been demonstrated that most patients regain the majority, if not all, of their weight loss over the next five years. If patients fail to achieve a 5% weight loss within six months, other treatment options should be explored. The addition of pharmacotherapy may represent one such option.

Drug therapy is recommended in patients with a BMI greater than or equal to 30 kg/m^2, or in patients with a BMI greater than or equal to 27 kg/m^2 and more than one obesity-related condition who are motivated to lose weight and have failed more standard behavioral interventions based on diet and exercise. Medications should be considered as an adjunct to a comprehensive lifestyle program. Medications must be approved by the Federal Drug Administration (FDA), and providers should weigh the potential risks and benefits (such as medication efficacy, potential for abuse, and undesirable side effects) prior to the initiation of a medication therapy program. Current pharmacologic therapies include pancreatic lipase inhibitors, serotonin-2C receptor agonists, GLP-1 agonists, noradrenergic sympathomimetics, and combination drugs. The approach to agent selection should be based on comorbidities and relevant contraindications for each individual.[101]

Metabolic and bariatric surgery is recommended for individuals with a BMI greater than or equal to 40 kg/m^2, or with a BMI greater than or equal to 35 kg/m^2 and at least one obesity-related disease. Metabolic and bariatric surgery is recognized by many as the only proven effective long-term solution to weight loss in the morbidly obese patient population. Many leading medical associations and professional organizations have outlined position statements in support of metabolic and bariatric surgery.[8,106,111] Patient selection for metabolic and bariatric surgery continues to be based on NIH guidelines dating back to 1991.[96] An individual is considered a candidate for surgery if the BMI is equal to or greater than 40 kg/m^2, or if the BMI is 35 to 39.9 kg/m^2 with significant documented comorbidity. Comorbidities include diabetes, hypertension, hyperlipidemia, sleep apnea syndrome, obesity hypoventilation syndrome, pseudotumor cerebri, degenerative joint dysfunction, disc disease, gastroesophageal reflux disease, and severe venous stasis disease. The patient must have an acceptable operative risk, must have attempted and failed nonsurgical therapy, must be well-informed, motivated, and willing to participate in treatment and long-term follow-up, and must be psychiatrically stable with no addictions. The NIH recommends that surgical candidates be evaluated by a interprofessional team comprising medical, surgical, psychiatric, and nutritional expertise prior to performing the surgical procedure.[96]

There is growing support for reevaluation of the 1991 NIH guidelines recommending the arbitrary cutoff of a BMI of 35 kg/m^2 (Class II obesity). The 2012 American Society for Metabolic and Bariatric Surgery (ASMBS) guidelines for Bariatric Surgery in Class I Obesity[13] made the following recommendations: Class I obesity is a well-defined disease process associated with various comorbid conditions, decreased life expectancy, and decreased quality of life. Individuals with a BMI of 30 kg/m^2 or higher have a 50% to 100% increased risk of premature death compared to the healthy individual with a lower BMI.[102] Additionally, this group has an increased risk of developing the following: type 2 diabetes, hypertension, CAD, congestive heart failure, asthma, stroke, pulmonary embolism, gall bladder disease, osteoarthritis, and certain types of cancer.[50] Nonsurgical treatment options are generally ineffective in the long-term. Metabolic and bariatric surgery should be made available for patients with a BMI of 30 to 35 kg/m^2.

Randomized control trials have demonstrated the effectiveness of gastric banding, sleeve gastrectomy, and gastric bypass in patients with a BMI of 30 to 35 kg/m^2. The Obesity Society (TOS), the American Association of Clinical Endocrinologists (AACE), and the International Diabetes Federation (IDF) all endorse guidelines recommending metabolic and bariatric surgery for patients with a BMI of 30 to 34.9 kg/m^2 who are suffering from diabetes or metabolic syndrome.[36,54,69]

Metabolic and Bariatric Procedures

The first true weight loss surgery was performed in the early 1950s by Dr. R. Varco. The procedure, known as *jejunoileal bypass,* consisted of dividing the proximal jejunum and creating a jejunoileal anastomosis just proximal to the ileocecal valve. In 1966, Dr. E. Mason designed a procedure to treat duodenal ulcers. He created a side-to-side anastomosis between the upper portion of the divided stomach and a loop of the jejunum. This procedure proved ineffective at treating duodenal ulcers, but Mason noted that it was associated with weight loss. This represented the beginnings of the gastric bypass procedure.[110] Since that time, the field of bariatric surgery has evolved, with several variations to and modifications of these original procedures. With the introduction of laparoscopic surgery in the early 1990s, the field of bariatric surgery was completely revolutionized. Minimally invasive surgery allows surgeons to perform complex gastrointestinal procedures on high-risk patients with dramatically reduced morbidity and mortality rates. The current likelihood of major complication ranges from 2.5% to 4%, with an overall 30-day mortality rate of 0.1%.[3,13,32,43]

In the United States, approximately 200,000 metabolic and bariatric surgeries are performed each year, representing approximately 1% of eligible candidates. Currently, the most commonly performed procedures in the United States are the Roux-en-Y gastric bypass (34%), the adjustable gastric band (14%), the sleeve gastrectomy (42%), and the biliopancreatic diversion/duodenal switch (1%).[12]

Metabolic and bariatric surgery is a proven long-term and effective therapy for the treatment of obesity and related comorbidities. The term *metabolic* was added to describe surgical procedures that are intended to not only treat obesity but also treat type 2 diabetes and other metabolic disease processes. In the past, weight loss procedures were classified as either restrictive or malabsorptive in nature. Research suggests that the underlying mechanisms of action are physiologic, and not merely based on nutrient restriction. Metabolic mechanisms of action that are being investigated include alterations

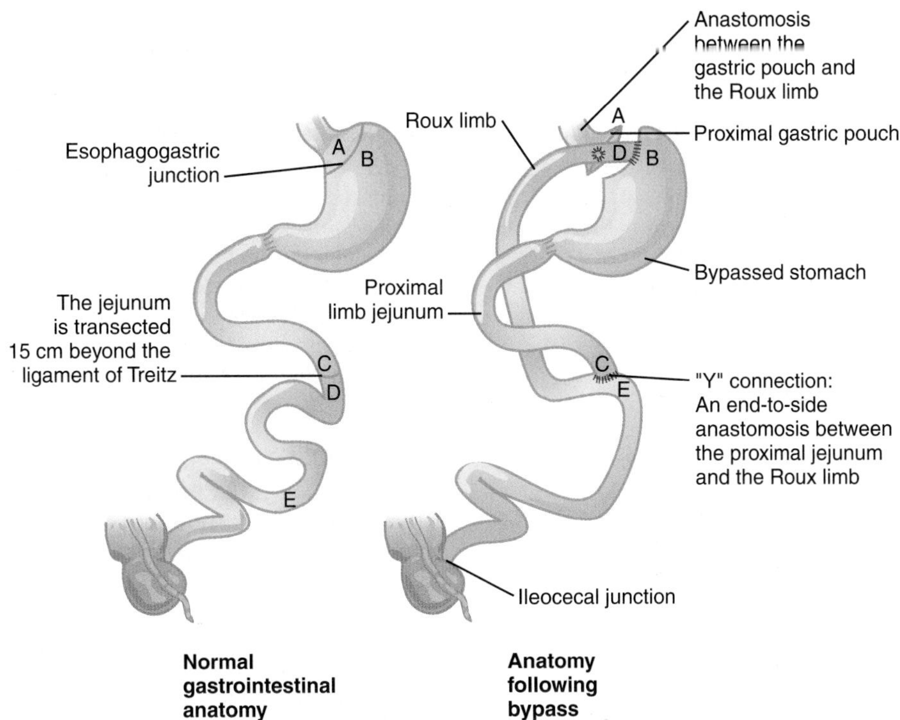

FIG. 38.2 Roux-en-Y gastric bypass.

in ghrelin, leptin, GLP-1, and cholecystokinin peptide YY levels, alterations in the gut microbiota, and changes in bile acid secretion.[18,71,120,128]

Roux-en-Y Gastric Bypass

The Roux-en-Y gastric bypass is considered the gold standard bariatric procedure. In this procedure, the stomach is divided into two sections. The upper part consists of a small gastric pouch capable of holding approximately 15 to 30 mL. The lower part consists of the remnant stomach. Although this remnant stomach no longer stores food, it continues to function and secrete digestive juices. The small intestine is divided. The jejunum is transected from the duodenum and then joined to the newly created gastric pouch. This limb of the jejunum is known as the *Roux limb* and can be 100 to 150 cm in length. The Roux limb is then attached downstream to the jejunum coming from the duodenum (i.e., the biliopancreatic limb). The biliopancreatic limb transports secretions from the gastric remnant, liver, and pancreas. This reconfiguration results in the "Y" shape of the Roux-en-Y gastric bypass. The newly created anatomy results in food passing through the gastric pouch and down the Roux limb with minimal digestion. Gastric and other digestive juices are delivered by the biliopancreatic limb. Digestion of food begins in the common channel past the joining of the Roux limb and the biliopancreatic limb (Fig. 38.2).[98]

Adjustable Gastric Band

With the adjustable gastric band procedure, an adjustable silicone ring is applied around the top part of the stomach. The band constricts the stomach, resulting in the creation of a small pouch with a narrow opening to the rest of the stomach. The constriction can be adjusted via tubing that is connected to a small port located underneath the skin. The band can be adjusted to increase or decrease restriction by injecting saline into or removing saline from the silicone ring.[98]

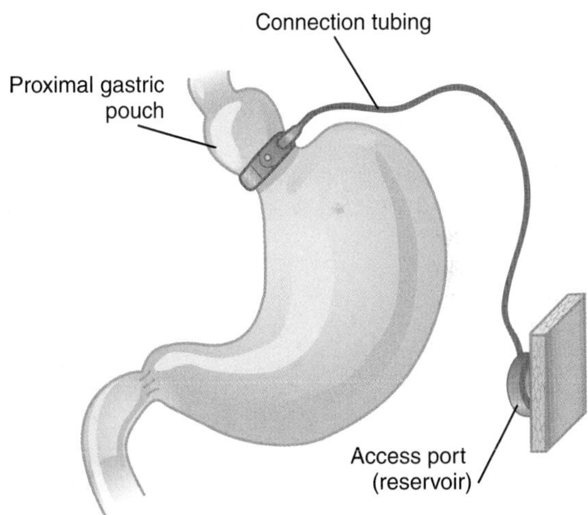

FIG. 38.3 Adjustable gastric band.

Recently, this procedure has fallen out of favor, due to poor long-term outcomes and the introduction of the sleeve gastrectomy. Failure has been described as poor weight loss, intolerable symptoms, and band malfunction, including erosion, slippage, and pouch and esophageal dilation.[60] Most studies demonstrate inadequate long-term weight loss, citing a mean excess weight loss of 30% to 45%.[72] It is difficult to determine the percentage of patients who have had their bands removed, because these patients often are lost to follow-up and difficult to track. However, one study reported that nearly 50% of patients have their bands removed, contributing to an overall reoperation rate of 60%.[60] In summary, the adjustable gastric band is a simple and safe procedure; however, its consistently high failure rates have left many patients seeking better quality long-term outcomes by requesting conversions to other procedures, such as the sleeve gastrectomy and gastric bypass (Fig. 38.3).

Sleeve Gastrectomy

The sleeve gastrectomy is the fastest growing bariatric procedure, and has become the most commonly performed bariatric procedure. This procedure was first introduced as the first stage of a two stage duodenal switch procedure. As a standalone procedure, the majority of the greater curvature of the stomach is removed, leaving a long banana-shaped stomach. The antrum is divided approximately 2 to 6 cm away from the pylorus, leaving it intact. The sleeve is created with the aid of a 35 to 40 French bougie. Most surgeons reinforce the staple line either by oversewing or by using buttress materials in order to decrease bleeding and leaks. There is no rerouting of the gastrointestinal tract in this procedure (Fig. 38.4).[98]

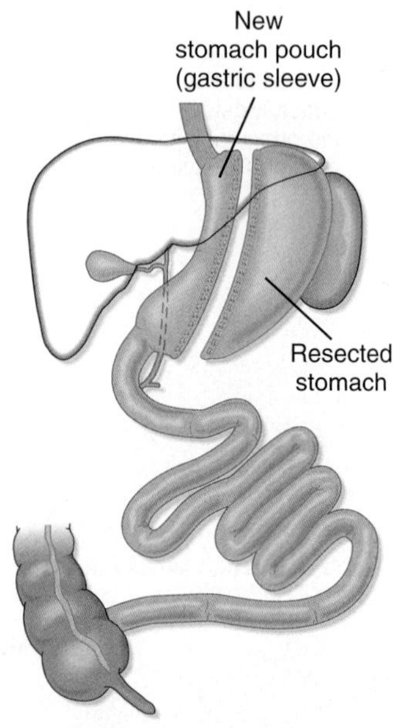

FIG. 38.4 Sleeve gastrectomy. (From Adams, J. G., et al. (2013). *Emergency medicine: clinical essentials* (2nd ed.). Philadelphia: Saunders.)

Biliopancreatic Diversion and Duodenal Switch

A sleeve gastrectomy is created by resecting two-thirds of the stomach. A narrow, vertical, tube-shaped stomach remains, with an intact pylorus. The duodenum is divided, and the proximal end is attached to a segment of the ileum. This becomes the new food limb. The food limb is then anastomosed to the part of the intestine coming from the duodenum at approximately 50 to 100 cm from the ileocecal valve. This results in a very short common channel, allowing for food digestion and absorption (Fig. 38.5).[98]

Perioperative Management of the Metabolic and Bariatric Surgery Patient

In 2013, the AACE, TOS, and the ASMBS updated their clinical practice guidelines for perioperative management of the bariatric surgery patient. Prior to considering a patient for metabolic or bariatric surgery, a comprehensive preoperative evaluation to assess surgical risk should be performed. Suggested elements are listed in Box 38.2.[90]

Postoperative management of the metabolic or bariatric surgical patient should involve a comprehensive interprofessional approach to ensure quality outcomes and safety. Box 38.3 lists key postoperative assessments to be considered.

Outcomes of Metabolic and Bariatric Surgery

Research into metabolic and bariatric surgery continues to demonstrate the efficacy of these procedures in producing long-term sustained weight loss, improvement or resolution of comorbid conditions, decreased mortality, and improved quality of life. On average, patients who undergo bariatric surgery decrease their risk of premature death by 30% to 40%. Patients who had

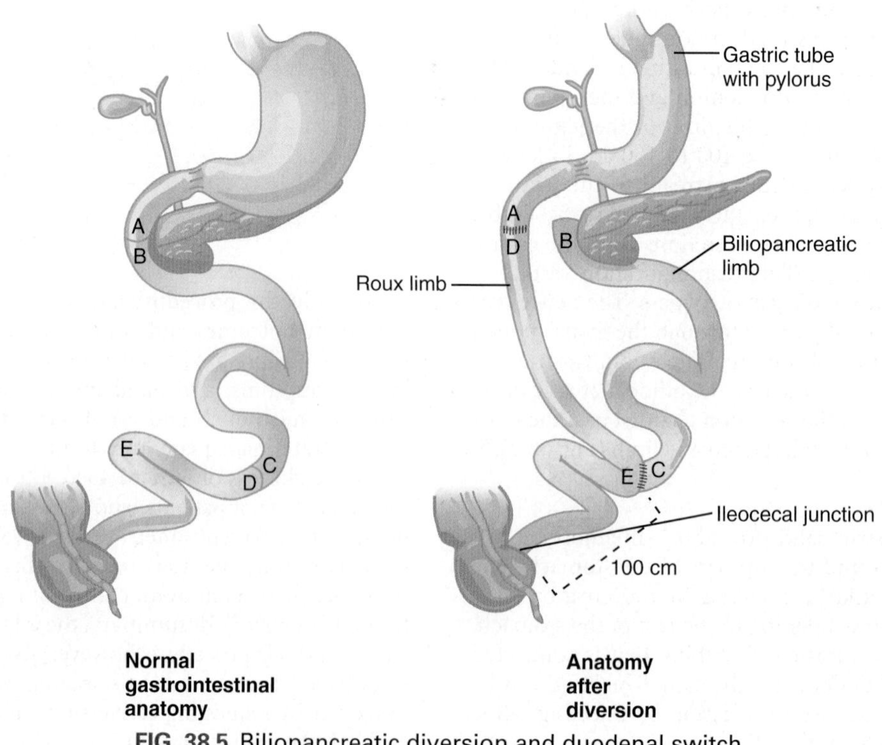

FIG. 38.5 Biliopancreatic diversion and duodenal switch.

surgery also saw their disease-specific mortality decrease by 56% for CAD, 92% for diabetes, and 60% for cancer.[7,119]

Most patients generally lose the majority of their weight within the first 2 years following metabolic and bariatric surgery. On average, patients may lose approximately 60% of their excess weight in the first 6 months following surgery, with many achieving greater than 75% excess weight loss within one year. A large meta-analysis of over 135,000 patients demonstrated that, on average, patients maintained a 60% excess weight loss at 2 years.[26] At five years, on average, patients maintain a 50% excess weight loss.[2]

Metabolic and bariatric surgery results in the improvement or resolution of many obesity-related diseases such as type 2 diabetes, heart disease, sleep apnea, gastroesophageal reflux disease, hypertension, hyperlipidemia, and certain cancers. A meta-analysis of over 22,000 patients demonstrated the improvement and/or resolution of type 2 diabetes mellitus, hypertension, OSA, and hyperlipidemia following bariatric surgery (Table 38.4).[75] A more recent review of Roux-en-Y gastric bypass patients showed similar outcomes, with percentages of patients who saw improvement or complete resolution as follows: 83% for type 2 diabetes, 87% for hypertension, 67% for dyslipidemia, and 76% for OSA.[59]

One of the most remarkable outcomes of metabolic and bariatric surgery is the resolution or improvement of type 2 diabetes, independent of weight loss. Bariatric surgeons have long witnessed this effect. In 1995, an article entitled: “Who would have thought it? An operation proves to be the most effective therapy for adult-onset diabetes mellitus,” was the first to describe how gastric bypass provided long-term control of both obesity and diabetes.[107] Since then, numerous studies have illustrated the same effect; however, it was not until 2012 that the first randomized control trials reported the superiority of surgery over medical treatment for diabetes.[91,113,114]

In one study, patients were randomly assigned to receive conventional medical treatment or undergo either gastric bypass or biliopancreatic diversion. At 2 years, the rate of diabetes remission was examined in both groups. Remission was defined as a fasting glucose level of less than 100 mg/dL and a glycated hemoglobin level of less than 6.5%, with no pharmacologic therapy. At 2 years, remission had not occurred in any of the patients in the medical treatment group. However, the surgical group saw a remission rate of 75% in the gastric bypass group and 95% in the biliopancreatic diversion group.[91]

In the STAMPEDE (Surgical Treatment and Medications Potentially Eradicate Diabetes Efficiently) clinical trial, patients were randomized to either an intensive medical therapy group or a surgical group (either gastric bypass or sleeve gastrectomy). The primary endpoint of this study was to examine the proportion of patients who achieved a glycated hemoglobin level of 6% or less at 12 months. This was achieved by 12% of the intensive medical therapy group, 42% of gastric bypass group, and 37% of the sleeve gastrectomy group. It was also noted that the use of medications to lower blood glucose, lipid levels, and blood pressure (BP) decreased significantly in the surgical groups but increased in the medical group. At 3 years, only 5% of the medical group achieved the endpoint, compared to 38% of the gastric bypass group and 24% of the sleeve gastrectomy group.[113,114]

The estimated yearly cost of treating a patient with diabetes is five times that of the patient without diabetes. In a study comparing bariatric surgery patients to diabetic and nonsurgical controls, only 28% of patients who underwent bariatric surgery still had a diagnosis of diabetes at 6 months following surgery. The average monthly prescription medication cost for the surgery patients was 64% lower than that for controls at 6 months following surgery, 69% lower at 1 year, and 72% lower at 2 years.[74] This illustrates not only the therapeutic benefit of bariatric surgery on diabetes, but also its economic impact.

BOX 38.2 Preoperative Evaluation

- Complete history and physical
- Routine laboratory testing
- Nutrient screening (iron, B12, folic acid, and 25-hydroxy vitamin D)
- Cardiopulmonary evaluation with sleep study
- Gastrointestinal evaluation
- Endocrine evaluation
- Nutrition evaluation by registered dietician
- 5% to 10% preoperative weight loss with energy-restricted diet to reduce liver size
- Elimination of alcohol consumption, especially in patients who will undergo a Roux-en-Y procedure, due to impaired alcohol metabolism and increased risk of alcohol disorders postoperatively
- Psychosocial behavioral evaluation that assesses environmental, familial, and behavioral factors
- Ongoing support group participation after discharge
- Smoking cessation at least 6 weeks prior to surgery; smoking should be avoided after surgery, given the increased risk for poor wound healing, anastomotic ulcers, and overall impaired health
- Women of reproductive age should be counseled to not become pregnant for 12–18 months following surgery

BOX 38.3 Postoperative Management

- Cardiovascular monitoring for patients with high perioperative risk of cardiac complications
- Pulmonary management to include incentive spirometry, supplemental oxygen, and continuous positive airway pressure (CPAP) for patients suffering from obstructive sleep apnea
- Deep venous thrombosis (DVT) prevention with sequential compression devices, prophylactic heparin, or enoxaparin and early ambulation
- Low-sugar, clear, liquid meal should be initiated within 24 hours of surgery, with diet progression at the discretion of the surgeon and dietitian
- Goal is to advance to 3 small meals per day, encouraging small bites, chewing thoroughly, and avoiding drinking with meals to avoid gastrointestinal symptoms
- Protein intake should be individualized, with the goal being a minimum 60 g/day
- Concentrated sweets should be eliminated to avoid dumping
- Extended release medications should be replaced with liquid, rapid-release, or crushed forms
- Minimum daily nutrient supplements for Roux-en-Y and sleeve gastrectomy include
  - Two adult multivitamins containing iron, thiamine, and folic acid
  - Elemental calcium
  - Vitamin D
  - Vitamin B12

TABLE 38.4 Outcomes of Metabolic and Bariatric Surgery

Condition/ Disease	Percentage Resolved or Improved	Percentage Resolved
Type 2 diabetes	86.0	76.8
Hypertension	78.5	61.7
Obstructive sleep apnea	85.7	83.6
Hyperlipidemia	78.5	61.7

Postoperative Complications

Significant improvements have been made in the field of metabolic and bariatric surgery, resulting in improved outcomes and patient safety. Mortality is an unlikely complication of metabolic and bariatric surgery. The overall mortality rate is approximately 0.1%.[3] Procedure-specific mortality rates are 0.02% for laparoscopic adjustable gastric band, 0.1% for gastric bypass, and 0.19% for sleeve gastrectomy.[99] A review by the Center for Medicare & Medicaid Services examined morbidity and mortality rates for gastric bypass in comparison to other procedures such as cholecystectomy, colectomy, and hip replacement.[35] Mortality rates for bypass were 0.2%; cholecystectomy, 0.9%; colectomy, 0.8%; and hip replacement, 0.2%. The most common cause of death in the perioperative period is pulmonary embolism, which accounts for nearly 50% of all deaths. Other causes include sepsis from anastomotic leaks, cardiac causes such as myocardial infarction or heart failure, and respiratory failure. The overall likelihood of a major complication following bariatric surgery is cited at approximately 2.5% to 4%.[40,43] A review of the Longitudinal Assessment of Bariatric Surgery (LABS) data illustrated that a prior history of deep venous thrombosis (DVT) or pulmonary embolism (PE), OSA, and decreased functional status were all independently predictive of a 30-day complication or adverse outcome, including death.[81]

Pulmonary Embolism

Obesity is an independent risk factor for the development of DVT and PE. The in-hospital VTE rate for bariatric surgery is 0.17%.[87] Interventions for the prevention of VTE include early ambulation, mechanical prophylaxis, and chemoprophylaxis. The ASMBS updated its position statement on perioperative VTE prophylaxis, supporting a combination approach; however, it did not recommend a standardized dosing protocol for chemoprophylaxis.[10] Signs and symptoms of VTE include hypoxia, tachycardia, hypotension, shortness of breath, and chest pain.

Anastomotic Leaks

Anastomotic leaks are by far the most dreaded of all potential complications following bariatric surgery. There are many potential causes for gastrointestinal leaks. Causes can be categorized as mechanical, tissue, or ischemic (where the intraluminal pressure exceeds the strength of the staple line or tissue). The incidence of occurrence can vary from 0% to 4%. In one study, the mean incidence of leaks following laparoscopic bypass was 0.8%.[65] The mean incidence following sleeve gastrectomy appears to be somewhat greater, at approximately 2.5%, given the higher pressure within the narrow sleeve.[45] In an effort to reduce the incidence of leaks, most surgeons either oversew or reinforce staple lines with either biological or synthetic materials. Intraoperative leak tests using air, dye, or endoscopy have also been used to reduce the incidence of leaks. Early recognition and management is crucial in order to prevent this life-threatening complication. However, recognition of leaks can be particularly challenging in the morbidly obese, as they can present with very subtle signs. Patients may present with sustained tachycardia, tachypnea, and fever. These symptoms often present before any abdominal pain, leukocytosis, oliguria, or hemodynamic instability. Another subtle sign may be the patient's reporting of a feeling of "impending doom." In the early postoperative period, a high index of suspicion is crucial, and any unexplained sustained tachycardia with a heart rate greater than or equal to 120 beats per minute is considered an anastomotic leak until proven otherwise.

Gastrointestinal Obstructions

Gastrointestinal obstructions can range from simple and spontaneously resolving to complex and life-threatening. When considering the possibility of obstruction post–bariatric surgery, it is imperative to have a clear understanding of the newly created anatomy. Some of the most common presentations of strictures and obstructions include: gastrojejunal stricture, internal hernia obstructions, obstructions due to intra-abdominal adhesions, incisional hernias, and intussusception. When diagnosing gastrointestinal obstructions, it is important to remember that the clinical presentation will vary depending on which area of the bowel is obstructed.[48]

Bleeding

Bleeding following bariatric surgery is classified according to bleeding site and time of onset. Bleeding can occur into the abdominal cavity (intra-abdominal) or into the gastrointestinal tract (intraluminal). Onset is defined as acute (1–7 days), early (1–6 weeks), late (6–12 weeks), and chronic (greater than 12 weeks).[98] Typically, intra-abdominal bleeds occur in the early postoperative phase, and are associated with staple lines and trocar sites. Intraluminal bleeds can occur at any time, and include both surgical and medical causes, such as ulcer disease and neoplasms. Bleeding can present as hematemesis or melena with intraluminal bleeding. If a surgical drain is in place, persistent bright red bloody output can represent an intra-abdominal bleed. Other signs and symptoms may include tachycardia, hypotension, oliguria, and a decrease in hemoglobin and hematocrit. Intraluminal bleeding is more common after gastric bypass, given the staple lines present at the gastrojejunostomy, the jejunojejunostomy, and the gastric remnant.[57]

Nutritional Deficiencies

A common misconception is that the obese patient is well-nourished. In fact, many obese patients who present for bariatric surgery are malnourished and have untreated nutrient deficiencies. With bariatric surgery, the gastrointestinal track is altered, leading to increased risk for nutritional deficiencies such as deficiencies in B12, iron, calcium, vitamin D, folate, thiamine, vitamin A/E/K, copper, selenium, and zinc. Protein deficiency is also common if patients do not adhere to the recommended daily protein intake.[67] Deficiencies may also develop as a result of prolonged vomiting, loss of appetite, and dehydration.

MANAGEMENT OF THE CRITICALLY ILL OBESE PATIENT

With the increasing obesity epidemic, it can be expected that greater numbers of obese individuals will be in critical care areas. One study demonstrated that nearly one-third of all intensive care unit (ICU) patients are obese, and 7% are morbidly obese.[63] Despite perceptions, multiple meta-analyses demonstrated no association between obesity and mortality in critically ill patients.[4,103] An international review of 355 ICUs demonstrated no association between extreme obesity and worse survival outcomes. However, patients with a BMI greater than or equal to 40 kg/m^2 had longer mechanical ventilation times and a longer ICU length of stay.[86] This patient population presents management challenges in the critical care setting. Simple tasks such as monitoring, catheterizing, turning, positioning, performing hygiene tasks, toileting, and ambulating can be more demanding with the obese patient. Safe care of the obese patient may require additional staff and specialized equipment. The body habitus of the obese patient may make physical assessments and diagnostic imaging more challenging. The healthcare team must be aware of these challenges and develop strategies for the safe care of the obese patient.

Airway Management

Anatomical and physiologic changes associated with obesity may make airway management more challenging, due to rapid oxygen desaturation and difficulty with mask ventilation, laryngoscopy, and intubation. Studies have looked into potential factors that may help to predict challenges in airway management in the obese. Despite the belief that morbid obesity and OSA are associated with difficult airway management, studies have not found a strong correlation between obesity, OSA, and failed laryngoscopy.[83,97] Excessive palatal and pharyngeal soft tissue, large tongue, mouth opening, and high anterior larynx may increase the difficulty of intubation.[68] Large neck circumference, Mallampati score of greater than or equal to three, and male gender have been cited as possible predictors of difficult laryngoscopy and tracheal intubation (Fig. 38.6).[83,97] Neck mobility may be limited due to short neck, large neck circumference, and possible posterior cervical fat pads preventing neck extension while in the supine position. Proper positioning of patients with the use of folded blankets or foam wedges will assist in achieving the "ramped" position. Correct positioning will ensure that the chin is above the chest and the external auditory meatus and the sternum are aligned along the same horizontal axis.[117] While in the supine position for intubation, the morbidly obese patient is at higher risk of rapid desaturation due to a lower FRC when in this position.[1,94] A position with the head of bed up at 25 degrees and a 30 degree reverse Trendelenburg position have been shown to be effective in limiting desaturation and increasing time for intubation.[94] The reverse Trendelenburg position has also been shown to reduce the risk of aspiration by lowering intra-abdominal pressures.

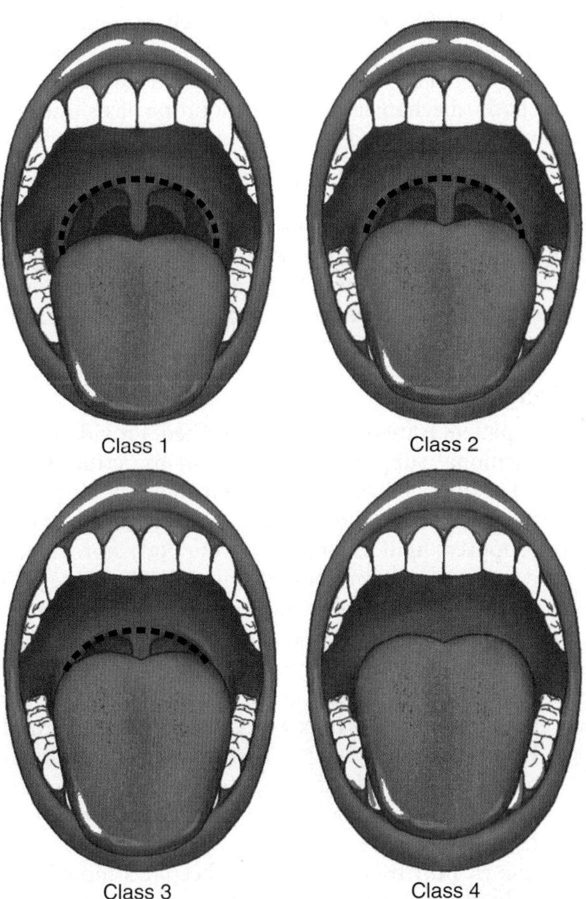

FIG. 38.6 Mallampati score. (In Beachey, W. (2010). *Respiratory care anatomy and physiology: Foundations for clinical practice* (3rd ed.). St. Louis: Mosby. Redrawn from Wilkins, R. L., et al. (2010). *Clinical assessment in respiratory care* (6th ed.). St Louis: Mosby.)

Obese patients requiring a tracheostomy may also present a challenge. Standard tracheostomy tubes are too curved and too short, given the increased distance between the skin and the trachea in the obese patient. This increases the likelihood of malpositioning or dislodgement. Custom-fit tracheostomy tubes may be used with this patient group. Traditionally, surgical tracheostomy has been considered the procedure of choice. However, some studies have shown success with bedside percutaneous tracheostomy in the morbidly obese.[84] Increased use of ultrasound technology has assisted in percutaneous tracheostomy. Ultrasound-guided percutaneous tracheostomy helps guide the tracheostomy procedure, decreasing complications and the risk of vascular puncture.[51]

Vascular Access

Securing vascular access, such as through the use of peripheral, arterial, and central venous catheters, can be difficult in the obese patient. With increased adiposity, the usual anatomic landmarks may be obscured, the distance from skin to vessel may be increased, and the angle of approach for insertion may be distorted.[118] Insertion of femoral lines can be complicated by impalpable pulses, a large pannus covering the groin area, and a high incidence of fungal infections in the groin area.[68] Access to the internal jugular may require multiple attempts and result in increased complication rates. Ultrasound-guided techniques facilitate successful access and reduce rates of complication. Ultrasound-guided insertion of peripherally inserted central catheters (PICC) presents an effective alternative to centrally placed catheters.

Respiratory

Obesity results in a restrictive lung pattern due to increased pulmonary blood volume and increased chest wall pressure from the effect of adipose tissue pressing on the thorax. The work of breathing is further exacerbated by the abnormal position of the diaphragm, increased upper airway resistance, and carbon dioxide (CO_2) production. Patient positioning helps to alleviate some of the effects of obesity on lung function. The reverse Trendelenburg position may prove beneficial for the obese patient. Studies have shown its effectiveness with obese intubated patients and those undergoing or recovering from surgery and anesthesia. This position improves ventilation and reduces the risk of aspiration by lowering intra-abdominal pressure.[1,94] This patient position results in larger tidal volumes and a lower respiratory rate. Various ventilation strategies have also been used for the improvement of respiratory function in the obese patient. The prophylactic use of bilevel positive airway pressure

(BiPAP) during the initial postoperative phase has been shown to reduce pulmonary dysfunction and promote preoperative function by improving FVC, FEV1, and peripheral capillary oxygen saturation (Spo_2). By affecting both inspiration and expiration, BiPAP serves to improve alveolar recruitment and prevent alveolar collapse upon expiration.[104]

OSA is highly correlated with obesity. Patients with OSA have excess oral and pharyngeal tissue, which is responsible for airway collapse during sleep. This results in periods of apnea with hypoxia. It is important to note that in the postoperative period, these patients are at increased risk, due to the residual effects of anesthesia and postoperative analgesia. The most common treatment for OSA is continuous positive airway pressure (CPAP). CPAP serves to displace the tongue and pharyngeal tissue, thereby preventing obstruction.

With reduced lung volumes and increased airway resistance, mechanical ventilation for the obese patient can be challenging. Ideal body weight should be used to calculate the delivered tidal volume. Actual body weight is not recommended, as it can result in high airway pressures, alveolar overdistention, and barotrauma. The use of end tidal CO_2 monitoring is not recommended, due to the widened alveolar-arterial gradients in the obese population. Providing the intubated patient positive end expiratory pressure (PEEP) can enhance alveolar recruitment and prevent atelectasis. Studies have demonstrated that 10 cm of PEEP results in better oxygenation with lower rates of atelectasis.[123]

Cardiology

Obesity causes various derangements in cardiac structure and performance. Most notably, obese patients often have left ventricular hypertrophy and dilatation, increased total blood volume, increasing resting cardiac output, and decreased ejection fraction. Fluid overload is not well tolerated in the obese critically ill patient; however, these patients may require a higher preload in order to maintain adequate renal perfusion.[118] In order to ensure proper fluid balance, the nurse must be alert to signs and symptoms of heart failure and pulmonary edema. Cardiovascular assessment can be challenging in the obese patient, as auscultation of heart and breath sounds may be difficult. Repositioning of the patient in a left lateral position or in a sitting position at a 45-degree angle may make sounds more audible, as the heart will be closer to the chest wall. With increased adiposity, it may be more difficult to palpate peripheral pulses. Larger BP cuffs are needed for accurate BP readings. Inappropriately small BP cuffs result in erroneously high systolic BP measurements. When accurate monitoring is needed for the determination of therapeutic interventions, an arterial line may be beneficial. Cardiac changes are evident in electrocardiography (EKG) findings. These may include prolonged PR, QRS, and QT intervals, left axis deviation, and low voltage QRS. Obese patients may experience various cardiac arrhythmias. Atrial fibrillation may occur with fluid overload and atrial dilation.[105]

Pharmacologic

Medication dosing in the obese patient can be complex. Currently, there are no universally accepted guidelines or evidence-based practices for determining the appropriate dosage in the obese patient. Obese subjects are often excluded from medication clinical trials, resulting in clinicians having limited information when deciding on medication dosing strategies.[39,55]

Many of the physiologic changes associated with obesity affect the distribution, binding, and clearance of medications. These altered mechanisms can result in either subtherapeutic underdosage or toxic medication levels due to overdose. Various weight descriptors are utilized for medication dosing regimens in an effort to limit toxicity and subtherapeutic levels. These include ideal body weight (IBW), total body weight (TBW), adjusted body weight (ABWadj), lean body weight (LBW), BMI, and body surface area (BSA).[55] IBW is considered the best suited for standard dosing of medications such as opioids, anticonvulsants, benzodiazepine, propofol, fluoroquinolones, digoxin, procainamide, beta blockers, H2 blockers, neuromuscular blockers, and long-course corticosteroids. For lidocaine and verapamil, it is recommended to use IBW for maintenance dose, but ABWadj for loading doses.[64,68] ABWadj is also used for unfractionated heparin, aminoglycosides, and short-term or emergent use of corticosteroids. TBW is used for vancomycin dosing. There are limited data for recommendations for beta lactams, amiodarone, vasopressors, and inotropes.[64] Clinicians should consult with a pharmacist when dosing medications for the obese critically ill patient.

Venous Thromboembolism Prophylaxis

Obesity is considered an independent risk factor for VTE.[121] Decreased mobility, increased venous stasis, and hypercoagulability predispose the morbidly obese patient to an increased risk of DVT and PE. Whereas this is a well-recognized risk in the obese, there is no consensus on optimal methods for the prevention of VTE.[47] Most accepted forms of prophylaxis include both mechanical and chemoprophylaxis measures. Chemoprophylaxis includes various medications such as low-dose heparin infusion, weight-based intermittent dosing of low molecular weight heparin, and unfractionated heparin. Fondaparinux has also been used as an alternative, but has limited research trials.[62] Many of the diagnostic imaging techniques used with normal weight patients can be compromised by the weight and girth of the obese patient, making diagnosis of VTE challenging.

Nutritional Support

The obese patient is frequently malnourished. Providing appropriate nutritional support, particularly in the critically ill, is essential. The obese ICU patient is prone to developing protein malnutrition as a result of metabolic stress. Elevated basal insulin levels suppress lipid mobilization from body stores, causing increased breakdown of protein into glucose. The obese patient is at increased risk for protein malnutrition, which involves a rapid decrease in lean body mass and increased production of urea.[68] Estimation of calorie requirements in the critically ill obese patient is complicated. Although impractical and not widely used, indirect calorimetry is considered the method of choice. If indirect calorimetry is unavailable, energy requirements should be determined using the Penn State University 2010 predictive equation, or the modified Penn State equation if the patient is over 60 years of age.[29]

Hypocaloric nutritional support has been recommended for the critically ill obese patient. A joint consensus statement by the Society for Critical Care Medicine and the American Society for Parenteral and Enteral Nutrition (ASPEN) in 2009 recommended providing no more than 60% to 70% of target caloric requirements or 11–14 kcal/kg actual body weight per day; for Class I-II obesity, a minimum of 2.0 g/kg of IBW as protein; for

Class III obesity, a minimum of 2.5 g/kg of IBW.[89] The 2013 ASPEN clinical guidelines state that clinical outcomes may be equivalent in patients with high protein feeding, hypocaloric high protein feeding, and eucaloric feeding. They suggest a trial of hypocaloric high protein feeding in patients who do not have severe renal or hepatic dysfunction, beginning with 50% to 70% of estimated energy needs or less than 14 kcal/kg actual weight or 2–2.5 g/kg of IBW, with adjustment of goal protein intake based on the results of nitrogen balance studies.[29]

Skin Integrity

With decreased perfusion to excess adipose tissue, the critically ill obese patient is at a 16.6% to 20.7% higher risk for skin breakdown than the normal weight ICU patient.[131] The prevalence of pressure ulcers has been shown to be higher in extremely obese patients.[130] In the ICU setting, patients with a BMI of greater than or equal to 40 kg/m^2 are at an increased risk of developing pressure ulcers.[66] The risk of developing a pressure ulcer is 1.5–3 times higher in the morbidly obese critically ill patient.[82] Factors increasing susceptibility to pressure ulcers include: comorbidities, hypotension, hypoxia, sedation, neuromuscular blocking agents, fluid overload, fever, incontinence, and increased difficulty with patient handling and positioning.[68] It can be challenging to reposition the obese patient while ensuring both patient and staff safety. Skin integrity must be protected against pressure, shearing, and pinching. Use of bariatric beds with low air loss surfaces or air fluidized mattresses with pressure relief, as well as bariatric equipment for lifting and transferring, is essential. The obese patient may also be at risk for atypical pressure ulcers related to skin folds and a large body habitus. Tubes and catheters can burrow into skin fold, resulting in skin ulcers. Pressure ulcers on the hips, trunk, and torso can also occur from increased pressure on skin from side rails or arm rests on inappropriately sized chairs and beds.[46] Skin folds also represent a high risk for skin breakdown, as the moist environment in skin folds encourages microbial infections. Skin should be protected by absorbing moisture with folded soft cloth placed in skin folds. A large abdominal pannus may also present a challenge in the care of the obese, with increased risk for skin breakdown and issues with mobility. In some patients, the pannus can weigh 40 to 50 pounds, requiring extra care when positioning and mobilizing the patient. Daily skin assessments with patient repositioning every 2 hours are required to maintain skin integrity. However, this can be quite difficult to accomplish in this patient population without the required resources of additional staff, patient handling equipment, and training.

Equipment

Size- and weight-appropriate equipment is required to deliver safe, quality care and promote patient participation, dignity, and mobility. In selecting appropriate equipment, staff should consider both patient weight and girth. Most regular hospital beds can accommodate patients with weights of 400 to 500 pounds, but may be too narrow, with a width of 36 inches. Bariatric beds should have a 1000-pound capacity and be at least 44 inches wide.[78] Other necessary pieces of equipment include bariatric wheelchairs, walkers, commodes, patient lifts, stretchers, and bedside chairs. Staff must be aware of all available equipment and have received proper training in how to use the equipment to prevent both patient and staff injury. This is especially important in patient handling with transfer devices and lifts. Most standard lifts can handle up to 600 pounds, whereas bariatric lifts are capable of handling 1000 pounds.[78] Wall-mounted toilets typically have a weight capacity of only 250 pounds. Floor-mounted toilets can support up to 1000 pounds. Toilet supports are available to provide additional support for wall-mounted toilets. These commercially available supports may increase the load capacity to 1000 pounds, depending on the model. In facilities with wall-mounted toilets but without commercially available supports, a bariatric commode should be used to ensure patient safety during toileting.

Diagnostic imaging may also pose a problem. The thickness of subcutaneous fat can make ultrasound and radiography more challenging. Computed tomography (CT) artifacts may also be more common in obese patients. To obtain higher quality images, adjustments may be required in scanning techniques and reconstruction methods. Prior to transfer from ICU to diagnostic imaging, scanner gantry aperture diameter and table load weight limit should be investigated to ensure the patient is within recommended limits.[92] A team approach utilizing appropriate equipment, trained staff, team communication, and planning will help to avoid some of the challenges in handling the obese patient.

Sensitivity: R-E-S-P-E-C-T Model of Care

The obese patient is often the victim of prejudice and discrimination. Discrimination against the obese has been labeled the last acceptable form of discrimination in our society. The obese individual may encounter discrimination in family, social, educational, and employment situations. Healthcare is not immune to this type of discrimination. Studies have shown that healthcare providers may have strong negative attitudes towards the obese, and often associate these patients with negative stereotypes, viewing the obese patient as lazy, unintelligent, undisciplined, weak-willed, over-indulgent, and noncompliant.[23] Unfortunately, this may negatively impact the quality of care delivered to the obese patient.

The position statement of the National Association of Bariatric Nurses (NABN) adopted the principles of advocacy, empathy, dignity, respect, responsibility, and safety to guide nurses in the care of the obese patient. The R-E-S-P-E-C-T Model of Care provides a framework for successful professional relationships by focusing on a culture of sensitivity towards the obese patient. R-E-S-P-E-C-T is the key to providing sensitive, patient-centered, quality care to the obese patient.[19] In establishing a respectful, caring, and compassionate environment of care, healthcare providers can develop a trusting relationship with the patient suffering from obesity. By developing strategies that ensure the availability and utilization of proper equipment, we can instill confidence in this patient population, as we are committed to caring for their unique needs in a safe and dignified manner. Society still views obesity as a personal choice. It is our role as healthcare providers to educate the public that obesity is not a choice, but rather a complex, poorly understood, chronic disease.

CONCLUSION

The current obesity epidemic has been described as the Black Plague of our modern day society. We continue to witness the detrimental effects of obesity and obesity-associated chronic diseases such as diabetes, cardiovascular disease, and respiratory conditions. With increasing numbers of individuals suffering from the disease of obesity, critical care units will inevitably witness a rise in the numbers of obese patients in their units. Healthcare providers will be caring for larger and more complex patients with multiple chronic conditions. It is therefore imperative for healthcare providers to anticipate the needs of these patients by developing a deeper understanding of how obesity alters their underlying physiology. Caring for the obese patient can present significant challenges with even the most basic of interventions. Nursing plays a key role in ensuring that the needs of obese patients are met and that they are cared for in a professional, caring, respectful, and compassionate manner. As nurses, we take pride in our role of patient advocates, and this must be especially true for the care of the obese patient. By anticipating and developing interprofessional plans of care to address the unique needs of this patient population, nurses can improve the comfort, safety, physical, and emotional well-being of obese patients, their families, and staff.

CASE STUDY 38.1

J.K. is a 57-year-old female who is 5'1" tall (154.9 cm) and weighs 351 pounds (159.5 kg), with an IBW of 47.7 and a BMI of 66.3. J.K. was found unconscious by her sister after she returned home from work (time of unconsciousness estimated at less than 12 hours). The patient was brought to the hospital by medics and was nonresponsive, with pinpoint pupils and a blood glucose level of 64 mg/dL. The patient's medical history includes: anemia, multiple PEs (4 in the last 10 years), depression, bipolar affective disorder, hypothyroid disease, OSA, asthma, arthritis in knees and ankles, chronic back pain, and chronic kidney disease (not requiring dialysis).

The patient's current medications include: cholecalciferol (vitamin D3); cholestyramine (Questran); divalproex (Depakote); gabapentin (Neurontin); levothyroxine (Synthroid); omeprazole (Prilosec); risperidone (Risperdal); rivaroxaban (Xarelto); tramadol (Ultram); and warfarin (Coumadin).

In the emergency department, the patient presented with heart rate (HR) 131, BP 56/34, mean arterial pressure (MAP) 39, Spo_2 86% on nonrebreather facemask, fraction of inspired oxygen (Fio_2) 0.30, respiratory rate (RR) 26, and temperature 36.6°C. She was difficult to arouse. Staff suspected potential pain medication overdose. Narcan and glucose failed to arouse her. The patient had significant skin breakdown. She was wheezing in both lung fields. The patient was intubated for airway protection. The laboratory was unable to draw blood, due to body habitus. The patient was transferred to the ICU for further management.

In the ICU, a right internal jugular central venous catheter was placed. Staff was unable to place arterial line despite several attempts in both right and left radial arteries. The patient's venous blood gas pH was 7.38, with partial pressure of carbon dioxide (Pco_2) 35.5, partial pressure of oxygen (Po_2) 54.6, HCO_3^- 20.6, base excess -3.5, and Spo_2 84.9%. Pulses were difficult to palpate, required use of Doppler. An EKG showed sinus tachycardia with no acute ST-T wave changes suggestive of ischemia; nonspecific changes with borderline left axis deviation were noted on the EKG. The patient's extremities were cold and mottled. BP measurements were unreliable, despite the use of a large BP cuff.

The laboratory results showed a normal white count and hematocrit, elevated potassium at 5.2, an international normalized ratio (INR) of 4.3, and elevated renal function tests with blood urea nitrogen (BUN) 28, creatine (Cr) 2.5, and creatine kinase (CK) 1392. Urinalysis was suggestive of urinary tract infection. A chest radiograph showed no obvious infiltrate or overt heart failure, with some mild diffuse interstitial markings. CT of the head showed no intracranial abnormality. The patient remained hypotensive despite fluid boluses, and was started on norepinephrine, phenylephrine, and vasopressin.

Staff had a very difficult time carrying out a thorough skin assessment given patient's body habitus, skin folds, and large pannus. Multiple deep tissue injuries were noted on the occiput, elbow, and coccyx. Further skin damage was noted on the buttocks, thighs, perineum, and labial folds, possibly from moisture due to incontinence of urine and stool. The patient was placed on a bariatric bed with a low air loss mattress. The patient was placed in ICU room with a ceiling lift to facilitate turning, positioning, and patient care.

The patient was hospitalized for a total of 41 days and then discharged to a skilled nursing facility, with a discharge diagnosis of septic shock, acute respiratory failure/acute respiratory distress syndrome, thrombocytopenia, acute chronic kidney disease (stage 3), generalized weakness, anemia, and severe morbid obesity.

Decision Point:

In reviewing the patient's medical history, identify obesity-related conditions.

Decision Point:

Identify challenges in the patient's care that were directly associated with her morbid obesity.

REFERENCES

1. Aceto, P., et al. (2013). Airway management in obese patients. *Surg Obes Relat Dis, 9*(5), 809–815.
2. Adams, T. (2007). Long Term mortality after gastric bypass surgery. *N Engl J Med, 357*(8), 753–761.
3. Agency for Healthcare Research and Quality (AHRQ). (2007). Statistical Brief #23 Bariatric Surgery Utilization and Outcomes in 1998 and 2004. http://www.hcup-us.ahrq.gov/reports/statbriefs/sb23.jsp.
4. Akinnusi, M. E., Pinea, L. A., & El Solh, A. A. (2008). Effect of obesity on intensive care morbidity and mortality: a meta-analysis. *Crit Care Med, 36*(1), 151–158.
5. Al-Benna, S. (2011). Perioperative management of morbid obesity. *J Perioper Pract, 21*(7), 225–233.
6. Allman-Farinelli, M. A. (2011). Obesity and venous thrombosis: a review. *Semin Thromb Hemost, 37*(8), 903–907.
7. American College of Obstetricians and Gynecologists. (2013). Obesity in Pregnancy. Committee Opinion No 549. American College of Obstetricians and Gynecologists. *Obstet Gynecol, 121*(1), 213–217.
8. American Diabetes Association. (2012). Position Statement-Standards of Medical Care in Diabetes-2012. *Diabetes Care, 35*(S1), S11–S63.
9. American Heart Association. Overweight and Obesity Statistics. (2009). Update 2009. http://www.heart.org/idc/groups/heart-public/@wcm/@sop/@smd/documents/downloadable/ucm_319588.pdf.
10. American Society for Metabolic and Bariatric Surgery Clinical Issues Committee. (2013). ASMBS updated position statement on prophylactic measures to reduce the risk of venous thromboembolism in bariatric surgery patients. *Surg Obes Relat Dis, 9*(4), 493–497.
11. Andrews, L. E., Liu, G. T., & Ko, M. W. (2014). Idiopathic intracranial hypertension. *Horm Res Paediatr, 81*(4), 217–225.
12. ASMBS. (2014). Fact Sheet. http://asmbs.org/resources/estimate-of-bariatric-surgery-numbers.
13. ASMBS Clinical Issues Committee. (2013). ASMBS statements/guidelines: bariatric surgery in class I obesity. *Surg Obes Relat Dis, 9*(1), e1–e10.
14. Atlantis, E., & Baker, M. (2008). Obesity effects on depression: systematic review of epidemiological studies. *Int J Obes, 32*(6), 881–891.
15. Bandaru, P., et al. (2013). The impact of obesity on immune response to infection and vaccine: an insight into plausible mechanisms. *Endocrinol Metab Synd, 2*(2), 113–121.
16. Barber, T. M., et al. (2006). Obesity and polycystic ovary syndrome. *Clin Endocrino (Oxf), 65*(2), 137–145.
17. Basen-Engquist, K., & Chang, M. (2011). Obesity and cancer risk: recent review and evidence. *Curr Oncol Rep, 13*(1), 71–76.
18. Basso, N., et al. (2011). First phase insulin secretion, insulin sensitivity, ghrelin, GLP-1 and PYY changes 72 hours after sleeve gastrectomy in obese diabetic patients: the gastric hypothesis. *Surg Endosc, 25*(11), 3540–3550.

19. Bejciy-Spring, S. (2008). R-E-S-P-E-C-T: a model for the sensitive treatment of the bariatric patient. *Bariatr Nurs Surg Patient Care, 8*(3), 47–57.
20. Berger, K. I., et al. (2009). Obesity hypoventilation syndrome. *Semin Respir Crit Care Med, 30*(3), 253–261.
21. Bjerkeset, O., et al. (2008). Association of adult BMI and height with anxiety, depression and suicide in the general population. *Am J Epidemio, 167*(2), 193–202.
22. Brewer, C. J., & Adam, H. B. (2010). The adverse effects of obesity on conception and implantation. *Reproduction, 140*(3), 347–364.
23. Brownell, K. D., Puhl, R. M., Schwartz, M. B., & Rudd, L. (2005). *Weight bias: nature consequences and remedies*. New York: The Guilford Press.
24. Bruffaerts, R., Scott, K. M., et al. (2008). Obesity and mental disorders in the general population: results from the world mental health surveys. *Int J Obes, 32*(1), 192–200.
25. Buchwald, H., et al. (2004). Bariatric surgery: a systematic review and meta-analysis. *JAMA, 292*(14), 1724–1737.
26. Buchwald, H., et al. (2009). Weight and type 2 diabetes after bariatric surgery: systematic review and meta-analysis. *Am J Med, 122*(3), 205–206.
27. Center for Disease Control and Prevention. (2013). Obesity Prevalence Maps. http://www.cdc.gov/obesity/data/prevalence-maps.html.
28. Centers for Disease Control. (2015). Exercise or Physical Activity. http://www.CDC.gov/nchs/fastats/exercise.htm.
29. Choban, P., Malone, A., Compher, C. (2013). The American Society for Parenteral and Enteral Nutrition. *JPEN J Parenter Enteral Nutr, 37*(6), 714–744.
30. Choquet, H., & Meyer, D. (2011). Genetics of obesity: what have we learned? *Curr Genomics, 12*(3), 169–179.
31. Collins, J. C., & Bentz, J. E. (2009). Behavioral and psychological factors in obesity. *The Journal of Lancaster General Hospital, 4*(4), 124–127.
32. DeMaria, E. J., et al. (2010). Baseline data from American Society for Metabolic and Bariatric Surgery-Designated Bariatric Surgery Centers of Excellence using BOLD. *Surg Obes Relat Dis, 6*(4), 347–355.
33. Despres, J. P., et al. (2008). Abdominal obesity and the metabolic syndrome: contribution to global cardiometabolic risk. *Arterioscler Thromb Vasc Biol, 28*(6), 1039–1049.
34. Diffee, P. D., Beach, M. M., & Cuellar, N. (2012). Caring for the patient with obstructive sleep apnea: implications for health care providers in post anesthesia care. *J Perianesth Nurs, 27*(5), 329–340.
35. Direct Research, LLC, Center for Medicare and Medicaid Services. (FY 2010). Med PAR, Medicare Fee for Service Inpatient Discharges with Selected Procedures.
36. Dixon, J. B., et al. (2011). Clinical practice bariatric surgery: an IDF statement for obese type 2 diabetes. *Diabet Med, 28*(6), 628–642.
37. Drewnowski, A. (2012). The economics of food choice behavior: why poverty and obesity are linked. *Nestle Nutr Inst Workshop Ser, 73*(1), 95–112.
38. Dubowitz, T., et al. (2013). Are our actions aligned with our evidence? The skinny on changing the landscape of obesity. *Obesity (Silver Spring), 21*(3), 419–420.
39. El Solh, A. A. (Ed.). (2012). *Critical care management of the obese patient*. Hoboken, New Jersey: Wiley-Blackwell.
40. Encinosa, W., et al. (2009). Recent improvements in bariatric surgery outcomes. *Med Care, 47*(5), 531–535.
41. Ernest, D., Vekic, T., & Bonanno, L. S. (2011). Evidence-based strategies to prevent postoperative respiratory dysfunction for patients with obstructive sleep apnea undergoing laparoscopic bariatric surgery. *Bariatr Nurs Surg Patient Care, 6*(2), 79–84.
42. Finkelstein, E. A., Cohen, J. W., et al. (2009). Annual medical spending attributable to obesity: payer and service specific estimates. *Health Aff, 28*(5), w822–w831.
43. Flum, D. R., et al. (2009). Perioperative safety in the longitudinal assessment of bariatric surgery. *N Engl J Med, 361*(5), 445–454.
44. Friedenberg, F. K., et al. (2008). The association between gastroesophageal reflux disease and obesity. *Am J Gastroenterol, 103*(8), 2111–2122.
45. Gagner, M., 5th (2015). International Consensus Summit for Sleeve Gastrectomy: is there a consensus? *Bariatric Times, 12*(4), A22–A23.
46. Gallagher, S. (2005). *The challenges of caring for the obese patient*. Edgemont, PA: Matrix Medical Communications.
47. Gould, M. K., Garcia, D. A., Wren, S. M., et al. (2012). Prevention of VTE in non-orthopedic surgical patients: antithrombotic therapy and prevention of thrombosis, 9th Ed: American College of Chest Physicians evidence-based clinical practice guidelines. *Chest, 141*(Suppl. 2), e227S–e277.
48. Griffith, P. S., et al. (2012). Managing complications associated with Roux en Y gastric bypass for morbid obesity. *Can J Surg, 55*(5), 329–336.
49. Grotle, M., Hagen, K. B., et al. (2008). Obesity and osteoarthritis in knee, hip and/or hand: an epidemiological study in the general population with 10 years follow up. *BMC Musculoskelet Disord, 9*(1), 132–136.
50. Guh, D. P., et al. (2009). The incidence of co-morbidities related to obesity and overweight: a systematic review and meta-analysis. *BMC Public Health, 9*(1), 88. http://dx.doi.org/10.1186/1471-2458-9-88.
51. Guinot, P. G., et al. (2012). Ultrasound-guided percutaneous tracheostomy in critically ill obese patients. *Crit Care, 16*(2), R40. http: doi:10.11861cc11233.
52. Hahler, B. (2006). An overview of dermatological conditions commonly associated with the patient with obesity. *Ostomy Wound Manage, 52*(6), 34–47.
53. Hamdallah, I. N., et al. (2013). Greater than expected prevalence of pseudotumor cerebri: a prospective study. *Surg Obes Relat Dis, 9*(1), 77–82.
54. Handelsman, Y., et al. (2015). American Association of Clinical Endocrinologists and American College of Endocrinology-Clinical practice guidelines for developing a diabetes mellitus comprehensive care plan. *Endocr Pract, 21*(1), 1–87.
55. Hanley, M. J., et al. (2010). Effect of obesity on the pharmacokinetics of drugs in humans. *Clin Pharmacokinet, 49*(2), 71–87.
56. Hartstra, A. V., Bouter, K. E. C., Backhed, F., & Nieuwdorp, M. (2015). Insights into the role of the microbiome in obesity and type 2 diabetes. *Diabetes Care, 38*(1), 159–165.
57. Heneghan, H., et al. (2012). Incidence and management of bleeding complications after gastric bypass surgery in the morbidly obese. *Surg Obes Relat Dis, 8*(6), 729–735.
58. Heredia, F. P., et al. (2012). Chronic and degenerative diseases—Obesity, inflammation and the immune system. *Proc Nutr Soc, 71*(2), 332–338.
59. Higa, K., et al. (2011). Laparoscopic RNY gastric bypass: 10-year follow-up. *Surg Obes Relat Dis, 7*(4), 516–525.
60. Himpens, J., et al. (2011). Long term outcomes of laparoscopic adjustable gastric banding. *Arch Surg, 146*(77), 802–807.
61. Hinney, A., Vogel, C., & Hebebrand, J. (2010). From monogenic to polygenic obesity: recent advances. *Eur Child Adolesc Psychiatry, 19*(3), 297–310.
62. Hirsh, J., et al. (2008). American College of Chest Physicians. Antithrombotic and thrombolytic therapy: american College of Chest Physicians evidence-based clinical practice guidelines (8th edition). *Chest, 133*(Suppl. 6), 110S–112S.
63. Hogue, C. W., et al. (2009). The impact of obesity on outcomes after critical illness: a meta-analysis. *Intensive Care Med, 35*(7), 1152–1170.
64. Honiden, S. (2012). Caring for the critically ill, obese patient. *CHEST, 25*(16). http://www.chestnet.org/Publications/CME-Publications/~/link.aspx?_id=827C7091290D4C9185C427275087B340&_z=z.
65. Hutter, M. M., et al. (2011). First report from the American College of Surgeons Bariatric Surgery Center Network: laparoscopic sleeve gastrectomy has morbidity and effectiveness positioned between the band and bypass. *Ann Surg, 254*(3), 410–420.
66. Hyun, S., et al. (2014). Body mass index and pressure ulcers: improved predictability of pressure ulcers in the intensive care patients. *Am J Crit Care, 23*(6), 494–501.
67. Jacques, J. (2006). *Micronutrition for the weight loss surgery patient*. Edgemont, PA: Matrix Medical Communications.
68. Jamadarkhana, S., Mallick, A., & Bodenham, A. (2014). Intensive care management of morbidly obese patients. *BJA Educ, 14*(2), 73–78.

69. Jensen, M. D., Ryan, D. H., et al. (2014). 2013 AHA/ACC/TOS Guidelines for the Management of Overweight and Obesity in Adults. *J Am Coll Cardiol, 63*(25), 3009–3023.
70. Kapur, V. K. (2010). Obstructive sleep apnea: diagnosis, epidemiology and economics. *Respir Care, 55*(9), 1155–1167.
71. Karamanakos, S., et al. (2008). Weight loss, appetite suppression and changes in fasting and postprandial ghrelin and peptide-YY levels after Roux-en-Y gastric bypass and sleeve gastrectomy: a prospective double blind study. *Ann Surg, 247*(3), 401–407.
72. Kindel, T., et al. (2014). High failure rate of the laparoscopic adjustable gastric band as a primary bariatric procedure. *Surg Obes Relat Dis, 10*(6), 1070–1075.
73. King, L. K., et al. (2013). Obesity and osteoarthritis. *Indian J Med Res, 138*(2), 185–193.
74. Klein, S., et al. (2011). Economic impact of the clinical benefits of bariatric surgery in diabetes patients with BMI≥35 kg/m^2. *Obesity (Silver Spring), 19*(3), 581–587.
75. Kraschnewski, J. L., et al. (2010). Long term weight loss maintenance in the United States. *Int J Obes (Lond), 34*(11), 1644–1654.
76. Lambert, D. M., Marceau, S., & Force, R. A. (2005). Intra-abdominal pressure in the morbidly obese. *Obes Surg, 15*(9), 1225–1232.
77. Landsberg, L., et al. (2012). Obesity-related hypertension: pathogenesis, cardiovascular risk and treatment. *J Clin Hypertens, 15*(1), 14–33.
78. Lautz, D. B., Jiser, M. E., et al. (2009). An update on best practice guidelines for specialized facilities and resources necessary for weight loss surgical programs. *Obesity (Silver Spring), 17*(5), 911–917.
79. Leblanc, E. S., et al. (2011). Effectiveness of primary care relevant treatments for obesity in adults: a systematic evidence review for the US Preventive Services Task Force. *Ann Intern Med, 155*(7), 434–447.
80. Lee, W. Y., & Mokhlesi, B. (2008). Diagnosis and management of obesity hypoventilation syndrome in the ICU. *Crit Care Clin, 24*(4), 533–549.
81. Longitudinal Assessment of Bariatric Surgery (LABS) Consortium. (2009). Perioperative Safety in the Longitudinal Assessment of Bariatric Surgery. *N Engl J Med, 361*(5), 445–454.
82. Lowe, J. R. (2009). Skin integrity in critically ill obese patients. *Crit Care Nurs Clin North Am, 21*(3), 311–322.
83. Lundstrom, L. H., et al. (2009). High body mass index is a weak predictor for difficult and failed tracheal intubation: a cohort study of 91,332 consecutive patients scheduled for direct laryngoscopy registered in the Danish Anesthesia Database. *Anesthesiology, 110*(2), 266–274.
84. Mallick, A., et al. (2010). Evaluation of a new tracheostomy technique for morbidly obese patients on an intensive care unit. *Crit Care, 14*(Suppl. I) 219.doi:10.11861cc8451.
85. Marchesini, G., et al. (2008). Obesity associated liver disease. *J Clin Endocrinol Metab, 93*(11), S74–S80.
86. Martino, J. L., et al. (2011). Extreme obesity and outcomes in critically ill patients. *Chest, 140*(5), 1198–1206.
87. Masoomi, H., et al. (2011). Factors predictive of venous thromboembolism in bariatric surgery. *Am Surg, 77*(10), 1403–1406.
88. Mathew, A. V., et al. (2011). Obesity related kidney disease. *Curr Diabetes Rev, 7*(1), 41–49.
89. McClave, S. A., Marinadale, R. G., & Vanek, C. W. (2009). ASPEN Board of Directors; American College of Critical Care Medicine; Society of Critical Care Medicine. Guidelines for the provision and assessment of nutrition a support therapy in the adult critically ill patient: society of Critical Care Medicine (SCCM) and American Society for Parenteral and Enteral Nutrition (ASPEN). *JPEN J Parenter Enteral Nutr, 33*(3), 277–316.
90. Mechanick, J. I., Jones, D. B., McMahon, M. M., Adams, T. D., Dixon, J. B., et al. (2013). Clinical practice guidelines for the perioperative nutritional, metabolic, and nonsurgical support of the bariatric surgery patient-2013 update: cosponsored by American Association of Clinical Endocrinologists, The Obesity Society and American Society for Metabolic and Bariatric Surgery. *Endocr Pract, 12*(2), e1–e36.
91. Mingrone, G., et al. (2012). Bariatric surgery vs. conventional medical therapy for type 2 diabetes. *N Engl J Med, 366*(17), 1577–1585.
92. Modica, M. J., & Kanal, K. M. (2011). The obese emergency patient: imaging challenges and solutions. *Radiographics, 31*(3), 811–823. doi http://dx.doi.org/10.1148/rg.313105138.
93. Morandi, A., & Maffeis, C. (2013). Urogenital complications of obesity. *Best Pract Res Clin Endocrinol Metab, 27*(2), 209–218.
94. Murphy, C., & Wong, D. T. (2013). Airway management and oxygenation in obese patients. *Can J Anesth, 60*(9), 929–945.
95. Naguib, M. T. (2014). Kidney disease in the obese patient. *South Med J, 107*(8), 481–485.
96. National Institutes of Health Consensus Development Panel. Gastrointestinal surgery for severe obesity. *Ann Intern Med, 115* (12), 956–961.
97. Neligan, P. J., et al. (2009). Obstructive sleep apnea is not a risk factor for difficult intubation in morbidly obese patients. *Anesth Analg, 109*(4), 1182–1186.
98. Nguyen, N. T., et al. (2015). *The ASMBS textbook of bariatric surgery* (Vol. 1). New York: Springer.
99. Nguyen, N. T., et al. (2011). Trends in use of bariatric surgery, 2003–2008. *J Am Coll Surg, 213*(2), 261–266.
100. Nguyen, N. T., Magno, C. P., Lane, K. T., et al. (2008). Association of hypertension, diabetes, dyslipidemia and metabolic syndrome with obesity: findings from the National Health and Nutrition Examination Survey, 1999–2004. *J Am Coll Surg, 207*(6), 928–934.
101. Obesity Society, American College of Cardiology and American Heart Association. (2014). Guidelines (2013) for managing overweight and obesity in adults–Executive Summary. *Obesity (Silver Spring), 7*(22), S1–S39 doi:10.10221oby20820.
102. Office of the Surgeon General-US Department of Health and Human Services. (2012). Overweight and obesity: health consequences. http://www.surgeongeneral.gov/topics/obesity/calltoaction/fact consequences.html.
103. Oliveros, H., & Villamor, E. (2008). Obesity and mortality in critically ill adults: a systematic review and meta-analysis. *Obesity (Silver Spring), 16*(3), 515–521.
104. Ortiz, V. E., et al. (2015). Strategies for managing oxygenation in obese patients undergoing laparoscopic surgery. *Surg Obes Relat Dis, 11*(3), 721–728.
105. Peavy, W. (2009). Cardiovascular effects of obesity: implications for critical care. *Crit Care Nurs Clin North Am, 21*(3), 293–300.
106. Poirer, P., Cornier, M. A., & Mazzone, T. (2011). Bariatric surgery and cardiovascular risk factors: a scientific statement from the American Heart Association. *Circulation, 123*(15), 1683–1701.
107. Poiries, M., et al. (1999). Who would have thought it? An operation proves to be the most effective therapy for adult-onset diabetes mellitus. *Ann Surg, 222*(3), 339–352.
108. Prentice, A. M. (2001). Fires of life: the struggles of an ancient metabolism in a modern world. *BNF Nutr Bull, 26*(1), 13–27.
109. Rabec, C., et al. (2011). Respiratory complications of obesity. *Arch Bronconeumol, 47*(5), 252–261.
110. Rosenthal, R. J., & Jones, D. B. (Eds.). (2008). *Weight loss surgery: a multidisciplinary approach*. Edgemont, PA: Matrix Medical Communications.
111. SAGES Guidelines Committee. (2008). SAGES guidelines for clinical application of laparoscopic bariatric surgery. *Surg Endosc, 22*(10), 2281–2300.
112. Samad, F., & Ruf, W. (2013). Inflammation, obesity and thrombosis. *Blood, 122*(20), 3415–3422.
113. Schauer, P., et al. (2014). Bariatric surgery vs. intensive medical therapy for diabetes-3 year outcomes. *N Engl J Med, 370*(21), 2002–2013.
114. Schauer, P., et al. (2012). Bariatric surgery vs. intensive medical therapy in obese patients with diabetes. *N Engl J Med, 366*(17), 1567–1576.
115. Shashaty, M. G., & Stapleton, R. D. (2014). Physiological and management implications of obesity in critical illness. *Annals ATS, 11*(8), 1286–1297.
116. Shawky, R. M., & Sadik, D. I. (2012). Genetics of obesity. *The Egyptian Journal of Medical Human Genetics, 13*(1), 11–17.
117. Sherwood, S. F., et al. (2012). Pulmonary considerations and management of the morbidly obese patient. *Bariatr Nurs Surg Patient Care, 7*(4), 160–166.
118. Sing Bajwa, S. J., Sehgal, V., & Bajwa, S. K. (2012). Clinical and critical care concerns in severely ill obese patient. *Ind J Endocrinol Metab, 16*(5), 740–748.
119. Sjostrom, L. (2007). Effects of bariatric surgery on mortality in Swedish obese subjects. *N Engl J Med, 8*(357), 741–752.

120. Stefater, M., et al. (2012). All bariatric surgeries are not created equal: insights from mechanistic comparisons. *Endocr Rev*, *33*(4), 595–622.
121. Stein, P. D., & Matta, F. (2010). Epidemiology and incidence: the scope of the problem and risk factors for the development of venous thromboembolism. *Clin Chest Med*, *31*(4), 611–628.
122. Subak, L. L., et al. (2009). Obesity and urinary incontinence: epidemiology and clinical research update. *J Urol*, *182*(6 Suppl), S2–S7.
123. Talab, H. F., et al. (2009). Intraoperative ventilator strategies for prevention of pulmonary atelectasis in obese patients undergoing laparoscopic bariatric surgery. *Anesth Analg*, *109*(5), 1511–1516.
124. Tchernof, A., & Despres, J. P. (2013). Pathophysiology of human visceral obesity: an update. *Physiol Rev*, *93*(1), 359–404.
125. Thorpe, K. (2009). America's Health Rankings: "The Future Cost of Obesity". http://www.americashealthrankings.org/.
126. Tilg, H., & Kaser, A. (2011). Gut microbiome, obesity, and metabolic dysfunction. *The Journal of Clinical Investigation*, *121*(6), 2126–2132.
127. Turnbaugh, P. J., et al. (2006). An obesity associated gut microbiome with increased capacity for energy harvest. *Nature*, *444*(7122), 1027–1031.
128. Tymitz, K., et al. (2011). Changes in ghrelin levels following bariatric surgery: review of the literature. *Obes Surg*, *21*(1), 125–130.
129. U.S. Department of Health and Human Services. (2013). Managing overweight and obesity in adults: a systematic evidence review from the obesity expert panel. http://www.nhlbi.nih.gov/files/obesity-evidence-review.pdf.
130. VanGilder, C., et al. (2009). Body mass index, weight, and pressure ulcer prevalence: an analysis of the 2006–2007 International Pressure Ulcer Prevalence Surveys. *J Nurs Care Qual*, *24*(2), 127–135.
131. VanGilder, C., et al. (2009). Results of the 2008–2009 International Pressure Ulcer Prevalence Survey and a 3-year, acute care, unit specific analysis. *Ostomy Wound Management*, *55*(11), 39–45.
132. Wang, Y. C., McPherson, K., Marsh, T., et al. (2011). Health and economic burden of the projected obesity trends in the USA and the UK. *Lancet*, *378*(9793), 815–825.
133. Weiss, E. C., et al. (2007). Weight regain in U.S. adults who experienced substantial weight loss 1999–2002. *Am J Prev Med*, *33*(1), 34–40.
134. World Health Organization, Media Centre. (2015). Obesity and overweight. Fact Sheet No. 311, Updated January 2015. http://www.who.int/mediacentre/factsheets/fs311/en/.
135. Wright, S. M., & Aronne, L. J. (2012). Causes of obesity. *Abdom Imaging*, *37*(5), 730–732.

39

Pain and Sedation

Sandra L. Siedlecki

Pain and discomfort are predictable consequences of injury, surgery, disease, and procedures common to critically ill patients. Yet pain and discomfort are frequently not anticipated, recognized, or managed well in the critical care population.[2,7,10,14] Common myths and misconceptions held by healthcare providers, both nurses and providers, are often the cause of poor pain management (Box 39.1). Attempting to correct these misconceptions through education is essential for improving pain management and patient outcomes.[81] Pain impacts all aspects of a person's life, impairing physical, psychological, social, and spiritual well-being[2,17,18,31] (Table 39.1). Pain and discomfort are sources of physical and emotional stress. In response to stress, the autonomic nervous system (ANS) and hypothalamic-pituitary-adrenal (HPA) axis are activated. This activation results in the release of epinephrine and norepinephrine, increasing the work of the cardiovascular and respiratory systems, and at the same time releasing cortisol and various cytokines, altering immune function.[18,31,49,51] Prolonged stress, such as that experienced by critically ill patients, is associated with higher rates of mortality and morbidity.[31,49,83]

Approximately 55,000 Americans will be admitted to critical care units each day this year;[6] nearly all will experience periods of discomfort and pain, and more than half will report their pain as moderate to severe.[80] Although knowledge by healthcare providers related to deleterious effects of uncontrolled pain has improved, nearly 71% of the five million patients admitted to an intensive care unit (ICU) each year remember being in severe pain.[16,80,86] Identification and management of pain in critically ill patients is a challenge complicated by the presence of symptoms associated with major organ damage, system dysfunction or failure, altered mental status, and/or impaired communication. However, few nursing interventions have the potential to improve patient outcomes more than providing comfort, minimizing discomfort, and managing pain.[81]

PATIENTS AT RISK

All critically ill patients are at risk for pain this risk is usually predictable. At increased risk are those who are aged, malnourished, confused, and nonresponsive, and those who have preexisting painful conditions (e.g., diabetic neuropathies or arthritis). Researchers found that more than half of patients were not medicated before or during painful procedures, and when analgesics were used, the amount was insufficient to adequately control pain.[36,66,84] Because pain and discomfort in critical care are often associated with predictable events, procedures, or conditions, they afford the nurse the opportunity to intervene preemptively (Table 39.2). Preemptive nursing interventions are those actions initiated by the nurse in an effort to prevent an anticipated and usually unpleasant situation or occurrence (i.e., pain or discomfort). Preemptive nursing interventions designed to promote comfort and to decrease pain should be initiated for all critically ill patients and continued throughout their hospitalization.

ACUTE VERSUS CHRONIC PAIN

Pain is most frequently classified by duration. Acute pain is a symptom that alerts the body to a potential threat, usually has an identifiable and treatable etiology, and diminishes with healing.[22,55,56] Critically ill patients often experience acute pain in several body locations simultaneously because of multiple injuries (e.g., trauma) or various insults (e.g., surgery, procedures) to the skin, bone, tissue, and/or organs. In addition, acute pain accompanies tissue injury that results in inflammation, complicating the nociceptive process and the body's response.[27,49,54,69]

BOX 39.1 Pain Myths

- Physical and behavioral symptoms are more reliable than self-report for assessing the presence of pain and its intensity.
- Pain rating scales are not reliable measures of pain in children, the older adult or those with any cognitive impairment.
- Complaints of pain that occur in the absence of tissue damage are probably psychosomatic or psychogenic in origin.
- Pain intensity is directly related to size of wound or amount of tissue damage, suggesting a uniform pain threshold.
- The more frequent and severe the pain, the more tolerant patients become.
- Analgesics should be withheld until a definitive diagnosis is made, to prevent the masking of important symptoms.
- Cancer pain is more severe than noncancer pain.
- Opioid abuse and addiction are common complications associated with the use of opioid analgesics to manage acute or chronic pain.
- Response to placebo analgesic is proof of malingering.
- Infants do not require analgesics, as their neurologic system is too immature to recognize and transmit nociceptive impulses.

From References 10, 21, and 65.

TABLE 39.1 Physiologic Consequences of Unrelieved Pain

System	Physiologic Effect	Clinical Manifestations
Endocrine/metabolic	Release of ADH, ACTH, cortisol, catecholamines (epinephrine and norepinephrine), and insulin	Weight loss, fever Increased respiratory and heart rates Fluid retention Shock
Cardiovascular	Sympathetic stimulation Increased vascular resistance Increased myocardial oxygen demand Hypercoagulation	Increased heart rate Increased blood pressure Unstable angina Myocardial ischemia Deep vein thrombosis
Respiratory	Decreased ventilatory effort	Atelectasis Pneumonia Acid-base disturbance
Gastrointestinal	Decreased gastric emptying Decreased gastric motility Hypermetabolic state	Anorexia Constipation/ileus Malnutrition
Musculoskeletal	Muscle spasm or cramping Muscle rigidity	Decreased range of motion Muscle weakness and/or fatigue
Genitourinary	Abnormal release of hormones (ADH, aldosterone) that affect urine output, fluid volume, and electrolyte balance	Decreased urine output Fluid retention Electrolyte disturbance Acid-base disturbance
Immune	Increased cortisol levels suppress inflammatory and immune response, decreasing number of circulating leukocytes and inhibiting their ability to migrate by decreasing capillary permeability Cortisol also inhibits release of histamine and prostaglandins, which depresses phagocyte activity High cortisol levels inhibit production of cytokines essential for mounting an immune response (IL-1)	Delayed wound healing Infection/sepsis

ACTH, Adrenocorticotropic hormone; *ADH*, antidiuretic hormone; *IL*, interleukin.

In contrast to acute pain, chronic pain is a syndrome rather than a symptom; it serves no useful purpose, persists for more than 6 months, and may or may not have a known cause.[69,73] Although the critically ill patient is most likely to experience acute pain during hospitalization, it should not be forgotten that many patients may have a preexisting chronic pain condition that also needs to be addressed. Of special concern are chronic pain patients who were using opioids for baseline pain management before admission and patients with a history of drug addiction or abuse. These patients may experience severe withdrawal symptoms if baseline levels of opioids are not maintained or if antagonists (e.g., naloxone hydrochloride [Narcan]) are administered. Collection of medical history information (from patient and/or family member) is essential to prevent this scenario. However, as prevention is not always possible, the nurse should be alert for symptoms of opioid withdrawal in all critically ill patients, because early recognition will prevent untoward complications (Box 39.2).

TABLE 39.2 Painful or Uncomfortable Conditions and Procedures

Conditions	Procedures
Environmental	**Line Placement**
Noise Odors Temperature	Arterial lines Central lines Peripheral lines
Musculoskeletal and/or Integument Trauma	**Tube or Drains (Insertion/Removal)**
Abrasions Burns Bruising Fractures Lacerations	Chest tubes Indwelling urinary catheters Nasogastric tubes
Thoracic and/or Abdominal Trauma	**Ventilation Support**
Blunt force injury Hemothorax Pneumothorax Rib fractures	Intubation Mechanical ventilation Suctioning Weaning
Disease	**Wound Care**
Arthritis Cancer Neuropathies Sickle cell anemia	Dressing changes Sutures or suture removal Wound irrigations
Side Effects of Treatment	**Surgery**
Constipation Ileus Nausea/vomiting	Emergency Routine
Physical	**Diagnostic Tests**
Hunger Shortness of breath Hygiene Immobility Positioning Thirst	Lab work Hemodynamic tests Radiologic tests

BOX 39.2 Symptoms Associated with Opioid Withdrawal

Mild Symptoms

- Restlessness
- Mydriasis (pupil dilation)
- Lacrimation
- Rhinorrhea
- Sneezing
- Piloerection
- Yawning
- Perspiration
- Restless sleep
- Aggressive behavior

Severe Symptoms

- Muscle spasm
- Back pain
- Abdominal pain (cramping)
- Hot and cold flashes (chills alternating with diaphoresis)
- Insomnia
- Nausea and vomiting
- Diarrhea
- Tachypnea
- Hypertension or hypotension
- Tachycardia, bradycardia, or other cardiac dysrhythmias

Peripheral Versus Central Pain

Because there is a high concentration of nerve endings in cutaneous tissue, injury to the skin produces a well-defined and localized pain. In contrast, somatic pain occurs in response to injury of ligaments, tendons, bones, and blood vessels. With few nociceptors located in these areas, pain is usually dull and poorly localized. Visceral pain is the result of activation of nociceptors located in organs and body cavities. Because of the scarcity of nociceptors in these areas, the pain is diffuse and poorly localized, and is described as a persistent aching.[52,53,55,73]

Pain can be classified as either peripheral or central in origin. Trauma to peripheral nerves results in neurogenic pain, whereas damage to the central nervous system (CNS) results in neuropathic pain. The main reason for distinguishing between origins of pain is to better understand the routes of transmission of painful stimuli. Nociceptive pain is a time-limited response to actual or potential tissue injury that serves as a protective mechanism (Table 39.3). In contrast, neurogenic pain and neuropathic pain are the result of a nervous system malfunction related to disease or injury to the peripheral or CNS (Table 39.4). Neurogenic or neuropathic pain can be caused by disorders such as diabetes, infiltration or compression of nerves by tumor or scar tissue, and inflammation attributable to infection.[8,22,27,51,55]

Pain Theory

The gate control theory (GCT), first described in 1968 by Melzack and Wall, identifies pain as a subjective experience composed of three components: (1) a sensory-discriminative component, described in terms of intensity, location, or quality of pain; (2) a motivational-affective component, characterized by feelings of anxiety, fear, or depression; and (3) a cognitive-evaluative component, responsive to thoughts about cause or meaning of the pain.[52,54,55] This multidimensional conceptualization of pain emphasizes the broad range of factors that contribute to the experience of pain.

Pain perception is dependent on a system of sensory neurons (nociceptors) and neural afferent pathways that respond to noxious stimuli (Fig. 39.1). In response to tissue damage, cells release neurochemical substances that stimulate nociceptors, causing them to discharge. Once discharged, the nociceptive impulse is transmitted by way of fast, myelinated A-delta fibers

TABLE 39.3 Characteristics of Nociceptive Pain

	Cutaneous	Somatic	Visceral
Nociceptors	Superficial: skin and mucous membranes	Deep: muscles, joints, and bones	Visceral organs*
Stimulus	External: mechanical, chemical, or thermal	External mechanical or internal chemical	Internal mechanical or chemical
Localization	Very specific; related to point of tissue injury	Diffuse or radiating but generally associated with area of injury	Generalized and poorly localized
Quality	Sharp, pinching, or burning	Dull, aching, cramping	Sharp, stabbing, and deep aching
Signs and symptoms	Tenderness, erythema, or edema to specific area of injury	Tenderness, spasm, or edema in and around general area Tachycardia, hypertension, diaphoresis, muscle tension, nausea and vomiting	General malaise, fever, diaphoresis, nausea, vomiting, and generalized pain and tenderness
Etiology	Burns, abrasions, lacerations	Sprains, strains, tendinitis, fractures, arthritis	Organ or system inflammation, blockage, or pressure on organ because of lesions or tumors

*Visceral organs are the heart, lungs, liver, bowels, and others.
From References 17, 16, 30, and 37.

TABLE 39.4 Characteristics of Neuropathic Pain

	PERIPHERAL NERVOUS SYSTEM			CENTRAL NERVOUS SYSTEM
	Neuropathies	**Deafferentation**	**Sympathetic**	**Central**
Explanation	Pain caused by peripheral nerve damage	Loss of sensory input from a portion of the body, caused by interruption of peripheral sensory nerve fibers	Pain caused by sympathetic activity	Pain caused by primary CNS lesion or dysfunction
Pain quality	Cutaneous: deep burning, aching Paroxysmal: lancing	Burning, cramping, crushing, aching, stabbing, shooting	Burning, throbbing, shooting	Burning, numbing, shooting, tingling
Associated symptoms	Abnormal skin sensation	Hyperalgesia,* hyperpathia*	Allodynia,* ANS dysregulation	Sensory loss, allodynia,* hyperalgesia*
Etiology	Diabetes, alcohol abuse, herpetic disorder, repetitive motion injury	Damage to peripheral nerve or nerve plexus	Damage to peripheral nerve with stimulation by circulating catecholamines	CNS damage caused by ischemia, tumors, injury, or demyelinating* disorders
Disorder examples	Diabetic and alcoholic neuropathies,* postherpetic neuralgia,* carpal tunnel syndrome	Phantom limb pain, postmastectomy pain	Complex regional pain syndromes, phantom limb pain, postherpetic neuralgia	Poststroke syndrome, multiple sclerosis

*Hyperalgesia, excessive sensitivity to pain; hyperpathia, a painful syndrome characterized by increased reaction to a stimulus, especially a repetitive stimulus, as well as an increased pain threshold; allodynia, condition in which normally nonpainful stimuli evoke pain; demyelinating disorders, diseases in which the myelin sheath of nerves is destroyed; neuropathy, a general term denoting functional or pathologic changes in peripheral nervous system. Involvement of one nerve is mononeuropathy, involvement of several nerves is polyneuropathy.
From Reference 85.

and slow, unmyelinated C-fibers to the dorsal horn of the spinal cord, where it is processed in the substantia gelatinosa (SG). In the SG, C-fibers release substance P, glutamate, aspartate, calcitonin gene-related peptide (CGRP), and nitric oxide, responsible for dorsal horn pain transmission. In the spinal cord, some impulses cross directly over to the anterior horn, where they stimulate sympathetic neurons and produce a reflex response (reflex arc). Other impulses cross the cord and ascend to the thalamus by way of the spinothalamic tract. The impulse is then transmitted to the cerebral cortex and the limbic system, where it is interpreted in light of physical, emotional, environmental, and personal factors that are unique to each person and each situation (Fig. 39.2).[27,52,54,55]

Nociception and Inflammation

Nociceptors are nonspecific nerve endings that lie adjacent to blood vessels and mast cells. These structures create a functional unit that efficiently responds to tissue injury by initiation of an inflammatory response (Fig. 39.3). In the presence of tissue damage, inflammation and physiologic changes occur that increase the sensation of pain.[52,54,55] The release of proinflammatory mediators (i.e., histamine, bradykinin, and prostaglandins) results in a lower sensory neuron threshold, leading to peripheral sensitization. Peripheral sensitization allows previously benign sensations, such as light touch, to cause pain (allodynia) by lowering the pain threshold. Inflammation also increases pain perception by altering properties and functions of neurons, through a process known as phenotypic switch or change, making more nociceptors available to transmit noxious stimuli.[51,52,54,55]

Central sensitization also affects pain impulse transmission. Central sensitization increases excitability and responsiveness of CNS neurons,[29,30,73] and has two major phases. The immediate nociceptive-dependent phase affects neurons in the dorsal horn, causing an effect similar to peripheral sensitization. In the delayed phase, inflammation results in hyperexcitability of CNS neurons, and blockage of descending inhibitory pain pathways. The combination of peripheral sensitization, phenotypic change, and central sensitization leads to a heightened response to painful stimuli, attributable to an increased response to stimuli (hyperalgesia) and a lowered pain threshold (allodynia).[29,30,73] Current research indicates that even a short period of persistent nociceptive activity can result in long-term changes in neural function that increase duration and intensity of pain.[29,30,55]

RESPONSE TO PAIN

The body responds to pain through the production of neurochemicals (i.e., serotonin, norepinephrine, zinc, endorphins) in the brain and spinal tract that work by blocking release of substance P at the synapse, or by blocking substance P receptor sites. GCT posits that, at each synapse, there is a gate either opened by release of substance P or closed by inhibition of substance P.[29,30,52,55] The mechanism of action for both pharmacologic and nonpharmacologic pain interventions is frequently explained through GCT. Because the perception of pain is influenced and directed by activity in the cerebral cortex and limbic system, interventions and environments that facilitate freedom from worry or stress, rest, and feelings of hope and control should close gates and raise the pain threshold.[29,30] In contrast, physical discomfort, fear, sadness, anxiety, isolation, and sleeplessness will lower the pain threshold, making patients more sensitive to pain and less sensitive to pain-inhibiting interventions.[49]

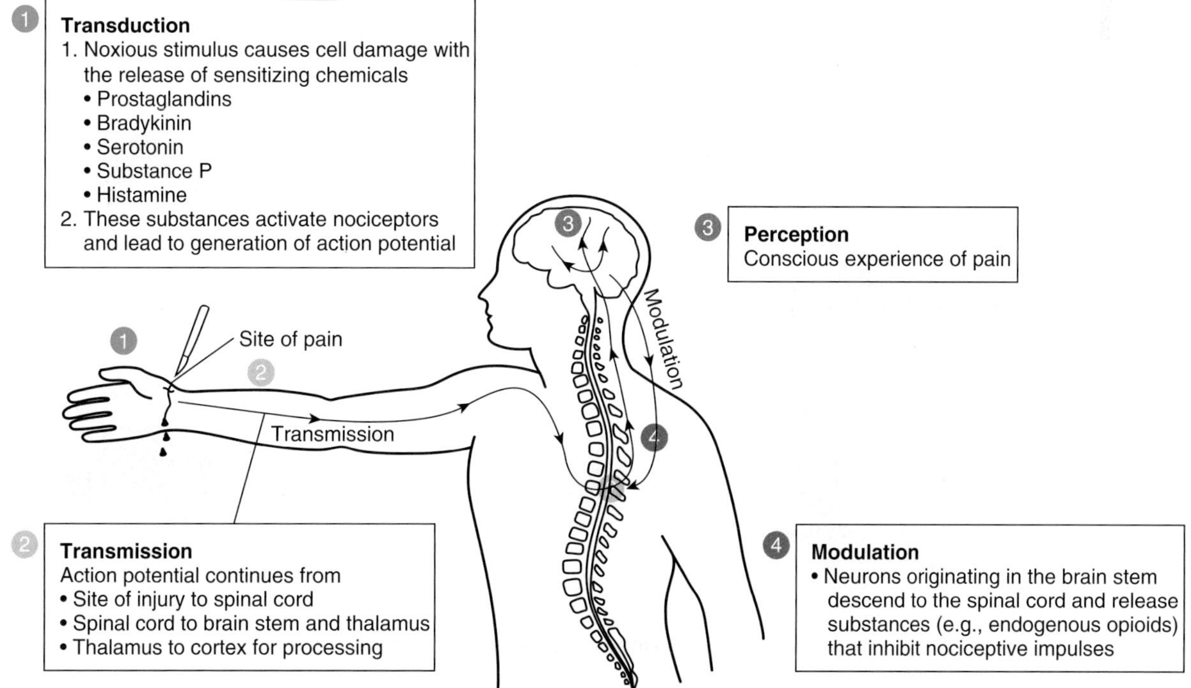

FIG. 39.1 **Pain transmission.** (From Lewis, S. L., Dirksen, S. R., Heitkemper, M. M., Bucher, L. (2014). *Medical surgical nursing: assessment and management of clinical problems* (9th ed.). St Louis: Elsevier.)

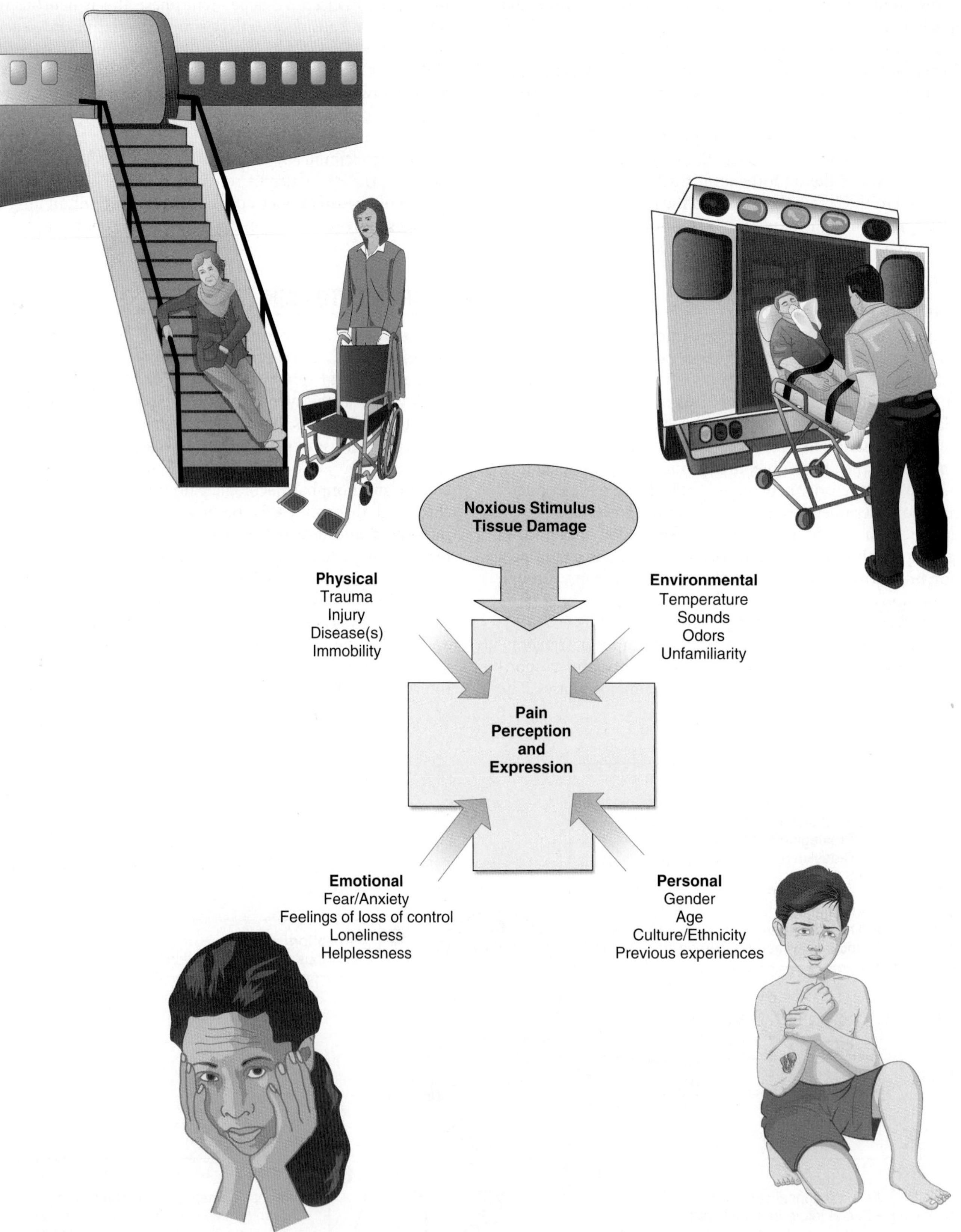

FIG. 39.2 Responses to noxious stimuli.

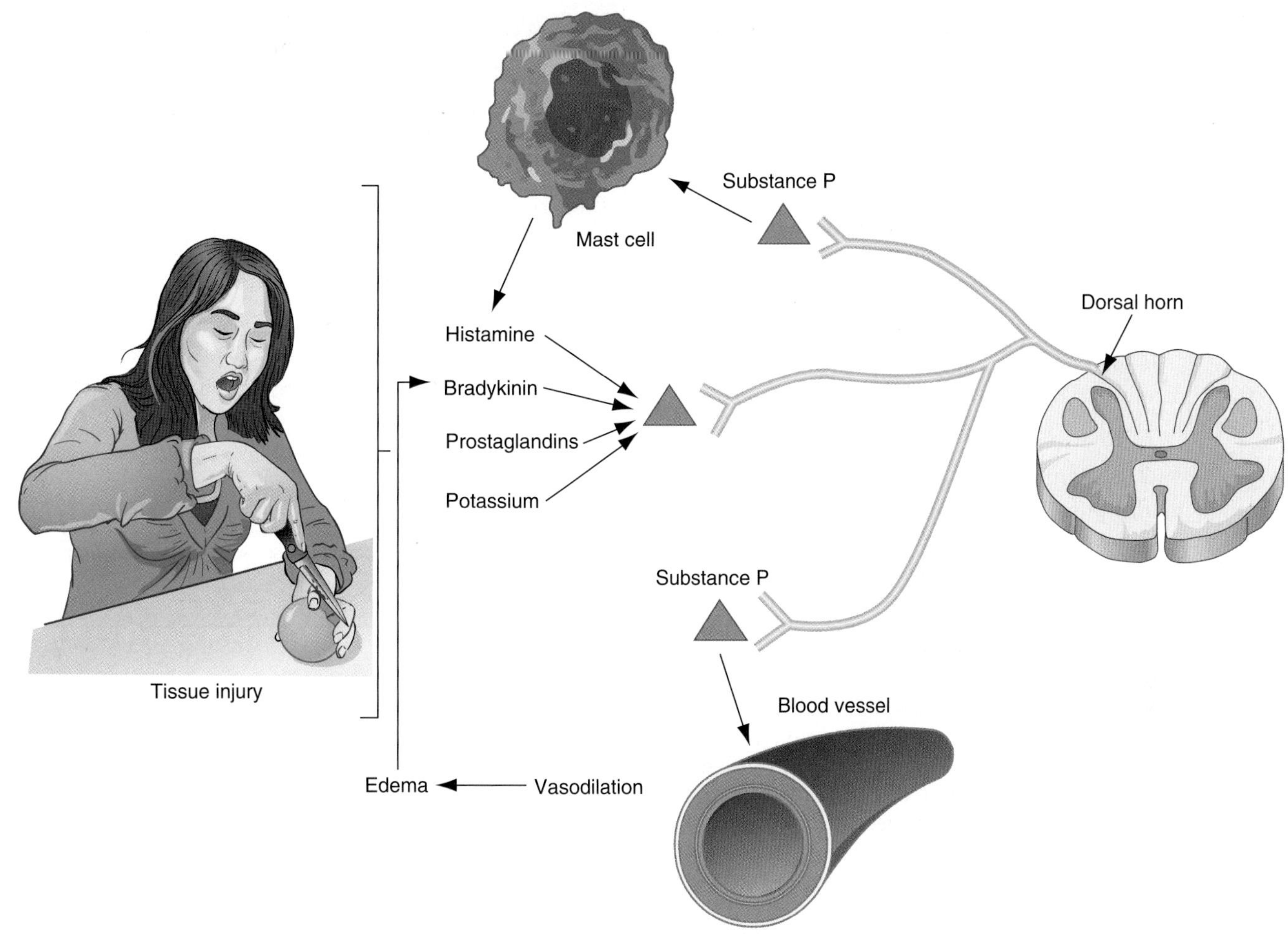

FIG. 39.3 Nociceptive chemical mediation.

The human body possesses its own analgesic system. In response to stress or injury, specific endogenous opioids (i.e., enkephalins, beta-endorphins, and dynorphins) are released, modulating pain impulses at multiple locations.[29,30,49] Distributed in the dorsal horn and periaqueductal gray (PAG) in the midbrain and brain stem, enkephalins are the most widely distributed endogenous opioids in the human body.[52,54,55] Of the three endogenous opioids, beta-endorphins produce the most morphine-like analgesic effect. The site of action and activation is the hypothalamus and pituitary gland. The most powerful of the endogenous opioids are dynorphins present in PAG and the spinal cord. These endogenous opioids moderate transmission of painful stimuli by altering release and activation of substance P.[52] To affect transmission of pain, endogenous opioids bind to opioid receptors. There are at least three types of receptors (i.e., mu, kappa, and delta) (Table 39.5). Enkephalins bind with delta receptors, dynorphins bind with kappa receptors, and endorphins bind with mu and delta receptor sites. Mu receptors are located in laminae III and IV of the cortex, thalamus, PAG, and substantia gelatinosa and when activated provide supraspinal analgesia. Kappa receptors, located in the hypothalamus, PAG, and substantia gelatinosa, provide spinal analgesia; delta receptors, located in the amygdala, olfactory bulbs, and deep cortex, provide general analgesia.[52,54,55]

TABLE 39.5 **Opioid Receptor Responses to Activation**

	RECEPTOR SITES		
Activation Response	**MU**	**KAPPA**	**DELTA**
Analgesia	X	X	X
Respiratory depression	X	X	
Miosis	X	X	
Mydriasis			X
Decreased gastrointestinal motility	X		
Hypothermia	X		
Hallucinations			X
Dysphoria		X	X
Euphoria	X		
Psychomimetic effects		X	

Modified from Reference 4.

Stress Response Theory

A discussion of the pathophysiology of pain in critically ill patients would be incomplete without inclusion of the psychoneuroimmune (PNI) response to stress. Critically ill patients experience significant and prolonged exposure to stress from multiple sources related to injury and/or interventions. Stress produces a nonspecific response to a perceived threat. The body reacts to acute physical, emotional, and environmental stressors through activation of a complex series of PNI responses.[17,18,27,49,51,83] Evidence also demonstrates that prolonged, unrelieved pain can lead to post traumatic stress syndrome and cause long-term complications.[40]

The HPA axis and the ANS are responsible for modulation of the stress response. Physiologic responses occur when signals are transmitted from the limbic system to sympathetic neurons in the spinal cord, causing postganglionic nerves to release catecholamines (i.e., epinephrine and norepinephrine) to the heart, peripheral vessels, lungs, adrenal medulla, and liver. Catecholamine release activates the sympathetic nervous system (SNS), resulting in increased blood pressure and heart rate.[49]

Activation of the HPA axis begins with hypothalamic stimulation of the pituitary through corticotropin-releasing hormone (CRH), causing release of adrenocorticotropic hormone (ACTH). In response to release of ACTH, the adrenal cortex releases cortisol and dehydroepiandrosterone (DHEA). Activation of the HPA axis inhibits immune and inflammatory responses through the activity of glucocorticoids. Glucocorticoids directly affect leukocyte movement and function, and alter production of cytokines that mediate the inflammatory process. At the same time, ANS activation induces release of interleukin-6 (IL-6). IL-6 helps to control inflammation by further stimulating secretion of glucocorticoids and suppressing secretion of IL-1 and tumor necrosis factor-alpha. Finally, catecholamines, released by activation of the ANS, inhibit IL-12 and stimulate IL-10, resulting in suppression of cellular immunity.[18,49]

The stress response was intended to protect the body from effects of acute stress. However, a prolonged response, as seen in critically ill patients, can affect wound healing, fluid balance, metabolism, and cardiac and respiratory workload. Each of these potential complications can become additional stressors for the critically ill patient. The goal of nursing care for critically ill patients should be to minimize the number of stressors, moderate the severity of stressors, and provide interventions that can counteract negative effects of stress.[10,17,18]

Guidelines Proposed by The Joint Commission

Recognizing that pain is a common component of nearly every patient's hospital experience and that unrelieved pain has negative physical and emotional consequences, in January, 2001, the Joint Commission on Accreditation of Healthcare Organizations (JCAHO) proposed pain assessment and management standards for hospitals.[60] This standard was updated in 2014 by The Joint Commission (TJC).[45] One of the standards directly impacting the critical care nurse is the right of all patients to have appropriate assessment of pain (Box 39.3). Pain assessment is used to evaluate the effectiveness of interventions, both pharmacologic and nonpharmacologic, and includes measures of pain intensity, quality, frequency, location, and duration, appropriate for the patient's age and condition.[60]

BOX 39.3 Principles of Pain Assessment and Management

- All patients have the right to appropriate assessment and management of their pain.
- Assess for pain in all patients at least with each set of vital signs and more often if indicated.
- Believe the patient's self-report. Pain is subjective and self-report is the most reliable indicator of pain.
- Do not rely on vital signs or behaviors. Physiologic signs (such as vital signs [e.g., tachycardia]) or behaviors (e.g., crying or grimacing) do not correlate well with pain and should not be used in place of self-report to assess pain.
- Assessment of pain should be appropriate to the patient population, taking into account language, culture, age, and cognitive and motor function.
- There are no neurophysiologic or laboratory tests that can be used to measure pain. Pain can exist even when no physiologic cause can be found.
- The same stimulus does not elicit the same response in different patients. There is no standard pain response.
- Chronic pain may make patients more sensitive to pain from other sources.
- Unrelieved pain has adverse physical and emotional consequences.

From References 10, 25, 42, and 45.

MEASURING AND ASSESSING PAIN

Pain is a subjective experience described as a hurt of varying intensity, whatever the experiencing person says it is, existing whenever the experiencing person says it does; or as an unpleasant sensory and emotional experience associated with actual or potential tissue damage, or described as such. As a subjective experience, there are no neurophysiologic or laboratory tests used to measure pain.[45] Research demonstrates perceptions of pain are poorly correlated with physiologic measures such as blood pressure, heart rate, and respiratory rate; therefore, pain is best assessed through self-report. However, obtaining self-report measures of pain from patients who are critically ill and often unable to communicate presents a major challenge for critical care nurses.[15,37,39,42,45,66,80]

There are numerous instruments available for assessing quantity of pain in patients who are able to provide self-report. The Visual Analog Scale (VAS) is one of the pain instruments used most frequently in research studies. However, patients often find it difficult to complete the VAS because it requires intact motor and cognitive function. The VAS consists of a 100-mm horizontal line with two anchors (Fig. 39.4). The anchor on the left side of the line is labeled *no pain* and the anchor on the right is labeled *worst pain imagined.*[23] Patients are instructed to make a mark through the horizontal line that corresponds to their current level of pain. The scale is interpreted by placing a 100-mm rule along the bottom of the line and reading from left to right, recording in millimeters the place where the patient's mark crossed the horizontal line.[17] For patients who must complete this scale lying down, it has been suggested that converting the VAS to a 100-mm vertical line, with *no pain* at the bottom and *worst pain imagined* at the top, would make it easier for patients to use. However, in clinical practice the VAS is at best difficult for patients to use, and cumbersome for nurses to interpret.

The more useful clinical pain assessment instruments, for patients who are able to provide self-report, are verbal rating scales (VRS), numerical rating scales (NRS), and the FACES scale. Of the three, the VRS is used most often in clinical settings. To use the VRS, the nurse asks the patient to rate the current level of pain on a scale from 0 to 10, in which 0 is *no pain* and 10 is the *worst pain imagined,* and then the nurse records

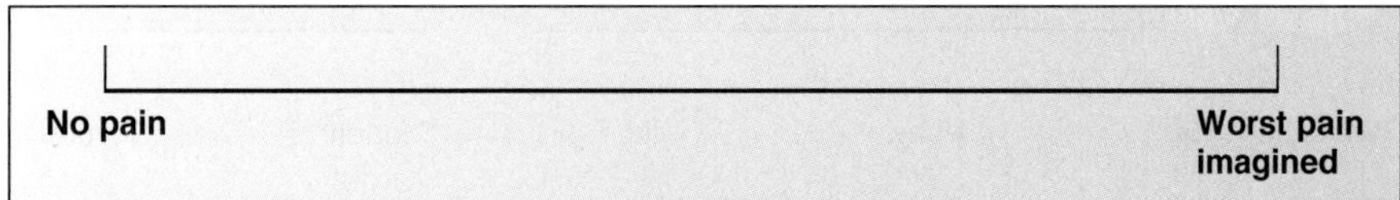

On the line below, indicate how much pain you are currently experiencing by placing a slash mark across the line.

FIG. 39.4 Visual analog scale.

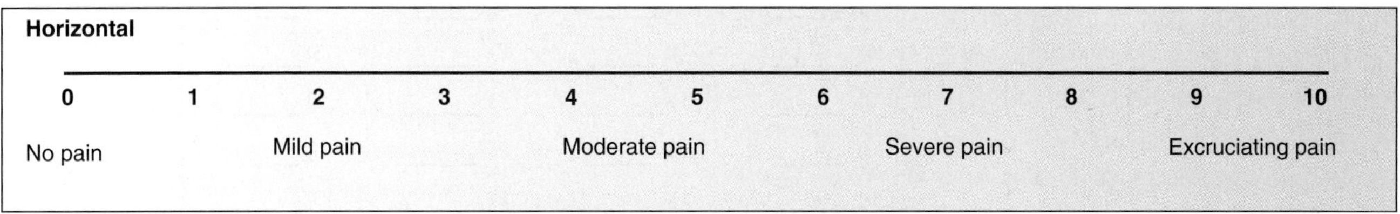

FIG. 39.5 Numerical pain rating scale.

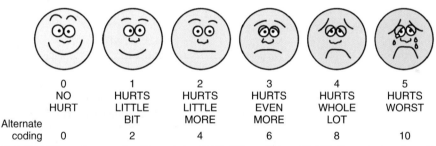

Brief word instructions: Point to each face using the words to describe the pain intensity. Ask the patient to choose the face that best describes own pain and record the appropriate number.

1 HURTS LITTLE BIT
2 HURTS LITTLE MORE

4 HURTS WHOLE LOT
5 HURTS WORST
Alternate coding 0 2 4 6 8 10

FIG. 39.6 FACES rating scale. (Copyright 1983, Wong-Baker FACES Foundation. http://www.WongBakerFACES.org. Used with permission. Originally published in *Whaley & Wong's nursing care of infants and children.* © Elsevier Inc.)

the patient's level of pain as the number (whole number and/or fraction) provided. In clinical practice, patients seem able to identify changes in pain halfway between two numbers, indicating that even small changes may be clinically significant. Although 0 to 10 is the most frequently used VRS, some facilities use a 0 to 5 VRS. The 0 to 10 scale offers more variability and therefore is theoretically more sensitive to change; however, the most important factor when using either the 0 to 10 or the 0 to 5 scale is consistency. It is recommended that a single or limited set of pain assessment tools with similar variability and end points be used consistently within a facility.

The NRS is a written version of the VRS and requires intact motor and cognitive function. Patients are usually instructed to circle the number that corresponds to their current level of pain (Fig. 39.5). The NRS score can vary from 0 to 5 or from 0 to 10. Anchor phrases that correspond to the numbers are no pain, mild pain, moderate pain, severe pain, and excruciating pain. Anchor phrases are labeled below a horizontal line or to the left of a vertical line, depending on the type of scale. Although instructed to circle a single number on the NRS, patients will often indicate a level of pain between pain categories. Because pain levels are recorded in whole numbers, the NRS may be less sensitive than the VAS to small, though clinically significant, changes in pain.

The FACES scale has several variations, and is useful for individuals who are able to self-report but may have communication limitations (Fig. 39.6). The FACES scale is often used with children, elderly, confused patients, or patients who speak a different language. Patients are presented a card with six faces that correspond to levels of pain, and asked to point to the face best describing their current level of pain.[44] For patients who are heavily sedated or for those with cognitive impairment, this scale may be the most useful. However, it is not as sensitive to small changes in pain as the VAS, VRS, and NRS.

In addition to assessing pain intensity, it is important to obtain a complete assessment including pain location, pain

Short-Form McGill Pain Questionnaire
Ronald Melzack

Patient's name: ______________________ Date: ____________

	Pain Rating Index	None	Mild	Moderate	Severe
1.	Throbbing	0) ____	1) ____	2) ____	3) ____
2.	Shooting	0) ____	1) ____	2) ____	3) ____
3.	Stabbing	0) ____	1) ____	2) ____	3) ____
4.	Sharp	0) ____	1) ____	2) ____	3) ____
5.	Cramping	0) ____	1) ____	2) ____	3) ____
6.	Gnawing	0) ____	1) ____	2) ____	3) ____
7.	Hot-burning	0) ____	1) ____	2) ____	3) ____
8.	Aching	0) ____	1) ____	2) ____	3) ____
9.	Heavy	0) ____	1) ____	2) ____	3) ____
10.	Tender	0) ____	1) ____	2) ____	3) ____
11.	Splitting	0) ____	1) ____	2) ____	3) ____
12.	Tiring-exhausting	0) ____	1) ____	2) ____	3) ____
13.	Sickening	0) ____	1) ____	2) ____	3) ____
14.	Fearful	0) ____	1) ____	2) ____	3) ____
15.	Punishing-cruel	0) ____	1) ____	2) ____	3) ____

Visual Analog Scale — No pain |————————| Worst possible pain

Present Pain Index

0. No pain ____
1. Mild ____
2. Discomforting ____
3. Distressing ____
4. Horrible ____
5. Excruciating ____

To complete the top of the questionnaire, the Pain Rating Index, the patient places a check mark in the column that represents the degree to which he or she feels each type of pain. Next, to indicate the overall pain experience, the patient places a tick mark on the Visual Analog Scale. The mark is interpreted as a number from 0 to 10. Finally, the patient selects the term on the Present Pain Index that best describes his or her current status. The clinician adds the numbers in each of the three sections to determine the patient's score.

FIG. 39.7 McGill pain questionnaire. (From Dr. Ronald Melzack, Department of Psychology, McGill University. Used with permission.)

quality (e.g., sharp, dull, burning, and aching) at each location, pain duration, and factors that increase or decrease the pain. Quality and location of pain may provide information related to pathophysiology of the patient's injury or disease, and changes may indicate changes in the patient's condition. Assessing duration of pain and factors the patient perceives to increase or decrease pain provides information that can assist the nurse in developing individualized strategies to maximize comfort. There are several instruments available for assessing location and/or quality of pain. The McGill Pain Questionnaire (MPQ), available in both long-form and short-form versions, can provide data on the sensory, affective, and evaluative nature of the pain experience[53] (Fig. 39.7). Another instrument commonly used for initial pain assessment is the Brief Pain Inventory (BPI), available in both long-form and short-form versions (Fig. 39.8). The BPI is especially useful for recording baseline pain assessment data, and covers location, quality, quantity, and duration of pain. Drawbacks to use of MPQ and BPI are

STUDY ID #:_________ DO NOT WRITE ABOVE THIS LINE HOSPITAL #:_________

Brief Pain Inventory (Short Form)

Date:____/____/____ Time: _______

Name: ________________ ________________ ____________
Last First Middle Initial

1. Throughout our lives, most of us have had pain from time to time (such as minor headaches, sprains, and toothaches). Have you had pain other than these everyday kinds of pain today?

   1. Yes 2. No

2. On the diagram, shade in the areas where you feel pain. Put an X on the area that hurts the most.

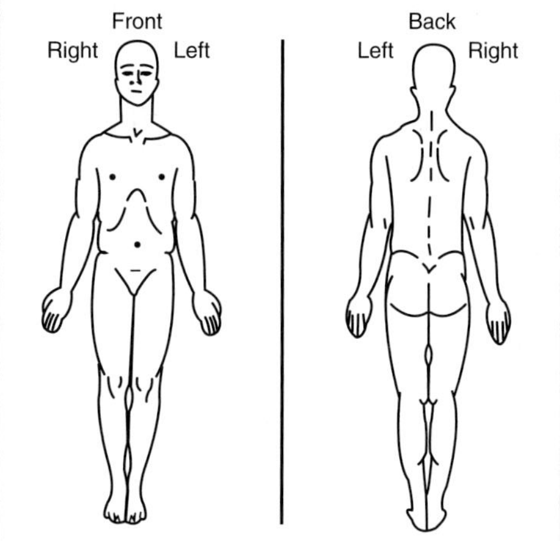

Front
Right Left

Back
Left Right

3. Please rate your pain by circling the one number that best describes your pain at its **worst** in the last 24 hours.

   0 1 2 3 4 5 6 7 8 9 10
   No Pain — Pain as bad as you can imagine

4. Please rate your pain by circling the one number that best describes your pain at its **least** in the last 24 hours.

   0 1 2 3 4 5 6 7 8 9 10
   No Pain — Pain as bad as you can imagine

5. Please rate your pain by circling the one number that best describes your pain on the **average**.

   0 1 2 3 4 5 6 7 8 9 10
   No Pain — Pain as bad as you can imagine

6. Please rate your pain by circling the one number that tells how much pain you have **right now**.

   0 1 2 3 4 5 6 7 8 9 10
   No Pain — Pain as bad as you can imagine

FIG. 39.8 Brief pain inventory. (Copyright 1991, Charles S. Cleeland, PhD, Pain Research Group. Used by permission.)

Continued

STUDY ID #:_________ DO NOT WRITE ABOVE THIS LINE HOSPITAL #:_________

Date:____/____/____ Time: _______

Name: ________________ ________________ ____________

Last First Middle Initial

7. What treatments or medications are you receiving for your pain?

____

8. In the last 24 hours, how much relief have pain treatments or medications provided? Please circle the one percentage that most shows how much **relief** you have received.

0% No Relief 10% 20% 30% 40% 50% 60% 70% 80% 90% 100% Complete Relief

9. Circle the one number that describes how, during the past 24 hours, pain has interfered with your:

A. General Activity

0 Does not Interfere 1 2 3 4 5 6 7 8 9 10 Completely Interferes

B. Mood

0 Does not Interfere 1 2 3 4 5 6 7 8 9 10 Completely Interferes

C. Walking Ability

0 Does not Interfere 1 2 3 4 5 6 7 8 9 10 Completely Interferes

D. Normal Work (includes both work outside the home and housework)

0 Does not Interfere 1 2 3 4 5 6 7 8 9 10 Completely Interferes

E. Relations With Other People

0 Does not Interfere 1 2 3 4 5 6 7 8 9 10 Completely Interferes

F. Sleep

0 Does not Interfere 1 2 3 4 5 6 7 8 9 10 Completely Interferes

G. Enjoyment of Life

0 Does not Interfere 1 2 3 4 5 6 7 8 9 10 Completely Interferes

FIG. 39.8, Cont'd

BOX 39.4 Guidelines for Assessing Pain in Patients Who Cannot Communicate

- Allow sufficient time to adequately assess patient's ability to respond to verbal or written communication.
- When in doubt, attempt use of rating scales appropriate for your population considering age, language, and functional ability.
- Follow the *Hierarchy of Indicators for Pain Assessment,* based on guidelines developed by the American Pain Society and recommended by TJC:[43,58]
  1. Patient self-report
  2. Exposure to pathologic conditions, injuries, or procedures known to be painful
  3. Reports from family members
  4. Pain-related behaviors, such as grimacing, restlessness, guarding, or crying out*
  5. Vital signs*

*Note that pain-related behaviors and vital signs are used as indicators of pain only when no other alternatives exist.

TABLE 39.6 Behavioral Pain Scale (BPS)

Item	Description	Score
Facial expression	Relaxed	1
	Partially tightened (e.g., brow lowering)	2
	Fully tightened (e.g., eyelid closing)	3
	Grimacing	4
Upper limb movements	No movement	1
	Partially bent	2
	Fully bent with finger flexion	3
	Permanently retracted	4
Compliance with mechanical ventilation	Tolerating movement	1
	Coughing but tolerating ventilation for the most of time	2
	Fighting ventilator	3
	Unable to control ventilation	4

BPS score ranges from 3 (no pain) to 12 (maximum pain).

that they require patients to have motor and cognitive function sufficient for providing self-report. In addition, unlike the VAS, VRS, and NRS, which take moments to complete and are sensitive to change over time, the MPQ and BPI take several minutes to complete and are less sensitive to small changes over brief periods.

The real challenge for critical care nurses is monitoring and assessing pain in patients who are not able to self-report (Box 39.4).[7,38,81] When patients are unable to provide self-report, the next consideration for the nurse is to assess the patient's risk for pain by considering that pain may be present because of pathologic conditions, disease, injury, equipment, positioning, or procedures.

Currently the Behavioral Pain Scale (BPS) and the Critical-Care Pain Observation Tool (CPOT) are recommended as the most valid and reliable of those available.[7,38] The BPS (Table 39.6) relies on observation of facial expressions, arm movement, and ventilation tolerance as indicators of pain.[7] The CPOT (Table 39.7) looks at facial expression and ventilator compliance, but it also looks at both general muscle movement and muscle tension.[7,38] Scores on the CPOT can range from 0 (no pain) to 8 (maximum pain), with scores greater than 2 considered as the cutoff score during nociceptive procedures.[38] One criticism or limitation of the CPOT is that there have been limited studies that have explored the use of the CPOT in critically ill patients with delirium.[38]

The nurse should be aware that because of altered levels of consciousness, sedation, and effects and side effects of many drugs used in critical care environments, critically ill patients may not exhibit physiologic indicators specific for pain (i.e., vital signs), nor will they be able to exhibit behaviors reflective of discomfort. The role of critical care nurses must be to anticipate and preempt pain whenever possible.

One of the most important variables associated with assessment of pain is appropriate timing of pain assessment. Pain should be assessed initially upon first contact with the patient; at intervals appropriate to the pharmacologic intervention, calculating onset and peak action of the drug; and at routine intervals based on knowledge of treatments or procedures scheduled for the patient. For critically ill patients, who by virtue of their injury, disease, or treatment regimen are at significant risk for pain and discomfort, pain assessment should be carried out with at least the same frequency as measurement of vital signs and hemodynamic parameters.

MANAGEMENT OF PAIN AND DISCOMFORT

All patients admitted to critical care have the potential to experience painful and uncomfortable events. Although often heavily sedated, as many as 54% of patients report pain and discomfort while in the intensive care unit.[87] Factors that affect comfort include presence of an endotracheal tube, medical procedures, pain, and noise.[87] As discussed earlier in this chapter, pain and discomfort are major stressors that ultimately affect the PNI system. Multiple stressors and prolonged periods of stress are common for critically ill patients and contribute to mortality and morbidity.[49] Interventions promoting comfort and decreasing discomfort and pain improve patient outcomes by decreasing the workload of the cardiovascular and respiratory systems and supporting immune system function.[49]

Nonpharmacologic Interventions

Pain and comfort measures for all patients, but especially for those who are critically ill, include both nonpharmacologic and pharmacologic interventions. Nonpharmacologic interventions should be started as soon as possible and continued throughout the duration of the patient's hospitalization. Both pharmacologic and nonpharmacologic interventions require continual assessment and reassessment to evaluate effectiveness. Treatment of pain, especially severe pain, is best accomplished through a multimodal approach that incorporates basic comfort measures, complementary therapies, and pharmacologic management[49] (Fig. 39.9). This approach maximizes analgesia while minimizing the side effects of pharmacologic agents and the consequences of prolonged stress, resulting in better patient outcomes.

Comfort Measures

Comfort measures are often thought of as basic nursing care. Basic comfort measures are fundamental to nursing, often undervalued by nurses and other healthcare providers and frequently overlooked in favor of high-tech skills or administration

TABLE 39.7 Critical-Care Observation Tool (CPOT)

Indicator	Description	Score	
Facial expression	No muscular tension observed	Relaxed, neutral	0
	Presence of frowning, brow lowering, orbit tightening, and levator contraction	Tense	1
	All of the above facial movements plus eyelid tightly closed	Grimacing	2
Body movements	Does not move at all (does not necessarily mean absence of pain)	Absence of movements	0
	Slow, cautious movements, touching or rubbing the pain site, seeking attention through movements	Protection	1
	Pulling tube, attempting to sit up, moving limbs/ thrashing, not following commands, striking at staff, trying to climb out of bed	Restlessness	2
Muscle tension	No resistance to passive movements	Relaxed	0
Evaluation by passive flexion and extension of upper extremities	Resistance to passive movements	Tense, rigid	1
	Strong resistance to passive movements, inability to complete them	Very tense or rigid	2
Compliance with the ventilator (intubated patients)	Alarms not activated, easy ventilation	Tolerating ventilator or movement	0
	Alarms stop spontaneously	Coughing but tolerating	1
OR	Asynchrony: blocking ventilation, alarms frequently activated	Fighting ventilator	2
Vocalization (extubated patients)	Talking in normal tone or no sound	Talking in normal tone or no sound	0
	Sighing, moaning	Sighing, moaning	1
	Crying out, sobbing	Crying out, sobbing	2
Total, range			0-8

of pharmacologic agents (Box 39.5). Yet to patients, these interventions are highly prized and welcomed ministrations providing comfort that minimize pain and suffering. Basic comfort measures include environment, hygiene, and positioning interventions.[59,82,86]

Complementary Therapies

Complementary therapies are nonpharmacologic interventions used to complement effects of traditional medical, surgical, or pharmacologic interventions. The list of complementary interventions is extensive (Box 39.6); however, for nurses in critical care, music, guided imagery, and massage are probably the easiest to use. Complementary therapies promote sleep and rest, induce muscle relaxation, strengthen immune function, and decrease anxiety, depression, and pain.[45,49] The use of complementary therapies has been shown to be analgesic sparing, translating into fewer analgesic-related complications.[45] Complementary interventions should be started as soon as possible, and should be thought of as first-line interventions for decreasing stress, pain, and discomfort while promoting comfort, relaxation, and rest.[45] Pain perception and response to noxious stimuli are influenced by multiple physical, emotional, and cognitive factors unique to each individual. Stress, anxiety, fear, and fatigue decrease the threshold for pain, making perceptions of pain more intense. Interventions that decrease stress, anxiety, fear, and fatigue will increase the pain threshold and inhibit transmission of noxious impulses. At the same time, complementary interventions promote immune function, minimizing the potential for iatrogenic complications of hospitalization (e.g., infection and poor wound healing).[34]

The selection of specific complementary nursing interventions should take into consideration the desires of the patient or family, knowledge of the nurse, and awareness of time constraints attributable to the environment or the patient's condition. Knowledge acquisition through special education is necessary to become proficient in the use of many of the complementary therapies, and some, such as acupressure, require coursework and certification.[34] However, the use of music, guided imagery, or simple hand and foot massage can easily be mastered through self-study.[1,33,50,58] Because time and cost are major constraints to the use of complementary therapies in critical care, it is important to select interventions that are cost-effective, easy for the nurse to administer, and usually well received by patients and their families.

Music therapy. Music is an easy, inexpensive, and safe complementary intervention taking a minimal amount of time on the part of the nurse, but has a significant impact on perceptions of pain and discomfort for patients.[19,20] Music has been found to be effective as a complementary intervention for management of acute pain, cancer pain, and procedural pain. Findings from previous music studies suggest that music facilitates relaxation, decreases anxiety, increases comfort and decreases perceptions of pain, and improves mood.[19,20,28]

Music interventions should be specific to patients' likes and dislikes; patient preference is the most important consideration. Ask the patient about his or her favorite music or have the family bring in a favorite selection. Many individuals will select calm, soothing, instrumental music to facilitate rest and relaxation, or to distract them from pain; however, some individuals will prefer more upbeat selections. Music can be fast or slow, loud or soft, or it may include the sounds of nature. To facilitate attention to music and to block out unpleasant environmental sounds, patients should be provided with personal headsets. Use music preemptively as you would pharmacologic interventions; and, as with any intervention, pain and comfort should be assessed before and after the intervention; effectiveness should be documented in the patient's hospital record.

Guided imagery. Like music, guided imagery is a mind-body intervention that can be provided in critical care settings to facilitate sleep, to promote relaxation, or to manage pain and discomfort. Guided imagery is a way to purposely focus a person's thoughts and divert attention away from unpleasant experiences. There are essentially four types of guided imagery: pleasant imagery, physiologic focused imagery, mental rehearsal and reframing imagery, and receptive imagery.[87] For critical care patients, pleasant or physiologic focused imagery may be most

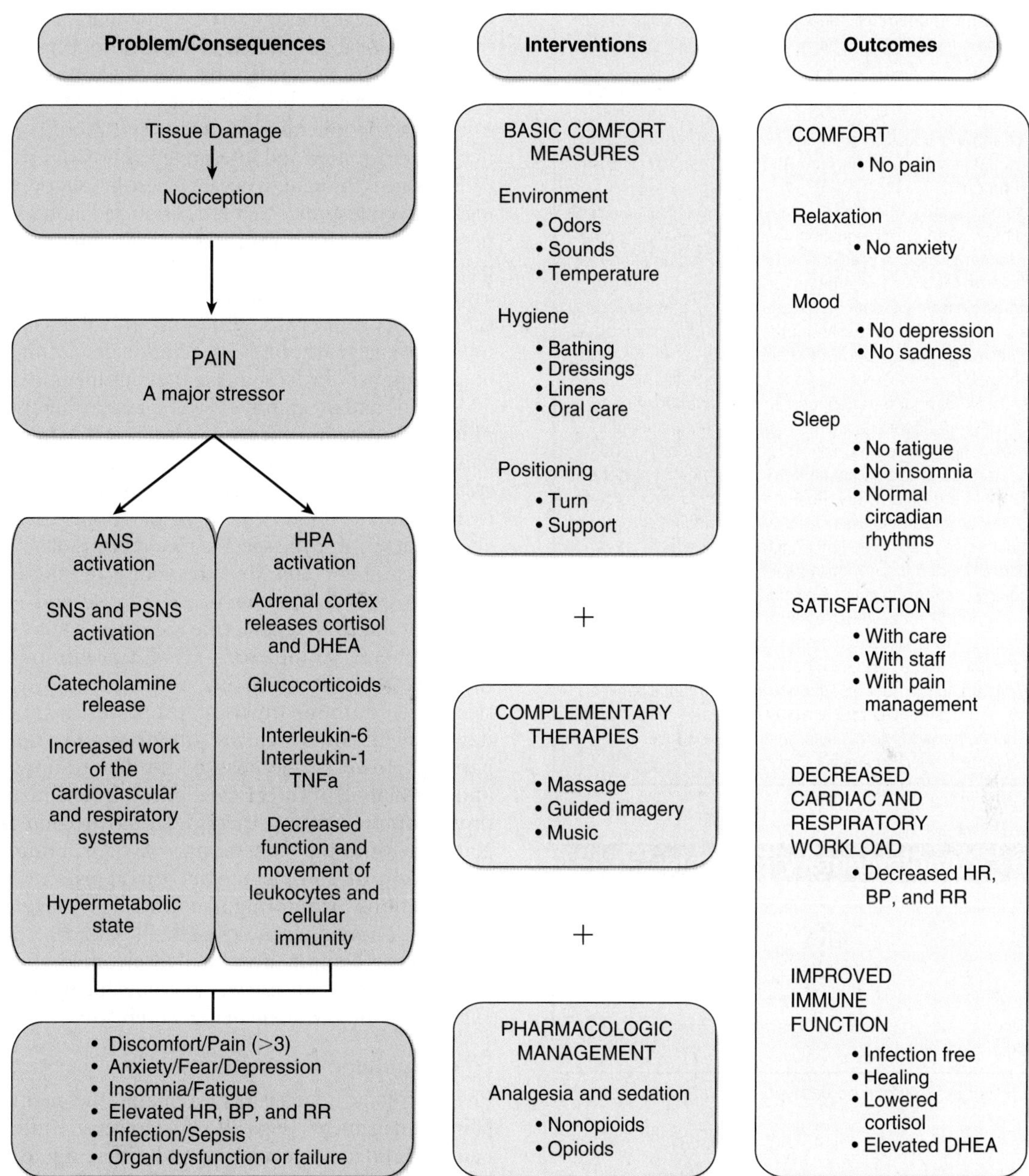

FIG. 39.9 Multimodal pain management model. *ANS,* Autonomic nervous system; *BP,* blood pressure; *DHEA,* dehydroepiandrosterone; *HPA,* hypothalamic-pituitary-adrenal axis; *HR,* heart rate; *PSNS,* parasympathetic nervous system; *RR,* respiratory rate, *SNS,* sympathetic nervous system; *TNF,* tumor necrosis factor.

BOX 39.5 Basic Comfort Measures

- Keep linens clean, dry, neat, and unwrinkled to minimize discomfort and prevent skin breakdown.
- Keep intravenous lines, catheters, or other tubing clear, so the patient is not lying on them.
- Assess dressings: loosen bandages that are constricting, and change wet or soiled bandages.
- If the patient has thromboembolic deterrent (TED) stockings or Ace wraps ordered, be sure to remove them and replace them every 4 to 8 hours.
- Be sure the environmental temperature is not too hot or too cold for the patient.
- Older patients and individuals with anemia will need extra blankets; patients with nausea or those who are short of breath may prefer cooler environments.
- Sounds should be kept to a minimum, but absolute quiet is usually not preferred and may contribute to agitation because of sensory deprivation. Loud and unfamiliar sounds are stressful; however, patients may like soft music or the television set left on.
- Keep odors to a minimum. If patients are nauseated, close the door when meals are served. Nurses and other healthcare personnel should avoid perfumes and colognes. For those who are nauseated, odors may increase their nausea and add to their distress.
- Patients who are NPO require frequent oral hygiene not only for comfort but also to prevent hospital-acquired respiratory tract infection.
- One of the most important comfort measures is positioning. This is especially important to critically ill patients who are unable to get out of bed because of surgery or injury. Positioning serves several functions: it prevents complications associated with immobility; promotes comfort; and decreases pain. Frequent position change (at least every 2 hours) is recommended for immobile patients.
- When positioning patients, have appropriate equipment. Correct alignment and support reduce muscle and skeletal strain. It takes at least four (preferably five) pillows to properly position a patient on his or her side. Place one at the head, two between the legs, at least one (preferably two) behind the patient, supporting the patient's back, and another pillow for the patient's upper arm to rest upon. When patients are trying to maintain a side-lying position without proper support, the extremities become fatigued, causing discomfort.

BOX 39.6 Complementary Therapies

- Aromatherapy
- Acupressure
- Acupuncture
- Biofeedback
- Distraction*
- Guided imagery*
- Massage therapy*
- Meditation
- Music therapy*
- Reiki
- Relaxation therapy
- Reflexology
- Therapeutic touch

*Denotes those therapies that can be easily incorporated into critical care nursing practice.
From References 1, 19, 20, 24, 28, 34, 45, 50, 58, and 87.

useful. Research suggests that guided imagery can strengthen the immune system, decrease feelings of anxiety and pain, and promote feelings of comfort. In addition, guided imagery was found to be a cost-effective and opioid-sparing intervention for cardiac surgery patients, resulting in decreased length of stay and reduced postoperative pain and anxiety. Finally, guided imagery was found to promote relaxation and facilitate sleep in critically ill adults.[87]

Although a personal one-on-one guided imagery session with a practitioner may be the most helpful, it is impractical in the critical care setting. However, guided imagery audiotapes or CDs can be purchased and used by nurses in critical care. As with music, headsets should be provided to facilitate attention and increase the ability of the patient to focus. Headsets also serve to block out unfamiliar or frightening sounds in the critical care environment, thereby further decreasing anxiety and stress.

Massage therapy. Massage is a complementary intervention that can promote relaxation, ease tension, and decrease fear.[1,24,50] Massage also promotes feelings of support and protection in the patient. Massage therapy refers to manual manipulation of soft tissue. In critical care, nurses can incorporate hand massage, foot massage, or back massage into routine care and hygiene (Fig. 39.10). However, caution is suggested if patients demonstrate evidence of peripheral or central sensitization, as even soft touch may be transmitted and interpreted as noxious stimuli.

Massage is thought to decrease perceptions of pain by providing competing stimuli that are conducted along faster neuronal networks, interfering with transmission and effectively closing pain gates before noxious stimuli can be processed. Massage is associated with a decreased release of substance P, which is associated with the release of serotonin, and inhibits transmission of noxious signals to the brain. In addition, it may impact the release of endorphins, which modulate the transmission of pain.[1,24,50]

Routine and preemptive use of massage therapy can have significant therapeutic effects. It can decrease stress, anxiety, and pain, resulting in less strain on the cardiovascular and immune systems; and improving patient outcomes. Future studies need to incorporate measurement of psychoneuroendocrine variables to determine the specific mechanisms of action associated with physical and emotional responses to massage therapy. In addition, the effectiveness of preemptive and routine use of massage therapy in critical care areas needs to be examined.

In general, complementary interventions are thought to decrease anxiety, pain, and discomfort, improve or strengthen immune function, promote relaxation, and facilitate rest, all of which are important for the critically ill patient. However, because of limited resources (i.e., time and personnel), critical care nurses must identify and use those complementary therapies that provide the best outcomes within the constraints of their limited resources. Integration of complementary therapies and basic nursing interventions promoting comfort may have a significant impact on outcomes of critically ill patients. Although complementary therapies are usually welcomed, the nurse should always discuss their use with patients, providing options and explaining the rationale behind their use.

Pharmacologic Interventions

Pharmacologic management remains the mainstay of acute pain management (Fig. 39.11). However, different types of pain and different people respond differently to specific pharmacologic agents. Mild pain may be managed with nonopioid analgesics, whereas moderate pain may require mild opioid analgesics. Severe pain is best managed by combining opioids and nonopioids to achieve the highest level of analgesia with the fewest side effects.[7,9,56]

Oral Nonopioid Analgesics

Oral acetylsalicylic acid (aspirin), acetaminophen (Tylenol), and nonsteroidal antiinflammatory drugs (NSAIDs) are useful and should be considered in management of patients with pain attributable to surgery, trauma, or cancer, unless contraindicated by the patient's condition. Nonopioids are more effective antiinflammatory agents than opioids. Aspirin (ASA), with its

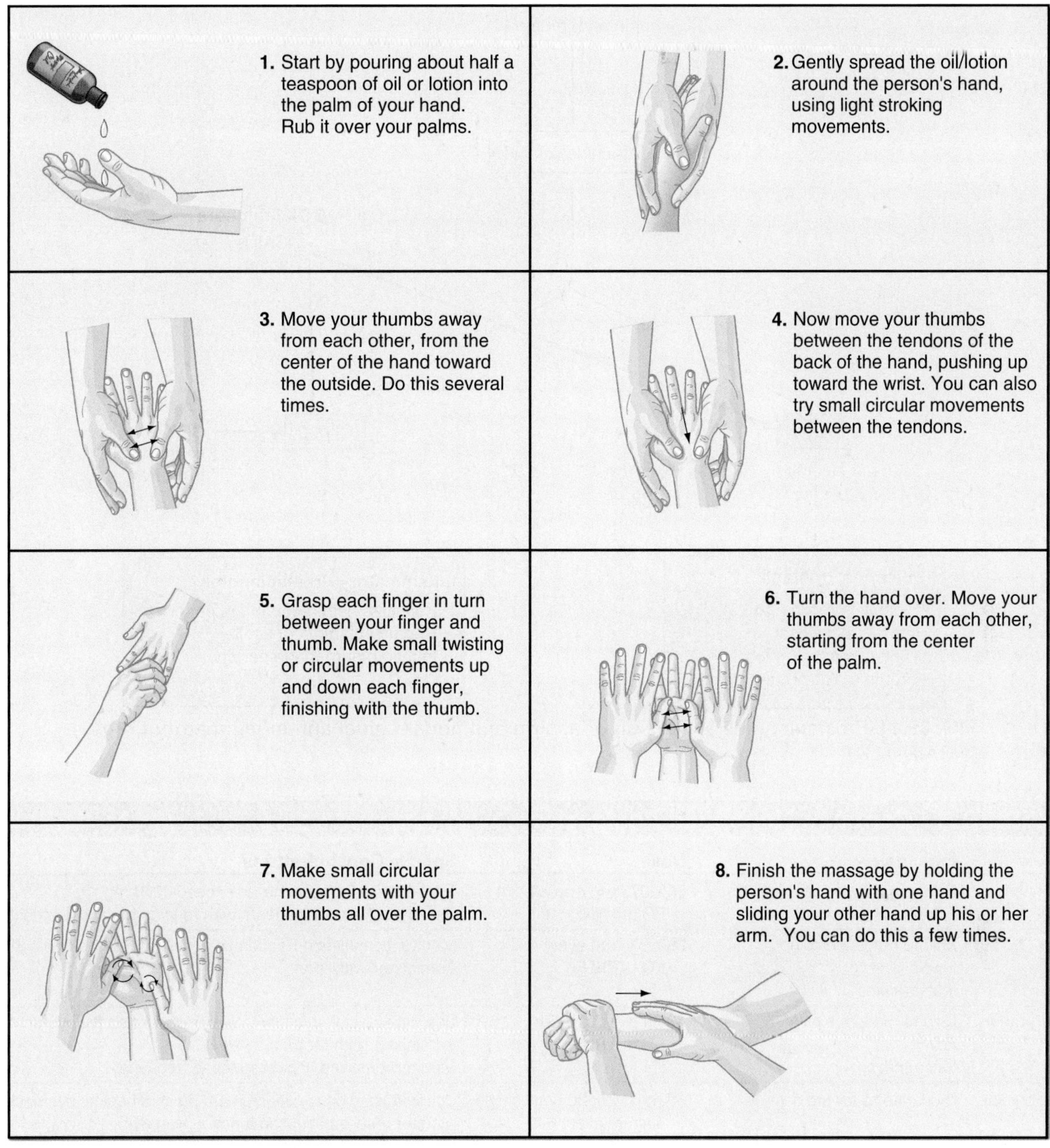

1. Start by pouring about half a teaspoon of oil or lotion into the palm of your hand. Rub it over your palms.
2. Gently spread the oil/lotion around the person's hand, using light stroking movements.
3. Move your thumbs away from each other, from the center of the hand toward the outside. Do this several times.
4. Now move your thumbs between the tendons of the back of the hand, pushing up toward the wrist. You can also try small circular movements between the tendons.
5. Grasp each finger in turn between your finger and thumb. Make small twisting or circular movements up and down each finger, finishing with the thumb.
6. Turn the hand over. Move your thumbs away from each other, starting from the center of the palm.
7. Make small circular movements with your thumbs all over the palm.
8. Finish the massage by holding the person's hand with one hand and sliding your other hand up his or her arm. You can do this a few times.

FIG. 39.10 Hand massage technique. (From Jane Ellwood, http://aromacaring.co.uk. Used with permission.)

analgesic, antiinflammatory, and antipyretic properties, is the oldest oral nonopioid analgesic agent. ASA acts in the periphery by inhibiting the production of prostaglandins. Because of its antiplatelet effect, gastrointestinal side effects, and association with Reye's syndrome, ASA has been largely replaced with acetaminophen and NSAIDs for management of pain and inflammation.[56]

Acetaminophen, another oral nonopioid analgesic, has analgesic and antipyretic properties similar to aspirin but lacks the antiinflammatory potency of ASA. Acetaminophen does not have an antiplatelet effect nor does it cause irritation to gastrointestinal mucosa. However, excessive doses of acetaminophen can cause fatal liver damage; patients with poor liver function or a history of alcoholism can develop hepatotoxicity, even at therapeutic doses. Acetaminophen has also been found to be a risk factor for excessive warfarin (Coumadin) anticoagulation. The mechanism of action for acetaminophen remains unclear, but it appears to work at the level of the CNS.[56]

NSAIDs work specifically by blocking release of the cyclooxygenase (COX) enzyme. Blocking COX inhibits production of prostaglandins. Prostaglandins produced by COX-1 enzymes protect the lining of the stomach, maintain normal platelet function, and maintain renal blood flow. Prostaglandins produced by COX-2 enzymes are inflammatory. The therapeutic effect of NSAIDs is a result of inhibition of COX-2, whereas side effects are attributable to inhibition of COX-1. As of 2016, celecoxib (Celebrex) is the only COX-2 inhibitor on the

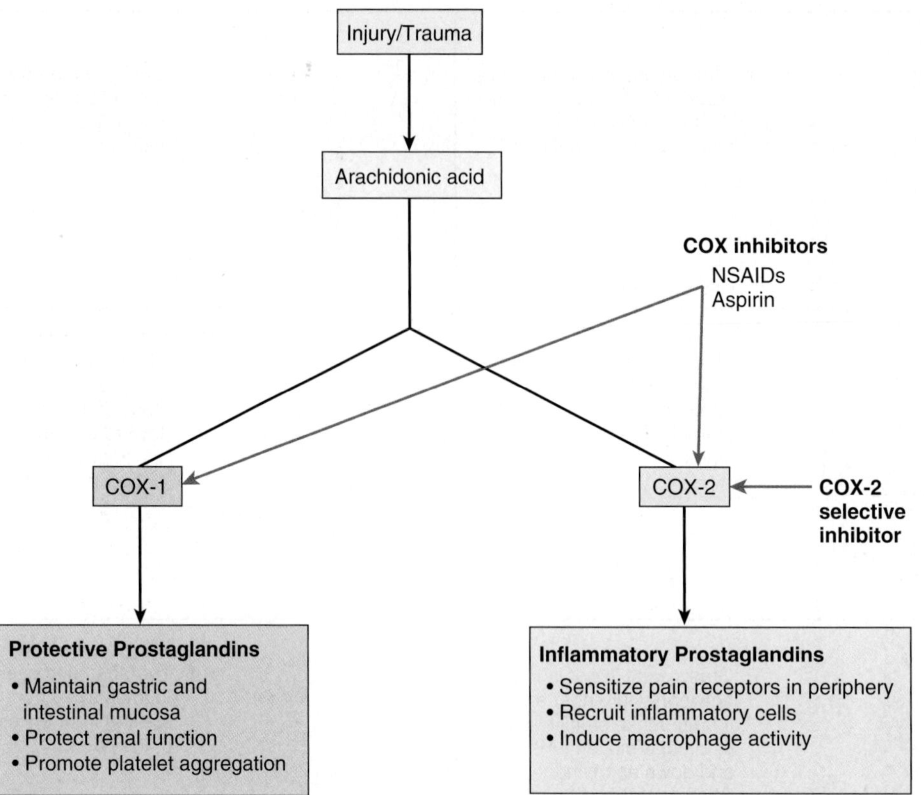

FIG. 39.11 Prostaglandins and action of aspirin and nonsteroidal anti-inflammatory drugs (NSAIDs).

TABLE 39.8 Common Nonopioid Analgesics

Medication	Indications	Dose	Special Considerations
Acetaminophen (Tylenol)	Mild to moderate pain Fever	650–975 mg every 4–6 h PO or PRN	Total dose in 24 hours not to exceed 4000 mg. Use with caution in patients with renal or hepatic dysfunction.
Aspirin	Mild to moderate pain Fever Inflammation	650–975 mg every 4–6 h PO or PRN	Monitor coagulation frequently; observe for signs of bleeding. Administer with food.
Ibuprofen (Motrin)	Mild to moderate pain Fever Inflammation	400 mg every 4–5 h PO or PRN	Use with caution in patients with renal or hepatic dysfunction. Administer with food. Monitor renal and hepatic function frequently.
Ketorolac (Toradol)	Moderate to severe pain	60 mg IM or 30 IV as single dose or every 6 h	Use with caution in patients with renal or hepatic dysfunction. Monitor renal and hepatic function frequently. Limit therapy to 5 days.
Naproxen (Naprosyn)	Mild to moderate pain caused by arthritis, tendinitis, or gout	500 mg (initial dose); 250 mg every 6–12 h PO	Use with caution in patients with renal or hepatic dysfunction. Administer with food. Monitor renal and hepatic function frequently

market. Several COX-2–selective NSAIDs were taken off the market due to an increased risk of heart attacks and strokes with longterm use.[56]

All NSAIDs (selective and nonselective COX inhibitors) can cause renal insufficiency. Risk factors associated with serious renal side effects (i.e., acute renal failure [ARF]) include heart failure, chronic renal insufficiency, cirrhosis, ascites, lupus, dehydration, multiple myeloma, or atherosclerotic disease. Symptoms of abrupt oliguria and sodium and water retention should be reported to the practitioner and NSAID treatment should be stopped. ARF secondary to NSAIDs usually reverses quickly once the drug is stopped. Common nonopioid analgesics are listed in Table 39.8.

Intravenous Nonopioids

The most recent nonopioid pharmacologic agent to be used to manage pain is intravenous acetaminophen, marketed under the name of Ofirmev. As with oral acetaminophen, its mechanism of action is not clearly understood, but it seems to act both centrally and peripherally. Intravenous acetaminophen provides a higher plasma concentration than either the oral or rectal route of administration, and has less variability in absorption. As with most drugs administered intravenously, intravenous (IV) acetaminophen has a rapid onset of action (5–10 minutes) and a relatively short duration of action (6 hours).[5,63,88,90] Recent studies suggest IV acetaminophen results in the need for less opioid and results

BOX 39.7 General Opioid Classification

Agonists: Activate All Opioid Receptor Sites
- Morphine
- Codeine
- Oxycodone
- Dihydrocodeine
- Oxymorphone
- Meperidine
- Levorphanol
- Hydromorphone
- Methadone
- Fentanyl
- Dextropropoxyphene
- Tramadol
- Dextromoramide

Partial Agonists: Activate Some Opioid Receptor Sites
- Buprenorphine

Agonist-Antagonists: Activate Some and Block Other Opioid Receptor Sites
- Pentazocine (Talwin)
- Butorphanol (Stadol)
- Nalbuphine (Nubain)

in fewer adverse side effects that are typically associated with opioids.[90] Because acetaminophen is processed by the liver, it is contraindicated for individuals with liver disease. Doses range from 650 mg to 1000 mg as a single dose or given every 4 to 6 hours. Because it can be hepatic toxic, the daily dose should not exceed 4000 mg/day.[61,63,69]

Opioid Analgesics

Opioid analgesics are the mainstay of pharmaceutical pain management.[35] Opioids act by binding to specific receptors (mu, delta, and kappa) in the brain and spinal cord. The specific site(s) of action determine(s) the effect of the analgesic agent (see Table 39.5). Opioids do not alter the pain threshold of afferent nerve endings and they do not affect conduction of impulses along peripheral nerves. Opioid analgesia is mediated instead at the spinal cord and CNS through modulation of the release of substance P, gamma-aminobutyric acid (GABA), dopamine, acetylcholine, and noradrenaline. Opioids also modulate the endocrine and immune systems, alter emotional responses to pain, and inhibit release of vasopressin, insulin, and glucagon. Opioid analgesic agents are classified as agonists, partial agonists, or mixed agonist-antagonists[3,43,74,79] (Box 39.7). Common opioids are summarized in Table 39.9.

TABLE 39.9 Dosing Data and Examples of Common Opioid Analgesics

Opioids	Indications	Routes of Administration	Approximate Equianalgesic Oral Dose*	Approximate Equianalgesic Parenteral Dose	Recommended Adult Starting Oral Dose	Recommended Adult Starting Parenteral Dose	Comments
Morphine	Severe pain caused by trauma, surgery, myocardial infarction, cancer, or chronic pain	Oral Intravenous bolus Infusion Intraspinal Subcutaneous Sublingual Rectal	30 mg every 3–4 h (around-the-clock dosing) 60 mg every 3–4 h (single dose or intermittent dosing)	10 mg every 3–4 h	30 mg every 3–4 h	4–10 mg every 3–4 h	Gold standard against which all other opioids are measured
Fentanyl (Sublimaze)	Moderate to severe pain	Oral Intravenous bolus Infusion Intraspinal Transmucosal Transdermal	NA		NA	Transdermal and intraspinal administration recommended	
Codeine	Mild to moderate pain	Oral	130 mg every 3–4 h	NA	30–60 mg every 3–4 h	NA	Doses higher than 65 mg increase constipation and other side effects without improving analgesic effect
Hydromorphone (Dilaudid)	Moderate to severe pain	Oral Intravenous Subcutaneous Rectal	7.5 mg every 3–4 h	1.5 mg every 3–4 h	6 mg every 3–4 h	1.5 mg every 3–4 h	Useful alternative to morphine
Meperidine (Demerol)†	Moderate to severe pain	Oral Intravenous Intramuscular Subcutaneous	300 mg every 2–3 h	75–100 mg every 3 h	Not recommended	100 mg every 3 h	Normeperidine, a by-product of meperidine metabolism, is neurotoxic

*Equianalgesic doses are compared to morphine. The equivalent of 30 mg of oral morphine is 130 mg of oral codeine.
†Meperidine is contraindicated for older patients, for individuals with renal or liver dysfunction, and for management of pain for more than 48 hours.
From References 9 and 74.

Agonists

Agonists are the most commonly used analgesic for critical care patients. The main effect of pure agonists occurs in the CNS, where agonists activate mu, delta, and kappa receptors located primarily in the limbic system, thalamus, midbrain, and spinal cord. Agonists have no ceiling effect, making side effects the dose-limiting factor in their administration. Morphine, first introduced more than 200 years ago, is a naturally occurring alkaloid derived from the poppy plant, and considered the preferred drug for opioid analgesia. Morphine is highly hydrophilic, so it crosses the blood-brain barrier poorly and diffuses slowly from the epidural space, increasing its general duration of action. Morphine, a potent agonist with both spinal and supraspinal actions, is available for oral, rectal, parenteral, and spinal administration.[74]

Fentanyl (Sublimaze), a semisynthetic opioid, is more potent than morphine. Fentanyl is a lipophilic opioid that has a very limited duration of action (30–60 minutes) when administered by parenteral or intraspinal routes. Fentanyl is available for parenteral, transdermal, transmucosal, and spinal administration.[74]

Meperidine (Demerol) is a synthetic opioid with analgesic properties similar to morphine and is primarily a kappa receptor agonist. Meperidine metabolizes into normeperidine (an active metabolite). Normeperidine is half as potent as meperidine but has nearly twice the side effects. In patients with impaired hepatic or renal function, the half-life of meperidine, which is normally 3 to 5 hours, is prolonged to 7 to 11 hours; and the half-life of normeperidine is even longer at 15 to 30 hours. The toxic effect of normeperidine causes anxiety, tremors, and seizures. Levels of normeperidine begin to accumulate with each dose. Patients with evidence of renal dysfunction, CNS disorders, and sickle cell disease; those receiving meperidine in doses greater than 600 mg in 24 hours; or those receiving meperidine for more than 48 hours are at risk for meperidine toxicity. Naloxone (Narcan) does not reverse the effects of normeperidine accumulation and is contraindicated because it may cause hyperexcitability. Because meperidine has been shown to be neurotoxic and has not been shown to be superior to morphine or other opioids in reducing spasm, it is no longer recommended for use as an analgesic.[12]

Partial Agonists

Partial agonists activate some but not all of the opioid receptor sites, have a ceiling effect, and produce less analgesia than full agonists, regardless of their concentration. Increasing doses of partial agonists beyond their ceiling would not increase the analgesic effect. When a partial agonist such as buprenorphine (Buprenex) is administered with a pure agonist, such as morphine, the partial agonist can displace the pure agonist at receptor sites, reducing analgesic action. If severe enough, this could cause opioid withdrawal. Therefore, caution is required when using multiple analgesics or when switching patients from a pure to a partial agonist.[74]

Mixed Agonist-Antagonists

Mixed agonist-antagonists block some sites and activate others. For example, pentazocine (Talwin) has a weak antagonist effect on mu receptor sites and an agonist effect on kappa sites. Therefore, in addition to analgesia, pentazocine is associated with psychotomimetic effects. Like partial agonists, agonist-antagonists have a ceiling effect, and when administered with a pure agonist, can produce withdrawal symptoms.[74]

Opioids are provided as individual or combination drugs. Caution should be taken when administering combination drugs, because their nonopioid component limits the dose. For example, agents such as oxycodone with acetaminophen (Percocet) or acetaminophen with codeine (Tylenol with codeine) may cause hepatotoxicity if the acetaminophen dose exceeds 4000 mg/day. Note that in the presence of liver disease, hepatotoxicity occurs at an even lower dose.[74]

Routes of Administration

One advantage of opioids is that they can be administered through a variety of routes. The oral route is preferred for long-term opioid treatment as it produces steady blood levels. The onset of action for oral morphine is usually 45 minutes with a peak effect in 1 to 2 hours. Because oral opioids (e.g., morphine) are deactivated during their first pass through the liver, a larger oral dose compared to the usual parenteral dose is required.[74] However, for patients with liver disease, dosage will need to be reduced to prevent overdose resulting from accumulation.

Intravenous opioid infusion. For rapid effect, IV bolus administration of opioids is recommended. Onset of action is nearly immediate, with a peak effect within 1 to 5 minutes for fentanyl, and 15 to 20 minutes for morphine. A second dose of opioid can be administered at expected peak times if severe pain persists and sedation level is within a safe range.[74] Managing continuous pain with repeated parenteral bolus is not recommended and may lead to a bolus effect, characterized by opioid toxicity at peak times and breakthrough pain at trough times.[74]

Continuous IV infusion of opioids avoids the bolus effect, providing relatively stable blood levels. However, prolonged use may increase risk of adverse effects. This has implications for patient-controlled analgesia (PCA), as research has not demonstrated an advantage in maintaining a basal infusion and has found that it may lead to opioid overdose.[74]

Transdermal opioid administration. Some opioids, like fentanyl, are easily absorbed through the dermis. Fentanyl is available as a patch providing continuous opioid delivery without need for IV access. Transdermal fentanyl is indicated for patients who require continuous opioid coverage; each patch provides a stable blood level for approximately 72 hours. This product is not indicated for acute procedural or postoperative pain, as onset of action is delayed by 12 to 18 hours, with a therapeutic lag time of up to 48 hours.[74]

It is important to note that skin integrity and heat can affect the rate of absorption from a fentanyl patch.[74] Patients with fever should be closely monitored for signs of excessive sedation or respiratory depression; use of warming blankets or heating pads should be avoided. Respiratory depression and excessive sedation may continue even after the patch has been removed; therefore, patients will require close monitoring and/or periodic administration of naloxone hydrochloride (to reverse effects of oversedation).

Transmucosal opioid administration. Fentanyl is also available in a transmucosal formulation that comes as a sucker (a lozenge with a handle). Through this route, 25% of the drug is absorbed quickly via oral mucosa, providing immediate analgesia; the remainder is absorbed slowly through the gastrointestinal tract, providing prolonged analgesia. Levels peak in approximately 15 minutes.[74,76,79] Although developed for children, lozenge-style drug delivery can be used with any age group and is especially useful for procedural analgesia.

Intramuscular and subcutaneous opioid administration. Additional routes of administration for opioids include subcutaneous (subQ), intramuscular (IM), and rectal. Opioids can be given through continuous or intermittent subcutaneous infusion, but the amount of infusate must be limited.[74] The IM route, although commonly used, is the least effective. Intramuscular administration of pain medications is painful, and absorption rates are unpredictable at best, with a peak effect lag time of up to 60 minutes. In addition, the fall-off effect for IM opioids is rapid, resulting in levels of severe pain followed by periods of excessive sedation. Repeated IM administration should be avoided, as frequent injections may result in sterile abscesses and muscle or tissue fibrosis.[74]

Rectal opioid administration. Rectal administration of opioids is an acceptable alternative when patients are unable to take oral medications. Rectal opioids are rapidly absorbed, and first-pass hepatic metabolism can be avoided if the suppository is inserted just past the rectal sphincter. If the suppository is inserted high into the rectum, there is danger of absorption into the superior renal vein, which empties into the portal vein, causing rapid hepatic metabolism.[74,76,79]

Intraspinal opioid administration. Opioid receptor sites are found in both the brain and dorsal horn of the spinal cord; thus it is possible to administer opioids directly to receptors in the spinal cord, minimizing supraspinal side effects and providing longer duration of analgesia with lower opioid doses than is possible with parenteral administration. Intraspinal routes of opioid administration are epidural and intrathecal.[43,74]

Epidural analgesia requires insertion of a catheter into the space just before the dura mater, and involves administration of an opioid or combination opioid and local anesthetic via a continuous infusion device. The opioid works at opioid receptor sites in the spinal cord, whereas the local anesthetic blocks sensory nerve fibers.[43,74]

Intrathecal analgesia requires insertion of a catheter into the space where the cerebral spinal fluid (CSF) is located. Administration of opioids directly into the CSF allows rapid binding to opioid receptor sites in the spinal cord. This route requires less opioid than the epidural route. However, because of the location of the catheter, the opportunity for significant infection is high.

Opioid analgesic doses vary significantly, with epidural doses approximately one-tenth the parenteral dose, and intrathecal doses one-tenth of epidural doses. For morphine, with a standard oral dose of 30 mg, the IV dose equivalent would be 10 mg, the epidural dose equivalent would be 1 mg, and the intrathecal dose equivalent would be 0.1 mg.[43,74,76,79]

Most often, morphine and fentanyl are the drugs chosen for intraspinal administration. It should be noted that morphine and fentanyl produce different levels of analgesia and side effects, due in part to variations in solubility.[74] Morphine, a hydrophilic opioid, diffuses poorly into capillaries and remains in cerebrospinal fluid for a longer time than fentanyl, a lipophilic opioid. Thus the duration of action for intraspinal morphine is longer than that of fentanyl, and intraspinal morphine is more likely to cause excess sedation and respiratory depression than fentanyl.[43,74]

Frequency and Titration of Opioids

As needed (PRN) administration of opioids for patients known to be in pain or at probable risk for pain is inappropriate. Opioid orders should include intermittent and continuous infusion orders, with specific provisions for breakthrough pain.[45] Opioid dosing should begin small and be increased routinely until an acceptable level of analgesia is reached without unwanted side effects. Once the optimal dose for a 24-hour period has been determined, around-the-clock administration should be started. Effectiveness of opioid dosing should be reevaluated frequently and readjusted based on assessment of pain and sedation.[45]

Recognizing and Managing Opioid Side Effects

Essential to management of pain with opioids is an understanding of side effects associated with their administration and knowledge of methods to minimize side effects (Table 39.10). The most common side effects are itching, constipation, nausea, vomiting, sedation, and respiratory depression.[9] When managing side effects, there are several options available: change dose, frequency, or route of administration; try a different opioid; consider addition of an opioid-sparing agent, such as an NSAID, to allow for a smaller dose of opioid; or add another drug that counteracts the troublesome side effects.[9,76,79] Changes in drug, dose, or route should be calculated using an equianalgesic table to determine starting doses (see Table 39.9). Equianalgesia refers to the relative potency of one opioid to another, using the parenteral dose of morphine (10 mg) as the standard for comparison. For example, to provide the same analgesia as 10 mg of parenterally administered morphine you would use the equianalgesic dose of 30 mg of oral morphine.[76,79]

Respiratory Depression

Adverse effects of most concern to healthcare providers are opioid toxicity and overdose. Overdose can lead to respiratory depression and/or respiratory arrest. To prevent this potentially fatal adverse effect, nurses should pay close attention to and frequently evaluate the patient's level of sedation, using a standard sedation scale. Because sedation precedes respiratory depression, monitoring sedation levels will allow the nurse to identify potential respiratory problems and prevent their occurrence. It is also important to recognize that respiratory depression or change in level of consciousness may be attributable to another problem (e.g., hypoxia or CNS insult). It is important to assess and treat the underlying condition appropriately. If respiratory depression (rate < 6 to 8 respirations /min) resulting from opioid toxicity occurs, an opioid antagonist (naloxone) may be administered in a dilute solution, made by mixing 0.4 mg of naloxone in 10 mL of saline. This solution can be administered at 0.5 mL every 2 minutes and titrated to response (increased rate and depth of respirations). Rapid administration of naloxone can precipitate withdrawal seizures, dysrhythmias, pulmonary edema, and severe pain.[9]

Tolerance and Dependence

Potential for problems should be monitored on a regular basis, including development of tolerance and physical dependence. Tolerance is an adaptive process that occurs in response to a drug and leads to a decrease in the effect of the drug over time. Tolerance to analgesics usually occurs in the first weeks of therapy. Patients who experience increased pain on a dose of opioid that previously kept them comfortable should be evaluated for tolerance by ruling out other potential causes of increased pain symptoms (e.g., new pathology, missed doses of pain

TABLE 39.10 Management of Analgesic Side Effects

Side Effect	Risk Factors	Interventions
Sedation	Elderly Analgesics and sedatives	Assess sedation level frequently. Assess for nonpharmacologic causes, such as hypoxia or increased intracranial pressure. Eliminate unnecessary analgesics or sedatives. Provide frequent physical stimulation. Decrease dose or change drugs for excessive sedation. Consider reversal for emergent sedation.
Confusion (delirium)	Elderly Other CNS condition Head injury Electrolyte imbalance	Eliminate unnecessary medications. Identify and treat cause of delirium. Consider neuroleptics for persistent delirium.
Respiratory depression	Opioid-naïve patient Head injury Chest injury Respiratory disorder	Monitor sedation level and respiratory rate. Hold or reduce dose of opioid. Consider reversal for severe respiratory depression.
Itching		Apply cool compresses. Consider diphenhydramine
Nausea/vomiting	May be dose or drug dependent	Control environmental odors. Assess cause; if caused by decreased gastric emptying, consider metoclopramide. Increase parenteral fluid intake. For chronic nausea, consider antiemetics.
Constipation	Elderly Immobility Dehydration	Maintain activity and encourage range-of-motion exercises. Monitor fluid balance; prevent dehydration. Administer stool softeners and stimulants as a preventive measure for all patients receiving opioids.
Ileus	Elderly Immobility Dehydration Constipation Surgery Analgesia and sedation	Maintain activity and encourage range-of-motion exercises. Monitor fluid balance; prevent dehydration. Administer stool softeners and stimulants as a preventive measure for all patients receiving opioids. Insert a nasogastric tube.
Altered hemodynamic status	Fluid imbalance Elderly Severity and length of illness Recurrent edema Sepsis CNS depression	Reduce analgesic. Administer parenteral fluids. Consider vasopressors. Administer antibiotics as indicated.

CNS, Central nervous system.

medications). Increasing the dose, adding an opioid-sparing agent, or changing to another medication may be needed to treat increased pain caused by tolerance.[9]

Another potential problem is risk of physical dependence that can occur with many medications. Physical dependence is not addiction; it actually occurs to some degree with any medication (e.g., antihypertensive medications or steroids). Physical dependence is an adaptive state; withdrawal symptoms can occur with abrupt cessation of the drug or, in the case of opioids, with administration of an opioid antagonist such as naloxone. Symptoms of withdrawal from opioids include anxiety, irritability, chills, excessive salivation, diaphoresis, nausea, abdominal cramps, and insomnia. Withdrawal symptoms are associated with drug half-life. Symptoms of morphine withdrawal may occur in as little as 6 to 12 hours and peak in 24 to 72 hours. Withdrawal symptoms from drugs with a longer half-life may not appear for several days. The role of the nurse is to anticipate and prevent withdrawal symptoms.[9] Patients treated with opioids for more than 2 weeks should have their medication gradually reduced before discontinuation. Reductions of 25% every day or two will generally prevent symptoms of withdrawal. If needed, clonidine (Catapres) can be used to treat withdrawal symptoms. The major drawback of clonidine therapy is the tendency towards hypotension.

Coanalgesics

In addition to nonopioid and opioid analgesics, a number of other drugs have the potential to improve analgesia or prevent side effects in special situations. Pharmacologic agents most commonly used as coanalgesics include tricyclic antidepressants (TCAs), antiepileptic drugs, local anesthetics, skeletal muscle relaxants, antihistamines, benzodiazepines, and topical agents.[45]

TCAs such as amitriptyline (Elavil), desipramine (Norpramin), imipramine (Tofranil), and nortriptyline (Pamelor) are useful for treatment of neuropathic pain related to surgery or trauma. Although studies have identified an analgesic effect for amitriptyline, occurring at relatively low doses (25 mg/day), anticholinergic side effects limit its tolerability. Sedation, hypotension, dry mouth, and urinary retention are common side effects associated with TCAs. In addition, TCAs may increase the incidence of ventricular dysrhythmias, making them risky for cardiovascular patients.[56]

BOX 39.8 Tardive Dyskinesia

Tardive dyskinesia, a neurologic syndrome associated with prolonged use of neuroleptic drugs, is characterized by repetitive, involuntary, purposeless movements. Tardive dyskinesia is treated by stopping the offending drug. However, the symptoms may remain even after the drug has been discontinued. When assessing the patient, look for the following:

- Repetitive grimacing
- Tongue protrusion
- Lip smacking, puckering, and pursing
- Rapid eye blinking
- Rapid movements of the arms and legs

Antiepileptic agents (e.g., gabapentin [Neurontin] and carbamazepine [Tegretol]) have been used to suppress the firing of sensory neurons. As with TCAs, these drugs are most often used to assist with management of neuropathic pain. The drawbacks to use of these drugs, especially gabapentin, are that they require dosing more than once a day and must be used with caution and at reduced doses for individuals with renal insufficiency.[56]

Local anesthetic agents can be used for nerve blocks or topical anesthesia. Skeletal muscle relaxants provide temporary management of pain related to muscle injury or strain. However, muscle relaxants in the benzodiazepine, sedative, or antihistamine family of agents may cause dependence if used for prolonged periods. Antihistamines may be used to treat itching and nausea associated with opioid therapy and because of their sedative effects they may be opioid sparing.[2,56]

Although phenothiazines, such as promethazine (Phenergan), have long been thought to potentiate analgesic effects of opioids, research demonstrates they only potentiate side effects, and prolonged use of phenothiazines can cause tardive dyskinesia, excessive sedation, and/or orthostatic hypotension. In addition, increased pain resulting from decreased analgesia can cause dysphoria, restlessness, and agitation (Box 39.8). Phenothiazines are contraindicated in patients receiving spinal or epidural anesthetics, and although they can be used to treat anxiety, benzodiazepines are recommended.[56]

ASSESSMENT AND MANAGEMENT OF SEDATION

Nearly 71% of patients in critical care experienced agitation as a result of sleep deprivation, anxiety, pain, immobility, or delirium, making it the most common reason for sedating critical care patients.[9] Both sedation and analgesia are essential tools for relieving pain, anxiety, fear, and stress in the critically ill patient and appear to have a synergistic effect.[9] A significant challenge for critical care nurses is to maintain balance between oversedation and undersedation. Oversedation is a dangerous event that leads to unnecessary tests, increased length of stay, and prolonged intubation and mechanical ventilation, whereas undersedation, costly in terms of human suffering (causing stress, anxiety, and agitation), has been associated with increased mortality and morbidity. Using an algorithm for sedation and analgesia is important for safe and effective management of critically ill patients[3,7,25,35,75,89] (Fig. 39.12).

Sedation may be indicated for patients who are mechanically ventilated and fighting the ventilator. Sedation for this purpose is appropriate only after attempting to manage the airway through adjustment of fraction of inspired oxygen (F_{IO_2}) and ventilator modification to flow, tidal volume, rate, and synchrony. For patients who must be sedated in order to maintain a functional airway and adequate ventilation, it is desirable to administer both analgesic and sedating pharmacologic agents, as analgesics potentiate effects of sedating agents, requiring lower doses of sedating agents.[47,48,64,65]

There are four levels of sedation: minimal, moderate, deep, and general anesthesia.[35,47] For each level of sedation, there are indications and end points (Table 39.11). Sedation used in critical care fits into the moderate sedation category. With moderate sedation, the patient maintains protective reflexes and the ability to maintain a patent airway and respond to verbal stimuli. Critically ill patients usually require special care and consideration when receiving moderate sedation.[3]

The need for sedation will vary throughout the patient's stay. Typically, sedation and analgesic requirements are highest upon arrival, plateau, and decrease over time, depending on the patient's condition. Although the Task Force of the Society of Critical Care Medicine recommended midazolam (Versed) and propofol (Diprivan) for short-term sedation and lorazepam (Ativan) for longer-term sedation, critical care sedation practices vary widely. A standard protocol is recommended to prevent under- and oversedation and polypharmacy problems.[25,35,47]

Once pharmacologic and nonpharmacologic interventions have been initiated, it is important to monitor the effectiveness of treatment by assessing changes in pain and sedation. When a patient who was previously alert and/or awake becomes somnolent or has difficulty staying awake while in conversation, the patient's level of sedation may require action (e.g., frequent physical stimulation or opioid reversal) to prevent subsequent respiratory depression. Because sedation precedes respiratory depression, if the sedation level is assessed at appropriate time intervals, the nurse will be able to detect excessive sedation related to pharmacologic interventions and prevent untoward events (e.g., respiratory depression or respiratory arrest).[25,35,47]

Assessing sedation levels in critical care is an important skill. Sedation scales are tools available to the nurse in assessing a patient's response to physical, auditory, or verbal stimuli.[72] The ideal scale would be easy to use and reliable, and able to distinguish between various degrees of sedation or agitation. Several scales have been developed, with the most common being observational scales, where nurses rate level of sedation based on patients' response to various stimuli. Scales differ in their approach to assessing sedation or sedation and agitation. The Ramsay Sedation Scale (Box 39.9) assesses sedation on a six-point asleep-awake scale. Although simple to use, it does not provide an adequate measure of agitation, and is therefore less useful for monitoring sedation in critically ill patients.[25,26,35,47]

A more useful instrument for assessing sedation in critically ill patients is the Riker Sedation-Agitation Scale (SAS), which rates sedation and agitation on a continuum from 1 to 7 (Box 39.10). Similarly, the Motor Activity Assessment Scale (MAAS) evaluates both sedation and agitation. However, the MAAS uses a continuum from 0 to 6 and includes behavioral clarifiers that may make it easier for use in critical care (Box 39.11). A more extensive instrument is the Richmond Agitation-Sedation Scale (RASS). The RASS uses a 10-point scale and measures sedation on a continuum from −5 to 0 and agitation from 1 to 4 (Box 39.12). Like the MAAS, the RASS

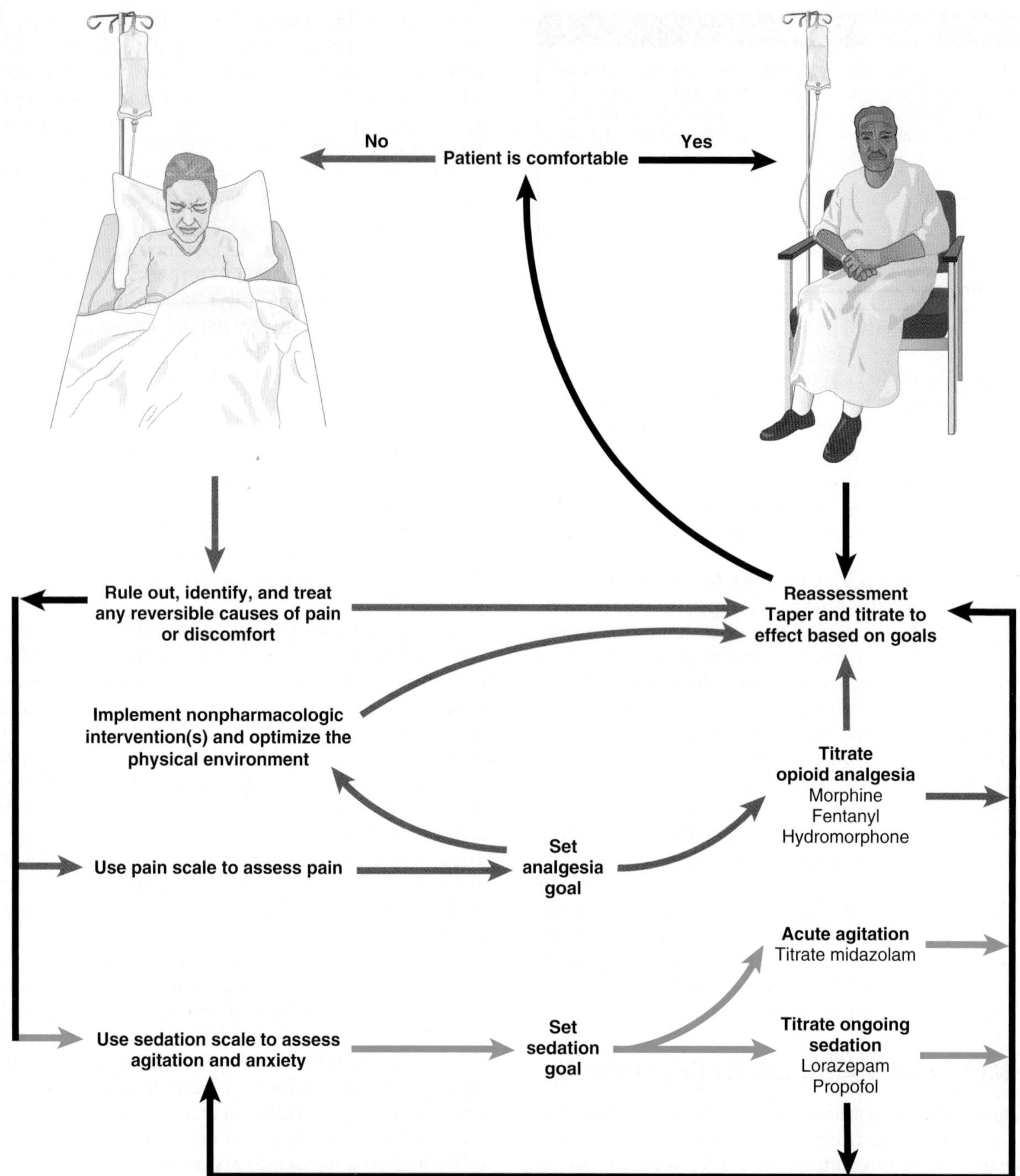

FIG. 39.12 Sedation and analgesia algorithm. (From Jacobi, J., Frase, G., Coursin, D., Riber, R., Fountaine, D., et al. (2002). Clinical practice guidelines for the sustained use of sedatives and analgesics in the critically ill adult. *Crit care med 30*(1): 119-141, with permission.)

includes specific behavioral clarifiers, making it easy to use in critical care.[62,64,68,70,72]

Scales reviewed so far focus on a single domain. De Jong[26] described the development of the American Association of Critical-Care Nurses' Sedation Scale for Critically Ill Patients (Table 39.12). This scale consists of five domains: consciousness, agitation, anxiety, sleep, and patient-ventilator synchrony. Because the domains in this scale were designed to parallel the most common sedation therapy goals, it may offer advantages over scales that focus on a single domain. However, clinical testing is needed to determine if this scale is a valid and reliable tool for measuring sedation in the critically ill population.[26]

Of note is that observational scales are not useful for assessing patients who are receiving neuromuscular blockade, and although vital signs (e.g., blood pressure and heart rate) may be objective indicators of sedation, they may also be indicators of other variables. Vital signs are affected by the patient's underlying condition and pharmaceutical agents, making their usefulness as a measure of sedation suspect.[62,64,68,70,72]

TABLE 39.11 Sedation End Points

Assessment Findings	Problem	Interventions	End Point	Outcome Measure
Chest movement that is poorly coordinated with ventilator cycling Extreme inspiratory or expiratory chest movement Frequent or sustained coughing Tightening of chest wall muscles during any phase of ventilator cycle Inadequate gas exchange Hemodynamic instability Increased peak airway pressure	Patient-ventilator dyssynchrony	Look for and correct any mechanical problems associated with ventilator or patient's airway. Look for and assess for metabolic, electrolyte, or cardiovascular cause of symptoms. Look for and correct any sources of discomfort. Assess sedation and pain levels. Titrate sedation and analgesia.	Patient-ventilator synchrony	Responds to ventilator breaths in coordinated manner Synchrony prevents excessive nonproductive muscle work Improved gas exchange Hemodynamic stability Normal peak airway pressure
Excessive restlessness Continuous nonpurposeful physical activity: fidgeting, thrashing side to side, pulling at clothing, bedding, and tubes Disorientation/confusion Unable to follow commands	Agitation	Differentiate between delirium and agitation and treat appropriately. Look for, correct, and/or treat physical (pain, hypoxia, drug reaction, hyperglycemia, hypoglycemia), emotional (fear, anxiety), or environmental causes (loud unfamiliar noises, bright lights, odors, uncomfortable room temperatures). Assess sedation and pain levels. Titrate sedation and analgesia.	Calm, nonagitated	No excessive nonpurposeful physical activity Orientation Ability to follow commands
Decreased level of consciousness Not aware of self or surroundings Unable to follow simple commands Stupor or coma Nonverbal Awake (opens eyes) but not aware (cannot carry out any cognitive functions) Persistent vegetative state	Altered level of consciousness	Look for, correct, and treat cause, which may include: Brain ischemia/lesions Metabolic disturbances Inflammatory conditions, infection, sepsis Neurodegenerative disorders Hypoxia Analgesic agents or sedatives Assess LOC and level of sedation. Titrate sedation and analgesia.	Baseline level of consciousness	Awake Aware of self and surroundings Able to follow simple commands Verbal Responds to verbal stimulus

LOC, Level of consciousness.
From References 34, 41, 46, 47, 48, and 62.

BOX 39.9 The Ramsay Sedation Scale

Response to Verbal Command	Numerical Score
Agitated	6
Responds readily to name in normal tone	5
Lethargic response to name in normal tone	4
Responds to name only if called loudly and repeatedly	3
Responds only after mild prodding or shaking	2
Does not respond to mild prodding or shaking	1
Does not respond to test stimulus	0

From References 57 and 67.

Because sedation-agitation tools have limited usefulness in chemically paralyzed patients, objective instruments have been developed that use neurologic monitoring with electroencephalography (EEG) and auditory-evoked potentials (AEPs).[32] Bispectral index (BIS) uses a mathematical technique to analyze EEG wave data. This analysis provides a number between 0 and 100, with higher numbers indicating less sedation (100 = awake) and lower numbers (0 = isoelectric EEG) indicating increased sedation. Although currently used in many critical care units, some studies have demonstrated a poor correlation between BIS and subjective measures of sedation and agitation. Because muscle activity affects EEG data, the nurse needs to

BOX 39.10 Riker Sedation-Agitation Scale (SAS)

Score	Term	Descriptor
7	Dangerous agitation	Pulling at endotracheal (ET) tube, trying to remove catheters, climbing over bed rail, striking at staff, thrashing side to side
6	Very agitated	Requiring restraint and frequent verbal reminding of limits, biting ET tube
5	Agitated	Anxious or physically agitated, calms to verbal instructions
4	Calm and cooperative	Calm, easily arousable, follows commands
3	Sedated	Difficult to arouse but awakens to verbal stimuli or gentle shaking; follows simple commands but drifts off again
2	Very sedated	Arouses to physical stimuli but does not communicate or follow commands; may move spontaneously
1	Unarousable	Minimal or no response to noxious stimuli; does not communicate or follow commands

From References 57 and 71.

BOX 39.11 Motor Activity Assessment Scale (MAAS)

Score	Description	Definition
0	Unresponsive	Does not move with noxious stimulus*
1	Responsive only to noxious stimuli	Opens eyes OR raises eyebrows OR turns head toward stimulus OR moves limbs with noxious stimulus*
2	Responsive to touch or name	Opens eyes OR raises eyebrows OR turns head toward stimulus OR moves limbs when touched or name is loudly spoken
3	Calm and cooperative	No external stimulus is required to elicit movement AND patient is adjusting sheets or clothes purposefully and follows commands
4	Restless and cooperative	No external stimulus is required to elicit movement AND patient is picking at sheet or tubes OR uncovering self and follows commands
5	Agitated	No external stimulus is required to elicit movement AND attempting to sit up OR moves limbs out of bed AND does not consistently follow commands (e.g., will lie down when asked but soon reverts back to attempts to sit up or move limbs out of bed)
6	Dangerously agitated, uncooperative	No external stimulus is required to elicit movement AND patient is pulling at tubes or catheters OR thrashing side to side OR striking at staff OR trying to climb out of bed AND does not calm down when asked

*Noxious stimulus, suctioning or 5 seconds of vigorous orbital, sternal, or nail bed pressure.
From Reference 57.

BOX 39.12 Richmond Agitation-Sedation Scale (RASS)

Score	Term	Description
+4	Combative	Overtly combative or violent: immediate danger to staff
+3	Very agitated	Pulls on or removes tube(s) or catheter(s) or has aggressive behavior toward staff
+2	Agitated	Frequent nonpurposeful movement or patient-ventilator dyssynchrony
+1	Restless	Anxious or apprehensive but movements not aggressive or vigorous
+0	Alert and calm	
−1	Drowsy	Not fully alert, but has sustained (more than 10 seconds) awakening, with eye contact to voice
−2	Light sedation	Briefly (less than 10 seconds) awakens with eye contact to voice
−3	Moderate sedation	Any movement (but no eye contact) to voice
−4	Deep sedation	No response to voice, but any movement to physical stimulation
−5	Unarousable	No response to voice or physical stimulation

From Reference 57.

use BIS with caution in patients who exhibit either voluntary or involuntary muscle activity.[32] In contrast to BIS, AEP uses auditory stimulation through headphones to elicit and measure cortical response to sound, with a decreased response associated with increased levels of sedation. AEPs have been correlated with subjective instruments such as the RASS.[32] However, these objective measures (BIS and AEP) are not yet universally used to assess levels of sedation and agitation; and because research is limited or conflicting related to their usefulness, they should be used only as adjuncts to subjective measures.[3,32]

Sedating Agents

Benzodiazepines, the most frequently used sedation agents, decrease anxiety and have amnesic and anticonvulsant properties. Benzodiazepines act by modulating GABA, an amino acid produced in the brain in response to stress.[76,79] GABA is our body's natural sedative. Unlike barbiturates, whose action mimics GABA, producing a pronounced CNS depressive effect, benzodiazepines potentiate the action of endogenous GABA, limiting the amount of CNS depression induced. As lipid-soluble agents, benzodiazepines cross the blood-brain barrier easily, and their effect (from decreasing anxiety to sedation to hypnosis) depends on the number of receptors occupied.[76,79] Benzodiazepines are easily absorbed and can be administered orally; however, the IV route is the most reliable. Benzodiazepines can be given intermittently (IV bolus) or by continuous infusion. Benzodiazepines should be used with caution in patients with signs of renal or hepatic dysfunction, and need for continuation should be evaluated at least daily.[76,79]

The most commonly used benzodiazepines are diazepam (Valium), lorazepam (Ativan), and midazolam (Versed). Onset and duration of action for these agents varies by drug; side effects such as respiratory depression and hypotension are dose dependent. Sedation guidelines prepared by the Task Force of the American College of Critical Care Medicine are shown in Box 39.13, and selected sedative agents are summarized in the Table 39.13.

Although not recommended at time of printing by the Task Force of the American College of Critical Care Medicine for reversal of prolonged benzodiazepine-induced sedation states, flumazenil (Romazicon), a competitive agonist, can be administered intravenously to reverse the sedative effect of short-term benzodiazepine use. As a benzodiazepine antagonist, flumazenil's duration of action is short; so once reversed, sedation may reoccur from longer-acting benzodiazepines. The critical care nurse should assess for and anticipate the possibility of withdrawal seizures with flumazenil administration, especially if the patient has been receiving benzodiazepines for a prolonged time.[71,74]

Another agent frequently used for sedation, when rapid onset of action is required, is propofol. Propofol is a general anesthetic at high doses but has sedative and hypnotic properties at lower doses. With rapid onset and short duration of action, propofol is frequently used in critical care. Propofol, which can cause pain with peripheral administration, may also affect blood pressure and cause respiratory depression. These adverse effects are typically dose and rate dependent; therefore the patient requires frequent monitoring of sedation level while receiving this agent. Propofol has a depressant effect on the cardiovascular system that can cause hypotension.[76,79] Of significant concern is the potential for patients receiving propofol for longer than 72 hours

TABLE 39.12 American Association of Critical-Care Nurses' Sedation Scale for Critically Ill Patients*

Domain Or Subscale	Indicator	Best 1	2	3	4	Worst 5
Consciousness	Awake and aware of self and environment	Spontaneously opens eyes and initiates interaction with others	Wakens and responds after light verbal or tactile stimuli May return to sleep when stimuli stop	Wakens and responds after strong or noxious verbal or tactile stimuli Returns to sleep when stimuli stop	Displays localization or withdrawal behaviors to noxious stimuli	Displays posturing or no response to strong or noxious stimuli
Agitation	Body movement, patient/staff safety*	Calm body movements and tolerance of treatments and restrictions Movements do not pose a significant risk for safety of patient or staff		Body movements or noncompliance with treatments or restrictions does not pose a significant risk for safety of patient or staff		Body movements or noncompliance with treatments or restrictions poses a significant risk for safety of patient or staff
	Noises of patient	No noises		Frequent moaning or calling out		Shouting, screaming, or other disruptive vocalizations
	Patient's statements	Very calm				Very restless
Anxiety	Patient's perceived anxiety† (Faces Anxiety Scale)‡	No anxiety				Extreme anxiety
Sleep	Observed sleep	Looks asleep, calm, resting (eyes closed, calm face and body)	Looks asleep; periodically wakens and returns to sleep easily	Awake; naps occasionally for brief periods		Unable to sleep or nap
	Patient's perceived quality of sleep	I slept well		I slept fair		I slept poorly
Patient-ventilator synchrony	Breathing pattern relative to ventilator	Synchrony of ventilator and patient at all times, patient cooperative and accepting ventilation Coordinated, relaxed chest movements		Occasional resistance to ventilation or spontaneous breathing is out of synchrony with the ventilator Chest movement occasionally not coordinated with ventilator		Frequent resistance to ventilation or spontaneous breathing not synchronous with the ventilator Uncoordinated chest and ventilator movements

*This component is assessed in all patients, regardless of the goal of sedation.
†Assumes the patient has the ability to understand directions and communicate his or her perceptions either verbally, in writing, or by pointing to words or pictures. If score is greater than 2 for this subscale, ask the patient if he or she needs something to help him or her relax.
‡Faces Anxiety Scale reprinted from McKinley et al., with permission of Blackwell Publishing.
From Reference 26. Used with permission.

to develop pancreatitis. Monitoring of triglyceride levels is also critical, as hypertriglyceridemia is seen in patients with infusions longer than 3 days.[76,79] Another significant precaution related to continuous infusions of propofol is risk for microbial contamination of the infusion. Propofol is a lipid emulsion, a rich medium for many organisms. Propofol infusions require a dedicated IV line to minimize incompatibility and infection problems. The infusion and setup should be replaced every 12 hours.[76,79]

Propofol is available as an emulsion and provides calories from fat (1 kcal/mL) that should be included in dietary calculations. Prolonged use of propofol has been associated with hypertriglyceridemia, elevated pancreatic enzymes, and pancreatitis. Long-term use or administration of high doses of propofol has also been linked to lactic acidosis, bradycardia, and lipidemia in pediatric patients, and to dysrhythmias and increased risk of cardiac arrest in adult patients. Patients given propofol for prolonged periods should be routinely monitored for both metabolic acidosis and cardiac dysrhythmias.[76,79]

Although new as a sedating agent in critical care, dexmedetomidine (Precedex), a selective alpha agonist, has been approved for use as a sedative. Dexmedetomidine can be used as a short-term (less than 24 hours) sedative in mechanically ventilated patients. An advantage this agent offers is that patients are sedated when left undisturbed, but arouse quickly with mild stimulus.[76,79] Dexmedetomidine is also analgesic sparing and has anxiolytic properties similar to benzodiazepines. Elevated blood pressure has been associated with rapid administration of dexmedetomidine. Prolonged administration is associated with bradycardia and hypotension, especially in patients with intravascular volume depletion.[76,79]

A possible complication of sedation and analgesia is that it may cause or exacerbate episodes of delirium.[7] Delirium is a reversible condition characterized by sudden onset of confusion and agitation, and a change in level of consciousness. All patients are at risk for development of delirium if they are extremely ill or taking medications that alter CNS function. However, sensory deprivation and sensory overload can also precipitate episodes of delirium. Factors that may contribute to delirium in critical care patients are social isolation, sedation, not wearing eyeglasses or hearing aids, sleep deprivation, and environmental noises and odors.[7] Just being admitted to the hospital, let alone critical care, contributes to delirium. Adverse effects of analgesics or sedatives are a frequent cause of delirium in critical care patients. However, abnormal levels of calcium, sodium, or magnesium can also cause delirium.[7] Before administering any drug to manage the symptoms of delirium, an attempt must be made to identify and treat the cause of delirium. Haloperidol (Haldol) is the drug most frequently used to treat critical care delirium. However, potential side effects require careful and critical monitoring to prevent untoward events. Patients should be monitored for prolonged Q-T intervals and cardiac dysrhythmias.[7,25]

BOX 39.13 Sedation Guidelines

- Midazolam and diazepam are useful for acutely agitated patients because of their rapid onset of action.
- When rapid awakening is essential for patient management, propofol is the preferred sedative.
- Midazolam is not recommended for prolonged use, and is associated with unpredictable waking times and prolonged intubation.
- Lorazepam, which can be given via continuous or intermittent infusion, is recommended for sedation in most patients.
- Sedative dosing should be titrated to a specific end point (using a sedation scale).
- Gradual tapering of sedative dose and daily drug interruption of sedation to assess underlying condition and reassess need for continued sedation are recommended for all sedating agents.

From References 47, 64, 65, and 68.

NEUROMUSCULAR BLOCKADE

In addition to administration of sedating and analgesic medications, critically ill patients may also require neuromuscular blockade. Neuromuscular blocking (NMB) agents are used only when analgesia and sedation have not been effective, or when needed to facilitate treatment.[41] Neuromuscular blockade may be indicated for patients who are mechanically ventilated, for those with tetanus, or for patients with increased intracranial pressure (ICP). The goal of neuromuscular blockade is to maximize oxygenation and ventilation by control of ineffective breathing patterns that might be caused by either agitation or hyperdynamic states related to disease or trauma.[39,37] NMB agents act by blocking the action of acetylcholine in postsynaptic receptor sites in neuromuscular junctions, causing muscle paralysis [41] (Fig. 39.13).

NMB agents reduce oxygen consumption, control ICP, and make intubation or procedures that require nonmovement by the patient safer and easier.[41] Because of the potential for very serious side effects, NMB agents should always be used with extreme caution. When continuous NMB is indicated (more than 48 hours), the infusion should be stopped daily to assess for its continued need.[46] Basic nursing care for patients receiving NMB is essential as patients are at increased risk for problems associated with immobility. In addition, long-lasting weakness may occur after NMB, with patients demonstrating elevated serum creatine kinase levels, muscle fiber atrophy, and muscle fiber necrosis. Prolonged weakness may be attributable to delayed clearing of the drug, or a synergistic effect that occurs when NMB agents are given with corticosteroids or aminoglycosides.[41] The actions of NMB agents are potentiated by aminoglycosides, antibiotics, hypothermia, hyperkalemia, and hypercalcemia.[76,79]

TABLE 39.13 Selected Sedative Agents

Medication	Actions	Dosage	Special Considerations
Diazepam (Valium)	Depresses CNS at limbic and subcortical levels by increasing effects of GABA	Bolus 0.03–0.1 mg/kg IV	Contraindicated in patients who are hypersensitive to benzodiazepines or have a history of narrow-angle glaucoma, psychosis, coma, or respiratory depression
Lorazepam (Ativan)	Probably stimulates GABA receptors in ascending RAS	Bolus 0.02–0.06 mg/kg IV followed by infusion at 0.01–0.1 mg/kg/h	Contraindicated in patients who are hypersensitive to benzodiazepines or have a history of narrow-angle glaucoma, psychosis, drug abuse, or chronic obstructive pulmonary disease
Midazolam (Versed)	Depresses CNS at limbic and subcortical levels by increasing effects of GABA	Bolus 0.02–0.08 mg/kg IV followed by infusion at 0.04–0.2 mg/kg/h	Contraindicated in patients who are hypersensitive to benzodiazepines or have a history of narrow-angle glaucoma, coma, or alcohol intoxication
Propofol (Diprivan)	Inhibits sympathetic nervous system activity; decreases vascular resistance	Initially 5 mcg/kg/min IV over 5 minutes; may give 5–10 mcg/kg/min over 5–10 minutes until desired response. For maintenance: infusion at 0.1–0.2 mg/kg/min (6–12 mcg/kg/min)	Do not give to patients who have hypersensitivity to eggs or soybean oil Do not leave hanging longer than 6 hours Strict sterile technique Sedation may be prolonged in obese patients

CNS, Central nervous system; *GABA*, gamma-aminobutyric acid.

NMB agents are classified as either depolarizing or nondepolarizing. Succinylcholine chloride (Anectine) is the only depolarizing agent. Succinylcholine chloride is given as a bolus (not as a continuous infusion) for rapid-sequence intubation. Because it can cause rapid elevation in serum potassium levels, risk of hyperkalemia and cardiac arrest is great. Succinylcholine works at the site of acetylcholine receptors and should only be used for short periods and with extreme caution.[76,79] Patients with acute spinal cord injuries, burns, and/or trauma are at highest risk for side effects and untoward events related to release of potassium and hyperkalemia. In addition, when succinylcholine is used in conjunction with sedating agents, it causes release of histamine, resulting in severe hypotension and bradycardia. Although rare, succinylcholine may cause a condition called malignant hyperthermia. Early recognition of malignant hyperthermia is essential to prevent muscle breakdown, acidosis, hyperthermia, and cardiac dysrhythmias. Warning symptoms include jaw spasms, muscle rigidity, increased heart and respiratory rates, and fever. Treatment includes discontinuation of the drug, correction of acid-base balance, treatment of fever, and cardiopulmonary support.[76,79] Overdose of succinylcholine chloride is treated by discontinuation of the drug, coupled with maintenance of airway and respiratory support. Anticholinesterase agents are not recommended to reverse NMB due to the action of depolarizing agents, and, if given, can increase the degree of NMB.[76,79]

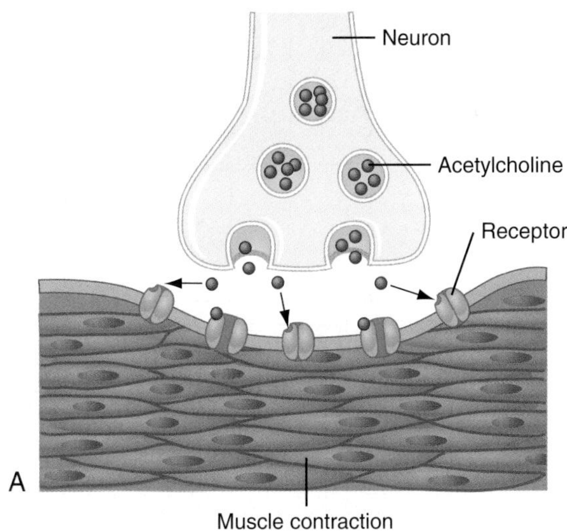

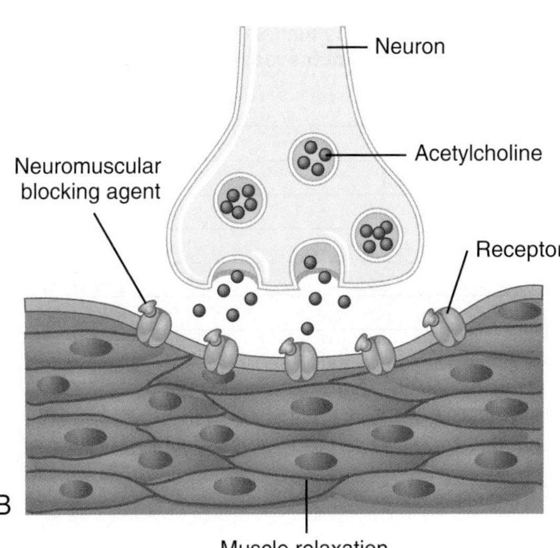

FIG. 39.13 A, Normal muscle contraction. B, Neuromuscular blockade.

Nondepolarizing agents, such as vecuronium bromide (Norcuron), atracurium (Tracrium), cisatracurium (Nimbex), and pancuronium bromide (Pavulon), are used most frequently in clinical practice and have an intermediate effect. Vecuronium, with an onset of action of 60 to 90 seconds (IV), peaks in 25 to 35 minutes and has few cardiovascular side effects. Thirty-five percent of vecuronium is excreted in the urine and fifty percent is excreted in bile; therefore patients with renal insufficiency or impaired hepatic function will need lower doses to prevent toxic accumulation.[76,79] Because prolonged blockade has been noticed more frequently with vecuronium than with other NMB agents, it has fallen out of favor and the frequency of its use in critical care has decreased.

An intermediate NMB agent with a duration of action of 30 to 40 minutes, atracurium is used for patients with renal and hepatic failure because it degrades rapidly, making its clearance independent of liver and renal elimination. Atracurium has cardiovascular side effects associated with histamine release at high doses. The most common side effects are hypotension and tachycardia, which can be prevented with administration of histamine blockers. Atracurium, like other NMB agents, can cause persistent or prolonged neuromuscular blockade.[72,76,79]

Cisatracurium has greater NMB potency than atracurium, with similar elimination, primarily via degradation; unlike atracurium, cisatracurium has fewer cardiovascular side effects, is administered in smaller doses, and has a duration of 45 minutes, compared to 30 to 40 minutes for atracurium.[76-79]

Pancuronium bromide, one of the first NMB agents used in critical care units, is long acting, with a 1- to 2-hour duration of action. Pancuronium bromide can be used for continuous infusion. Because of its vagolytic effect on the sinoatrial node and blocking of norepinephrine, the most common side effects are hypertension and tachycardia.[76,79] Pancuronium bromide should not be used in patients who cannot tolerate an increased heart rate.

When monitoring patients who are receiving NMB, paralysis and sedation level should be assessed frequently. Paralysis can be monitored through assessment of clinical indicators and by using a peripheral nerve stimulator (Fig. 39.14). Clinical indicators may be useful for detecting signs of inadequate sedation and paralysis. Clinical indicators include tachycardia, hypertension, diaphoresis, spontaneous breathing, and body movement.[76,79] However, these clinical indicators are not reliable indices of adequate sedation, nor can they be used to differentiate between adequate sedation and excessive sedation in patients with neuromuscular blockade. In general, visual, tactile, and electronic methods can be employed to assess muscle tone and neuromuscular blockade. The mainstay of assessment is nursing observation of movement (musculoskeletal) and respiratory effort. However, electronic tools are available to assist the nurse in monitoring neuromuscular blockade.[3]

Perhaps one of the most promising methods of assessing paralysis is peripheral nerve stimulation (PNS). To assess paralysis, a stimulus is applied to either the ulnar nerve

Education/Training/Certification of Nurses in Placement of TOF Monitoring Electrodes

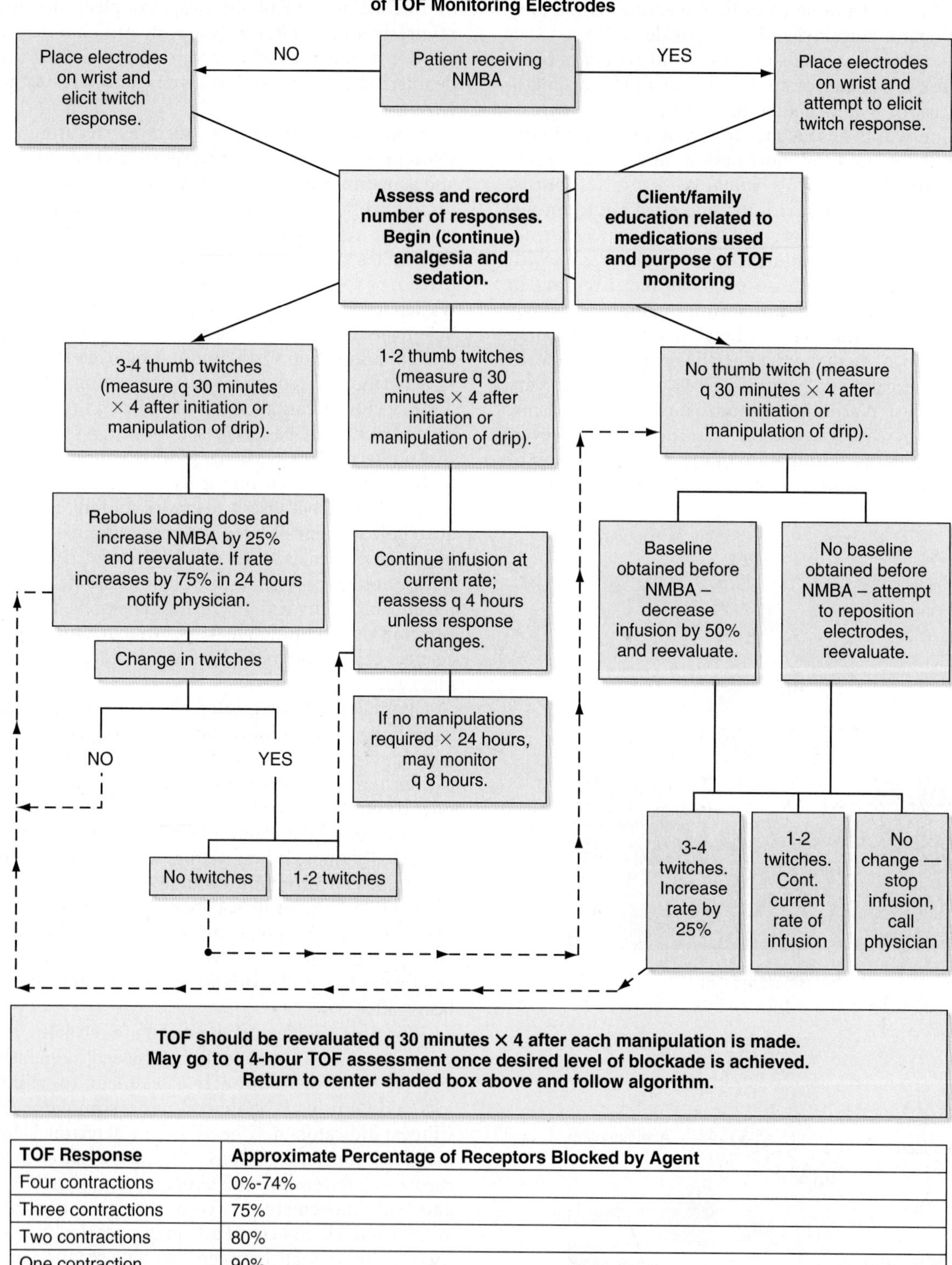
Patient receiving NMBA
NO
YES
Place electrodes on wrist and elicit twitch response.
Place electrodes on wrist and attempt to elicit twitch response.
Assess and record number of responses. Begin (continue) analgesia and sedation.
Client/family education related to medications used and purpose of TOF monitoring
3-4 thumb twitches (measure q 30 minutes × 4 after initiation or manipulation of drip).
1-2 thumb twitches (measure q 30 minutes × 4 after initiation or manipulation of drip).
No thumb twitch (measure q 30 minutes × 4 after initiation or manipulation of drip).
Rebolus loading dose and increase NMBA by 25% and reevaluate. If rate increases by 75% in 24 hours notify physician.
Change in twitches
NO
YES
No twitches
1-2 twitches
Continue infusion at current rate; reassess q 4 hours unless response changes.
If no manipulations required × 24 hours, may monitor q 8 hours.
Baseline obtained before NMBA – decrease infusion by 50% and reevaluate.
No baseline obtained before NMBA – attempt to reposition electrodes, reevaluate.
3-4 twitches. Increase rate by 25%
1-2 twitches. Cont. current rate of infusion
No change — stop infusion, call physician
TOF should be reevaluated q 30 minutes X 4 after each manipulation is made.
May go to q 4-hour TOF assessment once desired level of blockade is achieved.
Return to center shaded box above and follow algorithm.

TOF Response	Approximate Percentage of Receptors Blocked by Agent
Four contractions	0%-74%
Three contractions	75%
Two contractions	80%
One contraction	90%
Zero contractions	100%

FIG. 39.14 Algorithm for assessing neuromuscular blockade. *NMBA,* Neuromuscular blocking agents; *q,* every; *TOF,* train-of-four. (From Jones, S.K. (2003). An algorithm for train-of-four monitoring in patients receiving continuous neuromusclular blockade. *Dimens Crit Care Nurs, 22*(2), 50-57.)

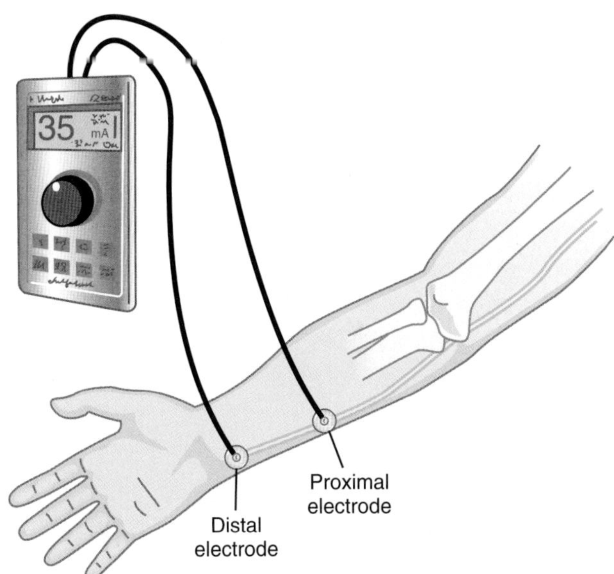
35
mA
Proximal
electrode
Distal
electrode

FIG. 39.15 Ulnar electrodes are placed along the ulnar nerve. This site is least affected by artifact.

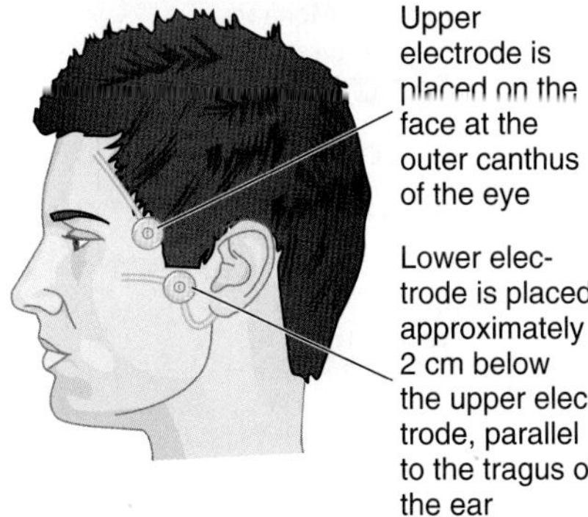
Upper
electrode is
placed on the
face at the
outer canthus
of the eye
Lower elec-
trode is placed
approximately
2 cm below
the upper elec-
trode, parallel
to the tragus of
the ear

FIG. 39.16 Facial electrodes are placed along the facial nerve.

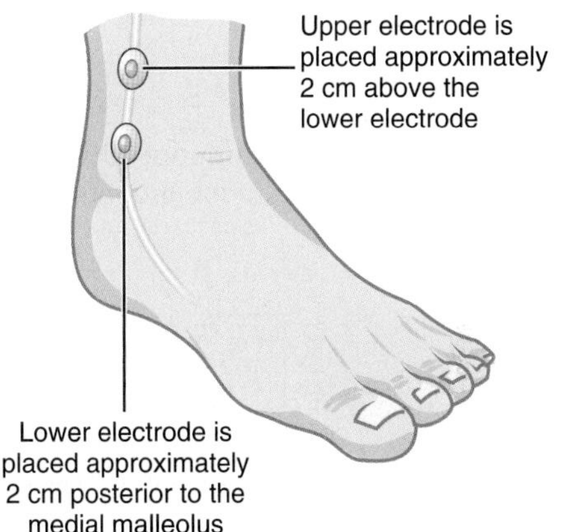
Upper electrode is
placed approximately
2 cm above the
lower electrode
Lower electrode is
placed approximately
2 cm posterior to the
medial malleolus

FIG. 39.17 Posterior tibial electrodes are placed along the posterior tibial nerve.

(Fig. 39.15), the facial nerve (Fig. 39.16), or the posterior tibial nerve (Fig. 39.17). The same site should be used consistently, with the ulnar nerve being preferred because it is least affected by artifact. In the absence of NMB, twitching should occur four times in response to four electrical impulses. The goal of neuromuscular blockade is 90%, which corresponds to one twitch for every four electrical stimuli. When using the stimulator, if no twitches are elicited, the tetanus mode, which delivers a 5-second stimulus, is used to generate a sustained twitch. This is followed by a repeat of the four stimuli. If no twitch occurs, the patient is overparalyzed and the NMB agent is stopped (intermittent dosing) or decreased (continuous dosing) until at least two twitches per four stimuli return. If the patient is receiving intermittent rather than continuous administration of NMB agents, then the four-sequence test should be performed every 30 to 60 minutes.

Another tool that can be used to assess adequacy of neuromuscular blockade is continuous airway pressure monitoring (CAPM), which uses a transducer cable, high-pressure tubing, and a transducer to display continuous airway pressures[7] (Fig. 39.18). CAPM can identify spontaneous diaphragmatic effort before any other signs of neurologic activity can be detected; thus it is a useful adjunct for assessing patients with NMB. For example, if a patient on a ventilator set as assist-control (AC) begins breakthrough breathing, it will be noted on the waveform and the nurse can adjust NMB[13] (Fig. 39.19).

In addition to assessing level of paralysis, nursing care centers on protecting the patient from untoward events associated with paralysis. Nursing management during NMB consists of protecting the airway, maintaining adequate ventilation, monitoring cardiac rhythm and blood pressure, treating pain and anxiety, protecting eyes, and maintaining skin integrity (Box 39.14).

When excessive NMB has been identified or when there is no longer a need for NMB, chemically induced paralysis can be reversed by administering an anticholinesterase agent, such as physostigmine (Antilirium), pyridostigmine (Mestinon), or neostigmine (Prostigmin). Anticholinesterase agents work by increasing the availability of acetylcholine at receptor sites. Although useful for reversing effects of nondepolarizing agents, use of anticholinesterase agents is contraindicated as a method of reversing the effects of succinylcholine chloride.[11]

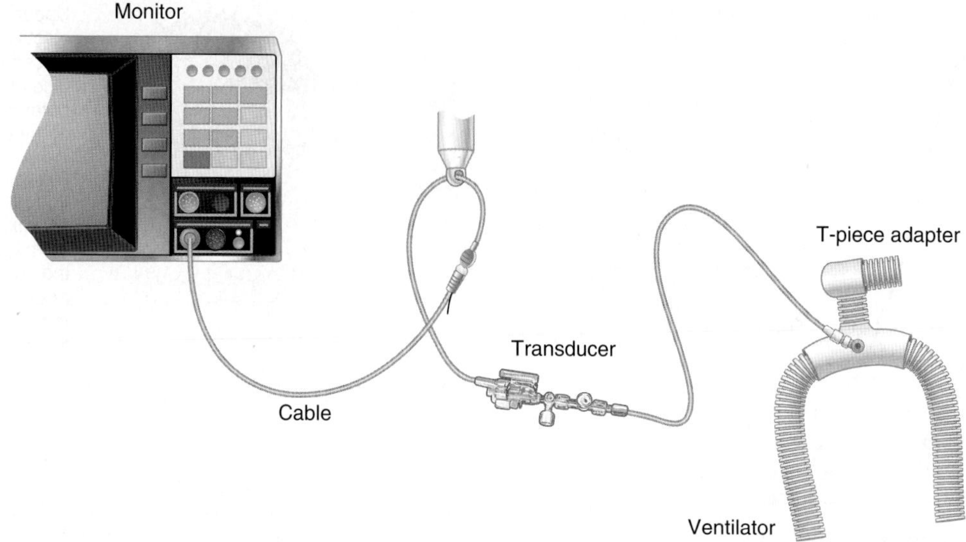

FIG. 39.18 Continuous airway pressure monitoring. (From Burns, S.M. (2004). Continuous airway pressure monitoring. *Crit Care Nurse 24*(6), 70-74. Used with permission.)

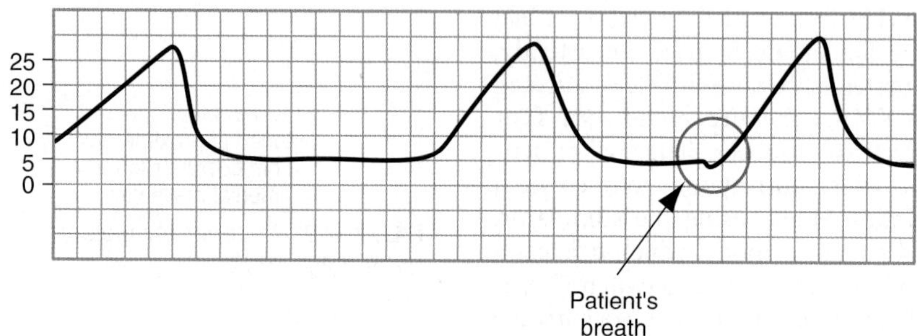

FIG. 39.19 Continuous airway pressure monitoring waveform in a patient on assist-control ventilation. (From Burns, S.M. (2004). Continuous airway pressure monitoring. *Crit Care Nurse 24*(6), 70-74. Used with permission.)

BOX 39.14 Caring for Patients Receiving Neuromuscular Blockade

Management of Airway, Breathing, and Circulation

- Establish and maintain a patent airway.
- Suction as indicated by patient's condition.
- Monitor ventilatory settings for accuracy.
- Evaluate oxygenation and ventilation through use of arterial blood gases and pulse oximetry.
- Maintain a manual resuscitation bag at the bedside at all times.
- Monitor for hemodynamic stability (blood pressure, heart rate and rhythm, temperature, peripheral pulses).
- Monitor and intervene as appropriate to maintain physiologic stability (acid-base status, electrolyte balance).
- Provide excellent physical assessment of cardiac and pulmonary systems to evaluate for effects of immobility.
- Observe skin for potential areas of breakdown.
- Reposition patient frequently.
- Consider use of a pressure-reducing mattress.
- Keep skin clean and dry. Consider use of massage to stimulate circulation as needed.
- Institute interventions to prevent deep vein thrombus.

Management of Eye Protection

- Close patient's eyes and cover with a soft eye pad.
- Use eye lubricants or artificial tears as ordered.

Management of Pain, Sedation, and Level of Neuromuscular Blockade

- Institute monitoring to evaluate level of neuromuscular blockade with frequency established by patient's condition.
  - Peripheral nerve stimulation.
  - Four-sequence testing.
  - Continuous airway pressure monitoring.
- Institute monitoring to evaluate patient's level of pain and sedation.
  - Administer adequate pain and sedation medications while patient is receiving neuromuscular blockade.

CONCLUSION

Pain is a common and usually predictable event for critically ill patients. Knowledge of and preemptive implementation of multimodal interventions that include basic comfort measures, the use of complementary therapies, and pharmacologic agents are essential to prevent the consequences of pain and to improve overall outcomes for critically ill patients. The interprofessional plan of care should include appropriate interventions for patients with varying levels of pain and anxiety. Nurses caring for critically ill patients must be aware of potential problems associated with pain management, sedation, and NMB that can impact patient outcomes. Research on management of pain and technology related to assessment of critically ill patients receiving sedative or NMB agents is rapidly changing the role of the nurse, requiring the acquisition of new knowledge and skills. Critical care nurses are in a unique position to monitor and assess the effectiveness of these innovations and provide important feedback on their usefulness for improving care of critically ill patients.

REFERENCES

1. Adams, R., White, B., & Beckett, C. (2010). The effects of massage on pain management in acute care setting. *Int J Ther Massage Bodywork, 3*(1), 4–11.
2. Alderson, S. M., & McKechnie, S. R. (2013). Unrecognized, undertreated, pain in ICU: causes, effects and how to do it better. *Open J Nurs, 3*, 108–113.
3. Alexander, E., & Sulsa, G. M. (2013). Update on the management and monitoring of deep analgesia and sedation in the intensive care unit. *AACN Adv Crit Care, 24*(2), 101–107.
4. Al-Hasani, R., & Bruchas, M. R. (2011). Molecular mechanisms of opioid receptor-dependent signaling and behavior. *Anesthesiology, 111*(6), 1363–1381.
5. Ammar, M. (2013). Intravenous acetaminophen – is it worth the cost? *Cleveland Clin Rx Forum, 1*(2), 1–7.
6. Angus, D. C., et al. (2006). Critical care delivery in the United States: distribution of services and compliance with leapfrog recommendations. *Crit Care Med, 34*(4), 1016–1024.
7. Barr, J., et al. (2013). Clinical practice guidelines for the management of pain, agitation, and delirium in adult patients in the intensive care unit. *Crit Care Med, 41*(1), 263–306.
8. Beers, J. M. H., & Berkow, R. (1999–2005). *The Merck manual of diagnosis and therapy: internet edition.* http://www.merck.com/mrkshared/mmanual/home.jsp.
9. Benyamin, R., et al. (2008). Opioid complications and side effects. *Pain Physician, 11*, S105–S120.
10. Bernhofer, E. (2011). Ethics: ethics and pain management in hospitalized patients. *Online J Issues Nurs, 17*(1), 11.
11. Brull, S. J., & Prielipp, R. C. (2015). Reversal of neuromuscular blockade: identification friend or foe. *Anesthesiology, 122*(6), 1183–1185.
12. Buck, M. L. (2011). Is meperidine the drug that just won't die? *J Pediatr Pharmacol Ther, 16*(3), 167–169.
13. Burns, S. M. (2004). Continuous airway pressure monitoring. *Crit Care Nurse, 24*(6), 70–74.
14. Buvanendran, A. (2015). The incidence and severity of postoperative pain following inpatient surgery. *Pain Med, 16*(12), 2277–2283.
15. Chanques, G., et al. (2010). The measurement of pain in intensive care unit: comparison of 5 self-report intensity scales. *Pain, 151*(3), 711–721.
16. Chanques, G., Sebbane, M., Barbotte, E., Viel, E., Eledjam, J. J., & Jaber, S. S. (2007). Prospective study of pain at rest: incidence and characteristics of an unrecognized symptom in surgical and trauma versus medical intensive care unit patients. *Anesthesiology, 107*(5), 858–860.
17. Chapman, C. R., Tuckett, R. P., & Song, C. W. (2008). Pain and stress in a systems perspective: reciprocal neural, endocrine and immune interactions. *J Pain, 9*(2), 122–145.
18. Charmandari, E., Tsigos, C., & Chrousos, G. (2005). Endocrinology of the stress response. *Annu Rev Physiol, 67*, 259–284.
19. Chlan, L. L., & Halm, M. A. (2013). Does music ease pain and anxiety in the critically ill? *Am J Crit Care, 22*(6), 528–532.
20. Chlan, L. L., Engeland, W. C., & Savik, K. (2013). Does music influence stress in mechanically ventilated patients? *Intensive Crit Care Nurs, 29*, 121–127.
21. Cowan, P. (2006). The myths of pain control. *ACPA*, 1–8.
22. Cox, D. S. (2002). Definitions pertaining to pain management. In B. St. Marie (Ed.), *Core curriculum for pain management nursing.* Philadelphia: Saunders.
23. Crichton, N. (2001). Information point: visual analogue scale (VAS). *J Clin Nurs, 10*(5), 697–706.
24. Cutshall, S. M., et al. (2010). Effect of massage therapy on pain, anxiety, and tension in cardiac surgery patients: a pilot study. *Complement Ther Clin Pract, 16*, 92–95.
25. Davidson, J. E., et al. (2015). Pain, agitation, and delirium guidelines: nurses' involvement in development and implementation. *Crit Care Nurs, 35*(3), 17–31.
26. De Jong, M. J., et al. (2005). Development of the American Association of Critical-Care Nurses' sedation assessment scale for critically ill patients. *Am J Crit Care, 14*(6), 531–544.
27. de Papathanassoglos, E. (2014). Recent advances in understanding pain: what lies ahead for critical care. *Nurs Crit Care, 19*(3), 110–112.
28. Dellavolpe, J. D., & Huang, D. T. (2015). Is there a role for music in the ICU? *Crit Care, 19*(1), 17. http://dx.doi.org/10.1186/s13054-0663-1.
29. Dickenson, A. H. (2002). Gate control theory of pain stands the test of time. *Brit J Anaesth, 88*, 755–757.
30. Dubin, A. E., & Patapoutian, A. (2015). Nociceptors: the sensors of the pain pathway. *J Clin Invest, 120*(11), 3760–3772.
31. Dunwoody, C. J., et al. (2008). Assessment, physiological monitoring, and consequences of inadequately treated acute pain. *J Perianesth Nurs, 23*(Suppl 1), S15–S27.
32. Fatovich, D. M., Gope, M., & Paech, M. J. (2004). A pilot trial of BIS monitoring for procedural sedation in the emergency department. *Emerg Med Australas, 16*, 103–107.
33. Field, T. (2014). Massage therapy research review. *Complement Ther Clin Pract, 20*, 224–229.
34. Fountaine, K. L. (2005). *Complementary and alternative therapies for nursing practice.* Upper Saddle River, NJ: Prentice Hall.
35. Fuchs, E. M., & Rueden, K. V. (2008). Sedation management in mechanically ventilated critically ill patients. *AACN Adv Crit Care, 19*(4), 421–432.
36. Gan, T. J., et al. (2014). Incidence, patient satisfaction, and perceptions of post-surgical pain: results from a US national survey. *Curr Med Res Opin, 30*(1), 149–160.
37. Gelinas, C., & Arbour, C. (2009). Behavioral and physiologic indicators during a nociceptive procedure in conscious and unconscious mechanically ventilated adults: similar or different? *J Crit Care, 24*, 228e7–228e17.
38. Gélinas, C., et al. (2013). A validated approach to evaluating psychometric properties of pain assessment tools for use in nonverbal critically ill adults. *Semin Respir Crit Care Med, 34*(2), 153–168.
39. Gélinas, C., & Johnston, C. (2007). Pain assessment in the critically ill ventilated adult: validation of the Critical-Care Pain Observation Tool and physiologic indicators. *Clin J Pain, 23*(6), 497–505.
40. Granja, C., et al. (2008). Understanding posttraumatic stress disorder-related symptoms after critical care: the early illness amnesia hypothesis. *Crit Care Med, 36*(10), 2801–2809.
41. Greenberg, S. B., & Vender, J. (2013). The use of neuromuscular blocking agents in the ICU: where are we now? *Crit Care Med, 41*(5), 1332–1344.
42. Herr, K., et al. (2011). Pain assessment in the patient unable to self-report: position statement with clinical practice recommendations. *Pain Manag Nurs, 12*(4), 230–250.
43. Hindle, A. (2008). Intrathecal opioids in the management of acute postoperative pain. *Contin Educ Anaesth Crit Care Pain, 8*(3), 81–85.
44. Hockenberry, M. J., Wilson, D., & Winklestein, M. L. (2005). *Wong's essentials of pediatric nursing* (7th ed.). St. Louis: Mosby.
45. Joint Commission. (2014). Clarification of new pain management standards. *Joint Commission Perspectives, 34*(11). http://www.jointcommission.org/assets/1/18/Clarification_of_the_Pain_Management__Standard.pdf.

46. Jones, K., et al. (2014). Achieving quality health outcomes through the implementation of spontaneous awakening and spontaneous breathing trial protocol. *AACN Adv Crit Care, 25*(1), 33–42.
47. Kweon, T. D. (2011). Sedation under JCI standards. *Korean J Anesthesiol, 61*(3), 190–194.
48. Lafleur, K. J. (2005). Will adequate sedation assessment include the use of actigraphy in the future? *Am J Crit Care, 14*(1), 61–62.
49. Lusk, B., & Lash, A. A. (2005). The stress response, psychoneuroimmunology, and stress among ICU patients. *Dimens Crit Care Nurs, 24*(1), 25–31.
50. Martorella, G., et al. (2014). Feasibility and acceptability of hand massage therapy for pain management of postoperative cardiac surgery patients in the intensive care unit. *Heart Lung, 43*, 437–444.
51. McCance, K. L., & Huether, S. E. (Eds.). (2006). *Pathophysiology: the biological basis for disease in adults and children*. St. Louis: Mosby.
52. Melzack, R., & Casey, K. L. (1968). Sensory, motivational and central control determinants of pain: a new conceptual model. In D. Kenshalo (Ed.), *The skin senses* (pp. 423–429). Springfield, Ill: Charles C. Thomas.
53. Melzack, R., & Katz, J. (1992). The McGill pain questionnaire: appraisal and current status. In D. C. Turk, & R. Melzack (Eds.), *Handbook of pain assessment*. New York: Guilford.
54. Melzack, R. (1968). Neurophysiologic foundation of pain. In R. A. Sternbach (Ed.), *The psychology of pain* (pp. 1–12). New York: Raven Press.
55. Melzack, R. (1999). Pain—an overview. *Acta Anaesthesiol Scand, 43*, 880–884.
56. Miaskowski, C., et al. (2008). *Principles of analgesic use in the treatment of acute pain and cancer pain* (6th ed.). Glenview, Ill: American Pain Society.
57. Mirski, M. A., LeDroux, N., Lewin, J. J., 3rd, et al. (2010). Validity and reliability of an intuitive conscious sedation scoring tool: the nursing instrument for the communication of sedation. *Crit Care Med, 38*(8), 1674–1684.
58. Moyer, C. A., Rounds, J., & Hannum, J. W. (2004). A meta-analysis of massage therapy research. *Psychol Bull, 130*(1), 3–18.
59. Munro, C. L., & Grap, M. J. (2004). Oral health and care in the intensive care unit: state of the science. *Am J Crit Care, 13*(1), 25–34.
60. National Pharmaceutical Councils and Joint Commission on Accreditation of Healthcare Organizations. (2001). *Pain: current understanding of assessment, management, and treatment*. Chicago: (Monograph) Author.
61. Ofirmev package insert. (2010). San Diego, CA: Cadence Pharmaceutical, Inc.
62. Olsom, D. M., Thoyre, S. M., & Auyong, D. B. (2007). Perspectives on sedation assessment in critical care. *AACN Adv Crit Care, 12*(4), 380–395.
63. Pasero, C., & Stannard, D. (2012). The role of intravenous acetaminophen in acute pain management: a case study-illustrated review. *Pain Manag Nurs, 13*(2), 107–124.
64. Patel, S. B., & Kress, J. P. (2012). Sedation and analgesia in the mechanically ventilated patient. *Am J Respir Crit Care Med, 185*(5), 486–497.
65. Peitz, G. J., et al. (2013). Top 10 myths regarding sedation and delirium in the ICU. *Crit Care Med, 41*(9), S46–S56.
66. Puntillo, K. A., et al. (2009). Evaluation of pain in ICU patients. *Chest, 135*(4), 1069–1074.
67. Ramsay Sedation Scale. http://www.frca.co.uk/article.aspx?articleid=100192. Anesthesia UK. Date: August 4, 2015.
68. Reade, M. C., & Finfer, S. (2015). Sedation and delirium in the intensive care unit. *N Engl J Med, 370*(5), 444–454.
69. Reichling, D. B., & Levine, J. D. (2009). Critical role of nociceptor plasticity in chronic pain. *Trends Neurosci, 32*(12), 611–618.
70. Riker, R. R., & Fraser, G. L. (2009). Altering intensive care sedation paradigms to improve patient outcomes. *Crit Care Clin, 25*, 527–538.
71. Riker Sedation-Agitation Scale (SAS). Accessed at http://www.icudelirium.org/docs/SAS.pdf.
72. Robinson, B. R. H., et al. (2008). Analgesia-delirium-sedation protocol for critically ill trauma patients reduces ventilator days and hospital length of stay. *J Trauma, 65*(3), 517–524.
73. Samad, T. A. (2004). New understandings of the link between acute pain and chronic pain: can we prevent long-term sequelae? In D. B. Carr, G. Novak, J. P. Rathmell, et al. (Eds.), *The spectrum of pain* (pp. 16–27). New York: McMahon.
74. Savage, S., Covington, E., Heit, H., et al. (2001). *Definitions related to the use of opioids for the treatment of pain: a consensus document from the American Academy of Pain Medicine, the American Pain Society, and the American Society of Addiction Medicine*. Glenview, IL.
75. Shehabi, Y., et al. (2012). Early intensive care sedation predicts long-term mortality in ventilated critically ill patients. *Am J Respir Crit Care Med, 186*(8), 724–731.
76. Skidmore-Roth, L. (2013). *Mosby's nursing drug reference*. St Louis: Mosby.
77. Skrobik, Y., & Ghanques, G. (2013). The pain, agitation, and delirium practice guidelines for adult critically ill patients: a post-publication perspective. *Ann Intensive Care, 3*(9), 1–9.
78. Smith, A., Farrington, M., & Mathews, G. (2014). Monitoring sedation in patients receiving opioids for pain management. *J Nurs Care Qual, 20*(4), 345–353.
79. Springhouse. (2008). *Nurse's drug guide 2008* (6th ed.). Philadelphia: Lippincott.
80. Stites, M. (2013). Observational pain scale in critically ill adults. *Crit Care Nurs, 33*(93), 68–78.
81. Subramanianet, P., et al. (2011). Challenges faced by nurses in managing pain in a critical care setting. *J Clin Nurs, 21*, 1254–1262.
82. Swanson, R. W., & Klein, D. G. (2005). Comfort and sedation. In M. L. Sole, D. G. Klein, & M. J. Moseley (Eds.), *Introduction to critical care nursing* (4th ed.). Philadelphia: Elsevier Saunders.
83. Tennant, F. (2013). The physiologic effects of pain on the endocrine system. *Pain Ther, 2*, 75–86.
84. Tocher, J., et al. (2012). Pain management and satisfaction in postsurgical patients. *J Clin Nurs, 21* 3361–2271.
85. Treede, R. D., et al. (2008). Neuropathic pain redefinition and a grading system for clinical and research purposes. *Neurology, 70*(18), 1630–1635.
86. Van de Leur, J. P., et al. (2004). Discomfort and factual recollection in intensive care unit patients. *Crit Care, 8*(6), R467–R473.
87. Van Kuiken, D. (2004). A meta-analysis of the effect of guided imagery practice on outcomes. *J Holist Nurs, 22*(2), 164–179.
88. Viscusi, E. R., et al. (2012). IV acetaminophen improves pain management and reduces opioid requirements in surgical patients: a review of the clinical data and case-based presentations. http://www.pharmacypracticenews.com/download/SR122_WM.pdf.
89. Woien, H., et al. (2012). Improving the systematic approach to pain and sedation management in the ICU by using assessment tools. *J Clin Nurs, 23*, 1552–1561.
90. Yeh, Y., & Reddy, P. (2012). Clinical and economic evidence for intravenous acetaminophen. *Pharmacotherapy, 32*(6), 559–579.

40

Comorbid Conditions

Paula McCauley

INTRODUCTION

Admission to critical care and the outcome of that admission are influenced by the patient's primary diagnosis and preexisting comorbidities. The presence of multi-organ involvement during critical illness plays a role in patient morbidity and mortality. For the purposes of this chapter, comorbid conditions refer to chronic conditions that exist prior to admission to critical care. Conditions that arise during hospitalization are considered to be acute conditions or complications, and are not discussed in this chapter.

CRITICAL CARE PREDICTIVE SCORING SYSTEMS

Critical care patients with preexisting comorbid conditions when they are admitted to the ICU have a 2% to 8.4% greater risk of mortality than patients with no comorbid conditions.[38,43,44,45] Predictive scoring systems in use in many critical care units attempt to calculate the mortality risk of the critical care patient on the basis of these comorbidities when the patient is admitted to critical care. Predictive scoring systems use a severity of illness score to adjust for mortality risk upon admission to critical care. The overall predictive patient score is calculated based on several factors including patient age, physiologic scoring, and preexisting conditions. The scoring systems described in this chapter are used solely as a starting point for understanding and comprehending the impact and importance of comorbidity in critical care.

The three most frequently used predictive scoring systems are the Acute Physiology and Chronic Health Evaluation (APACHE), the Simplified Acute Physiology Score (SAPS), and the Mortality Prediction Model (MPM). As changes in case mix and clinical practice occur, the scoring models must be revised to reflect clinical changes, resulting in different generations of these scoring systems (currently APACHE IV, SAPS 3, and MPM III). SAPS 3 is primarily used for international benchmarking; APACHE IV and MPM III require institutional or regional customization. These models allow facilities to make meaningful comparisons of current performance with past performance, identify opportunities in care processes, define interventions to address gaps in care processes, and evaluate the impact of process changes and new therapies.[22,24,37,46,60]

Scoring Systems Defined

The specific comorbidities present in scoring systems are listed in Table 40.1. APACHE IV considers the greatest number of comorbidities, whereas the SAPS 3 and MPM III only consider three comorbid conditions. The only comorbid condition found in all three scoring systems is the presence of metastatic disease. Acquired immunodeficiency syndrome (AIDS), cirrhosis, hematologic malignancies, and chronic kidney disease are found in two of the three scoring systems.

The APACHE IV model predicts mortality, ICU and hospital length of stay, duration of mechanical ventilation, and potential transfer from the ICU. Comorbid conditions are integrated into the scoring system, and include HIV/AIDS, hepatic failure, cirrhosis, lymphoma, metastatic cancer, leukemia or multiple myeloma, and immunosuppression.[13,38,60] The APACHE IV model equations were developed based on a contemporary database of US patients admitted to critical care units.

The MPM model, also developed in the United States, uses 15 variables to derive the severity score. The score is measured on admission, but can be updated at 24 hours after admission. The variables include several physiologic variables, type of admission, age, cardiopulmonary resuscitation, mechanical ventilation, and the presence or absence of three chronic disease states. The three chronic disease states impacting the score are: chronic renal insufficiency, cirrhosis, and metastatic cancer.[44,45,60]

The SAPS model was originally designed to streamline data collection. Data are collected, and a severity score is determined 24 hours after admission to the critical care unit. Data points include existing risk factors such as age, type of admission, 12 physiologic variables, and the presence or absence of three chronic diseases: AIDS, hematologic malignancy (such as lymphoma, acute leukemia, or multiple myeloma), and metastatic cancer.[43] As electronic health records improve, the SAPS will lend itself to automated scoring, decreasing the abstraction burden and the inter-rater variability that occur due to the manual data extraction required by current scoring systems.[60]

Impact of Comorbidities on Length of Stay and Treatment

Whereas most scoring systems use comorbidities to evaluate mortality risk (Table 40.2), there are several studies in which comorbidities have been used to predict factors such as length of stay (LOS) or length of time on a mechanical ventilator. Examples of these systems include the Charlson Comorbidity Index,[20] the Cumulative Illness Rating Scale (CIRS), and the Chronic Disease Score (CDS).[69]

The Charlson Comorbidity Index is a measure of the risk of 1-year mortality attributable to comorbidity in a longitudinal study of generalized hospitalized patients that was subsequently adapted for use with International Classification of Disease-9 (ICD-9) codes.[15] The comorbidities, which are given varying weights in the index, include the following: cardiovascular disease (myocardial infarction [MI], chronic heart failure [HF], peripheral vascular disease, and cerebrovascular disease), dementia, chronic pulmonary disease, connective tissue disease,

TABLE 40.1 Predictive Scoring Systems and the Comorbidities Identified

Apache II–IV	SAPS II	MPM II
Metastatic cancer	Metastatic cancer	Metastatic malignant neoplasm
Leukemia	Hematologic malignancies	
AIDS	AIDS	
Cirrhosis		Cirrhosis
Hepatic failure		
Lymphoma		
Multiple myeloma		
Immunosuppression		

APACHE, Acute Physiology and Chronic Health Evaluation; *MPM,* Mortality Prediction Model; *SAPS,* Simplified Acute Physiology Score.
From References 14, 39, 44, and 45.

TABLE 40.2 Elixhauser Comorbidities Affecting In-Hospital Mortality

Comorbidity	In-Hospital Mortality (Odds Ratio $p < 0.05$)
Heart failure	2.3
Cardiac dysrhythmias	1.4
Valvular disease	0.7
Pulmonary circulation disorders	1.9
Peripheral vascular disorders	1.2
Hypertension	0.6
Paralysis	1.7
Other neurologic disorders	2.8
Chronic pulmonary disease	1.2
Diabetes, complicated	1.1
Hypothyroidism	0.7
Renal failure	2.1
Liver disease	1.9
Peptic ulcer disease, excluding bleeding	0.8
AIDS	3.2
Lymphoma	1.8
Metastatic cancer	3.1
Coagulopathy	4.1
Obesity	0.5
Weight loss	3.2
Fluid and electrolyte disorders	2.7
Blood loss anemia	0.9
Alcohol abuse	1.1
Psychosis	1.2
Depression	0.6

Data from Reference 23.

ulcer disease, mild liver disease, diabetes, hemiplegia, moderate or severe renal disease, diabetes with end-organ damage, any tumor, leukemia, lymphoma, moderate or severe liver disease, metastatic solid tumor, and AIDS.[15]

The CIRS is one of the existing tools for measuring comorbidity. The CIRS measures the chronic illness burden, taking into consideration the severity of all chronic diseases present. The CIRS was developed and later revised to reflect common conditions in elderly patients, and renamed the Cumulative Illness Rating Scale for Geriatrics (CIRS-G).[50,51]

The CDS is a comorbidity measure based on medication utilization.[69] Medications used to treat the following diseases are weighted: heart disease, respiratory illness, asthma, rheumatism, rheumatoid arthritis, cancer, Parkinson's disease, hypertension, diabetes, epilepsy, ulcers, glaucoma, gout, hyperuricemia, high cholesterol, migraines, and tuberculosis. In a study conducted by Parker et al., the CDS was found to be a significant predictor of 30-day hospital readmission and LOS.[55] By combining pharmacy-based information with information abstracted from the patient's medical record modest improvement in predicting hospital outcomes was achieved.

Whereas multiple risk factors were studied in the development of all the previously mentioned scoring systems, other comorbidity risk factors are important in outcome and morbidity in critical illness. For example, in the past, diabetes mellitus (DM)—and its relationship to stress-induced hyperglycemia—emerged as a relevant risk factor. Other studies have demonstrated that elevated blood glucose levels during critical illness are a significant contributor to both morbidity and mortality in the nondiabetic patient.[40,64] Traditional scoring systems may not be adequate predictors in certain patient groups such as trauma patients, obstetrics patients, and AIDS patients.[15,67]

Trauma scores such as the Injury Severity Score or the Revised Trauma Score include age but exclude evaluation of other comorbidities. Predictors of mortality in geriatric trauma are not well-established.[41,42] Tan et al. found that comorbidities were common in trauma patients, especially those over 40 years of age.[67] They concluded that the outcome of trauma patients with comorbidities is difficult to predict using the traditional trauma scoring systems, and specifically the APACHE II system.[67] A systematic review conducted by Hashmi et al. concluded that trauma patients over 74 years of age have a higher risk of mortality.[30] The predictors considered in this review were the severity of injury, the Glasgow Coma Score, and age; comorbidities or frailty were not considered. Additional research is necessary in this population.

COMORBIDITIES USED IN SCORING SYSTEMS

Metastatic Cancer/Hematologic Malignancy

When oncology patients require admission to the critical care unit, their prognosis worsens. Advances in cancer care have improved short-term mortality, which may be attributable to advances in treatment of malignancies, earlier admission to the ICU, and perhaps better selection of patients who may benefit from critical care. The number of failed organ systems is prognostic of mortality, with hepatic and/or cardiovascular failure among the strongest associated independent predictors of mortality. Overall, critical care oncology patients have an average mortality rate of 30%, with higher rates (58%) for patients with a medical diagnosis, and lower rates (11%) for patients with scheduled surgical admission. In cancer patients admitted to critical care with respiratory failure and needing mechanical ventilation, critical care mortality exceeds 80%, and is even higher in those who have undergone marrow transplants.[24,39]

Multiple factors associated with increased mortality have been documented in patients with hematologic cancers. These patients are frequently admitted to the ICU with sepsis, bacteremia, vasopressor support, and mechanical ventilation. The mortality rate is high for patients with hematologic malignancy; 47% of these patients do not survive hospitalization, and there is a 75% mortality rate in patients with hematologic malignancy who require critical care. Central nervous system failure and hepatic failure are both independently associated with poor prognosis in this cohort.[7,24,39]

HIV, AIDS, and Immunosuppression

Similar to the critical care mortality rates of patients with cancer, the mortality rates of patients with HIV/AIDS are alarmingly high, although they have improved with advancements in care for this population. Previously, mortality was reported at 25% to 40%, whereas mortality is now reported in less than 10% of these patients; in addition, there has been a slight improvement in LOS. The development of highly active antiretroviral therapy (HAART) has altered outcomes, including the need for ICU care. Patients with HIV/AIDS are frequently admitted to the ICU due to illness related to infectious diseases, but noninfectious problems such as chronic disease states may negatively impact the LOS.[2] Patients with HIV/AIDS and severe sepsis have a higher mortality rate than patients with severe sepsis and no HIV/AIDS.[24,28] Other factors that appear to have an impact on outcomes include time since diagnosis with HIV/AIDS, number of previous opportunistic infections, weight loss, and nutritional status.

The use of HAART in the hospitalized critical care patient should be *continued* if prescribed prior to the admission, unless contraindicated. HAART should not be *initiated* in a hospitalized patient, unless the CD4 count is less than 200 or there is a prolonged LOS. Complications such as pancreatitis, lactic acidosis, hepatic failure, and renal failure can result from HAART therapy, and should be monitored closely.[2,24]

Chronic and End-Stage Liver Disease

Acute-on-chronic liver failure (ACLF) is an increasingly identified entity in critical care. The prognosis of patients who are critically ill with hepatic failure or cirrhosis is poor. The Child Turcotte Pugh (CTP) score for decompensated cirrhosis, the Chronic Liver Failure-Sequential Organ Failure Assessment (CLIF-SOFA), and the Model for End-Stage Liver Disease (MELD) scores have been developed to help define ICU mortality in these patients.[9,32,35,54,63,70,71]

Mortality in patients with chronic or end-stage liver disease admitted to a critical care unit exceeds 50%.[35,54] The high morbidity and mortality of end-stage liver disease (ESLD) are secondary to the associated complications. ESLD complications include infection, sepsis, variceal hemorrhage, ascites, spontaneous bacterial peritonitis, cirrhosis-associated acute kidney injury, hepatic encephalopathy, coagulation abnormalities, hepatopulmonary syndrome, and hepatocellular carcinoma. Acute kidney injury (AKI), mechanical ventilation, and shock are also associated with high mortality in this population.[35,54] The increased risk for infection associated with ESLD is felt to be due to the immunologic deficits that the syndrome produces. Vascular hyperactivity and hyperdynamic circulation may mask end-organ dysfunction and goal-directed therapy in sepsis.[35] Liver transplantation and palliative care are important considerations in this population. Careful consideration of whether to list the patient for transplantation or implement palliative care is necessary for improving outcomes, survival, and quality of life.[70]

The two most common causes of cirrhosis in the United States are alcoholic liver disease and hepatitis C, which together account for almost half of those patients undergoing liver transplantation.[35,54] The rates of morbidity and mortality in critical care are two to four times greater in patients with a history of chronic alcohol abuse than in patients with no history of alcohol abuse.[52,53]

Chronic Kidney Disease and End-Stage Renal Disease

Both acute and chronic renal diseases are associated with increased mortality in critical care. Similarly, both end-stage renal disease (ESRD) and chronic kidney disease (CKD) are associated with increased mortality in critical illness. The primary causes of death in patients with CKD are cardiovascular disease, infection, and respiratory failure. Other frequent complications in this population include gastrointestinal bleeding, malnutrition, and anemia.[6,19,33,66]

Defining and classifying CKD has standardized and enhanced the quality and effectiveness of care for this patient population. Published guidelines from Kidney Disease: Improving Global Outcomes (KDIGO) and the National Institute for Health and Care Excellence (NICE) have been adopted as the standard of care. Diabetes, hypertension, and proteinuria are all predictors of CKD progression.[66] CKD is an independent risk factor for developing AKI. AKI remains a significant clinical challenge in critical care, with a high mortality rate. Overall, 5% to 80% of all patients in the ICU have been reported to have AKI, with only 5% requiring renal replacement therapy (RRT).[19]

Patients with CKD and ESRD require critical care services at higher rates than the general population, but have relatively good outcomes when these factors are taken into account. Patients with ESRD carry a higher burden of comorbidities, which as a whole impacts illness severity and outcomes.[33] Critical care of these patients is complicated by the pathophysiology that impaired kidney function brings, which affects the pharmacokinetics of multiple medications, complicates fluid and electrolyte management, impairs hemostasis, and increases the risk of infectious complications. Major predictors of mortality include advanced age, sepsis, mechanical ventilation, and the number of failed organ systems.[24,33]

OTHER COMORBIDITIES AS PREDICTORS OF OUTCOME

Respiratory Conditions

Respiratory conditions, such as chronic obstructive pulmonary disease (COPD), interstitial lung disease, pulmonary fibrosis, and a history of smoking, lead to earlier intervention with mechanical ventilation and result in worse outcomes.[1,10,12,14,31,47,49,61,65]

ICU patients with diagnosis of COPD at admission have a higher incidence of complications and mortality. The diagnosis of COPD in hospitalized patients is associated with higher in-hospital mortality rates. COPD is associated with increased morbidity when combined with ischemic heart disease, pneumonia, thoracic malignancies, and respiratory failure.[8,17,65] Predictors of risk for rehospitalization and increased mortality include prior hospitalization for COPD, asthma, and pulmonary hypertension.[49] Mortality risk increases with advanced age, longer hospital LOS, and three or more acute COPD exacerbations.[8] The increased utilization of noninvasive ventilation has been associated with lower risk of hospital-acquired pneumonia and a shorter LOS.[47]

COPD is an independent risk factor for all-cause mortality and, when combined with cardiovascular disease, results in even greater mortality. Heart failure, dysrhythmias, shock, and hypotension occur more frequently in critically ill patients with a prior history of COPD. In a multivariate analysis, the APACHE II score, electrocardiograph (ECG) abnormalities (including supraventricular ectopy and right and/or left ventricular hypertrophy), and digoxin therapy were independent predictors of cardiovascular complications.[10,25,61]

Despite advances in infection control and antimicrobial therapy, patients with pneumonia (whether community-acquired or nosocomial) have greater morbidity and mortality during critical care hospitalization.[1,14] The appearance of multidrug-resistant organisms (MDROs) has increased the risk of mortality. The mortality rate for community-acquired pneumonia (CAP) in hospitalized patients can range from 20% to 54%. Factors that predict in-hospital mortality among patients who require hospitalization for the treatment of CAP include functional status at the time of hospital admission, as well as hyperkalemia, lymphopenia, and the type of antibiotic therapy.[28,59] Independent predictors of in-hospital mortality include: extent of lung injury (as assessed by the hypoxemia index), number of nonpulmonary organs that have failed, presence of immunosuppression, age greater than 80 years, and medical comorbidity with a prognosis for survival of less than five years.

There are various clinical decision tools available to assess CAP severity. These tools are useful in guiding antibiotic therapy and in determining disposition for admission and level of care for patients with CAP. They include the Pneumonia Severity Index (PSI), which is a score defined by 20 clinical variables; the CURB-65 score, which is a simple five-point score based on confusion (C), urea (U), respiratory rate (R), blood pressure (B), and age greater than 65; and the APACHE IV. These three tools predicted the 28-day mortality and in-hospital mortality of patients with CAP in the Recombinant Human Activated Protein C Worldwide Evaluation in Severe Sepsis (PROWESS) Phase 3 study.[58]

Pneumonia is the second most common type of infection acquired in the hospital, and 50% of cases are postoperative. The postoperative pneumonia risk index developed by Arozullah et al. identifies patients at risk for postoperative pneumonia, and may be helpful in guiding perioperative care (Table 40.3).[5] In this index, comorbidities and the type of surgery are ascribed a point value, which is then used to compute a total point score for the risk of pneumonia after surgery. Table 40.3 describes the point values and risk classes. Use of a risk tool such as this may be helpful in identifying patients at risk and targeting them for early intervention. Gupta et al. broadened the data used in this index to include variables from the American College of Surgeon's National Surgical Quality Improvement Program (NSQIP), and developed an interactive risk calculator.[29] Comorbidities were significant in both of these studies, and included age greater than 50 years, functional status (partially or totally dependent), COPD, and smoking within the year prior to surgery.

Ventilator-associated pneumonia (VAP) has substantial subsequent mortality, although the focus has been expanded to include ventilator-associated events (VAE) broadening the surveillance definition. The impact of VAP is controversial, but has been associated with increased LOS, greater economic impact, and mortality.[14]

Cardiovascular Disease

In the American College of Cardiology (ACC) and American Heart Association (AHA) guidelines for evaluating the cardiac risk of non–cardiac surgery patients, cardiovascular risk factors are considered to be major or intermediate clinical predictors for perioperative risk of MI, HF, or death.[4] The major clinical predictors are unstable coronary syndromes, decompensated HF, significant dysrhythmias, and severe valvular disease. Intermediate cardiovascular disease predictors include mild angina pectoris, prior MI, and compensated or prior HF. Two additional risk factors that are closely linked with known cardiac disease are also intermediate predictors: DM and renal insufficiency.[4] The stress of critical illness can increase the risk of cardiac sequelae. Scarduelli et al. demonstrated that 39% of patients admitted to respiratory ICUs with COPD developed cardiovascular complications, including hypotension, shock, HF, and/or dysrhythmias.[61] Patients who developed cardiovascular complications had a mortality rate of 15.5%, compared to a rate of 4.7% in patients without cardiovascular complications ($p = 0.0044$).[61] Studies have demonstrated that cardiac ischemia may develop during weaning from mechanical ventilation.[14,25] Detection of myocardial ischemia during critical

TABLE 40.3 Postoperative Pneumonia Risk Index

Variable	Risk Index Points*
Type of Surgery	
Abdominal aortic aneurysm repair	15
Thoracic	14
Upper abdominal	10
Neck	8
Neurosurgery	8
Vascular	3
Age (Years)	
≥ 80	17
70–79	13
60–69	9
50–59	4
Functional Status	
Totally dependent	10
Partially dependent	6
Weight loss > 10%	7
History of COPD	5
General anesthesia	4
Impaired sensorium	4
History of CVA	4
Blood Urea Nitrogen Level (mg/dL)	
< 8	4
22–30	2
≥ 30	3
Other Factors	
Transfusion > 4 units	3
Emergency surgery	3
Steroid use for chronic conditions	3
Current smoker within 1 year	3
Alcohol intake > 2 drinks/day in past 2 weeks	2

*To calculate risk of postoperative pneumonia, add the total points from the right column and use the following probabilities: (1) 0.24%, 0–15 points; (2) 1.19%, 16–25 points; (3) 4.0%, 26–40 points; (4) 9.4%, 41–55 points; (5) 15.8%, >55 points.

COPD, Chronic obstructive pulmonary disease; *CVA*, cerebrovascular accident.

From Reference 5.

illness and its impact on morbidity and mortality, especially in critically ill patients without a prior cardiac diagnosis, need further study.

Diabetes Mellitus

Patients with DM can be a challenge in critical care. Patients with DM are at greater risk for morbidity, including AKI, poor wound healing, infection, sepsis, and vascular events that ultimately may lead to worse outcomes. Surprisingly, diabetes is not a chronic condition that is taken into account in the APACHE IV, SAPS 3, or MPM III scoring systems. The importance of glycemic control in critically ill patients has been studied extensively in the literature since the early 1990s.[40,64] The earlier goal of controlling blood glucose levels between 80 and 110 mg/dL has been replaced by the goal of reducing glucose variability. Managing hyperglycemia is important, but avoiding hypoglycemia is equally important in the care of these patients. Avoiding significant hyperglycemia (>180 mg/dL) is now the standard in critical care.[24,57,64]

Age

Whereas age is not a true comorbidity, studies have examined the impact of age on outcomes in acute and critical care, with varying results. The rapid growth of the elderly as a population subgroup (referred to as the "silver tsunami") and the aging "epidemic," as well as the increase in chronic disease and identification of the specific physiologic needs of the elderly, have prompted increased emphasis on elder care.[66] Age is a predictor of mortality, when underlying disease and physiologic status are taken into account. Over 50% of older adults have three or more chronic diseases.[11,16,66] The most vulnerable patient subgroups are the frail elderly, patients over 85 years of age, patients with loss of functional status, and patients with cognitive impairment.[48] Prognostic models used to predict elderly mortality have been developed, but have not been sufficiently validated for use and credibility, and require further research.[36,50,51] Research has shown that elderly patients admitted to critical care with APACHE IV scores of greater than 25 have higher mortality rates than those with lower APACHE IV scores. The most important predictors of mortality in this group are the number of comorbid conditions, ESRD, and the severity of the acute illness.[30,33]

Obesity

Obesity is a major health problem in the United States. Obesity is associated with a chronic inflammatory state that affects several body systems, including the pulmonary, cardiovascular, gastrointestinal, hematologic, renal, immune, and metabolic systems.[56] Obesity is associated with an increased risk of multiple organ dysfunction, cardiovascular disease, DM, pulmonary disease, acute lung injury (ALI), sleep apnea, and obstructive airway disease.[24] Obesity has been associated with an increase in overall mortality, perioperative mortality, and mortality after trauma. Additionally, obesity is a risk factor for both morbidity and mortality during critical illness.[18,21,27,56] Morbid obesity presents a higher risk for prolonged mechanical ventilation, which exposes the patient to other risks such as ventilator-associated pneumonia, skin breakdown, and deep vein thrombosis from immobility.[62] Additional research has argued that morbid obesity is not a predictor of poor outcome in critical care. Further studies of both obese medical and surgical patients are warranted.[24,26,27,68]

Social and Psychological Comorbidities

Social comorbidities that may impact critical care illness include chronic alcohol and tobacco use. Iribarren et al. identified that there is a relationship between cigarette smoking and acute respiratory distress syndrome (ARDS) in ICU patients, with approximately 50% of ARDS cases being attributable to smoking.[34] As stated previously, morbidity and mortality in critical care are two to four times greater in patients with a history of chronic alcohol abuse. The literature suggests that the patient's overall psychological state may be a risk for increased mortality. A study conducted by Ely et al. showed that delirium was a predictor of mortality in the mechanically ventilated patient.[23] Many studies have validated the impact of delirium on morbidity and mortality. For greater detail on the standards of care related to the critically ill patient with a psychiatric disorder, see Chapter 37; for information about care of the patient with a chemical dependency, see Chapter 42.

CARE OF PATIENTS WITH MULTIPLE COMORBIDITIES

As critical care practitioners, it is evident that the addition of multiple comorbidities to an already critical condition increases the complexity of patient care, as well as the need for critical thinking in caring for these patients. The impact of comorbidities can be seen in several patient characteristics, as outlined in the American Association of Critical-Care Nurses (AACN) Synergy Model for Patient Care.[3] The model describes patient complexity as the intricate entanglement of two or more systems. These systems can be physiologic or emotional states of the body, family dynamics, or the environment. Resiliency is the patient's capacity to return to a restorative level of functioning, and can be affected by age, comorbidities, and compensatory mechanisms. Vulnerability is the level of susceptibility to adverse outcomes, and can be impacted by comorbidities. Predictability of the outcome or course of illness can be low if there are multiple comorbidities.[5] Because of the unpredictability and high complexity of illness, patients with multiple comorbidities need critical care nurses with strong clinical judgment and expertise. For example, care of a 40-year-old patient with no comorbidities with severe pneumonia requiring ventilator treatment is less complex than care of an 80-year-old patient with diabetes, COPD, angina with minimal activity, and severe pneumonia requiring ventilatory support. As the complexity of the critical care patient increases, so does the need for an advanced level of critical thinking and clinical expertise in the critical care nurse and advanced practitioner. For further information on the Synergy Model, refer to Chapter 1.

CONCLUSION

Patients with comorbidities, especially those of the severity listed earlier in this chapter, are at a higher opportunity for increased morbidity and mortality during critical care hospitalization. Risk-scoring systems are helpful in providing a starting point as to which comorbidities are important in treating the critically ill patient, but these scoring systems are not all-inclusive, and omit several important comorbidities. In an attempt to incorporate evidence-based medicine into clinical practice, it is necessary to have an understanding of the specific comorbidities that are the greatest predictors of poor outcome, as indicated by the literature. There is a paucity of data, as well as conflicting data, regarding some comorbid conditions such as age and obesity. These comorbidities are deserving of further attention and research to guide evidence-based practice in caring for these patients.

REFERENCES

1. Almirall, J., Mesalles, E., Klamburg, J., et al. (1995). Prognostic factors of pneumonia requiring admission to the intensive care unit. *Chest, 107*, 511–516.
2. Akgün, K. M., Pisani, M., & Crothers, K. (2011). The changing epidemiology of HIV-infected patients in the intensive care unit. *J Intensive Care Med, 26*(3), 151–164.
3. American Association of Critical-Care Nurses. (2006). *American Association of Critical-Care Nurses Synergy Model for Patient Care.*
4. American College of Cardiology and American Heart Association. (2005). *ACC/AHA guideline update for perioperative cardiovascular evaluation for noncardiac surgery.*
5. Arozullah, A., Khuri, S., Henderson, W., et al. (2001). Development and validation of a multifactorial risk index for predicting postoperative pneumonia after major noncardiac surgery. *Ann Intern Med, 135*(10), 847–857.
6. Arulkumaran, N., Annear, N., & Singer, M. (2013). Patients with end-stage renal disease admitted to the intensive care unit: systematic review. *Br J Anaesth, 110*(1), 13–20. http://dx.doi.org/10.1093/bja/aes401.
7. Azoulay, E., Thiery, G., Chevret, S., et al. (2004). The prognosis of acute respiratory failure in critically ill cancer patients. *Medicine, 83*(6), 360–370.
8. Batzlaff, C. M., Karpman, C., Afessa, B., et al. (2014). Predicting 1-year mortality rate for patients admitted with an acute exacerbation of chronic obstructive pulmonary disease to an intensive care unit: an opportunity for palliative care. *Mayo Clin Proc, 89*(5), 638–643. http://dx.doi.org/10.1016/j.mayocp.2013.12.00.
9. Bauer, M., Press, A. T., & Trauner, M. (2013). The liver in sepsis: patterns of response and injury. *Curr Opin Crit Care, 19*(2), 123–127. http://dx.doi.org/10.1097/MCC.0b013e32835eba6d.
10. Bi, H., Yanmin, Y., Jun, Z., et al. (2014). Clinical characteristics and prognostic significance of chronic obstructive pulmonary disease in patients with atrial fibrillation: results from a multicenter atrial fibrillation registry study. *J Am Med Dir Assoc, 15*(8), 576–581.
11. Bo, M., Massaia, M., Raspo, S., et al. (2003). Predictive factors of in-hospital mortality in older patients admitted to a medical intensive care unit. *J Am Geriatr Soc, 51*(4), 529–533.
12. Breen, D., Churches, T., Hawker, E., et al. (2002). Acute respiratory failure secondary to chronic obstructive pulmonary disease treated in the intensive care units: a long term follow up study. *Thorax, 57*(1), 29–33.
13. Cerner. (2006). APACHE IV scoring system. From http://www.cerner.com.
14. Chahoud, J., Semaan, A., & Almoosa, K. F. (2015). Ventilator-associated events prevention, learning lessons from the past: a systematic review. *Heart Lung, 44*(3), 251–259.
15. Charlson, M., Pompei, P., & MacKenzie, C. (1987). New method of classifying prognostic co-morbidity in longitudinal studies: development and validation. *J Chronic Dis, 40*, 373–383.
16. Chelluri, L., Pinsky, M., Donahoe, M., et al. (1993). Long-term outcome of critically ill elderly patients requiring intensive care. *J Am Med Assoc, 269*(24), 3119–3123.
17. Chronic obstructive pulmonary disease among adults - United States. (2011). *MMWR Morb Mortal Wkly Rep, 61*, 938–943 November 23, 2012.
18. Collins, J. (2014). Nutrition and care considerations in the overweight and obese population within the critical care setting. *Crit Care Nurs Clin North Am, 26*(2), 243–253. http://dx.doi.org/10.1016/j.ccell.2014.01.002.
19. Davies, H., & Leslie, G. (2012). Acute kidney injury and the critically ill patient. *Dimens Crit Care Nurs, 31*(3), 135–152.
20. Deyo, R., Cherkin, D., & Ciol, M. (1992). Adapting a clinical co-morbidity index for use with ICD-9-CM administrative databases. *J Clin Epidemiol, 45*(6), 613–619.
21. El-Solh, A., Sikka, P., Bozkanat, E., et al. (2001). Morbid obesity in the medical ICU. *Chest, 120*(6), 1989–1997.
22. Elixhauser, A., Steiner, C., Harris, D., et al. (1998). Comorbidity measures for use with administrative data. *Med Care, 36*(1), 8–27.
23. Ely, E., Shintani, A., Truman, B., et al. (2004). Delirium as a predictor of mortality in mechanically ventilated patients in the intensive care unit. *J Am Med Assoc, 291*(14), 1753–1762.
24. Esper, A., & Martin, G. (2011). The impact of comorbid conditions on critical illness. *Crit Care Med, 39*(12), 2728–2735.
25. Frazier, S. (2008). Cardiovascular effects of mechanical ventilation and weaning. *Nurs Clin North Am, 43*(1), 1–15.
26. Garrouste-Oregeas, M., Troche, G., Azoulay, E., et al. (2004). Body mass index: an additional prognostic factor in ICU patients. *Intensive Care Med, 30*, 437–443.
27. Goulenok, C., Monchi, M., Chiche, J., et al. (2004). Influence of overweight on ICU mortality. *Chest, 125*(1), 1441–1445.
28. Gross, P., DeMauro, P., Van Antwerp, C., et al. (1988). Number of comorbidities as a predictor of nosocomial infection acquisition. *Infect Control Hosp Epidemiol, 9*(11), 497–500.
29. Gupta, H., Gupta, P. K., Schuller, D., et al. (2013). Development and validation of a risk calculator for predicting postoperative pneumonia. *Mayo Clin Proc, 88*(11), 1241–1249.
30. Hashmi, A., Ibrahim-Zada, I., Rhee, P., et al. (2014). Predictors of mortality in geriatric trauma patients: a systematic review and meta-analysis. *J Trauma Acute Care Surg, 76*(3), 894–901.
31. Hilas, G., Perlikos, F., Tsiligianni, I., & Tzanakis, N. (2015). Managing comorbidities in COPD. *Int J Chron Obstruct Pulmon Dis, 10*, 95–109.
32. Ho, Y., Chen, C., Yang, C., et al. (2004). Outcome prediction for critically ill cirrhotic patients: a comparison of APACHE II and Child-Pugh scoring systems. *J Intensive Care Med, 19*(2), 105–110.
33. Hotchkiss, J. R., & Palevsky, P. M. (2012). Care of the critically ill patient with advanced chronic kidney disease or end-stage renal disease. *Curr Opin Crit Care, 18*(6), 599–606. http://dx.doi.org/10.1097/MCC.0b013e32835a1c59.
34. Iribarren, C., Jacobs, De, Sidney, S., et al. (2000). Cigarette smoking, alcohol consumption and risk of ARDS: a 15-year cohort study in a managed care setting. *Chest, 117*(1), 163–168.
35. Karvellas, C. J., & Bagshaw, S. M. (2014). Advances in management and prognostication in critically ill cirrhotic patients. *Curr Opin Crit Care, 20*(2), 210–217.
36. Kass, J. E., Castriotta, R., & Malakoff, F. (1992). Intensive care unit outcome in the very elderly. *Crit Care Med, 20*(1), 1666–1671.
37. Keegan, M., Gajic, O., & Afessa, B. (2011). Severity of illness scoring systems in the intensive care unit. *Crit Care Med, 39*(1), 163–169.
38. Knaus, W., Wagner, D., Draper, E., et al. (1991). The APACHE III prognostic system: risk prediction of hospital mortality for critically ill hospitalized adults. *Chest, 100*(1), 1619–1636.
39. Kostakou, E., Rovina, N., Kyriakopoulou, M., et al. (2014). Critically ill cancer patient in intensive care unit: issues that arise. *J Crit Care, 29*(5), 817–822.
40. Krinsley, J. (2004). Effect of an intensive glucose management protocol on the mortality of critically ill adult patients. *Mayo Clin Proc, 79*(8), 992–1000.
41. Lecky, F., Woodford, M., Edwards, A., et al. (2014). Trauma scoring systems and databases. *Br J Anaesth, 113*(2), 286–294.
42. Lefering, R. (2012). Trauma scoring systems. *Curr Opin Crit Care, 18*(6), 637–640.
43. LeGall, J., Lemeshow, S., & Saulnier, F. (1993). A new simplified acute physiology score (SAPS II) based on a European/North American multicenter study. *J Am Med Assoc, 270*, 2957–2963.
44. Lemeshow, S., & Le Gall, J. (1994). Modeling the severity of illness of ICU patients. A systems update. *J Am Med Assoc, 272*(13), 1049–1055.

45. Lemeshow, S., Teres, D., Klar, J., et al. (1993). Mortality probability models (MPM II) based on an international cohort of intensive care unit patients. *J Am Med Assoc, 270*(20), 2478–2486.
46. Lewis, A. (2009). How to measure the outcomes of chronic disease management. *Popul Health Manag, 12*(1), 47–54.
47. Lindenauer, P. K., Stefan, M. S., Shieh, M., et al. (2014). Outcomes associated with invasive and noninvasive ventilation among patients hospitalized with exacerbations of chronic obstructive pulmonary disease. *JAMA Intern Med, 174*(12), 1982–1993.
48. Mayer-Oakes, S., Oye, R., & Leake, B. (1991). Predictors of mortality in older patients following medical intensive care: the importance of functional status. *J Am Geriatr Soc, 39*(9), 862–868.
49. McGhan, R., Radcliff, T., Fish, R., et al. (2007). Predictors of rehospitalization and death after a severe exacerbation of COPD. *Chest, 132*(6), 1748–1755. CINAHL Plus with Full Text, Ipswich, MA. Accessed July 27, 2015.
50. Minne, L., Ludikhuize, J., de Rooij, S. E., & Abu-Hanna, A. (2011). Characterizing predictive models of mortality for older adults and their validation for use in clinical practice. *J Am Geriatr Soc, 59*(6), 1110–1115.
51. Minne, L., Ludikhuize, J., de Jonge, E., de Rooij, S., & Abu-Hanna, A. (2011). Prognostic models for predicting mortality in elderly ICU patients: a systematic review. *Intensive Care Med, 37*(8), 1258–1268.
52. Moss, M., & Burnham, E. (2003). Chronic alcohol abuse, acute respiratory distress syndrome and multiple organ dysfunction. *Crit Care Med, 31*(4), S207–S212.
53. Moss, M., Parsons, P., Steinberg, P., et al. (2003). Chronic alcohol abuse is associated with an increased incidence of ARDS and severity of multiple organ dysfunction in patients with septic shock. *Crit Care Med, 31*(3), 869–877.
54. Olson, J. C., & Kamath, P. S. (2011). Acute-on-chronic liver failure: concept, natural history, and prognosis. *Curr Opin Crit Care, 17*(2), 165–169.
55. Parker, J., McCombs, J., & Graddy, E. (2003). Can pharmacy data improve prediction of hospital outcomes? Comparisons with a diagnosis-based co-morbidity measure. *Med Care, 41*(3), 407–419.
56. Pieracci, F., Barie, P., & Pomp, A. (2006). Critical care of the bariatric patient. *Crit Care Med, 34*(6), 1796–1804.
57. Qaseem, A., Humphrey, L. L., Chou, R., Snow, V., Shekelle, P., Clinical Guidelines Committee of the American College of Physicians. (2011). Use of intensive insulin therapy for the management of glycemic control in hospitalized patients: a clinical practice guideline from the American College of Physicians. *Ann Intern Med, 154*(4), 260–267.
58. Richards, G., Levy, H., Laterre, P., et al. (2011). Curb-65, PSI, and APACHE II to assess mortality risk in patients with severe sepsis and community acquired pneumonia in process. *J Intensive Care Med, 26*(1), 34–40.
59. Rosenberger, L., Hranjec, T., McLeod, M., et al. (2013). Improvements in pulmonary and general critical care reduces mortality following ventilator-associated pneumonia. *J Trauma Acute Care Surg, 74*(2), 568–574.
60. Salluh, J. F., & Soares, M. (2014). ICU severity of illness scores: APACHE, SAPS and MPM. *Curr Opin Crit Care, 20*(5), 557–565.
61. Scarduelli, C., Ambrosino, N., Confalonieri, M., et al. (2004). Prevalence and prognostic role of cardiovascular complications in patients with exacerbation of chronic obstructive pulmonary disease admitted to Italian respiratory intensive care units. *Ital Heart J, 5*(12), 932–938.
62. Shashaty, M. S., & Stapleton, R. D. (2014). Physiological and management implications of obesity in critical illness. *Ann Am Thorac Soc, 11*(8), 1286–1297.
63. Singanayagam, A., & Bernal, W. (2015). Update on acute liver failure. *Curr Opin Crit Care, 21*(2), 134–141.
64. Smith, F. G., Sheehy, A. M., Vincent, J., et al. (2010). Critical illness-induced dysglycaemia: diabetes and beyond. *Crit Care, 14*(6), 327.
65. Soler-Cataluña, J., Martínez-García, M., Román Sánchez, P., et al. (2005). Severe acute exacerbations and mortality in patients with chronic obstructive pulmonary disease. *Thorax, 60*, 925–931.
66. Stevens, P. E., Lamb, E. J., & Levin, A. (2015). Integrating guidelines, CKD, multimorbidity, and older adults. *Am J Kidney Dis, 65*(3), 494–501.
67. Tan, C., Ng, A., & Civil, I. (2004). Comorbidities in trauma patients: common and significant. *N Z Med J, 117*(1201), U1044.
68. Tremblay, A., & Bandi, V. (2003). Impact of body mass index on outcomes following critical care. *Chest, 123*(4), 1202–1207.
69. Von Korff, M., Wagner, E., & Saunders, K. (1992). A chronic disease score from automated pharmacy data. *J Clin Epidemiol, 45*(2), 197–203.
70. Willars, C. (2014). Update in intensive care medicine: acute liver failure. Initial management, supportive treatment and who to transplant. *Curr Opin Crit Care, 20*(2), 202–209.
71. Zimmerman, J., Wagner, D., & Seneff, M. (1996). Intensive care unit admissions with cirrhosis: risk-stratifying patient groups and predicting individual survival. *Hepatology, 23*(6), 1393–1401.

41

Oncologic Emergencies

Roberta Kaplow

A diagnosis of cancer produces a number of physical and psychological responses in patients and their significant others. Additionally, serious conditions caused by treatment modalities, as well as the effects of disease itself, may complicate the patient's therapy. Although many patients have complication-free treatment following diagnosis, others experience treatment-associated complications. Some complications of treatment for cancer are life-threatening and require admission to critical care.

Six oncologic emergencies, as identified by the Oncology Nursing Society—hypercalcemia of malignancy (HCM), acute tumor lysis syndrome (ATLS), syndrome of inappropriate antidiuretic hormone secretion (SIADH), spinal cord compression (SCC), superior vena cava syndrome (SVCS), and cardiac tamponade—are discussed in this chapter. Three additional emergencies—sepsis, increased intracranial pressure, and disseminated intravascular coagulation—are discussed elsewhere in this text.

The development of oncologic emergencies may be subtle or rapid in onset. Given their life-threatening nature, prompt recognition and management are required for patient survival and quality of life.[21]

HYPERCALCEMIA OF MALIGNANCY

HCM is demonstrated by elevated serum calcium, and is defined as a total serum calcium level of greater than 10.4 mg/dL, corrected for low albumin levels.[2,8] It is considered to be a paraneoplastic syndrome, which is a clinical condition associated with cancer that is not directly related to the physical effects of the tumor or associated metastasis.[4]

Hypercalcemia occurs in up to 33% of patients with cancer.[1] Up to 40% of patients with breast or lung cancer, adult T-cell lymphoma, or multiple myeloma may be affected by HCM. Cases of HCM are usually mild but long-lasting.[9,21]

Patients at Risk

Cancers of the breast, lung (squamous cell), head and neck, kidney, esophagus, gastrointestinal tract, and cervix, as well as lymphomas, leukemia, multiple myeloma, sarcoidosis, renal cell carcinoma, and melanomas, are the most frequently reported malignancies associated with the development of HCM.[9,21] Tumors that cause release of parathyroid hormone-related peptide (PTHrP) into the systemic circulation are at risk. These include squamous cell carcinomas of the respiratory, upper digestive, and genitourinary tracts, and breast, kidney, cervical, endometrial, and ovarian cancers. Cancer that spreads to the bone (e.g., breast cancer, multiple myeloma) will cause stimulation of osteoclasts (cells that break down bone); this leads to bone resorption (the process of being reabsorbed), with subsequent hypercalcemia and destruction of bone.[2]

Additional risk factors for the development of HCM include dehydration, excessive intake of calcium and vitamin D, decreased parathyroid hormone levels, immobility, Paget's disease, vitamin A intoxication, hyperparathyroidism, and thiazide diuretic or lithium use.[2] Other therapies (e.g., estrogen, antiestrogen agents, all-trans retinoic acid) also have been associated with the development of transient HCM.[19,28]

Pathophysiology

HCM is an outcome of an aberration in calcium control; there is either excessive calcium entering the extracellular fluid or inadequate excretion of calcium by the kidneys. This most often results from bone metastasis (80% of cases), which causes osteoclastic bone resorption and the release of calcium.[2] This causes an imbalance between bone formation and resorption, resulting in additional calcium in the blood. HCM also can result from the tumor releasing substances with parathyroid hormone–like action or from inadequate calcium clearance by the kidney.[2]

There are two types of HCM: osteolytic and humoral. Osteolytic hypercalcemia is caused by direct bone destruction by a tumor or metastasis and bone resorption adjacent to the tumor tissue.[2] It arises when tumor growth in the bone results in calcium release into the blood. Humoral hypercalcemia, accounting for up to 80% of reported cases, results from circulating factors secreted by cancer cells (e.g., PTHrP, growth factors, interleukin-1, tumor necrosis factors, and interleukin-6), which cause calcium to be pumped out of the cells and into the bloodstream. It may also result from secretion of active vitamin D by some lymphomas or, rarely, from ectopic secretion of parathyroid hormone.[2]

Clinical Presentation

Clinical manifestations of HCM vary depending on the effects of calcium on different body systems, the rate of the rise in calcium levels, the patient's stage of disease and overall condition, renal function, and severity of the HCM (Table 41.1). Mild, moderate, and severe HCMs are defined as a corrected calcium level of 10.5–11.9 mg/dL (or ionized calcium 5.6–8 mg/dL), 12–13.9 mg/dL (or ionized calcium 5.6–8 mg/dL), and 14–16 mg/dL (or ionized calcium 10–12 mg/dL), respectively.[2] Symptoms may be nonspecific.[21] Patients with mild HCM can be asymptomatic; diagnosis may be made serendipitously when routine blood work is obtained. The history and physical assessment of a patient with any degree of HCM should focus on clinical manifestations,

TABLE 41.1 **Clinical Presentation of Hypercalcemia of Malignancy**

System	Findings
Cardiovascular	Hypertension, electrocardiogram changes (slowed conduction, prolonged PR interval, widened QRS complex, shortened QT interval, shortened or absent ST segments, widened T waves), dysrhythmias, bradycardia, bundle branch block, incomplete or complete atrioventricular block, increased myocardial contractility, myocardial irritability, increased sensitivity to effects of digitalis glycosides, syncope (from dysrhythmias), asystole, cardiac arrest
Gastrointestinal	Anorexia, nausea, vomiting, bowel hypomotility, increased gastric acid production, constipation/fecal impaction, abdominal pain, ileus, abdominal distention, dry mouth or throat, pancreatitis, peptic ulcer disease (from elevated gastrin levels from prolonged hypercalcemia)
Muscular	Fatigue, muscle weakness, hyporeflexia, muscle weakness, bone pain, ataxia
Neurologic	Restlessness, apathy, fatigue, depression, moodiness, irritability, confusion, somnolence, delirium, obtundation, visual disturbances, headache, lethargy, psychosis, symptoms of personality change, impaired concentration and memory, stupor (in severe hypercalcemia, i.e., > 14 mg/dL), weakness, paresis, hyporeflexia, disorientation, incoherent speech, hallucinations, delusions, coma
Renal	Nocturia, polyuria, polydipsia, distal renal tubular acidosis, acute and chronic renal insufficiency, azotemia, loss of urinary concentrating ability, decreased glomerular filtration rate, kidney stones, calcium phosphate crystals in renal tubules, renal failure, nephrogenic diabetes insipidus, dehydration
Skeleton	Osteopenia, osteoporosis, soft tissue calcification, arthritis, pathologic fractures
Other	Pruritus, keratitis, conjunctivitis

From References 2, 9, 20, and 21.

risk factors, causative agents, and a family history of hypercalcemia-associated conditions (e.g., kidney stones).[9,24]

Laboratory Findings

In addition to elevated calcium levels, laboratory findings associated with HCM include hypokalemia and hypomagnesemia if loop diuretics are administered. Hypophosphatemia and elevated serum creatinine may develop if the patient receives bisphosphonates.[7]

Diagnostic Evaluation

The diagnosis of HCM is based on serum calcium levels as compared with serum albumin levels. Patients with normal serum calcium levels and hypoalbuminemia may be considered to have HCM. Calcium levels should be corrected based on albumin levels, because 40% of calcium is bound to albumin. Two formulas are proposed:[2]

$$\text{Corrected calcium (mg/dL)} = \text{measured calcium (mg/dL)} + 0.8\,(4 - \text{measured albumin [g/dL]})$$

or

$$\text{Corrected calcium (mg/dL)} = \text{measured calcium (mg/dL)} - \text{measured albumin (g/dL)} + 4$$

Interprofessional Plan of Care

HCM management can be challenging, and is based on the severity of symptoms, underlying cause, the patient's quality of life, and options for cancer treatment.[2] The primary therapy for HCM is treatment of the underlying malignancy, which is the only effective long-term measure; this can entail chemotherapy, radiation therapy, hormonal therapy, surgical resection, or any combination of these. Irrespective of severity, management should include treatment of any underlying non–disease-related causes. This may include withholding any medications contributing to the condition.

Patients with mild HCM (corrected calcium level less than 12 mg/dL) may only require monitoring. Because some underlying tumors respond to cancer therapies more quickly than others, it may be necessary to initiate interventions to manage symptoms and stabilize the patient's metabolic status if the tumor will likely have a slower response to treatment.[9] Patients with moderate to severe HCM (greater than 14 mg/dL) require aggressive, immediate treatment to prevent further complications. Patients should be taught to avoid factors that can exacerbate HCM (e.g., thiazide diuretics, lithium carbonate, dehydration, immobility, calcium intake greater than 1000 mg/day).[9]

Rehydration

Rehydration is essential for patients with HCM, because most are volume-depleted. Patients with severe HCM will require aggressive volume resuscitation. As much as 300–500 mL/h of isotonic saline is administered until the patient is rehydrated.[21] Patients with moderate to severe HCM may require 5–10 L of fluid resuscitation to restore the extracellular fluid balance. Fluids should be administered at a rate of 200–300 mL/h to maintain urinary output at 100–150 mL/h. The volume needed for resuscitation depends on the severity of the symptoms and the amount of volume repletion required.[9] Patients usually show improvement within 24 hours of initiation of volume repletion. Therapeutic end points include sustained improvement of vital signs, hemodynamic status, mental status, and urinary output. Administration of loop diuretics (e.g., furosemide [Lasix]), which inhibits calcium resorption and enhances urinary calcium excretion, should be avoided until volume status has been restored, because further dehydration and a decrease in urinary calcium excretion may result.[2,9,21] Loop diuretics may be necessary in moderate doses once the patient has been rehydrated, to control volume overload (Table 41.7).[9,21]

Antiresorptive Therapy

In addition to rehydration, patients with HCM require administration of antiresorptive therapy with intravenous bisphosphonates, which inhibit bone resorption of calcium. Available agents include pamidronate (Aredia), zoledronic acid (Zometa), and etidronate (Didronel).[5,9] The former two are agents of choice. The latter agent reduces bone formation and does not affect calcium resorption by the renal tubules.[3,12] Although the precise mechanism of action of bisphosphonates on bone cells and bone resorption is not completely understood, it involves inhibition of the function of osteoclasts in a variety of ways; for example,

BOX 41.1 Antineoplastic Therapies Associated with the Development of Acute Tumor Lysis Syndrome

Chemotherapy
- amsacrine
- ara-C
- cisplatin (Platinol)
- cladribine (Leustatin)
- cytarabine (Cytosar-U)
- doxorubicin (Adriamycin)
- etoposide (Toposar)
- fludarabine (Fludara)
- hydroxyurea (Hydrea)
- intrathecal methotrexate (Folex)
- mitoxantrone (Novantrone)
- paclitaxel (Taxol)

Radiation Therapy (Less Often)

Immunotherapy/Biologic Response Modifiers
- alemtuzumab (Campath)
- bortezomib (Velcade)
- gemtuzumab (Mylotarg)
- imatinib mesylate (Gleevec)
- interferons
- interleukins
- rituximab (Rituxan)
- thalidomide (Thalomid)
- tumor necrosis factor

Corticosteroids

Hormonal Therapy
- tamoxifen (Nolvadex)

Data from References 11 and 21.

by producing a direct toxic effect on the resorbing osteoclasts, by promoting programmed cell death, or by inhibiting the differentiation of the osteoclasts into mature osteoclasts.[2] Antiresorptive therapy is not a replacement for volume repletion, as calcium levels do not decrease quickly enough with these agents.[21]

Calcitonin

Calcitonin (Fortical, Calcimar), a calcium-lowering hormone, is usually administered with a bisphosphonate. It increases renal excretion of calcium and decreases bone resorption by interfering with osteoclast function. Calcitonin's effectiveness is restricted to the first 48 hours, due to downregulation of the receptors. Calcitonin is most beneficial in patients with severe HCM when combined with volume resuscitation and bisphosphonates.[9]

Denosumab

For patients with severe HCM who are symptomatic and did not respond to zoledronic acid, subcutaneous administration of denosumab (Xgeva), a human monoclonal antibody, is indicated. Denosumab targets a protein that is required for the development, role, and survival of osteoclasts, and thus modifies calcium release from bone.[2]

Corticosteroid Therapy

Patients with HCM caused by steroid-responsive tumors such as lymphomas may benefit from corticosteroid therapy. Glucocorticoids work by enhancing calcium excretion in the urine and inhibiting calcium resorption in the gastrointestinal tract.[21]

Renal Replacement Therapies

If HCM results in renal failure (due to hypoperfusion from hypovolemia), dialysis therapy may be used. Peritoneal dialysis, hemodialysis, and ultrafiltration are effective methods of removing calcium. Patients receiving any of these therapies require careful monitoring of phosphorus levels. As phosphorus is lost, hypophosphatemia may develop and aggravate hypercalcemic conditions.[9]

Symptom Management

Management of hypercalcemia also may entail managing symptoms and increasing mobility, as clinically indicated. Immobility increases hypercalcemia; weight-bearing and mobilization are advised.[2] Collaboration with physical therapists may be indicated if patients have been immobile for long periods.

Treatment of HCM will likely palliate many of the distressing symptoms associated with the condition. Although polyuria, polydipsia, central nervous system symptoms, and some gastrointestinal symptoms may be relieved, other symptoms may not subside as readily.

Psychosocial Support

Patients with HCM may develop distressing changes in mental status, depending on the severity. Such changes include agitation, delirium, and confusion. Oral or intravenous neuroleptic agents like haloperidol (Haldol) with or without benzodiazepines may be indicated. The mental status of some patients will not resolve for several days or up to a week after normalization of serum calcium levels.

ACUTE TUMOR LYSIS SYNDROME

ATLS is an oncologic emergency that can develop from cancer itself or from treatment for cancer. It results from the release of intracellular components of destroyed cancer cells into the bloodstream.[21] Prompt treatment must occur to prevent renal failure, hemorrhage, multiple organ dysfunction syndrome, or death.[18] Patients with leukemia and lymphoma are reported to have an incidence rate of ATLS of 42% based on laboratory criteria, but the incidence of ATLS in all cancer patients is unknown.[11]

Patients at Risk

Patients with cancer and various preexisting conditions such as renal dysfunction, elevated serum creatinine levels, decreased glomerular filtration rate, anuria, oliguria, volume depletion, hyperuricemia, and elevated lactate dehydrogenase (LDH) levels are at risk for developing ATLS. Antineoplastic therapy places the patient at risk for ATLS. Some of the treatments implicated in its development include chemotherapy, biologic response modifiers, monoclonal antibodies, radiation therapy (less often), and corticosteroids (Box 41.1).[11]

ATLS occurs most frequently in patients with hematopoietic malignancies (e.g., leukemia and lymphoma) and in patients with bulky tumors made up of rapidly proliferating cells. Tumors

TABLE 41.2 **Clinical Presentation of Acute Tumor Lysis Syndrome**

	Hyperkalemia	Hyperphosphatemia	Hypocalcemia	Hyperuricemia
Cardiac	Tachycardia, bradycardia, pulseless electrical activity, ventricular tachycardia, ventricular fibrillation, asystole, peaked T waves, flattened P waves, widened QRS, sudden death	Hypertension, edema	Hypotension, prolonged QT interval, inverted T wave, ventricular dysrhythmias, heart block, cardiac arrest/sudden death	Edema, hypertension (if severe), endocarditis (if severe)
Gastrointestinal	Diarrhea, increased bowel sounds, nausea, vomiting		Nausea, vomiting, diarrhea, anorexia, cramps	Nausea, vomiting, diarrhea, anorexia
Neurologic	Tingling, paresthesias, twitching, paralysis, lethargy, syncope, weakness		Muscle twitching, tetany, paresthesias, depression, hallucinations, confusion, syncope, seizures, mental status changes, anxiety, carpopedal spasms, positive Chvostek's sign*, positive Trousseau's sign†, neuromuscular irritability, difficulty concentrating	
Renal		Oliguria, anuria, renal insufficiency/failure, azotemia, exacerbation of preexisting renal compromise		Compromised renal function, renal failure (if severe), oliguria, anuria, azotemia, flank pain, hematuria, colic (rare), metabolic acidosis, acute uric acid nephropathy
Other	Muscle cramps, muscle weakness	Muscle cramps	Muscle cramps, bronchospasm, laryngospasm, metallic taste, pruritus, restless legs	Gout, pruritus, fatigue, malaise, weakness

*Chvostek's sign is manifested with facial muscle twitching when the facial nerve is tapped.
†Trousseau's sign is manifested with carpopedal spasm that occurs when a blood pressure cuff is inflated. The spasm occurs when the cuff remains inflated at a level higher than the patient's systolic blood pressure for more than 3 minutes.
From References 11 and 21.

in which ATLS has been reported include Burkitt's lymphoma, acute lymphoblastic leukemia, acute lymphoblastic lymphoma, advanced non-Hodgkin's lymphoma, chronic leukemia, and rarely, solid tumors (e.g., small cell lung cancer [SCLC]). The solid tumors implicated in the development of ATLS include those that respond to chemotherapy (e.g., SCLC, metastatic medulloblastoma, inflammatory breast cancer, germ cell tumors, ovarian cancer, soft tissue sarcoma, thymoma, vulvar cancer, metastatic seminoma, rhabdomyosarcoma, hepatoblastoma, stage IV neuroblastoma, and metastatic melanoma).[21] Cancer that spreads to the liver also puts the patient at risk for ATLS.[11]

Pathophysiology

ATLS may occur when a large number of cancer cells are killed (or lysed) either spontaneously or via antineoplastic therapy. Normal intracellular components include potassium, phosphorus, and nucleic acids. When cancer cells are killed, these intracellular ions leave the cell and enter the bloodstream. The result is hyperkalemia and hyperphosphatemia, with secondary hypocalcemia, as calcium binds to phosphorus. Nucleic acids are converted to uric acid in the liver. When cells are destroyed, hyperuricemia results. In some patients, especially those with baseline renal insufficiency, the acute increase in electrolytes may exceed the kidneys' elimination abilities. This results in life-threatening levels of electrolytes in the blood (e.g., potassium levels greater than 6.5 mEq/L).[21]

Clinical Presentation

The signs and symptoms that a patient with ATLS manifests reflect the electrolyte imbalances and their respective effects on the body. Physical presentation findings appear in Table 41.2.

Laboratory Findings

Laboratory data indicative of ATLS are related to the pathophysiologic changes that occur when antineoplastic therapy kills cancer cells. Patients exhibit hyperuricemia, hyperkalemia, hyperphosphatemia, and hypocalcemia.[11,21] They also manifest decreased creatinine clearance, elevated blood urea nitrogen (BUN), elevated serum creatinine, decreased pH, and elevated bicarbonate levels. Urinalysis reveals uric acid crystals and hematuria.[11]

- Six to twelve hours after antineoplastic therapy, hyperkalemia is the first electrolyte abnormality to manifest.
- Hyperphosphatemia and the resultant hypocalcemia develop 24 to 48 hours after onset of treatment.
- Hyperuricemia occurs 24 to 48 hours after initiation of antineoplastic therapies, and can result in renal failure if uric acid levels are not controlled. Patients usually present with clinically significant findings when uric acid levels are greater than 10 mg/dL.[11]

Interprofessional Plan of Care

The primary goals of ATLS treatment are prevention and prompt management to correct any metabolic or electrolyte derangements that do occur despite preventive strategies. The interprofessional plan of care for ATLS incorporates preventing the syndrome from occurring, treating electrolyte abnormalities, and preventing complications.

Prevention of ATLS through several interventions is essential for all patients at risk. Collaboration among members of the interprofessional team is vital. Healthcare providers can identify patients at risk, including those with tumors with rapidly proliferating cells, those who will be receiving any of the treatment modalities that have been implicated in the development of this complication, and those with preexisting conditions that place them at risk.[11] Treatments that can cause electrolyte imbalances and factors compromising preexisting renal dysfunction should be eliminated, including nephrotoxic agents (e.g., aminoglycosides, amphotericin B, and nonsteroidal antiinflammatory agents).

A key preventive strategy is vigorous hydration 24 to 48 hours before initiating antineoplastic treatment, which should continue for up to 72 hours after chemotherapy administration is complete. Up to 4–5 L/day to achieve a urinary output of at least 3 L/day is recommended.[11] Once hydration has been initiated, further preventive strategies can continue with forced diuresis. This can be accomplished with either a loop or osmotic diuretic (i.e., furosemide [Lasix] or mannitol [Osmitrol], respectively). The furosemide dose is 1 to 2 mg/kg IV every 6 to 8 hours; the dose of mannitol is 0.5 g/kg IV every 6 to 8 hours if urine output is not maintained with fluids and furosemide. A specific gravity less than 1.010 is a good indicator of dilute urine.

Urinary alkalization is accomplished with the administration of sodium bicarbonate. Alkalization is started 24 to 48 hours before administration of antineoplastic therapy. This helps prevent precipitation and promotes excretion of uric acid. Concerns related to alkalization are the increased possibility of calcium phosphate precipitation in the renal tubules and enhanced hypocalcemia secondary to elevated pH.[11] Urinary alkalization should be stopped with urine pH levels greater than 7.0 or when normal uric acid levels have been attained. Administration of acetazolamide (Diamox) 250 to 500 mg/day to decrease bicarbonate resorption may be considered if bicarbonate does not adequately alkalize the urine.[11]

Allopurinol (Zyloprim, Aloprim), a xanthine oxidase inhibitor, is administered to decrease uric acid levels. Xanthine oxidase is the enzyme needed to help convert nucleic acids to uric acid. Patients should receive a loading dose of 600 to 900 mg and be placed on a maintenance dose of 100 to 300 mg given once or twice a day.[11,21] Rasburicase (Elitek), a recombinant form of the enzyme urate oxidase, also may be used to treat hyperuricemia.[11] Rasburicase is contraindicated for use in patients with glucose-6-phosphate dehydrogenase deficiency, because there is a risk for hemolytic anemia and methemoglobinemia.[11,21] The main side effect is hypersensitivity reaction (see Table 41.7).[11]

Following the initiation of antineoplastic therapy, laboratory data must be monitored to help ensure early detection of any metabolic derangements. A potassium level of 6 mEq/L or greater, phosphorus level greater than 10 mg/dL, uric acid level greater than 10 mg/dL, or BUN and creatinine levels twice the patient's baseline are all considered clinically significant.[11]

Hyperkalemia can be treated emergently with 50% dextrose with regular insulin, sodium bicarbonate, or an inhalation beta agonist. Any of these interventions will temporarily push potassium back into the cells. Removal of potassium from the body can be accomplished with the loop diuretic sodium polystyrene (Kayexalate) or renal replacement therapy, which is rarely needed. The clinician should minimize potassium administration. Medications such as potassium-sparing diuretics and angiotensin-converting enzyme inhibitors can increase potassium levels.[5] Enteral and parenteral nutrition and dietary and oral supplementation of potassium should be eliminated. Renal replacement therapies are rarely required for the acute management of hyperkalemia associated with ATLS.

Administration of oral or intravenous allopurinol helps prevent the development of hyperuricemia. Rasburicase may be indicated if the patient is unable to take or tolerate allopurinol. Rasburicase metabolizes uric acid into a soluble form and can be used to treat severe hyperuricemia.[11]

Calcium gluconate may be administered for cardioprotection to patients with a serum potassium level greater than 6.5 mEq/L. Calcium chloride may be administered if a patient's serum potassium level is greater than 6.0 mEq/L, particularly if electrocardiogram (ECG) changes are present. Calcium chloride has approximately three times more elemental calcium than calcium gluconate. Therefore, it is preferred in ATLS patients with hemodynamic compromise.

Dialysis

If unable to manage metabolic abnormalities of ATLS, consider initiating dialysis. Dialysis prevents the development of irreversible acute kidney injury and other life-threatening complications. Continuous renal replacement therapy may be used to correct fluid and electrolyte abnormalities. Hemodialysis is preferred, as there is more effective clearance of phosphorus and uric acid.[11]

SYNDROME OF INAPPROPRIATE ANTIDIURETIC HORMONE SECRETION

SIADH is a condition related to water intoxication. It is characterized by inappropriate production and secretion of antidiuretic hormone (ADH) (also known as arginine vasopressin, AVP), causing increased tubular water resorption with subsequent water retention, hyponatremia, decreased serum osmolality, and increased urine osmolality. The discernible secretion of ADH occurs despite adequate circulating fluid volume and urinary sodium excretion.[16]

Patients at Risk

SCLC is the most common cancer associated with the development of SIADH. Others include non–small cell lung cancer (NSCLC); carcinoid tumors; breast and brain tumors; squamous cell carcinoma of the head and neck, prostate, esophagus, pancreas, endometrium, ovaries, duodenum, bladder, and colon; thymoma; uterine cancer; Ewing's sarcoma; neuroblastoma; mesothelioma; Hodgkin's disease; non-Hodgkin's lymphoma; multiple myeloma; and leukemia. It also is associated by metastasis to the central nervous system.[16]

Administration of certain chemotherapeutic agents also places patients at risk for the development of SIADH. These agents include vincristine (Oncovin), vinblastine (Velban), high-dose cyclophosphamide (Cytoxan), ifosfamide (Ifex), cisplatin (Platinol), and melphalan (Alkeran). Each of these agents can cause elevated AVP levels.[16]

Pathophysiology

SIADH may result from an underlying tumor secreting a protein similar to ADH. This protein is not reactive to normal body feedback mechanisms. SIADH also may be caused by chemotherapy provoking the posterior pituitary to secrete ADH. Both of these mechanisms cause inappropriate and disproportionate secretion of ADH. ADH secretion stimulates water absorption in the distal tubules and collecting ducts. This results in decreased urinary excretion, urine concentration, plasma dilution, decreased serum osmolality, and dilutional serum hyponatremia.[16]

TABLE 41.3 Clinical Presentation of Syndrome of Inappropriate Antidiuretic Hormone

Body System	Associated Symptoms
Cardiac	Hypotension or normal blood pressure and heart rate, fluid retention
Central nervous system	Headache, lethargy, changes in behavior, ataxia, fatigue, malaise, mental status changes, irritability, disorientation, tremors, somnolence, hallucinations, confusion, hyporeflexia, weakness, myoclonus, agitation, obtundation, coma, unexplained seizures
Gastrointestinal	Anorexia, abdominal cramping, nausea, vomiting, diarrhea
Musculoskeletal	Muscle cramps, weakness
Renal	Thirst, incontinence, weight gain without edema, oliguria
Respiratory	Inability to mobilize secretions

From References 16 and 21.

Clinical Presentation

Patients present with a variety of symptoms, often related to their dilutional hyponatremia, hypocalcemia, or hypokalemia. Clinical presentation findings of SIADH are listed in Table 41.3.

Laboratory Findings

Laboratory data consistent with a diagnosis of SIADH include a urinary sodium level greater than 40 mEq/L, elevated urinary osmolality greater than 100 mOsm/L, decreased BUN (less than 10 mg/dL), serum hypo-osmolality (less than 280 mOsmo/kg), and serum hyponatremia (less than 134 mEq/L).[29]

Interprofessional Plan of Care

Ongoing assessment of the patient's neuromuscular, cardiac, gastrointestinal, and renal status is important in order to detect subtle changes in clinical status. Assessment of fluid and electrolyte status and assessment for side effects of cancer treatment are equally essential. Consultation with other members of the interprofessional team is typically not required. The interprofessional plan of care for SIADH entails treating the underlying cause, correcting sodium levels, and preventing complications.

When feasible, treatment of the underlying cause of SIADH should be implemented. Treatment modalities may include chemotherapy, radiation therapy, corticosteroids, or a combination of these.[16]

In addition to eradicating the underlying cause, the cornerstone of management is fluid restriction to 800–1000 mL/day until there is improvement in hyponatremia.[16] Administration of demeclocycline (Declomycin) at 600–1200 mg/day is recommended if fluid restriction is not effective. Demeclocycline, an oral antibiotic, causes nephrogenic diabetes insipidus by decreasing the tubular response to ADH. Side effects of demeclocycline include nausea, photosensitivity, and azotemia (see Table 42.7).[16]

If patients have acute hyponatremia and severe neurologic symptoms, an initial bolus of 100 mL of 3% saline is recommended. One or two additional doses in 10-minute intervals may be given if the patient's neurologic status does not recover or deteriorates.[16] Serum sodium should be corrected at a rate of no faster than 0.5 to 1 mEq/h for 3 to 4 hours. This should be followed by correcting serum sodium levels to less than 10 mEq/L in 24 hours and no more than 18 mEq/L in 48 hours to prevent complication of therapy (e.g., central pontine myelinolysis).[16,29]

For patients with mild symptoms, fluid restriction to 1000 mL/day is suggested in order to obtain a negative water balance.[16] In some cases, restriction to 500 mL/day may be required.[29] Diuretics may also need to be administered to prevent fluid overload.

SPINAL CORD COMPRESSION

SCC is compression of the thecal sac by a tumor in the epidural space. The tumor applies pressure on the spinal cord, affecting its vascular supply. The decreased blood flow to the spinal cord can lead to infarction or vertebral collapse. The compression can be located in the spinal cord or at the level of the cauda equina.[1] SCC incidence depends on the tumor's starting point; one study reported the probability of developing SCC at between 0.2% and 7.9%.[27]

Patients at Risk

SCC often results from metastatic tumors. The most frequently reported tumors with metastases to the skeleton are lung, breast, and prostate. Others include melanoma, sarcoma, neuroblastoma, myeloma, and renal cell carcinoma, and account for 5% to 10% of SCC cases.[21] Any tumor that spreads to the spinal cord or surrounding tissue can cause SCC.[10,27] The presence of SCC may be the initial presenting symptom of malignancy.[21]

Pathophysiology

SCC is usually caused by tumors that metastasize to the spine. SCC is classified as either intramedullary (within the spinal cord), intradural (within the dura mater), extramedullary (outside the spinal cord), or extradural (outside the dura mater).[10] Cancer can spread to specific areas on the spine. Lung, breast, and prostate cancers usually (70% of the time) metastasize to the thoracic area. Gastrointestinal and prostate tumors may metastasize to the lumbosacral spine.

Most tumors spread to the spinal cord as an embolic process through the paravertebral and extradural venous plexus to the bone marrow. This causes the vertebral body to collapse and an epidural mass to form.[21] Growth of a tumor in the epidural space may also result from adenopathy of the prevertebral lymph nodes. Central nervous system cancer can also spread to the cerebrospinal fluid. This results in spread to the subarachnoid space, brain, and spinal cord.[1] Most cases of SCC occur in the thoracic spine (60%), followed by the lumbosacral area (30%), and then the cervical spine (10%).[21]

Clinical Presentation

Patients with SCC may present in a variety of ways, depending on the location, extent, and etiology of the compression; blood supply involvement; and the speed at which the compression has developed. Effects can be sensory, motor, autonomic, or any combination of these.[21] Clinical presentation findings are listed in Table 41.4.

Back pain occurs in 90% of cases of SCC.[21] Pain may be localized at the site of the tumor, and is constant, dull, or aching. Pain may also be radicular (aggravated by movement or constant, and may be alleviated by sitting) or medullary. The pain may intensify when lying supine.[10] The patient may experience pain for three months before developing sensory deficits, and this pain usually intensifies with time. The pain may develop

TABLE 41.4 Clinical Presentation of Spinal Cord Compression

Motor Symptoms	Autonomic Symptoms	Sensory Symptoms
Ataxia	Bladder distention	Decrease in strength
Easy fatigue	Changes in bowel and bladder function	Decreased light touch, joint, and position sense, and proprioception
Gait disturbance	Constipation	Lhermitte's sign*
Hyporeflexia	Hesitancy	Loss of deep pressure sensation
Hypotonicity	Impotence	Loss of thermal sense
Leg pain	Lack of ability to bear down	Loss of vibration sensation
Loss of coordination	Lack of urge to defecate	Numbness
Motor weakness, usually in lower extremities	Obstipation	Paresthesia
Neck or back pain	Decreased anal sphincter tone	Sensory loss to level of compression
Paralysis	Urinary incontinence	Severe pain
Spasticity	Urinary overflow	Leg weakness
Weakness	Urinary retention	Valsalva maneuver may exacerbate radicular pain
Decreased or absent deep tendon reflexes		
Absent Babinski sign		

*Lhermitte's sign is a sudden, intermittent sensation of electric-like shocks that occur when the head is flexed. It is a symptom of compression of the cervical spine.
From References 3, 6, 13, 21, 25, and 26.

slowly over months before other neurologic symptoms appear, or quickly over hours before complete, irreversible damage to the spinal cord occurs.[21] Pain reports are varied, and may include pain upon coughing or sneezing, a sudden change in previous pain levels, pain that waxes and wanes, or unilateral or bilateral radiating leg pain.[10] Other symptoms of SCC depend on where the lesion(s) is/are located, degree of impingement, and how long impingement has existed.[21]

Sensory changes usually begin distally and rise to the level of the compression. Patients report weakness that usually occurs over some time, following pain.[10] Patients with compression of the cervical spine have quadriplegia. Patients with compression of the thoracic spine have paraplegia. When a patient has compression of the cauda equina, sensory loss is bilateral. Patients usually experience sensory and motor symptoms prior to autonomic dysfunction.

Early recognition of the signs and symptoms of SCC is essential. It is essential that a patient with reported back pain be thoroughly evaluated. Being able to ambulate after treatment for SCC is the most significant prognostic indicator. The most vital data to assist in the diagnosis of SCC are the patient history and clinical evaluation.[10] A comprehensive initial history, physical, and neurologic assessment, and evaluation of pain, sensory, motor, and autonomic functions are essential. Ongoing assessments include assessments of pain, sensory and motor function, and autonomic changes.[6]

The patient's history should include determining the characteristics of the symptoms (intensity, quality, onset, and duration) and the presence of sensory, motor, and autonomic symptoms. A thorough examination of the neurologic and musculoskeletal systems is imperative in any patient who is at risk for development of SCC and who is symptomatic, even if pain is the only presenting symptom.

Evaluation of pain, temperature, touch, vibration, and position should be conducted. The area of sensory or motor loss can determine the level of the compression; the level of motor loss is more reliable, except when the thoracic cord is affected.[13] The patient will usually report tenderness to percussion at the site of the compressed vertebrae.[20]

Once SCC causes symptoms, harm degrades from minimal to significant in an unpredictable but rapid manner. Sensory changes will progress if interventions are not initiated. Paresthesia will advance to sensory loss. Patients may report tingling in the arms or trunk that occurs with neck flexion. This is known as Lhermitte's sign.[13]

Motor changes progress without intervention. Initial weakness may advance to problems with coordination and finally, motor loss. Weakness usually begins in the feet and moves proximally. Patients should be evaluated for gait and reflex disturbances, muscle strength, involuntary movements, and coordination. Tendon reflexes are increased below the level of the compression, absent at the level of the compression, and normal above the level of the compression.[13] A patient displaying a positive Babinski sign likely has motor involvement. To assess for the presence of a positive Babinski sign, the sole of the foot should be stroked with a tool from the heel of the foot to the small toe. An arc is then drawn with the tool to under the big toe. A positive Babinski sign is manifested if there is dorsiflexion of the big toe with fanning of the other toes.[13]

Any reported autonomic dysfunction requires further evaluation, especially if the patient is at risk for developing SCC. Autonomic dysfunction is a poor prognostic indicator.[13]

Respiratory distress may occur if the compression is at the cervical level. Assessment for impaired oxygenation and ventilation is pivotal, especially in patients with tumor involvement at the C4 level or above. These patients require airway protection with intubation.[3]

Any findings on physical examination may help in the diagnosis of SCC. It should be noted, however, that a lack of signs and symptoms does not rule out the diagnosis. A patient at risk for SCC who reports sudden onset of back pain and leg weakness should be evaluated.[13]

Radiology Findings

Spinal radiograph is the initial diagnostic study for SCC. It may be normal, or may reveal fracture, damage, erosion, or a lesion in up to 85% of the vertebrae. Epidural metastasis is detected in the majority of cases.[10] Radiographs are limited, because 50% of bone must be destroyed for compression to be visible; in addition, radiographs have a false negative rate of up to 17%. These films also do not reveal all sources of SCC (e.g., soft tissue tumors). As such, they should not be used independently to rule out spinal cord impingement.[10,13,21]

Magnetic resonance imaging (MRI) with and without contrast is the most definitive tool (95% accuracy) for determining the exact location of the compression, evaluating the extent of disease, and determining the presence of vertebral tumors. It should be performed immediately in patients who have suspected SCC.[10,13,21] MRI visualizes the entire spine, including adjacent soft tissue and bone, the spinal cord, and cauda equine, and can thus identify metastasis and compression of the spinal cord at multiple sites. Either MRI or computed tomography (CT) scan may identify the location and extent of trauma to the spinal cord, as well as assess for bone destruction.[10] A myelogram may be done if MRI cannot be performed; however, MRI is preferable, because it is noninvasive and can image the entire spine.[10]

A myelogram is often performed concomitantly with CT scan with contrast. These two tests are often performed in patients who have contraindications for MRI (e.g., those with internal metal devices, implants, or shrapnel, or patients in severe pain who are unable to tolerate lying flat for the required extended period of time.)[13]

CT with contrast will detect paraspinal masses and early lesions, but does not image the entire spine.[10] CT scans are not endorsed because of poor exposure of the epidural space and spinal cord. Positron emission tomography (PET) can substantiate data received from MRI or CT.

A myelogram with or without concomitant CT scanning was formerly the diagnostic test of choice for SCC diagnosis. The results reveal data about the spine and provide a precise image of the areas of compression. However, a myelogram is invasive and distressing. It involves sampling of cerebrospinal fluid, which can augment the SCC or worsen neurologic deficits. This test is contraindicated in patients with a coagulopathy. Given these risks, CT scanning with high resolution essentially eliminates the need for a myelogram.[13]

Bone scans (radionuclide scintigraphy) have been used to help diagnose SCC. They are more accurate than plain radiology films, but less accurate than MRI. Data from bone scans do not reveal metastatic lesions. They lack spinal structure detail, and are associated with false positive results in patients with skeletal conditions not associated with a cancer diagnosis.

PET involves injection of a radioactive tracer. It provides information on bone metabolism and the tumor itself by evaluating uptake of the metabolites of the tracer. Diagnosis of SCC must be confirmed with MRI or CT scan prior to treatment for SCC, given the spatial resolution of the PET scan.[13]

Interprofessional Plan of Care

SCC is an oncologic emergency requiring immediate intervention to prevent permanent disability. Options for management include surgery, glucocorticoids, external beam radiation therapy, and chemotherapy (if caused by a chemosensitive tumor).[21] The goals of therapy are to provide pain relief, restore neurologic function, treat the underlying malignancy, and prevent permanent disability.[21] Treatment depends on the type of underlying tumor, location, and characteristics of the tumor.[25]

Radiation Therapy

Radiation therapy is the definitive treatment for SCC.[10] Doses of 30 Gray (Gy) in 10 fractions are administered.[21] The area that is radiated usually includes the affected vertebrae and one or two vertebral bodies above and below the compression.[21] Radiation therapy should be the first-line of therapy in ambulatory patients and for patients who are asymptomatic with epidural SCC. Radiation therapy is used to minimize the size of the tumor, decompress the spinal cord, and provide pain relief. Patients with significant pain who have a poor prognosis may receive a brief course of external beam radiation therapy (8 Gy for one or two fractions).[21]

Surgery

Surgery should be the first line of therapy in patients with spinal instability, bony compression, or paraplegia on initial presentation. The primary goals of surgery are to decrease pain and maintain neurologic function.[25] Surgical decompression may be used to alleviate pain and stabilize the spine, which can be accomplished by resection of a vertebral body with spinal immobilization. Surgery is considered when the underlying tumor does not respond to radiation therapy, or if the area has already been irradiated.[6]

Surgical intervention may include vertebroplasty or kyphoplasty.[1] These procedures may be used to stabilize the spine and provide pain management, and may be performed if the patient has indications and no contraindications.[6] With vertebroplasty, a needle is inserted under CT guidance to the vertebral body, and polymethyl methacrylate (PMMA) is injected. The vertebral body is straightened, resulting in pain relief and increased mobility. Kyphoplasty uses PMMA to strengthen the vertebral body. With this procedure, a balloon is introduced into the vertebral body and is inflated to reestablish the height of the vertebral body; PMMA is then injected to fill in the space.[6]

Corticosteroid Therapy

Steroids are commonly used in the initial management of SCC until treatment of the underlying cause (with radiation therapy or surgery) can be implemented.[21] It is essential that steroids be initiated as soon as possible if a patient is suspected of having SCC, so as to help prevent the development of permanent neurologic damage. Therapy should be initiated even before the diagnosis of SCC is confirmed.[13] Steroids are used to maintain neurologic function and decrease spinal cord edema, inflammation, and pain.[10,13] Dosing is typically based on the degree of neurologic symptoms.[13] Patients are given a loading dose of dexamethasone (Decadron) with subsequent tapering. Dosing recommendations vary in the literature.[13] Significant side effects, such as ulcers, bowel perforation, psychosis, and infection (including opportunistic infections with organisms such as *Pneumocystis jiroveci*) can occur with high-dose steroids, and patients should be closely monitored for these conditions. Maintenance therapy with steroids is associated with hyperglycemia, fluid retention, osteoporosis, depression, and adrenal insufficiency. Steroids are used for treatment until standard therapy (e.g., radiation therapy) is started. At that time, tapering of therapy can begin. If SCC is ruled out, steroids should be discontinued (see Table 41.7).[13]

Chemotherapy

Patients with lymphoma, neuroblastoma, or germ cell tumors may benefit from chemotherapy as a treatment for the underlying malignancy that led to SCC. It may also be used as an adjuvant therapy for patients with metastatic breast or prostate cancer or myeloma. Hormonal therapy may be indicated for patients with hormone-sensitive prostate cancer with paraplegia. Chemotherapy may be used in patients who are not candidates for radiation therapy or surgery. Patients with breast or prostate cancer may benefit from hormonal therapy.[25]

SUPERIOR VENA CAVA SYNDROME

SVCS occurs when a tumor constricts or metastasizes to the superior vena cava (SVC), or when a tumor develops in the chest region (e.g., lung cancer, breast cancer, lymphoma).[13] It can also occur when a thrombus develops within the SVC. With lung cancer, SVCS is a manifestation of cancer of the bronchus, and occurs in 5% to 10% of patients with an intrathoracic mass (primarily right-sided tumors).[23] Regardless of the etiology, blood return is obstructed to the head and upper body, causing venous congestion and decreased cardiac output. It is depicted by swelling of the neck and venous distention over the chest, and results from obstruction of the SVC. The obstruction may occur above or below the azygos vein due to an intravascular clot, a tumor in the right main upper lobe bronchus, or significant lymphadenopathy of the mediastinum, which is usually due to the right paratracheal or precarinal lymph node areas.[23]

Occlusion of the SVC occurs frequently because of its location and thin walls, and because it is surrounded by structures that do not compress. Because blood flow in the SVC is under low pressure, when regional lymph nodes or the aorta enlarge, the SVC constricts, and blood flow becomes sluggish, often resulting in occlusion.[23]

Patients at Risk

More than 80% of SVCS cases are a result of malignancy in the mediastinum. Of these, 75% are due to bronchogenic carcinoma; most of these cases are small cell carcinoma of the lung. Non-Hodgkin's lymphoma accounts for 10% to 15% of SVCS cases. A small number of cases of SVCS are due to Hodgkin's lymphoma, metastatic cancer, leiomyosarcoma of the mediastinal vessels, and plasmacytomas.[23] Some patients without cancer are at risk, such as those with tuberculosis; thrombosis of indwelling pacemaker wires; central venous, Silastic, or dialysis catheters; histoplasmosis; aneurysm of the aortic arch; or constrictive pericarditis. These account for almost 16% of SVCS cases.[21,23]

Pathophysiology

SVC obstruction is typically caused by compression of the SVC due to pressure from an invading mass. It may also be caused by tumor spread to the venous wall or by intravascular thrombosis. The obstruction impairs blood flow from the SVC to the right atrium, and venous drainage above the upper thorax is impaired. This results in a decreased venous return to the heart.[23]

Clinical Presentation

The clinical presentation of SVCS varies, and depends on the degree, severity, and location of the obstruction (i.e., above or below the azygos vein).[23] The more rapid the development of the obstruction, the more severe the symptoms will be, because of the body's inability to compensate. Clinical findings the patient may exhibit are listed in Table 41.5.

Radiology Findings

A CT scan is useful for identifying the site of the obstruction and the presence of associated thrombus. It can help reveal if the obstruction is secondary to a thrombosis or external compression and provide information about other vital anatomic structures.[23] A venogram, which is usually performed before stenting, can be used to determine if the obstruction of the SVC is a result of stenosis or obstruction, as well as the extent of a thrombus. It is the most definitive test for identifying the source of the obstruction.[23]

TABLE 41.5 Clinical Presentation of Superior Vena Cava Syndrome

Body System	Associated Symptoms
Cardiac	Edema of face, arm, and upper chest; congestion of collateral veins of neck and anterior chest wall; erythema of eyelids; dilated veins in upper torso, shoulders, and arms; jugular venous distention; tachycardia; chest pain; hypotension
Central nervous system	Headache, dizziness (especially if bending forward), confusion, anxiety, mental status changes, drowsiness, blurred vision, syncope
Respiratory	Dyspnea, shortness of breath, hoarseness, cyanosis, cough, dysphagia, stridor, epistaxis
Other	Tightness of neck (Stokes' sign), periorbital edema, head fullness, arm swelling, nausea, upper extremity edema

From References 21 and 23.

Chest radiograph may show a widened mediastinum or right chest mass. MRI allows for blood flow to be seen. Advantages of the MRI include no need for iodine-containing contrast media (a positive aspect if stent placement is indicated), and it is desirable for patients with renal failure or allergies to CT contrast.

Interprofessional Plan of Care

Treatment of SVCS is aimed at symptom management and treatment of the underlying cause. Symptom management may include elevating the head of bed and oxygen therapy.[23] Patients who have neurologic symptoms or cannot maintain a patent airway may require emergency interventions.[21] Customarily, treatment has consisted of steroids and either radiation therapy or chemotherapy.

Treatment of the underlying malignancy can relieve SVCS to varying degrees, depending on disease and treatment modality. Chemotherapy and radiation therapy are the two common treatments of choice. Radiation therapy is the standard treatment for SVCS. The radiation dose is based on the size of the tumor and whether the tumor is radiosensitive. Radiation therapy is helpful in alleviating obstruction symptoms in 70% of patients with lung cancer and over 95% of patients with lymphoma.[23]

Chemotherapy is indicated when the underlying malignancy is chemosensitive. It has been suggested that radiation therapy and chemotherapy should be withheld until the cause of the obstruction has been determined. If the patient's signs and symptoms are minimal, treatment may not be needed.[23]

Chemotherapy is indicated for chemosensitive tumor etiologies (e.g., SCLC or lymphoma). Patients have reported complete resolution of symptoms within two weeks.[23]

Data support the use of diuretic therapy in SVCS patients with edema of the upper airway. Diuretics may also decrease right-sided preload by decreasing venous return. This will decrease pressure on the SVC, resulting in symptom relief. Diuretics may also be helpful in alleviating cerebral edema (Table 41.6).[23]

Endovascular techniques such as thrombolysis, angioplasty, or stenting may be performed. Thrombolysis should be initiated if the cause of the obstruction is a thrombus. Administration of

TABLE 41.6 Clinical Presentation of Cardiac Tamponade

System	Signs And Symptoms
Cardiovascular	Tachycardia, jugular venous distention, *pulsus paradoxus*, pericardial friction rub, hypotension, cyanosis, narrowing pulse pressure (decreased systolic blood pressure, increased diastolic blood pressure), increased SVR, increased ventricular diastolic pressure, increased pulmonary venous pressure, distant or absent apical pulse, elevated CVP, palpitations, nonspecific chest pain that is relieved when leaning forward and worsens with deep inspiration, diaphoresis, edema, dysrhythmias (e.g., PACs, PVCs), decreased stroke volume, decreased cardiac output, muffled heart sounds, sharp stabbing chest pain that radiates to shoulder, back, or abdomen
Gastrointestinal	Hepatic enlargement/congestion, ascites, dysphagia, anorexia, hepatojugular reflux (elevation in jugular venous pressure by ≥ 1 cm), abdominal distention
Neurologic	Mental status changes, dizziness, drowsiness, restlessness, loss of consciousness, lightheadedness, fainting, anxiety
Respiratory	Shortness of breath, dyspnea on exertion that progresses to air hunger, tachypnea, crackles at base of lungs, hoarseness, cough, orthopnea
Other	Pallor, fatigue, weakness, malaise, low-grade fever, chills

CVP, Central venous pressure; *PACs*, premature atrial contractions; *PVCs*, premature ventricular contractions; *SVR*, systemic vascular resistance.
From References 14, 15, 21, 22, 30, and 31.

thrombolytics should be started within a few days of onset to be effective. Stenting of the SVC relieves symptoms within a few days. Some data suggest that stenting should be considered a first-line treatment for SVCS.[23]

Continuous monitoring and maintenance of a patent airway is essential for a patient with SVCS. Although rare, it is possible for the patient to develop airway compromise or obstruction.[23] Respiratory compromise from airway obstruction is potentially life-threatening. Monitoring of the respiratory status of a patient with SVCS is essential. Assessment should include monitoring of respiratory rate, blood oxygen saturation (Spo_2), and breath sounds, and evaluating for symptoms of distress (e.g., tachypnea, orthopnea, hoarseness, dyspnea, cyanosis, and cough). Respiratory compromise may be manifested with stridor. Should stridor occur, heliox (a mixture of helium and oxygen) may be administered. Heliox may be effective, because helium, being lighter than oxygen, may be able to pass through the obstructed airway. Patients may also receive bronchodilators, anxiolytics, analgesics, or any combination of these to help relieve associated dyspnea. Ideal positioning is in a semi-Fowler's or Fowler's position to decrease work of breathing.[13]

CARDIAC TAMPONADE

Cardiac tamponade is compression of the heart as a result of fluid accumulation in the pericardial sac. The fluid in the pericardial sac can cause enough pressure to prevent the atria and ventricles from filling completely during diastole. This results in a decreased cardiac output, decreased stroke volume, and hypotension. The body attempts to compensate with tachycardia. Eventually, the compensatory mechanisms fail, resulting in pulseless electrical activity or asystole. Cardiac tamponade occurs when the pericardial effusion results in hemodynamic instability, with compensatory mechanisms no longer being effective.[14,15]

Incidence/Prevalence

As many of the signs and symptoms of cardiac tamponade are often subtle, the diagnosis is often overlooked. Malignancies are the most common cause of cardiac tamponade, occurring in up to 65% of patients with cancer.[14]

Patients at Risk

Pericardial effusions, which can ultimately result in tamponade, may arise from direct expansion of a tumor or from metastasis through the lymphatic vessels of the mediastinum.[15] Cardiac tamponade occurs most often in patients with tumors that metastasize to the thoracic area.[14] Primary malignancies of the pericardium or myocardium, although rare, can put the patient at risk for development of a pericardial effusion. These include mesothelioma and sarcomas. Chemotherapeutic agents such as antitumor antibiotics (e.g., daunorubicin [Cerubidine], doxorubicin [Adriamycin], paclitaxel [Taxol], and docetaxel [Taxotere]) have been implicated.[15,21]

Cancers that metastasize to the heart put the patient at risk for developing cardiac tamponade. These cancers include lung, breast, and esophageal cancers; Hodgkin's and non-Hodgkin's lymphomas; chronic myeloid leukemia; melanoma; sarcoma; and liver, gastric, thymic, and pancreatic cancers.[15,22,30]

Cardiac tamponade can develop following surgery, radiation therapy, or chemotherapy, or from constriction of the pericardium by a tumor. Patients who have received mediastinal radiation therapy (more than 4000 cGy) are at risk because of the development of postradiation pericarditis.[15]

There are several noncancer causes of cardiac tamponade, including renal failure; myocardial infarction; viral, fungal, or bacterial infection; transvenous pacemaker insertion and other invasive cardiac procedures; pericarditis; chest trauma; immune disorders; hypoalbuminemia; hypothyroidism; aneurysm; improper central venous catheter insertion; complications from angioplasty; and any other cause of injury or inflammation to the pericardium. Other causes include anticoagulation, connective tissue disorders (e.g., systemic lupus erythematosus or rheumatoid arthritis), HIV infection, drugs (e.g., hydralazine [Apresoline], procainamide [Pronestyl], isoniazid [INH], minoxidil [Loniten]), postcoronary intervention, acupuncture, and percutaneous procedures (e.g., atrial septal defect closure or mitral valvuloplasty).[31]

Pathophysiology

The pericardial sac consists of the visceral and parietal layers. There is normally up to 50 mL of plasma-like fluid between the layers in the pericardial sac. The fluid lubricates the heart as it contracts.[15] When there is more than the normal amount of fluid in the pericardial sac, a pericardial effusion develops.

As cancer invades the pericardium, the cancer or the pericardium itself can produce excess fluid in response to the malignant process. Pericardial fluid can accumulate when lymphatic and venous flow is blocked by a tumor, thereby preventing fluid resorption. Tumors can bleed, causing accumulation that results in cardiac tamponade.[27]

As fluid accumulates in the pericardial sac, the pericardium stretches.[14] The pericardial sac can accommodate an approximate 1 to 2 L increase in fluid if the fluid accumulation occurs slowly; the hemodynamic effects occur gradually, because the body has a chance to compensate. If fluid accumulates rapidly, the pericardium is unable to stretch quickly enough to accommodate the excess fluid, and hemodynamic compromise will ensue.[15] As little as 200 mL of fluid accumulating over a short period of time can result in hemodynamic compromise. As fluid collects, the heart chambers become progressively smaller. The compression hinders blood flow from the right to left side, thus impairing ventricular filling, with a resultant decrease in stroke volume and cardiac output.[15]

Right ventricular filling is dependent on a gradient between central venous pressure and right ventricular diastolic pressure. The increased intrapericardial pressure that occurs with fluid accumulation in the pericardial sac affects this gradient, and the right ventricle is unable to fill adequately. A decrease in right ventricular preload and compression leads to a decrease in the amount of blood leaving that chamber. This decreases the amount of blood flowing to and from the left heart. As pressure in the pericardium increases, intrapericardial pressures increase, equalizing right and left ventricular end-diastolic pressures.[31]

The right atrium and ventricle may initially compensate by causing tachycardia in an effort to increase or maintain stroke volume. Eventually the compensatory mechanisms fail, and patients become symptomatic or develop cardiovascular collapse.[15]

Clinical Presentation

Early signs and symptoms of cardiac tamponade may be unremarkable and undetected.[15] The presentation of cardiac tamponade depends on a number of factors, including how quickly the fluid collects in the pericardium and the underlying cause. Symptom onset may be very impressive if the fluid accumulates quickly.

Patients most frequently present with progressive shortness of breath, chest pain, and cough. Other clinical presentation findings can be found in Table 41.7. Although rarely seen clinically, the three classic symptoms of cardiac tamponade, known as Beck's triad, include hypotension, distended neck veins, and distant heart sounds.[15]

Although not unique to cardiac tamponade, a *pulsus paradoxus* is a sign of this condition. This is a decrease of greater than or equal to 10 mm Hg in systolic blood pressure on inspiration. It may also be noted when more pulse beats are palpated on expiration than inspiration, or when a palpable pulse is lost on inspiration.[21] It is possible for patients with cardiac tamponade with severe hypotension or other cardiac conditions (e.g., atrial septal defect, severe aortic stenosis, or left ventricular dysfunction) to not have a *pulsus paradoxus*. A frequent finding on physical examination is pericardial friction rub. This is best auscultated at the left lower sternal border or the apex when the patient is sitting forward.[17]

Early signs and symptoms of cardiac tamponade include dyspnea and retrosternal chest pain that increases when the patient is in a supine position and is relieved when leaning forward. This is caused by compression on the heart. Patients also manifest dysphagia, hoarseness, or hiccoughs from mechanical compression on nerves of the esophagus, bronchi, or trachea; dizziness; lightheadedness or agitation due to hypoxia; and weakness, fatigue, or malaise related to decreased cardiac output. Gastrointestinal complaints include anorexia, nausea, or vomiting from visceral congestion and venous stasis.[15,21]

Late signs and symptoms include retrosternal chest pain, tachypnea, progressive dyspnea, hypoxia, and orthopnea related to decreased cardiac output; peripheral edema from venous congestion; and confusion, restlessness, and apprehension due to hypoxia and decreased cerebral perfusion. Hypotension and tachycardia will also be present.[15]

Several tests assist in the diagnosis of cardiac tamponade. These include chest radiograph, CT scan, MRI, pulmonary artery catheterization, echocardiogram, and ECG.[12,14,17,21,30]

Radiology Findings

Chest radiography of a patient with cardiac tamponade may reveal cardiac enlargement from the increased fluid in the pericardial sac and mediastinal widening, or hilar adenopathy. However, if the fluid accumulates rapidly, radiographic findings may be normal. If the fluid accumulates slowly, the pericardial sac may hold 1 to 2 L of fluid. In these cases, the radiograph reveals a "water bottle" heart.[14]

CT and MRI may be used in conjunction with clinical findings to help diagnose and manage cardiac tamponade.[15] CT reveals a pericardial effusion and differentiates this diagnosis from SVCS. MRI has partial value in the diagnosis of cardiac tamponade; it may show large pericardial effusions, and can be used to estimate the extent of an effusion.

Diagnostic Evaluation

Electrocardiogram

ECG findings are usually nonspecific. Excessive heart movement in the increased pericardial fluid causes electrical alternans, which is a change in the axis from beat to beat. Tachycardia, premature contractions, a change in the shape and amplitude of P waves, ST segment elevation or depression, and low voltage QRS complexes will also be noted.[15,17]

Echocardiogram

Echocardiogram is the quickest and most accurate method to diagnose cardiac tamponade. With an echocardiogram, ultrasonic waves that are produced with a probe create a picture of the heart and portray cardiac functioning. It will reveal fluid in the pericardial sac and compression of the heart chambers. Echocardiograms also provide an estimate of ejection fraction, and can detect a pericardial mass. An echocardiogram will further assess the hemodynamic sequelae of cardiac tamponade.[15]

Pulmonary Artery Catheterization

Insertion of a pulmonary artery catheter will reveal equalization of right- and left-sided heart pressures, decreased cardiac output, and elevated systemic vascular resistance (SVR), central venous pressure (CVP), left atrial pressure, pulmonary artery pressures, and pulmonary artery occlusive pressure (PAOP), also called pulmonary artery wedge pressure (PAWP). Pulmonary artery catheterization is an invasive procedure and is associated with several risks. Therefore, insertion as a diagnostic tool is not routinely done.[15]

Interprofessional Plan of Care

Overall management of cardiac tamponade centers on relieving pressure on the heart and enhancing cardiac function. Other goals include fluid removal, prevention of reaccumulation of fluid, and minimizing complications.[15]

Initial management strategies for the patient with cardiac tamponade should focus on stabilizing the patient. Patients may require maintenance of a patent airway and volume resuscitation to enhance right-sided preload and stroke volume. Maintaining adequate filling pressures and enhancing myocardial contractility and cardiac output are essential in managing the patient.[15] Treatment depends on cause and severity of the

TABLE 41.7 **Medications Used in Oncologic Emergencies**

Medication	Actions	Dosage	Special Considerations
Hypercalcemia of Malignancy			
Bisphosphonates	The precise mechanism of action of the bisphosphonates on bone cells and bone reabsorption is not completely understood. It involves inhibition of the function of osteoclasts in a variety of ways (e.g., by producing a direct toxic effect on the resorbing osteoclasts, by promoting programmed cell death, or by inhibiting the differentiation of the osteoclasts into mature osteoclasts). Inhibits calcium reabsorption and enhances urinary calcium excretion.	Pamidronate (Aredia): Serum calcium 12–13.5 mg/dL: 60–90 mg IV over 4 h; serum calcium > 13.5 mg/dL: 90 mg IV over 4 h. Zoledronic acid (Zometa): If serum calcium ≥ 12 mg/dL: 4 mg IV over at least 15 min.	Should be started when rehydration has been established.
Loop diuretics: Furosemide (Lasix)	Diureses excess fluid and calcium. Inhibits calcium reabsorption by the kidneys and protects against volume overload.	Up to 100 mg IV every 1–4 h.	Should be avoided until volume status has been restored. Carefully monitor magnesium and potassium levels.
Corticosteroids	Enhance calcium excretion in the urine and inhibit calcium resorption in the gastrointestinal tract. Part of treatment for the underlying malignancy.	Variable; depends on protocol used to treat the underlying malignancy.	Should be avoided until volume status has been restored. Carefully monitor magnesium and potassium values.
Acute Tumor Lysis Syndrome			
Sodium bicarbonate	Alkalizes urine to prevent uric acid crystal formation.	50–100 mEq added to each liter of hydration. Can be started 1–2 days prior to starting chemotherapy.	Maintain urine pH > 7.5.
Allopurinol (Zyloprim, Aloprim)	Xanthine oxidase inhibitor. Decreases uric acid formation.	PO: 100 mg daily. IV: 200–400 mg/m^2. Maximum of 600 mg/day.	Can be started 1–2 days prior to starting chemotherapy.
Rasburicase (Elitek)	Recombinant urate oxidase enzyme.	0.15–0.20 mg/kg IV over 30 min daily for 5 days.	Can cause severe hemolysis in patients with glucose-6-phosphate dehydrogenase deficiency. Can cause severe anaphylactic reactions. Has been associated with methemoglobinemia.
Syndrome of Inappropriate Antidiuretic Hormone Secretion			
Demeclocycline (Declomycin)	Causes nephrogenic diabetes insipidus.	600–1200 mg daily.	
Spinal Cord Compression			
Corticosteroids: Dexamethasone (Decadron)	Decreases inflammatory response to underlying tumor and edema surrounding the tumor that may damage the spinal cord.	Loading dose: 4–100 mg IV. Then 16–96 mg/day in divided doses.	Taper over several days.
Superior Vena Cava Syndrome			
Diuretics: Furosemide (Lasix)	Decreases right-sided preload (venous return), which will decrease pressure on the SVC.	20–80 mg PO; may repeat in 6–8 h.	
Corticosteroids: Methylprednisolone (Solu-Medrol)	Decreases inflammatory response to underlying tumor and edema surrounding the tumor.	Loading dose: 125–250 mg IV. Maintenance dose: 0.5–1 mg/kg IV every 6 h for up to 5 days.	

IV, Intravenous; *PO*, per os; SVC, superior vena cava.

tamponade. Patients with severe hemodynamic compromise require decompression with pericardiocentesis. Patients who are more stable may respond to supportive measures.[15]

Pericardiocentesis

Percutaneous pericardiocentesis entails insertion of a catheter into the pericardial space to drain the fluid. A pericardiocentesis is most often performed with 2-dimensional echocardiogram guidance, and may be performed at the bedside.[15]

In patients with significant hemodynamic compromise, removal of a small amount of pericardial fluid (50–100 mL) may improve the patient's condition. If possible, the catheter should remain in place to drain fluid. When less than 50 mL/day is draining, the catheter can be removed.[15]

Echocardiogram-Guided Pericardiocentesis

This is considered the procedure of choice to remove pericardial fluid. The direction and depth of needle advancement are confirmed with echocardiography. The needle tip is visualized with imaging, and the optimal point of penetration of the pericardium can be determined.[15]

Pericardial Window

Pericardial window procedures are performed on patients with recurrent tamponade who do not respond to other treatments. This procedure entails removing a section of the pericardium, which creates an opening for fluid to drain from the pericardial sac.[15]

Balloon Pericardiotomy

A pericardiocentesis will provide temporary relief of signs and symptoms until the underlying malignancy is treated. Balloon pericardiotomy is another option to prevent fluid accumulation. This procedure involves the insertion of a catheter with a balloon tip into the pericardial sac. This makes the size of the pericardial sac smaller.[15] The catheter tears the pericardium and creates a window for drainage of fluid. The chance of fluid reaccumulation is minimized, because the balloon decreases the space. Once the balloon is inserted, there is an opening in the pericardium that facilitates internal drainage and fluid resorption. When the balloon is in place, it is dilated to form a pericardial window, which allows fluid to drain.[12,15]

Sclerotherapy

Sclerotherapy may be indicated for patients with recurrent cardiac tamponade. It entails the insertion of a catheter into the pericardial sac with subsequent administration of a sclerosing agent. The effusion is resolved because of an inflammatory response from the agent, connecting the visceral and parietal layers of the pericardium.[15]

Common sclerosing agents include bleomycin (Blenoxane), doxycycline (Vibramycin), cisplatin (Platinol), fluorouracil (Adrucil), corticosteroids, mitomycin C (Mutamycin), thiotepa (Thioplex), and radioisotopes such as gold or chromic phosphate.[15]

Pericardiectomy

A pericardiectomy is the excision of part or all of the pericardium, and involves a thoracotomy or median sternotomy. The pericardium is resected to enhance drainage of fluid into the pleural space.[21] A pericardiectomy is indicated for patients with pericarditis or those with cancer with constriction due to radiation therapy. This surgical procedure can be used in patients with recurrent malignant cardiac tamponade.[15]

CONCLUSION

Patients undergoing treatment for cancer require ongoing support. This need is augmented when patients develop a potentially life-threatening complication of the disease or its treatments. When these emergencies occur, the interprofessional team plays a pivotal role in helping the patient and family cope. Focused monitoring and prompt intervention with preventive and management approaches are essential to promote quality of life and reduce morbidity and mortality. The knowledge of the critical care nurse regarding these oncologic emergencies is essential for attaining these quality patient outcomes.

CASE STUDY 41.1

A patient with a history of gout and Burkitt's lymphoma was admitted with R-Hyper CVAD (rituximab, high-dose cyclophosphamide, vincristine, doxorubicin, and dexamethasone). The patient received hydration and allopurinol for two days prior to admission. Once adequately hydrated, the patient was started on furosemide. On day 2 of therapy, the morning lab results revealed: potassium 5.7 mEq/L, phosphorus 8.2 mg/dL, calcium 6.8 mg/dL, and uric acid 18 mg/dL. An ECG was performed, and revealed elevated T waves. The patient reported nausea and was treated with the prescribed antiemetic regimen. Weakness, anorexia, and paresthesia were also reported. A diagnosis of acute tumor lysis syndrome was made.

The patient was started on aggressive intravenous fluid resuscitation, an oral phosphate binder, and calcium supplementation. Dextrose (50%, 25 g) and 10 units of regular insulin were administered intravenously. Rasburicase (0.2 mg/kg) was administered intravenously over 30 minutes. The allopurinol was discontinued at that time. No hypersensitivity reaction was noted from the rasburicase. The patient's electrolytes normalized over the course of the day, and the symptoms dissipated.

Decision Point:

What factors contributed to the patient's development of cardiac tamponade?

Decision Point:

Which disciplines would you collaborate with to help ensure optimal patient outcomes?

Decision Point:

Describe your role as a facilitator of learning for this patient. What patient education is required?

REFERENCES

1. Agency for Healthcare Research & Quality. (2012). Metastatic spinal cord compression. Diagnosis and management of adults at risk for and with metastatic spinal cord compression. https://www.guideline.gov/summaries/summary/14326/metastatic-spinal-cord-compression-diagnosis-and-management-of-adults-at-risk-of-and-with-metastatic-spinal-cord-compression.
2. Agraharkar, M. (2015). Hypercalcemia. http://emedicine.medscape.com/article/240681.
3. Austin, N., Krishnamoorthy, V., & Dagal, A. (2014). Airway management in cervical spine injury. *Int J Crit Illn Inj Sci, 4*(1), 50–56.
4. Bergman, P. J. (2012). Paraneoplastic hypercalcemia. *Top Companion Anim Med, 27*(14), 156–158.
5. Chemocare.com. (2002–2015). Hyperkalemia (High Potassium). http://chemocare.com/chemotherapy/side-effects/hyperkalemia-high-potassium.aspx.
6. Flaherty, A. M. (2011). Spinal cord compression. In C. H. Yarbro, D. Wujcik, & B. H. Gobel (Eds.), *Cancer nursing. Principles and practice* (10th ed.) (pp. 979–994). Sudbury, MA: Jones & Bartlett.
7. Glauser, J. M. (2014). Focus on…. Critical decisions: metabolic emergencies in cancer. https://www.acep.org/Education/Continuing-Medical-Education-(CME)/Focus-On/Focus-On----Critical-Decisions--Metabolic-Emergencies-in-Cancer-Patients/.
8. Green, T. (2014). Hypercalcemia in emergency medicine. http://emedicine.medscape.com/article/766373-overview.
9. Horowitz, M. J. (2014). Hypercalcemia of malignancy. http://www.uptodate.com/contents/hypercalcemia-of-malignancy.
10. Huff, J. S. (2015). Spinal cord neoplasms. http://emedicine.medscape.com/article/779872-overview.
11. Ikeda, A. K. (2014). Tumor lysis syndrome. http://emedicine.medscape.com/article/282171-overview.
12. Jones, D. A., & Jain, A. K. (2011). Percutaneous balloon pericardiotomy for recurrent malignant pericardial effusion. *J Thorac Oncol, 7*, 2138–2139.

13. Kaplan, M. (2012). Spinal cord compression. In M. Kaplan (Ed.), *Understanding and managing oncologic emergencies: a resource for nurses* (pp. 337–383). Pittsburgh, PA: Oncology Nursing Society.
14. Kaplow, R. (2011). Cardiac tamponade. In C. H. Yarbro, D. Wujcik, & B. H. Gobel (Eds.), *Cancer nursing. Principles and Practice* (7th ed.) (pp. 915–927). Sudbury, MA: Jones & Bartlett.
15. Kaplow, R. (2013). Cardiac tamponade. http://www.inpractice.com/Textbooks/oncology-Nursing/Oncologic-Emergencies/CardiacTamponade.aspx.
16. Kaplow, R. (2015). Syndrome of inappropriate antidiuretic hormone. In M. S. Baird, & S. Bethel (Eds.), *Manual of critical care nursing. Nursing interventions and collaborative management:* (7th ed.) St. Louis: Mosby (in press).
17. Khandaker, M. H., et al. (2010). Pericardial disease: diagnosis and management. *Mayo Clin Proc, 85*, 572–593.
18. Larson, R. A., & Phi, C.-H. (2015). Tumor lysis syndrome. *Prevention and treatment.* http://uptodate.com/contents/tumor-lysis-syndrome-prevention-and-treatment?source=search_result&search-tumor+lysis+syndrome&selectedTitle=1%7E150.
19. Leitman, A., Germain-Lee, E. L., & Levine, M. A. (2010). Hypercalcemia in children and adolescents. *Curr Opin Pediatr, 22*(4), 508–515.
20. Lewis, M. A., Hendrickson, A. W., & Moynihan, T. J. (2011). Oncologic emergencies: pathophysiology, presentation, diagnosis, and treatment. *CA Cancer J Clin, 61*, 287–314.
21. Maisch, B., Ristic, A., & Pankuweit, S. (2010). Evaluation and management of pericardial effusion in patients with neoplastic disease. *Prog Cardiovasc Dis, 53*, 157–163.
22. National Cancer Institute. (2011). Malignant pericardial effusion. http://www.cancer.gov/cancertopics/pdq/supportivecare/cardiopulmonary/HealthProfessional/page4.
23. Nickloes, T. A. (2014). Superior vena cava syndrome. http://emedicine.medscape.com/article/460865-overview.
24. Pelosof, L. C., & Gerber, D. E. (2010). Paraneoplastic syndromes. An approach to diagnosis and treatment. *Mayo Clin Proc, 85*(9), 838–854.
25. Raj, V. S., & Lofton, L. (2013). Rehabilitation and treatment of spinal cord tumors. *J Spinal Cord Med, 36*(1), 4–11.
26. Rubin, M. (2014). Compression of the spinal cord. http://www.merckmanuals.com/home/brain_spinal_cord_and_nerve_disorders/spinal_cord_disorders/compression_of_the_spinal_cord.html.
27. Schiff, D. (2014). Clinical features and diagnosis of neoplastic epidural spinal cord compression including cauda equine syndrome. http://www.uptodate.com/contents/clinical-features-and-diagnosis-of-neoplastic-epidural-spinal-cord-compression-including-cauda-equina-syndrome.
28. Shane, E. (2014). Etiology of hypercalcemia. http://www.uptodate.com/contents/etiology-of-hypercalcemia.
29. Simon, E. E. (2014). Hyponatremia workup. http://emedicine.medscape.com/article/242166-overview.
30. Story, K. T. (2013). Cardiac tamponade. In M. Kaplan (Ed.), *Understanding and managing oncologic emergencies: a resource for nurses.* (pp. 43–68). Pittsburgh, PA: Oncology Nursing Society.
31. Yarlagadda, C. (2015). Cardiac tamponade. http://emedicine.medscape.com/article/152083-overview.

42

Chemical Dependency

Andrea Efre

The chemically dependent patient presents a unique challenge in the acute and critical care setting. Successful management of these patients starts with the nursing team being well informed on abused substances in the local area, and having knowledge of their presenting symptoms, mechanism of action, side effects, and consequences. Monitoring subtle physical and behavioral changes of the intoxicated or withdrawing patient will ensure early intervention, avoid dangerous complications, and prevent further sequelae. The goal of this chapter is to provide a detailed description of factors that should be considered in caring for patients under the influence of drugs or alcohol, or those suffering from withdrawal.

Patients affected by drug or alcohol related conditions are treated in many acute and critical care settings. For example: (1) a teenager who is suffering from overdose of the street drug known as *Spice,* (2) a young adult in the trauma intensive care unit (ICU) who was struck by a car while running across a highway in a psychotic rage after using the street drug *Flakka,* (3) an older adult who had an acute myocardial infarction after using cocaine. These are just a handful of examples; many more exist throughout the United States.

Substance intoxication and withdrawal often involve several substances, used simultaneously or sequentially.[4] The signs and symptoms of substance withdrawal may be the reason for a hospital admission (meaning the patient presents with side effects of withdrawal); or withdrawal from a substance may occur as a side effect of being admitted. Symptoms of withdrawal may be a surprise to the patient as many do not recognize or acknowledge their dependency. It is important to ask questions and gather a detailed history on all patients; and to remain open minded and observant in anticipating withdrawal symptoms. If there is a preconceived image of what an addicted person looks like, then subtle findings may be missed. As an example: a person who drinks two glasses of wine a night may not think that is significant enough to mention upon admission, yet an extended hospital stay may induce alcohol withdrawal symptoms.

PREVALENCE OF SUBSTANCE USE DISORDERS

The development of substance use, abuse, or dependence is a process that appears to involve opportune exposure, drug availability, peer influences, and possibly genetic disposition.[84] It is estimated that 137 million Americans are drinkers of alcohol, and excessive drinking accounts for 1 in 10 deaths among working-age adults in the United States.[73] The highest rates of binge drinking and alcohol use disorders (AUD) occur between the ages of 18 and 29 years.[43] There is a gender difference in the consumption of alcohol, with women developing higher levels of intoxication by drinking the same amount as a male counterpart, making women more susceptible to alcoholic liver disease and complications.[65] It is believed that women have a smaller amount of body water and lower activity of alcohol dehydrogenase in the stomach, which assists with alcohol metabolism.[65] However, men have a greater prevalence of AUD than women, and the Native American population has greater rates of severe AUD than all other ethnicities, followed by Caucasians.[31] Genome-wide association studies link alcohol dependence and substance abuse to genetic risk factors.[2,84] However, choosing to engage in the behavior most likely depends on their environmental experiences.[84]

SUBSTANCE USE DISORDERS DEFINED

Substance use disorders are best defined by the American Psychiatric Association (APA) in the national resource for behavioral conditions, the *Diagnostic and Statistical Manual of Mental Disorders* (*DSM-5*). For diagnostic purposes, the APA separates substance use into 10 classifications: (1) alcohol, (2) caffeine, (3) cannabis, (4) hallucinogens (with separate categories for phencyclidine and other hallucinogens), (5) inhalants, (6) opioids, (7) sedatives, hypnotics, and anxiolytics, (8) stimulants (amphetamine-type substances, cocaine, and other stimulants), (9) tobacco, and (10) other/unknown substances.[4] Most of these categories will be covered in this chapter, with the focus being on alcohol and drugs that affect patients in critical care (Table 42.1).

ADDICTION

Addiction is a broad term used to describe many aspects of drug and alcohol use. The process involves the stimulation of the neurologic system involved in pleasure, and generates a positive or rewarding response. Repeated and frequent substance use induces adaptations in the brain associated with the acute rewarding effects of the drug, alcohol, or behavior. The neural pathways are affected (most notably enhancing dopamine release), including reward, motivation, and memory. The pattern of addiction depends on the substance being used. For example, cocaine, methamphetamine, and marijuana are related to drug induced euphoria and an obsessive desire to repeat the experience.[14] This reward (response) lasts until tolerance to the substance develops, at which time more substance is required to achieve the same reward. Withdrawal can induce negative emotions, anhedonia, and motivational deficits that may be due to decreased dopamine function (reward-deficiency), which drive the user to continue drug use in order to restore a normal dopamine level and reduce anxiety.[90]

TABLE 42.1 Definitions

Intoxication:	The presence of clinically significant and problematic behavioral or psychological changes following the recent use of a substance.
Abuse:	Substance affects the user's life and role, with maladaptive patterns of consumption that cause negative social, occupational, and legal consequences.
Craving:	An intense desire or urge for the substance and is associated with activation of specific reward structures in the brain.
Tolerance:	Repeated exposure to a substance results in a state of adaptation, or a loss of effect from the substances repeated exposure over time. Tolerance is reached by requiring an increased dose of the substance to achieve the desired effect, or responding to a reduced effect when the usual dose is consumed.
Sensitization:	Repeated exposure to stimulants results in an increased response.
Dependence:	Dependence suggests chronic or heavy use of a substance despite significant life problems related to its use. The body becomes accustomed (tolerant) to a substance used on a regular basis and, when lesser amounts are used than the body is accustomed to, withdrawal will occur.
Withdrawal:	Physiologic and psychologic effects that occur when blood or tissue concentrations decline caused by removal or cessation of the substance of abuse or dependence.
Alcohol Induced Disorder:	Includes intoxication, delirium, withdrawal, amnestic disorders, and fetal alcohol spectrum disorders related to the ingestion of alcohol.
Alcohol Withdrawal Syndrome (AWS):	Cessation or reduction in alcohol use that has been heavy and prolonged leading to autonomic hyperactivity of the central nervous system.
Alcohol Use Disorder (AUD):	Includes regular use, craving, abuse, tolerance, dependence, and harmful drinking of alcohol.

From References 4, 17, 61, and 74.

As part of the addiction process that leads to continued use and dependence, the mesolimbic dopamine system is activated by all major drugs of abuse.[90] Any act that increases the activity of the reward centers of the brain will lead to more activity that will achieve stimulation of the same craving pathway, which leads to drug-seeking behaviors. Addictive behaviors share the same core features as substance addictions. These include craving, tolerance, withdrawal, and compulsive use despite occupational, interpersonal, and financial adversity.[90] Many clinicians internationally use the word addiction to describe severe problems related to compulsive and habitual use of substances. However, it should be noted that the APA removed the term addiction from the *DSM-5* revision in favor of the term of substance use disorder, which they believe better describes the wide range of the disorder.[4]

Addiction affects biological, psychological, and social aspects of the user's life, and places large financial burdens on healthcare systems.[14] Many believe that addiction should be treated as a chronic disease such as diabetes or hypertension, and that medications may need to be continued indefinitely.[69] The Affordable Care Act requires that insurers provide treatment for addiction that is equal to that available for other chronic diseases such as diabetes or hypertension.[69]

PATHOPHYSIOLOGY OF CHEMICAL DEPENDENCE

It is important to understand the pathophysiology of how substances effect the body in order that effects of treatments may be more fully understood. The physiologic effects of alcohol and most drugs take place at the site of the neuron, by affecting the neurotransmitter balance, and thereby influencing the signals transmitted across the nerve junction. Neurotransmitters are biochemical messengers stored in the presynaptic side of the synapse in the axon terminal (belongs to the initiating neuron). They use ion channels to bind directly (like a lock and key mechanism) or indirectly (releasing secondary messengers to activate neighboring channels) at the post synaptic receptor site. Depending on the kind of neurotransmitter released, the effect can be either excitatory (depolarizing) or inhibitory (hyperpolarizing). The stimulation or depression of the neurons electrical excitability can be influenced by factors such as medications, recreational drugs, alcohol, caffeine, stress, poor diet, neurotoxins, disease states, or genetic predisposition.

Glutamate is the most prevalent neurotransmitter, is excitatory, involved in cognitive functions such as learning and memory, and in muscle strength. Changes in the glutamatergic neurotransmission are affected by alcohol and drug addiction.[66] Glutamate is an agonist to the N-methyl-D-aspartate (NMDA) receptor, and allows sodium (Na^+) and calcium (Ca^{2+}) ions into the cell and potassium (K^+) out of the cell. The NMDA receptor is modified by alcohol and many psychoactive drugs such as phencyclidine (PCP), dextromethorphan, methadone, and ketamine. It is glutamine imbalance that causes the physical symptoms of staggering, slurred speech, and memory blackouts. Excessive glutamate release can overstimulate the brain and lead to excitotoxicity, which may result in seizures.

Gamma-aminobutyric acid (GABA) is the primary inhibitory neurotransmitter, reducing excitation. With GABA cell activation there is a systemic calm, relaxed feeling of sedation, a decreased anxiety, relaxation of muscles, amnesia, and effects on visual acuity, which leads to blurred vision in the inebriated patient. When the GABA receptor cell is not activated, the body responds with a systemic nervous feeling. Benzodiazepine receptors are also located on the same GABA receptor, which is why alcohol withdrawal symptoms are treated with benzodiazepines. The mechanism of action of alcohol and many recreational drugs is to enhance the effects of GABA, specifically those with side effects of tranquilization, sedation, or anesthesia.

Monoamines are neurotransmitters that include dopamine, serotonin, epinephrine, norepinephrine, and histamine, which are all affected by substance use and withdrawal. Both recreational drugs and alcohol cause a release of dopamine in the reward pathway. Dopamine has a number of important functions in the brain, including regulation of motor behavior, pleasures, and the reward system. Serotonin regulates appetite, sleep, memory, learning, temperature, mood, behavior, and muscle contraction, all of which can be affected by drug or alcohol use. Epinephrine and norepinephrine have stimulatory qualities and play a role in sleep, alertness, and the fight-or-flight response. Histamines are slightly different from other neurotransmitters as they lack a specific reuptake transporter. They are involved in the homeostatic balance of the sleep-wake cycle, learning, body temperature, food and water intake, and influence drug addiction.[26]

Additional neurotransmitters affected by substance use and dependence include adenosine triphosphate (ATP) and adenosine, which play an important role in regulating neuronal activity and assisting in homeostasis of neurotransmitter systems such as GABA, glutamate, and dopamine. Adenosine exerts its function through several adenosine receptors and regulates glutamate levels in the brain. Adenosine is an endogenous sleep-promoting agent. Extracellular adenosine levels elevate in the presence of alcohol, which then affects the regulation of ataxic and hypnotic sleep.[66] Acetylcholine may be affected by some substances, and it may excite or inhibit internal organs in the autonomic system. It uses multiple receptors, but primarily the nicotinic and muscarinic, to connect motor nerves to muscles.

Physiologic Effects of Recreational Drug Use

Various substances affect physiology differently; some increase the dopamine activity in the upper centers of the brain, whereas others mimic the effects of neurotransmitters or block the reuptake of neurotransmitters such as dopamine. The physiologic effects of the drugs are determined purely by the substances' chemical structure, mechanism of action, and metabolism. For example, cocaine has a direct influence on the dopamine signaling in the brain, which then affects the reward pathways and plasticity mechanisms.[13] Alteration in the regulation of dopamine, norepinephrine, and glutamate occurs with cocaine use and dependence.[35] Cocaine blocks the presynaptic reuptake of dopamine and norepinephrine, resulting in enhanced dopamine (psychostimulant actions) and enhanced norepinephrine (cardiovascular symptoms, which increase myocardial oxygen demand). Cocaine also blocks the fast Na^+ channels in membranes, reducing action potential and inducing a local anesthetic effect.[48]

Narcotics such as heroin, morphine, and codeine activate endorphins and enkephalins.[42] The action of opioids is primarily at the mu receptors, resulting in diminished sensation of pain. The opioid receptors are termed mu, kappa, and sigma; the mu receptor mediates most of the opioid drug properties.[42] Repeated exposure to opioids causes molecular adaptations that result in up-regulation of the receptors and a lesser effectiveness of the drug at the previous repeated dose, leading to the requirement of an increased dose to achieve the desired effect. When the drug is abruptly stopped, the pain receptors fire at an abnormally high level, leading to the intense pain sensation. The pain then leads to use of more drugs, continuing the cycle of abuse.

Physiologic Effects of Alcohol Use

Alcohol has profound effects on medical, psychological, and social aspects of life, yet it is a small ambiguous molecule with a simple chemical structure (C_2H_5OH).[44] The systemic effects of alcohol use include sedation, decreased anxiety, relaxation of muscles, and amnesia, primarily due to the stimulation of the GABA receptor. Alcohol is a GABA agonist and reduces the flow of calcium into the cells. It stimulates GABA, releases opioid peptides, and influences norepinephrine and dopamine release. Alcohol exposure increases the number of binding sites for glutamate, and increases extracellular glutamate levels in the brain, affecting reward pathways.[66] Alcohol affects the endorphin system in a manner similar to opiates, acting as an analgesic and giving a rush of endorphins. Additional neurotransmitters affected by alcohol include adenosine, acetylcholine, and serotonin.

The immediate effects of alcohol cause central nervous system (CNS) depression due to the disruption of the inhibitory GABA and the excitatory NMDA glutamate pathways.[47,71,85] Acute ingestion of alcohol leads to augmentation of GABA activity and blocking of the excitatory action of glutamate at the NMDA receptor, leading to sedative and depressant effects.[61,71] The inhibition of the NMDA receptor induces an initial euphoria and reduced self-control. If alcohol is continued to be consumed it may progress to sedation, analgesia, and then an anesthetic type of effect, leading to loss of consciousness, a raised seizure threshold, and respiratory depression. This progression of symptoms is especially seen in binge drinkers.

The long-term effects of alcohol dependence relate to the struggle for balance in the GABA and NMDA receptors. GABA is consistently being activated by alcohol, which leads to down-regulation of the GABA receptors. In response there is an up-regulation (increase) in NMDA receptor activation to maintain neurotransmitter balance. As alcohol tolerance increases more alcohol must be taken in order to accomplish the GABA stimulation and induce the calming effects.[47,71,85] Chronic alcohol also affects the immune responses, inducing an overproduction of proinflammatory cytokines, leading to a detrimental effect on immune cells, organs, and tissues.[21] The cannabinoid genes and receptors may play a role in regulating this cytokine production and may limit alcohol-induced inflammation.[2]

Upon abrupt discontinuation or reduction of alcohol, these adaptive responses are unmasked. There is an overactivation of the NMDA pathway, resulting from up-regulation of NMDA receptors, and decreased inhibitory activity due to down-regulation of the GABA receptors.[47,71,85] It is this physiologic imbalance that results in the clinical signs and symptoms of alcohol withdrawal syndrome (AWS).[47]

KINDLING PHENOMENON

The kindling phenomenon refers to the neurologic condition caused by the dysregulation of neurotransmitters following repeated patterns of withdrawal in an alcohol or substance dependent patient. Chronic alcohol or substances use results in increased sensitization of glutamate receptors and reduced GABA function, leading to increased neuronal hyperexcitability with repeated withdrawal episodes, known as *the kindling effect*.[3,11,37,61,67,74]

Kindling is thought to explain the progressive risk of withdrawal symptoms from milder to more severe.[61,67] Each time the patient goes through withdrawal the symptoms worsen, and there is an increased risk of seizures with each withdrawal episode.[67,74] The symptoms also become increasingly resistant to treatment, particularly benzodiazepines, making pharmacologic management more difficult.[88] Therefore, obtaining a good history of past withdrawal symptoms is essential. Kindling is usually a result of withdrawal from sedative-hypnotic drugs such as benzodiazepines or alcohol, but it may also play a role in cocaine induced seizures.[74]

PATIENT ASSESSMENT (PHYSICAL EXAMINATION)

One of the most important aspects in the assessment of the patient is gathering information about the substances used, details of route, quantity, frequency, and last time of ingestion. Once substance information is known, it can be used to assist in the anticipation of side effects or withdrawal symptoms. This allows for earlier medical, nursing, and psychosocial management of the patient. New street drugs are being formulated constantly, and the substance used by the patient may be new or the street term used may make it difficult to determine the effects. Poison control will be able to assist in the most up to date information on toxicology and management of substance use and overdose. In addition, research on the internet is a fast and useful tool to determine origins and potential effects of substances. A thorough subjective and objective data collection is required to make an accurate diagnosis.

Interview (Subjective Data Collection)

A thorough assessment of the history of the patient's substance use is important in the diagnosis and management. However, patients may be reluctant to share out of shame, denial, or fear of social implications or legal consequences. The best way to obtain the information is to be nonjudgmental, supportive, and to inform the patient and family/support system of the importance of accurate information, both for predicting possible withdrawal and for personalizing a treatment plan. During the interview, remain neutral and be aware of nonverbal communication, both yours and that of the patient. When asking questions, do not act surprised or shocked by the answers. Be aware of your facial expressions and your responses to the answers received. Keep an open mind and use interview questions that can facilitate information flow and be redirected based on the patient's responses.

Subjective data collection begins with an investigation of the events that led up to the patient's arrival in your care. The history of present illness should be a clear, chronologic, complete account of what prompted the patient to seek care. It should include details of the onset of symptoms, manifestations, and treatments to date. Questions about the use of drug and alcohol should be specific; ask the patient to quantify: type, amount, time, frequency, previous use, immediate effects, and the events that took place following its use. The more detailed the history, the more accurate the treatment plan.

Subjective data collection includes medical, coexisting psychiatric conditions, surgical history, current medications, and allergies. Include questions of past withdrawal episodes, their severity (especially if seizures occurred), treatment, and if there have been periods of sobriety. Social history should include questions of lifestyle, daily habits, and living arrangements. When asking about tobacco, drug or alcohol use, ask about details (remembering that users may not be completely honest in the answer). It is also appropriate to ask about behavioral changes related to substance use, and if risky behaviors have been identified by the patient or family (this often involves promiscuity or sexually risky behaviors).

The review of systems should be comprehensive as many organ systems are affected by substance use. Beginning with the general constitution, questioning fatigue, fluctuations in weight, weakness, fevers, or difficulty sleeping. Inquire regarding changes in the skin, such as abscesses, discolorations, rash, or changes in texture. The head and neck review should include questions about visual disturbances and complaints of the nose, mouth, or teeth. Inquiry should include recent cough or shortness of breath, keeping in mind that heroin and alcohol use have long-term pulmonary effects.

If the patient has any chest pain or cardiac complaints there should be an immediate cardiac evaluation (including 12-lead electrocardiogram [ECG] and physical exam), as many substances affect the cardiovascular system in a negative way. The gastrointestinal system is often affected by substance use, including indigestion, nausea, vomiting, diarrhea, hematemesis, melena, or changes in bowel movements. The muscular skeletal system is usually unaffected but the neurologic and psychiatric systems are both significantly affected by drugs and alcohol. Determining if symptoms were induced by substance use, or prior to next use, will assist in determining if the substance causes them or if they may be related to withdrawal. If symptoms are experienced during long-term abstinence, they may be caused by an underlying medical or psychiatric condition. When the presenting complaint is syncope, near-syncope, dizziness, confusion, or altered level of consciousness, a cardiac and a neurologic examination should be performed. Hematologic, immunologic, and endocrine system symptoms may be present in a patient who has hepatic involvement, including bruising and bleeding.

Physical Exam (Objective Data Collection)

Physical manifestations of addiction are dependent on the type of substance used, its route, and the duration of use. The physical examination of the patient who is suspected to be under the influence, intoxicated, or suffering from withdrawal requires a thorough organized head to toe assessment. The acute versus chronic effects of the substance are based on the organs affected.

General Survey

The nurse should observe the general state of health, hygiene, nutritional status, signs of dehydration, diaphoresis, respiratory effort, alertness, interaction with the environment, and manner of speech. Constant monitoring of the cardiac and hemodynamic status is necessary. Elevation of systolic blood pressure of 20 to 30 mm Hg over baseline may occur in alcohol ingestion, dependence, or withdrawal. Tachycardia, hypertension, and hyperpyrexia are side effects of stimulants, psychedelics, and chemical synthetic drugs. Respiratory depression, decreased level of consciousness, and bradycardia are side effects of opioids, sedatives, and alcohol intoxication.

Skin

The skin is assessed for color, warmth, moisture, texture, and turgor. Jaundice may be seen in hepatic insufficiency (such as cirrhosis, toxicity, or hepatitis). The patient may hide intravenous drug use by using sites that are not suspected such as the feet, ankles, back of the arms, and between the fingers. Skin abscesses, cellulitis, discoloration, and scaring could be signs of previous needle marks, or could be related to skin popping, tweaking, or chemicals collecting in the skin from drugs such as methamphetamine. Inspect the fingers and hands for calluses, burns, discoloration, scars, and clubbing. Chronic alcohol use may lead to increased vascular skin changes, cutaneous telangiectasia, spider angiomas, flushing, rosacea, pruritus, and cutaneous stigmata of cirrhosis. Palmar erythema may be present in patients with advanced alcoholic liver disease.

HEENT

The head, eyes, ears, nose, and throat should be observed for changes in skin, mucous membranes, or structural anomalies. During the inspection of the eyes, observe jaundice to the sclera and nystagmus with extra ocular movement. Diplopia in the form of acute esotropia (a dysconjugate gaze) is a symptom of opioid withdrawal and is determined by inspection, extra ocular movements, and the cover-uncover test.[10,22] Evaluate pupils for size, shape, and responsiveness to light (changes may occur in both intoxication and withdrawal from multiple substances). For example, miosis (pinpoint pupils) may be seen in opiate use and mydriasis (dilated pupils) may be seen in cocaine use and opioid withdrawal. Look for sores or burns to the face, lips, mouth, or nose (from pipe use or smoking) and observe the nares for singed hair, epistaxis, septal deformity, or increased rhinorrhea (signs of insufflation). Observe the mouth for gum abscesses and rotten teeth noted from chemically manufactured drugs such as methamphetamine. Parotid gland enlargement is sometimes seen in extrahepatic toxicity related to alcohol abuse; additionally, cheilitis, glossitis, or bleeding gums may be a sign of alcohol-related harm.[46]

Neck

Neck veins are inspected for jugular venous distension (a sign of heart failure often found in chronic drug and alcohol users). Substance use may accelerate the development of atherosclerosis (e.g., cocaine); therefore, examine the carotid pulses and auscultate for bruits. Auscultation of the carotid arteries should be performed initially with the diaphragm of the stethoscope to detect higher frequency of the arterial bruits, followed with the bell to detect the low-pitched sounds of higher-grade stenosis.[10] A bruit suggests atherosclerosis and contraindicates carotid massage as a diagnostic tool or treatment option for tachycardia.

Thorax and Lungs

Inspect and palpate the chest for movement, depth, and rate. Slow shallow respirations may be related to opioid or sedative use. Percussion and voice sounds will identify dullness that could represent fluid or consolidation in pneumonia or infiltrates. Auscultate for adventitious sounds. Pulmonary complications may be found with drug and alcohol use (especially heroin) and alcoholics may experience pulmonary edema as a secondary effect of heart failure and portal hypertension.

Cardiovascular

Inspect the chest for vascular and skin changes, and palpate for parasternal lifts, heaves, and thrills. Palpation of the point of maximum impulse (PMI) and percussion of the left chest will establish the size and location of the heart. Enlargement of the cardiac silhouette may suggest ventricular hypertrophy or cardiomyopathies as a side effect of chronic chemical dependence. Heart sounds should be auscultated for regularity, rate, murmurs, clicks, or the presence of extra heart sounds. An audible S3 is a significant finding of increased ventricular filling and can be caused by fluid overload, heart failure, or decreased myocardial contractility, which may be end-points of chronic drug or alcohol use. An audible S4 is usually a pathologic finding related to resistance in ventricular filling and should be investigated. If a new heart murmur is present that has not previously been reported, establish which valvular region it is most audible over, and systolic or diastolic to indicate if caused by regurgitation or stenosis. Intravenous drug use can be a cause of infective endocarditis, which may be noted by a new valvular regurgitation.[40] Upon completion of the cardiovascular examination, the extremities should be examined for edema and peripheral pulses.

Abdomen

Inspect the abdomen for discoloration, scars, striae, rashes, ecchymosis, or venous collaterals. Dilated veins can be indicative of hepatic cirrhosis, and caput medusa may be found in advanced alcoholic liver disease.[10] The contour should be observed for asymmetry, signs of ascites such as protuberance, bulging flanks, or hernias. During auscultation for bowel sounds and bruits, listen over the liver and spleen for possible frictions rubs. Percussion of the abdomen, liver, and spleen will help to establish hepatosplenomegaly. The liver span is measured at the midclavicular line (normal 6–12 cm) and right midsternal line (normal 4–8 cm). Two techniques are used to detect enlargement of the spleen, the more accurate of which is thought to be percussion for dullness of the left lower anterior chest wall at Traube's space.[10] The percussion findings will be confirmed by palpation of both the liver and spleen. A large liver with a smooth tender edge suggests inflammation (such as hepatitis), whereas an enlarged liver with a firm or hardened irregular edge suggests nodules (such as hepatocellular carcinoma). An enlarged liver with firm edges (usually nontender) can suggest cirrhosis. However, the cirrhotic liver could be scarred and contracted.[10]

Genital

Assessment of the genital and rectal anatomy are often not a high priority of the critical care patient evaluation; but chronic drug or alcohol use could lead to sexual behavior that places the patient at risk for sexually transmitted infections, sexual abuse, or rape. Rape should be suspected if a patient has changes in level of consciousness or amnesia following a social event where drugs may have been used with or without the patient's knowledge (drugs such as MDMA, rohypnol, GHB, and some synthetic drugs) (Tables 42.2, 42.3 and 42.4). If rape is suspected, extra care must be taken to have a professional who is competent in the collection, handling, and preservation of the chain of evidence. Gynecomastia and hypogonadism are findings of advanced alcoholic liver disease.

Musculoskeletal

Evaluate range of motion, strength of joint and muscles, and observe for signs of trauma. A thickening and contraction of the palmar fascia known as Dupuytren's contracture may occur in severe liver disease. Muscle wasting and atrophy may be noted in chronic chemical dependence; muscle strength should be measured using a 0 to 5 scale (0 = no muscle contraction, 5 = normal strength).[10]

Neurologic

Assess the level of consciousness, orientation, and appropriateness of behavior based on environment, age, and cultural expectations. Signs or symptoms of dementia may be organic, related to withdrawal, or thiamine deficiency. Speech should be evaluated for fluidity, language, and ability to explain thoughts (for example, confabulation may indicate Korsakoff syndrome). Signs of intoxication may be present; for example: ataxia, slurred speech, mood lability, decreased concentration and memory, demonstrating poor judgment, dilated pupils, and nystagmus. If the patient is ambulatory, assess for gait abnormalities, ataxic gait, Parkinsonian gait, hemiparesis, or footdrop. Evaluate for postural changes, involuntary tremors, tics, chorea, hemiballismus, facial dyskinesias, or paraparesis. Assess reflexes; intoxication, chronic use, withdrawal, or the secondary effects of nutrition deficiencies and endocrine

TABLE 42.2 **Synthetic Drugs**

Drug Name	Street Name	Side Effects
Synthetic cannabinoid, Synthetic cannabis, Synthetic marijuana	Aroma, Banana Black Mamba, Bombay Blue, Cream, Crazy Clown, Fake weed, Genie, HU-210, JWH-018, JWH-073, K2, Moon Rocks, Nuke, Scooby Snax, Skunk, Spice, SpicyXXX, Yucatan Fire, Zohai	**HEENT:** Dilated pupils **Cardiac:** Chest pain, tachycardia, bradycardia **GI/GU:** Nausea and vomiting **Neuro:** Somnolence, confusion, tremors, muscle spasms, brisk reflexes, seizures, memory changes, and irritability **Psych:** Anxiety, severe agitation, paranoia, intense hallucinations, and psychotic episodes: including suicidal fixations
PCP PCP mixed with marijuana and laced with embalming fluid	Angel Dust Amp, Happy Sticks, Sherm, Wet, Wet Sticks	**General:** Overwhelmingly strong, no awareness of pain **GI/GU:** Nausea, vomiting **Neuro:** Dizziness, seizures, coma, and death **Psych:** Irrational, agitated, delusions, hallucinations, paranoia, catatonia, violent, homicidal, and suicidal tendencies
BATH SALTS AS A GROUP: INDUCE THE RELEASE OF SEROTONIN		**Note:** Date rape or rape drug: Observe for signs of sexual abuse, especially with Ethylone, which also reports similar effects to MDMA **General:** Hyperthermia, feelings of extreme heat, which can lead to renal failure and rhabdomyolysis. Weight loss after prolonged use **HEENT:** Visual disturbances, mydriasis, blurred vision, color and sound enhancements, dry mouth, sore mouth/throat, dry mouth, teeth grinding may be seen in mephedrone use **Skin:** Diaphoresis **Cardiac:** Tachycardia, hypertension chest pain palpitations, vasoconstriction myocarditis, cardiac arrest **GI/GU:** Nausea/vomiting, anorexia, abdominal pain **Neurologic:** Agitation, anxiety, prolonged panic attacks, psychosis, paranoia, hallucinations, seizures, disturbed sleep pattern and nightmares, insomnia, tremors, confusion, long-term cognitive impairment, mental fatigue, disorientation, loosening of association, paresthesias, falls, gait disturbance, limb and face dystonia, hypotonia, symmetric bradykinesia, headache, and dizziness **Psychiatric:** Irritability, aggression progressing to violent or even criminal behavior, anxiety, panic attacks, lack of motivation, anhedonia, depression, suicidal thoughts/actions, paranoid delusion, visual, and auditory hallucinations **Hematologic:** DIC, thrombocytopenia, anemia **Lab:** Hyponatremia, hyperkalemia, hyperuricemia, increased serum levels of creatinine and creatinine kinase, and metabolic acidosis
MDPV	Avalanch, Bath Salts, Bonsai Fertilizer, Cleaner, Energy-1, Ivory Wave, Jewelry Cleaner, Plant Fertilizer, Plant Food, Purple Wave, Shock Wave, Vanilla Sky	
Mephedrone	Bliss, Bounce, Drone, M-Cat, Mad Cow, Meow-Meow	
Mephedrone mixed with methylone	Bubbles	
Methylone	bk-MDMA, Explosion, Room Deodorizer, (may also be sold as "Molly" may or may not contain MDMA)	
Ethylone	MDEC, bk-MDEA	
Butylone	bk-MBDB	
Alpha PVP	Flakka/Flocka/Flocca, Gravel, Insanity	
DRUGS KNOWN AS RESEARCH CHEMICALS OR LEGAL HIGHS		**General:** Hyperthermia **Pulmonary:** Respiratory distress and arrest **Cardiac:** Tachycardia, hypertension, MI, cardiac arrest; vasoconstriction and extremity tissue necrosis associated with Bromo-DragonFly **GI/GU:** Hepatic and renal failure **Neuro/Psych:** Agitation, aggression, anxiety, panic, visual and auditory, hyper-reflexia, clonus, hallucinations, seizures **Lab:** Metabolic acidosis, elevated creatine kinase, and elevated white cell count with NBOMe
2C-I (India)	2C-I India	
Bromo Dragon Fly	2C-B-fly, 2's, B-Fly, Bromo, Fly, Nexus, Spectrum, Toonies, Venu	
25I-NBOMe	25I, 25C, 25B, Legal Acid, N-Bome, Smiles	
2C-T-7	Beautiful, Blue Mystic, Mescaline, Tripstay, Tweety-Bird, T7	

DIC, Disseminated intravascular coagulation; *GI,* gastrointestinal; *GU,* genitourinary; *HEENT,* head, eyes, ears, nose, and throat; *Lab,* laboratory; *MI,* myocardial infarction.
From References 82 and 97.

involvement in chronic substance use may affect responses. Evaluate the extremities for sensation, touch, vibration, proprioception, and discrimination (signs of peripheral neuropathy may indicate Korsakoff syndrome). Coordination/cerebellar function is evaluated (finger-nose test and rapid alternating movement). Romberg's test, seated balance, and pronator drift also evaluate coordination. Asterixis (a flapping motion of dorsiflexed hands) may be noted in the presence of hepatic encephalopathy.

Mental Health

Behavior, speech, orientation, and appropriate interaction with the environment should be evaluated. Mental status changes may occur from rapid rehydration or changes in electrolytes, particularly sodium. Patients can be undertreated or overtreated because of a misinterpretation of confusion symptoms. Confusion occurring in the absence of any other signs or symptoms of alcohol withdrawal is generally related to another mental status or cognitive change. Also note that associated mental health conditions and intimate partner violence injuries are highly associated with drug and alcohol use, and should be considered when evaluating the patient.[55]

DIAGNOSTIC TESTING

Blood and urine testing is used to quantify the presence of alcohol and some drugs, but many drugs are not detectable by current testing, or require specialty testing that may take days to

TABLE 42.3 Table of Sedatives

Drug Name	Street Name	Side Effects
GHB (gamma-hydroxybutyrate) GBL (gamma-butyrolactone, precursor of GHB) BD (1,4-butanediol, precursor of GHB)	Bodily Harm G, Gib, GBH, Grievous Bodily Harm, Liquid Ecstasy, Nitro, Scoop, Soap Blue Nitro, Gamma G, GH Revitalizer Revitalize Plus, Serenity, Thunder Nectar, Weight Belt Cleaner	**General:** Increased energy, happiness, talkative, feeling affectionate, sensuality, enhanced sexual experience and desire, and mild loss of inhibition **Note:** Date rape or rape drug: Observe for signs of sexual abuse **Pulmonary:** Respiratory arrest **GI/GU:** Nausea and vomiting, loss of gag reflex **Neuro/Psych:** Difficulty concentrating, somnolence, confusion, hallucinations, muscle relaxation, weakness, loss of coordination and muscle tone, deep sedation, seizures, coma, and death
Ketamine (Ketalar)	Blind Squid, Cat, Cat Valium, Green, K, Kit-Kat, Ket, Keets, Keller, Kelly's Day, Jet, Purple, Special La Coke, Super C, Special K, Super K, Super Acid, Valiums, Vitamin K	**General:** Feeling detached from your body (known as "k-hole") **Note:** Date rape or rape drug: Observe for signs of sexual abuse **HEENT:** Blurred vision **Pulmonary:** Respiratory depression **Cardiac:** Tachycardia, elevated BP, and increased cardiac output **GI/GU:** Intense upper abdominal colic type pain, known as "K-cramps," vomiting, frequency and urgency of urination, dysuria, urge incontinence and occasionally painful hematuria, and renal failure **Neuro/Psych:** Delirium, slurred speech, amnesia, long-term memory loss, depression, cognitive difficulties, psychosis, hallucinations, and panic attacks
Flunitrazepam (Rohypnol)	Circles, Forget-Me Pill, La Rocha, Mexican Valium, R2, Roche, Roofies, Rope, Rophies	**General:** Drowsiness, loss of motor control, lack of coordination **Note:** Date rape or rape drug: Observe for signs of sexual abuse **HEENT:** Visual disturbances **Pulmonary:** Decreased respirations **Cardiac:** Hypotension and bradycardia **GI/GU:** Gastrointestinal disturbances and urinary retention **Neuro/Psych:** Anterograde amnesia, slurred speech, confusion, and dizziness

GI, Gastrointestinal; *GU,* genitourinary; *HEENT,* head, eyes, ears, nose, and throat.

TABLE 42.4 Table of Hallucinogenics

Drug Name	Street Name	Side Effects
MDMA Ecstasy (usually pill) Molly (usually powder or capsule)	Adam, Beans, Clarity, E, Ectacy, Hug Drug, Lovers Speed, M, Rolls, X, XTC, Molly and Molly Water Molly is also sometimes used as a street name for some synthetic cathinones (Bath Salts or mixtures of ecstasy and methamphetamine)	**Note:** Excessive talking, enjoy touching others and being touched, reduced inhibitions, feelings of tingling and warmth **Note:** Date rape or rape drug: Observe for signs of sexual abuse **General:** Hyperthermia 107–109°F, chills/diaphoresis, and dehydration **HEENT:** Blurred vision, dilated pupils, and dry mouth **Cardiac:** Tachycardia and hypertension **GI:** Nausea and hepatic/renal failure **MS:** Muscle cramps, jaw muscle tension, teeth grinding and involuntary clenching, twitching, and tremors **Neuro/Psych:** Confusion, depression, faintness, loss of consciousness, panic attacks, problems sleeping, seizures, and death
LSD	Acid, Boomers, Doses, Hits, Microdot/Dots, Sugar Cubes, Tabs, Trips, Window Pane, Yellow Sunshine	**General:** Hyperthermia and elevated blood sugar **Skin:** Piloerection (gooseflesh) and perfuse perspiration **HEENT:** Dilated pupils (mydriasis) **Cardiac:** Tachycardia, palpitations, and hypertension **Neuro/Psych:** Hallucinations, delusions, paranoia, panic reactions, and tremors. Flashbacks are an unpredictable and dangerous side effect, occur spontaneously, vary in frequency and duration, and may occur days up to months after use
Salvia	Diviner's Sage, Lady Salvia, Magic Mint, Purple Sticky, Sage of the Seers, Shepherdess's Herb, Sister Salvia, Ska Maria Pastora, Ska Pastora	**General:** Altered behavior, dreamlike/childlike states, and increased in sensations **Skin:** Increased perspiration **HEENT:** Dilated pupils (mydriasis) **Cardiac:** Tachycardia and palpitations **Neuro/Psych:** Sense of fear or panic, psychedelic experience, closed and open eye visualizations, time distortion, social dissociation, altered thought patterns, and hallucinations
Khat		**General:** Excitement, talkative, hyperactivity, and insomnia **HEENT:** Dilated pupils (mydriasis) **Cardiac:** Tachycardia and hypertension **GI/GU:** Extreme thirst and loss of appetite, constipation **Neuro/Psych:** Euphoria, hyper-manic states, irritability, anger, delusions of grandeur, manic behavior paranoia, and hallucinations
Jimson Weed (*Datura stramonium*)	Angel's Trumpet, Crazy Tea, Devil's Seed, Devil's Snare, Devil's Trumpet, Ditch Weed, Locoweed, Mad Hatter, Stinkweed	**General:** Hyperthermia **HEENT:** Dilated pupils, blurred vision, dry mucous membranes, thirst, dysphagia, and dysphasia **Pulmonary:** Respiratory arrest **Cardiac:** Tachycardia **GI/GU:** Urinary retention **Neuro/psych:** Euphoria and delirium, confusion, hallucinations, and seizures

GI, gastrointestinal; *GU,* genitourinary; *HEENT,* head, eyes, ears, nose, and throat; *MS,* musculoskeletal.

BOX 42.2 Differential Diagnosis

- ☐ Alcohol intoxication or overdose
- ☐ Alcohol use disorder (AUD)
- ☐ Alcohol withdrawal syndrome (AWS)
- ☐ Alcohol-induced psychotic disorder
- ☐ Delirium
- ☐ Dementia
- ☐ Diabetic acidosis
- ☐ Hypoglycemia
- ☐ Hypoxia
- ☐ Neurologic conditions such as cerebellar ataxia or multiple sclerosis
- ☐ Substance abuse, intoxication, or overdose
- ☐ Substance use disorder (SUD)
- ☐ Substance withdrawal
- ☐ Traumatic brain injury

From Reference 4.

as constriction of coronary vessels, dysfunction of vascular endothelium, decreased aortic elasticity, hemodynamic disruptions, a hypercoagulable state, and direct toxicity to myocardial and vascular tissue.[1] Cocaine and methamphetamines are highlighted in Table 42.6.

Synthetic drugs are an emerging area for substance use and include synthetic cannabinoid, synthetic cathinones, and research chemicals. Synthetic cannabinoids are usually made with a dried plant base material that is sprayed or laced with synthetic tetrahydrocannabinol (THC) to produce a chemically enhanced version of cannabis (also known as synthetic marijuana) (Table 42.2). However, the amount of synthetic THC is much greater than a dose of natural THC in a marijuana cigarette, therefore multiple side effects are possible and unpredictable.

Synthetic cathinones, also known as "bath salts," are a chemically produced drug that mimic the effects of the khat plant, which is a naturally occurring cathinone (alkaloid), similar in structure and action to amphetamine.[30] The name bath salts originated in an attempt to evade law enforcement. The more commonly used synthetic cathinones are known as MDPV, mephedrone, methylone, ethylone, and butylone. The issues with regulation come from the ease of synthesis and modification of a specific functional group of the parent cathinone.[94] There are additional synthetic drugs that are made under the group name of "research chemicals." These drugs are also highly unpredictable in their effects and are sometimes referred to as "legal highs" because of their ease of availability and poor regulation.

The synthetic drugs and research chemicals produce many physiologic and behavioral changes, some of the worst being drug induced hyperthermia, hallucinations, and delusional paranoia. During the psychoactive phase, the user has a false sense of reality, and often times will have altered realities that place them in dangerous environments, whereas real threats to their well-being are not comprehended. The dangerous or risky behaviors tend to lead to traumatic injuries, which bring the user to the hospital. Admissions are most likely related to traumatic injury, so a thorough physical assessment of the musculoskeletal system is required. Synthetic cannabinoids, synthetic cathinones, and research chemicals are readily available on the internet, head shops, and convenience stores with packaging that states "not for human consumption," making them openly accessible for users.

Opiate drugs include heroin, morphine, fentanyl, hydrocodone (e.g., Vicodin), and oxycodone (e.g., OxyContin and Percocet) (Table 42.7). The adverse effects of opioid intoxication or overdose (including heroin) are known as an opioid triad and include altered mental status, pinpoint pupils, and respiratory depression. Timely administration of naloxone reverses respiratory depression from opioid overdose. Some states have expanded naloxone administration authority to nonparamedic first responders.[23] Many communities are offering training programs to nonmedical persons on how to use intranasal naloxone in the event of an opioid related emergency. Preliminary results of this practice are successful. If IV access is not available, intranasal naloxone is effective in reversing both respiratory depression and depressive effects on the central nervous system caused by opioid overdose[76,80] (Box 42.3). The national concern over opiate use, overdose, and deaths, has lead many states to adopt legislation that allows naloxone nasal spray over the counter without a prescription. Friends of family may be the first responders of an opiate overdose and use the reversal agent.

Intoxication may sometimes persist beyond the time when the substance is detectable in the body. This may be due to enduring central nervous system effects, the recovery of which takes longer than the time for elimination of the substance. There usually are no antidotes for substance use (unless opioid based), so treating symptoms, minimizing long-term effects, and attempting to protect organs from failure are the goals of management.

Alcohol Intoxication

Alcohol intoxication is the presence of clinically significant problematic behavioral or psychological changes following the ingestion of alcohol. Signs and symptoms include impaired judgment, aggressive or inappropriate sexual behavior, mood lability, and impaired social or occupational functioning[4] (Table 42.5). The legal limit for intoxication in most states within the United States is a blood alcohol level of 80 mg/dL (or 0.08%).[65,73] The effects of alcohol on an individual depend on a number of factors including gender, weight, tolerance, genetics, the speed with which the alcohol was consumed, and ingestion on empty stomach.[73] The average person is able to metabolize approximately one unit of alcohol per hour, and blood alcohol generally decreases at a rate of 15–20 mg/dL/hour.[4]

Heavy drinking leads to poor decision making (including initiating violence), incoordination, and poor performance of usual activities, which can interfere with driving abilities and lead to accidents.[4,44] Alcohol intoxication may cause memory lapses or periods of amnesia that are known as *blackouts*. This phenomenon is related to the presence of a high blood alcohol level or the rapidity with which this level is reached.[4] Higher blood alcohol levels (e.g., in excess of 300–400 mg/dL) can cause inhibition of respiration, pulse, and potentially death in nontolerant individuals.[4]

Alcohol Use Disorder

Approximately 2 billion people worldwide consume alcoholic beverages, and over 76 million people have alcohol use disorders (AUDs), which includes alcohol dependence, alcohol abuse and dependence, or harmful drinking (>14 drinks per week or >4 drinks per occasion for men; >7 drinks per week or >3 drinks per occasion for women).[17] Alcohol dependence is characterized by withdrawal, craving, impaired control, and tolerance of alcohol.[72] Individuals who are addicted to alcohol are likely to demonstrate a strong craving or urge to drink, and an inability to limit the amount of alcohol they consume.[70]

Alcohol dependence is associated with high rates of mental and physical illness and a wide range of social problems.[72]

TABLE 42.5 Diagnostic Criteria of Acute Intoxication

Alcohol Intoxication	Cannabis Intoxication (Marijuana, THC oil)	Sedative, Hypnotic, or Anxiolytic Intoxication	Stimulant Intoxication (Cocaine, Amphetamines)	Inhalant Intoxication (Solvents, Glues, Gases)	Phencyclidine Intoxication (PCP, Ketamine)	Hallucinogenic Intoxication (LSD, MDMA, Salvia, Synthetic Cannabinoid)	Opioid Intoxication (Heroin, Morphine, Oxycodone)
Behavioral or psychological changes such as: ■ Inappropriate sexual or aggressive behavior ■ Mood lability ■ Impaired judgment	Behavioral or psychological changes such as: ■ Impaired motor coordination ■ Euphoria ■ Anxiety ■ Sensation of slowed time ■ Impaired judgment ■ Social withdrawal	Maladaptive behavioral or psychological changes such as: ■ Inappropriate sexual or aggressive behavior ■ Mood lability ■ Impaired judgment	Behavioral or psychological changes such as: ■ Euphoria or affective blunting ■ Changes in sociability ■ Hypervigilance ■ Interpersonal sensitivity ■ Anxiety ■ Tension or anger ■ Stereotyped behaviors ■ Impaired judgment	Behavioral or psychological changes such as: ■ Belligerence ■ Violence ■ Apathy ■ Impaired judgment	Behavioral changes such as: ■ Belligerence ■ Violence ■ Impulsiveness ■ Unpredictability ■ Psychomotor agitation ■ Impaired judgment	Behavioral or psychological changes such as: ■ Marked anxiety or depression ■ Ideas of reference ■ Fear of "losing one's mind" ■ Paranoid ideation ■ Impaired judgment ■ Perceptual changes occurring in a state of full wakefulness and alertness ■ Subjective intensification of perceptions ■ Depersonalization ■ Derealization ■ Illusions ■ Hallucinations ■ Synesthesias	Problematic behavioral or psychological changes such as: ■ Initial euphoria followed by apathy ■ Dysphoria ■ Psychomotor agitation ■ Retardation impaired judgment
One or more: 1. Slurred speech 2. Incoordination 3. Unsteady gait 4. Nystagmus 5. Impairment in attention or memory 6. Stupor 7. Coma	Two or more: 1. Conjunctival injection 2. Increased appetite 3. Dry mouth 4. Tachycardia	One or more: 1. Slurred speech 2. Incoordination 3. Unsteady gait 4. Nystagmus 5. Impairment in cognition 6. Impaired attention 7. Impaired memory 8. Stupor 9. Coma	Two or more: 1. Tachycardia or bradycardia 2. Pupillary dilation 3. Elevated or lowered blood pressure 4. Diaphoresis or chills 5. Nausea/vomiting 6. Weight loss 7. Psychomotor agitation or retardation 8. Muscular weakness 9. Respiratory depression 10. Chest pain 11. Cardiac arrhythmias 12. Confusion 13. Seizures 14. Dyskinesias 15. Dystonias 16. Coma	Two or more: 1. Dizziness 2. Nystagmus 3. Incoordination 4. Slurred speech 5. Unsteady gait 6. Lethargy 7. Depressed reflexes 8. Psychomotor retardation 9. Tremor 10. Generalized muscle weakness 11. Blurred vision or diplopia 12. Stupor or coma 13. Euphoria	Two or more of the following within 1 hour of drug use: 1. Vertical or horizontal nystagmus 2. Hypertension 3. Tachycardia 4. Numbness or diminished responsiveness to pain 5. Ataxia 6. Dysarthria 7. Muscle rigidity 8. Seizures or coma 9. Hyperacusis	Two or more: 1. Pupillary dilation 2. Tachycardia 3. Sweating 4. Palpitations 5. Blurring of vision 6. Tremors 7. Incoordination	Pupillary constriction (or pupillary dilation due to anoxia from severe overdose) plus one of the following: 1. Drowsiness or coma 2. Slurred speech 3. Impairment in attention or memory

TABLE 42.6 Cocaine and Methamphetamine

Drug Name	Street Name	Most Common Side Effects
Cocaine and Crack Cocaine	Blow, Bump, C, Cain, Candy, Charlie, Coke, Dust, Flake, Girl, Line, Neurocain, Pony, Powder, Rock, Sneeze, Snow, The Lady, Toot, Tornado, White, Wicky Stick	• Hyperthermia • Tachycardia and hypertension • Arrhythmias, widened QRS/Q and prolonged QT segment • MI/ ACS/coronary artery spasms/V-Fib/cardiac arrest (high doses) • Aortic dissection • Anxiety, confusion, depression, agitation, and excitation • Tremors, hallucinations, and delirium • Seizures and convulsions • Rhabdomyolysis (from dopaminergic changes) • Respiratory arrest • Emboli may occur from injection
Methamphetamines	Amphetamines, Bikers Coffee, Black Beauties, Chalk, Crank, Crystal Meth, Crystal, Fire, Glass, Ice, Jibb, Meth, Poor Man's Cocaine, Speed, Tina, Tweak, Uppers, Yaba, Yellow Bam	• All of the same as cocaine (including seizures and hyperthermia) Plus: • Chronic fatigue and insomnia • Delusions, paranoia, aggression, hallucinations, and toxic psychosis • Toxic psychosis • Skin abscesses and rotting of gums and teeth

Note: Hyperthermia is thought to be related to the dopaminergic regulation of core temperature, and is a critical side effect that requires immediate rapid cooling methods.
ACS, Acute coronary syndrome; *MI,* myocardial infarction; *V-Fib,* ventricular fibrillation.
From References 1, 4, 13, 34, 35, 48, 87, and 93.

TABLE 42.7 Opioids

Drug Name	Street Name	Side Effects
Heroin	Big H, Boy, Dope, Dragon, H, Horse, Junk, Scat, Smack, Snow, Snowball, Tar, White Horse, White Lady	Opioid OD triad (observed in toxicity) • Coma • Respiratory depression and failure (prepare to intubate) • Depression of CNS – miosis – pinpoint pupils Additional side effects include: • Bradycardia • Cold and clammy skin • Constipation • Confusion and disorientation • Delirium • Hypotension • Hypoxia and cyanosis • Nausea • Organ complications (including liver disease) and vessel damage due to the additives with which the heroin was cut • Pulmonary complications - including pneumonia • Sedation • Seizures (convulsions) • Tolerance and addiction • Unconsciousness or coma Note: Death from overdose increases significantly with Fentanyl and Morphine combination.
Cocaine/Heroin mix	Belushi, Boy/Girl, Dynamite, Goofball, Speedball	
Codeine	Cody or Schoolboy	
Codeine syrup	'Sizzurp'	
Codeine with Acetaminophen	T and T-Threes	
Promethazine and Codeine cough syrup	"Purple Drank"	
Marijuana/Heroin mix	Atom Bomb, Woo-Woo	
Morphine/Heroin mix	New Jack Swing	
Fentanyl/Heroin mix	Chine White	
Fentanyl (Brand names: Actiq, Duragesic, and Sublimaze)	Apache, Cash, China Girl, China White, Dance Fever, Friend, Goodfella, Jackpot, Murder 8, Tango, TNT	
Oxycodone (OxyContin, Percodan,Percocet)	Blue, Hillbilly Heroin, Kickers, Killers, OC, Oxy, Oxy 80's, Oxycottons Percs, Percodoms	
Desomorphine (made from Codeine)	Krokodil, Crocodile	In addition to the opioid side effects: Krokodil is identified by: • Discolored, necrotic, and gangrenous flesh • Scabs and skin infections • Scaly and gray-green dead skin that forms at the site of an injection • Users often smell of iodine

CNS, Central nervous system; *OD,* overdose.

BOX 42.3 DSM-V Diagnostic Criteria for Opioid Withdrawal

A. Presence of either of the following:
  1. Cessation of (or reduction in) opioid use that has been heavy and prolonged (i.e., several weeks or longer).
  2. Administration of an opioid antagonist after a period of opioid use.

B. Three (or more) of the following developing within minutes to several days after Criterion A:
  1. Dysphoric mood.
  2. Nausea or vomiting.
  3. Muscle aches.
  4. Lacrimation or rhinorrhea.
  5. Pupillary dilation, piloerection, or sweating.
  6. Diarrhea.
  7. Yawning.
  8. Fever.
  9. Insomnia.

C. The signs or symptoms in Criterion B cause clinically significant distress or impairment in social, occupationally, or other important areas of functioning.

D. The signs or symptoms are not attributable to another medical condition and are not better explained by another mental disorder, including intoxication or withdrawal from another substance.

From American Psychiatric Association. (2013). *Diagnostic and statistical manual of mental disorders* (5th ed.). Washington, DC: APA.

Heavy, chronic alcohol use may induce psychiatric symptoms that mimic psychotic disorders, mood disorders, and anxiety disorders. The diagnosis of an independent co-occurring psychiatric disorder is difficult to discern in an individual who is actively drinking; therefore determination must wait until after the acute symptoms of use or withdrawal have passed. It is recommended that at least 4 weeks of sobriety be established prior to a diagnosis of an independent psychiatric disorder.[44]

It is estimated that approximately 50% of middle-class, highly functional individuals with AUD have experienced a full alcohol withdrawal syndrome.[4] It appears that AUDs affect 20% of adult patients in emergency rooms, with 50% of them experiencing withdrawal symptoms. However, the incidence of alcohol withdrawal in ICU patients varies from 8% to 40%, and appears to be associated with infectious complications and a higher mortality rate.[61]

Substance Withdrawal

In order to predict the severity of withdrawal symptoms, details of the substance use are needed. Identify the substances used, how much, how often, and what route. Gaining knowledge about the drug, its effects, side effects, and half-life will help predict how withdrawal symptoms will occur and how best to manage them. Many recreational drugs do not have a significant period of withdrawal that would require inpatient treatment. Sedatives and opioids have true withdrawal symptoms that last for a number of days.

Withdrawal syndrome involves both physical and neurologic symptoms when administration of a substance of abuse is abruptly stopped. This leads to intense craving, increased drug-seeking behaviors, and symptoms of withdrawal. The physical symptoms of abstinence syndrome from chronic cocaine or amphetamine use are less severe than the abstinence of a drug such as heroin or sedative-hypnotic drugs.[7]

For many, the treatment is determined to be detoxification (abstinence from the substance) and possibly some short-term medications for symptom control, as most insurance companies will not pay for long-term treatment plans, but will pay for detoxification.[69] Opioid withdrawal is reported to be painful and intense with multiple symptoms (Box 42.3). The more severe symptoms include severe dehydration and cardiovascular stress. Diplopia in the form of acute esotropia may manifest in up to 30% of individuals undergoing heroin withdrawal.[22] Opiate withdrawal by itself is usually not life threatening, but if combined with other substances such as alcohol, barbiturates, or benzodiazepines can be fatal. Usually the other substance will need to be removed first, and opioid medications continued until the patient is stable enough to withstand the opioid withdrawal.

MANAGEMENT OF SUBSTANCE USE DISORDERS AND WITHDRAWAL

As mentioned previously, each substance must be viewed individually, and there are no universal treatments and no universal antidotes, which makes treatment difficult. The goal of treatment is to stabilize hemodynamic status and prevent end-organ damage with all substance use, intoxications, or overdose. Treatment of substance use generally consists of stopping the offending drug and entering a detoxification program. Unfortunately, evidence-based treatment techniques are rarely used, and only 10% of individuals receive any treatment to assist their recovery.[69]

Cocaine use is associated with cardiac complication such as cocaine induced chest pain, coronary spasms, and myocardial infarction (Table 42.6). However, there are no specific pharmacologic medication therapies or treatment guidelines to manage cocaine associated chest pain. Nitroglycerin followed by calcium channel blockers are the first-line medications for cocaine-induced chest pain management.[1] However, the role of labetalol has been controversial and exacerbates cocaine-induced alpha-adrenergic stimulation.[1,87] Nicardipine is the better choice of dihydropyridine calcium channel blocker for vasospasms and high blood pressure as it is less likely to cause bradycardia or heart block.[87] Beta blockers should be avoided, as cocaine use results in stimulation of alpha-adrenergic receptors; if beta receptors are blocked, the alpha receptor actions are unopposed, and therefore may worsen cardiotoxicity.[87]

Many of the chemical drugs, such as synthetic cathinones, have a short half-life, and therefore stabilizing the patient until the effects of the drug have worn off is the best plan of care. Synthetic cannabinoids cause users to require emergency and critical care admission (Table 42.2). There are no antidotes for these substances; hemodynamic stabilization, cardiac and respiratory support, and protection of end organs is the best approach to management. Drugs that are classed as sedatives and hallucinogens tend to have no antidote and treatment is based on presenting symptoms (Table 42.3 and Table 42.4).

Heroin and opioid withdrawal is intense, and there are three types of medications most commonly used in the treatment of opioid withdrawal or dependence: methadone, buprenorphine, and naltrexone.[92] Using medication for long-term treatment is very controversial. Methadone has been used successfully for heroin dependence, but its use is considered by some to transfer the addiction to another opioid. Buprenorphine (also known as Suboxone or Subutex) has a higher affinity for the mu receptor than other opioids, and slowly dissociates from the receptor, leading to milder withdrawal symptoms upon discontinuation in patients who are addicted to drugs such as morphine, oxycodone, or heroin.[83] Buprenorphine is lipophilic and has a rapid onset of action via either the sublingual (30–60 minutes) or the IV (5–15 minutes) route.[83] Extended-release naltrexone (known as XRNT), an opioid receptor antagonist, is successfully used in the treatment of opioid dependence, but may reduce striatal dopamine transporter availability, causing depression and anhedonia as a side effect.[96] Upon discharge, prescription opioid dependency can be successfully managed with office-based buprenorphine/naloxone pharmacotherapy.[24] Diplopia in the form of acute esotropia occurs in 30% of heroin withdrawal and may be treated with pilocarpine eye drops or eye patching for symptomatic relief, but the resolution of this symptom may take 1 to 2 months.[22]

ALCOHOL WITHDRAWAL SYNDROME

Among individuals with AUD who are hospitalized or homeless, the rate of alcohol withdrawal may be greater than 80%.[4] However, less than 10% of individuals in withdrawal ever demonstrate alcohol withdrawal delirium or withdrawal seizures.[4] It is estimated that approximately 25% of patients with severe AWS require prolonged treatment in critical care, and are often complicated by respiratory failure, mechanical ventilation related to sedation, and nosocomial infection.[78] When alcohol is stopped suddenly, the GABA receptors are no longer stimulated and the up-regulated NMDA receptors are unopposed. This leads to excessive excitation and autonomic hyperactivity. If left untreated, the condition of hyperexcitability of the brain leads to seizures, delirium tremens (DTs), and can be fatal (see kindling phenomenon) (Box 42.4).

The symptoms of AWS are associated with falling or absent blood alcohol levels due to cessation or decrease in intake and usually begin within a few hours.[6,18,41,61,71,98] If the patient has been involved in trauma or surgery, the onset of symptoms may be delayed with exposure to anesthetic agents, analgesic, or sedative use, but usually develop within 36 to 48 hours.[6] However, symptoms have been reported in ICU patients up to 6 days from the alcohol-free period, with full blown withdrawal occurring approximately 50 to 60 hours after stopping alcohol use.[6] Following acute withdrawal, symptoms of anxiety, insomnia, and autonomic dysfunction may persist for up to 3 to 6 months at lower levels of intensity.[4]

The critical care patient presents an interesting challenge, as withdrawal symptoms may be similar to other causes such as pain, metabolic disturbances, toxicities, hypoxia, delirium, or dementia. It is also possible for some symptoms (such as tachycardia) to be masked by medications such as beta blockers, calcium channel blockers, or anesthetics used for procedures or surgeries. The symptoms may not be identified until the patient has progressed well into severe withdrawal. A common misconception is that the patient with positive testing for serum alcohol cannot be in withdrawal. However, the symptoms of AWS relate proportionately to the amount of alcohol consumed regularly, as well as the tolerance level. Therefore, symptoms are possible with dips in the blood alcohol level below the patient's usual range.

BOX 42.4 Diagnostic Criteria for Alcohol Withdrawal

Definition: Cessation or reduction in alcohol use that has been heavy and prolonged.

Diagnostic criteria: Two or more of the following:

1. Autonomic hyperactivity
   - Diaphoresis
   - Tachycardia (>100 bpm)
2. Increased hand tremor
3. Insomnia
4. Nausea or vomiting
5. Transient visual, tactile, or auditory hallucinations, or illusions
6. Psychomotor agitation
7. Anxiety
8. Generalized tonic–clonic seizures

From Reference 4.

Symptoms of Acute Alcohol Withdrawal Syndrome

Up to 50% of patients who use alcohol experience withdrawal symptoms, but only a minority of them require medical treatment.[61] Anxiety (related to the lack of GABA stimulation) and sleep disturbances are early signs of withdrawal to observe.[37] The onset and degree of symptoms can vary based on past consumption, past withdrawal episodes, and individual genetics. Minor withdrawal symptoms such as insomnia, tremulousness, anxiety, sleep disturbances, nausea, headache, diaphoresis, and palpitations may begin within the first few hours after cessation, and if they do not progress, they should resolve within 24 to 48 hours.[37,41,71] Symptoms may worsen to include restlessness, agitation, possible transient disorientation, moderate visible tremulousness, constant eye movement, marked diaphoresis, nausea, vomiting, diarrhea, tachycardia, and marked hypertension.[18,71] Severe symptoms are characterized by seizures, hallucinations, DTs, and coma.[61,65,88] Alcohol has a relatively fast metabolism and thus symptoms of AWS usually peak in intensity during the second day of abstinence and are likely to improve markedly by the fourth or fifth day.[4]

Alcoholic Withdrawal Seizures

Alcohol withdrawal seizures occur from CNS hyperexcitability, usually happen within the first 48 hours after the last drink, and may occur in up to 10% of AWS patients.[5,53,61,71,88] Seizures are generalized tonic–clonic seizures with little to no postictal period; they may occur once or be recurrent.[61,71] The risk of seizures increases in patients who have had previous seizures in withdrawal or in patients who have undergone repeated withdrawal episodes (see kindling phenomenon). Alcohol related seizures could occur with withdrawal or acute intoxication. An infectious disease work-up (to include compete blood count [CBC], lumbar puncture, and blood cultures) should be done if the seizure activity reoccurs or is prolonged.[53] Of the patients who present with AWS seizures, 33% will progress to DTs.[53]

Alcoholic Hallucinations

Alcoholic hallucinations may present as visual, auditory, or tactile and usually occur within 12 to 24 hours of the withdrawal. Patients often complain of lights being too bright, sounds being too loud, or hearing voices (noises within the ICU may be perceived as voices). The hallucinations may be persecutory and cause frank paranoia, leading to increased patient agitation, and if they change from transient to persistent, the patient has progressed to alcoholic hallucinosis.[61,88] Alcoholic hallucinosis is an uncommon alcohol-induced psychoactive disorder that may occur with acute intoxication or withdrawal, and consists of persistent hallucinations (usually acoustic verbal), delusions, and mood disturbances during clear consciousness, and may progress to chronic symptoms that mimic schizophrenia.[9]

When hallucinations occur in the absence of delirium (i.e., in a clear sensorium), a diagnosis of substance/medication-induced psychotic disorder should be considered.[4]

Delirium Tremens

DTs, also known as alcohol withdrawal delirium, is the most serious complication of alcohol withdrawal. The onset is typically rapid, beginning 3 to 5 days after the last drink, and may last up to 7 days.[71,81] Agitation related to autonomic hyperactivity and DTs may develop within 6 to 24 hours after the abrupt discontinuation or decrease of alcohol consumption.[61] DTs carry a mortality rate of 5% to 25% depending on the concomitant complications, or when preceding AWS symptoms were not recognized and appropriately managed.[53,71,81] It is unusual to see DT symptoms in hospitalized patients, but if they are observed it is most likely the result of poor symptom identification, undertreatment, or lack of timely treatment.[71] The symptoms usually consist of severe agitation, tremor, disorientation, hallucinations, and exacerbation of autonomic symptoms.[71] Causes of death associated with DTs include head trauma, cardiovascular complications, cardiac arrhythmias, infections, aspiration pneumonia, hyperthermia, withdrawal seizures, electrolyte abnormalities, low platelet counts, respiratory, cardiac, or gastrointestinal disease.[81] It is estimated that 3% to 5% of patients who are hospitalized for disturbances in attention and cognition from alcohol withdrawal meet the criteria for withdrawal delirium.[81]

Wernicke-Korsakoff Syndrome

Wernicke-Korsakoff syndrome refers to a combined syndrome of Wernicke encephalopathy mixed with Korsakoff syndrome, which are both are due to thiamine deficiency, and directly related to poor nutrition found in chronic alcoholics.

Wernicke's Encephalopathy

Wernicke's encephalopathy is an acute, neuropsychiatric emergency that is reversible with adequate thiamine replacement.[46] Clinical criteria for Wernicke's encephalopathy involve two of the following criteria: dietary deficiencies, oculomotor abnormalities, cerebellar dysfunction, or either altered mental state or mild memory impairment.[91] The subjective and objective findings include: tachycardia, hypotension, hypo- or hyperthermia, hearing loss, seizures, spastic paraparesis, delirium, coma, acute psychosis, miosis, anisocoria, papilledema, retinal hemorrhage, nystagmus, ophthalmoplegia, diplopia, gait ataxia, altered mental status, irritability, confusion, and memory impairment.[46] If undiagnosed or untreated, Wernicke's syndrome will progress to Korsakoff syndrome with irreversible brain damage, or may cause death.[46,91]

Korsakoff's Amnestic Syndrome

Korsakoff's amnestic syndrome is characterized by a profound anterograde amnesia (inability to form new memories) and retrograde amnesia (loss of memories), disorientation to place and time, and lack of insight. In addition, other findings include confabulation (making up stories), anxiety, apathy, ataxia, nystagmus, and peripheral neuropathy.[91] The best treatment for Korsakoff's syndrome is timely recognition of Wernicke's encephalopathy so that appropriate intervention and prevention occurs.[91]

TREATMENT OF ALCOHOL WITHDRAWAL SYNDROME

The treatment plan for AWS as an inpatient and outpatient are slightly different, and based on severity of dependence and symptoms. During the ICU management it is most likely necessary to treat the acute symptoms of AWS or intoxication, but, when selecting medication therapy, it is prudent to keep in mind how the patient will be managed in the community following discharge. The management of the critically ill patient with AWS is dependent on early recognition of symptoms and early initiation of medications to control those symptoms. The main treatment goal is to minimize the severity of symptoms and severe manifestations such as seizure, delirium, and death.[58,61,65,88]

Benzodiazepines

Benzodiazepines remain the gold standard pharmacologic agents of choice for optimal symptom control in AWS.[6,15,18,25,36,50,61,65,67,71,81] Diazepam, chlordiazepoxide, lorazepam, and oxazepam are currently approved to treat AWS[15] (Table 42.8). However, there are no data to support one benzodiazepine over another.[71] Chlordiazepoxide or diazepam are long-acting and may provide a smoother withdrawal period.[61,71] Diazepam has rapid onset of action and a long half-life, making it a good choice for seizure control and long-term relaxation, whereas shorter acting benzodiazepines such as midazolam or oxazepam may be a good option for milder symptoms of AWS, but less effective in controlling seizure activity.[73]

Care should be taken when selecting the benzodiazepine to individualize the therapy to the needs of the patient,

TABLE 42.8 Benzodiazepine Treatment for Alcohol Withdrawal

Generic Name	Trade Name	Onset	Duration	Half-Life	Usual Starting Dose
Chlordiazepoxide	Librium	Intermediate	Long	5–30 h	50–100 mg PO TID or QID (Max 300 mg/day)
Diazepam	Valium	Fast	Long	30–60 h	10 mg q 3–4h PRN (IV, IM, or PO)
Lorazepam	Ativan	Intermediate	Mid	10–20 h	2–4 mg BID-TID (IV, IM, or PO)
Oxazepam	Serax	Slow	Short	10 h	15–30 mg PO TID or QID
Midazolam	Versed	Fast	Short	2–5 h	0.02–0.1 mg/kg/h (IV, IM or PO)

Note: Lorazepam and oxazepam have no active metabolites; diazepam's metabolites can take up to 200 hours to clear.
BID, Twice per day; *IM*, intramuscular; *IV*, intravenous; *PO*, per os; *PRN*, when necessary; *q*, every; *QID*, four times per day; *TID*, three times per day.
From References 61, 73, and 85.

their presenting symptoms, age, and hepatic function. Benzodiazepines enhance GABA effects (inducing relaxation) by binding to the benzodiazepine receptors. They are hepatically metabolized (using the CYP450) but the conjugation or oxidation processes cause differences in the pharmacokinetic characteristics and a different half-life.[18] Lorazepam (Ativan) has the least effect on the liver, and is the safer option for some patients. Side effects, risks, and benefits should be considered when selecting a medication. Risks of benzodiazepine use include oversedation, respiratory depression, aspiration pneumonia, delirium, paradoxical agitation, and disinhibition.[29,50]

The benzodiazepine group has been well studied for use in the treatment of symptoms of AWS, and they remain the current standard of practice. However, managing the fine balance in the dosage can be difficult. If the dose is too small, symptoms may continue, putting the patient at risk for seizures. If the dose is too large, oversedation and respiratory depression may occur. Positive results seem to be achieved when symptom-triggered dosing is used. These include reduced duration of medication treatment, lower cumulative benzodiazepine dose, more rapid control of symptoms, and reduced length of ICU stay.[25,32,58,79] Some patients require additional medications for symptom control during withdrawal as the kindling phenomenon can result in benzodiazepine treatment resistance.[88]

Once benzodiazepines are used it is important that they are tapered slowly prior to discontinuation, and the patient should be monitored for secondary withdrawal symptoms throughout the discontinuation. The withdrawal from benzodiazepines will appear identical to that of alcohol withdrawal and will require treatment in the same symptomatic approach. Benzodiazepines are considered the first-line treatment choice in acute management. But following the acute management phase, subsequent dependency and danger if combined with alcohol makes benzodiazepines a less appropriate choice for outpatient therapy or maintenance of alcohol abstinence.[15,47] If benzodiazepines are unsuccessful as a monotherapy, adjunct therapies are used to provide supportive treatment.

Dexmedetomidine (Precedex)

Dexmedetomidine is a selective α_2 receptor agonist, useful in treating the hypersensitivity of the sympathetic nervous system caused by AWS, including hypertension and delirium. It is used as an adjunct to benzodiazepine-based therapy, not as a monotherapy, which may increase seizure risk.[20] In comparison to other pharmacologic agents used, dexmedetomidine quickly decreases autonomic hyperactivity while avoiding respiratory depression.[43] It also decreases delirium more effectively than benzodiazepines alone.[95] Dexmedetomidine has some similarities to clonidine, but is more selective, which may explain why it increases calmness with less sedative effects, and lessens the need for additional benzodiazepines.[43,61,63] Continuous cardiac monitoring will alert the team to the potential bradycardia (side effect of dexmedetomidine), but the occurrence may be lessened with low dosages.[63]

Propofol (Diprivan)

Propofol binds to the GABA-A receptor, causing an influx of chloride ions, resulting in anxiolysis, sedation, and impaired motor coordination.[85] Propofol activates the GABA receptors in a similar way to alcohol, inhibits the NMDA receptors, and makes it useful for sedation as an adjunct treatment in AWS for the ventilated patient. Mechanical ventilated AWS patients treated with propofol should experience similar symptom resolution, length of stay, days requiring mechanical ventilation, rates of reintubation, and in-hospital mortality as those treated with benzodiazepines.[85]

Phenobarbital

Phenobarbital may be used in a well-monitored environment such as the ICU, as an adjunct, or alternate therapy for symptom relief from AWS, but usually only if benzodiazepines are not controlling seizures or are contraindicated. Phenobarbital provides similar sedation to benzodiazepines, and should be symptom-adjusted. It has a long half-life and a narrow therapeutic window, which complicates dosage titration, and can lead to side effects such as respiratory depression.[18,39,59,78] Phenobarbital is a barbiturate, and increases the duration of the GABA chloride channel opening, and blocks the glutamate excitotoxicity observed in AWS.[78] This antiglutamatergic property may perhaps explain its efficacy in complicated alcohol withdrawal states.[67] The use of phenobarbital as adjunct to benzodiazepines has been shown in studies to be effective in enhancing therapeutic responsiveness to benzodiazepines and reducing the need for mechanical ventilation.[78]

Baclofen

Baclofen is a selective GABA receptor agonist generally used for muscle spasms and has been used (off-label) to reduce AWS symptoms in some patients.[18,51,69,77,86] The mechanism of action is not fully understood, but in addition to being a muscle relaxant, it is useful in treating alcohol withdrawal and dependence. Anxiety is a common symptom in patients being treated for alcohol withdrawal and alcohol dependence. As a GABA receptor agonist, baclofen plays a major role in regulating emotional behavior and control of anxiety.[86] Additionally, activation of GABA-B receptors by baclofen may result in local inhibition of surrounding dopamine neurons. This dopamine inhibition reduces the dopamine release that occurs from drinking alcohol, limiting the positive effect that alcohol consumption may have, therefore, aiding in abstinence from alcohol.[86]

It is possible that baclofen itself can cause withdrawal syndrome symptoms including confusion, agitation, seizures, and delirium.[77] These symptoms are similar to those of AWS and could lead to mistakes in diagnosis and treatment, so it is important to perform a thorough history and establish if baclofen has been used for AUD prior to admission. Although baclofen may reduce symptoms and improve CIWA-Ar scores, studies are limited, and there may be a possibility that it lowers the seizure threshold.[18] Baclofen is not currently indicated for AWS, but shows promise, and additional studies are currently underway in Europe.[86]

Anticonvulsants

Anticonvulsants can be effective in treating AWS as a nonaddictive option that has sedative-like properties and can be used following discharge into outpatient care and possibly extended to treating comorbid psychiatric disorders.[3] Carbamazepine, gabapentin, and topiramate have been used safely for treatment and prevention of alcohol withdrawal.[3] Phenytoin (Dilantin) does not treat withdrawal seizures, but can be considered in a patient with an underlying seizure disorder. As alternatives or adjuncts to benzodiazepines, anticonvulsants have anxiolytic, mood stabilizing, and anticonvulsant properties useful for their ability to inhibit kindling and to facilitate GABA inhibitory neurotransmission in AWS.[67]

Carbamazepine (Tegretol)

Carbamazepine is a tricyclic anticonvulsant that is not indicated for use in the United States for AWS, but has been widely used in Europe to successfully treat patients with mild to moderate AWS, and to suppress withdraw-induced kindling and alcohol withdrawal seizures.[3,18,67] Carbamazepine may assist in reducing the symptoms of AWS such as sleep disturbance, anxiety, and mood instability.[3]

Gabapentin (Neurontin)

Gabapentin, although not currently supported in the literature for AWS, may be useful in treating alcohol dependence. Some studies have determined its usefulness in treating seizures and anxiety.[47] As studies continue, there may be more indication for using gabapentin as a combination or adjunct therapy in treating AWS along with benzodiazepines.[15,18,47,55] The mechanism of action for gabapentin is not fully understood, and despite the name, it does not effect the GABA receptors directly. It may enhance GABA activity, increasing GABA concentrations via its interaction with voltage-dependent calcium channels, which assists in reducing the excitatory neurotransmitter release.[47] Gabapentin may be more useful in treating the milder symptoms of AUDs.[15,47,56,67] In treating AUDs, gabapentin normalizes the stress-induced GABA activation, and may assist with symptoms of insomnia, dysphoria, and craving, with a favorable safety profile.[56] It is especially useful when selecting a medication for prolonged therapy, as it is nonhabit forming, has low abuse potential, and appears to be nonlethal in overdose, making it beneficial in maintaining alcohol abstinence in alcoholics with psychiatric comorbidity.[3,15,47] Gabapentin is useful in the outpatient setting to reduce the risk of alcohol use relapse.[36,47,55,61]

Topiramate (Topamax)

Topiramate is an anticonvulsive approved for seizure disorders and has positive effects on alcohol dependence.[3,33,64,69] It can be prescribed for off-label use for relapse prevention in alcoholic individuals and is showing promise in the treatment of cocaine dependence.[69] Topiramate could be considered as a first-line treatment option for the management of AUDs, but there is still little evidence regarding its use in AWS.[33]

Alternate Medications in the Treatment of AWS and AUD

Other medications with GABA activity include valproic acid, clomethiazole, tiagabine, gamma-hydroxybutyric (GHB), pregabalin, and vigabatrin.[15,18] Pregabalin (Lyrica) was found to be safer and more effective than lorazepam or tiapride (not currently available in the United States).[54] Other medications that may be used in the treatment of AUD (but not indicated for withdrawal) are disulfiram, acamprosate, and naltrexone.[47] Clomethiazole is available in Europe as a sedative-hypnotic that enhances neurotransmission at GABA-A receptors and slows elimination of alcohol by inhibiting the enzyme alcohol dehydrogenase.[18] This medication is not currently prescribed in the United States.

Valproic Acid and Valproate Sodium

Valproic acid and valproate sodium are approved in the United States for use in epilepsy and bipolar disorder, but may be used as an adjunct for treatment of AWS. They have both anticonvulsant and antikindling properties, and act to enhance levels of GABA suppressing glutamate function via NMDA receptors.[67] They may also be helpful in reducing the risk of seizures in mild to moderate AWS, are frequently used as a post detoxification relapse-prevention agent, as well as maintaining alcohol abstinence in alcoholics with psychiatric comorbidity.[15] Valproate has been found to be effective in the treatment of alcoholic hallucinosis and is well tolerated.[9]

Gamma-hydroxybutyrate

Gamma-hydroxybutyrate (GHB) in its prescriptive form is known as sodium oxybate (Xyrem), and in its recreational form is most commonly known as GHB (a street drug). Its pharmacologic properties make it a viable treatment choice for alcohol withdrawal.[19,27,60,61] It is thought that GHB probably binds to the GABA receptor at high concentrations, and readily crosses the blood-brain barrier.[60] Several research studies have been carried out to test the efficacy and side effects of GHB, and it shows promise in symptom improvement and treatment of AWS.[19,27] GHB performed favorably in comparison with clomethiazole for AWS in ICU patients, with decreases in CIWA-Ar scores and improvement in symptomatology.[19] However, high doses seem to be the most successful, and side effects are increased in a history of poly-drug use, in addition to the AWS. This suggests that GHB treatment is contraindicated for patients with past or present substance use. GHB is not currently a recommendation in the United States. The United Kingdom guidelines on the treatment of AWS advise against its routine administration based on preliminary studies conducted in Europe.[19] Sodium oxybate may be as effective as oxazepam in the treatment of uncomplicated AWS (due to tolerability and absence of significant side effects) and may be considered a valid alternative choice in the treatment of AWS.[16]

Varenicline (Chantix)

Varenicline is a partial $\alpha 4\beta 2$ nicotinic acetylcholine agonist used for smoking cessation, but some studies are being conducted to evaluate its usefulness in alcohol dependence. It appears to significantly reduce alcohol consumption, craving, and drinking in both smokers and nonsmokers (or smokers who failed to stop smoking), with little to no adverse effects.[49]

Anticraving

The anticraving substances acamprosate and naltrexone, as well as the aversion therapeutic agent disulfiram (Antabuse), are currently available for pharmacotherapy of alcohol dependence.[49,64,69,86] Disulfiram blocks the metabolism of alcohol, and produces a flushing reaction if the patient consumes alcohol. Disulfiram should be administered when the patient is supervised by an adult or family member, which is necessary as disulfiram is rarely successful if self-medicated.[69] In Europe, nalmefene (an opioid receptor agonist) is also used to manage alcohol dependence and reduce alcohol consumption.[52,64,86] The medication was approved in the United States for opioid overdose, but is not currently approved for dependence on alcohol or other substances.

Adjunct Medications

Haloperidol (Haldol) may be required for the treatment of extreme, increasing agitation in the absence of any other withdrawal symptoms or in the patient experiencing increasing agitation despite adequate benzodiazepine therapy. It may also be used in the treatment of hallucinations. Haloperidol can prolong QT intervals and lower the seizure threshold; therefore, patients must be monitored during therapy. Beta blockers may be used in patients with coronary risk factors who may not tolerate the demands of withdrawal.

SUPPORTIVE CARE

In addition to pharmacologic agents, it is important to provide supportive care throughout the withdrawal period. Substance dependent patients are often nutritionally deficient, especially alcoholics who lack glycogen stores (which may lead to alcoholic ketoacidosis). In addition, opioid and AWS results in increased metabolic requirements and fluid losses. Therefore, it is important to monitor and manage hydration, electrolyte replacement, hyperthermia, hyperventilation, dehydration, diaphoresis, agitation, blood pressure, and renal function.[46,61,71,88,91] When hydration and electrolyte replacement is managed appropriately, it can prevent poor outcomes and decrease hospital length of stay.[88] Specific fluid and glucose treatments should be based on patient history (e.g., diabetes, cardiac dysfunction, or renal insufficiency). But most patients will likely need glucose supplementation for the increased metabolic requirements, and IV dextrose should be given for hypoglycemia, which should be considered in all cases of altered mental status.[88]

Electrolytes

Electrolytes should be evaluated and replaced as necessary.[46,61,88,91] Replacement of potassium, magnesium, phosphate, and glucose should all be calculated carefully.[71] Magnesium is an NMDA antagonist, and should be monitored and replaced. Symptomatic hypomagnesemia has some similarities to AWS and may affect the severity of DTs.[88] After verifying renal status, replace magnesium deficit at 2 mEq/kg.[91]

Thiamine

All patients in alcohol withdrawal should be treated with thiamine. Chronic alcohol use leads to malnutrition and results in thiamine deficiency. If left untreated, this deficiency places the patient at risk of Wernicke's encephalopathy or Wernicke-Korsakoff syndrome, which potentially results in permanent neurologic damage.[61,88] There are no universally accepted guidelines regarding optimal dose, mode of administration, frequency of administration, or duration of thiamine replacement.[46] Thiamine is usually dosed in 100 mL of normal saline intravenously over 30 minutes for 5 days.[46,91] It may also be given as 100 mg intramuscular (IM) or orally; and preferably before administration of oral or intravenous glucose, as glucose can precipitate or worsen Wernicke's syndrome.[61] Some clinicians recommend initial high doses of parenteral thiamine (500–1500 mg daily) to enable diffusion of thiamine across the blood brain barrier to prevent irreversible brain damage, restore vitamin status, improve clinical signs, and prevent death.[46,91]

Safety

Throughout the treatment period, it is important to remain alert to how AWS may affect the patient's behavior and emotional state. All healthcare workers must anticipate that substance use, intoxication, and withdrawal can lead to erratic and violent behavior, and should protect themselves from this danger.[8,38,98] In order to limit aggressive behavior and reduce violence, care should be taken to limit environmental stimulation. The patient's environment should be quiet, being aware of the volume of alarms and the loudness of voices. Patients may become paranoid and mistake general conversation as aggressive or attacking voices. Ensure the safety of the critical care team by preparing for potential agitation, hallucinations, and DTs. All staff members should be trained in deescalation techniques for the agitated patient. Additional supportive care should include frequent reassurance, reality orientation, and control of excessive environment stimulation such as bright lights, dark shadows, unusual noises, or other excessive stimuli.[61] The goal of withdrawal management is to provide safe withdrawal without harm to the patient or the critical care team.

MEDICAL SEQUELAE OF SUBSTANCE USE

Knowledge of the many comorbid conditions associated with chronic drug and alcohol use may be helpful in anticipation of possible withdrawal or may help explain conditions that can be exacerbated or complicated by continued substance exposure. Consideration of these conditions may assist in anticipating pending withdrawal in the patient with no apparent withdrawal symptoms on admission. For the vast amount of substances used, there are an equally large amount of potential medical sequelae, making it more of a challenge to identify drug related complications.

The medical sequelae of individuals who regularly use cannabis, or those who began using cannabis at an early age, include physiologic and psychosocial effects.[28] Users are at increased risk of advancing to more dangerous illicit drugs, jeopardizing educational, professional, and social achievements, increasing welfare dependence, and suffering from psychotic symptomatology.[28,92] The effects of long-term or heavy use of cannabis also include addiction, altered brain development, poor educational outcome, cognitive impairment, diminished life satisfaction and achievement, symptoms of chronic bronchitis, and increased risk of chronic psychosis disorders.[92]

The cardiovascular consequences of cocaine are well known, and related to changes in the sympathetic nervous system, cardiomyocytes, vasculature, endothelium, and the platelet system.[87] Chest pain is associated with a more severe acute cardiac syndrome, such as myocardial infarction, but mortality is relatively low.[87] Cocaine-positive patients with acute coronary syndrome are usually younger with fewer risk factors, less multivessel coronary artery disease, and lower drug-eluting stent and beta blocker usage.[34]

Regardless of the type of drug, intravenous drug use leads to complications. Some basic concerns of needle use are presented in Box 42.5. A noteworthy sequelae of ketamine use is ketamine-induced ulcerative cystitis and loss of bladder control.[62]

Chronic alcohol use leads to multiple medical sequelae, including cardiomyopathy, dysrhythmias, impaired liver function (affecting bleeding and clotting factors), portal hypertension, esophageal varices (contraindication for nasogastric tubes), and seizures (especially in alcohol withdrawal syndrome). If

BOX 42.5 Needle Use Risks and Complications

- Endocarditis
- Collapsed veins
- Abscesses
- Cellulitis
- Infected sites
- HIV, Hep B, and Hep C in needle users

intoxicated, there is a predisposition to aspiration and diminished pulmonary function. In addition, alcohol abuse has been identified as an independent risk factor for the development of adult respiratory distress syndrome (ARDS).[17] Alcohol has a profound impact on sleep and alcohol dependent patients suffer from a multitude of sleep disturbances both while drinking or during periods of abstinence.[66] Alcohol dependent patients have higher infection, sepsis, and septic shock rates. They are more likely to be admitted to the ICU, die in the hospital, and cost more in hospital resource dollars.[5] Critical comorbid conditions of alcohol dependence that require ICU management include trauma, severe sepsis, respiratory failure, ARDS, hemodynamic instability, gastrointestinal bleeding, hepatic failure, pancreatitis, rhabdomyolysis, cointoxication, coagulopathies, acute CNS process, cardiac arrhythmias, ischemia, or congestive failure, severe fluid or electrolyte defects, renal failure, persistent fever, complex acid-base imbalances, or persistent fever over 39° C.[18]

PSYCHIATRIC DISORDERS AND ADDICTION

A large percentage of addicted patients have one or more co-occurring psychiatric disorders impacting their behavior. There is a significant association between drug and alcohol dependence and psychiatric conditions, with the most prevalent psychiatric conditions being anxiety and depression.[73,75] Patients may present with demanding, manipulative, or emotionally unstable behavior. They may demonstrate behavioral changes such as interpersonal inappropriateness, aggressiveness, violence, tearfulness, anger, or nervousness. These behaviors may be exhibited as a response to intoxication, or may not be related to substance use or withdrawal, but may result from an underlying psychiatric disorder itself. Management of the difficult patient is not easy, but may be guided by several useful approaches, including pharmacologic psychoactive treatment, environmental adaptation (control of stimuli), and limiting engagement in hostile or argumentative conversations. For additional information on psychiatric disorders, see Chapter 37.

SPECIAL POPULATIONS

The Older Adult

Chemical dependence, addiction, and withdrawal in the older adult present a unique set of physiologic circumstances. It is estimated that 10% of the elderly drink excessively.[68] Up to 30% of older patients who are hospitalized in medical areas and up to 50% of those hospitalized in psychiatric units present with AUD.[17] Social isolation is often the contributing factor associated with the onset of a drinking problem in an older adult.[73] Illicit substance abuse is a less serious problem in the older adult than in younger individuals, but polypharmacy is a common problem in this population, and prescription medications are often used for medical and nonmedical reasons.[45]

Chemical dependence and AUDs have significant effects on multiple systems in the older adult, including glucose metabolism disorders, greater incidence of hypertension, and an increased risk of breast cancer.[17] Older age increases susceptibility to pulmonary infections due to a physiologic reduction of immune response, which is worsened by excessive alcohol intake, and increases the risk of ARDS.[17]

Signs and symptoms of chemical dependency could be mistaken for symptoms of depression or dementia, and substance use disorders, especially in the older adult, and are often ignored, unrecognized, or misdiagnosed.[45] Cognitive function declines with age, as does sensory perception, vision, hearing, tactile sensation, vibratory sensation, and ability to maintain balance. These changes, along with the change in environment, may result in significant confusion, depression, and risk of falls, but they also make identifying symptoms of withdrawal more complicated. Some older patients may have underlying dementia that becomes evident with the stress of withdrawal. Interestingly, the prevalence of dementia in the elderly is almost 5 times higher in alcoholics than in nonalcoholics; approximately 25% of elderly patients with dementia also have AUDs.[17] In addition, 90% of older adults with AUDs have a history of depression.[17]

As the body ages, there is a decrease in lean body mass and total body water with an increase in total body fat, which contributes to a negative impact of alcohol. The older patient has a greater loss of renal and hepatic function. Renal tubular function declines and the kidneys lose the ability to conserve sodium and excrete hydrogen ions. In addition, the older adult experiences less thirst, and therefore dehydration is a concern. The decrease in liver function permits maintenance of higher blood alcohol levels and influences the metabolism of benzodiazepines given for withdrawal. Using short to intermediate acting benzodiazepines, such as lorazepam or oxazepam, is a better option for these patients.[17,61,71]

Medical and neurologic complications increase during AWS in the elderly, and are more likely to have complex and potentially fatal effects.[18] Complications of AWS include myocardial ischemia, arrhythmias, orthostatic hypotension, aspiration pneumonia, hallucinations, DTs, dizziness, and seizures.[17] Neurotransmitter alterations associated with AWS may contribute to ICU delirium and cognitive defects in the elderly.[18] Wernicke–Korsakoff syndrome is also more prevalent in the older adult experiencing AWS, signs of which include peripheral neuropathy, ataxia, ocular paralysis, confusion, confabulation, and amnesia related to low magnesium. Therefore, it is recommended that administration of magnesium be added to the AWS treatment plan.[17]

Adolescents

Drugs and alcohol are typically initially tried by adolescents, which is when the brain undergoes enormous changes and functional reorganization, including executive cognitive function such as decision-making and effective regulation of behavior.[84] Habitual consumption of substances in adolescents seems to be related to adaptation failures, interpersonal conflicts, affiliation with other adolescents having similar psychological dysregulation, and the propensity to experience negative reinforcement.[84] Alcohol misuse is associated with multiple forms of disease and injury, and it is one of the leading causes of death among teenagers and young adults due to unintentional injuries, homicide, and suicide.[98] Although most adolescents use illicit substances, more adolescents appear to be using diverted medical marijuana than using medical marijuana legally, which results in higher odds of engaging in other types of substance use.[12]

Legal highs are substances that produce similar effects to those of illicit drugs (such as heroin, cocaine, and LSD), but they are not controlled under the Misuse of Drugs Act. These substances may contain some chemicals that are considered illegal is certain states, but the chemical formula can be changed to avoid state laws, and therefore continue to be sold. The contents of the substance may be considered illegal under current legislation, but if the packaging is adjusted to contain the words "not for human consumption," no laws appear to control the sale, supply, or advertisement of the drugs. The majority of these substances are purchased on the internet and shipped to the consumer directly.

When caring for adolescents in critical care it is often difficult to determine what substance was used prior to admission. One of the most important admission activities is gathering a history of events from the patient or friends to establish type of substance and timeline of use. Gaining the trust of the patient, or their friends, can be difficult; and generally their first concern is that law enforcement will be contacted, so one of the quickest and simplest things to tell them is that their health records are confidential and their privacy is protected. Many times this will be enough to establish a minimal history to help start the treatment plan.

Pregnant Patient

Recreational drugs and alcohol are teratogenic, and lead to fetal defects and fetal demise. Alcohol is possibly the worst substance to use during pregnancy. The effects of alcohol lead to fetal alcohol spectrum disorder, including morphologic abnormalities, low birth weight, and developmental and cognitive impairment.[73] Neonatal abstinence syndrome is a withdrawal syndrome that affects the newborn baby following delivery from a substance using mother. The severity of the withdrawal is influenced by the type of drug used during pregnancy, the amount used, and the gestational age upon delivery. These babies need immediate monitoring and management by a skilled neonatal team. Withdrawal of a pregnant patient from any drug or alcohol presents a dangerous situation for both the patient and the unborn child, and should be assessed and managed by specialists.

DISCHARGE PLANNING

Many times patients are discharged from critical care to a step-down unit or medical area, or may be discharged home from the unit following recovery of intoxications. Either way, the patient being discharged needs a strong discharge plan to include family, friends, and community support. Talking to the patient and their family about options for care after discharge should begin in the ICU, and may assist in preventing future admissions. Optimal therapy and plans for a successful discharge involve a coordinated interdisciplinary approach, including the medical and nursing teams, the social work department, dietitians, and various levels of specialty therapy that may be required based on severity of patient's condition and individual needs.

Once the acute treatment is completed, a plan must be developed to increase the patient's motivation for long-term substance use abstinence and facilitate entry into a relapse prevention program.[61] Discharge planning should include follow-up with primary care provider and counseling. Self-help groups such as Alcoholics Anonymous (AA) and Narcotics Anonymous (NA) provide additional support to both the patient and their loved ones. However, it is reported that AA and NA groups do not permit individuals who are taking prescribed medications such as methadone, buprenorphine, or naltrexone, to speak at meetings.[69] Continued care following discharge from the hospital is essential. Detoxification of many substances (drugs) will not resolve in the dependent patient unless followed by long-term treatment of at least 6 to 12 months and include prescribed medications in addition to therapy.[69]

CONCLUSION

Caring for the chemically dependent patient requires an understanding of the physiologic effects of the substance used. A detailed investigation into the history and a thorough physical examination will assist in recognition of the signs and symptoms of withdrawal. Anticipation of withdrawal symptoms will ensure that treatment plans are initiated early enough to prevent additional injury or negative sequelae.

The treatment of substance use, intoxication, or withdrawal is dependent on the type of substance used. Most research and medical management available focuses on AWS, recommending the use of benzodiazepines as the treatment of choice for AWS.[6,15,18,25,36,50,61,65,67,71,81] Protocol driven treatment involving symptom triggered and dose escalations of diazepam lead to decreased ICU length of stay, decreased duration on mechanical ventilation, and decreased benzodiazepine requirements in critically ill patients.[25]

An understanding of the chemical effects of drugs or alcohol on the brain and the subsequent tolerance and dependence is essential to understanding the clinical syndrome seen in acute withdrawal. Patients who have undergone repeated withdrawal episodes have a worsening of withdrawal with each subsequent detoxification and an increased risk of complications (e.g., seizures and DTs) due to the kindling phenomenon. Therefore, gathering a detailed history, being observant of early signs of withdrawal, and starting a preventative treatment plan is a large part of the patient's successful stay in critical care.

CASE STUDY 42.1

Opiates

B.B. is a 36-year-old male who is admitted to critical care from the emergency department (ED) at 1600 following a motor vehicle crash in which he sustained a fractured arm, fractured leg, and pneumothorax. A chest tube has been placed, and his arm and leg placed in immobilizers. He is scheduled for surgery later in the day. He is in excruciating pain on admission, profoundly diaphoretic, and begging for more pain medication. He states his pain is 10 out of 10 despite 40 mg of morphine in the ED. He is noted to be tremulous with his arms at his side. Vital signs include blood pressure 172/110 mm Hg, heart rate 143 beats/minute, and respiratory rate 26 breaths/minute with an oxygen saturation of 92% on 4 liters of oxygen per nasal cannula. He is nauseated with dry heaving, his pupils are slightly dilated, and he is profoundly diaphoretic. He is complaining that he is anxious and feeling panicked. He appears acutely ill. He reports drinking alcohol daily for many years, up to 10 drinks per day, predominantly gin and bourbon with some beer. He does get tremulous and very nauseated when he does not have regular alcohol. His last drink was 5 hours earlier. He also reports using opiates in the form of acetaminophen with hydrocodone and acetaminophen with oxycodone, obtained primarily from friends and the internet, with his daily use approximately 10 to 20 pills per day for the past 3 years. These are taken primarily orally. His last pill was this morning at 0600. He reports chewing oxycodone when he can get it. He also uses cocaine on a daily basis but is unable to quantify the amount. He further uses citalopram (Celexa), which he takes with alcohol to enhance the effects of both substances. He has also used amphetamines and diazepam on

Continued

an intermittent basis. He has not previously withdrawn from alcohol, but does experience opiate withdrawal if he does not take opiates every 4 hours. His labs in the ED were white blood cells (WBC) 14.6%, hemoglobin (Hgb) 12.4 g/dL, hematocrit (Hct) 35.7%, sodium 141 mEq/L, potassium 3.8 mEq/L, chloride 104 mEq/L, total CO_2 28 mEq/L, blood urea nitrogen (BUN) 9 mg/dL, creatinine 1.1 mg/dL, glucose 102 mg/dL, with a urine toxicology screen positive for cocaine and opiates. His blood alcohol level (BAL) is 0.28 mg/dL; he is a nonsmoker. He is started on morphine via patient-controlled analgesia.

Decision Point:

What potential withdrawal states may impact his critical care stay?

Decision Point:

Which withdrawal state can be fatal if untreated: alcohol or opiate?

Decision Point:

What substances will not result in withdrawal states?

Decision Point:

Would you anticipate seizure activity with this withdrawal?

Decision Point:

What are the potential signs of alcohol withdrawal present on the initial assessment?

REFERENCES

1. Agrawal, P. R., Scarabelli, T. M., Saravolatz, L., Kini, A., Jalota, A., Chen-Scarabelli, C., et al. (2015). Current strategies in the evaluation and management of cocaine-induced chest pain. *Cardiol Rev, 23*(6), 303–311.
2. Agudelo, M., Yndart, A., Morrison, M., Figueroa, G., Muñoz, K., Samikkannu, T., et al. (2013). Differential expression and functional role of cannabinoid genes in alcohol users. *Drug Alcohol Depend, 133*(2), 789–793.
3. Ait-Daoud, N. (2013). Anticonvulsant medications for the treatment of alcohol dependence. In *Interventions for addiction: comprehensive addictive behaviors and disorders, Vol. 3(pp. 391–396)*. San Diego: Academic Press.
4. American Psychiatric Association. (2013). *Diagnostic and statistical manual of mental disorders* (5th ed.).
5. Awissi, D. K., Lebrun, G., Coursin, D. B., Riker, R. R., & Skrobik, Y. (2013). Alcohol withdrawal and delirium tremens in the critically ill: a systematic review and commentary. *Intensive Care Med, 39*(1), 16–30.
6. Awissi, D. K., Lebrun, G., Fagnan, M., & Skrobik, Y. (2013). Alcohol, nicotine, and iatrogenic withdrawals in the ICU. *Crit Care Med, 41*(9), S57–S68.
7. Barceloux, D. G. (2012). *Medical toxicology of drug abuse: synthesized chemicals and psychoactive plants*. Hoboken, NJ: John Wiley & Sons.
8. Beck, A., Heinz, A. J., & Heinz, A. (2014). Translational clinical neuroscience perspectives on the cognitive and neurobiological mechanisms underlying alcohol-related aggression. In *Neuroscience of Aggression* (pp. 443–474). Springer Berlin Heidelberg.
9. Bhat, P. S., Ryali, V. S. S. R., Srivastava, K., Kumar, S. R., Prakash, J., & Singal, A. (2012). Alcoholic hallucinosis. *Ind Psychiatry J, 21*(2), 155.
10. Bickley, L., & Szilagyi, P. G. (2012). *Bates' guide to physical examination and history-taking*. Philadelphia: Lippincott Williams & Wilkins.
11. Bob, P., Jasova, D., Bizik, G., & Raboch, J. (2011). Epileptiform activity in alcohol dependent patients and possibilities of its indirect measurement. *PLoS One, 6*(4), e18678.
12. Boyd, C. J., Veliz, P. T., & McCabe, S. E. (2015). Adolescents' use of medical marijuana: a secondary analysis of monitoring the future data. *J Adolesc Health, 57*(2), 241–244.
13. Buchta, W. C., & Riegel, A. C. (2015). Chronic cocaine disrupts mesocortical learning mechanisms. *Brain Res, 1628*(PtA), 88–103.
14. Cadet, J. L., Bisagno, V., & Milroy, C. M. (2014). Neuropathology of substance use disorders. *Acta Neuropathol, 127*(1), 91–107.
15. Caputo, F., & Bernardi, M. (2010). Medications acting on the GABA system in the treatment of alcoholic patients. *Curr Pharm Des, 16*(19), 2118–2125.
16. Caputo, F., Vignoli, T., Grignaschi, A., Cibin, M., Addolorato, G., & Bernardi, M. (2014). Pharmacological management of alcohol dependence: from mono-therapy to pharmacogenetics and beyond. *Eur Neuropsychopharmacol, 24*(2), 181–191.
17. Caputo, F., Vignoli, T., Leggio, L., Addolorato, G., Zoli, G., & Bernardi, M. (2012). Alcohol use disorders in the elderly: a brief overview from epidemiology to treatment options. *Exp Gerontol, 47*(6), 411–416.
18. Carlson, R. W., Kumar, N. N., Wong-Mckinstry, E., Ayyagari, S., Puri, N., Jackson, F. K., et al. (2012). Alcohol withdrawal syndrome. *Crit Care Clin, 28*(4), 549–585.
19. Cooper, E., & Vernon, J. (2013). The effectiveness of pharmacological approaches in the treatment of alcohol withdrawal syndrome (AWS): a literature review. *J Psychiatr Ment Health Nurs, 20*(7), 601–612.
20. Crispo, A. L., Daley, M. J., Pepin, J. L., Harford, P. H., & Brown, C. V. (2014). Comparison of clinical outcomes in nonintubated patients with severe alcohol withdrawal syndrome treated with continuous-infusion sedatives: dexmedetomidine versus benzodiazepines. *Pharmacotherapy, 34*(9), 910–917.
21. Curtis, B. J., Zahs, A., & Kovacs, E. J. (2013). Epigenetic targets for reversing immune defects caused by alcohol exposure. *Alcohol Res, 35*(1), 97.
22. Czyz, C. N., Piehota, P. G., & Strittmatter, A. M. (2015). Acute onset esotropia after heroin withdrawal. *Am J Emerg Med, 33*(4), 598.e1–598.e2.
23. Davis, C. S., Ruiz, S., Glynn, P., Picariello, G., & Walley, A. Y. (2014). Expanded access to naloxone among firefighters, police officers, and emergency medical technicians in Massachusetts. *Am J Public Health, 104*(8), e7–e9.
24. Dreifuss, J. A., Griffin, M. L., Frost, K., Fitzmaurice, G. M., Potter, J. S., Fiellin, D. A., et al. (2013). Patient characteristics associated with buprenorphine/naloxone treatment outcome for prescription opioid dependence: results from a multisite study. *Drug Alcohol Depend, 131*(1), 112–118.
25. Duby, J. J., Berry, A. J., Ghayyem, P., Wilson, M. D., & Cocanour, C. S. (2014). Alcohol withdrawal syndrome in critically ill patients: protocolized versus nonprotocolized management. *J Trauma Acute Care Surg, 77*(6), 938–943.
26. Ellenbroek, B. A., & Ghiabi, B. (2014). The other side of the histamine H3 receptor. *Trends Neurosci, 37*(4), 191–199.
27. Elsing, C., Stremmel, W., Grenda, U., & Herrmann, T. (2009). Gamma--hydroxybutyric acid versus clomethiazole for the treatment of alcohol withdrawal syndrome in a medical intensive care unit: an open, single-center randomized study. *Am J Drug Alcohol Abuse, 35*(3), 189–192.
28. Fergusson, D. M., Boden, J. M., & Horwood, L. J. (2015). Psychosocial sequelae of cannabis use and implications for policy: findings from the Christchurch Health and Development Study. *Soc Psychiatry Psychiatr Epidemiol, 50*(9), 1317–1326.
29. Finn, K. M., & Greenwald, J. (2011). Hospitalists and alcohol withdrawal: yes, give benzodiazepines but is that the whole story? *J Hosp Med, 6*(8), 435–437.
30. German, C. L., Fleckenstein, A. E., & Hanson, G. R. (2014). Bath salts and synthetic cathinones: an emerging designer drug phenomenon. *Life Sci, 97*(1), 2–8.
31. Grant, B. F., Goldstein, R. B., Saha, T. D., Chou, S. P., Jung, J., Zhang, H., et al. (2015). Epidemiology of DSM-5 Alcohol Use Disorder: results from the National Epidemiologic Survey on Alcohol and Related Conditions III. *JAMA Psychiatry, 73*(10), 39–47.
32. Grgurich, P., Tulolo, A., Dargin, J., Sen, S., & Gray, A. (2014). 152: Evaluation of SAS-based symptom-triggered treatment of alcohol withdrawal in critically ill patients. *Crit Care Med, 42*(12), A1397.
33. Guglielmo, R., Martinotti, G., Quatrale, M., Ioime, L., Kadilli, I., Di Nicola, M., et al. (2015). Topiramate in alcohol use disorders: review and update. *CNS Drugs, 29*(5), 383–395.

34. Gupta, N., Washam, J. B., Mountantonakis, S. E., Li, S., Roe, M. T., de Lemos, J. A., et al. (2014). Characteristics, management, and outcomes of cocaine-positive patients with acute coronary syndrome (from the National Cardiovascular Data Registry). *Am J Cardiol, 113*(5), 749–756.
35. Haile, C. N., Mahoney, J. J., Newton, T. F., & De La Garza, R. (2012). Pharmacotherapeutics directed at deficiencies associated with cocaine dependence: focus on dopamine, norepinephrine and glutamate. *Pharmacol Ther, 134*(2), 260–277.
36. Hammond, C. J., Niciu, M. J., Drew, S., & Arias, A. J. (2015). Anticonvulsants for the treatment of alcohol withdrawal syndrome and alcohol use disorders. *CNS Drugs, 29*(4), 293–311.
37. Heilig, M., Egli, M., Crabbe, J. C., & Becker, H. C. (April 2010). Acute withdrawal, protracted abstinence and negative affect in alcoholism: are they linked? *Addict Biol, 15*(2), 169–184. http://dx.doi.org/10.1111/j.1369-1600.2009.00194.x PMC 3268458. PMID 20148778.
38. Heinz, A. J., Makin-Byrd, K., Blonigen, D. M., Reilly, P., & Timko, C. (2015). Aggressive behavior among military veterans in substance use disorder treatment: the roles of posttraumatic stress and impulsivity. *J Subst Abuse Treat, 50*, 59–66.
39. Hendey, G. W., Dery, R. A., Barnes, R. L., Snowden, B., & Mentler, P. (2011). A prospective, randomized, trial of phenobarbital versus benzodiazepines for acute alcohol withdrawal. *Am J Emerg Med, 29*(4), 382–385.
40. Hoen, B., & Duval, X. (2013). Infective endocarditis. *N Engl J Med, 368*(15), 1425–1433.
41. Jawa, R. S., Stothert, J. C., Shostrom, V. K., Yetter, D. L., Templin, H. R., Cemaj, S. K., et al. (2014). Alcohol withdrawal syndrome in admitted trauma patients. *Am J Surg, 208*(5), 781–787.
42. Julien, R. M. (2013). *A primer of drug action: a concise nontechnical guide to the actions, uses, and side effects of psychoactive drugs, revised and updated.* Holt Paperbacks.
43. Kalabalik, J., & Sullivan, J. B. (2015). Use of dexmedetomidine in the management of alcohol withdrawal syndrome in critically ill patients. *Int J Crit Care Emerg Med, 1*(1), 1–5.
44. Kennedy, A. P., Epstein, D. H., Jobes, M. L., Agage, D., Tyburski, M., Phillips, K. A., et al. (2015). Continuous in-the-field measurement of heart rate: correlates of drug use, craving, stress, and mood in polydrug users. *Drug Alcohol Depend, 151*, 159–166.
45. Koechl, B., Unger, A., & Fischer, G. (2012). Age-related aspects of addiction. *Gerontology, 58*(6), 540–544.
46. Latt, N., & Dore, G. (2014). Thiamine in the treatment of Wernicke encephalopathy in patients with alcohol use disorders. *Intern Med J, 44*(9), 911–915.
47. Leung, J. G., Hall-Flavin, D., Nelson, S., Schmidt, K. A., & Schak, K. M. (2015). The role of gabapentin in the management of alcohol withdrawal and dependence. *Ann Pharmacother, 49*(8), 897–906.
48. Liaudet, L., Calderari, B., & Pacher, P. (2014). Pathophysiological mechanisms of catecholamine and cocaine-mediated cardiotoxicity. *Heart Fail Rev, 19*(6), 815–824.
49. Litten, R. Z., Ryan, M. L., Fertig, J. B., Falk, D. E., Johnson, B., Dunn, K. E., et al. (2013). A double-blind, placebo-controlled trial assessing the efficacy of varenicline tartrate for alcohol dependence. *J Addict Med, 7*(4), 277.
50. Lizotte, R. J., Kappes, J. A., Bartel, B. J., Hayes, K. M., & Lesselyoung, V. L. (2014). Evaluating the effects of dexmedetomidine compared to propofol as adjunctive therapy in patients with alcohol withdrawal. *Clin Pharmacol, 6*, 171.
51. Lyon, J. E., Khan, R. A., Gessert, C. E., Larson, P. M., & Renier, C. M. (2011). Treating alcohol withdrawal with oral baclofen: a randomized, double-blind, placebo-controlled trial. *J Hosp Med, 6*(8), 469–474.
52. Mann, K., Bladström, A., Torup, L., Gual, A., & van den Brink, W. (2013). Extending the treatment options in alcohol dependence: a randomized controlled study of as-needed nalmefene. *Biol Psychiatry, 73*(8), 706–713.
53. Marik, P. E. (2015). Alcohol withdrawal syndrome. In *Evidence-based critical care* (pp. 751–757). New York, New York: Springer International Publishing.
54. Martinotti, G., Di Nicola, M., Frustaci, A., Romanelli, R., Tedeschi, D., Guglielmo, R., et al. (2010). Pregabalin, tiapride and lorazepam in alcohol withdrawal syndrome: a multi-centre, randomized, single-blind comparison trial. *Addiction, 105*(2), 288–299.
55. Marx, J., Walls, R., & Hockberger, R. (2013). *Rosen's emergency medicine-concepts and clinical practice.* Philadelphia, Pennsylvania: Elsevier Health Sciences.
56. Mason, B. J., Crean, R., Goodell, V., Light, J. M., Quello, S., Shadan, F., et al. (2012). A proof-of-concept randomized controlled study of gabapentin: effects on cannabis use, withdrawal and executive function deficits in cannabis-dependent adults. *Neuropsychopharmacology, 37*(7), 1689–1698.
57. McHugh, R. K., Fitzmaurice, G. M., Carroll, K. M., Griffin, M. L., Hill, K. P., Wasan, A. D., et al. (2014). Assessing craving and its relationship to subsequent prescription opioid use among treatment-seeking prescription opioid dependent patients. *Drug Alcohol Depend, 145*, 121–126.
58. Melson, J., Kane, M., Mooney, R., McWilliams, J., & Horton, T. (2014). Improving alcohol withdrawal outcomes in acute care. *Perm J, 18*(2), e141.
59. Michaelsen, I. H., Anderson, J. E., Fink-Jensen, A., Allerup, P., & Ulrichsen, J. (2010). Phenobarbital versus diazepam for delirium tremens–a retrospective study. *Dan Med Bull, 57*(8), A4169.
60. Miotto, K., Davoodi, P., & Maya, S. (2013). Background and history of club drugs. *Adolesc Psychiatry, 29*, 149.
61. Mirijello, A., D'Angelo, C., Ferrulli, A., Vassallo, G., Antonelli, M., Caputo, F., et al. (2015). Identification and management of alcohol withdrawal syndrome. *Drugs, 75*(4), 353–365.
62. Morgan, C. J., & Curran, H. V. (2012). Ketamine use: a review. *Addiction, 107*(1), 27–38.
63. Mueller, S. W., Preslaski, C. R., Kiser, T. H., Fish, D. N., Lavelle, J. C., Malkoski, S. P., et al. (2014). A randomized, double-blind, placebo-controlled dose range study of dexmedetomidine as adjunctive therapy for alcohol withdrawal. *Crit Care Med, 42*(5), 1131–1139.
64. Müller, C. A., Geisel, O., Banas, R., & Heinz, A. (2014). Current pharmacological treatment approaches for alcohol dependence. *Expert Opin Pharmacother, 15*(4), 471–481.
65. Myrick, H., Galanter, M., Kleber, H. D., & Brady, K. (Eds.). (2014). *The American Psychiatric Publishing textbook of substance abuse treatment* (5th ed.). Arlington, VA: American Psychiatric Publishing.
66. Nam, H. W., McIver, S. R., Hinton, D. J., Thakkar, M. M., Sari, Y., Parkinson, F. E., et al. (2012). Adenosine and glutamate signaling in neuron–glial interactions: implications in alcoholism and sleep disorders. *Alcohol Clin Exp Res, 36*(7), 1117–1125.
67. Nejad, S. H., Chuang, K., Hirschberg, R., Aquino, P. R., & Fricchione, G. L. (2014). The use of antiepileptic drugs in acute neuropsychiatric conditions: focus on traumatic brain injury, pain, and alcohol withdrawal. *Int J Clin Med, 5*, 724–736.
68. Noble, J. M., & Weimer, L. H. (2014). Neurologic complications of alcoholism. *Continuum (Minneap Minn), 20*(3), 624–641.
69. O'Brien, C. P. (2015). Science in the treatment of substance abuse. In *The American Psychiatric Publishing textbook of substance abuse treatment* (5th ed.).
70. Palmer, R. H. C., McGeary, J. E., Francazio, S., Raphael, B. J., Lander, A. D., Heath, A. C., et al. (2012). The genetics of alcohol dependence: advancing towards systems-based approaches. *Drug Alcohol Depend, 125*(3), 179–191.
71. Perry, E. C. (2014). Inpatient management of acute alcohol withdrawal syndrome. *CNS Drugs, 28*(5), 401–410.
72. Pilling, S., Yesufu-Udechuku, A., Taylor, C., & Drummond, C. (2011). Diagnosis, assessment, and management of harmful drinking and alcohol dependence: summary of NICE guidance. *BMJ, 342*.
73. Rastegar, D., & Fingerhood, M. (2015). *The American Society of Addiction Medicine handbook of addiction medicine.* New York: Oxford University Press.
74. Ries, R. K., Fiellin, D. A., Miller, S. C., & Saitz, R. (2014). *The ASAM principles of addiction medicine.* Philadelphia: Lippincott Williams & Wilkins.
75. Riper, H., Andersson, G., Hunter, S. B., Wit, J., Berking, M., & Cuijpers, P. (2014). Treatment of comorbid alcohol use disorders and depression with cognitive-behavioral therapy and motivational interviewing: a meta-analysis. *Addiction, 109*(3), 394–406.
76. Roberts, J. R. (2014). InFocus: intranasal naloxone for prehospital opioid overdose. *Emergency Medicine News, 36*(7), 4–6.

77. Rolland, B., Jaillette, E., Carton, L., Bence, C., Deheul, S., Saulnier, F., et al. (2014). Assessing alcohol versus baclofen withdrawal syndrome in patients treated with baclofen for alcohol use disorder. *J Clin Psychopharmacol, 34*(1), 153–156.
78. Roman, C., Gumbo, S., & Okuni, K. (2014). Phenobarbital use as adjunct to benzodiazepines in the treatment of severe alcohol withdrawal syndrome. *J Pharm Pharmacol, 2*, 551–557.
79. Russell, J., Richardson, N., & Dar, A. (2015). Use of a modified Clinical Institute Withdrawal Assessment (CIWA) for symptom-triggered management of alcohol withdrawal syndrome. *Clin Med, 15*(Suppl. 3), s20–s20.
80. Sabzghabaee, A. M., Eizadi-Mood, N., Yaraghi, A., & Zandifar, S. (2014). Naloxone therapy in opioid overdose patients: intranasal or intravenous? A randomized clinical trial. *Arch Med Sci, 10*(2), 309–314.
81. Schuckit, M. A. (2014). Recognition and management of withdrawal delirium (delirium tremens). *N Engl J Med, 371*(22), 2109–2113.
82. Seely, K. A., Lapoint, J., Moran, J. H., & Fattore, L. (2012). Spice drugs are more than harmless herbal blends: a review of the pharmacology and toxicology of synthetic cannabinoids. *Prog Neuropsychopharmacol Biol Psychiatry, 39*(2), 234–243.
83. Silverman, S. M. (2015). Buprenorphine for pain and opioid dependence. In A. D. Kaye, N. Vadievelu, & R. D. Urman (Eds.), *Substance abuse* (pp. 311–318). New York: Springer.
84. Sloboda, Z., Glantz, M. D., & Tarter, R. E. (2012). Revisiting the concepts of risk and protective factors for understanding the etiology and development of substance use and substance use disorders: implications for prevention. *Subst Use Misuse, 47*(8–9), 944–962.
85. Sohraby, R., Attridge, R. L., & Hughes, D. W. (2014). The use of propofol-containing versus benzodiazepine regimens for alcohol withdrawal requiring mechanical ventilation a retrospective chart review. *Ann Pharmacother, 48*(4), 456–461.
86. Soyka, M., & Lieb, M. (2015). Recent developments in pharmacotherapy of alcoholism. *Pharmacopsychiatry, 48*(4–5), 123–135.
87. Stankowski, R. V., Kloner, R. A., & Rezkalla, S. H. (2015). Cardiovascular consequences of cocaine use. *Trends Cardiovasc Med, 25*(6), 517–526.
88. Stehman, C. R., & Mycyk, M. B. (2013). A rational approach to the treatment of alcohol withdrawal in the ED. *Am J Emerg Med, 31*(4), 734–742.
89. Sullivan, J. T., Sykora, K., Schneiderman, J., Naranjo, C. A., & Sellers, E. M. (1989). Assessment of alcohol withdrawal: the revised clinical institute withdrawal assessment for alcohol scale (CIWA-Ar). *Br J Addict, 84*(11), 1353–1357.
90. Taber, K. H., Black, D. N., Porrino, L. J., & Hurley, R. A. (2012). Neuroanatomy of dopamine: reward and addiction. *J Neuropsychiatry Clin Neurosci, 24*(10), 1–4.
91. Thomson, A. D., Guerrini, I., & Marshall, E. J. (2012). The evolution and treatment of Korsakoff's syndrome. *Neuropsychol Rev, 22*(2), 81–92.
92. Volkow, N. D., Frieden, T. R., Hyde, P. S., & Cha, S. S. (2014). Medication-assisted therapies—tackling the opioid-overdose epidemic. *N Engl J Med, 370*(22), 2063–2066.
93. Weiss, R. D., Griffin, M. L., & Hufford, C. (1995). Craving in hospitalized cocaine abusers as a predictor of outcome. *Am J Drug Alcohol Abuse, 21*(3), 289–301.
94. Wood, M. R., Lalancette, R. A., & Bernal, I. (2015). Crystallographic investigations of select cathinones: emerging illicit street drugs known as 'bath salts'. *Acta Crystallogr C Struct Chem, 71*(1), 0–0.71(Pt1):32–38.
95. Woods, A. D., Giometti, R., & Weeks, S. M. (2015). The use of dexmedetomidine as an adjuvant to benzodiazepine-based therapy to decrease the severity of delirium in alcohol withdrawal in adult intensive care unit patients: a systematic review. *JBI Database System Rev Implement Rep, 13*(1), 224–252.
96. Zaaijer, E. R., van Dijk, L., de Bruin, K., Goudriaan, A. E., Lammers, L. A., Koeter, M. W., et al. (2015). Effect of extended-release naltrexone on striatal dopamine transporter availability, depression and anhedonia in heroin-dependent patients. *Psychopharmacology*, 1–11.
97. Zawilska, J. B., & Wojcieszak, J. (2013). Designer cathinones—an emerging class of novel recreational drugs. *Forensic Sci Int, 231*(1), 42–53.
98. Zerhouni, O., Bègue, L., Brousse, G., Carpentier, F., Dematteis, M., Pennel, L., et al. (2013). Alcohol and violence in the emergency room: a review and perspectives from psychological and social sciences. *Int J Environ Res Public Health, 10*(10), 4584–4606.

INTERNET RESOURCES

Note: These are not peer reviewed, scientific, or research-based sites.
http://www.drugabuse.gov.
http://www.justice.gov/dea/druginfo/factsheets.shtml.
http://www.justice.gov/dea/pr/top-story/SyntheticDesignerDrugs.shtml.
http://www.monitoringthefuture.org.
https://drugs-forum.com/index.php.
https://www.erowid.org/.

Palliative and End-of-Life Care

Debra L. Wiegand and Jooyoung Cheon

"You matter to the last moment of your life, and we will do all we can not only to help you die peacefully, but to live until you die."

Cicely Saunders

It is estimated that 2.5 million Americans die every year, with more than 60% of those deaths occurring in the acute care setting.[5,131] One in five deaths occurs during or within a short time after a stay in the intensive care unit (ICU).[5] The majority of patients who die in ICU do so after decisions are made to withhold and withdraw life-sustaining therapies.[8,34,55] The last phase of life varies based on each person's illness trajectory and clinical course.[85,86] Patients may die quite unexpectedly after a sudden illness or injury or after a prolonged, progressive illness. Among those with forewarning of death, some may steadily and predictably decline, whereas others may have fairly long periods of chronic illness with episodes of acute crises, one of which may prove fatal, although an entirely different problem may intervene to cause death.[48,63]

Palliative care is an important component of quality patient care and should be integrated along with life-sustaining therapy throughout a person's illness (Fig. 43.1). The goal of palliative care is to prevent and relieve suffering and support the best possible quality of life for patients and their families, regardless of the stage of the disease or the need for other therapies.[95] Palliative care interventions are used to relieve pain, dyspnea, and restlessness, and to facilitate the decision-making process while supporting patients and families. Palliative care expands traditional disease-model medical treatments and includes the goals of enhancing quality of life for patients and families, optimizing function, helping with decision making and providing opportunities for personal growth.[95] Refer to Box 43.1 for strategies for acute and critical care settings based on the National Consensus Guidelines.

At times it is clear to healthcare providers that patients will more than likely not survive their stay in critical care. However, at other times, predicting who will live and who will die is challenged by prognostic uncertainty. The Acute Physiology and Chronic Health Evaluation IV (APACHE IV) system, the Mortality Probability Admission Model-III (MPM-III), and the Simplified Acute Physiology Score 3 (SAP 3) are scoring systems used to measure the severity of illness.[57,75,146] Knowledge of the prognostic severity of illness score can be used by critical care providers as critical care survival predictions are made.[69]

END-OF-LIFE CONSIDERATIONS

Do Not Resuscitate Decisions

Do not resuscitate (DNR) or allow natural death (AND) decisions are commonly made in critical care. Usually resuscitation decisions occur as a patient is nearing death and are made within the overall context of goals of care and treatment. Patients and their families need accurate information about the patient's medical condition, prognosis, and what resuscitation is, in order to make informed decisions. Ideally, resuscitation decisions in critical care are made after the patient, family, and healthcare team discuss the possible need for cardiopulmonary resuscitation (CPR) and the use of further aggressive life-sustaining interventions (i.e., advanced cardiac life support). Before discussing resuscitation with the patient and family, the healthcare team should consider the following questions:

- What is the likelihood of the need for resuscitation?
- What is the potential success of resuscitation?
- What are the patient and family members' understandings of resuscitation?
- What does or would the patient want?

Defining Life-Sustaining Therapy

Life-sustaining therapy (LST) has been defined as encompassing "all healthcare interventions that have the effect of increasing the life span of the patient."[15,107] Examples of LST include CPR, mechanical ventilation, vasoactive agents, cardiac mechanical assist devices, renal replacement therapy, nutrition, hydration, antibiotics, and blood replacement products. Withholding LST involves deciding not to initiate treatment with the understanding that the patient will probably die without the treatment, whereas withdrawal of LST involves deciding to stop or remove treatment with the understanding that the patient will die following these actions.[15] Whether a treatment should be used depends on the balance of its usefulness or benefits for a particular patient and consideration of the burdens that the treatment would impose.[60] Technology should be used when necessary to accomplish goals of care; its use should be minimized when the primary goal is achievement of a peaceful death.[89]

Defining Death

The President's Commission for the Study of Ethical Problems in Medicine and Biomedical and Behavioral Research recommended that the Uniform Determination of Death Act (UDDA) serve as a model statute for state legislation defining death.[6] According to the UDDA, "an individual who has sustained either (1) irreversible cessation of circulatory and respiratory functions or (2) irreversible cessation of all functions of the entire brain, including the brain stem, is dead." In addition to clinical findings, "a determination of brain death always requires a formal apnea test; depending on the mechanism of injury, the determination of brain death may also involve corroborative evidence, such as a cerebral perfusion study or an electroencephalogram (EEG)."[105] Clinical findings in brain death include coma or

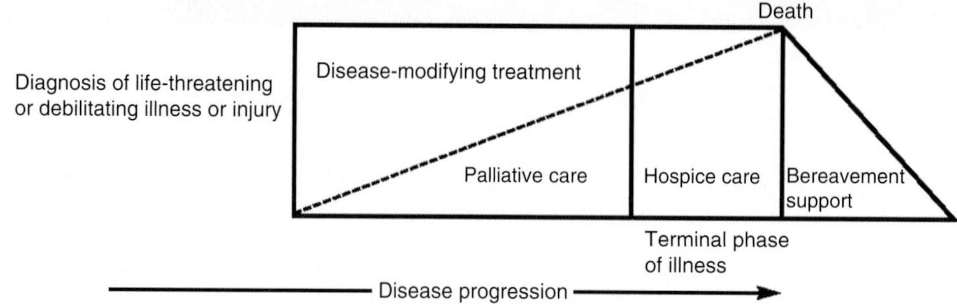

FIG. 43.1 Palliative care integrated with life-sustaining therapy throughout a person's illness trajectory. (From *A national framework and preferred practices for palliative and hospice care quality: a consensus report,* by the National Quality Forum, 2006 Washington, DC. Copyright 2015, National Quality Forum. Reproduced with Permission.)

BOX 43.1 Integration Strategies for Acute and Palliative Care

Clinical Practice Guidelines for Quality Palliative Care Critical Care Settings Based on the National Consensus Guidelines

Domain 1: Structure and Processes of Care

- An interprofessional team, including the patient and family, develops an overall plan of care.
- The plan of care is based on the identified and expressed values, goals, and needs of the patient and family and is developed with professional guidance and support for decision making.
- Critical care providers know both the patient's and the family's understandings of the patient's condition and prognosis.
- Treatment decisions are based on goals of care, assessment of risk and benefit, best evidence, and patient and family preferences.
- Hospital-based policies, procedures, and guidelines are related to palliative care.
- Quality improvement programs evaluating the effectiveness of palliative care are provided.
- Administration supports education and training regarding the integration of palliative care into critical care and is available to the interprofessional team.
- Relationships between palliative care and hospice services ensure continuity and the highest quality care across the illness trajectory.
- Resources are available to help the interprofessional team cope with the emotional impact of caring for dying patients and their families.

Domain 2: Physical Aspects of Care

- The interprofessional team is knowledgeable and skilled at efficiently and effectively preventing and managing potentially distressing symptoms.
- Pain, dyspnea, anxiety, agitation, and other signs and symptoms of discomfort are quickly assessed and managed.

Domain 3: Psychological and Psychiatric Aspects of Care

- Patients and families are assisted with psychological and psychiatric issues.
- Grief and bereavement services are offered to patients and families.
- Family members at risk for complicated grief and bereavement are referred to expert psychiatric practitioners.

Domain 4: Social Aspects of Care

- Family time together is encouraged.
- The healthcare team and the family meet regularly so that information can be shared, questions can be answered, and treatment goals can be discussed and reviewed.
- Discussions are focused on patient wishes and goals of care.
- Family meetings provide an opportunity to support the family and to facilitate the family decision-making process.

Domain 5: Spiritual, Religious, and Existential Aspects of Care

- The patient and family members' spiritual, religious, and existential concerns are assessed and addressed.
- Spiritual rituals are supported.
- Patients and families have access to pastoral care and to clergy of their own faith.

Domain 6: Cultural Aspects of Care

- Patient and family members' cultural concerns are assessed and addressed.
- Interpreter services facilitate communication among the patient, family, and the interprofessional healthcare team.
- Patient and family rituals are supported.

Domain 7: Care of the Imminently Dying Patient

- Signs and symptoms of impending death are recognized and communicated to the patient and family.
- Care during the active dying phase focuses on promotion of comfort and support of the patient and family.
- Patients die in the setting of their choice.

Domain 8: Ethical and Legal Aspects of Care

- Adults with decision-making capacity direct their course of treatment.
- Children with decision-making capacity are given appropriate weight in decision making.
- If patients do not have decision-making capacity, previously expressed wishes, values, and preferences guide the decision-making process.
- Consultants such as specialists in ethical and legal issues are available to help as needed.

Modified from a poster presented at the National Teaching Institute, May 2006, developed by P. Kalowes and D. Wiegand on behalf of AACN's Ethics Workgroup.

BOX 43.2 Checklist for Determination of Brain Death

Prerequisites (all must be checked)

- ☐ Coma, irreversible and cause known
- ☐ Neuroimaging explains coma
- ☐ CNS depressant drug effect absent (if indicated toxicology screen; if barbiturates given, serum level < 10 mcg/mL)
- ☐ No evidence of residual paralytics (electrical stimulation if paralytics used)
- ☐ Absence of severe acid-base, electrolyte, endocrine abnormality
- ☐ Normothermia or mild hypothermia (core temperature > 36°C)
- ☐ Systolic blood pressure ≥ 100 mm Hg
- ☐ No spontaneous respirations

Examination (all must be checked)

- ☐ Pupils nonreactive to bright light
- ☐ Corneal reflex absent
- ☐ Oculocephalic reflex absent (tested only if C-spine integrity ensured)
- ☐ Oculovestibular reflex absent
- ☐ No facial movement to noxious stimuli at supraorbital nerve, temporomandibular joint
- ☐ Gag reflex absent
- ☐ Cough reflex absent to tracheal suctioning
- ☐ Absence of motor response to noxious stimuli in all 4 limbs (spinally mediated reflexes are permissible)

Apnea Testing (all must be checked)

- ☐ Patient is hemodynamically stable
- ☐ Ventilator adjusted to provide normocarbia ($Paco_2$ 34–45 mm Hg)
- ☐ Patient preoxygenated with 100% Fio_2 for >10 minutes to Pao_2 >200 mm Hg
- ☐ Patient well-oxygenated with a PEEP of 5 cm of water
- ☐ Provide oxygen via a suction catheter to the level of the carina at 6 L/min or attach T-piece with CPAP at 10 cm H_2O
- ☐ Disconnect ventilator
- ☐ Spontaneous respirations absent
- ☐ Arterial blood gas drawn at 8–10 minutes, patient reconnected to ventilator
- ☐ Pco_2 ≥60 mm Hg, or 20 mm Hg rise from normal baseline value

OR:

- ☐ Apnea test aborted

Ancillary testing (only one needs to be performed; to be ordered only if clinical examination cannot be fully performed due to patient factors, or if apnea testing inconclusive or aborted)

- ☐ Cerebral angiogram
- ☐ HMPAO SPECT
- ☐ EEG
- ☐ TCD

Time of death (DD/MM/YY) ______________

Name of physician and signature ______________

CPAP, Continuous positive airway pressure; *EEG*, electroencephalogram; *Fio_2*, fraction of inspired oxygen; *HMPAO*, hexamethylpropyleneamine oxime; *H_2O*, water; *$Paco_2$*, partial pressure of carbon dioxide in arterial blood; *Pao_2*, partial pressure of arterial oxygen; *Pco_2*, partial pressure of carbon dioxide in the blood; *PEEP*, positive end-expiratory pressure; *SPECT*, single photon emission computed tomography; *TCD*, transcranial Doppler.

From Reference 145.

unresponsiveness, apnea, absence of cerebral motor responses to pain in all extremities, and absence of brain stem reflexes including pupillary signs, ocular movements, facial sensory and motor responses, and pharyngeal and tracheal reflexes.[21] State laws vary regarding requirements and criteria needed to determine brain death.[21,61,131] Refer to Box 43.2 for a checklist that can be used when determining brain death.[145]

Patients' families should be aware that brain death testing is being performed and must be informed as soon as brain death is determined. State laws vary with some states requiring that family members are informed of the intent to conduct brain death testing prior to initiating testing. When explaining brain death to families it is important to clearly and gently let them know that brain death is death, with no chance of recovery. Family members also should be told that their family member may have movements caused by activation of spinal motor neurons.[56,112] The family should be given the opportunity to notify additional family members and to say final goodbyes before removal of all treatments. The process is different from that of withdrawal of LST in that there is no decision for family members to make. If family members or surrogates do not understand the brain death declaration or need additional time, treatments may be continued for a limited time to help them accept their relative's death.[116,131]

Organ Donation

"Organ donation, with its ability to both improve the quality of life and potentially save lives, is a national healthcare priority."[39] The organ donation process is initiated when death is imminent. Many patients and families receive tremendous comfort knowing that they can help others through organ donation. All hospitals who receive Medicare and Medicaid reimbursement are required to determine if the patient or family would be willing to donate tissues or organs.[47] Every death or imminent death in a US hospital must be reported to an organ procurement organization (OPO) to meet the federal rules of the US Department of Health and Human Services.[54]

The OPO determines if the patient is an eligible donor. The OPO coordinator also assists with determining eligibility of a patient as a donor after cardiac death (non–heart beating organ donor). Donor criteria for non–heart beating organ donation include[22]:

- A patient is ventilator-dependent, does not meet brain death criteria, and decisions have been made to withdraw mechanical ventilation.
- Patient meets OPO designation for suitability for donation.
- Patient or surrogate has consented to donation.
- Cardiopulmonary death is likely to occur soon after withdrawal of mechanical support (i.e., less than 90 minutes); the time interval may vary according to the transplant surgical team and the organ.

First mention and decoupling are two concepts that are important components of the organ donation process.[108] First mention occurs when a healthcare provider brings to one's awareness the future possibility of donation. Decoupling refers to separating the end-of-life decision-making process from the organ donation process. Only the OPO coordinator or designated hospital requestor should approach the patient's family to discuss the patient or family's wishes concerning organ donation. If an organ donation decision is made, the entire process is coordinated by the OPO coordinator working collaboratively with the critical care team.

ETHICAL PALLIATIVE AND END-OF-LIFE CARE

Creating an ethical environment is important in the provision of quality palliative and end-of-life care. Related ethical considerations in critical care include a patient's right to self-determination, family advocacy and decision making, utility or benefit versus burden of therapy, medical futility, withholding and withdrawing LST, withdrawal of neuromuscular blockade, and the principle of double effect.

A Patient's Right to Self-Determination

Autonomy is an essential principle in decisions related to palliative care and end-of-life care. Autonomy is defined as the individual determining his or her course of action in accordance with a plan chosen by him or herself.[13] Respect for autonomy requires healthcare providers to obtain informed consent from patients before taking any action.[13] According to the President's Commission for the Study of Ethical Problems in Medicine and Biomedical and Behavioral Research,[107] the voluntary choice of a competent and informed patient should determine whether LST will be initiated, continued, or withdrawn, just as such choices provide the basis for other decisions about medical treatment.[107] Healthcare providers do not have the right to initiate and continue therapy that a patient does not desire.

Patients should be in control of all treatment decisions as long they have decision-making capacity. Lo suggests that the following criteria should be used when assessing decision-making capacity[81]:

- The patient can make and communicate decisions
- The patient is able to articulate an understanding of:
  - medical situation and prognosis
  - nature of the recommended care
  - alternative course of care
  - risks, benefits, and consequences of each alternative
- Decisions are consistent with known values and goals
- Patient uses reason to make choices

During admission to critical care, important information needs to be ascertained to determine if patients have made their treatment preferences known such as through a written advance directive. The Patient Self-Determination Act, part of the Omnibus Budget Reconciliation Act of 1990, was passed in an effort to encourage Americans to consider what they would and would not want toward life's end. It is estimated that less than 30% of Americans have completed an advance directive.[110,133] The advance directive may be in the form of a living will or a durable power of attorney for healthcare. If the patient has an advance directive, a copy of the document should be obtained and placed in the patient's chart. Hospitals often have a system in place for the patient's advance directive to automatically be placed in the front of the patient's medical records. Computerized patient health information systems have facilitated the process to retrieve advance directive information.

Many states have passed legislation regarding medical order sets, Medical Orders for Life-Sustaining Treatment (MOLST) or Physician/Provider Orders for Life-Sustaining Treatment (POLST). These portable medical orders were designed so that a patient's wishes would be honored regardless of setting.

The advance directive and MOLST/POLST documents should be reviewed with the patient to see if the information is current and accurate. Patients with decision-making capacity have the right to change their minds and should be encouraged to communicate changes in treatment preferences. Changes in treatment preferences can be communicated verbally or in writing.

Family Advocacy and Decision Making

Patients should be in control of all treatment decisions as long as they are able. Yet, at the end of life, patients frequently no longer have that capacity because of their illnesses, injuries, or treatments, and a surrogate decision maker is needed. If the patient has a written advance directive, the individual identified, who has durable power of attorney for healthcare (healthcare proxy), is the primary decision maker. All family members should be familiar with the designated healthcare proxy, and treatment decisions should be based on discussions the proxy has had with the patient.

If the patient does not have a living will and has not identified a durable power of attorney for healthcare, the family is turned to for input regarding the patient's desired wishes. Even though a written advance directive may not have been executed, patients have often had discussions with family members about what they would or would not want, should their sense of well-being or personhood be affected. The family in essence then provides substituted judgment, in which a designee makes a decision based on what decision the patient would make. If the family does not know what decision the patient would make, the family provides a best interest decision, based on what they think the patient would want.

If a patient is unable to participate in the decision-making process and has not previously identified a surrogate decision-maker, state laws and regulations should be followed to identify a decision maker. Typically, there is a tiered system with the spouse first, followed by adult children, parents, siblings, and others.

Treatment discussions should always focus on what goals of care the patient would want. Conversations using words such as, "If your mother could talk to us, what would she tell us?" should be asked. It is of utmost importance that the surrogate or family speaks from the patient's perspective, not from the perspective of the family members.

Families have found advance directives helpful when making decisions related to life-sustaining therapies.[50,66,84,88,99,120,126,127] Tilden et al. reported that written advance directives were most helpful to families making end-of-life decisions.[127]

Benefit Versus Burden of Therapy

Historically, treatments were discussed as if they were ordinary or extraordinary. Both the President's Commission for the Study of Ethical Problems in Medicine and Biomedical and Behavioral Research[107] and the Guidelines on the Termination of Life-Sustaining Treatment and the Care Near the End of Life recommended that all treatments, including nutrition, ventilation, dialysis, and others, should be determined based on the potential benefits versus burdens to the patient.[15,121]

Determination of benefit versus burden is not a unilateral decision. It is essential that the patient (if able to participate in decision making), the surrogate or family, and the healthcare providers discuss the utility of treatments. Instrumental to these discussions are patient values, advance directives, and choices. Furthermore, Sulmasy et al. distinguish between benefit and effectiveness of interventions.[118] They state that effectiveness relates to the impact of the intervention on the biomedical good of the patient and is an objective determination made by the healthcare team, whereas benefit is much broader, encompassing any positive change in the patient condition (as the patient perceives it); it is a subjective determination.[118] Whether a treatment is warranted depends on the balance of its usefulness or benefits for a particular patient and consideration of the burdens that the treatment would impose.[60]

Medical Futility

Medical futility is a complex issue that often arises in critical care. Medical futility is defined as "any clinical circumstance in which physicians and their consultants, consistent with the available medical literature, conclude that further treatment (except comfort care) cannot, within a reasonable possibility, cure, ameliorate, improve or restore a quality of life that would be satisfactory to the patient."[62] Another definition, suggested by Luce, is that treatment is considered futile when a patient cannot benefit from treatment, the patient's acute disorder is not reversible, it is projected that the patient will not survive the current hospitalization, or the quality of the patient's life following discharge will be poor.[83] Prendergast notes that there is no consensus definition of medical futility.[104]

Futility decisions come into play as goals of care increasingly become unachievable. As noted by Jecker, "Refraining from medically futile interventions is often the best way to care humanely for patients at the end of life."[68] The realization of medical futility is usually a process that evolves over time. It is important that the family is involved in the process. The family should be informed as soon as the interprofessional team determines medical futility. On occasion, the family is not in agreement with the medical team's determination of futility and recommendations regarding patient care.[67] Futility guidelines may serve to help with these situations.[129] Guidelines include information related to the process for conflict resolution and may help all involved reach a compromise. Resources such as the palliative care team and the ethics committee may be helpful with these complex situations.

Withholding and Withdrawing Life-Sustaining Therapy

The President's Commission for the Study of Ethical Problems in Medicine and Biomedical and Behavioral Research provided essential direction for healthcare providers by stating that there is no moral difference between withholding and withdrawing LST.[107] Additional experts and professional associations agree that there is no moral difference between withholding and withdrawing LST.[3,15,18,60,122]

The fundamental issue involved with both withholding and withdrawing is the efficacious use of the treatment and the patient's desire for the treatment. Each individual has the right to accept or refuse any treatment, including LST. There is no difference between deciding not to start a treatment or in deciding to stop a treatment. Consideration is given to the individual's desire for the treatment and the intended purpose of the treatment.

Time-limited interventions, especially in the face of uncertainty, can be trialed, in conjunction with palliative care interventions. Often a trial of treatment may be initiated for a patient with a plan for reevaluation and withdrawal of the treatment if it does not prove effective. From an ethical perspective, erring on the side of LST is a greater good than erring on the side of too little treatment or treatment that is withdrawn too quickly.[114] It is important to know that LSTs (i.e., intubation and ventilation) can be tried, but if they prove to be ineffective, they can be withdrawn. Thus if the appropriateness of LST is unclear, it should be initiated with the knowledge that if it proves to be futile, not beneficial, or disproportionately burdensome, it can later be stopped.[114]

Despite being ethically acceptable to withhold or withdraw LST, from a practical perspective it feels different to withhold it versus to withdraw it. Deciding not to start CPR if a patient's heart stops feels different than actually stopping mechanical ventilations and extubating a patient.[144] Withholding CPR is a passive process or natural process, whereas removing mechanical ventilation and extubating a patient is an active process.[144] End-of-life decisions are often made as a two-step process with decisions to withhold LST preceding decisions to withdraw LST.[139]

Neuromuscular Blockade

Neuromuscular blockade should play no role in the care of patients for whom LST is withheld or withdrawn. Neuromuscular-blocking agents should be discontinued and time allowed for their clearance from the body before withholding or withdrawing therapy. If a neuromuscular-blocking medication is infusing, the patient would not be able to exert any respiratory effort and may experience respiratory distress, anxiety, and pain that would not be able to be detected.

Healthcare providers have reported withdrawing LST from patients receiving paralytics.[45] "The use of paralytics in dying patients is disturbing as it is difficult, if not impossible, to adequately assess the comfort of patients who are paralyzed and a paralyzed patient, unable to exert respiratory effort, cannot compensate for hypoxia resulting from either terminal weaning or extubation, and while appearing comfortable, may experience respiratory distress or severe anxiety."[45] The use of paralytics compromises the ability to monitor a patient for distress, eliminates opportunities for patient and family interaction, and guarantees patient death.[26]

The Principle of Double Effect

The principle of double effect, sometimes referred to as the rule of double effect, is often invoked to justify claims that a single act having two foreseen effects, one good and one harmful, is not always morally prohibited if the harmful effect is not intended.[13] The principle of double effect is an issue that may arise when providing care to dying patients. For example, pain medication is usually titrated to promote comfort. A secondary effect of the pain medication may be a decrease in blood pressure or respiratory rate. During end-of-life care, nurses and providers administer pain medication to decrease discomfort; thus it is viewed as a beneficent act, even though death may be perceived as hastened. This double effect is recognized as ethically justified by ethicists and professional standards of care.[3,15] The US Supreme Court has also upheld the principle of double effect by supporting dying patients who obtain palliative care, where in some cases administration of analgesics may hasten death.[119]

PALLIATIVE SYMPTOM MANAGEMENT

Many seriously ill patients experience distressing symptoms. Family members from the Study to Understand Prognoses and Preferences for Outcomes and Risks of Treatments (SUPPORT) and the Hospitalized Elderly Longitudinal Project (HELP) studies reported that during the last 3 days of their lives, almost 40% of patients had severe pain, more than 50% of patients had severe dyspnea (excluding patients with colon cancer), and approximately 25% of patients had severe confusion.[87] In a study conducted by Tolle et al., family members reported that 34% of dying patients were in moderate to severe pain during the last week of life.[128] More specific data from this study demonstrated that more hospitalized patients experienced moderate to severe

TABLE 43.1 **Opioid Analgesics**

	Equivalent Dose (IV)*	Onset to Peak Effect (mins)	Duration of Effect (hrs)	Typical Adult Dose (IV)	Typical Infusion Rate
Morphine	10 mg	20–30	3–4	2–10 mg	0.05–0.5 mg/kg/h
Fentanyl	100 mcg	2–5	0.5–2	0.5–2 mcg/kg	0.5–10 mcg/kg/h
Hydromorphone	1.5–2 mg	20–30	3–4	0.5–2 mg	—

*Equivalent doses are approximations and are of limited value due to differences in onset and duration of effect.
IV, Intravenous.
Adapted from Reference 131.

pain during the final week of life (44%) as compared to individuals dying at home (34%) or dying in a nursing home (27%).[128] In a national study conducted by Puntillo et al., the majority of critical care nurses (78%) responded that in the unit where they worked, dying patients frequently (31%) or sometimes (47%) received inadequate pain medication.[109]

Managing symptoms is of primary importance in an effort to promote quality living to the very end and to promote peace and comfort during the dying process. Medications are administered and titrated to relieve symptoms. Anticipatory dosing is important. Anticipatory dosing refers to the initiation of medications in order to minimize symptoms that commonly occur at the end of life before the symptom is reported or displayed. If patients are already receiving continuous infusions of analgesics or sedatives (e.g., morphine, lorazepam [Ativan]), those medications are titrated to effect with consideration that patients may build up a tolerance, thus requiring higher doses.

Pain

Pain is an unpleasant sensory and emotional experience associated with actual or potential tissue damage, or described in terms of such damage. It is important to administer medications in anticipation of the possibility of pain and discomfort and titrate medications to effect. Pain can usually readily be assessed in an alert patient by using a numeric pain scale (0 to 10). Assessment of pain in the cognitively impaired or unconscious dying patient is more complex. Behavioral indicators such as agitation, restlessness, posturing, and facial expression, as well as physiologic indicators including tachycardia, hypertension, tachypnea, diaphoresis, and mydriasis, may indicate pain.[94] Instruments that can be used to assess pain in patients who cannot communicate pain include the Behavior Pain Scale[103] and the Critical Care Pain Observation Tool.[49]

Early, accurate detection of pain and quick management are essential.[25,41,42,92,137] A low-dose analgesic infusion can be administered to achieve patient comfort. Analgesic medications may include morphine, hydromorphone (Dilaudid), and fentanyl (Duragesic). The use of opioid analgesics is presented in Table 43.1. Opiates are preferred based on potency, lack of a ceiling effect, and their concomitant mild sedative and anxiolytic properties.[94] Morphine is most commonly given intravenously as a continuous infusion. Morphine produces analgesia and often sedation; its half-life is 3 to 4 hours. Hydromorphone is a synthetic highly soluble opioid; its half-life (2 to 3 hours) is a little shorter than that of morphine. Another synthetic opioid analgesic is fentanyl, a potent synthetic opiate with a short half-life of 1 to 2 hours.

The dose of the infusion can be increased based on signs and symptoms of pain. A low and slow titration is recommended.[25] There are no maximum doses. Increasing bolus doses by 50% to 100% and continuously monitoring for therapeutic effect is important.[25] At times two different medications may be needed to achieve patient comfort. Furthermore, there are a number of adjuvant analgesics that maximize patient comfort and distress, such as anticonvulsants, antidepressants, corticosteroids, local anesthetics, and even baclofen (Lioresal), which helps relieve spasm-associated pain.[7] Clinical pharmacists, pain, and palliative care specialists are invaluable resources and can assist in managing pain.

Promoting comfort during the dying process is essential. It is important to ensure that the patient is in a comfortable position and is repositioned as needed to maintain comfort. Skin and mouth care, massage, hot and cold therapies including cool moist towels, fans, and warm compresses may promote comfort. Management of a fever with antipyretics also may be comforting.

The titration of analgesia for the cognitively impaired or unconscious dying patient is best guided by careful assessment and observation. According to Rubenfeld, "Unconscious patients, by definition, cannot perceive pain and therefore may not require sedation or analgesia."[113] He also comments that "patients with diminished levels of consciousness also may not be able to manifest signs of discomfort."[113] However, despite this uncertainty, it is ethical to err on the side of administering analgesia and sedation in an attempt to promote comfort rather than not treat patient distress.

Dyspnea

Dyspnea is a subjective experience of breathing discomfort.[101] Alert patients can be asked to rate their perception of dyspnea, using a numeric scale (0 to 100) as a guide. Dyspnea in the cognitively impaired or unconscious patient can be assessed by observing the patient's respiratory rate, pattern, and use of accessory muscles, and by an auditory assessment of airway noises. Behavioral and physiologic indicators of respiratory distress may include tachycardia, tachypnea, use of accessory muscles, nasal flaring, paradoxical breathing pattern, fearful facial expression, grunting at end-expiration, and restlessness.[23] The Respiratory Distress Observation Scale is an instrument that can be used to assess patients who cannot self-report dyspnea.[28]

Dyspnea may occur during the dying process, or during or after withdrawal of LST. Prevention and quick relief of dyspnea are essential. Breathing changes at the end of life may include an increase or decrease in respiratory rate, an increase in respiratory secretions, an increase in airway noises, and changes in breathing patterns. An increase in the respiratory rate may occur as the body attempts to meet oxygen demands. A decrease in respiratory rate may result from the dying process. An increase in respiratory secretions may occur due to underlying pulmonary disease or may occur due to decreased contractility of the heart, resulting in a backup of fluid to the lungs. Airway noise may occur as muscles in the neck relax. Changes in a patient's breathing pattern may occur due to the dying process.

TABLE 43.2 **Sedative Agents**

	Onset to Peak Effect (min)	Duration of Effect (h)	Typical Initial Adult Dose (IV)	Typical Initial Infusion Dose (Adult)	Typical Initial Infusion Dose (Pediatric)
Sedatives					
Lorazepam	20–25	2–4	1–3 mg	0.5–4 mg/h	0.05–0.1 mg/kg/h
Midazolam	5–10	1.5–2	0.02–0.1 mg/kg	1–5 mg/h	0.05–0.1 mg/kg/h
Propofol	1–2	0.1–0.4	1 mg/kg	10–50 mcg/kg/h	10–50 mcg/kg/h
Neuroleptics					
Haloperidol	25–30	2–4	0.5–20 mg	3–5 mg/h	—

IV, Intravenous.
Adapted from Reference 131.

Preventing and managing dyspnea are important. Initiating an analgesic infusion (i.e., morphine) will physiologically promote pulmonary venodilation and may facilitate breathing at the end of life. An initial dose of morphine in a naïve patient to treat dyspnea is 2 mg intravenously and then slowly titrate as needed.[25] Reducing intravenous fluids, administering diuretics, and administrating anticholinergic medications will decrease pulmonary secretions. Bronchodilators and benzodiazepines may also be effective in relieving dyspnea. Ensure that the patient is in a comfortable position, with the head of the bed slightly elevated. Secretions may pool in the pharynx but can easily be suctioned to promote comfort. Oxygen use needs to be assessed on an individual basis.[17,20] Oxygen is not needed for patients who are actively dying and have no signs of respiratory distress.[29]

Anxiety

Anxiety is a subjective feeling of apprehension, tension, insecurity, and uneasiness.[44] An alert patient should be asked to rate anxiety as mild, moderate, or severe. Anxiety is difficult to assess in the cognitively impaired and may not be present in the unconscious patient. Behaviors associated with anxiety include restlessness, trembling, cold hands, diaphoresis, tachycardia, and hyperventilation.[25,44]

Support should be provided to the greatest extent possible. Involvement of the family and other members of the healthcare team can provide additional patient support. Sedatives can be started and titrated as needed. Refer to Table 43.2 for recommended sedative doses. Benzodiazepines (lorazepam, midazolam [Versed]) are commonly used to relieve anxiety. Tolerance can develop after several days; therefore, an increase in dosage may be needed to maintain symptom control.

Palliative sedation is defined as sedating a patient to the point of unconsciousness.[132] The intent of palliative sedation is to relieve suffering in dying patients.[60] Palliative sedation is indicated when distressing symptoms (e.g., hallucinations, severe pain, etc.) cannot be managed with traditional pharmacologic agents. Continuous infusions of benzodiazepines are most commonly used for palliative sedation. Sometimes a barbiturate may be added if the patient continues to experience distressing symptoms despite the continuous infusion of a benzodiazepine. Patients may still be aware of their environment while receiving palliative sedation; therefore, communication with the patient and support is important. In addition, analgesic and sedative infusions for managing pain and anxiety are essential.

Delirium, Agitation, and Confusion

Dying patients may develop delirium, agitation, and confusion. Patients with delirium manifest a disturbance of consciousness characterized by an acute onset and fluctuating courses of impaired cognitive function so that their ability to receive, process, store, and recall information is impaired.[74] Patients with delirium may experience disorientation, distorted sensations, hallucinations, illusions, and delusions. The Confusion Assessment Method for the intensive care unit (CAM-ICU)[43] and the Intensive Care Delirium Screening Checklist[14] can be used to assess delirium. Delirium may be accompanied by agitation and confusion.

Neuroleptic medications (i.e., haloperidol [Haldol]) have proven efficacy in the management of delirium.[82,131] Propofol (Diprivan) is a sedative and anesthetic medication that also can be considered. Table 43.2 includes recommended doses. As mentioned previously, barbiturates can be administered if other medications are ineffective.

Patients at end-of-life experience a multiplicity of symptoms and syndromes, regardless of their underlying medical condition. Pain is the most obvious example, but others include dyspnea, anxiety, agitation, confusion, and delirium. Taken together, these and other symptoms add significantly to the suffering of patients and their families but can be treated or prevented if recognized early. Hence, it is important for critical care clinicians to assess and manage the symptoms that are known to occur in dying patients in order to facilitate a peaceful and good death for patients and families.

CARING FOR AND SUPPORTING FAMILIES

Good communication is important between members of the interprofessional team and between the team and families. The President's Commission for the Study of Ethical Problems in Medicine and Biomedical and Behavioral Research identifies each patient's family as the best advocate for patients. Family members need to arrive at important patient decisions in collaboration with providers and other healthcare professionals.[107]

Patients, Families, and the Healthcare Team

Patients and families need information and support as they travel the end-of-life course. A consistent member of the healthcare team should be identified and be responsible for keeping the family informed.[98,141] It is important that members of the healthcare team are united and are communicating the same information.[16] Open communication is essential among the patient, family, and the interprofessional team.[2,9,12,35,51,79,80,93,98,99,116,140,142] As Levy notes, it is important that healthcare providers "communicate in an open, genuine manner about the truth of a patient's illness."[78]

Healthcare providers hold a key role in "planting seeds" by helping the patient and family understand the possibility that the patient might not survive.[97] Norton and Bowers also note the importance of the team presenting information together as a united group.[97] Family members need information that will help them to understand the patient's condition and prefer if healthcare providers are open, direct, honest, and realistic, even if prognosis is poor.[2,127,142] Treatment options should be discussed and the primary spokesperson for the interprofessional team should recommend a treatment option and explain the rationale behind the option. When discussing treatment options, it is important to focus on goals of treatment. Avoid directly asking family members, "What do you want us to do?" Instead consider, "Based on Mr. Lee's condition, and what you have told me about your father, I think we should consider this. What do you think?" Once a decision has been made, ask, "Do you think this is what your father would want?"

It often takes time for the patient's surrogate or family members to understand the information provided. As discussions progress, continue to keep the conversations focused on what the patient would want. Together with the surrogate or family determine a plan as well as a follow-up plan. If time permits (this depends on the severity of the patient's illness or injury) a gradual approach should be considered. This helps to avoid providing too much information or overwhelming the family.

Families often struggle with concern that they are doing the right thing. Healthcare providers can help families through shared decision making.[10,93,116,134,142] Shared decision making is a dynamic process with the responsibility for medical decisions shared between the patient or surrogate and the healthcare team.[116]

Tilden et al. found that when decisions were made related to withdraw of LST, family members tended to move through four phases that include (1) recognition of futility, (2) coming to terms, (3) shouldering the surrogate role, and (4) facing the question.[127] Family members usually came to terms when they realized that the ongoing medical treatments contributed to suffering.[127]

Families have reported frustrations related to the inability to interact enough with their family member's provider.[1,98,141] Nurses are uniquely positioned to promote family-centered care and to facilitate family and provider/healthcare team communication. Families need to be "aware of the possibility of death even as they are supported in their hope of recovery."[106] The healthcare team can help family members redirect their hope, moving from hoping for recovery to hoping for a comfortable death with as much dignity and meaning as possible.[2,12,36,97] Refer to Box 43.3 for strategies that can be used to improve family-centered end-of-life care in critical care.[142]

BOX 43.3 Strategies to Improve End-of-Life Care for Families in the ICU

1. Get to know the family
2. Assess the family's understanding of the patient's condition
3. Keep the family informed
4. Provide clear, honest information to the family
5. Maintain consistency of care providers
6. Coordinate early family meetings
7. Facilitate the decision-making process
8. Assist the family through shared decision making
9. Guide the family through the EOL process
10. Prepare the family for what to expect during the dying process

From Reference 142.

Conflict Within the Healthcare Team

Conflict may occur between members of the healthcare team. Team members may have different perspectives and expectations.[19,46,51] Conflicts may occur between providers, between nurses, and between providers and nurses and may be due to mistrust and poor communication.[8]

Prevention of conflict and developing mechanisms to facilitate conflict management is important. Team members need basic and ongoing education focused on palliative and end-of-life care, communication, and conflict management. Regular interprofessional forums, routine unit-level meetings, and the use of a daily goals sheet are strategies that may improve team communication.[11,51] In addition, ethics committees may be consulted for help in resolving conflict within the team.

Healthcare Provider Conflict with Family Choices

Healthcare providers do not always agree with family choices. Conflict often arises between family members and healthcare providers.[1,11,115] The values of healthcare providers may conflict with the values of the surrogate decision maker or the family. Acknowledgment of the value differences and maintaining open dialog with the family are important. Conflict can be constructive, uncovering differences in values and legitimate concerns that have been inadequately discussed.[136]

Disagreements may be effectively handled by negotiating with the family and the healthcare provider and at times by agreeing to a time-limited trial of therapy.[104] Consistently keeping discussions focused on patient preferences for treatment may be helpful. Palliative care experts, pastoral care, or ethics consultations can be extremely helpful to families and staff during these difficult situations.

Family Conflict

Conflict may also occur between patients and their family members. Koch et al. found that when the patient and family disagreed on medical treatment goals it was helpful for the provider to discuss the issue with the patient in the presence of the family in an effort to resolve conflict.[73] The capable patient's opinion always takes precedence over the opinion of the family. Some families may believe that the patient will not be able to cope with bad news or will not be able to participate in goals of care discussions, but the team needs to provide the patient with information and include him or her in treatment discussions.

Conflict can also occur between family members. Families or individual family members may not initially want to honor a patient's known wishes.[31] Although they have the patient's best interest at heart, they may be influenced by their own need to prolong the patient's life.[65]

Families may be too distressed or embarrassed to discuss dissention and hostility that exists within their family unit.[51,125] Some family members may want treatments continued, whereas others may not. It often takes time for families to reach consensus.[139] It is important to have early, frequent and open discussions with the family. Nurses can assess if conflict exists within the family and work with the family and the healthcare team to support and help families to resolve conflict.[51]

Family Meetings

Family meetings offer an opportunity for open dialog between the patient (if possible), the family, and the healthcare team. Family meetings should be set up in advance so that all key family members can be there. In addition, all key members of the interprofessional team should be present (primary nurse, physician, advance practice nurse, chaplain, social worker, member[s] of the palliative care team, etc.).

It is often a good idea for the members of the interprofessional team to meet briefly before the family meeting. This preconference provides time to discuss the purpose of the meeting, what will be discussed, who will facilitate the meeting, and share perspectives privately.

The critical care nurse or the social worker usually works with the patient's family and provider to coordinate a date and time for the meeting. The critical care nurse usually determines a location close to the critical care unit, usually a private room, with enough chairs for everyone to sit. It is important to make sure that everyone has their pagers and cell phones turned off. Healthcare providers (nurses, physicians, etc.) should prearrange for coverage by other members of the healthcare team so that the team's attention and time can focus on the meeting.

Usually the attending physician, intensivist, or advance practice nurse facilitates the meeting. Although residents may attend, they should not be responsible for facilitating a family meeting.[78] Family meetings should start by asking everyone to introduce themselves. The facilitator should review the purpose of the meeting. The family is asked about their understanding of their family member's condition. This offers an opportunity for the healthcare team members to clarify any misperceptions.

It is important to clarify patient wishes or anticipated wishes. Questions can be asked about the patient's values and preferences for healthcare. The family may give a good sense of what the patient was like and what things he or she enjoyed doing, and has the best sense of what the patient would want done. Families can be asked, "If your family member could speak to everyone right now, how would he or she guide us in our decision making?"[76]

McDonagh et al. studied family meetings and found that providers spoke 70% of the time and spent 30% of the time listening to families.[91] The researchers recommended giving families plenty of opportunity to talk during the meeting because the more time they had to speak, the more satisfied they were with the meeting. Family members should be asked to share their concerns and to ask questions.

At the end of the meeting, it is important to discuss what will likely happen next. The follow-up plan should include when the meeting facilitator or team will meet with the patient or family again and provide information as to how the patient or family can reach the facilitator if questions arise before the next meeting. It is also important that what happened at the family meeting is documented.

Family meetings should be held early in a patient's critical care stay.[38,142] Lilly found that early family meetings (held within 72 hours of patient admission to critical care) were effective in increasing family and healthcare provider consensus related to goals of patient care and early access to palliative care.[79] Early discussions of goals of care resulted in less CPR and decreased time from critical care admission to withdrawal of LST when death was determined to be inevitable.[52] Azoulay and Sprung recommended that "there should be a continuum of early information provision supplemented by intermittent family conferences when critical 'change in direction' decisions need to be made."[10]

PREPARING FOR THE END-OF-LIFE

Preparing for a patient's end-of-life is best done with thoughtful preparation. Preparation for the end-of-life begins as soon as goals of care transition from aggressive life-prolonging treatment to comfort care. At times, families need to be prepared quickly (as soon as it is clear to the interprofessional team) that a patient is actively dying despite continued aggressive interventions.[142] Particular attention should be given to the environment, the patient, and the patient's family. An important goal is to achieve the best possible death for the patient and the most compassionate care possible for the patient and family.[98,111,143]

Preparing the Environment

Ideally patients should die in a location of their choice. Most patients die in critical care; however, on occasion, arrangements can be made for a patient to die at home with the support of hospice services. Every effort should be made to honor this if requested. Someone from the palliative care team, social worker, or case manager can help with arranging patient transportation and coordinating care with the local hospice agency.

If possible, patients should die in the same setting where care was provided. Families prefer consistency in healthcare providers during the dying process.[141] Preparing for family privacy is important. Priority should be given to full access for family members to be with the patient. Prepare the room so that there are plenty of chairs for family members. Try to create a peaceful environment.

Preparing the Patient

Patients should be asked if they have any requests, which should be honored to the greatest extent possible. During the dying process comfort is the primary focus.

Patients should be clean and comfortable. Unnecessary tubes should be removed. The patient's bed should be lowered and at a minimum the bottom side rails should be lowered. Nonessential monitors and equipment should be removed from the room. Unnecessary catheters and tubes should be removed. All alarms should be shut off. Ensure that devices including implantable cardioverter defibrillators (ICDs) are inactivated. Planning ahead is essential as special equipment may be needed (i.e., a programmer to deactivate an ICD).

Assist as needed to arrange for the hospital chaplain or the patient's clergy to have a final opportunity for a visit and prayers. Also ensure that cultural and religious end-of-life practices are honored.

Preventing and Managing Distressing Symptoms

Critical care nurses administer and titrate analgesics, sedatives, and other medications prescribed to promote comfort. Anticipatory dosing of medications is essential. According to Truog et al., "As a general rule, any time an increase in an infusion dose is being considered due to reemergence of the signs or symptoms of suffering, intravenous bolus doses should be administered concurrently to achieve a rapid response."[131] The medications most commonly used to prevent and manage discomfort are opioids. A sedative is commonly initiated at the same time as an analgesic infusion. Refer to Tables 43.1 and 43.2.

The specific dose needed to relieve discomfort is unpredictable. Infusions are recommended because they are easier to manage and have the advantage of maintaining a steady level of medication. There is no maximum dose of opioids or sedatives.[89,131]

If a patient is receiving a neuromuscular-blocking agent it should be withdrawn before withdrawal of LST. A neuromuscular-blocking agent makes it impossible to assess patient discomfort.[24,89]

Critical care nurses and providers are sometimes uncomfortable titrating analgesics and sedatives at the end of life as they worry that increasing doses of these medications may hasten the patient's death. However, there is no evidence to support that analgesics and sedative hasten death.[24,102,131]

Preparing the Family

Education and support should be provided that focuses on the goal of providing comfort and reducing suffering. Reinforce that the dying process is unpredictable and varies greatly. Explain that the dying process may take minutes to hours to days.[102,143] If families do not want to be at the hospital during the dying process, set up a communication mechanism for keeping them informed. Families need to be prepared for what will happen to the patient, including changes in level of consciousness, breathing pattern, breathing sounds, coloration, changes in skin temperature, restlessness, and possible reflexive movement of the patient's arms or legs.[16,37,40,58,70,89,94,117,143]

The family may want to have children, extended family, and friends say final goodbyes. Prepare the children for what they will see. A pediatric clinical nurse specialist, child life specialist, palliative care specialist, or bereavement specialist may be a helpful resource in preparing children for visitation. Family members may even want the opportunity for visitation by a family pet. This process should be facilitated for the family if desired.

The family should be asked if they would like to participate in a final bath, massage, or rubbing lotion on the patient. They may want special music playing in the room. Let family members know they can talk, sing, read prayers, or tell their loved ones stories. Families should have unrestricted presence at the bedside. Ensure that plenty of tissues are in the patient's room. If space is available, designate an area for families to go to should they need a break or privacy.

Critical care nurses are well aware of the paramount role they hold in care of the dying: "We're with people in the most traumatic, beautiful, horrendous experiences in their lives but you can make a difference in someone's death."[4] How a person dies has a lasting memory for family and friends. As a critical care nurse described, "I know that's what they're going to remember. They're going to remember a lot about it for the rest of their lives and it's going to be really important."[4]

Preparing the Family for Withdrawal of Life-Sustaining Therapy

Critical care nurses play a pivotal role coordinating the withdrawal of the LST process. The patient's nurse can work with the family to determine the day and time that LST will be withdrawn. Once the day and time are determined, plans can be made by both the family and the healthcare team.[142] Families should be told what treatments will be stopped and how the patient will be prepared.

Families often want to wait for key family members to travel from out of town for final visits. Families may want to delay withdrawal of LST by a day or two to avoid a special anniversary, birthday, or holiday.

The critical care nurse should ask family members if they would like to be in the room when LSTs are discontinued or if they would like to come into the room immediately afterward. Family members may want to wait in the waiting room, a designated family room, or outside the patient's room. On occasion, family members want to be at the bedside; in this case, prepare them for what they might expect. Patients may gasp immediately after the endotracheal tube is removed. Assure the family that any signs of discomfort will be quickly treated. Families should be told that after LST is withdrawn, death is expected but not certain.[37,89,100,102,136,138] Some patients may die quickly (within minutes) and others may die gradually with the dying process extending for days.[30,71,140,141] Inform families that medications will be given to promote comfort.

CARE DURING THE DYING PROCESS

The patient and family may have preferences regarding which healthcare team members are present during the dying process. Nurses, providers, clergy, and other members of the healthcare team should do their best to honor patient and family wishes. Family end-of-life cultural and spiritual preferences should be respected.

If possible, avoid transferring dying patients from critical care. Families have reported feeling abandoned when their dying family member was transferred.[141] Throughout the dying process, the patient and family need to be assured that they will not be abandoned. The dying patient and the family need the utmost care and support throughout the process.

The critical care nurse plays an important role during active dying. The patient should be assessed frequently for signs or symptoms of pain, discomfort, or distressing symptoms. If symptoms develop, they should be treated quickly so that patient comfort is promoted. When this goal is achieved, further increases in sedation or analgesia are unnecessary and ethically problematic.[113]

Critical care nurses have reported that patients have a better quality of dying if they do not die alone.[10,59] Heyland et al. studied family members' satisfaction with care provided to dying patients in critical care.[55] Ninety-one percent of family members reported that the patient was comfortable in the final hours of life. The majority of family members (88%) also felt supported by the healthcare team. Levy et al. studied family members of patients who died in critical care and reported that pain was managed most or all of the time for 88% of patients, and 79% of patients died with dignity.[77,78]

BEREAVEMENT

Grief is a process that begins before the patient dies, continues after the loss, and is unpredictable. The combination of shock, grief, uncertainty, stress, and confusion may lead to varying emotional responses by family members.[71] How critical care nurses help families accept the death of a family member and deal with the initial stages of grief may influence their subsequent experience.[90] Critical care nurses should use available resources including pastoral care, palliative care, and bereavement specialists to help families.

Families should be sent home with information on how to access bereavement support services.[64] They also should be offered the opportunity to meet with a hospital provider, nurse, social worker, or clergy for a follow-up discussion.[32]

Consider sending condolence cards, conducting follow-up family telephone calls, and inviting family members to hospital memorial services. Family members have reported that it meant a lot to them to receive telephone calls and cards from hospital staff after the death of their loved one.[135] They were also helped by support they received by their pastor, family, and friends.[135]

END-OF-LIFE AND THE CRITICAL CARE NURSE

Providing quality palliative care and end-of-life care can be emotionally rewarding and draining. It is important that the members of the interprofessional team support each other by acknowledging and supporting the care provided. Time off, even if it is just for a short break, is important after providing care to a dying patient and his or her family. Taking time with other colleagues to discuss experiences can be invaluable. Memorial services can help critical care nurses and other members of the interprofessional team find important closure in end-of-life care. Bereavement specialists can provide needed support to the critical care team.

Professional resources are available to assist critical care nurses in providing quality, ethical palliative care and end-of-life care (Box 43.4). These resources can be used to develop hospital-based palliative and end-of-life care guidelines. Treece et al. found that a standardized order form for withdrawal of LST was helpful for critical care nurses and providers.[130] Protocols and guidelines can help guide palliative and end-of-life care.[27,33,53]

Palliative care specialists can also help to provide quality palliative and end-of-life care. In addition, ethics experts can assist with challenging end-of-life ethical dilemmas. Ethics committees can be consulted by the patient, family, or any member of the healthcare team if there are conflicts or dilemmas that need to be discussed.

BOX 43.4 Palliative Care and End-of-Life Resources

American Association of Critical-Care Nurses

http://www.aacn.org

AACN Protocol for Practice: Palliative Care and End-of-Life Issues in Critical Care, 2006

Resources for Palliative/End of Life

Promoting Excellence in Palliative and End-of-Life Care, 2015

American Nurses Association

http://www.ana.org

Position Statement: Nursing Care and Do-Not-Resuscitate (DNR) and Allow Natural Death (AND) Decisions

Position Statement: Forgoing Nutrition and Hydration

Position Statement: Euthanasia, Assisted Suicide and Aid in Dying

Hospice and Palliative Nurses Association

http://www.hpna.org

Position Statement: Palliative Sedation

Position Statement: The Ethics of Opioid Use at End-of-Life

Position Statement: Withholding and/or Withdrawing Life-Sustaining Therapies

American Association of Colleges of Nursing

http://www.aacn.nche.edu/elnec

End-of-Life Nursing Education Consortium (ELNEC) Project: Advancing End-of-Life Nursing Care

CONCLUSION

A good or painless death has been a major human concern throughout history.[124] The availability of the critical care nurse "to assess symptoms, administer medications, and provide other forms of support and comfort may be the single most important component of effective palliative care for a critically ill patient."[96] Critical care nurses have described good end-of-life care as having the following characteristics:

- Patient comfort and dignity is maintained
- Family members
  - are involved
  - are given time to go through the grieving process
  - are given opportunities for family rituals and goodbyes.[72]

As Nelson and Danis reported, "At one time, critical care and palliative care may have seemed to be inherently inconsistent. End-of-life care was simply a sequel to failed intensive care. This is no longer a workable paradigm. There is no reliable way to segregate patients who are dying from patients who will survive."[96] Thelen says that "Palliative care is not something that is offered because 'there is nothing we can do'; it is an active, aggressive plan of care designed to alleviate patients' symptoms and meet the diverse needs of patients and patients' families."[123]

REFERENCES

1. Abbott, K. H., Sago, J. G., Breen, C. M., Abernethy, A. P., & Tulsky, J. A. (2001). Families looking back: one year after discussion of withdrawal or withholding of life-sustaining support. *Crit Care Med, 29*(1), 197–201.
2. Adams, A., Mannix, T., & Harrington, A. (2015). Nurses' communication with families in the intensive care unit - a literature review. *Nurs Crit Care*. http://dx.doi.org/10.1111/nicc.12141 [doi].
3. American Nurses Association. (2010). Position statement: registered nurses' role and responsibilities in providing expert care and counseling at the end of life. http://www.nursingworld.org/MainMenuCategories/EthicsStandards/Ethics-Position-Statements/EndofLife-Position-Statement.pdf.
4. Andrew, C. M. (1998). Optimizing the human experience: nursing the families of people who die in intensive care. *Intensive Crit Care Nurs, 14*(2), 59–65.
5. Angus, D. C., Barnato, A. E., Linde-Zwirble, W. T., Weissfeld, L. A., Watson, R. S., Rickert, T., et al. (2004). Use of intensive care at the end of life in the United States: an epidemiologic study. *Crit Care Med, 32*(3), 638–643.
6. Anonymous. (1981). Guidelines for the determination of death. Report of the medical consultants on the diagnosis of death to the President's Commission for the Study of Ethical Problems in Medicine and Biomedical and Behavioral Research. *JAMA, 246*(19), 2184–2186.
7. Ashburn, M. A., Lipman, A. G., Carr, D., & Rubingh, C. (Eds.). (2003). *Principles of analgesic use in the treatment of acute pain and cancer pain* (5th ed.) Glenview, IL: American Pain Society.
8. Azoulay, E., Metnitz, B., Sprung, C. L., Timsit, J. F., Lemaire, F., Bauer, P., et al. (2009). End-of-life practices in 282 intensive care units: data from the SAPS 3 database. *Intensive Care Med, 35*(4), 623–630.
9. Azoulay, E., Pochard, F., Kentish-Barnes, N., Chevret, S., Aboab, J., Adrie, C., et al. (2005). Risk of post-traumatic stress symptoms in family members of intensive care unit patients. *Am J Respir Crit Care Med, 171*(9), 987–994.
10. Azoulay, E., & Sprung, C. L. (2004). Family-physician interactions in the intensive care unit. *Crit Care Med, 32*(11), 2323–2328.

11. Azoulay, E., Timsit, J. F., Sprung, C. L., Soares, M., Rusinova, K., Lafabrie, A., et al. (2009). Prevalence and factors of intensive care unit conflicts: the conflicus study. *Am J Respir Crit Care Med, 180*(9), 853–860.
12. Barnes, S., Gardiner, C., Gott, M., Payne, S., Chady, B., Small, N., et al. (2012). Enhancing patient-professional communication about end-of-life issues in life-limiting conditions: a critical review of the literature. *J Pain Symptom Manage, 44*(6), 866–879.
13. Beauchamp, T., & Childress, J. F. (2013). *Principles of biomedical ethics.* New York: Oxford University Press.
14. Bergeron, N., Dubois, M. J., Dumont, M., Dial, S., & Skrobik, Y. (2001). Intensive care delirium screening checklist: evaluation of a new screening tool. *Intensive Care Med, 27*(5), 859–864.
15. Berlinger, N., Jennings, B., & Wolf, S. M. (2013). *The Hastings center guidelines for decisions on life-sustaining treatment and care near the end of life* (2nd ed.). NY: Oxford University Press.
16. Bloomer, M. J., Morphet, J., O'Connor, M., Lee, S., & Griffiths, D. (2013). Nursing care of the family before and after a death in the ICU–an exploratory pilot study. *Aust Crit Care, 26*(1), 23–28.
17. Booth, S., Wade, R., Johnson, M., Kite, S., Swannick, M., Anderson, H., et al. (2004). The use of oxygen in the palliation of breathlessness. A report of the expert working group of the scientific committee of the association of palliative medicine. *Respir Med, 98*(1), 66–77.
18. Brody, H. (1995). Withdrawing versus withholding therapy: still a pernicious distinction. *J Am Geriatr Soc, 43*(6), 716–717.
19. Bruce, C. R., Miller, S. M., & Zimmerman, J. L. (2015). A qualitative study exploring moral distress in the ICU team: the importance of unit functionality and intrateam dynamics. *Crit Care Med, 43*(4), 823–831.
20. Campbell, M. L. (1998). *Foregoing life-sustaining therapy: how to care for the patient who is near death.* CA: American Association of Critical-Care Nurses.
21. Campbell, M. L. (2011a). Determination of death in adult patients. In D. L. Wiegand (Ed.), *AACN procedure manual for critical care* (6th ed.) (pp. 1211–1222). Philadelphia: Elsevier Saunders.
22. Campbell, M. L. (2011b). Donation after cardiac death. In D. L. Wiegand (Ed.), *AACN procedure manual for critical care* (6th ed.) (pp. 1229–1234). Philadelphia: Elsevier Saunders.
23. Campbell, M. L. (2004). Terminal dyspnea and respiratory distress. *Crit Care Clin, 20*(3), 403–417, viii–ix.
24. Campbell, M. L. (2007). How to withdraw mechanical ventilation: a systematic review of the literature. *AACN Adv Crit Care, 18*(4), 397–403, quiz 344–5.
25. Campbell, M. L. (2015). Caring for dying patients in the intensive care unit: managing pain, dyspnea, anxiety, delirium, and death rattle. *AACN Adv Crit Care, 26*(2), 110–120, quiz 121–2.
26. Campbell, M. L., & Carlson, R. W. (1992). Terminal weaning from mechanical ventilation: Ethical and practical considerations for patient management. *Am J Crit Care, 1*(3), 52–56.
27. Campbell, M. L., & Frank, R. R. (1997). Experience with an end-of-life practice at a university hospital. *Crit Care Med, 25*(1), 197–202.
28. Campbell, M. L., Templin, T., & Walch, J. (2010). A respiratory distress observation scale for patients unable to self-report dyspnea. *J Palliat Med, 13*(3), 285–290.
29. Campbell, M. L., Yarandi, H., & Dove-Medows, E. (2013). Oxygen is nonbeneficial for most patients who are near death. *J Pain Symptom Manage, 45*(3), 517–523.
30. Chan, J. D., Treece, P. D., Engelberg, R. A., Crowley, L., Rubenfeld, G. D., Steinberg, K. P., et al. (2004). Narcotic and benzodiazepine use after withdrawal of life support: association with time to death? *Chest, 126*(1), 286–293.
31. Cheon, J., Coyle, N., Wiegand, D. L., & Welsh, S. (2015). Ethical issues experienced by hospice and palliative nurses. *J Hosp Palliat Nurs, 17*(1), 7–15.
32. Cist, A. F., Truog, R. D., Brackett, S. E., & Hurford, W. E. (2001). Practical guidelines on the withdrawal of life-sustaining therapies. *Int Anesthesiol Clin, 39*(3), 87–102.
33. Clarke, E. B., Curtis, J. R., Luce, J. M., Levy, M., Danis, M., Nelson, J., et al. (2003). Quality indicators for end-of-life care in the intensive care unit. *Crit Care Med, 31*(9), 2255–2262.
34. Cook, D., Rocker, G., Marshall, J., Sjokvist, P., Dodek, P., Griffith, L., et al. (2003). Withdrawal of mechanical ventilation in anticipation of death in the intensive care unit. *N Engl J Med, 349*(12), 1123–1132.
35. Curtis, J. R., Engelberg, R. A., Wenrich, M. D., Nielsen, E. L., Shannon, S. E., Treece, P. D., et al. (2002). Studying communication about end-of-life care during the ICU family conference: development of a framework. *J Crit Care, 17*(3), 147–160.
36. Curtis, J. R., Patrick, D. L., Shannon, S. E., Treece, P. D., Engelberg, R. A., & Rubenfeld, G. D. (2001). The family conference as a focus to improve communication about end-of-life care in the intensive care unit: opportunities for improvement. *Crit Care Med, 29*(Suppl. 2), N26–N33.
37. Curtis, J. R., & Vincent, J. L. (2010). Ethics and end-of-life care for adults in the intensive care unit. *Lancet, 376*(9749), 1347–1353.
38. Cypress, B. S. (2011). Family conference in the intensive care unit: a systematic review. *Dimens Crit Care Nurs, 30*(5), 246–255.
39. Daly, B. J. (2006). End-of-life decision making, organ donation, and critical care nurses. *Crit Care Nurse, 26*(2), 78–86.
40. Davidson, J. E., Powers, K., Hedayat, K. M., Tieszen, M., Kon, A. A., Shepard, E., et al. (2007). Clinical practice guidelines for support of the family in the patient-centered intensive care unit: American College of Critical Care Medicine Task Force 2004–2005. *Crit Care Med, 35*(2), 605–622.
41. Desbiens, N. A., & Wu, A. W. (2000). Pain and suffering in seriously ill hospitalized patients. *J Am Geriatr Soc, 48*(Suppl. 5), S183–S186.
42. Desbiens, N. A., Wu, A. W., Broste, S. K., Wenger, N. S., Connors, A. F., Jr., Lynn, J., et al. (1996). Pain and satisfaction with pain control in seriously ill hospitalized adults: findings from the SUPPORT research investigations. for the SUPPORT investigators. study to understand prognoses and preferences for outcomes and risks of treatment. *Crit Care Med, 24*(12), 1953–1961.
43. Ely, E. W., Inouye, S. K., Bernard, G. R., Gordon, S., Francis, J., May, L., et al. (2001). Delirium in mechanically ventilated patients: validity and reliability of the confusion assessment method for the intensive care unit (CAM-ICU). *J AMA, 286*(21), 2703–2710.
44. End of Life Nursing Education Curriculum (ELNEC). (2007). *End of life nursing education consortium: promoting palliative care in critical care nursing: ELNEC-critical care training program.* City of Hope and the American Association of Colleges of Nursing.
45. Faber-Langendoen, K. (1994). The clinical management of dying patients receiving mechanical ventilation. a survey of physician practice. *Chest, 106*(3), 880–888.
46. Fassier, T., & Azoulay, E. (2010). Conflicts and communication gaps in the intensive care unit. *Curr Opin Crit Care, 16*(6), 654–665.
47. Conditions of participation for hospitals (42 CFR part 482.45). (2000). https://www.cms.gov/Regulations-and-Guidance/Guidance/Transmittals/downloads/R37SOMA.pdf.
48. Field, M. J., & Cassel, C. K. (1997). *Approaching death, improving care at the end of life.* Washington, D.C.: National Academy Press.
49. Gelinas, C., Fillion, L., Puntillo, K. A., Viens, C., & Fortier, M. (2006). Validation of the critical-care pain observation tool in adult patients. *Am J Crit Care, 15*(4), 420–427.
50. Gordy, S., & Klein, E. (2011). Advance directives in the trauma intensive care unit: do they really matter? *Int J Crit Illn Inj Sci, 1*(2), 132–137.
51. Grant, M. (2015). Resolving communication challenges in the intensive care unit. *AACN Adv Crit Care, 26*(2), 123–130.
52. Hall, R. I., Rocker, G. M., & Murray, D. (2004). Simple changes can improve conduct of end-of-life care in the intensive care unit. *Can J Anaesth, 51*(6), 631–636.
53. Hawryluck, L. A., Harvey, W. R., Lemieux-Charles, L., & Singer, P. A. (2002). Consensus guidelines on analgesia and sedation in dying intensive care unit patients. *BMC Med Ethics, 3*, E3.
54. Health Care Financing Administration. (1998). In Health Care Financing Administration (Ed.), *Medicare and Medicaid programs: hospital condition of participation; identification of potential organ, tissue and eye donors.* Washington, D.C.: Federal Register.
55. Heyland, D. K., Rocker, G. M., O'Callaghan, C. J., Dodek, P. M., & Cook, D. J. (2003). Dying in the ICU: perspectives of family members. *Chest, 124*(1), 392–397.

56. Heytens, L., Verlooy, J., Gheuens, J., & Bossaert, L. (1989). Lazarus sign and extensor posturing in a brain-dead patient. case report. *J Neurosurg, 71*(3), 449–451.
57. Higgins, T. L., Teres, D., Copes, W. S., Nathanson, B. H., Stark, M., & Kramer, A. A. (2007). Assessing contemporary intensive care unit outcome: an updated mortality probability admission model (MPM0-III). *Crit Care Med, 35*(3), 827–835.
58. Hinkle, L. J., Bosslet, G. T., & Torke, A. M. (2015). Factors associated with family satisfaction with end-of-life care in the ICU: a systematic review. *Chest, 147*(1), 82–93.
59. Hodde, N. M., Engelberg, R. A., Treece, P. D., Steinberg, K. P., & Curtis, J. R. (2004). Factors associated with nurse assessment of the quality of dying and death in the intensive care unit. *Crit Care Med, 32*(8), 1648–1653.
60. Hospice and Palliative Nurses Association. (2011). HPNA position statement: withholding and/or withdrawing life-sustaining therapies. http://hpna.advancingexpertcare.org/wp-content/uploads/2015/08/Withholding-and-or-Withdrawing-Life-Sustaining-Therapies.pdf.
61. Howard, R. J., Cornell, D. L., & Cochran, L. (2012). History of deceased organ donation, transplantation, and organ procurement organizations. *Prog Transplant, 22*(1), 6–16; quiz 17.
62. Hudson, T. (1994). Are futile-care policies the answer? Providers struggle with decisions for patients near the end of life. *Hosp Health Netw, 68*(4), 26–30, 32.
63. Institute of Medicine, I. o. M. (2015). *Dying in America: improving quality and honoring individual preferences near the end of life.* Washington, D.C.: The National Academies Press.
64. Jackson, I. (1992). Bereavement follow-up service in intensive care. *Intens Crit Care Nurs, 8*(3), 163–168.
65. Jacob, D. (1997). Family decision making for incompetent patients in the ICU. *Crit Care Nurs Clin North Am, 9*(1), 107–114.
66. Jacob, D. A. (1998). Family members' experiences with decision making for incompetent patients in the ICU: a qualitative study. *Am J Crit Care, 7*(1), 30–36.
67. Jacobs, B. B., & Taylor, C. (2005). Medical futility in the natural attitude. *ANS Adv Nurs Sci, 28*(4), 288–305.
68. Jecker, N. S. (1995). Medical futility and care of dying patients. *West J Med, 163*(3), 287–291.
69. Kalowes, P. (2015). Improving end-of-life care prognostic discussions: role of advanced practice nurses. *AACN Adv Crit Care, 26*(2), 151–166.
70. Kirchhoff, K. T., Conradt, K. L., & Anumandla, P. R. (2003). ICU nurses' preparation of families for death of patients following withdrawal of ventilator support. *Appl Nurs Res, 16*(2), 85–92.
71. Kirchhoff, K. T., Song, M. K., & Kehl, K. (2004). Caring for the family of the critically ill patient. *Crit Care Clin, 20*(3), 453–466, ix–x.
72. Kirchhoff, K. T., Spuhler, V., Walker, L., Hutton, A., Cole, B. V., & Clemmer, T. (2000). Intensive care nurses' experiences with end-of-life care. *Am J Crit Care, 9*(1), 36–42.
73. Koch, K. A., Rodeffer, H. D., & Wears, R. L. (1994). Changing patterns of terminal care management in an intensive care unit. *Crit Care Med, 22*(2), 233–243.
74. Kress, J. P., & Hall, J. B. (2004). Delirium and sedation. *Crit Care Clin, 20*(3), 419–433, ix.
75. Le Gall, J. R., Lemeshow, S., & Saulnier, F. (1993). A new simplified acute physiology score (SAPS II) based on a European/North American multicenter study. *J AMA, 270*(24), 2957–2963.
76. Levin, T. T., Moreno, B., Silvester, W., & Kissane, D. W. (2010). End-of-life communication in the intensive care unit. *Gen Hosp Psychiatry, 32*(4), 433–442.
77. Levy, C. R., Ely, E. W., Payne, K., Engelberg, R. A., Patrick, D. L., & Curtis, J. R. (2005). Quality of dying and death in two medical ICUs: perceptions of family and clinicians. *Chest, 127*(5), 1775–1783.
78. Levy, M. M. (2001). End-of-life care in the intensive care unit: can we do better? *Crit Care Med, 29*(Suppl. 2), N56–N61.
79. Lilly, C. M., De Meo, D. L., Sonna, L. A., Haley, K. J., Massaro, A. F., Wallace, R. F., et al. (2000). An intensive communication intervention for the critically ill. *Am J Med, 109*(6), 469–475.
80. Lilly, C. M., Sonna, L. A., Haley, K. J., & Massaro, A. F. (2003). Intensive communication: four-year follow-up from a clinical practice study. *Crit Care Med, 31*(Suppl. 5), S394–S399.
81. Lo, B. (2009). *Resolving ethical dilemmas: a guide for clinicians.* Philadelphia, PA: Lippincott Williams & Wilkins.
82. Lonergan, E., Britton, A. M., Luxenberg, J., & Wyller, T. (2007). Antipsychotics for delirium. *Cochrane Database Syst Rev, 2*(2), CD005594.
83. Luce, J. M. (1997). Withholding and withdrawal of life support from critically ill patients. *West J Med, 167*(6), 411–416.
84. Luce, J. M. (2010). End-of-life decision making in the intensive care unit. *Am J Respir Crit Care Med, 182*(1), 6–11.
85. Lunney, J. R., Lynn, J., Foley, D. J., Lipson, S., & Guralnik, J. M. (2003). Patterns of functional decline at the end of life. *JAMA, 289*(18), 2387–2392.
86. Lunney, J. R., Lynn, J., & Hogan, C. (2002). Profiles of older Medicare decedents. *J Am Geriatr Soc, 50*(6), 1108–1112.
87. Lynn, J., Teno, J. M., Phillips, R. S., Wu, A. W., Desbiens, N., Harrold, J., et al. (1997). Perceptions by family members of the dying experience of older and seriously ill patients. SUPPORT investigators study to understand prognoses and preferences for outcomes and risks of treatments. *Ann Intern Med, 126*(2), 97–106.
88. Mayer, S. A., & Kossoff, S. B. (1999). Withdrawal of life support in the neurological intensive care unit. *Neurology, 52*(8), 1602–1609.
89. McAdam, J., & Puntillo, K. (2010). The intensive care unit. In B. R. Ferrell, & N. Coyle (Eds.), *Oxford textbook of palliative nursing* (3rd ed.) (pp. 905–922). New York: Oxford University Press.
90. McClement, S. E., & Degner, L. F. (1995). Expert nursing behaviors in care of the dying adult in the intensive care unit. *Heart Lung, 24*(5), 408–419.
91. McDonagh, J. R., Elliott, T. B., Engelberg, R. A., Treece, P. D., Shannon, S. E., Rubenfeld, G. D., et al. (2004). Family satisfaction with family conferences about end-of-life care in the intensive care unit: increased proportion of family speech is associated with increased satisfaction. *Crit Care Med, 32*(7), 1484–1488.
92. Medina, J., & Puntillo, K. (2006). *AACN protocol for practice: palliative care and end-of-life care.* Boston: Jones and Bartlett.
93. Melhado, L. W., Byers, J., & Fowler. (2011). Patients' and surrogates' decision-making characteristics: withdrawing, withholding, and continuing life-sustaining treatments. *J Hosp Palliat Nurs, 13*(1), 16–30.
94. Mularski, R. A. (2004). Pain management in the intensive care unit. *Crit Care Clin, 20*(3), 381–401, viii.
95. National Consensus Project (Ed.). (2013). *Clinical practice guidelines for quality palliative care* (3rd ed.). Pittsburgh, PA: National Consensus Project for Quality Palliative Care. https://www.hpna.org/multimedia/NCP_Clinical_Practice_Guidelines_3rd_Edition.pdf.
96. Nelson, J. E., & Danis, M. (2001). End-of-life care in the intensive care unit: Where are we now? *Crit Care Med, 29*(Suppl. 2), N2–N9.
97. Norton, S. A., & Bowers, B. J. (2001). Working toward consensus: providers' strategies to shift patients from curative to palliative treatment choices. *Res Nurs Health, 24*(4), 258–269.
98. Norton, S. A., Tilden, V. P., Tolle, S. W., Nelson, C. A., & Eggman, S. T. (2003). Life support withdrawal: communication and conflict. *Am J Crit Care, 12*(6), 548–555.
99. O'Callahan, J. G., Fink, C., Pitts, L. H., & Luce, J. M. (1995). Withholding and withdrawing of life support from patients with severe head injury. *Crit Care Med, 23*(9), 1567–1575.
100. O'Mahony, S., McHugh, M., Zallman, L., & Selwyn, P. (2003). Ventilator withdrawal: procedures and outcomes. report of a collaboration between a critical care division and a palliative care service. *J Pain Symptom Manage, 26*(4), 954–961.
101. Parshall, M. B., Schwartzstein, R. M., Adams, L., Banzett, R. B., Manning, H. L., Bourbeau, J., et al. (2012). An official American Thoracic Society statement: update on the mechanisms, assessment, and management of dyspnea. *Am J Respir Crit Care Med, 185*(4), 435–452.
102. Paruk, F., Kissoon, N., Hartog, C. S., Feldman, C., Hodgson, E. R., Lipman, J., et al. (2014). The Durban world congress ethics round table conference report: III. Withdrawing mechanical ventilation–the approach should be individualized. *J Crit Care, 29*(6), 902–907.

103. Payen, J. F., Bru, O., Bosson, J. L., Lagrasta, A., Novel, E., Deschaux, I., et al. (2001). Assessing pain in critically ill sedated patients by using a behavioral pain scale. *Crit Care Med, 29*(12), 2258–2263.

104. Prendergast, T. J. (2000). Withholding or withdrawal of life-sustaining therapy. *Hosp Pract (1995), 35*(6), 91–92, 95–100,102.

105. Prendergast, T. J., Claessens, M. T., & Luce, J. M. (1998). A national survey of end-of-life care for critically ill patients. *Am J Respir Crit Care Med, 158*(4), 1163–1167.

106. Prendergast, T. J., & Puntillo, K. A. (2002). Withdrawal of life support: intensive caring at the end of life. *JAMA, 288*(21), 2732–2740.

107. President's Commission for the Study of Ethical Problems in Medicine and Biomedical and Behavioral Research. (1983). *Deciding to forgo life-sustaining treatment: Ethical, medical and legal issues in treatment decisions.* Washington, D.C.: US Government Printing Office.

108. Preuss, D. N. (2011). Organ donation: identification of potential organ donors, request for organ donation, and care of the organ donor. In D. L. Wiegand (Ed.), *AACN procedure manual for critical care* (6th ed.) (pp. 1223–1228). Philadelphia: Elsevier Saunders.

109. Puntillo, K. A., Benner, P., Drought, T., Drew, B., Stotts, N., Stannard, D., et al. (2001). End-of-life issues in intensive care units: a national random survey of nurses' knowledge and beliefs. *Am J Crit Care, 10*(4), 216–229.

110. Rao, J. K., Anderson, L. A., Lin, F. C., & Laux, J. P. (2014). Completion of advance directives among U.S. consumers. *Am J Prev Med, 46*(1), 65–70.

111. Rocker, G. M., & Curtis, J. R. (2003). Caring for the dying in the intensive care unit: in search of clarity. *JAMA, 290*(6), 820–822.

112. Ropper, A. H. (1984). Unusual spontaneous movements in brain-dead patients. *Neurology, 34*(8), 1089–1092.

113. Rubenfeld, G. D. (2004). Principles and practice of withdrawing life-sustaining treatments. *Crit Care Clin, 20*(3), 435–451, ix.

114. Schneiderman, L. J., & Spragg, R. G. (1988). Ethical decisions in discontinuing mechanical ventilation. *N Engl J Med, 318*(15), 984–988.

115. Schuster, R. A., Hong, S. Y., Arnold, R. M., & White, D. B. (2014). Investigating conflict in ICUs-is the clinicians' perspective enough? *Crit Care Med, 42*(2), 328–335.

116. Sprung, C. L., Truog, R. D., Curtis, J. R., Joynt, G. M., Baras, M., Michalsen, A., et al. (2014). Seeking worldwide professional consensus on the principles of end-of-life care for the critically ill. the consensus for worldwide end-of-life practice for patients in intensive care units (WELPICUS) study. *Am J Respir Crit Care Med, 190*(8), 855–866.

117. Steinhauser, K. E., Christakis, N. A., Clipp, E. C., McNeilly, M., Grambow, S., Parker, J., et al. (2001). Preparing for the end of life: preferences of patients, families, physicians, and other care providers. *J Pain Symptom Manage, 22*(3), 727–737.

118. Sulmasy, D. P., FitzGerald, D., & Jaffin, J. H. (1993). Ethical considerations. *Crit Care Clin, 9*(4), 775–789.

119. Vacco v. quill: 521 U.S. 793. (1997). https://supreme.justia.com/cases/federal/us/521/793/.

120. Swigart, V., Lidz, C., Butterworth, V., & Arnold, R. (1996). Letting go: family willingness to forgo life support. *Heart Lung, 25*(6), 483–494.

121. The Hastings Center. (1987). *Guidelines on the termination of life-sustaining treatment and the care of the dying.* Vriarcliff Manor, NY: The Hastings Center.

122. The Society of Critical Care Medicine Ethics Committee. (1997). Consensus statement of the society of critical care medicine's ethics committee regarding futile and other possibly inadvisable treatments. *Crit Care Med, 25*(5), 887–891.

123. Thelen, M. (2005). End-of-life decision making in intensive care. *Crit Care Nurse, 25*(6), 28–37; quiz 38.

124. Thompson, J. E., & Thompson, H. O. (1985). *Bioethical decision making for nurses.* Norwalk, CT: Appleton-Century-Crofts.

125. Tilden, V. P., Tolle, S. W., Garland, M. J., & Nelson, C. A. (1995). Decisions about life-sustaining treatment. impact of physicians' behaviors on the family. *Arch Intern Med, 155*(6), 633–638.

126. Tilden, V. P., Tolle, S. W., Nelson, C. A., & Fields, J. (2001). Family decision-making to withdraw life-sustaining treatments from hospitalized patients. *Nurs Res, 50*(2), 105–115.

127. Tilden, V. P., Tolle, S. W., Nelson, C. A., Thompson, M., & Eggman, S. C. (1999). Family decision making in foregoing life-extending treatments. *J Fam Nurs, 5*(4), 426–442.

128. Tolle, S. W., Tilden, V. P., Rosenfeld, A. G., & Hickman, S. E. (2000). Family reports of barriers to optimal care of the dying. *Nurs Res, 49*(6), 310–317.

129. Tomlinson, T., & Czlonka, D. (1995). Futility and hospital policy. *Hastings Cent Rep, 25*(3), 28–35.

130. Treece, P. D., Engelberg, R. A., Crowley, L., Chan, J. D., Rubenfeld, G. D., Steinberg, K. P., et al. (2004). Evaluation of a standardized order form for the withdrawal of life support in the intensive care unit. *Crit Care Med, 32*(5), 1141–1148.

131. Truog, R. D., Campbell, M. L., Curtis, J. R., Haas, C. E., Luce, J. M., Rubenfeld, G. D., et al. (2008). Recommendations for end-of-life care in the intensive care unit: a consensus statement by the American College [corrected] of Critical Care Medicine. *Crit Care Med, 36*(3), 953–963.

132. Truog, R. D., Cist, A. F., Brackett, S. E., Burns, J. P., Curley, M. A., Danis, M., et al. (2001). Recommendations for end-of-life care in the intensive care unit: the ethics committee of the Society of Critical Care Medicine. *Crit Care Med, 29*(12), 2332–2348.

133. Waite, K. R., Federman, A. D., McCarthy, D. M., Sudore, R., Curtis, L. M., Baker, D. W., et al. (2013). Literacy and race as risk factors for low rates of advance directives in older adults. *J Am Geriatr Soc, 61*(3), 403–406.

134. Walter, S. D., Cook, D. J., Guyatt, G. H., Spanier, A., Jaeschke, R., Todd, T. R., et al. (1998). Confidence in life-support decisions in the intensive care unit: a survey of healthcare workers. Canadian Critical Care Trials Group. *Crit Care Med, 26*(1), 44–49.

135. Warren, N. A. (2002). Critical care family members' satisfaction with bereavement experiences. *Crit Care Nurs Q, 25*(2), 54–60.

136. Way, J., Back, A. L., & Curtis, J. R. (2002). Withdrawing life support and resolution of conflict with families. *BMJ, 325*(7376), 1342–1345.

137. White, D. B., & Luce, J. M. (2004). Palliative care in the intensive care unit: barriers, advances, and unmet needs. *Crit Care Clin, 20*(3), 329–343, vii.

138. Wiegand, D. L., & Mahon, M. M. (2011). Withholding and withdrawing life-sustaining treatment. In D. L. Wiegand (Ed.), *AACN procedure manual for critical care* (6th ed.) (pp. 1235–1241). Philadelphia: Elsevier Saunders.

139. Wiegand, D. (2008). In their own time: the family experience during the process of withdrawal of life-sustaining therapy. *J Palliat Med, 11*(8), 1115–1121.

140. Wiegand, D. L. (2006a). Families and withdrawal of life-sustaining therapy: state of the science. *J Fam Nurs, 12*(2), 165–184.

141. Wiegand, D. L. (2006b). Withdrawal of life-sustaining therapy after sudden, unexpected life-threatening illness or injury: interactions between patients' families, healthcare providers, and the healthcare system. *Am J Crit Care, 15*(2), 178–187.

142. Wiegand, D. L., Grant, M. S., Cheon, J., & Gergis, M. A. (2013). Family-centered end-of-life care in the ICU. *J Gerontol Nurs, 39*(8), 60–68.

143. Wiegand, D. L., & Petri, L. (2010). Is a good death possible after withdrawal of life-sustaining therapy? *Nurs Clin North Am, 45*(3), 427–440.

144. Wiegand, D. L., & Grant, M. S. (2014). Bioethical issues related to limiting life-sustaining therapies in the intensive care unit. *J Hosp Palliat Nurs, 16*(2), 60–66.

145. Wijdicks, E. F., Varelas, P. N., Gronseth, G. S., Greer, D. M., & American Academy of Neurology (2010). Evidence-based guideline update: determining brain death in adults: report of the quality standards subcommittee of the American Academy of Neurology. *Neurology, 74*(23), 1911–1918.

146. Zimmerman, J. E., Kramer, A. A., McNair, D. S., & Malila, F. M. (2006). Acute physiology and chronic health evaluation (APACHE) IV: hospital mortality assessment for today's critically ill patients. *Crit Care Med, 34*(5), 1297–1310.

Answers to Decision Point Questions

CHAPTER 3 ACUTE CORONARY SYNDROMES

Decision Point:

What medication interventions should be instituted immediately on admission and prior to discharge?

Discussion:

Women derive the same treatment benefit as men from aspirin, $P2Y_{12}$ inhibitors (antiplatelet agents), anticoagulants, beta blockers, ACE inhibitors, and statins. Clinicians should pay close attention to weight and/or renally calculated doses of antiplatelet and anticoagulant agents to reduce bleeding risk in women.

Decision point:

Should Mrs. H. be taken for early interventional therapy versus ischemia-guided therapy?

Discussion:

Early intervention therapy.

Decision Point:

Why do women, more than men, have increased vascular complications with interventional revascularization?

Discussion:

These have been attributed to the smaller body surface area (BSA), smaller coronary arteries, sheaths that are too large for the vessel, and non–weight-adjusted anticoagulant dosing.

Decision Point:

Mrs. H has been taking HRT for her menopausal symptoms. What education should be provided to the patient on the continuation of the HRT treatment?

Discussion:

HRT should not be utilized as secondary prevention in individuals with ACS and should be discontinued if previously utilized.

CHAPTER 4 HEART FAILURE

Decision Point:

What signs and symptoms of heart failure was R.S. exhibiting?

Discussion:

The signs and symptoms R.S. exhibited were difficulty breathing at rest, So_2 of 82%, distended neck veins, S3 gallop, 4+ pedal edema, rales, and pulmonary congestion on chest X-ray.

Decision Point:

What causes, risk factors, and lifestyle choices does R.S. have for heart failure?

Discussion:

R.S. has a history of previous MI and poorly controlled hypertension. In addition, she has uncontrolled diabetes mellitus, is obese, and is African American. The lifestyle choices she has made that contribute to her decompensation are her nonadherence to prescribed medical therapy, including medications, and her continued consumption of a high-sodium, high-carbohydrate diet.

Decision Point:

What pathophysiologic mechanism contributed to the left ventricular hypertrophy and left ventricular dysfunction?

Discussion:

Ventricular remodeling was most likely triggered by the previous MI and then aggravated by neurohormone (norepinephrine, angiotensin II, and arginine vasopressin) release. Long-standing hypertension contributed to the increase in neurohormones, causing vasoconstriction and increased workload (and increased oxygen consumption) on the heart muscle.

Decision Point:

What pathophysiologic mechanism contributed to the fluid retention?

Discussion:

Activation of the renin-angiotensin-aldosterone system causes release of aldosterone from the adrenal cortex. Aldosterone promotes sodium and water retention. In addition, arginine vasopressin (or antidiuretic hormone) promotes water retention.

CHAPTER 5 CARDIAC SURGERY

Decision Point:

On admission, what problems required interventions for Ms. Smith?

Discussion:

1. Hypothermia: apply warm blankets or a forced warm air blanket.
2. Increased SVR: increased afterload requires a vasodilator. Due to a CVP of 7, a pure arterial vasodilator such as nicardipine is necessary so as not to decrease preload any further.
3. Hypovolemia: as Ms. Smith's temperature rises with the warming blankets, she will vasodilate, requiring fluids. Crystalloids should be administered during this time. BP should be monitored closely during the warming stage so that the vasodilators may be decreased.

Decision Point:

What do the updated parameters reveal, and what actions are necessary?

Discussion:

Mrs. Smith's CI is likely decreased due to her hypovolemia, which does not require blood transfusions at this point due to her adequate Hgb and decreasing chest tube drainage. Norepinephrine (Levophed) is initiated to vasoconstrict, along with continuing fluids. After 2 to 3 liters of crystalloid have been administered, it would be acceptable to switch to albumin 500 mL.

CHAPTER 6 VALVULAR DISEASE AND SURGERY

Decision Point:

When is the narrowed aortic valve considered to be critical?

Discussion:

Critical aortic stenosis is defined as a peak systolic pressure gradient > 50 mm Hg or a valve area < 0.8 cm^2, or < one-fourth of the normal aortic valve area (3.0–4.0 cm^2).

Decision Point:

What are key symptoms a patient with aortic stenosis should be taught to report to their healthcare provider?

Discussion:

Key symptoms the patient should report are increased shortness of breath with exertion, angina, syncope, and signs of heart failure.

Decision Point:

How frequently should a patient with aortic stenosis be seen by their healthcare provider once the aortic valve orifice is 1 cm^2?

Discussion:

Patients should be followed closely with echocardiograms at least yearly, and every 6 months if the aortic stenosis is severe.

Decision Point:

Is sinus tachycardia common following cardiac surgery? Why?

Discussion:

Valvular heart disease is associated with atrial hypertrophy and the development of electrophysiologic changes in the area of the pulmonary veins in the left atrium, contributing to atrial dysrhythmias. The postoperative incidence of atrial flutter and atrial fibrillation tends to be higher in these patients.

Decision Point:

What discharge instructions should be provided for this patient?

Discussion:

Discharge instructions should include similar information to that which other open heart surgery patients receive, as well as information on anticoagulation therapy and subacute bacterial endocarditis prophylaxis.

CHAPTER 7 VASCULAR EMERGENCIES AND SURGERY

Decision Point:

What interventions should be implemented at this time?

Discussion:

R.B. was started on a beta blocker to decrease BP, HR, and the force of contraction, with the goal of preventing further extension of the aortic dissection. The esmolol drip was titrated to achieve a HR < 60 bpm and a systolic BP 100–120 mm Hg. If beta-blocker therapy failed to achieve the target systolic BP, a vasodilator such as sodium nitroprusside (Nipride) could be added. An arterial line was inserted to help guide therapy. Morphine sulfate was administered intermittently to help decrease the pain associated with the dissection. Frequent serial assessments were performed to evaluate for potential extension of the dissection. Since R.B. was exhibiting ischemic complications related to his Type B dissection, arrangements were made for a surgical consult as soon as possible. Preferred treatment would be thoracic endovascular aortic repair (TEVAR) if feasible.

CHAPTER 8 HEART AND LUNG TRANSPLANTATION

Decision Point:

Is M.J. an appropriate heart transplant candidate?

Discussion:

M.J.'s history includes the typical presentation for heart transplant evaluation: multiple CAD risk factors and progressive symptoms. Early optimal control of his DM and hypertension may have prevented or at least prolonged the period before onset of his CAD. Despite maximal medical therapy, however, his disease has progressed. He has recurrent angina and end-stage heart failure. His social history reveals that he has stopped smoking and is not abusing alcohol. He has adequate social support, but a family meeting would be important to evaluate his financial support (because he is on disability) and to determine if his wife's rheumatoid arthritis will significantly limit her ability to assist him in his posttransplant recovery period.

Decision Point:

What is your assessment of his overall status?

Discussion:

M.J. is in fair condition despite relative bradycardia. His kidney function is probably a manifestation of relative ischemia intra- and postoperatively, plus exposure to tacrolimus.

Decision Point:

What interventions might be appropriate?

Discussion:

Adding AV pacing to maintain an HR of 100 beats/min would probably help and would allow the epinephrine to be weaned off. Consideration of holding the tacrolimus for 1 day may also help the kidneys to recover. Elevated WBC count could be infection; however, he is afebrile. The leukocytosis could also be from the high-dose steroids. This parameter will need to be monitored and he should be examined for any sign of infection. M.J. also has hyperglycemia and should be treated with an insulin drip until this is well controlled. The hyperglycemia may be related to his preexisting DM, high-dose steroids, physiologic stress response, or an infection. Again, the search for possible infectious causes should proceed. M.J. can probably be weaned from mechanical ventilation and, if possible, extubated and placed on 40% oxygen.

CHAPTER 9 ACUTE RESPIRATORY FAILURE AND ACUTE LUNG INJURY

Decision Point:

What is the patient's *A-a* gradient, what is normal, and why is this important to know?

Discussion:

The patient's *A-a* gradient is 156.18. His expected gradient is [(35 + 10)/4] = 11.25. The elevated *A-a* gradient indicates a lung etiology for the hypoxemia.

Decision Point:

What is the patient's P/F ratio, and does this patient have ALI or ARDS?

Discussion:

The patient's Pao_2/Fio_2 ratio is 58/0.36 = 161, which is < 200; indicative of ARDS.

Decision Point:

What signs does the patient exhibit that show continued respiratory compromise?

Discussion:

The patient is experiencing acute-onset, persistently decreased oxygen saturation with increasing Fio_2 and bilateral lung infiltrates on CXR, indicative of edema.

Decision Point:

What changes should occur to the plan of care?

Discussion:

The patient will need increased monitoring for respiratory failure, with transfer to a critical care unit. At this time, consider obtaining a pulmonary consultation. An assessment of nutritional status should occur. Nursing will need to provide assistance with activities of daily living, while monitoring for fatigue or respiratory failure. The nurse must be attentive to hydration needs and indicators of sepsis. The patient and family will need education on ARDS and the potential for intubation and mechanical ventilation.

CHAPTER 10 MECHANICAL VENTILATION AND WEANING

Decision Point:

What should be done to improve M.C.'s oxygenation status?

Discussion:

The refractory hypoxemia and chest X-ray findings suggest acute respiratory distress syndrome (ARDS). The management of ARDS should focus on recruiting the lung with PEEP and preventing volutrauma. In M.C.'s case, the PEEP level is too low and the tidal volume is too high. The team recognizes this, and the Vt is decreased to 300 mL (i.e., 6 mL/kg lean body weight) and the PEEP is increased over the next hour to 15 cm H_2O. M.C. is also sedated with lorazepam intravenous boluses and fentanyl for analgesia, which helps her tolerate the ensuing, anticipated hypercarbia. Her blood pressure is 110/60 mm Hg and heart rate 90 beats/min. The next ABG result is as follows: pH = 7.28, $Paco_2$ = 67 mm Hg, and Pao_2 = 150 mm Hg.

Decision Point:

What should be done next?

Discussion:

The hypercarbia is expected with these settings as a consequence of the reduced V_T. Oxygenation status is improved, suggesting lung recruitment. The next step is to decrease the Fio_2. The team's goal is to maintain an oxygen saturation at a minimum, of 90%. The PEEP level is maintained to ensure recruitment and prevent shear injury from repeated opening and closing of the lung during tidal breathing.

CHAPTER 11 THORACIC SURGERY

Decision Point:

What laboratory studies should be performed?

Discussion:

Alkaline phosphatase (ALP), alanine aminotransferase (ALT), aspartate aminotransferase (AST), total bilirubin, creatinine, and albumin laboratory studies should be considered for clinical evaluation.

Decision Point:

What diagnostic study should be performed?

Discussion:

Chest radiograph from 1 week ago demonstrated an abnormality in the apex of the right lung. Therefore, a CT scan of the chest and pelvis with intravenous contrast should be performed to further evaluate the abnormality noted on recent chest X-ray. A CT scan will show the size and shape of the mass and describe the lymph nodes. This marks the beginning of the staging process.

Decision Point:

Should a biopsy be scheduled at this time or should he be referred to an oncologist at this time?

Discussion:

Once a CT scan or PET scan is performed and lung cancer is of great suspicion, the patient should be referred to both a pulmonologist and an oncologist. A biopsy is then obtained either via a bronchoscopy, most commonly performed by a pulmonologist, or a needle biopsy performed by an interventional radiologist to confirm the diagnosis of lung cancer.

CHAPTER 12 HEAD INJURY AND DYSFUNCTION

Decision Point

What should the plan of care look like?

Discussion

M.P. will be placed on a ventilator initially on Fio_2 1.0 and weaned down to 0.40, PRVC mode, rate 16, tidal volume 650 mL,

PEEP 5 cm H_2O, pressure support 10 cm H_2O to maintain a $Pao_2 > 60$ mm Hg, $Paco_2$ 35–40 mm Hg and an oxygen saturation (Sao_2) > 90%. Avoid hypotension and fever. Perform serial neuroassessments at least hourly. Maintain head of the bed elevation (HOB) of 30 to 45 degrees and maintain neutral head alignment and no constriction of neck. Administer sedation and analgesia as needed. Insert orogastric tube and start nutrition, GI & DVT prophylaxes, maintain normal glucose, and monitor for seizure activity.

Decision point

What are the treatment options?

Discussion

Assess ICP waveform and CPP. Administer Mannitol or HTS as a bolus, monitoring osmolarity, tonicity, and sodium. Maintain all the previous interventions and adjust as needed. Adjust sedation and analgesia. Consider adding a continuous propofol infusion.

CHAPTER 13 CEREBROVASCULAR DISORDERS

Decision Point:

What pathophysiology is associated with this stroke?

Discussion:

Mrs. S.P. has had an aneurysmal SAH. The aneurysm has burst or leaked and blood has mixed with the CSF in the subarachnoid space. Her greatest risk during the first 24 hours is rebleeding, which could be fatal or cause loss of consciousness or major neurologic deficits. Her ventricles are most likely enlarged because the blood in the CSF has impaired the absorption of the CSF, resulting in hydrocephalus. In about 3 days, Mrs. S.P. will be at risk for vasospasm, which happens as a result of the blood surrounding the blood vessels, although the pathophysiology is not completely understood.

Decision Point:

What are the initial priorities for her care?

Discussion:

The initial priorities for Mrs. S.P.'s care are ongoing assessment and management of oxygenation, neurologic status, intracranial dynamics, blood pressure, and pain. To minimize the risk of secondary injury, a nasal cannula is needed to increase the Spo_2 to 95% or better. Her drowsiness may be related to hydrocephalus. A ventriculostomy may be needed to drain CSF and measure ICP. Initiation of nimodipine for the aneurysmal SAH, plus a low-dose intravenous opioid for pain, may decrease the blood pressure. However, if they are not effective, other antihypertensives may be needed. Dramatic increases or decreases in blood pressure are to be avoided. Mrs. S.P. needs minimal stimulation except for hourly assessments. She may also receive a loading dose of Dilantin as prophylaxis; however, the blood pressure must be monitored and the Dilantin given slowly to avoid hypotension. If Mrs. S.P. does not have a central venous catheter, fosphenytoin is preferable to phenytoin as it is less irritating to the tissues.

CHAPTER 14 TRAUMATIC SPINAL CORD INJURY

Decision Point:

What mechanisms of injury are likely to be associated with this injury?

Discussion:

Since the moving vehicle broke the guardrail, repeatedly rolled down the hill, stopped abruptly, and ejected J.G., the mechanism of his injury is likely acceleration-deceleration. However, a number of other mechanisms are possible, including hyperflexion, hyperextension, rotation, or axial loading. Based on J.G.'s clinical presentation, a hyperflexion injury may have fractured the vertebrae anteriorly, causing an anterior cord injury and disrupting posterior ligaments. Injury to the anterior cord results in damage to the corticospinal and spinothalamic tracts, the major voluntary movement, pain, and temperature pathways. With ligamentous injury, the injury is unstable.

Decision Point:

What associated injuries are likely?

Discussion:

With mechanisms of injury and traumatic SCI of this magnitude, a TBI is likely. J.G. remained conscious at the scene and during transport. Since he was found awake, talking, and confused following an acceleration-deceleration injury, he likely sustained a concussion. However, he needs to be closely monitored for deterioration in his level of consciousness that might occur with cerebral edema or hematoma formation. Other possible injuries, such as facial and skull fractures, long bone fractures, and organ damage, must be excluded.

Decision Point:

What are the initial priorities for his care?

Discussion:

The initial priorities for J.G.'s care are oxygenation and circulation while maintaining immobilization of his spine. The bradycardia and hypotension with poikilothermia reflect neurogenic shock, which will require resuscitation with fluids, vasopressors, and gradual rewarming. Atropine may be needed as well. Failure to provide adequate oxygenation and perfusion or any movement of the spine may result in further neurologic deterioration.

CHAPTER 17 LIVER DYSFUNCTION AND FAILURE

Decision Point:

Based on the onset of symptoms and clinical data, what type of liver failure does the patient have?

Discussion:

The patient has a rapid onset of jaundice, followed by mental alterations, and no prior history of liver disease, with severe hepatitis as evidenced by her elevated AST/ALT level. The patient has acute liver failure.

Decision Point:

What is the initial treatment plan for this patient?

Discussion:

The patient is in stage 3 hepatic encephalopathy, with imminent danger of loss of airway and onset of coma. Consider sedation with propofol (Diprivan) and elective intubation/ventilation. Initiate cooling measures for induction of mild hypothermia. Start lactulose administration. Monitor and replace serum glucose and electrolytes. Insert Foley catheter and monitor urine output and fluid status. Monitor serum laboratory values with liver function tests, complete blood count, and coagulation values. Consider radiographic tests: noncontrast CT of the head and ultrasound with Doppler evaluation of the abdomen to rule out alterations in hepatic or renal blood flow. Contact and refer to a tertiary liver treatment/transplant center for emergency evaluation and management of liver dysfunction, and possible listing for liver transplantation. Social work consultation should be provided for evaluation and support of family members.

CHAPTER 18 ACUTE PANCREATITIS

Decision Point:

What complications is J.D. likely experiencing?

Discussion:

Respiratory decompensation, SIRS versus sepsis, and renal compromise.

Decision Point:

What interventions are required for J.D.?

Discussion:

Improvement of oxygenation and decrease work of breathing with BiPAP versus intubation and mechanical ventilation, fluid resuscitation and monitoring for endpoints of resuscitation. He also requires pain management interventions.

CHAPTER 22 COMPLEX ACID-BASE DISORDERS AND ASSOCIATED: ELECTROLYTE IMBALANCES

Decision Point

Determine the etiology of the acid-base disorder from the original admission data.

Discussion

Patient has metabolic acidosis: normal Pao_2, low Pco_2 of 16, and has a positive anion gap (Na 140 – [Cl 100 + Co_2 8] = 140 – 108 = 32). Possible causes are lactate, uremia, and ketoacids. The patient is displaying signs of poor perfusion, low BP and altered mental status, which could result in anaerobic metabolism. He also has crush injuries which could result in rhabdomyolysis as well as altered perfusion to the areas again creating lactate. His abdomen is of concern, does he have an infarcted bowel from abdominal compartment syndrome which could lead to ischemic gut creating a lactic acidosis? The crush injuries and rhabdomyolysis can also cause acute tubular necrosis with AKI resulting in uremia.

Decision point

What are the manifestations of metabolic acidosis?

Discussion

Cardiovascular: decreased contractility, hypotension, increased PVR, dysrhythmia; Neurovascular: increased ICP, altered mental status; Respiratory: hyperventilation; Metabolic: increased metabolic demands, catabolism.

Decision point

Was it appropriate to treat the metabolic acidosis with $NaHCO_3$?

Discussion

Treating the underlying cause is the most important goal in addressing metabolic acidosis. Use of $NaHCO_3$ is considered in those with renal dysfunction and those with a pH of < 7.10 and HCO_3^- < 8.

Decision point

What is the acid-base disorder 12 hours after admission?

Discussion

The pH is normal but the $Paco_2$ is elevated indicating a mixed disorder. The elevated $Paco_2$ suggests a respiratory acidosis. In the setting or respiratory acidosis the predicted HCO_3^- increases by 1 meq for every 10 mm Hg increase in the $Paco_2$. This patient's $Paco_2$ is 10 mm above normal. Anion gap: 131 – (70 + 28) = 33 confirms a metabolic acidosis.

He has a triple disorder evident by the normal HCO_3^- : Respiratory acidosis possibly due to ALI and ARDS, a high anion gap metabolic acidosis from shock and lactic acid production, and metabolic alkalosis due to hydrochloric acid loss from the NGT.

Decision point

How should the acid-base disorders be treated?

Discussion

The metabolic acidosis should be treated by improving tissue perfusion with volume or vasopressor support, this in turn will increase renal perfusion and improve renal clearance of lactate. The metabolic alkalosis can be treated with volume replacement with normal saline with also includes chloride. KCL should also be included to replace both the potassium and chloride. The significant drainage from the NGT needs to be further evaluated to determine if there is obstruction or paralytic ileus. The respiratory acidosis can be addressed by improving minute ventilation and increased oxygenation. The title volume or rate could be increased to improve minute ventilation and the Fio_2 or PEEP adjusted to improve oxygenation. Additionally the underlying cause of the disorder needs to be addressed. Evaluation for pulmonary contusion or impending ALI, ARDS with CXR and evaluation of the *A-a* gradient.

CHAPTER 23 ACUTE KIDNEY INJURY

Decision Point:

What was the original insult that most likely led to R.F.'s developing acute kidney injury?

Discussion:

His age, the physiologic stress of a prolonged period of hypotension, and a CT scan are all risk factors for the development of acute kidney injury. In addition, his surgery for repair of an abdominal aortic aneurysm (AAA) can be associated with serious blood loss. R.F.'s early vital signs showed hypovolemic shock, which can lead to acute kidney injury if not treated aggressively with fluids.

Decision Point:

What measure would you expect to carry out in the immediate postoperative period to help minimize risk of developing acute kidney injury?

Discussion:

Insertion of a central venous access would allow for measurement of fluid volume status and monitoring of fluid resuscitation end points. R.F.'s early vital signs, flat neck veins, and tachycardia provide a high index of suspicion for hypovolemia.

The priority in critical care during the recovery period would be to maintain or improve the patient's fluid status in order to preserve cardiac output and thus maintain adequate renal perfusion.

Decision Point:

What are your treatment options for dialyzing this patient?

Discussion:

Collaboration with the clinical nurse specialist or acute care nurse practitioner as well as the nephrology team can yield helpful problem solving for this patient requiring renal replacement therapy. His hemodynamic status is unstable; therefore he is a better candidate for continuous renal replacement therapy (CRRT). CRRT corrects electrolyte and acid-base imbalances through a more gentle process.

CHAPTER 24 GLYCEMIC CONTROL

Decision Point:

How quickly should the patient's blood glucose be corrected and what is the risk associated with correcting the blood glucose value too quickly?

Discussion:

Blood glucose should be corrected no faster than 50–70 mg/dL/hour. If the blood glucose drops too rapidly, the patient is at risk of developing cerebral edema with electrolyte and fluid shifts.

Decision Point:

What changes in potassium level should be anticipated with initiation of the insulin infusion?

Discussion:

The potassium level will decrease as it shifts intracellularly in conjunction with insulin administration. Conversely, as the glucose level and insulin administration stabilizes, potassium will shift out of the cell and the patient may experience hyperkalemia in the DKA recovery phase.

Decision Point:

What are key interventions to avoid hypoglycemia when administering a continuous insulin infusion?

Discussion:

Blood glucoses should be checked hourly with initiation of the continuous insulin infusion until glucoses are stable and within target range for 4 hours. At that point, glucose checks can safely be changed to every 2 hours for the duration of the continuous infusion as long as glucose levels remain stable within range.

Decision Point:

What are the hallmark treatments of DKA?

Discussion:

Fluid replacements, continuous IV insulin therapy, and electrolyte stabilization.

Decision Point:

Briefly describe how to transition from IV administration to an SQ basal/bolus regimen.

Discussion:

The IV continuous infusion should continue to infuse for 2 hours after the first SQ dose of basal insulin dose is given. This avoids any gap in insulin availability during the transition from IV to SQ administration. If the insulin infusion was discontinued too quickly, a rapid rise in blood glucose could ensue, resulting in recurrence of DKA and/or elevated glucose.

CHAPTER 25 PITUITARY, THYROID, AND ADRENAL DISORDERS

Decision Point:

Discuss events of day 3 that place J.W. at risk for AI.

Discussion:

J.W. has a temperature of 103°F and he returned to the OR twice in 5 hours. J.W. experienced intermittent hypotension and hypoxia for several days.

Decision Point:

Discuss hemodynamic parameters as they relate to the diagnosis of AI.

Discussion:

J.W. has the following readings: decreased CVP, decreased PCWP, decreased SVR, increased CO, continued hypotension despite fluids and vasopressors. These readings are indicative of loss of the effects of cortisol (i.e., impaired pressor response to catecholamines, resulting in hypotension). Glucocorticoids are needed for the cardiovascular system to respond to epinephrine, norepinephrine, and angiotensin II. On the other hand, these readings could also be attributed to the systemic inflammatory response syndrome (SIRS) or early sepsis response.

Decision Point:

Discuss lab values as they pertain to AI.

Discussion:

Potassium level (5.8 mEq/L): decreased ability to excrete potassium; Na^+ (129 mEq/L): inability to conserve sodium and clear free water; calcium level (12 mg/dL): increased inability to form bone, allowing Ca to be reabsorbed into blood. Hypoglycemia related to impaired gluconeogenesis.

Decision Point:

Discuss the serum cortisol level.

Discussion:

J.W. has sustained pain, fever, hypovolemia, hypotension, hypoxia, and tissue damage resulting in continuous need for and release of ACTH and cortisol resulting in the loss of diurnal variation. Cortisol levels in critically ill and injured patients can be extremely variable and patient specific.

Decision Point:

Discuss why the provider ordered a vasopressin drip.

Discussion:

Vasopressin is an exogenous form of ADH. Catecholamine-resistant shock responds to this low-dose infusion that restores the physiologic concentration of vasopressin that may be depleted as a response to continuous stress.

Decision Point:

Why did the provider order dexamethasone before a corticotropin stimulation test?

Discussion:

The provider suspects that AI is responsible for the vasopressor-resistant hypotension. Dexamethasone can be given before the corticotropin stimulation test as it will not interfere with the results of the corticotropin test.

Decision Point:

Explain how a corticotropin stimulation test is performed and why the test was ordered.

Discussion:

This corticotropin test is performed by drawing a serum cortisol level. 250 mcg of synthetic corticotropin is administered IV. Serum cortisol levels are drawn at 30 and 60 minutes following the corticotropin administration. The corticotropin stimulation test is performed to determine if the HPA-adrenal axis is functioning. There should be a rise in the serum cortisol level following administration of exogenous ACTH. If no increase is noted, the diagnosis of primary adrenal insufficiency can be made, which reflects the inability of the adrenal gland to respond to ACTH.

Decision Point:

What would you expect the provider to order for the diagnosis of AI?

Discussion:

The provider's orders would include hydrocortisone 100 mg IV every 8 hours, which is considered to be a stress dose. Mineralocorticoids may need to be replaced in conjunction with hydrocortisone. Fludrocortisone can be given 0.1–0.2 mg every day. Aldosterone is secreted in response to renin-angiotensin system stimulation as a result of hypotension. In primary AI, serum aldosterone levels may be decreased despite elevated renin levels.

CHAPTER 26 BLOOD CONSERVATION AND BLOOD COMPONENT REPLACEMENT

Decision Point:

What laboratory studies should be obtained at this time? What investigations should be done to assist in determining the cause of her hemolysis?

Discussion:

A transfusion reaction workup was performed at the blood bank with negative results. A direct antiglobulin test (DAT)/Coombs' test was also negative. The testing pattern was not indicative of a warm-alloantibody or a drug-induced hemolytic anemia. Because of the absence of a previous transfusion history (other than transfusion during surgery) other causes of hemolysis should be entertained in patients who quickly become fatally ill with evidence of intravascular hemolysis.

Decision Point:

What blood components are indicated?

Discussion:

Since D.A. was hypotensive, the massive transfusion protocol was initiated: 4 units of RBCs, 4 units of FFP, 1 pool of cryoprecipitate, and an apheresis platelet were rapidly transfused. The FFP and the RBCs were transfused through a blood warmer/rapid infuser and another EHP was drawn. She continued to experience coagulopathy after these additional blood components were transfused (INR 1.9, PT 19 seconds, hematocrit 27%, fibrinogen level 104 mg/dL, platelet count 92,000 cells/mm^3, hypotensive, and hypothermic at 35.2°C).

Decision Point:

What is the nurse's role in assessing for an incompatible blood transfusion?

Discussion:

Acute hemolytic transfusion reactions may be complicated to discern by symptoms alone. The nurse's primary role is to assess whether an incompatible blood transfusion occurred by determining whether a clerical error occurred at the time that the blood bank specimen was drawn or while identifying the patient at the time of transfusion.

CHAPTER 27 COAGULOPATHIES

Decision Point:

What were this patient's risk factors for coagulopathy?

Discussion:

Preoperative anticoagulation with warfarin and no opportunity to plan for surgery. Previous heart surgery and adhesion formation. Use of cardiopulmonary bypass with hypothermia, heparin, and the potential to activate fibrinolysis. Complexity of the surgery with explant of devices and cardiac transplantation.

Decision Point:

What were his clinical indicators of postoperative coagulopathy?

Discussion:

Excessive chest tube drainage; hypotension; abnormal coagulation results: low hemoglobin, hematocrit, platelets, and fibrinogen; elevated INR.

Decision Point:

Explain the rationale and expected outcomes for the following interventions: DDAVP, PRBCs, cryoprecipitate, FFP, and platelets.

Discussion:

DDAVP stimulates the release of VWF, enhancing platelet function. PRBCs are given to increase blood volume and provide oxygen carrying capacity in patients who are anemic and actively bleeding. Cryoprecipitate replaces specific components; it supplies fibrinogen, factor VIII, and VWF. FFP supplies most active coagulation components and reverses elevated INR. Platelets are given for thrombocytopenia and disorders of platelet function.

The expected outcome for all of these interventions is to enhance Tom's ability to carry out effective hemostasis and to stop the bleeding.

CHAPTER 28 SHOCK AND END POINTS OF RESUSCITATION

Decision Point:

What parameters indicated incomplete resuscitation?

Discussion:

Initial review of patient data indicates ongoing shock and the need for further resuscitation. This conclusion is based on the persistence of a metabolic acidosis (pH 7.20) with significant base deficit (BD) of −11 and elevated lactate concentration of 8 mg/dL. Despite the "normal" BP, tachycardia is persistent and systemic vascular resistance (SVR) is elevated, consistent with the compensatory mechanisms of hypovolemic shock. The presence of a mild hypothermia along with metabolic acidosis places this patient at further risk for coagulopathic bleeding. Tissue oxygenation may be further compromised because of impaired pulmonary gas exchange related to the presence of pulmonary contusion and rib fractures. This is evidenced by the significant shunt on ABG noted previously. The Pao_2 is only 90 mm Hg on 100% Fio_2, resulting in a Pao_2/Fio_2 (P/F) ratio of 90.

Decision Point:

What physiologic and global parameters suggest that this patient is in septic shock?

Discussion:

In evaluating this patient, there are several physiologic and global parameters that indicate the presence of septic shock. The initial injuries, sustained shock, and resulting organ hypoperfusion place this patient at risk for infection. Most vulnerable are organs such as the intestine, where intramucosal ischemia may result in translocation of intestinal bacteria to the circulatory system, triggering sepsis. In addition, the presence of an open abdomen and the invasive medical devices place the patient at risk for infection. Review of the patient data revealed fever and tachycardia. The ABG indicated persistent metabolic acidosis and oxygenation abnormalities as the Pao_2/Fio_2 ratio is 75. Worsening static lung compliance is also noted with bilateral infiltrates on CXR. Laboratory data show elevated glucose level, elevated prothrombin time, and elevated renal function parameters. Although a specific organism has not been localized, the patient exhibits evidence of systemic inflammatory response syndrome with failure of multiple organ systems. These systems include pulmonary, cardiovascular, hematologic, and renal.

Decision Point:

What are the priorities of care for this patient?

Discussion:

Priorities of care for this patient are aimed at improving oxygenation of tissues compromised by hypoperfusion. Application of a lung-protective mode of ventilation may increase oxygenation through alveolar recruitment and reduction of pulmonary shunting while limiting the risks of alveolar shearing injury. Preload indicators such as right ventricular end-diastolic volume index, ejection fraction, and traditional indicators such as CVP and PAOP indicate adequate preload at this time. However, this must be considered in light of how much resuscitation volume has already been received and the fact that septic patients require significant volume resuscitation because of fluid shifts from the intravascular space attributable to capillary leakage. The initiation of vasopressor and inotropic agents is required in this patient as efforts to improve perfusion through volume resuscitation alone were insufficient.

CHAPTER 29 OPTIMIZING HEMODYNAMICS: STRATEGIES FOR FLUID AND MEDICATION TITRATION IN HYPOPERFUSION STATES

Decision Point:

To what do you attribute J.Q.'s hypotensive state?

Discussion:

The most likely reason for this change is warming and the reflexive fall in vascular tone. Without the high SVR, an occult hypovolemic state is uncovered, as seen by the drop in CVP and PAOP. Though both are within the "textbook normal" ranges, they are too low for a man of J.Q.'s age and cardiovascular status. Hypovolemia is common following surgical procedures, especially those requiring aortic cross-clamping. This finding is secondary to fluid shifting and cardiopulmonary bypass related to hyperosmolar priming solutions that cause diuresis.

Decision Point:

From this information, what is the source of J.Q.'s hypotension at this juncture and what treatments are indicated?

Discussion:

The lowered CVP and PAOP coupled with the abnormally low SVR (< 900 dynes) indicate a distributive form of shock. Coupled with the elevated temperature, J.Q. is likely septic. Early goal-directed therapy should be instituted.

CHAPTER 30 TRAUMA

Decision Point:

What are the likely explanations for her hemodynamic profile in the critical care unit?

Discussion:

The hemodynamic picture was confusing; while her filling pressures suggested hypovolemia, her Svo_2, Do_2I, Vo_2I, and EDVI suggested that she had more than adequate volume to support excellent oxygen delivery. In fact, her consumption was low because her otherwise young and healthy heart and lungs and adequate hemoglobin were able to deliver more oxygen than her tissues required. The cause of these interesting hemodynamics was not sepsis, as would seem most likely, but rather a lack of renal control of her blood pressure. Because of her unusual bilateral renal injuries, she was lacking renin-angiotensin-aldosterone influences on her blood pressure. She was profoundly vasodilated, but had enough volume and a healthy heart to support adequate oxygen delivery to her tissues. The low SVR was disconcerting, however, as it provided no physiologic safety net should she drop her blood pressure for any other reason, the surgeons ordered stress doses of IV hydrocortisone every 8 hours to simulate adrenal support, resulting in slight improvement of her SVR and blood pressure. (She required this support for several weeks before her adrenal function returned.)

Decision Point:

What are additional resuscitation and assessment priorities in the first hours following admission to critical care?

Discussion:

Reversal of hypothermia is critical because lower body temperature increases hemoglobin's affinity for oxygen and contributes to coagulopathy. This is most efficiently done with warm blankets and IV fluids, convective warming blankets, and CAVR. The source of acidosis must also be addressed; in this case it is probably the need for continued resuscitation with fluids and vasopressors to ensure adequate perfusion of all organ beds. Evaluation of interventions can be done by frequently assessing ABGs, LA, or BD. Coagulation tests should be conducted as necessary until Hgb, platelets, PT, PTT, and fibrinogen are within normal levels. Ventilator inspiratory pressures, pulmonary compliance, ABGs, and repeat chest X-rays will determine if fluid overload or ARDS.

CHAPTER 31 SEPSIS AND MULTIPLE ORGAN DYSFUNCTION SYNDROME

Decision Point:

Does L.M. show any signs of SIRS?

Discussion:

The patient has four SIRS criteria: heart rate 104 beats/min, systolic blood pressure below 90 mm Hg, respiratory rate > 20 breaths/min, and a WBC > 12,000/mm^3.

Decision Point:

What are appropriate interventions and further diagnostic tests for the patient at this time?

Discussion:

The patient demonstrates uncompensated metabolic acidosis despite hyperventilation (pH 7.33 with HCO_3^- 14), suggesting hypoperfusion that requires fluid resuscitation. In addition to the maintenance IV infusion, one bolus of NS 500–1000 mL is indicated to see if this will improve the tachycardia and hypotension. The patient's Pao_2 is only 79 mm Hg on 3 L/min via cannula. It would be important to know his baseline Pao_2 to determine if this value represents his baseline. However, in the face of his metabolic acidosis and general distressed appearance, more oxygen is warranted. The dramatic change in his WBC count suggests a rapid consumption of mature WBCs, which is a particular concern in a patient with longstanding hepatic failure. Underlying infection should be suspected, and he requires pan cultures with initiation of broad-spectrum antibiotics after the cultures have been obtained. He should also be typed and crossed for possible blood transfusion since his admitting diagnosis is GI bleed and his platelet count has now dropped. Consideration should be given for placement of a urine catheter and central venous catheter (CVC) to monitor fluid status. The CVC can also be used to track $Scvo_2$ as a resuscitation guide.

Decision Point:

What interventions should the critical care nurse anticipate in the event that the patient decompensates further?

Discussion:

If oxygenation or his ability to protect his airway decompensates, the patient will require intubation and mechanical ventilation. Low tidal volume ventilation should be considered to minimize secondary pulmonary injury from barotraumas. If the patient remains hypotensive and the $Scvo_2$ remains below 70% despite fluid resuscitation, the patient will require additional fluids and the addition of vasopressors to keep his MAP higher than 65 mm Hg. Blood and blood component transfusions may be needed if he develops ongoing blood loss or coagulopathy. Continued monitoring of ABGs, lactic acid, Hgb, electrolytes, glucose, and coagulation factors will also be necessary.

Decision Point:

What other interventions are needed to provide multisystem support of this critically ill patient with MODS?

Discussion:

An insulin infusion should be started to maintain the patient's glucose levels between 100 and 120 mg/dL. A general surgery consult should be requested to rule out necrotizing fasciitis as a source of his overwhelming inflammatory response. A steroid infusion could be started as well. If monitoring of his urine output and chemistries suggests further progression toward acute renal failure, then CVVH could be initiated. DVT and stress ulcer prophylaxis should also be initiated per protocols. The patient could be considered for APC therapy; he meets criteria for more than one organ system failure, his platelets are > 30,000/mm^3, and he does not have a recent history of surgery or intracranial hemorrhage. Of concern, however, is the initial diagnosis of GI bleed and demonstration of ongoing blood loss as noted by his low Hct and, therefore, this agent is contraindicated.

CHAPTER 32 CARING FOR THE IMMUNOCOMPROMISED PATIENT

Decision Point:

What does his admission lab work indicate?

Discussion:

Clearly, S.E. is experiencing an infectious process, although the physical findings and diagnostic test results are not clearly definitive for a source or microbe. There is an acidosis, primarily of metabolic origin, but an intrapulmonary disorder is also present as indicated by a high normal carbon dioxide level when compensatory hyperventilation should be occurring.

Decision Point:

Given his symptoms, what diagnosis would be made?

Discussion:

The presumed diagnosis is pneumonia.

Decision Point:

What are S.E.'s infection risks?

Discussion:

S.E.'s infection risks are multifactorial, involving both intrinsic and therapy-related abnormalities of immune function. At the core of his current health problems is the underlying chronic illness of diabetes mellitus that impairs granulocyte function. The presence of malignancy is indicative of immunosurveillance failure. Normal immunosurveillance should detect cell mutations that are the precursors to malignant cell transformation. This impairment is at least partly related to the immunosuppressive medications used to prevent graft rejection after S.E.'s kidney transplant. These agents suppress the T-lymphocytic recognition and rejection of transplanted tissue, but may also impair recognition of malignant cells. Lymphoma is a recognized complication associated with immunosuppressive medications, and its involvement of the hematopoietic cells and lymph nodes indicates an even greater lymphocyte defect.

Most chemotherapy agents destroy the rapidly dividing cells, which include tumor cells as well as bone marrow, skin, and mucous membranes. S.E.'s previous chemotherapy ending 9 days ago caused predictable bone marrow suppression predisposing him to infection. Chemotherapy-induced destruction of mucosal barriers has also resulted in oral mucositis. The open oral lesions may also contribute to a risk of infection for S.E., although his symptoms indicate that pneumonia is the predominant clinical problem. Most recently, S.E. received radiation therapy to the lung field, impairing normal alveolar macrophage function, and causing inflammation in the location of the tumor. Inflammation of the alveoli and bronchi can produce a chemical pneumonitis called "radiation pneumonitis," and also increase the risk for trapped secretions and development of infectious pneumonitis. The incidence of radiation pneumonitis peaks between 3 and 6 weeks after beginning therapy, matching the timing for S.E.'s symptoms.

The most important risk factor for infection is the granulocytic defects caused by S.E.'s diabetes and chemotherapy. The severity of neutropenia and its timing are chemotherapeutic agent and dose specific. S.E. received his last chemotherapy 9 days before admission and his particular treatment regimen produces moderate to severe neutropenia occurring between the 7th and 14th day after chemotherapy. The exact date of onset for S.E.'s neutropenia is unclear since he presented with his WBC count already depressed; however, clinicians should be prepared to aggressively support S.E.'s infection while awaiting recovery of the WBC count, realizing that the current symptoms reflect a reversible critical illness that is related to a short-term immune deficit associated with therapy. This patient presents with oral mucosal breakdown, also related to chemotherapy induced mucosal injury. This complication tends to clinically follow the same timing as bone marrow suppression, but in addition to causing pain, it may be a source of systemic infection or cause significant inflammation that interferes with breathing. The specific site of breath-sound and radiographic changes indicates predictable infection, given the existing tumor in the hilar lung region.

CHAPTER 33 CARING FOR THE PATIENT IN THE IMMEDIATE POSTOPERATIVE PERIOD

Decision Point:

What comorbid conditions influence her risk for anesthesia and surgery?

Discussion:

M.F. has a history of cardiovascular disease (hypertension), pulmonary disease (smoking), increased BMI (obesity), poor nutritional status, and an anticipated operative procedure lasting for greater than 3 hours.

Decision Point:

What information does the receiving nurse need to obtain during report?

Discussion:

A verbal handoff from the anesthesiologist and the surgical personnel should include information related to the procedure, type of anesthesia, airway management and plan, vascular access, fluids (I&Os) and replacement (crystalloid, colloids, blood), estimated blood loss, complications (anesthesia and operative), plan of care for ongoing pain management, and expectations for care (i.e., notification parameters, outcomes expected). Use of a standardized handoff tool, such as SBAR, is recommended.

Decision Point:

What complications are likely to arise in the immediate postoperative period?

Discussion:

Primary concerns include respiratory and hemodynamic status. Vigilant monitoring of these organ systems helps prevent significant complications.

Decision Point:

How should pain and sedation be managed postoperatively?

Discussion:

Because M.F. is not responding to verbal cues, a behavioral pain assessment using a validated tool, e.g., Critical Care Pain Observation Tool (CPOT), is recommended.

Decision Point:

When can she start to receive mobility?

Discussion:

Activity can begin upon completion of M.F.'s initial assessment and the handoff. To assess for skin alterations after prolonged surgery, M.F. should be turned to examine her head, back, and heels for any areas of redness or potential breakdown. If stable, M.F. can be repositioned to either side or tilted to reduce pressure and improve perfusion to underlying tissue.

CHAPTER 34 CARING FOR THE CRITICALLY ILL PREGNANT PATIENT

Decision Point:

Prior to the seizure, what initial stabilization measures should be taken?

Discussion:

Initial stabilization should include oxygen administration, positioning to relieve venacaval compression, initiation of magnesium sulfate infusion, administration of antihypertensive agents such as labetalol or hydralazine, and optimization of maternal fluid status. Assessment of fetal lung maturity should be undertaken, and consideration given to administration of betamethasone to enhance fetal lung maturity. The entire team, including obstetrics, critical care, anesthesia, and neonatal services should be consulted to provide a comprehensive patient care plan, including plans for location and type of delivery. MP's husband should be kept informed of his wife's condition and prognosis.

Decision Point:

What is the significance of the fetal heart rate tracing?

Discussion:

Fetal heart rate tracing is a Category II or indeterminate. Category II tracings require further assessment and evaluation. Category I tracings are predictive of normal fetal acid-base balance. Continuous monitoring should be employed, and consideration given to optimizing maternal stability with the therapies discussed previously.

Decision Point:

After the seizure, what are the current management priorities?

Discussion:

Current management priorities include prioritization of maternal stability, with initiation of cardiopulmonary resuscitation (CPR). Special care should be taken to ensure that uterine displacement occurs during compressions. Standard Advanced Cardiac Life Support (ACLS) guidelines should be followed for defibrillation and medication administration. Preparations for a perimortem cesarean section should be initiated so that everything is ready if return of spontaneous circulation does not occur within 5 minutes after initiation of CPR.

CHAPTER 35 CARING FOR THE PEDIATRIC PATIENT IN AN ADULT CRITICAL CARE UNIT

Decision Point:

Why is the treatment plan in this case study appropriate to the patient situation?

Discussion:

The use of nebulized albuterol or epinephrine may improve clinical symptoms but does not have a clear benefit in relation to decreased length of stay. Nebulized hypertonic saline treatments could be beneficial to increase mucociliary clearance in children whose length of stay is expected to be less than 3 days. Corticosteroid use in bronchiolitis has not been shown to decrease admission rates or improve clinical outcomes, and has been found to prolong viral shedding. The recommended supportive care of the child with bronchiolitis includes oxygen therapy, early nutrition, and hydration.

CHAPTER 36 CARING FOR THE CRITICALLY ILL ELDERLY PATIENT

Decision Point:

What are likely etiologies of R.S.'s initial episode of loss of consciousness?

Discussion:

Postural hypotension, cardiac dysrhythmias, a transient ischemic attack, head injury secondary to a fall, medication complications, and hypovolemia caused by diarrhea.

Decision Point:

What impact will routine beta-blocker use have on R.S.'s physiologic response to his injury and hospitalization?

Discussion:

Beta-blocking agents attenuate HR and other sympathetic responses to physiologic and psychologic stressors. Patients taking one of these drugs may be unable to mount an effective compensatory response despite the presence of hypotension or poor end-organ perfusion.

Decision Point:

What factors might be responsible for R.S.'s dwindling oxygen saturation?

Discussion:

Aspiration, narcotic administration, supine positioning, fluid boluses.

Decision Point:

What musculoskeletal changes of aging predispose this patient to fractures?

Discussion:

Aging is associated with osteoporosis, diminished muscular mass and strength, and drying of the joints. In addition, as a result of the changes in gait, balance, and righting reflexes, falls in the geriatric patient are a common event.

Decision Point:

What additional possible reason for R.S.'s hypotension, flushed skin, and altered level of consciousness is suggested by his cloudy, foul-smelling urine and moderate temperature elevation?

Discussion:

Urosepsis. Elderly patients have the highest incidence of sepsis of any age group. The respiratory and genitourinary tracts are the most common sources of infection.

CHAPTER 38 CARING FOR THE BARIATRIC PATIENT

Decision Point:

In reviewing her medical history, identify obesity related conditions.

Discussion:

Obesity affects virtually every organ in the body. The patient in this case review suffered from the following obesity related conditions: history of pulmonary emboli, obstructive sleep apnea, asthma arthritis in knees and ankles, chronic back pain, chronic kidney disease, and depression. In addition, while carrying out a skin assessment, the patient was noted to have extensive skin breakdown in skinfolds, under pannus and in perineal area due to moisture and incontinence.

Decision Point:

Identify challenges in the patient's care that were directly associated with her morbid obesity.

Discussion:

When caring for the obese individual, their physical size can complicate even the most basic care and interventions. For this patient, challenges included: physical assessment issues with being unable to palpate pulses and difficulty completing a thorough skin assessment; vascular access issues with lab unable to draw blood specimens, inability to place arterial line with multiple failed attempts in right and left radial and in the axilla; monitoring issues with unreliable blood pressure measurements from poorly fitting BP cuff and no arterial line for 4 days; airway management did not prove to be a problem in this scenario, but a fiberoptic scope had been made available in the event of a difficult intubation; hygiene and patient positioning; medication dosing; diagnostic imaging issues with less than ideal images with

X-ray, ultrasound and CT scan; nutritional deficiencies requiring high protein supplementation for optimal healing.

CHAPTER 41 ONCOLOGIC EMERGENCIES

Decision Point:

What factors contributed to the patient's development of cardiac tamponade?

Discussion:

The patient's diagnosis of Burkitt's lymphoma, an aggressive form of B-cell non-Hodgkin lymphoma, puts the patient at risk for development of ATLS. The patient's history of gout and three components of the treatment regimen (rituximab, doxorubicin, and corticosteroids) all place the patient at increased risk.

Decision Point:

With which disciplines would you collaborate to help ensure optimal patient outcomes?

Discussion:

Collaboration with the multidisciplinary hematology/oncology team to anticipate when the patient is at greatest risk for the development of ATLS will help assure that preventive strategies and early intervention are implemented. Collaboration with the oncology pharmacist and nephrologist is necessary if the patient develops renal insufficiency.

Decision Point:

Describe your role as a facilitator of learning for this patient. What patient education is required?

Discussion:

Educate patients and families on preventive measures to mitigate development of ATLS. Explain why the patient is at risk for development of this complication and the rationale for the lab and other diagnostic studies. Finally, education about signs and symptoms related to each of the electrolyte abnormalities may help with early recognition of problems.

CHAPTER 42 CHEMICAL DEPENDENCY

Decision Point:

What potential withdrawal states may impact his critical care stay?

Discussion:

He is at risk of both alcohol withdrawal and opiate withdrawal, both of which will impact his critical care stay.

Decision Point:

Which withdrawal state can be fatal if untreated, alcohol or opiate?

Discussion:

Alcohol can be fatal, even with treatment, if the patient goes into DTs. Opiate withdrawal, though excruciatingly painful and uncomfortable, will not place the patient at risk of death.

Decision Point:

What substances will not result in withdrawal states?

Discussion:

Amphetamines and cocaine have no physiologic withdrawal but have a very high psychological withdrawal that will result in intense drug craving. In this case, his benzodiazepine use will not result in significant withdrawal given his use of Valium is reported to be intermittent and not regular. It would be highly critical to validate this use pattern as more regular use would result in withdrawal that will likely result in seizure activity. Also, if benzodiazepines are used on a regular basis in the care of this patient, then, over time, he might be at risk of withdrawal.

Decision Point:

Would you anticipate seizure activity with this withdrawal?

Discussion:

You would not anticipate seizure activity based on his history of alcohol use and no reported prior withdrawals. If it was discovered that his benzodiazepine use was more frequent than intermittent or his urine toxicology screen was positive for benzodiazepines, then there would be a definite seizure risk.

Decision Point:

What are the potential signs of alcohol withdrawal present on the initial assessment?

Discussion:

Withdrawal symptoms could include nausea and dry heaves, profound diaphoresis, tremor with hands at rest, and elevated blood pressure and heart rate.

INDEX

Page numbers followed by b indicate boxes; f, figures; t, tables.

C

M

O

P

U